CARRANZA'S

Clinical PERIODONTOLOGY

CARRANZA'S

Clinical PERIODONTOLOGY

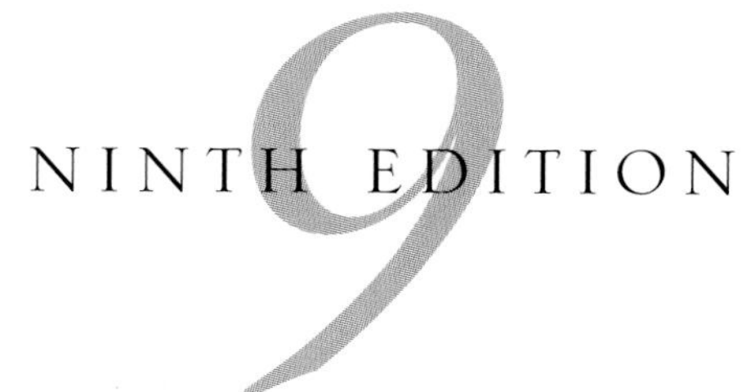

NINTH EDITION

Michael G. Newman, DDS
Adjunct Professor, Section of Periodontics
School of Dentistry, University of California, Los Angeles
Los Angeles, California

Henry H. Takei, DDS, MS
Clinical Professor, Section of Periodontics
School of Dentistry, University of California, Los Angeles
Los Angeles, California

Fermin A. Carranza, Dr Odont
Professor Emeritus, Section of Periodontics
School of Dentistry, University of California, Los Angeles
Los Angeles, California

W.B. SAUNDERS COMPANY
An Imprint of Elsevier Science
Philadelphia London New York St. Louis Sydney Toronto

W.B. SAUNDERS COMPANY
An Imprint of Elsevier Science

The Curtis Center
Independence Square West
Philadelphia, PA 19106

Library of Congress Cataloging-in-Publication Data

Carranza's clinical periodontology.—9th ed./ [edited by] Michael G. Newman, Henry H. Takei, Fermin A. Carranza.
p. ; cm.
Rev. ed. of: Clinical periodontology/ [edited by] Fermin A. Carranza, Jr., Michael G. Newman. 8th ed. ©1996.
Includes bibliographical references and index.
ISBN 0-7216-8331-2 (alk. paper)
1. Periodontics. I. Title: Clinical periodontology. II. Newman, Michael G. III. Takei, Henry H., 1938– IV. Carranza, Fermin A.
[DNLM: 1. Periodontal Diseases. 2. Oral Surgical Procedures. 3. Periodontal Prosthesis. WU 240 C641 2002]
RK361 .G58 2002
617.6′32—dc21

2001049984

Publishing Director: Linda L. Duncan
Senior Acquisitions Editor: Penny Rudolph
Developmental Editor: Jaime Pendill and Kimberly Alvis
Project Manager: Linda McKinley
Production Editor: Ellen Forest
Designer: Julia Ramirez
Cover Art: Imagineering

CARRANZA'S CLINICAL PERIODONTOLOGY ISBN: 0-7216-8331-2

Printed in the United States of America.

02 03 04 05 06 GW/KPT 9 8 7 6 5 4 3 2

Associate Editors

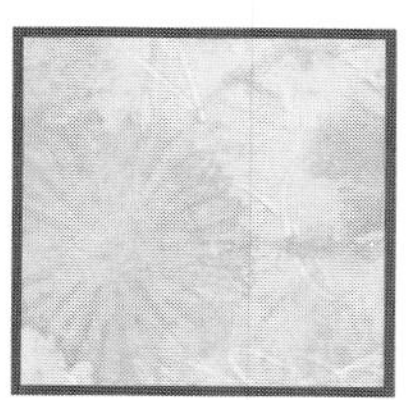

Sascha A. Jovanovic, DDS, MS
Research Associate and Director of Preceptorship Studies, Division of Oral Biology and Medicine, School of Dentistry, University of California, Los Angeles, Los Angeles, California

Susan Kinder Haake, DMD, MdentSc, PhD
Associate Professor, Section of Periodontics, Division of Associated Clinical Specialities, School of Dentistry, University of California, Los Angeles, Los Angeles, California

M. John Novak, BDS, LDS, MS, PhD
Professor, Department of Periodontics; Associate Director, Center for Oral Health Research, University of Kentucky, Lexington, Kentucky

Contributors

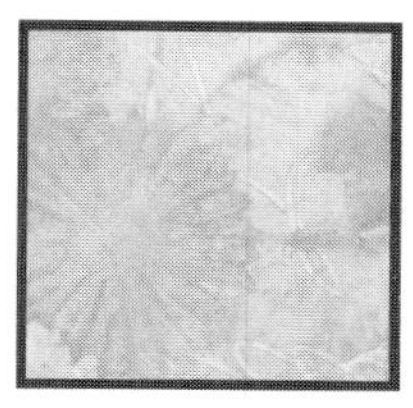

Alfredo Aguirre, DDS, MS
Director, Advanced Oral and Maxillofacial Pathology; Associate Professor, Department of Oral Diagnostic Sciences, State University of New York at Buffalo School of Dental Medicine, Buffalo, New York

William F. Ammons, Jr., DDS, MSD
Professor Emeritus, Department of Periodontics, University of Washington School of Dentistry, Seattle, Washington

Samuel J. Arbes, Jr., DDS, MPH, PhD
Clinical Fellow, Center for Oral and Systemic Diseases, University of North Carolina School of Dentistry, Chapel Hill, North Carolina

Robert R. Azzi, DDS
Clinical Associate Professor, Department of Periodontics, University of Paris VII School of Dentistry; Private Practice, Paris, France

James D. Beck, PhD
Kenan Professor, Department of Dental Ecology, University of North Carolina School of Dentistry, Chapel Hill, North Carolina

George W. Bernard, DDS, PhD
Professor, Department of Neurobiology, School of Dentistry, University of California, Los Angeles, Los Angeles, California

John Beumer, III, DDS
Chairman, Department of Advanced Prosthodontics, Biomaterials, and Hospital Dentistry, School of Dentistry, University of California, Los Angeles, Los Angeles, California

Carol A. Bibb, PhD, DDS
Adjunct Professor, Section of Oral Medicine and Orofacial Pain, School of Dentistry, University of California, Los Angeles, Los Angeles, California

Jaime Bulkacz, DrOdont, PhD
Lecturer, Section of Periodontics, School of Dentistry, University of California, Los Angeles, Los Angeles, California

Paulo M. Camargo, DDS, MS
Assistant Professor, Department of Periodontics, Division of Associated Clinical Specialties, School of Dentistry, University of California, Los Angeles, Los Angeles, California

Ting Ling Chang, DDS
Adjunct Assistant Professor, Department of Advanced Prosthodontics, Biomaterials, and Hospital Dentistry, School of Dentistry, University of California, Los Angeles, Los Angeles, California

Sebastian G. Ciancio, DDS, PhD
Distinguished Service Professor and Chair, Department of Periodontics, State University of New York at Buffalo School of Dental Medicine, Buffalo, New York

Joseph P. Cooney, BDS, MS
Clinical Professor and Director, Department of Advanced Prosthodontics, School of Dentistry, University of California, Los Angeles, Los Angeles, California

Denise J. Fedele, DMD, MS
Clinical Associate Professor, Department of Oral Health Care Delivery, Baltimore College of Dental Surgery Dental School, University of Maryland at Baltimore, Baltimore, Maryland; Chief, Professional Development and Research, Dental Care Clinical Center, Veterans Administration Maryland Healthcare System, Perry Point, Maryland

Thomas F. Flemmig, Dr. med. dent, Professor
Chairman, Clinic of Periodontology, Westfalian Wilhelm University, Münster, Germany

Stephen F. Goodman, BA, DDS
Former Clinical Professor, Division of Periodontics, Columbia University School of Dental and Oral Surgery, New York, New York; Past President, American Academy of Periodontology; Diplomate, American Board of Periodontology

Susan Kinder Haake, DMD, MDentSc, PhD
Associate Professor, Section of Periodontics, Division of Associated Clinical Specialties, School of Dentistry, University of California, Los Angeles, Los Angeles, California

Thomas J. Han, DDS, MS
Adjunct Associate Professor, Department of Periodontics, Section of Periodontics, School of Dentistry, University of California, Los Angeles, Los Angeles, California

Gerald W. Harrington, DDS, MSD
Professor Emeritus, Department of Endodontics, University of Washington School of Dentistry, Seattle, Washington

James E. Hinrichs, DDS, MS
Associate Professor and Director, Advanced Education Program in Periodontology, Department of Preventive Sciences, University of Minnesota School of Dentistry, Minneapolis, Minnesota

Eva L. Hogan, MD, DDS, MS
Lecturer, Section of Periodontics, School of Dentistry, University of California, Los Angeles, Los Angeles, California

George T.J. Huang, DDS, MSD, DSc
Graduate Program Director and Assistant Professor, Section of Endodontics, Division of Associated Clinical Specialties, School of Dentistry, University of California, Los Angeles, Los Angeles, California

Maria E. Itoiz, DrOdont
Professor and Chair, Department of Oral Pathology, Faculty of Dentistry, University of Buenos Aires, Buenos Aires, Argentina

David Jolkovsky, DMD, MS
Adjunct Assistant Professor, Section of Periodontics, School of Dentistry, University of California, Los Angeles, Los Angeles, California; Private Practice, Davis, California

Sascha A. Jovanovic, DDS, MS
Research Associate and Director of Preceptorship Studies, Division of Oral Biology of Medicine, School of Dentistry, University of California, Los Angeles, Los Angeles, California; President, European Association for Osseointegration, London, England

E. Barrie Kenney, BDSc, DDS, MS, FRACDS
Chair of Division of Associated Clinical Specialties and Periodontics, School of Dentistry, University of California, Los Angeles, Los Angeles, California

Perry R. Klokkevold, DDS, MS
Associate Professor and Clinical Director, Section of Periodontics, School of Dentistry, University of California, Los Angeles, Los Angeles, California

Vincent G. Kokich, DDS, MSD
Professor, Department of Orthodontics, University of Washington School of Dentistry, Seattle, Washington

Pamela K. McClain, DDS
Clinical Assistant Professor, Department of Surgical Dentistry, University of Colorado School of Dentistry, Denver, Colorado; Research Professor, Department of Periodontics, University of Maryland Dental School, Baltimore, Maryland

Michael J. McDevitt, DDS
Visiting Faculty, The Pankey Institute for Advanced Dental Education, Key Biscayne, Florida; Private Practice, Atlanta, Georgia

Brian L. Mealey, DDS, MS
Chairman and Program Director, Department of Periodontics, Wilford Hall Medical Center, Lackland Air Force Base, Texas; Clinical Assistant Professor, Department of Periodontics, University of Texas Health Science Center, San Antonio, Texas

Robert L. Merin, DDS
Private Practice, Woodland Hills, California; Diplomate, American Board of Periodontology

Bryan S. Michalowicz, DDS
Associate Professor, Department of Preventive Sciences, University of Minnesota School of Dentistry, Minneapolis, Minnesota

Kenneth T. Miyasaki, DDS, PhD
Associate Professor, Department of Oral Biology, School of Dentistry, University of California, Los Angeles, Los Angeles, California

Richard J. Nagy, DDS
Lecturer, Department of Periodontics, School of Dentistry, University of California, Los Angeles, Los Angeles, California; Staff Periodontist, Greater Los Angeles Veterans Administration Healthcare System, Los Angeles, California

Ian Needleman, BDS, MSc, PhD, MRD, RCS (Eng)
Department of Periodontology, Eastman Dental Institute for Oral Health Care Sciences, University of London, London, England

Mirdza E. Neiders, DDS
Professor, Department of Oral Diagnostic Sciences, State University of New York at Buffalo School of Dental Medicine, Buffalo, New York

Linda C. Niessen, DMD, MPH, MPP
Clinical Professor, Department of Public Health Sciences, Baylor College of Dentistry, Texas A&M Health Sciences Center, Dallas, Texas; Vice President of Clinical Education, Dentsply International, York, Pennsylvania

Russell J. Nisengard, DDS, PhD
Distinguished Teaching Professor and Associate Dean for Advanced Education and Research, Departments of Periodontics and Endodontics, State University of New York at Buffalo School of Dental Medicine, Buffalo, New York

Karen F. Novak, DDS, MS, PhD
Associate Professor, Department of Periodontics, Center for Oral Health Research, University of Kentucky, Lexington, Kentucky

M. John Novak, BDS, LDS, MS, PhD
Professor, Department of Periodontics; Associate Director, Center for Oral Health Research, University of Kentucky, Lexington, Kentucky

Joan Otomo-Corgel, DDS, MPH
Chair of Research, Department of Periodontics, Greater Los Angeles Veterans Administration Healthcare System, Los Angeles, California; Adjunct Assistant Professor in Residence, Department of Periodontics, School of Dentistry, University of California, Los Angeles, Los Angeles, California

Kwang-Bum Park, DDS, MS, PhD
Visiting Assistant Researcher in Periodontics, School of Dentistry, University of California, Los Angeles, Los Angeles, California; Director, Perio-Line Institute of Clinical Periodontics and Implantology, Taegu, Korea; Lecturer in Oral Anatomy and Histology, Kyung-Pook National University, Taegu, Korea

Anna Pattison, RDH, MS
Associate Professor, Department of Dental Hygiene, School of Dentistry, University of Southern California, Los Angeles, Los Angeles, California

Gordon Pattison, DDS
Lecturer in Periodontics, School of Dentistry, University of California, Los Angeles, Los Angeles, California

Dorothy A. Perry, RDH, PhD
Vice Chair, Department of Preventive and Restorative Dental Sciences; Chair, Division of Dental Hygiene, University of California–San Francisco School of Dentistry, San Francisco, California

Gregor Petersilka, Dr. med. dent
Assistant Professor, Clinic of Periodontology, Westfalian Wilhelm University, Münster, Germany

Bruce L. Pihlstrom, DDS, MS
Erwin Schaffer Periodontal Research Professor, Department of Preventive Sciences and Periodontology, University of Minnesota School of Dentistry, Minneapolis, Minnesota

John W. Rapley, DDS, MS
Director, Graduate Periodontics and Chairman, Department of Periodontics, University of Missouri–Kansas City School of Dentistry, Kansas City, Missouri

Terry D. Rees, DDS, MSD
Chairman and Professor, Department of Periodontics, Baylor College of Dentistry, Texas A&M Health Sciences Center, Dallas, Texas

Eleni Roumanas, DDS
Clinical Associate Professor, Department of Advanced Prosthodontics, Biomaterials, and Hospital Dentistry, School of Dentistry, University of California, Los Angeles, Los Angeles, California

Mariano Sanz, MD, DDS, PhD
Professor, Facultad de Odontologia, Universidad Complutense de Madrid, Madrid, Spain

Robert G. Schallhorn, DDS, MS
Clinical Professor, Department of Surgical Dentistry, University of Colorado School of Dentistry, Denver, Colorado; Research Professor, Department of Periodontics, Baltimore College of Dental Surgery Dental School, University of Maryland at Baltimore, Baltimore, Maryland

Max O. Schmid
Former Associate Professor of Periodontics, School of Dentistry, University of California, Los Angeles, Los Angeles, California; Private practice, Aarau, Switzerland

Dennis A. Shanelec, DDS
Director, Microsurgery Training Institute, Santa Barbara, California

Gerald Shklar, DDS, MS
Charles A. Brackett Professor of Oral Pathology, Harvard University School of Dental Medicine, Boston, Massachusetts

Thomas N. Sims, DDS
Senior Lecturer, Department of Periodontics, School of Dentistry, University of California, Los Angeles, Los Angeles, California

Frank M. Spear, DDS, MSD
Affiliate Professor, Graduate Prosthodontics, University of Washington School of Dentistry, Seattle, Washington; President Elect, American Academy of Esthetic Dentistry

Leonard S. Tibbetts, DDS, MSD
Visiting Assistant Professor, Graduate Periodontics, University of Washington School of Dentistry, Seattle, Washington

About the Authors

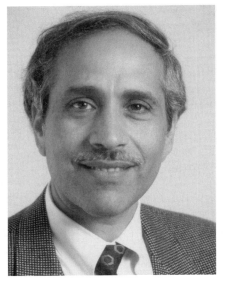

Michael G. Newman BA, DDS, FACD
Dr. Michael G. Newman graduated from the University of California–Los Angeles College of Letters and Sciences with a degree in Psychology. He completed his dental training at the School of Dentistry, University of California, Los Angeles in 1972. He is a Diplomate of the American Board of Periodontology and an Adjunct Professor of Periodontics at the School of Dentistry, University of California, Los Angeles. Dr. Newman is a Fellow and past President of the American Academy of Periodontology. In 1975, he won the Balint Orban Memorial Prize from the American Academy of Periodontology. He has been in the private practice of periodontics for more than 25 years.

Dr. Newman received a Certificate in Periodontics and Oral Medicine at the Harvard School of Dental Medicine and a Certificate in Oral Microbiology at the Forsyth Dental Center under the mentorship of Dr. Sigmund Socransky. Since that time, he has published more than 250 abstracts, journal articles, and book chapters and has coedited seven textbooks. Dr. Newman has served as an ad hoc reviewer for NIDCR, a consultant to the Council on Scientific Affairs of the American Dental Association, and a reviewer for numerous scientific and professional journals and governmental research organizations.

Dr. Newman has lectured throughout the world on microbiology, antimicrobials, evidence-based methodology, risk factors, and diagnostic strategies for periodontal disease. Dr. Newman has a strong interest in applied science and transfer of new technology for practical use. He has served as a consultant to many major dental and pharmaceutical companies throughout the world.

Dr. Newman is the Editor-in-Chief of the *Journal of Evidence-Based Dental Practice* and the Associate Editor of the *International Journal of Oral and Maxillofacial Implants.*

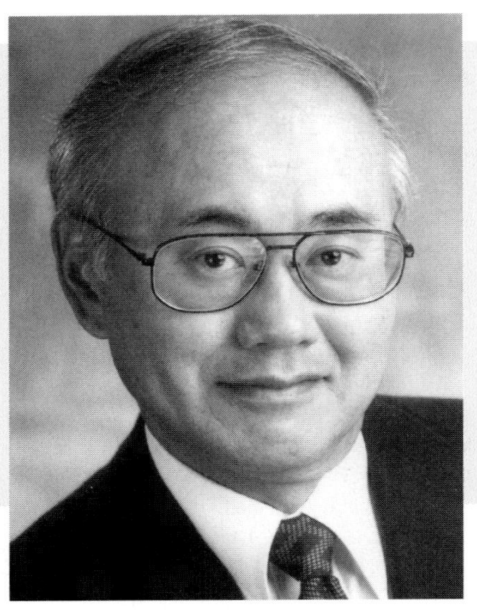

Henry H. Takei, DDS, MS, FACD
Dr. Henry H. Takei graduated from the Marquette University School of Dentistry in 1965. He completed his Periodontics Certificate and Master of Science Degree in 1967 at Marquette University and the Veterans Administration Hospital in Wisconsin.

Dr. Takei is a Clinical Professor of Periodontics at the School of Dentistry, University of California, Los Angeles, Consultant in Periodontics at the Veterans Administration Hospital in Los Angeles, and maintains a private practice limited to periodontics and implant surgery.

Dr. Takei has published numerous articles on periodontal surgery and has contributed chapters to five textbooks. He has received many teaching awards from both universities and dental organizations nationally and internationally. Dr. Takei has lectured throughout the world on periodontal and implant surgery and therapy.

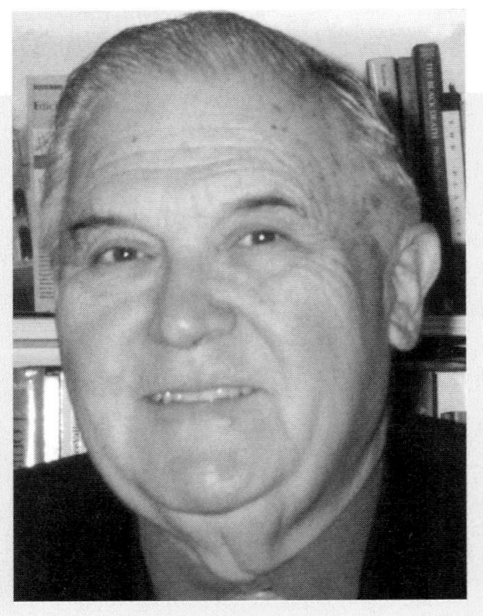

Fermin A. Carranza, Dr Odont, FACD
Dr. Fermin A. Carranza graduated from the University of Buenos Aires School of Dentistry in Argentina in 1948 and completed his postdoctoral training in Periodontics at Tufts University School of Dental Medicine in 1952 under the mentorship of Dr. Irving Glickman.

Dr. Carranza is Professor Emeritus of Periodontology at the School of Dentistry, University of California, Los Angeles. He was Head of the Department of Periodontics at the University of Buenos Aires from 1966 to 1974 and at University of California–Los Angeles from 1974 until his retirement in 1994.

Dr. Carranza has published more than 218 scientific papers and abstracts on basic and applied aspects of periodontics and eight books, including the last four editions of *Clinical Periodontology.* He has received numerous awards and recognition for his work, including the IADR Science Award in Periodontal Disease and the Gies Award of the American Academy of Periodontology.

Dr. Carranza has lectured throughout the world on clinical periodontology, pathology, and therapy.

Preface

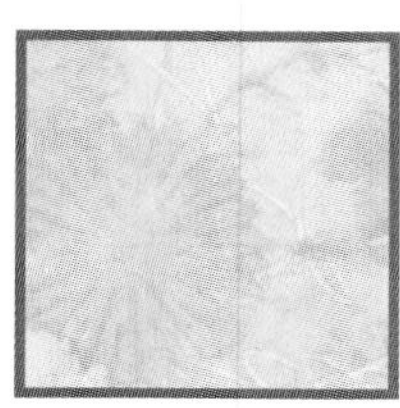

The originator of this book and author of its first four editions, published in 1953, 1958, 1964, and 1972, was Dr. Irving Glickman, Professor and Chairman of the Department of Periodontology at Tufts University School of Dental Medicine, in Boston, Massachusetts.

Dr. Glickman was a prominent researcher, superb teacher, gifted speaker, and brilliant writer whose concepts shaped periodontal thinking for many years. His style of writing and many of his original illustrations, ideas, and philosophy of dental practice can still be found in many areas of this book.

After Dr. Glickman's death in 1972 at 58 years of age, the responsibility for continuing this book was passed to Dr. Fermin A. Carranza, once a student and collaborator of Dr. Glickman. At the time Dr. Carranza was Professor and Chairman of Periodontics at the School of Dentistry, University of California–Los Angeles (UCLA). The following four editions were published in 1979, 1984, 1990, and 1996 under the guidance of Dr. Carranza, who is now Professor Emeritus at UCLA.

For this present edition, the task of maintaining the book's tradition of almost half a century has changed hands once again. Dr. Michael G. Newman and Dr. Henry H. Takei have joined Dr. Carranza to take major responsibility for this ninth edition.

In the 49 years that have elapsed since the first edition of this book, periodontology has made tremendous progress. The analysis of periodontal tissues and the mechanisms and causes of their involvement in various pathologic processes has gone beyond histology and physiology into cellular and molecular research. Therapeutic goals and techniques, based on the improved biologic foundation and multiple technologic advances, have surpassed the goal of attaining periodontal health and adequate function. Today, reconstruction of lost structures, replacement of teeth by implants, and achievement of esthetic results are integral parts of clinical periodontology.

All this development and growth has resulted in revisions of, additions to, and modifications in the book's content and organization throughout this latest edition. This multifaceted complex task has required the incorporation of numerous experts in the various fields that our discipline has entered.

This edition has also benefited by a number of technologic editorial advances that not only makes the book more attractive but also helps reading and understanding text and figures. The addition of a CD-ROM containing questions that may help teachers and students and an increased number of illustrations for each chapter will greatly enhance the usefulness of the book. The CD-ROM is a wonderful resource of illustrations, case studies, complex surgical procedures, implants, histopathology, and clinical photographs. The CD-ROM's slide show feature can be used to create your personal collection of images or to develop a presentation for your students or colleagues.

This book continues, however, to be primarily a textbook for practitioners of general dentistry and students preparing to become general practitioners. It contains abundant information of interest to periodontists, residents, and graduate students. It is our belief that the periodontal care of the public is primarily the concern of the general dentist, who cannot disregard his or her responsibility to examine, treat, or refer all periodontal problems. The high incidence of periodontal problems and the close relationship between periodontal and restorative dental therapies makes this an incontrovertible point. A well-trained group of periodontists who specialize in the diagnosis and treatment of severe or unusual problems should serve to supplement the general dental care available to our population.

It is our hope that this new edition will continue to be as useful to dentists, periodontists, and students as the previous editions and that it will contribute to the continuous progress of our profession.

Michael G. Newman
Henry H. Takei
Fermin A. Carranza

Acknowledgments

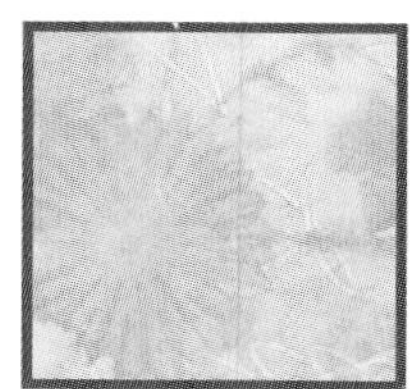

Many scientists and clinicians have shared their knowledge and expertise for the previous editions of this book, but their names no longer appear as contributors to the present one. We would like to express our deep gratitude to the following colleagues for their many valuable concepts and ideas that are still part of this book: *Drs. Donald F. Adams, Juan J. Carraro, Edmund Cataldo, Louis A. Cohn, John H. Flocken, Vojislav Lekovic, Vanessa Marinho, Francis McCarthy, Philip McCarthy, F. Reynaldo Saglie, Donald A. Seligman, William K. Solberg, Vladimir W. Spolsky, Angela Ubios,* and *Alfred Weinstock.*

For this edition, we again have been fortunate to obtain the valuable help of a group of scientists with remarkable expertise and knowledge in different clinical and research areas of periodontics.

We wish to gratefully acknowledge the valuable help of the following colleagues who contributed previously unpublished information or illustrations: *E. A. Albano, Beatriz Aldape, Carl Allen, D. C. Anderson, E. I. Ball, B. O. Barletta, Burton Becker, William Becker, Sol Bernick, Charles N. Bertolami, Gerald Bowers, A. Brendel, Raul G. Caffesse, Anand P. Chaudhry, Osvaldo Costa, Louis Cuccia, Douglas Damm, B. Ehmke, L. Roy Eversole, Terry Fiori, Stuart L. Fischman, J. Frontan, R. M. Frank, Steven I. Gold, M. Goodson, Robert J. Gorlin, A. Haffajee, T. J. Han, Fredrico Herrero, Stanley C. Holt, Joseph Hsiou, Steven Kwan, Linda Lee, J. Lindhe, Max Listgarten, Frank Lucatorto, Agusti Marfany, Philip Melnick, Robert Merin, David F. Mitchell, R. G. Oliver, Silvia Oreamuno, Joan Otomo-Corgel, Charles A. Palioca, Benjamin Patur, R. Earl Robinson, Ronald Rott, Joseph Schwartz, N. J. Selliseth, K. Selvig, Gerald Shklar, T. N. Sims, S. Socransky, John Sottosanti, Carlo Tinti, Sam Toll, Simon Wood, Spencer Woolfe,* and *Kim D. Zussman.*

We are grateful to the following UCLA postdoctoral periodontal residents who were very helpful in reviewing the literature and gathering illustrative material: *Drs. Claudia Lemus, Mark Redd, Afshen Salamati,* and *Nelson Yen;* and to *Dr. Rodrigo Lagos* for all his devoted effort on behalf of the book.

We are grateful to the following companies that have shared information, illustrations, or both with us: *T. B. Hartzell, Hu-Friedy, Nobel Biocare, Procter & Gamble,* and *3I Implants.*

We are indebted to *Imagineering* for their excellent artwork and their untiring efforts to follow our ideas.

Our thanks to W.B. Saunders and particularly to *Penny Rudolph, Ellen Forest, Kimberly Alvis,* and *Jaime Pendill.* Their expertise and detailed attention to every word and every concept contributed greatly to improving the quality of the book.

We also wish to express our gratitude to our mentors who guided our first steps in our profession and helped us develop our ideas in the field.

Dr. Newman: *Sigmund S. Socransky, Bernard Chaiken, Ed Loftus, Paul Goldhaber, Stephen Stone and J. D. Murray, F. A. Carranza,* and *Henry Takei* for directing and nurturing me. Special thanks to *E. Barrie Kenney* for his support in providing me the opportunity to manage this large, complex, and time-consuming project.

Dr. Takei: *Donald Van Scotter, Delbert P. Nachazel,* and *John Pfeiffer.* Special thanks also to *Rose Kitayama* for her administrative help.

Dr. Carranza: *Irving Glickman, Fermin Carranza, Sr.,* and *Romulo L. Cabrini.* My gratitude also to my coeditors who will continue the tradition of this book.

Last but not least, we wish to acknowledge the constant support of our parents, colleagues, and friends. Special gratitude goes to our wives and children: *Susan, Andrea,* and *Natalie; June, Scott,* and *Akemi;* and *Rita, Fermin, Patricia,* and *Laura,* who have always been so tolerant, encouraging, and understanding.

Michael G. Newman
Henry H. Takei
Fermin A. Carranza

Table of Contents

Content Associate Editor: M. John Novak

The Historical Background of Periodontology

Gerald Shklar and Fermin A. Carranza

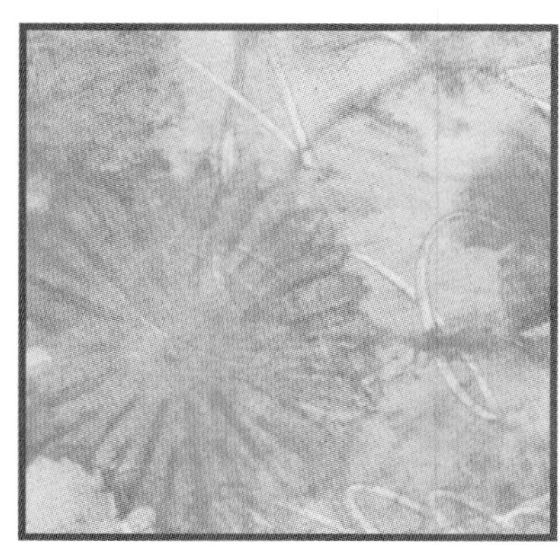

INTRODUCTION

CHAPTER OUTLINE

Gingival and periodontal diseases, in their various forms, have afflicted humans since the dawn of history, and studies in paleopathology have indicated that destructive periodontal disease as evidenced by bone loss affected early humans in such diverse cultures as ancient Egypt and early pre-Columbian America.[69] The earliest historical records dealing with medical topics reveal an awareness of periodontal disease and the need for treatment. Almost all the early writings that have been preserved have sections or chapters dealing with oral diseases, and periodontal problems comprise a significant amount of space in these writings. The relationship between calculus and periodontal disease often was considered, and underlying systemic disease often was postulated as a cause of periodontal disorders. However, methodic, carefully reasoned, therapeutic discussions did not exist until the Arabic surgical treatises of the Middle Ages; and modern treatment, with illustrated texts and sophisticated instrumentation, did not develop until the time of Pierre Fauchard in the 18th century.

EARLY CIVILIZATIONS

Oral hygiene was practiced by the Sumerians of 3000 BCE, and elaborately decorated gold toothpicks found in the excavations at Ur in Mesopotamia suggest an interest in cleanliness of the mouth. The Babylonians and Assyrians, like the earlier Sumerians, apparently suffered from periodontal problems, and a clay tablet of the period tells of treatment by gingival massage combined with various herbal medications.[36]

Periodontal disease was the most common of all diseases evidenced in the embalmed bodies of the ancient Egyptians. Thus it is not surprising that the problem received attention in medical and surgical writings of the time. The Ebers papyrus contains many references to gingival disease and offers a number of prescriptions for strengthening the teeth and gums. These remedies were made from various plants and minerals and were applied to the gums in the form of a paste with honey, vegetable gum, or residue of beer as a vehicle.[20]

Among the various medical papyri that have been preserved, the most sophisticated, in terms of modern medical practice, is the Edwin Smith surgical papyrus.[9] This remnant of a larger work presents 48 cases and discusses diagnosis, prognosis, and appropriate therapy. Mandibular fractures and dislocations are considered, but periodontal problems are not mentioned as diseases requiring surgical therapy.

The medical works of ancient India devote a significant amount of space to oral and periodontal problems. The *Susruta Samhita* contains numerous descriptions of severe periodontal disease with loose teeth and purulent discharge from the gingiva.[72] In a later treatise, the *Charaka Samhita,* toothbrushing and oral hygiene are stressed:

> *The stick for brushing the teeth should be either astringent or pungent or bitter. One of its ends should be chewed in the form of a brush. It should be used twice a day, taking care that the gums not be injured.*[15]

Ancient Chinese medical works also discussed periodontal disease. In the oldest book, written by Huang-Ti about 2500 BCE, a chapter is devoted to dental and gingival diseases. Oral diseases were divided into three types: *Fong Ya,* or inflammatory conditions; *Ya Kon,* or diseases of the soft investing tissues of the teeth; and *Chong Ya,* or dental caries.[17]

Gingival inflammations, periodontal abscesses, and gingival ulcerations are described in accurate detail. One gingival condition is described as follows:

> *The gingivae are pale or violet red, hard and lumpy, sometimes bleeding: the toothache is continuous.*

Herbal remedies *(Zn-hine-tong)* are mentioned for the treatment of these conditions. The Chinese were among the earliest people to use the "chewstick" as a toothpick and toothbrush to clean the teeth and massage the gingival tissues. Chewsticks were made of plant limbs or roots, with one end beaten into a soft fibrous condition and used for scrubbing and brushing the teeth. Chewsticks are still used by Asiatic and African peoples in underdeveloped regions.[39,47]

The importance of oral hygiene was recognized by the early Hebrews. Many pathologic conditions of the teeth and their surrounding structures are described in the Talmudic writings. Artifacts of the Phoenician civilization include a specimen of wire splinting, apparently constructed to stabilize teeth loosened by periodontal disease.[36]

GREECE

With the development of Greek culture and science came one of the golden ages of Western civilization. The Greeks attained preeminence in almost every field or discipline they attempted. Architecture, painting, sculpture, pottery, poetry, drama, philosophy, and history reached a degree of perfection rarely surpassed in succeeding ages. This was the age of Homer, Plato, and Aristotle; of Euripides, Aeschylus, and Sophocles; of Herodotus and Xenophon; of Phidias and Praxiteles. Modern science also had its birth in Greece, and medicine developed in terms of diagnostic approach and technical skill. Greek medicine continued into the succeeding Roman civilization and the early Byzantine Age.

Among the ancient Greeks, Hippocrates of Cos (460–377 BCE) was the father of modern medicine, the first to institute a systematic examination of the patient's pulse, temperature, respiration, excreta, sputum, and pulse.[13,39] He discussed the function and eruption of the teeth and the etiology of periodontal disease. He believed that inflammation of the gums could be caused by accumulations of pituita or calculus, with gingival hemorrhage occurring in cases of persistent splenic maladies. One splenic malady was described as follows:

> *The belly becomes swollen, the spleen enlarged and hard, the patient suffers from acute pain. The gums are detached from the teeth and smell bad.*[39]

ROME

Long before 735 BCE, the Etruscans were adept in the art of constructing artificial dentures, but no evidence exists that they were aware of periodontal disease or its treatment.

Among the Romans, Aulus Cornelius Celsus (25 BCE–50 CE) referred to diseases that affect the soft parts of the mouth and their treatment as follows:

> *If the gums separate from the teeth, it is beneficial to chew unripe pears and apples and keep their juices in the mouth.*

He described looseness of the teeth caused by the weakness of their roots or flaccidity of the gums and noted that it is necessary in these cases to touch the gums lightly with a red-hot iron and then smear them with honey.[14] The Romans were very interested in oral hygiene. Celsus believed that stains on the teeth should be removed and the teeth then rubbed with a dentifrice. The use of the toothbrush is mentioned in the writings of many of the Roman poets. Gingival massage was an integral part of oral hygiene.

Paul of Aegina (625–690 CE) differentiated between epulis, a fleshy excrescence of gums in the area of a tooth, and parulis, which he described as an abscess of the gums. He wrote that tartar incrustations must be removed with either scrapers or a small file and that the teeth should be carefully cleaned after the last meal of the day.[63]

THE MIDDLE AGES

The decline and eventual fall of the Roman Empire that plunged Europe into an age of darkness was accompanied by the rise of Islam and the golden age of Arabic science and medicine. The astonishing attainments of Islamic medicine provided for the rise of European medicine in the late Middle Ages and Renaissance. In the early medical schools of Salerno and Montpellier, the available texts were primarily the renowned Arabic treatises in adequate (but far from accurate) Latin translations.

Much of medieval and Renaissance stomatology and dentistry was derived directly from Arabic writings, particularly the treatises of Ibn Sina (Avicenna) and Abu'l-Qasim (Albucasis). The Arabic treatises derived much of their information from Greek medical treatises, but many refinements and novel approaches were added, particularly in surgical specialties.[70] Many of the Greek medical classics translated into Arabic in Baghdad during the Abbassid Caliphate were eventually retranslated into Latin after the destruction and virtual disappearance of scholarship in Europe during the Dark Ages. Baghdad, along with Córdoba in Spain, enjoyed both intellectual and medical eminence; these two cities represented the greatness of the Eastern and Western Caliphates, respectively.

Hunayn ibn-Ishaq (809–73) and his associates translated into Arabic the original Greek texts of Galen, Oribasius, Paul of Aegina, Dioscorides, and the Hippocratic corpus, as well as the philosophy of Plato and Aristotle and the mathematics of Archimedes. Abu Bakr Muhammed ibn Zakariya al Razi (Rhazes) (841–926) wrote an encyclopedic work on medicine and surgery in 25 books. He was also physician-in-chief at the great Baghdad hospital and taught medicine in terms of clinical cases. Ali ibn Abbas al Majousi (Haly Abbas) (930–94) described many dermatologic conditions and recommended such surgical advances as the suturing of blood vessels before the removal of tumors. He also wrote extensively on dental subjects.

Ibn Sina (Avicenna) (980–1037), born in Persia, was possibly the greatest of the Arabic physicians. His *Canon,* a comprehensive treatise on medicine, is probably the most famous medical text of all time and was in continuous use for almost 600 years. Avicenna used an extensive materia medica for oral and periodontal diseases and rarely resorted to surgery. Headings in the *Canon* on gingival disease include "Bleeding Gums," "Fissures of the Gums," "Ulcers of the Gums," "Separation of the Gums," "Recession of the Gums," "Looseness of the Gums," and "Epulis."[5]

Abu'l-Qasim (936–1013) was the preeminent physician and surgeon of the Western Caliphate at Córdoba. His contributions to dentistry and periodontology were among his outstanding achievements. He had a clear understanding of the major etiologic role of calculus deposits and described in detail the technique of scaling the teeth, using a sophisticated set of instruments that he developed. He also wrote in detail on the extraction of teeth, the splinting of loose teeth with gold wire, and the filing of gross occlusal abnormalities. The fame of his treatise spread through the Arab world and beyond. It was translated into Latin by Gerard of Cremona in the 12th century and greatly influenced the surgeons Guglielmo Saliceti (1201–77) and Guy de Chauliac (c. 1300–68)[59] in the 13th and 14th centuries and Fabricius of Aquapendente (1537–1619) in the 16th century. Abu'l-Qasim described the way to remove calculus from teeth:[2]

> *Occasionally there is deposited in the inner and outer surfaces of the teeth or between the gums, large and rough ugly concretion: the teeth take on a black, yellow or green color, following which the gums are altered and the teeth become unsightly.*

To treat this disease, seat the patient in front of you, placing the head in your lap. Scale [scrape] the teeth and molars that present the concretions or the gritty deposits until nothing remains. Scrape also throughout where the teeth are black, yellow, green or otherwise colored, until they [the calculus deposits] are gone. It is possible that one scaling will suffice. If not, begin a second, third or fourth time, until your purpose is completely attained.

You should know that the scaling of teeth is done with instruments of various shapes according to the use that is required for them. The scalers that one uses for scaling the inner surfaces of the teeth are different than those employed for the scaling of the exterior surfaces, and those that are used to scale the interdental surfaces. Here is an assortment of scalers all of which you have at your disposition (Fig. 1).

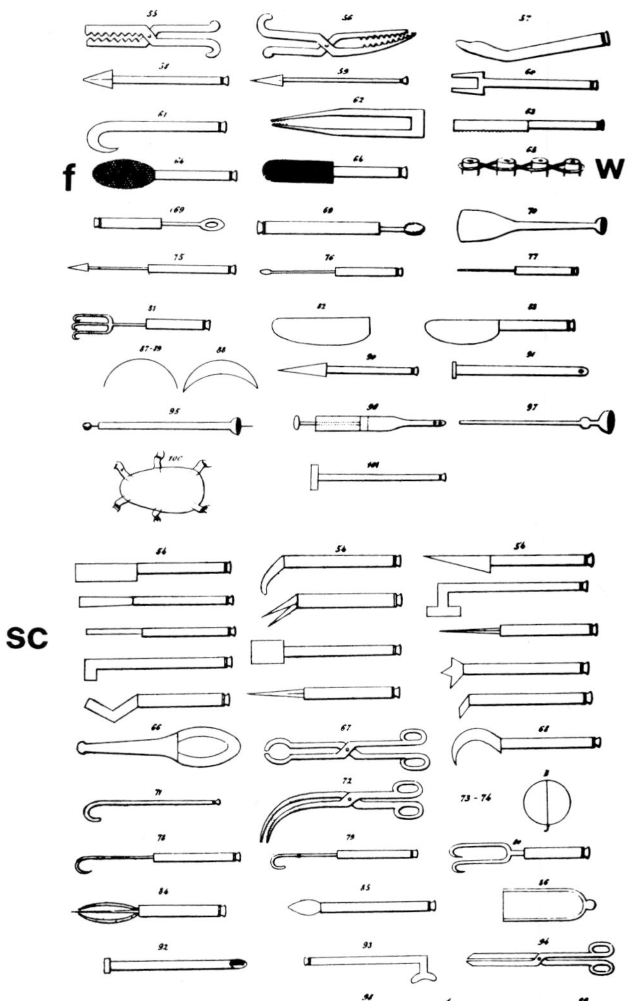

Fig. 1 Illustration of Abu'l-Qasim's periodontal instruments, showing scalers *(sc),* files *(f),* and the wiring of loose teeth *(w).*

In Japan in 984, a book by Yasuyori Tanba, entitled *I-Shin-Po,* which means "Essential Method of Medicine," was published.[26] *I-Shin-Po* consisted of 30 volumes, and in volume 5 the treatment of diseases of the mouth, teeth, throat, and nose was described. The author wrote that the teeth receive their nutrition from the bone marrow and that tooth mobility is caused by malnutrition.

RENAISSANCE

During the Renaissance, with the rebirth of classical scholarship and the development of scientific thought and medical knowledge in addition to the flowering of art, music, and literature, significant contributions were made to anatomy and surgery.

Paracelsus (1493–1541) continues to be a controversial figure of the Renaissance and Humanism. He wrote extensively on a large variety of subjects, and his collected works—14 large volumes in the fine modern edition of Sudhoff—are continuously being analyzed for an understanding of his ideas and often complex concepts, ranging from chemistry and the physical world to philosophy and the power of imagination.[61]

Paracelsus developed an interesting and unusual theory of disease among his special pathologic theories: the doctrine of calculus. He understood that pathologic calcification occurred in a variety of organs, and he considered these disease conditions to result from a metabolic disturbance whereby the body takes nourishment from food and discards the refuse as "tartarus," a material that cannot be broken down and the ultimate matter, or *materia ultima*. This tartar or ultimate material, consisting of gravel and gluelike components, was exogenous and came from barley and peas, milk, meat and fish, and drinks such as wine, beer, and fruit juice. This material in food could be eliminated by cooking and thus excreted in the feces. The tartar content of food was thought to vary in different geographic locations. Saliva served digestion in the mouth, as did other agents in the stomach. Tartar also could be precipitated by the action of salt, which dried up or coagulated mucoid matter in food. The amount of tartar formed depended on the region of the body. Paracelsus recognized the extensive formation of tartar on the teeth and related this to toothache. Toothache was thus comparable to the pain produced by calculus in other organs such as the kidneys.[61]

> *A specific digestive process already takes place in the mouth, and this process is potent enough to sustain life. Its waste products are deposited as tartar on the teeth with resulting decay of the gums, wearing down of teeth, pain due to acerbity with which tartarus is endowed. Toothache is thus comparable to the pain caused by calculus elsewhere.*[61]

Andreas Vesalius (1514–64), born in Brussels, taught at the University of Padua in the Venetian Republic, where he performed human dissections and wrote a magnificent book on anatomy with excellent illustrations throughout, which were drawn by Kalkar, a student of Titian.[75]

Bartholomaeus Eustachius (1520–74) of Rome was another outstanding anatomist and wrote a small book on dentistry, *Libellus de Dentibus* ("A Little Treatise on the Teeth"), in 30 chapters.[22]

In many ways, his anatomic studies were more detailed and comprehensive than those of his more famous contemporary, Vesalius, but his major studies remained unknown until their publication in 1722. This was the first original book on the teeth and offered many new descriptions and concepts based on research and clinical studies. In addition to the first clear description of the dental pulp and the root canal, Eustachius understood that the crowns of the teeth were composed of enamel overlying dentin, the first description of the two separate tissues of the tooth. Occlusion was described in detail in humans as well as animals. The permanent teeth were found to develop from dental follicles and not from the roots of deciduous teeth, as postulated by Vesalius. Eustachius' description of the periodontal tissues was a major advance:

> *At any rate, as I have already pointed out, the roots of all the teeth are so well attached to their respective sockets that the teeth can hardly be budged. Ligaments attached to each tooth provide added stability. Moreover, there are extremely strong fibers attached to the roots; these provide a firm connection to the socket. The manifold structure of the mouth created by the gingivae surrounds the teeth as soon as they emerge from their sockets. The structure of the gingivae themselves contributes in no small way to the strength of the teeth.*

Eustachius also described some diseases of the mouth in the last chapter of his book and offered treatment modalities as well as a rationale for treatment. His treatment of periodontitis was remarkably modern in that he advised both scaling of calculus and curettage of granulation tissue so that an actual reattachment of the gingival and periodontal tissues could take place.

> *The use of astringents to shrink the gum is of little value. But if the gums diminish and recede, and the teeth become covered with a hard, cuticle-like substance, reuniting the tooth and gum is as likely as joining the middle and index fingers unless the physician first scrapes the teeth and freshen the gums with a scalpel, and uses medicines that will encourage attachments.*

Artzney Buch-
lein/wider allerlei kran-
ckeyten vnd gebrechen der zeen/gezogen
auſs dem Galeno/Auicenna/Meſue/
Cornelio Celſo vnd andern mehr
der Artzney Doctorn/ſeher
nützlich zu
leſen.
M. D. XXX.

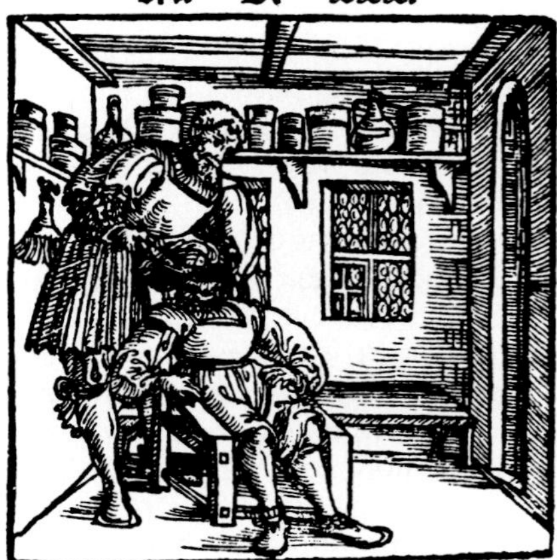

Fig. 2 Frontispiece of *Artzney Buchlein* (1530).

Ambroise Parè (1509–90), head surgeon at the Hôtel Dieu in Paris, was the outstanding surgeon of the Renaissance, and his contributions to dental surgery were substantial. He developed many oral surgical procedures in detail, including gingivectomy for hyperplastic gingival tissues.[62] He also understood the etiologic significance of calculus and used a set of scalers to remove the hard deposits on the teeth. Parè wrote in French rather than in Latin, and therefore his works could be widely read and understood.

The first book written in a common language (German) and specifically devoted to dental practice, entitled *Artzney Buchlein* or *Zene Artzney*[4] (Fig. 2), was published in Leipzig in 1530; 15 separate editions were published between that time and 1576. The author of this book remains unknown despite considerable historic research attempting to discover his identity.[11] The book was essentially a compendium of previous writings on oral and dental diseases and their management. Three chapters are devoted specifically to periodontal problems. In Chapter 7, "Concerning Yellow and Black Teeth," the author describes tartar as "a white, yellow, and black slime that settles on the lower part of the teeth and over the gums."

The author also suggests scraping black teeth and the use of toothpastes or powders to rub against the teeth. Recipes for several pastes and powders are offered.

Chapter 9, "Of Loose Teeth," describes periodontitis:

> *[Periodontitis] happens either through negligence or weakness or disease of the gums, or through the separation of those substances that hold the teeth in their places, which happens when humors from the head drop down upon the gums or roots of the teeth and loosen them by their noxious action.*

Thus a crude concept is presented of systemic and local factors in the etiology of periodontal disease. The presence of local infective agents, or "worms," also is mentioned. A variety of ointments, often astringent in nature, are suggested, and the binding of loose teeth to sound ones with silk or gold thread is recommended. Cauterizing the gingiva with a hot iron is mentioned, but "this burning is dangerous and needs an expensive skilled master." In Chapter 11, "Ulceration, Bad Smell, and Decay of the Gums," the management of necrotizing gingivitis with medicines containing vinegar and alum is discussed.

The Italian physician, mathematician, and philosopher Girolamo Cardano (1501–76) appears to have been the first to differentiate types of periodontal disease. In a publication dated 1562, he mentions one type of disease that occurs with advancing age and leads to progressive loosening and loss of teeth, as well as a second, very aggressive type that occurs in younger patients.[38] It was not until late in the 20th century that this classification was rediscovered and became widely accepted.

Anton van Leeuwenhoek (1632–1723) of Delft, Holland, contributed more to the development of modern biologic science than any classically trained scholar of his age. A layman with an inquisitive mind and a hobby of grinding lenses, he developed the microscope and used it to discover microorganisms, cellular structure, blood cells, sperm, and various other microscopic structures, including the tubular structure of dentin.[19] He was a strong opponent of the spontaneous generation concept, which was finally put to rest by Pasteur two centuries later. Leeuwenhoek described his findings in letters written originally in Dutch to the Royal Society of London, which translated them into English and published them in its *Philosophical Transactions*.

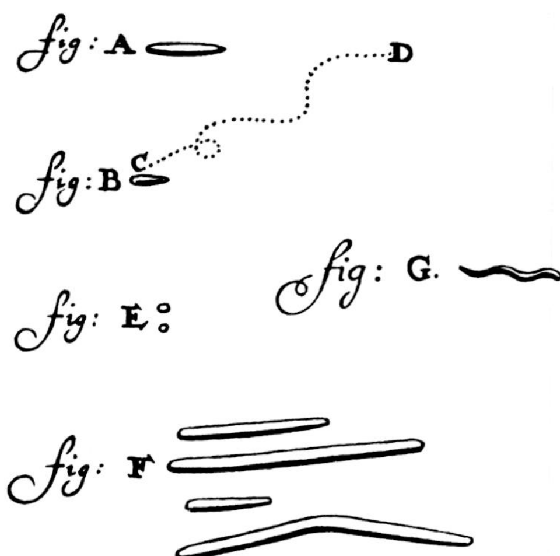

Fig. 3 Leeuwenhoek's drawing of oral spirochetes, bacilli, and other microorganisms.

Using material from his gingival tissues, Leeuwenhoek first described oral bacterial flora, and his drawings offered a reasonably good presentation of oral spirochetes and bacilli (Fig. 3).

> *I didn't clean my teeth (on purpose) for three days and then took the material that had lodged in small amounts on the gums above my front teeth. . . . I found a few living animalcules.*

He also described a great amount of bacteria in a man who had never cleaned his mouth.[50]

18TH CENTURY

Modern dentistry essentially developed in 18th-century Europe, particularly France and England. Pierre Fauchard, born in Brittany in 1678, is rightly regarded as the father of the profession as we know it. Although he was self-educated in dentistry, he was able to develop a systematic approach to dental practice based on contemporary knowledge. Fauchard significantly improved the instruments and technical skills required for dental treatment, and his book, *The Surgeon Dentist,* published in 1728 (Fig. 4), gave respectability to the profession and developed a wide appreciation for the technical and surgical skills of the dental practitioner.[23] Fauchard became the leading dentist in Paris and died in 1761 after a long life of service and achievement.

Fauchard's book not only transformed dental practice but also served to educate the succeeding generation

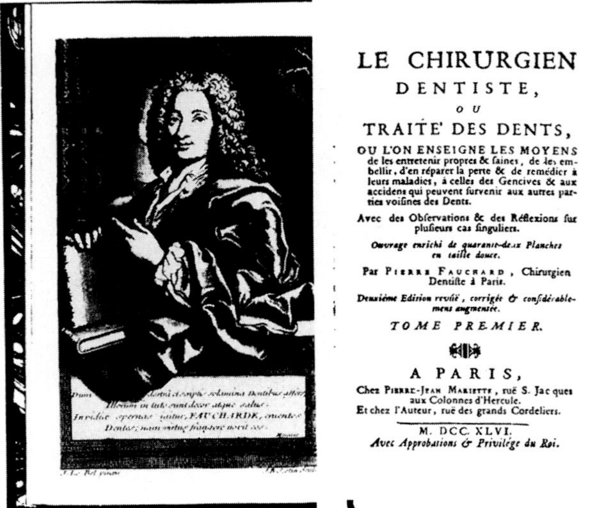

LE CHIRURGIEN
DENTISTE,
OU
TRAITE' DES DENTS,
OU L'ON ENSEIGNE LES MOYENS de les entretenir propres & saines, de les embellir, d'en réparer la perte & de remédier à leurs maladies, à celles des Gencives & aux accidens qui peuvent survenir aux autres parties voisines des Dents.
Avec des Observations & des Réflexions sur plusieurs cas singuliers.
Ouvrage enrichi de quarante-deux Planches en taille douce.
Par Pierre Fauchard, Chirurgien Dentiste à Paris.
Deuxième Edition revûë, corrigée & considérablement augmentée.
TOME PREMIER.
A PARIS,
Chez Pierre-Jean Mariette, ruë S. Jacques aux Colonnes d'Hercule.
Et chez l'Auteur, ruë des grands Cordeliers.
M. DCC. XLVI.
Avec Approbations & Privilége du Roi.

Fig. 4 Frontispiece of Fauchard's *The Surgeon Dentist* (1746).

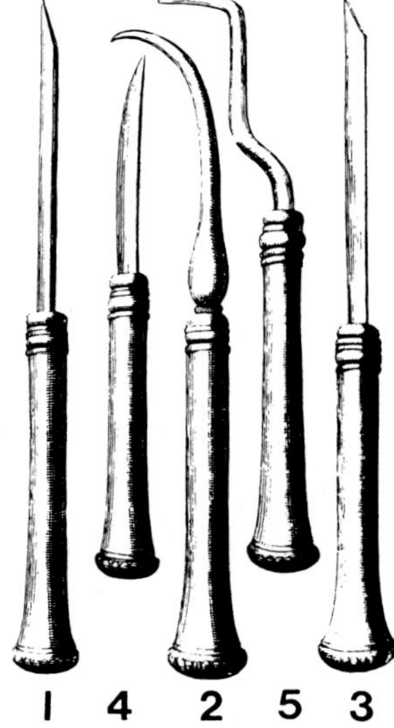

Fig. 5 The five types of instruments used by Fauchard for detaching tartar from the teeth: *1,* chisel; *2,* parrot beak; *3,* graver; *4,* convex blade; and *5,* Z-shaped hook.

of dentists, some of whom emigrated to America and practiced in the early years of the Republic. Some of George Washington's dentures were made with springs similar to those in the design illustrated by Fauchard. All aspects of dental practice are presented in his book (i.e., restorative dentistry, prosthodontics, oral surgery, periodontics, and orthodontics). Preventive dentistry is described in Chapter 4 ("The Regimen and Care Required for the Preservation of the Teeth") and in Chapter 5 ("How to Keep the Teeth White and Strengthen the Gums"). Fauchard wrote that confections and sweets destroy the teeth by sticking to their surfaces and producing an acid. He described in detail his periodontal instruments (Fig. 5) and the scaling technique to "detach hard matter or tartar from the teeth."

John Hunter (1728–93), the most distinguished anatomist, surgeon, and pathologist of 18th-century England, wrote an excellent treatise on dentistry entitled *The Natural History of the Human Teeth.*[42] He offered remarkably clear illustrations of the anatomy of the teeth and their supporting structures. He also described the features of periodontal diseases and enunciated the concept of active and passive eruption of teeth.

A contemporary of Hunter, Thomas Berdmore (1740–85), was considered the outstanding dentist in England and was known as "Dentist to His Majesty" (i.e., King George III). He published the *Treatise in the Disorders and Deformities of the Teeth and Gums* in 1770, with several chapters devoted to periodontal problems.[7] In Chapter 7, "Of Tartar of the Teeth, and the Recess of the Gums, and Toothache Occasioned by Tartarous Concretions Long Neglected," Berdmore offered detailed descriptions of instrumentation for tartar removal but stressed prevention. He also used surgery when necessary to remove hyperplastic gingival tissue once the tartar was removed:

> *For without this [surgery], the gums will not closely embrace a tooth which has been made smaller at the collar by the removal of its tartar.*

The first qualified American dentists were trained in England or France.[80] Robert Woffendale (1742–1828) was trained in London by Berdmore. Woffendale wrote one of the early dental books in America. In an advertisement in the *New York Weekly Journal* of 1766, he "begs Leave to inform the Public that he performs all Operations upon the Teeth, Gums, Sockets and Palate." Similar advertisements were placed by many contemporary dentists. John Baker (c. 1732–96) was one of George Washington's dentists and had a very successful career. He imparted his dental knowledge to Paul Revere, Isaac Greenwood, and Josiah Flagg. In an advertisement in the *New York Weekly Journal* of 1768, Baker tells the public that he

> *. . . cures the scurvy in the gums, be it ever so bad; first cleans and scales the teeth from that corrosive tartarous gritty substance, which hinders the gums from growing, infects the breath and is one of the principle causes of scurvy, and, if not timely prevented, eats away the gums so that many people's teeth fall out fresh. . . . His dentifrice with proper directions for preserving the teeth and gums is to be had at his lodgings.*

19TH CENTURY

Leonard Koecker (1785–1850) was a German-born dentist who practiced in Baltimore. In a paper in 1821 in the *Philadelphia Journal of Medicine and Physical Sciences,* he described inflammatory changes in the gingiva and the presence of calculus on teeth, leading to their looseness and exfoliation.[49] He mentioned the careful removal of tartar and the need for oral hygiene by the patient, which he recommended to be performed in the morning and after every meal, using an astringent powder and a toothbrush, placing "the bristles . . . into the spaces of the teeth." He also discouraged splinting because it loosened firm teeth, and he recommended that treatment of caries be postponed until after the gum treatment is completed and that placement of artificial teeth be avoided. Koecker was an early advocate of the odontogenic focal infection theory and recommended the extraction of all severely involved teeth and roots, including all unopposed molars, to prevent systemic infections.[49]

Levi Spear Parmly (1790–1859) was a New Orleans dentist who is considered the father of oral hygiene and the inventor of dental floss.[24] In a book published in 1819, he states that dental caries can be controlled by brushing and by using

> *. . . a waxen silken thread . . . which is to be passed through the interstices of the teeth, between their necks and the arches of the gum, to dislodge that irritating matter which no brush can remove and which is the real source of distress.*

The term *pyorrhea alveolaris* was used for the first time by Alphonse Toirac (1791–1863) in 1823, although some scholars dispute this.[41] It was introduced in the U.S. by F. H. Rehwinkel, a German physician who emigrated to the U.S. and attended the Baltimore College of Dental Surgery.[38]

In the mid-19th century, John W. Riggs (1811–85) (Fig. 6) was the leading authority on periodontal disease and its treatment in the U.S., to the point that periodontitis, or alveolar pyorrhea, was known as "Riggs' disease." He was born in Seymour, Conn., on October 25, 1811, and graduated from the Baltimore College of Dental Surgery in 1854. He practiced in Hartford, Conn., where he died on November 11, 1885. Riggs seems to have been the first individual to limit his practice to periodontics and therefore can be considered the first specialist in this field. Riggs was an associate of Horace Wells in Hartford, and he performed the first surgical operation under anesthesia, extracting a tooth of Dr. Wells' under nitrous oxide in 1844.

Riggs described his treatment of periodontal disease to an audience at the Connecticut Valley Dental Society at Northampton, Mass., in June 1867.[52] His publications, however, are very few. In a paper published in 1876 in the *Pennsylvania Journal of Dental Science,*[67] Riggs strongly advocated cleanliness of the mouth because he believed that "the teeth themselves, with their accumulated accretions and roughened surfaces . . . are the exciting cause of the disease." He strongly opposed surgery, which at the time consisted of resection of the gums.

Riggs and his disciples had great influence in the dental profession. They were the proponents of the so-called conservative approach to periodontal therapy, developing the concept of oral prophylaxis and prevention. Among his followers were L. Taylor, D. D. Smith, R. B. Adair, and W. J. Younger.[38] Many papers by followers and contemporaries of Riggs described clinical features and treatment of periodontal disease, the latter based mostly on hygienic measures.[52,66] Younger (1838–1920) considered periodontal disease a local infection and in 1893, he

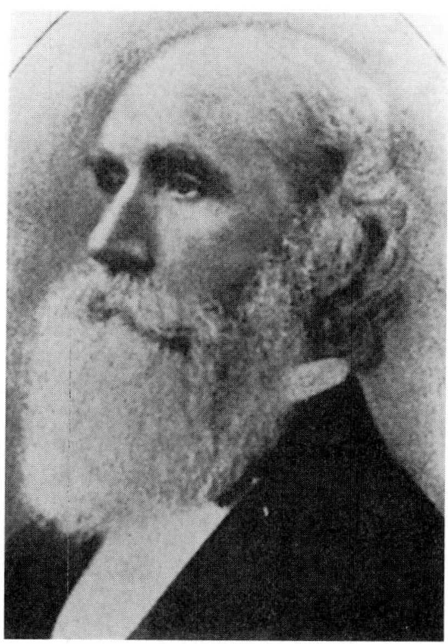

Fig. 6 John W. Riggs (1811–85). (From Hoffman-Axthelm W: History of Dentistry. Chicago, Quintessence, 1981.)

was the first to discuss the possibility of "reattachment." In 1902, Younger reported a case in which he grafted gingival tissue "from behind the third molar" to an extensive area of recession in an upper cuspid of the same patient. He first treated the root of the cuspid with lactic acid and then fixed the gum graft with "fine cambric needles," and he claims the operation to have been a success.[3]

Several major developments in medical science occurred in the second half of the 19th century, starting the era that can be called *modern medicine,* which of course includes dentistry.[12]

The first was the *discovery of anesthesia* by Horace Wells (1813–48) of Hartford, Conn. in 1845 and by William Morton (1819–1968) of Boston in 1846, who discovered the general anesthetic effects of nitrous oxide and ether, respectively. Four decades later, Sigmund Freud (1856–1939) experimented on the psychic effects of cocaine and noted its numbing effects on the tongue. He provided his friend Carl Koller (1857–1944), a Vienna ophthalmologist, with this drug, and he produced anesthesia of the eye with drops of cocaine. Further developments led to the discovery in 1905 of procaine (Novocaine) by the Munich chemists Alfred Einhorn and Richard Willstädter. Later, with the addition of adrenaline, discovered separately in the U.S. by Jokichi Takamine and Thomas Bell Aldrich, local anesthesia was born.[41]

The second scientific breakthrough was made by the French chemist Louis Pasteur (1822–95),[18,72] who finally proved that spontaneous generation of organisms does not exist and who established through his studies of the diseases of silk worms that one organism (a protozoa) can cause disease in another (the silk worm), thus establishing the *germ theory of disease*. Subsequently, the German physician Robert Koch (1843–1910), in a series of

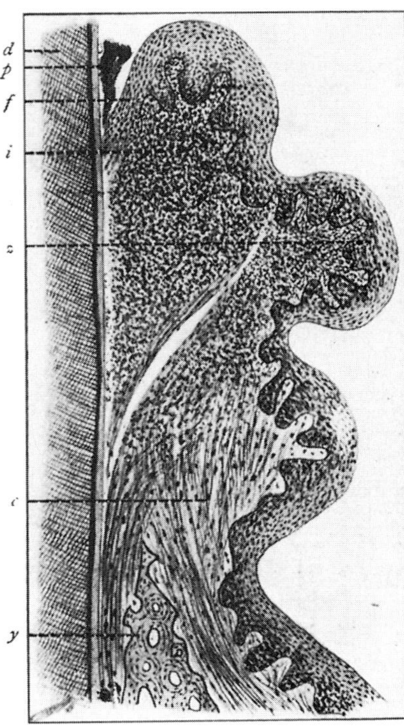

Fig. 7 Microscopic features of periodontal disease as presented by Znamensky.

brilliant investigations, discovered the microorganism that causes the cattle disease anthrax and the bacterial etiology of tuberculosis.[10]

The concepts of Pasteur were initially transferred to the clinical and surgical practice by Joseph Lister (1827–1912) of England, and thus the era of antisepsis (and later, asepsis) in surgery was born. Pasteur, Koch, and their collaborators and followers (Elie Metchnikoff, Emile Roux, Paul Ehrlich, Emil von Behring, Shibasaburo Kitasato, and many others) discovered the bacterial etiology of numerous diseases (e.g., pneumonia, cholera, puerperal fever, diphtheria, meningitis, plague, dysentery, syphilis) and gave birth to two sciences that became basic to periodontics: bacteriology and immunology.

A third scientific finding that changed the practice of dentistry in general and periodontics in particular was the *discovery of radiographs* by the German physicist Wilhelm Röntgen (1845–1923).[26] Röntgen's discovery was made in 1895 at the University of Würzburg and was purely a basic science finding, but it was immediately taken up by physicians and dentists and proved to be a crucial development in periodontics and many other areas of medicine and dentistry.

Also in the late 19th century, studies by Rudolph Virchow (1821–1902), Julius Cohnhein (1839–84), Elie Metchnikoff (1845–1916), and others had started to shed light on the microscopic changes occurring in inflammation.[1] This resulted in an understanding of the pathogenesis of periodontal disease based on histopathologic studies. N. N. Znamensky in Moscow understood the complex interaction of local and systemic factors in the etiology of periodontal disease (Fig. 7), and his observations and concepts were summarized in 1902 in a classic paper[87] in which he describes the presence in inflamed gingivae of a cellular infiltrate that extends deeper as the disease progresses, causing bone resorption associated to multinucleated cells (osteoclasts) and Howship's lacunae. Znamensky treated pyorrhea with removal of calculus and deep curettage of the pockets, using cocaine anesthesia.

The first individual to identify bacteria as the cause of periodontal disease appears to have been the German dentist Adolph Witzel (1847–1906),[31,84] who taught at the University of Jena, but the first true oral microbiologist was Willoughby D. Miller (1853–1907). Miller was born in Alexandria, Ohio and received training in basic sciences at the University of Michigan. He emigrated to Germany but later returned to the U.S. to receive his dental training at the Pennsylvania Dental College. Back in Berlin, he worked in Robert Koch's microbiology laboratory and embarked on a research career that introduced modern bacteriology principles to dentistry. His greatest accomplishments were in caries research, where he developed the chemicoparasitic theory of caries. In his classic book *The Microorganisms of the Human Mouth,* published in 1890, he described the features of periodontal disease and considered the role of predisposing factors, irritational factors, and bacteria in the etiology of pyorrhea alveolaris. He believed that the disease was not caused by a specific bacterium but by a complex array of various bacteria normally present in the oral cavity. This constitutes what was later known as the *nonspecific plaque hypothesis* that went unchallenged for seven decades.[31,54]

However, Miller did not recognize bacterial plaque. This was left to J. Leon Williams (1852–1932), an American dentist who practiced in London and who in 1897 described a gelatinous accumulation of bacteria adherent to the enamel surface in relation to caries;[83] and to G. V. Black (1836–1915), who in 1899 coined the term *gelatinous microbic plaque.*

Salomon Robicsek (1845–1928), born in Hungary, obtained his medical degree and practiced dentistry in Vienna. He developed a surgical technique consisting of a scalloped continuous gingivectomy excision, exposing the marginal bone for subsequent curettage and remodeling.[71] The first description (1901) of a possible role of trauma from occlusion and bruxism in periodontal disease is generally attributed to the Austrian dentist Moritz Karolyi (1865–1945),[46] who also recommended its correction by grinding occlusal surfaces and preparation of bite plates.

Acute Necrotizing Ulcerative Gingivitis

Acute necrotizing ulcerative gingivitis (ANUG) had been recognized in the 4th century BCE by Xenophon, who mentioned that Greek soldiers were affected with "sore mouth and foul-smelling breath." In 1778, Hunter had described the clinical features of this disease and differentiated it from scurvy and chronic periodontitis. ANUG occurred in epidemic form in the French army in the 19th century, and in 1886 the German pathologist Hersch discussed some of the features associated

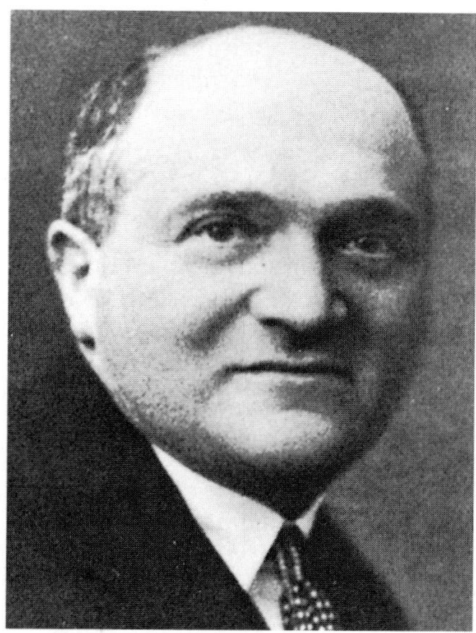

Fig. 8 Bernhard Gottlieb (1885–1950). (From Gold SI. Periodontics. The past. Part II. J Clin Periodontol 1985; 12:171.)

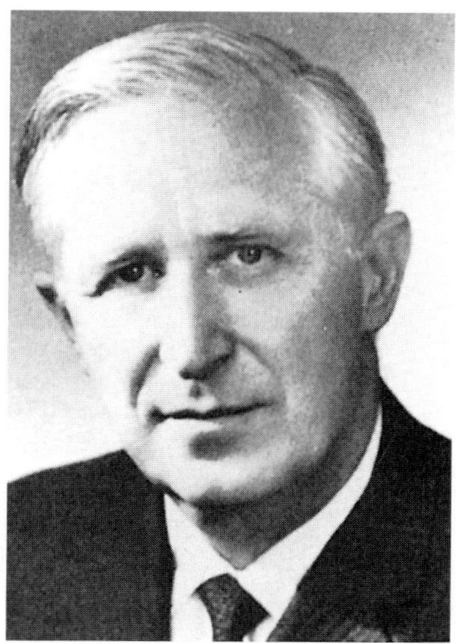

Fig. 9 Balint J. Orban (1899–1960). (From J Periodontol 1960; 31:266.)

with the disease, such as enlarged lymph nodes, fever, malaise, and increased salivation.

Hyacinthe Jean Vincent (1862–1950),[31,76] a French physician working at the Pasteur Institute in Paris, and Hugo Carl Plaut (1858–1928),[65] in Germany, described the spirillum and fusiform bacilli associated with what later became known as *Vincent's angina,* and in 1904 Vincent described these organisms in acute ulceronecrotic gingivitis.[77]

20TH CENTURY

In the first third of the 20th century, periodontics flourished in central Europe, with two major centers of excellence: Vienna and Berlin.

Vienna

The Vienna school developed the basic histopathologic concepts on which modern periodontics was built. The major representative from this group was Bernhard Gottlieb (1885–1950) (Fig. 8), who published extensive microscopic studies of periodontal disease in human autopsy specimens. His major contributions appeared in the German literature in the 1920s and described the attachment of the gingival epithelium to the tooth,[32] the histopathology of inflammatory and degenerative periodontal disease,[25,33,34] the biology of the cementum, active and passive tooth eruption, and traumatic occlusion. Gottlieb also carried out histologic studies on animal periodontal tissues in the laboratory of Julius Tandler. Reviews of Gottlieb's studies appeared in English in 1921 in *The Dental Cosmos* and in 1927 in the *Journal of the American Dental Association.* A book published in 1938 by Gottlieb and Orban, *Biology and Pathology of the Tooth and Its Supporting Mechanism,*[35] presented a complete review in English of the concepts developed by Gottlieb and his co-workers in Vienna.

A younger contemporary of Gottlieb's in Vienna was Balint J. Orban (1899–1960) (Fig. 9), who carried out extensive histologic studies on periodontal tissues that serve as the basis for much of current therapy. Other members of the Viennese school were Rudolph Kronfeld (1901–40), Joseph P. Weinmann (1889–1960), and Harry Sicher (1889–1974). All these scientists emigrated to the United States in the 1930s and contributed greatly to the progress of American dentistry.

Berlin

The Berlin group consisted mostly of clinical scientists who developed and refined the surgical approach to periodontal therapy. Prominent in this group were Oskar Weski and Robert Neumann.

Weski (1879–1952) (Fig. 10) carried out pioneering studies correlating radiographic and histopathologic changes in periodontal disease.[81] He also conceptualized the periodontium as formed by cementum, gingiva, periodontal ligament, and bone and gave it the name *paradentium,* which was later changed (owing to etymologic reasons) to *parodontium,* a term still used in Europe. The contributions of Alfred Kantorowicz (1880–1962) and Karl Haüpl (1893–1960), among others, to the histopathology of the periodontal tissues also deserve mention.

Neumann (1882–1958) (Fig. 11), in a book published in 1912[56] (with new editions in 1915, 1920, and 1924) described the principles of periodontal flap surgery, including osseous recontouring as it is currently known[28] (Fig. 12). Other clinicians who described flap surgery at the beginning of the century were Leonard Widman of Sweden (1871–1956)[82] and A. Cieszynski of Poland. A bitter controversy developed between Widman, Cieszynski, and Neumann in the 1920s over the priority in the description of the periodontal flap.[58]

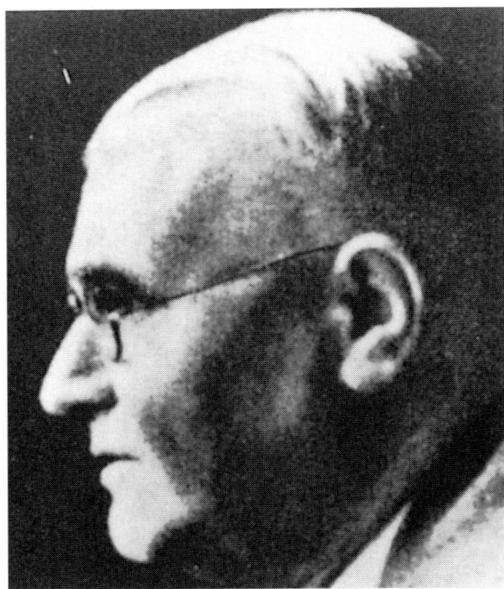

Fig. 10 Oskar Weski (1879–1952). (From Hoffman-Axthelm W: History of Dentistry. Chicago, Quintessence, 1981.)

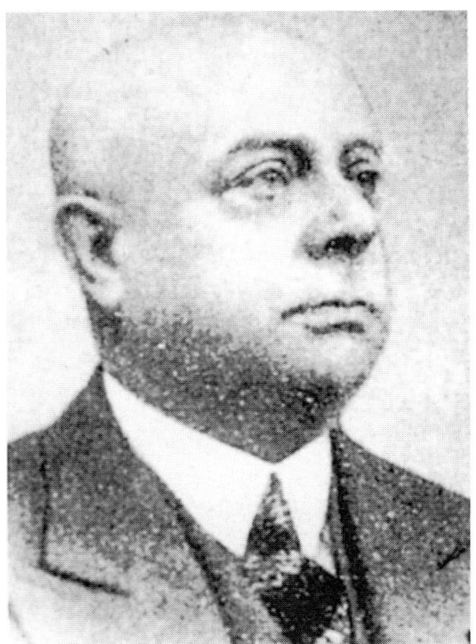

Fig. 11 Robert Neumann (1882–1958). (Courtesy Dr. Steven I. Gold, New York, N.Y.)

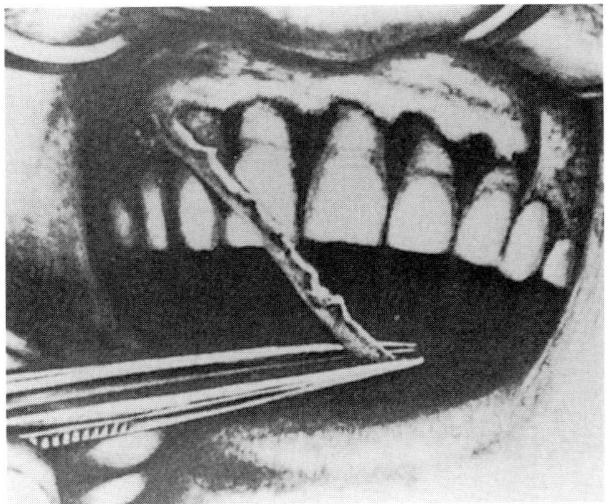

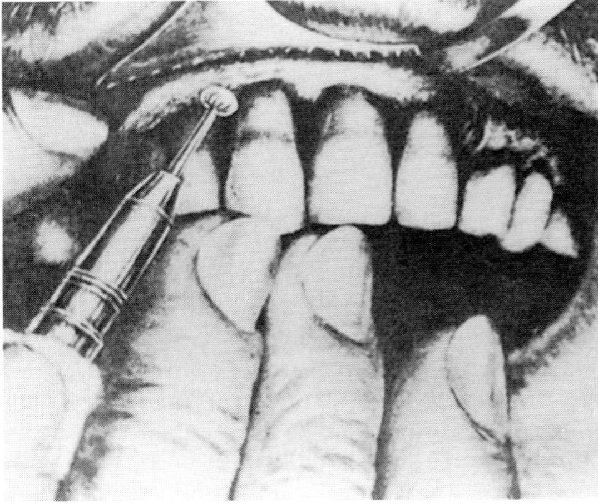

Fig. 12 Surgical procedure advocated by Robert Neumann in the early part of the 20th century. *Top,* After raising a mucoperiosteal flap, its edge is trimmed with scissors, leaving a scalloped outline. *Bottom,* Osseous recontouring with burs. (From Gold SI: Robert Neumann—a pioneer in periodontal flap surgery. J Periodontol 1982; 53:456.)

The United States and Other Countries

In the U.S., periodontal surgery developed in the first decades of the century. Early in the century, surgical techniques were developed for the coverage of denuded roots (W. J. Younger, 1902[3]; A. W. Harlan, 1906[6,37]; and P. Rosenthal, 1912[68]). However, these techniques did not attain wide usage. Before World War I, important contributions to periodontal surgery were made by A. Zentler,[86] J. Zemsky,[85] G. V. Black,[8] O. Kirkland,[48] A. W. Ward,[78] A. B. Crane and H. Kaplan,[16] and others. In 1923, Ward introduced the surgical pack under the trade name Wondr-Pak.[79]

The nonsurgical approach was championed by Isadore Hirschfeld (1882–1965) of New York, who wrote classic papers on oral hygiene,[40] local factors, and other topics. In 1913 the first school for dental hygienists was created by Alfred Fones (1869–1938) in Bridgeport, Conn.

In other countries, H. K. Box (Canada); M. Roy and R. Vincent (France); R. Jaccard and A.-J. Held (Switzerland); F. A. Carranza, Sr., and R. Erausquin (Argentina); W. W. James, A. Counsell, and E. W. Fish (Great Britain); and A. Leng (Chile) are well known for their important contributions. Probably the most comprehensive book on periodontics published in the first half of the 20th century was *El Paradencio, Su Patologia y Tratamiento,* by the Uruguayan F. M. Pucci, which appeared in 1939.

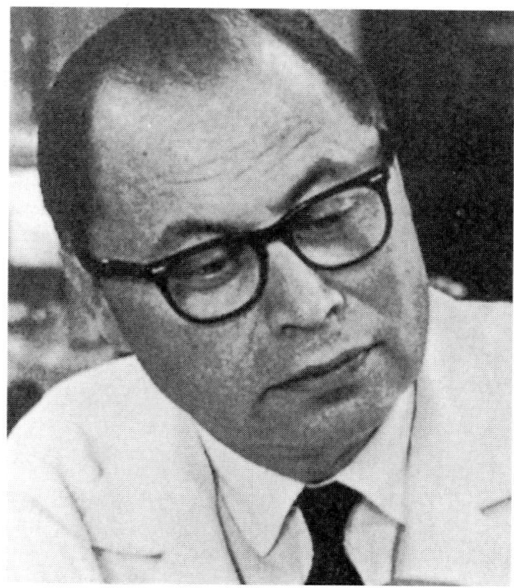

Fig. 13 Irving Glickman (1914–72).

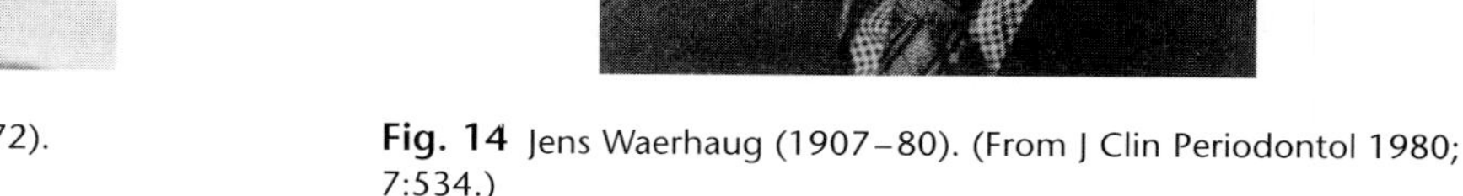

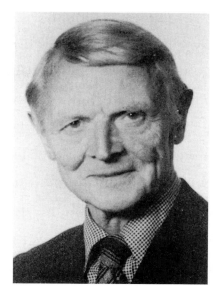

Fig. 14 Jens Waerhaug (1907–80). (From J Clin Periodontol 1980; 7:534.)

Focal Infection

The concept of systemic diseases originating in dental and oral infections had been mentioned in the Assyrian clay tablets (7th century BCE), by Hippocrates (460–370 BCE), in the Babylonian Talmud (3rd century CE), and by Girolamo Cardano and the German Walter Hermann Ryff in the 16th century.[41,60] In the 19th century, Benjamin Rush (famous physician and one of the signers of the American Declaration of Independence) in 1818 and Leonard Koecker in 1828 recognized the role of oral sepsis in rheumatic and other diseases. Later in the century, W. D. Miller also mentioned oral infections as the cause of many diseases.[54]

In a paper published in 1900[43] and a decade later, in a lecture at McGill University in Montreal,[43] Sir William Hunter (1861–1937), a British physician, indicted dentistry as being the cause of oral sepsis, which in turn caused rheumatic and other chronic diseases. This idea was taken up by Billings, Rosenow, and many others,[73] who advocated extractions of all teeth with periodontal or periapical infections to prevent systemic diseases. This led to wholesale extractions of teeth (and removal of tonsils).

The focal infection theory fell into disrepute when it was found that extractions failed to eliminate or reduce the systemic diseases to which the infected teeth were supposed to be linked.[21,60] However, the concept has been revisited in the 1990s, this time with a more solid research foundation (see Chapter 13).

After World War II

The U.S. and Scandinavia took a leading role in basic and clinical periodontal research from the 1950s on, with major advances in the fields of experimental pathology, microbiology, and immunology.

Animal models of periodontal disease were developed, and the role of local and systemic factors was studied by many investigators. Irving Glickman (1914–72) (Fig. 13) was a leading researcher of this period. Among other scientists who contributed to the knowledge of the experimental pathology of the periodontal tissues were Herman Becks (1897–1962), Paul Boyle (1901–80), Henry Goldman (1911–91), Balint Orban (1899–1960), Sigurd Ramfjord (1911–91), Isaac Schour (1900–64), Joseph Weinmann (1889–1960), and Helmut Zander (1912–91). In the clinical area, many authors expanded this knowledge, including Frank Beube (1904–95), Samuel Charles Miller (1902–57), Timothy O'Leary (1921–91), John Prichard (1907–90), Saul Schluger (1908–90), and Sidney Sorrin (1900–78).

The leading figure of the Scandinavian group was Jens Waerhaug (1907–80) (Fig. 14) of Oslo, whose dissertation, *The Gingival Pocket,* published in 1952, opened a new era in the understanding of the biology of the periodontium, challenging the ideas of the Vienna school on gingival attachment, and establishing the primary role of bacterial plaque in the etiology of periodontal disease.[51] Prominent members of the Scandinavian school include Harald Löe, Jan Lindhe, Sture Nyman, and Jan Egelberg.

At present, the role of microorganisms and the immunologic response are the center of attention of many research groups. Investigators such as Robert Genco, Roy Page, Sigmund Socransky, Max Listgarten, Walter Loesche, Jorgen Slots, and many others are carrying the torch into the future. This book documents their contributions.

Several workshops and international conferences have summarized the existing knowledge on the biologic and clinical aspects of periodontology. Worthy of mention are those conducted in 1951, 1966, 1977, 1989, and 1996 that were co-sponsored and published by the American Academy of Periodontology.

The American Academy of Periodontology, founded in 1914 by two female periodontists, Grace Rogers Spalding (1881–1953) and Gillette Hayden (1880–1929), has become the leader in organized periodontics. Its monthly scientific publication, *The Journal of Periodontology,* presents all the advances in this discipline. Other scientific periodontal journals include *Journal of Periodontal Research, Journal of Clinical Periodontology, Periodontology 2000,* and *International Journal of Periodontics and Restorative Dentistry.* In other languages, *Journal de Parodontologie* (France), *Periodoncia* (Spain), and *Journal of the Japanese Association of Periodontology* (Japan) deserve mention.

Periodontal education in the U.S. also has grown in the second half of the 20th century, and most dental schools have separate and independent units for teaching and research in this discipline. Periodontics was recognized as a specialty of dentistry by the American Dental Association in 1947. The first university-based programs for the training of specialists in periodontics were begun in several universities (Columbia, Michigan, Tufts) in the late 1940s; these 1-year programs expanded to 2-year programs about 10 years later. Currently, more than 50 periodontal graduate programs are based in universities and hospitals; all of these are 3-year programs.

REFERENCES

1. Ackernecht EH: Rudolf Virchow. New York, Arno Press, 1981.
2. Albucasis: La Chirurgie. Translated by L LeClere. Paris, Baillière, 1861.
3. American Dental Club of Paris: Meetings of December 1902 and January and March 1903. Dent Cosmos 1904; 46:39.
4. Artzney Buchlein. Leipzig, Michael Blum, 1530. English translation in Dent Cosmos 1887; 29:1.
5. Avicenna: Liber Canonis. Venice, 1507. Reprinted, Hildesheim, Georg Olms, 1964.
6. Baer PN, Benjamin SD: Gingival grafts; a historical note. J Periodontol 1981; 52:206.
7. Berdmore T: A Treatise on the Disorders and Deformities of the Teeth and Gums. London, B. White, 1786.
8. Black GV: Special Dental Pathology. Chicago, Medico-Dental Publishers, 1915.
9. Breasted JH: The Edwin Smith Surgical Papyrus. Chicago, University of Chicago Press, 1930.
10. Brock TD: Robert Koch. A Life in Medicine and Bacteriology. Washington, D.C., ASM Press, 1999.
11. Budjuhn K: The 1920 German commentary based on original sources regarding the history of the oldest printed book in dentistry. English translation by HE Cooper. In: The Classics of Dentistry Library. Zene Artzney, Birmingham, AL, 1981.
12. Carranza FA: Revolucionarios de la Ciencia. Ed. Vergara, Buenos Aires, 1998.
13. Castiglione A: History of Medicine, 2nd edition. New York, AA Knopf, 1941.
14. Celsus A: De Medicina. Translated by WG Spencer, London, Heinemann, 1935–1938.
15. Charaka Samhita. Edited, translated, and published by AC Kaviratna, Calcutta, 1892.
16. Crane A, Kaplan H: The Crane-Kaplan operation for pyorrhea alveolaris. Dent Cosmos 1931; 643.
17. Dabry P: La Medicine chez les Chinois. Paris, Plon, 1863.
18. Debré P: Louis Pasteur. Baltimore, Johns Hopkins University Press, 1994.
19. Dobell C: Anton van Leeuwenhoek and His "Little Animals." New York, Harcourt, 1932. Reprinted, New York, Dover Publications, 1960.
20. Ebbel B: The Papyrus Ebers. Copenhagen, Levin and Munksgaard, 1937.
21. Editorial. JAMA 1952; 150:490.
22. Eustachius B: A Little Treatise on the Teeth. Edited and introduced by DA Chernin and G Shklar. Translated by JH Thomas. Science History Pub/USA, 1999.
23. Fauchard P: Le Chirurgien Dentiste, ou Traite des Dents. Paris, J Maruiette, 1728. Reprinted in facsimile, Paris, Prèlat, 1961. English translation by Lillian Lindsay, London, Butterworth & Co., 1946.
24. Fischman SL: The history of oral hygiene: how far have we come in 6000 years? Periodontology 2000 1997; 15:7.
25. Fleischmann L, Gottlieb B: Beitrage zur Histologie und Pathogenese der Alveolarpyorrhoe. Z Stomatol 1920; 2:44.
26. Funakoshi M: Personal communication, 1993.
27. Glasser O: Röntgen, ed 2. Springfield, IL, Charles C. Thomas, 1972.
28. Gold SI: Robert Neumann: a pioneer in periodontal flap surgery. J Periodontol 1982; 53:456.
29. Gold SI: Periodontics. The past. Part I. Early sources. J Clin Periodontol 1985; 12:79.
30. Gold SI: Periodontics. The past. Part II. The development of modern periodontics. J Clin Periodontol 1985; 12:171.
31. Gold SI: Periodontics. The past. Part III. Microbiology. J Clin Periodontol 1985; 12:257.
32. Gottlieb B: Der Epithelansatz am Zahne. Dtsch Monatschr Zahn 1921; 39:142.
33. Gottlieb B: Die diffuse Atrophie der Alveolarknochen. Z Stomatol 1923; 21:195.
34. Gottlieb B: Schmutz Pyorrhöe, Paradental-pyorrhöe und Alveolar Atrophie. Fortschr d Zahnheilk 1925; 1:519.
35. Gottlieb B, Orban B: Biology and Pathology of the Tooth and Its Supporting Mechanism. Translated and edited by M Diamond. New York, Macmillan, 1938.
36. Guerini V: History of Dentistry. Philadelphia, Lea & Febiger, 1909.
37. Harlan AW: Restoration of gum tissue on the labial aspect of teeth. D Cosmos 1906; 48:927.
38. Held A-J: Periodontology. From its origins up to 1980: a survey. Birkhauser, Boston, 1989.
39. Hippocrates: Works. Edited and translated by WHS Jones and ET Withington. London, Heinemann, 1923, 1931.
40. Hirschfeld I: The Toothbrush: Its Use and Abuse. New York, Dent Items Interest Publishers, 1939.
41. Hoffman-Axthelm W: History of Dentistry. Chicago, Quintessence, 1981.
42. Hunter J: The Natural History of the Human Teeth. London, J Johnson, 1771. Reprinted as: Treatise in the natural history and diseases of the human teeth. In: Bell T (ed): Collected Works. London, Longman Rees, 1835.
43. Hunter W: Oral sepsis as a cause of disease. Br Med J 1900; 1:215.
44. Hunter W: An address on the role of sepsis and antisepsis in Medicine. Lancet 1911; 1:79.
45. Jastrow N: The medicine of the Babylonians and Assyrians. Proc Soc Med London 1914; 7:109.
46. Karolyi M: Beobachtungen ber Pyorrhea Alveolaris. Vjschr Zahnheilk 1901; 17:279.
47. Kimery MJ, Stallard RJ: The evolutionary development and contemporary utilization of various oral hygiene procedures. Period Abst 1968; 16:90.
48. Kirkland O: Surgical treatment of periodontoclasia. JADA 1936; 125.
49. Koecker A: An essay on the devastation of the gums and the alveolar processes. Philadelphia J Med Phys Sci 1821; 2:282.
50. Leeuwenhoek A van: Arcana Naturae. Delphis Bartavorum, 1695. Reprinted in facsimile, Brussels, Culture et Civilization, 1966.

51. Löe H: Periodontal diseases: A brief historical perspective. Periodontology 2000 1993; 2:7.
52. MacManus C: The makers of dentistry. Dent Cosmos 1902; 44:1105.
53. Major RHL: A History of Medicine. Springfield, IL, Charles C Thomas, 1954.
54. Miller WD: The human mouth as a focus of infection. Dent Cosmos 1891; 33:689, 789,913.
55. Mills GA: Some of the phases of Riggs' disease (so-called). Dent Cosmos 1877; 19:185,254,347.
56. Neumann R: Die Alveolarpyorrhoe und ihre Behandlung. Berlin, Meusser, 1912.
57. Neumann R: Die Radikal-Chirurgische Behandlung der Alveolarpyorrhoe. Vjschr Zahnheilk 1921; 37:113.
58. Neumann R: Erwiderung zu Widmans auffassungen¸ ber die Prioritatsfrage betreffs der radikalchirurgischen Behandlung der sogennanten Alveolarpyorrhoe. Vjschr Zahnheilk 1923; 39:170.
59. Nicaise E: La Grande Chirurgie de Guy de Chauliac. Paris, Alean, 1890.
60. O'Reilly PG, Claffey NM: A history of oral sepsis as a cause of disease. Periodontology 2000 2000; 23:13.
61. Paracelsus: Sämtliche Werke (Collected works in modern German). Ed. K. Sudhoff. 14 volumes. Munich, R Oldfenbourg, 1922-1933.
62. Parè A: Oeuvres Completes. Edited by JF Malgaigne. Paris, Baillière, 1840.
63. Paul of Aegina: The Seven Books. Translated by F Adams. London, Sydenham Society, 1844.
64. Pifteau P: Chirurgie de Guillaume de Salicet: Traduition et Commentaire. Toulouse, St Cyprien, 1989.
65. Plaut HC: Studien zur bakteriellen Diagnostik der Diphtherie und der Anginen. Dtsch Med Wochenschr 1894; 20:920.
66. Rawls AO: Pyorrhea alveolaris. D Cosmos 1885; 27:265.
67. Riggs JW: Suppurative inflammation of the gums and absorption of the gums and alveolar process. Pa J Dent Sci 1876; 3:99. Reprinted in Arch Clin Oral Pathol 1938; 2:423.
68. Rosenthal P: Recovering the exposed necks of teeth by autoplasty. Dent Cosmos 1912; 54:377.
69. Ruffer MA: Studies in the Paleopathology of Egypt. Chicago, University of Chicago Press, 1921.
70. Shklar G: Stomatology and dentistry in the golden age of Arabian medicine. Bull Hist Dent 1969; 17:17.
71. Stern IB, Everett FG, Robicsek K: S. Robicsek: a pioneer in the surgical treatment of periodontal disease. J Periodontol 1965; 36:265.
72. Susruta Samhita. Edited, translated, and published by KKL Bhishagratna, Calcutta, 1907.
73. Thoma KH: Oral Pathology. St Louis, Mosby, 1941.
74. Vallery-Radot M: Pasteur. Librairie Académique Perrin, Paris, 1994.
75. Vesalius S: De Humanis Corporis Fabrica, Basle, 1542. Reproduced in facsimile, Brussels, Culture et Civilisation, 1966.
76. Vincent JH: Sur l'etiologie et sur les lesions anatomopathologiques de la pourriture d'hospital. Ann de l'Inst Pasteur 1896; 10:448.
77. Vincent JH: Recherche sur l'etiologie de la stomatitis ulceromembraneuse primitive. Arch Int Laryngol 1904; 17:355.
78. Ward AW: The surgical eradication of pyorrhea. JADA 1928; 15:2146.
79. Ward AW: Inharmonius cusp relation as a factor in periodontoclasia. J Amer Dent Assoc 1923; 10:471.
80. Weinberger BW: An Introduction to the History of Dentistry. St Louis, Mosby, 1948.
81. Weski O: Roentgenographische-anatomische Studien auf dem Gebiete der Kieferpathologie. Vjrsch Zahnh 1921; 37:1.
82. Widman L: Surgical treatment of pyorrhea alveolaris. J Periodontol 1971; 42:571.
83. Williams JL: A contribution to the study of pathology of enamel. Dent Cosmos 1897; 39:169,269,353.
84. Witzel A: The treatment of pyorrhea alveolaris or infectious alveolitis. Br J Dent Sci 1882; 25:153,209,257.
85. Zemsky J: Surgical treatment of periodontal disease with the author's open view operation for advanced cases of dental periclasia. Dent Cosmos 1926; 68:465.
86. Zentler A: Suppurative gingivitis with alveolar involvement. A new surgical procedure. JAMA 1918; 71:1530.
87. Znamensky NN: Alveolar pyorrhoea; its pathological anatomy and its radical treatment. J Br Dent Assoc 1902; 23:585.

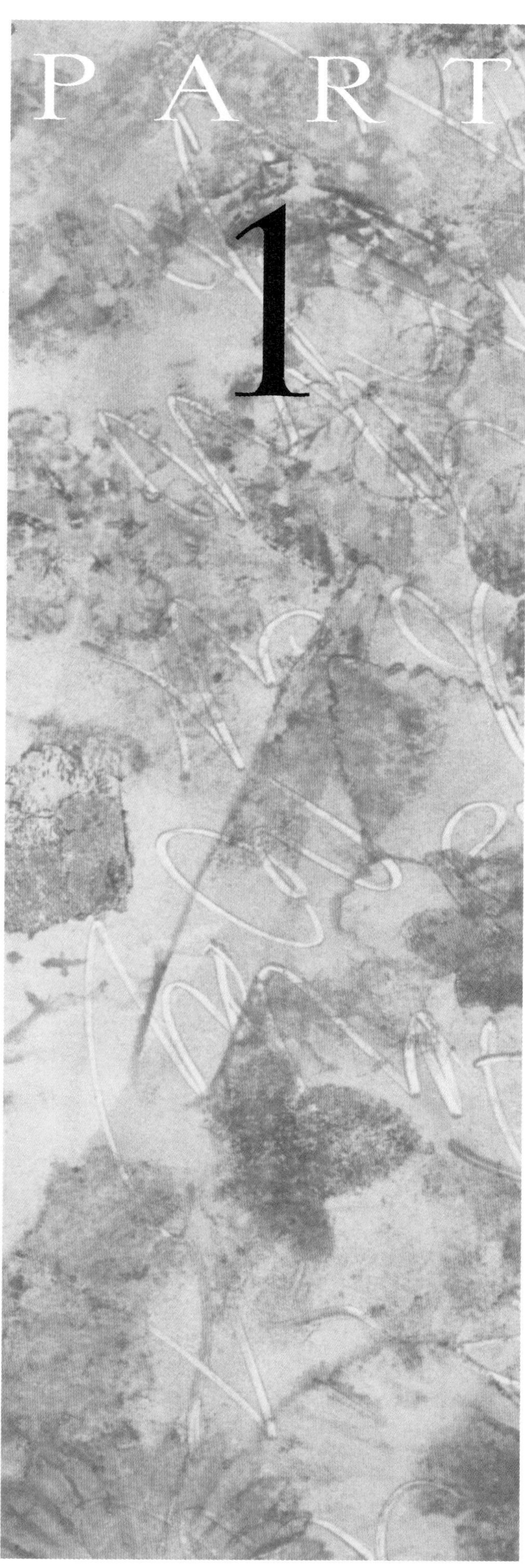

The Normal Periodontium

Michael G. Newman

The periodontium consists of the investing and supporting tissues of the tooth (gingiva, periodontal ligament, cementum, and alveolar bone). It has been divided into two parts: the gingiva, whose main function is protection of the underlying tissues, and the attachment apparatus, composed of the periodontal ligament, cementum, and alveolar bone.[1,2] The cementum is considered a part of the periodontium because, with the bone, it serves as the support for the fibers of the periodontal ligament.

The periodontium is subject to morphologic and functional variations as well as changes associated with age. This section deals with the normal features of the tissues of the periodontium, knowledge of which is necessary for an understanding of periodontal diseases.

The soft and hard tissues surrounding dental implants have many similar features and some important differences with the periodontal tissues. They are dealt with in Chapter 67.

The Gingiva

Maria E. Itoiz and Fermin A. Carranza

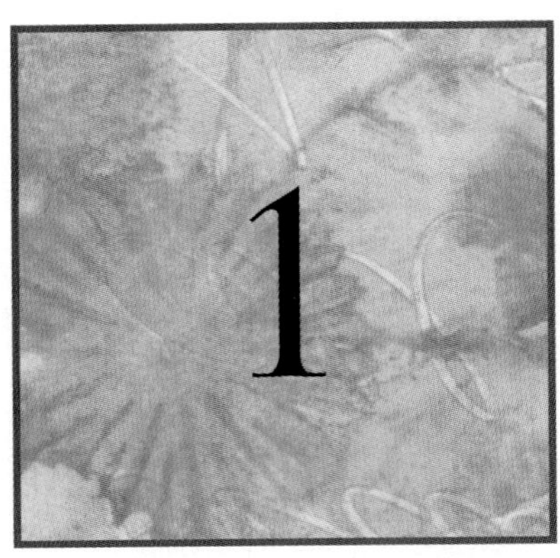

CHAPTER

CHAPTER OUTLINE

The *oral mucosa* consists of three zones: the gingiva and the covering of the hard palate, termed the *masticatory mucosa;* the dorsum of the tongue, covered by *specialized mucosa;* and the oral mucous membrane lining the remainder of the oral cavity. The *gingiva* is the part of the oral mucosa that covers the alveolar processes of the jaws and surrounds the necks of the teeth.

CLINICAL FEATURES

The gingiva is divided anatomically into marginal, attached, and interdental areas.

Marginal Gingiva

The marginal, or unattached, gingiva is the terminal edge or border of the gingiva surrounding the teeth in collarlike fashion (Figs. 1-1 and 1-2). In about 50% of cases, it is demarcated from the adjacent, attached gingiva by a shallow linear depression, the *free gingival groove.*[3] Usually about 1 mm wide, it forms the soft tissue wall of the gingival sulcus. It may be separated from the tooth surface with a periodontal probe.

Gingival Sulcus

The gingival sulcus is the shallow crevice or space around the tooth bounded by the surface of the tooth on one side and the epithelium lining the free margin of the gingiva on the other. It is V shaped and barely permits the entrance of a periodontal probe. The clinical determination of the depth of the gingival sulcus is an important diagnostic parameter. Under absolutely normal or ideal conditions, the depth of the gingival sulcus is or is about 0.[43] These strict conditions of normalcy can be produced experimentally only in germfree animals or after intense, prolonged plaque control.[8,23]

In clinically healthy gingiva in humans, a sulcus of some depth can be found. The depth of this sulcus, as determined in histologic sections, has been reported as 1.8 mm, with variations from 0 to 6 mm[81]; other studies have reported 1.5 mm[125] and 0.69 mm, respectively.[40] The clinical maneuver used to determine the depth of

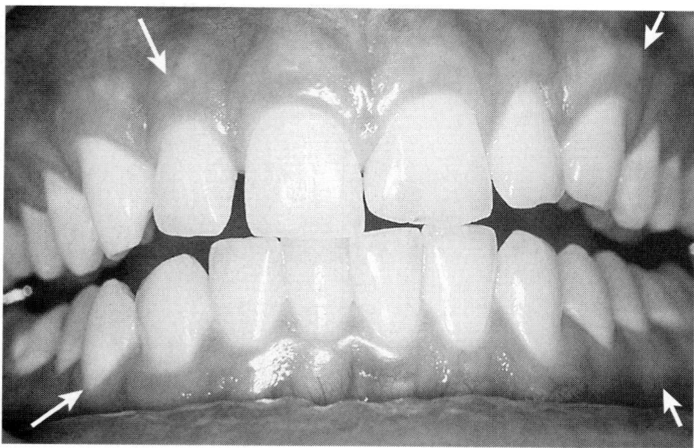

Fig. 1-1 Normal gingiva in a young adult. Note the demarcation (mucogingival line) *(arrows)* between the attached gingiva and the darker alveolar mucosa.

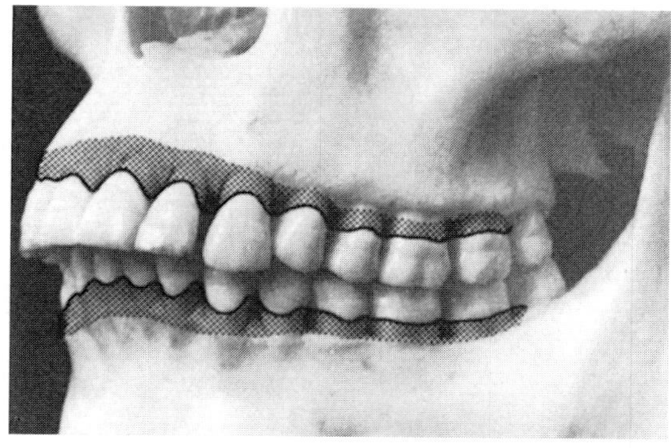

Fig. 1-3 Mean width of attached gingiva in human permanent dentition.

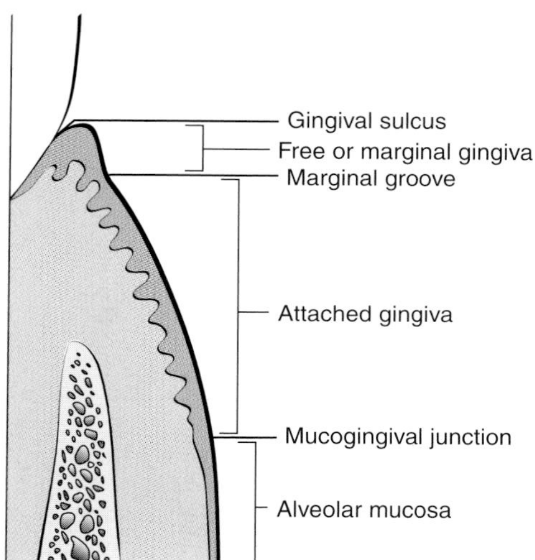

Fig. 1-2 Diagram showing anatomic landmarks of the gingiva.

the sulcus is the introduction of a metallic instrument—the periodontal probe—and the estimation of the distance it penetrates. The histologic depth of a sulcus need not be exactly equal to the depth of penetration of the probe. The so-called probing depth of a clinically normal gingival sulcus in humans is 2 to 3 mm (see Chapter 30).

Attached Gingiva

The attached gingiva is continuous with the marginal gingiva. It is firm, resilient, and tightly bound to the underlying periosteum of alveolar bone. The facial aspect of the attached gingiva extends to the relatively loose and movable alveolar mucosa, from which it is demarcated by the *mucogingival junction* (see Fig. 1-2).

The *width of the attached gingiva* is another important clinical parameter. It is the distance between the mucogingival junction and the projection on the external surface of the bottom of the gingival sulcus or the periodontal pocket. It should not be confused with the width of the keratinized gingiva because the latter also includes the marginal gingiva (see Fig. 1-2).

The width of the attached gingiva on the facial aspect differs in different areas of the mouth.[16] It is generally greatest in the incisor region (3.5 to 4.5 mm in the maxilla and 3.3 to 3.9 mm in the mandible) and less in the posterior segments, with the least width in the first premolar area (1.9 mm in the maxilla and 1.8 mm in the mandible)[3] (Fig. 1-3).

Because the mucogingival junction remains stationary throughout adult life,[1] changes in the width of the attached gingiva are caused by modifications in the position of its coronal end. The width of the attached gingiva increases with age[4] and in supraerupted teeth.[2] On the lingual aspect of the mandible, the attached gingiva terminates at the junction with the lingual alveolar mucosa, which is continuous with the mucous membrane lining the floor of the mouth. The palatal surface of the attached gingiva in the maxilla blends imperceptibly with the equally firm, resilient palatal mucosa.

Interdental Gingiva

The interdental gingiva occupies the gingival embrasure, which is the interproximal space beneath the area of tooth contact. The interdental gingiva can be pyramidal or have a "col" shape. In the former, the tip of one papilla is located immediately beneath the contact point; the latter presents a valleylike depression that connects a facial and lingual papilla and conforms to the shape of the interproximal contact[29] (Figs. 1-4 and 1-5).

The shape of the gingiva in a given interdental space depends on the contact point between the two adjoining teeth and the presence or absence of some degree of recession. (Fig. 1-6 depicts the variations in normal interdental gingiva.)

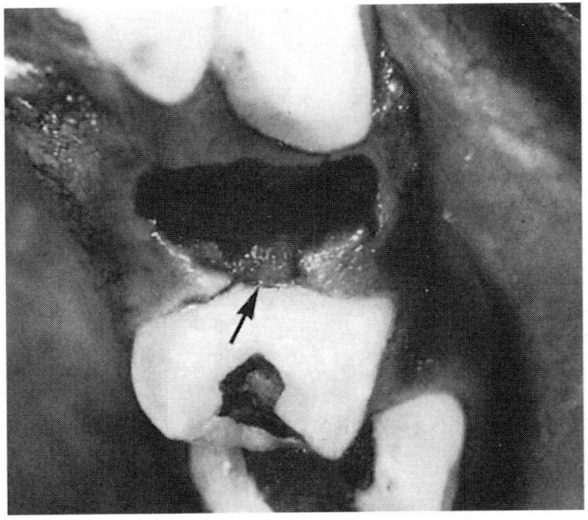

Fig. 1-4 Site of extraction showing the facial and palatal interdental papillae and the intervening col *(arrow)*.

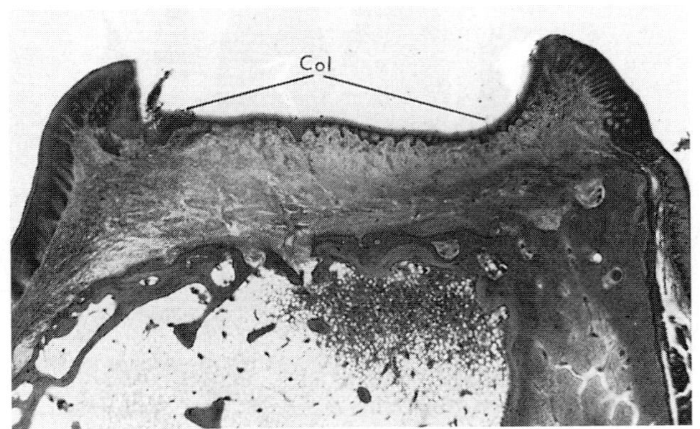

Fig. 1-5 Faciolingual section (monkey) showing col between the facial and lingual interdental papillae. The col is covered with nonkeratinized stratified squamous epithelium.

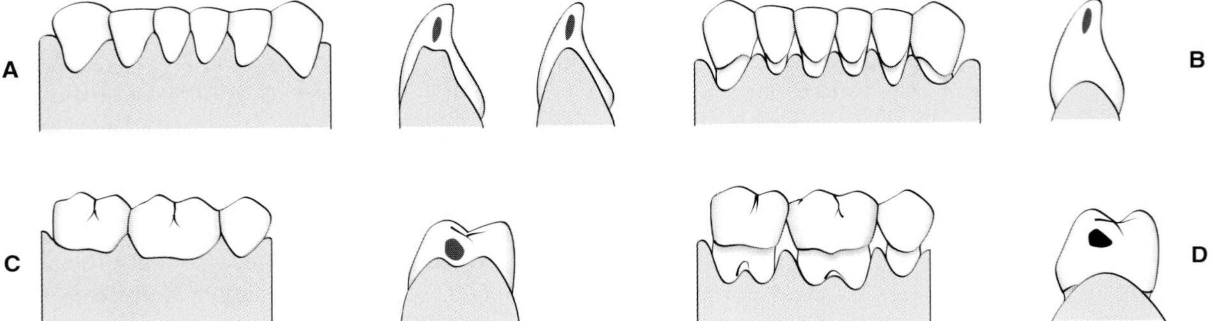

Fig. 1-6 Diagram comparing anatomic variations of the interdental col in the normal gingiva (left side) and after gingival recession (right side). **A, B,** Mandibular anterior segment, facial and buccolingual views, respectively. **C, D,** Mandibular posterior region, facial and buccolingual views, respectively. Tooth contact points are shown in **B** and **D**.

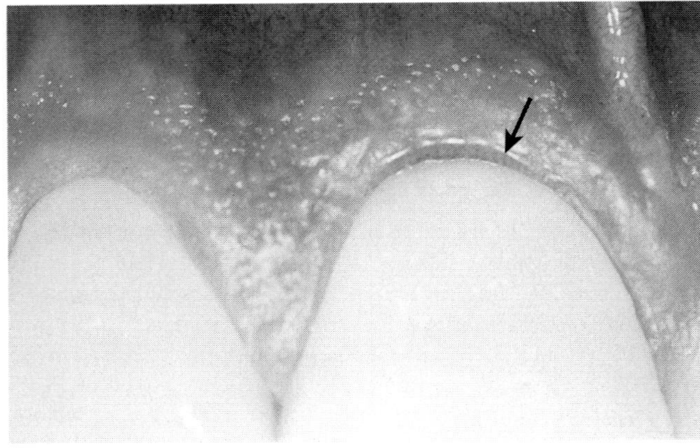

Fig. 1-7 Interdental papillae with central portion formed by attached gingiva. The shape of the papillae *(P)* varies according to the dimension of the gingival embrasure. (Courtesy Dr. Osvaldo Costa.)

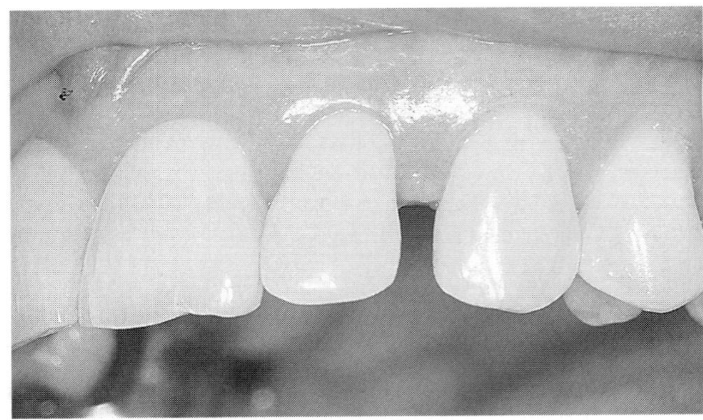

Fig. 1-8 Absence of interdental papillae and col where proximal tooth contact is missing. (Courtesy Dr. Osvaldo Costa.)

The facial and lingual surfaces are tapered toward the interproximal contact area, and the mesial and distal surfaces are slightly concave. The lateral borders and tips of the interdental papillae are formed by a continuation of the marginal gingiva from the adjacent teeth. The intervening portion consists of attached gingiva (Fig. 1-7).

If a diastema is present, the gingiva is firmly bound over the interdental bone and forms a smooth, rounded surface without interdental papillae (Fig. 1-8).

MICROSCOPIC FEATURES

The gingiva consists of a central core of connective tissue covered by stratified squamous epithelium. These two tissues will be considered separately.*

Gingival Epithelium

General Aspects of Gingival Epithelium Biology

Although it constitutes a continuous lining of stratified squamous epithelium, three different areas can be defined from the morphologic and functional points of view: the oral or outer epithelium, sulcular epithelium, and junctional epithelium.

The principal cell type of the gingival epithelium, as well as of other stratified squamous epithelia, is the *keratinocyte*. Other cells found in the epithelium are the clear cells or nonkeratinocytes, which include the Langerhans cells, Merkel cells, and melanocytes.

The main function of the gingival epithelium is to protect the deep structures while allowing a selective interchange with the oral environment. This is achieved by proliferation and differentiation of the keratinocyte.

Proliferation of keratinocytes takes place by mitosis in the basal layer and less frequently in the suprabasal layers, where a small proportion of cells remain as a proliferative compartment while a larger number begins to migrate to the surface.

Differentiation involves the process of keratinization, which consists of a sequence of biochemical and morphologic events that occur in the cell as it migrates from the basal layer (Fig. 1-9). The main morphologic change is a progressive flattening of the cell with an increasing prevalence of tonofilaments and intercellular junctions coupled to the production of keratohyaline granules and the disappearance of the nucleus. (See Schroeder[91] for further details.)

A complete keratinization process leads to the production of an *orthokeratinized* superficial horny layer similar to that of the skin with no nuclei in the stratum corneum and a well-defined stratum granulosum (Fig. 1-10). Only some areas of the outer gingival epithelium are orthokeratinized; the other gingival areas are covered by parakeratinized or nonkeratinized epithelium,[20] considered to be

* A detailed description of gingival histology can be found in Schroeder HE: The Periodontium, New York, Springer-Verlag, 1986; and in Biological structure of the normal and diseased periodontium, Periodontology 2000 1997; (13).

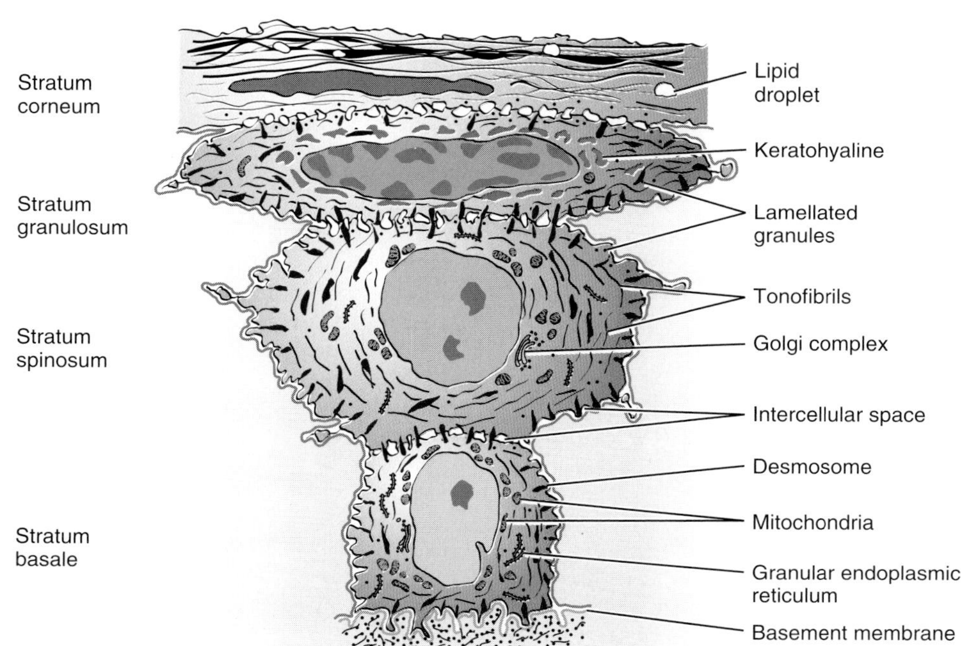

Fig. 1-9 Diagram showing representative cells from the various layers of stratified squamous epithelium as seen by electron microscopy. (Modified from Weinstock A. In: Ham AW: Histology, ed 7. Philadelphia, JB Lippincott, 1974.)

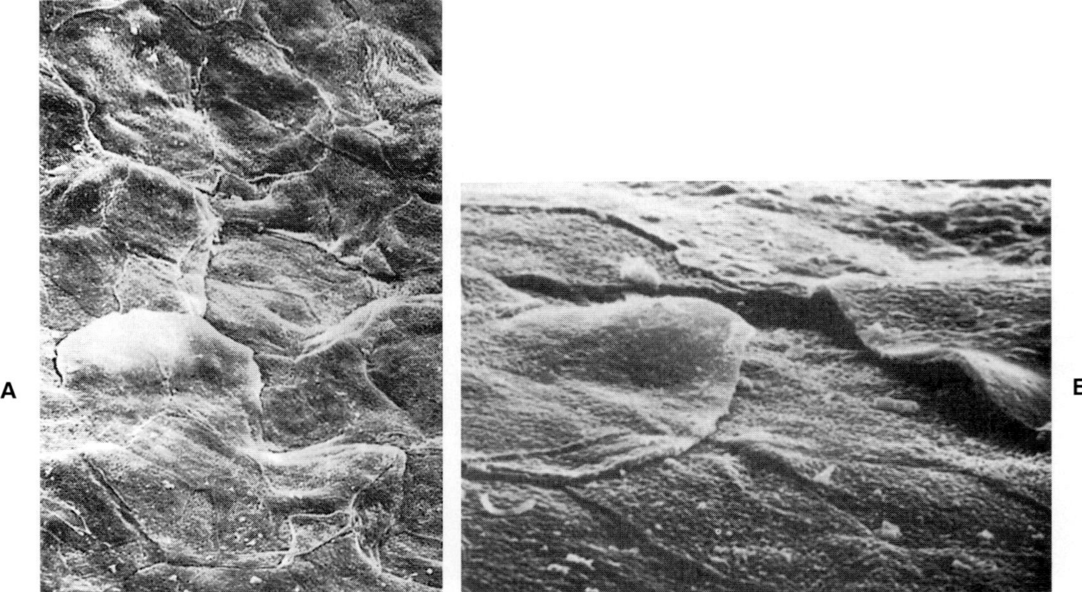

Fig. 1-10 A, Scanning electron micrograph of keratinized gingiva showing the flattened keratinocytes and their boundaries on the surface of the gingiva (×1000). **B,** Scanning electron micrograph of gingival margin at edge of gingival sulcus showing at close-up view several keratinocytes about to be exfoliated (×3000). (From Kaplan GB, Pameijer CH, Ruben MP: Scanning electron microscopy of sulcular and junctional epithelia correlated with histology [Part I]. J Periodontol 1977; 48:446.)

at intermediate stages of keratinization. These areas can progress to maturity or dedifferentiate under different physiologic or pathologic conditions.

In *parakeratinized epithelia,* the stratum corneum retains pyknotic nuclei and the keratohyalin granules are dispersed, not giving rise to a stratum granulosum. The *nonkeratinized epithelium* (although cytokeratins are the major component, as in all epithelia) has neither granulosum nor corneum strata, and superficial cells have viable nuclei.

Immunohistochemistry, gel electrophoresis, and immunoblot techniques have made identification of the characteristic pattern of cytokeratins possible in each epithelial type. The keratin proteins are composed of different polypeptide subunits characterized by their isoelectric points and molecular weights. They are numbered in a sequence contrary to their molecular weight. Generally, basal cells begin synthesizing lower molecular weight keratins (such as K19, 40 kd) and express other, higher molecular weight keratins as they migrate to the surface. K1 keratin polypeptide of 68 kd is the main component of the stratum corneum.[27]

Other proteins unrelated to keratins are synthesized during the maturation process. The most extensively studied are *keratolinin* and *involucrin,* which are precursors of a chemically resistant structure (the envelope) located below the cell membrane, and *filaggrin,* whose precursors are packed into the keratohyalin granules. In the sudden transition to the horny layer, the keratohyalin granules disappear and give rise to filaggrin, which forms the matrix of the most differentiated epithelial cell, the *corneocyte.*

Thus in the fully differentiated state, the corneocytes are mainly formed by bundles of keratin tonofilaments embedded in an amorphous matrix of filaggrin and surrounded by a resistant envelope under the cell membrane. The immunohistochemical patterns of the different keratin types, envelope proteins, and filaggrin, change under normal or pathologic stimuli, modifying the keratinization process.[51–53]

Electron microscopy reveals that keratinocytes are interconnected by structures on the cell periphery called *desmosomes.*[63] These desmosomes have a typical structure consisting of two dense attachment plaques into which tonofibrils insert and an intermediate, electron-dense line in the extracellular compartment. Tonofilaments, which are the morphologic expression of the cytoskeleton of keratin proteins, radiate in brushlike fashion from the attachment plaques into the cytoplasm of the cells. The space between the cells shows cytoplasmic projections resembling microvilli that extend into the intercellular space and often interdigitate.

Less frequently observed forms of epithelial cell connections are tight junctions *(zonae occludens),* where the membranes of the adjoining cells are believed to be fused.[114,123] Evidence suggests that these structures allow ions and small molecules to pass from one cell to another.

Cytoplasmic organelle concentration varies among different epithelial strata. Mitochondria are more numerous in deeper strata and decrease toward the surface of the cell. Accordingly, histochemical demonstration of succinic dehydrogenase, nicotinamide-adenine dinucleotide, cytochrome oxidase, and other mitochondrial enzymes revealed a more active tricarboxylic cycle in

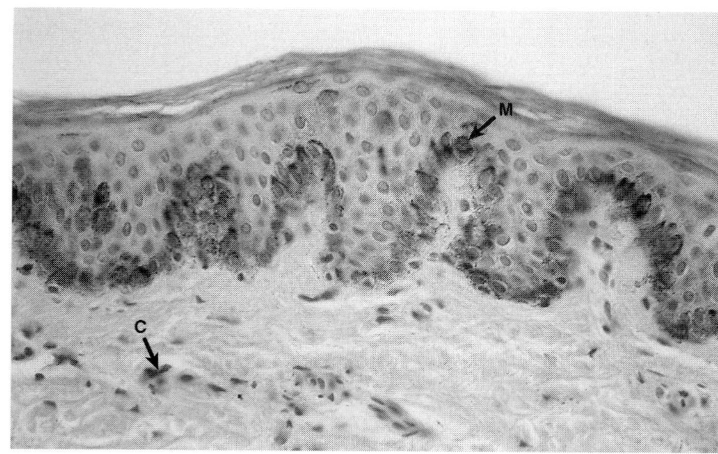

Fig. 1-11 Pigmented gingiva of dog, showing melanocytes *(M)* in the basal epithelial layer and melanophores *(C)* in the connective tissue (Glucksman technique).

basal and parabasal cells, where the proximity of the blood supply facilitates energy production through aerobic glycolysis.

Conversely, enzymes of the pentose shunt (an alternative pathway of glycolysis), such as glucose-6-phosphatase, increase their activity towards the surface. This pathway produces a larger amount of intermediate products for the production of ribonucleic acid (RNA), which in turn can be used for the synthesis of keratinization proteins. This histochemical pattern is in accordance with the increased volume and amount of tonofilaments observed in cells reaching the surface, and the intensity of activity is proportional to the degree of differentiation.[35,36,49,84]

The uppermost cells of the stratum spinosum contain numerous dense granules, *keratinosomes* or *Odland bodies*, which are modified lysosomes. They contain a large amount of acid phosphatase, an enzyme involved in the destruction of organelle membranes, which occurs suddenly between the granulosum and corneum strata and during the intercellular cementation of cornified cells. Thus acid phosphatase is another enzyme closely related to the degree of keratinization.[18,47,120]

Nonkeratinocyte cells are present in gingival epithelium as in other malpighian epithelia. *Melanocytes* are dendritic cells located in the basal and spinous layers of the gingival epithelium. They synthesize melanin in organelles called *premelanosomes* or *melanosomes*[30,90,107] (Fig. 1-11). These contain tyrosinase, which hydroxylates tyrosine to dihydroxyphenylalanine (dopa), which in turn is progressively converted to melanin. Melanin granules are phagocytosed and contained within other cells of the epithelium and connective tissue, called *melanophages* or *melanophores*.

Langerhans cells are dendritic cells located among keratinocytes at all suprabasal levels (Fig. 1-12). They belong to the mononuclear phagocyte system (reticuloendothelial system) as modified monocytes derived from the bone marrow. They contain elongated granules and are considered macrophages with possible antigenic properties.[32] Langerhans cells have an important role in the immune reaction as antigen-presenting cells for lymphocytes. They contain g-specific granules (Birbeck's granules) and have marked adenosine triphosphatase activity. They are found in oral epithelium of normal gingiva and in smaller amounts in the sulcular epithelium; they are probably absent from the junctional epithelium of normal gingiva.

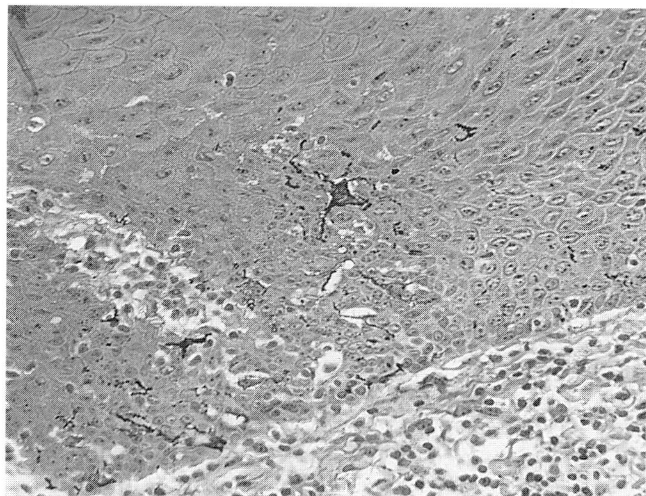

Fig. 1-12 Human gingival epithelium, oral aspect. Immunoperoxidase technique showing Langerhans cells.

Merkel cells are located in the deeper layers of the epithelium, harbor nerve endings, and are connected to adjacent cells by desmosomes. They have been identified as tactile perceptors.[78]

The epithelium is joined to the underlying connective tissue by a *basal lamina* 300 to 400 Å thick, lying approximately 400 Å beneath the epithelial basal layer.[59,96,108] The basal lamina consists of lamina lucida and lamina densa. Hemidesmosomes of the basal epithelial cells abut the lamina lucida, which is mainly composed of the glycoprotein laminin. The lamina densa is composed of type IV collagen. The basal lamina, clearly distinguishable at the ultrastructural level, is connected to a reticular condensation of the underlying connective tissue fibrils (mainly collagen type IV) by the anchoring fibrils.[77,85,111]

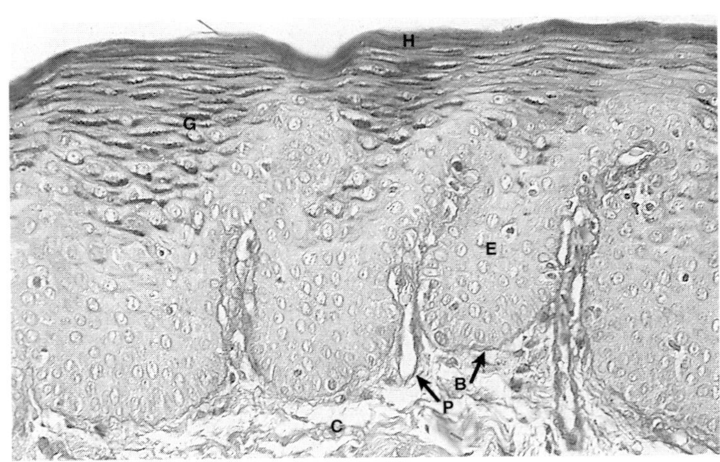

Fig. 1-13 Normal human gingiva stained with the periodic acid-Schiff (paS) histochemical method. The basement membrane *(B)* is seen between the epithelium *(E)* and the underlying connective tissue *(C)*. In the epithelium, glycoprotein material occurs in cells and cell membrane of the superficial hornified *(H)* and underlying granular layers *(G)*. The connective tissue presents a diffuse amorphous ground substance and collagen fibers. The blood vessel walls stand out clearly in the papillary projections of the connective tissue *(P)*.

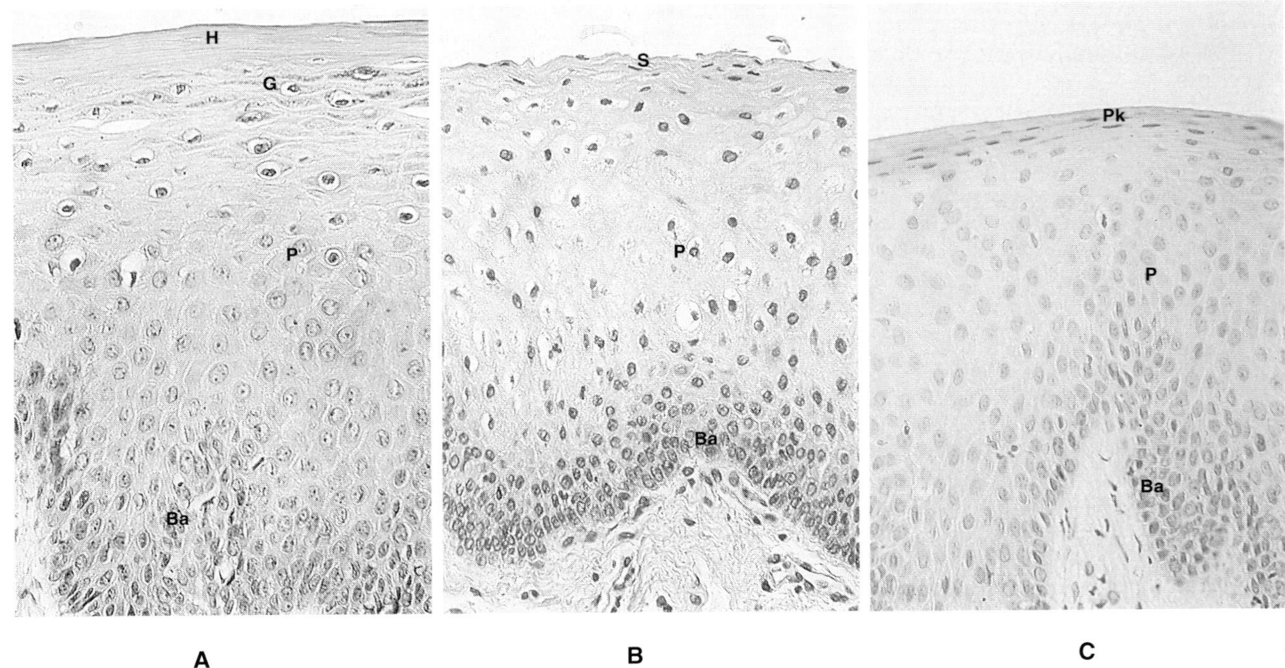

Fig. 1-14 Variations in gingival epithelium. **A,** Keratinized. **B,** Nonkeratinized. **C,** Parakeratinized. Horny layer *(H)*, granular layer *(G)*, prickle cell layer *(P)*, basal cell layer *(Ba)*, flattened surface cells *(S)*, parakeratotic layer *(Pk)*.

The complex of basal lamina and fibrils is the periodic acid-Schiff (paS) positive and argyrophilic line observed at the optical level[99,112] (Fig. 1-13). The basal lamina is permeable to fluids but acts as a barrier to particulate matter.

Structural and Metabolic Characteristics of the Different Areas of Gingival Epithelium

ORAL OR OUTER EPITHELIUM. The oral or outer epithelium covers the crest and outer surface of the marginal gingiva and the surface of the attached gingiva. It is keratinized (Fig. 1-14) or parakeratinized or presents various combinations of these conditions. The prevalent surface, however, is parakeratinized.[13,20,121]

The degree of gingival keratinization diminishes with age and the onset of menopause[83] but is not necessarily related to the different phases of the menstrual cycle.[54] Keratinization of the oral mucosa varies in different areas in the following order: palate (most keratinized), gingiva, ventral aspect of the tongue, and cheek (least keratinized).[74]

Keratins K1, K2, and K10 to K12, which are specific of epidermal-type differentiation, are immunohistochemically expressed with high intensity in orthokeratinized areas and less intensity in parakeratinized areas. K6 and K16, characteristic of highly proliferative epithelia, and K5 and K14, stratification-specific cytokeratins, also are present. Parakeratinized areas express K19, which is usually absent from orthokeratinized normal epithelia.[14,89]

In keeping with the complete or almost complete maturation, histoenzyme reactions for acid phosphatase and pentose-shunt enzymes are very strong.[19,49]

Glycogen can accumulate intracellularly when it is not completely degraded by any of the glycolytic pathways. Thus its concentration in normal gingiva is inversely related to the degree of keratinization[98,121] and inflammation.[31,116,119]

SULCULAR EPITHELIUM. The sulcular epithelium lines the gingival sulcus (Fig. 1-15). It is a thin, nonkeratinized stratified squamous epithelium without rete pegs and extends from the coronal limit of the junctional epithelium to the crest of the gingival margin (Fig. 1-16). It usually shows many cells with hydropic degeneration.[13]

As with other nonkeratinized epithelia, it lacks granulosum and corneum strata and K1, K2, and K10-K12 cytokeratins, but it contains K4 and K13, the so-called esophageal type cytokeratins. It also expresses K19 and normally does not contain Merkel cells.

Histochemical studies of enzymes have consistently revealed a lower degree of activity than in the outer epithelium, particularly in the case of enzymes related to keratinization. Glucose-6-phosphate dehydrogenase expressed a faint and homogeneous reaction in all strata, unlike the increasing gradient toward the surface observed in cornified epithelia.[49] Acid phosphatase staining is negative,[18] although lysosomes have been described in exfoliated cells.[60]

Despite these morphologic and chemical characteristics, the sulcular epithelium has the potential to keratinize if (1) it is reflected and exposed to the oral cavity[17,21] or (2) the bacterial flora of the sulcus is totally eliminated.[22] Conversely, the outer epithelium loses its keratinization when it is placed in contact with the tooth.[22] These findings suggest that the local irritation of the sulcus prevents sulcular keratinization.

The sulcular epithelium is extremely important because it may act as a semipermeable membrane through which injurious bacterial products pass into the gingiva and tissue fluid from the gingiva seeps into the sulcus.[113]

JUNCTIONAL EPITHELIUM. The *junctional epithelium* consists of a collarlike band of stratified squamous nonkeratinizing epithelium. It is three to four layers thick in early life, but the number of layers increases with age to 10 or even 20 layers. These cells can be grouped in two strata: basal and suprabasal. The length of the junctional epithelium ranges from 0.25 to 1.35 mm.

The junctional epithelium is formed by the confluence of the oral epithelium and the reduced enamel epithelium during tooth eruption (Fig. 1-17). However, the reduced enamel epithelium is not essential for its formation; in fact, the junctional epithelium is completely restored after pocket instrumentation or surgery and forms around an implant.[62]

Cell layers not juxtaposed to the tooth exhibit numerous free ribosomes and prominent membrane-bound structures, such as Golgi complexes, and cytoplasmic vacuoles, presumably phagocytic. Lysosomelike bodies also are present, but the absence of keratinosomes (Odland bodies) and histochemically demonstrable acid phosphatase, correlated with the low degree of differentiation, may reflect a low defense power against microbial plaque accumulation in the gingival sulcus. Similar morphologic findings have been described in the gingiva of germfree rats. Polymorphonuclear neutrophil leukocytes

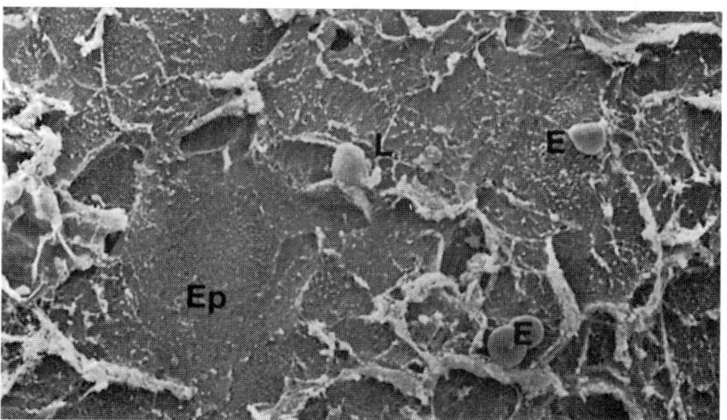

Fig. 1-15 Scanning electron microscopic view of epithelial surface facing the tooth in a normal human gingival sulcus. The epithelium *(Ep)* shows desquamating cells, some scattered erythrocytes *(E)*, and a few emerging leukocytes *(L)* (×1000).

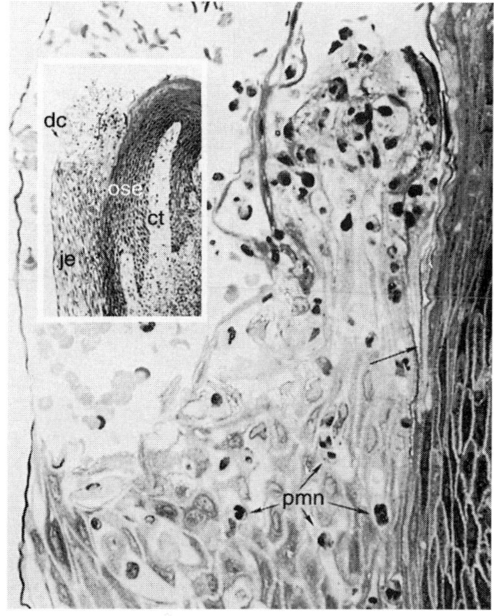

Fig. 1-16 An Epon-embedded human biopsy specimen showing a relatively normal gingival sulcus. The soft tissue wall of the gingival sulcus is made up of the oral sulcular epithelium *(ose)* and its underlying connective tissue *(ct)*, whereas the base of the gingival sulcus is formed by the sloughing surface of the junctional epithelium *(je)*. The enamel space is delineated by a dense cuticular structure *(dc)*. A relatively sharp line of demarcation exists between the junctional epithelium and the oral sulcular epithelium *(arrow)*, and several polymorphonuclear leukocytes *(pmn)* can be seen traversing the junctional epithelium. The sulcus contains red blood cells resulting from the hemorrhage occurring at the time of biopsy (×391; inset ×55). (From Schluger S, Youdelis R, Page RC: Periodontal Disease. Philadelphia, Lea & Febiger, 1977.)

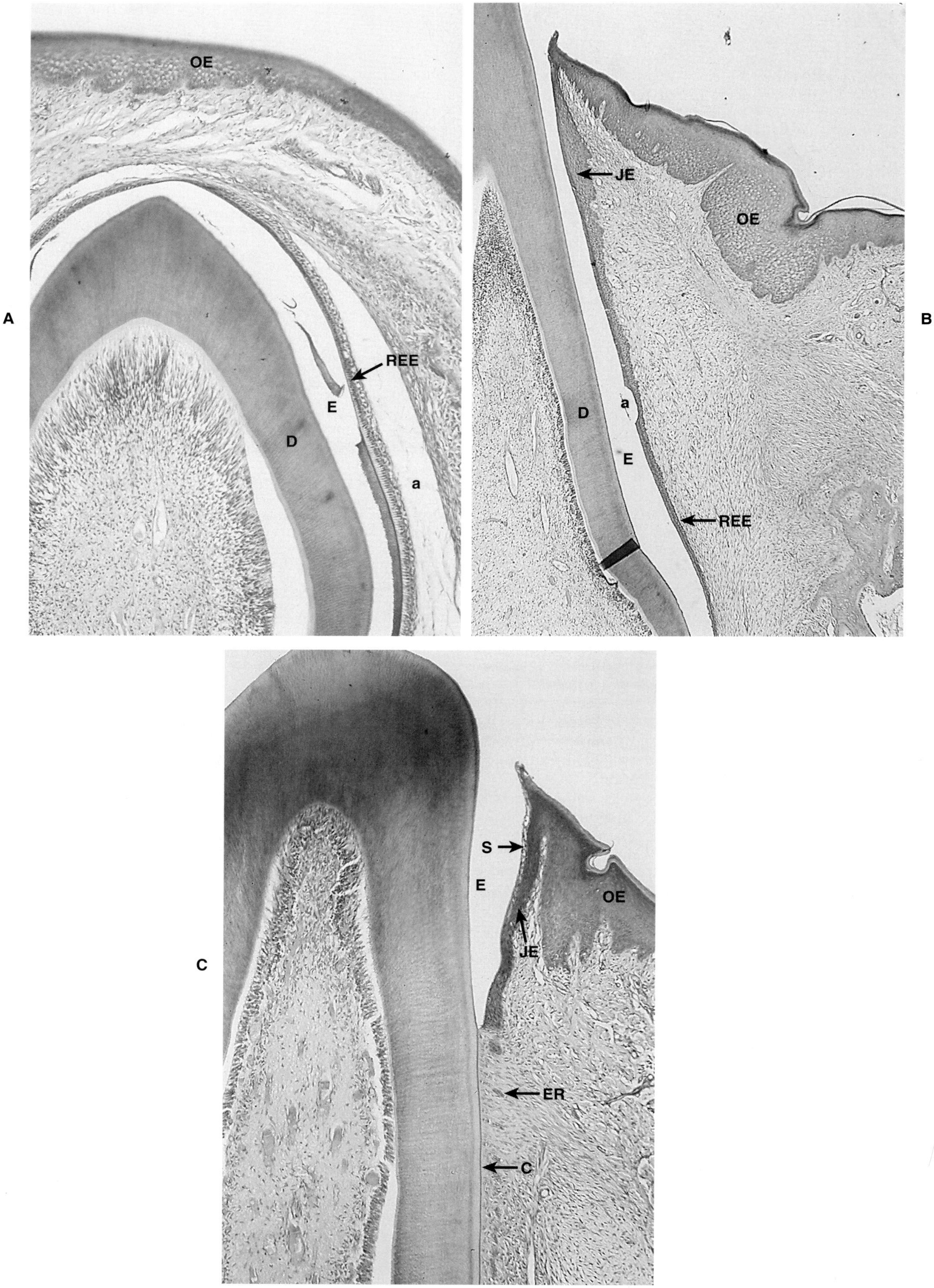

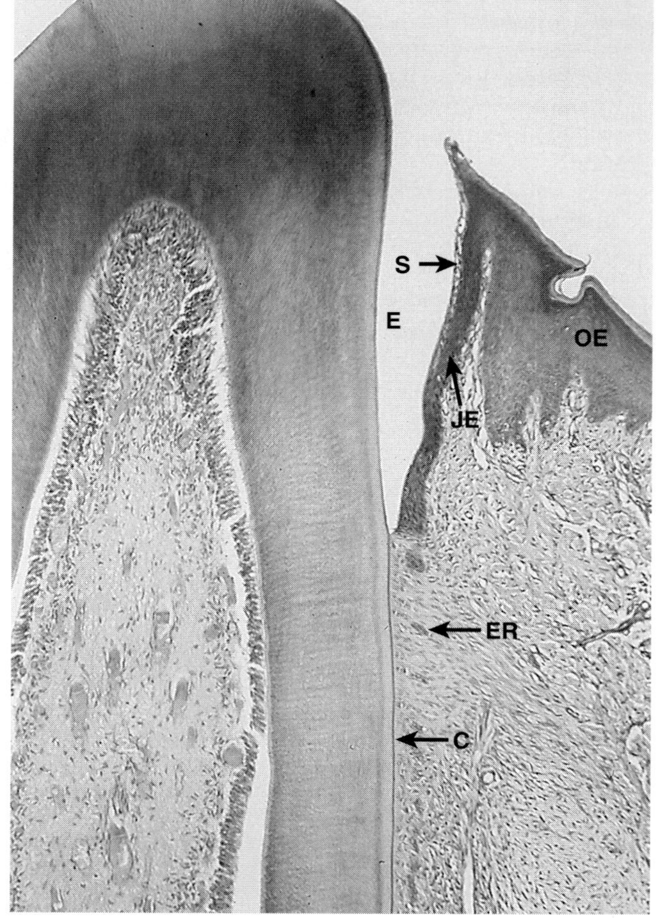
C
S
E
OE
JE
ER
C

are found routinely in the junctional epithelium of both conventional rats and germfree rats.[127]

The different keratin polypeptides of junctional epithelium have a particular histochemical pattern. It expresses K19, which is absent from keratinized epithelia, and the stratification-specific cytokeratins K5 and K14.[89] Morgan et al[75] reported that reactions to demonstrate K4 or K13 reveal a sudden change between sulcular and junctional epithelium, the junctional area being the only stratified nonkeratinized epithelium in the oral cavity that does not synthesize these specific polypeptides. Another particular behavior is the lack of expression of K6 and K16, which is usually linked to highly proliferative epithelia, although the turnover of the cells is very high.

Similar to sulcular epithelium, junctional epithelium exhibits lower glycolytic enzyme activity than outer epithelium and lacks acid phosphatase activity.[18,49]

The junctional epithelium is attached to the tooth surface (epithelial attachment) by means of an internal basal lamina and to the gingival connective tissue by an external basal lamina that has the same structure as other epithelial-connective tissue attachments elsewhere in the body.[64,69]

The internal basal lamina consists of a lamina densa (adjacent to the enamel) and a lamina lucida to which hemidesmosomes are attached. Organic strands from the enamel appear to extend into the lamina densa.[110] The junctional epithelium attaches to afibrillar cementum present on the crown (usually restricted to an area within 1 mm of the cementoenamel junction)[95] and root cementum in a similar manner.

Histochemical evidence for the presence of neutral polysaccharides in the zone of the epithelial attachment has been reported.[115] Data also have shown that the basal lamina of the junctional epithelium resembles that of endothelial and epithelial cells in its laminin content but differs in its internal basal lamina, which has no type IV collagen.[56,88] These findings indicate that the cells of the junctional epithelium are involved in the production of laminin and play a key role in the adhesion mechanism.

The attachment of the junctional epithelium to the tooth is reinforced by the gingival fibers, which brace the marginal gingiva against the tooth surface. For this reason, the junctional epithelium and the gingival fibers are considered a functional unit, referred to as the *dentogingival unit.*[66]

Development of the Gingival Sulcus

After enamel formation is complete, the enamel is covered with reduced enamel epithelium, which is attached to the tooth by a basal lamina and hemidesmosomes.[65,109] When the tooth penetrates the oral mucosa, the reduced enamel epithelium unites with the oral epithelium and transforms into the junctional epithelium. As the tooth erupts, this united epithelium condenses along the crown, and the ameloblasts, which form the inner layer of the reduced enamel epithelium (see Fig. 1-17), gradually become squamous epithelial cells. The transformation of the reduced enamel epithelium into a junctional epithelium proceeds in an apical direction without interrupting the attachment to the tooth. According to Schroeder and Listgarten, this process takes between 1 and 2 years.[95]

The junctional epithelium is a continually self-renewing structure with mitotic activity occurring in all cell layers.[65,109] The regenerating epithelial cells move toward the tooth surface and along it in a coronal direction to the gingival sulcus, where they are shed[11] (Fig. 1-18). The migrating daughter cells provide a continuous attachment to the tooth surface. The strength of the epithelial attachment to the tooth has not been measured.

The gingival sulcus is formed when the tooth erupts into the oral cavity. At that time, the junctional epithelium and reduced enamel epithelium form a broad band attached to the tooth surface from near the tip of the crown to the cementoenamel junction.

The gingival sulcus is the shallow, V-shaped space or groove between the tooth and gingiva that encircles the newly erupted tip of the crown. In the fully erupted

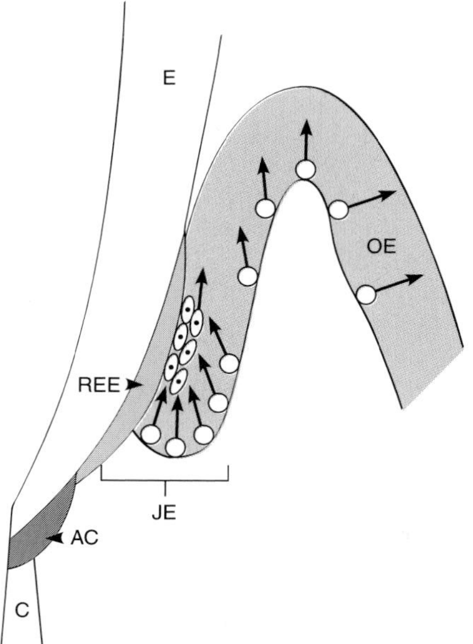

Fig. 1-18 Junctional epithelium on an erupting tooth. The junctional epithelium *(JE)* is formed by the joining of the oral epithelium *(OE)* and the reduced enamel epithelium *(REE)*. Afibrillar cementum, sometimes formed on enamel after degeneration of the REE, is shown at *AC*. The arrows indicate the coronal movement of the regenerating epithelial cells, which multiply more rapidly in the JE than in the OE. *E*, Enamel; *C*, root cementum. A similar cell turnover pattern exists in the fully erupted tooth. (Modified from Listgarten MA: Changing concepts about the dentogingival junction. J Can Dent Assoc 1970; 36:70.)

Fig. 1-17 Eruption process in cat's tooth. **A,** Unerupted tooth. Dentine *(D)*, remnants of enamel matrix *(E)*, reduced enamel epithelium *(REE)*, oral epithelium *(OE)*, artifact *(a)*. **B,** Erupting tooth forming junctional epithelium *(JE)*. **C,** Completely erupted tooth. Sulcus with epithelial debris *(S)*, cementum *(C)*, and epithelial rests *(ER)*.

tooth, only the junctional epithelium persists. *The sulcus consists of the shallow space that is coronal to the attachment of the junctional epithelium and bounded by the tooth on one side and the sulcular epithelium on the other. The coronal extent of the gingival sulcus is the gingival margin.*

Renewal of Gingival Epithelium

The oral epithelium undergoes continuous renewal. Its thickness is maintained by a balance between new cell formation in the basal and spinous layers and the shedding of old cells at the surface. The mitotic activity exhibits a 24-hour periodicity, with highest and lowest rates occurring in the morning and evening, respectively.[110] The mitotic rate is higher in nonkeratinized areas and is increased in gingivitis, without significant gender differences. Opinions differ as to whether the mitotic rate is increased[68,69,73] or decreased[10] with age.

The mitotic rate in experimental animals varies among different areas of the oral epithelium in descending order: buccal mucosa, hard palate, sulcular epithelium, junctional epithelium, outer surface of the marginal gingiva, and attached gingiva.[6,45,68,117] The following have been reported as turnover times for different areas of the oral epithelium in experimental animals: palate, tongue, and cheek, 5 to 6 days; gingiva, 10 to 12 days, with the same or more time required with age; and junctional epithelium, 1 to 6 days.[11,105]

Cuticular Structures on the Tooth

The term *cuticle* describes a thin, acellular structure with a homogeneous matrix, sometimes enclosed within clearly demarcated, linear borders.

Listgarten has classified cuticular structures into coatings of developmental origin and acquired coatings.[67] *Acquired coatings* include those of exogenous origin, such as saliva, bacteria, calculus, and surface stains (see Chapters 6 and 11). *Coatings of developmental origin* are those normally formed as part of tooth development. They include the reduced enamel epithelium, coronal cementum, and dental cuticle.

After enamel formation is completed, the ameloblastic epithelium is reduced to one or two layers of cells that remain attached to the enamel surface by hemidesmosomes and a basal lamina. This *reduced enamel epithelium* consists of postsecretory ameloblasts and cells from the stratum intermedium of the enamel organ.

In some animal species, the reduced enamel epithelium disappears entirely and very rapidly, thereby placing the enamel surface in contact with the connective tissue. Connective tissue cells then deposit a thin layer of cementum known as *coronal cementum* on the enamel. In humans, thin patches of afibrillar cementum sometimes may be seen in the cervical half of the crown.

Electron microscopy has shown a *dental cuticle* consisting of a layer of homogeneous organic material of variable thickness (approximately 0.25 micron) overlying the enamel surface. It is nonmineralized and not always present. In some instances near the cementoenamel junction, it is deposited over a layer of afibrillar cementum, which in turn overlies enamel. The cuticle may be present between the junctional epithelium and the tooth. Ultrastructural histochemical studies have shown the dental cuticle to be of proteinaceous nature,[57] and it may be an accumulation of tissue fluid components.[39,92]

Gingival Fluid (Sulcular Fluid)

The gingival sulcus contains a fluid that seeps into it from the gingival connective tissue through the thin sulcular epithelium. The gingival fluid is believed to 1) cleanse material from the sulcus, 2) contain plasma proteins that may improve adhesion of the epithelium to the tooth, 3) possess antimicrobial properties, and 4) exert antibody activity to defend the gingiva. (The gingival fluid and its significance in health and disease are discussed in detail in Chapter 15.)

Gingival Connective Tissue

The connective tissue of the gingiva is known as the *lamina propria* and consists of two layers: 1) a *papillary layer* subjacent to the epithelium, which consists of papillary projections between the epithelial rete pegs, and 2) a *reticular layer* contiguous with the periosteum of the alveolar bone. Connective tissue has a cellular and an extracellular compartment composed of fibers and ground substance.

The ground substance fills the space between fibers and cells, is amorphous, and has a high content of water. It is composed of proteoglycans, mainly hyaluronic acid and chondroitin sulfate, and glycoproteins, mainly fibronectin. Glycoproteins account for the faint paS positive reaction of the ground substance.[36] Fibronectin binds fibroblasts to the fibers and many other components of the intercellular matrix, helping mediate cell adhesion and migration. Laminin is another glycoprotein found in the basal laminae, which serves to attach it to epithelial cells.

The three types of connective tissue fibers are collagen, reticular, and elastic. Collagen type I forms the bulk of the lamina propria and provides the tensile strength to the gingival tissue. Type IV collagen (argyrophilic reticulum fiber) branches between the collagen type I bundles and is continuous with fibers of the basement membrane and blood vessel walls.[69]

The elastic fiber system is composed of oxytalan, elaunin, and elastin fibers distributed among collagen fibers.[26]

Gingival Fibers

The connective tissue of the marginal gingiva is densely collagenous, containing a prominent system of collagen fiber bundles called the *gingival fibers*. They consist of type I collagen.[85] The gingival fibers have the following functions:

1. To brace the marginal gingiva firmly against the tooth
2. To provide the rigidity necessary to withstand the forces of mastication without being deflected away from the tooth surface
3. To unite the free marginal gingiva with the cementum of the root and the adjacent attached gingiva

The gingival fibers are arranged in three groups: gingivodental, circular, and transseptal.[58]

GINGIVODENTAL GROUP. The gingivodental fibers are those on the facial, lingual, and interproximal surfaces. They are embedded in the cementum just beneath the epithelium at the base of the gingival sulcus. On the facial and lingual surfaces, they project from the cementum in fanlike conformation toward the crest and outer surface of the marginal gingiva, terminating short of the epithelium (Figs. 1-19 and 1-20). They also extend externally to the periosteum of the facial and lingual alveolar bones and terminate in the attached gingiva or blend with the periosteum of the bone. Interproximally, the gingivodental fibers extend toward the crest of the interdental gingiva.

CIRCULAR GROUP. The circular fibers course through the connective tissue of the marginal and interdental gingivae and encircle the tooth in ringlike fashion.

TRANSSEPTAL GROUP. Located interproximally, the transseptal fibers form horizontal bundles that extend between the cementum of approximating teeth into which they are embedded. They lie in the area between the epithelium at the base of the gingival sulcus and the crest of the interdental bone and are sometimes classified with the principal fibers of the periodontal ligament.

Page and co-workers[82] also have described (1) a group of *semicircular fibers*, which attach at the proximal surface of a tooth, immediately below the cementoenamel junction, go around the facial or lingual marginal gingiva of the tooth, and attach on the other proximal surface of the same tooth; and (2) a group of *transgingival fibers*, that attach in the proximal surface of one tooth, traverse the interdental space diagonally, go around the facial or lingual surface of the adjacent tooth, again traverse diagonally the interdental space, and attach in the proximal surface of the next tooth.

Cellular Elements

The preponderant cellular element in the gingival connective tissue is the *fibroblast*. Numerous fibroblasts are found between the fiber bundles. As in connective tissue elsewhere in the body, fibroblasts synthesize collagen and elastic fibers as well as the glycoproteins and glycosaminoglycans of the amorphous intercellular substance. Fibroblasts also regulate collagen degradation.

Mast cells, which are distributed throughout the body, are numerous in the connective tissue of the oral mucosa and the gingiva.[24,103,104,124] *Fixed macrophages* and *histiocytes* are present in the gingival connective tissue as components of the mononuclear phagocyte system (reticuloendothelial system) and are derived from blood monocytes. *Adipose cells* and *eosinophils*, although scarce, also are present in the lamina propria.

In clinically normal gingiva, *small foci* of plasma cells and lymphocytes are found in the connective tissue near the base of the sulcus (Fig. 1-21). Neutrophils can be seen in relatively high numbers in both the gingival connective tissue and the sulcus. These inflammatory cells usually are present in small amounts in clinically normal gingiva.

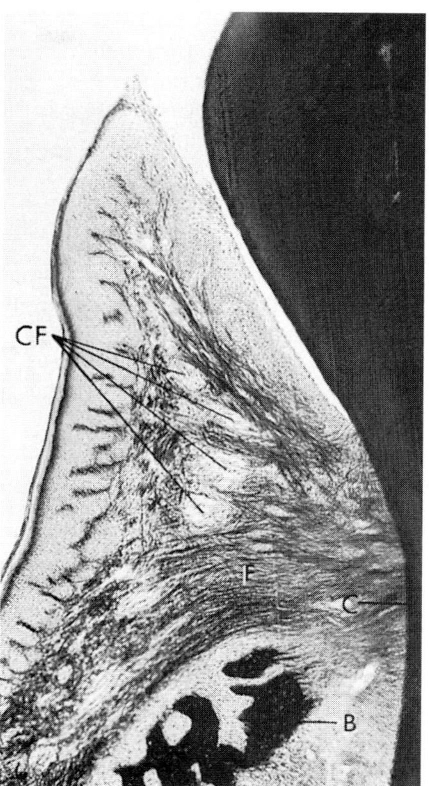

Fig. 1-19 Faciolingual section of marginal gingiva, showing gingival fibers *(F)* extending from the cementum *(C)* to the crest of the gingiva, to the outer gingival surface, and external to the periosteum of the bone *(B)*. Circular fibers *(CF)* are shown in cross-section between the other groups. (Courtesy Sol Bernick.)

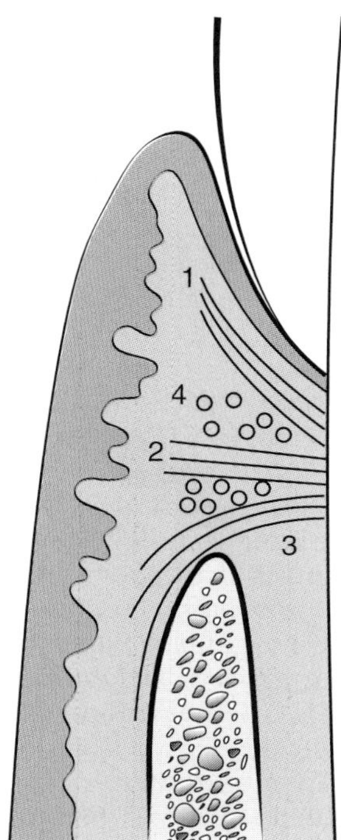

Fig. 1-20 Diagram of the gingivodental fibers extending from the cementum *(1)* to the crest of the gingiva, *(2)* to the outer surface, and *(3)* external to the periosteum of the labial plate. Circular fibers *(4)* are shown in cross-section.

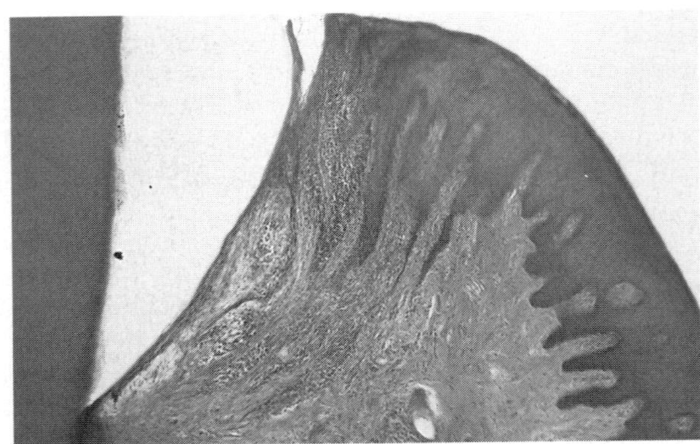

Fig. 1-21 Section of clinically normal gingiva, showing some degree of inflammation, which is almost always present near the base of the sulcus.

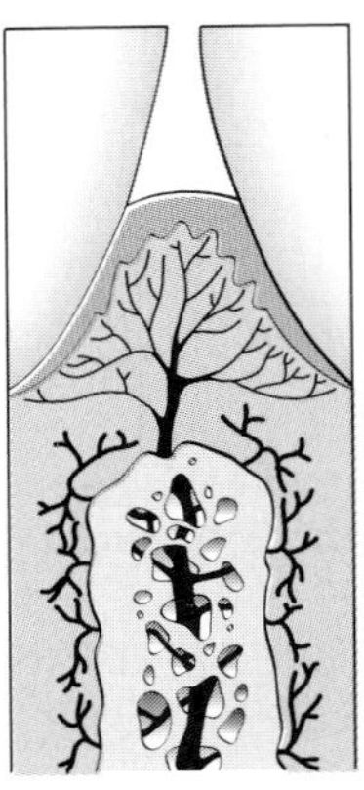

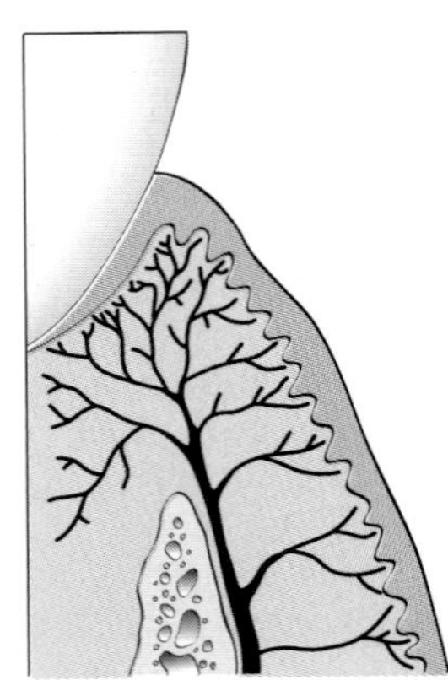

Fig. 1-22 Diagram of arteriole penetrating the interdental alveolar bone to supply the interdental tissues *(left)* and a supraperiosteal arteriole overlying the facial alveolar bone, sending branches to the surrounding tissue *(right)*.

Speculations about whether small amounts of leukocytes should be considered a normal component of the gingiva or an incipient inflammatory infiltrate without clinical expression are of theoretic rather than practical importance. Lymphocytes are absent when gingival normalcy is judged by very strict clinical criteria or under very special experimental conditions[8,80] but are practically constant in healthy normal gingiva, even before complete tooth eruption.[61,70,93] Immunohistochemical studies using monoclonal antibodies have identified the different lymphocyte subpopulations. The infiltrate in the area below the junctional epithelium of healthy gingiva in recently erupted teeth in children is mainly composed of T-lymphocytes (helper, cytotoxic, suppressor and natural killer)[7,41,102] and thus could be interpreted as a normal lymphoid tissue involved in the early defense recognition system. As time elapses, B-lymphocytes and plasma cells appear in greater proportions to elaborate specific antibodies against already recognized antigens that are always present in the sulcus of clinically normal gingiva.[97]

Blood Supply, Lymphatics, and Nerves

Blood vessels are easily evidenced in tissue sections by means of immunohistochemical reactions against proteins of endothelial cells (factor VIII and adhesion molecules). Before these techniques were developed, vascularization patterns of periodontal tissues had been described using histoenzymatic reactions for alkaline phosphatase and adenosine triphosphatase owing to the great activity of these enzymes in endothelial cells.[25,128] In experimental animals, the perfusion with India ink also was used to study vascular distribution. The injection and subsequent demonstration of peroxidase allows blood vessel identification and permeability studies.[101] The paS reaction also outlines vascular walls by a positive line in their basal membrane.[99] Endothelial cells also express 5-nucleotidase activity.[48] Scanning electron microscopy can be used after injection of plastic into the vessels through the carotid artery, followed by corrosion of the soft tissues.[37]

Three sources of blood supply to the gingiva are as follows (Figs. 1-22 and 1-23):

1. *Supraperiosteal arterioles* along the facial and lingual surfaces of the alveolar bone, from which capillaries extend along the sulcular epithelium and between the rete pegs of the external gingival surface.[34,46] Occasional branches of the arterioles pass through the alveolar bone to the periodontal ligament or run over the crest of the alveolar bone
2. *Vessels of the periodontal ligament,* which extend into the gingiva and anastomose with capillaries in the sulcus area.
3. *Arterioles,* which emerge from the crest of the interdental septa[37] and extend parallel to the crest of the bone to anastomose with vessels of the periodontal ligament, with capillaries in the gingival crevicular areas and vessels that run over the alveolar crest.

Beneath the epithelium on the outer gingival surface, capillaries extend into the papillary connective tissue between the epithelial rete pegs in the form of terminal hairpin loops with efferent and afferent branches, spirals, and varices[25,46] (Figs. 1-23 and 1-24). The loops are sometimes linked by cross-communications,[38] and flattened capillaries serve as reserve vessels when the circulation is increased in response to irritation.[42]

Along the sulcular epithelium, capillaries are arranged in a flat anastomosing plexus that extends parallel to the enamel from the base of the sulcus to the gingival margin.[25] In the col area, a mixed pattern of anastomosing capillaries and loops occurs.

The *lymphatic drainage of the gingiva* brings in the lymphatics of the connective tissue papillae.[100] It progresses into the collecting network external to the periosteum of the alveolar process and then to the regional lymph nodes (particularly the submaxillary group). In addition, lymphatics just beneath the junctional epithelium extend into the periodontal ligament and accompany the blood vessels.

Gingival innervation is derived from fibers arising from nerves in the periodontal ligament and from the labial,

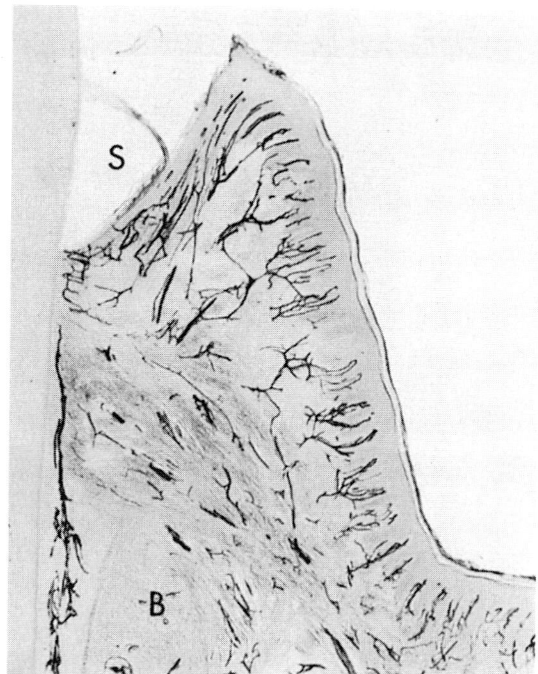

Fig. 1-23 Blood supply and peripheral circulation of the gingiva. Tissues perfused with India ink. Note the capillary plexus parallel to the sulcus *(S)* and the capillary loops in the outer papillary layer. Note also the supraperiosteal vessels external to the bone *(B)*, which supply the gingiva, and a periodontal ligament vessel anastomosing with the sulcus plexus. (Courtesy Sol Bernick.)

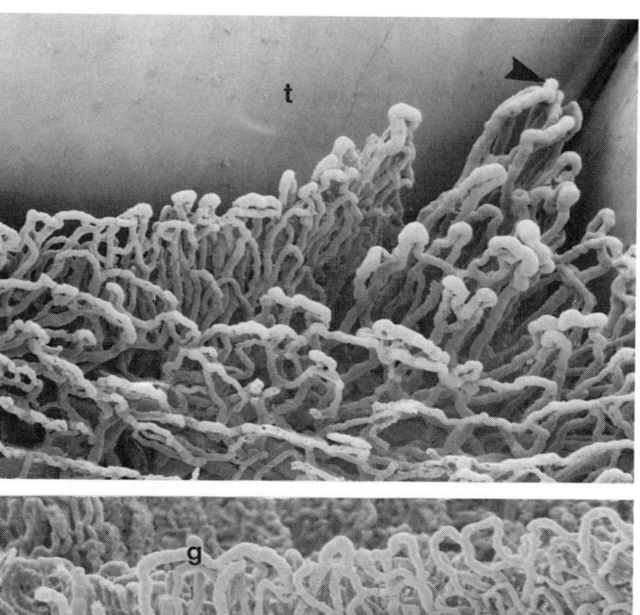

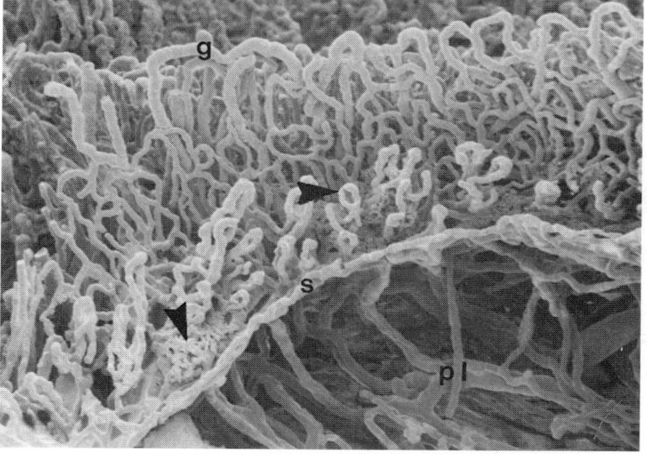

Fig. 1-24 Scanning electron microscopic view of gingival tissues of rat molar palatal gingiva after vascular perfusion of plastic and corrosion of soft tissue. **A,** Oral view of gingival capillaries: *t,* tooth; interdental papilla *(arrow)* (×180). **B,** View from the tooth side. Note the vessels of the plexus next to the sulcular and junctional epithelium. The arrowheads point to vessels in sulcus area with mild inflammatory changes. *G,* Crest of marginal gingiva; *s,* bottom of gingival sulcus; *pl,* periodontal ligament vessels (×150). (Courtesy NJ Selliseth and K Selvig, University of Bergen, Norway.)

buccal, and palatal nerves.[12] The following nerve structures are present in the connective tissue: a meshwork of terminal argyrophilic fibers, some of which extend into the epithelium; Meissner-type tactile corpuscles; Krause-type end bulbs, which are temperature receptors; and encapsulated spindles.[9]

CORRELATION OF CLINICAL AND MICROSCOPIC FEATURES

An understanding of the normal clinical features of the gingiva requires the ability to interpret them in terms of the microscopic structures they represent.

Color

The color of the attached and marginal gingivae is generally described as coral pink and is produced by the vascular supply, the thickness and degree of keratinization of the epithelium, and the presence of pigment-containing cells. The color varies among different persons and appears to be correlated with the cutaneous pigmentation. It is lighter in blond individuals with fair complexions than in swarthy, dark-haired individuals (Color Fig. 1-1).

The attached gingiva is demarcated from the adjacent alveolar mucosa on the buccal aspect by a clearly defined mucogingival line. The alveolar mucosa is red, smooth, and shiny rather than pink and stippled. Comparison of the microscopic structure of the attached gingiva with that of the alveolar mucosa affords an explanation for the difference in appearance. The epithelium of the alveolar mucosa is thinner, is nonkeratinized, and contains no rete pegs (Fig. 1-25). The connective tissue of the alveolar mucosa is loosely arranged, and the blood vessels are more numerous.

Physiologic Pigmentation (Melanin). Melanin, a non–hemoglobin-derived brown pigment, is responsible for the normal pigmentation of the skin, gingiva, and remainder of the oral mucous membrane. It is present in all normal individuals, often not in sufficient quantities to be detected clinically, but is absent or severely diminished in albinos. Melanin pigmentation in the oral cavity is prominent in black individuals (see Color Fig. 1-1).

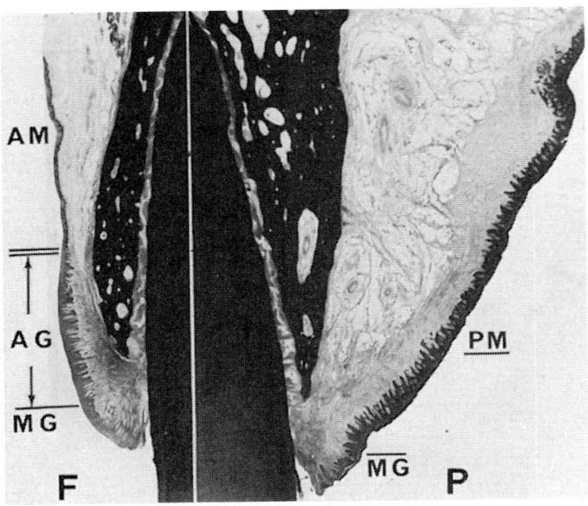

Fig. 1-25 Oral mucosa, facial, and palatal surfaces. The facial surface *(F)* shows the marginal gingiva *(MG)*, attached gingiva *(AG)*, and alveolar mucosa *(AM)*. The double line marks the mucogingival junction. Note the differences in the epithelium and connective tissue in the attached gingiva and alveolar mucosa. The palatal surface *(P)* shows the marginal gingiva *(MG)* and thick keratinized palatal mucosa *(PM)*.

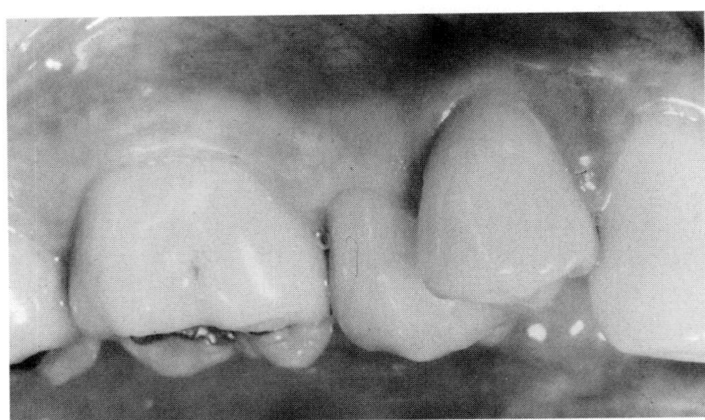

Fig. 1-26 Thickened shelflike contour of gingiva on tooth in lingual version aggravated by local irritation caused by plaque accumulation.

According to Dummett,[33] the distribution of oral pigmentation in black individuals is as follows: gingiva, 60%; hard palate, 61%; mucous membrane, 22%; and tongue, 15%. *Gingival pigmentation occurs as a diffuse, deep-purplish discoloration or as irregularly shaped brown and light brown patches*. It may appear in the gingiva as early as 3 hours after birth and often is the only evidence of pigmentation.[33]

Size

The size of the gingiva corresponds with the sum total of the bulk of cellular and intercellular elements and their vascular supply. Alteration in size is a common feature of gingival disease.

Contour

The contour or shape of the gingiva varies considerably and depends on the shape of the teeth and their alignment in the arch, the location and size of the area of proximal contact, and the dimensions of the facial and lingual gingival embrasures. The marginal gingiva envelops the teeth in collarlike fashion and follows a scalloped outline on the facial and lingual surfaces. It forms a straight line along teeth with relatively flat surfaces. On teeth with pronounced mesiodistal convexity (e.g., maxillary canines) or teeth in labial version, the normal arcuate contour is accentuated and the gingiva is located farther apically. On teeth in lingual version, the gingiva is horizontal and thickened (Fig. 1-26).

Shape

The shape of the interdental gingiva is governed by the contour of the proximal tooth surfaces and the location and shape of gingival embrasures. When the proximal surfaces of the crowns are relatively flat faciolingually, the roots are close together, the interdental bone is thin mesiodistally, and the gingival embrasures and interdental gingiva are narrow mesiodistally. Conversely, with proximal surfaces that flare away from the area of contact, the mesiodistal diameter of the interdental gingiva is broad (Fig. 1-27). The height of the interdental gingiva varies with the location of the proximal contact.

Consistency

The gingiva is *firm and resilient* and, with the exception of the movable free margin, tightly bound to the underlying bone. The collagenous nature of the lamina propria and its contiguity with the mucoperiosteum of the alveolar bone determine the firmness of the attached gingiva. The gingival fibers contribute to the firmness of the gingival margin.

Surface Texture

The gingiva presents a textured surface similar to an orange peel and is referred to as being stippled (see Color Fig. 1-1). Stippling is best viewed by drying the gingiva (see Color Fig. 1-1). *The attached gingiva is stippled; the marginal gingiva is not.* The central portion of the interdental papillae is usually stippled, but the marginal borders are smooth. The pattern and extent of stippling varies among individuals and different areas of the same mouth.[44,86] It is less prominent on lingual than facial surfaces and may be absent in some persons.

Stippling varies with age. It is absent in infancy, appears in some children at about 5 years of age, increases until adulthood, and frequently begins to disappear in old age.

Microscopically, stippling is produced by alternate rounded protuberances and depressions in the gingival surface. The papillary layer of the connective tissue projects into the elevations, and the elevated and depressed areas are covered by stratified squamous epithelium (Fig. 1-28). The degree of keratinization and the prominence of stippling appear to be related.

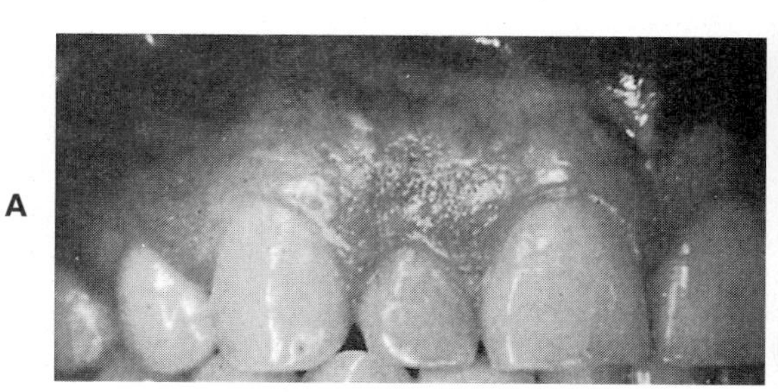

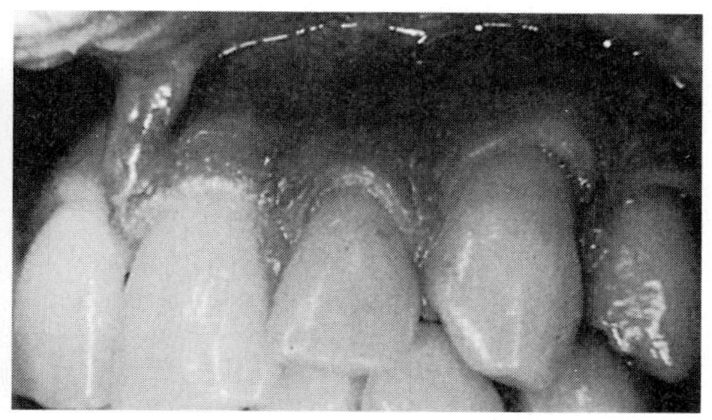

Fig. 1-27 Shape of interdental gingival papillae correlated with shape of teeth and embrasures. **A,** Broad interdental papillae. **B,** Narrow interdental papillae.

Scanning electron microscopy has shown considerable variation in shape but a relatively constant depth. At low magnification a rippled surface is seen, interrupted by irregular depressions 50 microns in diameter. At higher magnification, cell micropits are seen.[28]

Stippling is a form of adaptive specialization or reinforcement for function. It is a feature of healthy gingiva, and reduction or loss of stippling is a common sign of gingival disease. When the gingiva is restored to health after treatment, the stippled appearance returns.

The surface texture of the gingiva also is related to the presence and degree of epithelial keratinization. Keratinization is considered a protective adaptation to function. It increases when the gingiva is stimulated by toothbrushing. However, research on free gingival grafts (see Chapter 66) has shown that when connective tissue is transplanted from a keratinized area to a nonkeratinized area, it becomes covered by a keratinized epithelium.[55] This finding suggests a connective tissue–based genetic determination of the type of epithelial surface.

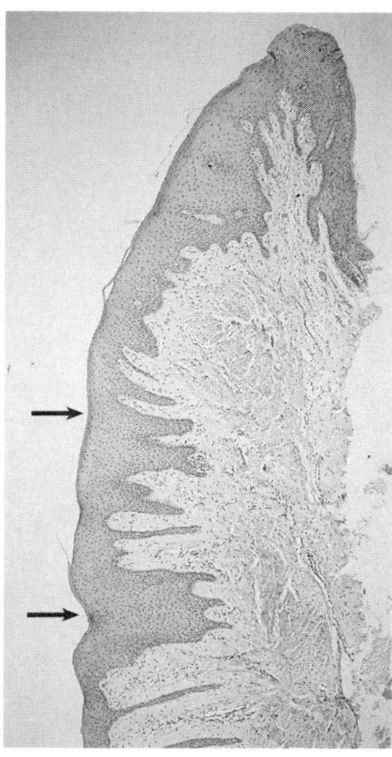

Fig. 1-28 Gingival biopsy of patient shown in Fig. 1-7, demonstrating alternate elevations and depressions *(arrows)* in the attached gingiva responsible for stippled appearance.

Position

The *position* of the gingiva refers to the level at which the gingival margin is attached to the tooth. When the tooth erupts into the oral cavity, the margin and sulcus are at the tip of the crown; as eruption progresses, they are seen closer to the root. During this eruption process, as described earlier, the junctional epithelium, oral epithelium, and reduced enamel epithelium undergo extensive alterations and remodeling, while at the same time maintaining the shallow physiologic depth of the sulcus. Without this remodeling of the epithelia, an abnormal anatomic relationship between the gingiva and the tooth would result.

Continuous Tooth Eruption. According to the concept of continuous eruption,[43] eruption does not cease when teeth meet their functional antagonists but continues throughout life. It consists of an active and a passive phase. *Active eruption* is the movement of the teeth in the direction of the occlusal plane, whereas *passive eruption* is the exposure of the teeth by apical migration of the gingiva.

This concept distinguishes between the *anatomic crown* (the portion of the tooth covered by enamel) and the *anatomic root* (the portion of the tooth covered by cementum) and between the *clinical crown* (the part of the tooth that has been denuded of its gingiva and projects into the oral cavity) and *clinical root* (the portion of the tooth covered by periodontal tissues). When the teeth reach their functional antagonists, the gingival sulcus and junctional epithelium are still on the enamel and the clinical crown is approximately two thirds of the anatomic crown.

Gottlieb believed that active and passive eruption proceed together. Active eruption is coordinated with attrition. The teeth erupt to compensate for tooth substance worn away by attrition. Attrition reduces the clinical crown and prevents it from becoming disproportionately

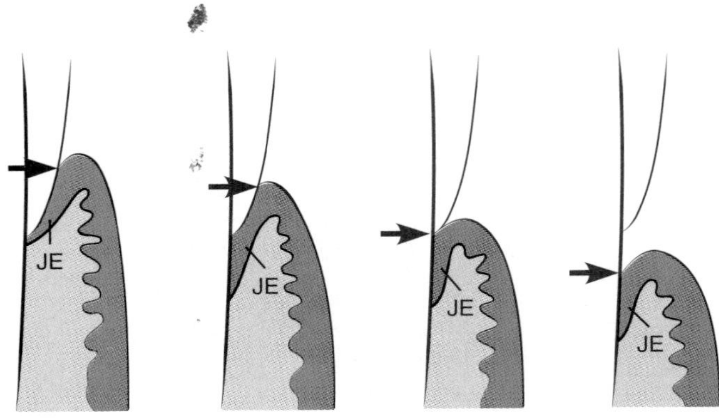

Fig. 1-29 Diagrammatic representation of the four steps in passive eruption according to Gottlieb and Orban.[45] *1,* Base of the gingival sulcus *(arrow)* and the junctional epithelium *(JE)* are on the enamel. *2,* Base of the gingival sulcus *(arrow)* is on the enamel, and part of the junctional epithelium is on the root. *3,* Base of the gingival sulcus *(arrow)* is at the cementoenamel line, and the entire junctional epithelium is on the root. *4,* Base of the gingival sulcus *(arrow)* and the junctional epithelium are on the root.

long in relation to the clinical root, thus avoiding excessive leverage on the periodontal tissues. Ideally, the rate of active eruption keeps pace with tooth wear, preserving the vertical dimension of the dentition.

As teeth erupt, cementum is deposited at the apices and furcations of the roots, and bone is formed along the fundus of the alveolus and at the crest of the alveolar bone. In this way, part of the tooth substance lost by attrition is replaced by lengthening of the root, and socket depth is maintained to support the root.

Passive eruption is divided into four stages (Fig. 1-29). Although this was originally thought to be a normal physiologic process, it is now considered a pathologic process.

Stage 1: The teeth reach the line of occlusion. The junctional epithelium and base of the gingival sulcus are on the enamel.

Stage 2: The junctional epithelium proliferates so that part is on the cementum and part is on the enamel. The base of the sulcus is still on the enamel.

Stage 3: The entire junctional epithelium is on the cementum, and the base of the sulcus is at the cementoenamel junction. As the junctional epithelium proliferates from the crown onto the root, it does not remain at the cementoenamel junction any longer than at any other area of the tooth.

Stage 4: The junctional epithelium has proliferated farther on the cementum. The base of the sulcus is on the cementum, a portion of which is exposed. Proliferation of the junctional epithelium onto the root is accompanied by degeneration of gingival and periodontal ligament fibers and their detachment from the tooth. The cause of this degeneration is not understood. At present, it is believed to be the result of chronic inflammation and therefore a pathologic process.

As noted previously, apposition of bone accompanies active eruption. The distance between the apical end of the junctional epithelium and the crest of the alveolus remains constant throughout continuous tooth eruption (1.07 mm).[40]

Exposure of the tooth by the apical migration of the gingiva is called *gingival recession,* or *atrophy.* According to the concept of continuous eruption, the gingival sulcus may be located on the crown, cementoenamel junction, or root, depending on the age of the patient and stage of eruption. Therefore some root exposure with age would be considered normal and referred to as *physiologic recession.* As mentioned previously, this concept is not accepted at present. Excessive exposure is termed *pathologic recession* (see Chapter 17).

REFERENCES

1. Ainamo A: Influence of age on the location of the maxillary mucogingival junction. J Periodont Res 1978; 13:189.
2. Ainamo A, Ainamo J: The width of attached gingiva on supraerupted teeth. J Periodont Res 1978; 13:194.
3. Ainamo J, Löe H: Anatomical characteristics of gingiva. A clinical and microscopic study of the free and attached gingiva. J Periodontol 1996; 37:5.
4. Ainamo J, Talari A: The increase with age of the width of attached gingiva. J Periodont Res 1976; 11:182.
5. Amstad-Jossi M, Schroeder HE: Age-related alterations of periodontal structures around the cementoenamel junction and of the gingival connective tissue composition in germfree rats. J Periodont Res 1978; 13:76.
6. Anderson GS, Stern I: The proliferation and migration of the attachment epithelium on the cemental surface of the rat incisor. Periodontics 1966; 4:15.
7. Armitt KL: Identification of T cell subsets in gingivitis in children. Periodontology 1986; 7:3.
8. Attstrom RM, Graf de Beer M, Schroeder HE: Clinical and histologic characteristics of normal gingiva in dogs. J Periodont Res 1975; 10:115.
9. Avery JK, Rapp R: Pain conduction in human dental tissues. Dent Clin North Am 1959; July:489.
10. Barakat MH, Toto PD, Choukas NC: Aging and cell renewal of oral epithelium. J Periodontol 1969; 40:599.
11. Beagrie GS, Skougaard MR: Observations on the life cycle of the gingival epithelial cells of mice as revealed by autoradiography. Acta Odontol Scand 1962; 20:15.
12. Bernick S: Innervation of the teeth and periodontium. Dent Clin North Am 1959; July:503.
13. Biolcati EL, Carranza FA Jr, Cabrini RL: Variaciones y alteraciones de la queratinizacion en encias humanas clinicamente sanas. Rev Asoc Odontol Argent 1953; 41:446.
14. Bosch FX, Ouyahoun JP, Bader BL, et al: Extensive changes in cytokeratin expression patterns in pathologically affected human gingiva. Arch VB Cell Path 1989; 58:59.
15. Bouchard P: La cellule de Langerhans: Un role immunitaire pour l'epithelium gingivale. J Parodontol 1987; 6:249.
16. Bowers, GM: A study of the width of the attached gingiva. J Periodontol 1963; 34:210.
17. Bral MM, Stahl SS: Keratinizing potential of human crevicular epithelium. J Periodontol 1977; 48:381.
18. Cabrini RL, Carranza FA Jr: Histochemical distribution of acid phosphatase in human gingiva. J Periodontol 1958; 29:34.
19. Cabrini RL, Carranza FA Jr: Histochemistry of periodontal tissues. A review of the literature. Int Dent J 1966; 16:476.
20. Cabrini R, Cabrini RL, Carranza FA Jr: Estudio histologico de la queratinizacion del epitelio gingival y de la adherencia epitelial. Rev Asoc Odontol Argent 1953; 41:212.
21. Caffesse RG, Karring T, Nasjleti CE: Keratinizing potential of sulcular epithelium. J Periodontol 1977; 48:140.

22. Caffesse RG, Nasjleti CE, Castelli WA: The role of the sulcular environment in controlling epithelial keratinization. J Periodontol 1979; 50:1.
23. Caffesse RG, Kornman KS, Nasjleti CE: The effect of intensive antibacterial therapy on the sulcular environment in monkeys. II. Inflammation, mitotic activity and keratinization of the sulcular epithelium. J Periodontol 1980; 5:155.
24. Carranza FA Jr, Cabrini RL: Mast cells in human gingiva. Oral Surg 1955; 8:1093.
25. Carranza FA Jr, Itoiz ME, Cabrini RL, et al: A study of periodontal vascularization in different laboratory animals. J Periodont Res 1966; 1:120.
26. Chavier C: Elastic fibers of healthy human gingiva. J Periodontol 1990; 9:29.
27. Clausen H, Moe D, Buschard K, Dabelsteen E: Keratin proteins in human oral mucosa. J Oral Path 1986; 15:36.
28. Cleaton Jones P, Buskin SA, Volchansky A: Surface ultrastructure of human gingiva. J Periodont Res 1978; 13:367.
29. Cohen B: Morphological factors in the pathogenesis of periodontal disease. Br Dent J 1959; 107:31.
30. Cohen L: ATPase and dopa oxidase activity in human gingival epithelium. Arch Oral Biol 1967; 12:1241.
31. Dewar MR: Observations on the composition and metabolism of normal and inflamed gingivae. J Periodontol 1955; 26:29.
32. DiFranco CF, Toto PD, Rowden G, et al: Identification of Langerhans cells in human gingival epithelium. J Periodontol 1985; 56:48.
33. Dummett CO: Physiologic pigmentation of the oral and cutaneous tissues in the Negro. J Dent Res 1946; 25:422.
34. Egelberg J: The topography and permeability of blood vessels at the dentogingival junction in dogs. J Periodont Res 1967; 2(Suppl. 1).
35. Eichel B, Shahrik HA, Lisanti VF: Cytochemical demonstration and metabolic significance of reduced diphosphopyridinenucleotide and triphosphopyridinenucleotide reductases in human gingiva. J Dent Res 1964; 43:92.
36. Engel MB: Water-soluble mucoproteins of the gingiva. J Dent Res 1953; 32:779.
37. Folke LEA, Stallard RE: Periodontal microcirculation as revealed by plastic microspheres. J Periodont Res 1967; 2:53.
38. Forsslund G: Structure and function of capillary system in the gingiva in man. Development of stereophotogrammetric method and its application for study of the subepithelial blood vessels in vivo. Acta Odontol Scand 1959; 17(Suppl. 26):9.
39. Frank RM, Cimasoni G: Ultrastructure de l'epithelium cliniquement normal du sillon et de la jonction gingivodentaire. Z Zellforsch 1970; 109:356.
40. Gargiulo AW, Wentz FM, Orban B: Dimensions and relations of the dentogingival junction in humans. J Periodontol 1961; 32:261.
41. Gillet R, Cruchley A, Johnson NW: The nature of the inflammatory infiltrates in childhood gingivitis, juvenile periodontitis and adult periodontitis. Immunohistochemical studies using monoclonal antibody to HLADR. J Clin Periodontol 1986; 13:281.
42. Glickman I, Johannessen L: Biomicroscopic (slitlamp) evaluation of the normal gingiva of the albino rat. J Am Dent Assoc 1950; 41:521.
43. Gottlieb B, Orban B: Active and passive eruption of the teeth. J Dent Res 1933; 13:214.
44. Greene AH: A study of the characteristics of stippling and its relation to gingival health. J Periodontol 1962; 33:176.
45. Hansen ER: Mitotic activity of the gingival epithelium in colchicinized rats. Odont T 1966; 74:229.
46. Hansson BO, Lindhe J, Branemark PI: Microvascular topography and function in clinically healthy and chronically inflamed dentogingival tissues. A vital microscopic study in dogs. Periodontics 1968; 6:265.
47. Itoiz ME, Carranza FA Jr, Cabrini RL: Histotopographic distribution of alkaline and acid phosphatase in periodontal tissues of laboratory animals. J Periodontol 1964; 35:470.
48. Itoiz ME, Carranza FA Jr, Cabrini RL: Histotopographic study of esterase and 5-nucleotidase in periodontal tissues of laboratory animals. J Periodontol 1967; 38:130.
49. Itoiz ME, Carranza FA Jr, Gimenez I, et al: Microspectrophotometric analysis of succinic dehydrogenase and glucose-6-phosphate dehydrogenase in human oral epithelium. J Periodont Res 1972; 7:14.
50. Itoiz ME, Carranza FA Jr, Neira V, et al: Fine structural localization of thiamine pyrophosphatase in normal human gingiva. J Periodontol 1974; 45:579.
51. Itoiz ME, Lanfranchi HE, Gimenez-Conti IB, et al: Immunohistochemical demonstration of keratins in oral mucosa lesions. Acta Odont Lat-Amer 1984; 1:47.
52. Itoiz ME, Conti CJ, Lanfranchi HE, et al: Immunohistochemical detection of filaggrin in preneoplastic and neoplastic lesions of the human oral mucosa. Oral Path 1986; 15:205.
53. Itoiz ME, Conti CJ, Gimenez-Conti IB, et al: Immunodetection of involucrin in lesions of the oral mucosa. J Oral Path 1986; 15:205.
54. Iusem R: A cytological study of the cornification of the oral mucosa in women. Oral Surg 1950; 3:1516.
55. Karring T, Lang NP, Löe H: The role of gingival connective tissue in determining epithelial differentiation. J Periodont Res 1975; 10:1.
56. Kobayashi K, Rose GG: Ultrastructural histochemistry of the dentoepithelial junction. II. Colloidal thorium and ruthenium red. J Periodont Res 1978; 13:164.
57. Kobayashi K, Rose GG: Ultrastructural histochemistry of the dentoepithelial junction. III. Chloramine T-silver methenamine. J Periodont Res 1979; 14:123.
58. Kronfeld R: Histopathology of the Teeth and Their Surrounding Structures. Philadelphia, Lea & Febiger, 1939.
59. Kurahashi Y, Takuma S: Electron microscopy of human gingival epithelium. Bull Tokyo Dent Col 1962; 3:29.
60. Lange D, Camelleri GE: Cytochemical demonstration of lysosomes in the exfoliated epithelial cells of the gingival cuff. J Dent Res 1967; 46:625.
61. Laurell L, Rylander H, Sundin Y: Histologic characteristics of clinically healthy gingiva in adolescents. Scand J Dent Res 1987; 95:456.
62. Lavelle CLB: Mucosal seal around endosseous dental implants. J Oral Implantol 1981; 9:357.
63. Listgarten MA: The ultrastructure of human gingival epithelium. Am J Anat 1964; 114:49.
64. Listgarten MA: Electron microscopic study of the gingivodental junction of man. Am J Anat 1966; 119:147.
65. Listgarten MA: Phase contrast and electron microscopic study of the junction between reduced enamel epithelium and enamel in unerupted human teeth. Arch Oral Biol 1966; 11:999.
66. Listgarten M: Changing concepts about the dentogingival junction. J Can Dent Assoc 1970; 36:70.
67. Listgarten MA: Structure and surface coatings on teeth. A review. J Periodontol 1976; 47:139.
68. Löe H, Karring T: Mitotic activity and renewal time of the gingival epithelium of young and old rats. J Periodont Res 1969; 4(Suppl.):18.
69. Löe H, Karring T: A quantitative analysis of the epithelium–connective tissue interface in relation to assessments of the mitotic index. J Dent Res 1969; 48:634.
70. Magnusson B: Mucosal changes at erupting molars in germ free rats. J Periodont Res 1969; 4:181.

71. McHugh WD: Keratinization of gingival epithelium in laboratory animals. J Periodontol 1964; 35:338.
72. McHugh WD, Zander HA: Cell division in the periodontium of developing and erupted teeth. Dent Pract 1965; 15:451.
73. Meyer J, Marwah AS, Weinmann JP: Mitotic rate of gingival epithelium in two age groups. J Invest Dermatol 1956; 27:237.
74. Miller SC, Soberman A, Stahl S: A study of the cornification of the oral mucosa of young male adults. J Dent Res 1951; 30:4.
75. Morgan PR, Leigh IM, Purkis PE, et al: Site variation in keratin expression in human oral epithelia. An immunocytochemical study of individual keratins. Epithelia 1987; 1:31.
76. Mori M, Kishiro A: Histochemical observation of aminopeptidase activity in the normal and inflamed oral epithelium. J Osaka Univ Dent Sch 1961; 1:39.
77. Moss ML: Phylogeny and comparative anatomy of oral ectodermal ectomesenchymal inductive interactions. J Dent Res 1969; 48:732.
78. Ness KH, Morton TH, Dale BA: Identification of Merker cells in oral epithelium using antikeratin and antineuroendocrine monoclonal antibodies. J Dent Res 1987; 66:1154.
79. Newcomb GM, Powell RN: Human gingival Langerhans cells in health and disease. J Periodont Res 1986; 21:640.
80. Oliver RC, Holm Pedersen P, Löe H: The correlation between clinical scoring, exudate measurements and microscopic evaluation of inflammation in the gingiva. J Periodontol 1969; 40:201.
81. Orban B, Kohler J: Die physiologische Zahn-fleischtasche, Epithelansatz und Epitheltiefenwucherung. Z Stomatol 1924; 22:353.
82. Page RC, Ammons WF, Schectman LR, et al: Collagen fibre bundles of the normal marginal gingiva in the marmoset. Archs Oral Biol 1972; 19:1039.
83. Papic M, Glickman I: Keratinization of the human gingiva in the menstrual cycle and menopause. Oral Surg 1950; 3:504.
84. Person P, Felton J, Fine A: Biochemical and histochemical studies of aerobic oxidative metabolism of oral tissues. III. Specific metabolic activities of enzymatically separated gingival epithelium and connective tissue components. J Dent Res 1965; 44:91.
85. Romanos GE, Bernimoulin J-P: Das Kollagen als Basiselement des Parodonts: Immunohistochemische Aspekte beim Menschen und bei Tieren. Parodontologie 1990; 4:363.
86. Rosenberg H, Massler MJ: Gingival stippling in young adult males. J Periodontol 1967; 38:473.
87. Saglie R, Sabag N, Mery C: Ultrastructure of the normal human epithelial attachment. J Periodontol 1979; 50:544.
88. Sawada T, Yamamoto T, Yanagisawa T, et al: Electron immunochemistry of laminin and type IV collagen in the junctional epithelium of rat molar gingiva. J Periodont Res 1990; 25:372.
89. Sawaf MH, Ouyahoun JP, Forest N: Cytokeratin profiles in oral epithelia: a review and new classification. J Biol Buccal 1991; 19:187.
90. Schroeder HE: Melanin containing organelles in cells of the human gingiva. J Periodont Res 1969; 4:1.
91. Schroeder HE: Differentiation of Human Oral Stratified Epithelia. New York, S. Karger, 1981.
92. Schroeder HE: The Periodontium. Springer-Verlag, Berlin, 1986.
93. Schroeder HE: Transmigration and infiltration of leukocytes in human junctional epithelium. Helv Odont Acta 1973; 17:6.
94. Schroeder HE, Amstad-Jossi M: Type and variability of the stratum corneum in normal and diseased human oral stratified epithelia. J Biol Buccale 1984; 12:101.
95. Schroeder HE, Listgarten MA: Fine structure of the developing epithelial attachment of human teeth. In: Monographs in Developmental Biology, vol 2. Basel, S. Karger, 1971.
96. Schroeder HE, Theilade J: Electron microscopy of normal human gingival epithelium. J Periodont Res 1966; 1:95.
97. Schroeder HE, Listgarten MA: The architecture of periodontal protection. Periodontology 2000 1997; 13:91.
98. Schultz-Haudt SD, From S: Dynamics of periodontal tissues. I. The epithelium. Odont T 1961; 69:431.
99. Schultz-Haudt SD, Paus S, Assev S: Periodic acid–Schiff reactive components of human gingiva. J Dent Res 1961; 40:141.
100. Schweitzer G: Lymph vessels of the gingiva and teeth. Arch Mik, Anat Ent 1907; 69:807.
101. Schwint AE, Itoiz ME, Cabrini RL: A quantitative histochemical technique for the study of vascularization using horseradish peroxidase. Histochem J 1984; 16:907.
102. Seymour GJ, Crouch MS, Powell RN, et al: The identification of lymphoid cell subpopulations in sections of human lymphoid tissue and gingivitis in children using monoclonal antibodies. J Periodont Res 1982; 17:247.
103. Shapiro S, Ulmansky M, Scheuer M: Mast cell population in gingiva affected by chronic destructive periodontal disease. J Periodontol 1969; 40:276.
104. Shelton L, Hall W: Human gingival mast cells. J Periodont Res 1968; 3:214.
105. Skougaard MR, Beagrie GS: The renewal of gingival epithelium in marmosets (*Callithrix jacchus*) as determined through autoradiography with thymidine-H3. Acta Ondontol Scand 1962; 20:467.
106. Soni NN, Silberkweit M, Hayes RL: Pattern of mitotic activity and cell densities in human gingival epithelium. J Periodontol 1965; 36:15.
107. Squier CA, Waterhouse LP: The ultrastructure of the melanocyte in human gingival epithelium. J Dent Res 1967; 46:112.
108. Stern IB: Electron microscopic observations of oral epithelium. I. Basal cells and the basement membrane. Periodontics 1965; 3:224.
109. Stern IB: The fine structure of the ameloblast-enamel junction in rat incisors, epithelial attachment and cuticular membrane. 5th International Congress for Electron Microscopy 1966; 2:6.
110. Stern IB: Further electron microscopic observations of the epithelial attachment. International Association for Dental Research Abstracts, 45th general meeting, 1967; 118.
111. Susi F: Histochemical, autoradiographic and electron microscopic studies of keratinization in oral mucosa. PhD thesis, Tufts University, 1967.
112. Swift JA, Saxton CA: The ultrastructural location of the periodate Schiff reactive basement membrane of the dermoepidermal junctions of human scalp and monkey gingiva. J Ultrastruct Res 1967; 17:23.
113. Thilander H: Permeability of the gingival pocket epithelium. Int Dent J 1964; 14:416.
114. Thilander H, Bloom GD: Cell contacts in oral epithelia. J Periodont Res 1968; 3:96.
115. Thonard JC, Scherp HW: Histochemical demonstration of acid mucopolysaccharides in human gingival epithelial intercellular spaces. Arch Oral Biol 1962; 7:125.
116. Trott JR: An investigation into the glycogen content of the gingivae. Dent Pract 1957; 7:234.
117. Trott JR, Gorenstein SL: Mitotic rates in the oral and gingival epithelium of the rat. Arch Oral Biol 1963; 8:425.

118. Turesky S, Crowley J, Glickman I: A histochemical study of protein-bound sulfhydryl and disulfide groups in normal and inflamed human gingiva. J Dent Res 1957; 36:225.
119. Turesky S, Glickman I, Litwin T: A histochemical evaluation of normal and inflamed human gingivae. J Dent Res 1951; 30:792.
120. Waterhouse JP: The gingival part of the human periodontium. Its ultrastructure and the distribution in it of acid phosphatase in relation to cell attachment and the lysosome concept. Dent Pract 1965; 15:409.
121. Weinmann JP, Meyer J: Types of keratinization in the human gingiva. J Invest Dermatol 1959; 32:87.
122. Weinstock A: Secretory function of postsecretory ameloblasts as shown by electron microscope radioautography. J Dent Res 1972; 50:82.
123. Weinstock A, Albright JT: Electron microscopic observations on specialized structures in the epithelium of the normal human palate. J Dent Res 1966; 45(Suppl.):79.
124. Weinstock A, Albright JT: The fine structure of mast cells in normal human gingiva. J Ultrastruct Res 1967; 17:245.
125. Weski O: Die chronische marginales Enzundungen des Alveolar-fortsatzes mit besonderer Berucksichtigung der Alveolarpyorrhoe. Vierteljahrschr. Zahnheilk 1922; 38:1.
126. Wilgram GF, Weinstock A: Advances in genetic dermatology: Acantholysis, hyperkeratosis, and dyskeratosis. Arch Dermatol 1966; 94:456.
127. Yamasaki A, Nikai H, Niitani K, et al: Ultrastructure of the junctional epithelium of germfree rat gingiva. J Periodontol 1979; 50:641.
128. Zander HA: The distribution of phosphatase in gingival tissue. J Dent Res 1941; 20:347.

The Tooth-Supporting Structures

Fermin A. Carranza and George W. Bernard

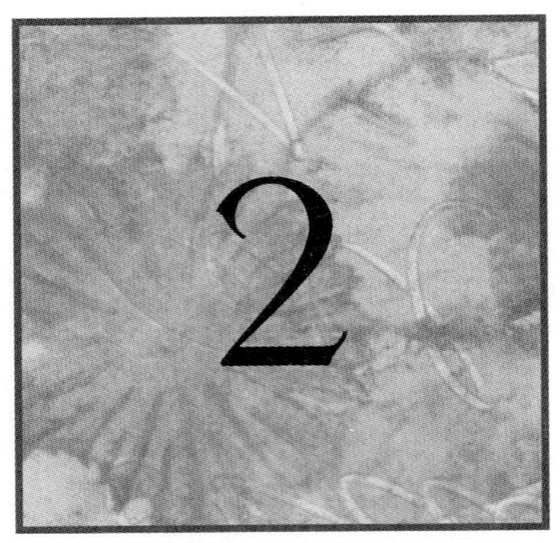

CHAPTER

CHAPTER OUTLINE

The attachment apparatus of the tooth includes the periodontal ligament, cementum, and alveolar bone. The structure of these tissues will be considered first, followed by a description of their development, vascularization, innervation, and functions.

PERIODONTAL LIGAMENT

The periodontal ligament is the connective tissue that surrounds the root and connects it to the bone. It is continuous with the connective tissue of the gingiva and communicates with the marrow spaces through vascular channels in the bone.

Periodontal Fibers

The most important elements of the periodontal ligament are the *principal fibers,* which are collagenous, are arranged in bundles, and follow a wavy course when viewed in longitudinal sections (Fig. 2-1). Terminal portions of the principal fibers that insert into cementum and bone are termed *Sharpey's fibers* (Fig. 2-2). The principal fiber bundles consist of individual fibers that form a continuous anastomosing network between tooth and bone.[9,26]

Collagen is a protein composed of different amino acids, the most important of which are glycine, proline, hydroxylysine, and hydroxyproline.[22] The amount of collagen in a tissue can be determined by its hydroxyproline content.

Collagen biosynthesis occurs inside the fibroblasts to form tropocollagen molecules. These aggregate into microfibrils that are packed together to form fibrils. Collagen fibrils have a transverse striation with a characteristic periodicity of 64 nm; this striation is caused by the overlapping arrangement of the tropocollagen

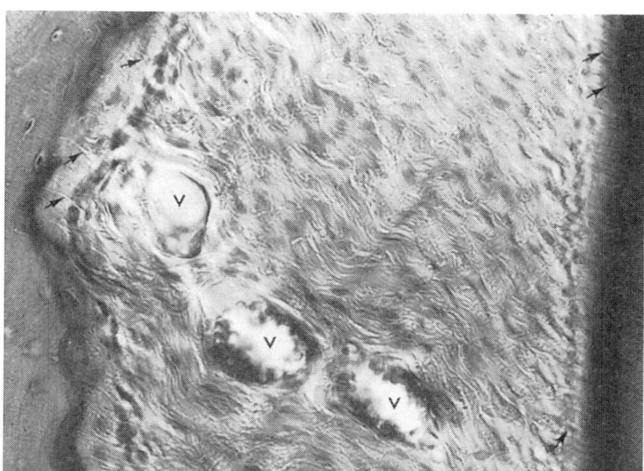

Fig. 2-1 Principal fibers of the periodontal ligament follow a wavy course when sectioned longitudinally. The formative function of the periodontal ligament is illustrated by the newly formed osteoid and osteoblasts along a previously resorbed bone surface *(left)* and the cementoid and cementoblasts *(right)*. Note the fibers embedded in the forming calcified tissues *(arrows)*. *V*, Vascular channels.

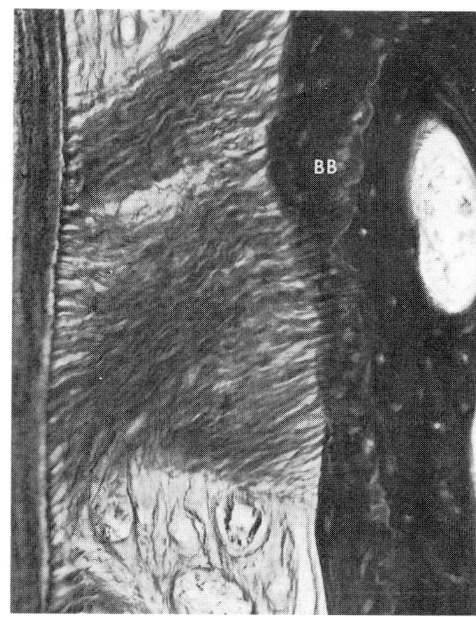

Fig. 2-2 Collagen fibers embedded in the cementum *(left)* and bone *(right)* (silver stain). Note Sharpey's fibers within the bundle bone *(BB)* overlying lamellar bone.

molecules. In collagen types I and III, these fibrils associate to form fibers, and in collagen type I the fibers associate to form bundles (Fig. 2-3).

Collagen is synthesized by fibroblasts, chondroblasts, osteoblasts, odontoblasts, and other cells. The several types of collagen are all distinguishable by their chemical composition, distribution, function, and morphology.[63] The principal fibers are composed mainly of collagen type I,[93] whereas reticular fibers are composed of collagen type III. Collagen type IV is found in the basal lamina.[94,95]

The molecular configuration of collagen fibers confers to them a tensile strength greater than that of steel. Consequently, collagen imparts a unique combination of flexibility and strength to the tissues wherein it lies.[63]

The principal fibers of the periodontal ligament are arranged in six groups that develop sequentially in the developing root: the transseptal, alveolar crest, horizontal, oblique, apical, and interradicular fibers (Fig. 2-4).

Transseptal group: Transseptal fibers extend interproximally over the alveolar bone crest and are embedded in the cementum of adjacent teeth (Fig. 2-5). They are a remarkably constant finding and are reconstructed even after destruction of the alveolar bone has occurred in periodontal disease. These fibers may be considered as belonging to the gingiva because they do not have osseous attachment.

Alveolar crest group: Alveolar crest fibers extend obliquely from the cementum just beneath the junctional epithelium to the alveolar crest (Fig. 2-6). Fibers also run from the cementum over the alveolar crest and to the fibrous layer of the periosteum covering the alveolar bone. The alveolar crest fibers prevent the extrusion of the tooth[24] and resist lateral tooth movements. Their incision does not significantly increase tooth mobility.[42]

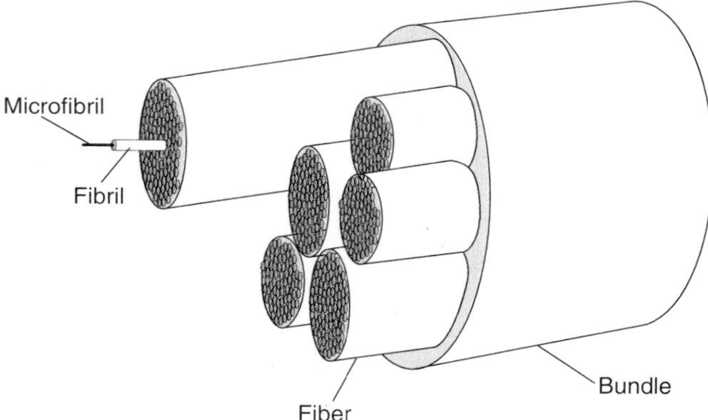

Fig. 2-3 Collagen microfibrils, fibrils, fibers, and bundles.

Horizontal group: Horizontal fibers extend at right angles to the long axis of the tooth from the cementum to the alveolar bone.

Oblique group: Oblique fibers, the largest group in the periodontal ligament, extend from the cementum in a coronal direction obliquely to the bone (see Fig. 2-4). They bear the brunt of vertical masticatory stresses and transform them into tension on the alveolar bone.

Apical group: The apical fibers radiate in a rather irregular fashion from the cementum to the bone at the apical region of the socket. They do not occur on incompletely formed roots.

Interradicular fibers: The interradicular fibers fan out from the cementum to the tooth in the furcation areas of multirooted teeth.

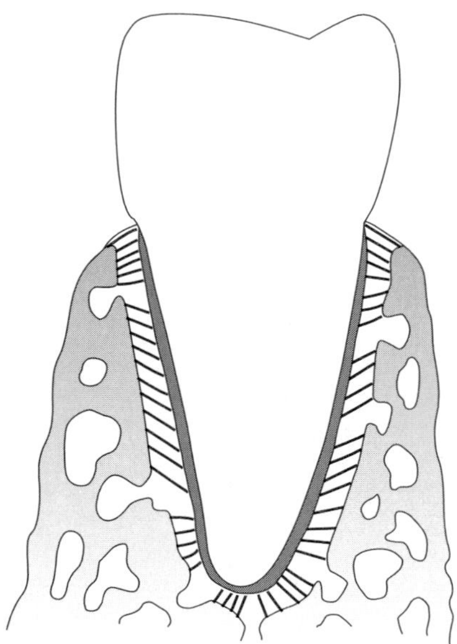

Fig. 2-4 Diagram of principal fiber groups.

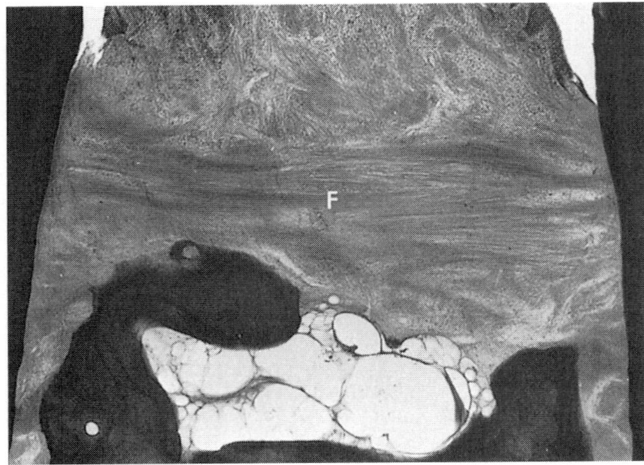

Fig. 2-5 Transseptal fibers *(F)* at the crest of the interdental bone.

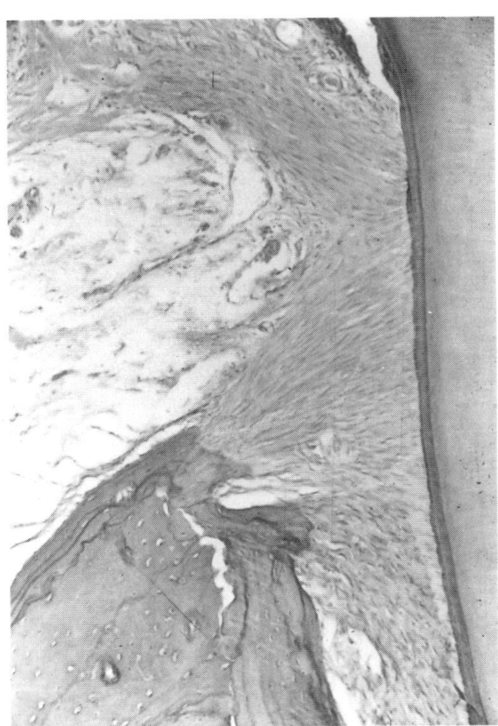

Fig. 2-6 Alveolar crest fibers in rat molar.

Other well-formed fiber bundles interdigitate at right angles or splay around and between regularly arranged fiber bundles. Less regularly arranged collagen fibers are found in the interstitial connective tissue between the principal fiber groups; this tissue contains the blood vessels, lymphatics, and nerves.

Although the periodontal ligament does not contain mature elastin, two immature forms are found—oxytalan and eluanin. The so-called *oxytalan fibers*[37,46] run parallel to the root surface in a vertical direction and bend to attach to cementum[37] in the cervical third of the root. They are thought to regulate vascular flow.[36] An elastic meshwork has been described in the periodontal ligament[59] as being composed of many elastin lamellae with peripheral oxytalan fibers and eluanin fibers. Oxytalan fibers have been shown to develop de novo in the regenerated periodontal ligament.[99]

The principal fibers are remodeled by the periodontal ligament cells to adapt to physiologic needs[108,125] and in response to different stimuli.[117]

In addition to these fiber types, small collagen fibers associated with the larger principal collagen fibers have been described. These fibers run in all directions, forming a plexus called the *indifferent fiber plexus.*[104]

Cellular Elements

Four types of cells have been identified in the periodontal ligament: connective tissue cells, epithelial rest cells, immune system cells, and cells associated with neurovascular elements.[8]

Connective tissue cells include fibroblasts, cementoblasts, and osteoblasts. Fibroblasts are the most common cells in the periodontal ligament and appear as ovoid or elongated cells oriented along the principal fibers and exhibiting pseudopodialike processes.[92] These cells synthesize collagen and also possess the capacity to phagocytose "old" collagen fibers and degrade them[108] by enzyme hydrolysis. Thus collagen turnover appears to be regulated by fibroblasts in a process of intracellular degradation of collagen not involving the action of collagenase.[7]

Phenotypically distinct and functionally different subpopulations of fibroblasts exist in the adult periodontal ligament. They look identical at both light and electron microscopic levels[51] but may have different

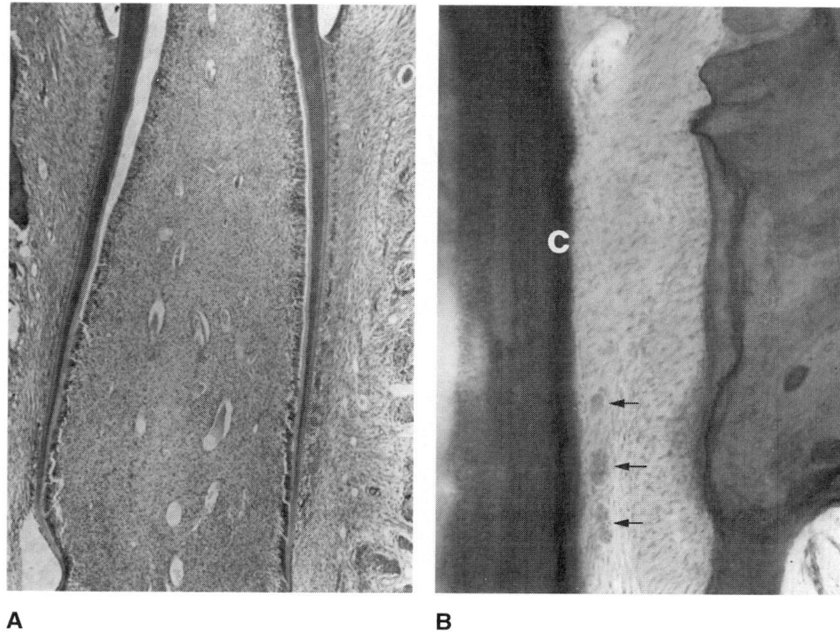

Fig. 2-7 Epithelial rests of Malassez. **A,** Erupting tooth in a cat. Fragmentation of Hertwig's epithelial root sheath giving rise to epithelial rests located along, and close to, the root surface. **B,** Human periodontal ligament with rosette-shaped epithelial rests *(arrows)* lying close to the cementum *(C)*.

functions such as secretion of collagen of different types or production of collagenase.

Osteoblasts and cementoblasts, as well as osteoclasts and odontoclasts, also are seen in the cemental and osseous surfaces of the periodontal ligament.

The *epithelial rests of Malassez* form a latticework in the periodontal ligament and appear as either isolated clusters of cells or interlacing strands (Fig. 2-7), depending on the plane in which the microscopic section is cut. Continuity with the junctional epithelium in experimental animals has been suggested.[48] The epithelial rests are considered remnants of Hertwig's root sheath, which disintegrates during root development.

Epithelial rests are distributed close to the cementum throughout the periodontal ligament of most teeth and are most numerous in the apical[88] and cervical areas.[119,120] They diminish in number with age[106] by degenerating and disappearing or undergoing calcification to become cementicles. The cells are surrounded by a distinct basal lamina, are interconnected by hemidesmosomes, and contain tonofilaments.[7] Epithelial rests proliferate when stimulated[109,112,116] and participate in the formation of periapical cysts and lateral root cysts.

The defense cells include neutrophils, lymphocytes, macrophages, mast cells, and eosinophils. These, as well as those cells associated with neurovascular elements, are similar to those in other connective tissues.

Ground Substance

The periodontal ligament also contains a large proportion of ground substance filling the spaces between fibers and cells. It consists of two main components: *glycosaminoglycans,* such as hyaluronic acid and proteoglycans, and *glycoproteins* such as fibronectin and laminin. It also has a high water content (70%).

The periodontal ligament also may contain calcified masses called *cementicles,* which are adherent to or detached from the root surfaces (Fig. 2-8). Cementicles may develop from calcified epithelial rests; around small spicules of cementum or alveolar bone traumatically displaced into the periodontal ligament; from calcified Sharpey's fibers; and from calcified, thrombosed vessels within the periodontal ligament.[75]

Functions of the Periodontal Ligament

The functions of the periodontal ligament are physical, formative and remodeling, nutritional, and sensory.

Physical Function. The physical functions of the periodontal ligament entail the following:

1. Provision of a soft tissue "casing" to protect the vessels and nerves from injury by mechanical forces
2. Transmission of occlusal forces to the bone
3. Attachment of the teeth to the bone
4. Maintenance of the gingival tissues in their proper relationship to the teeth
5. Resistance to the impact of occlusal forces (shock absorption)

RESISTANCE TO THE IMPACT OF OCCLUSAL FORCES (SHOCK ABSORPTION). Two theories relative to the mechanism of tooth support have been considered: the tensional and viscoelastic system theories.

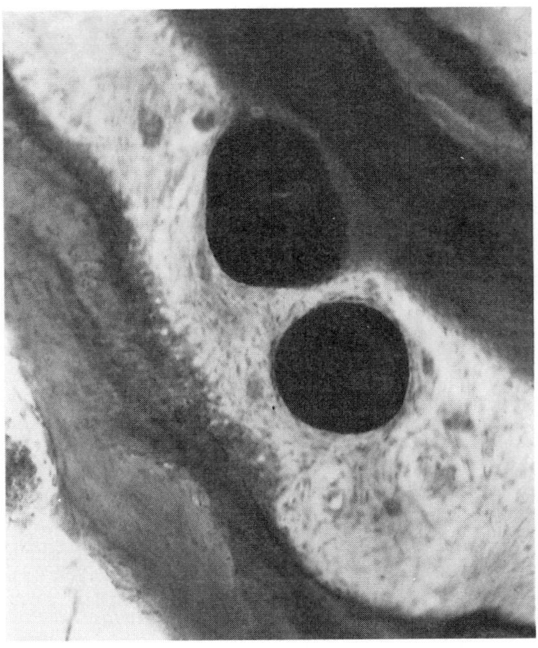

Fig. 2-8 Cementicles in the periodontal ligament, one lying free and the other adherent to the tooth surface.

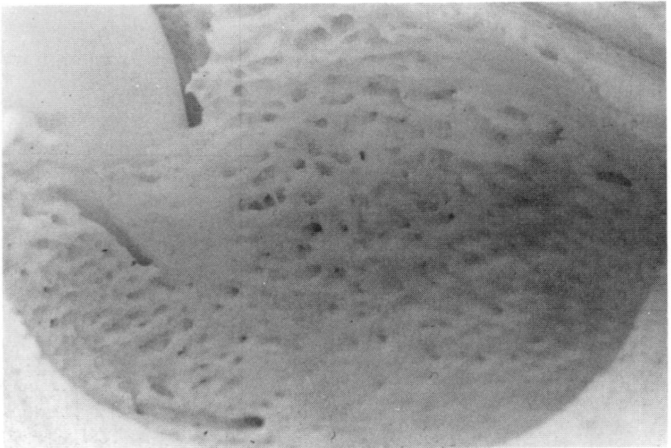

Fig. 2-9 Foramina perforating the lamina dura (dog jaw).

The *tensional theory* of tooth support ascribes to the principal fibers of the periodontal ligament the major responsibility in supporting the tooth and transmitting forces to the bone. When a force is applied to the crown, the principal fibers first unfold and straighten and then transmit forces to the alveolar bone, causing an elastic deformation of the bony socket. Finally, when the alveolar bone has reached its limit, the load is transmitted to the basal bone. Many investigators find this theory insufficient to explain available experimental evidence.

The *viscoelastic system theory* considers the displacement of the tooth to be largely controlled by fluid movements, with fibers having only a secondary role.[14,21]

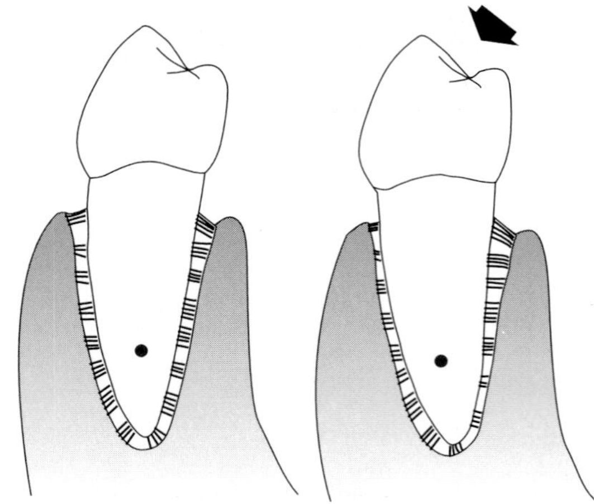

Fig. 2-10 *Right,* Distribution of faciolingual forces *(arrow)* around the axis of rotation *(black circle on root)* in a mandibular premolar. The periodontal ligament fibers are compressed in areas of pressure and tension. *Left,* The same tooth in a resting state.

When forces are transmitted to the tooth, the extracellular fluid passes from the periodontal ligament into the marrow spaces of bone through foramina in the cribriform plate. These perforations of the cribriform plate link the periodontal ligament with the cancellous portion of the alveolar bone and are more abundant in the cervical third than in the middle and apical thirds (Fig. 2-9).

After depletion of tissue fluids, the fiber bundles absorb the slack and tighten. This leads to blood vessel stenosis. Arterial back pressure causes ballooning of the vessels, and passage of blood ultrafiltrates into the tissues, thereby replenishing the tissue fluids.[14]

TRANSMISSION OF OCCLUSAL FORCES TO THE BONE. The arrangement of the principal fibers is similar to a suspension bridge or hammock. When an axial force is applied to a tooth, a tendency toward displacement of the root into the alveolus occurs. The oblique fibers alter their wavy, untensed pattern; assume their full length; and sustain the major part of the axial force. When a horizontal or tipping force is applied, two phases of tooth movement occur. The first is within the confines of the periodontal ligament, and the second produces a displacement of the facial and lingual bony plates.[31] The tooth rotates about an axis that may change as the force is increased.

The apical portion of the root moves in a direction opposite to the coronal portion. In areas of tension, the principal fiber bundles are taut rather than wavy. In areas of pressure, the fibers are compressed, the tooth is displaced, and a corresponding distortion of bone exists in the direction of root movement.[85]

In single-rooted teeth, the axis of rotation is located in the area between the apical third and the middle third of the root (Fig. 2-10). The root apex[78] and the coronal half of the clinical root have been suggested as other locations of the axis of rotation. The periodontal ligament, which is shaped like an hourglass, is narrowest in the region of the axis of rotation[29,65] (Table 2-1). In multirooted teeth, the axis of rotation is located in the bone

TABLE 2-1

Thickness of Periodontal Ligament of 172 Teeth from 15 Human Jaws

	Average of Alveolar Crest (mm)	Average of Mid-root (mm)	Average of Apex (mm)	Average of Tooth (mm)
Ages 11–16				
83 teeth from 4 jaws	0.23	0.17	0.24	0.21
Ages 32–50				
36 teeth from 5 jaws	0.20	0.14	0.19	0.18
Ages 51–67				
35 teeth from 5 jaws	0.17	0.12	0.16	0.15
Age 24 (1 case)				
18 teeth from 1 jaw	0.16	0.09	0.15	0.13

Modified from Coolidge ED: The thickness of the human periodontal membrane. J Am Dent Assoc 1937; 24:1260.

between the roots (Fig. 2-11). In compliance with the physiologic mesial migration of the teeth, the periodontal ligament is thinner on the mesial root surface than on the distal surface.

Formative and Remodeling Function. Cells of the periodontal ligament participate in the formation and resorption of cementum and bone, which occur in physiologic tooth movement; in the accommodation of the periodontium to occlusal forces; and in the repair of injuries. Variations in cellular enzyme activity[39-41] are correlated with the remodeling process.

Cartilage formation in the periodontal ligament, although unusual, may represent a metaplastic phenomenon in the repair of this ligament after injury.[4]

The periodontal ligament is constantly undergoing remodeling. Old cells and fibers are broken down and replaced by new ones, and mitotic activity can be observed in the fibroblasts and endothelial cells.[77] Fibroblasts form the collagen fibers, and the residual mesenchymal cells develop into osteoblasts and cementoblasts. Therefore the rate of formation and the differentiation of osteoblasts, cementoblasts, and fibroblasts affect the rate of formation of collagen, cementum, and bone.

Radioautographic studies with radioactive thymidine, proline, and glycine indicate a very high turnover rate of collagen in the periodontal ligament. The rate of collagen synthesis is twice as fast as that in the gingiva and four times as fast as that in the skin, as established in the rat molar.[107] A rapid turnover of sulfated glycosaminoglycans in the cells and amorphous ground substance of the periodontal ligament also occurs.[5]

It should be noted that most of these studies have been performed in rodents, and information on primates and humans is scarce.[100]

Nutritional and Sensory Functions. The periodontal ligament supplies nutrients to the cementum, bone, and gingiva by way of the blood vessels and provides lymphatic drainage (see later discussion).

The periodontal ligament is abundantly supplied

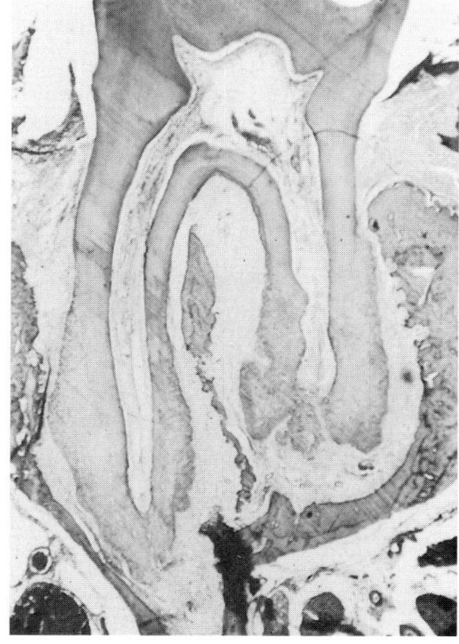

Fig. 2-11 Microscopic view of rat molar subjected to occlusohorizontal forces. Note the widened and narrowed areas of the periodontal ligament. The axis of rotation is in the interradicular space.

with sensory nerve fibers capable of transmitting tactile, pressure, and pain sensations by the trigeminal pathways.[3,13] Nerve bundles pass into the periodontal ligament from the periapical area and through channels from the alveolar bone that follow the course of the blood vessels. They divide into single myelinated fibers, which ultimately lose their myelin sheaths and end in one of four types of neural termination: free endings, which have a treelike configuration and carry pain sensation; Ruffini-like mechanoreceptors, located primarily in the apical area; coiled Meissner's corpuscles, also mechanoreceptors, found mainly in the midroot region; and spindlelike pressure and vibration endings, which are surrounded by a fibrous capsule and located mainly in the apex.[36,71]

CEMENTUM

Cementum is the calcified avascular mesenchymal tissue that forms the outer covering of the anatomic root. The two main types of cementum are acellular (primary) and cellular (secondary) cementum.[47] Both consist of a calcified interfibrillar matrix and collagen fibrils.

The two sources of collagen fibers in cementum are Sharpey's (extrinsic) fibers, which are the embedded portion of the principal fibers of the periodontal ligament[94] and are formed by the fibroblasts, and fibers that belong to the cementum matrix per se (intrinsic) and are produced by the cementoblasts.[102] Cementoblasts also form the noncollagenous components of the interfibrillar ground substance, such as proteoglycans, glycoproteins, and phosphoproteins.

Acellular cementum is the first to be formed and covers approximately the cervical third or half of the root; it does not contain cells (Fig. 2-12). This cementum is formed before the tooth reaches the occlusal plane, and its thickness ranges from 30 to 230 μm.[100] Sharpey's fibers comprise most of the structure of acellular cementum, which has a principal role in supporting the tooth. Most fibers are inserted at approximately right angles into the root surface and penetrate deep into the cementum, but others enter from several different directions. Their size, number, and distribution increase with function.[57] Sharpey's fibers are completely calcified, with the mineral crystals oriented parallel to the fibrils as in dentin and bone, except in a 10- to 50-μm-wide zone near the cementodentinal junction, where they are only partially calcified. The peripheral portions of Sharpey's fibers in actively mineralizing cementum tend to be more calcified than the interior regions, according to evidence obtained by scanning electron microscopy.[61] Acellular cementum also contains intrinsic collagen fibrils that are calcified and irregularly arranged or parallel to the surface.[100]

Cellular cementum, formed after the tooth reaches the occlusal plane, is more irregular and contains cells (cementocytes) in individual spaces (lacunae) that communicate with each other through a system of anastomosing canaliculi (Fig. 2-13). Cellular cementum is less calcified than the acellular type.[58] Sharpey's fibers occupy a smaller portion of cellular cementum and are separated by other fibers that are arranged either parallel to the root surface or at random. Sharpey's fibers may be completely or partially calcified or have a central, uncalcified core surrounded by a calcified border.[60,102]

Both acellular cementum and cellular cementum are arranged in lamellae separated by incremental lines parallel to the long axis of the root (see Figs. 2-12 and 2-13). These lines represent rest periods in cementum formation and are more mineralized than the adjacent cementum.[96] In addition, loss of the cervical part of the reduced enamel epithelium at the time of tooth eruption may place portions of mature enamel in contact with the connective tissue, which then will deposit over it an acellular afibrillar type of cementum.[69]

Based on these findings, Schroeder[100] has classified cementum as follows:

Acellular afibrillar cementum (AAC) contains neither cells nor extrinsic or intrinsic collagen fibers, apart from a mineralized ground substance. It is a product of cementoblasts and is found as coronal cementum in humans, with a thickness of 1 to 15 μm.

Acellular extrinsic fiber cementum (AEFC) is composed almost entirely of densely packed bundles of Sharpey's fibers and lacks cells. It is a product of fibroblasts and cementoblasts and is found in the cervical third of roots in humans but may extend further apically. Its thickness is between 30 and 230 μm.

Cellular mixed stratified cementum (CMSC) is composed of extrinsic (Sharpey's) and intrinsic fibers and may contain cells. It is a co-product of fibroblasts and cementoblasts, and in humans it appears primarily in the apical third of the roots and apices and in furcation areas. Its thickness ranges from 100 to 1000 μm.

Cellular intrinsic fiber cementum (CIFC) contains cells but no extrinsic collagen fibers. It is formed by cementoblasts, and in humans it fills resorption lacunae.

Intermediate cementum is an ill-defined zone near the cementodentinal junction of certain teeth that appears to contain cellular remnants of Hertwig's sheath embedded in calcified ground substance.[33,68]

The inorganic content of cementum (hydroxyapatite; $Ca_{10}[Po_4]_6[OH]_2$) is 45% to 50%, which is less than that of bone (65%), enamel (97%), or dentin (70%).[127] Opinions differ about whether the microhardness increases[79] or decreases with age,[122] and no relationship has been established between aging and the mineral content of cementum.

Permeability of Cementum

In very young animals, cellular and acellular cementum are very permeable and permit the diffusion of dyes from the pulp and external root surface. In cellular cementum, the canaliculi in some areas are contiguous with the dentinal tubuli. The permeability of cementum diminishes with age.[17]

Cementoenamel Junction

The cementum at and immediately subjacent to the cementoenamel junction is of particular clinical importance in root scaling procedures. Three types of relationships involving the cementum may exist at the cementoenamel junction.[80] In about 60% to 65% of cases, cementum overlaps the enamel (Fig. 2-14); in about 30% an edge-to-edge butt joint exists; and in 5% to 10% the cementum and enamel fail to meet. In the last instance, gingival recession may result in accentuated sensitivity because the dentin is exposed.

Thickness of Cementum

Cementum deposition is a continuous process that proceeds at varying rates throughout life. Cementum

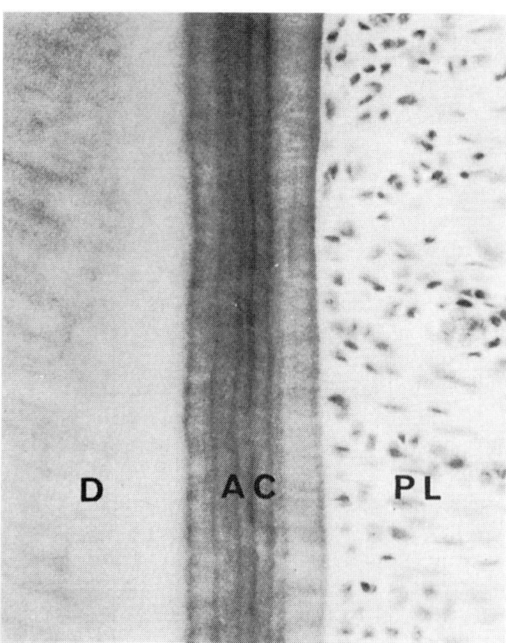

Fig. 2-12 Acellular cementum *(AC)* showing incremental lines running parallel to the long axis of the tooth. These lines represent the appositional growth of cementum. Note the thin, light lines running into the cementum perpendicular to the surface; these represent Sharpey's fibers of the periodontal ligament *(PL)*. *D,* Dentin. (Magnification ×300.)

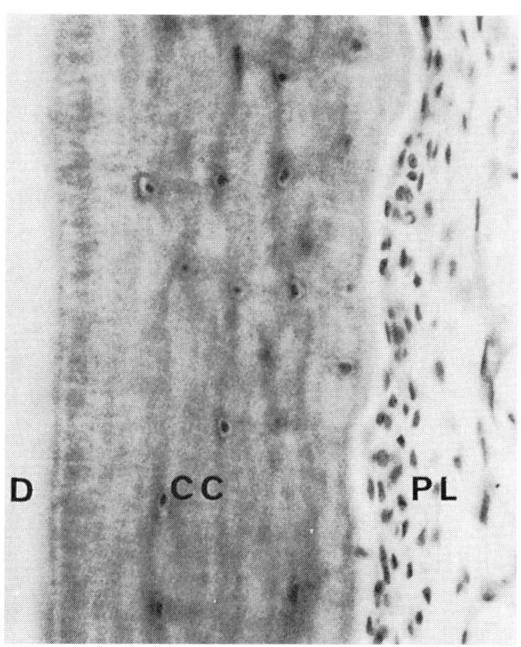

Fig. 2-13 Cellular cementum *(CC)* showing cementocytes lying within lacunae. Cellular cementum is thicker than acellular cementum (cf. Fig. 2-16). Evidence of incremental lines also exists, but they are less distinct than in acellular cementum. The cells adjacent to the surface of the cementum in the periodontal ligament *(PL)* space are cementoblasts. *D,* Dentin. (Magnification ×300.)

formation is most rapid in the apical regions, where it compensates for tooth eruption, which itself compensates for attrition. The thickness of cementum on the coronal half of the root varies from 16 to 60 μm, or about the thickness of a hair. It attains its greatest thickness (up to 150 to 200 μm) in the apical third and in the furcation areas. It is thicker in distal surfaces than in mesial surfaces, probably because of functional stimulation from mesial drift over time.[30] Between the ages of 11 and 70, the average thickness of the cementum increases threefold, with the greatest increase in the apical region. Average thicknesses of 95 μm at age 20 and 215 μm at age 60 have been reported.[126]

The term *hypercementosis* (cementum hyperplasia) refers to a prominent thickening of the cementum. It may be localized to one tooth or affect the entire dentition. Because of considerable physiologic variation in the thickness of cementum among different teeth in the same person and also among different persons, distinguishing between hypercementosis and physiologic thickening of cementum is sometimes difficult.

Hypercementosis occurs as a generalized thickening of the cementum, with nodular enlargement of the apical third of the root. It also appears in the form of spikelike excrescences (cemental spikes) created by either the coalescence of cementicles that adhere to the root or the calcification of periodontal fibers at the sites of insertion into the cementum.[68]

The etiology of hypercementosis varies and is not completely understood. The spikelike type of hypercementosis generally results from excessive tension from orthodontic appliances or occlusal forces. The generalized type occurs in a variety of circumstances. In teeth without antagonists, hypercementosis is interpreted as an effort to keep pace with excessive tooth eruption. In teeth subject to low-grade periapical irritation arising from pulp disease, it is considered compensation for the destroyed fibrous attachment to the tooth. The cementum is deposited adjacent to the inflamed periapical tissue. Hypercementosis of the entire dentition may occur in patients with Paget's disease.[98]

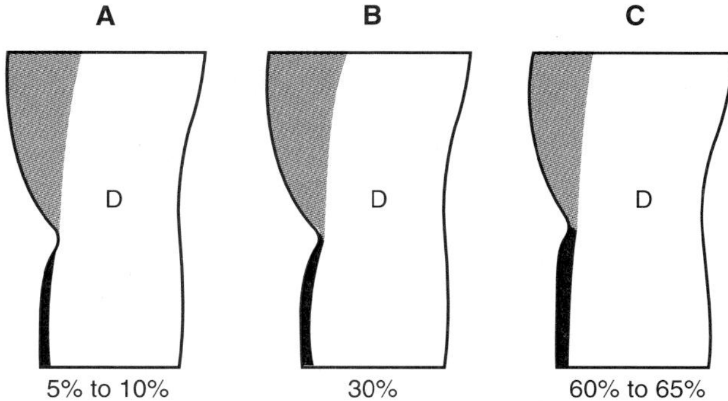

Fig. 2-14 Normal variations in tooth morphology at the cementoenamel junction. **A,** Space between enamel and cementum with dentin *(D)* exposed. **B,** End-to-end relationship of enamel and cementum. **C,** Cementum overlapping the enamel.

Cementum Resorption and Repair

Permanent teeth do not undergo physiologic resorption as do primary teeth. However, the cementum of erupted as well as unerupted teeth is subject to resorptive changes that may be of microscopic proportion or sufficiently extensive to present a radiographically detectable alteration in the root contour. Microscopic cementum resorption is extremely common. In one study, it occurred in 236 of 261 teeth (90.5%).[54] The average number of resorption areas per tooth was 3.5. Of the 922 areas of resorption, 708 (76.8%) were located in the apical third of the root, 177 (19.2%) in the middle third, and 37 (4.0%) in the gingival third. Approximately 70% of all resorption areas were confined to the cementum without involving the dentin.

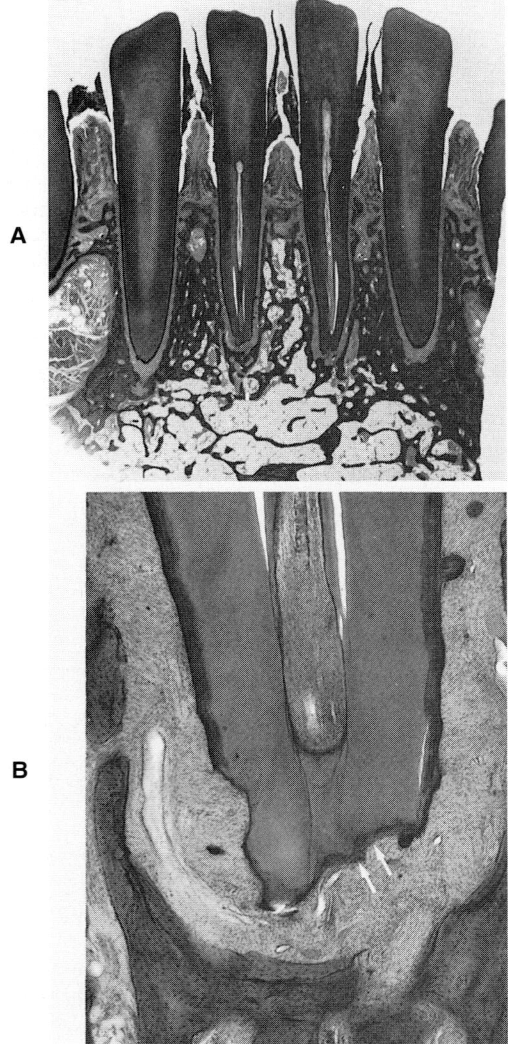

Fig. 2-15 Cemental resorption associated with excessive occlusal forces. **A,** Low-power histologic section of mandibular anterior teeth. **B,** High-power micrograph of apex of left central incisor shortened by resorption of cementum and dentin. Note partial repair of the eroded areas *(arrows)* and cementicle at upper right.

Cementum resorption may be caused by local or systemic causes or may occur without apparent etiology (i.e., idiopathic). Among the local conditions in which it occurs are trauma from occlusion[82] (Fig. 2-15); orthodontic movement;[53,81,97] pressure from malaligned erupting teeth, cysts, and tumors;[66] teeth without functional antagonists; embedded teeth; replanted and transplanted teeth;[1,60] periapical disease; and periodontal disease. Among the systemic conditions mentioned as predisposing to or inducing cemental resorption are calcium deficiency,[62] hypothyroidism,[6] hereditary fibrous osteodystrophy,[114] and Paget's disease.[98]

Cementum resorption appears microscopically as baylike concavities in the root surface (Fig. 2-16). Multinucleated giant cells and large mononuclear macrophages are generally found adjacent to cementum undergoing active resorption (Fig. 2-17). Several sites of resorption may coalesce to form a large area of destruction. The resorptive process may extend into the underlying dentin and even into the pulp, but it is usually painless. Cementum resorption is not necessarily continuous and may alternate with periods of repair and the deposition of new cementum. The newly formed cementum is demarcated from the root by a deeply staining irregular line, termed a *reversal line,* which delineates the border of the previous resorption (Fig. 2-18). Embedded fibers of the periodontal ligament reestablish a functional relationship in the new cementum. Cementum repair requires the presence of viable connective tissue. If epithelium proliferates into an area of resorption, repair will not take place. Cementum repair can occur in devitalized as well as in vital teeth.

Ankylosis. Fusion of the cementum and alveolar bone with obliteration of the periodontal ligament is termed *ankylosis*. Ankylosis occurs in teeth with cemental resorption, which suggests that it may represent a form of abnormal repair. Ankylosis also may develop

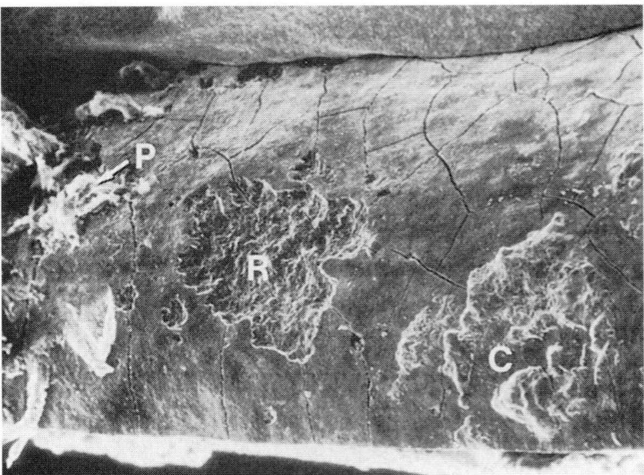

Fig. 2-16 Scanning electron micrograph of root exposed by periodontal disease showing large resorption bay *(R)*. Remnants of the periodontal ligament *(P)* and calculus *(C)* are visible. Cracking of the tooth surface occurs as a result of the preparation technique. (Magnification ×160.) (Courtesy John Sottosanti, San Diego, Calif.)

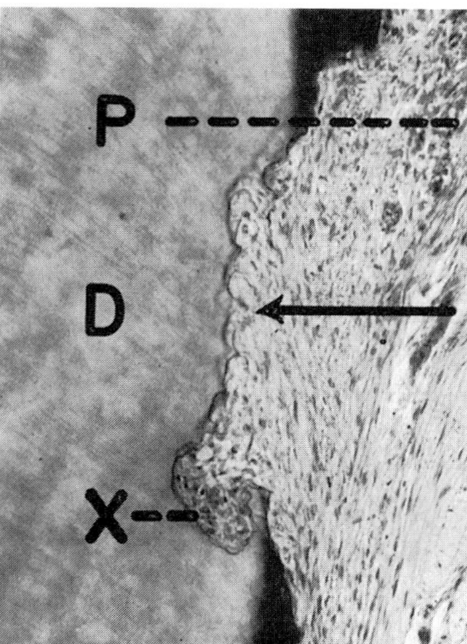

Fig. 2-17 Resorption of cementum and dentin. A multinuclear osteoclast is seen at *X*. The direction of resorption is indicated by the arrow. Note the scalloped resorption front in the dentin *(D)*. The cementum is the darkly stained band at the upper and lower right. *P*, Periodontal ligament.

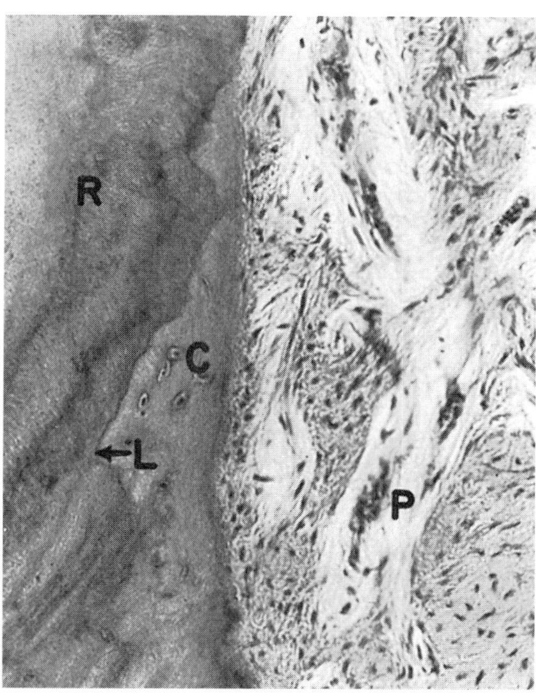

Fig. 2-18 Section showing repair of previously resorbed root. The defect is filled in with cellular cementum *(C)*, which is separated from the older cementum *(R)* by an irregular line *(L)* that indicates the preexisting outline of the resorbed root. *P*, Periodontal ligament.

after chronic periapical inflammation, tooth replantation, and occlusal trauma and around embedded teeth.

Ankylosis results in resorption of the root and its gradual replacement by bone tissue. For this reason, reimplanted teeth that ankylose will lose their roots after 4 to 5 years and exfoliate.

When titanium implants are placed in the jaw, healing results in bone formed in direct apposition to the implant without any intervening connective tissue. This may be interpreted as a form of ankylosis. Because resorption of the metallic implant cannot occur, the implant remains indefinitely "ankylosed" to the bone. Also, a true periodontal pocket will not form because apical proliferation of the epithelium along the root, a key element of pocket formation, is not possible owing to the ankylosis.

Exposure of Cementum to the Oral Environment

Cementum becomes exposed to the oral environment in cases of gingival recession and as a consequence of loss of attachment in pocket formation. The cementum is sufficiently permeable to be penetrated in these cases by organic substances, inorganic ions, and bacteria. Bacterial invasion of the cementum occurs commonly in periodontal disease (see Chapter 22). Caries of the cementum also can develop (see Chapter 30).

ALVEOLAR PROCESS

The *alveolar process* is the portion of the maxilla and mandible that forms and supports the tooth sockets (alveoli). It forms when the tooth erupts to provide the osseous attachment to the forming periodontal ligament; it disappears gradually after the tooth is lost.

The alveolar process consists of the following:

1. An external plate of cortical bone formed by haversian bone and compacted bone lamellae
2. The inner socket wall of thin, compact bone called the *alveolar bone proper*, which is seen as the lamina dura in radiographs. Histologically, it contains a series of openings *(cribriform plate)* through which neurovascular bundles link the periodontal ligament with the central component of the alveolar bone, the cancellous bone.
3. Cancellous trabeculae, between these two compact layers, which act as supporting alveolar bone. The *interdental septum* consists of cancellous supporting bone enclosed within a compact border (Fig. 2-19).

In addition, the jaw bones consist of the *basal bone*, which is the portion of the jaw located apically but unrelated to the teeth (Fig. 2-20).

The alveolar process is divisible into separate areas on an anatomic basis, but it functions as a unit, with all parts interrelated in the support of the teeth. Figs. 2-21 and 2-22 show the relative proportions of cancellous bone and compact bone that form the alveolar process. Most of the facial and lingual portions of the sockets are formed by compact bone alone; cancellous bone surrounds the lamina dura in apical, apicolingual, and interradicular areas.

Cells and Intercellular Matrix

Osteoblasts, the cells that produce the organic matrix of bone, are differentiated from pluripotent follicle cells.

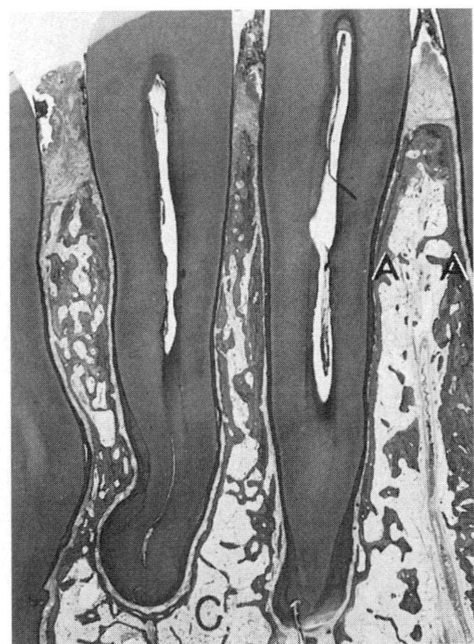

Fig. 2-19 Mesiodistal section through mandibular canine and premolars showing interdental bony septa. The dense bony plates *(A)* represent the alveolar bone proper (cribriform plates) and are supported by cancellous bony trabeculae *(C)*. Note the vertical blood vessels within a nutrient canal in the interdental septum at the right.

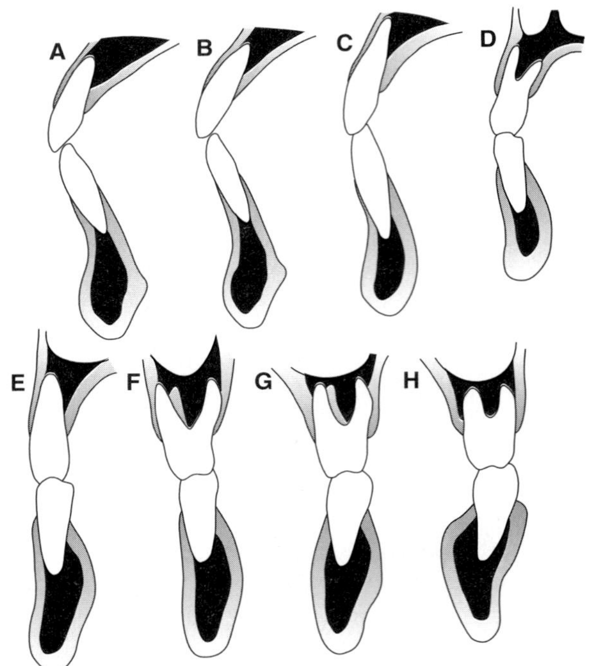

Fig. 2-21 Relative proportions of cancellous bone and compact bone in a longitudinal faciolingual section of central incisors *(A)*, lateral incisors *(B)*, canines *(C)*, first premolars *(D)*, second premolars *(E)*, first molars *(F)*, second molars *(G)*, and third molars *(H)*.

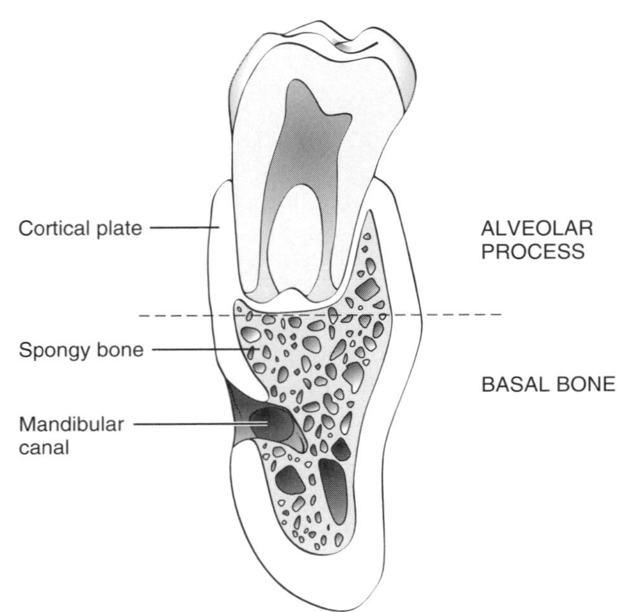

Fig. 2-20 Section through human jaw with tooth in situ. The dotted line indicates the separation between basal bone and alveolar bone. (Redrawn from Ten Cate AR: Oral Histology. Development, Structure, and Function, ed 4. St Louis, Mosby, 1994.)

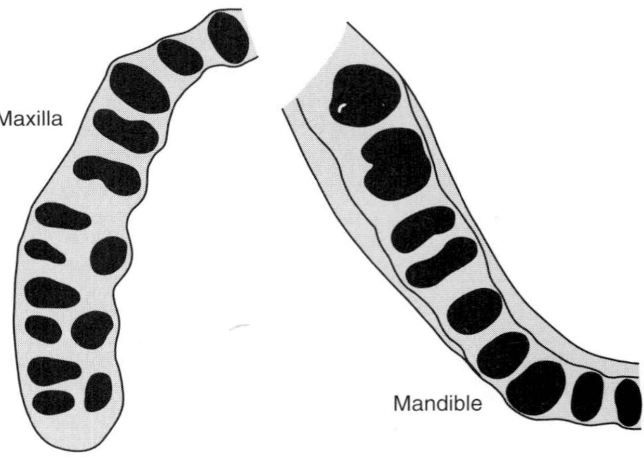

Fig. 2-22 Shape of roots and surrounding bone distribution in a transverse section of maxilla and mandible at mid-root level.

Alveolar bone is formed during fetal growth by intramembranous ossification and consists of a calcified matrix with osteocytes enclosed within spaces called *lacunae.* The osteocytes extend processes into canaliculi that radiate from the lacunae. The canaliculi form an anastomosing system through the intercellular matrix of the bone, which brings oxygen and nutrients to the osteocytes through the blood and removes metabolic waste products. Blood vessels branch extensively and travel through the periosteum. The endosteum lies adjacent to the marrow vasculature. Bone growth occurs by apposition of an organic matrix that is deposited by osteoblasts. Haversian systems (osteons) are the internal mechanisms that bring a vascular supply to bones too thick to be supplied only by surface vessels. These are found primarily in the outer cortical plates and the alveolar bone proper.

Bone consists of two-thirds inorganic matter and one-third organic matrix. The inorganic matter is composed principally of the minerals calcium and phosphate, along with hydroxyl, carbonate, citrate, and trace amounts of other ions[44] such as sodium, magnesium, and fluorine. The mineral salts are in the form of hydroxyapatite crystals of ultramicroscopic size and constitute approximately two thirds of the bone structure.

The organic matrix[32] consists mainly (90%) of collagen type I,[76] with small amounts of noncollagenous proteins such as osteocalcin, osteonectin, bone morphogenetic protein, phosphoproteins, and proteoglycans.[87]

Although the alveolar bone tissue is constantly changing in its internal organization, it retains approximately the same form from childhood through adult life. Bone deposition by osteoblasts is balanced by resorption by osteoclasts during tissue remodeling and renewal.

Remodeling is the major pathway of bony changes in shape, resistance to forces, repair of wounds, and calcium and phosphate homeostasis in the body.

Bone contains 99% of calcium ions of the body and therefore is the major source for calcium release when the calcium blood levels decrease; this is monitored by the parathyroid gland. Blood calcium decrease is mediated by receptors on the chief cells of the parathyroid glands, which then release parathyroid hormone (PTH). PTH stimulates osteoblasts to release interleukin 1 and 6, which stimulates monocytes to migrate into the bone area. Leukemia inhibiting factor (LIF), secreted by osteoblasts, coalesce monocytes into multinucleated osteoclasts, which then resorb bone, releasing calcium ions from hydroxyapatite into the blood. This release normalizes the blood level of calcium. A feedback mechanism of normal blood levels of calcium turns off the parathyroid gland secretion of PTH. In the meantime, osteoclasts have resorbed organic matrix along with hydroxyapatite. The breakdown of collagen from the organic matrix releases various osteogenic substrates, which are covalently bound to collagen, and this in turn stimulates the differentiation of osteoblasts, which ultimately deposit bone. This interdependency of osteoblasts and osteoclasts in remodeling is called *coupling.*

The bone matrix that is laid down by osteoblasts is nonmineralized *osteoid.* While new osteoid is being deposited, the older osteoid located below the surface becomes mineralized as the mineralization front advances.

Bone resorption is a complex process morphologically related to the appearance of eroded bone surfaces (Howship's lacunae) and large, multinucleated cells (osteoclasts) (Fig. 2-23). Osteoclasts originate from hematopoietic tissue[25,50,70] and are formed by the fusion of mononuclear cells of asynchronous populations.[10,64,84,113] When osteoclasts are active as opposed to resting, they possess an elaborately developed ruffled border from which hydrolytic enzymes are believed to be secreted.[118] These enzymes digest the organic portion of bone. The activity of osteoclasts and morphology of the ruffled border can be modified and regulated by hormones such as parathormone (indirectly) and calcitonin, which has receptors on the osteoclast membrane.

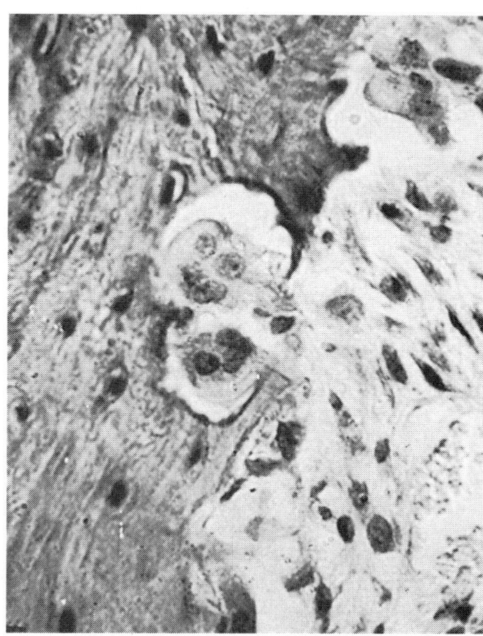

Fig. 2-23 Rat alveolar bone. Histologic view of two multinucleated osteoclasts in a Howship lacuna.

Another mechanism of bone resorption consists of the creation of an acidic environment on the bone surface, leading to the dissolution of the mineral component of bone. This event can be produced by different conditions, among them a proton pump through the cell membrane of the osteoclast,[16] bone tumors, or local pressure,[70] translated through the secretory activity of the osteoclast.

Ten Cate[113] described the sequence of events in the resorptive process as follows:

1. Attachment of osteoclasts to the mineralized surface of bone
2. Creation of a sealed acidic environment through action of the proton pump, which demineralizes bone and exposes the organic matrix
3. Degradation of the exposed organic matrix to its constituent amino acids by the action of released enzymes, such as acid phosphatase and cathepsine
4. Sequestering of mineral ions and aminoacids within the osteoclast

Socket Wall

The socket wall consists of dense, lamellated bone, some of which is arranged in haversian systems, and bundle bone. *Bundle bone* is the term given to bone adjacent to the periodontal ligament that contains a great number of Sharpey's fibers (Fig. 2-24).[123] It is characterized by thin lamellae arranged in layers parallel to the root, with intervening appositional lines (Fig. 2-25). Bundle bone is localized within the alveolar bone proper. Some

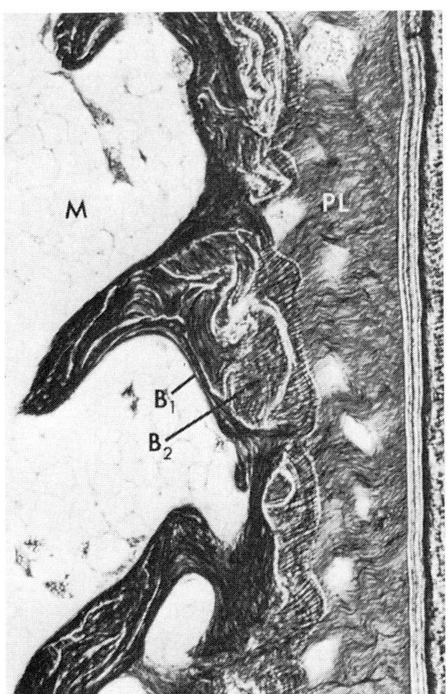

Fig. 2-24 Deep penetration of Sharpey's fibers into bundle bone. The darkly stained bone *(B_1)* is lamellar bone. Bundle bone *(B_2)* takes up less stain and shows numerous white lines running more or less parallel to each other; these lines correspond to Sharpey's fibers. *M,* Fatty marrow; *PL,* periodontal ligament.

Sharpey's fibers are completely calcified, but most contain an uncalcified central core within a calcified outer layer.[102] Bundle bone is not unique to the jaws; it occurs throughout the skeletal system wherever ligaments and muscles are attached.

The cancellous portion of the alveolar bone consists of trabeculae that enclose irregularly shaped marrow spaces lined with a layer of thin, flattened endosteal cells. Wide variation occurs in the trabecular pattern of cancellous bone,[83] which is affected by occlusal forces. The matrix of the cancellous trabeculae consists of irregularly arranged lamellae separated by deeply staining incremental and resorption lines indicative of previous bone activity, with an occasional haversian system.

Cancellous bone is found predominantly in the interradicular and interdental spaces and in limited amounts facially or lingually, except in the palate. In the adult human, more cancellous bone exists in the maxilla than in the mandible.

Bone Marrow

In the embryo and newborn, the cavities of all bones are occupied by red hematopoietic marrow. The red marrow gradually undergoes a physiologic change to the fatty or yellow inactive type of marrow. In the adult, the marrow of the jaw is normally of the latter type, and red marrow is found only in the ribs, sternum, vertebrae, skull, and humerus. However, foci of red bone marrow are occasionally seen in the jaws, often accompanied by resorption of bony trabeculae.[19] Common locations are the maxillary tuberosity (Fig. 2-26), the maxillary and mandibular molar and premolar areas, and the mandibular symphysis and ramus angle, which may be visible radiographically as zones of radiolucency.

Periosteum and Endosteum

All bone surfaces are covered by layers of differentiated osteogenic connective tissue. The tissue covering the outer surface of bone is termed *periosteum,* whereas the tissue lining the internal bone cavities is called *endosteum.*

The periosteum consists of an inner layer composed of osteoblasts surrounded by osteoprogenitor cells, which have the potential to differentiate into osteoblasts, and an outer layer rich in blood vessels and nerves and composed of collagen fibers and fibroblasts. Bundles of periosteal collagen fibers penetrate the bone, binding the periosteum to the bone. The endosteum is composed of a single layer of osteoblasts and sometimes a small amount of connective tissue. The inner layer is the osteogenic layer and the outer is the fibrous layer.

Interdental Septum

The interdental septum consists of cancellous bone bordered by the socket wall cribriform plates (lamina dura or alveolar bone proper) of approximating teeth and the facial and lingual cortical plates (Fig. 2-27). If the interdental space is narrow, the septum may consist of only the cribriform plate. For example, the space between mandibular second premolars and first molars consists of cribriform plate and cancellous bone in 85% of the cases and only cribriform plate in the remaining 15%.[52] If roots are too close together, an irregular "window" can appear in the bone between adjacent roots (Fig. 2-28). Between maxillary molars, the septum consists of cribriform plate and cancellous bone in 66.6% of cases, is composed of only cribriform plate in 20.8% of cases, and has a fenestration in 12.5% of cases.[52] Determining root proximity radiographically is important (see Chapter 31). The mesiodistal angulation of the crest of the interdental septum usually parallels a line drawn between the cementoenamel junctions of the approximating teeth.[91] The distance between the crest of the alveolar bone and the cementoenamel junction in young adults varies between 0.75 and 1.49 mm (average 1.08 mm).[38] This distance increases with age to an average of 2.81 mm.[38] However, this phenomenon may not be as much a function of age as of periodontal disease.

The mesiodistal and faciolingual dimensions and shape of the interdental septum are governed by the size and convexity of the crowns of the two approximating teeth, as well as by the position of the teeth in the jaw and their degree of eruption.[91]

Osseous Topography

The bone contour normally conforms to the prominence of the roots, with intervening vertical depressions that taper toward the margin (Fig. 2-29). Alveolar bone anatomy varies among patients and has important

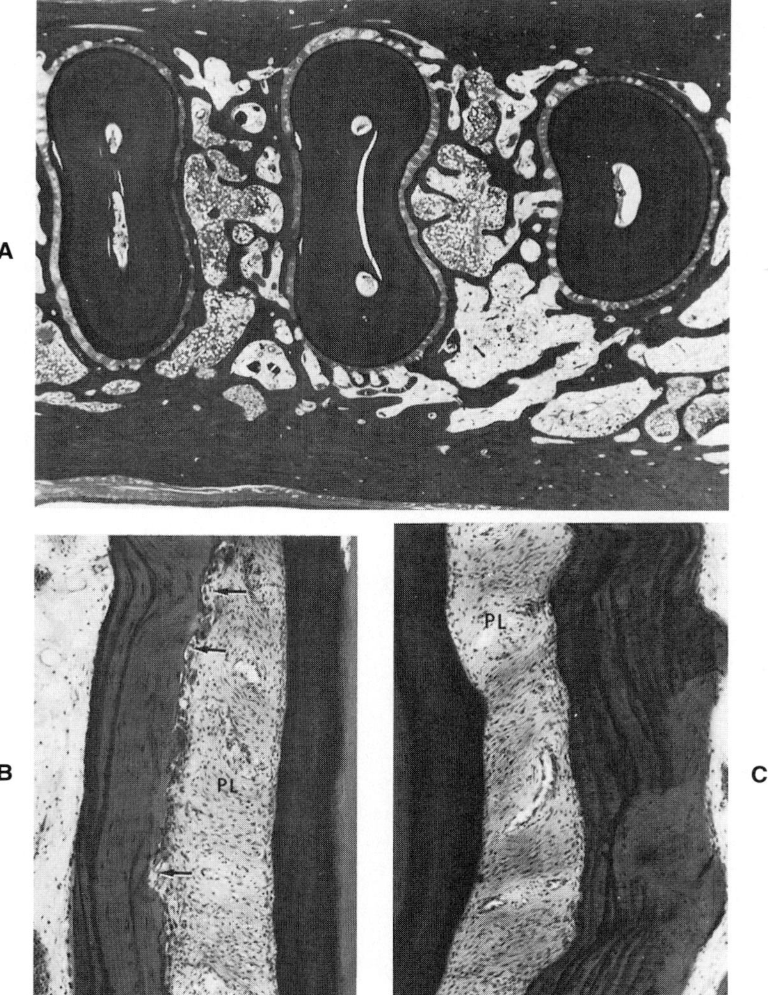

Fig. 2-25 Bundle bone associated with physiologic mesial migration of the teeth. **A,** Horizontal section through molar roots in the process of mesial migration (*left,* mesial; *right,* distal). **B,** Mesial root surface showing osteoclasis of bone *(arrows).* **C,** Distal root surface showing bundle bone that has been partially replaced with dense bone on the marrow side. *PL,* Periodontal ligament.

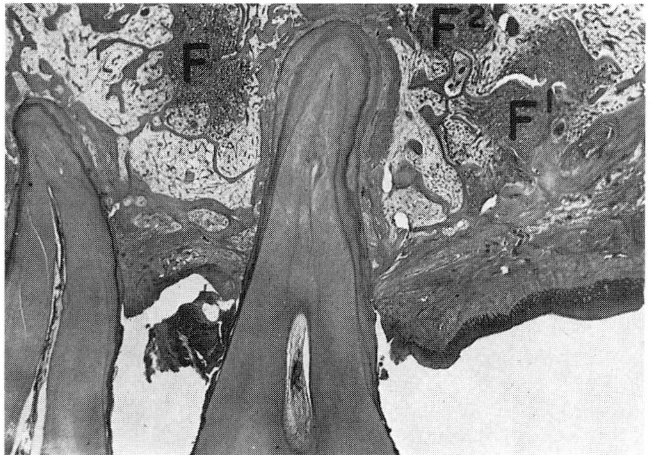

Fig. 2-26 Mesiodistal section in the molar area of the maxilla of a 59-year-old male, showing foci of hematopoiesis in the marrow *(F, F^1, F^2).*

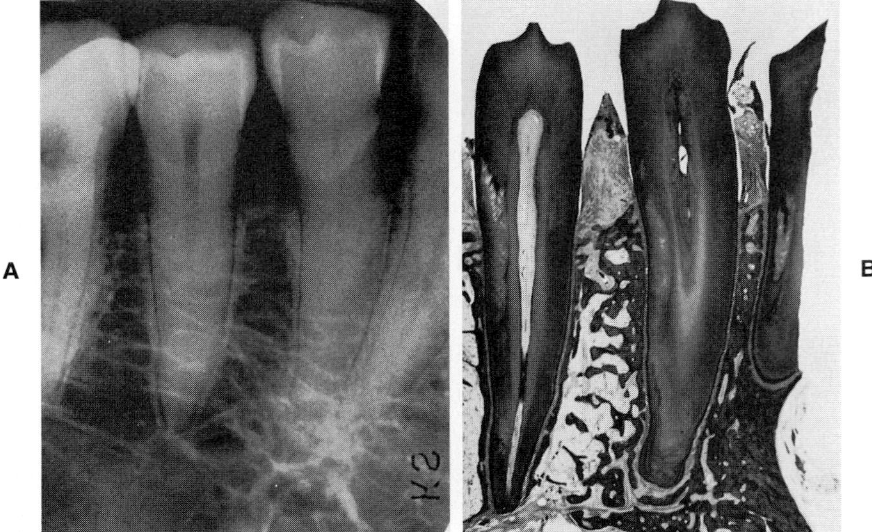

Fig. 2-27 Interdental septa. **A,** Radiograph of mandibular premolar area. Note the prominent lamina dura. **B,** Interdental septa between the canine *(right)* and premolars. The central cancellous portion is bordered by the dense bony cribriform plates of the socket. (This forms the lamina dura around the teeth in the radiograph.)

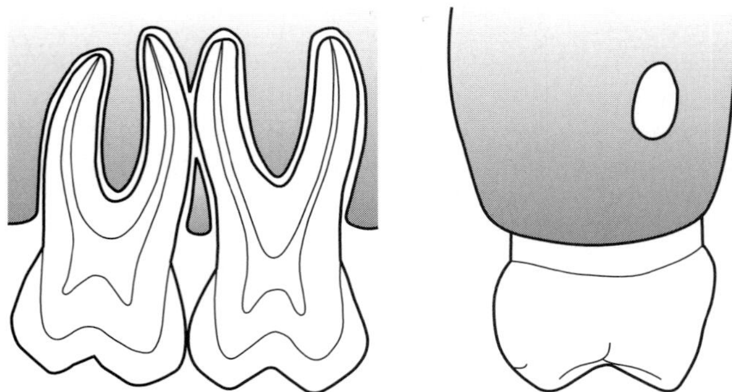

Fig. 2-28 Boneless "window" between adjoining close roots of molars.

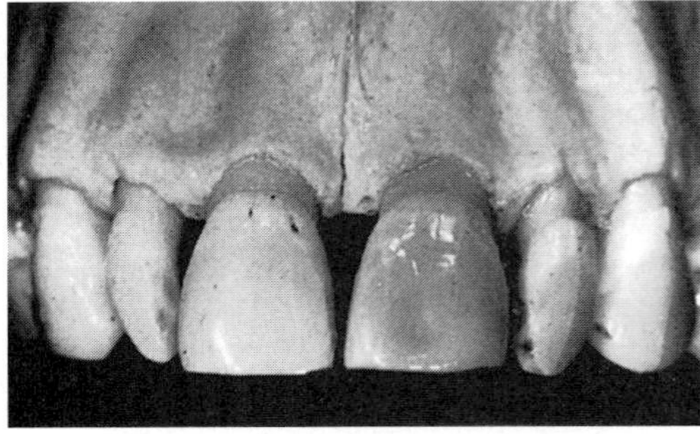

Fig. 2-29 Normal bone contour conforms to the prominence of the roots.

clinical implications. The height and thickness of the facial and lingual bony plates are affected by the alignment of the teeth, angulation of the root to the bone, and occlusal forces.

On teeth in labial version, the margin of the labial bone is located farther apically than on teeth in proper alignment. The bone margin is thinned to a knife edge and presents an accentuated arc in the direction of the apex. On teeth in lingual version, the facial bony plate is thicker than normal. The margin is blunt and rounded and horizontal rather than arcuate. The effect of the root-to-bone angulation on the height of alveolar bone is most noticeable on the palatal roots of maxillary molars. The bone margin is located farther apically on the roots, which form relatively acute angles with the palatal bone.[56] The cervical portion of the alveolar plate is sometimes considerably thickened on the facial surface, apparently as reinforcement against occlusal forces (Fig. 2-30).

Fenestrations and Dehiscences

Isolated areas in which the root is denuded of bone and the root surface is covered only by periosteum and overlying gingiva are termed *fenestrations*. In these instances the marginal bone is intact. When the denuded areas extend through the marginal bone, the defect is called a *dehiscence* (Fig. 2-31). Such defects occur on approximately 20% of the teeth; they occur more often on the facial bone than on the lingual, are more common on anterior teeth than on posterior teeth, and are frequently bilateral. Microscopic evidence of lacunar resorption may be

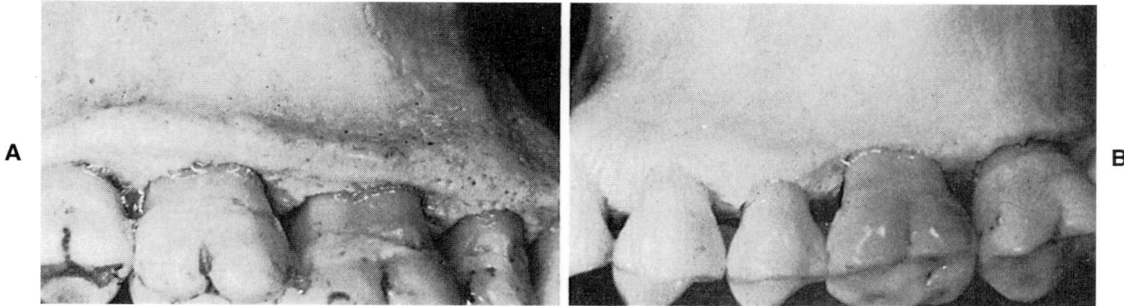

Fig. 2-30 Variation in the cervical portion of the buccal alveolar plate. **A,** Shelflike conformation. **B,** Comparatively thin buccal plate.

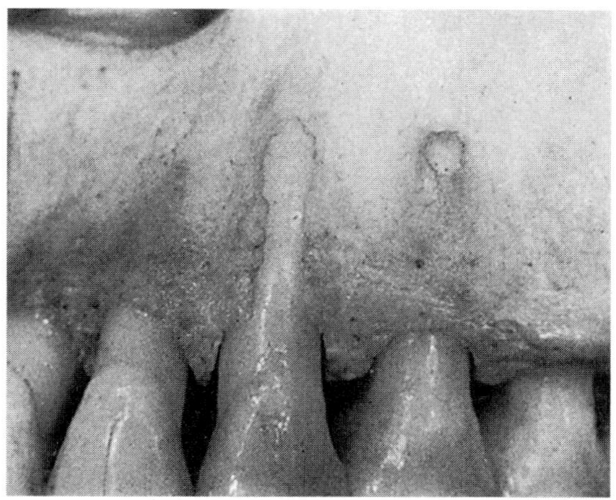

Fig. 2-31 Dehiscence on the canine and fenestration of the first premolar.

present at the margins. The cause of these defects is not clear. Prominent root contours, malposition, and labial protrusion of the root combined with a thin bony plate are predisposing factors.[34] Fenestration and dehiscence are important because they may complicate the outcome of periodontal surgery.

Remodeling of Alveolar Bone

In contrast to its apparent rigidity, alveolar bone is the least stable of the periodontal tissues because its structure is in a constant state of flux. A considerable amount of internal remodeling takes place by means of resorption and formation, which are regulated by local and systemic influences. Local influences include functional requirements on the tooth and age-related changes in bone cells. Systemic influences are probably hormonal (e.g., parathyroid hormone, calcitonin, or vitamin D_3).

The remodeling of the alveolar bone affects its height, contour, and density, and it is manifested in the following three areas: adjacent to the periodontal ligament, in relation to the periosteum of the facial and lingual plates, and along the endosteal surface of the marrow spaces.

DEVELOPMENT OF THE ATTACHMENT APPARATUS

After the crown has formed, the stratum intermedium and the stellate reticulum of the enamel organ disappear. The outer and inner epithelia of the enamel organ remain and form the so-called *reduced enamel epithelium.* The apical portion of this constitutes *Hertwig's epithelial root sheath,* which will continue to grow apically and determines the shape of the root. Before the beginning of root formation, the root sheath bends horizontally at the future cementoenamel junction, narrowing the cervical opening and forming the *epithelial diaphragm.* The epithelial diaphragm separates the dental follicle from the dental papilla.

After root dentin formation starts, Hertwig's root sheath breaks up and partially disappears; the remaining cells form the epithelial clusters or strands known as *epithelial rests of Malassez* (see Fig. 2-7, *A*). In multirooted teeth, the epithelial diaphragm grows in such a way that tonguelike extensions develop horizontally, leaving spaces for each of the future roots to form.

Cementum

The rupture of Hertwig's root sheath allows the mesenchymal cells of the dental follicle to contact the dentin, where they start forming a continuous layer of cementoblasts. Based on immunochemical and ultrastructural studies, Thomas[115] and others[18,73] have speculated that cementoblasts also can be of epithelial origin (Hertwig's root sheath), which would undergo an epithelial mesenchymal transformation.

Cementum formation begins by deposition of a meshwork of irregularly arranged collagen fibrils sparsely distributed in a ground substance or matrix called *precementum* or *cementoid.* This is followed by a phase of matrix maturation, which subsequently mineralizes to form cementum. Cementoblasts, which are initially separated from the cementum by uncalcified cementoid, sometimes become enclosed within the matrix and are trapped. Once they are enclosed, they are referred to as *cementocytes* and will remain viable in a fashion similar to that of osteocytes.

The enamel organ—including the epithelial root sheath as it develops—is surrounded by a layer of connective tissue known as the *dental sac.* The zone immediately in contact with the dental organ and continuous with the ectomesenchyme of the dental papilla is called the *dental follicle*[109-111] and consists of undifferentiated fibroblasts.

Periodontal Ligament

As the crown approaches the oral mucosa during tooth eruption, these fibroblasts become active and start producing collagen fibrils. These initially lack orientation, but they soon acquire an orientation oblique to the tooth. The first collagen bundles then appear in the region immediately apical to the cementoenamel junction and give rise to the gingivodental fiber groups. As tooth eruption progresses, additional oblique fibers appear and become attached to the newly formed cementum and bone. The transseptal and alveolar crest fibers develop when the tooth merges into the oral cavity. Alveolar bone deposition occurs simultaneously with periodontal ligament organization.[107]

Studies of the squirrel monkey[49] have shown that during eruption, cemental Sharpey's fibers appear first, followed by Sharpey's fibers emerging from bone. Sharpey's fibers are fewer in number and more widely spaced than those emerging from the cementum. At a later stage, alveolar fibers extend into the middle zone to join the lengthening cemental fibers and attain their classic orientation, thickness, and strength when occlusal function is established.

Early investigators had suggested that the individual fibers, rather than being continuous, consisted of two separate parts spliced together midway between the cementum and the bone in a zone that is called the *intermediate plexus.* The plexus has been reported in the periodontal ligament of continuously growing incisors but not in the posterior teeth of rodents[55,74,128] and in actively erupting human and monkey teeth,[49] but not after they reach occlusal contact. Rearrangement of the fiber ends in the plexus is supposed to accommodate tooth eruption without necessitating the embedding of new fibers into the tooth and the bone.[74] The existence of such a plexus, however, has not been confirmed by radioautographic data and other studies, and it is considered a microscopic artifact.[100]

Alveolar Bone

Just before mineralization, osteoblasts start producing matrix vesicles.[12] These vesicles contain enzymes such as alkaline phosphatase that help jump-start the nucleation of hydroxyapatite crystals. As these crystals grow and develop, they form coalescing bone nodules, which, with fast-growing nonoriented collagen fibers, are the substructure of woven bone, the first bone formed in the alveolus. Later, through bone deposition, remodeling, and the secretion of oriented collagen fibers in sheets, mature lamellar bone is formed.[12]

The hydroxyapatite crystals are generally aligned with their long axes parallel to the collagen fibers and appear to be deposited on and within the collagen fibers in mature lamellar bone. In this fashion, bone matrix is able to withstand the heavy mechanical stresses applied to it during function.

The alveolar bone develops around each tooth follicle during odontogenesis. When a deciduous tooth is shed, its alveolar bone is resorbed. The succedaneous permanent tooth moves into place, developing its own alveolar bone from its own dental follicle. As the tooth root forms and the surrounding tissues develop and mature, alveolar bone merges with the separately developing basal bone and the two become one continuous structure. Although alveolar bone and basal bone have different intermediate origins, both are ultimately derived from neural crest ectomesenchyme.

Mandibular basal bone begins mineralization at the exit of the mental nerve from the mental foramen, whereas the maxillary basal bone begins at the exit of the infraorbital nerve from the infraorbital foramen.

Physiologic Migration of the Teeth

Tooth movement does not end when active eruption is completed and the tooth is in functional occlusion. With time and wear, the proximal contact areas of the teeth are flattened and the teeth tend to move mesially. This is referred to as *physiologic mesial migration.* By age 40, it results in a reduction of about 0.5 cm in the length of the dental arch from the midline to the third molars. Alveolar bone is reconstructed in compliance with the physiologic mesial migration of the teeth. Bone resorption is increased in areas of pressure along the mesial surfaces of the teeth, and new layers of bundle bone are formed in areas of tension on the distal surfaces (Fig. 2-32; see also Fig. 2-25).

EXTERNAL FORCES AND THE PERIODONTIUM

The periodontium exists for the purpose of supporting teeth during function and depends on the stimulation it receives from function for the preservation of its structure. Therefore a constant and sensitive balance is present between external forces and the periodontal structures.

Alveolar bone undergoes constant physiologic remodeling in response to external forces, particularly occlusal forces. Bone is removed from areas where it is no longer needed and added to areas where it is presently needed. The socket wall reflects the responsiveness of alveolar bone to external forces. Osteoblasts and newly formed osteoid line the socket in areas of tension; osteoclasts and bone resorption occur in areas of pressure. Forces exerted on the tooth also influence the number, density, and alignment of cancellous trabeculae. The bony trabeculae are aligned in the path of the tensile and compressive stresses to provide maximal resistance to the occlusal force with a minimum of bone substance (Fig. 2-33).[43,105] When forces are increased, the cancellous bony trabeculae increase in number and thickness, and bone may be added to the external surface of the labial and lingual plates.

The periodontal ligament also depends on stimulation provided by function to preserve its structure.

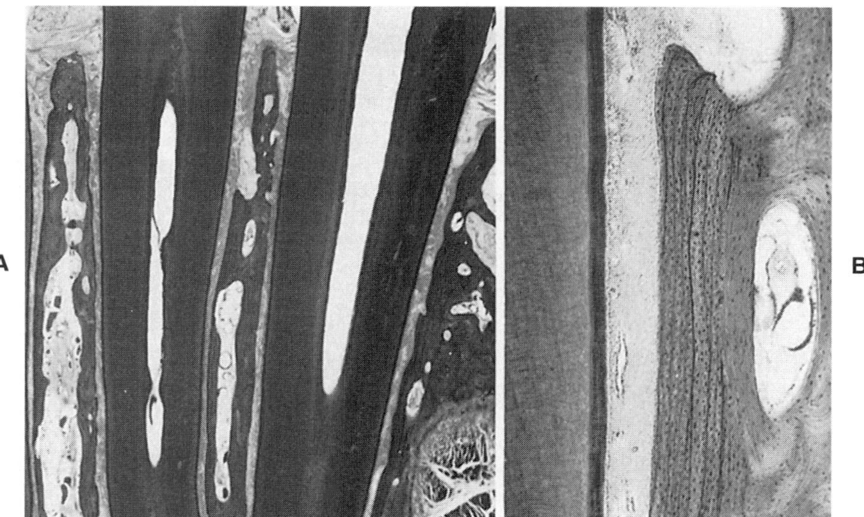

Fig. 2-32 Bone response to physiologic mesial migration. **A,** Interdental septa between the canine *(left)* and first and second premolars. **B,** Interdental septum between the first and second premolars, showing lamellae of newly apposed bone opposite the distal of the first premolar *(left)* and resorption opposite the mesial of the second premolar *(right).*

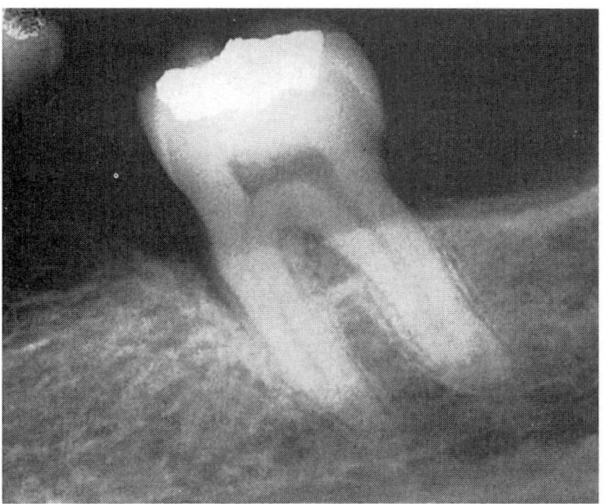

Fig. 2-33 Bony trabeculae realigned perpendicular to the mesial root of tilted molar.

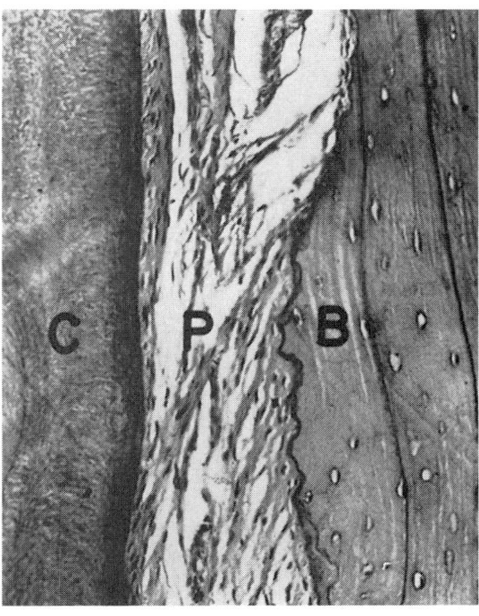

Fig. 2-34 Atrophic periodontal ligament *(P)* of a tooth devoid of function. Note the scalloped edge of the alveolar bone *(B),* indicating that resorption has occurred. *C,* Cementum.

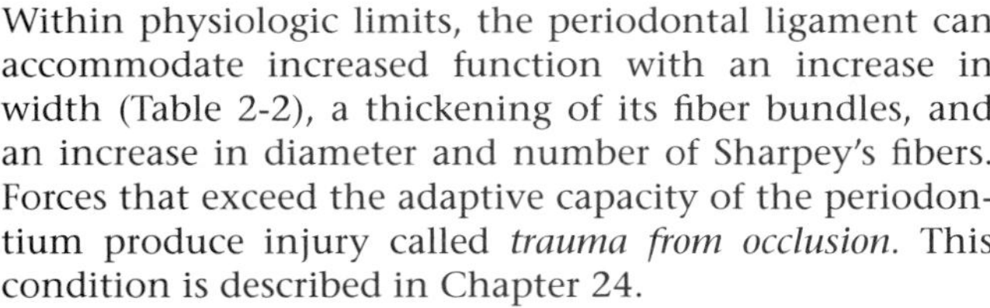

Within physiologic limits, the periodontal ligament can accommodate increased function with an increase in width (Table 2-2), a thickening of its fiber bundles, and an increase in diameter and number of Sharpey's fibers. Forces that exceed the adaptive capacity of the periodontium produce injury called *trauma from occlusion.* This condition is described in Chapter 24.

When occlusal forces are reduced, the number and thickness of the trabeculae are reduced.[28] The periodontal ligament also atrophies, appearing thinned, and the fibers are reduced in number and density, disoriented,[2,90] and ultimately arranged parallel to the root surface (Fig. 2-34). This is termed *disuse* or *afunctional atrophy.* In this condition, the cementum is either unaffected[28] or thickened and the distance from the cementoenamel junction to the alveolar crest is increased.[86]

VASCULARIZATION OF THE SUPPORTING STRUCTURES

The blood supply to the supporting structures of the tooth is derived from the inferior and superior alveolar arteries to the mandible and maxilla, respectively, and

TABLE 2-2

Comparison of Periodontal Width of Functioning and Functionless Teeth in a 38-Year-Old Man

	Average Width of Periodontal Space at Entrance of Alveolus (mm)	Average Width of Periodontal Space at Middle of Alveolus (mm)	Average Width of Periodontal Space at Fundus of Alveolus (mm)
Heavy Function: Left upper 2nd bicuspid	0.35	0.28	0.30
Light Function: Left lower 1st bicuspid	0.14	0.10	0.12
Functionless: Left upper 3rd molar	0.10	0.06	0.06

Modified from Kronfeld R: Histologic study of the influence of function on the human periodontal membrane. J Am Dent Assoc 1931; 18:1242.

reaches the periodontal ligament from three sources: apical vessels, penetrating vessels from the alveolar bone, and anastomosing vessels from the gingiva.[27] The branches of the apical vessels supply the apical region of the periodontal ligament before the vessels enter the dental pulp. The transalveolar vessels are branches of the intraseptal vessels that perforate the lamina dura and enter the ligament. The intraseptal vessels continue to vascularize the gingiva; these gingival vessels in turn anastomose with the periodontal ligament vessels of the cervical region.[35]

The vessels within the periodontal ligament are contained in interstitial spaces of loose connective tissue between the principal fibers and are connected in a netlike plexus that runs longitudinally and closer to the bone than the cementum[23] (Figs. 2-35 and 2-36). The blood supply increases from the incisors to the molars; is greatest in the gingival third of single-rooted teeth, less in the apical third, and least in the middle; is equal in the apical and middle thirds of multirooted teeth; is slightly greater on the mesial and distal surfaces than on the facial and lingual; and is greater on the mesial surfaces of mandibular molars than on the distal.[15]

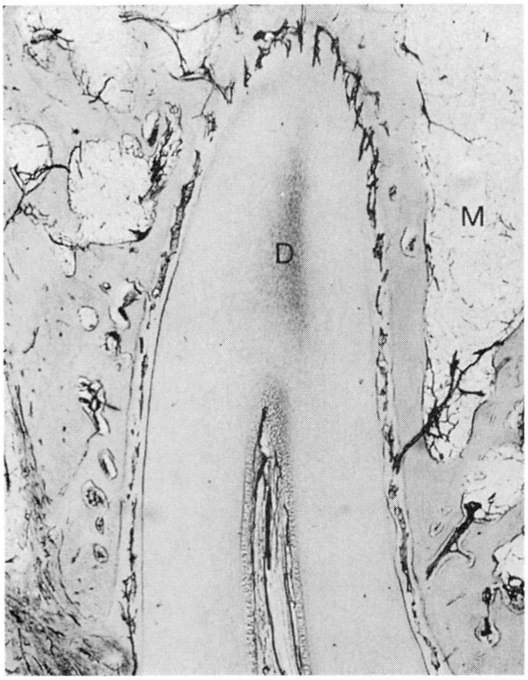

Fig. 2-35 Vascular supply of monkey periodontium (perfused with India ink). Note the longitudinal vessels in the periodontal ligament and alveolar arteries passing through channels between the bone marrow *(M)* and periodontal ligament. *D,* Dentin. (Courtesy Sol Bernick, Los Angeles, Calif.)

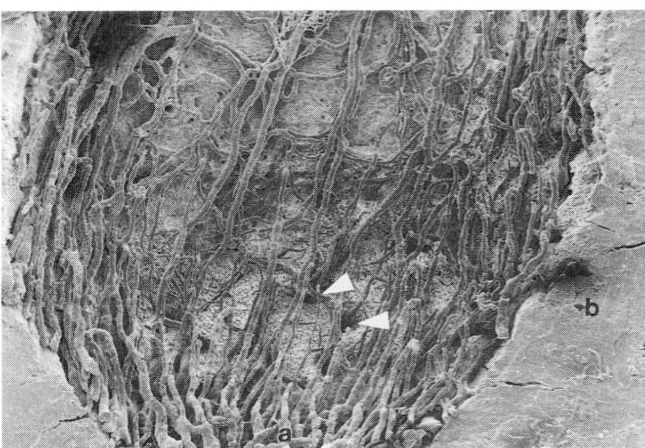

Fig. 2-36 Vascular supply to the periodontal ligament in rat molar, as viewed by scanning electron microscopy after perfusion with plastic and tissue corrosion. Middle and apical areas of the periodontal ligament are shown with longitudinal blood vessels from apex *(below)* to gingiva *(above),* perforating vessels entering the bone *(b),* and many transverse connections *(arrowheads).* Apical vessels *(a)* form a cap that connects with the pulpal vessels. (Courtesy NJ Selliseth and K Selvig, University of Bergen, Norway.)

The vascular supply to the bone enters the interdental septa through nutrient canals together with veins, nerves, and lymphatics. Dental arterioles, which also branch off the alveolar arteries, send tributaries through the periodontal ligament, and some small branches enter the marrow spaces of the bone through the perforations in the cribriform plate. Small vessels emanating from the facial and lingual compact bone also enter the marrow and spongy bone.

The **venous drainage** of the periodontal ligament accompanies the arterial supply. Venules receive the blood through the abundant capillary network; also, arteriovenous anastomoses bypass the capillaries. These are more frequent in apical and interradicular regions, and their significance is unknown.

Lymphatics supplement the venous drainage system. Those draining the region just beneath the junctional epithelium pass into the periodontal ligament and accompany the blood vessels into the periapical region.[20] From there they pass through the alveolar bone to the inferior dental canal in the mandible or the infraorbital canal in the maxilla and then to the submaxillary lymph nodes.

REFERENCES

1. Agnew RG, Fong CC: Histologic studies on experimental transplantation of teeth. Oral Surg 1956; 9:18.
2. Anneroth G, Ericsson SG: An experimental histological study of monkey teeth without antagonist. Odont Revy 1967; 18:345.
3. Avery JK, Rapp R: Pain conduction in human dental tissues. Dent Clin North Am July 1959, p. 489.
4. Bauer WH: Effect of a faultily constructed partial denture on a tooth and its supporting tissue, with special reference to formation of fibrocartilage in the periodontal membrane as a result of disturbed healing caused by abnormal stresses. Am J Orthod Oral Surg 1941; 27:640.
5. Baumhammers A, Stallard R: S35 sulfate utilization and turnover by connective tissues of the periodontium. J Periodont Res 1968; 3:187.
6. Becks H: Root resorptions and their relation to pathologic bone formation. Int J Orthod Oral Surg 1936; 22:445.
7. Beertsen W, McCullough CAG, Sodek J: The periodontal ligament: a unique, multifunctional connective tissue. Periodontology 2000 1997; 13:20.
8. Berkovitz BKB, Shore RC: Cells of the periodontal ligament. In: Berkovitz BKB, Moxham BJ, Newman HE (eds): The Periodontal Ligament in Health and Disease. London, Pergamon Press, 1982.
9. Berkovitz BKB: The structure of the periodontal ligament: an update. Eur J Orthod 1990; 12:51.
10. Bernard GW, Ko JS: Osteoclast formation *in vitro* from bone marrow mononuclear cells in osteoclast-free bone. Amer J Anat 1981; 161:415.
11. Bernard GW, Marvaso V: Matrix vesicles as an assay for primary tissue calcification *in vivo* and *in vitro*. In: Ascenzi A, Bonucci B, DeBernard B (eds): Matrix Vesicles, Proceedings of the 3rd International Conference on Matrix Vesicles. Milano, Wichtig, 1981.
12. Bernard GW, Pease DC: An electron microscopic study of initial intramembranous osteogenesis. Amer J Anat 1969; 125:271.
13. Bernick S: Innervation of the teeth and periodontium. Dent Clin North Am 1959; 503.
14. Bien SM: Hydrodynamic damping of tooth movement. J Dent Res 1966; 45:907.
15. Birn H: The vascular supply of the periodontal membrane. J Periodont Res 1966; 1:51.
16. Blair HC, Teitelbaum SC, Ghiselli R, et al: Osteoclastic bone resorption by a polarized vacuolar proton pump. Science 1989; 245:855.
17. Blayney JR, Wasserman F, Groetzinger G, et al: Further studies on mineral metabolism of human teeth by the use of radioactive isotopes. J Dent Res 29:559, 1941.
18. Bosshardt AL, Schroeder HE: Cementogenesis reviewed: a comparison between human premolars and rodent molars. Anat Rec 1996; 245:267.
19. Box HK: Bone resorption in red marrow hyperplasia in human jaws. Can Dent Res Found 1936; Bulletin 21.
20. Box KF: Evidence of lymphatics in the periodontium. J Can Dent Assoc 1949; 15:8.
21. Boyle PE: Tooth suspension. A comparative study of the paradental tissues of man and of the guinea pig. J Dent Res 1938; 17:37.
22. Carneiro J, Fava de Moraes F: Radioautographic visualization of collagen metabolism in the periodontal tissues of the mouse. Arch Oral Biol 1955; 10:833.
23. Carranza FA Jr, Itoiz ME, Cabrini RL, et al: A study of periodontal vascularization in different laboratory animals. J Periodont Res 1966; 1:120.
24. Carranza FA Sr, Carranza FA Jr: The management of the alveolar bone in the treatment of the periodontal pocket. J Periodontol 1956; 27:29.
25. Chambers TJ: The cellular basis of bone resorption. Clin Orthop 1980; 251:283.
26. Ciancio SC, Neiders ME, Hazen SP: The principal fibers of the periodontal ligament. Periodontics 1967; 5:76.
27. Cohen L: Further studies into the vascular architecture of the mandible. J Dent Res 1960; 39:936.
28. Cohn SA: Disease atrophy of the periodontium in mice. Arch Oral Biol 1965; 10:909.
29. Coolidge ED: The thickness of the human periodontal membrane. J Am Dent Assoc 1937; 24:1260.
30. Dastmalchi R, Polson A, Bouwsma O, et al: Cementum thickness and mesial drift. J Clin Periodontol 1990; 17:709.
31. Davies WI, Picton DC: Dimensional changes in the periodontal membrane of monkey's teeth with horizontal thrusts. J Dent Res 1967; 46:114.
32. Eastoe JE: The organic matrix of bone. In: Bourne GH (ed): The Biochemistry and Physiology of Bone. New York, Academic Press, 1956.
33. El Mostehy MR, Stallard RE: Intermediate cementum. J Periodont Res 1968; 3:24.
34. Elliot JR, Bowers GM: Alveolar dehiscence and fenestration. Periodontics 1963; 1:245.
35. Folke LEA, Stallard RE: Periodontal microcirculation as revealed by plastic microspheres. J Periodont Res 1967; 2:53.
36. Freeman E: The periodontium. In: Ten Cate R (ed): Oral Histology, ed 4. St Louis, Mosby, 1994.
37. Fullmer HM, Sheetz JH, Narkates AJ: Oxytalan connective tissue fibers: a review. J Oral Pathol 1974; 3:291.
38. Gargiulo AW, Wentz FM, Orban B: Dimensions and relations of the dentogingival junction in humans. J Periodontol 1961; 32:261.
39. Gibson W, Fullmer H: Histochemistry of the periodontal ligament. I. The dehydrogenases. Periodontics 1966; 4:63.
40. Gibson W, Fullmer H: Histochemistry of the periodontal ligament. II. The phosphatases. Periodontics 1967; 5:226.
41. Gibson W, Fullmer H: Histochemistry of the periodontal ligament. III. The esterases. Periodontics 1968; 6:71.

42. Gillespie BR, Chasens AF, Brownstein CN, et al: The relationship between the mobility of human teeth and their supracrestal fiber support. J Periodontol 1979; 50:120.
43. Glickman I, Roeber FW, Brion M, et al: Photoelastic analysis of internal stresses in the periodontium created by occlusal forces. J Periodontol 1970; 41:30.
44. Glimcher MJ, Friberg U, Levine P: The identification and characterization of a calcified layer of coronal cementum in erupted bovine teeth. J Ultrastruct Res 1964; 10:76.
45. Glimcher MJ: The nature of the mineral component of bone and the mechanism of calcification. In: Avioli LV, Krane SM (eds): Metabolic Bone Disease and Clinical Related Disorders. Philadelphia, WB Saunders, 1990.
46. Goggins JF: The distribution of oxytalan connective tissue fibers in periodontal ligaments of deciduous teeth. Periodontics 1966; 4:182.
47. Gottlieb B: Biology of the cementum. J Periodontol 1942; 17:7.
48. Grant D, Bernick S: A possible continuity between epithelial rests and epithelial attachment in miniature swine. J Periodontol 1969; 40:87.
49. Grant D, Bernick S: The formation of the periodontal ligament. J Periodontol 1972; 43:17.
50. Hagel-Bradway S, Dziak R: Regulation of bone cell metabolism. J Oral Pathol Med 1989; 18:344.
51. Hassell TM, Stanek EJ: Evidence that healthy human gingiva contains functionally heterogenous fibroblast subpopulations. Arch Oral Biol 1983; 28:617.
52. Heins PJ, Wieder SM: A histologic study of the width and nature of interradicular spaces of human adult premolars and molars. J Dent Res 1986; 65:948.
53. Hemley S: The incidence of root resorption of vital permanent teeth. J Dent Res 1941; 20:133.
54. Henry JL, Weinmann JP: The pattern of resorption and repair of human cementum. J Am Dent Assoc 1951; 42:271.
55. Hindle MC: Quantitative differences in periodontal membrane fibers. J Dent Res 1964; 43:953.
56. Hirschfeld I: A study of skulls in the American Museum of Natural History in relation to periodontal disease. J Dent Res 1923; 5:241.
57. Inoue M, Akiyoshi M: Histologic investigation on Sharpey's fibers in cementum of teeth in abnormal function. J Dent Res 1962; 41:503.
58. Ishikawa J, Yamamoto H, Ito K, et al: Microradiographic study of cementum and alveolar bone. J Dent Res 1964; 43:936.
59. Johnson RB, Pylypas SP: A reevaluation of the distribution of the elastic meshwork within the periodontal ligament of the mouse. J Periodont Res 1992; 27:239.
60. Jones ML, Alfred MJ, Hardy P: Tooth resorption in the two-stage transplantation technique. Br J Orthodont 1983; 10:157.
61. Jones SJ, Boyde A: A study of human root cementum surfaces as prepared for and examined in the scanning electron microscope. Z Zellforsch 1972; 130:318.
62. Jones MR, Simonton FV: Mineral metabolism in relation to alveolar atrophy in dogs. J Am Dent Assoc 1928; 15:881.
63. Junqueira LC, Carneiro J, Kelley RO: Basic Histology, ed 6. Norwalk, CT, Appleton & Lange, 1989.
64. Ko JS, Bernard GW: Osteoclast formation in vitro from bone marrow mononuclear cells in osteoclast-free bone. Am J Anat 1981; 161:415.
65. Kronfeld R: Biology of the cementum. J Am Dent Assoc 1938; 25:1451.
66. Kronfeld R: Histologic study of the influence of function on the human periodontal membrane. J Am Dent Assoc 1931; 18:1242.
67. Kronfeld R: Histopathology of the Teeth and Their Surrounding Structures. Lea & Febiger, Philadelphia, 1933.
68. Lester K: The incorporation of epithelial cells by cementum. J Ultrastruct Res 1969; 27:63.
69. Listgarten MA: A light and electron microscopic study of coronal cementogenesis. Arch Oral Biol 1968; 13:93.
70. Lopez Otero R, Parodi RJ, Ubios AM, et al: Histologic and histometric study of bone resorption after tooth movement in rats. J Periodont Res 1973; 8:327.
71. Maeda T, Kannari K, Sato O, et al: Nerve terminals in human periodontal ligament as demonstrated by immunohistochemistry for neurofilament protein (NFP) and S-100 protein. Arch Histol Cytol 1990; 53:259.
72. Marks CS Jr: The origin of osteoclasts: Evidence, clinical implications and investigative challenges of an extraskeletal source. J Pathol 1983; 12:226.
73. MacNeil RL, Thomas HF: Development of the murine periodontium. II. Role of the epithelial root sheath in formation of the periodontal membrane. J Periodontol 1993; 64:285.
74. Melcher AH: Remodeling of the periodontal ligament during eruption of the rat incisor. Arch Oral Biol 1967; 12:1649.
75. Mikola OJ, Bauer WH: Cementicles and fragments of cementum in the periodontal membrane. Oral Surg 1949; 2:1063.
76. Miller EJ: A review of biochemical studies on the genetically distinct collagens of the skeletal system. Clin Orthop 1973; 92:260.
77. Mühlemann HR, Zander HA, Halberg F: Mitotic activity in the periodontal tissues of the rat molar. J Dent Res 1954; 33:459.
78. Mühlemann HR: The determination of tooth rotation centers. Oral Surg 1954; 7:392.
79. Nihei I: A study of the hardness of human teeth. J Osaka Univ Dent Soc 1959; 4:1.
80. Noyes FB, Schour I, Noyes HJ: A Textbook of Dental Histology and Embryology, ed 5. Philadelphia, Lea & Febiger, 1938.
81. Oppenheim A: Human tissue response to orthodontic intervention of short and long duration. Am J Orthodont Oral Surg 1942; 28:263.
82. Orban B: Tissue changes in traumatic occlusion. J Am Dent Assoc 1928; 15:2090.
83. Parfitt GJ: An investigation of the normal variations in alveolar bone trabeculation. Oral Surg 1962; 15:1453.
84. Parodi RJ, Ubios AM, Mayo J, et al: Total body irradiation effects on the bone resorption mechanism in rats subjected to orthodontic movement. J Oral Pathol 1973; 2:1.
85. Picton DC, Davies WI: Dimensional changes in the periodontal membrane of monkeys (Macaca irus) due to horizontal thrusts applied to the teeth. Arch Oral Biol 1967; 12:1635.
86. Pihlstrom BL, Ramfjord SP: Periodontal effects of nonfunction in monkeys. J Periodontol 1971; 42:748.
87. Raisz LG, Rodan GA: Cellular basis for bone turnover. In: Avioli LV, Krane SM (eds): Metabolic Bone Disease and Clinical Related Disorders. Philadelphia, WB Saunders, 1990.
88. Reeve CM, Wentz FJ: The prevalence, morphology and distribution of epithelial rests in the human periodontal ligament. Oral Surg 1962; 15:785.
89. Riffle AB: Cementoenamel junction. J Periodontol 1952; 23:41.
90. Rippin JW: Collagen turnover in the periodontal ligament under normal and altered functional forces. II. Adult rat molars. J Periodont Res 1978; 13:149.
91. Ritchey B, Orban B: The crests of the interdental alveolar septa. J Periodontol 1953; 24:75.

92. Roberts WE, Chamberlain JG: Scanning electron microscopy of the cellular elements of rat periodontal ligament. Arch Oral Biol 1978; 23:587.
93. Romaniuk K: Some observations of the fine structure of human cementum. J Dent Res 1967; 46:152.
94. Romanos GE, Schroter-Kermani C, Bernimoulin J-P: Das Kollagen als Basis-element des Parodonts: Immunohistochemische Aspekte bein Menschen und bei Tieren. Parodontologie 1991; 1:47.
95. Romanos GE, Schroter-Kermani C, Hinz N, et al: Immunohistochemical distribution of the collagen types IV, V and VI and glycoprotein laminin in the healthy rat, marmoset (Callithrix jacchus) and human gingiva. Matrix 1991; 11:125.
96. Romanos GE, Schroter-Kermani C, Hinz N, et al: Immunohistochemical localization of collagenous components in healthy periodontal tissues of the rat and marmoset (Callithrix jacchus). I. Distribution of collagens type I and III. J Periodont Res 1992; 27:101.
97. Rudolph CE: An evaluation of root resorption occurring during orthodontic therapy. J Dent Res 1940; 19:367.
98. Rushton MA: Dental tissues in osteitis deformans. Guys Hosp Rep 1938; 88:163.
99. Saffar J-L, Lasfargues J-J, Cherruau M: Alveolar bone and the alveolar process: the socket that is never stable. Periodontology 2000 1997; 13:76.
100. Schroeder HE: The Periodontium. Berlin, Springer-Verlag, 1986.
101. Sculean A, Karring T, Theilade J, et al: The regenerative potential of oxytalan fibers. J Clin Periodontol 1997; 24:932.
102. Selvig KA: The fine structure of human cementum. Acta Odontol Scand 1965; 23:423.
103. Sequeira P, Domenicucci C, Wasi S, et al: Specific immunohistochemical localization of osteonectin and collagen types I and III in fetal and adult porcine dental tissues. J Histochem Cytochem 1985; 33:531.
104. Shackleford JM: The indifferent fiber plexus and its relationship to principal fibers of the periodontium. Am J Anat 1971; 131:427.
105. Sicher H, DuBrul EL: Oral Anatomy, ed 6. St Louis, Mosby, 1975.
106. Simpson HE: The degeneration of the rests of Malassez with age as observed by the apoxestic technique. J Periodontol 1965; 36:288.
107. Sodek J: A comparison of the rates of synthesis and turnover of collagen and non-collagen proteins in adult rat periodontal tissues and skin using a microassay. Arch Oral Biol 1977; 22:655.
108. Ten Cate AR, Deporter DA: The degradative role of the fibroblast in the remodeling and turnover of collagen in soft connective tissue. Anat Rec 1975; 182:1.
109. Ten Cate AR, Mills C, Solomon G: The development of the periodontium. A transplantation and autoradiographic study. Anat Rec 1971; 170:365.
110. Ten Cate AR: Formation of supporting bone in association with periodontal ligament organization in the mouse. Arch Oral Biol 1975; 20:137.
111. Ten Cate AR: The development of the periodontium. In: Melcher AH, Bowen WH (eds): Biology of the Periodontium. New York, Academic Press, 1969.
112. Ten Cate AR: The histochemical demonstration of specific oxidative enzymes and glycogen in the epithelial cell of Malassez. Arch Oral Biol 1965; 10:207.
113. Ten Cate AR: Hard tissue formation and destruction. In: Ten Cate AR (ed): Oral Histology—Development, Structure, and Function, ed 4. St Louis, Mosby, 1994.
114. Thoma KH, Sosman MC, Bennett GA: An unusual case of hereditary fibrous osteodystrophy (fragilitas ossium) with replacement of dentine by osteocementum. Am J Orthodont Oral Surg 1943; 29:1.
115. Thomas HE: Root formation. Int J Develop Biol 1995; 39:231.
116. Trowbridge HO, Shibata F: Mitotic activity in epithelial rests of Malassez. Periodontics 1967; 5:109.
117. Ubios AM, Cabrini RL: Tritiated thymidine uptake in periodontal tissues subjected to orthodontic movement. J Dent Res 1971; 50:1160.
118. Vaes G: Cellular biology and biochemical mechanism of bone resorption. Clin Orthop 1988; 231:239.
119. Valderhaug JP, Nylen MU: Function of epithelial rests as suggested by their ultrastructure. J Periodont Res 1966; 1:69.
120. Valderhaug JP, Zander H: Relationship of epithelial rests of Malassez to other periodontal structures. Periodontics 1967; 5:254.
121. Vilmarin H: Characteristics of growing bone surfaces. Scand J Dent Res 1979; 87:65.
122. Warren EB, Hansen NM, Swartz ML, et al: Effects of periodontal disease and of calculus solvents on microhardness of cementum. J Periodontol 1964; 35:505.
123. Weinmann JP, Sicher H: Bone and Bones. Fundamentals of Bone Biology, ed 2. St Louis, Mosby, 1955.
124. Yamamoto H, et al: Microradiographic and histopathological study of the cementum. Bull Tokyo Dent Univ 1962; 9:141.
125. Yamamoto T, Wakita M: Bundle formation of principal fibers in rat molars. J Periodont Res 1992; 27:20.
126. Zander HA, Hurzeler B: Continuous cementum apposition. J Dent Res 1958; 37:1035.
127. Zipkin J: The inorganic composition of bones and teeth. In: Schraer H (ed): Biological Calcification. New York, Appleton-Century-Crofts, 1970.
128. Zwarych PD, Quigley MB: The intermediate plexus of the periodontal ligament: History and further observations. J Dent Res 1965; 44:383.

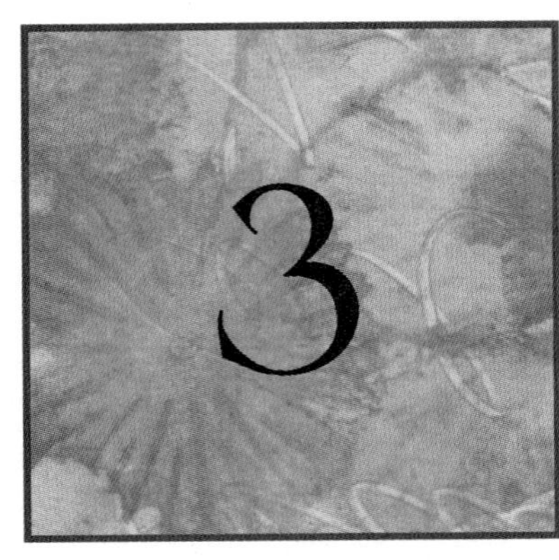

CHAPTER

Aging and the Periodontium

Ian Needleman

CHAPTER OUTLINE

The successes of both increased health awareness and preventive dentistry have led to decreasing tooth loss for all age groups. The effects of this shift in tooth retention on the periodontal needs of a population with increased life expectancy and oral health expectations need to be considered carefully. It is important not only to review aging effects in isolation but also from the perspectives of their clinical significance to the disease process and their possible effects on treatment outcomes.

The evidence base is not without problems, many of which make it difficult to draw conclusions on the effects of aging. Some of these problems include inconsistency in the definition of a true "aged" group, inadequate exclusion of adults with systemic diseases that can modify study findings, and attempts to extrapolate results from animal research. For the purposes of this chapter, the effects of aging will be limited to a narrow review of possible biologic and microbiologic changes.* The reader should be fully aware that this excludes many important age-associated phenomena, including the reduction in an individual's cognitive or motor function skills, which may have a direct impact on periodontal management (see Chapter 39).

* For further reading on the effects of aging on the dental and periodontal patient, the reader should consult P. Holm-Pederson's *Textbook of Geriatric Dentistry,* ed 2; and Ellen EP (ed): Periodontal disease among older adults, Periodontology 2000 1998; 16.

EFFECTS OF AGING ON THE PERIODONTIUM

Gingival Epithelium

Thinning and decreased keratinization of the gingival epithelium have been reported with age.[31] The significance of these findings could mean an increase in epithelial permeability to bacterial antigens, a decreased resistance to functional trauma, or both, which might influence long-term periodontal outcomes. However, other studies have found no age-related differences in the gingival epithelium of humans or dogs.[7,16] Other reported changes with aging include the flattening of rete pegs and altered cell density. Conflicting data regarding surgical regeneration times for gingival epithelium have been ascribed to problems in research methodology.[33]

The effect of aging on the location of the junctional epithelium has been the subject of much speculation.

Some reports show migration of the junctional epithelium from its position in healthy individuals (i.e., on enamel) to a more apical position on the root surface with accompanying gingival recession.[7] However, in other animal studies, no apical migration has been noted.[19] With continuing gingival recession, the width of the attached gingiva would be expected to decrease with age, but the opposite appears to be true.[2,3] Alternatively, the migration of the junctional epithelium to the root surface could be caused by the tooth erupting through the gingiva in an attempt to maintain occlusal contact with its opposing tooth (passive eruption) as a result of tooth surface loss from attrition (Fig. 3-1). The consensus is that gingival recession is not an inevitable physiologic process of aging but is explained by cumulative effects of inflammation or trauma on the periodontium[6,7] (see later discussion) (Fig. 3-2).

Gingival Connective Tissue

Increasing age results in coarser and more dense gingival connective tissues.[36] Qualitative and quantitative changes to collagen have been reported. These include an increased rate of conversion of soluble to insoluble collagen, increased mechanical strength, and increased denaturing temperature. These results indicate increased collagen stabilization caused by changes in the macromolecular conformation.[23] Not surprisingly, a greater collagen content has been found in the gingiva of older animals despite a lower rate of collagen synthesis decreasing with age.[7,23,33]

Periodontal Ligament

Changes in the periodontal ligament that have been reported with aging include decreased numbers of fibroblasts and a more irregular structure, paralleling the changes in the gingival connective tissues.[7,23,33] Other findings include decreased organic matrix production and epithelial cell rests and increased amounts of elastic fiber.[33] Conflicting results have been reported for changes in the width of periodontal ligament in human and animal models. Although true variation might exist, this finding probably reflects the functional status of the teeth in the studies because the width of the space will decrease if the tooth is unopposed (hypofunction) or will increase with excessive occlusal loading.[23,33] Both scenarios might be anticipated as a result of tooth loss in this population. These effects also might explain the variability in studies reporting qualitative changes within the periodontal ligament.

Cementum

Some consensus regarding aging effects on cementum exists. An increase in cemental width is a common finding; this increase may be 5 to 10 times with increasing age.[7] This finding is not surprising because deposition continues after tooth eruption. The increase in width is greater apically and lingually.[33] Although cementum has limited capacity for remodeling, an accumulation of resorption bays explains the finding of increasing surface irregularity.[13]

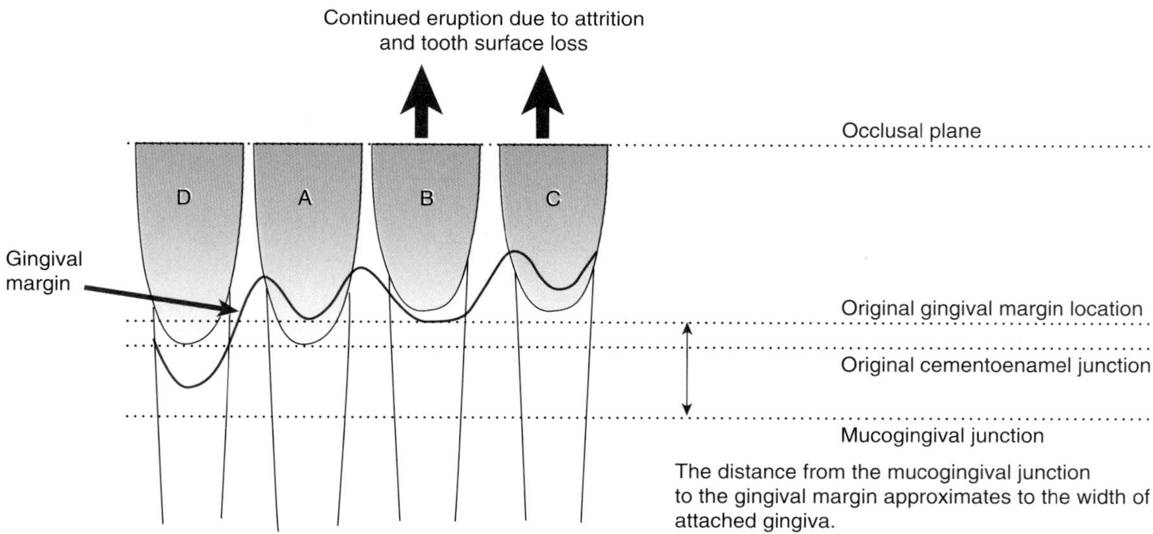

Fig. 3-1 Diagram showing the relationship of the gingival margin with the crown and root surface. **A,** Normal relationship with the gingival margin 1 to 2 mm above the cementoenamel junction. **B,** Wear of the incisal edge and continued tooth eruption. The gingival margin remains in the same position as in **A,** therefore the root surface is exposed and clinical recession is evident. The width of the attached gingiva has not changed. **C,** Wear of the incisal edge and continued tooth eruption. The gingival margin has moved with the tooth, therefore the entire dentogingival complex has moved coronally with a resulting increase in the width of the attached gingiva. **D,** No wear of incisal edge is evident. Gingiva has moved apically, and clinical recession is evident. The width of attached gingiva is reduced.

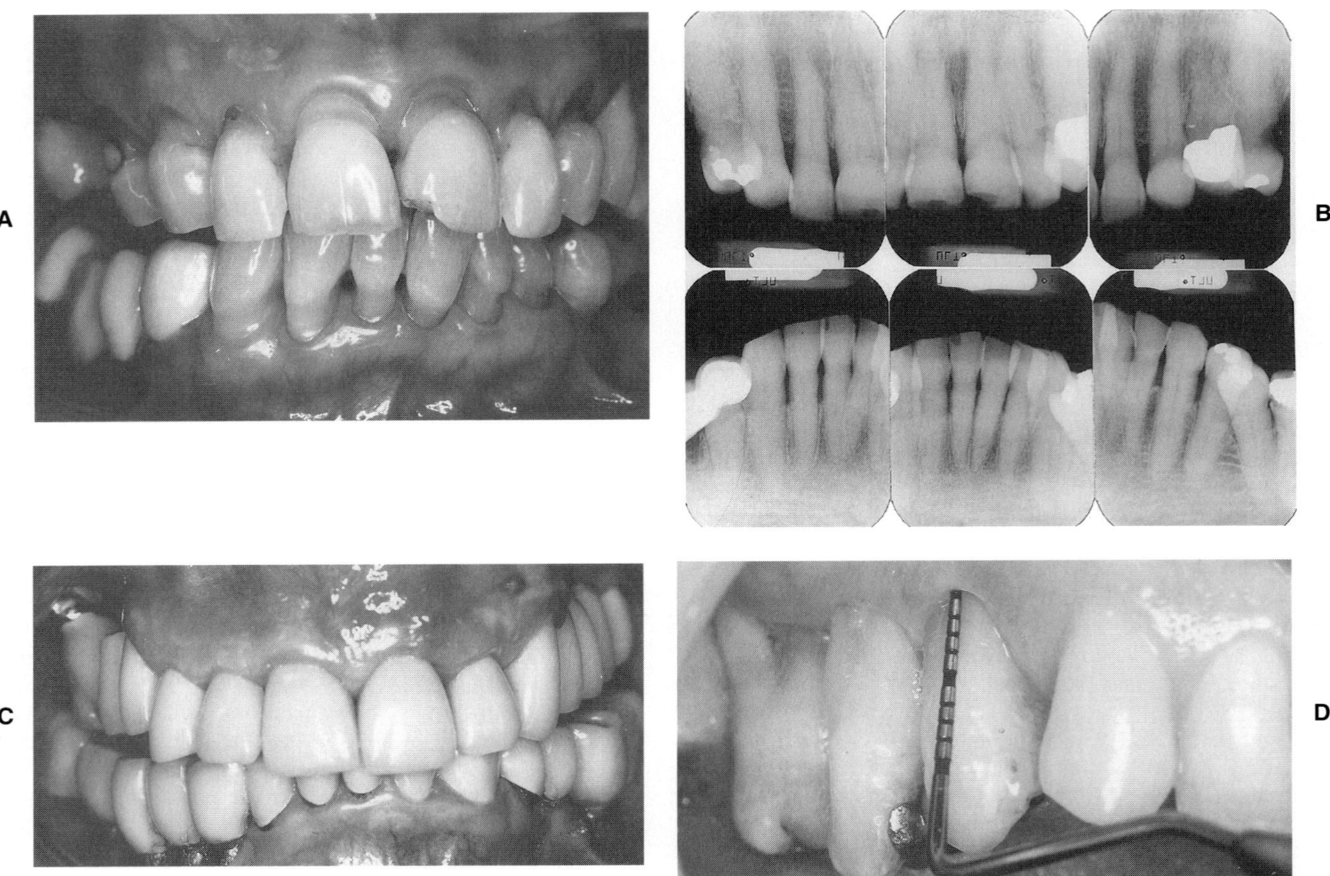

Fig. 3-2 Three scenarios illustrating the variation of the position of the gingival margin with age. **A,** Overeruption with recession in older individual (68-year-old woman) with generalized recession and previous (treated) history of periodontitis. Note some overeruption of lower anterior teeth and wear of teeth related to oral hygiene measures. **B,** Radiographs of the patient in **A**. **C,** Overeruption without recession in an older individual (72-year-old woman) with no periodontitis but marked lower incisor tooth wear and overeruption. Note how the gingival margin has migrated coronally with the erupting teeth. **D,** Extensive recession in young individual (32-year-old man) with marked recession and no history of periodontitis. The recession has resulted from a combination of anatomically thin tissues and toothbrush-related trauma.

Alveolar Bone

Reports of morphologic changes in alveolar bone mirror age-related changes in other bony sites. Specific to the periodontium are findings of a more irregular periodontal surface of bone and less regular insertion of collagen fibers.[33] Although age is a risk factor for the bone mass reductions in osteoporosis, it is not causative and therefore should be distinguished from physiologic aging processes.[15] Overriding the diverse observations of bony changes with age is the important finding that the healing rate of bone in extraction sockets appears to be unaffected by increasing age.[4] Indeed, the success of osseointegrated dental implants, which relies on intact bone healing responses, does not appear to be age related.[8] However, balancing this view is the recent observation that bone graft preparations (decalcified freeze-dried bone) from donors more than 50 years old possessed significantly less osteogenic potential than graft material from younger donors.[30] The possible significance of this phenomenon on normal healing responses needs to be investigated.

Bacterial Plaque

Dentogingival plaque accumulation has been suggested to increase with age.[14] This might be explained by the increase in hard tissue surface area as a result of gingival recession and the surface characteristics of the exposed root surface as a substrate for plaque formation compared with enamel. Other studies have shown no difference in plaque quantity with age. This contradiction might reflect the different age ranges of experimental groups as variable degrees of gingival recession and root surface exposure. For supragingival plaque, no real qualitative differences have been shown for plaque composition.[14] For subgingival plaque, one study has shown similar subgingival flora to a normal flora, whereas another study reported increased numbers of enteric rods and pseudomonads in older adults.[27,32] Mombelli suggests caution in the interpretation of this finding because of increased oral carriage of these species among older adults.[26] It has been speculated that a shift occurs in the importance of certain periodontal pathogens with age, specifically including an increased role for *Porphyromonas gingivalis* and a decreased role for *Actinobacillus actinomycetemcomitans.* However, differentiating true age effects from the changes in ecological determinants for periodontal bacteria will be difficult. This topic is considered in more detail in a recent review.[26]

Immune Responses

Recent advances in the study of the effects of aging on the immune response (immunosenescence) have altered the understanding of this phenomenon. In particular, more recent studies have set tighter controls on excluding individuals with systemic conditions known to affect the immune response. As a result, age has been recognized as having much less effect in altering the host response than previously thought.[17,24] Differences between young and older individuals can be demonstrated for T and B cells, cytokines, and natural killer cells but not for polymorphonuclear cells and macrophage activity. McArthur concludes, "Measurement of indicators of immune and inflammatory competency suggested that, within the parameters tested, there was no evidence for age-related changes in host defenses correlating with periodontitis in an elderly (65 to 75 years) group of individuals, with and without disease."[24] Age-related differences in the inflammatory response in gingivitis have been clearly demonstrated and are discussed later in this textbook.

In summary, although many contradictions exist, a survey of the literature demonstrates that some age-related changes are evident in the periodontium and host response. Whether these changes are significant in altering the progression of periodontal diseases or the response of an older adult to periodontal treatment will be examined next.

EFFECTS OF AGING ON THE PROGRESSION OF PERIODONTAL DISEASES

In a classic experimental gingivitis study, subjects were rendered plaque free and inflammation free through frequent professional cleaning. Once this was achieved, the subjects abstained from oral hygiene measures for periods of 3 weeks to allow gingivitis to develop.[22] In this experimental model, a comparison of developing gingivitis between young and older individuals demonstrated a greater inflammatory response in older subjects, both in humans and dogs.[7,11,12,14] In the older age group (65 to 80 years), the findings included a greater size of infiltrated connective tissue, increased gingival crevicular fluid flow, and increased gingival index.[11,12] Other studies have not demonstrated differences between subjects; this may be related to smaller differences between the ages of the younger and older experimental groups.[37] Intriguingly, even at the baseline level of excellent gingival health before commencing plaque accumulation, differences may exist between groups, with older individuals demonstrating more inflammation.[11,12]

The phrase "getting long in the tooth" expresses a widespread belief that age is inevitably associated with an increased loss of connective tissue attachment. However, this observation might equally well reflect a cumulative exposure to a number of potentially destructive processes. These exposures might include plaque-associated periodontitis, chronic mechanical trauma from tooth brushing, and iatrogenic damage from unfavorable restorative dentistry or repeated scaling and root planing. The effects of these exposures act in one direction only (i.e., increased loss of attachment).[34]

In an attempt to differentiate the effects of age from these other processes, several studies have been designed to eliminate confounding issues and address more clearly the question of age as a risk factor for periodontitis. A *risk factor* is defined as an exposure or factor that increases the probability that the disease (periodontitis) will occur.[28] The conclusions from these studies are strikingly consistent and show that the effect of age is either nonexistent or provides a small and clinically insignificant increased risk of loss of periodontal support.[9,21,28,29] Indeed, in comparison with the odds ratio of 20.52 for poor oral hygiene status and periodontitis, the odds ratio for age was only 1.24.[1] Therefore age has been suggested to be not a true risk factor but a background or an associated factor for periodontitis.[28] In addition, the recent reports of a genetic basis for susceptibility to severe forms of periodontitis underline the overriding importance of plaque, smoking, and susceptibility in explaining most of the variation in periodontal disease severity between individuals.[18,25]

EFFECTS OF AGING ON THE RESPONSE TO TREATMENT OF THE PERIODONTIUM

The successful treatment of periodontitis requires both meticulous home-care plaque control by the patient and meticulous supragingival and subgingival debridement by the therapist.[10] Unfortunately, only a few studies have directly compared such an approach among patients of different age groups. The few studies that have done so clearly demonstrate that despite the histologic changes in the periodontium with aging, no differences in response to nonsurgical or surgical treatment have been shown for periodontitis.[5,20,35] However, if plaque control is not ideal, continued loss of attachment is inevitable.

A purely biologic or physiologic review indicates that the effects of aging on the structure of the periodontium, function of the immune response, and nature of either supragingival or subgingival plaque have a negligible impact on an individual's experience of periodontal diseases. Aging might affect other aspects of managing the periodontal diseases (see Chapter 39), and the resulting difficulties should not be underestimated.

REFERENCES

1. Abdellatif HM, Burt BA: An epidemiological investigation into the relative importance of age and oral hygiene status as determinants of periodontitis. J Dent Res 1987; 66:13.
2. Ainamo A, Ainamo J, Poikkeus R: Continuous widening of the band of attached gingiva from 23 to 65 years of age. J Periodontal Res 1981; 16:595.
3. Ainamo J, Talari A: The increase with age of the width of attached gingiva. J Periodontal Res 1976; 11:182.
4. Amler MH: Age factor in human alveolar bone repair. J Oral Impl 1993; 19:138.
5. Axelsson P, Lindhe J, Nystrom B: On the prevention of caries and periodontal disease. Results of a 15-year longitudinal study in adults. J Clin Periodontol 1991; 18:182.
6. Baker DL, Seymour GJ: The possible pathogenesis of gingival recession. A histological study of induced recession in the rat. J Clin Periodontol 1976; 3:208.
7. Berglundh T: Clinical and structural characteristics of periodontal tissues in young and old dogs. J Clin Periodontol 1991; 18:616.
8. Bryant SR, Zarb GA: Osseointegration of oral implants in older and younger adults. Int J Maxillofac Impl 1998; 13:492.
9. Burt BA: Periodontitis and aging: Reviewing recent evidence. JADA 1994; 125:273.
10. Cobb CM: Nonsurgical pocket therapy: mechanical. Ann Periodontol 1996; 1:443.
11. Fransson C, Berglundh T, Lindhe J: The effect of age on the development of gingivitis. J Clin Periodontol 1996; 23:379.
12. Fransson C, Mooney J, Kinane DF, et al: Differences in the inflammatory response in young and old human subjects during the course of experimental gingivitis. J Clin Periodontol 1999; 26:453.
13. Grant D, Bernick S: The periodontium of aging humans. J Periodontol 1972; 43:660.
14. Holm-Pedersen P, Agerbaek N, Theilade E: Experimental gingivitis in young and elderly individuals. J Clin Periodontol 1975; 2:14.
15. Jeffcoat MK: Osteoporosis: a possible modifying factor in oral bone loss. Ann Periodontol 1998; 3:312.
16. Karring T, Loe H: A computerized method for quantitative estimation of the epithelium-connective tissue interface applied to the gingiva of various age groups. Acta Odontol Scand 1973; 31:241.
17. Kay MMB: Immunology and aging. In: Holm-Pedersen P (ed): Textbook of Geriatric Dentistry, ed 2. Copenhagen, Munksgaard, 1996.
18. Kornman KS, Crane A, Wang HY, et al: The interleukin-1 genotype as a severity factor in adult periodontal disease. J Clin Periodontol 1997; 24:72.
19. Lindhe J, Hamp SE, Loe H: Plaque induced periodontal disease in beagle dogs. A 4-year clinical, roentgenographical and histometrical study. J Perio Res 1975; 10:243.
20. Lindhe J, Socransky S, Nyman S, et al: Effect of age on healing following periodontal therapy. J Clin Periodontol 1985; 12:774.
21. Locker D, Slade GD, Murray H: Epidemiology of periodontal disease among older adults: A review. Periodontol 2000 1999; 16:16.
22. Loe H, Theilade E, Jensen SB: Experimental gingivitis in man. J Periodontol 1965; 36:177.
23. Mackenzie IC, Holm-Pedersen P, Karring T: Age changes in the oral mucous membranes and periodontium. In: Holm-Pedersen P (ed): Textbook of Geriatric Dentistry, ed 2. Copenhagen, Munksgaard, 1996.
24. McArthur WP: Effect of aging on immunocompetent and inflammatory cells. Periodontol 2000 1999; 16:53.
25. McGuire MK, Nunn ME: Prognosis versus actual outcome. IV. The effectivenesss of clinical parameters and IL-1 genotype in accurately predicting prognoses and tooth survival. J Periodontol 1999; 70:49.
26. Mombelli A: Aging and the periodontal and periimplant microbiota. Periodontol 2000 1999; 16:44.
27. Newman MG, Grinenco V, Weiner M, et al: Predominant microbiota associated with periodontal health in the aged. J Periodontol 1978; 49:553.
28. Page RC, Beck JD: Risk assessment for periodontal diseases. Int Dent J 1997; 47:61.
29. Papapanou PN, Lindhe J, Sterrett JD, et al: Considerations on the contribution of ageing to loss of periodontal tissue support. J Clin Periodontol 1991; 18:611.
30. Schwartz Z, Somers A, Mellonig JT, et al: Ability of commercial demineralized freeze-dried bone allograft to induce new bone formation is dependent on donor age but not gender. J Periodontol 1998; 69:470.
31. Shklar G: The effects of aging upon oral mucosa. J Invest Dermatol 1966; 47:115.
32. Slots J, Feik D, Rams TE: Age and sex relationships of superinfecting microorganisms in periodontitis patients. Oral Microbiol Immunol 1990; 5:305.
33. van der Velden U: Effect of age on the periodontium. J Clin Periodontol 1984; 11:81.
34. Waerhaug J: Epidemiology of periodontal disease-review of the literature. In: Ramfjord SP, Kerr DA, Ash MM (eds): World Workshop in Periodontics. Ann Arbor, American Academy of Periodontology, 1966.
35. Wennstrom JL, Serino G, Lindhe J, et al: Periodontal conditions of adult regular dental care attendants. A 12-year longitudinal study. J Clin Periodontol 1993; 20:714.
36. Wentz FM, Maier AW, Orban B: Age changes and sex differences in the clinically "normal" gingiva. J Periodontol 1952; 23:13.
37. Winkel EG, Abbas F, der Van V, et al: Experimental gingivitis in relation to age in individuals not susceptible to periodontal destruction. J Clin Periodontol 1987; 14:499.

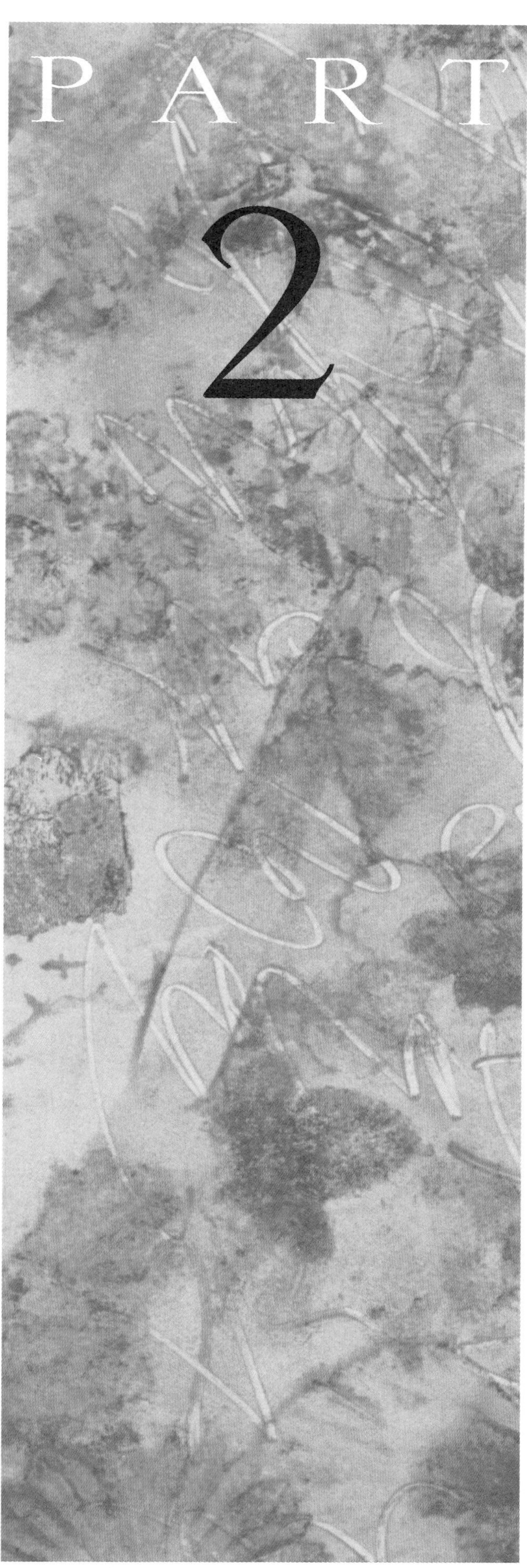

Classification and Epidemiology of Periodontal Diseases

Michael G. Newman

Disease classifications are useful for the purpose of diagnosis, prognosis, and treatment planning. Different classifications of periodontal diseases have been used over the years and have been replaced as new knowledge has improved our understanding of the etiology and pathology of the diseases of the periodontium.

Part 2 also includes information about the epidemiology of periodontal diseases that will aid the student and the clinician to analyze a disease and base their diagnostic and therapeutic decisions on its prevalence, incidence, and distribution in large populations or groups. Knowledge of the epidemiology of a disease improves our understanding and sharpens our decisions on individual cases.

Classification of Diseases and Conditions Affecting the Periodontium

M. John Novak

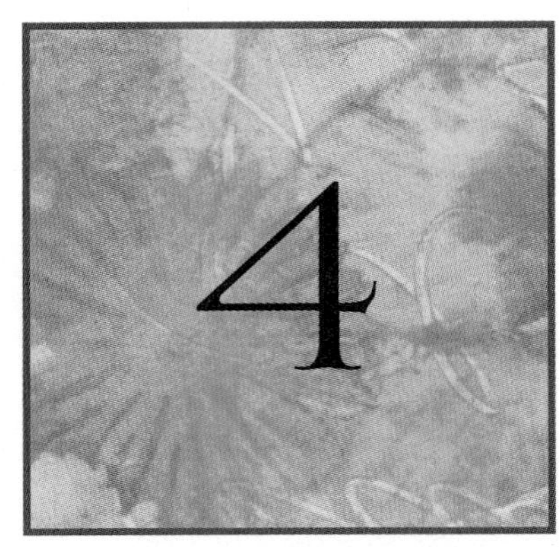

CHAPTER

CHAPTER OUTLINE

Our understanding of the etiology and pathogenesis of oral diseases and conditions is continually changing with increased scientific knowledge. In light of this, a classification can be most consistently defined by the differences in the clinical manifestations of diseases and conditions because they are clinically consistent and require little, if any, clarification by scientific laboratory testing. The classification presented in this chapter is based on the most recent, internationally accepted, consensus opinion of the diseases and conditions affecting the tissues of the periodontium and was presented and discussed at the 1999 International Workshop for the Classification of the Periodontal Diseases organized by the American Academy of Periodontology (AAP).[2] The overall classification system is presented in Box 4-1 and each of the diseases or conditions are discussed where clarification is needed. In each case, the reader is referred to pertinent reviews on the subject and specific chapters within this book that discuss the topics in more detail.

GINGIVAL DISEASES

Dental Plaque–Induced Gingival Diseases

Gingivitis that is associated with dental plaque formation[1] is the most common form of gingival disease (Box 4-2), and its epidemiology (Chapter 5), its etiology (Chapters 6 through 15), and its clinical characteristics (Chapters 16 through 21) are discussed elsewhere in this textbook and in other sources.[7,10,12,19,20] Gingivitis has been previously characterized by the presence of clinical signs of inflammation that are confined to the gingiva and associated with teeth showing no attachment loss. Gingivitis also has been observed to affect the gingiva of periodontitis-affected teeth that have previously lost attachment but have received periodontal therapy to stabilize any further attachment loss. In these treated cases, plaque-induced gingival inflammation may reoccur but without any evidence of further attachment loss. In light of this evidence, it has been concluded that *plaque-induced gingivitis may occur on a periodontium with no*

BOX 4-1

Classification of Periodontal Diseases and Conditions[2]

Gingival Diseases
Plaque-induced gingival diseases*
Non–plaque-induced gingival lesions

Chronic Periodontitis**
Localized
Generalized

Aggressive Periodontitis
Localized
Generalized

Periodontitis as a Manifestation of Systemic Diseases

Necrotizing Periodontal Diseases
Necrotizing ulcerative gingivitis (NUG)
Necrotizing ulcerative periodontitis (NUP)

Abscesses of the Periodontium
Gingival abscess
Periodontal abscess
Pericoronal abscess

Periodontitis Associated with Endodontic Lesions
Endodontic–periodontal lesion
Periodontal–endodontic lesion
Combined lesion

Developmental or Acquired Deformities and Conditions
Localized tooth-related factors that predispose to plaque-induced gingival diseases or periodontitis
Mucogingival deformities and conditions around teeth
Mucogingival deformities and conditions on edentulous ridges
Occlusal trauma

* These diseases may occur on a periodontium with no attachment loss or on a periodontium with attachment loss that is stable and not progressing.

** Aggressive periodontitis can be further classified on the basis of extent and severity. As a general guide, extent can be characterized as localized ($<$30% of sites involved) or generalized ($>$30% of sites involved). Severity can be characterized on the basis of the amount of clinical attachment loss (CAL) as follows: Slight = 1 or 2 mm CAL; moderate = 3 or 4 mm CAL; and severe $\geq$ 5 mm CAL.

attachment loss or on a periodontium with previous attachment loss that is stable and not progressing. This implies that gingivitis may be the diagnosis for inflamed gingival tissues associated with a tooth with no previous attachment loss or with a tooth that has previously undergone attachment and bone loss (reduced periodontal support) but is not currently losing attachment or bone even though gingival inflammation is present. For this diagnosis to be made, longitudinal records of periodontal status, including clinical attachment levels, should be available.

Gingivitis Associated with Dental Plaque Only

Plaque-induced gingival disease is the result of an interaction between the microorganisms found in the dental plaque biofilm and the tissues and inflammatory cells of the host. The plaque–host interaction can be altered by the effects of local factors, systemic factors, or both; medications; and malnutrition that can influence the severity and duration of the response. Local factors that may contribute to gingivitis, in addition to plaque-retentive calculus formation on crown and root surfaces, are discussed in "Developmental or Acquired Deformities and Conditions." These factors are contributory because of their ability to retain plaque microorganisms and inhibit their removal by patient-initiated plaque control techniques.

Gingival Diseases Modified by Systemic Factors

Systemic factors[10,12,19] contributing to gingivitis, such as the endocrine changes associated with puberty, the menstrual cycle, pregnancy, and diabetes, may be exacerbated because of alterations in the gingival inflammatory response to plaque. This appears to be caused by the effects of the systemic conditions on the cellular and immunologic functions of the host. These changes are most apparent during pregnancy, when the prevalence and severity of gingival inflammation may increase even in the presence of low levels of plaque. Blood dyscrasias such as leukemia may alter immune function by disturbing the normal balance of immunologically competent white blood cells supplying the periodontium. Gingival enlargement and bleeding are common findings and may be associated with swollen, spongy gingival tissues caused by excessive infiltration of blood cells.

Gingival Diseases Modified by Medications

Gingival diseases modified by medications[7,12,20] are increasingly prevalent because of the increased use of anticonvulsant drugs known to induce gingival enlargement, such as phenytoin, immunosuppressive drugs such as cyclosporine A, and calcium channel blockers such as nifedipine, verapamil, diltiazem, and sodium valproate. The development and severity of gingival enlargement in response to medications is patient specific and may be influenced by uncontrolled plaque accumulation. The increased use of oral contraceptives by premenopausal women has been associated with a higher incidence of gingival inflammation and development of gingival enlargement that may be reversed by discontinuation of the oral contraceptive.

Gingival Diseases Modified by Malnutrition

Gingival diseases modified by malnutrition[12] have received attention because of clinical descriptions of bright red, swollen, and bleeding gingiva associated with severe ascorbic acid (vitamin C) deficiency or scurvy. Nutritional deficiencies are known to affect immune function and may have an impact on the host's ability to protect

BOX 4-2

Gingival Diseases[9,12]

Dental Plaque–Induced Gingival Diseases

These diseases may occur on a periodontium with no attachment loss or on one with attachment loss that is stable and not progressing.

- I. Gingivitis associated with dental plaque only
  - A. Without local contributing factors
  - B. With local contributing factors (see Box 4-4)
- II. Gingival diseases modified by systemic factors
  - A. Associated with the endocrine system:
    - 1. Puberty-associated gingivitis
    - 2. Menstrual cycle–associated gingivitis
    - 3. Pregnancy associated
      - a. Gingivitis
      - b. Pyogenic granuloma
    - 4. Diabetes mellitus–associated gingivitis
  - B. Associated with blood dyscrasias
    - 1. Leukemia-associated gingivitis
    - 2. Other
- III. Gingival diseases modified by medications
  - A. Drug-influenced gingival diseases
    - 1. Drug-influenced gingival enlargements
    - 2. Drug-influenced gingivitis
      - a. Oral contraceptive–associated gingivitis
      - b. Other
- IV. Gingival diseases modified by malnutrition
  - A. Ascorbic acid deficiency gingivitis
  - B. Other

Non–Plaque-Induced Gingival Lesions

- I. Gingival diseases of specific bacterial origin
  - A. *Neisseria gonorrhea*
  - B. *Treponema pallidum*
  - C. Streptococcal species
  - D. Other
- II. Gingival diseases of viral origin
  - A. Herpesvirus infections
    - 1. Primary herpetic gingivostomatitis
    - 2. Recurrent oral herpes
    - 3. Varicella zoster
  - B. Other
- III. Gingival diseases of fungal origin
  - A. *Candida*-species infections: Generalized gingival candidosis
  - B. Linear gingival erythema
  - C. Histoplasmosis
  - D. Other
- IV. Gingival lesions of genetic origin
  - A. Hereditary gingival fibromatosis
  - B. Other
- V. Gingival manifestations of systemic conditions
  - A. Mucocutaneous lesions
    - 1. Lichen planus
    - 2. Pemphigoid
    - 3. Pemphigus vulgaris
    - 4. Erythema multiforme
    - 5. Lupus erythematosus
    - 6. Drug induced
    - 7. Other
  - B. Allergic reactions
    - 1. Dental restorative materials
      - a. Mercury
      - b. Nickel
      - c. Acrylic
      - d. Other
    - 2. Reactions attributable to
      - a. Toothpastes or dentifrices
      - b. Mouthrinses or mouthwashes
      - c. Chewing gum additives
      - d. Foods and additives
    - 3. Other
- VI. Traumatic lesions (factitious, iatrogenic, or accidental)
  - A. Chemical injury
  - B. Physical injury
  - C. Thermal injury
- VII. Foreign body reactions
- VIII. Not otherwise specified

itself against some of the detrimental effects of cellular products such as oxygen radicals. Unfortunately, little scientific evidence is available to support a role for specific nutritional deficiencies in the development or severity of gingival inflammation or periodontitis in humans.

Non–Plaque-Induced Gingival Lesions

Oral manifestations of systemic conditions that produce lesions in the tissues of the periodontium are rare. They are observed in lower socioeconomic groups, developing countries, and immunocompromised individuals.[9]

Gingival Diseases of Specific Bacterial Origin

Gingival diseases of specific bacterial origin[21,23] are increasing in prevalence especially as a result of sexually transmitted diseases such as gonorrhea *(Neisseria gonorrhoeae)* and to a lesser degree, syphilis *(Treponema pallidum)*. Oral lesions may be secondary to systemic infection or may occur through direct infection. Streptococcal gingivitis or gingivostomatitis also is a rare condition that may present as an acute condition with fever, malaise, and pain associated with acutely inflamed, diffuse, red, and swollen gingiva with increased bleeding and occasional gingival abscess formation. The gingival infections usually are preceded by tonsillitis and have been associated with group A β-hemolytic streptococcal infections.

Gingival Diseases of Viral Origin

Gingival diseases of viral origin[9,21,23] may be caused by a variety of deoxyribonucleic acid (DNA) and ribonucleic acid (RNA) viruses, the most common being the herpes viruses. Lesions are frequently related to reactivation of latent viruses, especially as a result of reduced immune function. The oral manifestations of viral infection have been comprehensively reviewed.[9,21,23]

Gingival Diseases of Fungal Origin

Gingival diseases of fungal origin[9,23,25] are relatively uncommon in the immunocompetent individual but occur more frequently in individuals who are immunocompromised or in whom the normal oral flora has been disturbed by the long-term use of broad-spectrum antibiotics. The most common oral fungal infection is candidiasis caused by infection with *Candida albicans,* which also can be seen under prosthetic devices, in individuals using topical steroids, and in individuals with decreased salivary flow, increased salivary glucose, or decreased salivary pH. A generalized candidal infection may manifest as white patches on the gingiva, tongue, or oral mucous membrane that can be removed with gauze, leaving a red, bleeding surface. In HIV-infected individuals, candidal infection may present as erythema of the attached gingiva and has been referred to as *linear gingival erythema* or *HIV-associated gingivitis* (see Chapter 29). Diagnosis of candidal infection can be made by culture, smear, and biopsy. Several less-common fungal infections, in addition to candidal infections, have been previously described.[23,25]

Gingival Diseases of Genetic Origin

Gingival diseases of genetic origin may involve the tissues of the periodontium and have been previously described in detail.[1] One of the most clinically evident conditions is hereditary gingival fibromatosis that exhibits autosomal dominant or (rarely) autosomal recessive modes of inheritance. The gingival enlargement may completely cover the teeth, delay eruption, and present as an isolated finding or be associated with several more generalized syndromes.

Gingival Manifestations of Systemic Conditions

Gingival manifestations of systemic conditions[9,18,24] may appear as desquamative lesions, ulceration of the gingiva, or both. These conditions, including those listed in Box 4-2, have been previously described in detail.[18,24] Allergic reactions that manifest with gingival changes are uncommon but have been observed in association with several restorative materials, toothpastes, mouthwashes, chewing gum, and foods (see Box 4-2). The diagnosis of these conditions may prove difficult and may require an extensive history and selective elimination of potential culprits.

Traumatic Lesions

Traumatic lesions[9] may be factitial (produced by artificial means; unintentionally produced) as in the case of toothbrush trauma resulting in gingival ulceration, recession or both; iatrogenic (trauma to the gingiva induced by the dentist or health professional) as in the case of preventive or restorative care that may lead to traumatic injury of the gingiva; or accidental as in the case of damage to the gingiva through minor burns from hot foods and drinks.

Foreign Body Reactions

Foreign body reactions[9] lead to localized inflammatory conditions of the gingiva and are caused by the introduction of foreign material into the gingival connective tissues through breaks in the epithelium. Common examples are the introduction of amalgam into the gingiva during the placement of a restoration or extraction of a tooth, leaving an amalgam tattoo, or the introduction of abrasives during polishing procedures.

PERIODONTITIS

Periodontitis is defined as "an inflammatory disease of the supporting tissues of the teeth caused by specific microorganisms or groups of specific microorganisms, resulting in progressive destruction of the periodontal ligament and alveolar bone with pocket formation, recession, or both." The clinical feature that distinguishes periodontitis from gingivitis is the presence of clinically detectable attachment loss. This often is accompanied by periodontal pocket formation and changes in the density and height of subjacent alveolar bone. In some cases, recession of the marginal gingiva may accompany attachment loss, thus masking ongoing disease progression if pocket depth measurements are taken without measurements of clinical attachment levels. Clinical signs of inflammation, such as changes in color, contour, and consistency and bleeding on probing, may not always be positive indicators of ongoing attachment loss. However, the presence of continued bleeding on probing at sequential visits has proven to be a reliable indicator of the presence of inflammation and the potential for subsequent attachment loss at the bleeding site. The attachment loss associated with periodontitis has been shown to progress either continuously or in episodic bursts of disease activity.

Although many classifications of the different clinical manifestations of periodontitis have been presented over the past 20 years, consensus workshops in North America in 1989[5] and in Europe in 1993[3] (Table 4-1) identified that periodontitis may present in early onset, adult-onset, and necrotizing forms. In addition, the AAP consensus concluded that periodontitis may be associated with systemic conditions such as diabetes and HIV infection and that some forms of periodontitis may be refractory to conventional therapy. Early onset disease was distinguished from adult-onset disease by the age of onset (35 years of age was set as an arbitrary separation of diseases), the rate of disease progression, and the presence of alterations in host defenses. The early onset diseases were more aggressive, occurred in individuals younger than 35 years old, and were associated with defects in host defenses, whereas adult forms of disease were slowly progressive, began in the fourth decade of life, and were not associated with defects in host defenses. In addition, early onset periodontitis was subclassified into prepubertal, juvenile, and rapidly progressive forms with localized or generalized disease distributions. Extensive clinical and basic scientific research of these disease entities has been performed in many countries, and some disease characteristics outlined 10 years ago no longer stand up to rigid scientific scrutiny.[6,11,26] In particular, supporting evidence was lacking for the distinct classifications of adult periodontitis, refractory periodontitis, and the various different forms of early onset periodontitis as outlined by the America Academy of Periodontology (AAP) Workshop for the International Classification of Periodontal Diseases in 1999[2] (see Table 4-1). It has been observed that chronic periodontal destruction, due to the accumulation of local factors such as plaque and calculus, can occur prior to the age of 35 years and that the aggressive disease seen in young patients may be independent of age but has a familial (genetic) association. With respect to refractory periodontitis, little evidence supports that this is indeed a distinct clinical entity because the causes of continued loss of clinical attachment and alveolar bone after periodontal therapy are currently poorly defined and apply to many disease entities. In addition, the clinical and etiologic manifestations of the different diseases outlined in North America in 1989 and in Europe in 1993 were not consistently observed in different countries around the world and did not always fit the models presented. As a result, the AAP held an International Workshop for the Classification of Periodontal Diseases in 1999[2] to further clarify a classification system based on current clinical and scientific data. The resulting classification of the different forms of periodontitis was simplified to describe three general clinical manifestations of periodontitis: chronic periodontitis, aggressive periodontitis, and periodontitis as a manifestation of systemic diseases (see Table 4-1 and Box 4-3).

Chronic Periodontitis

Chronic periodontitis[6] is the most common form of periodontitis and the characteristics of this form of periodontitis are outlined in Box 4-3. Chronic periodontitis is most prevalent in adults but can be observed in children;

TABLE 4-1

Classification of the Various Forms of Periodontitis

Classification	Forms of Periodontitis	Disease Characteristics
AAP World Workshop in Clinical Periodontics, 1989[5]	Adult periodontitis	Age of onset >35 years Slow rate of disease progression No defects in host defenses
	Early onset periodontitis (may be prepubertal, juvenile, or rapidly progressive)	Age of onset <35 years Rapid rate of disease progression Defects in host defenses Associated with specific microflora
	Periodontitis associated with systemic disease	Systemic diseases that predispose to rapid rates of periodontitis Diseases: diabetes, Down syndrome, HIV infection, and Papillon-Lefevre syndrome
	Necrotizing ulcerative periodontitis	Similar to acute necrotizing ulcerative gingivitis but with associated clinical attachment loss
	Refractory periodontitis	Recurrent periodontitis that does not respond to treatment
European Workshop on Periodontology, 1993[3]	Adult periodontitis	Age of onset: fourth decade of life Slow rate of disease progression No defects in host response
	Early onset periodontitis	Age of onset: prior to fourth decade of life Rapid rate of disease progression Defects in host defenses
	Necrotizing periodontitis	Tissue necrosis with attachment and bone loss
AAP International Workshop for Classification of Periodontal Diseases, 1999[2]	Chronic periodontitis	See Box 4-3
	Aggressive periodontitis	See Box 4-3
	Periodontitis as a manifestation of systemic diseases	See Box 4-3

therefore the age range of >35 years previously designated for the classification of this disease has been discarded. Chronic periodontitis is associated with the accumulation of plaque and calculus and generally has a slow to moderate rate of disease progression, but periods of more rapid destruction may be observed. Increases in the rate of disease progression may be caused by the impact of local, systemic, or environmental factors that may influence the normal host–bacterial interaction. Local factors may influence plaque accumulation (Box 4-4); systemic diseases such as diabetes mellitus and HIV infection may influence the host defenses; environmental factors such as cigarette smoking and stress also may influence the response of the host to plaque accumulation.

BOX 4-3

Periodontitis

The disease periodontitis can be subclassified into the following three major types based on clinical, radiographic, historical, and laboratory characteristics.[6,11,26]

Chronic Periodontitis

The following characteristics are common to patients with chronic periodontitis:

- Prevalent in adults but can occur in children
- Amount of destruction consistent with local factors
- Associated with a variable microbial pattern
- Subgingival calculus frequently found
- Slow to moderate rate of progression with possible periods of rapid progression
- Possibly modified by or associated with the following:
  Systemic diseases such as diabetes mellitus and HIV infection
  Local factors predisposing to periodontitis (see Box 4-3)
  Environmental factors such as cigarette smoking and emotional stress

Chronic periodontitis may be further subclassified into localized and generalized forms and characterized as slight, moderate, or severe based on the common features described above and the following specific features:

Localized form: <30% of sites involved
Generalized form: >30% of sites involved
Slight: 1 to 2 mm of clinical attachment loss
Moderate: 3 to 4 mm of clinical attachment loss
Severe: ≥5 mm of clinical attachment loss

Aggressive Periodontitis

The following characteristics are common to patients with aggressive periodontitis:

- Otherwise clinically healthy patient
- Rapid attachment loss and bone destruction
- Amount of microbial deposits inconsistent with disease severity
- Familial aggregation of diseased individuals

The following characteristics are common but not universal:

- Diseased sites infected with *Actinobacillus actinomycetemcomitans*
- Abnormalities in phagocyte function
- Hyperresponsive macrophages, producing increased PGE_2 and IL-1β
- In some cases, self-arresting disease progression

Aggressive periodontitis may be further classified into localized and generalized forms based on the common features described here and the following specific features:

Localized form:

- Circumpubertal onset of disease
- Localized first molar or incisor disease with proximal attachment loss on at least two permanent teeth, one of which is a first molar
- Robust serum antibody response to infecting agents

Generalized form:

- Usually affecting persons under 30 years of age (however, may be older)
- Generalized proximal attachment loss affecting at least three teeth other than first molars and incisors
- Pronounced episodic nature of periodontal destruction
- Poor serum antibody response to infecting agents

Periodontitis as a Manifestation of Systemic Diseases

Periodontitis may be observed as a manifestation of the following systemic diseases:

1. Hematologic disorders
   a. Acquired neutropenia
   b. Leukemias
   c. Other
2. Genetic disorders
   a. Familial and cyclic neutropenia
   b. Down syndrome
   c. Leukocyte adhesion deficiency syndromes
   d. Papillon-Lefévre syndrome
   e. Chediak-Higashi syndrome
   f. Histiocytosis syndromes
   g. Glycogen storage disease
   h. Infantile genetic agranulocytosis
   i. Cohen syndrome
   j. Ehlers-Danlos syndrome (Types IV and VIII AD)
   k. Hypophosphatasia
   l. Other
3. Not otherwise specified

Chronic periodontitis may occur as a localized disease wherein <30% of evaluated sites demonstrate attachment and bone loss, or as a more generalized disease wherein >30% of sites are affected. The disease also may be described by the severity of disease as slight, moderate, or severe based on the amount of clinical attachment loss (see Box 4-3).

Aggressive Periodontitis

Aggressive periodontitis[15,26] differs from the chronic form primarily by the rapid rate of disease progression seen in an otherwise healthy individual, an absence of large accumulations of plaque and calculus, and a family history of aggressive disease suggestive of a genetic trait (see Box 4-3). This form of periodontitis was previously classified as early onset periodontitis (see Table 4-1) and therefore still includes many of the characteristics previously identified with the localized and generalized forms of early onset periodontitis. Although the clinical presentation of aggressive disease appears to be universal, the etiologic factors involved are not always consistent. Additional clinical, microbiologic, and immunologic characteristics of aggressive disease that may be present are outlined in Box 4-3. As was previously described for early onset disease, aggressive forms of disease usually affect young individuals at or after puberty and may be observed during the second and third decade of life (i.e., 10 to 30 years of age). The disease may be localized as previously described for localized juvenile periodontitis (LJP) or generalized as previously described for generalized juvenile periodontitis (GJP) and rapidly progressive periodontitis (RPP) (see Table 4-1). The common features of the localized and generalized forms of aggressive periodontitis are outlined in Box 4-3.

BOX 4-4

Developmental or Acquired Deformities and Conditions[4,8,17]

Localized Tooth-Related Factors That Modify or Predispose to Plaque-Induced Gingival Diseases or Periodontitis

1. Tooth anatomic factors
2. Dental restorations or appliances
3. Root fractures
4. Cervical root resorption and cemental tears

Mucogingival Deformities and Conditions around Teeth

1. Gingival or soft tissue recession
   A. Facial or lingual surfaces
   B. Interproximal (papillary)
2. Lack of keratinized gingiva
3. Decreased vestibular depth
4. Aberrant frenum or muscle position
5. Gingival excess
   A. Pseudopocket
   B. Inconsistent gingival margin
   C. Excessive gingival display
   D. Gingival enlargement (see Box 4-2)
   E. Abnormal color

Mucogingival Deformities and Conditions on Edentulous Edges

1. Vertical and/or horizontal ridge deficiency
2. Lack of gingiva or keratinized tissue
3. Gingival or soft tissue enlargements
4. Aberrant frenum or muscle position
5. Decreased vestibular depth
6. Abnormal color

Occlusal Trauma

1. Primary occlusal trauma
2. Secondary occlusal trauma

Periodontitis as a Manifestation of Systemic Diseases

Several hematologic and genetic disorders have been associated with the development of periodontitis in affected individuals[10,11] (see Box 4-3). The majority of these observations of effects on the periodontium are the result of case reports, and few research studies have been performed to investigate the exact nature of the effect of the specific condition on the tissues of the periodontium. It is speculated that the major effect of these disorders is through alterations in host defense mechanisms that have been clearly described for disorders such as neutropenia and leukocyte adhesion deficiencies but are less well understood for many multifaceted syndromes. The clinical manifestation of many of these disorders appears at an early age and may be confused with aggressive forms of periodontitis with rapid attachment loss and the potential for early tooth loss. With the introduction of this form of periodontitis in this and previous classification systems (see Table 4-1), the potential exists for overlap and confusion between periodontitis as a manifestation of systemic disease and both the aggressive and chronic forms of disease when a systemic component is suspected. At present, periodontitis as a manifestation of systemic disease is the diagnosis to be used when the systemic condition is the major predisposing factor and local factors such as large quantities of plaque and calculus are not clearly evident. In the case where periodontal destruction is clearly the result of local factors but has been exacerbated by the onset of such conditions as diabetes mellitus or HIV infection, then the diagnosis should be chronic periodontitis modified by the systemic condition.

NECROTIZING PERIODONTAL DISEASES

The clinical characteristics of necrotizing periodontal diseases may include but are not limited to ulcerated and necrotic papillary and marginal gingiva covered by a yellowish-white or grayish slough or pseudomembrane, blunting and cratering of papillae, bleeding on provocation or spontaneous bleeding, pain, and fetid breath. These diseases may be accompanied by fever, malaise, and lymphadenopathy, although these characteristics are not consistent. Two forms of necrotizing periodontal disease have been described: necrotizing ulcerative gingivitis (NUG) and necrotizing ulcerative periodontitis (NUP). NUG has been previously classified under gingival diseases or gingivitis because clinical attachment loss is not a consistent feature, whereas NUP has been classified as a form of periodontitis because attachment loss is present. Recent reviews of the etiologic and clinical characteristics of NUG and NUP have suggested that the two diseases represent clinical manifestations of the same disease, except that distinct features of NUP are clinical attachment and bone loss. As a result, both NUG and NUP have been determined as a separate group of diseases that has tissue necrosis as a primary clinical feature (see Box 4-1).

Necrotizing Ulcerative Gingivitis

The clinical and etiologic characteristics of NUG[22] are described in detail in Chapter 21. The defining characteristics of NUG are its bacterial etiology, its necrotic lesion, and predisposing factors such as psychologic stress, smoking, and immunosuppression. In addition, malnutrition may be a contributing factor in developing countries. NUG is usually seen as an acute lesion that responds well to antimicrobial therapy combined with professional plaque and calculus removal and improved oral hygiene.

Necrotizing Ulcerative Periodontitis

NUP[16] differs from NUG in that loss of clinical attachment and alveolar bone is a consistent feature. All other characteristics appear to be the same between the two forms of necrotizing disease. The characteristics of NUP are described in detail in Chapter 27. NUP may be observed among patients with HIV infection and manifests as local ulceration and necrosis of gingival tissue with exposure and rapid destruction of underlying bone, spontaneous bleeding, and severe pain. HIV-infected patients with NUP are 20.8 times more likely to have CD4+ cell counts below 200 cells/mm^3 of peripheral blood than HIV-infected patients without NUP, suggesting that immunosuppression is a major contributing factor. In addition, the predictive value of NUP for HIV-infected patients with CD4+ cell counts below 200 cells/mm^3 was 95.1%, and a cumulative probability of death within 24 months of a NUP diagnosis in HIV-infected individuals had a 72.9% cumulative probability of death within 24 months of NUP diagnosis. In developing countries, NUP also has been associated with severe malnutrition that in some instances may lead to immunosuppression.

ABSCESSES OF THE PERIODONTIUM

A periodontal abscess[13] is a localized purulent infection of periodontal tissues and is classified by its tissue of origin. The clinical, microbiologic, immunologic, and predisposing characteristics are discussed in detail in Chapters 4–6.

PERIODONTITIS ASSOCIATED WITH ENDODONTIC LESIONS

Classification of lesions affecting the periodontium and pulp is based on the disease process sequence.[4]

Endodontic–Periodontal Lesions

In endodontic–periodontal lesions, pulpal necrosis precedes periodontal changes. A periapical lesion originating in pulpal infection and necrosis may drain to the oral cavity through the periodontal ligament, resulting in destruction of the periodontal ligament and adjacent alveolar bone. This may present clinically as a localized, deep, periodontal pocket extending to the apex of the tooth. Pulpal infection also may drain through accessory canals, especially in the area of the furcation, and may lead to furcal involvement through loss of clinical attachment and alveolar bone.

Periodontal–Endodontic Lesions

In periodontal–endodontic lesions, bacterial infection from a periodontal pocket associated with loss of attachment and root exposure may spread through accessory canals to the pulp, resulting in pulpal necrosis. In the case of advanced periodontal disease, the infection may reach the pulp through the apical foramen. Scaling and root planing removes cementum and underlying dentin and may lead to chronic pulpitis through bacterial penetration of dentinal tubules. However, many periodontitis-affected teeth that have been scaled and root planed show no evidence of pulpal involvement.

Combined Lesions

Combined lesions occur when pulpal necrosis and a periapical lesion occur on a tooth that also is periodontally involved. A radiographically evident intrabony defect is seen when infection of pulpal origin merges with infection of periodontal origin.

In all cases of periodontitis associated with endodontic lesions, the endodontic infection should be controlled before beginning definitive management of the periodontal lesion, especially when regenerative or bone-grafting techniques are planned.

DEVELOPMENTAL OR ACQUIRED DEFORMITIES AND CONDITIONS

Localized Tooth-Related Factors That Modify or Predispose to Plaque-Induced Gingival Diseases or Periodontitis

In general, these factors[4] are considered to be those local factors that contribute to the initiation and progression of periodontal disease through an enhancement of plaque accumulation or the prevention of effective plaque removal by normal oral hygiene measures (see Box 4-4). These factors fall into three subgroups.

Tooth Anatomic Factors

These factors are associated with malformations of tooth development or tooth location. Anatomic factors such as cervical enamel projections and enamel pearls have been associated with clinical attachment loss, especially in furcation areas. Cervical enamel projections are found on 15% to 24% of mandibular molars and 9% to 25% of maxillary molars, and strong associations have been observed with furcation involvement. Palatogingival grooves, found primarily on maxillary incisors, are observed in 8.5% of individuals and are associated with increased plaque accumulation, clinical attachment, and bone loss. Proximal root grooves on incisors and maxillary premolars also predispose to plaque accumulation, inflammation, and loss of clinical attachment and bone. Tooth location is considered important in the initiation and development of disease. Tooth malalignment predisposes to plaque accumulation and inflammation in children and may predispose to clinical attachment loss in adults, especially when associated with poor oral hygiene. In addition, open contacts have been associated with increased loss of alveolar bone, most probably through food impaction.

Dental Restorations or Appliances

Dental restorations or appliances are frequently associated with the development of gingival inflammation, especially when they are located subgingivally. This may apply to subgingivally placed onlays, crowns, fillings, and orthodontic bands. Restorations may impinge on the biologic width by being placed deep in the sulcus or within the junctional epithelium. This may promote inflammation and loss of clinical attachment and bone with apical migration of the junctional epithelium and reestablishment of the attachment apparatus at a more apical level.

Root Fractures

Root fractures caused by traumatic forces or restorative or endodontic procedures may lead to periodontal involvement through an apical migration of plaque along the fracture when the fracture originates coronal to the clinical attachment and is exposed to the oral environment.

Cervical Root Resorption and Cemental Tears

Cervical root resorption and cemental tears may lead to periodontal destruction when the lesion communicates with the oral cavity and allows bacteria to migrate subgingivally.

Mucogingival Deformities and Conditions around Teeth

Mucogingival is defined as "a generic term used to describe the mucogingival junction and its relationship to the gingiva, alveolar mucosa, frenula, muscle attachments, vestibular fornices, and the floor of the mouth." A *mucogingival deformity* may be defined as "a significant departure from the normal shape of gingiva and alveolar mucosa" and may involve the underlying alveolar bone. *Mucogingival surgery* is defined as "periodontal surgical procedures designed to correct defects in the morphology, position, and/or amount of gingiva" and is described in detail in Chapter 66. The surgical correction of mucogingival deformities may be performed for esthetic reasons, to enhance function, or to facilitate oral hygiene.[17]

Mucogingival Deformities and Conditions on Edentulous Ridges

Mucogingival deformities and conditions on edentulous ridges usually require corrective surgery to restore form and function before the prosthetic replacement of missing teeth or implant placement.[17]

Occlusal Trauma

The etiology of trauma from occlusion and its effects on the periodontium is discussed in detail in Chapters 24, 25, and 52.[8]

REFERENCES

1. Aldred MJ, Bartold PM: Genetic disorders of the gingivae and periodontium. Periodontol 2000 1998; 18:7.
2. Armitage GC: Development of a classification system for periodontal diseases and conditions. Ann Periodontol 1999; 4:1.
3. Attstrom R, Vander Velden U: Summary of session 1. In Lang N, Karring T (eds): Proceedings of the 1st European workshop in periodontology. Berlin, Quintessence, 1993.
4. Blieden TM: Tooth-related issues. Ann Periodontol 1999; 4:91.
5. Caton J: Periodontal diagnosis and diagnostic aids; consensus report. In: Proceedings of the world workshop in clinical periodontics, American Academy of Periodontology, 1989, pp. 1-32.
6. Flemmig TF: Periodontitis. Ann Periodontol 1999; 4:32.
7. Hallmon WW, Rossmann JA: The role of drugs in the pathogenesis of gingival overgrowth. Periodontol 2000 1999; 21:176.
8. Hallmon WW: Occlusal trauma: effect and impact on the periodontium. Ann Periodontol 1999; 4:102.
9. Holmstrup P: Non–plaque-induced gingival lesions. Ann Periodontol 1999; 4:20.
10. Kinane DF: Blood and lymphoreticular disorders. Periodontol 2000 1999; 21:84.
11. Kinane DF: Periodontitis modified by systemic factors. Ann Periodontol 1999; 4:54.
12. Mariotti A: Dental plaque-induced gingival diseases. Ann Periodontol 1999; 4:7.
13. Meng HX: Periodontal abscess. Ann Periodontol 1999; 4:79.
14. Meng HX: Periodontic–endodontic lesions. Ann Periodontol 1999; 4:84.
15. Novak MJ, Novak KF: Early onset periodontitis. Curr Opinion 1996; 3:45.
16. Novak MJ: Necrotizing ulcerative periodontitis. Ann Periodontol 1999; 4:74.
17. Pini Prato GP: Mucogingival deformities. Ann Periodontol 1999; 4:98.
18. Plemons JM, Gonzalez TS, Burkhart NW: Vesiculobullous diseases of the oral cavity. Periodontol 2000 1999; 21:158.

19. Porter SR: Gingival and periodontal aspects of diseases of the blood and blood-forming organs and malignancy. Periodontol 2000 1998; 18:102.
20. Rees TD: Drugs and oral disorders. Periodontol 2000 1998; 18:21.
21. Rivera Hidalgo F, Stanford TW: Oral mucosal lesions caused by infective microorganisms I. Viruses and bacteria. Periodontol 2000 1999; 21:106.
22. Rowland RW: Necrotizing ulcerative gingivitis. Ann Periodontol 1999; 4:65.
23. Scully C, Monteil R, Sposto MR: Infectious and tropical diseases affecting the human mouth. Periodontol 2000 1998; 18:47.
24. Scully C, Laskaris G: Mucocutaneous disorders. Periodontol 2000 1998; 18:81.
25. Stanford TW, Rivera-Hidalgo F: Oral mucosal lesions caused by infective microorganisms II. Fungi and parasites. Periodontol 2000 1999; 21:125.
26. Tonetti MS, Mombelli A: Early-onset periodontitis. Ann Periodontol 1999; 4:39.

Epidemiology of Gingival and Periodontal Diseases

James D. Beck and Samuel J. Arbes, Jr.

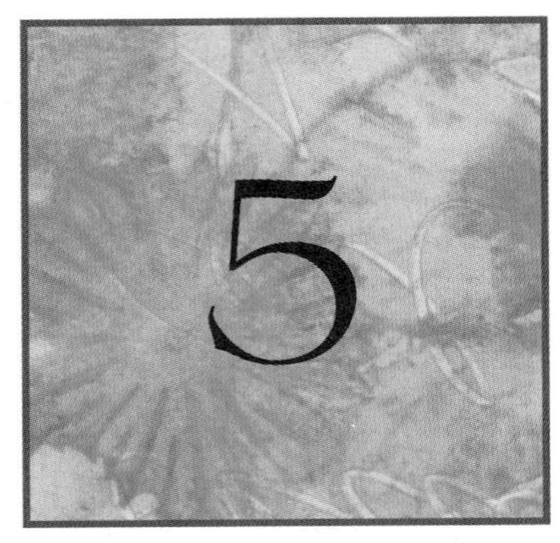

CHAPTER

CHAPTER OUTLINE

Although information about the epidemiology of a disease is based on groups of people, whereas clinicians are primarily interested in the individual patient being treated, thoughtful clinicians understand the value of epidemiologic information for the decisions they must make about the philosophy of their practice and the treatment of each patient. Questions that frame the diagnosis of an individual patient include "Is this a rare or common condition? Does my patient fit the profile of people likely to have this disease? Where on the continuum of normality to disease are the signs and symptoms I see in my patient?" Epidemiologic studies identifying risk factors for diseases provide guidance for primary prevention recommendations, and newer molecular epidemiology studies help identify where to intervene in the disease process. Treatment-related questions such as "What is the natural history of the disease that I am treating?" lead to decisions about whether to treat now or continue to evaluate the condition. Similarly, much of our knowledge about the prognosis for an individual patient under a specific treatment comes from epidemiologic studies of treatment outcomes.

The focus of this chapter is on the clinician, which is the reason that many of the topic headings address clinical issues such as abnormality, definition of a case, diagnosis, and risk for new disease and disease progression. A short review of epidemiology and study designs used in epidemiologic and clinical studies precedes discussion of these clinical issues. (For those who are well versed in these matters, the authors recommend skipping the next section and using it as a reference for the remainder of the chapter.)

WHAT IS EPIDEMIOLOGY?

Epidemiology is "the study of the distribution and determinants of health-related states or events in specified populations, and the application of this study to control health problems."[42] Epidemiology traditionally has been considered a basic science of public health. What distinguishes public health practice from clinical practice is that public health practice emphasizes the health of population groups, whereas clinical practice is concerned with the health of individual patients. The determinants of disease in an individual patient may be quite different from the determinants of disease in a population. For example, a periodontist may attribute a patient's periodontal disease to the accumulation of plaque and calculus (factors that can be addressed in a practice), whereas a public health practitioner may attribute the high prevalence of periodontal disease in a given population to low socioeconomic status or the lack of access to preventive dental services.

As the definition implies, epidemiology has three purposes: 1) to determine the amount and distribution of a disease in a population, 2) to investigate causes for the disease, and 3) to apply this knowledge to the control of the disease. Perhaps the most basic question in public health and clinical practice is "How much disease is present?" Descriptive studies are used to measure the amount of disease in a population. Disease often is described in terms of the percentage of persons affected and its distribution among subgroups (defined by age, gender, ethnicity, education levels, or other characteristics) in the population. The underlying assumption in epidemiology is that the distribution of disease among members of a population is not random.[32] Some members or subgroups of the population have characteristics that make them more susceptible to disease. These characteristics include the physical, biologic, behavioral, cultural, and social factors that determine health.[42] Epidemiologists use analytic studies such as case-control or cohort studies to investigate factors associated with a disease. The final purpose of epidemiology is to apply the knowledge gained from studies to "promote, protect, and restore health."[42] Epidemiologic data are the foundation for much of our public health policy. One of the most successful public health interventions has been the fluoridation of public drinking water to prevent dental caries. Epidemiologic data also have been the foundation for much of clinical practice.[32] Diagnostic tests, prognoses, and selection of appropriate therapies are based on studies of groups of people. The practice of evidence-based dentistry requires clinical practitioners to use the best available scientific information in making decisions about the care of individual patients. Much of this scientific information comes from epidemiologic studies and randomized clinical trials in particular.

Epidemiologic Measures of Disease

Prevalence

Prevalence is the proportion of persons in a population who have the disease of interest at a given point or period of time.[33] It is calculated by dividing the number of persons in the population who have the disease by the number of persons in the population.

$$\text{Prevalence} = \frac{\text{Number of persons with the disease}}{\text{Number of persons in the population}}$$

Prevalence, which can be reported as a proportion or percentage, is a measure of the burden of disease in a population. Information about prevalence can be useful for estimating the need for health care resources. For example, prevalence data on dental disease is used for estimating the number of new general dentists and specialists that dental schools should train.

Several factors influence the prevalence of disease. The prevalence of a disease at a given point in time is the result of the dynamic situation between the addition of new cases (incidence), which increases prevalence, and the removal of cases through death or cure, which decreases prevalence.[32] Ironically, the introduction of more sensitive diagnostic tests or new treatments that enhance survival increases prevalence.[32] Also, the prevalence of a nonfatal chronic disease, such as adult periodontitis, tends to increase with increasing age. This increase in prevalence with age, which is simply caused by the accumulation of cases, often is misinterpreted as meaning that older adults are at higher risk for the disease.

Incidence

Incidence—also referred to as *risk* or *cumulative incidence*—is the average percentage of unaffected persons who will develop the disease of interest during a given period of time.[3] Incidence can be viewed as the risk or probability that a person will become a case. It is calculated by dividing the number of new cases of disease by the number of persons in the population who are at risk for the disease.

$$\text{Incidence} = \frac{\text{Number of new cases}}{\text{Number of persons at risk}}$$

Whereas prevalence is a measure of the amount of disease existing in a population, incidence is a measure of the occurrence of new disease. The numerator of the incidence equation is the number of persons who transition from a nondiseased state to a diseased state during the period of observation. The denominator in the equation must contain only those persons in the population who are at risk for but do not have the disease at the start of observation. For example, in a study of oral cancer, only individuals who are free of oral cancer at the beginning of the study could be included in the population at risk. In the expression of incidence, specifying the period of observation is necessary. Without a specified time period, such as per month or per year, incidence has little meaning.

In the study of periodontal disease, rarely, if ever, does *incident periodontal disease* refer strictly to the onset of disease in previously periodontitis-free adults. Instead, it usually refers to the development of new periodontal lesions in people who may have had other periodontal lesions at baseline and to the progression of existing lesions (see later discussion). Incident periodontal disease is typically measured as a change in attachment level over time, and studies rarely differentiate between the development of new lesions and the progression of existing ones.

Epidemiologic Study Designs

To investigate the prevalence and incidence of disease, risk factors associated with disease, and the effectiveness and efficacy of interventions, researchers conduct epidemiologic studies. Most epidemiologic studies are observational. In these studies, the researchers observe natural occurrences in the population. The most common observation studies are cross-sectional, cohort, and case-control studies. In addition to observational studies, epidemiologists also conduct experimental studies in which they manipulate exposures, such as in drug trials when one group of subjects receives the study drug and another group receives a placebo. Experimental studies are useful in studying the efficacy of preventive interventions, treatments, and drugs. Community intervention trials and randomized clinical trials are two types of experimental studies. Because researchers can control the exposures, these studies provide the strongest evidence for cause and effect. For more information of community intervention and clinical trials, the interested reader is referred to texts by Hulley and Cummings, Lilienfeld, and Friedman et al.[30,38,43] Features of the most common observational study designs are reviewed here.

Cross-Sectional Studies

In cross-sectional studies, the presence or absence of disease and characteristics of the members of a population are measured at a point in time. These studies are useful for providing prevalence data on a disease, comparing the characteristics of persons with and without disease, and generating hypotheses regarding the etiology of a disease. Whereas cohort and case-control studies are considered analytic study designs, cross-sectional studies are considered descriptive. Cross-sectional studies also are referred to as *disease frequency surveys* or *prevalence studies.* Depending on the size of the population and the resources available to the researchers, the entire population or a representative sample of the population can be studied. Cross-sectional studies repeated at regular intervals can provide information on trends in disease over time or the effectiveness of prevention or treatment programs.

Cross-sectional studies have two major limitations. First, cross-sectional studies can only identify prevalent cases of disease. Because these studies do not follow a population at risk of the disease over time, incidence cannot be determined. Second, although cross-sectional studies may show that a certain characteristic is associated with having the disease, determining whether the characteristic preceded the disease is not always possible. For example, a cross-sectional study may reveal that people with periodontal disease are more likely to be smokers; however, it cannot always be determined whether the smoking or the disease occurred first. Establishing the temporal relationship between a particular characteristic and the onset of disease is an important criterion for determining whether the characteristic is a cause of the disease. Cohort studies that observe people over time are required to calculate incidence and establish temporality. The advantages of cross-sectional studies are that they are generally less expensive than longitudinal studies and quicker to conduct.

Cohort Studies

Unlike cross-sectional studies, cohort studies follow subjects over time. The purpose of a cohort study is to determine whether an exposure or characteristic is associated with the development of a disease or condition. At the beginning of the study, all subjects must be free of the disease of interest. Subjects are classified into exposed and unexposed groups and then followed over time and monitored for the development of the disease. Incidence can be calculated because new cases of disease are assessed. If the incidence of disease is greater in the exposed group than in the unexposed group, then the study provides evidence that the exposure is a risk factor for the disease. Because a cohort study can demonstrate that an exposure preceded a disease, it provides strong support for an association. The disadvantages of cohort studies are that they can require long periods of follow-up and can be expensive to conduct. Also, if the disease of interest is rare, large numbers of subjects will need to be followed. The preferred study design for investigating rare diseases is the case-control study.

Case-Control Studies

Case-control studies provide an efficient way to investigate the association between an exposure and a disease, especially a rare disease. In a case-control study, persons with the disease (cases) and persons without the disease (controls) are recruited into the study and assessed for the exposure of interest. If an association exists between the exposure and the disease, then the proportion of exposed persons would be expected to be greater among the cases than the controls.

Because case-control studies do not follow subjects through time, they require fewer resources and can be conducted more quickly than cohort studies. For rare diseases such as oral cancer, recruiting existing cases is much more efficient than enrolling a large, cancer-free cohort and observing the subjects over time. The major disadvantage of the case-control study is that the temporal relationship between the exposure and the onset of disease cannot always be determined because the exposure is usually assessed when the disease status is established. Also, the prevalence or incidence of a disease cannot be determined from a case-control study because the subjects are recruited into the study based on their disease status.

More information on the basics of epidemiology can be found in texts by Gordis and Greenberg et al.[32,33]

DIAGNOSIS

Normal versus Abnormal; Health versus Disease

For epidemiologists to study disease in populations or for clinicians to care for individual patients, they have to be able to identify individuals with disease. For some conditions, the distinction between health and disease is apparent. For example, if a teenager has extensive bone loss around the first molars and lower incisors, the clinical diagnosis of localized, aggressive periodontitis (formerly localized juvenile periodontitis) is obvious. Yet for many conditions, a gray area exists between health and disease. Does a patient with a diastolic blood pressure of 90 mm Hg have hypertension? If the tip of a dental explorer "sticks" on the occlusal surface of a molar with no obvious cavitation, is dental caries present? Does a patient with 3 mm of periodontal attachment loss on only one tooth have periodontitis? The consequences of making the wrong decision could be significant. In clinical practice, misdiagnosing diseased and disease-free patients could mean that persons without disease would face the costs and risks of unnecessary treatment while persons with disease go untreated. In epidemiologic studies, the misclassification of subjects would result in the underestimation or overestimation of the prevalence of disease. It also could lead to invalid conclusions about the association between a disease and some exposure or characteristic.

When making diagnoses, clinicians assimilate information from a variety of sources, such as patient interviews, clinical examinations, radiographs, and laboratory data. From this information, the clinician has to distinguish between normal and abnormal findings. One approach for making this distinction is to consider abnormal as unusual.[28] In clinical practice, this refers to the unexpected or infrequent finding or test result. What is unexpected or infrequent is sometimes based on statistically defined thresholds such as two standard deviations from the mean or the 95th percentile (those in the upper 5%). However, thresholds based on statistical considerations are not adequate for all diseases. As Fletcher et al point out, if the same statistical threshold was chosen for all clinical tests, then the prevalence of all diseases would be the same.[28] Another approach is to establish the threshold using observations associated with an increased risk of disease. For example, 90 mm Hg is chosen as the threshold for hypertension because observations that are above that value are associated with greater risk for developing cardiovascular disease. For a more in-depth discussion of the criteria for abnormality, the interested reader is referred to *Clinical Epidemiology: The Essentials*.[28]

Principles of Diagnostic Testing

Practitioners use diagnostic tests to increase the probability of making correct diagnoses. In dentistry, the diagnosis of periodontal disease is made by the assimilation of clinical and radiographic information, such as bleeding on probing, pocket depth, attachment loss, and bone loss. However, progress is being made in the development of diagnostic tests for periodontal disease. Because periodontal disease is a chronic, infectious disease, microbiologic tests have been developed to detect the presence of specific periodontal pathogens in the gingival sulcus or pockets. These tests are useful for planning treatment for new patients, selecting appropriate recall intervals, monitoring periodontal therapy, determining appropriate antibiotic therapy for patients who do not respond to conventional therapy, and screening patients before extensive restorative or implant therapy.[80] Also, immunologic and biochemical tests to measure the individual's response to periodontal pathogens are being developed. As more of these tests become available, it will become increasingly important for dental practitioners to understand the principles of diagnostic testing.

Sensitivity and Specificity

When a diagnostic test for a disease or condition gives a positive result, the result can be correct (true positive) or incorrect (false positive). When a test gives a negative result, the result can be true (true negative) or false (false negative) (Table 5-1). The ability of a test to give a correct answer is indicated by its sensitivity and specificity.

The sensitivity of a test is the proportion of subjects with the disease who test positive.

$$\text{Sensitivity} = \frac{\text{Number of subjects who test positive}}{\text{Number of subjects with disease}} = \frac{A}{A + C}$$

A highly sensitive test is unlikely to be negative when someone has the disease (false negative). A clinician should choose a highly sensitive test when the consequences of not identifying a person with a disease could be severe, such as during testing for human immunodeficiency virus (HIV) infection. Another example would be a microbiologic test for active periodontal disease.

TABLE 5-1

Comparison of Diagnostic Test Results with True Disease Status

	TRUE DISEASE STATUS	
Test Result	**Disease**	**No Disease**
Positive	A (true positive)	B (false positive)
Negative	C (false negative)	D (true negative)
Sensitivity	A ÷ (A + C)	
Specificity	D ÷ (B + D)	
Positive predictive value	A ÷ (A + B)	
Negative predictive value	D ÷ (C + D)	

Although the consequences would not be as potentially severe as in the HIV example, a false-negative result for active periodontal disease could mean that appropriate therapy would not be prescribed. Sensitive tests also are useful when a clinician wants to rule out possible diseases during the early stages of diagnostic work-ups or screen for diseases during routine physical examinations.[28] Because sensitive tests rarely give false-negative results, sensitive tests are most informative when the results are negative.[28] That is, if the results are negative, the clinician can be reasonably sure the person does not have the disease.

The specificity of a test is the proportion of subjects without the disease who test negative.

$$\text{Specificity} = \frac{\text{Number of subjects who test negative}}{\text{Number of subjects without disease}} = \frac{D}{B + D}$$

A highly specific test is unlikely to be positive when a person does not have the disease (false positive). Specific tests are especially indicated when the misdiagnosis of disease in the absence of disease could harm a person either emotionally, physically, or financially.[28] For example, a false-positive screening test for HIV could cause significant emotional stress until more definitive testing could be performed. Although a false-positive microbiologic test for active periodontal disease could mean unnecessary treatment and expense, it also could mean that a person who desires extensive restorative treatment or dental implants would inappropriately be considered as too high-risk for such care. Because highly specific tests rarely give false-positive results, specific tests are most informative to clinicians when the results are positive.[28]

Ideally, a diagnostic test would be highly sensitive and specific; however, for most tests, sensitivity comes at the expense of specificity and vice versa. This is because most diagnostic test results take on values distributed over a range of values. In such cases, a threshold, or cut-off point, has to be established to distinguish between positive and negative results. As the threshold is moved higher or lower, the sensitivity and the specificity change in opposite directions. Currently, the threshold for hypertension is a diastolic blood pressure of 90 mm Hg. However, if the threshold for hypertension were increased to 100 mm Hg, the number of false positives would decrease (increased specificity) while the number of false negatives would increase (decreased sensitivity). The decision of where to place a threshold for a test depends on the penalty for making the wrong decision. If the penalty for a false-negative result is higher than the penalty for a false positive, then a threshold that makes the test more sensitive should be selected. But if the penalty for a false positive result is higher, a threshold that makes the test more specific should be selected. Because diagnostic tests are rarely both sensitive and specific, a highly sensitive test is sometimes administered first to rule out people who do not have the disease. Then the people who test positive are given a highly specific test to rule in people who have the disease.

Predictive Value

Sensitivity and specificity are characteristics of a diagnostic test that are useful in choosing an appropriate test. However, once a clinician has received the test result, the most relevant question becomes "Given this test result, what is the probability that it is right?" The answer to this question is the predictive value of the test. The probability that a person with a positive test has the disease is called the *positive predictive value of the test* (A ÷ A + B, as shown in Table 5-1). The probability that a person with a negative test does not have the disease is referred to as the *negative predictive value* (D ÷ C + D). For a given diagnostic test, the predictive values are influenced by the prevalence of the disease in the population tested.[28] As the prevalence of disease in the population decreases, a higher proportion of the positive tests are false. As the prevalence of disease increases, a higher proportion of negative tests are false. This situation is better explained by looking at the extremes of prevalence:

> *Imagine a population in which no one has the disease. In such a group, all positive results, even for a very specific test, will be false positives. Therefore as the prevalence of disease in a population approaches zero, the positive predictive value of a test also approaches zero. Conversely, if everyone in a population tested has the disease, all negative results will be false negatives, even for a very sensitive test. As prevalence approaches 100%, negative predictive value approaches zero.*[28]

Because of the influence of prevalence on the predictive values of tests, clinicians have to be aware of the patient's probability of having disease.

RISK VERSUS PROGNOSIS

Risk, Risk Factors, and Risk Assessment

In addition to determining who has a disease at a given point in time, clinicians and epidemiologists are also interested in predicting who will get the disease. The likelihood that a person will get a disease in a specified time period is called *risk*. For any given disease, the risk of developing the disease differs among individuals. The characteristics of individuals that place them at increased risk for getting a disease are called *risk factors*. As the definition implies, exposure to a risk factor must occur before the onset of disease. Exposure to a risk factor may have been at a single point in time, episodic, or continuous. Removal of a risk factor or a reduction in exposure should reduce an individual's risk of getting the disease, but once a person has the disease, removal of the risk factor may not make the disease disappear. And rarely does a single risk factor explain a person's entire risk for a disease. The identification and importance of risk factors for a disease are based on current knowledge, and as knowledge about relationships between factors and disease changes, new factors may become important while previously identified factors become less important or irrelevant.

The process of predicting an individual's probability of disease is called *risk assessment.* Clinicians use risk assessment in several ways. One way is to predict which patients are at risk for disease. For example, people who smoke cigarettes or have diabetes are at a higher risk of developing periodontal disease than nonsmokers or nondiabetics. This information may be important for scheduling the frequency of hygiene appointments. Another way clinicians use risk assessment is to aid in the diagnosis of disease. In adolescent patients with localized bone loss on the lower first molars, the detection of significant numbers of *Actinobacillus actinomycetemcomitans* can help in the diagnosis of early onset periodontitis. Finally, clinicians often use risk assessment to prevent disease by identifying and modifying risk factors. For example, dental providers commonly identify cigarette smokers within their practices and offer smoking cessation services. The amount of disease prevented depends on the success of the intervention in reducing the risk and the number of risk factors associated with the disease.

Prognosis, Prognostic Factors, and Prognosis Assessment

Once disease is identified, the patient's and clinician's attentions usually turn to the course of disease. Unlike risk, which deals with the prediction of new disease, prognosis is the prediction of the course or outcome of the disease. Depending on the disease, important outcomes may include death, survival, or quality of life issues, such as pain and disability. For periodontal disease, important outcomes include tooth loss, recurrent disease, and loss of function. The characteristics or factors that predict the outcome of a disease once disease is present are known as *prognostic factors,* and the process of using prognostic factors to predict the course of a disease is called *prognosis assessment.* In periodontics, factors often considered in the generation of a prognosis include but are not limited to tooth type, furcation involvement, bone loss, pocket depth, tooth mobility, occlusal force, patient's home dental care, presence of systemic disease, and cigarette smoking (see Chapter 32).

As discussed earlier, measures of disease incidence commonly include new periodontal lesions in sites without previous disease and progression of disease in already diseased sites. In reality, the latter event is actually disease progression, not disease incidence. While this distinction may not be extremely important when considering the incidence of disease, the difference between risk factors and prognostic factors should be remembered. Some factors such as smoking may be both risk factors and prognostic factors, while others are either risk factors or prognostic factors. Thus once a person has the disease, two processes must be considered: reducing the risk in healthy sites and increasing the risk for a positive prognosis in the sites with disease.

GINGIVAL DISEASE

Obviously, a gingivitis case involves a person with gingivitis. The more difficult part involves deciding when a person has gingivitis. An early definition of gingivitis simply stated that gingivitis was inflammation of the gingiva.[51] Another definition in the literature states that gingivitis is inflammation of the gingiva in which the junctional epithelium remains attached to the tooth at its original level.[31] This definition implies that gingivitis does not exist if the tooth has periodontitis. In other words, if the inflammatory process involves the gingiva and the periodontium and loss of periodontal attachment has occurred, then according to this definition, the condition should be called *periodontitis,* not gingivitis. The presence of plaque-induced gingivitis in a patient with existing but nonprogressing attachment loss has recently been classified (see Box 4-2). Whether the presence or absence of gingivitis is conditional on the presence of attachment loss has important implications for the estimation of the prevalence of gingivitis.

Although the clinical signs of gingivitis are easy to detect, it is not clear how much inflammation a person must have to be considered a gingivitis case. A universally accepted threshold for the amount or severity of gingival inflammation that must be present in an individual does not exist. In studies of gingivitis, a variety of indices have been used. Because different indices have different clinical criteria for establishing the presence or absence of gingivitis, the definition of a gingivitis case varies across studies. In general, however, a gingivitis case is a person with at least mild inflammation in at least one of the gingival units that are assessed. Depending on the study, a gingival unit may be an anatomic structure of the gingiva, such as the interdental papilla, marginal gingiva, or attached gingiva, or it may be a gingival site defined in relation to a tooth, such as the facial, lingual, mesial, or distal gingiva.

How Is Gingivitis Measured?

Gingivitis is measured by gingival indices. Indices are methods for quantifying the amount and severity of diseases or conditions in individuals or populations. Indices are used in clinical practice to assess the gingival status of patients and follow any changes in gingival status over time. Gingival indices are used in epidemiologic studies to compare the prevalence of gingivitis in population groups. In clinical studies, gingival indices are used to test the efficacy of therapeutic agents or devices. The ideal index is simple and quick to use, accurate, reproducible, and quantitative. All gingival indices measure one or more of the following: gingival color, gingival contour, gingival bleeding, extent of gingival involvement, and gingival crevicular fluid flow.[24] Most indices assign numbers on an ordinal scale (0, 1, 2, 3, and so on) to represent the extent and severity of the gingival condition. These numbers usually can be summarized to represent the gingival status in an individual or a population. The first quantitative methods for assessing gingivitis appeared around the end of World War II. Many gingival indices have been introduced since that time, and no single index has universal application or acceptance.[45]

TABLE 5-2

Criteria for the Gingival Index

Score	Criteria
0	Normal gingiva
1	Mild inflammation: slight change in color and slight edema. *No bleeding on probing.*
2	Moderate inflammation: redness, edema, and glazing. *Bleeding on probing.*
3	Severe inflammation: marked redness and edema. Ulceration. *Tendency toward spontaneous bleeding.*

From Löe H: The gingival index, the plaque index, and the retention index systems. J Periodontol 1967; 38:610(suppl).

TABLE 5-3

Criteria for the Modified Gingival Index

Score	Criteria
0	Absence of inflammation
1	Mild inflammation: slight change in color, little change in texture of any portion of but not the entire marginal or papillary gingival unit
2	Mild inflammation: criteria as above but involving the entire marginal or papillary gingival unit
3	Moderate inflammation: glazing, redness, edema, and/or hypertrophy of the marginal or papillary gingival unit
4	Severe inflammation: marked redness, edema, and/or hypertrophy of the marginal or papillary gingival unit; spontaneous bleeding, congestion, or ulceration

From Lobene RR, Weatherfor T, Ross NM, et al: A modified gingival index for use in clinical trials. Clin Prevent Dent 1986; 8(1):3.

Gingival Index. The gingival index (GI) was proposed in 1963 as a method for assessing the severity and quantity of gingival inflammation in individual patients or among subjects in large population groups (Table 5-2).[47,49] Only gingival tissues are assessed with the GI. According to this method, each of the four gingival areas of the tooth (facial, mesial, distal, and lingual) is assessed for inflammation and given a score from 0 to 3. The criteria for quantifying the severity of gingival inflammation are shown in Table 5-2. Bleeding is assessed by running a periodontal probe along the soft tissue wall of the gingival crevice. The scores for the four areas of the tooth can be totaled and divided by four to give a tooth score. By adding the tooth scores together and dividing by the number of teeth examined, an individual's GI score can be obtained. The gingival areas of all teeth or selected teeth can be assessed. A GI score of 0.1 to 1.0 indicates mild inflammation, 1.1 to 2.0 indicates moderate inflammation, and 2.1 to 3.0 indicates severe inflammation.[47]

Modified Gingival Index. The modified gingival index (MGI) introduced two important changes to the GI: 1) elimination of gingival probing to assess the presence or absence of bleeding and 2) redefinition of the scoring system for mild and moderate inflammation (Table 5-3).[46] The developers of the MGI decided to eliminate probing, which could disturb plaque and irritate the gingiva.[46] A noninvasive index would allow for repeated evaluations and permit intracalibration and intercalibration of examiners.[46] Also, the developers wanted an index that would be more sensitive to earlier, more subtle changes in gingival inflammation.[46] To achieve this, they assigned a score of 1 to mild inflammation that involved only a portion of the marginal or papillary gingival unit and a score of 2 to mild inflammation that involved the entire marginal or papillary gingival unit. Scores of 3 and 4 correspond with the original scores of 2 and 3, respectively, of the GI. The scoring criteria for the MGI can be found in Table 5-3. As with the GI, four gingival units per tooth (two marginal, two papillary) are assessed. Either a full or partial mouth assessment can be performed. A mean score for an individual can be calculated by summing the gingival unit scores and dividing by the number of gingival units examined.

The MGI is perhaps the most widely used index in clinical trials of therapeutic agents.[24] Like its predecessors, the MGI does not assess the presence of periodontal pockets or attachment loss. Thus these indices cannot identify gingivitis in the absence of periodontitis.

Gingival Bleeding Indices. Whereas the clinical assessment of gingival color, form, and texture is subjective in nature, gingival bleeding is an objective diagnostic sign of inflammation. Research suggests that bleeding upon the gentle probing of the gingival sulcus may occur before changes in color, form, or texture are apparent.[34,37,53] Since 1974, numerous indices that measure bleeding only, such as the gingival bleeding index and the Eastman interdental bleeding index, have been published and reviewed elsewhere.[21,23,56] Periodontal probes are used with most indices; however, toothpicks and dental floss are used to elicit bleeding with some indices.[56] Among the indices that require the use of periodontal probes, the type of probe and the angulation, depth, and force of probing vary. Even though gingival bleeding is a sign of inflammation, the bleeding from the gingival sulcus may be associated with other forms of periodontal disease, not just gingivitis. For indices that require insertion of the periodontal probe to the bottom of the gingival sulcus, bleeding may be a sign of periodontitis rather than gingivitis. Gingival bleeding indices are used in clinical practice, surveys of population groups, and clinical trials of antiplaque and antigingivitis agents.

NIDCR Protocol for the Assessment of Gingival Bleeding. In several of its national surveys, such as the NIDR National Survey of Oral Health in U.S. Employed Adults and Seniors (1985–86) and the Third National Health and Nutrition Examination Survey (1988–94), the

National Institute of Dental and Craniofacial Research (NIDCR) has used the presence or absence of gingival bleeding as an indication of gingival health. The gingival assessment is just one of several components of the NIDCR protocol for the assessment of periodontal disease. For this approach, the facial and mesiofacial sites of teeth in two randomly selected quadrants, one maxillary and one mandibular, are assessed for bleeding. A special probe known as the *NIDR probe* is used in these assessments. The NIDR probe is color coded and is graduated at 2, 4, 6, 8, 10, and 12 mm. To begin the assessment, the examiner dries a quadrant of teeth with air. Then, starting with the most posterior tooth in the quadrant (excluding the third molar), the examiner places a periodontal probe 2 mm into the sulcus at the facial site and carefully sweeps the probe into the mesial interproximal area. After probing the sites in the quadrant, the examiner assesses the presence or absence of bleeding at each probed site. The same procedure is repeated for the remaining quadrant. For an individual, the number or percent of teeth or sites with bleeding can be calculated. For population groups, the prevalence of gingival bleeding, usually defined as bleeding at one or more sites, can be determined.

How Much Gingivitis Is Present?

The most recent data on the dental health of the U.S. population come from the third National Health and Nutrition Examination Survey (NHANES III), conducted from 1988 to 1994. The survey was the seventh in a series of national surveys designed to provide estimates of the health status of the U.S. population. This survey used the NIDCR protocol for gingival bleeding, which involves placing the probe in the gingival sulcus at a depth of 2 mm and sweeping the probe from the mesiofacial to the mesial interproximal area. According to data from NHANES III, 54% of the noninstitutionalized civilian U.S. population aged 13 years and older had gingival bleeding in at least one gingival site.[75] Gingival bleeding was most prevalent in the 13- to 17-year-old age group (63%) and declined gradually through the 35- to 44-year-old age group (Fig. 5-1). The prevalence increased again at the 45- to 54-year-old age group but remained fairly constant in older age groups. On average per person, 10% of all sites had gingival bleeding; however, among persons with gingival bleeding, an average of 18% of sites had gingival bleeding. The extent of gingival bleeding among persons with gingival bleeding was higher in the younger and older age groups than in the middle age groups (Fig. 5-2).

A study of U.S. school children ages 14 to 17 years reported that the prevalence of gingival bleeding was 61.5%, essentially identical to the prevalence reported among 13- to 17-year-olds in the NHANES III study.[15] Both surveys used the NIDCR gingival sweep method for eliciting gingival bleeding. The prevalence decreased with age from a high of 65% in 14-year-olds to a low of 57% in 17-year-olds. On average per child, 6% of sites measured had gingival bleeding with probing.

In NHANES III, gingival bleeding was assessed at periodontal sites without regard to the periodontal status of the tooth. One definition of gingivitis states that gingivitis is inflammation of the gingiva in which the junctional epithelium remains attached to the tooth at its original level.[31] If the prevalence of gingival bleeding from NHANES III data is recalculated using only periodontal sites without attachment loss (<1 mm), the prevalence of one or more sites per person with gingival bleeding decreases slightly from 54% to 47%. This indicates that about 7% of the people had bleeding only in sites with attachment loss. The remainder of individuals either did not have any bleeding in sites with

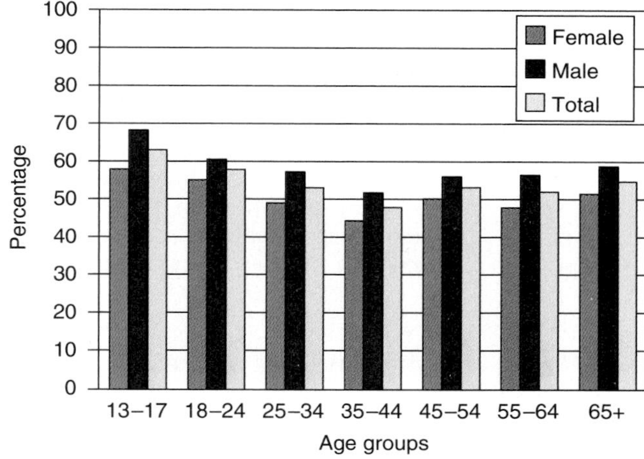

Fig. 5-1 Percentage of persons in the United States with one or more sites of gingival bleeding. (Courtesy U.S. Department of Health and Human Services: National Center for Health Statistics. Third National Health and Nutrition Examination Survey, 1988–1994, NHANES III Examination Data File [CD-ROM]. Public Use Data File Documentation Number 76200. Hyattsville, MD, Centers for Disease Control and Prevention, 1996.)

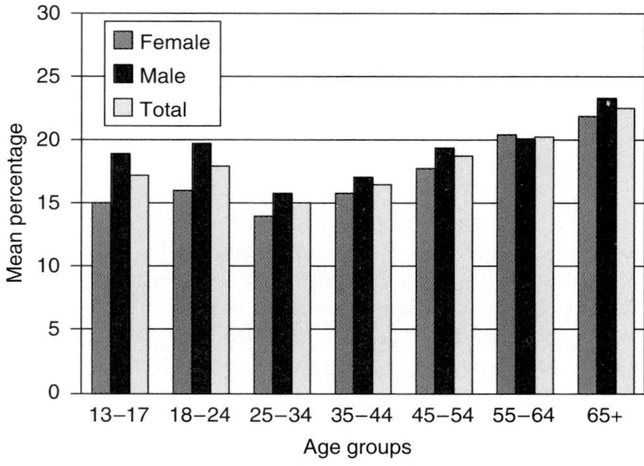

Fig. 5-2 The mean percentage of sites per person with gingival bleeding among persons in the United States with gingival bleeding. (Courtesy U.S. Department of Health and Human Services: National Center for Health Statistics. Third National Health and Nutrition Examination Survey, 1988–1994, NHANES III Examination Data File [CD-ROM]. Public Use Data File Documentation Number 76200. Hyattsville, MD, Centers for Disease Control and Prevention, 1996.)

attachment loss or had bleeding in sites with and without attachment loss.

Is More or Less Gingivitis Present Now than Previously?

Although it is generally believed that the prevalence of gingivitis is declining in the U.S., the epidemiologic data needed to make that claim do not exist.[8] Since 1960, several national health surveys have assessed periodontal health—the Health Examination Survey (HES) (1960–62), NHANES I (1971–74), the Health Resources and Services Administration (HRSA) survey of households (1981), the National Institute of Dental Research (NIDR) study of employed adults (1985–86), and NHANES III (1988–94). However, because of differences in populations, sampling methods, and periodontal measurement methods, comparisons of results between these surveys are difficult, if not impossible, to make. Table 5-4 summarizes periodontal findings from studies based on data from these surveys. Even if results from these studies could be compared, they do not support the view that the prevalence of gingivitis is declining.

Does My Patient with Gingivitis Fit the Typical Profile?

Gingivitis is so common that any patient presenting with gingivitis could be considered typical; however, gingivitis is more prevalent among certain groups. Adolescents have a higher prevalence of gingivitis than prepubertal children or adults. The rise of sex hormones during adolescence is suspected to be the cause of the increased prevalence. Studies suggest that the increase in sex hormones during puberty affects the composition of the subgingival microflora.[35,52,54] One study found that increased serum levels of testosterone in boys and estradiol and progesterone in girls was associated with increased levels of the periodontal pathogens *Prevotella intermedia* and *Prevotella nigrescens*.[54] Hormonal effects also may be responsible for the increased prevalence during pregnancy and among women using oral contraceptives. Estimates of the prevalence of gingivitis during pregnancy range from 30% to 100%.[29]

As shown in Fig. 5-1, males in all age groups are more likely to have gingivitis than females. The prevalence of gingivitis is especially high for males aged 13 to 17 years. Also, males with gingivitis have more involved sites than females (see Fig. 5-2), especially in the younger age groups. Although the reason for the existence of these gender differences is not known, poorer plaque control among males could likely explain much of their higher prevalence and extent of disease.

Why Do Patients Have Gingivitis, and What Puts Them at Risk?

It is clear from experimental and epidemiologic studies that microbial plaque is the direct cause of gingivitis.[44,50,59,65] The cause and effect relationship between plaque and gingival inflammation was demonstrated in a classic study by Löe et al.[50] In that study, 12 individuals (9 dental students, 1 instructor, and 2 laboratory technicians) were asked to abstain from all measures of oral hygiene. Dental plaque began to form quickly, and the amount of plaque increased with time. All subjects developed gingivitis within 10 to 21 days. The mean GI score increased from 0.27 at baseline to 1.05 at the end of the "no-brushing" period. Gingival inflammation resolved in all subjects within 1 week of resuming hygiene measures. The authors concluded that bacterial plaque was essential in the production of gingival inflammation.

Because bacterial plaque is the cause of the most common form of gingivitis, factors that influence the oral hygiene status of individuals would likely influence the prevalence of gingivitis. The generally poorer oral hygiene status of males may explain the higher prevalence and extent among males.[3] Poorer oral hygiene also may explain the higher prevalence of gingivitis among adolescents. Even though the increased levels of circulating sex hormones have been implicated in the higher prevalence, the influence of plaque control on gingivitis may be more important than the rising levels of hormones.[74] The conversion of bleeding gingival sites to nonbleeding sites with oral hygiene interventions alone provide string evidence for the role of poor oral hygiene in the etiology of gingivitis.[7,16,22]

Few population-based studies of the association between oral hygiene status and gingivitis have been published. In NHANES I, information on toothbrushing frequency and oral hygiene status were collected. A study that investigated the associations between these factors and the periodontal index (PI) reported that increased toothbrushing frequency and better oral hygiene scores were associated with lower PI scores.[76] These associations remained statistically significant after controlling for age, race, socioeconomic status, alcohol consumption, smoking habits, and dental visits. Although this study was based on the PI, an index of periodontal disease, gingivitis is a component of all but the most severe category. In NHANES III, information on the presence or absence of calculus was collected. However, this study has not reported any association between calculus and gingival health.

Although smoking is one of the most important risk factors for adult periodontitis, its role in gingivitis is unclear. Several studies have indicated that gingival bleeding is reduced among smokers.[14,66] Plaque levels in the smokers were either similar to or greater than plaque levels in nonsmokers. This reduction in gingival bleeding among smokers is perhaps the result of the vasoconstrictive effects of nicotine in cigarette smoke. In clinical practice, the smoking status of patients should be considered when gingival bleeding is assessed.

CHRONIC PERIODONTITIS

Periodontitis is inflammation of the periodontium that extends beyond the gingiva and produces destruction of the connective tissue attachment of the teeth.[68] No longer considered a single disease, periodontitis is now considered to exist in three primary forms: chronic, aggressive, and as a manifestation of systemic diseases (see Box 4-4). Chronic periodontitis is the most common

TABLE 5-4

U.S. Population–Based Prevalence Studies* of Periodontal Disease

Survey	Year(s) Conducted	Population Sampled	Age at Periodontal Assessment	Method of Periodontal Assessment	Prevalence of Gingivitis	Prevalence of Periodontal Pockets	Prevalence of Attachment Loss
HES[26]	1960–62	Total civilian, noninstitutionalized population aged 18 to 79 years	18 to 79 years	Periodontal index; no probing	48.5%	25.4% with pockets Average PI per person: 1.13	Not assessed
HANES I[27]	1971–74	Total civilian, noninstitutionalized population aged 1 to 74 years	6 to 74 years	Periodontal index; no probing	25%	4.5% with 1 to 3 pockets 12.1% with ≥4 pockets Average PI per person: 0.83	Not assessed
HRSA[28]	1981	Households (including military personnel and their families)	19 years of age and older	Periodontal index (with modifications) Pocket depth measured in mm at mesial of every permanent erupted tooth	50% with gingivitis without any pockets ≥4 mm	28% with 1 or more teeth with pockets 4 to 6 mm 8% with 1 or more teeth with a pocket ≥6 mm	Not assessed
NIDR[29]	1985–86	Employed persons aged 18 to 64 years	18 to 64 years	Bleeding on probing. Ramfjord probing technique: Measured mesiofacial and midfacial sites in one upper and one lower quadrant (maximum of 28 sites in 14 teeth)	44% with one or more sites with bleeding	13.4% with one or more sites with pockets 4 to 6 mm 0.6% with one or more sites with pockets ≥ 7 mm	43.8% with one or more sites with attachment loss ≥ 3mm
NHANES III[30]	1988–1994	Total civilian, noninstitutionalized population aged 2 months and older	13 years and older	Bleeding on probing. Ramfjord probing technique: Measured mesofacial and midfacial sites in one upper and one lower quadrant (maximum of 28 sites in 14 teeth)	54% with one or more sites with bleeding	21.0% with one or more sites with pockets ≥4 mm	38.1% with one or more sites with attachment loss ≥ 3 mm

* References refer to published studies that analyzed data from these surveys. Periodontal findings in any given column are from the study referenced in the second column.

form. Chronic periodontitis progresses slowly and generally becomes clinically significant in adults but may be observed in children. For epidemiologic purposes, a case of chronic periodontitis is a person with the disease. As with gingivitis, methods to measure periodontitis and the amount of disease necessary to consider a person a case vary widely across studies.

How Is Periodontitis Measured?

Periodontal Index. In the early 1950s, gingivitis indices were gaining in popularity; however, no index was available to measure more advanced stages of periodontal disease. Motivated by the lack of valid indices for measuring the prevalence of periodontal disease in population groups, Russell developed the PI (Table 5-5).[69] Use of the PI requires a minimum of equipment—a light source, a mouth mirror, and an explorer. The supporting tissues for each tooth in the mouth are scored according to a progressive scale that gives little weight to gingival inflammation and relatively great weight to advanced periodontal disease.[69] The scoring criteria for the PI are shown in Table 5-5. An individual's score is the sum of the tooth scores divided by the number of teeth examined. The population score is the sum of the individual scores divided by the number of persons examined. Periodontal probing was not recommended because, according to Russell, it "added little and proved to be a troublesome focus of examiner disagreement."[69]

TABLE 5-5

Criteria for the Periodontal Index

Score	Criteria and Scoring for Field Studies
0	Negative: There is neither overt inflammation in the investing tissues nor loss of function due to destruction of supporting tissues.
1	Mild gingivitis: There is an overt area of inflammation in the free gingiva, but this area does not circumscribe the tooth.
2	Gingivitis: Inflammation completely circumscribes the tooth, but there is no apparent break in the epithelial atachment.
6	Gingivitis with pocket formation: The epithelial attachment has been broken, and there is a pocket (not merely a deepened gingival crevice due to swelling in the free gingiva). There is no interference with normal masticatory function, the tooth is firm in its socket, and it has not drifted.
8	Advanced destruction with loss of masticatory function: The tooth may be loose, may have drifted, may sound dull on percussion with a metallic instrument, or may be depressible in its socket.

Modified from Russell AL: A system of classification and scoring for prevalence surveys of periodontal disease. J Dent Res 1954; 35(3):350.

The PI is fast and easy to use. However, one important criticism of the index is that it underestimates the prevalence of disease.[67]

Periodontal Disease Index. As a consultant to the World Health Organization for a 1957 study of periodontal disease in India, Ramfjord was faced with the inadequacies of the available indices for measuring periodontal disease.[67] Taking the most valuable features of existing indices and adding new features to compensate for their shortcomings, Ramfjord developed his own system for measuring periodontal disease.[67] This system became known as the *periodontal disease index (PDI)*. One unique aspect of the PDI was the examination of six preselected teeth in the mouth—the maxillary right first molar, maxillary left central incisor, maxillary left first premolar, mandibular left first molar, mandibular right central incisor, and mandibular right first premolar. This selection of teeth became known as the *Ramfjord teeth*. Another unique aspect of the PDI was the use of the cementoenamel junction as a fixed landmark for measuring periodontal attachment loss.

To begin an assessment using the PDI, the examiner dries the areas around the six teeth. Next, the examiner assesses the severity of gingival inflammation around the six teeth. Gingival scores for a tooth range from G0 for absence of inflammation to G3 for severe gingivitis. At the mesial, facial, distal, and lingual side of each of the six teeth, the distance from the free gingival margin to the cementoenamel junction and the distance from the free gingival margin to the bottom of the gingival sulcus are measured in millimeters with a periodontal probe. If the free gingival margin is on the cementum, its distance from the cementoenamel junction is recorded as a negative number. The distance from the cementoenamel junction to the bottom of the gingival sulcus is the difference between these two measurements. The distance from the cementoenamel junction to the bottom of the gingival sulcus is a measurement of periodontal attachment loss. Ramfjord's method for measuring this distance is commonly referred to as the *indirect method for measuring periodontal attachment loss*. The PDI score for each tooth is based on the assessment of gingival inflammation and the depth of the gingival sulcus in relation to the cementoenamel junction (Table 5-6). If the gingival sulcus does not extend apically to the cementoenamel junction in any of the measured areas, then the PDI score for the tooth is the gingival score. If the gingival sulcus extends below the cementoenamel junction in any of the measured areas by 3 mm or less, then the PDI score is 4. Teeth with sulcus measurements of 3 to 6 mm and greater than 6 mm are given scores of 5 and 6, respectively. The PDI for the individual is the sum of the tooth scores divided by the number of teeth examined. If any of the six preselected teeth are missing, another tooth is not substituted in its place. In addition to the PDI score for periodontal disease, the PDI provides a method for calculating tooth scores for calculus, occlusal attrition, mobility, and proximal contacts.

Although the PDI is rarely used today, two aspects of the index are commonly used: selection of the six Ramfjord teeth and the method for measuring pocket depth and loss of periodontal attachment. Ramfjord's technique for measuring pocket depth and periodontal attachment loss has been used in national surveys such as the National Health and Nutritional Examination Surveys.

Extent and Severity Index. The PI and the PDI yield scores that represent the severity of periodontal disease in individuals or populations, but these scores do not provide information on the extent of disease. The extent and severity index (ESI) of periodontal disease was developed to provide separate estimates of the extent and severity of periodontal disease in individuals and populations.[20] Unlike the PI and PDI, the ESI does not assess gingival inflammation. Instead, it estimates the loss of periodontal attachment using the periodontal probing method developed by Ramfjord for the PDI.[67] A threshold of disease has to be established to calculate the extent score for an individual. In their initial study of the ESI, Carlos et al considered a site to be diseased when attachment loss exceeded 1 mm.[20] (Because the measurements are always rounded down to the next lowest millimeter, greater than 1 mm means ≥2 mm.) For an individual, the extent score is the percentage of sites examined that have attachment loss greater than 1 mm. The severity score for an individual is the average loss of attachment per site among the disease sites. The ESI is expressed as a bivariate statistic: ESI = (Extent, Severity). For example, an individual's ESI of (20, 3.0) would be interpreted as 20% of sites examined had disease, and of the diseased sites, the average loss of attachment was 3.0 mm. The ESI for a population would be the average extent and severity scores for the individuals examined.

When ESI scores from two sites per tooth in the whole mouth were compared with an assessment of one upper and one lower quadrant, the developers of the ESI found that little information was lost from the half-mouth assessment.[20] However, the ESI has been used for full-mouth examinations on as many as six sites per tooth.

NIDCR Protocol for Periodontal Disease Assessment. The NIDCR periodontal disease assessment, as used in NHANES III, contains three parts: a periodontal destruction assessment, gingival assessment, and calculus assessment.[55] The gingival assessment was previously described in the section on gingivitis. The periodontal destruction examination involves an assessment of loss of periodontal attachment and furcation involvement. Loss of attachment is the distance (in millimeters) from the cementoenamel junction to the bottom of the gingival sulcus. This distance is measured at the facial and mesiofacial sites of teeth in two randomly selected quadrants, one maxillary and one mandibular, using the indirect measurement method developed by Ramfjord.[67] Probing is carried out with the use of the NIDCR probe, which is color coded and has markings at 2, 4, 6, 8, 10, and 12 mm. In NHANES III, loss of attachment was reported in millimeters for each site measured. Periodontal pocket depth, which is the distance from the free gingival margin to the bottom of the sulcus, also was reported in millimeters for each site.

Furcation involvement is assessed on eight teeth: the maxillary first and second molars, the maxillary first premolars, and the mandibular first and second molars. The assessment requires the use of a #17 dental explorer for the maxillary teeth and a #3 cowhorn explorer for the mandibular teeth. The extent of furcation involvement is assessed at the mesial, facial, and distal of the maxillary molars, the mesial and distal of the premolars, and the facial and lingual of the mandibular molars. If furcation involvement does not exist, the site is scored as 0.

TABLE 5-6

Criteria for the Periodontal Disease Index

GINGIVAL ASSESSMENT

Score	Criteria
G0	Absence of inflammation
G1	Mild to moderate inflammatory gingival changes not extending all around the tooth
G2	Mild to moderate severe gingivitis extending all around the tooth
G3	Severe gingivitis characterized by marked redness, tendency to bleed, and ulceration

RECORD POCKETS

The distance from the free gingival margin to the cementoenamel junction and the distance from the free gingival margin to the bottom of the gingival crevice or pocket should be recorded for the mesial, facial, distal, and lingual aspects of each tooth examined. The interproximal recording should be secured at the buccal aspect of the interproximal contact areas with the probe pointing in the direction of the long axis of the tooth.

If the gingival margin is on the enamel:

1. Measure from the gum margin to the cementoenamel junction, and record the measurement on the crown of the schematic tooth. If the epithelial attachment is on the crown and the cementoenamel junction cannot be felt by the probe, record the depth of the gingival crevice on the crown.
2. Measure from the gingival margin to the bottom of the pocket when the crevice extends apically to the cementoenamel junction. The measurement should be recorded on the root of the schematic tooth. (The distance from the cementoenamel junction to the bottom of the pocket can then be found by subtracting measurement 1 from measurement 2.)

If the gingival margin is on the cementum:

1. Measure from the cementoenamel junction to the gingival margin. Record as minus value on the root of the schematic tooth.
2. Measure from the cementoenamel junction to the bottom of the gingival crevice. Record value on the root.

Modified from Ramfjord SP: Indices for prevalence and incidence of periodontal disease. J Periodontol 1959; 30:51.

If partial involvement exists but the probe cannot pass through the furcation, the site is scored as 1. If the explorer can pass between the roots (through involvement), the site is scored as 2.

At each site assessed for loss of attachment, the presence or absence of supragingival and subgingival calculus is assessed. Subgingival calculus is detected using the NIDCR probe. A score of 0 is recorded for the site if no calculus is present, a score of 1 is recorded if only supragingival calculus is present, and a score of 2 is recorded if supragingival and subgingival calculus are present.

Radiographic Assessment of Bone Loss. The radiographic assessment of bone loss is an important part of the clinical diagnosis of periodontal disease. However, for the purposes of estimating the prevalence or incidence of periodontitis in population groups, radiographs are rarely used because of ethical and practical considerations. In studies in which radiographic bone loss is used as a measure of periodontitis, bone loss is usually measured from bite-wing radiographs as the distance from the cementoenamel junction to the alveolar crest. Bone loss can be expressed as this distance in millimeters or as a percentage of the root length. Various studies have used bone loss thresholds ranging from >1 mm to >3 mm.[10] Bone loss measurements from radiographs are highly correlated with measurements of attachment loss taken with periodontal probes.[10] The three main sources of error in the assessment of bone loss are 1) variations in projection geometry, 2) variations in film contrast and density, and 3) obstruction of the view by other anatomic structures.[10] Computerized programs can detect bone changes as small as 0.5 mm when measuring bone loss from sequential radiographs.[40] Also, advanced image-processing techniques such as digital subtraction radiography and computer-assisted densitometric image analysis can enhance the ability to detect bone loss over time.[40]

How Much Chronic Periodontitis Is Present?

The most recent data for the prevalence of periodontal disease in the U.S. comes from NHANES III (1988–94). Because the assessment of periodontitis in a cross-sectional survey such as NHANES III is a cumulative measure of periodontal destruction, separating chronic periodontitis in adults from other forms is not possible. However, an analysis of NHANES III data for adults aged 30 years and older was recently reported.[4] The prevalence of periodontal attachment loss is greatly dependent on the threshold chosen, ranging from a high of 99% for a threshold of >1 mm to a low of 7% for a threshold of >7 mm (Fig. 5-3). At a threshold of >3 mm, the prevalence of attachment loss in at least one site in the mouth was 53.1%. The prevalence of attachment loss increased steadily with age, from a low of 35.7% for the 30- to 39-year-old age group to a high of 89.2% for the 80- to 90-year-old age group (Fig. 5-4). On average per person, 19.6% of the teeth had attachment loss of >3 mm. Among people with at least one site of attachment loss of >3 mm, an average of 36.6% of the teeth per person were affected. The mean percentage of teeth affected also increased with age (Fig. 5-5). Maxillary molars and mandibular incisors were more likely than other teeth to have attachment loss of >3 mm, whereas maxillary central incisors were the least likely.

As with attachment loss, the prevalence of periodontal pockets is greatly dependent on the threshold chosen (Fig. 5-6). Generally, pockets greater than 3 mm are considered to reflect disease. The prevalence of periodontal pockets >4 mm was 23.1%. The increase in the prevalence of attachment loss with increasing age is not seen with pocket depth (Fig. 5-7). The average extent of pockets >4 mm was 5.2% of teeth per person, and the extent varied little with age (Fig. 5-8).

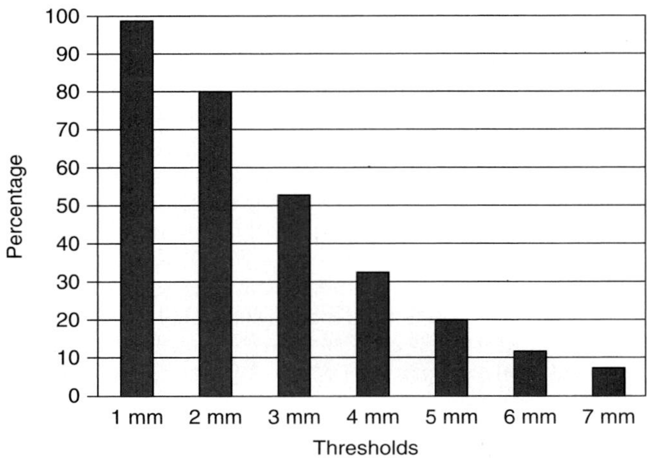

Fig. 5-3 Percentage of persons in the United States with periodontal attachment loss according to different thresholds of attachment loss. (From Albandar JM, Brunelle JA, Kingman A: Destructive periodontal disease in adults 30 years of age and older in the United States, 1988–1994. J Periodontol 1999; 70[1]:13.)

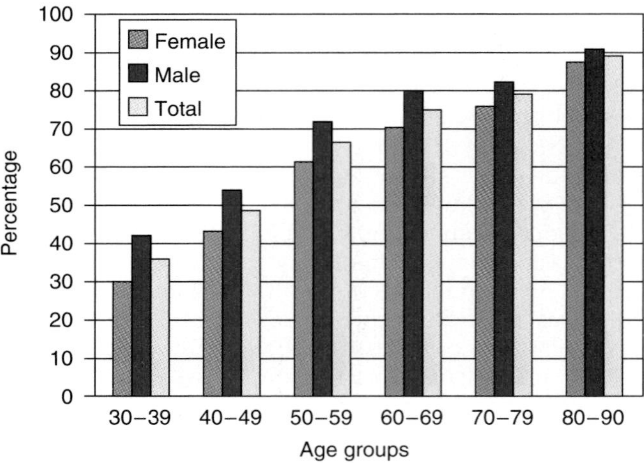

Fig. 5-4 Percentage of persons in the United States with periodontal attachment loss of >3 mm. (From Albandar JM, Brunelle JA, Kingman A: Destructive periodontal disease in adults 30 years of age and older in the United States, 1988–1994. J Periodontol 1999; 70[1]:13.)

The answer to the question "How much adult periodontitis is out there?" must be "It depends on the case definition used."

Is More or Less Chronic Periodontitis Present Now than Previously?

It is frequently stated that the prevalence of periodontal disease has decreased in the U.S. over the past 30 years. However, because of methodologic differences in the national surveys conducted over the years, making any conclusions about changes in the prevalence of periodontal disease is difficult. Drawing any conclusions about trends in the chronic form of periodontitis is even more difficult. A comparison of the methodologies and results from five national surveys conducted in the U.S. can be found in Table 5-4. The first two surveys, the HES (1960–62) and HANES I (1971–74), used the PI to measure periodontal disease. The PI relies only on visible signs of inflammation to determine the severity of periodontal disease. The presence of periodontal pockets was estimated by the presence of clinical signs, and clinical attachment loss was not measured. The HRSA survey of U.S. households (1981) was the first national survey to directly measure the depth of periodontal pockets with a periodontal probe; however, periodontal attachment loss was not measured. The last two national surveys, the NIDR survey of employed persons (1985–86) and the

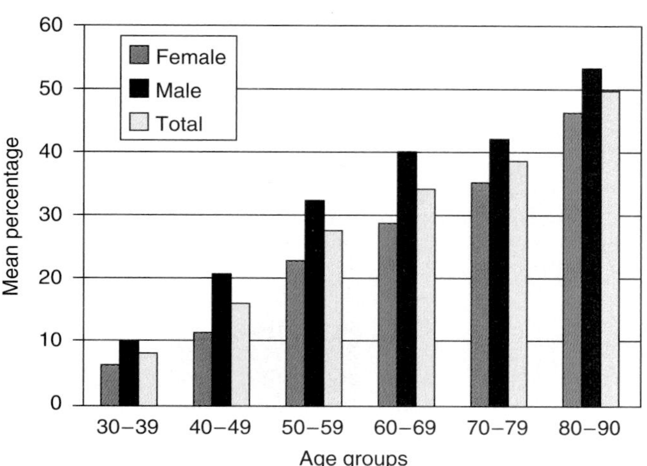

Fig. 5-5 Mean percentage of teeth per person in the United States with attachment loss of >3 mm. (From Albandar JM, Brunelle JA, Kingman A: Destructive periodontal disease in adults 30 years of age and older in the United States, 1988–1994. J Periodontol 1999; 70[1]:13.)

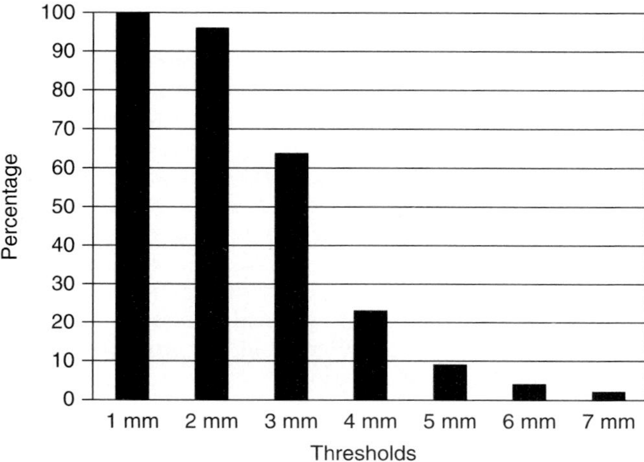

Fig. 5-6 Percentage of persons in the United States with periodontal pockets according to different thresholds of pocket depth. (From Albandar JM, Brunelle JA, Kingman A: Destructive periodontal disease in adults 30 years of age and older in the United States, 1988–1994. J Periodontol 1999; 70[1]:13.)

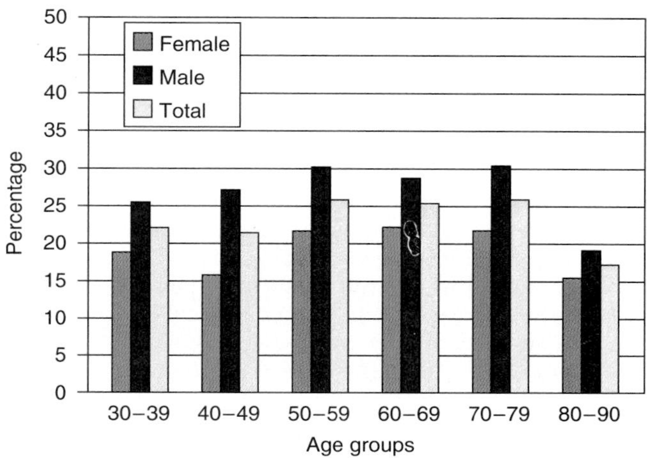

Fig. 5-7 Percentage of persons in the United States with periodontal pockets of >4 mm. (From Albandar JM, Brunelle JA, Kingman A: Destructive periodontal disease in adults 30 years of age and older in the United States, 1988–1994. J Periodontol 1999; 70[1]:13.)

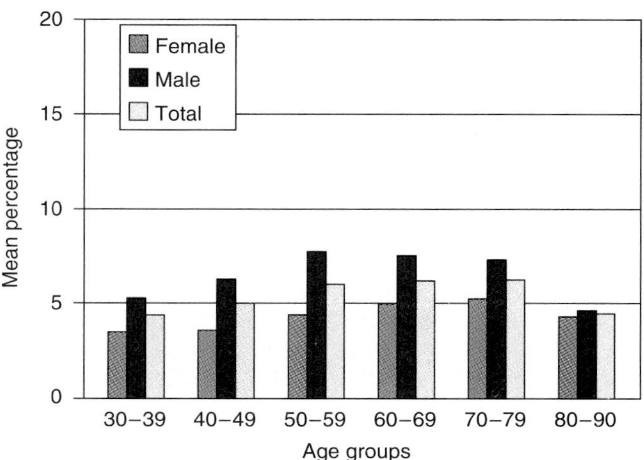

Fig. 5-8 Mean percentage of teeth per person in the United States with pocket depths of >4 mm. (From Albandar JM, Brunelle JA, Kingman A: Destructive periodontal disease in adults 30 years of age and older in the United States, 1988–1994. J Periodontol 1999; 70[1]:13.)

NHANES III (1988–94), used the Ramfjord technique for measuring pocket depth and attachment loss, but the NIDR survey only included employed persons, thereby excluding major groups in the U.S.

Conclusions about trends in periodontal disease will not be available until a series of national surveys that similarly measure periodontal disease are conducted. However, as Douglas and Fox concluded in their study of trends in periodontal disease, "Even if the prevalence and severity of periodontal disease are seen as declining over the next 30 years, it would seem that a substantial proportion of this decline will be counterbalanced by the sizable increase in number of persons and number of teeth per person at risk of disease."[26] In fact, Douglas and Fox estimated that for U.S. adults who are over the age of 25 years, the number of adults with some manifestation of periodontal disease would increase at least through the year 2010.[26]

How Much New or Progressing Chronic Periodontitis Is Present?

In contrast to prevalence data, no nationally representative longitudinal studies are available in the U.S. The incidence rates must be taken from studies representative of local or regional groups in the U.S. and other countries.

A 10-year follow-up study among Chinese individuals aged 20 to 80 years found that 79.8% of all sites measured (4 sites per tooth) experienced attachment loss.[11] Approximately 48% of the sites measured lost >2 mm, 21.8% of the sites lost >3 mm, and 9% of the sites lost >4 mm. The average attachment level change per person was between 1.45 and 1.86 mm during the follow-up period, corresponding with 0.15 to 0.19 mm per year. Because very little difference in mean attachment loss by age groups existed, the researchers concluded that the influence of age on the rate of periodontal disease progression might be minimal. According to the researchers, the rate of disease progression in this group of Chinese individuals, who had limited access to dental care and poor dental hygiene, was similar to the rate of progression found in other populations around the world.

The Chinese study made no distinction between attachment level changes in sites without disease at the baseline examination and in sites that had existing disease. One study that made a distinction between disease onset and disease progression was a study of community-dwelling older adults (age 65 years and older) living in five contiguous North Carolina counties.[13] The subjects, who were followed for 36 months, were categorized into four groups according to their type of periodontal attachment loss: 1) those who only had attachment loss in previously nondiseased sites, 2) those with only progression of attachment loss in previously diseased sites, 3) those who experienced both types of attachment loss, and 4) those who had no new sites with attachment loss. The researchers considered change to be 3 or more mm of attachment loss over the 3-year period. The researchers found that 40% of the people had no change in their baseline attachment level, 27.5% of the people experienced only new lesions, 11.1% of the people only had attachment loss in sites that had attachment loss at baseline, and 20.1% of the people had both kinds of attachment loss.

Table 5-7 summarizes four other cohort studies—one from Japan, one from the U.S., and two from Sweden. Follow-up times for the four studies ranged from 1 year to 28 years. The two Swedish studies used radiographs to assess changes in alveolar bone height, whereas the studies from the U.S. and Japan used periodontal probing to assess changes in clinical attachment levels. Mean annual loss of bone or attachment loss per person, ranging from approximately 0.03 mm to 0.14 mm, was fairly consistent across the three studies that reported this information. Each study shows that attachment loss or alveolar bone loss progressed in only a small percentage of periodontal sites and subjects. In the study by Ismail et al, 59.3% of the periodontal sites present at baseline showed no change in attachment loss over the 28 years of follow-up. Only 13.3% of the subjects had a mean change in attachment loss of 2 mm or greater. Approximately 90% of the sites followed in the study by Albandar et al showed no change in bone height in the 6 years that passed between baseline and reexamination. In that study, 70% of the subjects had few or no sites with additional bone loss. From the results in these studies, adult periodontitis appears to progress fairly slowly and in only a minority of the adult population.

Does My Patient with Chronic Periodontitis Fit the Typical Profile?

Chronic periodontitis generally becomes clinically significant after age 30.[68] The disease is characterized by a slow progression of attachment loss over time. With 53% of U.S. adults having at least one periodontal site with attachment loss of 3 mm or more, periodontitis is a common disease. Among adults, the prevalence of attachment loss and periodontal pockets are higher in males than females (see Figs. 5-4 and 5-7). Males also are more likely than females to have more teeth with attachment loss and more teeth with pockets (see Figs. 5-5 and 5-8). Typically, the prevalence and extent of periodontal attachment loss increases with age (see Figs. 5-4 and 5-5). This increased prevalence with age is more likely a reflection of the cumulative effect of attachment loss over time as opposed to an increased susceptibility to periodontitis. Unlike attachment loss, the prevalence or extent of periodontal pocketing does not show much variation with age (see Figs. 5-7 and 5-8). The increase in attachment loss with age without a corresponding increase in pocket depth may result from the increasing prevalence of gingival recession with age. In the U.S., the prevalence of >1 mm of gingival recession increases from 38% in the 30- to 39-year-old age group to 90% in the 80- to 90-year-old age group.[6]

Why Do Patients Have Chronic Periodontitis, and What Puts Them at Risk?

Periodontitis is an infectious disease associated with a group of mainly gram-negative bacteria.[79] The pathogenesis of periodontal disease and the role of microbial factors was extensively reviewed at the 1996 World

TABLE 5-7

Other Studies of Periodontal Disease Progression among Adults

Study	Length	Subjects	Methodology	Results
Haffajee et al[52]	1 year	Random sample of 271 residents of Ushiku, Japan, ages 20 to 79 years.	Clinical attachment loss measured at six sites on all teeth. Change defined as attachment loss of ≥3 mm in 1 year.	27.3% of persons had attachment loss at one or more sites. Older subjects had greater risk of disease progression than younger subjects. Persons with attachment loss at baseline were more likely to have progression.
Ismail et al[53]	28 years	526 residents of Techumseh, MI, ages 5 to 60, examined at baseline in 1959. 167 reexamined in 1987.	Clinical attachment loss measured at four sites per tooth on all teeth present. Calculated mean attachment loss per person over 28 years.	13.3% of persons had mean loss ≥2 mm. 3.0% of persons had mean loss ≥3 mm. 1.2% of persons had mean loss ≥4 mm. 59.3% of all sites did not change. Mean annual attachment loss per person was 0.04 mm. Only 10.9% of teeth were lost during follow-up.
Albandar et al[54]	6 years	293 employees of an industrial plant in Oslo, Sweden, examined at baseline (ages 18 to 67 years). 142 were reexamined at 2 and 6 years.	Radiographic alveolar bone height measured from periapical films. Change defined as ≥1 mm of bone loss during 2 consecutive exams.	70% of subjects had few or no sites with bone loss. 25% of subjects had moderate progression. 5% had high rates of progression. 90% of all sites did not change. Mean annual bone loss per person ranged by age from 0.03 to 0.05 mm.
Papapanou et al[55]	10 years	531 Swedes examined at baseline in 1974–76 (ages 25 to 70). 201 Swedes reexamined in 1985–86.	Radiographic alveolar bone height measured at the mesial and distal of each tooth. Reported mean bone loss per person over the 10 years.	17% of persons had mean loss of ≥2 mm. Mean annual bone loss per person was 0.07 to 0.14 mm in ages 25 to 65 years (age at baseline), 0.28 mm in 70-year-olds.

Workshop in Periodontics.[57,79] After reviewing the scientific literature, the section members concluded by consensus that sufficient evidence exists to consider three microorganisms as etiologic agents: *A. actinomycetemcomitans, Porphyromonas gingivalis,* and *Bacteriodes forsythus.*[8] Of these bacteria, *P. gingivalis* and *B. forsythus* often are found in chronic periodontitis, whereas *A. actinomycetemcomitans* often is found in cases of aggressive periodontitis. Evidence suggests that other microorganisms also may be involved in the development of periodontitis.

Although these pathogens are necessary to cause periodontitis, their presence is not sufficient to cause disease. Epidemiologic studies have shown that the presence of microorganisms in the subgingival plaque explains only a small portion of the cases of periodontitis. To explain these findings, periodontal researchers recently have begun to talk about a "new paradigm" for the etiology of adult periodontitis.[61] This paradigm indicates that microorganisms are the cause of periodontitis but that the clinical expression of the disease (extent and severity) depends on how the host responds to the extent and virulence of the microbial burden. In response to periodontal pathogens and their endotoxins, immune cells in the periodontium, particularly monocytes, secrete proinflammatory mediators such as prostaglandin E, interleukin 1, and tumor necrosis factor. The body's inflammatory response is an attempt to protect itself from the pathogens, but at the same time the inflammation can lead to periodontal connective tissue destruction and bone degeneration as the body attempts to rid itself of the infectious tooth. Further understanding of the role of differences in immune response should help in understanding an individual's susceptibility to periodontal disease.

Much epidemiologic research has focused on the identification of environmental and host factors that are involved in the initiation and progression of periodontal disease. Of all the environmental factors known to be associated with periodontitis, cigarette smoking may be the most important. Evidence for the role of smoking in periodontitis includes 1) a higher prevalence of disease among smokers in cross-sectional studies, 2) a higher incidence of periodontitis among smokers in longitudinal studies, 3) a statistically significant association even after controlling for other risk factors, 4) increased prevalence and incidence of disease with increased amounts of smoking, and 5) biologically plausible mechanisms that can explain how smoking is involved in the destruction of periodontal tissues.[63] Cigarette smokers are up to 5 times more likely than nonsmokers to develop severe periodontitis, and the risk of the disease increases with the amount of cigarettes smoked.[60]

Diabetes is another factor that enhances an individual's susceptibility to periodontis. The prevalence and severity of periodontitis is significantly higher in Type 1 (formally called *insulin-dependent* but now called *immune-mediated*) diabetics and Type 2 (formally called *noninsulin–dependent*) diabetics than in nondiabetics.[27,73] Type 1 diabetes typically occurs during childhood or adolescence, whereas Type 2 diabetes usually occurs after age 45. Approximately 9 of 10 individuals with diabetes have Type 2 diabetes. Much of clinicians' understanding of the epidemiologic association between diabetes and periodontitis comes from studies of the Pima Indians of the Gila River Indian Community in Arizona. The Pimas have the highest incidence of Type 2 diabetes ever recorded.[41] Among the Pimas, diabetics have a threefold risk of developing periodontitis.[27] The effects of diabetes appears to be similar among individuals with Type 1 and Type 2 diabetes as long as the duration of their disease is similar. However, individuals with Type 1 diabetes often have had diabetes longer than Type 2 diabetics and therefore may be at risk of developing more periodontitis.[58] In addition to the duration of diabetes, the long-term metabolic control of diabetes is an important factor in periodontitis. Compared with well- and moderately controlled diabetics, the prevalence, severity, and extent of periodontitis are increased among poorly controlled diabetics.[72] The encouraging news is that well-controlled diabetics have similar levels of periodontal disease as nondiabetics, and diabetics treated for moderate to advanced adult periodontitis are able to maintain a healthy periodontium.[58,78]

Although numerous cross-sectional studies indicate that the prevalence and severity of periodontitis increases with age, the current opinion is that aging does not cause periodontitis. In cross-sectional studies, indicators of periodontitis such as attachment loss and bone loss are cumulative measures of disease over an individual's lifetime. The greater prevalence and severity of periodontitis among older persons in these studies is due to the cumulative effects of the disease over time rather than a greater susceptibility of older people.[18] In fact, studies support the view that if a person is susceptible to severe periodontal destruction, the tendency will be seen early.[19] Longitudinal studies examining the association between age and periodontitis have been inconclusive.[12] One longitudinal study indicated that when good oral hygiene is maintained throughout a lifetime, periodontal disease progression is negligible.[2] In that study, oral hygiene was shown to be the most important predictor for periodontitis, and in all age groups, more than 95% of individuals with good oral hygiene did not have periodontitis. The authors concluded "The effect of age on the progression of periodontitis could therefore be considered negligible when good oral hygiene is maintained."[2] Finally, the profitability of continuing the debate of whether age is a risk factor is unclear because whether the risk for periodontal disease is reduced by intervention cannot be tested (i.e., people cannot become younger).

Several other characteristics have been investigated as possible risk factors for adult periodontitis. The following list, adapted from Page and Beck, summarizes many of those characteristics in terms of the current status of the evidence to support their candidacy as risk factors.[60]

- Nutrition: Most information regarding nutrition and periodontal diseases is dated and primarily based on animal studies that involved severe nutritional deficiencies. Minor nutritional deficiencies or imbalances failed to demonstrate an effect on periodontal disease in these animal models. Longitudinal studies that control for possible confounders meeting our stated criteria for evaluation of nutrition as a risk factor are lacking.
- Low socioeconomic and educational status: Periodontal disease is more severe in individuals of lower socioeconomic status and poorer education. However, when periodontal status is adjusted for oral hygiene and smoking, the associations between lower socioeconomic and educational status and severe periodontal disease are not seen. Thus socioeconomic and educational statuses do not appear to directly affect the pathogenesis.
- Osteoporosis: Longitudinal data are scarce, and multivariate analyses produce inconsistent results.
- HIV infection and AIDS: Longitudinal data are scarce. Multivariable analyses generally are lacking. HIV infection and AIDS appear to elevate risk for severe periodontitis.
- Infrequent dental visits: Longitudinal data are available. However, multivariate analyses are inconsistent, and risk assessments and intervention studies have not been completed.
- Bacteria: Longitudinal data are available. Multivariate analyses implicate certain bacteria, and assessments and some interventions have been completed. Bacteria are generally considered to be causal. However, whether the presence of putative pathogenic species can be used as a strong indicator for future clinical

attachment loss remains controversial. Although some reports claim that the presence of these species is a good predictor, others observed an association with disease progression but found that the presence of putative pathogenic species was unreliable as a predictor for future clinical attachment loss in individual patients and at specific sites. Subject prediction usually is more accurate than site prediction. The absence of any of the group of five to seven putative periodontal pathogens is a reliable indicator for the absence of future clinical attachment loss for most patients.

- Bleeding on probing: Longitudinal data are available. Multivariate analyses implicate bleeding on probing in combination with increasing pocket depth. At present, bleeding on probing is widely used as an indication for needed treatment. However, bleeding on probing alone is not a predictor of elevated risk for future loss of clinical attachment. On the other hand, a lack of bleeding on probing, especially on two or more occasions, is an excellent indicator of periodontal health, with a predictive value of 0.972.
- Previous periodontal disease: Longitudinal data are available. Multivariate analyses implicate past disease. The risk for future periodontal deterioration in a given individual is strongly associated with the presence and severity of existing periodontitis. In other words, individuals with the most advanced existing periodontitis are at greatest risk for future clinical attachment loss. Individuals who are currently free of periodontitis are less likely to experience future clinical attachment loss than those with periodontitis. However, past disease is only a good clinical predictor. It is not likely to be causal, and it is unclear whether past disease is predictive of both incidental attachment loss and progression of current disease.
- Genetic factors: Longitudinal data are available. Multivariate analyses implicate genetic factors. Genetic factors are strongly associated with the aggressive forms and, to a lesser extent, with the chronic form.
- Stress: Most studies involve necrotizing ulcerative gingivitis (NUG). Case control and a few short-term longitudinal studies indicate associations. Multivariate and intervention studies are needed. Biologic mechanisms are known.

AGGRESSIVE PERIODONTITIS

Aggressive periodontitis (formerly known as *early onset periodontitis*) is periodontal destruction that becomes clinically significant around adolescence or early adulthood. The disease has been classified into two types—localized and generalized.[68] Other terms found in the literature that have been used to describe aggressive forms of periodontitis include juvenile, localized juvenile, generalized juvenile, rapidly progressive, severe, and prepubertal periodontitis (see Table 4-3).[68] The distinction between the localized and generalized forms is based on the distribution of the periodontal destruction in the mouth. Localized aggressive periodontitis is characterized by bone loss around the first molars and incisors. As the name implies, generalized aggressive periodontitis is characterized by a more widespread pattern of periodontal destruction.

Although aggressive periodontitis is characterized by age at onset and pattern of periodontal destruction, case definitions for early onset disease or its subtypes have varied across epidemiologic studies. In a national survey of the oral health of U.S. school children, three case definitions were used for aggressive periodontitis, as follows:[48]

- Localized aggressive periodontitis: At least one first molar and at least one incisor or second molar and two or fewer canines or premolars had >3 mm of attachment loss.
- Generalized aggressive periodontitis: Criteria for localized disease were not met, four or more teeth had >3 mm of attachment loss, and at least 2 affected teeth were second molars, canines, or premolars.
- Incidental loss of periodontal attachment: Criteria for localized or generalized were not met, and one or more teeth had >3 mm of attachment loss.

Other studies have based case definitions on various combinations of disease patterns and the extent and severity of pocket depth, attachment loss, and bone loss. A thorough review of studies that have investigated aggressive forms of periodontitis in childhood and adolescence can be found in an article by Papapanou.[62] As our understanding of aggressive periodontitis changes, the nomenclature for the disease and case definitions will likely continue to evolve.

How Much Aggressive Periodontitis Is Present?

Most studies from the U.S. and other countries that have examined localized aggressive periodontitis in adolescents have reported prevalence estimates below 1%.[62] In the U.S., the prevalence of localized and generalized aggressive periodontitis were estimated to be 0.53% and 0.13%, respectively.[48] Another 1.61% of the adolescents had incidental attachment loss—attachment loss that did not fit the study's case definitions for localized or generalized disease.[73] Although these prevalence estimates are small, together they represented almost 300,000 U.S. adolescents at the time of the study (1986–87).[48]

How Much New Aggressive Periodontitis Is Present?

Very few longitudinal studies of aggressive periodontitis have been conducted. One longitudinal study conducted in the United Kingdom followed 167 subjects from ages 14 to 19.[25] Periodontal attachment loss was measured on the mesiofacial surfaces of the first molars, first premolars, and central incisors. During the 5 years of follow-up, the percentage of subjects with attachment loss on one or more of the examined teeth increased dramatically—from 3% to 77% for attachment loss of >1 mm and from 0% to 14% for attachment loss of >2 mm. By age 19, 31% of the sites examined had attachment loss of >1 mm, and 3.1% had attachment loss of >2 mm. The teeth most commonly affected were the maxillary first molars and the mandibular central incisors. In the 19-year-old subjects, 9% of the maxillary molars had attachment loss of >2 mm. The presence of subgingival calculus and plaque at baseline were significant predictors of loss of attachment at 5 years. Although this study provides useful information on the change in prevalence of aggressive periodontitis, its authors pointed out that the cohort was not a randomly selected group of 14-year-olds, and therefore the results cannot be generalized to the population at large.

Another study that followed a cohort of 14-year-old subjects was conducted among Norwegians.[1] Of the 2767 subjects examined at baseline (14 years old) in 1984, 215 were reexamined in 1992 (they were also examined in 1986 and 1988). At each examination, the prevalence of radiographic alveolar bone loss was assessed on sets of bite-wing radiographs. Bone loss was measured on the mesial and distal of fully erupted teeth (distal of the canines to the mesial of the second molars) and was defined as the distance from the cemento-enamel junction to the alveolar crest. The distance had to exceed 2 mm for bone loss to be present. At baseline, the prevalence of subjects with one or more lesions was approximately 3.5%. By 1992 the prevalence of subjects with bone loss had doubled. The percentage of subjects with 3 or more sites with bone loss also increased during that time from 2.5% to 33.3%.

A review of the available longitudinal studies of periodontitis in childhood and adolescence concluded that subjects with signs of periodontal disease at a young age are likely to have further periodontal deterioration. Progression is more extensive at initially infected sites and among subjects of low socioeconomic status.[62]

Does My Patient with Aggressive Periodontitis Fit the Typical Profile?

The prevalence of aggressive periodontitis is higher in African-Americans than in whites. In a study of aggressive periodontitis among adolescents in the U.S., it was estimated that 2.05% of African-Americans had localized periodontitis, compared with 0.14% of whites.[48] For generalized disease, the prevalence was 0.59% for African-Americans and 0.03% for whites. The prevalence of incidental attachment loss was much higher among African-Americans than whites—4.63% versus 0.91%.

Whether or not the prevalence of aggressive periodontitis differs by gender is unclear. Early case reports and small studies often found the condition to be more prevalent among women; however, findings from larger studies have suggested the distribution of the disease is fairly equal between the genders.[70] The 1986–87 survey of U.S. schoolchildren indicated that males had slightly higher but statistically insignificant prevalence of localized and generalized aggressive periodontitis and incidental attachment loss.[48] However, when the distribution of the disease by gender was examined among race groups, differences by gender became much more evident. Among African-Americans, males were 2.9 times more likely than females to have localized disease. Among whites, the association was reversed. White females were 2.5 times more likely than white males to have localized disease.

Why Do Patients Have Aggressive Periodontitis, and What Puts Them at Risk?

The bacterium *A. actinomycetemcomitans* is found in high numbers in localized aggressive periodontal lesions and is the primary pathogen associated with the disease.[79] Elimination of the pathogen is associated with clinical improvement.[79] The bacterium produces a strong leukotoxin that kills neutrophils, which provide an important defense against periodontal infections. Different strains of *A. actinomycetemcomitans* produce different levels of leukotoxin. Highly toxic strains produce 10 to 20 times the levels of leukotoxin as do minimally toxic strains.[81] Patients with localized aggressive periodontitis are more likely to harbor the highly leukotoxic strains than periodontally healthy persons or persons with chronic periodontitis.[81] In a study of 21 families with at least one family member with localized disease, children infected with the highly leukotoxic strains of *A. actinomycetemcomitans* were more likely to develop localized aggressive periodontitis.[17] Persons with African backgrounds have been found more likely to be infected with the more virulent strains of *A. actinomycetemcomitans,* which may explain the elevated risk of localized juvenile periodontitis among African-Americans.[71] Although infection with *A. actinomycetemcomitans* is strongly associated with cases of localized disease, not all individuals infected with *A. actinomycetemcomitans* develop localized aggressive periodontitis, and not all individuals with localized disease have detectable levels of *A. actinomycetemcomitans.*

Another factor believed to be involved in the pathogenesis of aggressive periodontitis is defective neutrophil function. Depressed neutrophil chemotaxis is a consistent finding among patients with localized or generalized forms of the disease.[77] Studies have shown that 70% to 75% of patients with localized disease have depressed neutrophil chemotaxis.[77] Localized aggressive periodontitis tends to occur in families, and this neutrophil chemotaxic abnormality is genetic in origin and may predispose individuals to localized disease.[77] However, not all individuals with localized disease have depressed neutrophil chemotaxis, and not all individuals with depressed neutrophil chemotaxis develop localized disease. Other, currently unidentified host factors are likely involved in the pathogenesis of the disease.

REFERENCES

1. Aass AM, Tollefsen T, Gjermo P: A cohort study of radiographic alveolar bone loss during adolescence. J Clin Periodontol 1994; 21:133.
2. Abdellatif HM, Burt BA: An epidemiological investigation into the relative importance of age and oral hygiene status as determinants of periodontitis. J Dent Res 1987; 66:13.
3. Addy M, Hunter ML, Kingdon A, et al: An 8-year study of changes in oral hygiene and periodontal health during adolescence. Int J Paediatr Dent 1994; 4:75.
4. Albandar JM: A 6-year study on the pattern of periodontal disease progression. J Clin Periodontol 1990; 17:467.
5. Albandar JM, Brunelle JA, Kingman A: Destructive periodontal disease in adults 30 years of age and older in the United States, 1988–1994. J Periodontol 1999; 70:13.

6. Albandar JM, Kingman A: Gingival recession, gingival bleeding, and dental calculus in adults 30 years of age and older in the United States, 1988–1994. J Periodontol 1999; 70:30.
7. Amato R, Caton J, Polson A, et al: Interproximal gingival inflammation related to the conversion of a bleeding to a nonbleeding state. J Periodontol 1986; 57:63.
8. Anonymous: Consensus report. Periodontal diseases: pathogenesis and microbial factors. Ann Periodontol 1996; 1:926.
9. Anonymous: Position paper: epidemiology of periodontal diseases. American Academy of Periodontology [see comments]. J Periodontol 1996; 67:935.
10. Armitage GC: Periodontal diseases: diagnosis. Ann Periodontol 1996; 1:37.
11. Baelum V, Luan WM, Chen X, et al: A 10-year study of the progression of destructive periodontal disease in adult and elderly Chinese. J Periodontol 1997; 68:1033.
12. Beck JD: Periodontal implications: older adults. Ann Periodontol 1996; 1:322.
13. Beck JD, Koch GG, Offenbacher S: Incidence of attachment loss over 3 years in older adults—new and progressing lesions. Community Dent Oral Epidemiol 1995; 23:291.
14. Bergstrom J: Oral hygiene compliance and gingivitis expression in cigarette smokers. Scand J Dent Res 1990; 98:497.
15. Bhat M: Periodontal health of 14–17-year-old US schoolchildren. J Public Health Dent 1991; 51:5.
16. Bouwsma O, Caton J, Polson A, et al: Effect of personal oral hygiene on bleeding interdental gingiva. Histologic changes. J Periodontol 1988; 59:80.
17. Bueno LC, Mayer MP, DiRienzo JM: Relationship between conversion of localized juvenile periodontitis-susceptible children from health to disease and *Actinobacillus actinomycetemcomitans* leukotoxin promoter structure [see comments]. J Periodontol 1998; 69:998.
18. Burt BA: Periodontitis and aging: reviewing recent evidence. J Am Dent Assoc 1994; 125:273.
19. Burt BA, Eklund SA: Dentistry, Dental Practice, and the Community, ed 5. Philadelphia, Saunders, 1999.
20. Carlos JP, Wolf MD, Kingman A: The extent and severity index: a simple method for use in epidemiologic studies of periodontal disease. J Clin Periodontol 1986; 13:500.
21. Carter HG, Barnes GP: The gingival bleeding index. J Periodontol 1974; 45:801.
22. Caton J, Bouwsma O, Polson A, et al: Effects of personal oral hygiene and subgingival scaling on bleeding interdental gingiva. J Periodontol 1989; 60:84.
23. Caton JG, Polson AM: The interdental bleeding index: a simplified procedure for monitoring gingival health. Compend Contin Educ Dent 1985; 6:88.
24. Ciancio S: Current status of indices of gingivitis. J Clin Periodontol 1986; 13:375.
25. Clerehugh V, Lennon MA, Worthington HV: 5-year results of a longitudinal study of early periodontitis in 14- to 19-year-old adolescents. J Clin Periodontol 1990; 17:702.
26. Douglass CW, Fox CH: Cross-sectional studies in periodontal disease: current status and implications for dental practice. Adv Dent Res 1993; 7:25.
27. Emrich LJ, Shlossman M, Genco RJ: Periodontal disease in non–insulin-dependent diabetes mellitus [see comments]. J Periodontol 1991; 62:123.
28. Fletcher RH, Fletcher SW, Wagner EH: Clinical Epidemiology: The Essentials, ed 2. Baltimore, Williams & Wilkins, 1988.
29. Folkers SA, Weine FS, Wissman DP: Periodontal disease in the life stages of women. Compendium 1992; 13:852.
30. Friedman LM, Furberg CD, DeMets DL: Fundamentals of Clinical Trials, ed 3. St Louis, Mosby, 1996.
31. Genco RJ: Classification and clinical and radiographic features of periodontal disease. In: Genco RJ, Goldman HM, Cohen DW (eds): Contemporary Periodontics. St Louis, Mosby, 1990.
32. Gordis L: Epidemiology. Philadelphia, Saunders, 1996.
33. Greenberg RS: Medical Epidemiology, ed 2. Norwalk, CT, Appleton & Lange, 1996.
34. Greenstein G: The role of bleeding upon probing in the diagnosis of periodontal disease. A literature review. J Periodontol 1984; 55:684.
35. Gusberti FA, Mombelli A, Lang NP, et al: Changes in subgingival microbiota during puberty. A 4-year longitudinal study. J Clin Periodontol 1990; 17:685.
36. Haffajee AD, Socransky SS, Lindhe J, et al: Clinical risk indicators for periodontal attachment loss. J Clin Periodontol 1991; 18:117–125.
37. Hirsch RS, Clarke NG, Townsend GC: The effect of locally released oxygen on the development of plaque and gingivitis in man. J Clin Periodontol 1981; 8:21.
38. Hulley SB, Cummings SR, Browner WS: Designing Clinical Research: An Epidemiologic Approach. Baltimore, Williams & Wilkins, 1988.
39. Ismail AI, Morrison EC, Burt BA, et al: Natural history of periodontal disease in adults: findings from the Tecumseh Periodontal Disease Study, 1959–87. J Dent Res 1990; 69:430.
40. Jeffcoat MK, Wang IC, Reddy MS: Radiographic diagnosis in periodontics. Periodontol 2000 1995; 7:54.
41. Knowler WC, Pettitt DJ, Savage PJ, et al: Diabetes incidence in Pima Indians: contributions of obesity and parental diabetes. Am J Epidemiol 1981; 113:144.
42. Last JM, Abramson JH, International Epidemiological Association: A Dictionary of Epidemiology, ed 3. New York, Oxford University Press, 1995.
43. Lilienfeld DE, Stolley PD, Lilienfeld AM: Foundations of Epidemiology, ed 3. New York, Oxford University Press, 1994.
44. Lindhe J, Hamp S, Löe H: Experimental periodontitis in the beagle dog. J Periodontal Res 1973; 8:1.
45. Lobene RR: Discussion: clinical status of indices for measuring gingivitis. J Clin Periodontol 1986; 13:381.
46. Lobene RR, Weatherford T, Ross NM, et al: A modified gingival index for use in clinical trials. Clin Prev Dent 1986; 8:3.
47. Löe H: The gingival index, the plaque index and the retention index systems. J Periodontol 1967; 38:610 (supplement).
48. Löe H, Brown LJ: Early onset periodontitis in the United States of America. J Periodontol 1991; 62:608.
49. Löe H, Silness J: Periodontal disease in pregnancy. I. Prevalence and severity. Acta Odontol Scand 1963; 21:533.
50. Löe H, Theilade E, Jensen SB: Experimental gingivitis in man. J Periodontol 1965; 36:177.
51. Lyons H, Kerr DM, Hine MK: Report from the 1949 Nomenclature Committee of the American Academy of Periodontology. J Periodontol 1950; 21:40.
52. Mombelli A, Lang NP, Burgin WB, et al: Microbial changes associated with the development of puberty gingivitis. J Periodontal Res 1990; 25:331.
53. Muhlemann HR, Son S: Gingival sulcus bleeding—A leading symptom in initial gingivitis. Helv Odontol Acta 1971; 15:107.
54. Nakagawa S, Fujii H, Machida Y, et al: A longitudinal study from prepuberty to puberty of gingivitis. Correlation between the occurrence of *Prevotella intermedia* and sex hormones. J Clin Periodontol 1994; 21:658.
55. National Center for Health Statistics: Third National Health and Nutrition Examination Survey, 1988–1994, NHANES III Examination Data File (CD-ROM). Public Use Data File Doc-

umentation Number 76200. Hyattsville, MD, National Center for Health Statistics and Centers for Disease Control and Prevention, 1996. Available from National Technical Information Service (NTIS), Springfield, VA.
56. Newbrun E: Indices to measure gingival bleeding. J Periodontol 1996; 67:555.
57. Offenbacher S: Periodontal diseases: pathogenesis. Ann Periodontol 1996; 1:821.
58. Oliver RC, Tervonen T: Diabetes—A risk factor for periodontitis in adults? J Periodontol 1994; 65:530.
59. Page RC: Gingivitis. J Clin Periodontol 1986; 13:345.
60. Page RC, Beck JD: Risk assessment for periodontal diseases. Int Dent J 1997; 47:61.
61. Page RC, Offenbacher S, Schroeder HE, et al: Advances in the pathogenesis of periodontitis: summary of developments, clinical implications and future directions. Periodontol 2000 1997; 14:216.
62. Papapanou PN: Periodontal diseases: epidemiology. Ann Periodontol 1996; 1:1.
63. Papapanou PN: Risk assessments in the diagnosis and treatment of periodontal diseases. J Dent Educ 1998; 62:822.
64. Papapanou PN, Wennstrom JL, Grondahl K: A 10-year retrospective study of periodontal disease progression. J Clin Periodontol 1989; 16:403.
65. Payne WA, Page RC, Ogilvie AL, et al: Histopathologic features of the initial and early stages of experimental gingivitis in man. J Periodontal Res 1975; 10:51.
66. Preber H, Bergstrom J: Occurrence of gingival bleeding in smoker and non-smoker patients. Acta Odontol Scand 1985; 43:315.
67. Ramfjord SP: Indices for prevalence and incidence of periodontal disease. J Periodontol 1959; 30:51.
68. Ranney R: Classification of periodontal diseases. Periodontol 2000 1993; 2:13.
69. Russell AL: A system of classification and scoring for prevalence surveys of periodontal disease. J Dent Res 1956; 35:350.
70. Saxby MS: Sex ratio in juvenile periodontitis: the value of epidemiological studies. Community Dent Health 1984; 1:29.
71. Schenkein HA: Etiology of localized juvenile periodontitis [editorial; comment]. J Periodontol 1998; 69:1068.
72. Tervonen T, Oliver RC: Long-term control of diabetes mellitus and periodontitis. J Clin Periodontol 1993; 20:431.
73. Thorstensson H, Hugoson A: Periodontal disease experience in adult long-duration insulin-dependent diabetics. J Clin Periodontol 1993; 20:352.
74. Tiainen L, Asikainen S, Saxen L: Puberty-associated gingivitis. Community Dent Oral Epidemiol 1992; 20:87.
75. U.S. Department of Health and Human Services (DHHS): National Center for Health Statistics. Third National Health and Nutrition Examination Survey, 1988–1994, NHANES III Examination Data File (CD-ROM). Public Use Data File Documentation Number 76200. Hyattsville, MD, Centers for Disease Control and Prevention, 1996.
76. U.S. Public Health Service, National Center for Health Statistics: Diet and dental health, a study of relationships, United States, 1971–74. DHEW Publ. no. (PHS) 82-1645, Vital and Health Statistics, Series 11 no. 225. Washington, D.C., Government Printing Office, 1982.
77. Van Dyke TE, Schweinebraten M, Cianciola LJ, et al: Neutrophil chemotaxis in families with localized juvenile periodontitis. J Periodontal Res 1985; 20:503.
78. Westfelt E, Rylander H, Blohme G, et al: The effect of periodontal therapy in diabetics. Results after 5 years. J Clin Periodontol 1996; 23:92.
79. Zambon JJ: Periodontal diseases: microbial factors. Ann Periodontol 1996; 1:879.
80. Zambon JJ, Haraszthy VI: The laboratory diagnosis of periodontal infections. Periodontol 2000 1995; 7:69.
81. Zambon JJ, Haraszthy VI, Hariharan G, et al: The microbiology of early onset periodontitis: association of highly toxic *Actinobacillus actinomycetemcomitans* strains with localized juvenile periodontitis. J Periodontol 1996; 67:Suppl:282.

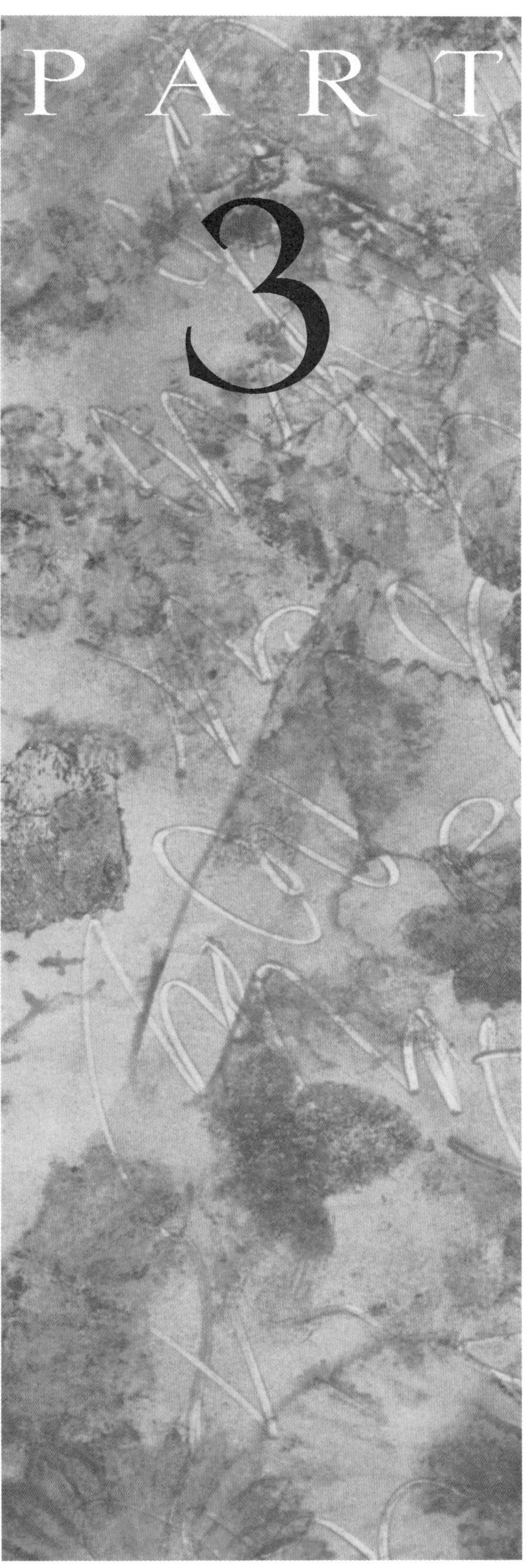

Etiology of Periodontal Diseases

Susan Kinder Haake

The clinical manifestations of periodontal disease result from a complex interplay between the etiologic agents, in this case specific bacteria found in dental plaque, and the host tissues. This part describes the many different factors, locally or systemically, that can influence the course of disease by modifying the processes inherent in the bacterial-host interaction.

Inflammation is the central pathologic feature of periodontal disease, and bacterial plaque is the etiologic factor responsible for inducing the host inflammatory processes. In a healthy host, small but variable amounts of bacterial plaque are controlled by the body's defense mechanisms with no net destruction. Specific bacteria in plaque are more likely to be associated with periodontal destruction. Specific strains of a pathogenic species may be more virulent than other strains. Increased plaque accumulation results from ineffective oral hygiene and is further complicated by the presence of local factors such as calculus overhanging dental restorations or crowded and malaligned teeth.

The host response to bacterial plaque is influenced by the individual's genotype, or genetic makeup, and by environmental influences. Genetic variation or mutations that modulate the individual's response to bacterial insult have been identified and in some cases are associated with severe forms of periodontal disease. Individuals who have diabetes or smoke are more susceptible to periodontal destruction than comparable nondiabetic or nonsmoking individuals. Host factors are also critical in the processes of tissue repair inherent in the successful treatment of periodontal diseases. The influence of systemic host factors on periodontal diseases has long been recognized. More recent data indicate that periodontal diseases may have significant impact on systemic conditions such as the occurrence of heart disease, stroke, or preterm, low-birth-weight infants. Thus host factors may act locally in reducing resistance to periodontal tissue destruction as a result of bacterial challenge, and the bacterial challenge may produce local or systemic responses that contribute to a systemic disease.

Periodontal Microbiology

Susan Kinder Haake, Michael G. Newman, Russell J. Nisengard, and Mariano Sanz

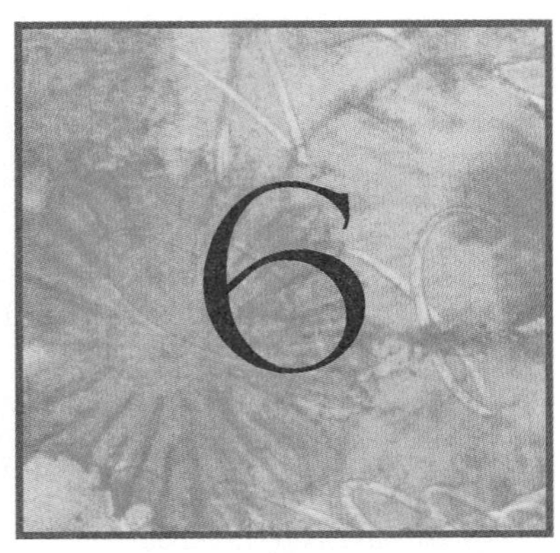

CHAPTER

CHAPTER OUTLINE

Periodontal disease comprises a group of inflammatory conditions of the supporting tissues of the teeth that are caused by bacteria. Our understanding of the etiology of periodontal diseases has undergone major advances in recent decades.[94,95] In the mid-1900s, all bacterial species found in dental plaque were believed to be equally capable of causing disease, and periodontitis was believed to be the result of cumulative exposure to dental plaque. The association of specific bacterial species with disease came about in the early 1960s, when microscopic examination of plaque revealed that different bacterial morphotypes were found in periodontally healthy versus periodontally diseased sites. In the 1960s and 1970s, technical improvements were made in the procedures used to isolate, cultivate, and identify periodontal microorganisms. This resulted in refinements in bacterial taxonomy (Table 6-1) and clarification of the specific groups of microorganisms present with diseases of the periodontium. In the 1990s, the application of molecular approaches to the identification of microorganisms furthered this process, indicating a substantially greater diversity of species in the periodontal environment than was previously recognized.[46] As our understanding of periodontal microbial ecology continues to advance, so will our understanding of the etiology of periodontal diseases.

The identification of bacterial pathogens in periodontal diseases has been difficult because of a number of factors.[94] The periodontal microbiota is a complex community of microorganisms, many of which are still difficult or impossible to isolate in the laboratory. Currently, it is apparent that multiple species function as pathogens, and species that function as pathogens in one site also may be present in low numbers in healthy sites. The chronic nature of periodontal disease has complicated the search for bacterial pathogens. It was previously thought that periodontal diseases progressed at a slow but steady rate. However, epidemiologic studies have established that the disease progresses at different rates, with alternating episodes of rapid tissue destruction and periods of remission. Identification of the microorganisms found during the different phases of the disease process is technically challenging. Furthermore, the interpretation of microbiologic data is greatly influenced by the clinical classification of disease status, an area that has undergone a number of recent revisions.[2] Previous and perhaps current classifications involve the grouping of potentially different disease states because of

TABLE 6-1

Selected Identification and Reclassifications of Periodontal Bacteria

Current Classification	Previous Status
Campylobacter rectus	*Wolinella recta*
Campylobacter showae	New species
Porphyromonas endodontalis	*Bacteroides endodontalis*
Porphyromonas gingivalis	*Bacteroides gingivalis*
Prevotella denticola	*Bacteroides denticola*
Prevotella intermedia	*Bacteroides intermedius*
Prevotella loescheii	*Bacteroides loescheii*
Prevotella melaninogenica	*Bacteroides melaninogenicus*
Prevotella nigrescens	New species
Prevotella pallens	New species
Treponema amylovorum	New species
Treponema lecithinolyticum	New species
Treponema maltophilum	New species
Treponema medium	New species

Based on: Etoh Y, Dewhirst FE, Paster BJ, et al: *Campylobacter showae* sp. nov., isolated from the human oral cavity. Int J Syst Bacteriol 1993; 43:631; Kononen E, Eerola E, Frandsen EV, et al: Phylogenetic characterization and proposal of a new pigmented species to the genus *Prevotella*: *Prevotella pallens* sp. nov. Int J Syst Bacteriol 1998; 48:47; Shah HN, Collins MD: Proposal for reclassification of *Bacteroides asaccharolyticus, Bacteroides gingivalis,* and *Bacteroides endodontalis* in a new genus, *Porphyromonas.* Int J Syst Bacteriol 1988; 38:128; Shah HN, Collins DM: Prevotella, a new genus to include *Bacteroides melaninogenicus* and related species formerly classified in the genus *Bacteroides.* Int J Syst Bacteriol 1990; 40:205; Shah HN, Gharbia SE: Biochemical and chemical studies on strains designated *Prevotella intermedia* and proposal of a new pigmented species, *Prevotella nigrescens* sp. nov. Int J Syst Bacteriol 1992; 42:542; Umemoto T, Nakazawa F, Hoshino E, et al: *Treponema medium* sp. nov., isolated from human subgingival dental plaque. Int J Syst Bacteriol 1997; 47:67; Vandamme P, Falsen E, Rossau R, et al: Revision of *Campylobacter, Helicobacter,* and *Wolinella* taxonomy: Emendation of generic descriptions and proposal of *Arcobacter* gen. nov. Int J Syst Bacteriol 1991; 41:88; 108. Wyss C, Choi BK, Schupbach P, et al: *Treponema maltophilum* sp. nov., a small oral spirochete isolated from human periodontal lesions. Int J Syst Bacteriol 1996; 46:745; Wyss C, Choi BK, Schupbach P, et al: *Treponema amylovorum* sp. nov., a saccharolytic spirochete of medium size isolated from an advanced human periodontal lesion. Int J Syst Bacteriol 1997; 47:842; Wyss C, Choi BK, Schupbach P, et al: *Treponema lecithinolyticum* sp. nov., a small saccharolytic spirochaete with phospholipase A and C activities associated with periodontal diseases. Int J Syst Bacteriol 1999; 49:1329.

the difficulties in accurately distinguishing them clinically. It is important to recognize that these types of groupings may obscure microbiologic associations.

Despite the difficulties inherent in characterizing the microbiology of periodontal diseases, a small group of pathogens is recognized because of their association with disease. The properties of these microorganisms that enable them to function as pathogens in the periodontal environment are currently under investigation and promise to provide much information about the basic mechanisms involved in the disease process. Technologic advances in molecular microbiology have improved the ability to detect specific bacteria and their products, which may serve as markers of ongoing disease or predictors of future disease. Some of these technologies have led to commercial products that are currently available for use in clinical therapy. However, although considerable advances have been made toward understanding the bacterial etiology of periodontal diseases, a complete answer to the question "What causes periodontal diseases?" is not known.

DENTAL PLAQUE: A HOST-ASSOCIATED BIOFILM

Dental plaque is a host-associated biofilm. The significance of the biofilm environment has been increasingly recognized in recent years because the environment itself may alter properties of the microorganisms. The biofilm community is initially formed through bacterial interactions with the tooth and then through physical and physiologic interactions among different species within the microbial mass. Furthermore, the bacteria found in the plaque biofilm are strongly influenced by external environmental factors that may be host mediated. Periodontal health can be considered to be a state of balance when the bacterial population coexists with the host and no irreparable damage occurs to either the bacteria or the host tissues. Disruption of this balance causes alterations in both the host and biofilm bacteria and results ultimately in the destruction of the connective tissues of the periodontium.

Macroscopic Structure and Composition of Dental Plaque

Dental plaque can be defined as the soft deposits that form the biofilm adhering to the tooth surface or other hard surfaces in the oral cavity, including removable and fixed restorations.[3] Plaque is differentiated from other deposits that may be found on the tooth surface such as materia alba and calculus (Color Fig. 6-1). *Materia alba* refers to soft accumulations of bacteria and tissue cells that lack the organized structure of dental plaque and are easily displaced with a water spray. *Calculus* is a hard deposit that forms by mineralization of dental plaque and is generally covered by a layer of unmineralized plaque.

Dental plaque is broadly classified as supragingival or subgingival based on its position on the tooth surface. *Supragingival plaque* is found at or above the gingival margin; the supragingival plaque in direct contact with the gingival margin is referred to as *marginal plaque.*

Subgingival plaque is found below the gingival margin, between the tooth and the gingival sulcular tissue. Morphologic studies indicate a differentiation of tooth-associated and tissue-associated regions of subgingival plaque,[52,69] and in certain cases bacteria are found within the host tissues.[81,82] The different regions of plaque are significant to different processes associated with diseases of the teeth and periodontium. For example, marginal plaque is of prime importance in the development of gingivitis. Supragingival plaque and tooth-associated subgingival plaque are critical in calculus formation and root caries, whereas tissue-associated subgingival plaque is important in the soft tissue destruction that characterizes different forms of periodontitis.

Dental plaque is composed primarily of microorganisms (Fig. 6-1). One gram of plaque (wet weight) contains approximately 2×10^{11} bacteria.[91] Because 1 g of pure streptococcal cells packed by centrifugation contains 2.3×10^{11} bacteria, bacteria account for most of the plaque weight.[91] Cultivation studies, in which bacteria are isolated and characterized in the laboratory, indicate that more than 500 distinct microbial species are found in dental plaque.[68] Recent studies have focused on molecular approaches to bacterial identification, which rely on analysis of ribosomal DNA sequences rather than cultivation. Data using these approaches suggest that as much as 30% of the microorganisms found associated with gingivitis may represent previously uncultivated species.[46] Thus it is apparent that substantial numbers of plaque microorganisms are yet to be identified. Nonbacterial microorganisms that are found in plaque include *Mycoplasma* species, yeasts, protozoa, and viruses.[12] The microorganisms exist within an intercellular matrix that also contains a few host cells such as epithelial cells, macrophages, and leukocytes (Fig. 6-2).

The intercellular matrix, estimated to account for 20% to 30% of the plaque mass, consists of organic and inorganic materials derived from saliva, gingival crevicular fluid, and bacterial products. Organic constituents of the matrix include polysaccharides, proteins, glycoproteins, and lipid material. Glycoproteins from saliva are an important component of the pellicle that initially coats a clean tooth surface (see later discussion), but they also become incorporated into the developing plaque biofilm. Polysaccharides produced by bacteria, of which dextran is the predominant form, contribute to the organic portion of the matrix. Albumin, probably originating from crevicular fluid, has been identified as a component of the plaque matrix. The lipid material consists of debris from the membranes of disrupted bacterial and host cells and possibly food debris.

The inorganic component of plaque is predominately calcium and phosphorus, with trace amounts of other minerals such as sodium, potassium, and fluoride. The source of inorganic constituents of supragingival plaque is primarily saliva; as the mineral content increases, the plaque mass becomes calcified to form calculus. Calculus is frequently found in areas of the dentition adjacent to salivary ducts (e.g., the lingual surface of the mandibular anteriors and the buccal surface of the maxillary first molars), reflecting the high concentration of minerals available from saliva in those regions.

The inorganic component of subgingival plaque is derived from crevicular fluid, which is a serum transudate. Calcification of subgingival plaque also results in calculus formation. Subgingival calculus is typically dark green or dark brown, probably reflecting the presence of subgingival matrix components distinct from those of supragingival calculus (e.g., blood products associated with subgingival hemorrhage). The fluoride component of plaque is largely derived from external sources such as fluoridated toothpastes and rinses. Fluoride is used therapeutically to aid in remineralization of tooth structure, prevention of demineralization of tooth structure, and inhibition of the growth of many plaque microorganisms.[79]

Studies using traditional histologic methods suggested a relatively uniform dense structure to dental plaque. However, these approaches are subject to artifacts from the processes of dehydration, fixation, embedding, and staining. Recent studies using newly developed microscopic techniques have enabled examination of plaque structure without these processing requirements. In contrast with earlier findings, studies using these newer microscopy techniques reveal that plaque is actually heterogeneous in structure, with clear evidence of open fluid-filled channels running through the plaque mass.[13,14,107] (Fig. 6-3). These channels may provide for circulation within plaque to facilitate movement of soluble molecules such as nutrients or waste products. The bacteria exist and proliferate within the intercellular matrix through which the channels course. This matrix confers a specialized environment, which distinguishes bacteria that exist within the biofilm from those that are free-floating in solutions such as saliva or crevicular fluid. For example, the biofilm matrix functions as a barrier. Substances produced by bacteria within the biofilm are retained and essentially concentrated, which fosters metabolic interactions among the different bacteria (see later discussion of physiologic properties).

Formation of Dental Plaque

Dental plaque may be readily visualized on teeth after 1 to 2 days with no oral hygiene measures. Plaque is white, grayish, or yellow and has a globular appearance. Movement of tissues and food materials over the teeth results in mechanical removal of plaque; such removal is particularly effective on the coronal two thirds of the tooth surface. Thus plaque is typically observed on the gingival third of the tooth surface, where it accumulates without disruption by the movement of food and tissues over the tooth surface during mastication. Plaque deposits also form preferentially in cracks, pits, and fissures in the tooth structure; under overhanging restorations; and around malaligned teeth. The location and rate of plaque formation vary among individuals, and determining factors include oral hygiene as well as host factors such as diet or salivary composition and flow rate.[60]

Small amounts of plaque that are not discernible on the tooth surface may be detected by running a periodontal probe or explorer along the gingival third of the tooth. Another common method of detecting small amounts of plaque is the use of disclosing solutions (see Color Fig. 6-1). Interproximal plaque formation is less evident visually but also may be monitored with an explorer or probe.

In the absence of oral hygiene measures, plaque continues to accumulate until a balance is reached between the forces of plaque removal and those of plaque formation. The formation of dental plaque at the microscopic level represents a highly ordered and predictable ecologic succession. The process of plaque formation can be

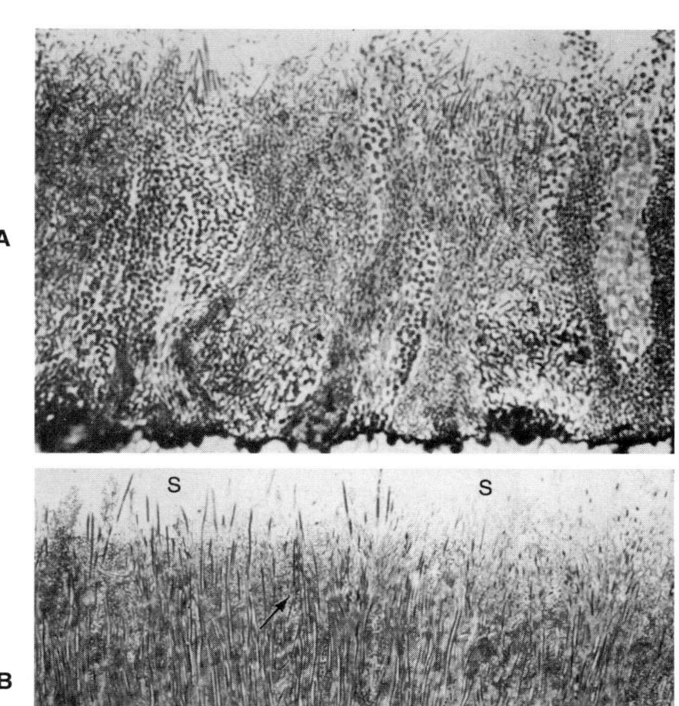

Fig. 6-1 **A,** One-day-old plaque. Microcolonies of plaque bacteria extend perpendicularly away from tooth surfaces. **B,** Developed supragingival plaque showing overall filamentous nature and microcolonies *(arrows)* extending perpendicularly away from tooth surface. Saliva-plaque interface shown *(S)*. (**A,** From Listgarten M: Development of dental plaque on epoxy resin crowns in man. A light and electron microscopic study. J Periodontol 1975; 46:10. **B,** Courtesy Dr. Max Listgarten, Philadelphia, Penn.)

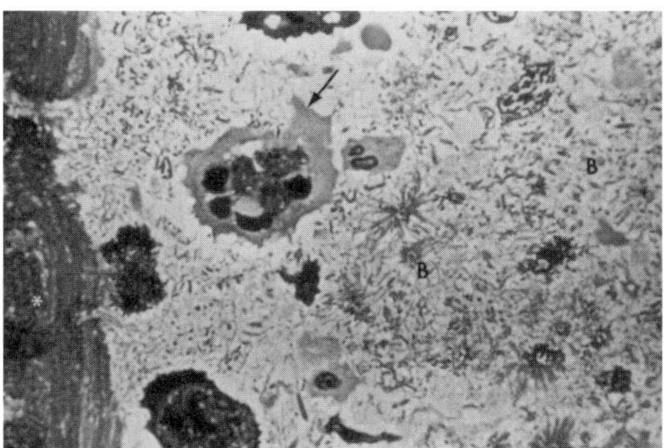

Fig. 6-2 Histologic section of plaque showing nonbacterial components such as white blood cells *(arrow)* and epithelial cells *(asterisk)*, interspersed among bacteria *(B)*. (Courtesy Dr. Max Listgarten, Philadelphia, Penn.)

divided into three phases: formation of the pellicle coating on the tooth surface, initial colonization by bacteria, and secondary colonization and plaque maturation.

Formation of the Dental Pellicle. Formation of the dental pellicle on the tooth surface is the initial phase of plaque development. All surfaces of the oral cavity, including all tissue surfaces as well as surfaces of teeth and fixed and removable restorations, are coated with a glycoprotein pellicle. This pellicle is derived from components of saliva and crevicular fluid as well as bacterial and host tissue cell products and debris.

The specific components of pellicles on different surfaces vary in composition. Studies of early (2-hour) enamel pellicle reveal that its amino acid composition differs from that of saliva,[83] indicating that the pellicle forms by *selective adsorption of the environmental macromolecules.* The mechanisms involved in enamel pellicle formation include electrostatic, van der Waals, and hydrophobic forces. The hydroxyapatite surface has a predominance of negatively charged phosphate groups that interact directly or indirectly with positively charged components of salivary and crevicular fluid macromolecules.[78]

Pellicles function as a protective barrier, providing lubrication for the surfaces and preventing tissue desiccation. However, they also provide a substrate to which bacteria in the environment attach. Because the epithelial tissue cells are continually sloughed, the bacterial population on the tissue surfaces is continually disrupted. In contrast, pellicle on the nonshedding hard surfaces provides a substrate on which bacteria progressively accumulate to form dental plaque.

Initial Colonization of the Tooth Surface. Within a few hours, bacteria are found on the dental pellicle.

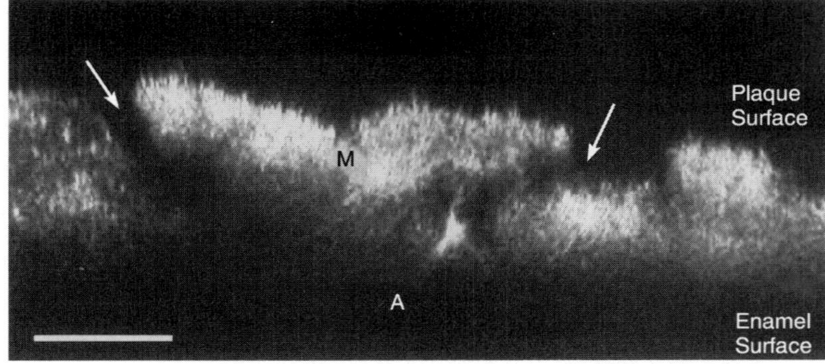

Fig. 6-3 Vertical section through a 4-day human plaque sample. An intraoral device designed for in vivo generation of plaque biofilms on enamel was used. Confocal microscopy enabled visualization of the section of plaque without the dehydration steps used in conventional histologic preparations. Notice the channels *(white arrows)* that traverse from the plaque surface through the bacterial mass (*M*; grey-white areas) to the enamel surface. An area in which the bacterial mass appears to attach to the enamel surface *(A)* is indicated. Scale bar = 25 μm. (From Wood et al: Architecture of intact natural human plaque biofilms studied by confocal laser scanning microscopy. J Dent Res 2000; 79:21. Courtesy Dr. Simon Wood, Leeds, England.)

The initial bacteria colonizing the pellicle-coated tooth surface are predominantly gram-positive facultative microorganisms such as *Actinomyces viscosus* and *Streptococcus sanguis.* These initial colonizers adhere to the pellicle[23,24,63] through specific molecules, termed *adhesins,* on the bacterial surface that interact with receptors in the dental pellicle. For example, cells of *A. viscosus* possess fibrous protein structures called *fimbriae* that extend from the bacterial cell surface. Protein adhesins on these fimbriae specifically bind to proline-rich proteins that are found in dental pellicle,[63] resulting in the attachment of the bacterial cell to the pellicle-coated tooth surface.

The plaque mass then matures through the growth of attached species, as well as the colonization and growth of additional species. *In this ecologic succession of the biofilm, there is a transition from the early aerobic environment characterized by gram-positive facultative species to a highly oxygen-deprived environment in which gram-negative anaerobic microorganisms predominate.*

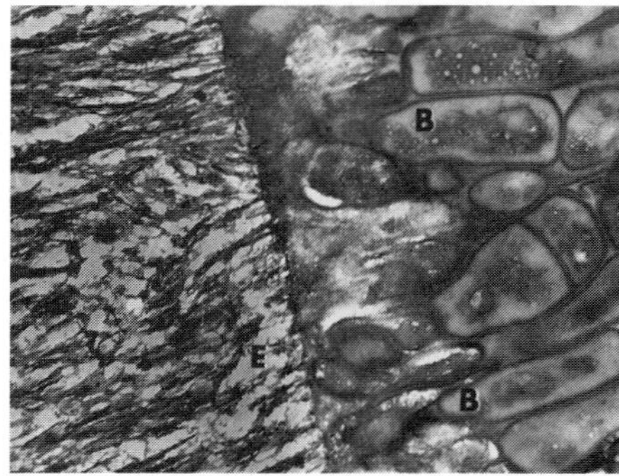

Fig. 6-4 Plaque formed directly on enamel surface. Electron micrograph of decalcificed, noncarious enamel surface showing remnants of enamel matrix *(E)* and gram-positive bacteria *(B)* in attached plaque. (Courtesy Dr. R.M. Frank and Dr. A. Brendel, Strasbourg, France.)

Secondary Colonization and Plaque Maturation. Secondary colonizers are the microorganisms that do not initially colonize clean tooth surfaces, including *Prevotella intermedia, Prevotella loescheii, Capnocytophaga* spp., *Fusobacterium nucleatum,* and *Porphyromonas gingivalis.*[39] These microorganisms adhere to cells of bacteria already in the plaque mass. Extensive laboratory studies have documented the ability of different species and genera of plaque microorganisms to adhere to one another, a process known as *coaggregation.* This process occurs primarily through the highly specific stereochemical interaction of protein and carbohydrate molecules located on the bacterial cell surfaces[37,39] in addition to the less specific interactions resulting from hydrophobic, electrostatic, and van der Waals forces.[18,25]

The significance of coaggregation in oral colonization has been documented in studies of biofilm formation in vitro[4] as well as in animal model studies.[62] Well-characterized interactions of secondary colonizers with early colonizers include the coaggregation of *F. nucleatum* with *S. sanguis,*[35] *P. loescheii* with *A. viscosus,*[103,104] and *Capnocytophaga ochracea* with *A. viscosus.*[105] Most studies of coaggregation have focused on interactions among different gram-positive species and between gram-positive and gram-negative species. In the latter stages of plaque formation, coaggregation between different gram-negative species is likely to predominate. Examples of these types of interactions are the coaggregation of *F. nucleatum* with *P. gingivalis*[36,38] or *Treponema denticola.*[40]

Microscopic Structure and Physiologic Properties of Dental Plaque

A high degree of specificity is found in the interactions between bacteria in dental plaque, as demonstrated by the studies of coaggregation. This is further evident from light and electron microscopic studies of the structure of

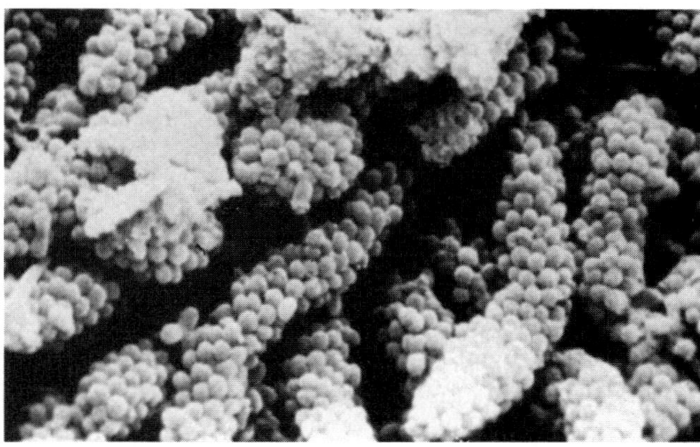

Fig. 6-5 Long-standing supragingival plaque near the gingival margin demonstrates "corncob" arrangement. A central gram-negative filamentous core supports the outer coccal cells, which are firmly attached by interbacterial adherence or coaggregation.

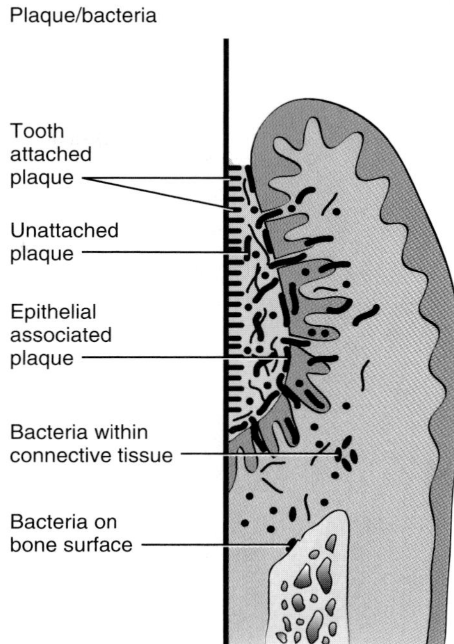

Fig. 6-6 Diagram depicting the plaque–bacteria association with tooth surface and periodontal tissues.

dental plaque formed in vivo.[52] Supragingival plaque typically demonstrates a stratified organization of the bacterial morphotypes. Gram-positive cocci and short rods predominate at the tooth surface (Fig. 6-4), whereas gram-negative rods and filaments (see Fig. 6-1) as well as spirochetes predominate in the outer surface of the mature plaque mass. Highly specific cell-to-cell interactions are also evident from the "corncob" structures[51] often observed (Fig. 6-5). Corncob formations have been observed between rod-shaped bacterial cells (e.g., *Bacterionema matruchotii* or *F. nucleatum*) that form the inner core of the structure and coccal cells (e.g., streptococci or *P. gingivalis*) that attach along the surface of the rod-shaped cell.[37,48]

The environmental parameters of the subgingival region differ from those of the supragingival region. The gingival crevice or pocket is bathed by the flow of crevicular fluid, which contains many substances that the bacteria may use as nutrients (see later discussion). Host inflammatory cells and mediators are likely to have considerable influence on the establishment and growth of bacteria in this region. Morphologic and microbiologic studies of subgingival plaque reveal distinctions between the tooth-associated and tissue-associated regions of subgingival plaque (Figs. 6-6 and 6-7).

The tooth-associated (attached) plaque (Figs. 6-8 and 6-9) is characterized by gram-positive rods and cocci, including *Streptococcus mitis, S. sanguis, A. viscosus, Actinomyces naeslundii,* and *Eubacterium* spp. *The apical border of the plaque mass is separated from the junctional epithelium by a layer of host leukocytes, and the bacteria of this apical tooth-associated region show an increased concentration of gram-negative rods.* The portion of plaque adjacent to the tissue surfaces (Figs. 6-10 and 6-11) is more loosely organized than the very dense tooth-associated region. It contains primarily gram-negative rods and cocci, as well as large numbers of filaments, flagellated rods, and spirochetes. Host tissue cells (e.g., white blood cells and epithelial cells) also may be found in this region. Studies of tissue-associated plaque indicate a predominance of species such as *S. oralis, S. intermedius, P. micros, P. gingivalis, P. intermedia, Bacteroides forsythus,* and *F. nucleatum.*[16,21] Bacteria found in tissue-associated plaque (e.g., *P. gingivalis*) also have been found in host tissues.[82] Thus the physical proximity of these bacteria to the host tissues in the plaque mass may be important in the process of tissue invasion (see Chapter 8).

The transition from gram-positive to gram-negative microorganisms observed in the structural development of dental plaque is paralleled by a physiologic transition in the developing plaque. The early colonizers (e.g., streptococci and *Actinomyces* species) use oxygen and lower the reduction-oxidation potential of the environment, which then favors the growth of anaerobic species.[15,102] Gram-positive species use sugars as an energy source and saliva as a carbon source. The bacteria that predominate in mature plaque are anaerobic and asaccharolytic, and use amino acids and small peptides as energy sources.[56]

Laboratory studies have demonstrated many physiologic interactions among the different bacteria found in dental plaque (Fig. 6-12). Lactate and formate are byproducts of the metabolism of streptococci and *Actinomyces* species and may be used in the metabolism of other plaque microorganisms. The growth of *P. gingivalis* is enhanced by metabolic byproducts produced by other microorganisms, such as succinate from *C. ochracea* and protoheme from *Campylobacter rectus*.[27,28,61]

The host also functions as an important source of nutrients. For example, the bacterial enzymes that degrade host proteins result in the release of ammonia, which may be used by bacteria as a nitrogen source.[7] Hemin iron from the breakdown of host hemoglobin may be im-

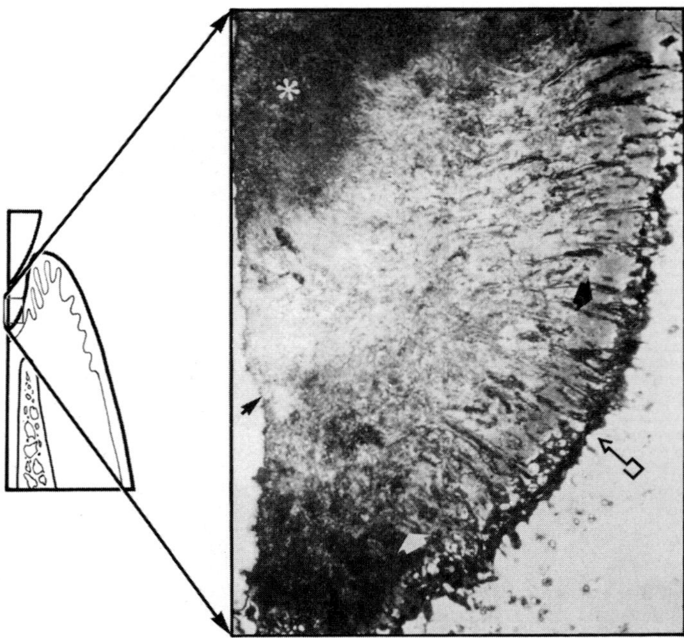

Fig. 6-7 *Left,* Diagrammatic representation of the histologic structure of subgingival plaque. *Right,* Histologic section of subgingival plaque. *Arrow with box,* Sulcular epithelium. *White arrow,* Predominantly gram-negative unattached zone. *Black arrow,* Tooth surface. *Asterisk,* Predominantly gram-positive attached zone. (From Listgarten M: Development of dental plaque on epoxy resin crowns in man. A light and electron microscopic study. J Periodontol 1975; 46:10.)

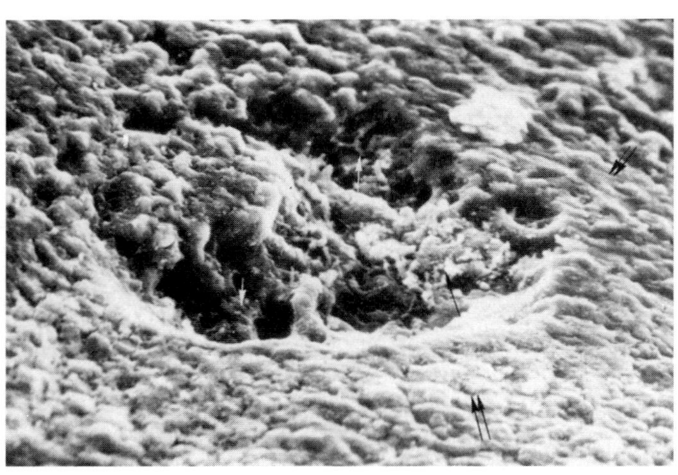

Fig. 6-8 Minute lesion on surface of root (resorption cavity) previously covered by attached plaque. Note microorganisms *(single arrows)* within resorption cavity. Cemental mounds can easily be identified *(double arrows).* (Courtesy Dr. J. Sottosanti, La Jolla, Calif.)

portant in the metabolism of *P. gingivalis.*[5] Increases in steroid hormones are associated with significant increases in the proportions of *P. intermedia* found in subgingival plaque.[42] Physiologic interactions occur both between different microorganisms in plaque and between the host and plaque microorganisms. These nutritional interdependencies are probably critical to the growth and survival of microorganisms in dental plaque and may partly explain the evolution of highly specific structural interactions observed among bacteria in plaque.

Significance of the Biofilm Environment

Studies of oral microbial communities as biofilms in vitro further highlight the significance of structural and physiologic interactions between bacterial species in plaque. For example, the presence of *F. nucleatum* in experimental mixed biofilm communities is critical to the survival of high numbers of the anaerobic species *P. nigrescens* and *P. gingivalis.* The ability of *F. nucleatum* to coaggregate with both the facultative and anaerobic species may facilitate the survival of the anaerobes.[4] In addition, *F. nucleatum* can reduce the reduction-oxidation potential of its environment so that it may function to provide a protective econiche for other anaerobic species.[15] Similar effects have been observed in other biofilm model systems using different combinations of anaerobic and facultative species.[74] Recent analyses of more than 13,000 plaque samples of 40 subgingival microorganisms using a DNA-hybridization methodology was used to define "complexes" of periodontal microorganisms. The composition of the different complexes is based on the frequency with which microorganisms are recovered together.[96] Interestingly, the early colonizers are either independent of defined complexes *(A. naeslundii, A. viscosus)* or members of the yellow (*Streptococcus* spp.) or purple

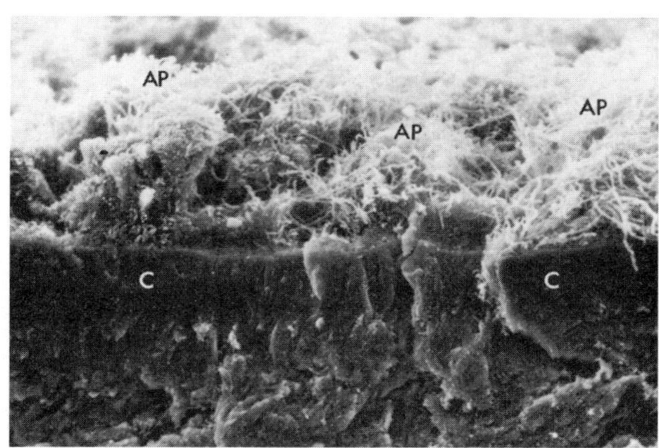

Fig. 6-9 Scanning electron photomicrograph of cross section of cementum *(C)* with attached subgingival plaque *(AP)*. Area shown is within a periodontal pocket. (Courtesy Dr. J. Sottosanti, La Jolla, Calif.)

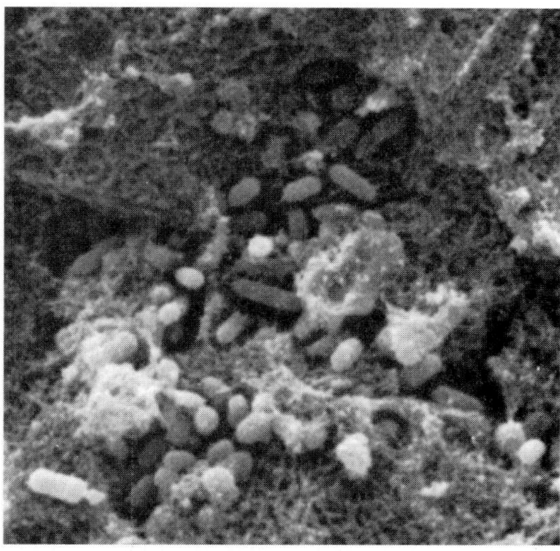

Fig. 6-11 Scanning electron micrograph of frontal view of pocket wall showing short rods on epithelial surface. (Magnification ×10,000.)

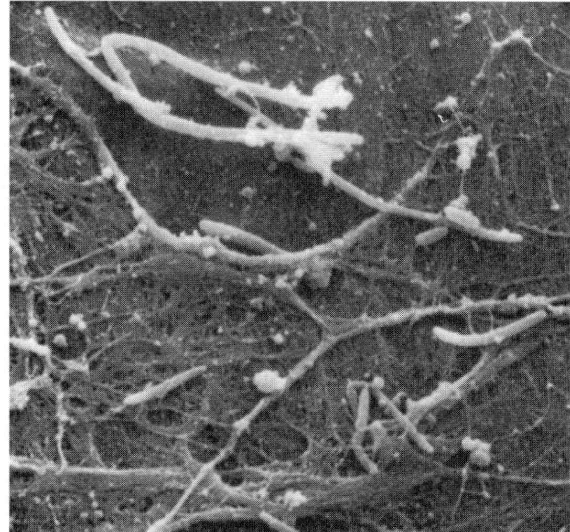

Fig. 6-10 Scanning electron micrograph of cocci and filaments associated with surface of pocket epithelium in a case of marginal gingivitis. (Magnification ×3000.)

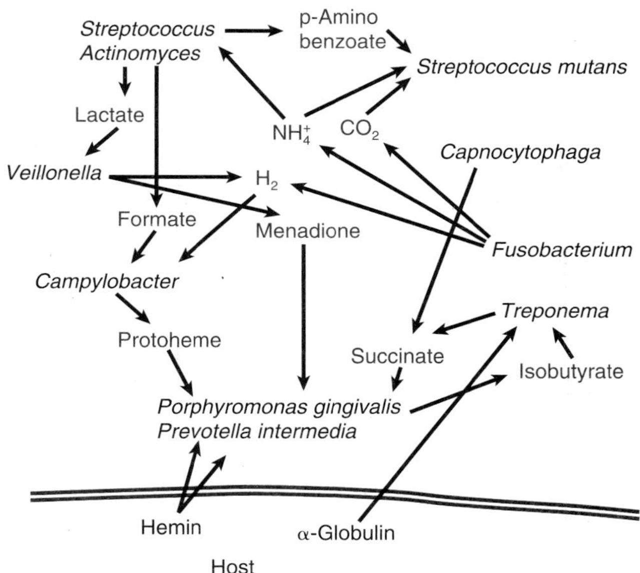

Fig. 6-12 Schematic illustration of metabolic interactions among different bacterial species found in plaque, as well as between the host and plaque bacteria. These interactions are likely to be important to the survival of bacteria in the periodontal environment. (Based on Carlsson,[7] Grenier,[28] Loesche,[56] and Walden and Hentges.[102])

complexes (*A. odontolyticus*) (Fig. 6-13). The microorganisms primarily considered secondary colonizers fell into the green, orange or red complexes. The green complex includes *E. corrodens, Actinobacillus actinomycetemcomitans* serotype a, and *Capnocytophaga* spp. The orange complex includes *Fusobacterium, Prevotella,* and *Campylobacter* spp. The green and orange complexes include species recognized as pathogens in periodontal and nonperiodontal infections. The red complex consists of *P. gingivalis, B. forsythus,* and *T. denticola*. The red complex is of particular interest because it is associated with bleeding on probing, which is an important clinical parameter of destructive periodontal diseases.[96] The existence of complexes of species in plaque is another reflection of bacterial interdependency in the biofilm environment.

It has been recognized for some time that bacteria growing in microbial communities adherent to a surface do not "behave" the same as bacteria growing suspended in a liquid environment. For example, the resistance of bacteria to antimicrobial agents is significantly increased in the biofilm environment.[1,14,31,74] The resistance to antimicrobials inherent to biofilm bacteria may relate to limited diffusion of substances into the biofilm matrix,

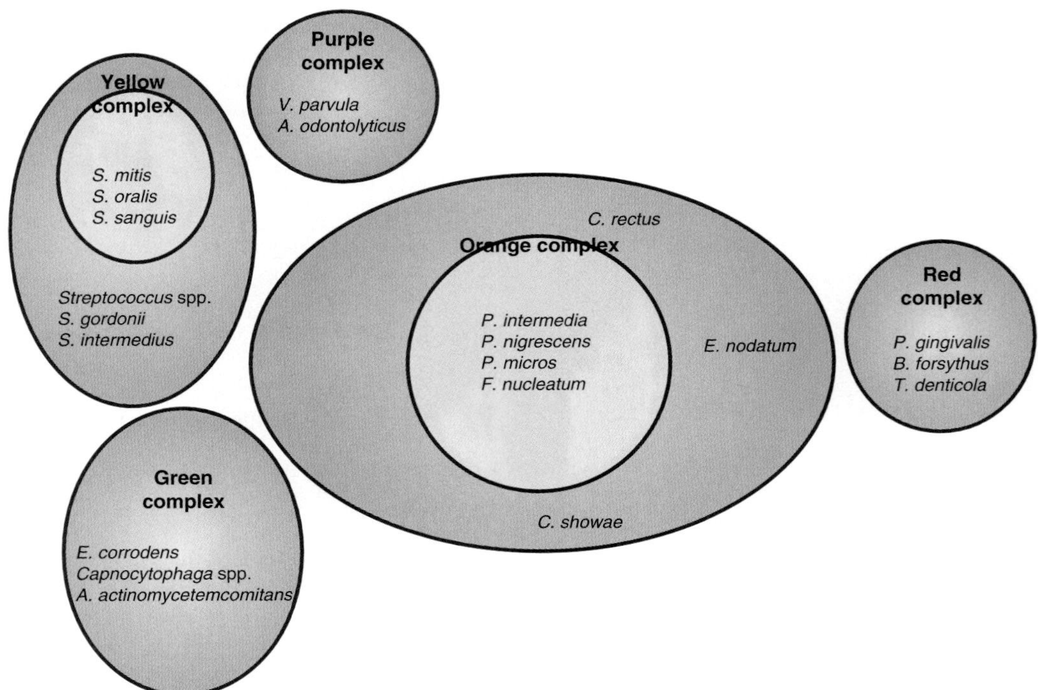

Fig. 6-13 Diagrammatic representation of selected species in the microbial complexes identified in the subgingival microbiota. Each defined grouping is identified by a color. The red complex species, as a group and individually, are found more often in periodontal sites demonstrating bleeding on probing. (Adapted from Socransky et al: Microbial complexes in subgingival plaque. J Clin Periodontol 1998; 25:134.)

the slow rate of cell growth in the biofilm environment, and possibly to altered properties of bacteria in response to growth on a surface.[14] This is a critical issue in the use of antimicrobials to manage periodontal infections or other biofilm associated infections, and it is currently a very active area of research.

ASSOCIATION OF PLAQUE MICROORGANISMS WITH PERIODONTAL DISEASES

Microbial Specificity of Periodontal Diseases

In the mid-1900s, periodontal disease was believed to result from an accumulation of plaque over time in conjunction with a diminished host response and increased host susceptibility with age. This thinking was supported by epidemiologic studies that correlated both age and the amount of plaque with evidence of periodontitis.[59,80,84] Periodontal disease was clearly associated with plaque, and all plaque was thought to be alike and equally capable of causing disease.

However, several observations contradicted these conclusions. First, some individuals with considerable amounts of plaque and calculus, as well as gingivitis, never developed destructive periodontitis. Furthermore, individuals who did present with periodontitis demonstrated considerable site specificity in the pattern of disease. Some sites were unaffected, whereas advanced disease was found in adjacent sites. In the presence of a uniform host response, these findings were inconsistent with the concept that all plaque was equally pathogenic. Recognition of the differences in plaque at sites of different clinical status (i.e., disease versus health)[54,89,91] led to a renewed search for specific pathogens in periodontal diseases and a conceptual transition from the nonspecific to the specific plaque hypothesis.

Nonspecific Plaque Hypothesis

The nonspecific and specific plaque hypotheses were delineated in 1976 by Walter Loesche, a researcher at the University of Michigan. The nonspecific plaque hypothesis maintains that periodontal disease results from the "elaboration of noxious products by the entire plaque flora."[57] According to this thinking, when only small amounts of plaque are present, the noxious products are neutralized by the host. Similarly, large amounts of plaque would produce large amounts of noxious products, which would essentially overwhelm the host's defenses. Inherent in the nonspecific plaque hypothesis is the concept that control of periodontal disease depends on control of the amount of plaque accumulation. Treatment of periodontitis by debridement (nonsurgical or surgical) and oral hygiene measures focuses on the removal of plaque and its products and is founded in the nonspecific plaque hypothesis. Thus although the nonspecific plaque hypothesis has been discarded in favor of the specific plaque hypothesis, much clinical treatment is still based on the nonspecific plaque hypothesis.

Specific Plaque Hypothesis

The specific plaque hypothesis states that only certain plaque is pathogenic, and its pathogenicity depends on the presence of or increase in specific microorganisms.[57] This concept predicts that plaque harboring specific bacterial pathogens results in periodontal disease because these organisms produce substances that mediate the destruction of host tissues.

At about the same time that Loesche proposed the specific plaque hypothesis, major advances were made in techniques used to isolate and identify periodontal microorganisms. These included improvements in procedures to sample subgingival plaque, handling of samples to prevent killing the bacteria, and media used to grow the bacteria in the laboratory.[94] The result was a tremendous increase in the ability to isolate periodontal microorganisms and considerable refinement in bacterial taxonomy. Acceptance of the specific plaque hypothesis was spurred by the recognition of *A. actinomycetemcomitans* as a pathogen in localized aggressive periodontitis.[71,89] These advances led to a series of association studies focused on identifying specific periodontal pathogens by examining the microbiota associated with states of health and disease in cross-sectional and longitudinal studies.

Microorganisms Associated with Specific Periodontal Diseases

The microbiota associated with periodontal health and disease has been studied with a wide variety of techniques for sampling, cultivation, and/or detection of bacteria by DNA hybridization.[11,20,58,68,71,96,97,111] Further, the classification of periodontal diseases has undergone a number of changes during the time that association studies have been conducted.[2,75] The following material is discussed in the context of the recently revised classification system[2] with reference to earlier classification schemes as necessitated by the population studied. These evolving variables make direct comparisons of the association studies difficult. However, comparisons do reveal the general characteristics of the microbial populations found in the presence of different clinical states and implicate a discrete group of bacteria that function as periodontal pathogens.

Early studies that used appropriate microbiologic procedures clearly demonstrated that the number and proportions of different subgingival bacterial groups varied in periodontal health when compared with the disease state.[53,89,91] The total number of bacteria, determined by microscopic counts per gram of plaque, are twice as high in periodontally diseased sites than in healthy sites.[91] Because considerably more plaque is found at diseased sites, this suggests that the total bacterial load is much greater than that at healthy sites.

The differences between periodontal health and disease also are evident when the morphotypes of the bacteria from healthy and diseased sites are examined. Fewer coccal cells and more motile rods and spirochetes are found in diseased sites than in healthy sites (Fig. 6-14).[53] The bacteria cultivated from periodontally healthy sites[89] consist predominantly of gram-positive facultative rods and cocci (approximately 75%). The recovery of this group of microorganisms is decreased proportionally in gingivitis (44%) and periodontitis (10% to 13%). These decreases are accompanied by increases in the proportions of gram-negative rods, from 13% in health to 40% in gingivitis and 74% in advanced periodontitis (Fig. 6-15).

Periodontal Health. The recovery of microorganisms from periodontally healthy sites is meager when compared with that from diseased sites. The bacteria associated with periodontal health are primarily gram-positive facultative species and members of the genera *Streptococcus* and *Actinomyces* (e.g., *S. sanguis, S. mitis, A. viscosus,* and *A. naeslundii*). Small proportions of gram-negative species are also found, most frequently *P. intermedia, F. nucleatum,* and *Capnocytophaga, Neisseria,* and *Veillonella* spp. Microscopic studies indicate that a few spirochetes and motile rods also may be found.

Certain bacterial species have been proposed to be protective or beneficial to the host, including *S. sanguis, Veillonella parvula,* and *C. ochracea.* They are typically found in high numbers at periodontal sites that do not demonstrate attachment loss (inactive sites) but in low numbers at sites where active periodontal destruction occurs.[19,94] These species probably function in preventing the colonization or proliferation of pathogenic microorganisms. One example of a mechanism by which this may occur is the production of H_2O_2 by *S. sanguis*; H_2O_2 is known to be lethal to cells of *A. actinomycetemcomitans.* Clinical studies have shown that sites with high levels of *C. ochracea* and *S. sanguis* are associated with a greater gain of attachment level after therapy,[94] further supporting this concept. A better understanding of plaque ecology and the interactions between bacteria and their products in plaque will undoubtedly reveal many other examples.

Gingivitis. The development of gingivitis has been extensively studied in a model system referred to as *ex-*

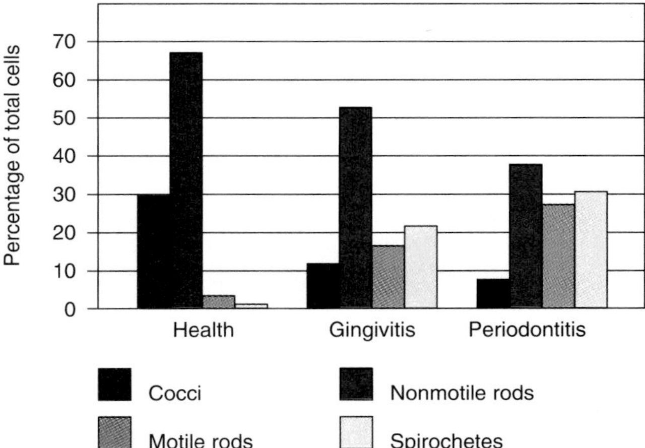

Fig. 6-14 Bacterial morphotypes in the subgingival microbiota associated with periodontal health and disease based on direct microscopic examination. (Adapted from Slots J, Rams TE: Microbiology of periodontal disease. In: Slots J, Taubman MA (eds): Contemporary Oral Microbiology and Immunology. St. Louis, Mosby, 1992.)

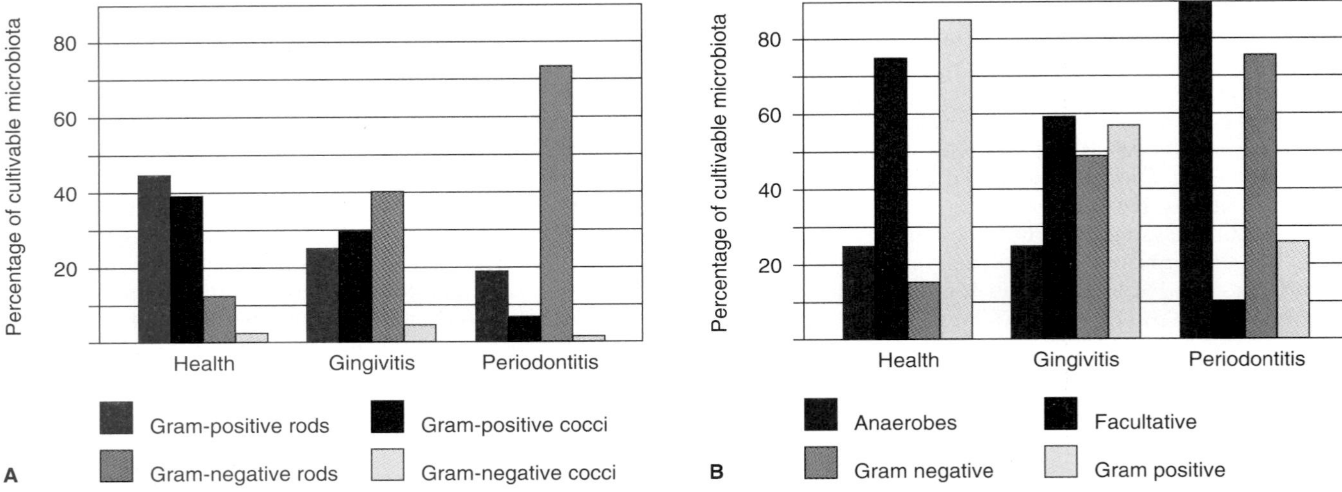

Fig. 6-15 Cultivable subgingival microbiota associated with periodontal health and disease. **A,** Distribution of gram-positive and gram-negative rods and cocci. **B,** Distribution of anaerobic, facultative, gram-positive and gram-negative species. (Adapted from Slots J, Rams TE: Microbiology of periodontal disease. In: Slots J, Taubman MA (eds): Contemporary Oral Microbiology and Immunology. St Louis, Mosby, 1992.)

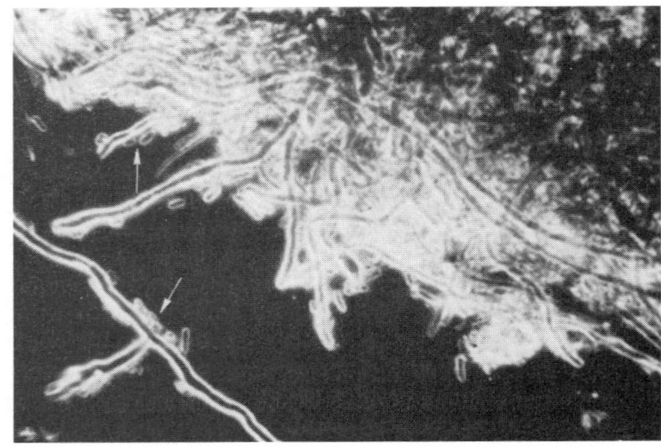

Fig. 6-16 Darkfield photomicrograph demonstrating the filamentous nature of plaque associated with gingivitis. Note attachment of smaller bacteria to filaments *(arrows).*

perimental gingivitis and initially described by Harald Löe and coworkers.[54,98] Periodontal health is first established in human subjects by cleaning and rigorous oral hygiene measures, followed by abstinence from oral hygiene for 21 days. After 8 hours without oral hygiene, bacteria may be found at concentrations of 10^3 to 10^4 per square millimeter of tooth surface and will increase in number by a factor of 100 to 1000 in the next 24-hour period.[92]

The initial microbiota of experimental gingivitis consists of gram-positive rods, gram-positive cocci, and gram-negative cocci. The transition to gingivitis is evident by inflammatory changes observed in the gingival tissues and is accompanied first by the appearance of gram-negative rods and filaments (Fig. 6-16), then by spirochetal and motile microorganisms.[98]

The bacteria found in naturally occurring *dental plaque-induced gingivitis (chronic gingivitis)* consist of roughly equal proportions of gram-positive (56%) and gram-negative (44%) species, as well as facultative (59%) and anaerobic (41%) microorganisms (see Fig. 6-15).[89] Predominant gram-positive species include *S. sanguis, S. mitis, S. intermedius, S. oralis, A. viscosus, A. naeslundii,* and *Peptostreptococcus micros.* The gram-negative microorganisms are predominantly *F. nucleatum, P. intermedia, V. parvula,* as well as *Hemophilus, Capnocytophaga* and *Campylobacter* spp.[65,68,89]

Pregnancy-associated gingivitis is an acute inflammation of the gingival tissues associated with pregnancy. This condition is accompanied by increases in steroid hormones in crevicular fluid and dramatic increases in the levels of *P. intermedia,* which use the steroids as growth factors.[42]

Studies of gingivitis support the conclusion that disease development is associated with selected alterations in the microbial composition of dental plaque and are not simply the result of an accumulation of plaque. Gingivitis is generally believed to precede the development of chronic periodontitis; however, many individuals demonstrate long-standing gingivitis that never advances to destruction of the periodontal attachment.[6,55]

Chronic Periodontitis. The hallmark of periodontitis is the loss of connective tissue attachment to the tooth. Numerous forms of periodontal disease are found in adult populations; these forms are characterized by different rates of progression (Fig. 6-17) and different responses to therapy.[2] Studies in which untreated populations were examined over long time intervals indicate disease progression at mean rates ranging from 0.05 to 0.3 mm of attachment loss per year (i.e., the gradual model).[6] When populations are examined over short time intervals, individual sites demonstrated short phases of attachment destruction interposed by periods of no disease activity (i.e., the burst model).[26] It is unclear from recent studies whether the gradual or burst

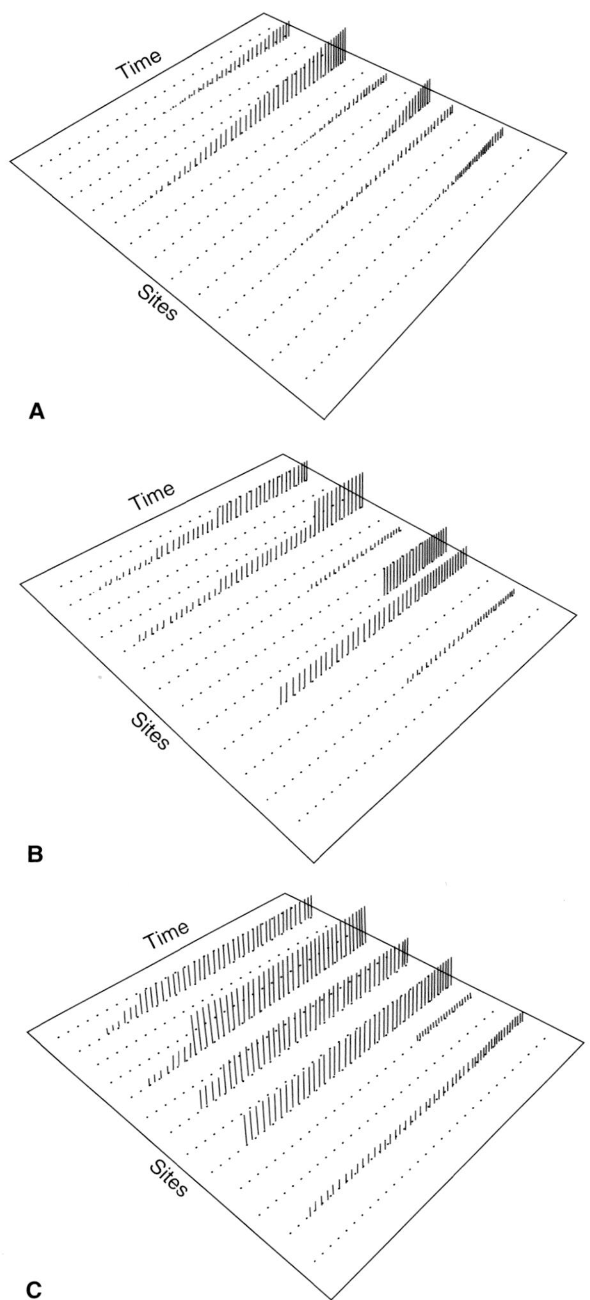

Fig. 6-17 Diagrammatic representation of different possible modes of progression of chronic destructive periodontal disease. Sites on the x-axis are plotted against time on the y-axis, and activity is shown on the z-axis. **A,** Some sites show progressive loss of attachment over time, whereas others show no destruction. The time of onset and the extent of destruction vary among sites. **B,** Random burst model. Activity occurs at random at any site. Some sites show no activity, whereas others show one or several bursts of activity. The cumulative extent of destruction varies among sites. **C,** Asynchronous multiple burst model. Several sites show bursts of activity over a finite period, followed by prolonged periods of inactivity. Occasional bursts may occur infrequently at certain sites at later periods. Other sites show no periodontal disease activity at any time. The difference from the model shown in **B** is that in **C,** the majority of destructive disease activity takes place within a few years of the individual's life. (Courtesy Drs. S. Socransky, A. Haffajee, M. Goodson, and J. Lindhe, Boston, Mass., and Göteborg, Sweden.)

model of disease progression, or some other model, is correct.[6]

Microbiologic examinations of chronic periodontitis have been carried out in both cross-sectional and longitudinal studies; the latter have been conducted with and without treatment. These studies support the concept that chronic periodontitis is associated with specific bacterial agents. Microscopic examination of plaque from sites with chronic periodontitis have consistently revealed elevated proportions of spirochetes (see Fig. 6-14).[53,58] Cultivation of plaque microorganisms from sites of chronic periodontitis reveals high percentages of anaerobic (90%) gram-negative (75%) bacterial species (see Fig. 6-15).[88,89]

In *chronic periodontitis,* the bacteria most often cultivated at high levels include *P. gingivalis, B. forsythus, P. intermedia, C. rectus, Eikenella corrodens, F. nucleatum, A. actinomycetemcomitans, P. micros,* and *Treponema* and *Eubacterium* spp.[45,47,56,68,89,93,94,97] When periodontally active sites (i.e., with recent attachment loss) were examined in comparison with inactive sites (i.e., with no recent attachment loss), *C. rectus, P. gingivalis, P. intermedia, F. nucleatum,* and *B. forsythus* were found to be elevated in the active sites.[20] Furthermore, detectable levels of *P. gingivalis, P. intermedia, B. forsythus, C. rectus,* and *A. actinomycetemcomitans* are associated with disease progression,[20,106] and elimination of specific bacterial pathogens with therapy is associated with an improved clinical response.[10,29,90] Both *P. gingivalis* and *A. actinomycetemcomitans* have been shown to invade host tissue cells, which may be significant in aggressive forms of adult periodontitis.[8,9,82] Recent studies have documented an association between chronic periodontitis and viral microorganisms of the herpesviruses group, most notably Epstein-Barr Virus-1 (EBV-1) and human cytomegalovirus (HCMV).[12] Further, the presence of subgingival EBV-1 and HCMV are associated with high levels of putative bacterial pathogens, including *P. gingivalis, B. forsythus, P. intermedia,* and *T. denticola.* These data support the hypothesis that viral infection may contribute to periodontal pathogenesis, but the potential role of viral agents remains to be determined.

Localized Aggressive Periodontitis. Several forms of periodontitis are characterized by rapid and severe attachment loss occurring in individuals during or before puberty. Localized aggressive periodontitis (previously referred to as *localized juvenile periodontitis [LJP]*) (see Chapter 28) develops around the time of puberty, is observed in females more often than in males, and typically affects the permanent molars and incisors. This condition is almost uniformly seen in individuals who demonstrate some systemic defect in immune regulation, and most affected individuals demonstrate defective neutrophil function.

The microbiota associated with localized aggressive periodontitis is predominantly composed of gram-negative, capnophilic, and anaerobic rods.[70,71,89] Microbiologic studies indicate that almost all LJP sites harbor *A. actinomycetemcomitans,* which may comprise as much as 90% of the total cultivable microbiota.[43,67] Other organisms found in significant levels include *P. gingivalis, E. corrodens, C. rectus, F. nucleatum, B. capillus, Eubacterium brachy,* and *Capnocytophaga* spp. and spirochetes.[43,64,66,67] Herpesviruses, including EBV-1 and HCMV, also have been associated with localized aggressive periodontitis.[12,64,99]

A. actinomycetemcomitans is generally accepted as the primary etiologic agent in most, but not all, cases of localized aggressive periodontitis (see discussion of virulence factors in Chapter 8).[44,94] Studies of therapy indicate that both mechanical debridement and systemic antibiotic treatment are necessary to control the levels of *A. actinomycetemcomitans* in this disease.[43,76,77] The failure of mechanical therapy alone may relate to the ability of this organism to invade host tissues.[8,9,82]

Periodontitis as a Manifestation of Systemic Disease. Previous classification schemes delineated "prepubertal periodontitis" as a rare form of periodontitis found to affect the primary dentition. This group has now been reclassified under the heading of periodontitis as a manifestation of systemic disease because most children with severe periodontal destruction also demonstrate profound immunologic abnormalities. The underlying immune deficiency may vary and includes neutrophil defects and leukocyte adhesion defects, for example.[17,34] Recent studies have demonstrated that some cases of severe periodontal destruction are associated with a mutation in the cathepsin C gene in afflicted children (see Chapter 10, "Genetic Factors Associated with Periodontal Disease"). Studies of patients with "prepubertal periodontitis" indicate that subgingival bacteria associated with other forms of periodontal disease also are found in these patients.[68,73] This is consistent with the concept that the occurrence of severe destruction at an early age is a reflection of an increased host susceptibility, in this case resulting from systemic disease. Identification of severe periodontal destruction in a child may be one of the first signs of systemic disease.

Necrotizing Periodontal Diseases. Necrotizing periodontal diseases present as acute inflammation of the gingival and periodontal tissues characterized by necrosis of the marginal gingival tissue and interdental papillae. Clinically, these conditions often are associated with stress or human immunodeficiency virus (HIV) infection. They may be accompanied by malodor, pain, and possibly systemic symptoms including lymphadenopathy, fever, and malaise. Microbiologic studies indicate that high levels of *P. intermedia* and spirochetes are found in necrotizing ulcerative gingivitis lesions. Spirochetes are found to penetrate necrotic tissue and apparently unaffected connective tissue.[49,50]

Abscesses of the Periodontium. Periodontal abscesses are acute lesions that may result in very rapid destruction of the periodontal tissues. They often occur in patients with untreated periodontitis but also may be found in patients during maintenance or after scaling and root planing. Periodontal abscesses also may occur in the absence of periodontitis; for example, associated with impaction of a foreign object (e.g., a popcorn kernel or dental floss) or with endodontic problems.[33] Typical clinical symptoms of periodontal abscesses include pain, swelling, suppuration, bleeding on probing, and mobility of the involved tooth. Signs of systemic involvement may be present, including cervical lymphadenopathy and an elevated white blood cell count.[32] Investigations reveal that bacteria recognized as peri-

TABLE 6-2

Evidence Supporting a Role for *A. actinomycetemcomitans* and *P. gingivalis* as Pathogens in Periodontal Disease: Socransky's Criteria

Criterion	*A. actinomycetemcomitans*	*P. gingivalis*
Association	Increased in localized aggressive periodontitis (LAP) lesions	Increased in periodontitis lesions
	Increased in some chronic periodontitis lesions Detected in the tissues of LAP lesions	Found associated with crevicular epithelium
Elimination	Suppressed or eliminated in successful therapy Found in recurrent lesions	Suppressed or eliminated in successful therapy Found in recurrent lesions
Host response	Increased serum and local antibody levels in LAP	Increased systemic and local antibody levels in periodontitis
Animal studies	Capable of inducing disease in gnotobiotic rats	Found to be important in experimental mixed infections and in periodontitis in the cynomolgus monkey
Virulence factors	Host tissue cell invasion, leukotoxin, collagenase, endotoxin (LPS), epitheliotoxin, fibroblast inhibiting factor, bone resorption-inducing factor	Host tissue cell adherence and invasion, collagenase, trypsin-like enzyme, fibrinolysin, phospholipase A, phosphatases, endotoxin (LPS), H_2S, NH_3, fatty acids, factors that affect PMN function

Adapted from Socransky SS, Haffajee AD: The bacterial etiology of destructive periodontal disease: Current concepts. J Periodontol 1992; 63:322.

odontal pathogens are commonly found in significant numbers in periodontal abscesses. These microorganisms include *F. nucleatum, P. intermedia, P. gingivalis, P. micros,* and *B. forsythus.*[30,32,72]

Conclusions from Studies of the Association of Microorganisms with Periodontal Diseases

Studies examining the microbiota associated with periodontal diseases versus the healthy state suggest that a discrete number of microorganisms may function as pathogens in the disease processes. However, conclusions based on these studies must be considered in light of several limitations. One limitation is our inability to identify and isolate a substantial proportion of the microorganisms found in the subgingival environment. Even with improvements in cultivation, the relative occurrence of the newly described species in health and disease needs to be addressed. For example, little information is available on the newly described spirochetal microorganisms (*Treponema* spp., Table 6-2). Another limitation is that association, although important, is only one aspect of demonstrating an etiologic role for a particular bacterium (see following discussion). The periodontal microbiota is a very complex ecologic system with many structural and physiologic interactions among the resident bacteria and between the bacteria and the host. It is clearly possible that levels of a particular species may be elevated as a result of environmental changes produced by the disease process and may not be a causative agent. A possible example of this comes from studies on the development of gingivitis in humans at the time of puberty. It was found that the proportions of *Capnocytophaga* spp. increased before the development of gingivitis, whereas *P. intermedia* was recovered after the onset of gingivitis.[65] This suggests a causative role for the *Capnocytophaga* spp., in contrast to the emergence of *P. intermedia* associated with environmental changes upon the development of gingivitis. Similarly, recent studies have demonstrated an association of herpesviruses with periodontal diseases, but the possible role of these microorganisms in the disease process is yet to be determined. Thus association studies represent an important, but only a first, step in critically identifying pathogens in periodontal diseases.

CRITERIA FOR IDENTIFICATION OF PERIODONTAL PATHOGENS

In the 1870s, Robert Koch developed the classic criteria by which a microorganism can be judged to be a causative agent in human infections. These criteria, known as *Koch's postulates,* stipulate that the causative agent must:

1. Be routinely isolated from diseased individuals
2. Be grown in pure culture in the laboratory
3. Produce a similar disease when inoculated into susceptible laboratory animals
4. Be recovered from lesions in a diseased laboratory animal

Streptococcus mutans, for example, has been shown to fulfill Koch's postulates as an etiologic agent of dental caries. However, difficulties exist in the application of these criteria to other types of diseases, and the applicability of Koch's postulates has been increasingly challenged in recent years. In the case of periodontitis, three primary problems are the inability to culture all the organisms that have been associated with disease (e.g., many of the oral spirochetes), the difficulties inherent in defining and culturing sites of active disease, and the lack of a good animal model system for the study of periodontitis.[94]

Sigmund Socransky, a researcher at the Forsyth Dental Center in Boston, proposed criteria by which periodontal microorganisms may be judged to be potential pathogens.[94] According to these criteria, a potential pathogen must:

1. Be associated with disease, as evident by increases in the number of organisms at diseased sites
2. Be eliminated or decreased in sites that demonstrate clinical resolution of disease with treatment
3. Demonstrate a host response, in the form of an alteration in the host cellular or humoral immune response
4. Be capable of causing disease in experimental animal models
5. Demonstrate virulence factors responsible for enabling the microorganism to cause destruction of the periodontal tissues

Data supporting the role of *A. actinomycetemcomitans* and *P. gingivalis* as periodontal pathogens, based on these criteria, are presented in Table 6-2. The association and elimination criteria are discussed in the preceding sections. The latter three criteria focus on the host parasite interaction, which is discussed in Chapter 8 (Microbial Interactions with the Host in Periodontal Diseases).

FUTURE ADVANCES IN PERIODONTAL MICROBIOLOGY

Scientific progress at the end of the 20th century, particularly in the field of molecular biology, has led to advances in our approach to the study of periodontal microbiology. DNA-based methodology for the identification and detection of specific bacteria and viruses represents a remarkable advantage in time and cost as compared with cultivation techniques. This has led to a dramatic increase in the number of samples that can be examined and the number of microorganisms enumerated. Perhaps even more profound, the ability to detect microorganisms that cannot be cultivated has underscored the limitations of our knowledge of this complex ecologic niche. The use of these approaches to continue the study of the periodontal region will undoubtedly refine our current understanding of the microbial ecology and etiology of diseases.

REFERENCES

1. Allison DG, Gilbert P: Modification by surface association of antimicrobial susceptibility of bacterial populations. J Ind Microbiol 1995; 15:311.
2. Armitage GC: Development of a classification system for periodontal diseases and conditions. Ann Periodontol 1999; 4:1.
3. Bowen WH: Nature of plaque. Oral Sci Rev 1976; 9:3.
4. Bradshaw DJ, Marsh PD, Watson GK, et al: Role of *Fusobac-*

terium nucleatum and coaggregation in anaerobe survival in planktonic and biofilm oral microbial communities during aeration. Infect Immun 1998; 66:4729.
5. Bramanti TE, Holt SC: Roles of porphyrins and host iron transport proteins in regulation of growth of *Porphyromonas gingivalis* W50. J Bacteriol 1991; 173:7330.
6. Brown LJ, Löe H: Prevalence, extent, severity and pro gression of periodontal disease. Periodontol 2000 1993; 2:57.
7. Carlsson J: Microbiology of plaque associated periodontal disease. In: Lindhe J (ed): Textbook of Clinical Periodontology, ed 1. Munksgaard, Munksgaard International Publishers, 1983.
8. Carranza FA Jr, Saglie R, Newman MG, et al: Scanning and transmission electron microscopic study of tissue-invading microorganisms in localized juvenile periodontitis. J Periodontol 1983; 54:598.
9. Christersson LA, Albini B, Zambon JJ, et al: Tissue localization of *Actinobacillus actinomycetemcomitans* in human periodontitis. I. Light, immunofluorescence and electron microscopic studies. J Periodontol 1987; 58:529.
10. Christersson LA, Zambon JJ, Genco RJ: Dental bacterial plaques. Nature and role in periodontal disease. J Clin Periodontol 1991; 18:441.
11. Colombo AP, Haffajee AD, Dewhirst FE, et al: Clinical and microbiological features of refractory periodontitis subjects. J Clin Periodontol 1998; 25:169.
12. Contreras A, Slots J: Herpesviruses in human periodontal disease. J Periodontal Res 2000; 35:3.
13. Costerton JW, Lewandowski Z, Caldwell DE, et al: Microbial biofilms. Ann Rev Microbiol 1995; 49:711.
14. Costerton JW, Stewart PS, Greenberg EP: Bacterial biofilms: a common cause of persistent infections. Science 1999; 284:1318.
15. Diaz PI, Zilm PS, Rogers AH: The response to oxidative stress of *Fusobacterium nucleatum* grown in continuous culture. FEMS Microbiol Lett 2000; 187:31.
16. Dibart S, Skobe Z, Snapp KR, et al: Identification of bacterial species on or in crevicular epithelial cells from healthy and periodontally diseased patients using DNA-DNA hybridization. Oral Microbiol Immunol 1998; 13:30.
17. Dougherty N, Gataletto MA: Oral sequelae of chronic neutrophil defects: case report of a child with glycogen storage disease type 1b. Pediatr Dent 1995; 17:224.
18. Doyle RJ, Rosenberg M, Drake D: Hydrophobicity of oral bacteria. In: Doyle RJ, Rosenberg M (eds): Microbial Cell Surface Hydrophobicity. Washington, DC, American Society for Microbiology, 1990.
19. Dzink JL, Tanner AC, Haffajee AD, et al: Gram-negative species associated with active destructive periodontal lesions. J Clin Periodontol 1985; 12:648.
20. Dzink JL, Socransky SS, Haffajee AD: The predominant cultivable microbiota of active and inactive lesions of destructive periodontal diseases. J Clin Periodontol 1988; 15:316.
21. Dzink JL, Gibbons RJ, Childs WCd, et al: The predominant cultivable microbiota of crevicular epithelial cells. Oral Microbiol Immunol 1989; 4:1.
22. Etoh Y, Dewhirst FE, Paster BJ, et al: *Campylobacter showae* sp. nov., isolated from the human oral cavity. Int J Syst Bacteriol 1993; 43:631.
23. Fachon-Kalweit S, Elder BL, Fives-Taylor P: Antibodies that bind to fimbriae block adhesion of *Streptococcus sanguis* to saliva-coated hydroxyapatite. Infect Immun 1985; 48:617.
24. Fives-Taylor PM, Thompson DW: Surface properties of *Streptococcus sanguis* FW213 mutants nonadherent to saliva-coated hydroxyapatite. Infect Immun 1985; 47:752.
25. Fletcher M: The physiological activity of bacteria attached to solid surfaces. Adv Microbiol Physio 1991; 32:53.
26. Goodson JM, Tanner AC, Haffajee AD, et al: Patterns of progression and regression of advanced destructive periodontal disease. J Clin Periodontol 1982; 9:472.
27. Grenier D, Mayrand D: Etudes d'infections mixtes anaerobies comportant *Bacteroides gingivalis*. Can J Microbiol 1983; 29:612.
28. Grenier D: Nutritional interaction between two suspected periodontopathogens, *Treponema denticola* and *Porphyromonas gingivalis*. Infect Immun 1992; 60:5298.
29. Haffajee AD, Cugini MA, Dibart S, et al: Clinical and microbiological features of subjects with adult periodontitis who responded poorly to scaling and root planing. J Clin Periodontol 1997; 24:767.
30. Hafstrom CA, Wikstrom MB, Renvert SN, et al: Effect of treatment on some periodontopathogens and their antibody levels in periodontal abscesses. J Periodontol 1994; 65:1022.
31. Helmerhorst EJ, Hodgson R, van 't Hof W, et al: The effects of histatin-derived basic antimicrobial peptides on oral biofilms. J Dent Res 1999; 78:1245.
32. Herrera D, Roldan S, Gonzalez I, et al: The periodontal abscess (I). Clinical and microbiological findings. J Clin Periodontol 2000; 27:387.
33. Herrera D, Roldan S, Sanz M: The periodontal abscess: a review. J Clin Periodontol 2000; 27:377.
34. Kamma JJ, Lygidakis NA, Nakou M: Subgingival microflora and treatment in prepubertal periodontitis associated with chronic idiopathic neutropenia. J Clin Periodontol 1998; 25:759.
35. Kaufman J, DiRienzo JM: Isolation of a corncob (coaggregation) receptor polypeptide from *Fusobacterium nucleatum*. Infect Immun 1989; 57:331.
36. Kinder SA, Holt SC: Characterization of coaggregation between *Bacteroides gingivalis* T22 and *Fusobacterium nucleatum* T18. Infect Immun 1989; 57:3425.
37. Kolenbrander PE: Surface recognition among oral bacteria: multigeneric coaggregations and their mediators. Crit Rev Microbiol 1989; 17:137.
38. Kolenbrander PE, Andersen RN: Inhibition of coaggregation between *Fusobacterium nucleatum* and *Porphyromonas (Bacteroides) gingivalis* by lactose and related sugars. Infect Immun 1989; 57:3204.
39. Kolenbrander PE, London J: Adhere today, here tomorrow: oral bacterial adherence. J Bacteriol 1993; 175:3247.
40. Kolenbrander PE, Parrish KP, Andersen RN, et al: Intergeneric coaggregation of oral *Treponema* spp. with *Fusobacterium* spp. and intrageneric coaggregation among *Fusobacteriium* spp. Infect Immun 1995; 63:4584.
41. Kononen E, Eerola E, Frandsen EV, et al: Phylogenetic characterization and proposal of a new pigmented species to the genus *Prevotella*: *Prevotella pallens* sp. nov. Int J Syst Bacteriol 1998; 48:47.
42. Kornman KS, Loesche WJ: Effects of estradiol and progesterone on *Bacteroides melaninogenicus* and *Bacteroides gingivalis*. Infect Immun 1982; 35:256.
43. Kornman KS, Robertson PB: Clinical and microbiological evaluation of therapy for juvenile periodontitis. J Periodontol 1985; 56:443.
44. Kornman KS, Löe H: The role of local factors in the etiology of periodontal diseases. Periodontol 2000 1993; 2:83.
45. Kremer BH, Loos BG, van der Velden U, et al; *Peptostreptococcus micros* smooth and rough genotypes in periodontitis and gingivitis. J Periodontol 2000; 71:209.
46. Kroes I, Lepp PW, Relman DA: Bacterial diversity within the human subgingival crevice. Proc Natl Acad Sci USA 1999; 96:14547.
47. Lai CH, Listgarten MA, Shirakawa M, et al: *Bacteroides*

forsythus in adult gingivitis and periodontitis. Oral Microbiol Immunol 1987; 2:152.
48. Lancy P, DiRienzo JM, Appelbaum B, et al: Corncob formation between *Fusobacterium nucleatum* and *Streptococcus sanguis*. Infect Immun 1983; 40:303.
49. Listgarten MA, Socransky SS: Ultrastructural characteristics of a spirochete in lesions of acute necrotizing ulcerative gingivostomatitis (Vincent's infection). Arch Oral Biol 1964; 9:95.
50. Listgarten MA: Electron microscopic observations on the bacterial flora of acute necrotizing ulcerative gingivitis. J Periodontol 1965; 36:328.
51. Listgarten MA, Mayo H, Amsterdam M: Ultrastructure of the attachment device between coccal and filamentous microorganisms in "corn cob" formations of dental plaque. Arch Oral Biol 1973; 18:651.
52. Listgarten MA: Structure of the microbial flora associated with periodontal health and disease in man. J Periodontol 1976; 47:1.
53. Listgarten MA, Hellden L: Relative distribution of bacteria at clinically healthy and periodontally diseased sites in humans. J Clin Periodontol 1978; 5:115.
54. Löe H, Theilade E, Jensen SB: Experimental gingivitis in man. J Periodontol 1965; 36:177.
55. Löe H: Periodontal diseases: a brief historical perspective. Periodontol 2000 1993; 2:7.
56. Loesche WJ: Importance of nutrition in gingival crevice microbial ecology. Periodontics 1968; 6:245.
57. Loesche WJ: Chemotherapy of dental plaque infections. Oral Sci Rev 1976; 9:65.
58. Loesche WJ, Syed SA, Schmidt E, et al: Bacterial profiles of subgingival plaques in periodontitis. J Periodontol 1985; 56:447.
59. Lovdal A, Arno A, Waerhaug J: Evidence of clinical manifestations of periodontal disease in light of oral hygiene and calculus formation. J Am Dent Assoc 1958; 56:21.
60. Manganiello AD, Socransky SS, Smith C, et al: Attempts to increase viable count recovery of human supragingival dental plaque. J Periodontal Res 1977; 12:107.
61. Mayrand D, McBride BC: Ecological relationships of bacteria involved in a simple, mixed anaerobic infection. Infect Immun 1980; 27:44.
62. McBride BC, van der Hoeven JS: Role of interbacterial adherence in colonization of the oral cavities of gnotobiotic rats infected with *Streptococcus mutans* and *Veillonella alcalescens*. Infect Immun 1981; 33:467.
63. Mergenhagen SE, Sandberg AL, Chassy BM, et al: Molecular basis of bacterial adhesion in the oral cavity. Rev Infect Dis 1987; 9:S467.
64. Michalowicz BS, Ronderos M, Camara-Silva R, et al: Human herpesviruses and *Porphyromonas gingivalis* are associated with juvenile periodontitis. J Periodontol 2000; 71:981.
65. Mombelli A, Lang NP, Burgin WB, et al: Microbial changes associated with the development of puberty gingivitis. J Periodontal Res 1990; 25:331.
66. Moore WE, Holdeman LV, Cato EP, et al: Comparative bacteriology of juvenile periodontitis. Infect Immun 1985; 48:507.
67. Moore WE: Microbiology of periodontal disease. J Periodontal Res 1987; 22:335.
68. Moore WE, Moore LV: The bacteria of periodontal diseases. Periodontol 2000 1994; 5:66.
69. Newman HN: The approximal apical border of plaque on children's teeth. 1. Morphology, structure and cell content. J Periodontol 1979; 50:561.
70. Newman MG, Socransky SS, Savitt ED, et al: Studies of the microbiology of periodontosis. J Periodontol 1976; 47:373.
71. Newman MG, Socransky SS: Predominant cultivable microbiota in periodontosis. J Periodontal Res 1977; 14:120.
72. Newman MG, Sims TN: The predominant cultivable microbiota of the periodontal abscess. J Periodontol 1979; 50:350.
73. Page RC, Schroeder H: Periodontitis in Man and Other Animals. Basal, Karger, 1982.
74. Pratten J, Barnett P, Wilson M: Composition and susceptibility to chlorhexidine of multispecies biofilms of oral bacteria. Appl Environ Microbiol 1998; 64:3515.
75. Ranney RR: Classification of periodontal diseases. Perio 2000 1993; 2:13.
76. Renvert S, Wikstrom M, Dahlen G, et al: On the inability of root debridement and periodontal surgery to eliminate *Actinobacillus actinomycetemcomitans* from periodontal pockets. J Clin Periodontol 1990; 17:351.
77. Renvert S, Wikstrom M, Dahlen G, et al: Effect of root debridement on the elimination of *Actinobacillus actinomycetemcomitans* and *Bacteroides gingivalis* from periodontal pockets. J Clin Periodontol 1990; 17:345.
78. Rolla G: Pellicle formation. In Lazzari EP (ed): CRC Handbook of Experimental Aspects of Oral Biochemistry. Boca Raton, FL, CRC Press, 1983.
79. Rolla G, Ogaard B, Cruz RA: Topical application of fluorides on teeth. New concepts of mechanisms of interaction. J Clin Periodontol 1993; 20:105.
80. Russel AL: Epidemiology of periodontal disease. Int Dent J 1967; 17:282.
81. Saglie FR, Carranza FA Jr, Newman MG, et al: Identification of tissue-invading bacteria in human periodontal disease. J Periodontal Res 1982; 7:452.
82. Saglie FR, Marfany A, Camargo P: Intragingival occurrence of *Actinobacillus actinomycetemcomitans* and *Bacteroides gingivalis* in active destructive periodontal lesions. J Periodontol 1988; 9:259.
83. Scannapieco FA, Levine MJ: Saliva and dental pellicles. In: Genco RJ, Goldman HM, Cohen DW (eds): Contemporary Periodontics. St Louis, Mosby, 1990.
84. Schei O, Waerhaug J, Lovdal A, et al: Alveolar bone loss as related to oral hygiene and age. J Periodontol 1959; 30:7.
85. Shah HN, Collins MD: Proposal for reclassification of *Bacteroides asaccharolyticus, Bacteroides gingivalis,* and *Bacteroides endodontalis* in a new genus, *Porphyromonas*. Int J Syst Bacteriol 1988; 38:128.
86. Shah HN, Collins DM: *Prevotella,* a new genus to include *Bacteroides melaninogenicus* and related species formerly classified in the genus *Bacteroides*. Int J Syst Bacteriol 1990; 40:205.
87. Shah HN, Gharbia SE: Biochemical and chemical studies on strains designated *Prevotella intermedia* and proposal of a new pigmented species, *Prevotella nigrescens* sp. nov. Int J Syst Bacteriol 1992; 42:542.
88. Slots J: The predominant cultivable microflora of advanced periodontitis. Scand J Dent Res 1977; 85:114.
89. Slots J: Subgingival microflora and periodontal disease. J Clin Periodontol 1979; 6:351.
90. Slots J, Listgarten MA: *Bacteroides gingivalis, Bacteroides intermedius,* and *Actinobacillus actinomycetemcomitans* in human periodontal diseases. J Clin Periodontol 1988; 15:85.
91. Socransky SS, Gibbons RJ, Dale AC, et al: The microbiota of the gingival crevice area of man. I. Total microscopic and viable counts of specific microorganisms. Arch Oral Biol 1953; 8:275.
92. Socransky SS, Manganiello AD, Propas D, et al: Bacteriological studies of developing supragingival dental plaque. J Periodontal Res 1977; 12:90.
93. Socransky SS, Haffajee AD: Microbial mechanisms in the pathogenesis of destructive periodontal diseases: a critical assessment. J Periodontal Res 1991; 26:195.

94. Socransky SS, Haffajee AD: The bacterial etiology of destructive periodontal disease: current concepts. J Periodontol 1992; 63:322.
95. Socransky SS: Evidence of bacterial etiology: a historical perspective. Periodontol 2000 1994; 5:7.
96. Socransky SS, Haffajee AD, Cugini MA, et al: Microbial complexes in subgingival plaque. J Clin Periodontol 1998; 25:134.
97. Tanner AC, Haffer C, Bratthall GT, et al: A study of the bacteria associated with advancing periodontitis in man. J Clin Periodontol 1979; 6:278.
98. Theilade E, Wright WH, Jensen SB, et al: Experimental gingivitis in man. II. A longitudinal clinical and bacteriological investigation. J Periodontal Res 1966; 1:1.
99. Ting M, Contreras A, Slots J: Herpesvirus in localized juvenile periodontitis. J Periodontal Res 2000; 35:17.
100. Umemoto T, Nakazawa F, Hoshino E, et al: *Treponema medium* sp. nov., isolated from human subgingival dental plaque. Int J Syst Bacteriol 1997; 47:67.
101. Vandamme P, Falsen E, Rossau R, et al: Revision of *Campylobacter, Helicobacter,* and *Wolinella* taxonomy: emendation of generic descriptions and proposal of *Arcobacter* gen. nov. Int. J. Syst. Bacteriol. 1991; 41:88.
102. Walden WC, Hentges DJ: Differential effects of oxygen and oxidation-reduction potential on the multiplication of three species of anaerobic intestinal bacteria. Appl Microbiol 1975; 30:781.
103. Weiss EI, London J, Kolenbrander PE, et al: Characterization of monoclonal antibodies to fimbria-associated adhesins of *Bacteroides loescheii* PK1295. Infect Immun 1988; 56:219.
104. Weiss EI, London J, Kolenbrander PE, et al: Localization and enumeration of fimbria-associated adhesins of *Bacteroides loescheii.* J Bacteriol 1988; 170:1123.
105. Weiss EI, Eli I, Shenitzki B, et al: Identification of the rhamnose-sensitive adhesin of *Capnocytophaga ochracea* ATCC 33596. Arch Oral Biol 1990; 35:127S.
106. Wennstrom JL, Dahlen G, Svensson J, et al: *Actinobacillus actinomycetemcomitans, Bacteroides gingivalis* and *Bacteroides intermedius*: predictors of attachment loss? Oral Microbiol Immunol 1987; 2:158.
107. Wood SR, Kirkham J, Marsh PD, et al: Architecture of intact natural human plaque biofilms studied by confocal laser scanning microscopy. J Dent Res 2000; 79:21.
108. Wyss C, Choi BK, Schupbach P, et al: *Treponema maltophilum* sp. nov., a small oral spirochete isolated from human periodontal lesions. Int J Syst Bacteriol 1996; 46:745.
109. Wyss C, Choi BK, Schupbach P, et al. *Treponema amylovorum* sp. nov., a saccharolytic spirochete of medium size isolated from an advanced human periodontal lesion. Int J Syst Bacteriol 1997; 47:842.
110. Wyss C, Choi BK, Schupbach P, et al: *Treponema lecithinolyticum* sp. nov., a small saccharolytic spirochaete with phospholipase A and C activities associated with periodontal diseases. Int J Syst Bacteriol 1999; 49:1329.
111. Zambon JJ, Reynolds HS, Slots J: Black-pigmented *Bacteroides* spp. in the human oral cavity. Infect Immun 1981; 32:198.

Immunity and Inflammation: Basic Concepts

Kenneth T. Miyasaki, Russell J. Nisengard, and Susan Kinder Haake

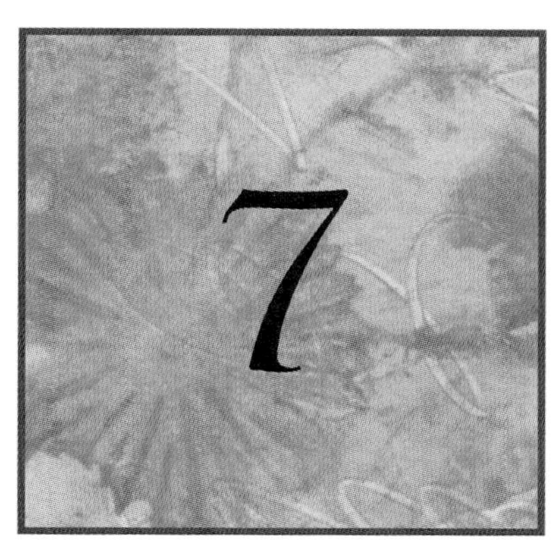

CHAPTER

CHAPTER OUTLINE

The common periodontal diseases found in humans are gingivitis and periodontitis. These are inflammatory responses in the periodontal tissues induced by microorganisms in dental plaque, which may lead to tissue destruction. This chapter focuses on the role of the immune system in inflammation. The immune system is a network designed for the homeostasis of large molecules (oligomers) and cells based on specific recognition processes. Recognition of the structural features of an oligomer by receptors on immune cells is an important component of the **specificity** of the immune system.

Immune responses are categorized as either innate or adaptive. **Innate immune responses** do not adapt with repeated exposure to the same pathogen. An example of innate immunity is phagocytic cells (i.e., monocytes, macrophages, and neutrophils), which possess a number of inherently antimicrobial peptides and proteins that kill many different, rather than one specific, pathogen. In contrast, the specific adaptive immune responses will increase after exposure to a pathogen. Lymphocytes (e.g., T-cells and B-cells) are important in the fundamental form of specific adaptive immunity referred to as the **specific immune response.** The ability of T-cells and B-cells to recognize specific oligomeric structures on a pathogen and generate progeny that also recognize the structure enables the immune system to respond more rapidly and effectively when exposed to that pathogen again.

Inflammation is an observable alteration in tissues associated with changes in vascular permeability and dilation, often with the infiltration of leukocytes into affected tissues. These changes result in the erythema, edema, heat, pain, and loss of function that are the "cardinal signs" of inflammation. Typically, inflammation can progress through three stages: immediate, acute, and chronic. **Leukocytes,** the white blood cells, control all three stages of inflammation (Table 7-1, Fig. 7-1).

Leukocytes originate in the bone marrow and exit from the blood by **transendothelial migration** under normal conditions, accounting for the **resident leukocytes** (or nonelicited leukocytes) found in tissues. Among the most important resident leukocytes are mast cells, peripheral dendritic cells (DC), and monocyte-derivatives such as dermal dendrocytes (histiocytes). These resident leukocytes transmit information that

TABLE 7-1

Cells of the Immune System

Leukocyte	Normal Blood Levels (per mm³)	Notable Properties (Cell Diameter in Blood)	Key Receptors in Interactions with Antigen*	Important Functions in Inflammation
Myeloid Cells				
Neutrophil	4000 to 8000	Terminally differentiated in blood, granular cytoplasm (9 to 10 μm)	CR1, CR3 (Mac-1) CR4 FcγRII C5aR(CD88)	Phagocytic killing of microorganisms
Monocyte	200 to 800	Immature in blood (9 to 10 μm)	CR1, CR3 (Mac-1) CR4, CD1 FcγRI, FcγRII MHC Class II C5aR (CD88)	Can differentiate to macrophages with diameters $>$ 20 μm Functions in phagocytosis and antigen processing and presentation
Peripheral dendritic cell	N/A	Immature in blood (9 to 10 μm)	ICAM-1, LFA-1 MHC Class II CD1	Resident in parabasilar epithelium Function in processing and presentation of antigen
Eosinophil	50 to 300	Terminally differentiated in blood, granular cytoplasm (9 to 10 μm)	FCϵRII (low affinity) FcγRII C5aR (CD88) CR1, CR3 (Mac-1) CR4	Antiparasitic and antihelminthic activity, mediated by IgE
Basophil	0 to 100	Terminally differentiated in blood, granular cytoplasm (9 to 10 μm)	FcϵRI (high affinity) CR1, CR3, CR4 C5aR (CD88)	Receptor profile suggests that cells may respond to bacterial and parasitic infections
Mast cell	N/A	N/A	FcϵRI (high affinity) C3aR C5aR (CD88) CR4, no CR3	Resident in perivascular connective tissue Anaphylactic effects in response to C3a and C5a Antigen recognized by IgE
Lymphoid Cells				
CD4+ cells	400 to 1600	(8 to 10 μm)	TCR, CD4	Scanning antigen presented by professional antigen-presenting cells In inflammation, this may result in clonal expansion of B-cells and T-cells
CD8+ cells	200 to 800	(8 to 10 μm)	TCR, CD8	Scanning antigen presented by all cells In inflammation, this may result in clonal expansion and killing of the cell presenting antigen
B-cell	200 to 800	(8 to 10 μm)	BCR MHC Class II	Binding soluble antigen, antigen processing and presentation In inflammation, this may result in clonal expansion and antibody secretion
NK-cell	100 to 500	(8 to 15 μm)	KIR, KAR	Scanning cell antigens, target cell killing if KAR scans antigen, no killing if KIR scans antigen

N/A, Not applicable.

* All cells present self-derived antigens using MHC Class I molecules. See text for explanation of receptor designations.

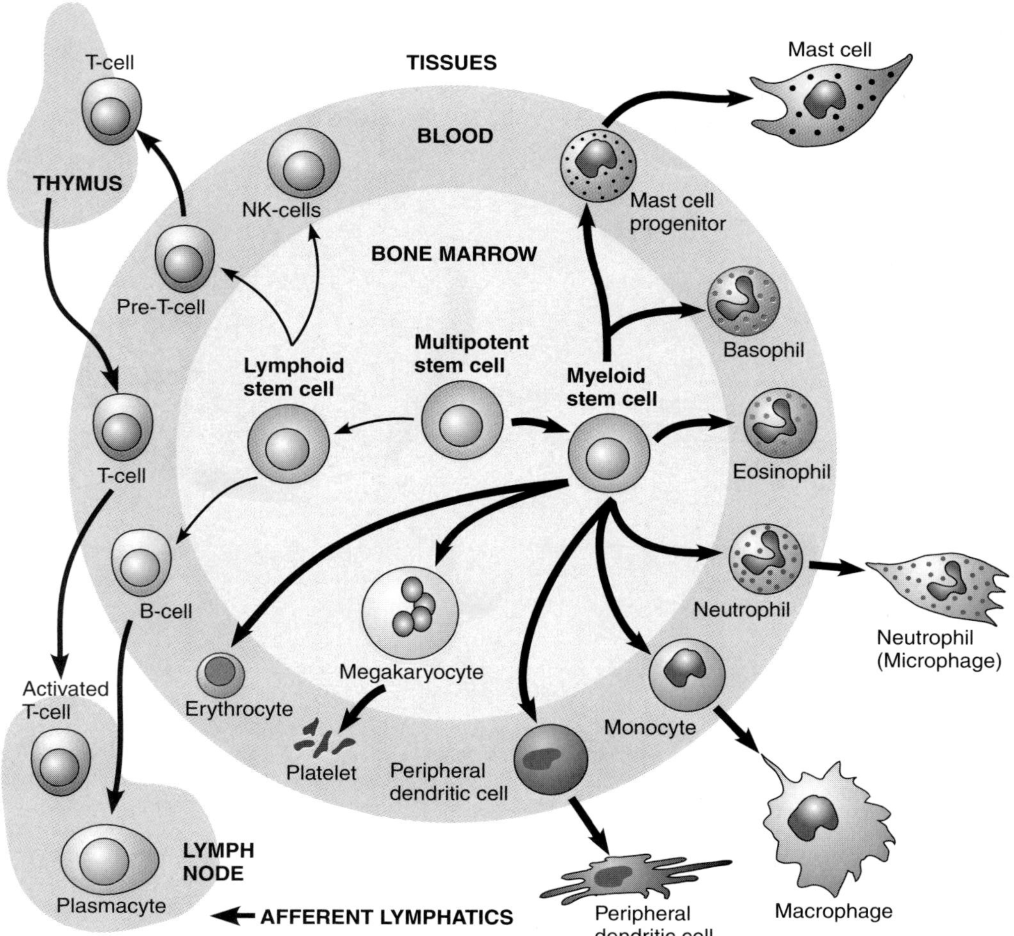

Fig. 7-1 The main cells of the immune system are derived from the lymphoid and myeloid arms of the hematopoietic system. In the bone marrow, the myeloid arm gives rise to peripheral dendritic cells, phagocytes (neutrophils and monocytes), mast cell precursors, basophils, eosinophils, platelets, and erythrocytes. In the tissues, peripheral dendritic cells, monocytes, and mast cell precursors further differentiate. The monocyte can become a macrophage. In the bone marrow, the lymphoid arm gives rise to NK-cells, B-cells, and pre-T-cells. The pre-T-cells differentiate to T-cells in the thymus. Secondary lymphoid organs, including lymph nodes and the spleen, are areas where antigen presenting cells, B-cells, and dendritic cells, present antigen to T-cells. Terminal differentiation of B- and T-cells also occurs in these organs.

initiates the processes of **immediate inflammation** (Fig. 7-2). Immediate inflammation is followed within minutes by a short-lived period (up to several hours) of **acute inflammation** that is characterized by an influx of neutrophils to the area after they exit the blood. If the problem is not resolved, acute inflammation gives way to a potentially unending period of **chronic inflammation** dominated by the migration of lymphocytes and macrophages to the local tissues. The leukocytes recruited into tissues in acute and chronic inflammation are termed **inflammatory leukocytes.**

CELLS OF IMMUNITY AND INFLAMMATION

Cells of the immune system that are important in inflammation and host defenses include in mast cells, dermal dendrocytes (histiocytes), peripheral dendritic cells, neutrophils, monocytes/macrophages, T-cells, B-cells, and NK-cells (see Table 7-1, Fig. 7-1). Other hematopoietic leukocytes (i.e., basophils, eosinophils, erythrocytes, and platelets) also participate in certain forms of inflammation or immune function but will not be described here.

Cells possess receptors, which are molecules on the cell surfaces that enable the cell to interact with other molecules or cells. Receptors reflect and dictate the function of cells. Historically, the names given to receptors often related to function. In addition to these common names, a systematic nomenclature known as the **CD (cluster of differentiation) system** has been developed. Under this system, receptors are identified as CD1, CD2, and so on. In this chapter, multiple designations are provided for specific receptors when the different designations have been commonly used.

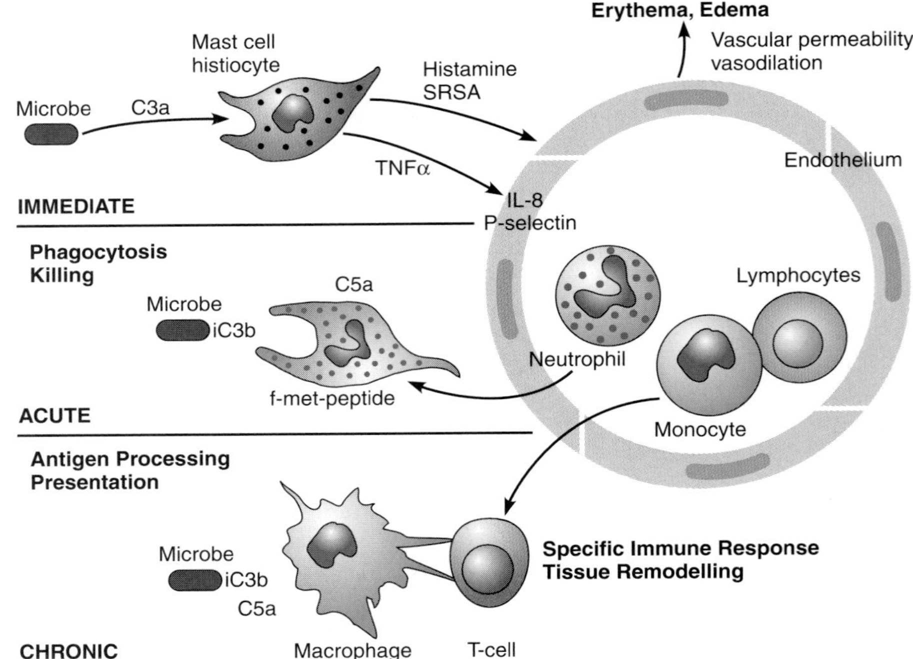

Fig. 7-2 The natural history of inflammation actually starts before an irritant exists, with the transendothelial migration of resident leukocytes, especially the mast cell. Mast cells are among the most effective cells in alerting the endothelium of a local problem. Mast cell interaction with the vascular system leads to erythema and edema, which are two of the five cardinal signs of inflammation. Mast cells also signal the endothelial cells to recruit inflammatory leukocytes. The inflammatory leukocytes are active in phagocytosis, killing, antigen processing and presentation, specific immune responses, and tissue remodeling. They cause the infiltrated area to lose function (the fifth cardinal sign of inflammation) as a side effect of their intense focus on resolving the problem and remodeling the tissue. Also depicted are the complement metabolites, iC3b, C3a, and C5a. These molecules are important in allowing the immune system to "see" substances for which they do not possess receptors.

Mast Cells

Mast cells are important in immediate inflammation (see Table 7-1 and Fig. 7-1). They possess receptors for complement components (C3a and C5a) as well as receptors for the Fc portion of the antibody molecules IgE and IgG (FcϵR and FcγR, respectively). The stimulation of these receptors can result in activation and secretion of vasoactive substances that increase vascular permeability and dilation, two important signs of **anaphylaxis.** Anaphylaxis can be life threatening if it is widespread (systemic), but it is usually localized and is important in initiating inflammatory responses against local microbial invasion.[22] Mast cells feature prominent cytoplasmic granules, termed **lysosomes,** which store inflammatory mediators such as histamine, eosinophil chemotactic factor, neutrophil chemotactic factor, and heparin. Mast cells can synthesize, *de novo,* other inflammatory mediators, such as the slow-reacting substances of anaphylaxis (SRS-A), tumor necrosis factor-α (TNF-α), and leukotriene C4.

Dermal Dendrocytes

Dermal dendrocytes (histiocytes) are widely distributed and form a large system of collagen-associated dendritic cells of myeloid origin. These cells are distributed near blood vessels and possess receptors for the complement component C3a, by which they participate in immediate inflammation. They express the major histocompatibility complex (MHC; see discussion below) Class II molecules.[32]

Peripheral Dendritic Cells

Peripheral dendritic cells (DC) are leukocytes with cytoplasmic projections, or dendrites (see Table 7-1).[8] **Langerhans cells** are DCs that reside in the suprabasilar portions of squamous epithelium. DCs ingest antigen locally and transport the antigen to the lymph nodes through the afferent lymphatics. DCs express high levels of MHC Class II molecules and CD1 as well as cell adhesion molecules (intercellular adhesion molecule-1 [ICAM-1]; leukocyte function associated antigen-3 [LFA-3]), and **costimulatory factors** (B7-1, B7-2; discussed below).

Neutrophils and Monocytes/Macrophages

Neutrophils and monocytes are closely related phagocytic leukocytes. The fundamental difference between these two cells is that neutrophils differentiate almost completely within the bone marrow (14 days), whereas monocytes exit the bone marrow after 2 days in a relatively immature state and may differentiate in the tissues. Neutrophils and monocytes are the same size (10-μm diameter) in the blood.

Neutrophils (also known as *polymorphonuclear leukocytes,* or *PMNs*) are the predominant leukocyte in blood, accounting for about two thirds of all blood leukocytes (4000 to 8000 cells/mm^3; see Table 7-1). They possess many lysosomes within their cytoplasm. Because neutrophils do not need to differentiate substantially to function, they are suited for rapid responses. When neutrophils leave the blood, they always retain their small size and hence were once called *microphages*. Neutrophils possess receptors for metabolites of the complement molecule C3, designated complement receptor 1, 3, and 4 (CR1, CR3, CR4); and C5 (C5aR). They also possess receptors for IgG antibody (FcγR). These receptors enable neutrophils to participate in the inflammatory response and to ingest foreign molecules and cells in the process of phagocytosis.

By convention, monocytes are referred to as *macrophages* when they leave the blood. They complete their differentiation in the local tissues and may become greater than 22 μm diameter; hence the macrophage designation (see Table 7-1). Because macrophages differentiate and live in the local tissues, they are suited for communicating with lymphocytes and other surrounding cells. Macrophages live long enough to present antigen to T-cells. Together, macrophages and lymphocytes (discussed below) orchestrate the chronic immune response. Monocytes/macrophages possess CR1, CR3, CR4, C5aR receptors, several classes of Fcγ receptors (FcγRI, FcγRII, FcγRIII), and molecules important in antigen presentation (MHC Class II receptor, CD1).

Lymphocytes

The three main types of lymphocytes are distinguished on the basis of their receptors for antigens: T- and B-lymphocytes and natural killer (NK) cells. In the blood, B-cells and T-cells are inactive and exhibit a fairly small size (8 to 10 μm). NK-cells may differentiate extensively in the bone marrow and appear in blood as a large, granular lymphocyte. With a diameter of 15 μm or greater, these cells are larger than any other leukocyte in the blood.

T-Cells

T-cells recognize diverse antigens using a low-affinity transmembranous complex, the **T-cell antigen receptor (TCR).** Antigens are recognized by T-cells in association with either MHC Class I or Class II molecules on the surface of the antigen presenting cell. T-cells are subdivided based on whether they possess the coreceptors CD4 or CD8. The CD4 coreceptor reversibly binds (scans for) MHC Class II molecules (HLA-DR, HLA-DP, HLA-DQ) that are found on dendritic cells, macrophages, and B-cells. CD4+ T-cells initiate and help with immune responses by providing proliferative and differentiative signals. The CD8 coreceptor scans for MHC Class I molecules, which are found on all cells. The CD8+ T-cells are predominantly cytotoxic T-cells involved in controlling intracellular antigens (e.g., certain bacteria, hyphal fungi, viruses).

B-Cells

B-cells help control extracellular antigens such as bacteria, fungal yeast, and virions. B-cells recognize diverse antigens using the **B-cell antigen receptor (BCR),** which is a high-affinity antigen receptor. The high-affinity interaction between BCR and antigen enables the B-cell to bind and ingest the antigen without antigen presentation. The antigen is tightly bound, not scanned. Ingested antigen is degraded and presented to T-cells.

Before antigen exposure, B-cells express IgM as part of the BCR. After antigen exposure, some B-cells differentiate to form **plasma cells** dedicated to the production and secretion of antibodies of the IgM isotype. Others in the presence of T-cells may differentiate along the memory pathway, forming **memory B-cells.** Memory B-cells give rise to plasma cells upon secondary exposure to antigen and produce high-affinity antibodies of the appropriate isotype.

Natural Killer (NK) Cells

NK-cells recognize and kill certain tumor and virally infected cells. The NK-cells possess several classes of antigen receptors, including **killer inhibitory receptors (KIR)** and **killer activating receptors (KAR).** These receptors will recognize antigens associated with MHC Class I molecules, MHC Class I molecules themselves, or certain other surface glycoproteins. Normal cells possess MHC Class I molecules that present antigens recognized as "self"; these interact with KIR and protect the cells from NK-cell mediated killing. Alterations in antigens presented by the MHC Class I molecules, occurring in tumor- and virally infected cells, may result in NK-cell activation because the KIR do not detect sufficient self antigens. Additionally, cells can present self-antigens in response to stress or other alteration, which are recognized by the KAR. KAR activation can override KIR inhibition and cause the NK-cell to kill the target cell.

COMPLEMENT

Complement (C) is an interacting network of about 30 membrane-associated cell receptors and soluble serum glycoproteins (Table 7-2). Soluble components of this system account for about 5% (3 to 4 mg/mL) of the total serum protein. Most soluble components are synthesized in the liver, but many also may be produced by macrophages (C1, C2, C3, C4, C5, Factor B, C1–INA, Factor D, and Factor H). The soluble components of the complement system were first observed to cause bacteriolysis and cytolysis in association with antibody (a "complement" of antibody), and later in the absence of antibody. These lytic effects are famous but represent only one function of complement.

The complement system is a central component of inflammation that enables endothelium and leukocytes to recognize and bind foreign substances for which they lack receptors. Complement promotes inflammation by generating the following:

- A vasoactive substance, termed *kinin-like,* C2a, which induces pain, increases vascular permeability and dilation
- Molecules, termed *anaphylatoxins,* C3a and C5a, which produce anaphylaxis by inducing mast cell secretion
- A chemotaxin, C5a, which attracts leukocytes and stimulates phagocyte secretion
- An opsonin, iC3b, covalently bound to molecular aggregates, particles, or cells, which enables phagocytes to ingest them

C3 is the most important component of complement (Fig. 7-3, *A*). It also is the predominant component, accounting for about one third of the total complement (1.6 mg/mL). A sequestered, internal thioester bond is the essential feature of C3, and it shares this feature with

TABLE 7-2

Complement Components

Component	Molecular Weight (kd)	Serum Concentration (μg/ml)*
Classical Pathway Initiators		
C1q†	410	150 to 180
C1r	85	50
C1s	85	100
Mannose-binding lectin (MBL)	400	1.5 to 1.8
MASP1	93 (proform)	1.5 to 12
MASP2	90 (proform)	Undetermined
C3 Convertase and C3/C5 Convertase Formation		
C2	110	30
C3	195	1200 to 1300
C4	210	400 to 450
Factor B	93	200 to 225
Factor D	25	1.5
Membrane Attach Complex Formation		
C5	205	80
C6	128	75
C7	121	55
C8	155	80
C9	79	200
C1-INA	109	180
Factor I	88 to 93	25 to 35
Anaphylatoxin inactivator	310	30
Soluble Regulators of Complement Activation		
Factor H	150	500 to 520
C4BP	570	200
Membrane Regulators of Complement Activation		
		Location
MCP (CD46)	45 to 70	All cells
DAF (CD55)	75 to 80	All cells
CR1 (CD35)	250	Phagocytes, B-cells, erythrocytes
CR2 (CD21)	140	B-cells
Opsonic Receptors of iC3b		
CR3 (Mac-1; CD11b/CD18)	165/95‡	Phagocytes, dendritic cells
CR4 (p150/95; CD11c/CD18)	150/95‡	Phagocytes

* Normal serum protein concentration range is 60 to 78 mg/ml.

† See text for explanation of abbreviations.

‡ Molecular weights of individual subunits of the receptors are provided.

the related molecule, C4. Splitting of C3 forms C3a and C3b and exposes the internal thioester bond residing within the C3b fragment. Two main pathways result in the splitting of C3, the **alternative** and the **classical** pathways (Fig. 7-3, *B*). The outcome of C3b generation is dictated by the presence or absence of the **regulators of complement activation** (discussed below).

Both the alternative pathway and classical pathway lead to inflammation and phagocytosis through an enzyme that is designated a **bound C3 convertase.** The alternative pathway is initiated without provocation by a spontaneous hydrolysis of the internal thioester bond of C3 by water. This pathway leads to the hydrolysis of C3b by larger structures (designated R), including the hydroxyls and amines on macromolecules and bacterial cell surfaces. The resulting covalent structure, C3b-R, leads to the bound C3 convertase (R-C3bBb).

The classical pathway is initiated in response to the presence of some irritant. Irritants include antibody-antigen complexes, certain membranes, or suspicious polymers (e.g., mannans). This pathway involves the activation of a serine protease (e.g., C1qrs) which has attached to an irritant. The protease serves as a C4/C2 convertase and leads to formation of a C3 convertase covalently bound to R (R-C4bC2b), with release of the vasoactive kinin-like substance C2a. The classical pathway also may be activated in the absence of such irritants, but this is controlled by an inactivator, C1-Inactivator (C1-INA). A deficiency of C1-INA (often occurring secondary to infection) can result in swollen lips or eyelids (angioedema) due to such spontaneous activation of the classical pathway.

Two main processes can occur with the formation of bound C3 convertase in the absence of regulators, such as in the presence of bacterial cells (Fig. 7-4). First, amplification occurs; second, the membrane attack complex is formed. **Amplification** is an exponential increase in the formation of C3b. This results because the bound C3 convertase (either R-C3bBb or R-C4bC2b) forms more C3b, and the resultant C3b may form more C3 convertases (R-C3bBb). Formation of C3b also is associated with the production of the anaphylatoxin C3a.

Formation of the **membrane attack complex** is initiated after approximately 100 molecules of C3b are formed, when the thioester of one C3b is hydrolyzed by the C3 convertase (R-C3bBb or R-C4bC2b) itself at a specific site on the C3b (or C4b) subunit of the convertase.[20] This results in the formation of the structure R-C3b-C3bBb or R-C3b-C4bC2b. These new complexes can bind and cleave both C3 and C5; thus they are called **C3/C5 convertases.** The C5 convertase activity is monumentally slow (in fact, one of the slowest enzymatic activities in the known universe); at best, one C5 is converted every four minutes by one C5 convertase.[27] Nonetheless, the cleavage of C5 produces two important fragments, C5a and C5b. The C5a fragment is the main leukocyte chemoattractant derived from complement and is an important anaphylatoxin. The C5b component associates with C6, C7, C8, and C9, forming a membrane attack complex that can lyse certain bacteria and cells by forming a large pore in the target cell membrane.

The six **regulators of complement activation** are encoded in a tight cluster on chromosome 1: **Factor H, membrane cofactor protein (MCP), complement receptor 1 (CR1), complement receptor 2 (CR2), decay accelerating factor (DAF), and C4-binding protein (C4BP).** Four of these regulators are cofactors working with the proteolytic soluble enzyme, **Factor I,** including Factor H, MCP, CR1, and C4bp.

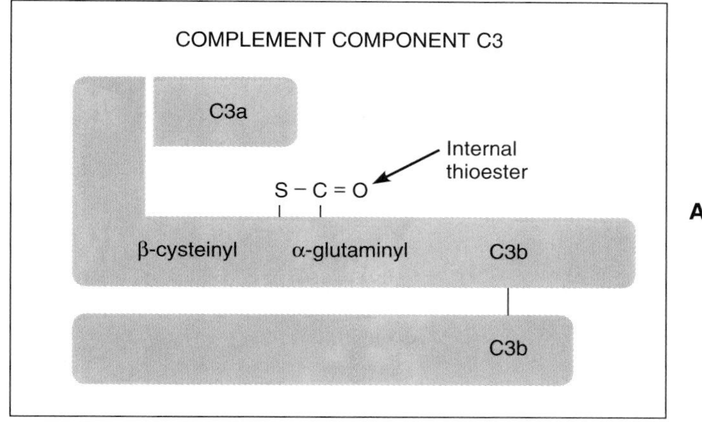

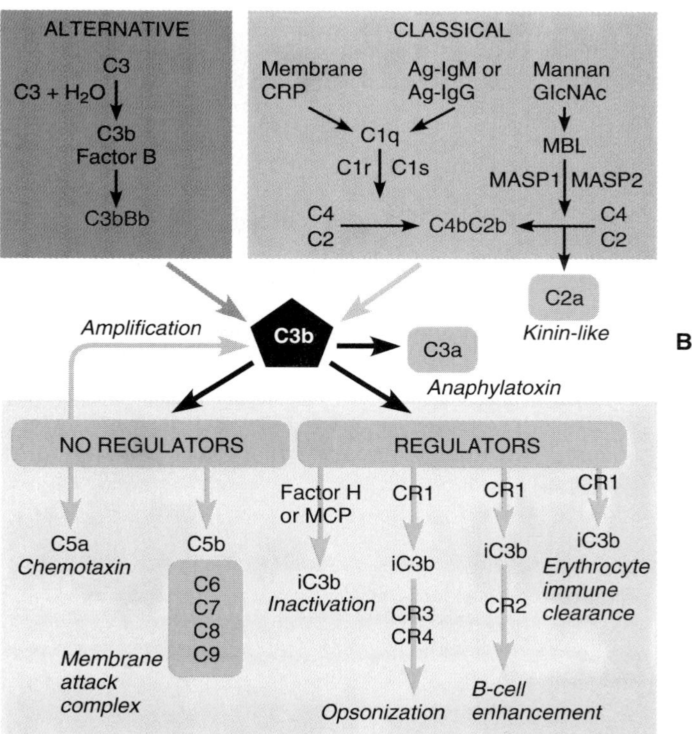

Fig. 7-3 **A,** The central component of complement is C3. See the text for details of the importance and function of C3. **B,** The central goal of the complement system is the formation of C3b. Both the alternative and classical pathways lead to formation of C3 convertase enzymes (C3bBb, C4bC2b) and the generation of C3b. The biologic consequences of C3b formation depend on the presence or absence of regulators. See the text for details of the complement pathways.

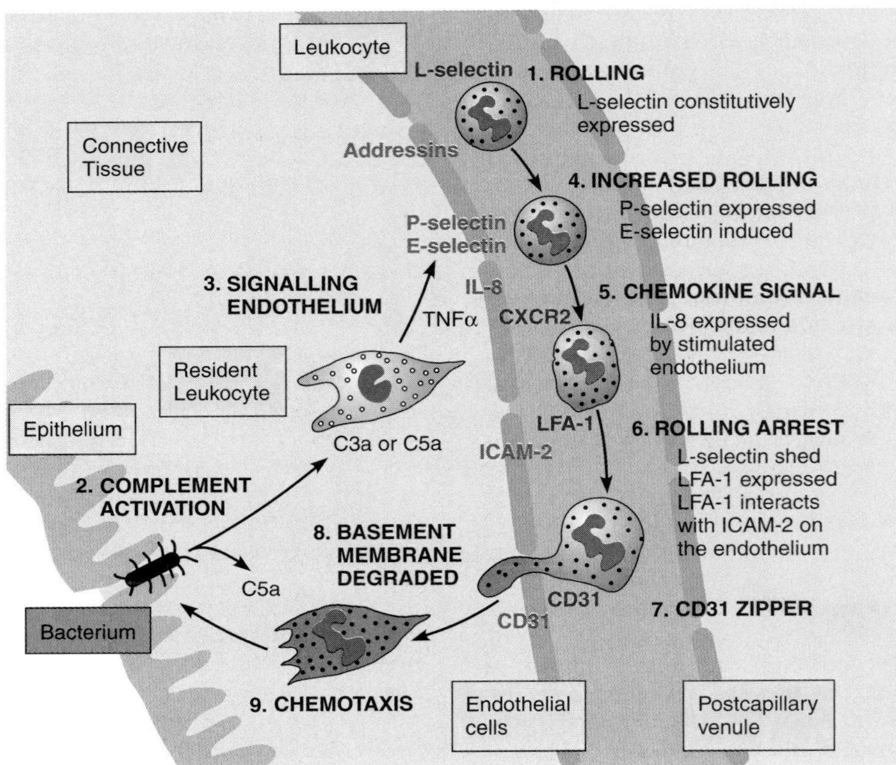

Fig. 7-4 Inflammation is a result of the interaction between complement, resident leukocytes, endothelium, and the recruited inflammatory leukocytes. Endothelial components are indicated in gray type; leukocyte components are indicated in red type. See the text for a discussion of the events involved in transendothelial migration.

Factor H and C4BP are serum cofactors that are most important in the inactivation of fluid phase C3b and C4b respectively. Factor H enables Factor I to inactivate C3b by clipping out a small piece, forming inactivated C3b (iC3b). The iC3b is inactive because it no longer can bind Factor G and thus can no longer generate C3 convertases. MCP and DAF are widely distributed on host cells and are mainly designed to protect the host cell against C3b and C3 convertase, respectively, which have bound to the same host cell. MCP binds to R-C3b, and enables Factor I to convert the R-C3b to R-iC3b. This halts further amplification. Eventually, iC3b is further metabolized and destroyed.

CR1 is a transmembrane molecule expressed by phagocytes (neutrophils and macrophages), B-cells, and red blood cells. CR1 binds C3b that is attached covalently to the surface of another particle, and it attracts Factor I, leading to the inactivation of amplification by the formation of iC3b. Phagocytes possess receptors for iC3b and will efficiently ingest the iC3b-bound cell or particle in a process known as opsonic phagocytosis (discussed further below), with subsequent destruction of the ingested material. Thus whereas MCP protects host cells, CR1 targets foreign or altered cells or molecules in the area for destruction.

In summary, the complement system is important in identifying and neutralizing substances for which the host does not possess specific receptors. Complement can be considered to be the fire of the immune system. When this fire ignites, it radiates the local area with molecules (C2a, C3a, and C5a) that enhance the inflammatory response and enable the endothelium and leukocytes to "see" and "find" the problem. The complement system additionally facilitates phagocytosis and destruction of foreign substances or direct destruction of cells or microorganisms via the membrane attack complex.

TRANSENDOTHELIAL MIGRATION

The directed movement of leukocytes from the blood into the local tissues is central to inflammation. Transendothelial migration is a selective interaction between leukocytes and endothelium that results in the leukocyte pushing its way between endothelial cells to exit the blood and enter the tissues. Defects in transendothelial migration are associated with aggressive periodontitis; reflecting the importance of this process in periodontal diseases.

Neutrophils and monocytes spend less than 12 hours in circulation. B-cells and T-cells stay in the blood for only about 30 minutes at a time. B-cells and T-cells require the additional influence of lymphoid organs (lymph nodes, spleen, tonsils, Peyer's patches, adenoids) to function properly. Thus they constantly exit the blood, pass through lymphatics and secondary lymphoid organs, and re-enter the blood in a perpetual process known as **lymphocyte recirculation.** The blood contains only 2% of all lymphocytes at any given time, and lymphocytes are estimated to recirculate as much as 50 times a day.[30]

In a local inflammatory response, transendothelial migration occurs in the following sequential phases: rolling (Step 1), an insult to local tissue (Step 2), signaling the endothelium (Step 3), increased rolling (Step 4), signal for rolling arrest (Step 5), strong adhesion (arrested rolling) (Step 6), and the zipper phase (Step 7). These processes are illustrated in Figure 7-4 and discussed below.

Leukocytes use the lectin (a nonenzymatic carbohydrate-binding protein), designated **L-selectin,** to interact with carbohydrate molecules known as *vascular addressins* (e.g., sialomucin CD34)[4] on the lumenal surface of endothelial cells (Step 1, Fig. 7-4). This brief interaction manifests itself as the **rolling** of the leukocyte along the lumenal surface of the endothelium, a process whereby the leukocyte essentially pauses to inspect the endothelium.

A local insult (Step 2, Fig. 7-4) triggers the release of a variety of inflammatory signals (such as interleukin-1β [IL-1β], tumor necrosis factor α [TNF-α]) from cells in the tissue, especially from resident leukocytes such as mast cells.[33] Mast cells are crucial in initiating neutrophil recruitment against bacteria[22] and respond to anaphylatoxins such as C3a and C5a (Step 3, Fig. 7-4).

IL-1β, TNF-α, C5a, and lipopolysaccharides can stimulate endothelial cells to express **P-selectin** and **E-selectin** on their lumenal surfaces.[14,34] Either of these selectins can bind carbohydrate molecules found on the leukocyte,[5] resulting in an increase in the time the leukocyte remains associated with the endothelium. This appears microscopically as an increase in number of leukocytes attached to the lumenal surface of the endothelium, or **increased rolling.** Notice that endothelial cells, not inflammatory leukocytes, initially respond to local inflammatory signals from the resident leukocytes.

The stimulated endothelium also releases **chemokines.** Chemokines are small peptide cytokines, first recognized for their chemoattractant activities, which play a fundamental role as selective signals for leukocytes to exit the blood (Step 5, Fig. 7-4). Chemokines function as a **signal for rolling arrest.** As illustrated in Fig. 7-4, the interaction of a chemokine, interleukin-8 (IL-8), with the leukocyte receptor, CXCR2 causes the leukocyte to shed L-selectin and upregulate the integrin, leukocyte function–associated antigen-1 **(LFA-1).**[17] Integrins are transmembrane adhesins, some of which have been adapted for use by the immune system. LFA-1 binds intercellular adhesion molecule-2 (ICAM-2), which is expressed constitutively by endothelium (Step 6, Fig. 7-4). This results in **rolling arrest** because the phagocyte becomes firmly associated with the endothelium. Prolonged or severe disturbances of the endothelium can upregulate ICAM-1, which is a more efficient ligand for LFA-1.

Because leukocytes differ with respect to their chemokine receptors, the chemokines dictate which leukocytes (e.g., neutrophils, macrophages, lymphocytes, eosinophils, basophils) dominate the leukocyte infiltrate. Different stimuli (e.g., cytokines, tissue injury, viral or microbial insults) can lead to expression of different chemokines.[11,13,21] For example, hypoxia, a condition in which only neutrophils can function successfully, favors endothelial release of IL-8,[19] a chemokine to which neutrophils are responsive. The integrin phase of transendothelial migration (i.e., the interaction of LFA-1 with ICAM-2) also can be somewhat selective. Thus chronic inflammatory leukocytes (monocytes and lymphocytes) possess integrins that are not expressed by neutrophils. One such integrin, "very late antigen-4 (VLA-4)," binds endothelial vascular cell adhesion molecule-1 (VCAM-1). Endothelium expresses VCAM-1 after prolonged inflammation, thus providing a mechanism for the selection of chronic inflammatory cells.

CD31 (Platelet-Endothelial Cell Adhesion Molecule-1) is a 130-kd transmembrane glycoprotein present at the intercellular borders of endothelial cells facing into lumen and on all leukocytes. CD31 is a homophilic adhesion molecule because CD31 molecules bind to one another. The binding of CD31 on endothelium with CD31 on leukocytes guides leukocytes to the boundaries between endothelial cells (Step 7, Fig. 7-4). Once the leukocyte locates the interendothelial junction, it uses its own CD31 like a zipper **(CD31 zipper)** with the CD31 of the endothelial cells.[6] This zipper effect has been proposed as a mechanism of minimizing the leakage of fluid. As the endothelium unzips its CD31, the leukocyte rapidly "zips" between the endothelial cells.

Leukocytes accumulate briefly between the basement membrane and the endothelial cell. This pause may reflect a period of secretion of proteases to degrade the basement membrane (Step 8, Fig. 7-4). Leukocytes possess several proteases, including urokinase plasminogen activator receptor (uPAR). The uPAR leads to the activation of collagenase, which then may degrade the basement membrane and enable the leukocyte to enter the connective tissues.

LEUKOCYTE FUNCTIONS

Chemotaxis

Once the leukocyte enters the connective tissue, it must be able to locate and migrate to the site of insult. This is accomplished by **chemotaxis,** which depends on the leukocyte's ability to sense a chemical gradient across its cell body and migrate in the direction of increasing concentration (Step 9, Fig. 7-4). The phagocyte senses only a limited number of chemicals—chemotaxins for which it has receptors, or chemotaxin receptors. Table 7-3 lists some molecules that can serve as chemotaxins and their sources. The receptors for chemotaxis belong to a family called the *G-protein coupled family* (Fig. 7-5, *A*). This family of receptors also includes the various light receptors in our retinas; thus in some ways, leukocytes "see" a chemotactic gradient much as we see light. The only class of chemotaxins derived directly from bacteria are formyl-methionyl peptides.

To migrate toward a target, leukocytes assume an asymmetric or polarized shape rather than the rounded morphology evident in blood (Fig. 7-5, *B*). Even under ideal experimental conditions, neutrophil migration has been observed to be primarily random until the neutrophil is 1 to 2 body lengths (10 to 20 μm) away from a recognizable target particle.[16]

Phagocytosis

Phagocytosis is the process by which cells ingest particles of a size visible to light microscopy. Neutrophils and monocytes/macrophages are the only cells efficient enough at phagocytosis to be considered "professional phagocytes." Phagocytosis results in the eventual containment of a pathogen within a membrane-delimited structure, the **phagosome** (Figs. 7-6 and 7-7, *A*). The immune system has evolved mechanisms of coating the pathogen with a few recognizable ligands, which enable the phagocyte to bind and ingest the pathogen. This is referred to as **opsonization.** A selected list of opsonins and the molecules with which they interact is presented in Table 7-4.

Once a microbe has been ingested, it may be killed. Phagocytes kill bacteria by two broad categories of **killing mechanisms.** One category is based on the reduction of oxygen and is referred to as *oxidative*. **Oxidative mechanisms** require 1) the presence of oxygen and 2) an oxidation-reduction potential, Eh, at or above −160 mV. Both variables may be suboptimal within the gingival crevice. Neutrophils do not require oxygen for energy and can function under anaerobic conditions. Thus phagocytes also must possess the second category of killing mechanisms, the **nonoxidative mechanisms.**

Nonoxidative killing requires **phagosome-lysosome fusion.** This process involves the movement toward and subsequent membrane fusion of the lysosome with the phagosome, forming a **phagolysosome.** This results in the secretion of lysosomal components into the phagolysosome. Each neutrophil possesses two main types of lysosomes, or granules: specific granules, designed for both extracellular and intraphagolysosomal secretion, and azurophil granules, designed mainly for intraphagolysosomal secretion. Less than 30 seconds after phagocy-

TABLE 7-3

Chemotaxins for Neutrophils

Chemotaxin*	Source
Tumor necrosis factor (TNF)	Macrophage/monocytes
IL-8	Neutrophils (PMN), endothelium
Platelet activating factor	Many cells
Leukotriene B4	
C5a	Serum/plasma
Neutrophil chemotactic factor	Mast cells
IL-1	B-cells, macrophage
IFNγ	Activated T-cells
N-formyl-methionyl peptides	Bacteria

* See text for explanation of abbreviations.

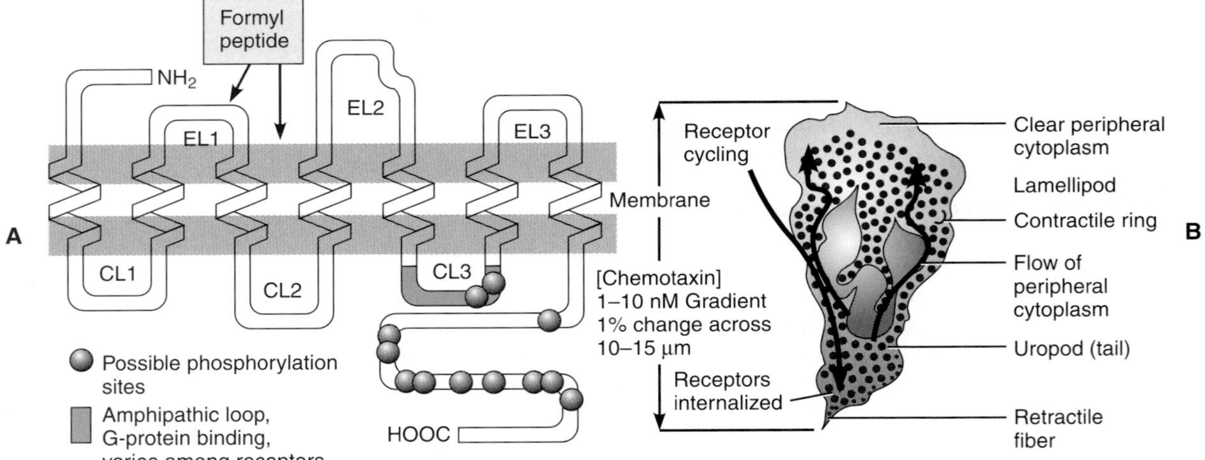

Fig. 7-5 Leukocytes can "hone in" on various irritants, such as a microorganism, by chemotaxis. This requires a chemotaxin receptor **(A).** The chemotaxin receptors are members of the G-protein coupled family. Seven transmembranous domains, three extracellular loops (EL1-3), and three cytosolic loops (CL1-3) characterize this family of molecules. **B,** Neutrophils polarize, forming an anterior lamellipod and a posterior uropod. Cytoplasm appears to squirt through a contractile ring. Neutrophils exhibit strikingly sensitive chemotaxis and can detect a 1% gradient over the length of its cell body at nanomolar concentrations.

tosis, neutrophils secrete specific granule components into the phagolysosome. Specific granules contain several microbiocidal components including lysozyme and lactoferrin. Lysozyme is an enzyme that possesses enzyme-dependent bactericidal activity and enzyme-independent bactericidal and fungicidal activity. Lactoferrin is a bacteriostatic compound that contains a bactericidal peptide domain, lactoferricin. Neutrophils secrete azurophil granule components into the phagolysosome minutes after the secretion of the specific granules. Among the microbicidal compounds are small antimicrobial peptides known as **α-defensins** (e.g., HNP-1, HNP-2, HNP-3, and HNP-4), serprocidins (elastase, proteinase 3, azurocidin), cathepsin G, and lysozyme. These nonoxidative mechanisms of neutrophil killing may be of particular importance in periodontal diseases because of the highly anaerobic conditions in the subgingival environment.

In the presence of oxygen, phagocytes additionally possess mechanisms of **oxidative killing.** In particular, neutrophils exert intense microbicidal activity by forming toxic, reduced oxygen metabolites such as superoxide anion (O_2^-) using the **NADPH oxidase system.** The superoxide anion also contributes to the formation of hydrogen peroxide (H_2O_2), which is capable of diffusing across membranes. Inside a target cell, H_2O_2 may be further reduced to the hydroxyl radical, which can cause DNA damage. More importantly, H_2O_2 is a substrate for **myeloperoxidase (MPO).** In the presence of H_2O_2 and chloride, MPO catalyzes the formation of hypochlorous acid (HOCl). This molecule is the acidic form of the laundry bleach salt, sodium hypochlorite (NaOCl), which also is used as an antimicrobialcleansing irrigant in endodontics. Deficiencies in the NADPH oxidase system result in chronic granulomatous disease, a severe, recurrent, focal infection by organisms which do not release H_2O_2 on their own. Chronic granulomatous disease has been associated inconsistently with aggressive periodontal disease, suggesting that oxidative microbicidal mechanisms are of some importance in periodontal infections.

In summary, phagocytosis is of primary importance in the ability of a host to resist or combat infection. Once a pathogenic microorganism is ingested, several mechanisms of killing are possible. Because of the highly anaerobic conditions in the periodontal environment, nonoxidative mechanisms of killing are of particular importance.

Antigen Processing and Presentation

The **major histocompatibility complex (MHC)** is a locus on the short arm of chromosome 6 (6p21.3) that encodes a number of molecules, including MHC Classes I, II, and III molecules, which are involved with antigen uptake, processing, and presentation. All cells process and present self-derived antigens (intracellular antigens) in association with MHC Class I molecules. MHC Class I molecules are used to present intracellular antigens to CD8+ T-cells and NK-cells. MHC Class III molecules include complement factors B, C2, and C4.

Antigens derived from extracellular sources are presented by professional **antigen-presenting cells (APC)** in association with MHC Class II molecules. The three main professional APC are peripheral dendritic cells, monocyte-derivatives, and B-cells. These cells are

A. Chemotaxis

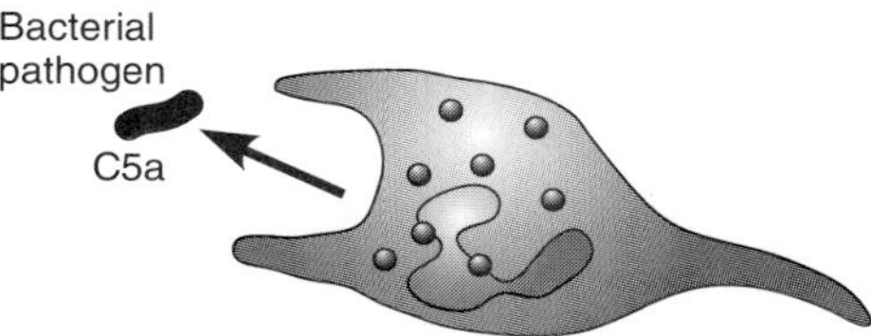

B. Initiate Phagocytosis

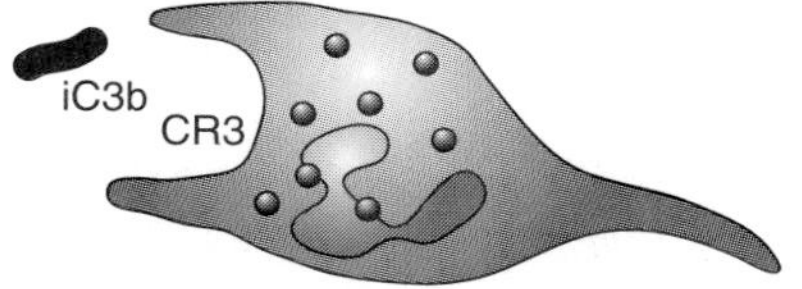

C. Oxygen Reduction

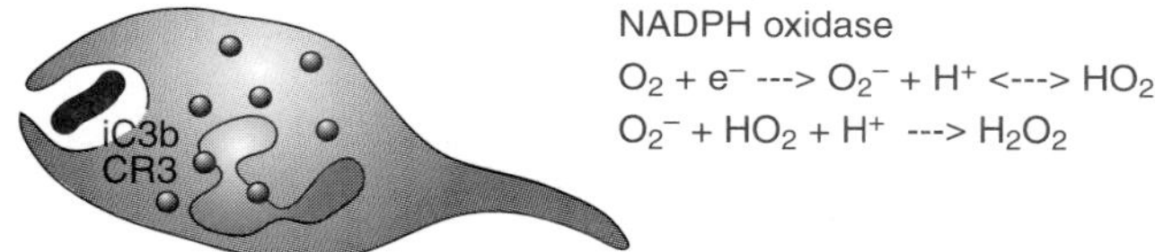

D. Killing

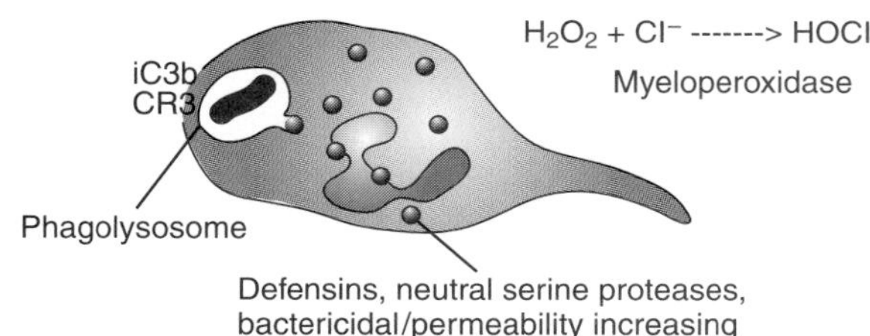

Fig. 7-6 After neutrophils exit the blood, they must kill the offending pathogens. This process consists of overlapping steps, which are illustrated in this diagram. **A,** *Chemotaxis* refers to directed motility that enables the leukocyte to locate its target. C5a is a chemotaxin, which may be generated by any target that activates complement. **B,** Phagocytosis also requires the interaction of receptors with a few ligands. The diagram illustrates the important interaction between the opsonin iC3b, which will coat an offending particle or cell, and the opsonic receptor CR3. **C,** Oxygen reduction requires the presence of oxygen and a certain redox potential, both of which can vary in the gingival crevice. The formation of several oxygen metabolites can kill some bacteria. **D,** "Killing" involves several processes. First, phagocytosis traps the microorganism in the stringent environment of the phagosome. Second, the phagosome and lysosomes (granules) fuse to form the phagolysosome. In this step, all the toxic compounds of the lysosome (e.g., defensins, neutral serine proteases) are dumped into the phagolysosome. Third, myeloperoxidase in the phagolysosome can convert hydrogen peroxide to hypochlorous acid.

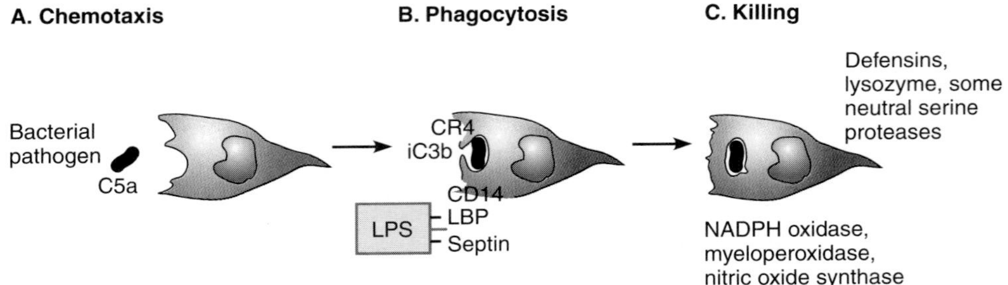

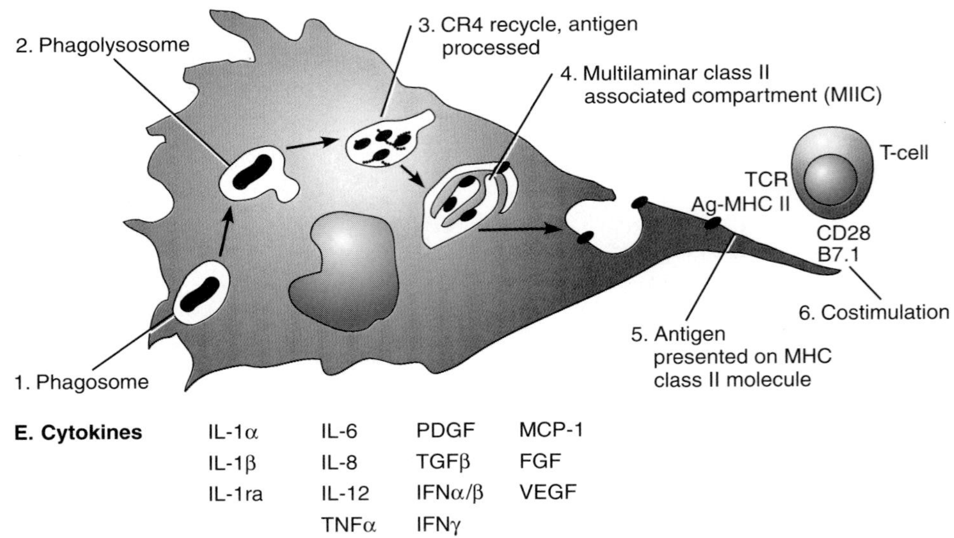

Fig. 7-7 Mononuclear phagocytes (monocytes in blood, macrophages in tissues) are closely related to neutrophils. Their activities are similar, and they exhibit chemotaxis **(A)**, phagocytosis **(B)**, and killing **(C)**, similar to neutrophils. Mononuclear phagocytes are particularly adept at processing and presenting antigen to T-cells **(D)**, a process that may require more than 20 hours. Note that antigen is presented in association with MHC Class II molecules along with a costimulatory signal (B7-1). Mononuclear phagocytes also release cytokines **(E)** that direct lymphocyte differentiation. See the text for details of the interactions illustrated.

TABLE 7-4

Opsonins and Opsonic Receptors

Target	Opsonin	Opsonic Receptor	Cell Possessing Opsonic Receptor
Gram-negative bacteria	LPS-binding protein (LBP) or septin	CD14	Macrophages Neutrophils (if primed with TNFα)
Any particle or cell	iC3b	CR3 (Mac1)	Neutrophils Macrophages
		CR4	Macrophages
Any particle or cell	IgG1, IgG2, IgG3	FcγRI FcγRII	Macrophages Macrophages Neutrophils

See text for explanation of abbreviations.

specialized to present antigen to CD4+ T-cells, which recognize antigen in association with the MHC Class II molecule. This is important because CD4+ T-cells control the proliferation of other T- and B-cells.

The professional APC express MHC Class II molecules (i.e., HLA-DP, HLA-DQ, HLA-DR) constitutively. Externally derived antigens are processed by phagocytosis, and the resulting peptide molecules associate with the MHC Class II molecules on the cell surface. As shown in Fig. 7-7, *D,* antigen associates with the MHC Class II molecule within the multilaminar Class II-associated compartment (MIIC). Oligomeric peptide fragments derived from extracellular polymers are bound by as many as four specificity pockets found in the MHC Class II molecule. Because the binding specificity is not for the entire peptide sequence, MHC Class II molecules are somewhat promiscuous and may bind to many different peptides.

Members of MHC Class I, II, and III molecules are among the most pleomorphic molecules in man. **Pleomorphism** refers to stable variations among individuals within a species, based on the occurrence of variants of certain genes. Pleomorphism in the MHC is particularly high near the specificity pockets. This means that the antigens bound by one person's MHC Class I or II molecules may not bind exactly the same peptides as those from a different individual. The existence of such pleomorphism may be important in species survival (as opposed to individual survival) and has become a significant consideration in transplantation (hence the term *histocompatibility*). If the donor tissue is not well matched in the MHC, it will present a multitude of new antigens that are recognized as foreign, and the donor tissue will be rejected by the resulting immune response.

The interaction between two cells permits a high level of sophistication unattainable by the simple interaction of two molecules, enabling the APC to present antigen to the T-cell with a second signal. The most important second signal is called *costimulation.* **Costimulation** reaffirms to the T-cell that it has recognized an undesirable antigen. In the absence of costimulation, T-cells may become unresponsive or apoptotic and die. Costimulation is mediated by a variety of transmembrane molecules of the tumor necrosis factor superfamily (Table 7-5), a family of molecules that deals with issues of cellular life and death. Costimulation does three things: 1) it makes the T-cell resistant to **apoptosis** (a programmed cell death); 2) it upregulates growth factor receptors on the T-cell, thereby stimulating its proliferation; and 3) it decreases the amount of time needed to trigger the T-cell (also referred to as *amplification*).[7,18]

Increases in the expression of costimulatory molecules occur in the presence of certain environmental stimuli. Macrophages increase the expression of costimulatory molecules if they are exposed to bacterial LPS[31,36] as well as particulate and occasionally soluble antigen. B-cells exposed to antigen to which they are specific, to selected bacterial membrane components (e.g., specific proteins, LPS), or to a B-cell activator molecule produced by T-cells (Gp39), respond by increasing the expression of the costimulatory molecules B7-1, B7-2, or both.[10,35] In addition, viral infection or certain chemical irritants can upregulate B7-1 or B7-3 on nonprofessional APCs.[12] A receptor molecule named Toll, first identified in fruit flies (*Drosophila* spp.), was shown to be important in certain responses to injury or infection. The human **Toll-like receptors (TLRs)** are stimulated by highly conserved bacterial components such as LPS.[26] The IL-1 receptor also is a TLR. TLRs cause APCs to upregulate the costimulatory B7 molecules.[23,24] Although T-cells may constantly interact with antigen, costimulation enables this interaction to progress to T-cell proliferation.

SPECIFIC IMMUNE RESPONSES

Chronic inflammation, if protracted, can result in an adaptation called the *specific immune response.* The specific immune response requires lymphocytes, which use two types of receptors to generate specific immune responses, the B-cell antigen receptor (BCR) and the T-cell antigen receptor (TCR). Four phases are involved in the generation of specific immunity: 1) **clonal selection,** the selection of lymphocytes that bear receptors (BCRs or TCRs) recognizing the specific antigen; 2) **clonal expansion,** the proliferation of those lymphocytes; 3) **clonal contraction,** the death of "effector" lymphocytes; and 4) **memory,** the maintenance of an expanded clone of cells that bears the specific receptors (BCRs or TCRs) recognizing the antigen (Fig. 7-8). As long as a sufficient number of lymphocytes are maintained to provide protection against a specific antigen, the individual is said to be immune.

TABLE 7-5

Selected TNF Superfamily Molecules Involved in Costimulation

Stimulating Cell (Antigen Presentor)	Costimulatory Factor	Stimulated Cell	Costimulatory Receptor on Stimulated Cell
APC	B7-2 (CD86)	CD4+ and CD8+ T-cells	CD28
APC	B7-2 (CD80)	Activated T-cells	CD28
Nonprofessional APC	B7-3	T-cells	CD28
Stimulated B-cells	CD70 (TNFSF7)	CD4+ T-cells	CD27

See text for explanation of abbreviations.

T-cells are selected when their TCR interacts with antigen presented by MHC Class I or II molecules. B-cell clonal selection requires only the multivalent binding of antigen by the BCR. A proliferation of the antigen-specific cells occurs after this clonal selection. This process is called *clonal expansion* and results in a 100- to 5000-fold increase in these cells.[1] In B-cell responses, some antigen-specific receptors are produced as soluble **antibodies.** The increase in antibody concentration and the strength of antibody binding is referred to as an increase in **titer.** Titer is operationally defined as the reciprocal dilution of antibody required to detect a standardized amount of antigen. Clonal contraction occurs by apoptosis at a rate equal to that of clonal expansion. More than 95% of antigen-specific T-cells are lost during the contraction phase,[1] usually occurring over several weeks. After clonal contraction, an increased population of memory T-cells or B-cells are maintained; this is the essence of the specific immune response.

The increase in antibody titer or antigen-specific T-cells resulting from the exposure of a host to an antigen for the first time is referred to as the **primary response.** The **secondary response** develops after a subsequent exposure to that same antigen. Because of the generation of memory (i.e., the expanded pool of cells recognizing antigen), the secondary response 1) is more rapid in onset, 2) is longer in duration, 3) is greater in strength due to higher titers, and 4) for B-cells, may have greater specificity against the antigen compared to the primary response. The expanded pool of memory cells provides a reservoir of cells that is sustained for years by constant stimulation of antigen maintained by follicular dendritic cells (non-hematopoetic cells found in the lymphoid tissues). The primary response takes slightly more than 1 week (8 to 14 days) to become measurable and biologically or clinically useful. Secondary responses are measurable within 1 to 3 days and are so effective that an individual may not be aware of the infection. **Vaccination** is the development of immunity, or resistance to infection, after a secondary response (the booster) that is adequate to consider the individual **immune** to a subsequent infection.

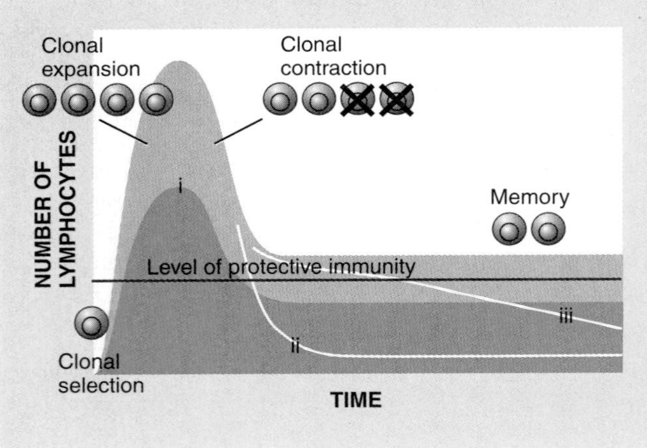

Fig. 7-8 Schematic illustration of the four phases of the specific immune response in relation to the occurrence of protective immunity. See the text for details of the four phases: clonal selection, clonal expansion, clonal contraction, and memory. Protective immunity is achieved if an adequate number of the lymphocytes are maintained in the memory phase, and the individual is said to be "immune". However, this does not always happen, as an individual may i) not undergo sufficient clonal expansion, ii) undergo excessive clonal contraction, or iii) be unable to maintain memory. (Adapted from Ahmed R, Gray D: Immunological memory and protective immunity: Understanding their relation. Science 1996; 272:54.)

T-CELL RESPONSES

To obtain a specific immune response, the T-cell must interact with the antigen-presenting cell (APC). This is a complex process requiring that the T-cell recognize the antigen on the APC, receive costimulation, activate growth cytokine receptors, and produce cytokines, which signal and support growth and differentiation. Once activated, the T-cell undergoes proliferation and differentiation, leading to one of several possible mature T-cell phenotypes.

T-cell antigen recognition is a function of the T-cell antigen receptor, a low-affinity receptor of the immunoglobulin superfamily. T-cells may express 3000 to 50,000 TCRs on their surface. Antigens are presented to the TCR by MHC Class I or II molecules on the APC. CD1 is a related antigen-presenting molecule that presents specific antigens to NKT-cells, a unique subpopulation of CD4- and CD8- T-cells. The TCR recognizes and binds the MHC-peptide complex.[28] Antigen (Ag) is contacted by the TCR using variable domains found at the N-terminus of the TCR α and β subunits. TCR-peptide binding is more specific than that of the MHC-peptide, which is based on recognition of a smaller number of discontinuous amino acids. Thus the T-cell may recognize fewer antigens than those presented by the MHC.

The TCR consists of a number of components in addition to those that bind antigen. These include components that form the **CD3 transductory apparatus** (TCR-CD3), which is important in the activation of the TCR and the eventual transmission or transduction of the signal into the cell. **CD8** and **CD4** are **T-cell coreceptors** whose recognition of MHC Class I and II molecules, respectively, on APC is essential for T-cell function and subsequent TCR activation. Activation of these coreceptors 1) increases the excitability of the TCR and 2) increases the binding between the T-cell and the antigen-presenting cell.

The low affinity of the TCR enables the T-cell to bind antigen presenting cells in a reversible manner, which occurs between multiple TCRs and one or a few antigens over time. This time-dependent interaction of many TCRs with a few antigens is referred to as **scanning.** Scanning that leads to T-cell activation is called **serial triggering.** To fully activate T-cells, multiple TCR engagement must be sustained for 2 to 20 hours.

Activation of T-cells leads to proliferative differentiation. This process begins with activation of the protein tyrosine kinases lck, fyn and ZAP, which activate the TCR, phospholipase C (PLC), and CD28 respectively (Fig. 7-9). Activation of CD28 prepares the T-cell to receive the costimulatory signals, which are important in T-cell survival and function. Activation of phospholipase C

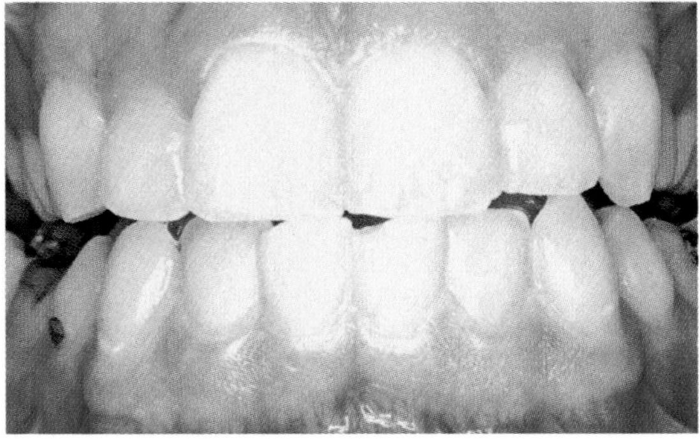

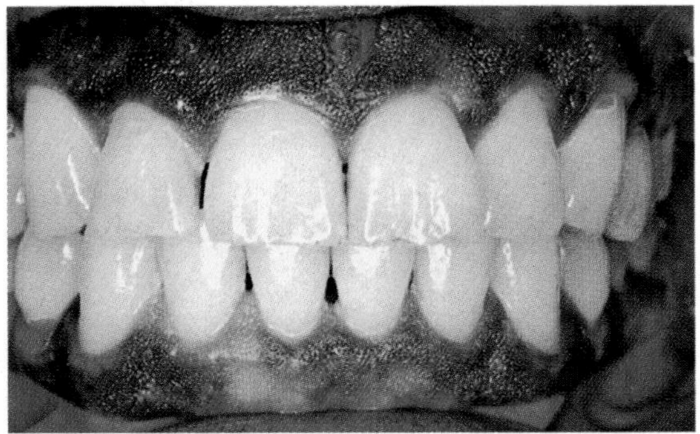

Color Fig. 1-1 *Left,* Clinically normal gingiva in a young adult. *Right,* Heavily pigmented (melanotic) gingiva in a middle-aged adult. (From Glickman I, Smulow JB: Periodontal Disease: Clinical, Radiographic, and Histopathologic Features. Philadelphia, Saunders, 1974.)

A B

C D

E F

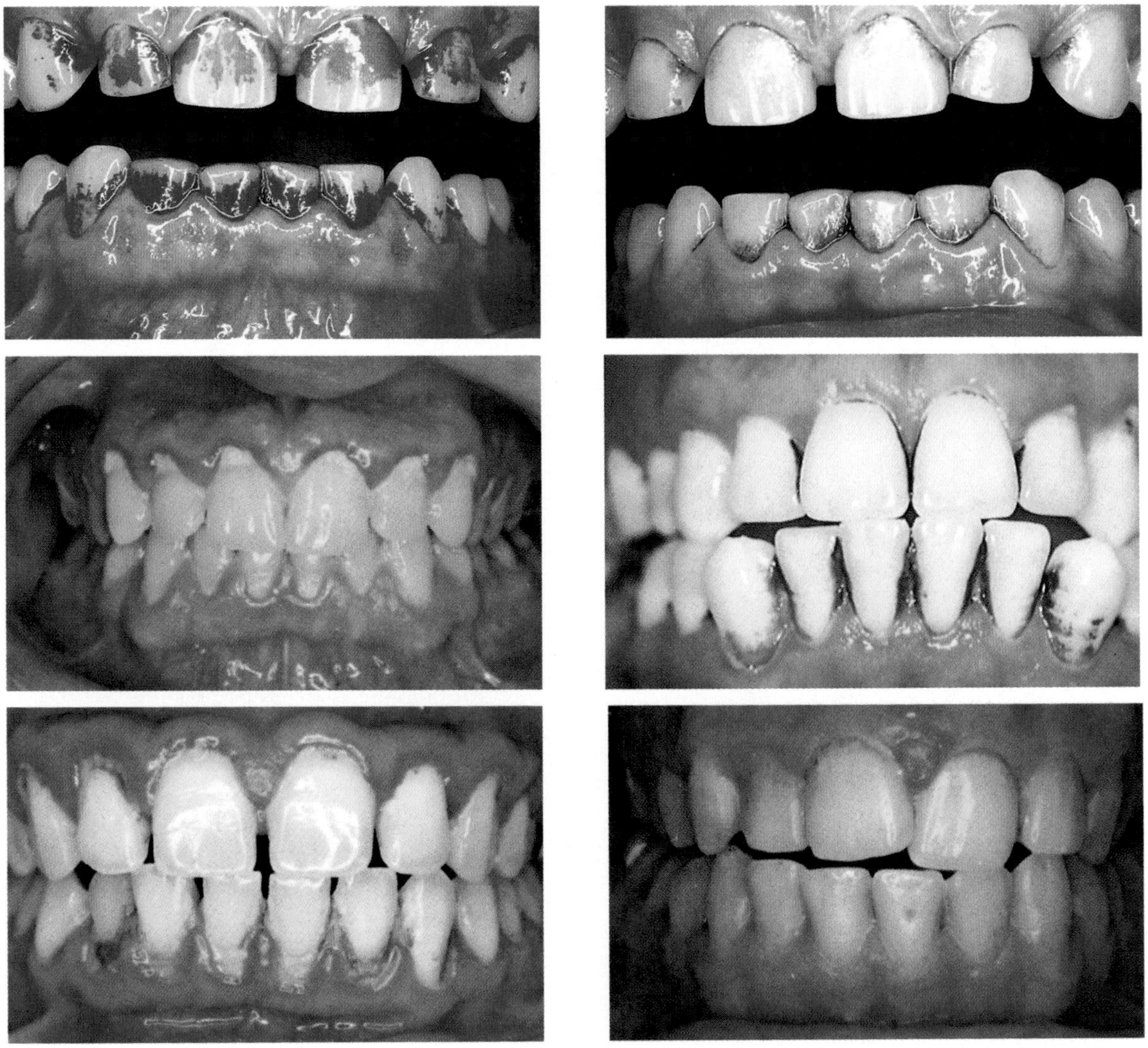

Color Fig. 6-1 **A,** Disclosed supragingival plaque covering one half to two thirds of the clinical crowns. **B,** Same patient as in **A.** Supragingival plaque disclosed with an oxidation-reduction dye that indicates reduced (anaerobic) areas of plaque. The supragingival anaerobic areas (purple stain) are located interproximally and along the gingival margin. **C,** *Materia alba* generalized throughout the mouth, with heaviest accumulation near the gingiva. Note the gingiva present. **D,** Teeth stained by several weeks of mouthrinses with alexidine. This stain can be easily removed. **E,** Supragingival calculus in a patient with gingival inflammation. **F,** Green stain on anterior teeth. Note the inflamed, enlarged interdental papilla between the maxillary central incisors. (**A** and **B,** courtesy Dr. S. Socransky, Boston, Mass.)

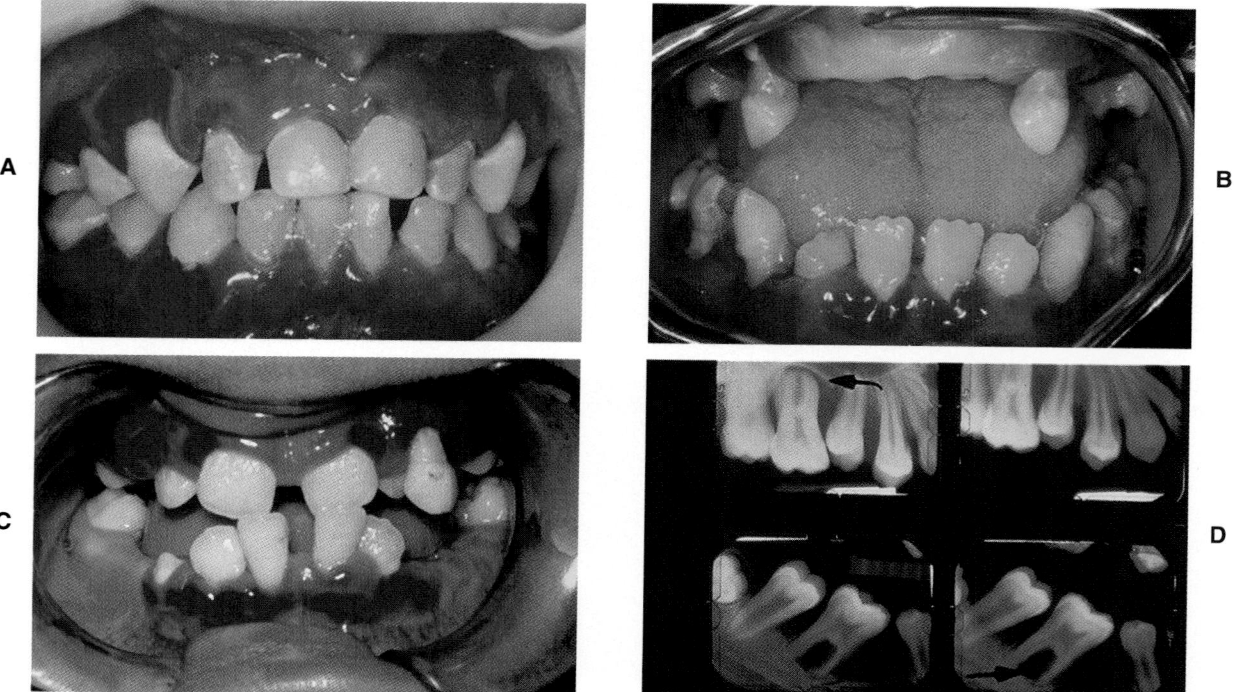

Color Fig. 8-1 Periodontal manifestations of disorders affecting neutrophil function. **A and B,** Clinical appearance of patients with cyclic neutropenia, a condition that involves reduction in the number of circulating neutrophils (blood neutrophil levels <1500/mm³). **A,** 5-year-old boy with cyclic neutropenia. Note the aggressive and extensive inflammation in the gingival tissues. **B,** A 7-year-old boy with cyclic neutropenia demonstrating acute and extensive gingival inflammation and advanced attachment loss with recession evident. **C and D,** Clinical and radiographic appearances of patients with leukocyte adhesion deficiency (LAD type 1). This disorder involves defects in neutrophil transendothelial migration, resulting in a lack of extravascular neutrophils in periodontal lesions. However, dense infiltrates of mononuclear leukocytes are found in the periodontal lesions.[170] Note the tissue inflammation evident clinically **(C)** and the extensive bone loss seen in these patients (**D,** *arrows*). For additional information, see text and Table 8-5. (Courtesy Dr. Max Listgarten [A and B] and Dr. D. C. Anderson [C and D]).

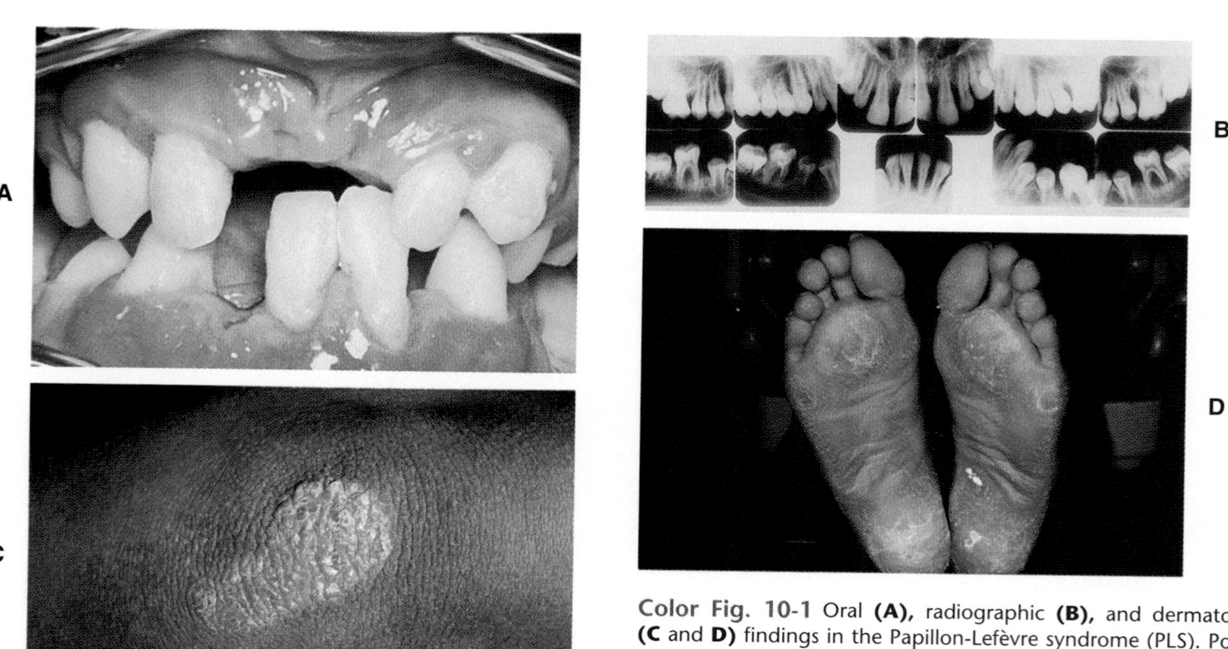

Color Fig. 10-1 Oral **(A),** radiographic **(B),** and dermatologic **(C** and **D)** findings in the Papillon-Lefèvre syndrome (PLS). Pocketing and bone loss usually affects the primary and secondary teeth shortly after eruption. Although numerous palmoplantar keratodermas have been described, the hyperkeratotic lesions of PLS can affect the elbows **(C)** and knees and the palms and plantar surfaces of the feet **(D).** (Courtesy Dr. Robert J. Gorlin.)

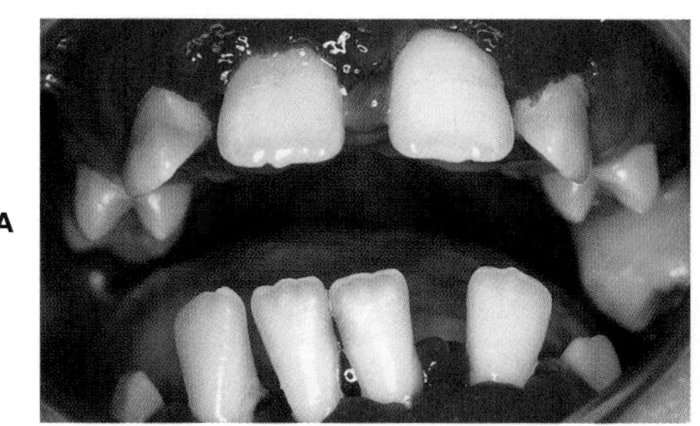

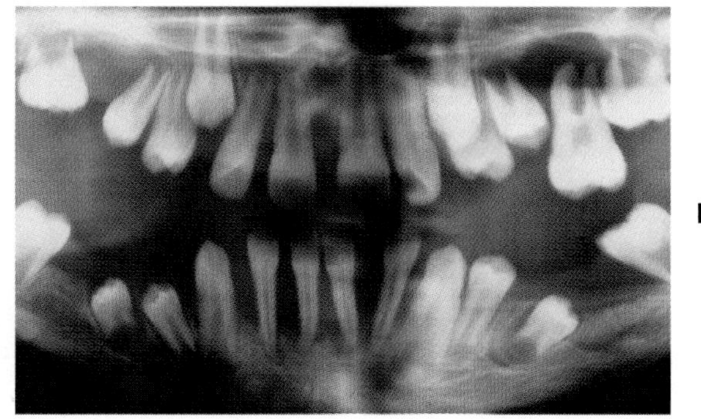

Color Fig. 10-2 Oral **(A)** and radiographic **(B)** appearance of a patient with leukocyte adhesion deficiency (LAD). The child was deficient in CD18 (i.e., LAD type I), which results in absent or severely reduced levels of the β-2 integrin molecule. The patient suffered from recurrent infections of the middle ear, tongue, and perirectal areas as well as the periodontium. (From Majorana A, Notarangelo LD, Savoldi E, et al: Leukocyte adhesion deficiency in a child with severe oral involvement. Oral Surg Oral Med Oral Pathol Oral Radiol Endod 1999; 87:691.)

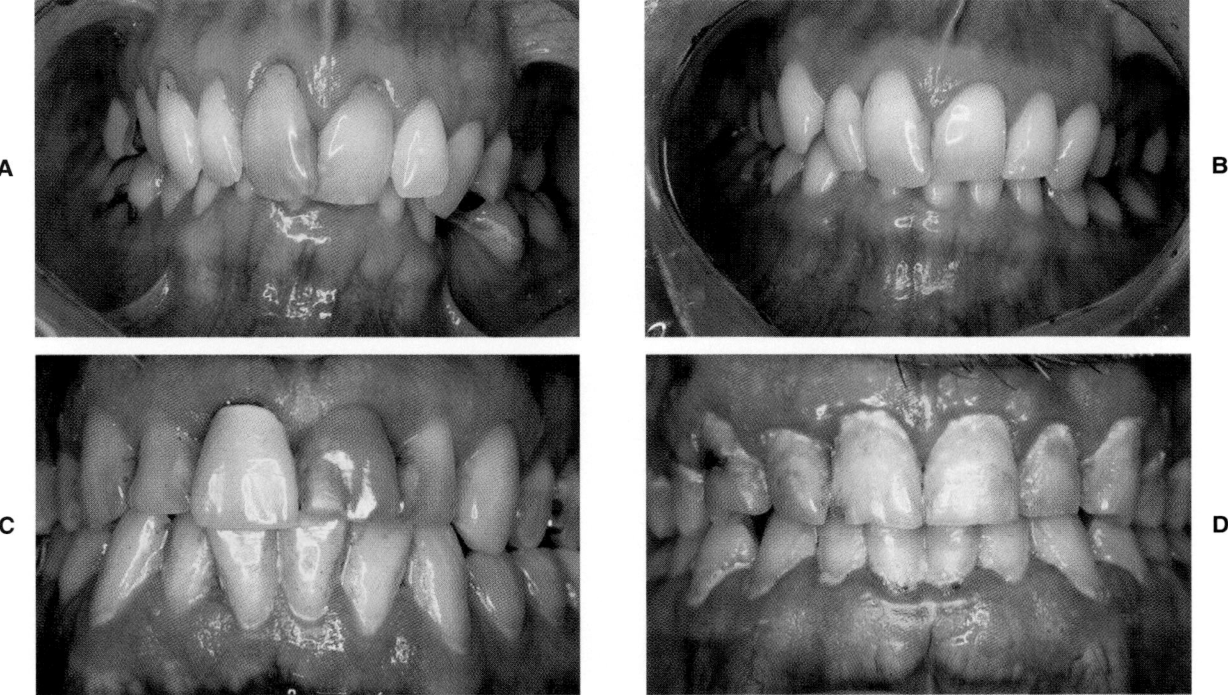

Color Fig. 10-3 Reared-apart twin pairs. **A,** 37-year-old female identical twins. Note the similarity in tooth and arch forms in the twins. **B,** 40-year-old male fraternal twins. (From Pihlstrom B, Michalowicz B: Genetic risk for periodontal disease: A clinical perspective. Journal de Paradontologie d'Implantologie Orale 1998; 17:123.)

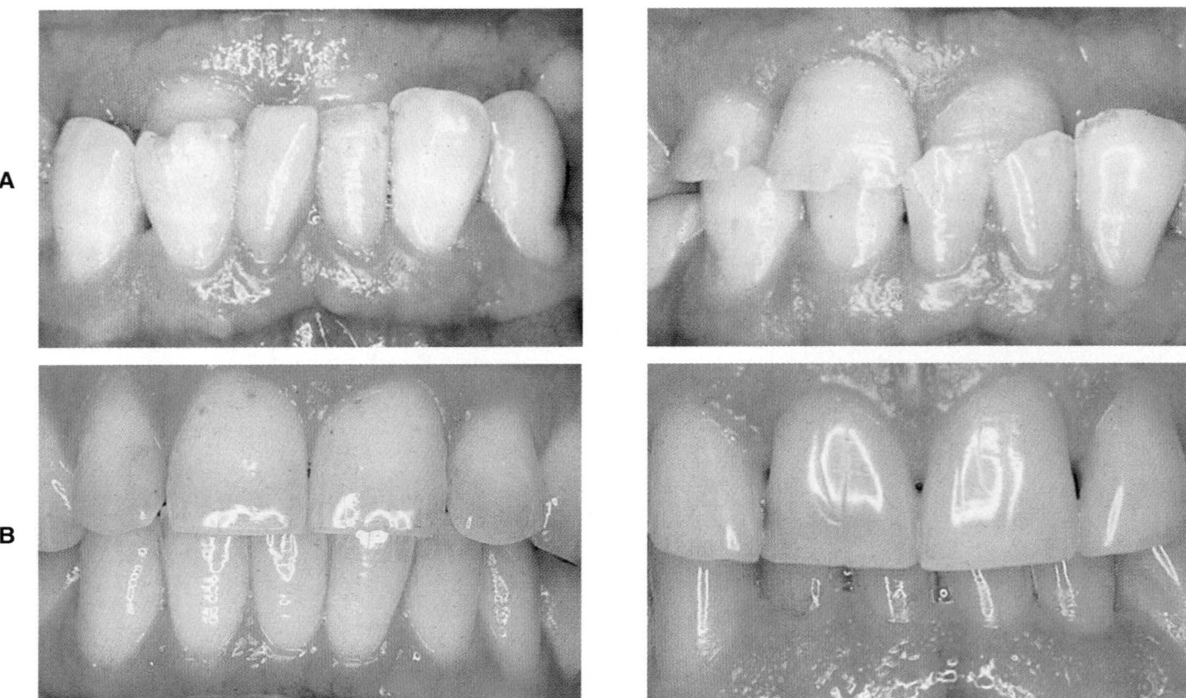

Color Fig. 10-4 Reared-together twin pairs. **A,** 70-year-old male identical twins. **B,** 67-year-old male fraternal twins. (From Pihlstrom B, Michalowicz B: Genetic risk for periodontal disease: A clinical perspective. Journal de Paradontologie d'Implantologie Orale 1998; 17:123.)

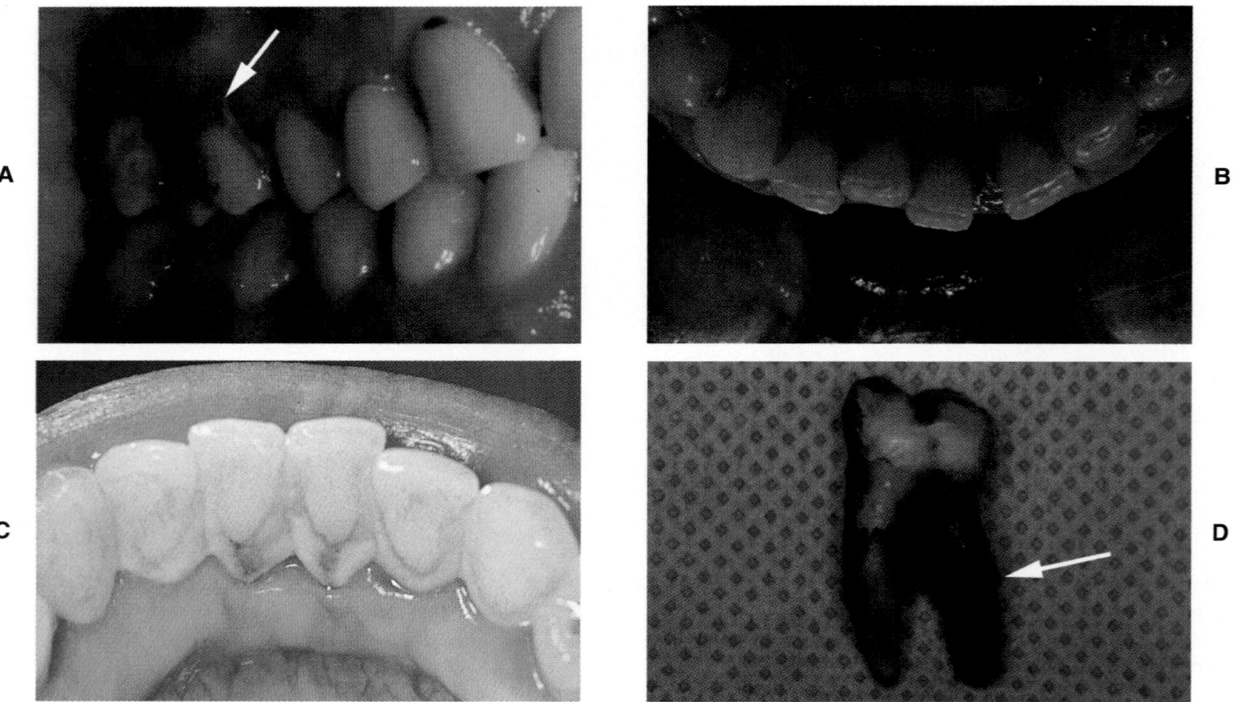

Color Fig. 11-1 **A,** Supragingival calculus is depicted on the buccal surfaces of maxillary molars adjacent to orifice for Stenson's duct. **B and C,** Extensive supragingival calculus is present on the lingual surfaces of lower anterior teeth. **D,** Dark pigmented deposits of subgingival calculus are shown on the distal root of an extracted lower molar.

Continued

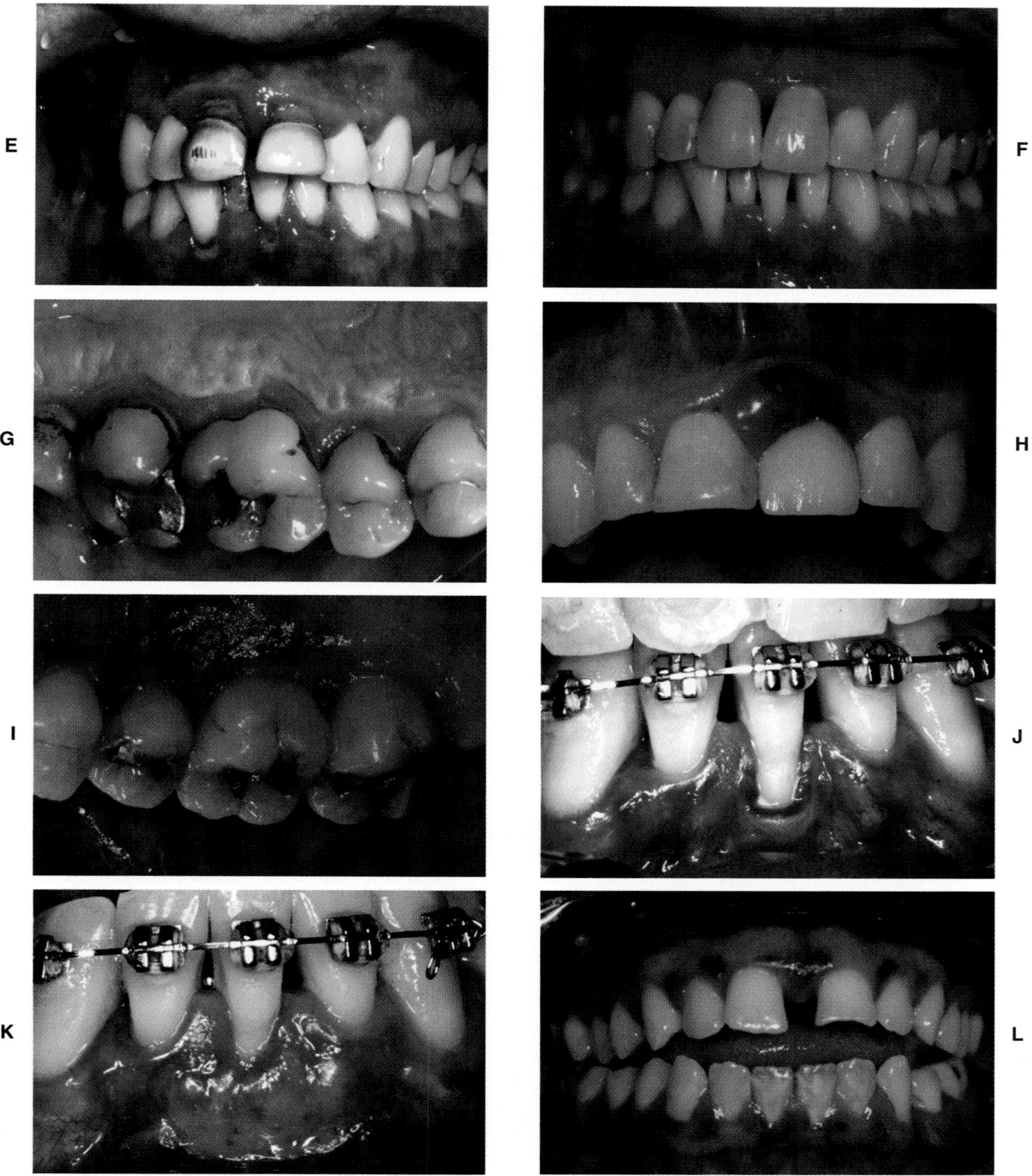

Color Fig. 11-1 cont'd **E,** A 31-year-old Caucasian man is shown with extensive supragingival and subgingival calculus deposits throughout his dentition. **F,** The same patient as shown in **E,** 1 year after receiving thorough scaling and root planing to remove supragingival and subgingival calculus deposits followed by restorative care. Note the substantial reduction in gingival inflammation. **G,** Tobacco stains on the apical third of the clinical crown due to cigarette smoking. **H,** Inflamed marginal and papillary gingiva adjacent to an overcontoured porcelain-fused to metal crown on the maxillary left central. **I,** Inflamed palatal gingiva associated with a maxillary provisional acrylic partial denture. Note the substantial difference in color of the inflamed gingiva adjacent to the premolars and first molar compared with the gingiva adjacent to the second molar. **J,** A lower incisor depicting a prominent root without any attached gingiva and accompanying gingival recession. **K,** The same patient as shown in **J,** following the placement of a soft tissue graft to gain attached gingiva and treat the gingival recession. **L,** Anterior open bite with flared incisors as observed in association with a habit of tongue thrusting.

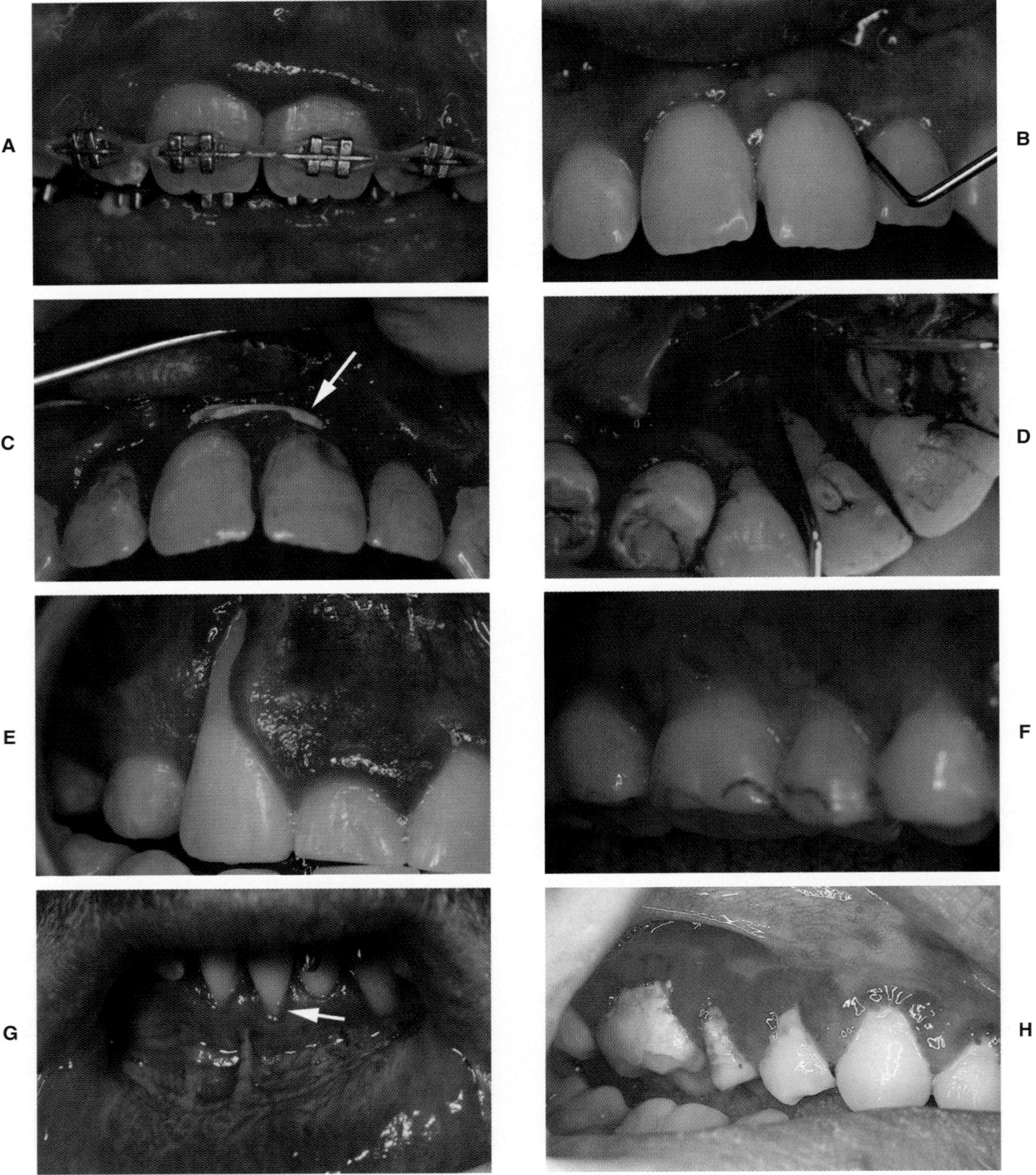

Color Fig. 11-2 **A,** Gingival inflammation and enlargement associated with orthodontic appliance and poor oral hygiene. **B,** Maxillary central incisors in which an elastic ligature was used to close a midline diastema. Note inflamed gingival and deep probing depths. **C,** The same patient as shown in **B.** A full-thickness mucoperiosteal flap has been reflected to expose the elastic ligature and angular intrabony defects around the central incisors. **D,** Palatal flap reflected to reveal bony dehiscence on the maxillary lateral incisor shown in Fig. 11-30. **E,** A maxillary canine that illustrates gingival recession due to self-inflicted trauma by the patient's fingernail. **F,** The overzealous use of a toothbrush may denude the gingival epithelial surface, leaving the underlying connective tissue exposed as a painful ulcer. **G,** Gingival recession and hyperkeratosis of the vestibular mucosa have developed as a consequence of using chewing tobacco. **H,** Heavy calculus deposits on facial surfaces of the upper first molar and second premolar. Note the severe gingival inflammation in the entire quadrant.

Continued

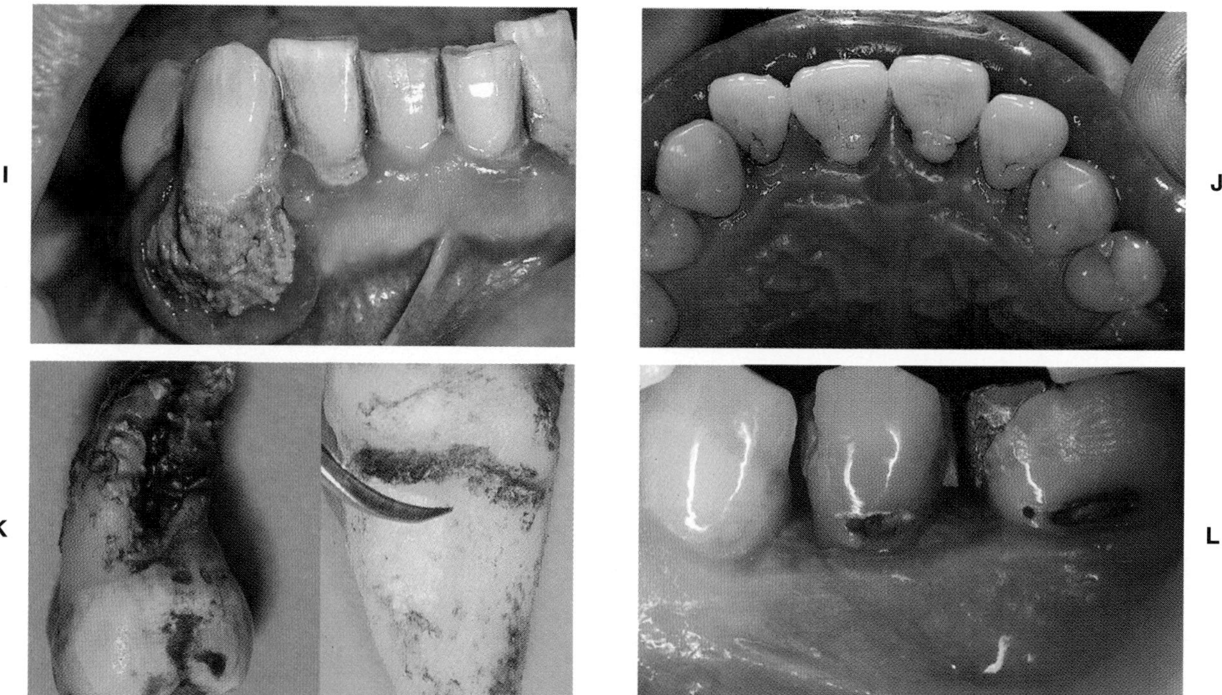

Color Fig. 11-2 cont'd **I,** Heavy calculus deposit on the facial surface of the lower cuspid with associated gingival recession. **J,** Palatal view of upper anterior teeth with heavy calculus deposits, particularly in interdental spaces. **K,** Different shapes of calculus on extracted teeth. **L,** Overhanging margin of restoration and atrophied and inflamed gingival papilla.

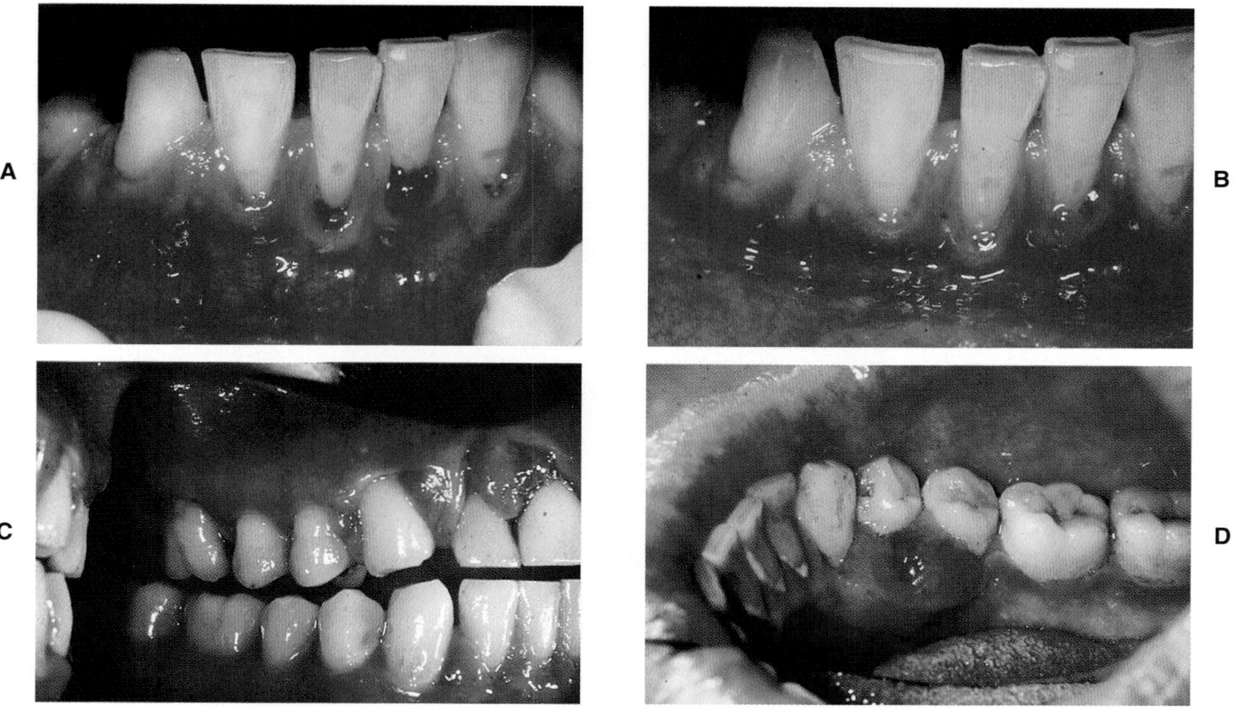

Color Fig. 12-1 Diabetes and periodontal disease. **A,** An adult patient with diabetes (blood glucose level of 400 mg/100 ml). Note the gingival inflammation, spontaneous bleeding, and edema. **B,** Same patient as in **A** after 4 days of insulin therapy (glucose level less than 100 mg/100 ml). The clinical periodontal picture has improved in the absence of local therapy. **C,** An adult patient with uncontrolled diabetes. Note the enlarged, smooth red gingiva with initial enlargement in the anterior area. **D,** Lingual view of right mandibular area in the same case as in **C.** Note the inflamed enlarged area around teeth #27–30.

Continued

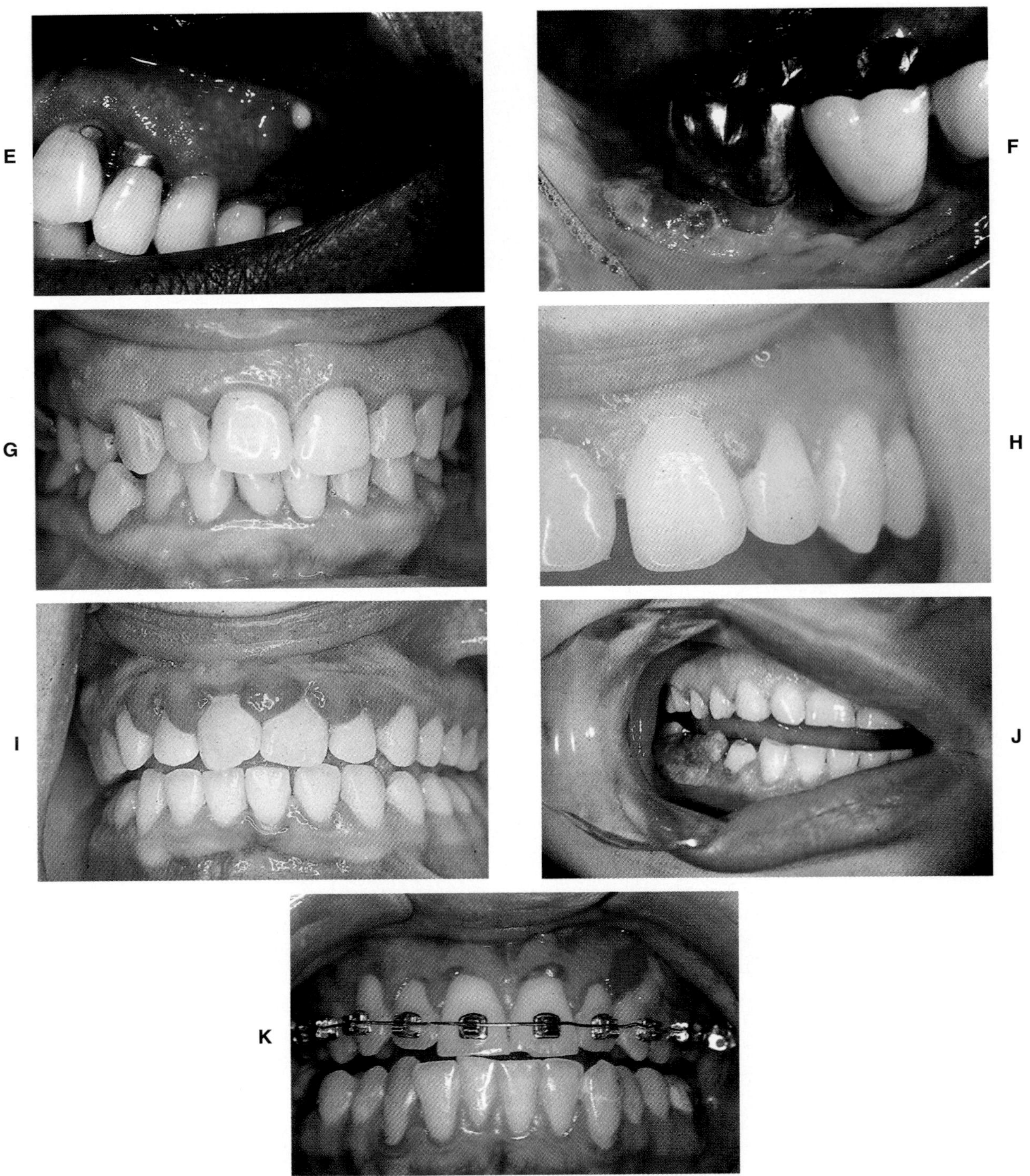

Color Fig. 12-1 cont'd **E,** Suppurating abscess, facial of upper left area, in a patient with uncontrolled diabetes. **F,** An adult patient with uncontrolled diabetes, showing delayed healing 7 weeks after surgery in tooth #31. **G,** Marginal redness and easily bleeding gingivae in a 5-month-pregnant woman. **H,** Incipient gingival enlargement in the papilla between teeth #9 and 10 in a 4-month-pregnant woman. **I,** Generalized gingival enlargement in pregnancy, especially noticeable in the upper anterior area. **J,** Localized discrete gingival enlargement in area facial of teeth #28–30 in a pregnant woman. **K,** Easily bleeding, marginal erythema with a diffuse erythematous area between the upper left lateral incisor and canine. Marginal edematous changes are seen, as well as easily bleeding around lower anterior teeth. The patient is 7 months pregnant. (**A** and **B,** courtesy Dr. Joan Otomo-Corgel; **C–F,** courtesy Dr. T. N. Sims; **K,** courtesy Dr. Philip Melnick.)

results in the generation of diacylglycerol **(DAG)** and 1,4,5-inositol triphosphate **(IP3).** DAG signals the activation of a transcription activating cofactor, NF-ATn. IP3 stimulates the release of Ca^{++}, which results in the activation of a calmodulin-calcineurin A/B phosphatase. This phosphatase dephosphorylates NF-ATc and enables it to enter the nucleus, where it combines with NF-ATn to form active **NF-AT (nuclear factor of activated T-cells).** NF-AT then upregulates transcription of genes, such as those for IL-2 and IL-2Rα, which support T-cell growth and differentiation. The latent cytoplasmic transcription factor NF-$\kappa\beta$ also is activated and is important in delaying apoptosis. One of the most important proliferative differentiation signals is the cytokine interleukin-2. The activated transcription factors are required for the T-cell to express one of the subunits of the heterotrimeric receptor for IL-2 and the IL-2Rα and also produce IL-2.[9] Thus IL-2 produced by the activated T-cell interacts

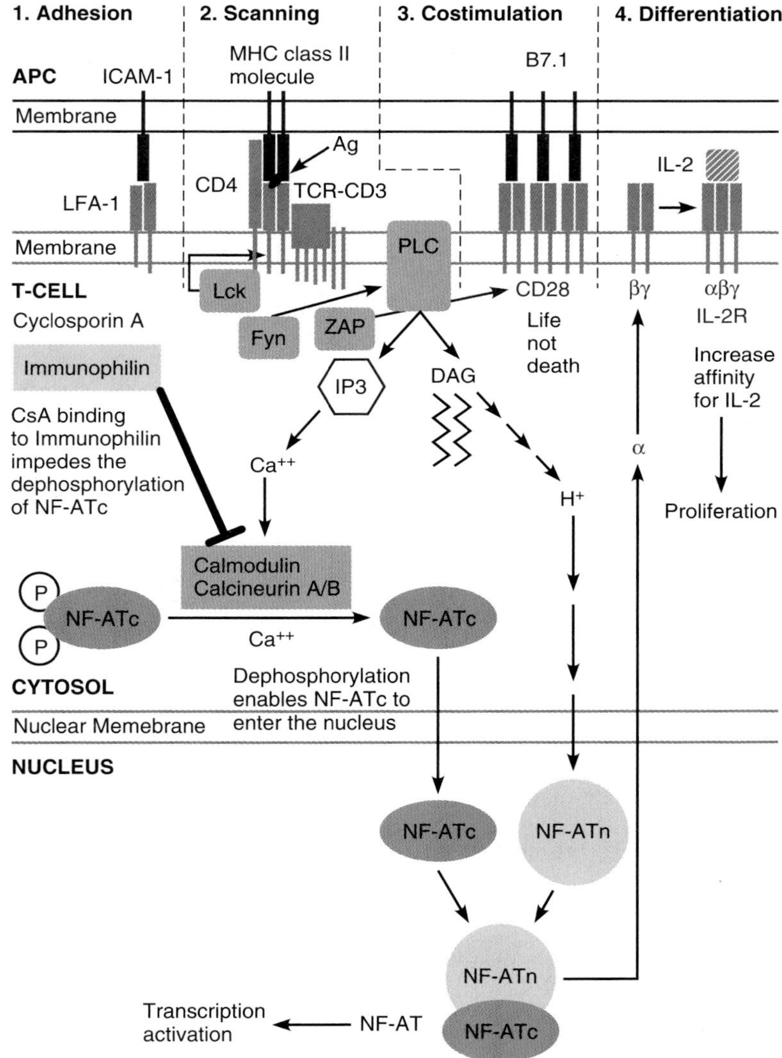

Fig. 7-9 Schematic illustration of receptor-mediated events leading to T-cell activation. *1,* Adhesion between the T-cell and the antigen presenting cell (APC) is mediated by adhesins such as LFA-1 and ICAM-1. *2,* Scanning of the APC by the T-cell coreceptors, CD4 or CD8, helps activate the TCR using the kinase Lck. Recognition of antigen by the TCR results in activation of phospholipase C (PLC) and CD28 by Fyn and ZAP, respectively. *3,* Activated CD28 binds costimulatory factors such as B7-1. The costimulatory factors are upregulated by environmental cues and reinforce the activation signal. *4,* The scanning of antigen results in transcription of an important growth harmone receptor subunit, the IL-2 receptor α subunit. This increases the affinity of the IL-2 receptor. Later, the T-cell produces IL-2, which interacts with the IL-2 receptor to stimulate its own proliferation.

with the IL-2R on the same cell to stimulate proliferative differentiation.

Clinically important immunosuppressants block the intracellular processes of T-cell activation. Immunophilins are regulatory factors that diminish the action of calcineurin. Immunosuppressants such as **cyclosporin A** and **tacrolimus** bind and activate immunophilins, resulting in their immunosuppressive effects.

CD4+ T-cells mature to form phenotypic subpopulations that are distinguishable on the basis of their cytokine production[25,29] (Fig. 7-10). In addition to antigen and costimulation, professional APCs provide immature **Th T-cells** with the maturational signal **interleukin 1β (IL-1β),** which induces T-cell maturation to a multifaceted **Th0 T-cell** phenotype. Th0 T-cells produce cytokines, which can stimulate both B-cells and CD8+ T-cells. Other cells in the area—especially macrophages, dendritic cells, other T-cells, and NK-cells—provide further differentiation signals. High or low concentrations of interleukin-12 (IL-12) or cytokines such as interferon-γ (IFNγ, IL-2, IL-4, IL-10, and TGF-β) then can induce T-cells to mature to the Th1, Th2, or Th3 phenotypes. The Th1 phenoytpe is important in controlling altered cells and intracellular molecules, the Th2 phenotype is important in proinflammatory responses against extracellular antigens, and the Th3 phenotype is important in antiinflammatory responses against extracellular antigens. These later T-cell maturational subpopulations are important in B-cell development.

B-CELL RESPONSES AND ANTIBODIES

B-cells produce immunoglobulin. An immunoglobulin that binds a known antigen is an antibody. Once antigen is bound, a number of consequences can occur, as dictated by the type (isotype) of immunoglobulin involved (Table 7-6). Immunoglobulin accounts for about 20% to 25% (15 mg/mL) of the total serum protein (60 to 70 mg/mL). Humans possess 9 genetically distinct isotypes of immunoglobulins: **IgM, IgD, IgG1, IgG2, IgG3, IgG4, IgA1, IgA2,** and **IgE.** When B-cells exit the bone marrow, they possess receptors bearing only IgM and the cells are capable of producing soluble IgM. IgM functions in the primitive agglutination reactions that facilitate antigen clearance. Secondary imunoglobulin response classes permit a more discriminating response. To form secondary response isotypes, B-cells must enter a pathway of differentiation. In this memory pathway, B-cells undergo the process of isotype switching. One example of the significance of this process to periodontal diseases is that certain pathogens, such as *Actinobacillus actinomycetemcomitans,* can only be con-

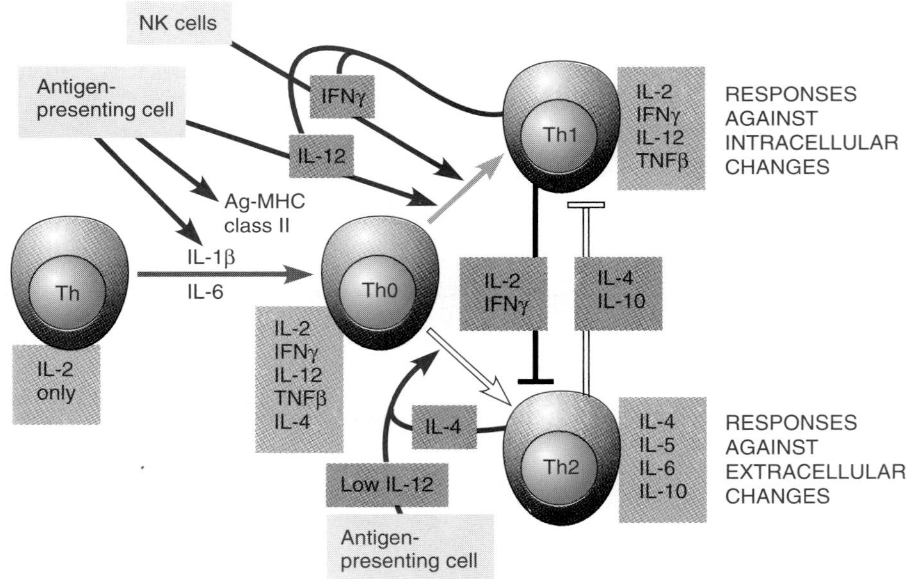

Fig. 7-10 Schematic illustration of T-cell differentiation. Early inflammatory signals from macrophages and peripheral dendritic cells such as IL-1β activate the CD4+ T-helper (Th) T-cell. The Th cell then produces many cytokines, including IL-2, INFγ and IL-4, and is referred to as a *Th0 T-cell.* The Th0 T-cell further differentiates to form Th1 or Th2 T-cells, which regulate immune responses against intracellular and extracellular antigens, respectively. A key signal determining which pathway the T-cell follows is the level of IL-12 provided by the antigen presenting cell. High levels of IL-12 favor the Th1 pathway, and low levels of IL-12 favor the Th2 pathway. Subsequently, the Th1 phenotype is favored in the presence of Th1 cytokines such as IFNγ, which stimulates Th1 differentiation and blocks Th2 differentiation. Similarly, the Th2 cytokines such as IL-4 block Th1 differentiation while promoting Th2 differentiation. The Th3 T-cell, which produces IgA and functions in mucosal defense, is not illustrated here.

trolled by neutrophils when opsonized by antibody of the IgG isotype. Complement, LPS-binding protein (LBP), and any other immunoglobulin isotypes are not effective.

The ability of B-cells to respond to antigen is dependent on the B-cell antigen receptor (BCR). The BCR is formed partly by immunoglobulin molecules on the B-cell surface, which serve as highly specific antigen receptors, and partly by transductory elements of the immunoglobulin superfamily. The BCR binds antigen with a high affinity and is designed for binding. This contrasts with the low-affinity binding of the TCR, which is ideal for scanning. B-cells are capable of responding to certain antigens in the absence of T-cells. This is referred to as *T-independent B-cell antibody response.* However, these B-cell responses do not mature (i.e., they do not enter the memory pathway). The cells maintain an IgM isotype, and their antibody products retain a relatively low affinity for antigen binding. B-cells must interact with T-cells to enter the memory pathway, thus the memory pathway is considered to be T-cell dependent.

B-cells bind soluble antigens using the BCR. If enough antigen is bound, they then are ingested and processed, and parts of the antigen are presented to specific CD4+ T-cells using MHC Class II molecules. After antigen presentation, the T-cells provide an **activation** signal to the B-cell. T-cell activators are transmembranous molecules, analogous to the costimulatory factors for T-cells discussed previously. Activators include T-cell-derived Gp39 and Gp34, which interact with the B-cell receptors, CD40 or OX40, respectively. Mutations in the gene for Gp39 lead to a condition called *X-linked hyperimmunoglubulinemia M syndrome,* characterized by a deficiency in most immunoglobulin isotypes and a compensatory increase in IgM.[2] T-cell Gp39 enables B-cell entry into the memory pathway, whereas the absence of Gp39 leads to terminal differentiation of the B-cells toward IgM, producing plasma cells.[3] B-cells upregulate B7-1 and B7-2 if activated by Gp39. These costimulatory factors enable the T-cells to differentiate, both with respect to proliferation and in the production of cytokines. Some T-cell cytokines are **switch factors;** these cytokines fall into three classes: TH1 (IL-2, IFNγ), TH2 (IL-4, IL-10), or TH3 (TGFβ). TH1 and TH2 switch signals generally promote switching to inflammatory immunoglobulins (IgG or IgE). The TH3 signal promotes a switch to an antiinflammatory isotype (IgA).[15] Unlike the activator, switch factors are usually soluble rather than membrane associated. Some effects of various combinations of activators and switch factors are shown in Fig. 7-11.

B-cells that differentiate to become plasma cells no longer express surface immunoglobulin and CD40; however, they do express secreted immunoglobulin. IgM is a primordial, all-purpose, **primary response immunoglobulin.** IgM is capable of complement activation but not direct opsonization (i.e., no Fc receptors exist for IgM). IgD is often coexpressed on B-cells with IgM, and it is believed to help increase B-cell responses to antigen. The memory B-cells give rise to the **secondary response immunoglobulins.** These B-cells produce immunoglobulin isotypes that can be divided into the IgE or IgG mediated inflammatory isotype responses, or the IgA mediated anti-inflammatory isotype responses. IgA is considered antiinflammatory because it does not stimulate complement activation, tends to antagonize IgE and IgG, and does not serve as a direct opsonin. Daily, humans produce about three times more IgA than all other immunoglobulin isotypes combined. IgA protects mucosal surfaces above and below the epithelium and is an important molecule in mucosal immunity.

TABLE 7-6

Selected Properties of Immunoglobulin Isotypes

Immunoglobulin Isotype	IgG1	IgG2	IgG3	IgG4	IgM	IgA1	IgA2	IgD	IgE
Concentration in serum (mg/ml)	9	3	1	0.5	1.5	3	0.5	0.03	0.00005
Molecular weight (kilodaltons)	146	146	170	146	970	160	160	184	188
Present on naïve B cells	–	–	–	–	+	–	–	+	–
Activation of complement (classical pathway)	++	+	+++	–	+++	–	–	–	–
Functions as opsonin without complement	+	–	+	+	–	–	–	–	–
With antigen stimulates mast cells	–	–	–	–	–	–	–	–	++++
With antigen stimulates eosinophils	–	–	–	–	–	–	–	–	++
Functions in mucosal immunity	–	–	–	–	–	+	+	–	–

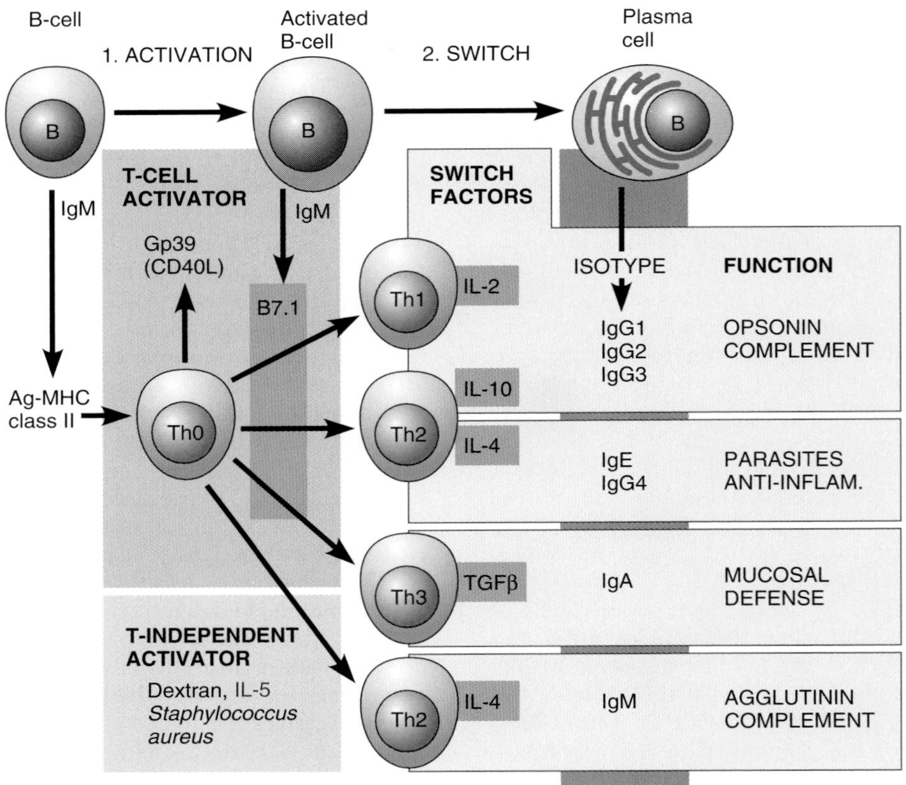

Fig. 7-11 Schematic illustration of B-cell differentiation. The essential signals in B-cell differentiation are activator and switch factors. *1,* The activator signal often requires cell contact because T-cell activators (Gp37, Gp34) are transmembranous. T-cells express Gp39 after antigen has been scanned. In the absence of T-cell switch signals, T-independent activation can result in an IgM response. Once the B-cell is activated, it can provide costimulation to the T-cells, which allows them to respond to differentiation signals (see Fig. 7-10). *2,* Switch signals also are derived from T-cells, and T-cells are required for isotype switching. Notice that IgG1-IgG3 can function in responses against both extracellular (Th2) and intracellular (Th2) pathogens. In contrast, Th1 responses are not that important for generation of IgA and IgE, which function in mucosal defenses.

SUMMARY

This chapter focused on the role of the immune system in inflammation, which is the host response to injury or insult and a central feature of the majority of periodontal diseases. Innate immunity provides critical early phase defenses against invading microorganisms. Adaptive immunity, including the development of the specific immune response, provides mechanisms by which the host can become more efficient in protecting against specific pathogens. Chapter 8 will discuss the interaction of the immune system with microbial pathogens involved in periodontal diseases.

REFERENCES

1. Ahmed R, Gray D: Immunological memory and protective immunity: understanding their relation. Science 1996; 272:54.
2. Allen RC, Armitage RJ, Conley ME, et al: CD40 ligand gene defects responsible for X-linked hyper-IgM syndrome. Science 1993; 259:990.
3. Arpin C, Dechanet J, Van Kooten C, et al: Generation of memory B cells and plasma cells in vitro. Science 1995; 268:720.
4. Baumheter S, Singer MS, Henzel W, et al: Binding of L-selectin to the vascular sialomucin CD34. Science 1993; 262:436.
5. Bevilacqua MP, Stengelin S, Gimbrone MA, Jr, et al: Endothelial leukocyte adhesion molecule 1: an inducible receptor for neutrophils related to complement regulatory proteins and lectins. Science 1989; 243:1160.
6. Bianchi E, Bender JR, Blasi F, et al: Through and beyond the wall: late steps in leukocyte transendothelial migration. Immunol Today 1997; 18:586.
7. Carroll RG, Riley JL, Levine BL, et al: Differential regulation of HIV-1 fusion cofactor expression by CD28 costimulation of CD4+ T cells. Science 1997; 276:273.
8. Caux C, Liu YJ, Banchereau J: Recent advances in the study of dendritic cells and follicular dendritic cells. Immunol Today 1995; 16:2.
9. Cerdan C, Martin Y, Courcoul M, et al: CD28 costimulation up-regulates long-term IL-2R B expression in human T cells through combined transcriptional and post-transcriptional regulation. J Immunol 1995; 154:1007.
10. Constant S, Schweitzer N, West J, et al: B lymphocytes can be competent antigen-presenting cells for priming CD4+ T cells to protein antigens in vivo. J Immunol 1995; 155:3734.
11. Craigen JL, Yong KL, Jordan NJ, et al: Human cytomegalovirus infection up-regulates interleukin-8 gene expression

and stimulates neutrophil transendothelial migration. Immunology 1997;92:138.

12. Dezzutti CS, Rudolph DL, Lal RB: Infection with human T-lymphotropic virus types I and II results in alterations of cellular receptors, including the up-modulation of T-cell counterreceptors CD40, CD54, and CD80 (B7-1). Clin Diagn Lab Immunol 1995; 2:349.
13. Ebnet K, Simon MM, Shaw S: Regulation of chemokine gene expression in human endothelial cells by proinflammatory cytokines and Borrelia burgdorferi. Ann N Y Acad Sci 1996; 797:107.
14. Gaboury JP, Johnston B, Niu XF, et al: Mechanisms underlying acute mast cell-induced leukocyte rolling and adhesion in vivo. J Immunol 1995; 154:804.
15. Harriman W, Volk H, Defranoux N, et al: Immunoglobulin class switch recombination. Annu Rev Immunol 1993; 11:361.
16. Hirsch JG: Cinemicrographic observations on granule lysis in polymorphonuclear leukocytes during phagocytosis. J Exp Med 1962; 116:827.
17. Huber AR, Kunkel SL, Todd RF, et al: Regulation of transendothelial neutrophil migration by endogenous interleukin-8. Science 1991; 254:99.
18. Iezzi G, Karjalainen K, Lanzavecchia A: The duration of antigenic stimulation determines the fate of naive and effector T cells. Immunity 1998; 8:89.
19. Karakurum M, Shreeniwas R, Chen J, et al: Hypoxic induction of interleukin-8 gene expression in human endothelial cells. J Clin Invest 1994; 93:1564.
20. Kozono H, Kinoshita T, Kim YU, et al: Localization of the covalent C3b-binding site on C4b within the complement classical pathway C5 convertase, C4b2a3b. J Biol Chem 1990; 265:14444.
21. Lloyd AR, Oppenheim JJ, Kelvin DJ, et al: Chemokines regulate T cell adherence to recombinant adhesion molecules and extracellular matrix proteins. J Immunol 1996; 156:932.
22. Malaviya R, Ikeda T, Ross E, et al: Mast cell modulation of neutrophil influx and bacterial clearance at sites of infection through TNF-alpha. Nature 1996; 381:77.
23. Medzhitov R, Preston-Hurlburt P, Janeway CA, Jr: A human homologue of the Drosophila Toll protein signals activation of adaptive immunity. Nature 1997; 388:394.
24. Medzhitov R, Preston-Hurlburt P, Kopp E, et al: MyD88 is an adaptor protein in the hToll/IL-1 receptor family signaling pathways. Mol Cell 1998; 2:253.
25. Mosmann TR, Coffman RL: Heterogeneity of cytokine secretion patterns and functions of helper T cells. Adv Immunol 1989; 46:111.
26. O'Neill LA, Greene C: Signal transduction pathways activated by the IL-1 receptor family: ancient signaling machinery in mammals, insects, and plants. J Leukoc Biol 1998; 63:650.
27. Rawal N, Pangburn MK: C5 convertase of the alternative pathway of complement. Kinetic analysis of the free and surface-bound forms of the enzyme. J Biol Chem 1998; 273:16828.
28. Reinherz EL, Tan K, Tang L, et al: The crystal structure of a T cell receptor in complex with peptide and MHC class II. Science 1999; 286:1913.
29. Romagnani S: Human TH1 and TH2 subsets: doubt no more. Immunol Today 1991; 12:256.
30. Rosenberg YJ, Anderson AO, Pabst R: HIV-induced decline in blood CD4/CD8 ratios: viral killing or altered lymphocyte trafficking? Immunol Today 1998; 19:10.
31. Schmittel A, Scheibenbogen C, Keilholz U: Lipopolysaccharide effectively up-regulates B7-1 (CD80) expression and costimulatory function of human monocytes. Scand J Immunol 1995; 42:701.
32. Sontheimer RD, Matsubara T, Seelig LL, Jr: A macrophage phenotype for a constitutive, class II antigen-expressing, human dermal perivascular dendritic cell. J Invest Dermatol 1989; 93:154.
33. Thorlacius H, Raud J, Rosengren-Beezley S, et al: Mast cell activation induces P-selectin-dependent leukocyte rolling and adhesion in postcapillary venules in vivo. Biochem Biophys Res Commun 1994; 203:1043.
34. Walsh LJ: Ultraviolet B irradiation of skin induces mast cell degranulation and release of tumor necrosis factor-α. Immunol Cell Biol 1995; 73:226.
35. Wetzler LM, Ho Y, Reiser H, et al: Neisserial porins induce B lymphocytes to express costimulatory B7-2 molecules and to proliferate. J Exp Med 1996; 183:1151.
36. Zhao J, Freeman GJ, Gray GS, et al: A cell type-specific enhancer in the human B7.1 gene regulated by NF-$\kappa\beta$. J Exp Med 1996; 183:777.

Microbial Interactions with the Host in Periodontal Diseases

Susan Kinder Haake, Russell J. Nisengard, Michael G. Newman, and Kenneth T. Miyasaki

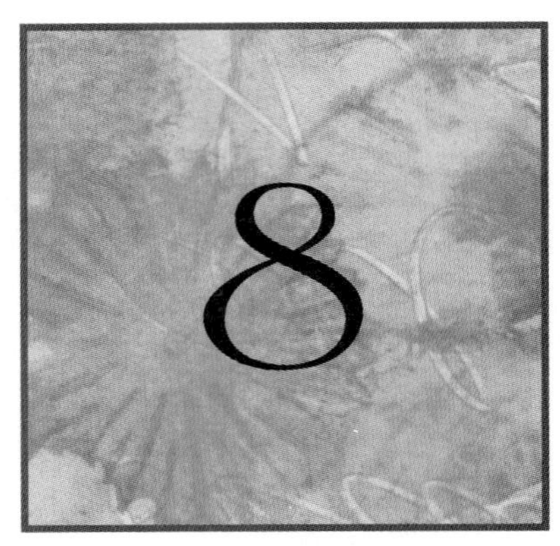

CHAPTER

CHAPTER OUTLINE

Gingivitis and periodontitis, as well as other less common periodontal diseases, are chronic infectious diseases. The interaction of the microorganism with the host determines the course and extent of the resulting disease. Microorganisms may exert pathogenic effects directly by causing tissue destruction itself or indirectly by stimulating and modulating the host response. The host response is mediated by the microbial interaction and inherent characteristics of the host, including genetic factors that vary among individuals. In general, the host response functions in a protective capacity, preventing the local infection from progressing to a systemic, life-threatening infection. However, local alteration and destruction of host tissues, which is evident as periodontal disease, may result. The varying balance between locally harmful and beneficial effects of the pathogenic microorganisms and the host accounts for the wide variety of patterns of tissue changes observed among patients.

MICROBIOLOGIC ASPECTS OF THE MICROBIAL-HOST INTERACTION

The specific microorganisms that have been found to be associated with differing states of health and disease are discussed in Chapter 6. In general, gram-negative facultative or anaerobic bacteria appear to represent the predominant microorganisms associated with disease. Predominant bacterial species that have been implicated in the disease processes include *Porphyromonas gingivalis, Actinobacillus actinomycetemcomitans, Treponema denticola, Bacteroides forsythus, Fusobacterium nucleatum, Prevotella intermedia, Campylobacter rectus, Peptostreptococcus micros,* and *Eikenella corrodens*. This chapter focuses on how the interaction of bacterial pathogens with host tissues results in disease. These issues relate to three of the criteria established by Socransky to identify periodontal pathogens (see Chapter 6). Studies of microbial interactions with the host involve analysis of the *host response* as well as the ability of a microorganism to cause disease in an *animal model* system. The properties of a microorganism that enable it to cause disease are referred to as *virulence factors*.

Considerable research is currently focused on defining the **virulence factors** of periodontal pathogens. From a simplistic viewpoint, to function as a pathogen, a bacterium must colonize the appropriate host tissue site and then cause destruction of the host tissues. In periodontitis, the initial step in the disease process is the colonization of the periodontal tissues by pathogenic species. Entry of the bacterium itself (invasion) or of bacterial products into the periodontal tissues may be important in the disease process. Furthermore, inherent in successful colonization of host tissues is the ability of the bacterium to evade host defense mechanisms aimed at eliminating the bacterium from the periodontal environment. The process of tissue destruction results from the interaction of bacteria or bacterial substances with host cells, which directly or indirectly lead to degradation of the periodontal tissues. Thus virulence properties can be broadly categorized into two groups: factors that enable a bacterial species to colonize and invade host tissues, and factors that enable a bacterial species to directly or indirectly cause host tissue damage.

TABLE 8-1

Selected Bacterial Adhesins and Target Substrates

Probable Attachment Surface	Substrate	Bacterial Species	Bacterial Adhesin	Substrate Receptor
Tooth	Saliva-coated mineralized surfaces	*A. viscosus*	Fimbriae	Saliva-treated hydroxyapatite
		A. viscosus	Fimbriae	Proline-rich proteins
	Saliva-coated surfaces	*S. mitis*	70-, 90-kd protein	Sialic acid residues
		F. nucleatum	300- to 330-kd outer membrane protein	Glactosyl residue
Tissue	Epithelial cells	*P. gingivalis*	Fimbriae	Galactosyl residues
		A. viscosus *A. naeslundii*	Fimbriae	Galactosyl residues
	Fibroblasts	*T. denticola*	Surface protein	Galactosyl or mannose residues
	Polymorphonuclear leukocytes	*A. viscosus* *A. naeslundii*	Fimbriae	Galactosyl residues
		F. nucleatum	Protein	Galactosyl residues
	Connective tissue components	*P. gingivalis*	Membrane protein	Fibrinogen/Fibronectin
		P. intermedia	Membrane protein	Fibrinogen
Preexisting plaque mass	*S. sanguis*	*A. viscosus*	Fimbriae	Repeating heptasaccharide on polysaccharide
	S. sanguis *A. naeslundii* *A. israelii*	*C. ochracea*	Heat-sensitive protein	Rhamnose, fucose, or *N-acetylneuraminic* acid residue
	S. sanguis *A. israelii*	*P. loescheii*	75- to 45-kd fimbrial proteins	Galactosyl residues
	P. gingivalis *T. denticola* *P. micros*	*F. nucleatum*	Heat and protease sensitive protein	Galactosyl residues

Adapted from Socransky SS, Haffajee AD: Microbiol mechanisms in the pathogenesis of destructive periodontal diseases: A critical assessment. J Periodontal Res 1991; 26:195; Lantz MS, Allen RD, Bounelis P, et al: *Bacteroides gingivalis* and *Bacteroides intermedius* recognize different sites on human fibrinogen. J Bacteriol 1990; 172:716; and Lantz MS, Allen RD, Duck LW, et al: Identification of *Porphyromonas gingivalis* components that mediate its interactions with fibronectin. J Bacteriol 1991; 173:4263; Bas HA, van Steenbergen M: *Peptostreptococcus micros* coaggregates with *Fusobacterium nucleatum* and non-encapsulated *Porphyromonas gingivalis*. FEMS Microbiol Lett 2000; 182:57; and Kolenbrander PE, Parrish KD, Andersen, RN, et al: Intergeneric coaggregation of oral *Treponema* spp. with *Fusobacterium* spp. and intrageneric coaggregation among *Fusobacterium* spp. Infect Immun 1995; 63:4584.

Bacterial Colonization and Survival in the Periodontal Region

Bacterial Adherence in the Periodontal Environment. The gingival sulcus and periodontal pocket are bathed in gingival crevicular fluid, which flows outward from the base of the pocket. Bacterial species that colonize this region must attach to available surfaces to avoid displacement by the fluid flow. Therefore adherence represents a virulence factor for periodontal pathogens.

The surfaces available for attachment include the tooth or root, tissues, and preexisting plaque mass. Numerous interactions between periodontal bacteria and these surfaces have been characterized, and in some cases the molecules responsible for mediating these highly specific interactions have been determined (Table 8-1). Bacteria that initially colonize the periodontal environment most likely attach to the pellicle- or saliva-coated tooth surface. A relevant example is the adherence of *Actinomyces viscosus* through fimbriae on the bacterial surface to proline-rich proteins found on saliva-coated tooth surfaces.[114]

Bacterial attachment to preexisting plaque is studied by examining the adherence between different bacterial strains (coaggregation). One of the best-characterized interactions is the adherence of *A. viscosus* through surface fimbriae to a polysaccharide receptor on cells of *Streptococcus sanguis*.[112] These types of interactions are thought to be of primary importance in the colonization of the periodontal environment. In addition, the adherence of bacteria to host tissues is likely to play a role in colonization and may be a critical step in the process of bacterial invasion. Thus the ability of *P. gingivalis* to attach to other bacteria,[82–84] epithelial cells,[28] and the connective tissue components fibrinogen and fibronectin[93,94] are all likely to be important in the virulence of this microorganism.

Host Tissue Invasion. The presence of bacteria in host tissues in patients with necrotizing ulcerative gingivitis (NUG) has been recognized for years, based on histologic studies.[97] Investigations carried out largely in the 1980s demonstrated the presence of bacteria in periodontal tissues in gingivitis,[42] advanced chronic adult periodontitis,[45,143] and juvenile periodontitis.[19,22] Both gram-positive and gram-negative bacteria, including cocci, rods, filaments, and spirochetes, have been observed in gingival connective tissue and in proximity to alveolar bone. Bacteria may enter host tissues through ulcerations in the epithelium of the gingival sulcus or

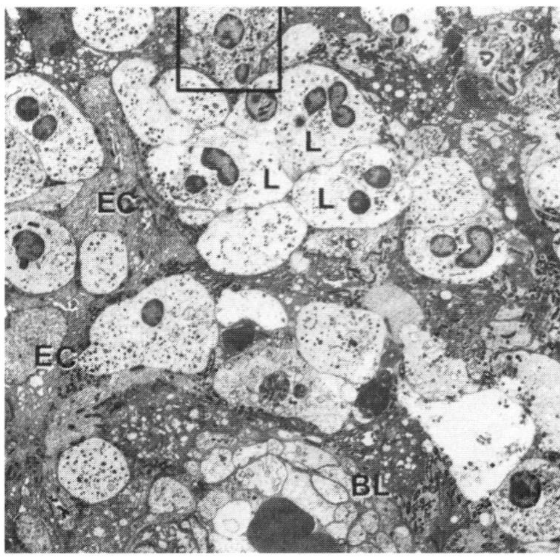

Fig. 8-2 Interface between pocket epithelium and connective tissue separated by the basement lamina *(BL)*. Abundant bacteria can be seen in the intercellular spaces. Numerous infiltrating polymorphonuclear leukocytes *(L)* are seen between epithelial cells *(EC)*. Some leukocytes show engulfed bacteria. (Magnification ×3908.)

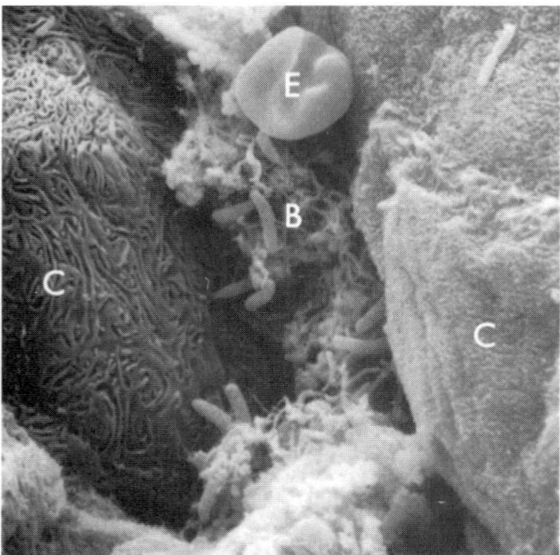

Fig. 8-1 Scanning electron micrograph of epithelial intercellular spaces containing bacterial plaque *(B)* enmeshed in a fibrin-like material. *C,* Epithelial cells; *E,* erythrocyte. The cells to the left show signs of necrosis. (Magnification ×4000.)

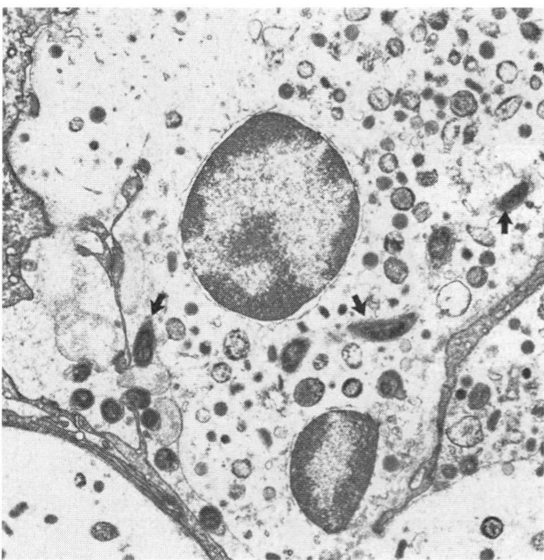

Fig. 8-3 Higher magnification of the polymorphonuclear leukocyte in square in Fig. 8-2 with engulfed bacteria *(arrows)*. (Magnification ×15,000.)

pocket and have been observed in intercellular spaces of the gingival tissues (Figs. 8-1 to 8-4). Another means of tissue invasion may involve the direct penetration of bacteria into host epithelial or connective tissue cells. Laboratory investigations have demonstrated the ability of *A. actinomycetemcomitans*,[156] *P. gingivalis* (Fig. 8-5),[144] *F. nucleatum*,[58] and *Treponema denticola*[173] to directly invade host tissue cells.

The clinical significance of bacterial invasion is not clear. Bacterial species that have been identified as capa-

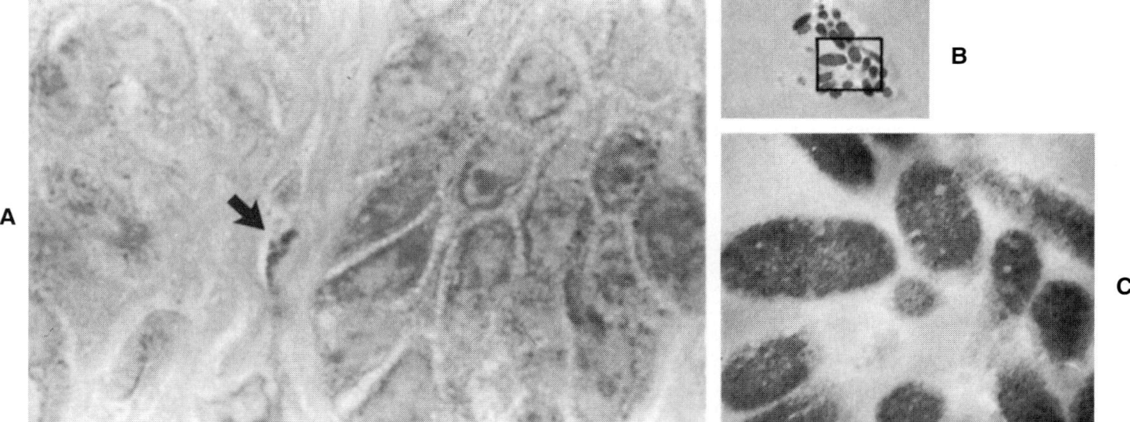

Fig. 8-4 **A,** Gingival tissue of a patient with localized juvenile periodontitis showing granular positive (dark gray) staining in the connective tissue for *Actinobacillus actinomycetemcomitans (arrow).* Formalin paraffin section, peroxidase antiperoxidase method, anti-*A. actinomycetemcomitans,* counterstained with hematoxylin. (Magnification ×1200.) **B,** Electron micrograph of the same paraffin section showing the area indicated by the arrow in **A,** which was reembedded in plastic (modified "pop-off" technique). (Magnification ×40,000.) **C,** Higher magnification of the rectangle in **B** showing the short coccobacillary rod with approximately the size and shape of *A. actinomycetemcomitans.* (Magnification ×80,000.)

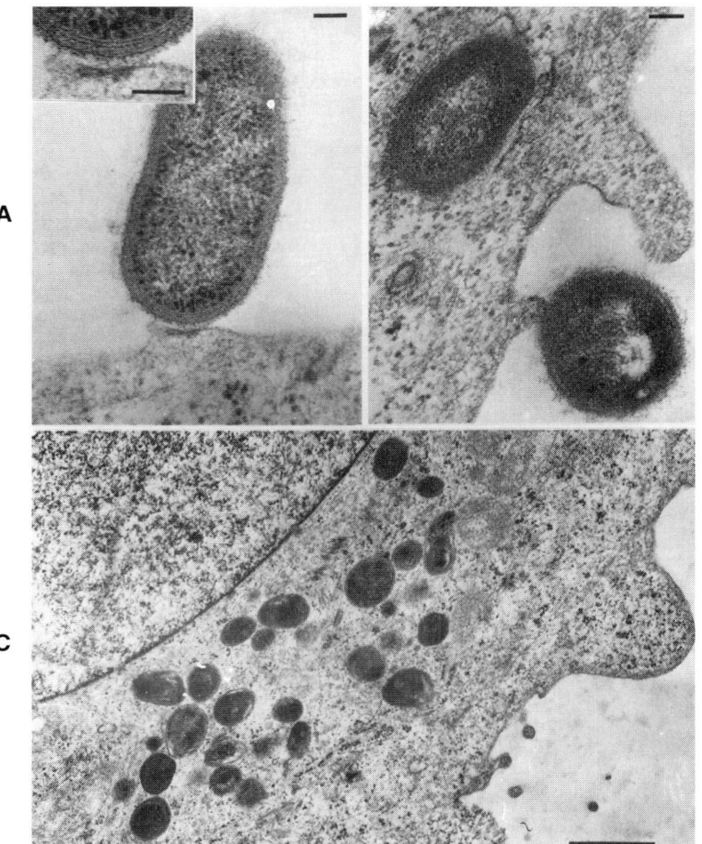

Fig. 8-5 High-magnification electron photomicrographs of the interaction of *Porphyromonas gingivalis* strain W50 with the epithelial cell HEp-2. **A,** *P. gingivalis* is attached to the HEp-2 plasma membrane by its tip. *Insert*: Note the electron-dense region juxtaposed to the site of interaction, possibly an early stage of clatherin pit formation. **B,** *P. gingivalis* is seen in transverse section attached to a microvillus extension. An internalized *P. gingivalis* also is apparent in the cell section. **C,** Numerous *P. gingivalis* W50 cells are seen in the HEp-2 cytoplasm. (Courtesy Dr. Stanley C. Holt, Boston, Mass.)

ble of tissue invasion are strongly associated with disease, and the ability to invade has been proposed as a key factor distinguishing pathogenic from nonpathogenic gram-negative species or strains.[102] Certainly, localization of bacteria to the tissues provides an ideal position from which the organism can effectively deliver toxic molecules and enzymes to the host tissue cells, and this may be the significance of invasion as a virulence factor. Indeed, some investigators have speculated that the "bursts of disease activity" observed in periodontitis may be related to phases of bacterial invasion of the tissues.[142] An additional possibility is that bacteria in the tissues may enable persistence of that species in the periodontal pocket by providing a reservoir for recolonization. Consistent with this hypothesis is the observation that mechanical debridement alone is insufficient, and that systemic antibiotics in combination with surgical therapy are required, to eliminate *A. actinomycetemcomitans* from lesions in patients with localized aggressive periodontitis (LJP).[21,86]

Bacterial Evasion of Host Defense Mechanisms. To survive in the periodontal environment, bacteria must neutralize or evade the host mechanisms involved in bacterial clearance and killing. Bacterial adherence and invasion are representative strategies by which microorganisms accomplish this task. The ability to adhere allows bacteria to avoid displacement by host secretions, and eukaryotic cell invasion disrupts the natural barriers formed by host tissue cells. Periodontal bacteria neutralize or evade host defenses via numerous other mechanisms; selected examples are presented in Table 8-2. For

TABLE 8-2

Selected Bacterial Properties Involved in Evasion of Host Defense Mechanisms

Host Defense Mechanism	Bacterial Species	Bacterial Property	Biologic Effect
Specific antibody	*P. gingivalis* *P. intermedia* *P. melaninogenica* *Capnocytophaga* sp.	IgA and IgG degrading proteases	Degradation of specific antibody
Polymorphonuclear leukocytes	*A. actinomycetemcomitans*	Leukotoxin	Inhibition of PNM function
	F. nucleatum	Heat-sensitive surface protein	Apoptosis (programmed cell death) of PMN
	P. gingivalis	Capsule	Inhibition of phagocytosis
	P. gingivalis *T. denticola*	Inhibition of superoxide production	Decreased bacterial killing
Lymphocytes	*A. actinomycetemcomitans*	Leukotoxin	Killing of mature B and T cells; nonlethal suppression of activity
	A. actinomycetemcomitans	Cytolethal distending toxin	Impairment of function by arresting of lymphocyte cell cycle
	F. nucleatum	Heat-sensitive surface protein	Apoptosis of mononuclear cells
	B. forsythus	Cytotoxin	Apoptosis of lymphocytes
	P. intermedia *T. denticola* *A. actinomycetemcomitans*	Suppression	Decreased response to antigens and mitogens
Release of IL-8	*P. gingivalis*	Inhibition of IL-8 production by epithelial cells	Impairment of PMN response to bacteria

Adapted from Socransky SS, Haffejee AD: Microbial mechanisms in the pathogenesis of destructive periodontal diseases: A critical assessment. J Periodontal Res 1991; 26:195; Jewett A, Hume WR, Le H, et al: Induction of apoptotic cell death in peripheral blood mononuclear and polymorphonuclear cells by an oral bacterium, *Fusobacterium nucleatum.* Infect Immun 2000; 68:1893; Shenker BJ, McKay T, Datar S, et al: *Actinobacillus actinomycetemcomitans* immunosuppressive protein is a member of the family of cytolethal distending toxins capable of causing a G2 arrest in human T cells. J Immunol 1999; 162:4773; Arakawa S, Nakajima T, Ishikura H, et al: Novel apoptosis-inducing activity in *Bacteroides forsythus:* a comparative study with three serotypes of *Actinobacillus actinomycetemcomitans.* Infect Immun 2000; 68:4611; Darveau RP, Belton CM, Reife RA, et al: Local chemokine paralysis, a novel pathogenic mechanism for *Porphyromonas gingivalis.* Infect Immun 1998; 66:1660; and Huang GT, Haake SK, Kim JW, et al: Differential expression of interleukin-8 and intercellular adhesion molecule-1 by human gingival epithelial cells in response to *Actinobacillus actinomycetemcomitans* or *Porphyromonas gingivalis* infection. Oral Microbiol Immunol 1998; 13:301.

example, immunoglobulins might function to facilitate phagocytosis of bacteria by opsonization or block adherence by binding to the bacterial cell surface and restricting access to bacterial adhesins. The production of immunoglobulin-degrading proteases by specific microorganisms may counteract these host defenses. Similarly, bacteria produce substances that suppress the activity of or kill polymorphonuclear leukocytes and lymphocytes normally involved in host defenses. An example of this is the production by *A. actinomycetemcomitans* of two toxins (a leukotoxin and cytolethal distending toxin) that may be important in the virulence of this microorganism in aggressive periodontitis and possibly in chronic periodontitis (see Chapter 9). Similarly, *B. forsythus*[2] and *F. nucleatum*[69] have been shown to induce apoptosis, a form of cellular "suicide," in lymphocytes. Many periodontal pathogens stimulate the production of interleukin-8 (IL-8), a proinflammatory chemokine that provides a signal for the recruitment of neutrophils (PMNs) to a local site (see discussion below). *P. gingivalis* is able to inhibit the production of IL-8 by epithelial cells, which may provide the microorganism with an advantage in evading PMN-mediated killing (see Chapter 9).

Microbial Mechanisms of Host Tissue Damage

Research on virulence factors has focused on the properties of bacteria related to the destruction of host tissues. These bacterial properties can be broadly categorized as those resulting directly in degradation of host tissues and those causing the release of biologic mediators from host tissue cells that lead to host tissue destruction.

Some bacterial products inhibit the growth or alter the metabolism of host tissue cells; these include a number of metabolic by-products such as ammonia; volatile sulfur compounds; and fatty acids, peptides, and indole.[149,170] An important class of molecules in tissue destruction is the variety of enzymes produced by periodontal microorganisms (Table 8-3). These enzymes appear to be capable of degrading essentially all host tissue and intercellular matrix molecules.[24,90] In particular, a wide range of proteolytic enzymes have been identified from *P. gingivalis* (see Chapter 9), including a trypsin-like enzyme and those that degrade collagen, fibronectin, and immunoglobulins. Bacterial enzymes may facilitate tissue destruction and invasion of bacteria into host tissues. However, the exact role of bacterially derived proteases in the disease process has not been determined because similar enzymes (e.g., collagenases) in the periodontal environment originate from host tissue cells. Indeed, one mechanism by which bacteria may indirectly cause tissue damage is by induction of host tissue proteinases such as elastase and matrix metalloproteinases (see discussion below).[29,30]

The host immune system involves a complex network of interactions among cells and regulatory molecules. Bacterial products may perturb the system, resulting in tissue destruction (Table 8-4). Well-characterized interactions involve the release of interleukin-1 (IL-1), tumor necrosis factor (TNF), and prostaglandins from monocytes, macrophages, and PMNs exposed to bacterial endotoxin (lipopolysaccharide).[137,180] These host-derived mediators have the potential to stimulate bone resorption and activate or inhibit other host immune cells. Many additional examples of this type of interaction exist, and the mechanisms underlying their manipulation of the host response is the focus of the next section.

TABLE 8-3

Bacterial Enzymes Capable of Degrading Host Tissues

Bacterial Enzyme	Species
Collagenase	*P. gingivalis* *A. actinomycetemcomitans*
Trypsin-like enzyme	*P. gingivalis* *A. actinomycetemcomitans* *T. denticola*
Keratinase	*P. gingivalis* *T. denticola*
Arylsulfatase	*C. rectus*
Neuraminidase	*P. gingivalis* *B. forsythus* *P. melaninogenica*
Fibronectin-degrading enzyme	*P. gingivalis* *P. intermedia*
Phospholipase A	*P. intermedia* *P. melaninogenica*

Adapted from Socransky SS, Haffajee AD: Microbial mechanisms in the pathogenesis of destructive periodontal diseases: A critical assessment. J Periodontal Res 1991; 26:195; and Loesche WJ: Bacterial mediators in periodontal disease. Clin Infect Dis 1993; 16(suppl 4):S203.

IMMUNOLOGIC ASPECTS OF THE MICROBIAL INTERACTION WITH THE HOST

Periodontal disease is dependent on bacteria, as discussed previously, and bacteria may directly interact with the host tissues in mediating tissue destruction. In addition, many tissue changes associated with periodontal diseases appear to be well-orchestrated responses, suggesting the influence of host regulation. Among the orchestrated responses are the antimicrobial activities by acute inflammatory cells (neutrophils) and the adaptive activities brought about by monocytes/macrophages and lymphocytes. Adaptive responses include the epithelial alterations, angiogenesis, episodic remodeling of the underlying of hard and soft connective tissues, and antigen-specific immune responses. Remodeling of the connective tissues appears to be episodic and occurs in cycles of destruction and reconstruction. Excessive destruction or inadequate reconstruction can result in periodontal disease.

In this section, a paradigm for the role of the immune system in periodontal pathogenesis is presented. The paradigm is consistent with the specific plaque hypothesis, current concepts in immunology, and the classic clinical and histologic observations (see Chap-

TABLE 8-4

Examples of the Effects of Bacteria and their Products on Production of Biologically Active Molecules by Host Tissues

Effect on Cytokine Levels	Bacterial Species	Bacterial Component Involved	Target Host Tissue
Increased release of Interleukin-1	*A. actinomycetemcomitans*	Lipopolysaccharide (LPS)	PMNs
	F. nucleatum		
	A. actinomycetemcomitans	37 kDa protein	Macrophages
	P. gingivalis	LPS	Monocytes
Increased release of Interleukin-6	*A. actinomycetemcomitans*	37 kDa protein	Macrophages
	A. actinomycetemcomitans	Whole cells	Gingival fibroblasts
	C. rectus		
	E. corrodens	Whole cells	Epithelial cells
Increased release of Interleukin-8	*A. actinomycetemcomitans*	Whole cells	Epithelial cells
	E. corrodens		
	F. nucleatum		
	A. actinomycetemcomitans	Whole cells	Gingival fibroblasts
	C. rectus		
	A. actinomycetemcomitans	LPS	PMNs
	F. nucleatum		
Increased release of TNF	*A. actinomycetemcomitans*	LPS	PMNs
	F. nucleatum		
	A. actinomycetemcomitans	37 kDa protein	Macrophages
Stimulated release of Prostaglandin E2	*C. rectus*	LPS	Monocytes
	A. actinomycetemcomitans		
	P. intermedia		
	P. gingivalis		

Adapted from Socransky SS, Haffajee AD: Microbial mechanisms in the pathogenesis of destructive periodontal diseases: A critical assessment. J Periodontal Res 1991; 26:195; and data compiled from references[26,31,47,58,65,66,137,161,180,181].

ters 15 and 21) regarding periodontal diseases. *The paradigm is that in response to bacterial infection, 1) innate factors such as complement, resident leukocytes, and especially mast cells play an important role in signaling endothelium, thus initiating inflammation; 2) acute inflammatory cells (i.e., neutrophils) protect local tissues by controlling the periodontal microbiota within the gingival crevice and junctional epithelium; and finally, 3) chronic inflammatory cells, macrophages, and lymphocytes protect the entire host from within the subjacent connective tissues and do all that is necessary to prevent a local infection from becoming systemic and life threatening, including the sacrifice of local tissues.*

In this paradigm, periodontal disease represents a well-regulated response to protracted bacterial infection directed by the inflammatory cells of the host immune system (Fig. 8-6). Neutrophils function primarily as antimicrobial cells, and chronic inflammatory cells orchestrate adaptive responses. Neutrophils function to contain the microbial challenge through phagocytosis and killing and may contribute to local tissue changes by the release of tissue-degrading enzymes. The chronic inflammatory cells, the lymphocytes and monocytes, orchestrate connective tissue changes associated with both periodontal infection and periodontal repair and healing. They also function to assist the neutrophils in controlling bacterial infection by forming specific opsonic antibodies. The host response in the connective tissues may result in local destruction of the tissue, which is evident as periodontal disease. In recent years, the potential systemic impact of periodontal disease has been increasingly recognized (see Chapters 12 and 13). However, the end result of the periodontal host response is largely successful for the host in preventing progressive spread of the infection despite local tissue destruction.

Innate Factors and the Initiation of Inflammation

The onset of inflammation involves the development of edema and erythema, which are signs of vascular changes. Complement activation in response to bacterial infection results in generation of the complement-derived anaphylatoxins C3a and C5a. Anaphylatoxins are substances that stimulate vascular changes indirectly by causing degranulation of the resident leukocytes, the mast cells. Degranulated mast cells increase within the gingival connective tissue as gingival inflammation increases. Mast cells constitutively transcribe TNF-α, transforming growth factor β (TGFβ), interleukin 4 (IL-4), and interleukin 6 (IL-6); when stimulated, they induce transcription of proinflammatory cytokines such as IL-1, IL-6, IFNγ, and others.[115] The stimulation of endothelial cells by C5a, IL-1β, TNF-α, and bacterial LPS results in the expression of selectins on the lumenal surface of the endothelial cells and release of chemokines from the endothelial cells. These processes are central in transendothelial migration of leukocytes (see Fig. 7-4), which results in the movement of leukocytes into the local tissues.

In healthy individuals, complement levels in gingival crevicular fluid (GCF) are about 3% of that in serum. As periodontal inflammation increases, a concomitant increase in the levels of complement components occurs. The levels of C3 and C4, for example, can increase to 25% and 85% of that in serum.[145] The level of complement components in GCF are more than adequate to support the recruitment of acute and chronic inflammatory cells, opsonization and neutralization of pathogens or pathogenic substances, and local regulation of connective tissue changes.

Controlling the Bacterial Challenge: A Primary Role for Neutrophils

Neutrophils are believed to play an important role in controlling the periodontal microbiota. They are the first leukocytes to arrive at the site of inflammation and are always the dominant cell type within the junctional epithelium and the gingival crevice. (See Chapters 15 and 21.) For neutrophils to effectively control bacterial infections, their functions—including transendothelial migration, chemotaxis, transepithelial migration, opsonization, phagocytosis and intraphagolysosomal killing—must be intact. Disorders of neutrophils are associated with invasive periodontal infection and aggressive periodontitis (Table 8-5). For example, severe periodontal destruction involving both the primary dentition and

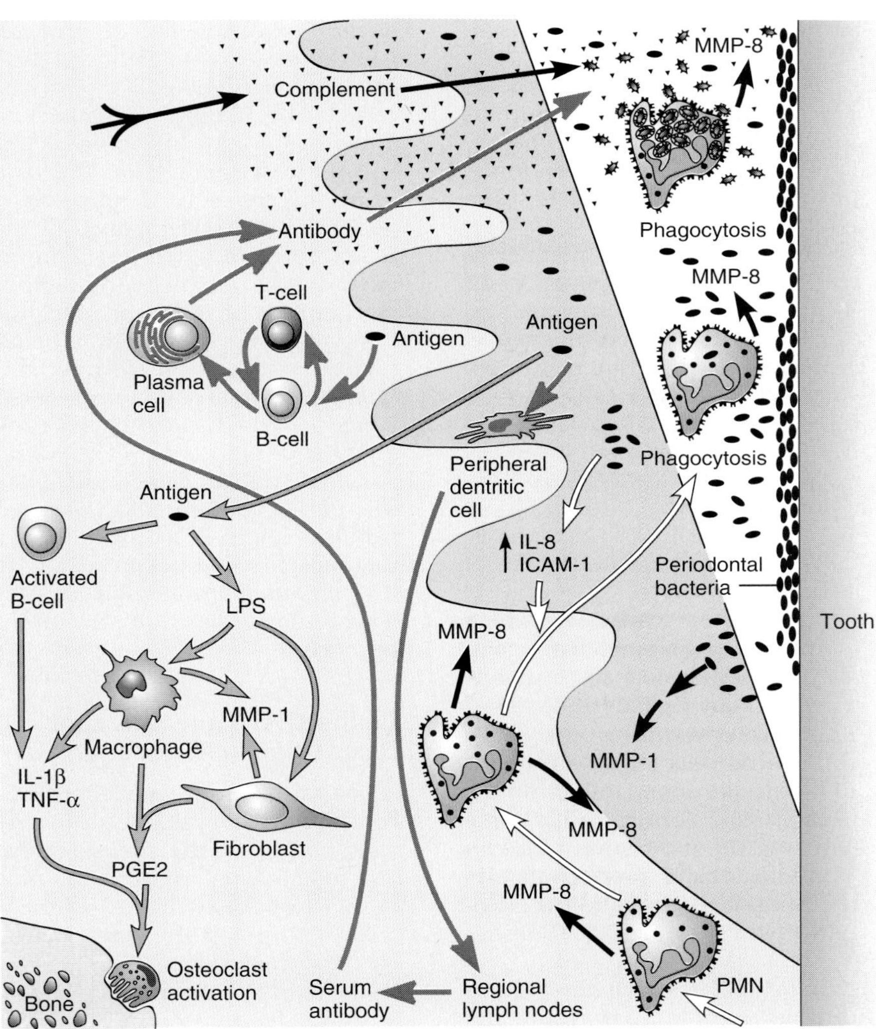

Fig. 8-6 Schematic illustration of key processes of the host bacterial interaction in periodontal diseases. Interactions of the bacteria or bacterial antigen with host tissues leads to neutrophil recruitment *(white arrows),* antibody production *(gray arrows),* and bone resorption *(light gray arrows with black outlines).* IL-8 and ICAM-1 production in the epithelial cells in response to periodontal bacteria provides a chemotactic signal for neutrophils (PMN). Neutrophils function to control the bacterial assault by phagocytosis but also secrete matrix metalloproteinases (MMP-8), which may contribute to tissue destruction. The interaction of bacterial antigens with peripheral dendritic cells leads to the generation of systemic antibody, whereas interaction with local B-cells leads to production of local antibody. Antibody specific to many of the periodontal microorganisms is essential for phagocytosis. Complement components also may contribute to efficient bacterial phagocytosis. The production of IL-1β, TNF-α, and PGe_2 in response to bacterial LPS leads to bone resorption through osteoclast activation, proliferation, and differentiation.

permanent dentition is evident in individuals with disorders affecting neutrophil chemotaxis and phagocytosis (Color Fig. 8-1). Also, otherwise healthy individuals with severe periodontal problems may have subtle defects in neutrophil function (discussed further below).

About 1% to 2% of all neutrophils migrate across the junctional epithelium on a daily basis. This transepithelial migration requires a chemotaxin gradient (see Fig. 8-6). The junctional epithelium expresses the chemotactic cytokine (chemokine) IL-8 and intercellular cell adhesion molecule 1 (ICAM-1). A gradient of the membrane-bound ICAM-1 and the soluble IL-8 molecules is formed, with increased expression toward the outer surface of the tissue.[165] This distribution is ideal for the migration of neutrophils into the gingival sulcus. Neutrophils may use their adhesins LFA-1, Mac-1, or both to bind ICAM-1 on the epithelial cell in the process of epithelial transmigration.

In vitro studies have shown that *P. gingivalis* impedes transepithelial migration of neutrophils[107] and prevents epithelial cells from secreting IL-8 in response to bacterial challenge.[26,65] These properties may contribute to the virulence of *P. gingivalis* by interfering with the host immune response (see Chapter 9).

Opsonization refers to the coating of particles, such as bacteria, with host proteins that facilitate phagocytosis (see Fig. 8-6 and Fig. 8-7). For example, a bacterial cell may be coated with molecules derived from complement components (e.g., iC3b) for which the neutrophil has receptors (CR3). Similarly, bacterial cells may be coated with specific antibody that fixes complement and results in surface deposition of C3b that is recognized by the CR3 neutrophil receptor when converted to iC3b. Specific antibody of the IgG isotype also facilitates phagocytosis directly by binding with the neutrophil Fc receptor and appears to be essential for phagocytosis of certain periodontal pathogens (see below).

Patients with periodontitis often exhibit very high serum titers of IgG to specific periodontal pathogens. Although B-cells are directly responsible for antibody production, T-cells are required to regulate the isotype switch from IgM to IgG. Antigen-presenting cells (APCs) such as the peripheral dendritic cells (e.g., Langerhans cells, macrophages, and B-cells) are abundant within the gingival tissues[127] and can transport antigen to regional lymph nodes, thus promoting the production of serum IgG antibody. Local immunoglobulin production also has been documented within the gingiva, and the gingival tissues are impregnated with very high levels of immunoglobulins.

Scaling and root planing stimulates antibody production against microorganisms such as *P. gingivalis* and *A. actinomycetemcomitans*.[20,150] Variability in the levels, types, and strength of binding of the antibody is evident in different patients, and the significance of the antibody depends on its functional capabilities.[81] Antibody may function to facilitate host clearance of periodontal pathogens. For example, antibody appears to be essential for opsonization and phagocytosis of *A. actinomycetemcomitans*[10] and virulent strains of *P. gingivalis*.[25] Antibody also may function to neutralize bacterial components important in colonization or host cell interactions. A monoclonal antibody preparation specific for a hemagglutinin of *P. gingivalis* has been shown to prevent recolonization of deep periodontal pockets in vivo in periodontitis patients.[14,74] More information is needed to clarify the role of antibody to specific bacterial epitopes in disease progression and resolution. It is noteworthy that in LJP, the absence of a host antibody response has been postulated to contribute to disease progression (see discussion below).

Once the bacterial cell is bound to the neutrophil, ingestion (phagocytosis) results in entrapment of the bacterial cell into the membrane-delimited structure known as the *phagosome*. Bacteria within the phagosome and phagolysosome may be killed by oxidative or nonoxidative mechanisms. The gingival sulcus is characterized by a diminished level of oxygen, and the reduction-oxidation potential of the periodontal pocket is more reduced than the gingival sulcus. This is indicated by measurements of crevicular oxygen levels and reduction-oxidation potential[75] and reflected by the growth of strictly anaerobic bacteria such as *P. gingivalis* and the oral spirochetes. The oxidative killing mechanisms of crevicular neutrophils may be intact in a healthy sulcus but impaired in the periodontal pocket. A shutdown of oxidative killing may be an important factor in the progression to periodontitis. Nonoxidative mechanisms of killing involve phagosome-lysosome fusion, resulting in secretion of bactericidal substances such as lysozyme, cathepsin G, and α-defensins into the phagolysosome containing the ingested bacterium. Some periodontal pathogens evade phagocytic cells as a virulence mechanism. For example, the leukotoxin of *A. actinomycetemcomitans* kills phagocytes by binding to the LFA-1 adhesin and subsequently lysing the eukaryotic cell.[92] Recently it was demonstrated *in vitro* that specific antibodies to *A. actinomycetemcomitans* or antileukotoxin serum protects neutrophils from leukotoxin-mediated injury and enables phagocytosis to proceed.[70]

Connective Tissue Alterations: Tissue Destruction in Periodontitis

A central feature of periodontitis is the remodeling of connective tissues that leads to a net loss of local soft tissues, bone, and the periodontal attachment apparatus. The fundamental event in the transition from gingivitis to periodontitis is the loss of the soft tissue attachment to the tooth and the subsequent loss of alveolar bone. Bacterial components that contribute directly or indirectly to tissue destruction have been discussed previously. Mediators produced as a part of the host response that contribute to tissue destruction include proteinases, cytokines, and prostaglandins.

Proteinases. Matrix metalloproteinases (MMPs) are considered to be primary proteinases involved in periodontal tissue destruction by degradation of extracellular matrix molecules. MMPs are a family of proteolytic enzymes that degrade extracellular matrix molecules, such as collagen, gelatin, and elastin. MMP-8 and MMP-1 are both collagenases; MMP-8 is released by infiltrating neu-

TABLE 8-5

Systemic Neutrophil Abnormalities Associated with Aggressive Periodontitis

Condition	Neutrophil Abnormality	Periodontal Manifestations
Neutropenia, agranulocytosis	Decreased number of neutrophils	Severe aggressive periodontitis
Chediak-Higashi syndrome	Decreased neutrophil chemotaxis and secretion. Neutrophil granules fuse to form characteristic giant granules called *megabodies.*	Aggressive periodontitis and oral ulceration. The syndrome is caused by a mutation in the vesicle trafficking regulator gene, LYST.
Papillon-LeFevre syndrome	Multiple functional neutrophil defects, including myeloperoxidase deficiency as well as defective chemotaxis and phagocytosis	Severe aggressive periodontal destruction at an early age, which may involve the primary and permanent dentition. Recently associated in affected individuals with a mutation in the cathepsin C gene (see Chapter 10).
Leukocyte adhesion deficiency Type I	Defects in leukocyte function due to lack of integrin $\beta 2$ subunit (CD18). Neutrophil defects include impaired migration and phagocytosis. Histologically, almost no extravascular neutrophils are evident in periodontal lesions.	Aggressive periodontitis, at an early age and affecting primary and permanent dentition, in individuals who are homozygous for the defective gene.
Leukocyte adhesion deficiency Type II	Neutrophils fail to express the ligand (CD15) for P- and E-selectins, resulting in impaired transendothelial migration in response to inflammation	Aggressive periodontitis at a young age

Data compiled from references[11,27,49,59,60,120,135,148,171]

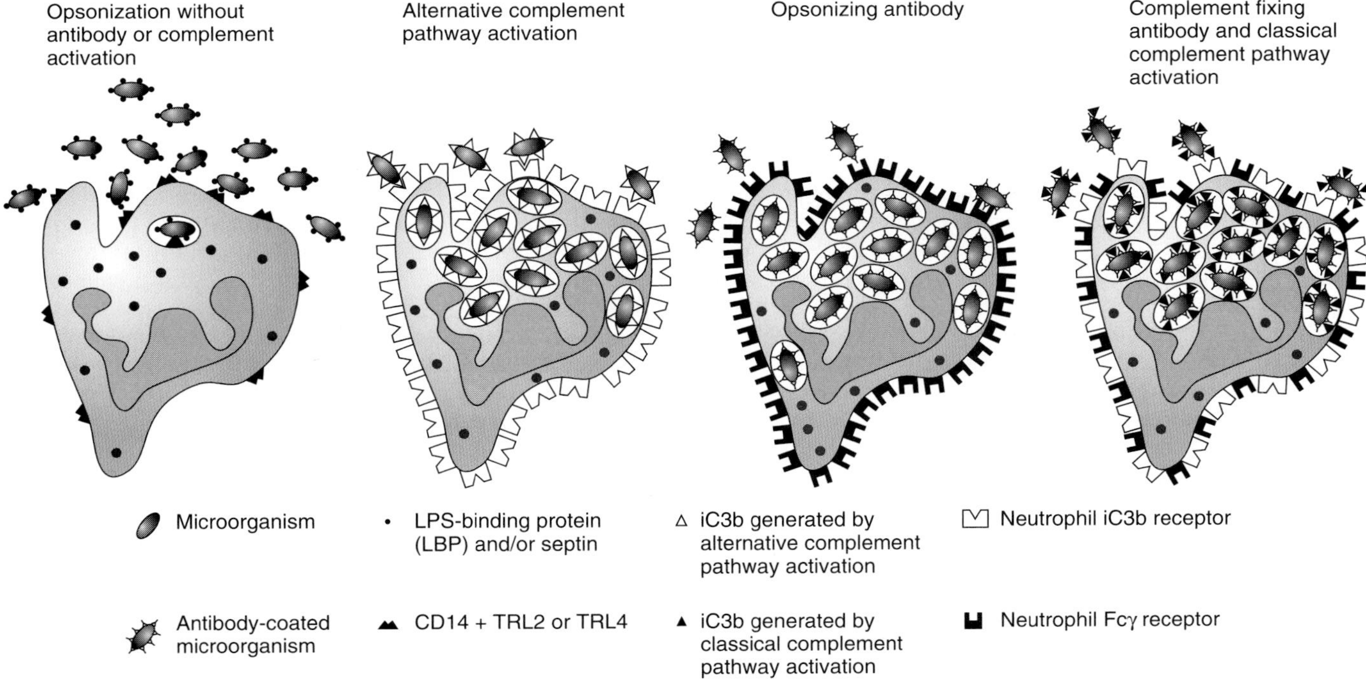

Fig. 8-7 Schematic illustration of some routes of opsonization and phagocytosis. Bacterial control in the periodontal environment is achieved largely by opsonization, phagocytosis, and killing of the bacteria by neutrophils. *Opsonization* refers to the coating of the bacterial cell with host-derived proteins such as LPS-binding protein (LBP), specific antibody, or the complement component iC3b. Opsonization with specific antibody of the IgG subclass is required for phagocytosis of certain bacteria, such as *Actinobacillus actinomycetemcomitans.* See text for further details.

trophils whereas MMP-1 is expressed by resident cells including fibroblasts, monocytes/macrophages, and epithelial cells (see Fig. 8-6). Collagenase is elevated in tissues and GCF associated with periodontitis, as compared with gingivitis or healthy controls.[68,138]

MMPs are secreted in an inactive (latent) form. Enzyme activity in the tissues is partly controlled by activation of the latent enzyme and the level of enzyme inhibitors present. One mechanism of MMP activation involves the proteolytic cleavage of a portion of the latent enzyme. Proteases capable of activation MMPs include bacterial enzymes such as the chymotrypsin-like protease produced by *T. denticola,* as well as host cell enzymes such as neutrophil cathepsin G. MMPs are inactivated by α-macroglobulins that are found in serum and gingival crevicular fluid, and tissue inhibitors of MMPs (TIMPs) that are produced by many cell types and are common in host tissues and fluids.[13]

Other proteinases associated with periodontitis include the neutrophil serine proteinases, elastase and cathepsin G. Elastase is capable of degrading a wide range of molecules including elastin, collagen, and fibronectin. Cathepsin G is a bactericidal proteinase that also may function in the activation of MMP-8. Endogenous inhibitors of elastase and cathepsin G (e.g., α1-proteinase inhibitor, α1-antichymotrypsin, and α2 macroglobulin) are found in plasma and GCF.[67] The role of these enzymes in pathogenesis is likely to depend on the balance of enzyme and enzyme inhibitor in the local tissue. Cathepsin G is elevated in the gingival tissues and GCF in adult periodontitis.[163] Elevated levels of elastase in GCF are associated with active periodontal attachment loss,[3] and elastase may provide a convenient clinical marker of disease progression.

Cytokines. Two proinflammatory cytokines, IL-1 and tumor necrosis factor (TNF), appear to have a central role in periodontal tissue destruction (see Fig. 8-6).[53,132] IL-1 is found in two active forms, IL-1α and IL-1β, encoded by separate genes. Both are potent proinflammatory molecules and are the main constituents of what was once called "osteoclast activating factor." The IL-1 family also includes the IL-1 receptor antagonist (IL-1ra), which will bind the IL-1 receptor without stimulation of the host cell. TNF also is found in two forms, TNF-α and TNF-β. TNF-α shares many of the same biologic activities as IL-1, including the stimulation of bone resorption.

IL-1 is produced primarily by activated macrophages or lymphocytes but also may be released by other cells, including mast cells, fibroblasts, keratinocytes, and endothelial cells. Bacterial LPS is a potent activator of macrophage IL-1 production, whereas TNF-α and IL-1 itself also can activate macrophage IL-1 production. The ability of IL-1 to upregulate its own production may provide a significant amplification mechanism. TNF-α also is produced by activated macrophages, particularly in response to bacterial LPS. TNF-β is primarily produced by the Th1 subset of CD4+ T-cells that have been activated by antigen or mitogen. The proinflammatory effects of IL-1 and TNF-α include stimulation of endothelial cells to express selectins that facilitate recruitment of leukocytes, activation of macrophage IL-1 production, and induction of prostaglandin E_2 (PGE_2) by macrophages and gingival fibroblasts.[132]

The properties of these cytokines that relate to tissue destruction involve stimulation of bone resorption and induction of tissue-degrading proteinases. IL-1 is a potent stimulant of osteoclast proliferation, differentiation, and activation. TNF-α has similar effects on osteoclasts but is far less potent than IL-1. Both IL-1 and TNF-α induce production of proteinases in mesenchymal cells, including MMPs, which may contribute to connective tissue destruction.[53,132]

Substantial data from *in vivo* studies support the concept that IL-1 and TNF-α are key molecules in the pathogenesis of periodontitis. IL-1 and TNF-α are found in significant concentrations in GCF from periodontally diseased sites, and reductions in IL-1 concentration are associated with successful treatment.[110,157] Increasing severity of periodontitis is associated with increased concentrations of IL-1 and decreasing concentrations of IL-1ra.[136] In a primate model of experimental periodontitis, application of antagonists to IL-1 and TNF resulted in an 80% reduction in recruitment of inflammatory cells in proximity to the alveolar bone and a 60% reduction in bone loss.[8]

Prostaglandins. Prostaglandins are arachidonic acid metabolites generated by cyclooxygenases (COX-1, COX-2). Arachidonic acid is a 20-carbon polyunsaturated fatty acid found in the plasma membrane of most cells. COX-2 is upregulated by IL-1β, TNF-α, and bacterial LPS and appears to be responsible for generating the prostaglandin PGE_2 that is associated with inflammation. The primary cells responsible for PGE_2 production in the periodontium are macrophages and fibroblasts. PGE_2 is increased in periodontal sites demonstrating inflammation and attachment loss.[88,129] Induction of MMPs and osteoclastic bone resorption is induced by PGE_2 (see Fig. 8-6).

PGE_2 appears to be partly responsible for the bone loss associated with periodontitis. Studies in vitro demonstrated that bone loss associated with several periodontal pathogens was inhibited in part by inhibitors of prostaglandin synthesis.[184] In addition, use of a nonsteroidal antiinflammatory agent as an inhibitor of prostaglandin synthesis in human subjects with advanced periodontitis resulted in significantly less bone loss as compared to placebo.[174] PGE_2 release from monocytes from patients with severe or aggressive periodontitis is greater than that from patients with little to no periodontal destruction.[48,129] It has been postulated that high-risk periodontal patients have a "monocyte hypersecretory trait" that results in an exaggerated response both locally and systemically to bacterial LPS.[129]

Summary. The production of these proteinases and mediators as well as their inhibitors by host tissue cells are influenced by bacteria and regulatory molecules produced by host cells that are resident within, or recruited to, the periodontal tissues. In normal tissue turnover, a balance exists such that no net loss of tissue occurs. In disease, tissue loss occurs, suggesting that this balance is disrupted. In addition, although bacterial proteinases do not appear predominant in this environment, their effects locally within the periodontal econiche may be significant. Loss of bone in periodontal diseases appears to occur in part through the action of regulatory molecules, including IL-1, TNF-α, and PGE_2.

Connective Tissue Alterations: Healing Processes in Periodontitis

The chronic immune system plays an important role in healing processes, which consist of regeneration and repair. **Regeneration** involves the replacement of tissues with new, identical tissues that function like the original tissues. Periodontal tissues are limited in their regenerative capacity, and considerable research is being devoted to developing techniques and materials to augment host processes that facilitate regeneration (see Chapters 63 and 71).

Repair involves replacement of one tissue with another tissue, such as fibrous connective tissue, which may not function like the tissue replaced. After traumatic or surgical injury, healing is initiated as part of the immediate and acute inflammatory responses. A clot that usually provides hemostasis almost immediately after injury also forms a matrix rich in platelet-derived cytokines that stimulates and facilitates healing. In contrast, periodontal infections do not normally produce the massive, platelet-rich clot observed in traumatic injury. Thus the periodontal "healing" cycle during the pathogenesis of periodontal disease is primarily postinflammatory; and cellular elements other than platelets provide important signals in this process. Periodontal repair occurs in overlapping phases of inflammation shutdown, angiogenesis and fibrogenesis.

In the postinflammatory healing process, the shutdown of inflammatory processes and initiation of postinflammatory healing is orchestrated by leukocytes. Some of the important antiinflammatory signals generated by leukocytes include **IL-1 receptor antagonist (IL-1ra)** and **transforming growth factor β (TGF-β).**[50] In inflamed periodontal tissues, macrophages are a source of IL-1ra,[71] whereas neutrophils, macrophages, and mast cells and lymphocytes produce TGF-β.[158]

Angiogenesis and fibrogenesis, as well as cytokines such as IL-1β and TNF-β that help to induce these processes, participate in both inflammation and healing. IL-1β and IL-1α are indirectly involved in inducing fibroblast proliferation and collagen synthesis by stimulating the production of PGE_2 or the release of "secondary" cytokines such as **platelet-derived growth factor (PDGF)** and TGF-β. PDGF is a protein complex formed by different combinations of α and β chains, resulting in three isoforms, PDGF-AA, PDGF-AB and PDGF-BB. It is produced by numerous cells and tissues, including endothelium, vascular smooth muscle, and macrophages. PDGF activates fibroblasts and osteoblasts, resulting in the induction of protein synthesis.[51] The PDGFs are related structurally and functionally to **vascular endothelial growth factor (VEGF),** an important factor in endothelial proliferation. VEGF is a glycoprotein produced by many cells, including monocytes/macrophages, and it is induced by antiinflammatory factors such as TGF-β.

TGF-β is a multifunctional peptide that stimulates osteoblasts and fibroblasts and inhibits osteoclasts, epithelial cells, and most immune cells. Receptors for TGF-β are found in almost all cells. TGF-β is produced as a propeptide, and activation requires acidic conditions. TGF-β is known for its ability to promote the elaboration of fibroblast extracellular matrix adhesion.

Other fibrogenic cytokines that may play a role include basic fibroblast growth factor (bFGF), TGF-α, and TNF-α. TGF-α and TNF-α are produced mainly by cells of the monocyte lineage, and within the periodontium, bFGF is produced primarily by PDL cells and endothelium.[46]

In the healing of alveolar bone, regeneration of bone within a defect clearly can occur. The immune system can induce regenerative bone healing by preventing osteoclast formation and activation and by activating osteoblasts. By blocking osteoclast formation or increasing osteoclast death, it is possible to cause a marked decrease in osteoclastic activity. TGF-β is a potent inhibitor of osteoclast formation. Bone matrix itself contains TGF-β, which is released by osteoclastic resorption,[119] and osteoclasts may provide the acidic conditions necessary for TGF-β activation. Osteoclast differentiation and activation are inhibited by interferon-γ (IFN-γ), which is secreted by NK-cells, Th1 T-cells, and macrophages. The main effect of IFN-γ appears to be inhibition of IL-1 and TNF-α–induced osteoclast activation. IL-1ra also is effective in blocking IL-1 and TNF-α–induced osteoclast activation.

Much research in bone healing has focused on activation of osteoblasts and PDL cells as a means of promoting regenerative healing. Two substances, insulinlike growth factor I (IGF-I) and PDGF, have been shown to induce or augment regenerative repair.[64,104,133] The insulinlike growth factors induce osteoblast growth, differentiation, and synthesis of collagen. Several studies in nonhuman primates indicate that the combination of IGF-1 and PDGF effectively and significantly enhances regeneration of periodontal structures, including new bone and cementum.[51,140]

MICROBIOLOGY AND IMMUNOLOGY IN GINGIVAL HEALTH

The gingival crevice harbors bacteria in both health and disease. In a clinically healthy periodontium, the microbial flora is largely composed of gram-positive facultative microorganisms, predominately species such as *Actinomyces* and *Streptococcus* spp. Gram-negative species and spirochetal forms also may be found, but they are considerably less prevalent and occur in much smaller numbers. Serum antibodies to microorganisms are usually in low titers, suggesting the minimal systemic antigenic stimulation by plaque during gingival health. The gingival tissues typically demonstrate some evidence of inflammation. Tissues are usually infiltrated with chronic inflammatory cells, generally lymphocytes. Neutrophils also are common within the junctional epithelium and in the gingival crevice. The infiltration of inflammatory cells is thought to be a response to bacterial plaque, and host defense mechanisms in a healthy individual are effective in managing the bacterial challenge. Physical mechanisms of host defense include the integrity of the epithelial cell layer, as well as the shedding of epithelial cells and the flow of crevicular fluid that may function to clear bacteria and their products from the subgingival environment. It is likely that the complement, neutrophils, and antibody production contribute to controlling the sulcular microbiota.

MICROBIOLOGY AND IMMUNOLOGY IN PERIODONTAL DISEASES

Gingivitis

The most common form of gingivitis is **plaque-induced gingivitis.**[108] Common clinical findings in gingivitis include erythema, edema, tissue enlargement, and bleeding. Two forms of plaque-induced gingivitis have been investigated: a naturally occurring gingivitis and experimental gingivitis. Experimental gingivitis is a longitudinal clinical model that has been widely used in human and animal studies.[98] In humans, experimental gingivitis is induced through abstinence from oral hygiene measures; in animal studies a soft diet favoring plaque accumulation is instituted. The studies of experimental gingivitis have provided a clear demonstration that plaque accumulation invariably causes gingivitis and that gingivitis is reversible with removal of the plaque deposits.

Page and Schroeder reviewed the histopathology of human and animal experimental gingivitis in a classic article[130] that delineated three temporal stages of gingivitis, including the initial, early, and established lesions (see Chapter 15). Central to the histopathologic changes are the vascular inflammation and infiltration of neutrophils and then lymphocytes in the early stages. The early lymphocytic infiltrate is dominated by T-cells, but eventually B-cells become dominant. The established lesion is characterized by a predominance of B-cells that have transformed into plasma cells in the connective tissues. Neutrophils continue to dominate the junctional epithelium and gingival crevice with a marked increase in crevicular fluid flow. It is noteworthy that collagen loss in the involved tissues is evident in the earliest stages of gingivitis. Page and Schroeder report a predominance of plasma cells in the established lesion. Several studies of human experimental gingivitis have failed to demonstrate plasma cell dominance[15,16,146]; however, increases in the proportions of plasma cells are evident with long-standing gingivitis.[15]

The development of experimental gingivitis occurs in parallel with a tremendous increase in the number of bacteria present in plaque. A distinct shift in the bacterial composition of the plaque also occurs, with increasing proportions of gram-negative anaerobes.[159] Studies on the microbiology of naturally occurring gingivitis indicate relatively equal proportions of gram-positive facultative and gram-negative anaerobic bacteria,[151] with evidence of a greater shift as compared with experimental gingivitis. The host response to plaque bacteria is fundamentally an inflammatory response involving the processes described previously. Although gingivitis is not associated with loss of connective tissue attachment, it is evident histologically that some loss of collagen occurs within the connective tissues.

Specialized forms of gingivitis include those associated with hormonal changes, with medications, and with systemic disease.[108] In these instances, evidence exists of an altered host environment that appears to contribute to an increase in host susceptibility to gingivitis. For example, the inflammatory response to plaque during pregnancy appears to be exaggerated, with an increased prevalence and severity of gingivitis beyond that expected for the level of plaque accumulation.[107] Alterations in the subgingival microbiota and the host immune response to bacterial antigens during pregnancy have been reported.[85,103] For example, increases in hormone levels appear to correlate with increases in the subgingival proportions of *P. intermedia,* a microorganism that can substitute progesterone or estradiol for vitamin K as an essential bacterial growth factor.[85] These alterations, as well as the increased clinical susceptibilty to gingivitis, resolve postpartum.

Chronic Periodontitis

Gingivitis and periodontitis share the clinical feature of inflammation. In contrast, periodontitis involves clinically detectable levels of host tissue destruction that are not found in gingivitis. These include clinical attachment loss, periodontal pocketing, and alveolar bone loss. In the common form of periodontitis, chronic periodontitis, the amount of tissue destruction is consistent with the local etiologic factors of plaque and calculus[44] and associated with a variable microbial pattern. The clinical course of disease follows a slow to moderate rate of progression, but periods of rapid progression may occur.[52]

Bacterial Etiology in Chronic Periodontitis. Despite a remarkable diversity of bacteria found in the periodontal microbiota, only a few species have been associated with periodontitis (see Chapter 6). These include *P. gingivalis, B. forsythus, P. intermedia, C. rectus, E. corrodens, F. nucleatum, A. actinomycetemcomitans, P. micros,* and *T. denticola.*[89,91,100,106,117,151,153,154,162] Studies of the microbiologic **responses to periodontal therapy** support a role for these species in the disease process. Decreases in the prevalence and numbers of *P. gingivalis, B. forsythus,* and *T. denticola* are associated with successful clinical treatment of disease.[23,57,101] When diseased sites with recent attachment loss are compared with inactive sites, increases in the recovery of *P. gingivalis, F. nucleatum, P. intermedia, B. forsythus, E. corrodens, A. actinomycetemcomitans,* and *C. rectus* is evident in the active sites.[32,33,36] In addition, when treatment results are compared with microorganisms detected before treatment, poorly responding sites demonstrate higher levels of *F. nucleatum* and *P. micros.*[55]

Alterations in the **host response** associated with specific periodontal pathogens are clearly evident. Increases in serum and crevicular fluid antibody specific to putative pathogens,[35,36,81,125] including *P. gingivalis, A. actinomycetemcomitans, P. intermedia, E. corrodens, F. nucleatum,* and *C. rectus,* are evident in patients with periodontitis. Therapy itself is associated with initial increases in serum antibody levels, which return to pretreatment levels by 8 to 12 months posttreatment.[9,34]

Studies in **animal models** have been used to demonstrate the pathologic potential of periodontal microorganisms in vivo. A commonly used animal model involves abscess formation in mice, and *P. gingivalis, C. rectus, P. micros, P. intermedia, P. nigrescens, A. actinomycetemcomitans, F. nucleatum,* and *T. denticola* are pathogenic in this system.[38,77,78,121,167] Differences in the virulence of distinct strains of the same species also are evident in the abscess model.[121] Furthermore, *P. gingivalis, C. rectus,* and *A. actinomycetemcomitans* demonstrate increased virulence in mice that are depleted of neutrophils, indicating an important role for neutrophils in responding to the bacterial challenge.[38]

Synergistic interactions between microbial pathogens appear to be important in bacterial virulence. In the mouse model, simultaneous infection with *P. gingivalis* and *F. nucleatum* enhanced virulence as compared with infection with *P. gingivalis* alone.[41] In a rabbit abscess model, *B. forsythus* in combination with either *P. gingivalis* or *F. nucleatum* produces abscesses, whereas none of the microorganisms alone causes abscess formation.[160] Evidence of synergy in virulence, exemplified by these data, is an important consideration in infections that are polymicrobial.

Another area that has been addressed using animal model systems is the generation of immunity to infection. Inoculation with a specific microorganism or specific bacterial component that results in protective immunity suggests that the microorganism or molecule may be important in the disease process. Studies in which *P. gingivalis* outer membrane or fimbriae were used as immunogens have demonstrated a protective effect in a rodent model.[12,40] Using a nonhuman primate model of periodontal disease, immunization with whole cells of *P. gingivalis* or the cysteine protease of *P. gingivalis* has resulted in decreased periodontal destruction.[118,134] Although these investigations are useful in assessing microbial interactions in the disease process, much more investigation is needed for consideration of vaccine therapy in humans, particularly with regard to the polymicrobial nature of periodontitis.

Immunologic Considerations in Chronic Periodontitis. Considerable information is available regarding components of the host immune response that are not specific to a given microbial pathogen but occur in response to the infection and are likely to contribute to pathogenesis. Chronic periodontitis is characterized primarily as involving alternative pathway activation of complement, with C3 and B cleavage in gingival fluids observed. This suggests that even though pathogen-specific antibodies are formed in chronic periodontitis, activation of the classical complement pathway by processes involving antibody-antigen binding does not predominate. It also is possible that specific cleavage products in crevicular fluid result from the action of bacterial enzymes. *P. gingivalis,* for example, produces an enzyme that can cleave C5 to its active metabolite, C5a.[178]

Collagenase activity is associated with active periodontal destruction.[96] MMP-8 is elevated in chronic periodontitis, whereas the levels of TIMP (TIMP-1) are not.[68] The ability of the chymotrypsin-like enzyme of *T. denticola* to activate MMPs may contribute to MMP-mediated tissue destruction at periodontitis sites with high levels of this microorganism.[155] In addition, studies of GCF in chronic periodontitis reveal that collagenase activity is as much as sixfold greater than that of gingivitis. Most of the collagenase activity associated with chronic periodontitis is due to the neutrophil collagenase MMP-8.[138] Some microorganisms may modulate neutrophil secretion of collagenase. For example, the phagocytosis of *F. nucleatum* and *T. denticola* are associated with the release of high levels of elastase and MMP-8 from neutrophils.[29,30]

Clear evidence of variations exists among individuals in their susceptibility to periodontitis. Despite considerable accumulation of bacterial plaque including the presence of putative pathogens, some individuals appear to be resistant to the disease process whereas others develop disease. These differences relate primarily to variability in the host immunoinflammatory response to the infectious challenge, but the underlying basis for varying susceptibility may be **genetic** or **environmental** in nature.

Systemic factors that modify susceptibility to periodontitis include conditions such as diabetes or HIV infection and environmental influences such as smoking and stress.[80] Epidemiologic studies indicate that the prevalence and severity of periodontitis are increased in diabetics, and poorly controlled diabetics appear to be particularly susceptible.[141] Periodontitis has been recently recognized as one of six primary complications of diabetes.[99] HIV infection is associated with alterations in the CD4+ T-cells and monocytes/macrophages. HIV patients may exhibit acute necrotizing periodontal conditions, particularly when CD4+ T-cell levels are very low.[80,126] Smoking is strongly associated with periodontitis in epidemiologic studies. Smoking affects the vasculature, immune system, and inflammatory processes and is an important risk factor for development of periodontitis.[80] Stress is associated with necrotizing ulcerative gingivitis (NUG) and an increased prevalence of periodontitis. The effects of stress may be mediated by alterations in the immune response and inflammatory processes.[80] Diminished wound healing is associated with stress, and thus diminished reparative processes may play a role in periodontal pathogenesis.[79,109] Although the specific mechanisms behind the association of these conditions with periodontitis are not clear (see discussions in Chapter 13), a central role of alterations in the host inflammatory processes appears to be a consistent theme.

A **genetic** basis for variations in periodontal disease susceptibility is indicated by recent studies demonstrating an association between a composite genotype involving the IL-1 genes and the occurrence of chronic periodontitis. The composite genotype consists of a variant of the IL-1β gene with a single base pair alteration in the DNA sequence at the +3953 position, in combination with similar alterations at the −889 and the +4845 positions of the IL-1α gene.[39,87] Studies indicate that individuals, primarily those of Caucasian European decent, carrying the composite genotype are at significantly increased odds (odds ratio of approximately 5 to 7) of having moderate to severe periodontitis.[87,111] The occurrence of these alleles in the IL-1 genes are considerably lower in individuals of Chinese and African-American heritage.[5,172] Thus these genetic polymorphisms may not contribute to variations in susceptibility and may be less useful as markers in these populations. The IL-1β allele (+3953) of the composite genotype is known to be associated with a twofold to fourfold increase in IL-1β production. Individuals negative for the composite genotype undergoing periodontal treatment demonstrate decreases in GCF levels of IL-1β, whereas those with the composite genotype do not demonstrate this response to treatment.[39] These data provide some information as to the molecular basis for variations in host susceptibility, and it is likely that additional genetic loci will be identified that also influence these processes.

Refractory Periodontitis. The majority of patients with chronic periodontitis are successfully managed with conventional treatment regimes. However, a small proportion of patients do not respond to treatment and demonstrate continued clinical periodontal destruction. These individuals are referred to as **refractory periodontitis** patients. Prominent periodontal pathogens such as *P. gingivalis, B. forsythus, F. nucleatum, P. micros, E. corrodens,* and *S. intermedius* have been found to be elevated in patients who do not respond to treatment.[55,56] Often, patients identified as refractory to treatment have other factors, particularly smoking, that may contribute to the disease process.[72,73] The impact of smoking on the response to treatment may relate to alterations in neutrophil chemotaxis and phagocytosis, as well as altered levels of cytokines (e.g., IL-1, IL-6) at the local sites.[61,76,95,105]

Aggressive Periodontitis

A primary characteristic of aggressive periodontitis that differentiates it from chronic periodontitis is the rapid progression of attachment and bone loss evident.[166] Other consistent features of patients with aggressive periodontitis are that they are otherwise healthy and that the disease demonstrates a familial pattern of occurrence. A number of features are generally, but not universally, associated with aggressive periodontitis. These include inconsistencies between the amount of microbial deposits and the severity of periodontal destruction; the presence of elevated levels of *A. actinomycetemcomitans;* and evidence of phagocyte abnormalities and hyperresponsive monocytes/macrophages, leading to elevations in PGE_2 and IL-1β. Furthermore, the disease process is self-limiting in some cases of aggressive periodontitis.

Aggressive periodontitis may be localized or generalized. The classic form of localized aggressive periodontitis was initially referred to as "periodontosis"[122] and then as *localized juvenile periodontitis (LJP).* Classic LJP was defined by several distinguishing characteristics: onset around the time of puberty, aggressive periodontal destruction localized almost exclusively to the incisors and first molars, and a familial pattern of occurrence. The incidence of LJP is low, ranging between 0.1% to 2.3% of juveniles and adolescents.[43] However, studies of this distinctive disease process have provided a window into the processes underlying periodontal pathogenesis. **Localized aggressive periodontitis (LAP)** is the new classification designated to replace LJP. Thus in the following discussions, LAP will be used synonymously with LJP. **Generalized aggressive periodontitis** is differentiated from the localized form by the extent of involvement of the permanent teeth, and it is considered to include some of the individuals previously categorized as having rapidly progressive periodontitis.[4]

Bacterial Etiology of Localized Aggressive Periodontitis. Early microbiologic studies of LAP provided clear evidence of a strong association between disease and a unique bacterial microbiota predominated by a microorganism later identified as *A. actinomycetemcomitans.*[122–124] Other microorganisms that have been associated with LAP include *P. gingivalis, E. corrodens, C. rectus, F. nucleatum, B. capillus,* and *Capnocytophaga* spp. and spirochetes.[86,116,122,123] However, subsequent research has continued to provide support for a primary etiologic role of *A. actinomycetemcomitans* in LAP. These findings are summarized as follows:

1. The prevalence of a humoral immune response to this organism is elevated in patients with LAP. *A. actinomycetemcomitans* has been isolated in up to 97% of LAP patients, compared with 21% of adult periodontitis patients and 17% of healthy subjects.[182] Not only is the prevalence of *A. actinomycetemcomitans* six times greater in LAP than in healthy patients, but its proportion of the cultivable subgingival flora also is elevated. Among the three serotypes, serotype B is the most common, followed by serotype A.
2. The incidence of *A. actinomycetemcomitans* is greater in younger LAP patients than in older LAP patients.[6] If age is considered relative to the duration of the disease, younger patients have more destructive disease developing within a shorter period. This suggests that the presence of this organism correlates with disease activity.
3. A large number of *A. actinomycetemcomitans* organisms occur in lesions in LAP patients, but such organisms are absent or occur in low numbers in healthy sites.[43]
4. *A. actinomycetemcomitans* can be identified by electron microscopy, immunofluorescence, and culture from LAP lesions within the gingival connective tissues.[183]
5. *A. actinomycetemcomitans* is quite virulent, producing a leukotoxin, collagenase, phosphatases, and bone-resorbing factors, as well as other factors important in invasion of host tissue cells, evasion of host defenses, immunosuppression, and destruction of periodontal tissues.[43,70]
6. A positive correlation exists between the elimination of this organism from the subgingival flora and successful clinical treatment of LAP.[21,152]

A primary focus of studies on the virulence properties of *A. actinomycetemcomitans* has been on the leukotoxin produced by this bacterium. The ability of this molecule to bind to and lyse phagocytes is considered to be an important mechanism of host defense.[70,92] Early studies revealed that the levels of leukotoxin produced by different strains varied considerably. More recent investigations have linked the strains producing high levels of leukotoxin with a deletion in the promoter region of the leukotoxin gene[17] and further linked the onset of LAP in a high-risk population with the presence of these high leukotoxin-producing strains.[18] The molecular basis of leukotoxin expression is discussed further in Chapter 9. Another potentially important virulence determinant is the production of an immunosuppressive factor[147] capable of inhibiting lymphocyte functions.

The familial occurrence of LAP raises the question as to whether transmission of specific strains of *A. actinomycetemcomitans* between family members could contribute to the disease process. Recognition of variations in virulence between different strains further suggests that this could be important. Genetic analyses of *A. actinomycetemcomitans* strains isolated from family members suggest that transmission of a strain between spouses or from parent to child occurred in approximately one third of the families investigated.[7]

Therapeutic approaches to infections involving *A. actinomycetemcomitans* must take into account the host parasite interaction. Mechanical methods alone do not predictably control this microorganism. The ability of *A. actinomycetemcomitans* to invade and reside within the gingival tissues appears to provide a reservoir by which the bacterium can rapidly repopulate the pocket, and sites that continue to deteriorate after treatment harbor substantial levels of the microorganism. Clinical studies suggest that surgery and antibiotic therapy may be required to control *A. actinomycetemcomitans*.[21,86,152]

Immunologic Considerations in Localized Aggressive Periodontitis. Numerous mechanisms of serum-mediated bacterial killing are available, including lysis by the membrane attack complex of complement and antimicrobial substances such as lysozyme. However, some bacteria, including all known strains of *A. actinomycetemcomitans* as well as some strains of most putative periodontal pathogens, are resistant to serum-mediated killing mechanisms.[10] For serum-resistant bacteria, the neutrophil is the primary host response mechanism of bacterial control. Studies of LAP have revealed a number of aspects of neutrophil function that may result in a compromised bacterial killing and have been key in demonstrating the importance of neutrophil function in periodontal health and disease.

Approximately 75% of patients with LAP have dysfunctional neutrophils, involving a decreased expression of G-protein coupled receptors. The defect is evident as a decrease in the chemotactic response to several chemotactic agents, including the complement component C5a, N-formyl-methionyl leucyl phenylalanine (FMLP), and leukotriene B4.[128] The defect is associated with a 40% deficiency in a 110-kilodalton membrane glycoprotein, GP110, on the neutrophil surface.[169] The function of GP110 is unknown, but diminished GP110 expression is associated with diminished surface expression of all G-protein coupled receptors. For this reason, this neutrophil defect has been called a *global membrane receptor defect.* The precise dysfunction caused by the G-protein coupled receptor deficiency responsible for disease has not been identified. However, neutrophil transendothelial migration, transepithelial migration, chemotaxis, secretion, and priming can be effected. The molecular basis for the receptor defect is postulated to be inherited as an intrinsic cellular defect or a modulation of neutrophil receptor expression by elevated levels of proinflammatory cytokines including IL-1 and TNF-α.[1,168] LAP patients (25%) that do not have the G-protein coupled receptor deficiency present have the same clinical picture as those with this neutrophil defect. This suggests that the G-protein coupled receptor deficiency is sufficient but not essential for LAP, and other alterations of the host bacterial interaction may yield a similar clinical outcome.

In LAP the predominant collagenase found in tissues and crevicular fluid is MMP-1, and elevated levels of TIMP-1 are present.[68] This contrasts the situation found in chronic periodontitis, in which the collagenous activity is due to MMP-8 from neutrophils. The differences in MMPs may relate to altered neutrophil functions and further underscore the evidence that varying mechanisms of tissue destruction occur in these different forms of periodontal destruction.

Patients with LAP demonstrate elevated antibodies to *A. actinomycetemcomitans*,[37] and antibody as well as complement is essential for opsonization and efficient phagocytosis.[10] In LAP the dominant serum antibody isotype IgG2 is specific for surface antigens of *A. actinomycetemcomitans*, including LPS and at least one major outer membrane protein.[176,177] Some individuals possess a variant of the Fc receptor on neutrophils (R131 allele of FcγRII-α) that does not efficiently bind IgG2, and this is one possible basis for disease susceptibility.[175] It has been hypothesized that because this binding is less efficient, an antibody response more vigorous than normal is necessary to control the *A. actinomycetemcomitans* infection in LAP and that the progression in LAP is limited by the development of a strong antibody response. In comparison, individuals with generalized early onset periodontitis do not develop a strong antibody response,[54,164] which supports the hypothesis that antibodies function to limit the disease process.

Summary of Localized Aggressive Periodontitis. The evidence indicates that LAP is a form of periodontitis that is clearly distinct from chronic periodontitis. The pathogenesis of LAP is characterized by a highly specific infection involving predominantly *A. actinomycetemcomitans*. This bacterium is capable of tissue destruction and inhibition of host defenses through the production of a leukotoxin and an immunosuppressive factor. The host response is characterized by the high prevalence of neutrophil chemotaxis defects in affected individuals as well as a selective antibody response dominated by high titers of IgG2. This antibody response may necessitate particularly high levels of antibody for efficient opsonization and phagocytosis of *A. actinomycetemcomitans*.

Generalized Aggressive Periodontitis. The recent reclassifications limit the information available pertinent to this group of patients. Some but not all of the individuals previously classified as having rapidly progressive periodontitis (RPP) would likely be considered to have generalized aggressive periodontitis. Studies of RPP indicate a diverse microbial pattern that includes microorganisms associated with chronic periodontitis and a host response often characterized by defects in either neutrophils or monocytes.[131]

Necrotizing Periodontal Diseases

Two forms of necrotizing ulcerative periodontal diseases are **necrotizing ulcerative gingivitis (NUG)** and **necrotizing ulcerative periodontitis (NUP).** These conditions represent acute forms of periodontal destruction typically associated with some form of host compromise.

The essential components of NUG are interdental gingival necrosis, pain, and bleeding; variable features include lymphadenopathy, fever, and malaise.[139] The tissue necrosis results in an appearance often described as "punched-out" papillae. Microbiologic studies indicate that predominant species associated with NUG include *P. intermedia, Fusobacterium* spp., and spirochetal microorganisms. Electron microscopic studies of NUG reveal a zone of tissue infiltration of spirochetal microorganisms in advance of the region of tissue necrosis.[97] NUG is normally associated with predisposing host factors including stress, immunosuppression, and malnutrition.[139]

NUP is distinguished from NUG by the loss of clinical attachment and bone in affected sites, but the clinical presentation and etiologic factors are similar to that of NUG in the absence of systemic disease.[126] In the presence of systemic immunosuppression, exemplified by HIV infection, NUP may result in rapid and extensive necrosis to the tissues and underlying alveolar bone.[179]

Periodontal Abscesses

Periodontal abscesses are purulent infections localized to the gingival, periodontal, or pericoronal regions. In the presence of periodontitis, a periodontal abscess represents an acute infectious process with active tissue and bone destruction. Microorganisms that are prevalent in periodontal abscesses are *P. intermedia, F. nucleatum,* and *P. gingivalis*; but other periodontal pathogens also are found, including *B. forsythus, P. micros, Prevotella melaninogenica,* and *C. rectus*.[62,124] Histologic studies indicate the presence of neutrophils and macrophages surrounding an internal region of dead leukocytes and tissue debris. In the absence of periodontitis, abscesses are typically associated with impaction of foreign objects such as dental floss or a popcorn kernel.[63,113]

SUMMARY

The pathogenesis of periodontal destruction involves a complex interplay between bacterial pathogens and the host tissues. For some time it has been recognized that "not all dental plaque is equal" and that specific bacterial pathogens appear to be responsible for the changes resulting in disease. It also has been recognized for some time that in the process of effectively limiting the bacterial assault of the periodontal tissues, host defense mechanisms contribute to the destruction of tissues locally.

Recent investigations have revealed that not all strains of a specific microbial species are equal in their capacity to cause disease, and not all hosts are equal in their susceptibility to disease. The challenge for the future is to be able to better identify the more virulent bacterial strains and the more susceptible hosts. In this manner it may be possible to accurately predict the individuals at risk for future disease and to develop more effective strategies to prevent the onset and progression of periodontitis.

REFERENCES

1. Agarwal S, Suzuki JB, Riccelli AE: Role of cytokines in the modulation of neutrophil chemotaxis in localized juvenile periodontitis. J Periodontal Res 1994; 29:127.
2. Arakawa S, Nakajima T, Ishikura H, et al: Novel apoptosis-inducing activity in *Bacteroides forsythus*: a comparative study with three serotypes of *Actinobacillus actinomycetemcomitans*. Infect Immun 2000; 68:4611.
3. Armitage GC, Jeffcoat MK, Chadwick DE, et al: Longitudinal evaluation of elastase as a marker for the progression of periodontitis. J Periodontol 1994; 65:120.
4. Armitage GC: Development of a classification system for periodontal diseases and conditions. Ann Periodontol 1999; 4:1.
5. Armitage GC, Wu Y, Wang HY, et al: Low prevalence of a periodontitis-associated interleukin-1 composite genotype in individuals of Chinese heritage. J Periodontol 2000; 71:164.
6. Asikainen S: Occurrence of *Actinobacillus actinomycetemcomitans* and spirochetes in relation to age in localized juvenile periodontitis. J Periodontol 1986; 57:537.
7. Asikainen S, Chen C, Slots J: Likelihood of transmitting *Actinobacillus actinomycetemcomitans* and *Porphyromonas gingivalis* in families with periodontitis. Oral Microbiol Immunol 1996; 11:387.
8. Assuma R, Oates T, Cochran D, et al: IL-1 and TNF antagonists inhibit the inflammatory response and bone loss in experimental periodontitis. J Immunol 1998; 160:403.
9. Aukhil I, Lopatin DE, Syed SA, et al: The effects of periodontal therapy on serum antibody (IgG) levels to plaque microorganisms. J Clin Periodontol 1988; 15:544.
10. Baker PJ, Wilson ME: Opsonic IgG antibody against *Actinobacillus actinomycetemcomitans* in localized juvenile periodontitis. Oral Microbiol Immunol 1989; 4:98.
11. Barbosa MD, Nguyen QA, Tchernev VT, et al: Identification of the homologous beige and Chediak-Higashi syndrome genes. Nature 1996; 382:262.
12. Bird PS, Gemmell E, Polak B, et al: Protective immunity to *Porphyromonas gingivalis* infection in a murine model. J Periodontol 1995; 66:351.
13. Birkedal-Hansen H: Role of matrix metalloproteinases in human periodontal diseases. J Periodontol 1993; 64:474.
14. Booth V, Ashley FP, Lehner T: Passive immunization with monoclonal antibodies against *Porphyromonas gingivalis* in patients with periodontitis. Infect Immun 1996; 64:422.
15. Brecx MC, Frohlicher I, Gehr P, et al: Stereological observations on long-term experimental gingivitis in man. J Clin Periodontol 1988; 15:621.
16. Brecx MC, Lehmann B, Siegwart CM, et al: Observations on the initial stages of healing following human experimental gingivitis. A clinical and morphometric study. J Clin Periodontol 1988; 15:123.
17. Brogan JM, Lally ET, Poulsen K, et al: Regulation of *Actinobacillus actinomycetemcomitans* leukotoxin expression: analysis of the promoter regions of leukotoxic and minimally leukotoxic strains. Infect Immun 1994; 62:501.

18. Bueno LC, Mayer MP, DiRienzo JM: Relationship between conversion of localized juvenile periodontitis-susceptible children from health to disease and *Actinobacillus actinomycetemcomitans* leukotoxin promoter structure. J Periodontol 1998; 69:998.
19. Carranza FA, Jr, Saglie R, Newman MG, et al: Scanning and transmission electron microscopic study of tissue-invading microorganisms in localized juvenile periodontitis. J Periodontol 1983; 54:598.
20. Chen HA, Johnson BD, Sims TJ, et al: Humoral immune responses to *Porphyromonas gingivalis* before and following therapy in rapidly progressive periodontitis patients. J Periodontol 1991; 62:781.
21. Christersson LA, Slots J, Rosling BG, et al: Microbiological and clinical effects of surgical treatment of localized juvenile periodontitis. J Clin Periodontol 1985; 12:465.
22. Christersson LA, Albini B, Zambon JJ, et al: Tissue localization of *Actinobacillus actinomycetemcomitans* in human periodontitis. I. Light, immunofluorescence and electron microscopic studies. J Periodontol 1987; 58:529.
23. Cugini MA, Haffajee AD, Smith C, et al: The effect of scaling and root planing on the clinical and microbiological parameters of periodontal diseases: 12-month results. J Clin Periodontol 2000; 27:30.
24. Curtis MA, Kuramitsu HK, Lantz M, et al: Molecular genetics and nomenclature of proteases of *Porphyromonas gingivalis*. J Periodontal Res 1999; 34:464.
25. Cutler CW, Kalmar JR, Arnold RR: Phagocytosis of virulent *Porphyromonas gingivalis* by human polymorphonuclear leukocytes requires specific immunoglobulin G. Infect Immun 1991; 59:2097.
26. Darveau RP, Belton CM, Reife RA, et al: Local chemokine paralysis, a novel pathogenic mechanism for *Porphyromonas gingivalis*. Infect Immun 1998; 66:1660.
27. Delcourt-Debruyne EM, Boutigny HR, Hildebrand HF: Features of severe periodontal disease in a teenager with Chediak-Higashi syndrome. J Periodontol 2000; 71:816.
28. Dickinson DP, Kubiniec MA, Yoshimura F, et al: Molecular cloning and sequencing of the gene encoding the fimbrial subunit protein of *Bacteroides gingivalis*. J Bacteriol 1988; 170:1658.
29. Ding Y, Uitto VJ, Haapasalo M, et al: Membrane components of *Treponema denticola* trigger proteinase release from human polymorphonuclear leukocytes. J Dent Res 1996; 75:1986.
30. Ding Y, Haapasalo M, Kerosuo E, et al: Release and activation of human neutrophil matrix metallo- and serine proteinases during phagocytosis of *Fusobacterium nucleatum, Porphyromonas gingivalis,* and *Treponema denticola*. J. Clin. Periodontol 1997; 24:237.
31. Dongari-Bagtzoglou AI, Ebersole JL: Production of inflammatory mediators and cytokines by human gingival fibroblasts following bacterial challenge. J Periodontal Res 1996; 31:90.
32. Dzink JL, Tanner AC, Haffajee AD, et al: Gram negative species associated with active destructive periodontal lesions. J Clin Periodontol 1985; 12:648.
33. Dzink JL, Socransky SS, Haffajee AD: The predominant cultivable microbiota of active and inactive lesions of destructive periodontal diseases. J Clin Periodontol 1988; 15:316.
34. Ebersole JL, Taubman MA, Smith DJ, et al: Effect of subgingival scaling on systemic antibody responses to oral microorganisms. Infect Immun 1985; 48:534.
35. Ebersole JL, Taubman MA, Smith DJ, et al: Human immune responses to oral microorganisms: Patterns of systemic antibody levels to *Bacteroides* species. 1986; 51:507.
36. Ebersole JL, Taubman MA, Smith DJ, et al: Human serum antibody responses to oral microorganisms. IV. Correlation with homologous infection. Oral Microbiol Immunol 1987; 2:53.
37. Ebersole JL: The protective nature of host responses in periodontal diseases. 1994; 5:112.
38. Ebersole JL, Kesavalu L, Schneider SL, et al: Comparative virulence of periodontopathogens in a mouse abscess model. Oral Dis 1995; 1:115.
39. Engebretson SP, Lamster IB, Herrera-Abreu M, et al: The influence of interleukin gene polymorphism on expression of interleukin-1β and tumor necrosis factor-α in periodontal tissue and gingival crevicular fluid. J Periodontol 1999; 70:567.
40. Evans RT, Klausen B, Sojar HT, et al: Immunization with *Porphyromonas (Bacteroides) gingivalis* fimbriae protects against periodontal destruction. Infect Immun 1992; 60:2926.
41. Feuille F, Ebersole JL, Kesavalu L, et al: Mixed infection with *Porphyromonas gingivalis* and *Fusobacterium nucleatum* in a murine lesion model: Potential synergistic effects on virulence. 1996; 64:2095.
42. Fillery ED, Pekovic DD: Identification of microorganisms in immunopathological mechanisms on human gingivitis. J Dent Res 1982; 61:253.
43. Fives-Taylor PM, Meyer DH, Mintz KP, et al: Virulence factors of *Actinobacillus actinomycetemcomitans*. Periodontol 2000; 20:136.
44. Flemmig TF: Periodontitis. Ann Periodontol 1999; 4:32.
45. Frank RM: Bacterial penetration in the apical wall of advanced human periodontitis. J Periodontal Res 1980; 15:563.
46. Gao J, Jordan TW, Cutress TW: Immunolocalization of basic fibroblast growth factor (bFGF) in human periodontal ligament (PDL) tissue. J Periodontal Res 1996; 31:260.
47. Garrison SW, Holt SC, Nichols FC: Lipopolysaccharide-stimulated PGE_2 release from human monocytes. Comparison of lipopolysaccharides prepared from suspected periodontal pathogens. J Periodontol 1988; 59:684.
48. Garrison SW, Nichols FC: LPS-elicited secretory responses in monocytes: altered release of PGE_2 but not IL-1β in patients with adult periodontitis. J Periodontal Res 1989; 24:88.
49. Genco RJ, Wilson ME, De Nardin E: Periodontal complications and neutrophil abnormalities. In: Genco RJ, Goldman HM, Cohen DW (eds): Contemporary Periodontics. St Louis, 1990, Mosby.
50. Genco RJ: Host responses in periodontal diseases: current concepts. J Periodontol 1992; 63:338.
51. Giannobile WV, Hernandez RA, Finkelman RD, et al: Comparative effects of platelet-derived growth factor-BB and insulin-like growth factor-I, individually and in combination, on periodontal regeneration in *Macaca fascicularis*. J Periodontal Res 1996; 31:301.
52. Goodson JM, Tanner AC, Haffajee AD, et al: Patterns of progression and regression of advanced destructive periodontal disease. J Clin Periodontol 1982; 9:472.
53. Graves DT: The potential role of chemokines and inflammatory cytokines in periodontal disease progression. Clin Infect Dis 1999; 28:482.
54. Gunsolley JC, Burmeister JA, Tew JG, et al: Relationship of serum antibody to attachment level patterns in young adults with juvenile periodontitis or generalized severe periodontitis. J Periodontol 1987; 58:314.
55. Haffajee AD, Socransky SS, Ebersole JL: Survival analysis of periodontal sites before and after periodontal therapy. J Clin Periodontol 1985; 12:553.
56. Haffajee AD, Socransky SS, Dzink JL, et al: Clinical, microbiological and immunological features of subjects with refractory periodontal diseases. J Clin Periodontol 1988; 15:390.
57. Haffajee AD, Cugini MA, Dibart S, et al: Clinical and microbiological features of subjects with adult periodontitis

who responded poorly to scaling and root planing. J Clin Periodontol 1997; 24:767.

58. Han YW, Shi W, Huang GT, et al: Interactions between periodontal bacteria and human oral epithelial cells: *Fusobacterium nucleatum* adheres to and invades epithelial cells. Infect Immun 2000; 68:3140.
59. Hart TC, Stabholz A, Meyle J, et al: Genetic studies of syndromes with severe periodontitis and palmoplantar hyperkeratosis. J Periodontal Res 1997; 32:81.
60. Hart TC, Hart PS, Bowden DW, et al: Mutations of the cathepsin C gene are responsible for Papillon-Lefèvre syndrome. J Med Genet 1999; 36:881.
61. Hernichel-Gorbach E, Kornman KS, Holt SC, et al: Host responses in patients with generalized refractory periodontitis. J Periodontol 1994; 65:8.
62. Herrera D, Roldan S, Gonzalez I, et al: The periodontal abscess (I). Clinical and microbiological findings. J Clin Periodontol 2000; 27:387.
63. Herrera D, Roldan S, Sanz M: The periodontal abscess: a review. J Clin Periodontol 2000; 27:377.
64. Howell TH, Fiorellini JP, Paquette DW, et al: A phase I/II clinical trial to evaluate a combination of recombinant human platelet-derived growth factor-BB and recombinant human insulin-like growth factor-I in patients with periodontal disease. J Periodontol 1997; 68:1186.
65. Huang GT-J, Kinder Haake S, Kim J-W, et al: Differential expression of interleukin-8 and intercellular adhesion molecule-1 by human gingival epithelial cells in response to *Actinobacillus actinomycetemcomitans* or *Porphyromonas gingivalis* infection. Oral Microbiol Immunol 1998; 13:301.
66. Huang GT-J, Kinder Haake S, Park N-H: Gingival epithelial cells increase interleukin-8 secretion in response to *Actinobacillus actinomycetemcomitans* challenge. J Periodontol 1998; 69:1105.
67. Ingman T, Sorsa T, Kangaspunta P, et al: Elastase and α1–proteinase inhibitor in gingival crevicular fluid and gingival tissue in adult and juvenile periodontitis. J Periodontol 1994; 65:702.
68. Ingman T, Tervahartiala T, Ding Y, et al: Matrix metalloproteinases and their inhibitors in gingival crevicular fluid and saliva of periodontitis patients. J Clin Periodontol 1996; 23:1127.
69. Jewett A, Hume WR, Le H, et al: Induction of apoptotic cell death in peripheral blood mononuclear and polymorphonuclear cells by an oral bacterium, *Fusobacterium nucleatum*. Infect Immun 2000; 68:1893.
70. Johansson A, Sandstrom G, Claesson R, et al: Anaerobic neutrophil-dependent killing of *Actinobacillus actinomycetemcomitans* in relation to the bacterial leukotoxicity. Eur J Oral Sci 2000; 108:136.
71. Kabashima H, Nagata K, Hashiguchi I, et al: Interleukin-1 receptor antagonist and interleukin-4 in gingival crevicular fluid of patients with inflammatory periodontal disease. J Oral Pathol Med 1996; 25:449.
72. Kaldahl WB, Johnson GK, Patil KD, et al: Levels of cigarette consumption and response to periodontal therapy. J Periodontol 1996; 67:675.
73. Kaldahl WB, Kalkwarf KL, Patil KD, et al: Long-term evaluation of periodontal therapy: II. Incidence of sites breaking down. J Periodontol 1996; 67:103.
74. Kelly CG, Booth V, Kendal H, et al: The relationship between colonization and haemagglutination inhibiting and B cell epitopes of *Porphyromonas gingivalis*. Clin Exp Immunol 1997; 110:285.
75. Kenney EB, Ash MM, Jr: Oxidation reduction potential of developing plaque, periodontal pockets and gingival sulci. J Periodontol 1969; 40:630.
76. Kenney EB, Kraal JH, Saxe SR, et al: The effect of cigarette smoke on human oral polymorphonuclear leukocytes. J Periodontal Res 1977; 12:227.
77. Kesavalu L, Holt SC, Crawley RR, et al: Virulence of *Wolinella recta* in a murine abscess model. Infect Immun 1991; 59:2806.
78. Kesavalu L, Ebersole JL, Machen RL, et al: *Porphyromonas gingivalis* virulence in mice: Induction of immunity to bacterial components. Infect Immun 1992; 60:1455.
79. Kiecolt-Glaser JK, Marucha PT, Malarkey WB, et al: Slowing of wound healing by psychological stress. Lancet 1995; 346:1194.
80. Kinane DF: Periodontitis modified by systemic factors. Ann Periodontol 1999; 4:54.
81. Kinane DF, Mooney J, Ebersole JL: Humoral immune response to *Actinobacillus actinomycetemcomitans* and *Porphyromonas gingivalis* in periodontal disease. Periodontol 2000 1999; 20:289.
82. Kinder SA, Holt SC: Characterization of coaggregation between *Bacteroides gingivalis* T22 and *Fusobacterium nucleatum* T18. Infect Immun 1989; 57:3425.
83. Kinder SA, Holt SC: Carbohydrate receptor on *Porphyromonas gingivalis* T22 mediating coaggregation with *Fusobacterium nucleatum* T18. J Dent Res 1991; 70:275.
84. Kolenbrander PE, Andersen RN: Inhibition of coaggregation between *Fusobacterium nucleatum* and *Porphyromonas (Bacteroides) gingivalis* by lactose and related sugars. Infect Immun 1989; 57:3204.
85. Kornman KS, Loesche WJ: Effects of estradiol and progesterone on *Bacteroides melaninogenicus* and *Bacteroides gingivalis*. Infect Immun 1982; 35:256.
86. Kornman KS, Robertson PB: Clinical and microbiological evaluation of therapy for juvenile periodontitis. J Periodontol 1985; 56:443.
87. Kornman KS, Crane A, Wang HY, et al: The interleukin-1 genotype as a severity factor in adult periodontal disease. J Clin Periodontol 1997; 24:72.
88. Kornman KS: Host modulation as a therapeutic strategy in the treatment of periodontal disease. Clin Infect Dis 1999; 28:520.
89. Kremer BH, Loos BG, van der Velden U, et al: *Peptostreptococcus micros* smooth and rough genotypes in periodontitis and gingivitis. J Periodontol 2000; 71:209.
90. Kuramitsu HK: Proteases of *Porphyromonas gingivalis*: what don't they do? Oral Microbiol Immunol 1998; 13:263.
91. Lai CH, Listgarten MA, Shirakawa M, et al: *Bacteroides forsythus* in adult gingivitis and periodontitis. Oral Microbiol Immunol 1987; 2:152.
92. Lally ET, Kieba IR, Sato A, et al: RTX toxins recognize a β-2 integrin on the surface of human target cells. J Biol Chem 1997; 272:30463.
93. Lantz MS, Rowland RW, Switalski LM, et al: Interactions of *Bacteroides gingivalis* with fibrinogen. Infect Immun 1986; 54:654.
94. Lantz MS, Allen RD, Duck LW, et al: Identification of *Porphyromonas gingivalis* components that mediate its interactions with fibronectin. J Bacteriol 1991; 173:4263.
95. Lee HJ, Kang IK, Chung CP, et al: The subgingival microflora and gingival crevicular fluid cytokines in refractory periodontitis. J Clin Periodontol 1995; 22:885.
96. Lee W, Aitken S, Sodek J, et al: Evidence of a direct relationship between neutrophil collagenase activity and periodontal tissue destruction in vivo: role of active enzyme in human periodontitis. J Periodontal Res 1995; 30:23.
97. Listgarten MA: Electron microscopic observations on the bacterial flora of acute necrotizing ulcerative gingivitis. J Periodontol 1965; 36:328.
98. Löe H, Theilade E, Jensen SB: Experimental gingivitis in man. J Periodontol 1965; 36:177.

99. Löe H: Periodontal disease. The sixth complication of diabetes mellitus. Diabetes Care 1993; 16:329.
100. Loesche WJ: Importance of nutrition in gingival crevice microbial ecology. Periodontics 1968; 6:245.
101. Loesche WJ, Syed SA, Schmidt E, et al: Bacterial profiles of subgingival plaques in periodontitis. J Periodontol 1985; 56:447.
102. Loesche WJ: Bacterial mediators in periodontal disease. Clin Infect Dis 1993; 16(Suppl 4):S203.
103. Lopatin DE, Kornman KS, Loesche WJ: Modulation of immunoreactivity to periodontal disease-associated microorganisms during pregnancy. Infect Immun 1980; 28:713.
104. Lynch SE, Nixon JC, Colvin RB, et al: Role of platelet-derived growth factor in wound healing: synergistic effects with other growth factors. Proc Natl Acad Sci U S A 1987; 84:7696.
105. MacFarlane GD, Herzberg MC, Wolff LF, et al: Refractory periodontitis associated with abnormal polymorphonuclear leukocyte phagocytosis and cigarette smoking. J Periodontol 1992; 63:908.
106. Macuch PJ, Tanner AC: Campylobacter species in health, gingivitis, and periodontitis. J Dent Res 2000; 79:785.
107. Madianos PN, Papapanou PN, Sandros J: *Porphyromonas gingivalis* infection of oral epithelium inhibits neutrophil transepithelial migration. Infect Immun 1997; 65:3983.
108. Mariotti A: Dental plaque-induced gingival diseases. Ann Periodontol 1999; 4:7.
109. Marucha PT, Kiecolt-Glaser JK, Favagehi M: Mucosal wound healing is impaired by examination stress. Psychosom Med 1998; 60:362.
110. Masada MP, Persson R, Kenney JS, et al: Measurement of interleukin-1α and -1β in gingival crevicular fluid: implications for the pathogenesis of periodontal disease. J Periodontal Res 1990; 25:156.
111. McDevitt MJ, Wang HY, Knobelman C, et al: Interleukin-1 genetic association with periodontitis in clinical practice. J Periodontol 2000; 71:156.
112. McIntire FC, Bush CA, Wu SS, et al: Structure of a new hexasaccharide from the coaggregation polysaccharide of *Streptococcus sanguis* 34. Carbohydr Res 1987; 166:133.
113. Meng HX: Periodontal abscess. Ann Periodontol 1999; 4:79.
114. Mergenhagen SE, Sandberg AL, Chassy BM, et al: Molecular basis of bacterial adhesion in the oral cavity. Rev Infect Dis 1987; 9:S467.
115. Metcalfe DD, Costa JJ, Burd PR: Mast cells and basophils. In: Gallin JI, Goldstein IM, Snyderman R (ed): Inflammation: basic principals and clinical correlates, ed 2. New York, Raven Press, 1992.
115. Moore WE, Holdeman LV, Cato EP, et al: Comparative bacteriology of juvenile periodontitis. Infect Immun 1985; 48:507.
117. Moore WE, Moore LV: The bacteria of periodontal diseases. Periodontol 2000 1994; 5:66.
118. Moritz AJ, Cappelli D, Lantz MS, et al: Immunization with *Porphyromonas gingivalis* cysteine protease: effects on experimental gingivitis and ligature-induced periodontitis in *Macaca fascicularis*. J Periodontol 1998; 69:686.
119. Mundy GR: Inflammatory mediators and the destruction of bone. J Periodontal Res 1991; 26:213.
120. Nagle DL, Karim MA, Woolf EA, et al: Identification and mutation analysis of the complete gene for Chediak-Higashi syndrome. Nat Genet 1996; 14:307.
121. Neiders ME, Chen PB, Suido H, et al: Heterogeneity of virulence among strains of *Bacteroides gingivalis*. J Periodontal Res 1989; 24:192.
122. Newman MG, Socransky SS, Savitt ED, et al: Studies of the microbiology of periodontosis. J Periodontol 1976; 47:373.
123. Newman MG, Socransky SS: Predominant cultivable microbiota in periodontosis. J Periodontal Res 1977; 14:120.
124. Newman MG, Sims TN: The predominant cultivable microbiota of the periodontal abscess. J Periodontol 1979; 50:350.
125. Nisengard RJ: The role of immunology in periodontal disease. J Periodontol 1977; 48:505.
126. Novak MJ: Necrotizing ulcerative periodontitis. Ann Periodontol 1999; 4:74.
127. Nunes IP, Johannessen AC, Matre R, et al: Epithelial expression of HLA class II antigens and Fc gamma receptors in patients with adult periodontitis. J Clin Periodontol 1994; 21:526.
128. Offenbacher S, Scott SS, Odle BM, et al: Depressed leukotriene B4 chemotactic response of neutrophils from localized juvenile periodontitis patients. J Periodontol 1987; 58:602.
129. Offenbacher S, Salvi GE: Induction of prostaglandin release from macrophages by bacterial endotoxin. Clin Infect Dis 1999; 28:505.
130. Page RC, Schroeder HE: Pathogenesis of inflammatory periodontal disease. A summary of current work. Lab Invest 1976; 34:235.
131. Page RC, Altman LC, Ebersole JL, et al: Rapidly progressive periodontitis. A distinct clinical condition. J Periodontol 1983; 54:197.
132. Page RC: The role of inflammatory mediators in the pathogenesis of periodontal disease. J Periodontal Res 1991; 26:230.
133. Park JB, Matsuura M, Han KY, et al: Periodontal regeneration in class III furcation defects of beagle dogs using guided tissue regenerative therapy with platelet-derived growth factor. J Periodontol 1995; 66:462.
134. Persson GR, Engel D, Whitney C, et al: Immunization against *Porphyromonas gingivalis* inhibits progression of experimental periodontitis in nonhuman primates. Infect Immun 1994; 62:1026.
135. Price TH, Ochs HD, Gershoni-Baruch R, et al: In vivo neutrophil and lymphocyte function studies in a patient with leukocyte adhesion deficiency type II. Blood 1994; 84:1635.
136. Rawlinson A, Dalati MH, Rahman S, et al: Interleukin-1 and IL-1 receptor antagonist in gingival crevicular fluid. J Clin Periodontol 2000; 27:738.
137. Roberts FA, Richardson GJ, Michalek SM: Effects of *Porphyromonas gingivalis* and *Escherichia coli* lipopolysaccharides on mononuclear phagocytes. Infect Immun 1997; 65:3248.
138. Romanelli R, Mancini S, Laschinger C, et al: Activation of neutrophil collagenase in periodontitis. Infect Immun 1999; 67:2319.
139. Rowland RW: Necrotizing ulcerative gingivitis. Ann Periodontol 1999; 4:65.
140. Rutherford RB, Niekrash CE, Kennedy JE, et al: Platelet-derived and insulin-like growth factors stimulate regeneration of periodontal attachment in monkeys. J Periodontal Res 1992; 27:285.
141. Safkan-Seppala B, Ainamo J: Periodontal conditions in insulin-dependent diabetes mellitus. J Clin Periodontol 1992; 19:24.
142. Saglie FR, Marfany A, Camargo P: Intragingival occurrence of *Actinobacillus actinomycetemcomitans* and *Bacteroides gingivalis* in active destructive periodontal lesions. J Periodontol 1988; 59:259.
143. Saglie R, Newman MG, Carranza FA, Jr, et al: Bacterial invasion of gingiva in advanced periodontitis in humans. J Periodontol 1982; 53:217.
144. Sandros J, Papapanou P, Dahlen G: *Porphyromonas gingi-*

valis invades oral epithelial cells in vitro. J Periodontal Res 1993; 28:219.
145. Schenkein HA: The role of complement in periodontal diseases. Crit Rev Oral Biol Med 1991; 2:65.
146. Seymour GJ, Powell RN, Aitken JF: Experimental gingivitis in humans. A clinical and histologic investigation. J Periodontol 1983; 54:522.
147. Shenker BJ, Hoffmaster RH, McKay TL, et al: Expression of the cytolethal distending toxin (Cdt) operon in *Actinobacillus actinomycetemcomitans*: evidence that the CdtB protein is responsible for G2 arrest of the cell cycle in human T cells. J Immunol 2000; 165:2612.
148. Shibutani T, Gen K, Shibata M, et al: Long-term follow-up of periodontitis in a patient with Chediak-Higashi syndrome. A case report. J Periodontol 2000; 71:1024.
149. Singer RE, Buckner BA: Butyrate and propionate: Important components of toxic dental plaque extracts. Infect Immun 1981; 32:458.
150. Sjostrom K, Ou J, Whitney C, et al: Effect of treatment on titer, function, and antigen recognition of serum antibodies to *Actinobacillus actinomycetemcomitans* in patients with rapidly progressive periodontitis. Infect Immun 1994; 62:145.
151. Slots J: Subgingival microflora and periodontal disease. J Clin Periodontol 1979; 6:351.
152. Slots J, Rosling BG: Suppression of the periodontopathic microflora in localized juvenile periodontitis by systemic tetracycline. J Clin Periodontol 1983; 10:465.
153. Socransky SS, Haffajee AD: Microbial mechanisms in the pathogenesis of destructive periodontal diseases: a critical assessment. J Periodontal Res 1991; 26:195.
154. Socransky SS, Haffajee AD: The bacterial etiology of destructive periodontal disease: Current concepts. J Periodontol 1992; 63:322.
155. Sorsa T, Ding YL, Ingman T, et al: Cellular source, activation and inhibition of dental plaque collagenase. J Clin Periodontol 1995; 22:709.
156. Sreenivasan PK, Meyer DH, Fives-Taylor PM: Requirements for invasion of epithelial cells by *Actinobacillus actinomycetemcomitans*. Infect Immun 1993; 61:1239.
157. Stashenko P, Jandinski JJ, Fujiyoshi P, et al: Tissue levels of bone resorptive cytokines in periodontal disease. J Periodontol 1991; 62:504.
158. Steinsvoll S, Halstensen TS, Schenck K: Extensive expression of TGF-beta1 in chronically-inflamed periodontal tissue. J Clin Periodontol 1999; 26:366.
159. Syed SA, Loesche WJ: Bacteriology of human experimental gingivitis: Effect of plaque age. 1978; 21:821.
160. Takemoto T, Kurihara H, Dahlen G: Characterization of *Bacteroides forsythus* isolates. J Clin Microbiol 1997; 35:1378.
161. Tani Y, Tani M, Kato I: Extracellular 37–kDa antigenic protein from *Actinobacillus actinomycetemcomitans* induces TNF-alpha, IL-1 beta, and IL-6 in murine macrophages. J Dent Res 1997; 76:1538.
162. Tanner AC, Haffer C, Bratthall GT, et al: A study of the bacteria associated with advancing periodontitis in man. J Clin Periodontol 1979; 6:278.
163. Tervahartiala T, Konttinen YT, Ingman T, et al: Cathepsin G in gingival tissue and crevicular fluid in adult periodontitis. J Clin Periodontol 1996; 23:68.
164. Tew JG, Zhang JB, Quinn S, et al: Antibody of the IgG2 subclass, *Actinobacillus actinomycetemcomitans,* and early-onset perioodontitis. J Periodontol 1996; 67:317.
165. Tonetti MS, Imboden MA, Lang NP: Neutrophil migration into the gingival sulcus is associated with transepithelial gradients of interleukin-8 and ICAM-1. J Periodontol 1998; 69:1139.
166. Tonetti MS, Mombelli A: Early-onset periodontitis. Ann Periodontol 1999; 4:39.
167. van Dalen PJ, van Deutekom-Mulder EC, de Graaff J, et al: Pathogenicity of *Peptostreptococcus micros* morphotypes and *Prevotella* species in pure and mixed culture. J Med Microbiol 1998; 47:135.
168. Van Dyke TE, Schweinebraten M, Cianciola LJ, et al: Neutrophil chemotaxis in families with localized juvenile periodontitis. J Periodontal Res 1985; 20:503.
169. Van Dyke TE, Wilson-Burrows C, Offenbacher S, et al: Association of an abnormality of neutrophil chemotaxis in human periodontal disease with a cell surface protein. Infect Immun 1987; 55:2262.
170. van Steenbergen TJ, van der Mispel LM, de Graaff J: Effects of ammonia and volatile fatty acids produced by oral bacteria on tissue culture cells. J Dent Res 1986; 65:909.
171. Waldrop TC, Anderson DC, Hallmon WW, et al: Periodontal manifestations of the heritable Mac-1, LFA-1, deficiency syndrome. Clinical, histopathologic and molecular characteristics. J Periodontol 1987; 58:400.
172. Walker SJ, Van Dyke TE, Rich S, et al: Genetic polymorphisms of the IL-1alpha and IL-1beta genes in African-American LJP patients and an African-American control population. J Periodontol 2000; 71:723.
173. Wang B, Holt SC: Interaction of *Treponema denticola* with HEp-2 cells. J Dent Res 1993; 72:324.
174. Williams RC, Jeffcoat MK, Howell TH, et al: Altering the progression of human alveolar bone loss with the non-steroidal anti-inflammatory drug flurbiprofen. J Periodontol 1989; 60:485.
175. Wilson M, Kalmar JR: FcgRIIa (CD32): A potential marker defining susceptibility to localized juvenile periodontitis. J Periodontol 1996; 67:323.
176. Wilson ME, Hamilton RG: Immunoglobulin G subclass response of localized juvenile periodontitis patients to *Actinobacillus actinomycetemcomitans* Y4 lipopolysaccharide. Infect Immun 1992; 60:1806.
177. Wilson ME, Hamilton RG: Immunoglobulin G subclass response of juvenile periodontitis subjects to principal outer membrane proteins of *Actinobacillus actinomycetemcomitans*. Infect Immun 1995; 63:1062.
178. Wingrove JA, DiScipio RG, Chen Z, et al: Activation of complement components C3 and C5 by a cysteine proteinase (gingipain-1) from *Porphyromonas (Bacteroides) gingivalis*. J Biol Chem 1992; 267:18902.
179. Winkler JR, Robertson PB: Periodontal disease associated with HIV infection. Oral Surg Oral Med Oral Pathol 1992; 73:145.
180. Yoshimura A, Hara Y, Kaneko T, et al: Secretion of IL-1 beta, TNF-alpha, IL-8 and IL-1ra by human polymorphonuclear leukocytes in response to lipopolysaccharides from periodontopathic bacteria. J Periodontal Res 1997; 32:279.
181. Yumoto H, Nakae H, Fujinaka K, et al: Interleukin-6 (IL-6) and IL-8 are induced in human oral epithelial cells in response to exposure to periodontopathic *Eikenella corrodens*. Infect Immun 1999; 67:384.
182. Zambon JJ, Christersson LA, Slots J: *Actinobacillus actinomycetemcomitans* in human periodontal disease. Prevalence in patient groups and distribution of biotypes and serotypes within families. J Periodontol 1983; 54:707.
183. Zambon JJ: *Actinobacillus actinomycetemcomitans* in human periodontal disease. 1985; 12:1.
184. Zubery Y, Dunstan CR, Story BM, et al: Bone resorption caused by three periodontal pathogens in vivo in mice is mediated in part by prostaglandin. Infect Immun 1998; 66:4158.

Molecular Biology of the Host-Microbe Interaction in Periodontal Diseases: Selected Topics

Susan Kinder Haake and George T.-J. Huang

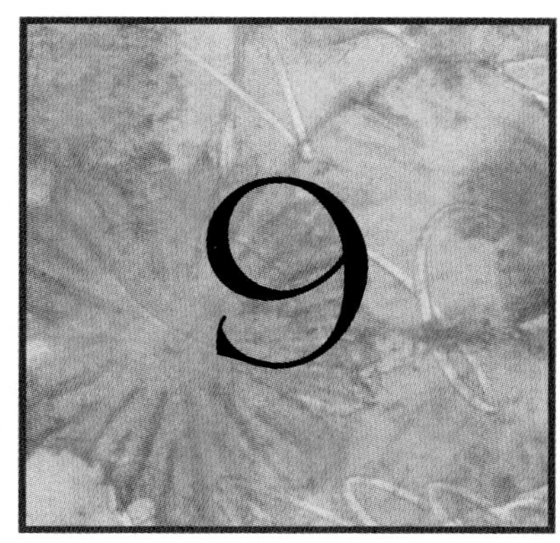

CHAPTER

CHAPTER OUTLINE

It was only in the mid-1900s that deoxyribonucleic acid (DNA) was recognized as the molecule that carries genetic information. Subsequent work has clarified the fundamental processes of DNA replication as well as the transcription and translation processes leading to expression of gene products. The advent of recombinant DNA technology was possible only after the discovery and isolation of restriction endonucleases, enzymes produced by bacteria that cleave DNA at highly specific sites. The subsequent development of cloning technologies allowed the study of genes in the laboratory and furthered the development of genetic transfer of DNA into living organisms. These advances in molecular biology achieved in the latter half of the 20th century have revolutionized the study of biologic systems.

Utilization of molecular approaches in the study of periodontal diseases has followed on the heels of these developments. Periodontal diseases represent the outcome of a complex interaction between the host and the pathogenic microorganism in the unique environment of the tooth-to-tissue interface. Chapter 10 focuses on the association of human genetics with periodontal diseases. In this chapter, selected topics illustrate areas of progress in understanding the molecular basis of the host-parasite interaction in periodontal diseases. The work summarized in this chapter is at the very forefront of scientific investigation, and in some cases it challenges earlier paradigms of bacterial pathogenesis and host susceptibility.

NOT ALL *ACTINOBACILLUS ACTINOMYCETEMCOMITANS* ARE CREATED EQUAL: THE SPECIFIC PLAQUE HYPOTHESIS REVISITED

The gram-negative facultative anaerobe *Actinobacillus actinomycetemcomitans* is implicated as a pathogen in several forms of aggressive and chronic periodontitis, most notably localized aggressive periodontitis. It is one of a few periodontal microorganisms that are strongly implicated in the etiology of periodontitis, providing support for the Specific Plaque Hypothesis (see Chapter 6). *A. actinomycetemcomitans* possesses the ability to kill human leukocytes through the production of a 116-kDa protein toxin termed a *leukotoxin*. Because leukocytes are critical to an effective host response against periodontal pathogens, the ability of this microorganism to kill leukocytes is an important mechanism in evading host defenses. Early studies indicated that not all strains of *A. actinomycetemcomitans* demonstrated the leukotoxic properties.[2] Recent investigations have revealed a molecular basis for this variability in leukotoxin expression and led to new insights on the role of specific strains of *A. actinomycetemcomitans* in periodontitis.

The Leukotoxin of *A. actinomycetemcomitans*

The *A. actinomycetemcomitans* leukotoxin (LtxA) is a member of a family of pore-forming toxins, characterized by a series of glycine-rich repeats in the C-terminal portion of the protein that are involved in cation binding and appear to be essential to toxin activity. This family of toxins has been designated as RTX (repeat in toxin) toxins, and they are produced by several pathogenic, gram-negative species. Other RTX toxins include the leukotoxin of *Pasturella haemolytica,* a respiratory pathogen of cattle, as well as hemolysins of pathogenic *Escherichia coli* and *Bordetella pertussis,* the causative agent of whooping cough. A high degree of specificity in the cells affected by the *A. actinomycetemcomitans* LtxA was evident in early studies. The affected target cells include human polymorphonuclear leukocytes (neutrophils or PMNs), monocytes and lymphocytes. Human platelets, fibroblasts, and endothelial and epithelial cells are resistant to the effects of the LtxA.[71,78] The target cell susceptibility is a result of cell surface expression of the β2-integrin molecule, lymphocyte function-associated antigen 1 (LFA-1).[44,79] The identification of LFA-1 as the receptor for LtxA suggests that killing is a receptor-mediated process.

Mechanism of Leukotoxin Action

Evidence exists for two LtxA-mediated mechanisms of cell death: necrosis and apoptosis. Exposure of neutrophils and monocytes/macrophages to strains that produce large amount of LtxA results in killing within a relatively short period of time (Fig. 9-1, panels A–C).[2] This cell death is thought to result from the ability of LtxA to form pores in the membrane of target cells, leading to osmotic lysis caused by water influx into the cell.[45] In contrast, prolonged exposure of lymphocytes and NK cells to LtxA results in the induction of apoptosis, a programmed sequence of cellular alteration progressing to cell death.[40,49,66] There is evidence that lower concentrations of LtxA result in apoptosis whereas higher concentrations result in necrosis.[39] It has been hypothesized that the LtxA molecules in high concentration fuse to form large pores in the target cell membrane, resulting in more rapid necrotic destruction.

Molecular Characterization of the Leukotoxin Genes

The gene encoding the *A. actinomycetmecomitans* leukotoxin, *ltx*A, is part of an operon of four genes in the sequence *ltx*C, *ltx*A, *ltx*B, and *ltx*D (Fig. 9-2). This operon structure of C, A, B, and D genes in sequence is characteristic of the RTX family of toxins. Considerable sequence homology exists between the individual genes from these different organisms, suggesting a common evolutionary origin and function.[41,43] As is characteristic of genes clustered in an operon, these genes are all related to leukotoxin function. The A gene encodes the leukotoxin itself and is produced in an inactive "protoxin" state. The C gene product, *ltx*C, is required to activate the pro-toxin. In the case of the *E. coli* hemolysin, this process involves a chemical modification in which fatty acids are linked to two sites on the leukotoxin protein.[69] Based on the similarity between the C genes and gene products, the *ltx*C gene product of *A. actinomycetemcomitans* also is thought to function in leukotoxin activation. The B and D genes are typically involved in secretion of the leukotoxin from the bacterial cell, and studies of the *ltx*B and *ltx*D genes of *A. actinomycetemcomitans* suggest similar functions.[22,43] For many years, it was thought that the leukotoxin of *A. actinomycetemcomitans* remained associated with the bacterial cell and was not secreted into the external environment. Recent studies have revealed that certain strains in their early growth phases secrete an abundant amount of leukotoxin into the environment.[33] Further studies of the factors governing the cellular retention or release of the leukotoxin may shed more light on the role of these properties in pathogenesis.

Molecular Basis of Variability in Leukotoxin Production

It has been long recognized that some strains of *A. actinomycetemcomitans* are highly toxic and produce high levels of leukotoxin, whereas other strains are weak or minimally toxic and produce low levels of leukotoxin. A key discovery in the study of the leukotoxin production in *A. actinomycetemcomitans* was the variation in the DNA sequence of the leukotoxin promoter region.[9,25] Bacterial promoters consist of specific segments of DNA that provide a recognition and binding site for the enzyme RNA polymerase, which is responsible for RNA (ribonucleic acid) synthesis. Different promoters vary in their level of transcription, leading to differences in the level of mRNA and thus differences in the amount of protein product generated. The regulation of gene expression based on the amount of mRNA produced is referred to as *transcriptional control.* Investigation of the DNA sequence upstream of the *ltx*C gene revealed that the highly toxic strains have a deletion of 530 base pairs (bp) of DNA as compared with the minimally toxic strains (see Fig. 9-2). Analysis of mRNA revealed the presence of two promoters functioning in the highly toxic strains (see Fig. 9-2, *A,* P1 and P2), but in the minimally toxic strains a single promoter is responsible for initiating transcription (Fig. 9-2, *B,* P3). This latter promoter (P3) resides within the 530 base pair region that is missing in the highly toxic

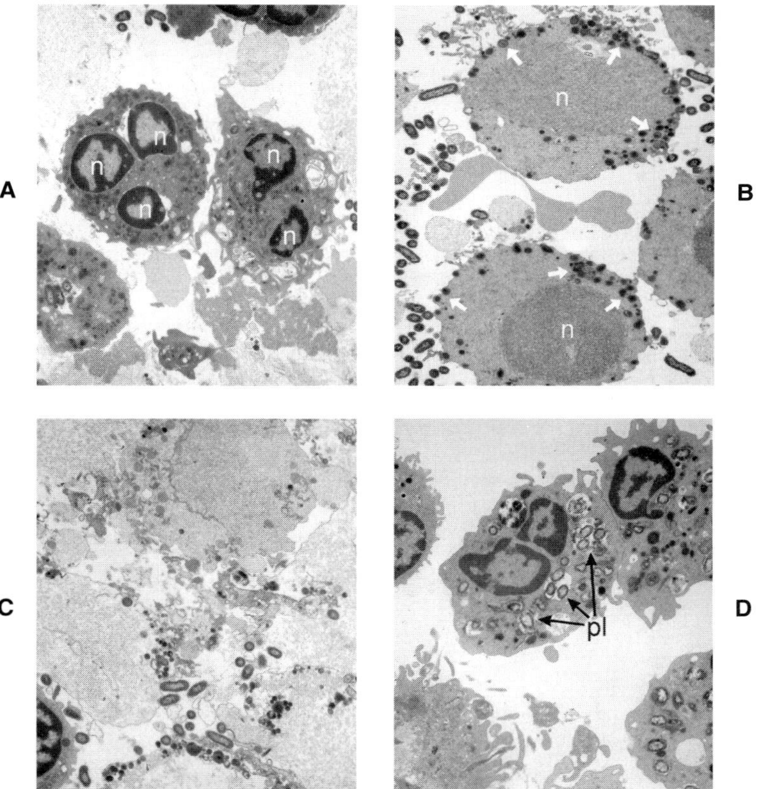

Fig. 9-1 Highly leukotoxic *A. actinomycetemcomitans* evasion of neutrophil phagocytosis. Electron micrographs of neutrophils challenged with the highly leukotoxic strain *A. actinomycetemcomitans* HK1519 for **(A)** 0 minute, **(B)** 7 minutes, and **(C)** 45 minutes. Cell morphology of the neutrophils initially appears normal, including the nuclei *(n)*. By 7 minutes' incubation, nuclear degeneration and peripheralization of the neutrophil granules *(white arrows)* are evident. Further incubation reveals complete lysis of the neutrophils. In contrast, challenge with the minimally leukotoxic strain NCTC 9710 for 60 minutes **(D)** does not result in cytopathic alterations of the neutrophils. Rather, uptake of bacterial cells into phagolysosomes *(pl)* is evident. (From Johansson A, et al: Anaerobic neutrophil-dependent killing of *Actinobacillus actinomycetemcomitans* in relation to the bacterial leukotoxicity. Eur J Oral Sci 2000; 108:136. Figure courtesy of A. Johansson.)

strains. Studies of the regulation of transcription further differentiate the different promoters. The P3 promoter is regulated by the level of oxygen present during bacterial growth, with increased mRNA, increased leukotoxin expression, and a 3- to 4-fold increase in toxicity when the bacterium is grown under anaerobic conditions. In contrast, oxygen concentrations have no effect on the P1 or P2 promoters. The amount of mRNA and leukotoxin produced and the resulting toxicity are substantially greater in the highly toxic strains using the P1 and P2 promoters, regardless of the environmental conditions, as compared with the minimally toxic strains using the P3 promoter. It is hypothesized that the highly toxic strains may have evolved from a minimally toxic strain by the deletion of this DNA in the promoter region.

The leukotoxin is considered an important virulence determinant of *A. actinomycetemcomitans* because it allows the microorganism to neutralize host defense mechanisms. The interaction of highly versus minimally toxic strains with neutrophils is demonstrated in Fig. 9-1. The highly toxic strain rapidly induces degenerative changes and then lysis of the neutrophils (see Fig. 9-1, panels A–C). In contrast, the minimally toxic strain does not induce lysis of the neutrophil, but rather the bacterial cells are phagocytosed and phagolysosomes containing the bacterial cells are evident microscopically (see Fig. 9-1, panel D). The presence of the 530-bp deletion in the DNA sequence has provided a marker for distinguishing the highly versus minimally leukotoxic strains, which can be easily detected using PCR techniques. The occurance of the highly leukotoxic strain varies widely in different geographic regions as well as in different racial groups.[23] In addition, in a population of children at risk for the development of localized aggressive periodontitis, those who harbored the highly leukotoxic strain were found to be more likely to develop disease.[10]

Summary

The significance of the findings related to leukotoxin expression ranges from theoretic to practical.[64] The theoretic implications relate to the clear demonstration that not all *A. actinomycetemcomitans* are created equal, but rather that some strains are more virulent than others.

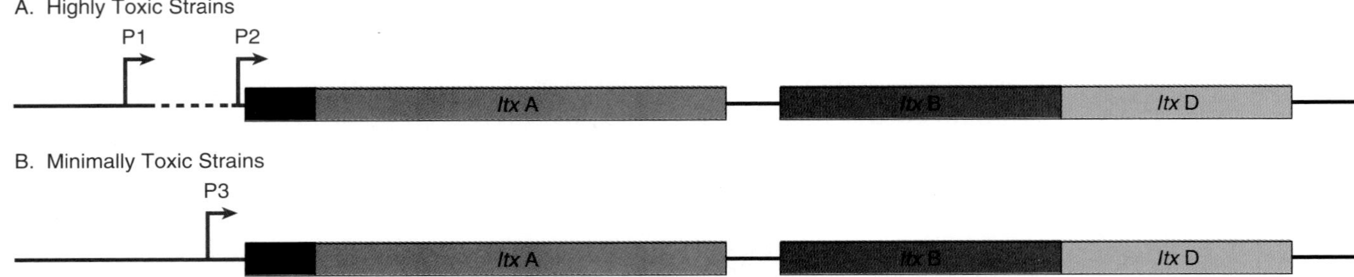

Fig. 9-2 Schematic illustration of the leukotoxin operon in highly and minimally toxic strains of *A. actinomycetemcomitans.* The leukotoxin operon consists of the four genes *ltx*C, *ltx*A, *ltx*B, and *ltx*D, arranged in tandem. The leukotoxin itself is encoded by the *ltx*A gene. See the text for descriptions of the functions of the remaining gene products. The position of the 530 bp DNA deletion in the highly toxic strains is indicated by the dotted line. The positions of the promoters (P1, P2, and P3) functioning in the highly versus minimally toxic strains are indicated.

The specific plaque hypothesis (see Chapter 6) states that disease is associated with specific bacterial species. The findings described here suggest that the specific plaque hypothesis should be revised to state that disease is associated with specific strains of a given species. It is likely that most, if not all, recognized periodontal pathogens demonstrate differences in phenotypic properties related to their ability to cause disease. Further investigation at a molecular level will undoubtedly continue to reveal the genetic basis for variability in virulence properties among pathogenic strains. Practical implications relate to microbial monitoring of periodontitis patients as well as assessments of risk in susceptible individuals. Current practices of microbial testing do not differentiate the highly toxic versus minimally toxic *A. actinomycetemcomitans* strains. This can lead to a situation where an individual with a minimally toxic strain might be inappropriately considered at high risk for disease development or progression. Furthermore, in clinical trials in which the presence of *A. actinomycetemcomitans* is evaluated as a risk factor for development or progression of disease, the inclusion of minimally toxic strains may dilute and essentially mask a stronger association of the highly leukotoxic strain with disease. Clarification of specific bacterial virulence factors that contribute to pathogenesis and development of the tools or probes needed to identify strains possessing virulence factors will enhance our ability to both prevent and manage periodontal diseases.

DESTRUCTION AT THE HOST TISSUE INTERFACE: THE PROTEASES OF *PORPHYROMONAS GINGIVALIS*

P. gingivalis is a periodontal microorganism that is strongly associated with chronic and aggressive forms of periodontal disease in humans (see Chapter 6). In addition, this gram-negative anaerobe has been shown to be pathogenic in nonhuman primate and rodent models of periodontitis.[19,24] Investigations in the laboratory have identified numerous properties of *P. gingivalis* that may account for its ability to cause disease, and preeminent among these is the ability of *P. gingivalis* to elaborate a variety of proteolytic enzymes. Investigations during the last 2 decades demonstrated that a wide variety of protein substrates are degraded by *P. gingivalis* proteases. This led to a period of considerable confusion regarding the number and activity of different proteases. Molecular analyses have now confirmed the presence of a relatively limited number of protease genes (Table 9-1) and clarified the relationships among genes characterized from different strains.[12]

It is noteworthy that *P. gingivalis* proteases are not inactivated by host proteinase inhibitors. Rather, evidence exists that the *P. gingivalis* proteases inactivate or degrade the host proteinase inhibitors.[57] This may lead to an imbalance in the normal host mechanisms of tissue turnover, contributing further to host tissue destruction. The proteases of *P. gingivalis* are important in the metabolism and ecology of the bacterium itself, but they additionally act at the host-parasite interface to contribute to pathogenesis through host tissue degradation and modulation of host defense mechanisms. Molecular analyses have been used to define the genetic basis of protease production and delineate the mechanisms by which the proteases may contribute to host tissue destruction. In addition, genetic approaches to specifically inactivate protease genes have been used to demonstrate that proteases play an important role in the virulence of *P. gingivalis.*

P. gingivalis Proteolytic Activity

P. gingivalis is unable to break down or degrade sugar substrates as a source of energy or to take up and use free amino acids as metabolic building blocks.[14] Rather, *P. gingivalis* relies on its ability to degrade proteins into short peptides that are taken in and used metabolically in the generation of energy and as sources of carbon and nitrogen. In the periodontal environment, the host tissues provide an abundant source of proteins. For example, a major protein constituent of the periodontal tissues is collagen, and *P. gingivalis* possesses the proteolytic activity to degrade collagen into peptide components that it can use. The bacterial collagenase produced by *P. gingivalis* (PrtC), host cell collagenases, or probably both contribute to collagen degradation. Several peptidases found on the cell surface of *P. gingivalis* are suffi-

TABLE 9-1

Selected Proteases Produced by *P. gingivalis*

Enzyme	Gene	Molecular Weight of Protein Product	Enzyme Class	Cleavage Specificity	Comments on Function	References
Arg-gingipain (RgpA)	*rgp*A	50 to 110 kDa	Cysteine	Cleaves peptide bonds following an arginine residue	Gene also encodes an adhesin domain that appears to improve proteolytic efficiency	1, 18, 37, 58, 62
Arg-gingipain (RgpB)	*rgp*B	48 to 90 kDa	Cysteine	Cleaves peptide bonds following an arginine residue	Gene is homologous to *rgp*A but lacks the adhesin domain	53, 55, 68
Lys-gingipain (Kgp)	*kgp*	60 to 180 kDa	Cysteine	Cleaves peptide bonds following a lysine residue	Gene also encodes an adhesin domain	7, 62
Periodontain	N/A	75 kDa heterodimer	Cysteine	Only cleaves denatured proteins; 55 kDa fragment possesses catalytic domain	Rapidly inactivates host plasma proteinase inhibitors, such as α-1-protease inhibitor, the primary inhibitor of human neutrophil elastase	57
Prolyl tripeptidase PtpA	*ptp*A	82 kDa	Serine	Cleaves tripeptides from the amino-terminal end, where proline is the third residue from the amino-terminal end	Enzyme is cell associated and may be important in generating tri-peptides used in bacterial nutrition	5
Prolyl dipeptidyl peptidase IV	*dpp*	78 kDa	Serine	Cleaves dipeptides from the amino-terminal end, where proline is the second residue from the amino-terminal end	Enzyme is cell associated and may be important in generating di-peptides used in bacterial nutrition as well as host molecules	3, 38, 42
Collagenase	*prt*C	38 kDa	Metallo-protease	Degrades type I collagen but cleavage specificity not determined	Differs from other bacterial collagenases in that it does not degrade gelatin	36

N/A, Not applicable.

cient to completely degrade the collagen fragments. These include dipeptidyl peptidase IV (DPPIV) and prolyl tripeptidyl peptidases (PtpA), proteases that generate di- and tri-peptide fragments, which may be transported into the bacterial cell. Another group of *P. gingivalis* proteases, the gingipains (discussed below), also are capable of degrading collagen fragments. The degradation of collagen and other host tissue molecules supports *P. gingivalis* metabolically but also contributes to pathogenesis because of the resulting host tissue damage.

Molecular Characterization of the Gingipain Protease Genes

The most intensely studied enzymes of *P. gingivalis* are a group of related proteases known as *gingipains*. These proteases occur in multiple forms that are found extracellularly or on the bacterial cell surface and in some cases are associated with protein regions or "domains" involved in adherence properties (Fig. 9-3). The gingipains specifically cleave proteins at the peptide bond following arginine residues (Arg-gingipains or Rgps) or lysine residues (Lys-gingipain or Kgp). Molecular studies revealed that the Arg-gingipains are encoded by two genes, *rgp*A and *rgp*B, whereas the Lys-gingipain is encoded by a single gene, *kgp*A. Analysis of the *rgp*A DNA sequence indicates that the protein product initially consists of three distinct domains: a propeptide domain at the amino-terminal end of the protein that is cleaved off when the protease is activated, a protease domain, and a carboxy-terminal adhesin domain (see Fig. 9-3). The propeptide and protease domains are very closely related to those of the second Arg-gingipain gene, *rgp*B. In contrast, *rgp*B lacks the adhesin domain. The Lys-gingipain gene *kgp* is similar in organization to *rgp*A, with propeptide, protease, and adhesin domains. The amino acid sequence of the Kgp protease domain demonstrates only 22% identity to that of RgpA, with key catalytic regions that are identical and substantial regions of unrelated sequence that may account for the differences in substrate specificity between

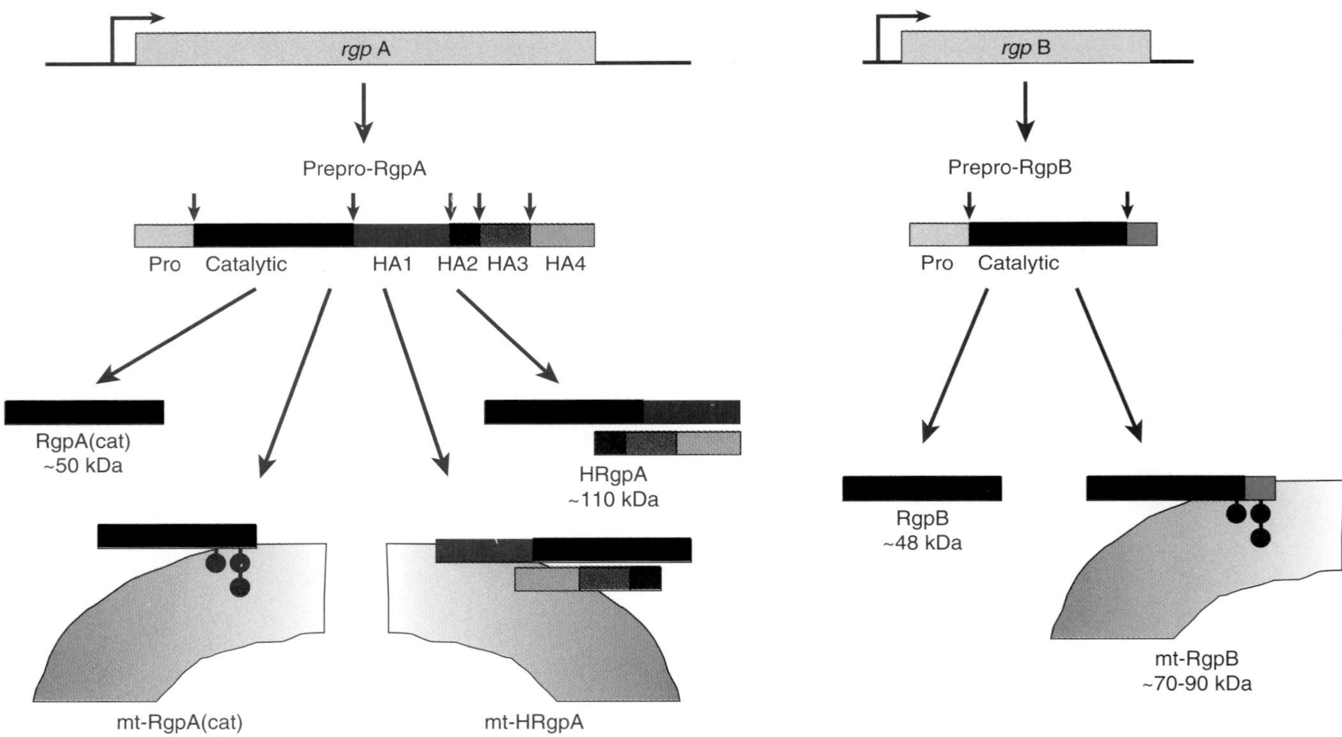

Fig. 9-3 Schematic illustration of the posttranslational processing of the initial translational products of the *rgp*A and *rgp*B genes. The initial translational products (prepro-RgpA and prepro-RgpB) of the genes include propeptide domains (pro) and catalytic domains. RgpA possesses an adhesin domain consisting of a number of defined regions related to hemagglutination genes (HA1, HA2, etc.). These initial protein products undergo posttranslational processing that involves cleavage of the protein *(small arrows)* and addition of carbohydrate groups *(black circles)* to generate multiple isoforms. The propeptide is cleaved off and is not present in the final protein products. A high molecular weight form of RgpA consists of the catalytic and adhesin domains and is designated HrgpA. Note that either the catalytic domain (RgpA[cat]) alone or the HrgpA may be associated with the bacterial cell membrane. The membrane-associated forms are designated as "mt-" forms; for example, mt-RgpA(cat). The posttranslational processing of prepro-RgpB is less complex in that the *Rgp*B gene lacks the adhesin domain. (Adapted from Travis J, Potempa J: Bacterial proteinases as targets for the development of second-generation antibiotics. Biochimica et Biophysica Acta 2000; 1477:35.)

the two enzymes.[61] The translational protein products of the *rgp* genes undergo posttranslational modifications, including cleavage and addition of carbohydrate groups, to yield multiple forms (termed *isoforms*) of the protease (see Fig. 9-3). Interestingly, the adhesin domains found in RgpA and Kgp share stretches of sequence that are closely related to adhesin domain sequences found in a hemagglutinin (HagA) and an outer membrane receptor protein (Tla) of *P. gingivalis*. It has been demonstrated that the adhesin domain mediates adherence of the protease-adhesin complex to connective tissue molecules, including fibrinogen, fibronectin, and laminin.[63] Furthermore, the adhesin-protease complex is about twice as effective in degrading fibrinogen and fibrin as compared with the protease lacking the adhesin.[31] Adherence is an important component of pathogenesis, and the combination of adherence and protease activity is likely to facilitate the process of tissue degradation.

Functional Studies of the Gingipain Proteases

The gingipains of *P. gingivalis* are capable of disrupting normal host systems in a way that contributes to the growth and virulence of the bacterium and destruction of the host tissues (Table 9-2). The ability of gingipains to stimulate the release of bradykinin, resulting in increased vascular permeability, provides a mechanism to explain the increased crevicular fluid flow evident at sites of inflammation, a condition that improves the nutrient supply for resident microorganisms. The host immune response may be neutralized by the gingipains because they degrade the host cell receptor for LPS (CD14), the proinflammatory cytokines such as IL-1β, IL-6, and the chemokine IL-8. In addition, the effects on neutrophil function and degradation of host inflammatory mediators alter the normal host inflammatory responses to the bacterial assault. The gingipains appear to both stimulate and inhibit the host immune response with re-

TABLE 9-2

Effects of *P. gingivalis* Gingipains on Host Biologic Systems: Selected Examples

Host Biologic System	*P. gingivalis* Protease	Mechanism of Action	Effect	References
PMN phagocytosis of bacteria	Rgps	Cleavage of complement component C5 to form C5a	Increased PMN recruitment to site of infection	16, 80
	Rgps, Kgp	Specific cleavage of the cytokine IL-8, making it more active in PMN recruitment	Increased PMN recruitment to site of infection	52
	Membrane-associated Rgps	Degradation of IL-8	Decreased PMN recruitment to the site of infection	52
	Kgp (also membrane-associated serine proteases)	Cleavage of PMN cell surface receptor for C5a (C5aR)	Decreased phagocytosis	32
	Rgps	Degradation of the complement factor C3 and immunoglobulin IgG	Decreased opsonization and phagocytosis	64, 80
Innate immune response	Rgps, Kgp	Degradation of monocyte CD14, the receptor for LPS and activation of toll-like receptors	Inability of host cells to recognize and respond to bacteria	70
Host cytokine network	Rgps, Kgp	Degradation of Il-1β, IL-6, IL-8, and TNF-α	Disrupted host inflammatory response to infection	4, 11, 20
Kallikrein/kinin system	Rgps, Kgp	Activation with release of bradykinin, a potent inducer of vascular permeability	Increased vascular permeability, resulting in increased crevicular fluid flow, tissue edema, and increased supply of nutrients for bacterial growth and virulence	29, 76
Coagulation/ fibrinosysis systems	Rgps, Kgp	Paradoxical effects involved in activation of clot formation and clot (fibrinogen) degradation	Local dysregulation may relate to increased bleeding on probing at sites of periodontal disease	6, 30

gard to neutrophil function. For example, the soluble Rgps and Kgp cleave IL-8 in a manner that makes this proinflammatory cytokine more active in the recruitment of neutrophils. However, the membrane-associated Rgps are able to abolish IL-8 activity by completely degrading the molecule. This has led to the hypothesis that *P. gingivalis* has proinflammatory effects at long distances mediated by soluble proteases but antiinflammatory effects at close range mediated by membrane-associated proteases (Fig. 9-4).[52] Inherent in this hypothesis is the premise that *P. gingivalis* benefits from the presence of neutrophils in the area because the neutrophils release a wealth of proteolytic enzymes that undoubtedly contribute to tissue protein degradation and thus assist in the acquisition of nutrients for the bacterium. However, neutrophil function is thought to be inhibited in close proximity to *P. gingivalis* cells, by virtue of the membrane-associated proteases on the bacterial cells or vesicles released into the bacterial cell's immediate surroundings, to protect the bacterium from phagocytosis. Mechanisms for the inhibition of neutrophil function include the degradation of IL-8 by membrane-associated Rgps as well as molecules (e.g., complement component C3) and receptors (neutrophil C5a receptors) involved in opsonization and phagocytosis.

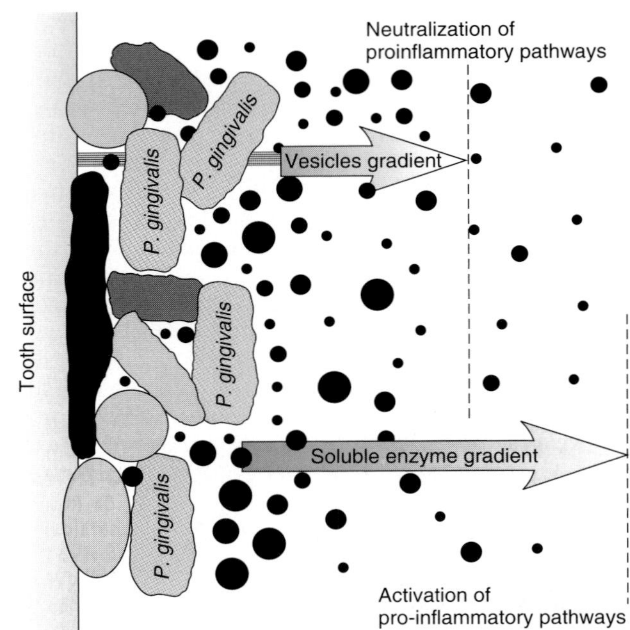

Fig. 9-4 Schematic illustration of the putative compartmentalization of pro- and anti-inflammatory effects of *P. gingivalis* gingipains. The proinflammatory pathways are hypothesized to be mediated by soluble gingipains whose effects include activation of IL-8, which is involved in recruitment of neutrophils. The antiinflammatory effects are hypothesized to be mediated by membrane-associated gingipains such as vesicles *(small filled circles)* released by the bacterium. The antiinflammatory effects focus on an inhibition of neutrophil function as a means of bacterial evasion of host defenses. (Reprinted by permission of the Federation of the European Biochemical Societies. From Mikolajczyk-Pawlinska J, Travis J, Potempa J, et al: Modulation of interleukin-8 activity by gingipains from *Porphyromonas gingivalis*: implications for pathogenicity of periodontal disease. FEBS Lett 1998; 440:282.)

Inactivation of the Gingipain Genes

Molecular studies often focus initially on isolating a particular gene of interest by cloning and expressing that gene in a foreign bacterial host system such as *E. coli.* This approach has been invaluable in isolating and characterizing genes and their products. Another powerful tool in molecular studies is to inactivate, or "knock out," specific target genes at the molecular level. This is typically achieved by inserting an unrelated "marker" gene, such as an antibiotic resistance gene, into the coding sequence of the target gene on the chromosome of the native microorganism. Transcription of the target gene is disrupted, and the presence of the "marker" antibiotic resistance gene is easily assessed by growth of the bacterium on media containing the relevant antibiotic. The resulting bacterial strain is termed an *isogenic mutant.* These mutants differ from the parental strain by the disruption of one, or in some cases several, defined gene(s) and provide an important technique for assessing the role of the gene product in the native host cell. *P. gingivalis* mutants in the *rgp*A and *rgp*B genes confirmed that both genes encode Arg-gingipains (Table 9-3). A mutant strain in which both the genes have been inactivated indicates that these two genes account for all of the Arg-gingipain activity found in *P. gingivalis.*[53] Similarly, the properties of an isogenic mutant in *kgp* indicates that this gene accounts for the Lys-gingipain activity.[59] The loss of hemagglutination in mutants with the *rgp*A or *kgp* genes inactivated supports a role for the protease-associated adhesin domains in hemagglutination.[53]

Analysis of the gingipain isogenic mutants further confirms studies on the role of these proteases in bacterial nutrition, tissue destruction, and modulation of the host immune response. The mutant with all three gingipain genes (*rgp*A, *rgp*B, and *kgp*) inactivated demonstrated a complete loss of extracellular proteolytic activity and diminished growth on complex media, presumably because of an inability to degrade proteins for use in bacterial metabolism.[67] Inactivation of the *rgp*A gene specifically resulted in loss of the ability of the bacterium to degrade type I collagen, a major component of the periodontal tissues.[73] Mutations in both *rgp*A and *rgp*B were associated with alterations in the bacterial-neutrophil interaction. The supernatants taken from cultures of *P. gingivalis* normally inhibit neutrophil function. Strains with either *rgp*A or *rgp*B inactivated partially lose the ability to inhibit neutrophil function, whereas inactivation of both *rgp*A and *rgp*B results in almost complete loss of the ability to inhibit neutrophil function. In addition, the *rgp*A mutant is less resistant to neutrophil phagocytosis.[65] This mutant demonstrated a loss in the ability to degrade the complement factor C3 and an increase in the accumulation of iC3b on the bacterial cell surface. Thus the loss of Arg-gingipain activity is associated with a loss in the ability of the bacterium to disrupt the processes of opsonization and phagocytosis.

Several unexpected findings also have emerged from the studies of the gingipain isogenic mutant strains (see Table 9-3). Inactivation of the *rgp* genes is associated with altered expression or loss of the bacterial fimbriae normally found on the *P. gingivalis* cell surface. The fimbriae are important in adherence of the bacterial cells, as reflected in the alterations in adherence properties observed in the *rgp* mutant strains. Subsequent investigation revealed that Arg-gingipain plays an important role in the processing of prefimbrilin to form fimbrilin, a major component of the bacterial fimbriae.[34] Fimbrial expression is important in the virulence of *P. gingivalis*,[48] underscoring again the role of Arg-gingipain activity in pathogenesis. A second unexpected finding was that inactivation of *kgp* results in a loss of the black pigmentation of the *P. gingivalis* colonies as well as altered adsorption of hemoglobin and heme accumulation. *P. gingivalis* colonies normally turn black when grown on blood agar as the cells accumulate an oxidized form of heme, hemin. The hemin appears to be derived from hemoglobin and provides an important nutritional source of iron for the bacterium.[8] Subsequent studies revealed that Lys-gingipain is able to cleave human hemoglobin and thus appears to function as a hemoglobinase in the acquisition of heme and iron.[46] Interestingly, the hemoglobin receptor protein of *P. gingivalis* is encoded as part of the adhesin domain associated with the *kgp*, *rgp*A, and *hag*A genes.[54] The physical proximity of the hemoglobin receptor and the hemoglobinase in the protein product presumably facilitates this aspect of nutrient aquisition. Hemin levels are known to be important in the virulence properties of *P. gingivalis*.[51] The unexpected findings described here illustrate the importance of investigating gene function, not just in a foreign host system such as *E. coli* but in the native host cell (in this case, *P. gingivalis*), to fully understand the role of any particular gene or gene product in pathogenesis.

TABLE 9-3

Phenotypic Alterations Resulting from Inactivation of Gingipain Genes in *P. gingivalis*

Protease Inactivated	Protease Gene Inactivated	Phenotypic Properties of Mutant Strain in Comparison with Parental Strain	References
Arg-gingipain (RgpA)	*rgp*A	Partial loss of Arg-gingipain activity • Loss of resistance to PMN phagocytosis Partial loss of ability to inhibit PMN function[1] Partial loss of adherence properties • Decrease in hemagglutination • Loss or altered expression of bacterial fimbriae • Deficient in adherence to other bacteria and type I collagen Loss of ability to degrade type I collagen Partial loss of virulence in mouse model of bacterial invasiveness	19, 53, 64, 73
Arg-gingipain (RgpB)	*rgp*B	Partial loss of Arg-gingipain activity Partial loss of ability to inhibit PMN function[1] Partial loss of adherence properties • Altered expression of bacterial fimbriae • Decreased adherence to other bacteria, as well as host epithelial cells, connective tissue matrix proteins, and type I collagen	56, 72
Arg-gingipain (RgpA and RgpB)	*rgp*A, *rgp*B	Complete loss of Arg-gingipain activity Loss of ability to inhibit PMN function[1] Loss of bacterial fimbriae Defective maturation of bacterial cell surface components	53, 56, 67
Lys-gingipain (Kgp)	*kgp*	Complete loss of Lys-gingipain activity Decreased hemagglutination • Loss of colony pigmentation • Decreased adsorption of hemoglobin and accumulation of heme Decreased fibrinogen degradation No loss of ability to inhibit PMN function[1] Partial loss of virulence in mouse model of bacterial invasiveness	46, 47, 59
Arg-gingipain and Lys-gingipain	*rgp*A, *rgp*B, *kgp*	Complete loss of Arg-gingipain and Lys-gingipain activity Complete loss of extracellular protease activity • Growth limitations on complex media Loss of hemagglutination • Loss of hemoglobin binding • Loss of colony pigmentation	67

[1] PMN function assessed by chemiluminescence.

Summary

Molecular studies have been instrumental in delineating the different proteolytic activities of *P. gingivalis* and their respective contributions to bacterial virulence. These findings are important to our understanding of the mechanisms of periodontal pathogenesis but also may provide a useful therapeutic approach to controlling periodontal diseases. Although the bacterial proteases are related to host-encoded enzymes, they are sufficiently different such that the development of inhibitors specifically targeting bacterial proteases has been proposed as a strategy for the development of a new generation of antibiotics.[77] An example of this approach is the very successful use of inhibitors targeting proteases of the HIV virus in the treatment of AIDS patients.[21,77] The increasing resistance of microorganisms to conventional antibiotics has fostered considerable interest in new microbial targets.

DISRUPTION OF HOST CELL COMMUNICATIONS: EPITHELIAL EXPRESSION OF INTERLEUKIN-8 (IL-8) AND INTERCELLULAR ADHESION MOLECULE-1 (ICAM-1)

Epithelium has traditionally been considered a mechanical barrier, providing protection to the underlying connective tissues. However, in recent years, mucosal epithelium has been increasingly recognized as a dynamic component in the communication network involved in recognizing and responding to microbial pathogens in the host environment.[35] In essence, the mucosal epithelium functions as a sensor of the adjacent bacterial population and sends signals to the underlying tissues to activate inflammatory and immune responses. This signaling process thus activates host systems that are central to host defenses.

The periodontal region is a unique mucosal interface. Bacterial populations accumulate on the nonshedding surface of the tooth adjacent to the sulcular and junctional epithelium that cover the underlying connective tissues. The responsiveness of periodontal tissues to the adjacent bacterial load is clearly evident in the inflammation of gingivitis and periodontitis. The first leukocyte to arrive at the site of infection is the neutrophil, which is the host immune cell that consistently predominates in the junctional epithelium and periodontal pocket in close proximity to the periodontal bacteria. The critical role of the neutrophil also is evident in that individuals with defects in neutrophil function suffer severe forms of periodontal disease (see Chapter 8). The processes leading to recruitment of neutrophils to the site of infection involve a series of events (see Chapter 7), many of which involve molecules generated by host cells in response to their recognition of bacteria. Two key molecules in the recruitment and localization of neutrophils are the chemokine interleukin-8 (IL-8) and the cell adhesion molecule known as *intercellular adhesion molecule-1 (ICAM-1)*. Over the last decade, molecular analyses have enabled a better understanding of the mechanisms by which these molecules control neutrophil distribution and function, as well as the role of periodontal bacteria in regulating these processes.

Distribution of IL-8 and ICAM-1 in the Periodontal Tissues

IL-8 is a proinflammatory chemokine, a potent chemoattractant and activator of neutrophils. IL-8 induces the neutrophil to express the integrin molecules, LFA-1 or Mac-1, on its cell surface and upregulates neutrophil binding activity. These integrin molecules, LFA-1 and Mac-1, bind to ICAM-1, an immunoglobulin-related glycoprotein found on host tissue cells.[15,50] The ability of neutrophils to migrate across epithelium is dependent on LFA-1 and Mac-1.[60] Thus IL-8 and ICAM-1 appear to be key molecules in the recruitment, localization, and activation of neutrophils.

IL-8 and ICAM-1 are produced in the epithelium of the lung, intestine, urinary tract, and gingival tissues in response to bacterial exposure. Histologic studies indicate that IL-8 and ICAM-1 are present in gingival tissues in both health and disease. IL-8 is localized to the epithelium, including the sulcular and junctional epithelium (Fig. 9-5).[17,27,74,75] ICAM-1 is strongly expressed in the junctional epithelium (Fig. 9-6), but minimal evidence of ICAM-1 has been found elsewhere in the gingival tissues.[27] The pattern of ICAM-1 distribution in particular indicates an increase in concentration toward the sulcular surface of the junctional epithelium. This pattern of distribution is closely matched by the tissue localization of neutrophils.[74,75] Thus studies of tissue localization are consistent with the role of IL-8 and ICAM-1 in recruiting neutrophils and facilitating their migration across the junctional epithelium.

Bacterial Modulation of IL-8 and ICAM-1 Protein Expression

A common approach to evaluating the effects of bacteria on epithelial cells is to incubate the bacteria with the host cells for an initial time period and then wash the cells and evaluate parameters of interest over time. Under these conditions, *A. actinomycetemcomitans* and *F. nucleatum,* as well as most other oral bacteria that have been examined, induce pronounced increases in oral epithelial cell secretion of IL-8 and expression of ICAM-1.[13,26,28] For example, when oral epithelial cells are challenged with *F. nucleatum,* increased secretion of IL-8 is evident at 2 hours after infection with a rapid accumulation of IL-8 in culture fluids (Fig. 9-7, *A*). In contrast to other bacteria, *P. gingivalis* induces a decrease of both IL-8 secretion and ICAM-1 expression in oral epithelial cells.[13,28] The decrease, or attenuation, in IL-8 in the extracellular fluids is observed by 2 hours after the initial epithelial challenge with the bacterial cells (Fig. 9-7, *B*). This distinctive effect of *P. gingivalis* has been of particular interest because of its potential role in bacterial evasion of the normal host response.

The attenuation of IL-8 levels by *P. gingivalis* may be accounted for in part by degradation of the IL-8 protein by the bacterial gingipains. However, *P. gingivalis* strains in which the gingipain genes *rgp*A, *rgp*B, or *kgp* are inactivated

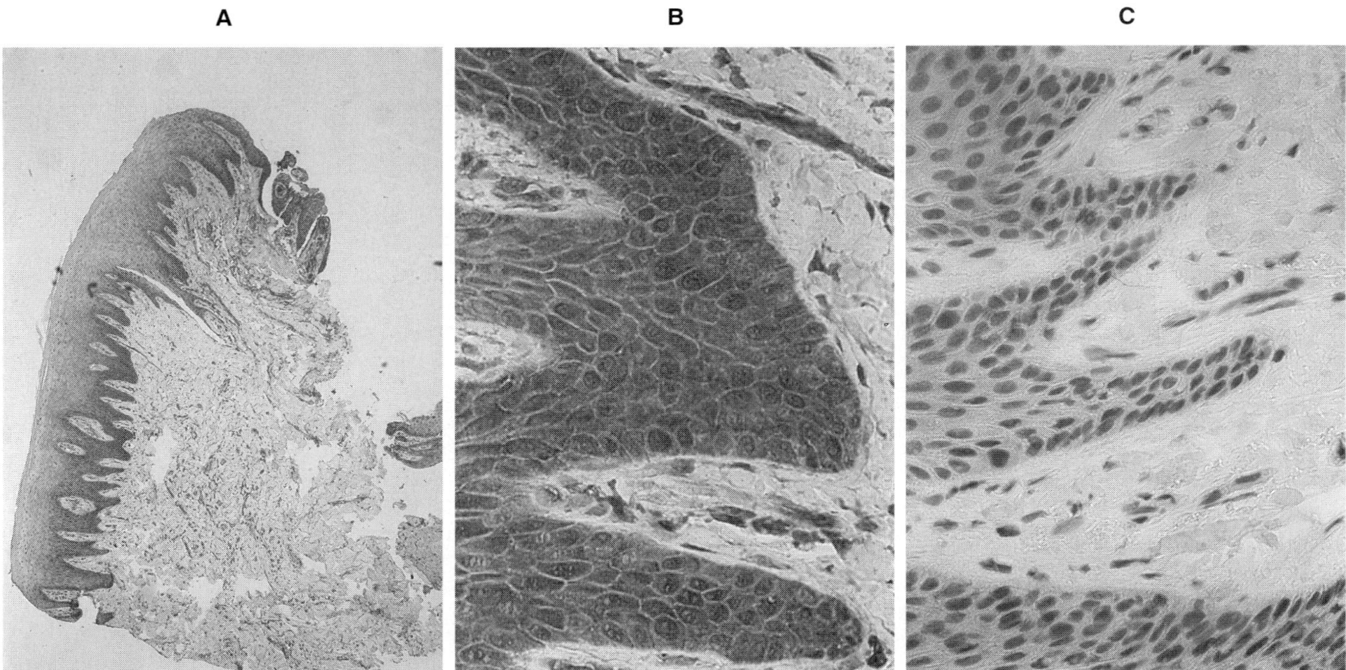

Fig. 9-5 IL-8 Immunohistochemical analysis of a diseased human gingival sample. The tissue samples were stained with antibody specific for human IL-8, or as a negative control nonimmune antibody. **A,** The diseased tissue demonstrates IL-8 staining in the basal and prickle cell layers of the gingival epithelium and in the junctional epithelium. Magnification ×40. **B,** Higher magnification of the basal layers of the epithelium demonstrating IL-8 staining. Magnification ×400. **C,** Control tissue from the same sample stained with nonimmune immunoglobulin. In comparison with **B,** this section demonstrates complete negative staining. Magnification ×400. (From Huang GT, Zhang X: Immunohistochemical analysis of interleukin-8 and intercellular adhesion molecule-1 in human gingival epithelium. Internat J Oral Biol 1999; 24:7.)

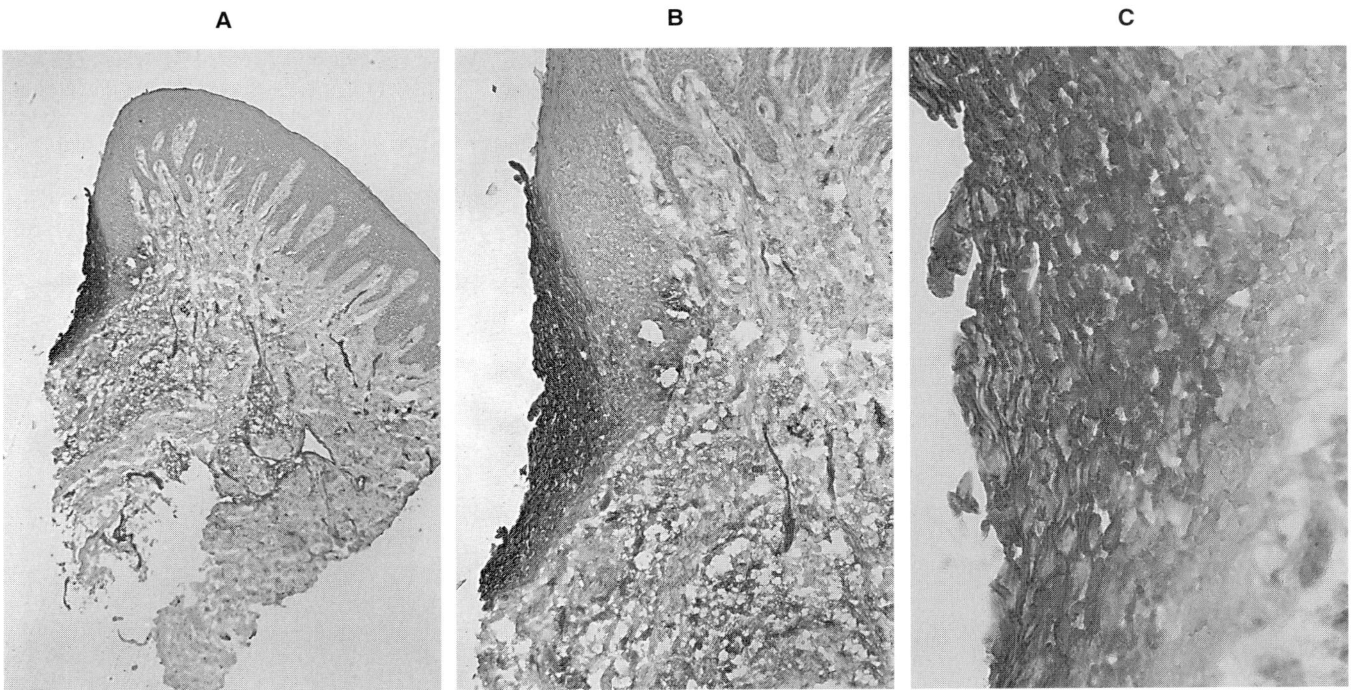

Fig. 9-6 ICAM-1 immunohistochemical analysis of a human gingival sample. The tissue samples were stained with a monoclonal antibody specific for human ICAM-1, or as a negative control nonimmune antibody. **A,** The tissues demonstrate no ICAM-1 in external gingival epithelium, but strong ICAM-1 staining is evident in the junctional epithelium. Magnification ×40. **B and C,** Higher-power views of the sulcular and junctional epithelium indicate increased ICAM-1 staining in the cells towards the sulcus or tooth surface. Magnification ×100 **(B)** and ×400 **(C).** (From Huang GT, Zhang X: Immunohistochemical analysis of interleukin-8 and intercellular adhesion molecule-1 in human gingival epithelium. Internat J Oral Biol 1999; 24:7.)

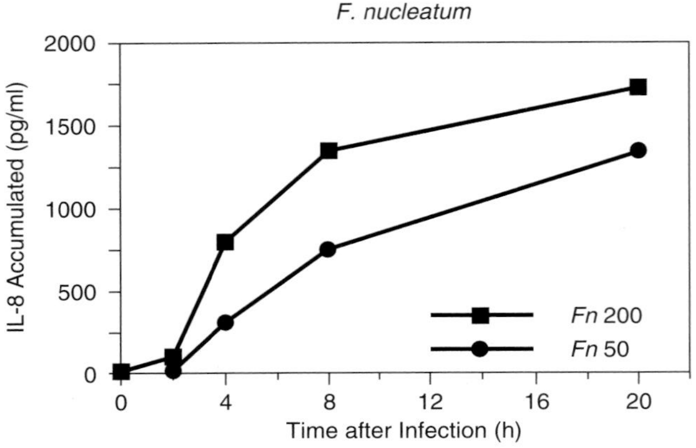

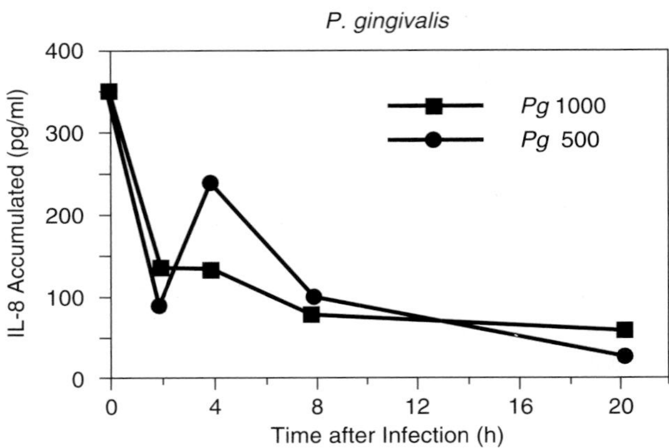

Fig. 9-7 Release of IL-8 by gingival epithelial cells following bacterial challenge. Epithelial cells were challenged by incubation with suspensions of either *F. nucleatum* or *P. gingivalis* for 2 hours. The cells then were washed and incubated with media containing antibiotics to kill any attached bacteria. At various time points, supernatant fluids were collected for measurement of IL-8 by enzyme-linked immunosorbant assay (ELISA). The ratio of bacterial cells per epithelial cell is indicated in the graph. For example, Fn 200 indicates that the results are from an assay using approximately 200 *F. nucleatum* cells per epithelial cell. *F. nucleatum* induced an increase in the secretion of IL-8 from the epithelial cells, whereas *P. gingivalis* causes an attenuation, or loss, of IL-8 from the supernatant. (From Huang GT, Kim D, Lee JK, et al: Interleukin-8 and intercellular adhesion molecule 1 regulation in oral epithelial cells by selected periodontal bacteria: Multiple effects of *Porphyromonas gingivalis* via antagonistic mechanisms. Infect Immun 2001; 69:1364.)

also produce the same IL-8 attenuation as the parental strains.[26] These findings suggest that proteases alone may not account for the alterations evident in IL-8 levels.

Bacterial Modulation of IL-8 mRNA Levels

Control of the level of protein expression can be regulated by degradation of the protein product, in this case IL-8. However, regulation also may occur via processes that govern the level of transcription and translation leading to the final protein product, and the level of specific mRNA in the cells is of interest in this regard. A Northern blot analysis used to evaluate IL-8 and ICAM-1 mRNA levels is presented in Fig. 9-8. The analysis involved probing mRNA samples isolated from the epithelial cells with radiolabeled IL-8- and ICAM-1-specific DNA. The DNA probe binds to complementary sequences in the mRNA sample, and the density of the labeled band reflects the concentration of the specific mRNA present. When oral epithelial cells are treated initially with either *F. nucleatum* or *P. gingivalis,* an increase occurs in IL-8 mRNA levels, peaking 2 to 4 hours after bacterial exposure, and then a decrease occurs in background levels. The levels of epithelial IL-8 mRNA from cells challenged with *F. nucleatum* (Fig. 9-8, panel B) is elevated over a 4-hour time period, regardless of whether the cells are challenged continuously (C) or only initially and then washed (W), as compared with untreated cells (mock). It can be seen that ICAM-1 mRNA levels also increase after *F. nucleatum* challenge. The human glyceraldehyde-3-phosphate dehydrogenase (GAPDH) mRNA levels are stable in the epithelial cells, so this probe provides a control to verify that equal amounts of total mRNA have been analyzed.

Northern analyses of mRNA samples from epithelial cells treated with *P. gingivalis* (Fig. 9-8, panel A) indicate that ICAM-1 mRNA levels are increased with either continuous (C) or initial (W) bacterial challenge. IL-8 mRNA levels also are elevated when epithelial cells are treated initially with the *P. gingivalis* cells (W). However, continuous incubation (C) of *P. gingivalis* with the epithelial cells results in a pronounced decrease of IL-8 mRNA levels (Fig. 9-8, panel A). Thus the *P. gingivalis* interaction with epithelial cells results in an initial increase or upregulation of IL-8 mRNA, followed by a decrease or downregulation of IL-8 mRNA. The mechanism of initial IL-8 mRNA upregulation may be similar to that used by other bacteria. The downregulation of IL-8 mRNA could result from either decreased transcription or an increased rate of IL-8 mRNA breakdown. The downregulation of IL-8 mRNA may be an important factor in the ability of *P. gingivalis* to attenuate IL-8 levels.

Summary

IL-8 and ICAM-1 are important molecules produced by epithelial cells in response to bacterial challenge. Most oral bacteria induce expression of these molecules, which function in the recruitment, localization, and activation of neutrophils. *P. gingivalis* possesses the novel ability to downregulate the expression of IL-8 and ICAM-1. The attenuation of IL-8 expression appears to result from a downregulation of IL-8 mRNA, probably in combination with degradation of the IL-8 protein. The regulation of IL-8 at the mRNA levels suggests that *P. gingivalis* is able to modulate the intercellular signaling pathways of the host epithelial cells, which govern gene

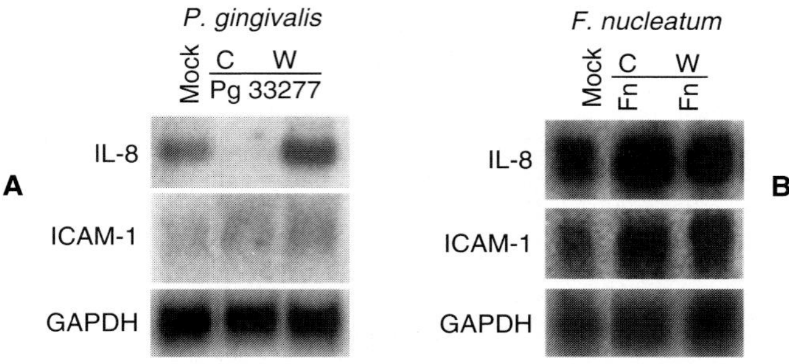

Fig. 9-8 Regulation of mRNA levels by gingival epithelial cells following bacterial challenge. Epithelial cells were challenged with *P. gingivalis* **(panel A)** or *F. nucleatum* **(panel B),** either continuously (C) for 4 hours or initially for 2 hours followed by washing and 2 hours of incubation with media without added bacterial cells (W). Control samples were incubated with media only for 4 hours (mock). RNA was isolated from the epithelial cells at 4 hours, and samples were probed with radiolabeled DNA probes specific for IL-8, ICAM-1, or human glyceraldehyde-3-phosphate dehydrogenase (GAPDH; a control for the amount of mRNA per sample). Initial and continuous incubation of *F. nucleatum* with the epithelial cells resulted in increases in the IL-8 and ICAM-1 mRNA, as reflected by the increased density of the reactive bands **(panel B).** Initial and continuous incubation of *P. gingivalis* with the epithelial cells resulted in increases in the ICAM-1 mRNA. In contrast, the level of IL-8 mRNA was increased with initial incubation, but greatly decreased with continuous incubation with *P. gingivalis.* (From Huang GT, Kim D, Lee JK, et al: Interleukin-8 and intercellular adhesion molecule 1 regulation in oral epithelial cells by selected periodontal bacteria: Multiple effects of *Porphyromonas gingivalis* via antagonistic mechanisms. Infect Immun 2001; 69:1364.)

regulation at either the transcriptional or posttranscriptional levels.

Understanding the molecular mechanisms involved in regulation provides insight into ability of bacteria to manipulate the host response. However, the goal is to understand the effects in the context of the host environment. In healthy individuals, large numbers of neutrophils are present at the site of periodontal lesions, and it is unlikely that *P. gingivalis* could block entirely neutrophil recruitment to the site. The ability of *P. gingivalis* to downregulate IL-8 may slow the recruitment of neutrophils sufficiently to provide an advantage for the bacterium in terms of host tissue degradation. In addition, the local levels of IL-8 may be diminished sufficiently to lessen neutrophil activation, thus lessening neutrophil-mediated phagocytosis of the local bacteria. The phenomena of *P. gingivalis* attenuation IL-8 expression has been referred to as *chemokine paralysis,*[13] and it provides a powerful approach by which the bacterium may be able to subvert host defenses. Further clarification of the mechanisms underlying these effects may lead to new strategies to counteract the effects of *P. gingivalis* on the periodontal tissues.

SUMMARY

As we enter the 21st century, a notable achievement in molecular biology has been the completion of genomic sequencing projects involving the human and bacterial genomes. Information on the genomes of human and periodontal microorganisms will open new avenues to investigate the molecular basis of the host-parasite interaction. It is important to recognize, however, that knowledge of DNA sequence is only one step in identifying and understanding genes that may be relevant to a disease such as periodontitis. A fundamental understanding of how a specific gene and its gene product participate in pathogenesis, and how that information can be used in assessment of risk and development of therapeutics, requires considerably more investigation. The examples discussed in this chapter represent some types of molecular approaches to the study of periodontal pathogenesis as well as potential prognostic and therapeutic implications that may result. Progress in delineating the molecular basis of periodontal pathogenesis in coming years will be greatly increased due to the tremendous advances in DNA sequence information and techniques for its use in molecular analyses.

REFERENCES

1. Aduse-Opoku J, Muir J, Slaney JM, et al: Characterization, genetic analysis, and expression of a protease antigen (PrpRI) of *Porphyromonas gingivalis* W50. Infect Immun 1995; 63:4744.
2. Baehni PC, Tsai CC, McArthur WP, et al: Leukotoxic activity in different strains of the bacterium *Actinobacillus actinomycetemcomitans* isolated from juvenile periodontitis in man. Arch Oral Biol 1981; 26:671.
3. Banbula A, Bugno M, Goldstein J, et al: Emerging family of proline-specific peptidases of *Porphyromonas gingivalis*: purification and characterization of serine dipeptidyl peptidase, a structural and functional homologue of mammalian prolyl dipeptidyl peptidase IV. Infect Immun 2000; 68:1176.
4. Banbula A, Bugno M, Kuster A, et al: Rapid and efficient inactivation of IL-6 gingipains, lysine- and arginine-specific proteinases from *Porphyromonas gingivalis*. Biochem Biophys Res Commun 1999; 261:598.
5. Banbula A, Mak P, Bugno M, et al: Prolyl tripeptidyl peptidase from *Porphyromonas gingivalis*. A novel enzyme with possible pathological implications for the development of periodontitis. J Biol Chem 1999; 274:9246.
6. Barkocy-Gallagher GA, Foley JW, Lantz MS: Activities of the *Porphyromonas gingivalis* PrtP proteinase determined by construction of *prt*P-deficient mutants and expression of the gene in *Bacteroides* species. J Bacteriol 1999; 181:246.
7. Barkocy-Gallagher GA, Han N, Patti JM, et al: Analysis of the prtP gene encoding porphypain, a cysteine proteinase of *Porphyromonas gingivalis*. J Bacteriol 1996; 178:2734.
8. Bramanti TE, Holt SC: Roles of porphyrins and host iron transport proteins in regulation of growth of *Porphyromonas gingivalis* W50. J Bacteriol 1991; 173:7330.
9. Brogan JM, Lally ET, Poulsen K, et al: Regulation of *Actinobacillus actinomycetemcomitans* leukotoxin expression: analysis of the promoter regions of leukotoxic and minimally leukotoxic strains. Infect Immun 1994; 62:501.
10. Bueno LC, Mayer MP, DiRienzo JM: Relationship between conversion of localized juvenile periodontitis-susceptible children from health to disease and *Actinobacillus actinomycetemcomitans* leukotoxin promoter structure. J Periodontol 1998; 69:998.
11. Calkins CC, Platt K, Potempa J, et al: Inactivation of tumor necrosis factor-alpha by proteinases (gingipains) from the periodontal pathogen, *Porphyromonas gingivalis*. Implications of immune evasion. J Biol Chem 1998; 273:6611.

12. Curtis MA, Kuramitsu HK, Lantz M, et al: Molecular genetics and nomenclature of proteases of *Porphyromonas gingivalis*. J Periodontal Res 1999; 34:464.
13. Darveau RP, Belton CM, Reife RA, et al: Local chemokine paralysis, a novel pathogenic mechanism for *Porphyromonas gingivalis*. Infect Immun 1998; 66:1660.
14. Dashper SG, Kandasamy S, O'Brien-Simpson N, et al: Amino acid and peptide uptake by *Porphyromonas gingivalis*. J Dent Res 1998; 77:1133.
15. Diamond MS, Staunton DE, de Fougerolles AR, et al: ICAM-1 (CD54): a counter-receptor for Mac-1 (CD11b/CD18). J Cell Biol 1990; 111:3129.
16. Discipio RG, Daffern PJ, Kawahara M, et al: Cleavage of human complement component C5 by cysteine proteinases from *Porphyromonas (Bacteroides) gingivalis*. Prior oxidation of C5 augments proteinase digestion of C5. Immunology 1996; 87:660.
17. Fitzgerald JE, Kreutzer DL: Localization of interleukin-8 in human gingival tissues. Oral Microbiol Immunol 1995; 10:297.
18. Fletcher HM, Schenkein HA, Macrina FL: Cloning and characterization of a new protease gene (*prtH*) from *Porphyromonas gingivalis*. Infect Immun 1994; 62:4279.
19. Fletcher HM, Schenkein HA, Morgan RM, et al: Virulence of a *Porphyromonas gingivalis* W83 mutant defective in the *prtH* gene. Infect Immun 1995;63:1521.
20. Fletcher J, Nair S, Poole S, et al: Cytokine degradation by biofilms of *Porphyromonas gingivalis*. Curr Microbiol 1998; 36:216.
21. Flexner C: HIV-protease inhibitors. N Engl J Med 1998; 338:1281.
22. Guthmiller JM, Kolodrubetz D, Kraig E: Mutational analysis of the putative leukotoxin transport genes in *Actinobacillus actinomycetemcomitans*. Microb Path 1995; 18:307.
23. Haraszthy VI, Hariharan G, Tinoco EM, et al: Evidence for the role of highly leukotoxic *Actinobacillus actinomycetemcomitans* in the pathogenesis of localized juvenile and other forms of early-onset periodontitis [In Process Citation]. J Periodontol 2000; 71:912.
24. Holt SC, Ebersole J, Felton J, et al: Implantation of *Bacteroides gingivalis* in nonhuman primates initiates progression of periodontitis. Science 1988; 239:55.
25. Hritz M, Fisher E, Demuth DR: Differential regulation of the leukotoxin operon in highly leukotoxic and minimally leukotoxic strains of *Actinobacillus actinomycetemcomitans*. Infect Immun 1996; 64:2724.
26. Huang GT, Kim D, Lee JK, et al: Interleukin-8 and intercellular adhesion molecule 1 regulation in oral epithelial cells by selected periodontal bacteria: Multiple effects of *Porphyromonas gingivalis* via antagonistic mechanisms. Infect Immun 2001; 69:1364.
27. Huang GT, Zhang X: Immunohistochemical analysis of interleukin-8 and intercellular adhesion molecule-1 in human gingival epithelium. Int J Oral Biol 1999; 24:7.
28. Huang GT-J, Kinder Haake S, Kim J-W, et al: Differential expression of interleukin-8 and intercellular adhesion molecule-1 by human gingival epithelial cells in response to *Actinobacillus actinomycetemcomitans* or *Porphyromonas gingivalis* infection. Oral Microbiol Immunol 1998; 13:301.
29. Imamura T, Pike RN, Potempa J, et al: Pathogenesis of periodontitis: a major arginine-specific cysteine proteinase from *Porphyromonas gingivalis* induces vascular permeability enhancement through activation of the kallikrein/kinin pathway. J Clin Invest 1994; 94:361.
30. Imamura T, Potempa J, Tanase S, et al: Activation of blood coagulation factor X by arginine-specific cysteine proteinases (gingipain-Rs) from *Porphyromonas gingivalis*. J Biol Chem 1997; 272:16062.
31. Imamura T, Potempa J, Travis J, et al: Comparison of pathogenic properties between two types of arginine-specific cysteine proteinases (gingipains-R) from *Porphyromonas gingivalis*. Microb Pathog 2000; 29:155.
32. Jagels MA, Travis J, Potempa J, et al: Proteolytic inactivation of the leukocyte C5a receptor by proteinases derived from *Porphyromonas gingivalis*. Infect Immun 1996; 64:1984.
33. Kachlany SC, Fine DH, Figurski DH: Secretion of RTX leukotoxin by *Actinobacillus actinomycetemcomitans*. Infect Immun 2000; 68:6094.
34. Kadowaki T, Nakayama K, Yoshimura F, et al: Arg-gingipain acts as a major processing enzyme for various cell surface proteins in *Porphyromonas gingivalis*. J Biol Chem 1998; 273:29072.
35. Kagnoff MF, Eckmann L: Epithelial cells as sensors for microbial infection. J Clin Invest 1997; 100:6.
36. Kato T, Takahashi N, Kuramitsu HK: Sequence analysis and characterization of the *Porphyromonas gingivalis prt*C gene, which expresses a novel collagenase activity. J Bacteriol 1992; 174:3889.
37. Kirszbaum L, Sotiropoulos C, Jackson C, et al: Complete nucleotide sequence of a gene *prtR* of *Porphyromonas gingivalis* W50 encoding a 132 kDa protein that contains an arginine-specific thiol endopeptidase domain and a haemagglutinin domain. Biochem Biophys Res Comm 1995; 207:424.
38. Kiyama M, Hayakawa M, Shiroza T, et al: Sequence analysis of the *Porphyromonas gingivalis* dipeptidyl peptidase IV gene. Biochim Biophys Acta 1998; 1396:39.
39. Korostoff J, Wang JF, Kieba I, et al: *Actinobacillus actinomycetemcomitans* leukotoxin induces apoptosis in HL-60 cells. Infect Immun 1998; 66:4474.
40. Korostoff J, Yamaguchi N, Miller M, et al: Perturbation of mitochondrial structure and function plays a central role in *Actinobacillus actinomycetemcomitans* leukotoxin-induced apoptosis. Microb Pathog 2000; 29:267.
41. Kraig E, Dailey T, Kolodrubetz D: Nucleotide sequence of the leukotoxin gene from *Actinobacillus actinomycetemcomitans*: homology to the alpha-hemolysin/leukotoxin gene family. Infect Immun 1990; 58:920.
42. Kumagai Y, Konishi K, Gomi T, et al: Enzymatic properties of dipeptidyl aminopeptidase IV produced by the periodontal pathogen *Porphyromonas gingivalis* and its participation in virulence. Infect Immun 2000; 68:716.
43. Lally ET, Golub EE, Kieba IR, et al: Analysis of the *Actinobacillus actinomycetemcomitans* leukotoxin gene. Delineation of unique features and comparison to homologous toxins. J Biol Chem 1989; 264:15451.
44. Lally ET, Kieba IR, Sato A, et al: RTX toxins recognize a beta2 integrin on the surface of human target cells. J Biol Chem 1997; 272:30463.
45. Lear JD, Furblur UG, Lally ET, et al: *Actinobacillus actinomycetemcomitans* leukotoxin forms large conductance, voltage-gated ion channels when incorporated into planar lipid bilayers. Biochim Biophys Acta 1995; 1238:34.
46. Lewis JP, Dawson JA, Hannis JC, et al. Hemoglobinase activity of the lysine gingipain protease (Kgp) of *Porphyromonas gingivalis* W83. J Bacteriol 1999; 181:4905.
47. Lewis JP, Macrina FL: IS195, an insertion sequence-like element associated with protease genes in *Porphyromonas gingivalis*. Infect Immun 1998; 66:3035.
48. Malek R, Fisher JG, Caleca A, et al: Inactivation of the *Porphyromonas gingivalis fim*A gene blocks periodontal damage in gnotobiotic rats. J Bacteriol 1994; 176:1052.
49. Mangan DF, Taichman NS, Lally ET, et al: Lethal effects of *Actinobacillus actinomycetemcomitans* leukotoxin on human T lymphocytes. Infect Immun 1991; 59:3267.
50. Marlin SD, Springer TA: Purified intercellular adhesion mol-

ecule-1 (ICAM-1) is a ligand for lymphocyte function-associated antigen 1 (LFA-1). Cell 1987; 51:813.

51. Marsh PD, McDermid AS, McKee AS, et al: The effect of growth rate and haemin on the virulence and proteolytic activity of *Porphyromonas gingivalis* W50. Microbiol 1994; 140:861.
52. Mikolajczyk-Pawlinska J, Travis J, Potempa J, et al: Modulation of interleukin-8 activity by gingipains from *Porphyromonas gingivalis*: implications for pathogenicity of periodontal disease. FEBS Lett 1998; 440:282.
53. Nakayama K, Kadowaki T, Okamoto K, et al: Construction and characterization of arginine-specific cysteine proteinase (Arg-gingipain)–deficient mutants of *Porphyromonas gingivalis*. Evidence for significant contribution of Arg-gingipain to virulence. J Biol Chem 1995; 270:23619.
54. Nakayama K, Ratnayake DB, Tsukuba T, et al: Haemoglobin receptor protein is intragenically encoded by the cysteine proteinase-encoding genes and the haemagglutinin-encoding gene of *Porphyromonas gingivalis*. Mol Microbiol 1998; 27:51.
55. Nakayama K, Slakeski N, Bhogal PS, et al: Domain-specific rearrangement between the two Arg-gingipain-encoding genes in *Porphyromonas gingivalis*: possible involvement of nonreciprocal recombination. Microbiol Immunol 1997; 41:185.
56. Nakayama K, Yoshimura F, Kadowaki T, et al: Involvement of arginine-specific cysteine proteinase (Arg-gingipain) in fimbriation of *Porphyromonas gingivalis*. J Bacteriol 1996; 178:2818.
57. Nelson D, Potempa J, Kordula T, et al: Purification and characterization of a novel cysteine proteinase (periodontain) from *Porphyromonas gingivalis*. Evidence for a role in the inactivation of human alpha1-proteinase inhibitor. J Biol Chem 1999; 274:12245.
58. Okamoto K, Misumi Y, Kadowaki T, et al: Structure characterization of argingipain, a novel arginine-specific cysteine proteinase as a major periodontal pathogenic factor from *Porphyromonas gingivalis*. Arch Biochem Biophy 1995; 316:917.
59. Okamoto K, Nakayama K, Kadowaki T, et al: Involvement of a lysine-specific cysteine proteinase in hemoglobin adsorption and heme accumulation by *Porphyromonas gingivalis*. J Biol Chem 1998; 273:21225.
60. Parkos CA, Delp C, Arnaout MA, et al: Neutrophil migration across a cultured intestinal epithelium. Dependence on a CD11b/CD18-mediated event and enhanced efficiency in physiological direction. J Clin Invest 1991; 88:1605.
61. Pavloff N, Pemberton PA, Potempa J, et al: Molecular cloning and characterization of *Porphyromonas gingivalis* lysine-specific gingipain. A new member of an emerging family of pathogenic bacterial cysteine proteinases. J Biol Chem 1997; 272:1595.
62. Pavloff N, Potempa J, Pike RN, et al: Molecular cloning and structural characterization of the Arg-gingipain proteinase of *Porphyromonas gingivalis*. Biosynthesis as a proteinase-adhesin polyprotein. J Biol Chem 1995; 270:1007.
63. Pike RN, Potempa J, McGraw W, et al: Characterization of the binding activities of proteinase-adhesin complexes from *Porphyromonas gingivalis*. J Bacteriol 1996; 178:2876.
64. Schenkein HA: Etiology of localized juvenile periodontitis. J Periodontol 1998; 69:1068.
65. Schenkein HA, Fletcher HM, Bodnar M, et al: Increased opsonization of a *prt*H-defective mutant of *Porphyromonas gingivalis* W83 is caused by reduced degradation of complement-derived opsonins. J Immunol 1995; 154:5331.
66. Shenker BJ, Vitale LA, Keiba I, et al: Flow cytometric analysis of the cytotoxic effects of *Actinobacillus actinomycetemcomitans* leukotoxin on human natural killer cells. J Leukoc Biol 1994; 55:153.
67. Shi Y, Ratnayake DB, Okamoto K, et al: Genetic analyses of proteolysis, hemoglobin binding, and hemagglutination of *Porphyromonas gingivalis*. Construction of mutants with a combination of *rgp*A, *rgp*B, *kgp*, and *hag*A. J Biol Chem 1999; 274:17955.
68. Slakeski N, Bhogal PS, O'Brien-Simpson NM, et al: Characterization of a second cell-associated Arg-specific cysteine proteinase of *Porphyromonas gingivalis* and identification of an adhesin-binding motif involved in association of the *prt*R and *prt*K proteinases and adhesins into large complexes. Microbiol 1998; 144:1583.
69. Stanley P, Koronakis V, Hughes C: Acylation of *Escherichia coli* hemolysin: a unique protein lipidation mechanism underlying toxin function. Microbiol Mol Biol Rev 1998; 62:309.
70. Sugawara S, Nemoto E, Tada H, et al: Proteolysis of human monocyte CD14 by cysteine proteinases (gingipains) from *Porphyromonas gingivalis* leading to lipopolysaccharide hyporesponsiveness. J Immunol 2000; 165:411.
71. Taichman NS, Dean RT, Sanderson CJ: Biochemical and morphological characterization of the killing of human monocytes by a leukotoxin derived from *Actinobacillus actinomycetemcomitans*. Infect Immun 1980; 28:258.
72. Tokuda M, Duncan M, Cho MI, et al: Role of *Porphyromonas gingivalis* protease activity in colonization of oral surfaces. Infect Immun 1996; 64:4067.
73. Tokuda M, Karunakaran T, Duncan M, et al: Role of Arg-gingipain A in virulence of *Porphyromonas gingivalis*. Infect Immun 1998; 66:1159.
74. Tonetti MS: Molecular factors associated with compartmentalization on gingival immune responses and transepithelial neutrophil migration. J Periodontal Res 1997; 32:104.
75. Tonetti MS, Imboden MA, Gerber L, et al: Localized expression of mRNA for phagocyte-specific chemotactic cytokines in human periodontal infections. Infect Immun 1994; 62:4005.
76. Travis J, Banbula A, Potempa J: The role of bacterial and host proteinases in periodontal disease. In: Langer J, Ansorge S (eds): Cellular Peptidases in Immune Functions and Diseases 2. New York, Kluwer Acedemic/Plenum, 2000.
77. Travis J, Potempa J: Bacterial proteinases as targets for the development of second-generation antibiotics. Biochim Biophys Acta 2000; 1477:35.
78. Tsai CC, McArthur WP, Baehni PC, et al: Extraction and partial characterization of a leukotoxin from a plaque-derived Gram-negative microorganism. Infect Immun 1979; 25:427.
79. Wang JF, Kieba IR, Korostoff J, et al: Molecular and biochemical mechanisms of *Pasteurella haemolytica* leukotoxin-induced cell death. Microb Pathog 1998; 25:317.
80. Wingrove JA, DiScipio RG, Chen Z, et al: Activation of complement components C3 and C5 by a cysteine proteinase (gingipain-1) from *Porphyromonas* (*Bacteroides*) *gingivalis*. J Biol Chem 1992; 267:18902.

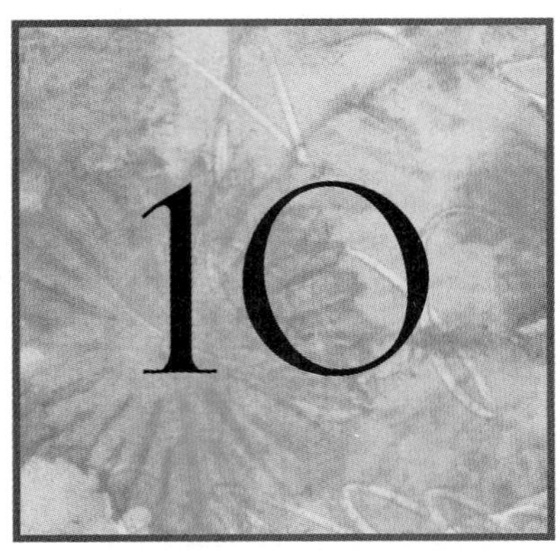

CHAPTER

Genetic Factors Associated with Periodontal Disease

Bryan S. Michalowicz and Bruce L. Pihlstrom

CHAPTER OUTLINE

Traditionally, periodontitis was thought to be strictly environmental in origin. Despite this belief, it was recognized that only a portion of the variability of disease in the population could be explained by environmental factors alone. In a classic longitudinal study of the natural history of periodontitis, Löe et al[51] found that among individuals with poor oral hygiene and no access to dental care, some developed disease at a rapid rate whereas others experienced little or no disease. This variation must have been attributable to either unrecognized components of the environment or differences among individuals in their susceptibilities to disease. Because host susceptibility may be defined in terms of genetic variation, a relatively recent focus in periodontology has been to quantify genetic risk and identify specific gene variants that determine disease susceptibility. At present, the specific role that genes play in defining susceptibility remains largely unknown. The purpose of this chapter is to provide the reader with a brief overview of some approaches used to ascertain genetic risk and to discuss genetic risk factors for the various forms of periodontal disease.

The American Academy of Periodontology recently established a new diagnostic scheme for the periodontal diseases (see Chapter 4). Diagnoses are now based primarily on the rate of disease progression. The terms *localized juvenile periodontitis* and *generalized juvenile periodontitis* have been replaced with *localized aggressive periodontitis* and *generalized aggressive periodontitis*, respectively. Although aggressive periodontitis, by definition, can occur at any age, it usually has a circumpubertal onset. Previously, juvenile periodontitis was defined within a relatively narrow age range—from puberty to the early 20s. The term *chronic periodontitis* is now used to describe any slow or moderately progressing disease. Previously, *adult periodontitis* referred to chronic disease in patients 35 years of age or older. Because the studies described in this chapter were based on the previous diagnostic classifications, which included these important age restrictions, the former terminology is used when referring to diseases.

Portions of this chapter were adapted from: Pihlstrom BL, Michalowicz BS: Genetic risk for periodontal diseases: A clinical perspective. Journal de Paradontologie D'Implantologie Orale, 1998; 17:123.

OVERVIEW OF GENETIC STUDY DESIGNS

A person's unique genetic code is contained in the sequences of nucleotide bases (adenine, thymine, cytosine, and guanine), which make up deoxyribonucleic acid (DNA). The human genome consists of more than 3 billion pairs of bases contained in 22 pairs of chromosomes, termed *autosomes,* and two sex chromosomes (Fig. 10-1). Genes are sequences of nucleotide bases contained in noncontiguous segments called *exons.* The exons provide the DNA template for the subsequent synthesis of polypeptides that regulate all developmental, physiologic, and immunologic processes in the body. Recent estimates indicate that the human genome contains about 25,000 to 35,000 genes.[95]

The genetic composition of an organism is termed the *genotype,* and the collection of traits or characteristics is termed the *phenotype.* The phenotype is determined by the interaction of genes and the environment.[50] Traits and diseases might be caused by a single gene (monogenic), several genes (oligogenic), or many genes (polygenic). Diseases whose etiologies include both genetic and environmental factors are referred to as *multifactorial.* Most common diseases are multifactorial.

Specific locations on chromosomes are referred to as **loci,** and variations in the nucleotide sequence at a locus are termed **alleles.** At a given locus, an individual is considered homozygous if the alleles are identical on homologous chromosomes or heterozygous if the alleles are different. Some alleles are associated with profound changes in the phenotype, whereas others have no measurable effects. Phenotypic differences in the population may be caused by the effects of alleles in the coding region of a gene or in flanking noncoding regions that control gene transcription or expression.

The term **genetic marker** refers to any gene or nucleotide sequence that can be mapped to a specific location or region on a chromosome. From a genetic epidemiologic viewpoint, any marker that is sufficiently polymorphic, or variable, in the population can be used to map or locate disease alleles. Finally, there is an important distinction between the role of genes in monogenic disorders such as Huntington's disease and their role in complex multifactorial diseases such as periodontitis. In monogenic disorders, genes are referred to as *causative* because nearly everyone with the mutation develops the condition. Environmental factors generally play a minor role in determining the phenotype. In contrast, genes involved in complex multifactorial diseases are often referred to as *susceptibility genes* (or more correctly, *susceptibility alleles*). For these diseases, individuals who inherit susceptibility alleles will not develop disease unless they are exposed to deleterious environments. For the periodontal diseases, important environmental risk factors include gram-negative anaerobic microorganisms, cigarette smoking, and poor oral hygiene.

The theory that genes influence susceptibility to common diseases such as periodontitis is not new or revolutionary. Given its complex etiology and pathogenesis, variations in any number or combination of genes that control the development of the periodontal tissues or the competency of the cellular and humoral immune systems could affect an individual's risk for disease. In

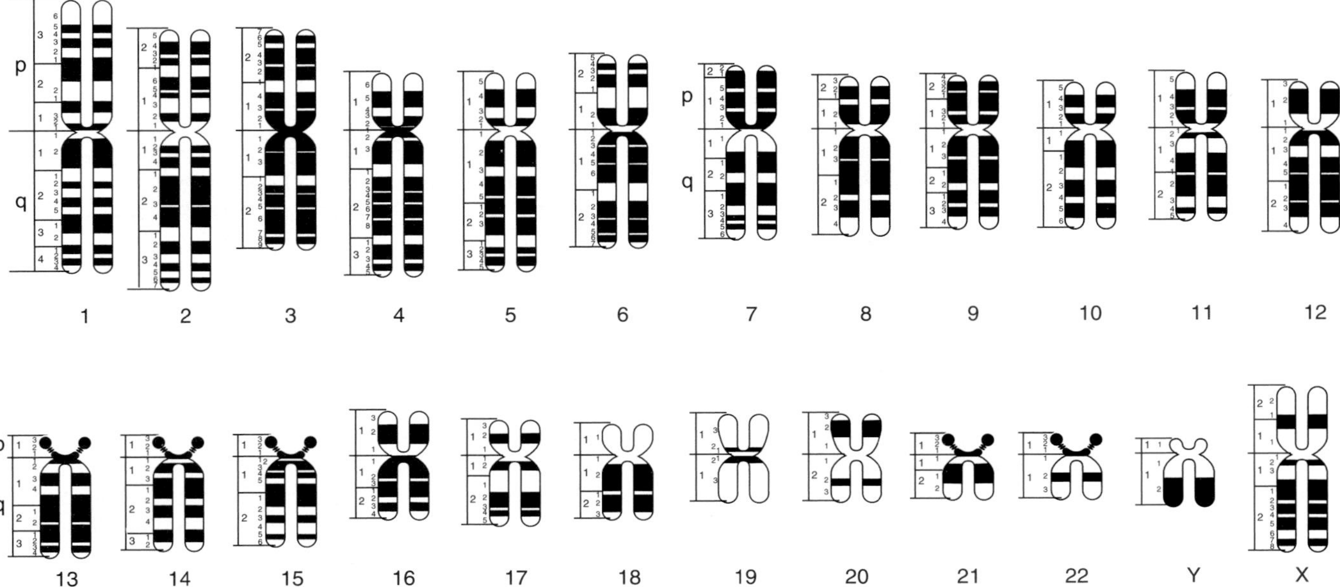

Fig. 10-1 The nomenclature used to locate positions along chromosomes is based on the physical appearance and staining patterns of chromosomes viewed during prophase or early metaphase. Each chromosome contains a short arm (p, or petite) and long arm (q). In this schematic, termed an *ideogram,* the chromosomes are depicted as they appear following Giemsa staining (hence the term *G banding patterns*). Genes are located based on their positions within these bands. For example, 11q23 denotes a position in the third band of the second region on the long arm of chromosome 11. Sub-bands are designated by decimal points (e.g., 11q23.2). (From Jorde LB, Carey JC, White RL [eds]: Medical Genetics. St Louis, Mosby, 1995.)

fact, critics might argue that every trait and disease likely has some genetic variation and that merely confirming this fact has little or no practical value. Once the genetic basis for a disease has been established, it is equally important to determine which alleles have a measurable effect on the phenotype and whether the prevention, diagnosis, or treatment of the disease can be improved once disease alleles are identified. The former issue can be addressed in a systematic but nontrivial manner. The latter issue is more complex and involves debate on scientific, ethical, and public health grounds.

Segregation Analyses

Inherited diseases "run" in families. The pattern in which the disease is transmitted across generations depends on whether the disease alleles lie on autosomes or sex chromosomes, whether they are dominant or recessive, and whether they are fully or partially penetrant. Generally, a **dominant** allele determines the phenotype in a heterozygote with another recessive allele. A **recessive** allele determines the phenotype only when present at both loci on homologous chromosomes. **Penetrance** refers to the probability that a particular phenotype will result from a genotype. **Partially penetrant** means that only a fraction of individuals who inherit the disease alleles will be affected.

In segregation analyses, the observed pattern of disease in families is compared with patterns expected under various models of inheritance. The statistical power of this design depends on the number and composition of the families and the heterogeneity of the disease. **Heterogeneity** means that there are different causes of disease among families. Generally, segregation analyses have low power to resolve heterogeneity. Segregation analyses also cannot distinguish between genetic effects and unmeasured environmental causes of disease, such as the transmission of pathogenic organisms within families.[21]

Twin Studies

The relative influence of genetic and environmental factors on complex diseases can be estimated using twin data. **In the classic twin study, reared-together monozygotic and dizygotic twins are compared to estimate the effects of shared genes. Monozygotic (MZ)** twins are genetically identical, whereas **dizygotic (DZ)** or fraternal twins share on average 50% of their genes by descent. For binary traits (present or absent) a genetic effect is inferred if the positive **concordance rate,** or percentage of twin pairs in which both twins are affected, is greater for MZ than DZ twins. For continuous measures, such as periodontal probing depth or attachment loss, intraclass correlations are calculated. These correlations reflect the variation between twin pairs relative to the variation within pairs. Typically, twin data are used to estimate **heritability,** which is the proportion of phenotypic variation attributed to genetic variation. A heritability estimate of 50% means that one half of the variance in the population is attributed to genetic variance. It does not mean that there is a 50% chance that offspring of affected parents will be affected. Very large samples of reared-together twins are needed to estimate heritability with precision.

Heritability also can be estimated from MZ twins who are separated at birth and raised apart. Because they do not share a common environment, similarities between such twins may be attributed to the effects of shared genes. (Raised-apart twins also share an environment in utero. To the extent that this environment affects the disease, heritability estimates from MZ twins raised apart may be artificially inflated.) Although more powerful than the classic twin design, few such studies have been conducted because of the scarcity of such twins.

Regardless of the method of estimation, heritability pertains to populations and not individuals. Furthermore, such estimates describe the impact of genes on specific populations exposed to a particular range of environments. Finally, twin studies alone cannot be used to determine the mode of inheritance of a disorder or the number or location of disease alleles.

Linkage and Association Studies

Linkage and association studies are used to map disease alleles to specific regions on chromosomes. These studies exploit a unique feature of the way in which alleles segregate during meiosis. During gametogenesis, diploid cells (containing 2N copies of each allele) divide to become haploid (containing only one copy of each parental allele). The probability that two alleles at different loci will recombine (termed a *recombination* or *crossover event*) is generally proportional to the distance between them. Two alleles selected at random from the genome will likely recombine, and the chance that any two maternal or paternal alleles will be transmitted together to an offspring is 50%. Alleles at nearby loci, however, tend to segregate together; that is, they are linked. By identifying genetic markers that segregate with disease, researchers can infer the location of putative disease alleles. It is not necessary for the same marker allele to be transmitted with the disease allele in all affected families, and a marker that is linked to the disease allele within a family may not be associated with disease in the population. **Allelic associations (linkage disequilibrium) occur when the *same* marker allele is linked to disease in multiple families** (Fig. 10-2).

Linkage studies use sets of families, or pedigrees, with multiple affected individuals. Genotypes are determined for affected and unaffected family members, and complex statistical models are used to determine whether the marker allele(s) and disease cosegregate in the families under a given inheritance model. Parameters that must be specified in the model include the mode of inheritance, frequency of the marker allele in the population, and disease penetrance. The summary statistic used to assess linkage is the **logarithm of the odds (LOD) score,** which is a measure of the likelihood that the marker and disease alleles are linked versus not linked at a given recombination rate. Although linkage analyses are typically conducted for qualitative traits or diseases, methods to evaluate linkage for quantitative traits or

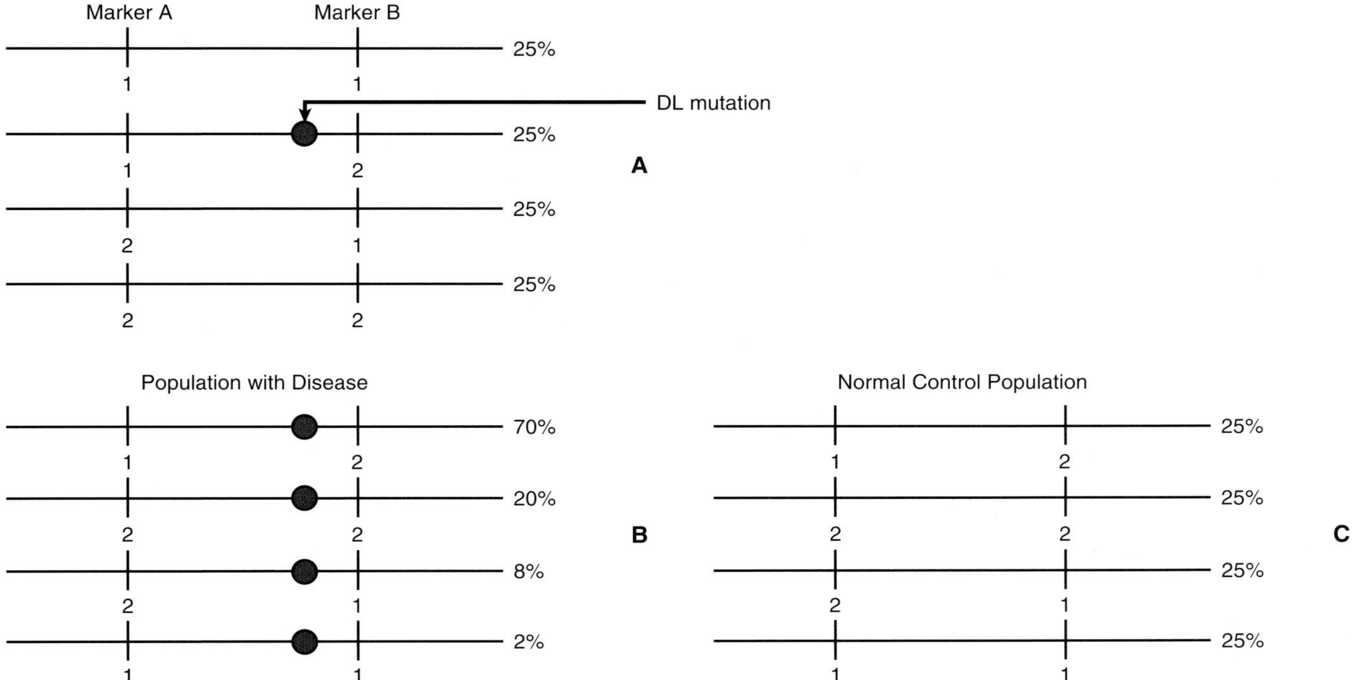

Fig. 10-2 Linkage disequilibrium between a disease locus (DL) and two linked loci, **A** and **B.** The DL mutation first arises on the chromosome with the A_1B_2 haplotype. After a number of generations, most chromosomes carrying the DL mutation still have the A_1B_2 haplotype, but as a result of recombination the DL mutation is also found on other haplotypes. Because the A_1B_2 haplotype is seen in 70% of DL chromosomes but only 25% of normal chromosomes, there is linkage disequilibrium between the DL and loci A and B. Because locus B is closer to DL, it is in greater linkage disequilibrium with DL than is locus A. (Modified from Jorde LB, Carey JC, White RL [eds]: Medical Genetics. St Louis, Mosby, 1995.)

measures have been developed. Once linkage to a particular region has been established, the task of identifying the actual disease allele or mutation is far from trivial. Linkage can be detected if the marker and disease alleles are within 20 to 30 centiMorgans (cM) of one another. In humans, 1 cM represents approximately 1 million nucleotide bases. Because sequencing 20 million to 30 million base pairs in search of mutations remains a daunting task at present, fine marker mapping is used to further refine the regions of interest. Fortunately, given the rapid progress in decoding the human genome, it will soon be possible to identify all nearby candidate genes for study once linkage is established.

To test for associations (linkage disequilibrium), the frequency of alleles at a given locus is compared between subjects with disease (cases) and healthy controls sampled from the same population. Although commonly used in genetic epidemiology, results from case-control studies should be interpreted with caution. An association does not necessarily imply a biologic link between the disease and an allele. It may be due to some environmental component causing both the marker and the disease to increase in the population, an unrecognized difference in the racial or ethnic makeup of the cases and controls, or chance alone.[13] The finding of true linkage disequilibrium in an outbred and random mating population implies that the disease and marker alleles lie very close to one another on a chromosome.

Associations (linkage disequilibrium) suggest that the presence of an allele confers risk for disease within a defined environment. This later qualification is essential when discussing common multifactorial diseases such as periodontitis. Alleles that can be used to predict disease in one population may not be useful in other populations or even in the same population when exposed to markedly different environments. For example, suppose a gene that influences the humoral response to a particular class of bacterial antigens is polymorphic in the population. Individuals with the low-response, or "disease," allele cannot effectively suppress the growth of pathogenic microorganisms that express these antigens. In the presence of the pathogens, individuals with the low-response allele develop disease. On the other hand, no relationship may exist between the disease and this allele in populations where the particular bacteria are either never or only rarely present. Therefore the notion of "high-risk" alleles may be specific to an environment.

EARLY ONSET PERIODONTAL DISEASES

The early onset periodontal diseases (EOP) are a group of diseases—prepubertal, juvenile, and rapidly progressive periodontitis—that occur in children, adolescents, and young adults. The rate of periodontal destruction is greater in EOP than in the more common adult or chronic form. Although diagnoses are based on clinical and radiographic criteria, the immunologic and microbiologic profiles can vary substantially within the subforms. This variability complicates the search for disease alleles because multiple causes of the same phenotype (etiologic heterogeneity) and different genetic risk factors acting in different subpopulations (genetic heterogeneity) may exist. Most studies of the EOP to date have had inadequate statistical power to resolve substantial genetic heterogeneity. The variability in the clinical presentation of these diseases and the limited criteria used to establish disease diagnoses also have made the search for susceptibility genes more difficult. Nonetheless, evidence from a variety of sources suggests that the risk for EOP may be substantially heritable.[83]

Associations with Genetic and Inherited Conditions

Early onset periodontitis is a consistent feature in a number of inherited or genetic disorders (Table 10-1). These disorders, which have been discussed in detail by Soafer[87] and Hart,[39] demonstrate the ways in which major genes can affect risk for EOP. The disorders have been grouped according to the resultant protein or biochemical defect(s)—the mutant alleles may affect the function of phagocytic immune cells or the structure of epithelia, connective tissue, or the teeth themselves. For some conditions, the specific gene or tissue defect responsible for the condition has been identified; for others, it has not.

Hypophosphatsia is a rare disorder caused by mutations in the tissue-nonspecific alkaline phosphatase gene (1p36.1-p34).[77] These mutations lead to a deficiency in alkaline phosphatase that results in abnormal bone mineralization, skeletal anomalies, and cementum hypoplasia. Both autosomal dominant forms and recessive forms have been reported. Although the infantile form is usually fatal, milder forms can occur in children and adults. The condition leads to the premature loss of the primary and occasionally the permanent teeth.[14]

Papillon-Lefèvre Syndrome (PLS) is a rare autosomal recessive disorder characterized by palmoplantar hyperkeratosis and early onset periodontitis (Color Fig. 10-1).[28,38] Both the primary dentitions and secondary dentitions can be affected. PLS is caused by mutations in the cathepsin C gene, located on chromosome 11 (11q14-q21).[33,93]

Cathepsin C is a cysteine protease normally expressed at high levels in various tissues, including epithelium and immune cells such as polymorphonuclear leukocytes (PMNs).[75] It appears to function in protein degradation and activation of proenzymes in immune and inflammatory cells. PLS patients, who lack almost all cathepsin C activity,[93] are either mutant homozygotes (i.e., they inherited the same mutation from both parents) or compound heterozygotes (i.e., they inherited a different mutation from each parent).[32]

In some PLS patients, EOP is associated with the virulent microorganism *Actinobacillus actinomycetemcomitans*. The periodontal destruction in PLS patients can be arrested by eradicating *A. actinomycetemcomitans*,[73] which raises the possibility that EOP is not a direct result of the genetic mutation but rather the consequence of a specific bacterial infection in a highly susceptible host.

Inherited disorders such as acatalasia, leukocyte adhesion deficiency, and the Chediak-Higashi syndrome highlight the importance of competent phagocytes in the defense against periodontal infections. Many, but not all, patients with prepubertal periodontitis also have some inherited or congenital defect in phagocytic cell function. The immunologic defects associated with these syndromes can be profound, and patients generally suffer from systemic infections in addition to periodontitis. Although the mutant alleles responsible for these syndromes may be uncommon, other, more common alleles at the same loci may serve as candidate markers for nonsyndromic forms of EOP. Very recently, nonsyndromic prepubertal periodontitis-affected individuals in a Jordanian family were found to be homozygous for a cathepsin C gene mutation (Fig. 10-3).[34]

To reach the periodontal tissues, blood-borne phagocytes must adhere to and then traverse the blood vessel wall. Surface molecules present on both the phagocyte and endothelium mediate this adhesion. Three adhesion

TABLE 10-1

Genetic and Inherited Disorders Associated with Early Onset Periodontitis

Disorder	Protein or Biochemical Defect
Leukocyte adhesion deficiency Type I	CD18 (β-2 integrin chain of the LFA molecule)
Leukocyte adhesion deficiency Type II	CD15 (neutrophil ligand for E and P selectins); inborn error in fucose metabolism
Acatalasia	Catalase enzyme
Chronic and cyclic neutropenias	Unknown
Chediak-Higashi syndrome	Abnormal transport of vesicles to and from neutrophil lysosomes caused by mutations in the lysosomal trafficking regulator gene
Ehler-Danlos syndrome [Type IV, VIII, IX]	Type III collagen
Papillion-Lefèvre syndrome	Cathepsin C (dipeptidyl aminopeptidase I)
Hypophosphatsia	Tissue–nonspecific alkaline phosphatase
Trisomy 21	Multiple; critical trisomic region is at least 5 Mb long
Prepubertal periodontitis (nonsyndromic)	Cathepsin C

molecules expressed on leukocytes are composed of a unique α subunit (CD11a, b, or c) and a common β subunit (CD18). When too few of these molecules are present, cells cannot adhere to endothelium and an important component of the cellular immune response is compromised. Patients with inherited deficiencies in leukocyte adhesion molecules are at high risk for EOP and especially prepubertal periodontitis in particular. Two inherited forms of leukocyte adhesion deficiency (LAD) have been described, each of which affects a different adhesion molecule. Homozygotes carrying two copies of the mutant allele experience a dramatic reduction in the number of leukocyte adhesion molecules and develop recurrent infections including periodontitis (Color Fig. 10-2). Expression is about half of normal in heterozygotes carrying one mutant and one nonmutant allele. Although cell adherence is usually normal in heterozygotes, they may be at increased risk for adult-onset disease.[96]

Segregation Analyses of Early Onset Periodontitis

It has been recognized for years that juvenile periodontitis (JP) aggregates in families.[8,12] This finding suggests but does not prove that the disease has a genetic basis. Clustering within families can occur because of shared environmental factors. Evidence for a heritable basis for JP, however, comes from a variety of sources.

In most studies of JP, the localized and generalized forms (LJP and GJP, respectively) have been considered variants of the same disorder. This theory is supported by the observation that both forms frequently occur in the same family[52,54,57]; the probability of two rare diseases occurring in the same family is exceedingly small. Prepubertal periodontitis and JP also have been observed in the same family,[88] which again suggests that these diseases have shared genetic risk factors. Also, different forms of EOP diseases have been observed to occur sequentially in the same individual.[86]

Many case reports of multiplex families (containing more than one affected member) with EOP are available. The patterns of disease in these families have led investigators to propose both dominant inheritance and recessive modes of inheritance. However, few formal segregation analyses have been conducted, and the results have been varied (Table 10-2). Melnick et al[57] proposed X-linked inheritance due to the preponderance of female probands (the initially identified disease-afflicted individual in the family) and affected family members. Later, this preponderance was attributed to ascertainment bias because women are more likely than men to seek dental care and participate in family studies.[37] Also, father-to-son transmissions, which were not seen in earlier studies (the lack of such transmissions suggested X-linked inheritance) were observed in later studies. The autosomal recessive mode was clearly favored in Finnish populations because parents of probands were not affected.[80,81] In the largest study conducted in the U.S. to date, the autosomal dominant mode was favored in African-American and Caucasian families.[54] The estimated frequency of the disease allele, however, was significantly higher in African-Americans and reflects the higher prevalence of EOP in this group.

Segregation analyses consistently have supported the role of a major gene in the etiology of the EOP. Multifactorial or polygenic models alone cannot adequately account for the patterns of disease observed in families. Results from these studies, however, are prone to error due to the difficulty in correctly diagnosing older individuals, the variable clinical appearance of disease, and the likely etiologic and genetic heterogeneity of these diseases.[10,72] Beaty et al[5] recognized that the narrow age range in which EOP can reliably be diagnosed increases the chance that an incorrect model of inheritance is favored over the true one.

Schenkein[82] proposed a model of inheritance that distinguishes between the etiologies of localized and generalized EOP and allows for family clustering. He theorized that EOP and immunoglobulin (Ig) G2 responsiveness to bacterial lipopolysaccharides (LPS) segregate independently as dominant and codominant traits, respectively. Under this model, subjects with one EOP allele and two copies of the high IgG2 response allele would develop only localized disease. In contrast, subjects who carry the EOP allele and only one copy of the IgG2 allele would develop more widespread disease because their IgG2 response to LPS would be less robust. This model, although appealing, requires more rigorous testing, and the work needed to resolve the confounding effects of race and smoking on IgG2 levels and disease is far from trivial.

Linkage Studies of Early Onset Periodontitis

To date, few linkage studies of EOP have been performed. Boughman et al[11] was the first to report linkage between

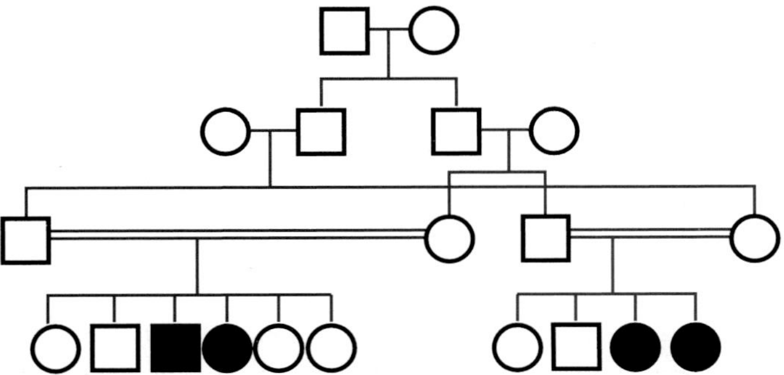

Fig. 10-3 Pedigree of a family segregating for prepubertal periodontitis. Filled squares and circles denote affected males and females, respectively. The double lines between the parents of affected individuals indicate they are blood relatives (in this case, first cousins), which is a frequent finding in rare autosomal recessive disorders. Affected individuals were homozygous by descent for a mutation in the cathepsin C gene. The four parents of the affected individuals were heterozygous for the mutation, as were the two unaffected siblings. None of these heterozygotes had clinical evidence of the disease. (From Hart TC, Hart PS, Michalec MD, et al: Localization of a gene for prepubertal periodontitis to chromosome 11q14 and identification of a cathepsin C gene mutation. J Med Genet 2000; 37:95.)

TABLE 10-2

Segregation Analyses of the Early Onset Periodontal Diseases

Racial/Ethnic Groups	Number of Families (Individuals)	Favored Model	Comments	Reference
Caucasian and African-American	19 (88)	X-linked dominant	Reviewed cases in the literature plus 2 new ones. Recognized paucity of males in families. Penetrance estimated at 75%.	57
Finnish	31 (158)	Autosomal recessive	Genetic ratio 0.26 for complete and 0.17 for very incomplete ascertainment. No affected parents observed.	81
	30 (142)	Autosomal recessive	Genetic ratios highly consistent with AR[1] mode. No affected parents observed.	80
Triracial isolate	1 (50)	Autosomal dominant	One five-generation family. JP[2] cosegregated with dentinogenesis imperfecta. Disease allele linked to chromosome 4.	11
African-American, Caucasian, Asian	32 (199)	Autosomal recessive	Tested AR, XD[3], and sporadic models. XD mode favored in 8 of 33 kindreds.	52
Not specified, US sample	28 (157)	Autosomal recessive	High type II error realized for mistakenly accepting AR over AD[4] model. Tested AR, XD, and sporadic models.	5
African-American, Caucasian	100 (631)	Autosomal dominant	Evidence of racial heterogeneity. Disease allele more frequent in African-Americans than Caucasians.	54

[1] *AR,* Autosomal recessive.
[2] *JP,* Juvenile periodontitis.
[3] *XD,* X-linked dominant.
[4] *AD,* Autosomal dominant.

JP and a specific chromosomal region. These researchers studied an extended family in which an autosomal dominant form of JP was found to cosegregate with dentinogenesis imperfecta (DGI). A putative JP gene was localized to the long arm of chromosome 4 (4q11-13) near the gene for DGI. In the general population, however, juvenile periodontitis does not cosegregate with DGI and linkage to this same region has been excluded.[36]

Saxen and Koskimies[79] typed a small number of multiplex Finnish families for the HLA antigens and concluded it was unlikely that JP was linked to this region. In a Virginia family study, genome-wide searches identified two chromosomal regions suggestive of linkage but failed to identify any that were statistically significant.[98] Again, disease heterogeneity appeared to be a complicating factor because this sample provided sufficient power to detect linkage to a major gene if the disease were genetically homogeneous.

Association Studies of Early Onset Periodontitis

Rather than conducting random searches of the genome for alleles associated with EOP, researchers have focused on candidate regions. These regions lie within or near genes that code for enzymes or regulatory molecules that are likely to be involved in the pathogenesis of disease. The number and variety of candidates for EOP are vast. Polymorphisms in genes encoding the immunoglobulin receptors, LPS binding proteins, prostaglandins, and cytokines are all suitable markers for study.[35,99] Polymorphisms in the vitamin D receptor[40] and mutations in the N-formyl-1-methionyl-1-leucyl-1-phenylalanine (FMLP) receptor[30] have been associated with localized forms of EOP.

The human leukocyte antigens (HLA) have been considered to be candidate markers for EOP because they are involved in regulating immune responses. More than 40 diseases, most of which are autoimmune in nature, have been associated with various HLA antigens.[92] Genes for the class I and II antigens are located on chromosome 6 in humans. Nearby genes encode for complement fragments and the proinflammatory cytokine, tumor necrosis factor-α. Currently, more than 150 HLA antigens have been defined serologically. Dissection of the coding sequences has revealed even more impressive variation at the genotype level. More than 220 alleles that code for the β-1 molecule of the dimeric class II DR antigen (DRB1 alleles) have been identified. Although this variation is desirable for linkage studies (because most individuals will be heterozygotes for a given marker), it can hinder the search for allelic associations (linkage disequilibrium). With so many antigens and alleles, the chance of obtaining an adequate number of subjects with any particular HLA type is small except in large, homogeneous samples. Also, the possibility that an association will be found due to chance alone increases with the number of tests conducted. For example, consider a study that tests for associations between periodontal disease and all known HLA antigens. At a standard significance level of 5%, approximately 7 antigens (150 antigens multiplied by 0.05) would be expected to be associated with the disease by chance alone. Although statistical methods to adjust for multiple hypotheses testing are available, such corrections have not always been made.

Despite the many case-control studies of HLA antigens in the periodontal literature, few consistent findings are available (Table 10-3). This inconsistency may be due to false-positive findings, differences in the racial or ethnic makeup of the study groups, differences in the clinical criteria used to define patient groups, or true heterogeneity. **Two antigens that appear to be consistently associated with EOP are HLA-A9 and B15.** The risk of disease in subjects with HLA-A9 or B15 is about 1.5 to 3.5 times greater than in those lacking these antigens.[87] In contrast, the HLA-A2 antigen appears to be less prevalent in juvenile periodontitis patients than controls, suggesting that this antigen somehow may be protective.[42,43,91] The class II DR4 antigen has been of particular interest in periodontology because of its association with insulin-dependent diabetes mellitus (IDDM). IDDM patients with the DR4 antigen are at increased risk for diabetes-related complications,[78] including periodontitis. It has been suggested that the HLA-D antigens may mediate the association between periodontal disease and IDDM.[22] Although the number of cases was small, Katz et al[44] found the DR4 antigen to be more prevalent in EOP cases than controls. Others, however, have found no association with this antigen (see Table 10-3).

The interleukin (IL)-1 gene has been studied because of its role in the initiation and progression of the periodontal lesion. Produced primarily by activated monocytes, its actions are pleiotropic; it stimulates bone resorption, inhibits collagen synthesis, and upregulates matrix metalloproteinase activity and prostaglandin synthesis.[48,90] IL-1 exists in two forms, IL-1α and IL-1β. An IL-1 antagonist (IL-1 ra) blocks the activity of IL-1 by competitively binding to IL-1 receptors. In humans, genes encoding IL-1α, IL-1β, and IL-1 ra are clustered on the long arm of chromosome 2.[65] Although several polymorphisms have been identified in this region, not all correlate to differences in IL-1 activity. However, one variant, due to a single nucleotide base-pair substitution in a coding region, has been associated with a four-fold increase in IL-1β production.[35] Because the magnitude of the IL-1 response may correlate to the levels of tissue destruction, functional polymorphisms in the IL-1 gene region could influence susceptibility to periodontitis.[48]

An IL-1β allele has been reported to be in linkage disequilibrium with generalized EOP,[21] suggesting that at least one disease allele is at or very close to this Il-1β polymorphism (2q13). In this study, linkage disequilibrium was detected using the transmission disequilibrium test, which contrasts the number of marker alleles transmitted versus not transmitted from heterozygous parents to affected offspring. The probability that an unlinked marker allele will be transmitted is 50%. If the marker and disease allele are in linkage disequilibrium, however, the marker will be transmitted more than 50% of the time. The number of nuclear families in this report was small, however, and sibling pair analyses of the same population provided only little if any evidence of linkage to this region.[21] However, this "high-risk" Il-1β allele may be too common in African-Americans—who are at higher risk than Caucasians for these diseases—to be of diagnostic value for JP.[97]

PERIODONTITIS IN ADULTS

Clinicians have long suspected that susceptibility to periodontitis differs among racial and ethnic groups. In the U.S., African-Americans have more severe disease than Caucasians.[7,68] Elsewhere, Sri Lankans and South Pacific islanders appear to be more prone to disease than other groups with similar environments.[4] Although these differences may be due to unrecognized environmental factors, they also may be the result of differences in genetic makeup.

Measures of periodontitis and gingivitis are correlated within families.[6,94] The basis of this similarity—whether it be shared environmental factors or genes—has been investigated in several large family studies. Initially, studies of Japanese and Hawaiian children suggested that gingivitis was due to recessive genes.[84] Later, correlations within families (e.g., sibling, parent-offspring) were used to estimate genetic and environmental variances for periodontitis among various racial groups in Hawaii. It was concluded that similarities within families were attributable to cultural inheritance and the common family environment, but not shared genes.[15,74] Beaty et al[6] reported similar results in a sample primarily of African-Americans. The correlations in clinical periodontal measures were greater between mothers and offspring than between fathers and offspring. Sibling correlations in this study were generally low, and the hypothesis of no familial correlation (and hence no genetic effect) could not be rejected.

Twin Studies of Adult Periodontitis

As early as 1940, Novack[66] recognized that the periodontal conditions of identical twins were often similar. Independent twin studies in Minnesota and Virginia concluded that a significant heritable component to adult periodontitis exists. The Minnesota group[58,59,61,62] studied both reared-together and reared-apart adult twins. Examples of twins in this study are depicted in Color Figs. 10-3 and 10-4. Between 38% and 82% of the population variance for gingivitis, probing depth, and clinical attachment loss could be attributed to genetic variation. A significant heritable influence on radiographic crestal alveolar bone height was found in these same twins. Moreover, reared-apart MZ twins were no less similar than reared-together MZ twins, indicating that the family environment had no significant influence on clinical measures of disease. The latter finding was surprising because it is within this environment that oral hygiene behaviors are learned and pathogenic bacteria may be acquired from other family members.

TABLE 10-3

HLA Antigens and Alleles in the Periodontal Disease: Summary of Association Studies

Disease	Ages of Cases (Years)	Racial/Ethnic Group	Number of Cases	Number of Controls	Associations with Disease	Comments	References
JP and non-JP EOP	13–30	Caucasians	19 JP, 28 non-JP	41[1] 267[2]	↓ A2, A5 in non-JP	Trend for ↓ A2 in JP. No associations with ANUG.	42, 91
RPP	23–39 Median 31	Caucasians	44	2041[2]	↑ A9 (A24)	Subjects had no evidence of past JP. No significant ↑ in B15 or DR antigens although trend for DR5.	45
JP and non-JP EOP	13–30	Caucasians	33 JP, 41 Non-JP	53	↓ A2 in non-JP	Similar trend for JP. No difference in A9, A28, Bw15. Also tested ABO blood groups.	43
JP	11–29 Mode 21	Caucasians	39	1967[2]	↑ A9, A28, Bw15	No significant associations with AP. Trend for ↓ A2 in JP group.	76
JP	≤25	Caucasians & African-Americans	30	341	↑ Bw15 in blacks (Class I only)	Trend for ↑ B12 in whites. Small samples. No evidence of linkage to HLA region in collection of 8 families.	20
EOP	Mean 26.5	Japanese	24	47	None (Class II only)	Trend for ↑ DRB1 ×1401, ×1501, & DQB1 ×0503, ×0602. DR association thought to be due to linkage disequilibrium with DQ alleles.	67
JP	15–25	Afro-Caribbeans	38	42	↑ A1, B22, A28, DR7 ↓ A68 (28), B5, DR2	None remained significant following corrections for multiple comparisons.	64
RPP	21–35	Ashkenazi and non-Ashkenazi Jews	10	120	↑ DR4	Small sample size. Borderline and uncorrected P value.	44
JP	Puberty to 35	Non-Ashkenazi Jews	26	113[2]	↑ A9, B15	Associations in GJP but not LJP group. No association with DR antigens.	87
RPP	20–35	6 ethno-geographic groups	12	55	↑ DRB1 ×0401, ×0404, ×0405, or ×0408	Small sample of EOP. No significant association for all patients (n = 48) or for all DR alleles combined.	9

LJP & RPP	LJP: puberty–24; RPP: puberty–35	Turkish citizens	30 LJP, 30 RPP	3731[2]	↑ A9 (A24), DR4	↑ DR4 in both patient groups.	24
EOP + AP (?)	25–40 Mean 33.0	Not specified	49	70[1] 600[2]	↑ A9; ↓ A10	↑ A9 in patients versus resistant group, ↓ A10 in resistant group versus undiagnosed controls.	2
EOP & AP	Mean 34.9	Japanese	55	26	None (Class II only)	Atypical enzyme restriction site in DQB1 gene detected in a subgroup of patients.	89
Generalized EOP	Not reported	European Caucasians	90	88	None (DQB1 gene only)	Tested for association with restriction site (described in Reference 90).	41
Not specified	Mean 35.9	Caucasians	30[3]	30[3]	↑ DR4, DR53, DQ3 (Class II only)	Association between diabetes and periodontitis may be mediated by D antigens.	1, 22
EOP + AP	20–49	Not specified	50	257[2]	↑ A9, B44 (12), Bw35, Cw4	Cw4 and Bw35 in strong disequilibrium (gametic association).	55
AP	40–73 Mean 49.9	Caucasians and African-Americans	25	25[1] 22,000[2]	↓ A28, B5	Significant ↓ in A28 in African-Americans and B5 in Caucasians when compared with undiagnosed controls.	29

1 Resistant group.
2 Population-based controls, disease status not determined.
3 15 subjects with insulin-dependent diabetes mellitus.
EOP, Early onset periodontitis; *JP*, juvenile periodontitis; *RPP*, rapidly progressive periodontitis; *AP*, adult periodontitis.

Despite the usefulness of the twin study design, very large sample sizes are needed to estimate heritability precisely. For example, heritability for clinical attachment loss in the preceding study was estimated to be 48%.[58] The 90% confidence interval for this estimate was quite large, ranging from 21% to 71%.

A questionnaire survey of several thousand adult twin pairs provided further evidence of the heritable component to periodontitis.[19] The concordance rate for disease was significantly greater in MZ twins (23%) than DZ twins (8%). Although the assessment method is questionable—twins may not be aware of their own or their twin's periodontal condition—the findings were confirmed in a more recent clinical study from the same population.[60] Heritability estimates for the extent and severity of disease were approximately 50%, which were consistent with previous estimates. The heritable component for periodontitis was not associated with behaviors such as smoking, utilization of dental care, and oral hygiene habits. This implies that genes controlling biologic mechanisms, and not behaviors, mediate the genetic influence on disease.

The twin design also has been used to study whether host genes affect the composition of the oral microbiota. Oral bacteria are transmitted within families,[3] a finding that could partly explain why periodontitis can cluster in families. Although the introduction of a bacterium into the oral cavity is an environmental event, long-term colonization of the host may be determined by both host genetic factors and environmental factors. Adolescent twins have been found to be more similar in their oral microbiota than pairs of unrelated individuals.[63] In adults, however, neither host genes nor the early family environment appear to significantly influence the presence of periodontal bacteria in subgingival plaque.[61] Together, these findings suggest that although host genes may influence initial colonization, this effect does not persist into adulthood.

Association Studies of Adult Periodontitis

Many of the same genes considered candidates for EOP are suitable for study in AP. The association between AP and the HLA antigens has been examined using the case-control design; however, the results of these studies have been equivocal (see Table 10-3). In one study, the HLA-B5 antigen was found to be more prevalent in adults resistant to disease.[29]

Kornman et al[47] reported that a "composite" IL-1 genotype—consisting of at least one copy of the more rare allele at both an IL-1α and IL-1β loci—was associated with severe periodontitis in Northern European adults. Nonsmokers with the composite genotype were 6.8 times more likely to have severe (as opposed to mild) periodontal disease. No association in smokers was found, which supports the theory that some environmental components are such strong risk factors that they overwhelm any genetically determined susceptibility or resistance to disease. In contrast, Gore et al[27] found the more rare IL-1β allele, but not the composite genotype, to be more prevalent in patients with advanced AP. The IL-1 and IL-1β sites were in linkage disequilibrium, which meant that the apparent role of the IL-1α allele could be due to its association with the IL-1β allele and not with the disease itself. Similar evidence that risk for EOP is conferred more by the IL-1β than IL-1α allele is available.[21]

Galbraith et al[26] found no association between AP and TNF-α polymorphisms, although one genotype was correlated with elevated TNF-α production by oral PMNs in patients with advanced disease. Similarly, Engebretson et al[23] reported a difference in the amount of IL-1 in the gingival crevicular fluid of patients with periodontitis who were positive for the composite IL-1 genotype. The TNF-α and IL-1 variants are examples of functional polymorphisms. In other words, they are variations in coding sequences that affect either the structure (and hence function) or production of the final protein product. The identification of additional functional polymorphisms, especially within genes that regulate immune responsiveness, should facilitate the discovery of alleles that determine host susceptibility to periodontitis.

Patients who respond poorly to periodontal treatment by continuing to lose clinical attachment are said to have refractory periodontitis. Both EOP and AP can be refractory to treatment. Neutrophils from refractory disease patients usually display some functional defect.[53,69] Kobayashi et al[46] tested the association between neutrophil immunoglobulin G receptor (FcγR) polymorphisms and AP in a Japanese population. These polymorphisms, which reside in genes that encode receptors for the IgG isotypes, correlate with how efficiently PMNs are able to phagocytose opsonized antigens. The frequency of FcγR genotypes did not differ between AP patients and healthy controls. Among patients, however, one allele (FcγRIIIb-NA2) was found to be more prevalent in those who experienced recurrent disease. Others studies have not confirmed the association between FcγR genotypes and refractory disease.[18]

CLINICAL IMPLICATIONS OF GENETIC STUDIES

The role of host genes in the etiology and pathogenesis of the periodontal diseases is just beginning to be understood. Genetic tests may prove useful for identifying patients who are most likely to develop disease, suffer from recurrent disease, or suffer tooth loss as a result of disease. The utility of any screening tool, however, must be evaluated in diverse populations. Given the complex etiology of the periodontal diseases, it is likely that any genetic test will be useful in only a subset of patients or populations. Genetic testing to determine risk for complex diseases (e.g., cancer) is becoming increasingly more common. With the availability of such tests, practitioners have the responsibility to fully inform the demanding public what genetic tests can do, act on the results, and advise and support individuals before and after testing.[71]

Knowledge of specific genetic risk factors could enable clinicians to direct environmentally based prevention and treatments to individuals who are most susceptible to disease. For example, early and aggressive efforts to prevent pathogenic microorganisms from colonizing the oral cavity may be effective in preventing disease in highly susceptible individuals. At present, however, the efficacy of specific preventive and treatment strategies in susceptible patients has yet to be clearly established.

Genetic information also may prove to be useful in predicting treatment outcomes. A retrospective cohort study of periodontal maintenance patients suggests that a patient's periodontal prognosis may depend in part on his or her IL-1 genotype.[56] In this study, the composite genotype described earlier was found to increase an individual's risk of tooth loss 2.7 times. The combined effect of a positive genotype and heavy smoking increased the risk of tooth loss nearly eightfold. Although prospective studies are needed to control for other known risk factors, this study demonstrated that a patient's Il-1 genotype might be an important factor for predicting future disease.

The identification of genetic risk factors for periodontitis in no way mitigates the importance of recognizing and controlling important environmental risk factors. For example, tobacco use is a major risk factor in AP. The risk of disease attributed to smoking appears to override any genetic susceptibility or resistance to disease.[47] For patients who smoke, preventive strategies must address the overwhelming environmental factor: tobacco use. It also is possible that new treatment strategies will be developed to directly counter the deleterious effects of certain risk allele(s). A simple theoretic example is the use of select antiinflammatory drugs in patients who are genetically programmed to be hyperresponders to bacterial antigens.

FUTURE OF GENETIC STUDIES IN PERIODONTOLOGY

At present, the search for risk alleles for periodontitis must focus on candidate gene regions. Genome-wide searches for risk alleles are not feasible due to the limited number of genetic markers currently available for typing. Single nucleotide polymorphisms (SNPs) are likely to be valuable tools in the search for disease alleles. SNPs are single base-pair substitutions that occur very frequently (i.e., every 1000 or so base pairs) throughout the genome. Few SNPs alter the amino acid sequences of proteins or even reside in exons. From an epidemiologic viewpoint, however, they are useful because they represent variation in the population. Currently, tens or even hundreds of thousands of such markers are thought to be required to detect associations for most common, complex disorders.[49] With the continual and rapid progress in the human genome project, however, it soon will become feasible to identify all alleles that confer even a moderate risk for disease. Even today, more than 800 SNPs have been identified within the 75 genes thought to be candidates for hypertension.[31] A similar number of candidate SNPs probably exists for the periodontal diseases, especially in genes whose products regulate humoral or cellular immune responses.[35]

To date, very few alleles have been consistently associated with any specific periodontal disease and the number of subjects studied has been relatively small. Therefore the risk associated with any one allele or genotype has not been precisely estimated. As the number of candidate genes available for study increases, the potentially large number of false-positive findings could lead researchers to pursue many erroneous leads. Associations between the disease and the gene(s) should be confirmed in multiple studies, and the gene(s) should have a biologically plausible relationship with the periodontal disease.

Periodontitis is clearly multifactorial, and researchers also need to design studies that examine the role of important environmental and genetic factors simultaneously. Given the large numbers of genes in the human genome and bacteria in the oral cavity, it is likely that genes and the environment interact in important yet unrecognized ways to alter disease risk. Most importantly, identifying specific genetic risk factors may be academically appealing but is of little use unless it leads to improvements in the prevention or treatment of disease.

REFERENCES

1. Alley CS, Reinhardt RA, Maze CA, et al: HLA-D and T lymphocyte reactivity to specific periodontal pathogens in type 1 diabetic periodontitis. J Periodontol 1993; 64:974.
2. Amer A, Singh G, Darke C, et al: Association between HLA antigens and periodontal disease. Tissue Antigens 1988; 31:53.
3. Asikainen S, Chen C, Alaluusua S, et al: Can one acquire periodontal bacteria and periodontitis from a family member? J Am Dent Assoc 1997; 128:1263.
4. Baelum V, Chen X, Manji F, et al: Profiles of destructive periodontal disease in different populations. J Periodontol Res 1996; 31:17.
5. Beaty TH, Boughman JA, Yang P, et al: Genetic analysis of juvenile periodontitis in families ascertained through an affected proband. Am J Hum Genet 1987; 40:443.
6. Beaty TH, Colyer CR, Chang YC, et al: Familial aggregation of periodontal indices. J Dent Res 1993; 72:544.
7. Beck JD, Koch GG, Rozier RG, et al: Prevalence and risk indicators for periodontal attachment loss in a population of older community dwelling blacks and whites. J Periodontol 1990; 61:521.
8. Benjamin SD, Baer PN: Familial patterns of advanced alveolar bone loss in adolescence (periodontosis). Periodontics 1967; 5:82.
9. Bonfil JJ, Dillier FL, Mercier P, et al: A "case control" study on the role of HLA DR4 in severe periodontitis rapidly progressive periodontitis. Identification of types and subtypes using molecular biology (PCR.SSO). J Clin Periodontol 1999; 26:77.
10. Boughman JA, Beaty TH, Yang P, et al: Problems of genetic model testing in early onset periodontitis. J Periodontol 1988; 59:332.
11. Boughman JA, Halloran SL, Roulston D, et al: An autosomal-dominant form of juvenile periodontitis: its localization to chromosome 4 and linkage to dentinogenesis imperfecta and Gc. J Craniofac Genet Dev Biol 1986; 6:341.
12. Butler JH: A familial pattern of juvenile periodontitis (periodontosis). J Periodontol 1969; 40:115.
13. Cantor RM, Rotter JI: Analysis of genetic data: Methods and interpretation. In: King RA, Rotter JI, Motulsky AG (eds): The Genetic Basis of Common Diseases. Oxford University Press, New York, 1992.
14. Chapple IL: Hypophosphatasia: dental aspects and mode of inheritance. J Clin Periodontol 1993; 20:615.
15. Chung CS, Kau MCW, Chung SSC, et al: A genetic and epidemiologic study of periodontal disease in Hawaii. II. Genetic and environmental influence. Am J Hum Genet 1977; 29:76.

16. Chung CS, Runck DW, Niswander JD, et al: Genetic and epidemiologic studies of oral characteristics in Hawaii's school children: I. Caries and periodontal disease. J Dent Res 1970; 49:1374.
18. Colombo AP, Eftimiadi C, Haffajee AD, et al: Serum IgG2 level, Gm(23) allotype and Fc gammaRIIa and Fc gamma RIIIb receptors in refractory periodontal disease. J Clin Periodontol 1998; 25:465.
19. Corey LA, Nance WE, Hofstede P, et al: Self-reported periodontal disease in a Virginia twin population. J Periodontol 1993; 64:1205.
20. Cullinan MP, Sachs J, Wolf E, et al: The distribution of HLA-A and -B antigens in patients and their families with periodontosis. J Periodontal Res 1980; 15:177.
21. Diehl SR, Wang YF, Brooks CN, et al: Linkage disequilibrium of interleukin-1 genetic polymorphisms with early onset periodontitis. J Periodontol 1999; 70:418.
22. Dyer JK, Peck MA, Reinhardt RA, et al: HLA-D types and serum IgG responses to Capnocytophaga in diabetes and periodontitis. J Dent Res 1997; 76:1825.
23. Engebretson SP, Lamster IB, Herra-Abreu M, et al: The influence of interleukin polymorphisms on expression of interleukin-1 and tumor necrosis factor-a in periodontal tissue and gingival crevicular fluid. J Periodontol 1999; 70:567.
24. Firatli E, Kantarci A, Cebeci I, et al: Association between HLA antigens and early onset periodontitis. J Clin Periodontol 1996; 23:563.
25. Fischer J, Blanchet-Bardon C, Prud'homme J-F, et al: Mapping of Papillon-Lefévre syndrome to the chromosome 11q14 region. Europ J Hum Genet 1997; 5:156.
26. Galbraith GM, Steed RB, Sanders JJ, et al: Tumor necrosis factor alpha production by oral leukocytes: Influence of tumor necrosis factor genotype. J Periodontol 1998; 69:428.
27. Gore EA, Sanders JJ, Pandey JP, et al: Interleukin-1 beta+ 3953 allele 2: association with disease status in adult periodontitis. J Clin Periodontol 1998; 25:781.
28. Gorlin RJ, Sedano H, Anderson VF: The syndrome of palmar-plantar hyperkeratosis and premature periodontal destruction of the teeth. J Pediatr 1964; 65:985.
29. Goteiner D, Goldman MJ: Human lymphocyte antigen haplotype and resistance to periodontitis. J Periodontol 1984; 55:155.
30. Gwinn MR, Sharma A, De Nardin E: Single nucleotide polymorphisms of the N-formyl peptide receptor in localized juvenile periodontitis. J Periodontol 1999; 70:1194.
31. Halushka MK, Fan JB, Bentley K, et al: Patterns of single-nucleotide polymorphisms in candidate genes for blood-pressure homeostasis. Nat Genet 1999; 22:239.
32. Hart PS, Zhang Y, Firatli E, et al: Identification of cathepsin C mutations in ethnically diverse Papillon-Lefévre syndrome patients. J Med Genet 2000; 37:927.
33. Hart TC, Hart PS, Bowden DW, et al: Mutations of the cathepsin C gene are responsible for Papillon-Lefévre syndrome. J Med Genet 1999; 36:881.
34. Hart TC, Hart PS, Michalec MD, et al: Localisation of a gene for prepubertal periodontitis to chromosome 11q14 and identification of a cathepsin C gene mutation. J Med Genet 2000; 37:95.
35. Hart TC, Kornman KS: Genetic factors in the pathogenesis of periodontitis. Periodontol 2000 1997; 14:202.
36. Hart TC, Marazita ML, McCanna KM, et al: Reevaluation of the chromosome 4q candidate region for early onset periodontit s. Hum Genet 1993; 91:416.
37. Hart TC, Marazita ML, Schenkein HA, et al: No female preponderance in juvenile periodontitis after correction for ascertainment bias. J Periodontol 1991; 62:745.
38. Hart TC, Stabholz A, Meyle J, et al: Genetic studies of syndromes with severe periodontitis and palmoplantar hyperkeratosis. J Periodontal Res 1997; 32(1 Pt 2):81.
39. Hart TC: Genetic considerations of risk in human periodontal disease. Current Opinions Periodontol 1994; 3.
40. Hennig BJ, Parkhill JM, Chapple IL, et al: Association of a vitamin D receptor gene polymorphism with localized early onset periodontal diseases. J Periodontol 1999; 70:1032.
41. Hodge PJ, Riggio MP, Kinane DF: No association with HLA-DQB1 in European Caucasians with early onset periodontitis. Tissue Antigens 1999; 54(2):205.
42. Kaslick RS, West TL, Chasens AI, et al: Association between HL-A2 antigen and various periodontal diseases in young adults. J Dent Res 1975; 54:424.
43. Kaslick RS, West TL, Chasens AI: Association between ABO blood groups, HL-A antigens and periodontal diseases in young adults: a follow-up study. J Periodontol 1980; 51:339.
44. Katz J, Goultschin J, Benoliel R, et al: Human leukocyte antigen (HLA) DR4. Positive association with rapidly progressing periodontitis. J Periodontol 1987; 58:607.
45. Klouda PT, Porter SR, Scully C, et al: Association between HLA-A9 and rapidly progressive periodontitis. Tissue Antigens 1986; 28:146.
46. Kobayashi T, Westerdaal NA, Miyazaki A, et al: Relevance of immunoglobulin G Fc receptor polymorphism to recurrence of adult periodontitis in Japanese patients. Infect Immun 1997; 65:3556.
47. Kornman KS, Crane A, Wang HY, et al: The interleukin-1 genotype as a severity factor in adult periodontal disease. J Clin Periodontol 1997; 24:72.
48. Kornman KS, di Giovine FS: Genetic variations in cytokine expression: a risk factor for severity of adult periodontitis. Ann Periodontol 1998; 3:327.
49. Kruglyak L: Prospects for whole-genome linkage disequilibrium mapping of common disease genes. Nat Genet 1999; 22:139.
50. Lewin B: Genes, ed 4. Oxford, Oxford University Press, 1994.
51. Löe H, Anerud A, Boysen H, et al: Natural history of periodontal disease in man. Rapid moderate, and no loss of attachment in Sri Lankan laborers 14 to 46 years of age. J Clin Periodontol 1986; 13:431.
52. Long JC, Nance WE, Waring P, et al: Early onset periodontitis: a comparison and evaluation of two proposed modes of inheritance. Genet Epidemiol 1987; 4:13.
53. MacFarlane GD, Herzberg MC, Wolff LF, et al: Refractory periodontitis associated with abnormal polymorphonuclear leukocyte phagocytosis and cigarette smoking. J Periodontol 1992; 63:908.
54. Marazita ML, Burmeister JA, Gunsolley JC, et al: Evidence for autosomal dominant inheritance and race-specific heterogeneity in early onset periodontitis. J Periodontol 1994; 65:623.
55. Marggraf E, von Keyserlingk-Eberius HJ, Komischke B, et al: Association of histocompatibility antigens (HLA antigens) with deep periodontopathies [in German]. Dtsch Zahnarztl Z 1983; 38:585.
56. McGuire MK, Nunn ME: Prognosis versus actual outcome. IV. The effectiveness of clinical parameters and IL-1 genotype in accurately predicting prognoses and tooth survival. J Periodontol 1999; 70:49.
57. Melnick M, Shields ED, Bixler D: Periodontosis: a phenotypic and genetic analysis. Oral Surg Oral Med Oral Pathol 1976; 42:32.
58. Michalowicz BS, Aeppli D, Virag JG, et al: Periodontal findings in adult twins. J Periodontol 1991; 62:293.
59. Michalowicz BS, Aeppli DM, Kuba RK, et al: A twin study of genetic variation in proportional radiographic alveolar bone height. J Dent Res 1991; 70:1431.

60. Michalowicz BS, Diehl SR, Gunsolley JC, et al: Evidence of a substantial genetic basis for risk of adult periodontitis. J Periodontol 2000; 71:1699.
61. Michalowicz BS, Wolff LF, Klump, D, et al: Periodontal bacteria in adult twins. J Periodontol 1999; 70:263.
62. Michalowicz BS: Genetic and heritable risk factors in periodontal disease. J Periodontol 1994; 65(5 Suppl):479.
63. Moore WE, Burmeister JA, Brooks CN, et al: Investigation of the influences of puberty, genetics, and environment on the composition of subgingival periodontal floras. Infect Immun 1993; 61:2891.
64. Moses JH, Tsichti H, Donaldson P, et al: HLA and susceptibility to juvenile periodontitis in Afro-Caribbeans. Tissue Antigens 1994; 43:316.
65. Nicklin MJ, Weith A, Duff GW: A physical map of the region encompassing the human interleukin-1 alpha, interleukin-1 beta, and interleukin-1 receptor antagonist genes. Genomics 1994; 19:382.
66. Noack B: Die Parodontoseätiologie im Lichte der Vererbung. Untersuchungen an erbverschiedenen und erbgleichen Zwillingspaaren. Osterr Zschr Stomat 1940; 38:267, 369, 395.
67. Ohyama H, Takashiba S, Oyaizu K, et al: HLA Class II genotypes associated with early onset periodontitis: DQB1 molecule primarily confers susceptibility to the disease. J Periodontol 1996; 67:888.
68. Oliver RC, Brown LJ, Löe H: Variations in the prevalence and extent of periodontitis. J Amer Dent Assoc 1991; 122:43.
69. Oshrain IB, Telsey B, Mandel ID: Neutrophil chemotaxis in refractory cases of periodontitis. J Clin Periodontol 1987; 14:52.
70. Pihlstrom BL, Michalowicz BS: Genetic risk for periodontal diseases: A clinical perspective. Journal De Paradontologie & D'Implantologie Orale 1998; 17:123.
71. Ponder BA: Costs, benefits and limitations of genetic testing for cancer risk. Br J Cancer 1999; 80 Suppl 1:46.
72. Potter RH: Guest Editorial. Etiology of periodontitis: the heterogeneity paradigm. J Periodontol 1989; 60:593.
73. Preus HR: Treatment of rapidly destructive periodontitis in Papillon-Lefevre syndrome. Laboratory and clinical observations. J Clin Periodontol 1988; 15:639.
74. Rao DC, Chung CS, Morton NE: Genetic and environmental determinants of periodontal disease. Am J Med Genet 1979; 4:39.
75. Rao NV, Rao GV, Hoidal JR: Human dipeptidyl-peptidase I: Gene characterization, localization, and expression. J Biol Chem 1997; 272:10260.
76. Reinholdt J, Bay I, Svejgaard A: Association between HLA-antigens and periodontal disease. J Dent Res 1977; 56:1261.
77. Root AW: Recent advances in the genetics of disorders of calcium homeostasis. Adv Pediatr 1996; 43:77.
78. Rotter JR, Vadheim CM, Rimoin DL: Diabetes mellitus. In: King RA, Rotter JI, Motulsky AG (eds): The Genetic Basis of Common Diseases. New York, Oxford University Press, 1992.
79. Saxen L, Koskimies S: Juvenile periodontitis—no linkage with HLA-antigens. J Periodontal Res 1984; 19:441
80. Saxen L, Nevanlinna HR: Autosomal recessive inheritance of juvenile periodontitis: test of a hypothesis. Clin Genet 1984; 25:332.
81. Saxen L: Heredity of juvenile periodontitis. J Clin Periodontol 1980; 7:276.
82. Schenkein HA: Genetics of early onset periodontal diseases. In: Genco R, et al (eds): Molecular Pathogenesis of Periodontal Disease. Washington, D.C., American Society for Microbiology, 1994.
83. Schenkein HA: Inheritance as a determinant of susceptibility for periodontitis. J Dent Educ 1998; 62:840.
84. Schull WJ, Neel JV: Effects of Inbreeding on Japanese Children. New York, Harper and Row, 1965.
85. Shapira L, Eizenburg S, Sela MN, et al: HLA A9 and B15 are associated with generalized form, but not the localized form, of early onset periodontal diseases. J Periodontol 1994; 65:219.
86. Shapira L, Smidt A, Van Dyke TE, et al: Sequential manifestation of different forms of early onset periodontitis. A case report. J Periodontol 1994; 65:631.
87. Sofaer JA: Genetic approaches in the study of periodontal diseases. J Clin Periodontol 1990; 17:401.
88. Spektor MD, Vandesteen GE, Page RC: Clinical studies of one family manifesting rapidly progressive, juvenile and prepubertal periodontitis. J Periodontol 1985; 56:93.
89. Takashiba S, Noji S, Nishimura F, et al: Unique intronic variations of HLA-DQ beta gene in early onset periodontitis. J Periodontol 1994; 65:379.
90. Tatakis DN: Interleukin-1 and bone metabolism: a review. J Periodontol 1993; 64(5 Suppl):416.
91. Terasaki PI, Kaslick RS, West TL, et al: Low HL-A2 frequency and periodontitis. Tissue Antigens 1975; 5:286.
92. Thomson G: HLA disease associations: models for the study of complex human genetic disorders. Crit Rev Clin Lab Sci 1995; 32:183.
93. Toomes C, James J, Wood AJ, et al: Loss-of-function mutations in the cathepsin C gene result in periodontal disease and palmoplantar keratosis. Nat Genet 1999; 23:421.
94. van der Velden U, Abbas F, Armand S, et al: The effect of sibling relationship on the periodontal condition. J Clin Periodontol 1993; 20:683.
95. Venter JC, Adams MD, Myers EW, et al: The sequence of the human genome. Science 2001; 291:1304.
96. Waldrop TC, Anderson DC, Hallmon WW, et al: Periodontal manifestations of the heritable Mac-1, LFA-1, deficiency syndrome. Clinical, histopathologic and molecular characteristics. J Periodontol 1987; 58:400.
97. Walker SJ, Van Dyke TE, Rich S, et al: Genetic polymorphisms of the IL-1alpha and IL-1beta genes in African-American LJP patients and an African-American control population. J Periodontol 2000; 71:723.
98. Wang S, Sun C, Gillanders E, et al: Evidence for susceptibility genes for early onset periodontitis. J Dent Res 1997; 76:151 (Abstract).
99. Wilson ME, Kalmar JR: Fc-gamma-RIIA (CD32)—a potential marker defining host susceptibility to localized juvenile periodontitis. J Periodontol 1996; 67:323.

The Role of Dental Calculus and Other Predisposing Factors

James E. Hinrichs

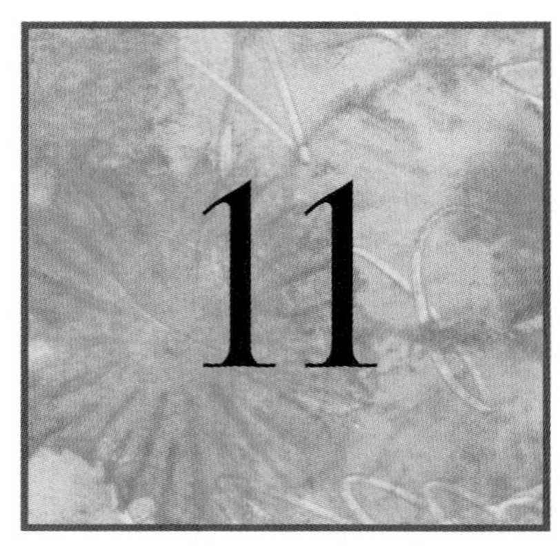

CHAPTER

CHAPTER OUTLINE

The primary cause of gingival inflammation is bacterial plaque (see Chapters 6 and 8), along with other predisposing factors. These predisposing factors include calculus, faulty restorations, complications associated with orthodontic therapy, self-inflicted injuries, use of tobacco, and others.

CALCULUS

Calculus consists of mineralized bacterial plaque that forms on the surfaces of natural teeth and dental prostheses. Calculus is classified as supragingival or subgingival, according to its relation to the gingival margin.

Supragingival and Subgingival Calculus

Supragingival calculus is located coronal to the gingival margin and therefore is visible in the oral cavity. It is usually white or whitish yellow in color, hard with claylike consistency, and easily detached from the tooth surface. After removal, it may rapidly recur, especially in the lingual area of the mandibular incisors. The color is influenced by contact with such substances as tobacco and food pigments. It may localize on a single tooth or group of teeth, or it may be generalized throughout the mouth.

The two most common locations for supragingival calculus to develop are the buccal surfaces of the maxillary molars (Fig. 11-1) (Color Figs. 11-1 and 11-2) and the lingual surfaces of the mandibular anterior teeth.[50] Saliva from the parotid gland flows over the facial surfaces of upper molars via Stensen's duct, whereas the orifices of Wharton's duct and Bartholin's duct empty onto the lingual surfaces of the lower incisors from the submaxillary and sublingual glands, respectively. In extreme cases, calculus may form a bridgelike structure over the interdental papilla of adjacent teeth or cover the occlusal surface of teeth without functional antagonists (Fig. 11-2).

Subgingival calculus is located below the crest of the marginal gingiva and therefore is not visible on routine clinical examination. The location and extent of subgingival calculus may be evaluated by careful tactile perception with a delicate dental instrument such as an explorer. Clerehugh et al used a World Health Organization #621 probe to detect and score subgingival calculus.[45] Subsequently, these teeth were extracted and visually scored for subgingival calculus. An agreement of 80% was found between these two scoring methods. Subgingival calculus is typically hard and dense and frequently appears dark brown or greenish black in color (Fig. 11-3) while being firmly attached to the tooth surface. Supragingival calculus and subgingival calculus generally occur together, but one may be present without the other. Microscopic studies demonstrate that deposits of subgingival calculus usually extend nearly to the base of periodontal pockets in chronic periodontitis but do not reach the junctional epithelium.

When the gingival tissues recede, subgingival calculus becomes exposed and is therefore reclassified as supragingival (Fig. 11-4). Thus supragingival calculus can be composed of both supragingival calculus and previous subgingival calculus. A reduction in gingival inflammation and probing depths and a gain in clinical attachment can be observed after the removal of subgingival plaque and calculus (Fig. 11-5) (see Chapter 47).

Prevalence

Anerud and co-workers observed the periodontal status of a group of Sri Lankan tea laborers and a group of Norwegian academicians for a 15-year period.[6] The Norwegian population had ready access to preventive dental care throughout their lives, whereas the Sri Lankan tea laborers did not. The formation of supragingival calculus was observed early in life in the Sri Lankan individuals, probably shortly after the teeth erupted. The first areas to exhibit calculus deposits were the facial aspects of maxillary molars and the lingual surfaces of mandibular incisors. Deposition of supragingival calculus continued as individuals aged, reaching a maximal calculus score around 25 to 30 years of age. At this time, most of the teeth were covered by calculus, although the facial surfaces had less calculus than the lingual or palatal surfaces. Calculus accumulation appeared to be symmetric, and by age 45 only a few teeth, typically the premolars, were without calculus. Subgingival calculus appeared first either independently or on the interproximal aspects of areas where supragingival calculus already existed.[6] By age 30, all surfaces of all teeth had subgingival calculus without any pattern of predilection.

The Norwegian academicians received oral hygiene instructions and frequent preventive dental care throughout their lives. The Norwegians exhibited a marked reduction in the accumulation of calculus as compared with the Sri Lankan group. However, despite the fact that 80% of teenagers formed supragingival calculus on the facial surfaces of the upper molars and the lingual surfaces of lower incisors, no additional calculus formation occurred on other teeth, nor did it increase with age.[6]

More recently, the third National Health and Nutrition Examination Survey (NHANES III) evaluated 9689 adults in the United States between 1988 and 1994.[4] This survey revealed that 91.8% of the subjects had detectable calculus and 55.1% had subgingival calculus.

Both supragingival calculus and subgingival calculus may be seen on radiographs (see Chapter 31). Highly calcified interproximal calculus deposits are readily detectable as radioopaque projections that protrude into the interdental space (Fig. 11-6). However, the sensitivity level of calculus detection by radiographs is low.[37] The location of calculus does not indicate the bottom of the periodontal pocket because the most apical plaque is not sufficiently calcified to be visible on radiographs.

Composition

Inorganic Content. Supragingival calculus consists of inorganic (70% to 90%[68]) and organic components. The inorganic portion consists of 75.9% calcium phosphate, $Ca_3(PO_4)_2$; 3.1% calcium carbonate, $CaCO_3$; and traces of magnesium phosphate, $Mg_3(PO_4)_2$, and other metals.[214] The percentage of inorganic constituents in calculus is similar to that in other calcified tissues of the body. The principal inorganic components are calcium, 39%; phosphorus, 19%; carbon dioxide, 1.9%; magnesium, 0.8%; and trace amounts of sodium, zinc, strontium, bromine, copper, manganese, tungsten, gold, aluminum, silicon, iron, and fluorine.[140]

At least two thirds of the inorganic component is

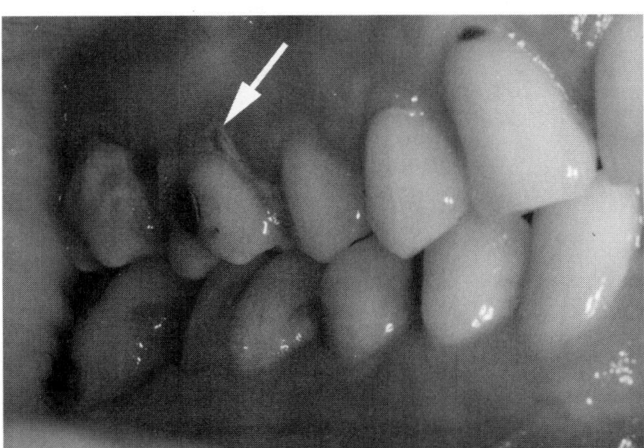

Fig. 11-1 Supragingival calculus is depicted on the buccal surfaces of maxillary molars adjacent to orifice for Stenson's duct.

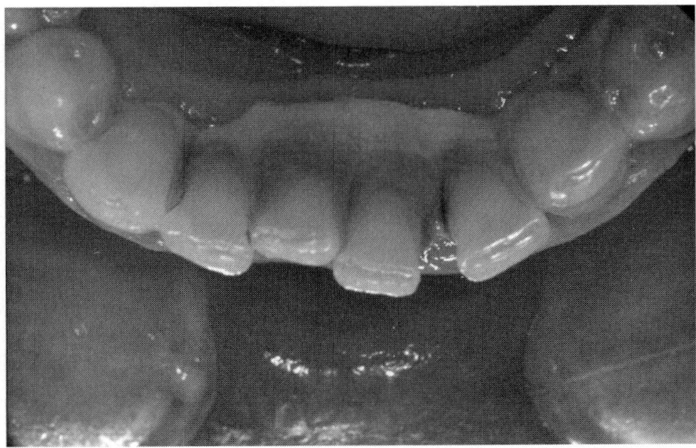

Fig. 11-2 Extensive supragingival calculus is present on the lingual surfaces of lower anterior teeth.

crystalline in structure.[110] The four main crystal forms and their percentages are as follows:

Hydroxyapatite, approximately 58%
Magnesium whitlockite, approximately 21%
Octacalcium phosphate, approximately 12%
Brushite, approximately 9%

Generally, two or more crystal forms are typically found in a sample of calculus. Hydroxyapatite and octacalcium phosphate are detected most frequently (i.e., in 97% to 100% of all supragingival calculus) and constitute the bulk of the specimen. Brushite is more common in the mandibular anterior region and magnesium whitlockite in the posterior areas. The incidence of the four crystal forms varies with the age of the deposit.[26]

Organic Content. The organic component of calculus consists of a mixture of protein-polysaccharide complexes, desquamated epithelial cells, leukocytes, and various types of microorganisms.[125] Between 1.9% and 9.1% of the organic component is carbohydrate, which consists of galactose, glucose, rhamnose, mannose, glucuronic acid, galactosamine, and sometimes arabinose, galacturonic acid, and glucosamine.[114,124,195] All these organic components are present in salivary glycoprotein with the exception of arabinose and rhamnose. Salivary proteins account for 5.9% to 8.2% of the organic component of calculus and include most amino acids. Lipids account for 0.2% of the organic content in the form of neutral fats, free fatty acids, cholesterol, cholesterol esters, and phospholipids.[115]

The composition of subgingival calculus is similar to that of supragingival calculus, with some differences. It has the same hydroxyapatite content, more magnesium whitlockite, and less brushite and octacalcium phosphate.[177,201] The ratio of calcium to phosphate is higher subgingivally, and the sodium content increases with the depth of periodontal pockets.[116] Salivary proteins present in supragingival calculus are not found subgingivally.[16] Dental calculus, salivary duct calculus, and calcified dental tissues are similar in inorganic composition.

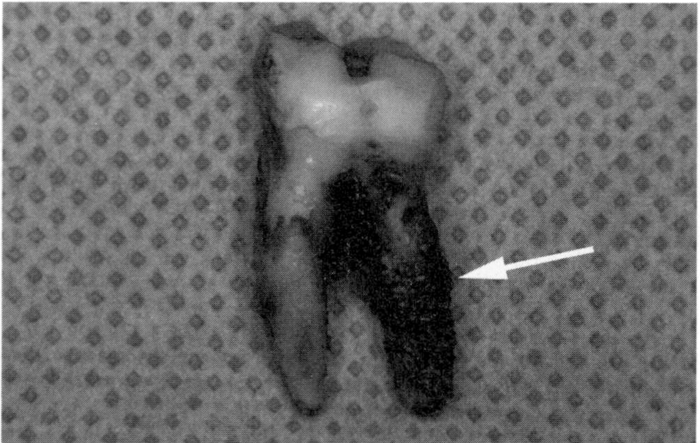

Fig. 11-3 Dark pigmented deposits of subgingival calculus are shown on the distal root of an extracted lower molar.

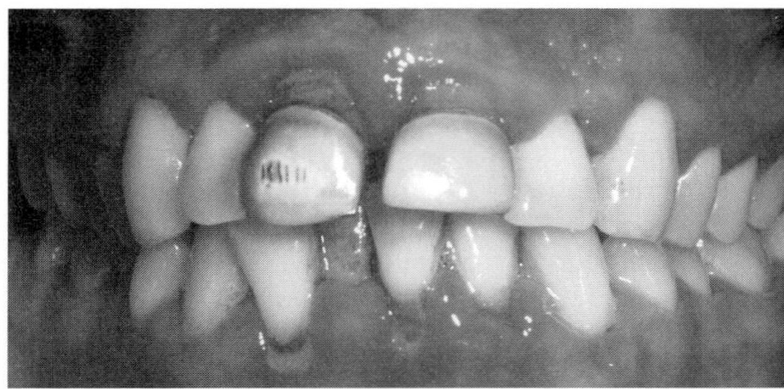

Fig. 11-4 A 31-year-old Caucasian male is shown with extensive supragingival and subgingival calculus deposits throughout his dentition.

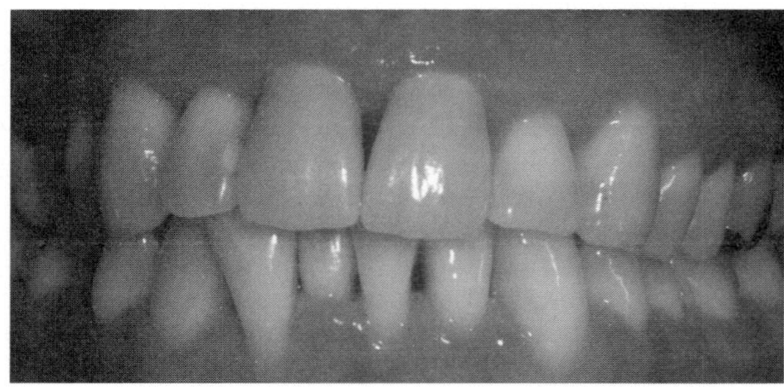

Fig. 11-5 The same patient as shown in Fig. 11-4, 1 year after receiving thorough scaling and root planing to remove supragingival and subgingival calculus deposits followed by restorative care. Note the substantial reduction in gingival inflammation.

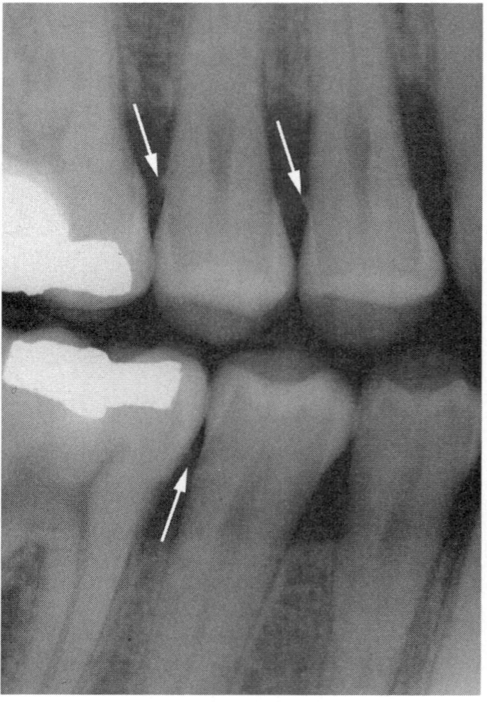

Fig. 11-6 A bitewing radiograph illustrating extensive subgingival calculus deposits that are depicted as interproximal spurs.

Attachment to the Tooth Surface

Differences in the manner in which calculus is attached to the tooth surface affect the relative ease or difficulty encountered in its removal. Four modes of attachment have been described[106,179,220]: attachment by means of an organic pellicle (Fig. 11-7, *A*); mechanical locking into surface irregularities such as resorption lacunae and caries (Figs. 11-7, *B* and 11-8); close adaptation of calculus undersurface depressions to the gently sloping mounds of the unaltered cementum surface[196] (Fig. 11-9); and penetration of calculus bacteria into cementum. However, not all investigators universally acknowledge this forth mode of attachment (Fig. 11-10).[106] Calculus embedded deeply in cementum may appear morphologically similar to cementum and thus has been termed *calculocementum*.[186]

Formation

Calculus is dental plaque that has undergone mineralization. The soft plaque is hardened by the precipitation of mineral salts, which usually starts between the 1st and 14th days of plaque formation. However, calcification has been reported to occur in as little as 4 to 8 hours.[202] Calcifying plaques may become 50% mineralized in 2 days and 60% to 90% mineralized in 12 days.[139,180,190] All plaque does not necessarily undergo calcification. Early plaque contains a small amount of inorganic material, which increases as the plaque develops into calculus. Plaque that does not develop into calculus reaches a plateau of maximal mineral content within 2 days.[181] Microorganisms are not always essential in calculus formation because calculus occurs readily in germ-free rodents.[78]

Saliva is the source of mineralization for supragingival calculus, whereas the serum transudate called *gingival crevicular fluid* furnishes the minerals for subgingival calculus.[93,197] Plaque has the ability to concentrate calcium at 2 to 20 times its level in saliva.[26] Early plaque of heavy calculus formers contains more calcium, three times more phosphorus, and less potassium than that of non-calculus formers, suggesting that phosphorus may be more critical than calcium in plaque mineralization.[125] Calcification entails the binding of calcium ions to the carbohydrate-protein complexes of the organic matrix and the precipitation of crystalline calcium phosphate salts.[123] Crystals form initially in the intercellular matrix and on the bacterial surfaces and finally within the bacteria.[69,221]

Calcification begins along the inner surface of the supragingival plaque and in the attached component of subgingival plaque adjacent to the tooth. Separate foci of calcification increase in size and coalesce to form solid masses of calculus (Fig. 11-11). Calcification may be accompanied by alterations in the bacterial content and staining qualities of the plaque. As calcification progresses, the number of filamentous bacteria increases and foci of calcification change from basophilic to eosinophilic. There is a reduction in the staining intensity of groups exhibiting a positive periodic acid-Schiff reaction. Sulfhydryl and amino groups also are reduced and instead stain with toluidine blue, which is initially orthochromatic but becomes metachromatic and disappears.[210] Calculus is formed in layers, which are often

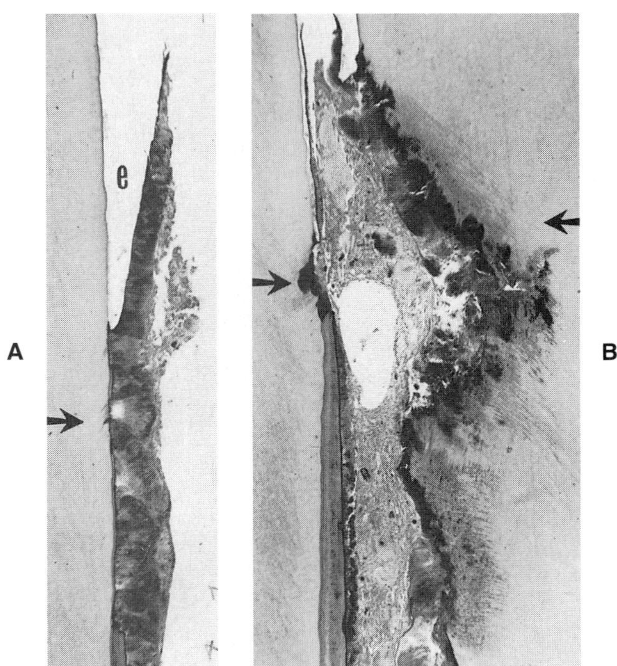

Fig. 11-7 Calculus. **A,** Calculus attached to pellicle on enamel surface *(e)*. The enamel was removed in the preparation of the specimen. Also note calculus attached to dentin and associated penetration of dental tubules *(arrows)*. **B,** Interproximal area with early and advanced root caries of adjacent teeth and with calculus attached to carious surfaces *(arrows)*.

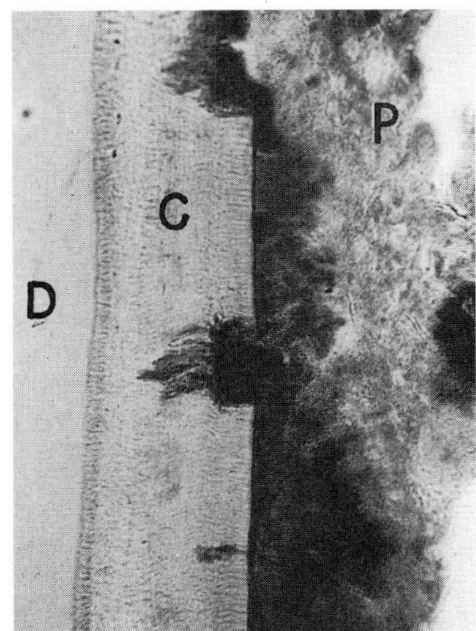

Fig. 11-8 Calculus on tooth surface embedded within the cementum *(C)*. Note the early stage of penetration shown in the lower portion of the illustration. *D,* Dentin; *P,* plaque attached to calculus.

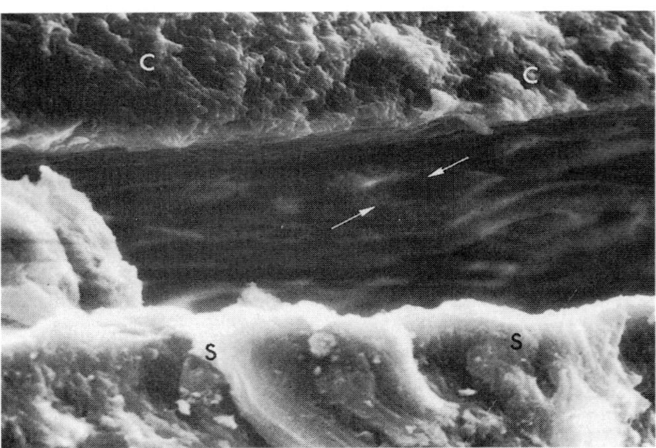

Fig. 11-9 Undersurface of subgingival calculus *(C)* previously attached to the cementum surface *(S)*. Note impression of cementum mounds in calculus *(arrows)*. (Courtesy Dr. John Sottosanti, La Jolla, Calif.)

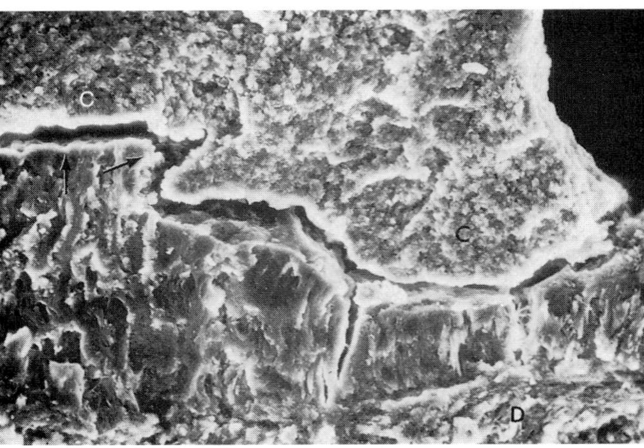

Fig. 11-10 Subgingival calculus *(C)* embedded beneath the cementum surface *(arrows)* and penetrating to the dentin *(D)*, making removal difficult. (Courtesy Dr. John Sottosanti, La Jolla, Calif.)

separated by a thin cuticle that becomes embedded in the calculus as calcification progresses.[127]

The initiation of calcification and the rate of calculus accumulation vary from person to person, for different teeth, and at different times in the same person.[140,206] On the basis of these differences, persons may be classified as heavy, moderate, or slight calculus formers or as noncalculus formers. The average daily increment in calculus formers is from 0.10% to 0.15% of dry weight.[190,206] Calculus formation continues until it reaches a maximum, after which it may be reduced in amount. The time required to reach the maximal level has been reported as 10 weeks[46] and 6 months.[208] The decline from maximal calculus accumulation, referred to as *reversal phenomenon,* may be explained by the vulnerability of bulky calculus to mechanical wear from food and from the cheeks, lips, and tongue.

Anticalculus (antitartar) dentifrices claim to reduce the quantity and quality of calculus formed, making it easier for removal by the clinician. These products appear to be helpful for some patients.

Theories Regarding the Mineralization of Calculus. The theoretic mechanisms by which plaque becomes mineralized can be stratified into two principal categories.[141]

1. *Mineral precipitation results from a local rise in the degree of saturation of calcium and phosphate ions,* which may be brought about in several ways:

   A rise in the pH of the saliva causes precipitation of calcium phosphate salts by lowering the precipitation constant. The pH may be elevated by the loss of carbon dioxide and the formation of ammonia by dental plaque bacteria or by protein degradation during stagnation.[25,88]

   Colloidal proteins in saliva bind calcium and phosphate ions and maintain a supersaturated solution with respect to calcium phosphate salts. With stagnation of saliva, colloids settle out and the supersaturated state is no longer maintained, leading to precipitation of calcium phosphate salts.[164,183]

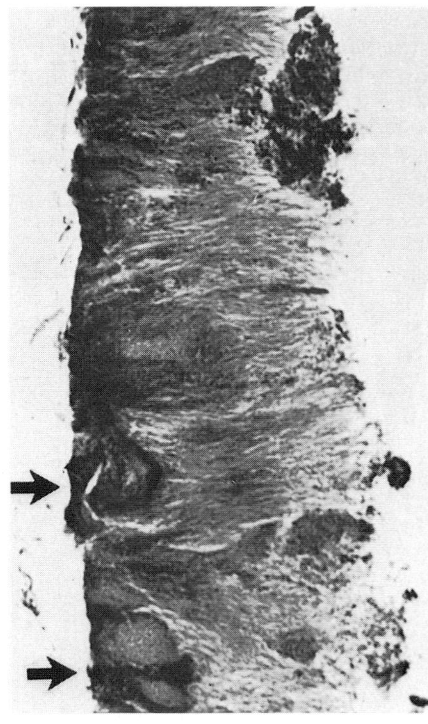

Fig. 11-11 Five-day plaque, showing spherical calcification foci *(arrows)* and perpendicular alignment of filamentous organisms along the inner surface and colonies of cocci on the outer surface. (From Turesky S, Renstrup G, Glickman I: Histologic and histochemical observations regarding early calculus formation in children and adults. J Periodontol 1961; 32:7.)

   Phosphatase liberated from dental plaque, desquamated epithelial cells, or bacteria precipitate calcium phosphate by hydrolyzing organic phosphates in saliva, thus increasing the concentration of free phosphate ions.[212] Esterase is another enzyme that is present in the cocci and filamentous organisms, leukocytes, macrophages, and desquamated epithelial cells of dental plaque.[10] Esterase may initiate calcification by hydrolyzing fatty esters into free fatty acids. The fatty acids form soaps with calcium and magnesium that are later converted into the less-soluble calcium phosphate salts.

2. *Seeding agents induce small foci of calcification that enlarge and coalesce to form a calcified mass.*[143] This concept has been referred to as the *epitactic concept* or more appropriately, *heterogeneous nucleation.* The seeding agents in calculus formation are not known, but it is suspected that the intercellular matrix of plaque plays an active role.[126,139,221] The carbohydrate-protein complexes may initiate calcification by removing calcium from the saliva (chelation) and binding with it to form nuclei that induce subsequent deposition of minerals.[123,209]

Role of Microorganisms in the Mineralization of Calculus. Mineralization of plaque starts extracellularly around both gram-positive organisms and gram-negative organisms[108]; it may also start intracellularly. Filamentous organisms, diphtheroids, and *Bacterionema* and *Veillonella* species have the ability to form intracellular apatite crystals (Fig. 11-12). Calculus formation spreads until the matrix and bacteria are calcified.[69,221]

Bacterial plaque may actively participate in the mineralization of calculus by forming phosphatases, which changes the pH of the plaque and induces mineralization,[55,123] but the prevalent opinion is that these bacteria are only passively involved[69,173,212] and are simply calcified with other plaque components. The occurrence of calculus-like deposits in germ-free animals supports this opinion.[78] However, other experiments suggest that transmissible factors are involved in calculus formation and that penicillin in the diets of some of these animals reduces calculus formation.[11]

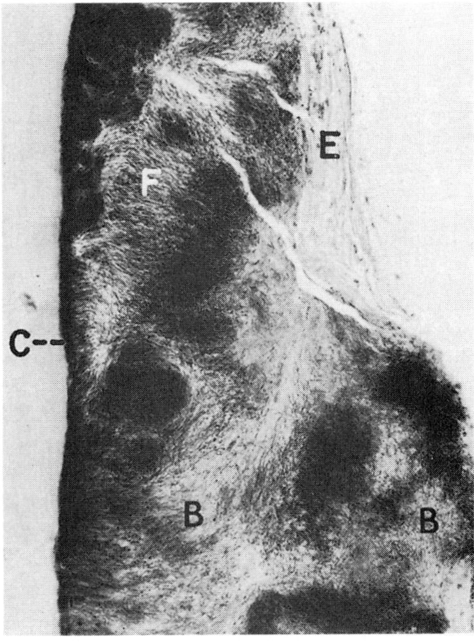

Fig. 11-12 Detailed microscopic examination of calculus showing an inner structure *(C),* filamentous organisms *(F),* other bacteria *(B),* and desquamated epithelial cells *(E).*

Etiologic Significance

Distinguishing between the effects of calculus and plaque on the gingiva is difficult because calculus is always covered with a nonmineralized layer of plaque.[181] A positive correlation between the presence of calculus and the prevalence of gingivitis exists,[167] but this correlation is not as great as that between plaque and gingivitis.[72] In young persons, periodontal condition is more closely related to plaque accumulation than to calculus, but the situation is reversed with age.[72,111] The incidence of calculus, gingivitis, and periodontal disease increases with age. It is extremely rare to find periodontal pockets in adults without subgingival calculus, although subgingival calculus may be of microscopic proportion in some cases.

The nonmineralized plaque on the calculus surface is the principal irritant, but the underlying calcified portion may be a significant contributing factor (Fig. 11-13). It does not irritate the gingiva directly but provides a fixed nidus for the continued accumulation of plaque and retains it in close proximity to the gingiva. Subgingival calculus may be the product rather than the cause of periodontal pockets. Plaque initiates gingival inflammation, which starts pocket formation, and the pocket in turn provides a sheltered area for plaque and bacterial accumulation. The increased flow of gingival fluid associated with gingival inflammation provides the minerals that convert the continually accumulating plaque into subgingival calculus. Over a 6-year period, Albander et al observed 156 teenagers with histories of aggressive periodontitis.[4] They noted that areas with detectable subgingival calculus at the initiation of the study were much more likely to experience loss of periodontal attachment than sites that did not initially exhibit subgingival calculus.

While the bacterial plaque that coats the teeth is the main etiologic factor in the development of periodontal disease, the removal of subgingival plaque and calculus constitute the cornerstone of periodontal therapy. Calculus plays an important role in maintaining and accentuating periodontal disease by keeping plaque in close contact with the gingival tissue and creating areas where plaque removal is impossible. Therefore *the clinician must not only possess the clinical skill to remove the calculus and other irritants that attach to the teeth but also be very conscientious about performing this task.*

Materia Alba, Food Debris, and Dental Stains

Materia alba is a concentration of microorganisms, desquamated epithelial cells, leukocytes, and a mixture of salivary proteins and lipids, with few or no food particles, and it lacks the regular internal pattern observed in plaque.[182] It is a yellow or grayish-white, soft, sticky

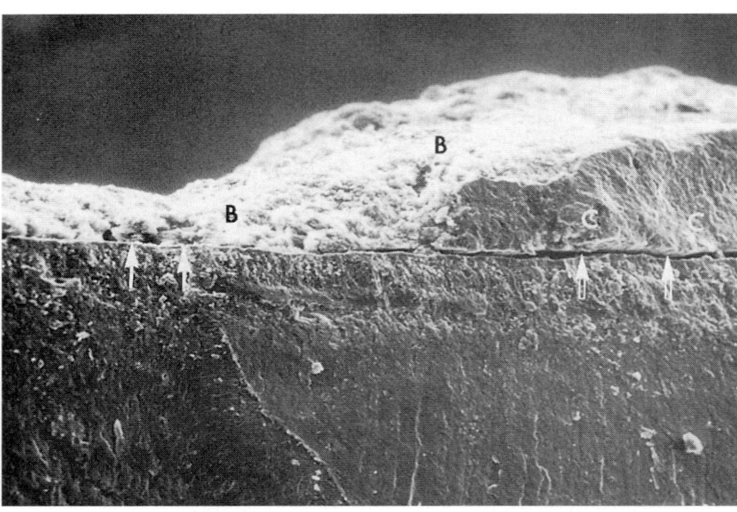

Fig. 11-13 Scanning electron microscope view of an extracted human tooth, fractured experimentally, showing a cross-section of subgingival calculus *(C)* that is not firmly attached to the cemental surface *(arrows).* Note bacteria *(B)* attached to calculus and cemental surface. (Courtesy Dr. John Sottosanti, La Jolla, Calif.)

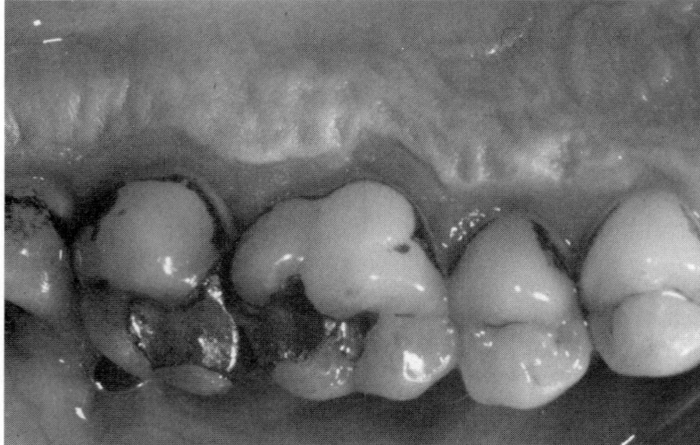

Fig. 11-14 Tobacco stains on the apical third of the clinical crown due to cigarette smoking.

deposit and is somewhat less adherent than dental plaque. The irritating effect of materia alba on the gingiva is caused by bacteria and their products.

Most food debris is rapidly liquefied by bacterial enzymes and cleared from the oral cavity by salivary flow and the mechanical action of the tongue, cheeks, and lips. The rate of clearance from the oral cavity varies with the type of food and the individual. Aqueous solutions are typically cleared within 15 minutes, whereas sticky foods may adhere for more than 1 hour.[99,207] Dental plaque is not a derivative of food debris, nor is food debris an important cause of gingivitis.[54] Although the oral microflora is the main determinant of the gingival status, recent research indicates that short-chain carboxylic acids found in retained food particles may also have an impact on the periodontal status.[99]

Pigmented deposits on the tooth surface are called *dental stains.* Stains are primarily an aesthetic problem and do not cause inflammation of the gingiva. The use of tobacco products (Fig. 11-14), coffee, tea, certain mouthrinses, and pigments in foods can contribute to stain formation.[117]

OTHER PREDISPOSING FACTORS

Iatrogenic Factors

Deficiencies in the quality of dental restorations or prostheses are contributing factors to gingival inflammation and periodontal destruction. Inadequate dental procedures that contribute to the deterioration of the periodontal tissues are referred to as *iatrogenic factors.* Characteristics of dental restorations and removable partial dentures that are important to the maintenance of periodontal health include: the location of the gingival margin for the restoration, the space between the margin of the restoration and the unprepared tooth, the contour of restorations, the occlusion, materials used in the restoration, the restorative procedure itself, and the design of the removable partial denture. These characteristics are described in this chapter as they relate to the etiology of periodontal disease. A more comprehensive review with special emphasis on the interrelationship between restorative procedures and the periodontal status is presented in Chapter 75.

Margins of Restorations. Overhanging margins of dental restorations contribute to the development of periodontal disease by 1) changing the ecologic balance of the gingival sulcus to an area that favors the growth of disease-associated organisms (predominately gram-negative anaerobic species) at the expense of the health-associated organisms (predominately gram-positive facultative species)[109] and 2) inhibiting the patient's access to remove accumulated plaque.

The frequency of overhanging margins of proximal restorations varies in different studies from 16.5% to 75%.[28,66,92,149] A highly significant statistical relationship has been reported between marginal defects and reduced bone height.[28,83,92] Removal of overhangs permits more effective control of plaque, resulting in a reduction of gingi-

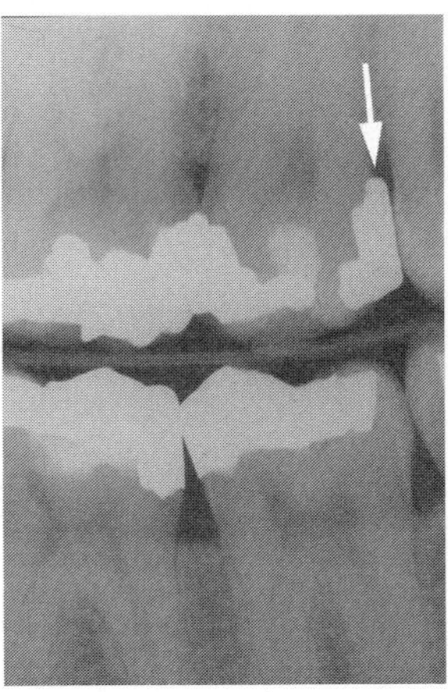

Fig. 11-15 Radiograph of amalgam overhang on the distal surface of maxillary second molar, which is a source of plaque retention and gingival irritation.

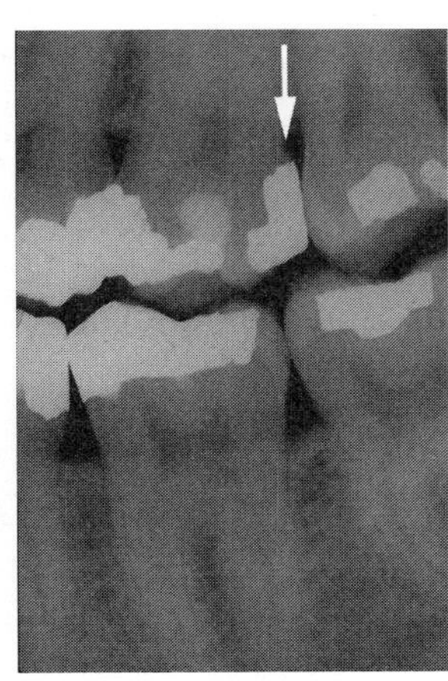

Fig. 11-16 Radiograph showing same patient as in Fig. 11-15 after the excessive amalgam has been removed.

val inflammation and a small increase in radiographic alveolar bone support[71,85,193] (Figs. 11-15 and 11-16).

The location of the gingival margin for a restoration is directly related to the health status of adjacent periodontal tissues.[191] Numerous studies[66,89,98,169,193] have shown a positive correlation between margins located apical to the marginal gingiva and the presence of gingival inflammation. Subgingival margins are associated with large amounts of plaque, more severe gingivitis, and deeper pockets. Even high-quality restorations, if placed subgingivally, will increase plaque accumulation, gingival inflammation[107,109,138,170] and the rate of gingival fluid flow.[19,74] Margins placed at the level of the gingival crest induce less severe inflammation, whereas supragingival margins are associated with a degree of periodontal health similar to that seen with non-restored interproximal surfaces.[62,191]

Roughness in the subgingival area is considered to be a major contributing factor to plaque build-up and subsequent gingival inflammation.[191] The subgingival zone is composed of the margin of the restoration, the luting material, and the prepared as well as the unprepared tooth surface. Sources of marginal roughness include[191] grooves and scratches in the surface of carefully polished acrylic resin, porcelain, or gold restorations (Fig. 11-17); separation of the restoration margin and luting material from the cervical finish line, thereby exposing the rough surface of the prepared tooth (Fig. 11-18); dissolution and disintegration of the luting material between the preparation and the restoration, leaving a space (Fig. 11-19); and inadequate marginal fit of the restoration. Subgingival margins typically have a gap of 20 to 40 microns between the margin of the restoration and the unprepared tooth.[189] Colonization of this gap by bacterial plaque undoubtedly contributes to the detrimental effect of margins placed in a subgingival environment.

Contours/Open Contacts. Overcontoured crowns and restorations tend to accumulate plaque and possibly prevent the self-cleaning mechanisms of the adjacent cheek, lips, and tongue.[7,104,136,218] (Figs. 11-20 and 11-21) Restorations that fail to reestablish adequate interproximal embrasure spaces are associated with papillary inflammation. Undercontoured crowns that lack a protective height of contour may not be as detrimental during mastication as once thought.[218]

The contour of the occlusal surface as established by the marginal ridges and related developmental grooves normally serves to deflect food away from the interproximal spaces. The optimal cervicoocclusal location for a posterior contact is at the longest mesiodistal diameter of the tooth, which is generally just apical to the crest of the marginal ridge. The integrity and location of the proximal contacts along with the contour of the marginal ridges and developmental grooves typically prevent interproximal food impaction. *Food impaction* is the forceful wedging of food into the periodontium by occlusal forces. As the teeth wear down, their originally convex proximal surfaces become flattened and the wedging effect of the opposing cusp is exaggerated. Cusps that tend to forcibly wedge food into interproximal embrasures are known as *plunger cusps*. The interproximal plunger cusp effect may also be observed when missing teeth are not replaced and the relationship between proximal contacts of adjacent teeth is altered. An intact, firm proximal contact precludes the forceful wedging of food into the interproximal embrasure space, whereas a light or open contact is conducive to impaction.

The classic analysis of the factors leading to food impaction was made by Hirschfeld,[87] who recognized the following factors: uneven occlusal wear, opening of the contact point as a result of loss of proximal support or from extrusion, congenital morphologic abnormalities, and improperly constructed restorations.

The presence of the previously mentioned abnormalities does not necessarily lead to food impaction and periodontal disease. A study of interproximal contacts and marginal ridge relationships[109] in three groups of periodontally healthy males revealed that 0.7% to 76% of

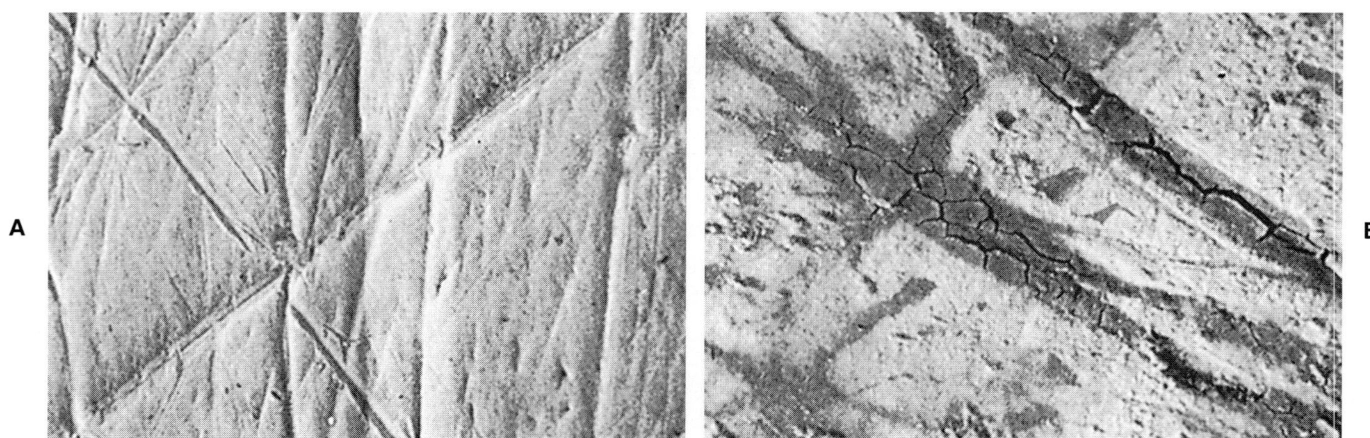

Fig. 11-17 **A,** A polished gold alloy crown demonstrates surface scratches. **B,** A gold alloy crown that had been in the mouth for several years has scratches filled with deposits. (From Silness J: Fixed prosthodontics and periodontal health. Dent Clin North Am 1980; 24:317.)

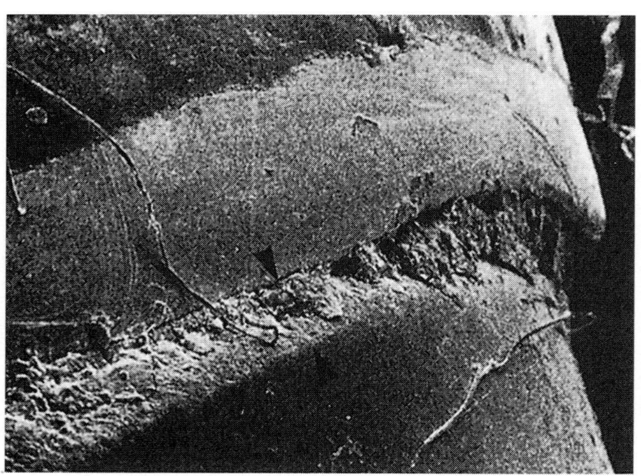

Fig. 11-18 After cementation, luting material prevents approximation of the crown margin and the finishing line, leaving part of the prepared tooth uncovered (area between arrowheads). (From Silness J: Fixed prosthodontics and periodontal health. Dent Clin North Am 1980; 24:317.)

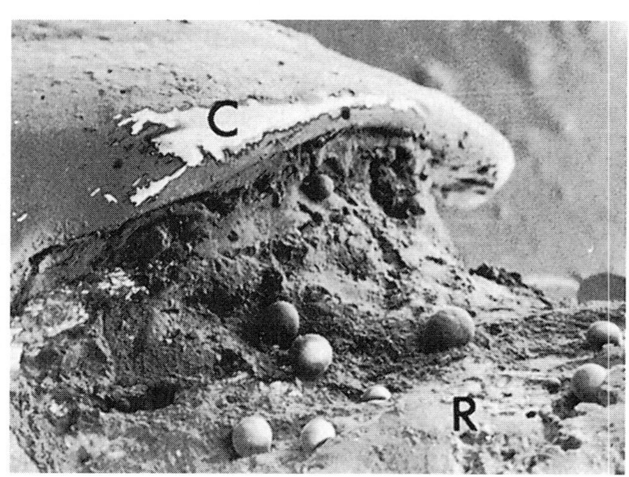

Fig. 11-19 Craters have formed after dissolution and disintegration of the luting material. Spherical bodies are not identified. *C,* Crown; *R,* root. (From Silness J: Fixed prosthodontics and periodontal health. Dent Clin North Am 1980; 24:317.)

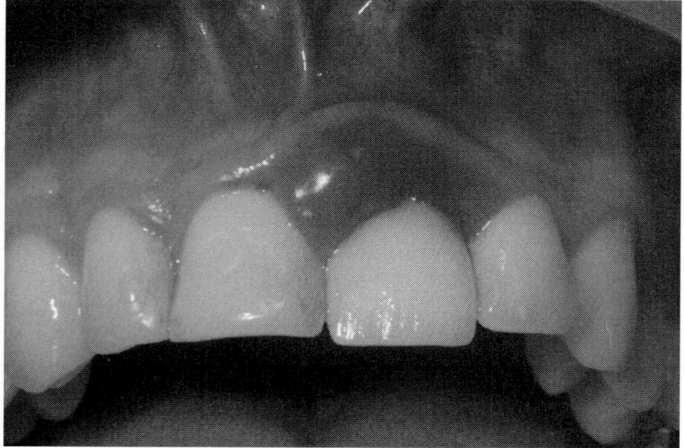

Fig. 11-20 Inflamed marginal and papillary gingiva adjacent to an overcontoured porcelain–fused to metal crown on the maxillary left central.

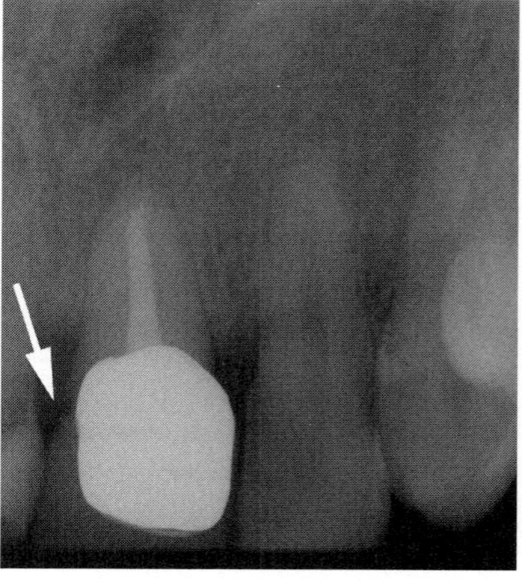

Fig. 11-21 Radiograph of ill-fitting porcelain fused to metal crown shown in Fig. 11-20.

the proximal contacts were defective and 33.5% of adjacent marginal ridges were uneven.[148] However, greater probing depth and loss of clinical attachment have been reported for sites that exhibited both an open contact and food impaction as compared with contralateral control sites without open contacts or food impaction.[94] Excessive anterior overbite is a common cause of food impaction on the lingual surfaces of the maxillary anterior teeth and the facial surfaces of the opposing mandibular teeth. These areas may be exemplified by attachment loss with gingival recession.

Materials. In general, restorative materials are not in themselves injurious to the periodontal tissues.[7,100] One exception to this may be self-curing acrylics[211] (Fig. 11-22).

Plaque that forms at the margins of restorations is similar to that founded on adjacent nonrestored tooth surfaces. The composition of plaque formed on all types of restorative materials is similar, with the exception of that formed on silicate.[145] Although surface textures of restorative materials differ in their capacity to retain plaque,[211,215] all can be adequately cleaned if they are polished[145,178] and accessible to methods of oral hygiene. The undersurface of pontics in fixed bridges should barely touch the mucosa. Access for oral hygiene is inhibited with excessive pontic to tissue contact, thereby contributing to plaque accumulation that will cause gingival inflammation and possibly formation of pseudopockets.[61,192]

Design of Removable Partial Dentures. Several investigations have shown that after the insertion of partial dentures, the mobility of the abutment teeth, gingival inflammation, and periodontal pocket formation increases.[27,38,185] This is because partial dentures favor the accumulation of plaque, particularly if they cover the gingival tissue. Partial dentures that are worn during both night and day induce more plaque formation than those worn only during the daytime.[27] These observations emphasize the need for careful and personalized oral hygiene instruction to avoid harmful effects of partial dentures on the remaining teeth and periodontium.[19] The presence of removable partial dentures induces not only quantitative changes in dental plaque[64] but also qualitative changes, promoting the emergence of spirochetal microorganisms.[65]

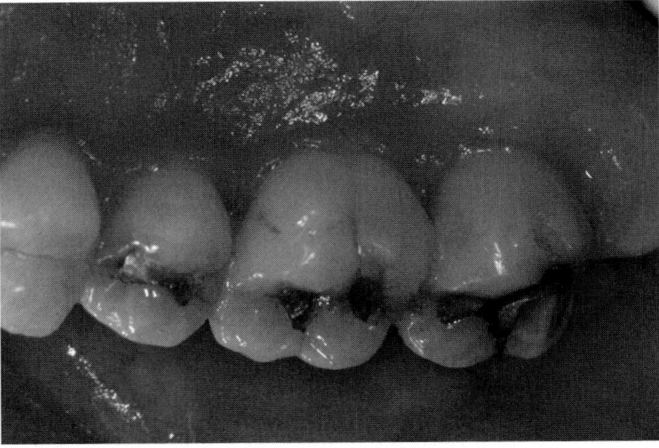

Fig. 11-22 Inflamed palatal gingiva associated with a maxillary provisional acrylic partial denture. Note the substantial difference in color of the inflamed gingiva adjacent to the premolars and first molar compared with the gingiva adjacent to the second molar.

Restorative Dentistry Procedures. The use of rubber dam clamps, matrix bands, and burs in such a manner as to lacerate the gingiva results in varying degrees of mechanical trauma and inflammation. Although such transient injuries generally undergo repair, they are needless sources of discomfort to the patient. Forceful packing of a gingival retraction cord into the sulcus to prepare subgingival margins on a tooth or for the purpose of obtaining an impression may mechanically injure the periodontium and leave behind impacted debris capable of causing a foreign body reaction. (See Chapter 75 for a more detailed explanation.)

Malocclusion

Irregular alignment of teeth as found in cases of malocclusion may make plaque control more difficult. Several authors have found a positive correlation between crowding and periodontal disease[36,151,199] whereas other investigators did not find any correlation.[63] Uneven marginal ridges of contiguous posterior teeth have been found to have a low correlation with pocket depth, loss of attachment, plaque, calculus, and gingival inflammation.[103] Roots of teeth that are prominent in the arch (Figs. 11-23 and 11-24), such as in buccal or lingual version, or that are associated with a high frenal attachment and small quantities of attached gingiva frequently exhibit recession.[2,133]

Failure to replace missing posterior teeth may have adverse consequences on the periodontal support for the remaining teeth.[42] The following scenario illustrates the possible ramifications of not replacing a missing posterior tooth. When the mandibular first molar is extracted, the initial change is a mesial drifting and tilting of the mandibular second and third molars with extrusion of the maxillary first molar. As the mandibular second molar tips mesially, its distal cusps extrude and act as plungers. The distal cusps of the mandibular second molar wedge between the maxillary first and second molars and open the contact by deflecting the maxillary second molar distally. Subsequently, food impaction may occur and be accompanied by gingival inflammation with eventual loss of the interproximal bone between the maxillary first and second molars. The preceding example does not occur in all cases where mandibular first molars are not replaced. However, drifting and tilting of the remaining teeth with an accompanying alteration of the proximal contacts is generally a consequence of not replacing posterior teeth that have been extracted.

Tongue thrusting exerts excessive lateral pressure on the anterior teeth, which may result in spreading and tilting of the anterior teeth (Figs. 11-25 and 11-26). Tongue thrusting is an important contributing factor in

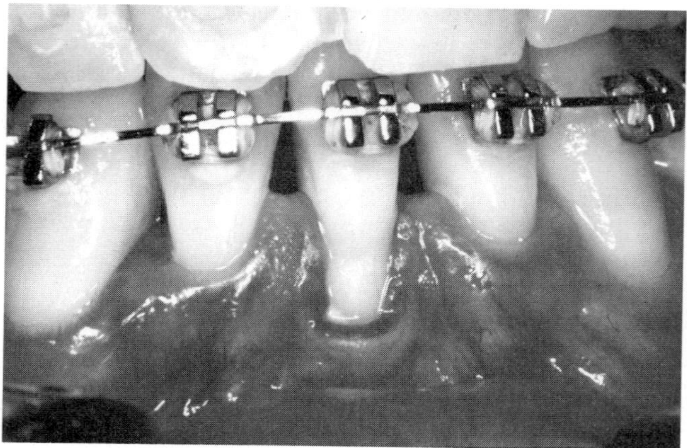

Fig. 11-23 A lower incisor depicting a prominent root without any attached gingiva and accompanying gingival recession.

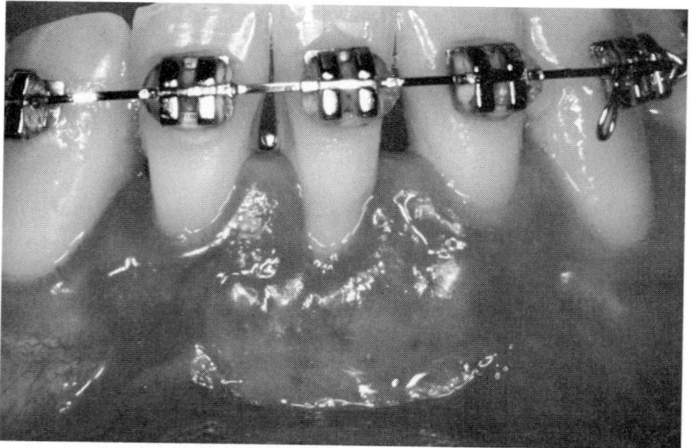

Fig. 11-24 The same patient as shown in Fig. 11-23 following the placement of a soft tissue graft to gain attached gingiva and treat the gingival recession.

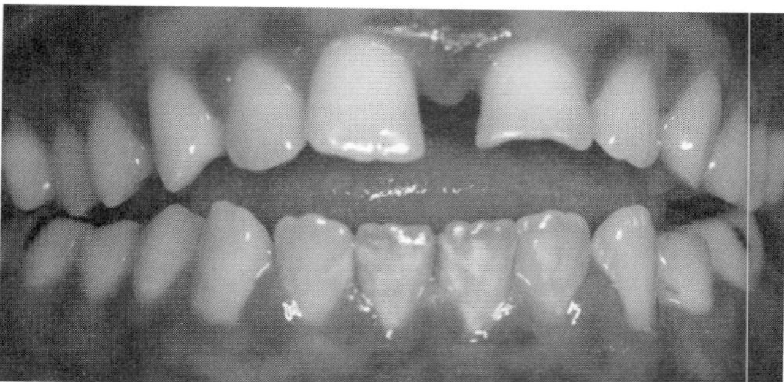

Fig. 11-25 Anterior open bite with flared incisors as observed in association with a habit of tongue thrusting.

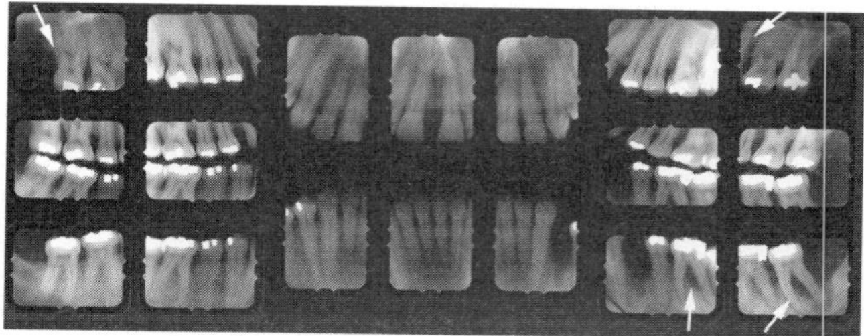

Fig. 11-26 Radiographs of patient shown in Fig. 11-25 with anterior open bite. Note severe periodontal destruction *(arrows)* in molar regions.

pathologic tooth migration and the development of an anterior open bite.[39] Mouth breathing may be observed in association with a habit of tongue thrusting and an anterior open bite. Marginal and papillary gingivitis is frequently encountered in the maxillary anterior sextant in cases involving an anterior open bite with mouth breathing. However, the role of mouth breathing as a local etiologic factor is unclear because conflicting evidence has been reported, including the following:

1. Mouth breathing has no effect on the prevalence or extent of gingivitis, except when considerable amounts of calculus are present.[5]
2. Mouth breathers have more severe gingivitis than non-mouth breathers with similar plaque scores.[90]
3. There is no relationship between mouth breathing and prevalence of gingivitis, except a slight increase in severity.[199]
4. Crowding of teeth is associated with gingivitis only in mouth breathers.[91]

Restorations that do not conform to the occlusal pattern of the mouth result in occlusal disharmonies that may cause injury to the supporting periodontal tissues. Histologic features of the periodontium for a tooth subjected to traumatic occlusion include a widened subcrestal periodontal ligament space, a reduction in collagen content of the oblique and horizontal fibers, an increase in vascularity and leukocyte infiltration, and an increase in the number of osteoclasts on bordering alveolar bone.[24] However, these observations are generally apical and separate from the bacterial-induced inflammation that occurs at the base of the sulcus. On the basis of current human trials, it is still impossible to definitively answer the question, "Does occlusal trauma modify the progression of periodontal attachment loss associated with sulcular inflammation?"[188] (See Chapter 24 for a more detailed explanation of periodontal trauma from occlusion and the periodontal response to external forces.)

Periodontal Complications Associated with Orthodontic Therapy

Orthodontic therapy may affect the periodontium by favoring plaque retention, by directly injuring the gingiva as a result of overextended bands, and by creating excessive forces, unfavorable forces, or both on the tooth and supporting structures.

Plaque Retention and Composition. Orthodontic appliances not only tend to retain bacterial plaque and food debris, resulting in gingivitis (Fig. 11-27), but also are capable of modifying the gingival ecosystem. An increase in *Prevotella melaninogenica, Prevotella intermedia,* and *Actinomyces odontolyticus* and a decrease in the proportion of faculative microorganisms was detected in the gingival sulcus following the placement of orthodontic bands.[52] More recently, *Actinobacillus actinomycetemcomitans* was found in at least one site for 85% of children wearing orthodontic appliances compared with only 15% of the control subjects who were positive for *A. actinomycetemcomitans.*[150]

Gingival Trauma and Alveolar Bone Height. Orthodontic treatment is often started soon after eruption of the permanent teeth, when the junctional epithelium is still adherent to the enamel surface. Orthodontic bands should not be forcefully placed beyond the level of attachment because this will detach the gingiva from the tooth and result in apical proliferation of the junctional epithelium with an increased incidence of gingival recession.[152]

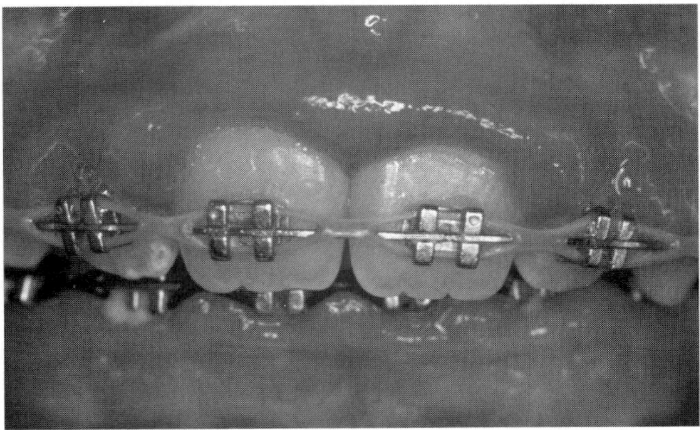

Fig. 11-27 Gingival inflammation and enlargement associated with orthodontic appliance and poor oral hygiene.

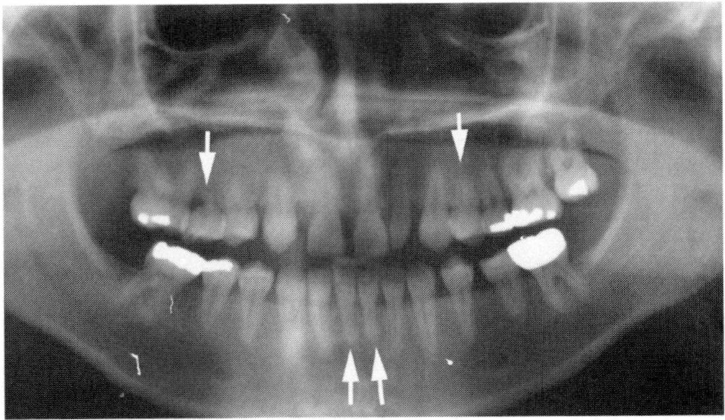

Fig. 11-28 Panoramic radiograph illustrating that a limited degree of pretreatment root resorption existed before orthodontic care was initiated.

The mean alveolar bone loss per patient for adolescents who underwent 2 years of orthodontic care during a 5-year observation period ranged between 0.1 and 0.5 mm.[31] This small magnitude of alveolar bone loss was also noted in the control group and therefore considered to be of little clinical significance. However, the degree of bone loss during adult orthodontic care may be higher than that observed in adolescents,[119] especially if the periodontal condition is not treated before initiating orthodontic therapy.

Tissue Response to Orthodontic Forces. Orthodontic tooth movement is possible because the periodontal tissues are responsive to externally applied forces.[168,184] Alveolar bone is remodeled by osteoclasts inducing bone resorption in areas of pressure and osteoblasts forming bone in areas of tension. Although moderate orthodontic forces ordinarily result in bone remodeling and repair, excessive force may produce necrosis of the periodontal ligament and adjacent alveolar bone.[156–158] Excessive orthodontic forces also increase the risk of apical root resorption.[34,35] The prevalence of severe root resorption, as indicated by resorption of more than one third of the root length, during orthodontic therapy in adolescents has been reported at 3%.[97] The incidence of moderate to severe root resorption for incisors among adults ranging in age from 20 to 45 years has been reported as 2% pretreatment and 24.5% posttreatment[119] (Figs. 11-28 to 11-30). *It is important to avoid excessive force and too rapid tooth movement in orthodontic treatment.*

The use of elastics to close a diastema may result in severe attachment loss with possible tooth loss as the elastics migrate apically along the root (Figs. 11-31 and 11-32). Surgical exposure of impacted teeth and orthodontic-assisted eruption has the potential to compromise the periodontal attachment on adjacent teeth (Figs. 11-33 and 11-34). However, the majority of impacted teeth that are surgically exposed and aided in their eruption by orthodontic treatment subsequently exhibited ≥90% of their attachment intact.[86]

It has been reported that the dentoalveolar gingival fibers that are located within the marginal and attached gingiva are stretched when teeth are rotated during orthodontic therapy.[53] Surgical severing or removal of these gingival fibers in combination with a brief period of retention may reduce the incidence of relapse after orthodontic treatment intended to realign rotated teeth.[33,135]

Extraction of Impacted Third Molars

Numerous clinical studies have reported that the extraction of impacted third molars often results in the creation of vertical defects distal to the second molars.[8] This iatrogenic effect is unrelated to flap design[43] and appears to occur more often when third molars are extracted in individuals older than 25 years.[8,105,130] Other factors that appear to play a role in the development of lesions on the distal surface of second molars, particularly in those

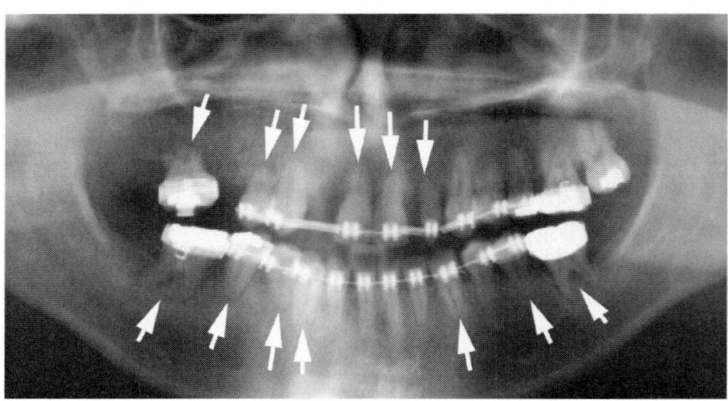

Fig. 11-29 Panoramic radiograph of the same patient as shown in Fig. 11-28 after 4 years of intermittent orthodontic treatment. Note that several roots have undergone severe resorption (see arrows) during orthodontic care.

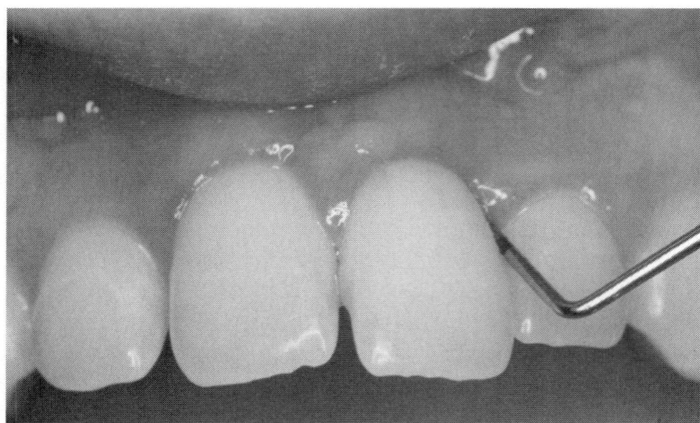

Fig. 11-31 Maxillary central incisors in which an elastic ligature was used to close a midline diastema. Note inflamed gingival and deep probing depths.

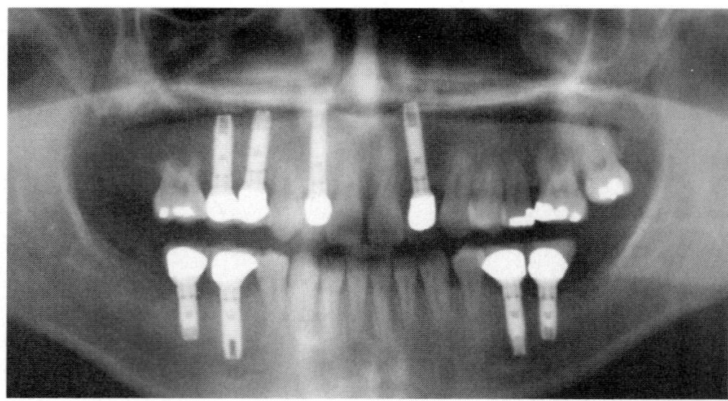

Fig. 11-30 Panoramic radiograph of the same patient as depicted in Fig. 11-29. Note the teeth that had developed extensive root resorption with accompanying hypermobility have been extracted and replaced by implant supported bridgework.

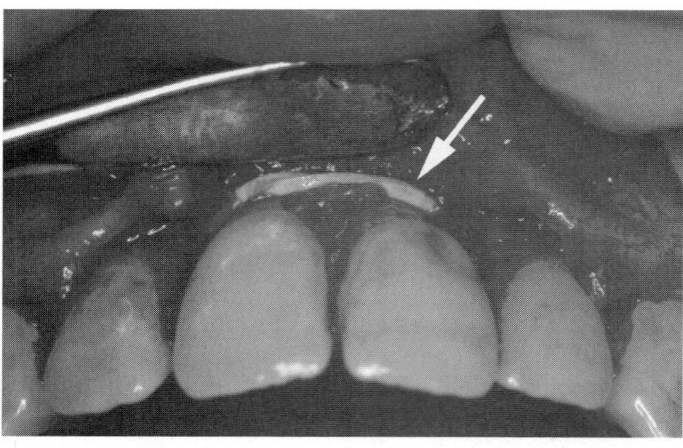

Fig. 11-32 The same patient as shown in Fig. 11-31. A full thickness mucoperiosteal flap has been reflected to expose the elastic ligature and angular intrabony defects around the central incisors.

older than 25 years, include the presence of visible plaque, bleeding on probing, root resorption in the contact area between second and third molars, presence of a pathologically widened follicle, inclination of the third molar, and close proximity of the third molar to the second molar (Fig. 11-35).[105]

Habits and Self-Inflicted Injuries

Patients might not be aware of their self-inflicted injurious habits that may be important to the initiation and progression of their periodontal disease. Mechanical forms of trauma can stem from improper use of a toothbrush, wedging of toothpicks between the teeth, application of fingernail pressure against the gingiva, pizza burns, and others[29] (Fig. 11-36). Sources of chemical irritation include topical applications of caustic medications such as aspirin or cocaine, allergic reactions to toothpaste and chewing gum, use of chewing tobacco and concentrated mouthrinses, and others.[187]

Toothbrush Trauma. Abrasions of the gingiva as well as alterations in tooth structure may result from aggressive brushing in a horizontal or rotary fashion. The deleterious effect of abusive brushing is accentuated when highly abrasive dentifrices are used. The gingival changes attributable to toothbrush trauma may be acute or chronic. The acute changes vary in their appearance and duration from scuffing of the epithelial surface to denudation of the underlying connective tissue with the formation of a painful gingival ulcer (Fig. 11-37). Diffuse erythema and denudation of the attached gingiva throughout the mouth may be a striking sequelae of overzealous brushing. Signs of acute gingival abrasion are frequently noted when the patient first uses a new brush. Puncture lesions may be produced when heavy pressure is applied to firm bristles that are aligned perpendicular to the surface of the gingiva. A forcibly embedded toothbrush bristle may be retained in the gingiva and cause an acute gingival abscess (see Chapter 19).

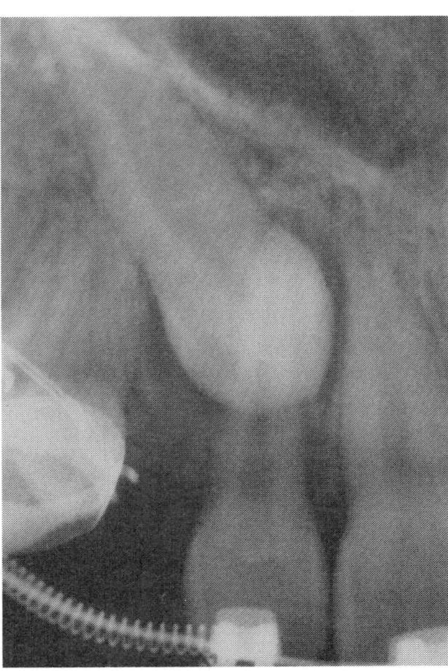

Fig. 11-33 Radiograph of an impacted maxillary canine that required surgically exposed and orthodontic assistance to erupt.

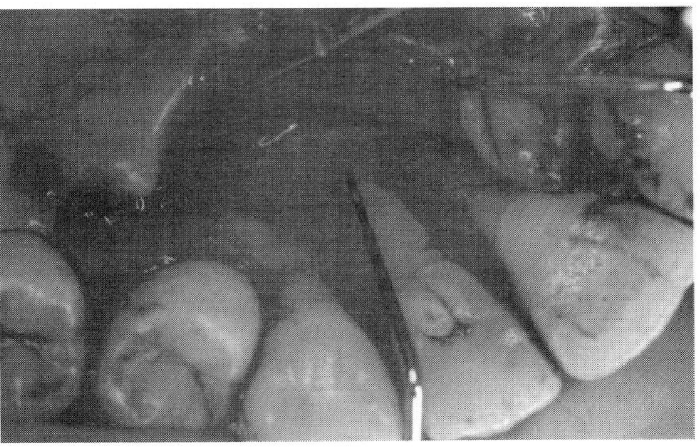

Fig. 11-34 Palatal flap reflected to reveal bony dehiscence on the maxillary lateral incisor shown in Fig. 11-33.

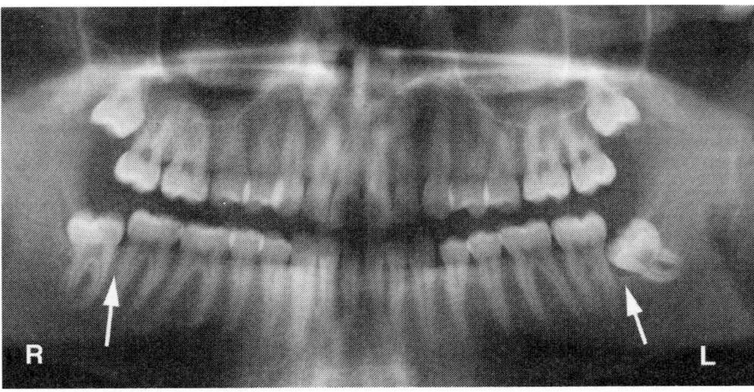

Fig. 11-35 Panoramic radiograph illustrating a mesial impacted lower left third molar with a widened follicle and no apparent bone on the distal interproximal surface of the second molar. Alternatively, the lower right third molar is vertically impacted and exhibits interproximal bone between distal to the second molar and the mesial surface of the third molar.

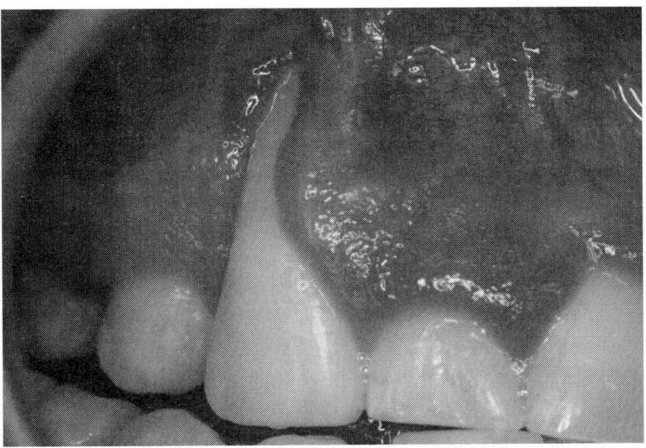

Fig. 11-36 A maxillary canine that illustrates gingival recession due to self-inflicted trauma by the patient's fingernail.

Chronic toothbrush trauma results in gingival recession with denudation of the root surface. Interproximal attachment loss is generally a consequence of bacteria-induced periodontitis, whereas buccal and lingual attachment loss is frequently the result of toothbrush abrasion.[194] Improper use of dental floss may result in lacerations of the interdental papilla.

Chemical Irritation. Acute gingival inflammation may be caused by chemical irritation resulting from either sensitivity or nonspecific tissue injury. In allergic inflammatory states, the gingival changes range from simple erythema to painful vesicle formation and ulceration. Severe reactions to ordinarily innocuous mouthwashes, dentifrices, or denture materials are often explainable on this basis.

Acute inflammation with ulceration may be produced by the nonspecific injurious effect of chemicals on the gingival tissues. The indiscriminate use of strong mouthwashes (Figs. 11-38 and 11-39), topical application of corrosive drugs such as aspirin or cocaine, and accidental contact with drugs such as phenol or silver nitrate are common examples of chemicals that cause irritation of the gingiva.

Tobacco Use

Approximately 25% of the U.S. population smokes cigarettes,[40] and in other portions of the world the percentage of smokers appears to be even higher.[15,121] Smoking was associated with the prevalence of necrotizing ulcerative gingivitis (NUG) as early as 1947.[154,155] In investigations in which plaque levels were kept to a minimum for both smoking and nonsmoking groups or the data were adjusted for this difference, smokers had more sites with deeper pockets[21,23,112] and greater attachment loss.[9,17,77,112] The prevalence of furcation involvement

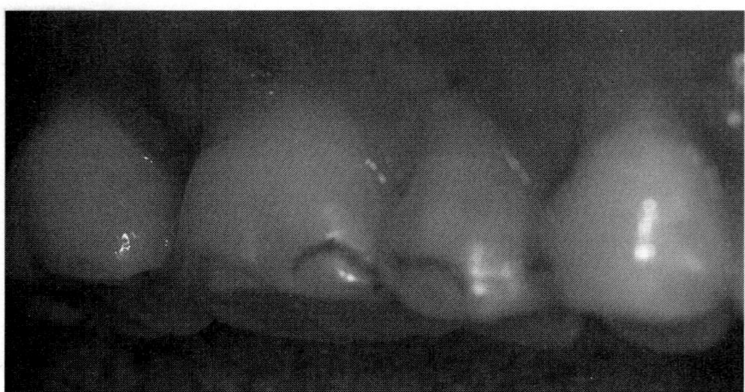

Fig. 11-37 The overzealous use of a toothbrush may denude the gingival epithelial surface, leaving the underlying connective tissue exposed as a painful ulcer.

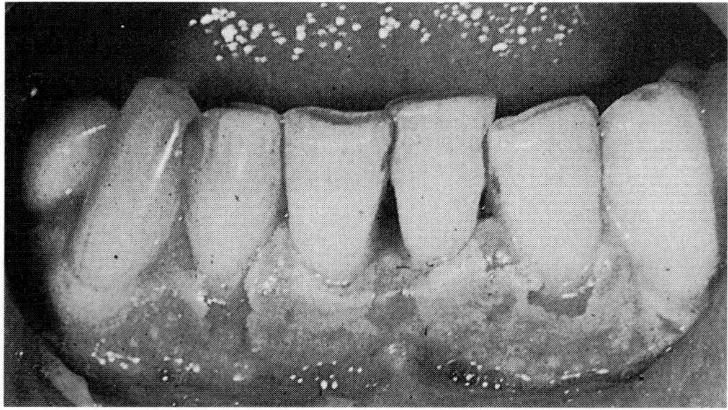

Fig. 11-38 The use of a concentrated mouthwash caused a chemical burn with accompanying necrosis and sloughing of the marginal gingiva.

among smokers was higher[9,142] as was the degree of alveolar bone loss.[20,74,216] It can be concluded that smokers have greater attachment loss and bone loss, an increased number of deep pockets and amount of calculus formation. However, smokers demonstrate varied levels of plaque and inflammation with a bias toward decreased inflammation.

Depending on which clinical parameters are used to assess periodontal disease, smokers are 2.6 to 6 times more likely to develop periodontal disease than nonsmokers.[18,22,77,79,198] The odds ratio for a moderate smoker (15 to 30 pack years) to have periodontal disease is 2.77 times that of a nonsmoker, and a heavy smoker (≥30 pack years) is 4.75 times more likely to have periodontal disease than a nonsmoker.[21] Pack years can be defined as the number of cigarettes smoked per day multiplied by the number of years that an individual smoked. Smoking also appears to be a contributing factor for periodontitis.[1,120,122] MacFarlane and coworkers reported that greater than 90% of their refractory periodontitis patients were smokers as compared with approximately 30% of the general population being smokers.[120] Periodontal maintenance patients who smoke are reported to be twice as likely to lose teeth over a 5-year period as compared with periodontal maintenance patients who do not smoke.[132] Smoking is one of the most significant risk factors currently available to predict the development and progression of periodontitis.[17,18,77]

Two possible explanations for smokers experiencing more prevalent and severe periodontal disease might be that they harbor more pathogenic subgingival microflora or their flora might be more virulent. However, several investigations failed to find any significant difference in the percentage of periodontal pathogens recovered from

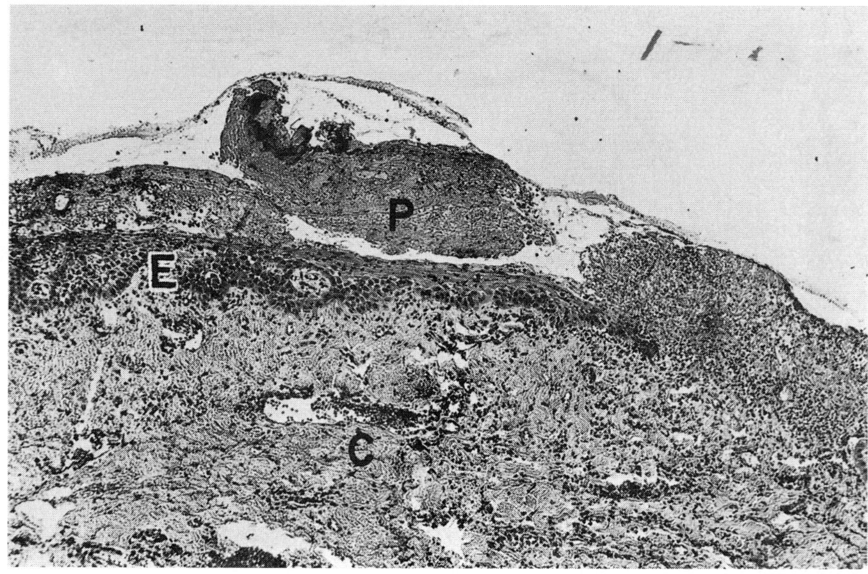

Fig. 11-39 Biopsy specimen of a necrotic area produced by chemical burn. Note the inflamed connective tissue *(C)* and surface pseudomembrane *(P)*. Of particular clinical importance is the newly formed sheet of epithelial cells *(E)*, which undermines the necrotic pseudomembrane and separates it from the underlying connective tissue. This is an important feature of the healing process.

deep pockets in smokers and nonsmokers.[160,163,198] The analysis of subgingival plaque samples collected from a large cross-sectional population in Erie County, New York[219] revealed that smokers were more likely to be infected with *A. actinomycetemcomitans, Porphyromonas gingivalis,* and *Bacteroides forsythus* than nonsmokers. However, the elevated values for these putative pathogens were not statistically higher than those found in nonsmokers. A diminished response to nonsurgical therapy has been reported for smokers. Recent research has indicated that it is more difficult to suppress certain bacteria such as *A. actinomycetemcomitans,*[171] *P. gingivalis,*[76,82] and *B. forsythus*[76] in smokers than in nonsmokers, which may partially explain a diminished response.

Although bacteria are the primary etiologic factors of periodontal disease, a patient's diminished host response may contribute to increased disease susceptibility. Smokers exhibit depressed numbers of helper T-lymphocytes, which are important to stimulate B-cell function for antibody production,[14,48,67] thereby reducing serum levels of IgG.[14] Smoking has been shown to decrease serum IgG2 levels in adult Caucasian subjects[165] and correlate with a dramatic reduction in levels of serum IgG2 anti-*A. actinomycetemcomitans* in African-American smokers with generalized, aggressive periodontitis.[200] Smokers have also been reported to exhibit reduced serum IgG antibodies to *P. intermedia* and *F. nucleatum.*[81] Neutrophils from smokers with refractory periodontitis exhibit impaired phagocytosis.[120] Neutrophils with diminished chemotaxis, phagocytosis, or both[102] may be a consequence of a lower antibody titer, which curtails opsonization. Nicotine has been shown to decrease gingival blood flow.[44] Periodontal wound healing may be adversely affected by exposure to tobacco or nicotine, which may impair revascularization in soft[137] and hard tissues.[172]

Smoking has been identified as a significant variable to predict the response to periodontal treatment.[132,144] Most investigations that evaluated the effect of smoking on nonsurgical therapy have demonstrated less reduction in probing depth[3,75,76,82,96,162,171] and smaller gains in attachment levels in smokers as compared with nonsmokers.[3,82] Smokers who were treated with surgical periodontal therapy and subsequently followed with maintenance care exhibited less probing depth reduction,[3,96,161] smaller gains in clinical attachment levels[3,96] and less gain in bone height[32] than nonsmokers. Heavy cigarette smoking decreases the amount of root coverage obtainable with thick free gingival grafts,[133] whereas the effect of smoking on subepithelial connective tissue grafts is not conclusive.[84,222] Gains in clinical attachment were less in smokers as compared with nonsmokers when guided tissue regenerative procedures were employed.[47,118,175,204,205] Several studies have found implant success rates to be lower in smokers.[12,51,70,95] Implant success rate in excess of 95% have been reported among nonsmokers as compared with less than 89% in smokers during a 6-year period.[12] Patients who quit smoking 1 week before surgery and abstained for 8 weeks following the surgical placement of their implants had only one third as many failures as compared with those individuals who continued to smoke.[13] Implant failure rates in these subjects were similar to nonsmokers. However,

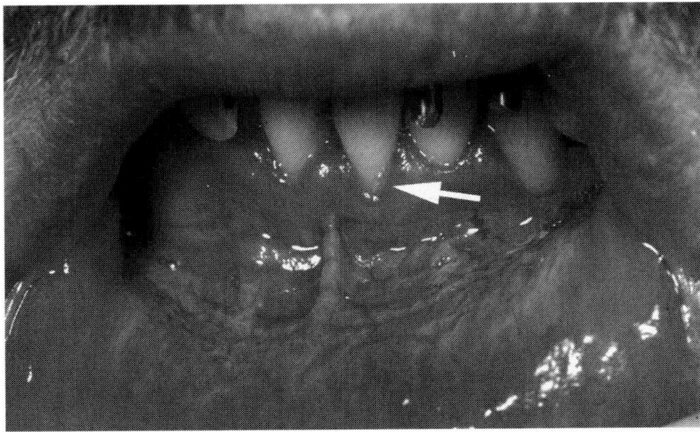

Fig. 11-40 Gingival recession and hyperkeratosis of the vestibular mucosa have developed as a consequence of using chewing tobacco.

other retrospective implant studies have failed to identify smoking as a variable associated with failure.[134,213] A 15-year longitudinal study[113] detected a slightly greater amount of marginal bone loss around implants supporting mandibular fixed prosthesis in smokers as compared with nonsmokers. In summary, smoking has a negative effect on periodontal therapy. However, periodontal therapy did result in an improvement in the periodontal condition of both smokers and nonsmokers when compared with their pretreatment status.

The prevalence and severity of periodontal disease in former smokers is between that of nonsmokers and current smokers.[30,79,80] This implies that once the patients stop smoking, additional adverse effects attributed to smoking may be minimized. However, previous damage is not reversed. Both nonsmokers and former smokers respond more favorably to periodontal therapy than current smokers, whereas no significant difference in response was noted between former smokers and nonsmokers.[76,96] The benefits of terminating smoking on periodontal treatment do not appear to be related to the number of years since smoking was halted.[76] Therefore a past history of smoking does not appear to be deleterious to the response of current periodontal treatment.

Feldman and co-workers reported that plaque, calculus, probing depth, and bone loss measurements for cigar smokers were intermediate to those for nonsmokers and cigarette smokers while exhibiting a tendency to be closer to nonsmoker values.[59]

Approximately 9% of the U.S. high school population currently use smokeless tobacco products such as snuff and chewing tobacco.[41] The relationship between the use of smokeless tobacco and squamous cell carcinoma in the oral cavity is well established.[217] A strong relationship has been established between white oral mucosal lesions and the use of smokeless tobacco by athletes[57,174] and adolescents.[49,147,203] These white mucosal lesions occur in approximately 50% to 60% of smokeless tobacco users, whereas 25% to 30% exhibit localized attachment loss in the form of gingival recession on the facial surfaces of mandibular anterior teeth (Fig. 11-40).[73,159,174] A recent publication demonstrated that 97.5% of these leukoplakia lesions are clinically resolved after abstaining from smokeless tobacco for 6 weeks.[131]

Radiation Therapy

Radiation therapy has cytotoxic effects on both normal cells and malignant cells. A typical total dose of radiation for head and neck tumors is in the range of 5000 to 8000 centiGrays (cGy = 1 rad).[153] The total dose of radiation is generally given in partial incremental doses referred to as *fractionation.* Fractionation helps minimize the adverse effects of the radiation while maximizing the death rate for the tumor cells.[60] Fractionated doses are typically administered in the range of 100 to 1000 cGys per week.

Radiation treatment induces an obliterative endarteritis that results in soft tissue ischemia and fibrosis while irradiated bone becomes hypovascular and hypoxic.[128] Adverse affects of head and neck radiation therapy include dermatitis and mucositis of the irradiated area as well as muscle fibrosis and trismus, which may restrict access to the oral cavity.[176] The mucositis typically develops 5 to 7 days after radiation therapy is initiated. The severity of the mucositis can be reduced by asking the patient to avoid secondary sources of irritation to the mucous membrane, such as smoking, alcohol, and spicy foods. Use of a chlorhexidine digluconate mouthrinse may help reduce the mucositis.[166] However, all chlorhexidine mouthrinses currently available in the U.S. have a high alcohol content that may act as an astringent, which dehydrates the mucosa, thereby intensifying the pain. Saliva production is permanently impaired when salivary glands that are located within the portal of radiation receive ≥6000 cGy.[129] Xerostomia results in greater plaque accumulation and a reduced buffering capacity from what saliva is left. The use of effective oral hygiene, professional dental prophylactic cleanings, fluoride applications, and frequent dental examinations are essential to control caries and periodontal disease. The use of customized trays appears to be a more effective method of fluoride application as compared with the toothbrush.[101]

Periodontal attachment loss and tooth loss was greater in cancer patients who were treated with high-dose unilateral radiation as compared with the nonradiated control side of the dentition.[56] Irradiated patients should be covered with prophylactic antibiotics before receiving appropriate nonsurgical periodontal therapy following the patient's initial recovery from radiation therapy.[58] Dental and periodontal infections have the potential to be a severe risk to a patient who has been treated with head and neck radiation. Therefore the dental therapist may choose to consult with the patient's oncologist before initiating therapy. The risk of osteoradionecrosis must be evaluated before extracting a tooth or performing periodontal surgery in an irradiated site. Precautions must be taken regarding prophylactic antibiotics, atraumatic surgical technique, microbiologic culture and sensitivity, restricted use of local anesthetic with vasoconstrictor, and the need for hyperbaric oxygen therapy. (Refer to Chapter 38 for more detail on the periodontal management of medically compromised patients.)

REFERENCES

1. Adams D: Diagnosis and treatment of refractory periodontitis. Curr Opin Dent 1992; 2:33.
2. Addy M, Dummer P, Hunter M, et al: A study of the association of fraenal attachment, lip coverage and vestibular depth with plaque and gingivitis. J Periodontol 1987; 58:752.
3. Ah M, Johnson G, Kaldahl W, et al: The effect of smoking on the response to periodontal therapy. J Clin Periodontol 1994; 21:91.
4. Albandar J, Kingman A, Brown L, et al: Gingival inflammation and subgingival calculus as determinants of disease progression in early-onset periodontitis. J Clin Periodontol 1998; 25:231.
5. Alexander A: Habitual mouth breathing and its effect on gingival health. Parodontologie 1970; 24:49.
6. Anerud A, Löe H, Boysen H: The natural history and clinical course of calculus formation in man. J Clin Periodontol 1991; 18:160.
7. App G: Effect of silicate, amalgam and cast gold on the gingiva. J Prosthet Dent 1961; 11:522.
8. Ash M, Costich E, Hayward J: A study of periodontal hazards of third molars. J Periodontol 1962; 33:209.
9. Axelsson P, Paulander J, Lindhe J: Relationship between smoking and dental status in 35-, 50-, 65-, and 75-year old individuals. J Clin Periodontol 1998; 25:297.
10. Baer P, Burstone M: Esterase activity associated with formation of deposits on teeth. Oral Surg 1959; 12:1147.
11. Baer P, Keyes P, White C: Studies on experimental calculus formation in the rat. XII. On the transmissibility of factors affecting dental calculus. J Periodontol 1968; 39:86.
12. Bain C, Moy P: The association between the failure of dental implants and cigarette smoking. Int J Oral Maxillofac Implants 1993; 8:609.
13. Bain C: Smoking and implant failure—Benefits of a smoking cessation protocol. Int J Oral Maxillofac Implants 1996; 11:756.
14. Barbour S, Nakashim K, Zhang J, et al: Tobacco and smoking: Environmental factors that modify the host response (immune system) and have an impact on periodontal health. Crit Rev Oral Biol Med 1997; 8:437.
15. Bartecchi C, MacKenzie T, Schrier R: The human costs of tobacco use. I. N Engl J Med 1994; 331:907.
16. Baumhammers A, Stallard R: A method for the labeling of certain constituents in the organic matrix of dental calculus. J Dent Res 1966; 45:1568.
17. Beck J, Koch C, Offenbacher S: Incidence of attachment loss over 3 years in older adults—new and progressing lesions. Community Dent Oral Epidemiol 1995; 23:291.
18. Beck J, Koch G, Rozier R, et al: Prevalence and risk indicators for periodontal attachment loss in a population of older community-dwelling blacks and whites. J Periodontol 1990; 61:521.
19. Bergman B, Hugoson A, Olsson C: Periodontal and prosthetic conditions in patients treated with removable partial dentures and artificial crowns. Acta Odontol Scand 1971; 29:621.
20. Bergström J, Eliasson S: Cigarette smoking and alveolar bone height in subjects with high standard of oral hygiene. J Clin Periodontol 1987; 14:466.
21. Bergström J, Eliasson S: Noxious effect of cigarette smoking on periodontal health. J Periodont Res 1987; 22:513.
22. Bergström J, Preber H: Tobacco use as a risk factor. J Periodontol 1994; 65:545.
23. Bergström J: Cigarette smoking as risk factor in chronic periodontal disease. Community Dent Oral Epidemiol 1989; 17:245.

24. Biancu S, Ericsson I, Lindhe J: Periodontal ligament tissue reactions to trauma and gingival inflammation. An experimental study in beagle dogs. J Clin Periodontol 1995; 22:772.
25. Bibby B: The formation of salivary calculus. Dent Cosmos 1935; 77:668.
26. Birkeland J, Jorkjend L: The effect of chewing apples on dental plaque and food debris. Commun Dent Oral Epidemiol 1974; 2:161.
27. Bissada N, Ibrahim S, Barsoum W: Gingival response to various types of removable partial dentures. J Periodontol 1974; 45:651.
28. Bjorn AL, Bjorn H, Grcovic B: Marginal fit of restorations and its relation to periodontal bone level. Odont Revy 1969; 20:311.
29. Blanton P, Hurt W, Largent M: Oral factitious injuries. J Periodontol 1977; 48:33.
30. Bolin A, Eklund G, Frithiof L, et al: The effect of changed smoking habits on marginal alveolar bone loss. Swed Dent J 1993; 17:211.
31. Bondemark L: Interdental bone changes after orthodontic treatment: a 5-year longitudinal study. Am J Orthod Dentofac Orthop 1998; 114:25.
32. Bostrom L, Linder L, Bergstrom J: Influence of smoking on the outcome of periodontal surgery. A 5-year follow-up. J Clin Periodontol 1998; 25:194.
33. Brain W: The effect of surgical transsection of free gingival fibers on the regression of orthodontically rotated teeth in the dog. Am J Orthod 1969; 55:50.
34. Brezniak N, Wasserstein A: Root resorption after orthodontic treatment: Part 1. Literature review. Am J Orthod Dentofac Orthop 1993; 103:62.
35. Brezniak N, Wasserstein A: Root resorption after orthodontic treatment: Part 2. Literature review. Am J Orthod Dentofac Orthop 1993; 103:138.
36. Buckley L: The relationship between malocclusion and periodontal disease. J Periodontol 1972; 43:415.
37. Buchanan S, Jenderseck R, Granet M, et al: Radiographic detection of dental calculus. J Periodontol 1987; 58:747.
38. Carlsson G, Hedegard B, Koivumaa K: Studies in partial dental prosthesis. IV. Final results of a four-year longitudinal investigation of dentogingivally supported partial dentures. Acta Odontol Scand 1965; 23:443.
39. Carranza F, Sr, Carraro J: El empuje lingual como factor traumatizante en periodoncia. Rev Asoc Odontol Argent 1959; 47:105.
40. Centers for Disease Control and Prevention: Cigarette smoking among adults. MMWR Morb Mort Wkly Rep 1997; 48:1217.
41. Centers for Disease Control: Tobacco use among high school students—United States. MMWR Morb Mort Wkly Rep 1998; 47:229.
42. Chaikin B: Anterior periodontal destruction due to the loss of one or more unreplaced molars. Dent Items Int 1939; 61:17.
43. Chin Quee T, Gosselin D, Millar E, et al: Surgical removal of the fully impacted mandibular third molar. The influence of flap design and alveolar bone height. J Periodontol 1985; 56:625.
44. Clarke N, Shephard B, Hirsch R: The effects of intra-arterial epinephrine and nicotine on gingival circulation. Oral Surg Oral Med Oral Pathol 1981; 52:577.
45. Clerehugh V, Abdeia R, Hull P: The effect of subgingival calculus on the validity of clinical probing measurements. J Dentistry 1996; 24:329.
46. Conroy C, Sturzenberger O: The rate of calculus formation in adults. J Periodontol 1968; 39:142.
47. Cortellini P, Pini Prato G, Tonetti M: Long-term stability of clinical attachment following guided tissue regeneration and conventional therapy. J Clin Periodontol 1996; 23:106.
48. Costabel U, Bross K, Reuter C, et al: Alterations in immunoregulatory T-cell subsets in cigarette smokers. A phenotypic analysis of bronchoalveolar and blood lymphocytes. Chest 1986; 90:39.
49. Creath C, Cutter G, Bradley D, et al: Oral leukoplakia and adolescent smokeless tobacco use. Oral Surg Oral Med Oral Pathol 1991; 72:35.
50. Dawes C: Recent research on calculus. N Zealand Dent J 1998; 94:60.
51. De Bruyn H, Collaert B: The effect of smoking on early implant failure. Clin Oral Impl Res 1994; 5:260.
52. Diamanti-Kipioti A, Gusberti F, Lang N: Clinical and microbiological effects of fixed orthodontic appliances. J Clin Periodontol 1987; 14:326.
53. Edwards J: A study of the periodontium during orthodontic rotation of teeth. Am J Orthod 1968; 54:441.
54. Egelberg J: Local effect of diet on plaque formation and development of gingivitis in dogs. III. Effect of frequency of meals and tube feeding. Odontol Revy 1965; 16:50.
55. Ennever J: Microbiologic mineralization: A calcifiable cell-free extract from a calcifiable microorganism. J Dent Res 1983; 41:1383.
56. Epstein J, Lunn R, Le N, et al: Periodontal attachment loss in patients after head and neck radiation therapy. Oral Surg Oral Med Oral Pathol 1998; 86:673.
57. Ernster V, Grady DG, Greene JC, et al: Smokeless tobacco use and health effects among baseball players. JAMA 1990; 264:218.
58. Fattore L, Strauss R, Bruno J: The management of periodontal disease in patients who have received radiation therapy for head and neck cancer. Spec Care Dentist 1987; 7:120.
59. Feldman R, Alman J, Chauncey H: Periodontal disease indexes and tobacco smoking in healthy aging men. Gerodontics 1987; 3:43.
60. Fletcher G: The role of irradiation in the management of squamous-cell carcinomas of the mouth and throat. Head Neck Surg 1979; 1:441.
61. Flemmig T, Sorensen J, Newman M, et al: Gingival enhancement in fixed prosthodontics. Part II. Microbiologic findings. J Prosthet Dent 1991; 65:365.
62. Flores-de-Jacoby L, Zafiropoulos G, Ciancio S: The effect of crown margin location on plaque and periodontal health. Int J Periodont Restor Dent 1989; 9:197.
63. Geiger A, Wasserman B, Turgeon L: Relationship of occlusion and periodontal disease. VIII. Relationship of crowding and spacing to periodontal destruction and gingival inflammation. J Periodontol 1974; 45:43.
64. Ghamrawy E: Quantitative changes in dental plaque formation related to removable partial dentures. J Oral Rehabil 1976; 3:115.
65. Ghamrawy E: Qualitative changes in dental plaque formation related to removable partial dentures. J Oral Rehabil 1979; 6:183.
66. Gilmore N, Sheiham A: Overhanging dental restorations and periodontal disease. J Periodontol 1971; 42:8.
67. Ginns L, Goldenheim P, Miller L: T-lymphocyte subsets in smoking and lung cancer. Analyses of monoclonal antibodies and flow cytometry. Am Rev Res Dis 1982; 126:265.
68. Glock G, Murray M: Chemical investigation of salivary calculus. J Dent Res 1938; 17:257.
69. Gonzales F, Sognnaes R: Electromicroscopy of dental calculus. Science 1960; 131:156.
70. Gorman L, Lambert P, Morris H, et al: The effect of smoking on implant survival at second stage surgery: DICRG

interim report No. 5. Dental implant clinical research group. Implant Dent 1994; 3:165.
71. Gorzo I, Newman H, Strahan J: Amalgam restoration, plaque removal and periodontal health. J Clin Periodontol 1979; 6:98.
72. Greene J: Oral hygiene and periodontal disease. Am J Public Health 1963; 53:913.
73. Greer R, Poulson T: Oral tissue alterations associated with the use of smokeless tobacco by teen-agers, Part I. Clinical findings. Oral Surg Oral Med Oral Pathol 1983; 56:275.
74. Grossi S, Genco R, Machtei E, et al: Assessment of risk for periodontal disease. II Risk indicators for alveolar bone loss. J Periodontol 1995; 66:23.
75. Grossi S, Skrepcinski F, DeCaro T, et al: Response to periodontal therapy in diabetics and smokers. J Periodontol 1996; 67:1094.
76. Grossi S, Zambon J, Machtei E, et al: Effects of smoking and smoking cessation on healing after mechanical therapy. J Amer Dent Assoc 1997; 128:599.
77. Grossi S, Zambon J, Ho A, et al: Assessment of risk for periodontal disease. I. Risk indicators for attachment loss. J Periodontol 1994; 65:260.
78. Gustafsson B, Krasse B: Dental calculus in germ free rats. Acta Odontol Scand 1962; 20:135.
79. Haber J, Kent RL: Cigarette smoking in periodontal practice. J Periodontol 1992; 63:100.
80. Haber J, Wattles J, Crowley M, et al: Evidence for cigarette smoking as a major risk factor for periodontitis. J Periodontol 1993; 64:16.
81. Haber J: Cigarette smoking: A major risk factor for periodontitis. Compendium Cont Educ Dent 1994; 15:1002.
82. Haffajee A, Cugini M, Dibart S, et al: The effect of SRP on the clinical and microbiological parameters of periodontal diseases. J Clin Periodontol 1997; 24:324.
83. Hakkarainen K, Ainamo J: Influence of overhanging posterior tooth restorations of alveolar bone height in adults. J Clin Periodontol 1980; 7:114.
84. Harris R: The connective tissue with partial thickness double pedicle graft. The results of 100 consecutively treated defects. J Periodontol 1994; 65:448.
85. Highfield J, Powell R: Effects of removal of posterior overhanging metallic margins of restorations upon the periodontal tissues. J Clin Periodontol 1978; 5:169.
86. Hinrichs J, ElDeeb M, Waite D, et al: Periodontal evaluation of canines erupted through grafted alveolar cleft defects. J Oral Maxillofac Surg 1984; 42:717.
87. Hirschfeld I: Food impaction. J Am Dent Assoc 1930; 17:1504.
88. Hodge H, Leung S: Calculus formation. J Periodontol 1950; 21:211.
89. Huttner G: Follow-up study of crowns and abutments with regard to the crown edge and the marginal periodontium. Dtsch Zahnarztl Z 1971; 26:724.
90. Jacobson L: Mouth breathing and gingivitis. J Periodont Res 1973; 8:269.
91. Jacobson L, Linder-Aronson S: Crowding and gingivitis: A comparison between mouth breathers and non-mouth breathers. Scand J Dent Res 1972; 80:500.
92. Jeffcoat M, Howell T: Alveolar bone destruction due to overhanging amalgam in periodontal disease. J Periodontol 1980; 51:599.
93. Jenkins G: The Physiology of the Mouth. Oxford, Blackwell Scientific Publications, 1966.
94. Jernberg G, Bakdash B, Keenan K: Relationship between proximal tooth open contact and periodontal disease. J Periodontol 1983; 54:529.
95. Jones J, Triplett R: The relationship of cigarette smoking to impaired intraoral wound healing: A review of evidence and implications for patient care. J Oral Maxillofac Surg 1992; 50:237.
96. Kaldahl W, Johnson G, Patil K, et al: Levels of cigarette consumption and response to periodontal therapy. J Periodontol 1996; 67:675.
97. Kaley J, Phillips C: Factors related to root resorption in edgewise practice. Angle Orthod 1991; 61:125.
98. Karlsen K: Gingival reactions to dental restorations. Acta Odontol Scand 1970; 28:895.
99. Kashket S, Zhang J, Niederman R: Gingival inflammation induced by food and short-chain carboxylic acids. J Dent Res 1998; 77:412.
100. Kawakara H, Yamagani A, Nakamura M, Jr: Biological testing of dental materials by means of tissue culture. Int Dent J 1968; 18:443.
101. Keene H, Fleming T, Toth B: Cariogenic microflora in patients with Hodgkin's disease before and after mantle field radiotherapy. Oral Surg Oral Med Oral Pathol 1994; 78:577.
102. Kenney EG, Kraal JH, Saxe SR, et al: The effect of cigarette smoke on human oral polymorphonuclear leukocytes. J Periodont Res 1977; 12:227.
103. Kepic T, O'Leary T: Role of marginal ridge relationships as an etiologic factor in periodontal disease. J Periodontol 1978; 49:570.
104. Koivumaa K, Wennstrom A: A histological investigation of the changes in gingival margins adjacent to gold crowns. Odont T 1960; 68:373.
105. Kugelberg C: Third molar surgery. Curr Opin Dent 1992; 2:9.
106. Kupczyk L, Conroy M: The attachment of calculus to root planed surfaces. Periodontics 1968; 6:78.
107. Lang N, Kiel R, Anderhalden K: Clinical and microbiological effect of subgingival restorations with overhanging or clinically perfect margins. J Clin Periodontol 1983; 10:563.
108. Leach S, Saxton C: An electron microscopic study of the acquired pellicle and plaque formed on the enamel of human incisors. Arch Oral Biol 1966; 11:1081.
109. Leon A: Amalgam restorations and periodontal disease. Br Dent J 1976; 140:377.
110. Leung S, Jensen A: Factors controlling the deposition of calculus. Int Dent J 1958; 8:613.
111. Lilienthal B, Amerena V, Gregory G: An epidemiological study of chronic periodontal disease. Arch Oral Biol 1965; 10:553.
112. Linden G, Mullally B: Cigarette smoking and periodontal destruction in young adults. J Periodontol 1994; 65:718.
113. Lindquist L, Carlsson G, Jemt T: A prospective 15-year follow-up study of mandibular fixed prosthesis supported by osseeointegrated implants. Clinical results and marginal bone loss. Clin Oral Impl Res 1996; 7:329.
114. Little M, Bowman L, Casciani C, et al: The composition of dental calculus. III. Supragingival calculus. The amino acid and saccharide component. Arch Oral Biol 1966; 11:385.
115. Little M, Bowman L, Dirksen T: The lipids of supragingival calculus. J Dent Res 1964; 43:836.
116. Little M, Hazen S: Dental calculus composition. 2. Subgingival calculus: Ash, calcium, phosphorus, and sodium. J Dent Res 1964; 43:645.
117. Löe H, Schiott C: The effect of mouth rinses and topical application of chlorhexidine on the development of dental plaque and gingivitis in man. J Periodont Res 1970; 5:79.
118. Luepke P, Mellonig J, Brunvold M: A clinical evaluation of a bioresorbable barrier with and without decalcified freeze-dried bone allograft in the treatment of molar furcations. J Clin Periodontol 1998; 24:440.

119. Lupi J, Handelman C, Sadowsky C: Prevalence and severity of apical root resorption and alveolar bone loss in orthodontically treated adults. Am J Orthod Dentofac Orthop 1996; 109:28.
120. MacFarlane G, Herzberg M, Wolff L, et al: Refractory periodontitis associated with abnormal polymorphonuclear leukocyte phagocytosis and cigarette smoking. J Periodontol 1992; 63:908.
121. MacKenzie T, Bartecchi C, Schrier, R: The human costs of tobacco use. II. N Engl J Med 1994; 331:975.
122. Magnusson I, Walker C: Refractory periodontitis or recurrence of disease. J Clin Periodontol 1996; 23:289.
123. Mandel I: Calculus formation. The role of bacteria and mucoprotein. Dent Clin North Am 1960; 4:731.
124. Mandel I: Histochemical and biochemical aspects of calculus formation. Periodontics 1963; 1:43.
125. Mandel I: Biochemical aspects of calculus formation. J Periodont Res 1969; 4(suppl):7.
126. Mandel I, Levy B, Wasserman B: Histochemistry of calculus formation. J Periodontol 1957; 28:132.
127. Manly R: A structureless recurrent deposit on teeth. J Dent Res 1973; 22:479.
128. Marciani R, Ownby H: Osteoradionecrosis of the jaw. J Oral Maxillofac Surg 1986; 44:218.
129. Markitziu A, Zafiropoulos G, Tsalkis L, et al: Gingival health and salivary function in head and neck-irradiated patients. A five year follow-up. Oral Surg Oral Med Oral Pathol 1992; 73:427.
130. Marmary Y, Brayer L, Tzukert A, et al: Alveolar bone repair following extraction of impacted mandibular third molars. Oral Surg Oral Med Oral Pathol 1986; 61:324.
131. Martin G, Brown J, Eifler C, et al: Oral leukoplakia status six weeks after cessation of smokeless tobacco use. J Amer Dent Assoc 1999; 130:945.
132. McGuire M, Nunn M: Prognosis versus actual outcome. III. The effectiveness of clinical parameters in accurately predicting tooth survival. J Periodontol 1996; 67:666.
133. Miller P: Root coverage with the free gingival graft. Factors associated with incomplete coverage. J Periodontol 1987; 58:674.
134. Minsk L, Polson A, Weisgold A, et al: Outcome failures of endosseous implants from a clinical training center. Compend Cont Ed 1996; 17:849.
135. Moffett B: Remodeling changes of the facial sutures, periodontal and temporomandibular joints produced by orthodontic forces in Rhesus monkeys. Bull Pac Coast Soc Ortho 1969; 44:46.
136. Morris M: Artificial crown contours and gingival health. J Prosthet Dent 1962; 12:1146.
137. Mosely L, Finseth F, Goody M: Nicotine and its effects on wound healing. Plast Rectonr Surg 1978; 61:570.
138. Mueller H: The effect of artificial crown margins on the periodontal conditions in a group of periodontally supervised patients treated with fixed bridges. J Clin Periodontol 1986; 13:97.
139. Mühlemann H, Schroeder H: Dynamics of supragingival calculus formation. Adv Oral Biol 1964; 1:175.
140. Mühler J, Ennever J: Occurrence of calculus through several successive periods in a selected group of subjects. J Periodontol 1962; 33:22.
141. Mukherjee S: Formation and prevention of supragingival calculus. J Periodont Res 1968; 3(suppl 2):1.
142. Mullally B, Linden G: Molar furcation involvement associated with cigarette smoking in periodontal referrals. J Clin Periodontol 1996; 23:658.
143. Neuman W, Neuman M: The Chemical Dynamics of Bone Mineral. Chicago, University of Chicago Press, 1958.
144. Newman M, Kornman K, Holtzman S: Association of clinical risk factors with treatment outcomes. J Periodontol 1994; 65:489.
145. Norman R, Mehia R, Swartz M, et al: Effect of restorative materials on plaque composition. J Dent Res 1972; 51:1596.
146. Normann W, Regolati B, Renggli H: Gingival reaction to well-fitted subgingival proximal gold inlays. J Clin Periodontol 1974; 1:120.
147. Offenbacher S, Weathers D: Effects of smokeless tobacco on the periodontal, mucosal and caries status of adolescent males. J Oral Pathol 1985; 14:169.
148. O'Leary T, Badell M, Bloomer R: Interproximal contact and marginal ridge relationships in periodontally healthy young males classified as to orthodontic status. J Periodontol 1975; 46:6.
149. Pack A, Coxhead L, McDonald B: The prevalence of overhanging margins in posterior amalgam restorations and periodontal consequences. J Clin Periodontol 1990; 17:145.
150. Paolantonio M, Girolamo G, Pedrazzoli V, et al: Occurrence of *Actinobacillus actinomycetemcomitans* in patients wearing orthodontic appliances. A cross-sectional study. J Clin Periodontol 1996; 23:112.
151. Paunio K: The role of malocclusion and crowding in the development of periodontal disease. Int Dent J 1973; 23:420.
152. Pearson L: Gingival height of lower central incisors, orthodontically treated and untreated. Angle Orthod 1968; 38:337.
153. Peterson D, D'Ambrosio J: Nonsurgical management of head and neck cancer patients. Dent Clin North Am 1994; 38:425.
154. Pindborg J: Tobacco and gingivitis. I. Statistical examination of the significance of tobacco in the development of ulceromembranous gingivitis and in the formation of calculus. J Dent Res 1947; 26:261.
155. Pindborg J: Tobacco and gingivitis. II. Correlation between consumption of tobacco, ulceromembranous gingivitis and calculus. J Dent Res 1949; 28:460.
156. Polson A, Reed BE: Long-term effect of orthodontic treatment on crestal alveolar bone levels. J Periodontol 1984; 55:28.
157. Polson A, Adams R, Zander H: Osseous repair in the presence of active tooth hypermobility. J Clin Periodontol 1983; 10:370.
158. Polson A: The relative importance of plaque and occlusion in periodontal disease. J Clin Periodontol 1986; 13:923.
159. Poulson T, Lindenmuth J, Greer R: A comparison of the use of smokeless tobacco in rural and urban teenagers. CA: A Cancer Journal for Clinicians 1984; 34:248.
160. Preber H, Bergström J, Linder L: Occurrence of periopathogens in smoker and non-smoker patients. J Clin Periodontol 1992; 19:667.
161. Preber H, Bergström J: Effect of cigarette smoking on periodontal healing following surgical therapy. J Clin Periodontol 1990; 17:324.
162. Preber H, Bergström J: The effect of non-surgical treatment on periodontal pockets in smokers and non-smokers. J Clin Periodontol 1986; 13:319.
163. Preber H, Linder L, Bergstrom J: Periodontal healing and periopathogenic microflora in smokers and non-smokers. J Clin Periodontol 1995; 22:946.
164. Prinz H: The origin of salivary calculus. Dent Cosmos 1921; 63:231, 369, 503, 619.
165. Quinn S, Zhang J, Gunsolley J, et al: The influence of smoking and race on adult periodontitis and serum IgG2 levels. J Periodontol 1998; 69:171.
166. Raether D, Walker P, Bostrum B, et al: Effectiveness of oral chlorhexidine for reducing stomatitis in a pediatric bone marrow transplant population. Pediatr Dent 1989; 11:37.

167. Ramfjord S: The periodontal status of boys 11 to 17 years old in Bombay, India. J Periodontol 1961; 32:237.
168. Reitan K: Tissue changes following experimental tooth movement as related to the time factor. Dent Record 1953; 73:559.
169. Renggli H: The influence of subgingival proximal filling borders on the degree of inflammation of the adjacent gingiva. A clinical study. Schweiz Monatsschr Zahnheilkd 1974; 84:181.
170. Renggli H, Regolati B: Gingival inflammation and plaque accumulation by well-adapted supragingival and subgingival proximal restorations. Helv Odontol Acta 1972; 16:99.
171. Renvert S, Dahlen G, Widstrom M: The clinical and microbiological effects of non-surgical periodontal therapy in smokers and non-smokers. J Clin Periodontol 1998; 25:153.
172. Riebel G, Boden S, Whitesides T, et al: The effect of nicotine on incorporation of cancellous bone graft in an animal model. Spine 1995; 20:2198.
173. Rizzo A, Martin G, Scott D, et al: Mineralization of bacteria. Science 1962; 135:439.
174. Robertson P, Walsh M, Greene J, et al: Periodontal effects associated with the use of smokeless tobacco. J Periodontol 1990; 61:438.
175. Rosen P, Marks M, Reynolds M: Influence of smoking on long-term clinical results of intrabony defects treated with regenerative therapy. J Periodontol 1996; 67:1159.
176. Rothwell B: Prevention and treatment of the orofacial complications of radiotherapy. J Am Dent Assoc 1987; 114:316.
177. Rowles S: The inorganic composition of dental calculus. In: Blackwood HJ (ed): Bone and Tooth. Oxford, Pergamon Press, 1964.
178. Sanchez-Sotres L, Van Huysen G, Gilmore H: A histologic study of gingival tissue response to amalgam, silicate and resin restorations. J Periodontol 1969; 42:8.
179. Schoff F: Periodontia: An observation on the attachment of calculus. Oral Surg 1955; 8:154.
180. Schroeder H: Inorganic content and histology of early dental calculus in man. Helv Odontol Acta 1963; 7:17.
181. Schroeder H: Crystal morphology and gross structures of mineralizing plaque and of calculus. Helv Odontol Acta 1965; 9:73.
182. Schroeder H: Formation and inhibition of dental calculus. Berne, Hans Huber, 1969.
183. Schroeder H, Bambauer H: Stages of calcium phosphate crystallization during calculus formation. Arch Oral Biol 1966; 11:1.
184. Schwartz A: Tissue changes incidental to orthodontic tooth movement. Ortho Oral Surg Rad Int J 1932; 18:331.
185. Scoman S: Study of the relationship between periodontal disease and the wearing of partial dentures. Aust Dent J 1963; 8:206.
186. Selvig J: Attachment of plaque and calculus to tooth surfaces. J Periodont Res 1970; 5:8.
187. Serio F, Siegel M, Slade B: Plasma cell gingivitis of unusual origin. J Periodontol 1991; 62:390.
188. Serio F, Hawley C: Periodontal trauma and mobility. Diagnosis and treatment planning. Dent Clin North Am 1999; 43:37.
189. Setz J, Diehl J: Gingival reaction on crowns with cast and sintered metal margins: a progressive study. J Prosthet Dent 1994; 71:442.
190. Sharawy A, Sabharwal K, Socransky S, et al: A quantitative study of plaque and calculus formation in normal and periodontally involved mouths. J Periodontol 1966; 37:495.
191. Silness J: Fixed prosthodontics and periodontal health. Dent Clin North Am 1980; 24:317.
192. Sorensen J, Doherty F, Newman M, et al: Gingival enhancement in fixed prosthodontics. Part I. Clinical findings. J Prosthet Dent 1991; 65:100.
193. Sorensen J, Larsen I, Jorgensen K: Gingival and alveolar bone response to marginal fit of subgingival crown margins. Scand J Dent Res 1986; 94:109.
194. Spieler E: Preventing toothbrush abrasion and the efficacy of the Alert toothbrush. Comp Continu Edu Dent 1996; 17:478.
195. Standford J: Analysis of the organic portion of dental calculus. J Dent Res 1966; 45:128.
196. Stanton G: The relation of diet to salivary calculus formation. J Periodontol 1969; 40:167.
197. Stewart R, Ratcliff P: The source of components of subgingival plaque and calculus. Periodont Abstr 1966; 14:102.
198. Stoltenberg J, Osborn J, Pihlstrom B, et al: Association between cigarette smoking, bacterial pathogens, and periodontal status. J Periodontol 1993; 64:1225.
199. Sutcliffe P: Chronic anterior gingivitis: An epidemiological study in school children. Br Dent J 1968; 125:47.
200. Tangada S, Califano J, Nakashima K, et al: The effect of smoking on serum IgG2 reactive with *Actinobacillus actinomycetemcomitans* in early-onset periodontitis patients. J Periodontol 1997; 68:842.
201. Theilade J, Schroeder H: Recent results in dental calculus research. Int Dent J 1966; 16:205.
202. Tibbetts L, Kashiwa H: A histochemical study of early plaque mineralization. Abstract No. 616, J Dent Res 1970; 19:202.
203. Tomar S, Winn D, Swango P, et al: Oral mucosal smokeless tobacco lesions among adolescents in the United States. J Dent Res 1997; 76:1277.
204. Tonetti M, Pini-Prato G, Cortellini P: Effect of cigarette smoking on periodontal healing following GTR in infrabony defects. A preliminary retrospective study. J Clin Periodontol 1995; 22:229.
205. Trombelli L, Kim C, Zimmerman G, et al: Retrospective analysis of factors related to clinical outcome of guided tissue regeneration procedures in intrabony defects. J Clin Periodontol 1997; 24:366.
206. Turesky S, Renstrup G, Glickman I: Effects of changing the salivary environment on progress of calculus formation. J Periodontol 1962; 33:45.
207. Volker J, Pinkerton D: Acid production in saliva carbohydrates. J Dent Res 1947; 26:229.
208. Volpe A, Kupczak L, King W, et al: In vivo calculus assessment. Part IV. Parameters of human clinical studies. J Periodontol 1969; 40:76.
209. Von der Fehr F, Brudevold F: In vitro calculus formation. J Dent Res 1960; 39:1041.
210. Waerhaug J: The source of mineral salts in subgingival calculus. J Dent Res 1955; 34:563.
211. Waerhaug J, Zander H: Reaction of gingival tissue to self-curing acrylic restorations. J Am Dent Assoc 1957; 54:760.
212. Wasserman B, Mandel J, Levy BM: In vitro calcification of calculus. J Periodontol 1958; 29:145.
213. Weyant R: Characteristics associated with the loss and peri-implant tissue health of endosseous dental implants. Int J Oral Maxillofac Implants 1994; 9:95.
214. White D: Dental calculus: recent insights into occurrence, formation, prevention, removal and oral health effects of supragingival and subgingival deposits. Eur J Oral Sci 1997; 105:508.
215. Wise M, Dykema R: The plaque retaining capacity of four dental materials. J Prosthet Dent 1975; 33:178.
216. Wouters F, Salonen L, Frithiof L, et al: Significance of some variables on interproximal alveolar bone height based on cross-sectional epidemiologic data. J Clin Periodontol 1993; 20:199.

217. Wray A, McGuirt F: Smokeless tobacco usage associated with oral carcinoma. Incidence, treatment, outcome. Arch Otolaryngol Head Neck Surg 1993; 119:929.
218. Yuodelis R, Weaver J, Sapkos S: Facial and lingual contours of artificial complete crowns and their effect on the periodontium. J Prosthet Dent 1973; 29:61.
219. Zambon J, Grossi S, Machtei E, et al: Cigarette smoking increases the risk for subgingival infection with periodontal pathogens. J Periodontol 1996; 67:1050.
220. Zander H: The attachment of calculus to root surfaces. J Periodontol 1953; 24:16.
221. Zander H, Hazen S, Scott D: Mineralization of dental calculus. Proc Soc Exp Biol Med 1960; 103:257.
222. Zucchelli G, Clauser C, De Sanctis M, et al: Mucogingival versus guided tissue regeneration procedures in the treatment of deep recession type defects. J Periodontol 1998; 69:138.

Influence of Systemic Disease and Disorders on the Periodontium

Perry R. Klokkevold, Brian L. Mealey, and Fermin A. Carranza

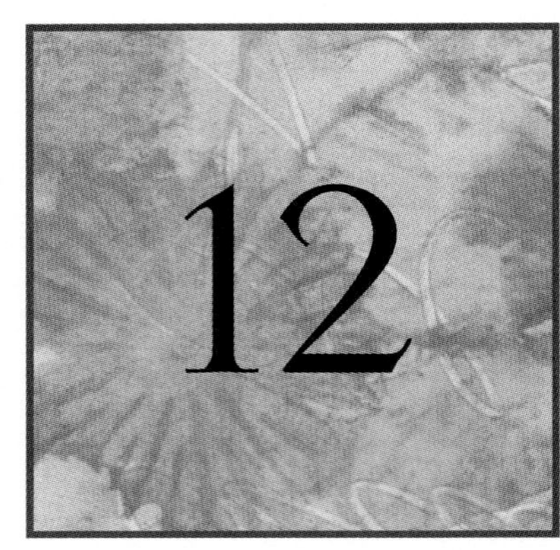

CHAPTER

CHAPTER OUTLINE

Many systemic disorders have been implicated as risk indicators or risk factors for adverse periodontal conditions. Clinical and basic science research over the past several decades has unveiled a much better understanding of the complexity and pathogenesis of periodontal diseases.[153] Clearly, there is an *essential* bacterial cause, and there are *specific* bacteria (periodontal pathogens) associated with destructive periodontal disease. These pathogens do not cause disease simply by their presence alone, but their absence appears to be consistent with periodontal health. The role of bacteria in disease etiology and pathogenesis are discussed in Chapters 6 and 8. Perhaps one of the most revealing recent discoveries about periodontitis is that the host response varies between individuals and that either an inadequate host immune response or an exaggerated host immune response to bacterial pathogens leads to more severe forms of the disease. In other words the host response to periodontal pathogens is very important and likely explains the differences in disease severity from one individual to another. Recent evidence is also beginning to shed light on the role of periodontal infections on systemic health problems such as coronary heart disease, stroke, diabetes, preterm labor, low-birth-weight delivery, and respiratory disease.[138] The potential role of periodontal infections on systemic health are discussed in Chapter 13. In addition to the interrelationships between periodontal infections and host immune response, a number of environmental, physical, and psychosocial stress factors affect periodontal tissues and modify disease expression. In general, these disorders do not initiate chronic destructive periodontitis, but they may predispose, accelerate, or otherwise increase its progression toward periodontal tissue destruction. This chapter discusses the influence of systemic disease and disorders on the periodontium.

NUTRITIONAL INFLUENCES

Some clinicians enthusiastically adhere to the theory in periodontal disease that assigns a key role to nutritional deficiencies and imbalances. Research conducted up to the present in general does not support this view, but numerous problems in experimental design and data interpretation may render these research findings inadequate.[5] The majority of opinions and research findings on the effects of nutrition on oral and periodontal tissues point to the following:

1. *There are nutritional deficiencies that produce changes in the oral cavity.* These changes include alterations of the lips, oral mucosa, and bone, as well as the periodontal tissues. These changes are considered to be periodontal or oral manifestations of nutritional disease.
2. *There are no nutritional deficiencies that by themselves can cause gingivitis or periodontal pockets.* However, nutritional deficiencies can affect the condition of the periodontium and thereby can aggravate the injurious effects of local factors and excessive occlusal forces. Theoretically, it can be assumed that there may be a "border zone" in which local factors of insufficient severity can cause gingival and periodontal disorders, if their effect on the periodontium is aggravated by nutritional deficiencies.

This section analyzes the existing knowledge in the field of nutrition as it relates to periodontal disease, with reference also made to other oral changes of nutritional origin.

Physical Character of the Diet

Numerous experiments in animals have shown that the physical character of the diet may play some role in the accumulation of plaque and the development of gingivitis.[156] Soft diets, although nutritionally adequate, may lead to plaque and calculus formation.[33,123,156] Hard, fibrous foods provide surface cleansing action and stimulation, which results in less plaque and gingivitis, even if the diet is nutritionally inadequate.[55,94,109,213]

In humans, however, studies have been unable to demonstrate reduced plaque formation when hard foods are consumed.[114] The discrepancy may be related to differences in tooth anatomy and to the fact that hard foods are fed to experimental animals as the only diet, whereas humans also consume soft foods. Human diets also have a high sucrose content, which favors the production of a thick plaque.

Effect of Nutrition on Oral Microorganisms

Although dietary intake is generally thought of in terms of sustaining the individual, it is also the source of nutrients for bacteria.[17] Through its effects on the oral bacteria, the diet may influence relative distribution of types of organisms, their metabolic activity, and their pathogenic potential, which in turn affect the occurrence and severity of oral disease.

Sources of nutrients for the microorganisms can be endogenous and exogenous. Among the exogenous factors, the influence of the sugar content of the diet has been extensively studied, and it has been demonstrated that the amount and type of carbohydrates in the diet and the frequency of intake can influence bacterial growth.[38] Attachment and subsequent colonization of the tooth surface by certain microorganisms also may be made possible by components of the diet.

Fat-Soluble Vitamin Deficiency

Vitamins A, D, and E are fat-soluble vitamins required in the human diet. This section describes observations of deficiency of these vitamins.

Vitamin A Deficiency. A major function of vitamin A is to maintain the health of epithelial cells of the skin and mucous membranes. Deficiency of vitamin A results in dermatologic, mucosal, and ocular manifestations. In the absence of vitamin A, degenerative changes occur in epithelial tissues, resulting in a keratinizing metaplasia. Since epithelial tissues provide a primary barrier function to protect against invading microorganisms, vitamin A also plays an important role in maintaining epithelial.

Little information is available regarding the effects of vitamin A deficiency on the oral structures in humans. Several epidemiologic studies have failed to demonstrate any relation between this vitamin and periodontal disease in humans.[206]

In experimental animals, vitamin A deficiency results in hyperkeratosis and hyperplasia of the gingiva with a tendency for increased periodontal pocket formation. The following periodontal changes have been reported in vitamin A–deficient rats: hyperplasia and hyperkeratinization of the gingival epithelium with proliferation of the junctional epithelium and retardation of gingival wound healing.[29,64] In the presence of local factors, vitamin A–deficient rats develop periodontal pockets that are deeper than those in animals not deficient in vitamin A and exhibit associated epithelial hyperkeratosis.[28,77]

Vitamin D Deficiency. Vitamin D, or calciferol, is essential for the absorption of calcium from the gastrointestinal tract and the maintenance of the calcium-phosphorus balance. Deficiency in vitamin D and/or imbalance in calcium-phosphorus intake results in rickets in the very young and osteomalacia in adults.

The effect of such deficiency or imbalance on the periodontal tissues of young dogs results in osteoporosis of alveolar bone; osteoid that forms at a normal rate but remains uncalcified; failure of osteoid to resorb, which leads to its excessive accumulation; reduction in the width of the periodontal ligament space; a normal rate of cementum formation, but defective calcification and some cementum resorption; and distortion of the growth pattern of alveolar bone.[14,208]

In osteomalacic animals, there is rapid, generalized, severe osteoclastic resorption of alveolar bone, proliferation of fibroblasts that replace bone and marrow, and new bone formation around the remnants of unresorbed bony trabeculae.[53] Radiographically, there is generalized partial to complete disappearance of the lamina dura and reduced density of the supporting bone, loss of trabeculae, increased radiolucence of the trabecular interstices, and increased prominence of the remaining trabeculae. Microscopic and radiographic changes in the periodontium are almost identical with those seen in experimentally induced hyperparathyroidism.

Vitamin E Deficiency. Vitamin E serves as an antioxidant to limit free-radical reactions and to protect cells from lipid peroxidation. Cell membranes, which are high in polyunsaturated lipids, are the major site of damage in vitamin E deficiency.

No relationship has been demonstrated between deficiencies in vitamin E and oral disease, but systemic vitamin E appears to accelerate gingival wound healing in the rat.[107,144,155]

Water-Soluble Vitamin Deficiency

Vitamins B and C are water-soluble vitamins required in the human diet. The function of these vitamins and the clinical manifestations of their deficiency are described in this section.

B-Complex Deficiency. The vitamin B complex includes thiamin, riboflavin, niacin, pyridoxine (B_6), biotin, folic acid, and cobalamin (B_{12}). Oral disease is rarely due to a deficiency in just one component of the B-complex group; the deficiency is generally multiple.

Oral changes common to B-complex deficiencies are gingivitis, glossitis, glossodynia, angular cheilitis, and inflammation of the entire oral mucosa. The gingivitis in vitamin B deficiencies is nonspecific, as it is caused by bacterial plaque rather than by the deficiency, but it is subject to the modifying effect of the latter.[2]

The human manifestations of **thiamin deficiency,** called *beriberi,* are characterized by paralysis; cardiovascular symptoms, including edema; and loss of appetite. Frank beriberi is rare in the United States. Oral disturbances that have been attributed to thiamin deficiency include hypersensitivity of the oral mucosa; minute vesicles (simulating herpes) on the buccal mucosa, under the tongue, or on the palate; and erosion of the oral mucosa.[83,130]

The symptoms of **riboflavin deficiency (ariboflavinosis)** include glossitis, angular cheilitis, seborrheic dermatitis, and a superficial vascularizing keratitis. The glossitis is characterized by a magenta discoloration and atrophy of the papillae. In mild to moderate cases, the dorsum exhibits a patchy atrophy of the lingual papillae and engorged fungiform papillae, which project as pebble-like elevations.[2,99] In severe deficiency, the entire dorsum is flat, with a dry and often fissured surface.

Angular cheilitis begins as an inflammation of the commissure of the lips, followed by erosion, ulceration, and fissuring. Riboflavin deficiency is not the only cause of angular cheilitis. Loss of vertical dimension, together with drooling of saliva into the angles of the lips, may produce a condition similar to angular cheilitis. Candidiasis may develop in the commissures of debilitated persons; this lesion has been termed *perlèche.*[81]

Changes observed in riboflavin-deficient animals include severe lesions of the gingivae; periodontal tissues; and oral mucosa, including noma.[41,199]

Niacin deficiency results in pellagra, which is characterized by dermatitis; gastrointestinal disturbances; neurologic and mental disturbances (dermatitis, diarrhea, and dementia); glossitis, gingivitis; and generalized stomatitis.

Glossitis and stomatitis may be the earliest clinical signs of niacin deficiency.[131] The gingiva may be involved in aniacinosis with or without tongue changes.[108] The most common finding is necrotizing ulcerative gingivitis, usually in areas of local irritation.

Oral manifestations of vitamin B-complex and niacin deficiency in experimental animals include black tongue and gingival inflammation with destruction of the gingiva, periodontal ligament, and alveolar bone.[2,15,50] Necrosis of the gingiva and other oral tissues, as well as leukopenia, are terminal features of niacin deficiency in experimental animals.

Folic acid deficiency results in macrocytic anemia with megaloblastic erythropoiesis, accompanied by oral changes, gastrointestinal lesions, diarrhea, and intestinal malabsorption.[52] Folic acid–deficient animals demonstrate necrosis of the gingiva, periodontal ligament, and alveolar bone without inflammation.[182] The absence of inflammation is the result of deficiency-induced granulocytopenia. In humans with sprue and other folic acid deficiency states, generalized stomatitis occurs, which may be accompanied by ulcerated glossitis and cheilitis. Ulcerative stomatitis is an early indication of the toxic effect of folic acid antagonists used in the treatment of leukemia.

In a series of human studies, a significant reduction of gingival inflammation has been reported after systemic or local use of folic acid, when compared with placebo.[203,204] This reduction occurred with no change in plaque accumulation. The same authors have postulated that the gingival changes associated with pregnancy and oral contraceptives may be partly related to suboptimal levels of folic acid in the gingiva.[202] In a clinical study of pregnant women, a reduction in gingival inflammation occurred with the use of topical folate mouth rinses; no change was found with systemic folic acid.[152] A relationship has also been assumed between phenytoin-induced gingival overgrowth and folic acid, based on the interference of folic acid absorption and utilization of phenytoin.[201]

Vitamin C (Ascorbic Acid) Deficiency. Severe vitamin C deficiency in humans results in **scurvy,** a disease characterized by hemorrhagic diathesis and retardation of wound healing. Vitamin C is required in the human diet but not in that of other animals except other primates, guinea pigs, and some rare flying mammals.[48] Vitamin C is abundant in fruits and vegetables. Scurvy is uncommon in countries that have adequate food supplies, but it may appear in infants in their first year of life if formulas are not fortified with vitamins and in the very old, especially those living alone and on restricted diets.[48] Alcoholism also may predispose an individual to scurvy.

Clinical manifestations of scurvy include hemorrhagic lesions into the muscles of the extremities, the joints, and sometimes the nail beds; petechial hemorrhages, often around hair follicles; increased susceptibility to infections; and impaired wound healing.[48] Bleeding, swollen gingiva and loosened teeth are also common features of scurvy.

Vitamin C deficiency (scurvy) results in defective formation and maintenance of collagen, retardation or cessation of osteoid formation, and impaired osteoblastic function.[61,212] Vitamin C deficiency is also characterized by increased capillary permeability, susceptibility to traumatic hemorrhages, hyporeactivity of the contractile elements of the peripheral blood vessels, and sluggishness of blood flow.[116]

POSSIBLE ETIOLOGIC RELATIONSHIPS BETWEEN ASCORBIC ACID AND PERIODONTAL DISEASE. It has been suggested that ascorbic acid may play a role in periodontal disease by one or more of the following mechanisms[213]:

1. *Low levels of ascorbic acid influence the metabolism of collagen within the periodontium, thereby affecting the ability of the tissue to regenerate and repair itself.* No experimental evidence supports this view of the role of ascorbic acid; furthermore, it has been shown that collagen fibers in the periodontal ligament of scorbutic monkeys are the last affected before death of the animals.[205]
2. *Ascorbic acid deficiency interferes with bone formation, leading to loss of periodontal bone.* Changes that do occur in alveolar bone and other bones as a result of failure of the osteoblasts to form osteoid take place very late in the deficiency state.[72] Osteoporosis of alveolar bone in scorbutic monkeys occurs as a result of increased osteoclastic resorption and is not associated with periodontal pocket formation.[205]
3. *Ascorbic acid deficiency increases the permeability of the oral mucosa to tritiated endotoxin and tritiated inulin and of normal human crevicular epithelium to tritiated dextran.*[6,7] Optimal levels of this vitamin, therefore, would maintain the epithelium's barrier function to bacterial products.
4. *Increasing levels of ascorbic acid enhance both the chemotactic and migratory action of leukocytes without influencing their phagocytic activity.*[79] Megadoses of vitamin C seem to impair the bactericidal activity of leukocytes.[183] The significance of these findings for the pathogenesis and treatment of periodontal diseases is not understood.
5. *An optimal level of ascorbic acid is apparently required to maintain the integrity of the periodontal microvasculature, as well as the vascular response to bacterial irritation and wound healing.*[36]
6. *Depletion of vitamin C may interfere with the ecologic equilibrium of bacteria in plaque and thus increase its pathogenicity.* However, there is no evidence that demonstrates this effect.

Epidemiologic Studies. Several studies in large populations have analyzed the relationship between gingival or periodontal status and ascorbic acid levels.[206] These studies used different methods for the biochemical analysis of ascorbic acid and various indices for the assessment of periodontal changes; they were made in persons of different socioeconomic status, different races, and various ages. All the epidemiologic surveys failed to establish a causal relationship between the levels of vitamin C and the prevalence or severity of periodontal disease.[35,58,172] Megadoses of ascorbic acid have also been found to be unrelated to better periodontal health.[97,214]

Gingivitis. The legendary association of severe gingival disease with scurvy led to the presumption that vitamin C deficiency is an etiologic factor in gingivitis, which is common at all ages.

Gingivitis with enlarged, hemorrhagic, bluish-red gingiva is described as one of the classic signs of vitamin C deficiency, but *gingivitis is not caused by vitamin C deficiency per se.* Vitamin C–deficient patients do not necessarily have gingivitis. Acute vitamin C deficiency does not cause or increase the incidence of gingival inflammation, but it does increase its severity.[42,72,73] Gingivitis in vitamin C–deficient patients is caused by bacterial plaque. Vitamin C deficiency may aggravate the gingival response to plaque and worsen the edema, enlargement, and bleeding. In addition, although correcting the deficiency may reduce the severity of the disorder, gingivitis will remain as long as bacterial factors are present.

Periodontitis. Changes in the supporting periodontal tissues and gingiva in vitamin C deficiency have been documented extensively in experimental animals.[72,94,205] Acute vitamin C deficiency results in edema and hemorrhage in the periodontal ligament, osteoporosis of the alveolar bone, and tooth mobility; hemorrhage, edema, and degeneration of collagen fibers occur in the gingiva. Vitamin C deficiency also retards gingival healing. The periodontal fibers that are least affected by vitamin C deficiency are those just below the junctional epithelium and above the alveolar crest, which explains the infrequent apical downgrowth of the epithelium.[205]

Vitamin C deficiency does not cause periodontal pockets; local bacterial factors are required for pocket formation to occur. However, acute vitamin C deficiency accentuates the destructive effect of gingival inflammation on the underlying periodontal ligament and alveolar bone.[73]

The exaggerated destruction results partly from an inability to marshal a defensive delimiting connective tissue barrier reaction to the inflammation and partly from destructive tendencies caused by the deficiency itself, including inhibition of fibroblast formation and differentiation to osteoblasts, as well as impaired formation of collagen and mucopolysaccharide ground substance.

Experimental studies conducted in humans failed to show the dramatic clinical changes that have traditionally been described in scurvy.[49,93,165] A case report published by Charbeneau and Hurt showed worsening of a preexisting moderate periodontitis with the development of scurvy.[42]

In a retrospective analysis of 12,419 adults studied in the Third National Health and Nutrition Examination Survey (NHANES III), Nishida et al found that there was a weak but statistically significant dose-response relationship between the levels of dietary vitamin C intake and periodontal disease in current and former smokers as measured by clinical attachment.[146] This suggests that vitamin C deficiency has its greatest impact on periodontal disease when preexisting disease and other codestructive factors are present.

In summary, analysis of the literature indicates that the microscopic signs of vitamin C deficiency are quite different from those that occur in plaque-induced periodontal disease in humans. Patients with acute or chronic vitamin C–deficient states and no plaque accumulation show minimal, if any changes in their gingival health status.

Protein Deficiency

Protein depletion results in hypoproteinemia with many pathologic changes, including muscular atrophy, weakness, weight loss, anemia, leukopenia, edema, impaired lactation, decreased resistance to infection, slow wound healing, lymphoid depletion, and reduced ability to form certain hormones and enzyme systems.[38] Protein deprivation also causes changes in the periodontium of experimental animals.[43] The following observations have been made in protein-deprived animals: degeneration of the connective tissue of the gingiva and periodontal ligament, osteoporosis of alveolar bone, retardation in the deposition of cementum, delayed wound healing, and atrophy of the tongue epithelium.[39,190,191] Similar changes occur in the periosteum and bone in other non-oral areas. Osteoporosis results from reduced deposition of osteoid, reduction in the number of osteoblasts, and retardation in the morphodifferentiation of connective tissue cells to form osteoblasts, rather than from increased osteoclastic activity.

These observations are of interest in that they reveal a loss of alveolar bone that is the result of the inhibition of normal bone-forming activity rather than of the introduction of destructive factors. Protein deficiency also accentuates the destructive effects of local factors and occlusal trauma on the periodontal tissues, but the initiation of gingival inflammation and its severity depend on the local factors.[140,191] In other words, protein deprivation results in periodontal tissues that lack integrity and, as a result, are more vulnerable to breakdown when challenged by bacteria.

Starvation

Starvation is the ultimate nutritional challenge. Without any food intake, there is a total lack of nutrients, no physical stimulation and no fuel for energy. In a study of controlled semistarvation in young adults, there were no changes in the oral cavity or skeletal system, despite a 24% loss of body weight.[106] Another study, however, showed a reduction in Plaque Index scores and a considerable increase in Gingival Index scores as the fasting period lengthened.[189]

In experimental animals, acute starvation results in osteoporosis of alveolar bone and other bones, reduction in the height of alveolar bone, and accentuated bone loss associated with gingival inflammation.[74]

ENDOCRINE DISORDERS

Endocrine disorders, such as diabetes, and hormonal fluctuations that are associated with puberty and pregnancy are well known examples of systemic conditions that adversely affect the health of the periodontium. Endocrine disturbances and hormone fluctuations affect the periodontal tissues directly, modify the tissue response to local factors, and produce anatomic changes in the gingiva that may favor plaque accumulation and disease progression. This section describes the evidence supporting the relationship between endocrine disorders and periodontal disease.

Diabetes Mellitus

Diabetes mellitus is an extremely important disease from a periodontal standpoint. It is a complex metabolic disease characterized by chronic hyperglycemia. Diminished insulin production, impaired insulin action, or a combination of both result in the inability of glucose to be transported from the bloodstream into the tissues, which in turn, results in high blood glucose levels and excretion of sugar in the urine. Lipid and protein metabolism is also altered in diabetes. Uncontrolled diabetes (chronic hyperglycemia) is associated with several long-term complications, including microvascular diseases (retinopathy, nephropathy, neuropathy); macrovascular diseases (cardiovascular and cerebrovascular); an increased susceptibility to infections; and poor wound healing.

An estimated 15.7 million individuals, or 5.9% of the population in the United States, have diabetes.[143] Nearly half of these individuals are unaware that they have the disease. The two major types of diabetes are types 1 and 2, with several less common secondary types of diabetes.

Type 1 diabetes mellitus, formerly insulin-dependent diabetes mellitus (IDDM), is caused by a cell-mediated autoimmune destruction of the insulin-producing beta cells of the islets of Langerhans in the pancreas, which results in insulin deficiency. Type 1 diabetes accounts for 5% to 10% of all cases of diabetes and most often occurs in children and young adults. This type of diabetes results from a lack of insulin production and is very unstable and difficult to control. It has a marked tendency toward ketosis and coma, is not preceded by obesity, and requires injected insulin to be controlled. Patients with type 1 diabetes mellitus present with the symptoms traditionally associated with diabetes, including polyphagia, polydipsia, polyuria and predisposition to infections.

Type 2 diabetes mellitus, formerly non-insulin dependent diabetes mellitus (NIDDM) is caused by peripheral resistance to insulin action, impaired insulin secretion, and increased glucose production in the liver. The insulin-producing beta cells in the pancreas are not destroyed by cell-mediated autoimmune reaction. Type 2 diabetes is the most common form of diabetes accounting for 90% to 95% of all cases. This form of the disease most often has an adult onset. Many times individuals are not aware they have the disease until severe symptoms or complications occur. It generally occurs in obese individuals and can often be controlled by diet and/or oral hypoglycemic agents. The development of ketosis and coma is not common. Type 2 diabetes can present with the same symptoms as type 1 diabetes but typically in a less severe form.

An additional category of diabetes is hyperglycemia secondary to other diseases or conditions. A prime example of this type of hyperglycemia is gestational diabetes associated with pregnancy. Gestational diabetes develops in 2% to 5% of all pregnancies but disappears after delivery. Women who have had gestational diabetes are at increased risk of developing type 2 diabetes later in life. Other secondary types of diabetes are those associated with diseases that involve the pancreas and destruction of the insulin-producing cells. Endocrine diseases such as acromegaly and Cushing's syndrome, tumors, pancreatectomy, and drugs or chemicals that cause altered insulin levels are included in this group. Experimentally induced types of diabetes generally belong in this category rather than in one of the two classic categories of disease.

Oral Manifestations of Diabetes

Numerous oral changes have been described in diabetics, including cheilosis, mucosal drying and cracking, burning mouth and tongue, diminished salivary flow, and alterations in the flora of the oral cavity, with greater predominance of *Candida albicans,* hemolytic streptococci, and staphylococci.[1,23,82,133] An increased rate of dental caries has also been observed in poorly controlled diabetes.[59,67] It should be noted that these changes are not always present, are not specific, and are not pathognomonic for diabetes.[136] Furthermore, these changes are less likely to be observed in well-controlled diabetics. Individuals with controlled diabetes have a normal tissue response, a normally developed dentition, a normal defense against infections and no increase in the incidence of caries.[197]

The influence of diabetes on the periodontium has been thoroughly investigated. Although it is difficult to make definitive conclusions about the specific effects of diabetes on periodontium, a variety of changes have been described, including a tendency toward enlarged gingiva, sessile or pedunculated gingival polyps, polypoid gingival proliferations, abscess formation, periodontitis, and loosened teeth[92] (Color Fig. 12-1). Perhaps the most striking changes in uncontrolled diabetes are the reduction in defense mechanisms and the increased susceptibility to infections leading to destructive periodontal disease.

Periodontitis in type 1 diabetes appears to start after age 12.[44] The prevalence of periodontitis has been reported as being 9.8% in 13 to 18 year olds, increasing to 39% in those 19 years and older.

The extensive literature on this subject and the overall impression of clinicians point to the fact *that periodontal disease in diabetics follows no consistent or distinct pattern.* Very severe gingival inflammation, deep periodontal pockets, rapid bone loss, and frequent periodontal abscesses often occur in diabetic patients with poor oral hygiene (see Color Fig. 12-1).[3] Children with type 1 diabetes tend to have more destruction around the first molars and incisors than elsewhere, but this destruction becomes more generalized at older ages.[44] In juvenile diabetics, extensive periodontal destruction often occurs due to the age of these patients.

Other investigators have reported that the rate of periodontal destruction appears to be similar for those with diabetes and without, up to the age of 30.[70,195] After age 30, there is a greater degree of destruction in individuals with diabetes. This may be related to disease destruction over time. Patients showing overt diabetes over a period of more than 10 years have greater loss of periodontal structures than those with a diabetic history of less than 10 years.[70] It may also be related to the diminished tissue integrity that continues to deteriorate over time. See the following description of altered collagen metabolism in diabetics.

Despite the fact that some studies have not found a correlation between the diabetic state and the periodontal condition, the majority of well-controlled studies show a higher prevalence and severity of periodontal disease in individuals with diabetes than without, with similar local factors.[10,23,37,45,89,96,145,147,149,174,209] Findings include a greater loss of attachment, increased bleeding on probing, and increased tooth mobility (Fig. 12-1). Perhaps the different degrees of diabetic involvement and control of the disease in patients examined and the diversity of indices and patient sampling are responsible for this lack of consistency.

Recent studies suggest that uncontrolled or poorly controlled diabetes is associated with an increased susceptibility and severity of infections including periodontitis.[12,174] Diabetes does not cause gingivitis or periodontal pockets, but there are indications that it alters the response of the periodontal tissues to local factors (see Color Fig. 12-1, *A, B*), hastening bone loss and retarding postsurgical healing of the periodontal tissues. Frequent periodontal abscesses appear to be an important feature of periodontal disease in diabetics.

Approximately 40% of adult Pima Indians in Arizona have type 2 diabetes. A comparison of individuals with or without diabetes in this Native American tribe has shown a clear increase in prevalence of destructive periodontitis, as well as a 15% increase in edentulousness, in individuals with diabetes.[51] The risk of developing destructive periodontitis increases threefold in these individuals.[57]

Bacterial Pathogens

The glucose content of gingival fluid and blood is higher in individuals with diabetes than without, with similar Plaque and Gingival Index scores.[60] The increased glucose in the gingival fluid and blood of individuals with diabetes could change the environment of the microflora, inducing qualitative changes in bacteria that could account for the severity of periodontal disease observed in poorly controlled individuals with diabetes.

Patients with type 1 diabetes with periodontitis have been reported to have a subgingival flora composed mainly of *Capnocytophaga,* anaerobic vibrios, and *Actinomyces* species. *Porphyromonas gingivalis, Prevotella intermedia,* and *Actinobacillus actinomycetemcomitans,* which are common in periodontal lesions of individuals without diabetes, are present in low numbers in those with the disease.[88,134] Other studies, however, found scarce *Capnocytophaga* and abundant *A. actinomycetemcomitans* and black-pigmented *Bacteroides,* as well as *P. intermedia, P. melaninogenica,* and *Campylobacter rectus.*[133,175] Black-pigmented species, especially *P. gingivalis, P. intermedia,* and *C. rectus,* are prominent in severe periodontal lesions of Pima Indians with type 2 diabetes.[68,215] These results point to an altered flora in the periodontal pockets of patients with diabetes. The exact role of these microorganisms has not been determined.

Polymorphonuclear Leukocyte Function

The increased susceptibility of diabetics to infection has been hypothesized as being due to polymorphonuclear leukocyte deficiencies resulting in impaired chemotaxis, defective phagocytosis, or impaired adherence.[69,137,158] No alteration of immunoglobulins A, G, or M has been found in diabetics.[169]

Altered Collagen Metabolism

Increased collagenase activity and decreased collagen synthesis is found in individuals with diabetes with chronic hyperglycemia. Decreased collagen synthesis, osteoporosis, and reduction in the height of alveolar bone occur in diabetic animals, with comparable osteoporosis in other bones.[71,178] The periodontal ligament and cementum are not affected, but glycogen is depleted in the gingiva. Other investigators report that gingival inflammation and bone destruction associated with local factors are more severe in diabetic than in nondiabetic animals.[25] Generalized osteoporosis, resorption of the alveolar crest, and gingival inflammation and periodontal pocket formation associated with calculus have been described in Chinese hamsters with hereditary diabetes under insulin replacement therapy.[186]

Chronic hyperglycemia adversely affects the synthesis, maturation, and maintenance of collagen and extracellular matrix. In the hyperglycemic state, numerous proteins and matrix molecules undergo a nonenzymatic glycosylation, resulting in advanced glycation end products (AGEs). The formation of AGEs can occur at normal glucose levels, but in hyperglycemic environments, AGE formation is excessive. AGE formation cross-links collagen, making it less soluble and less likely to be normally repaired or replaced. As a result, collagen in the tissues of poorly controlled diabetics is aged and more susceptible to breakdown.

AGEs play a central role in the classic complications of diabetes.[31] They may play a significant role in the

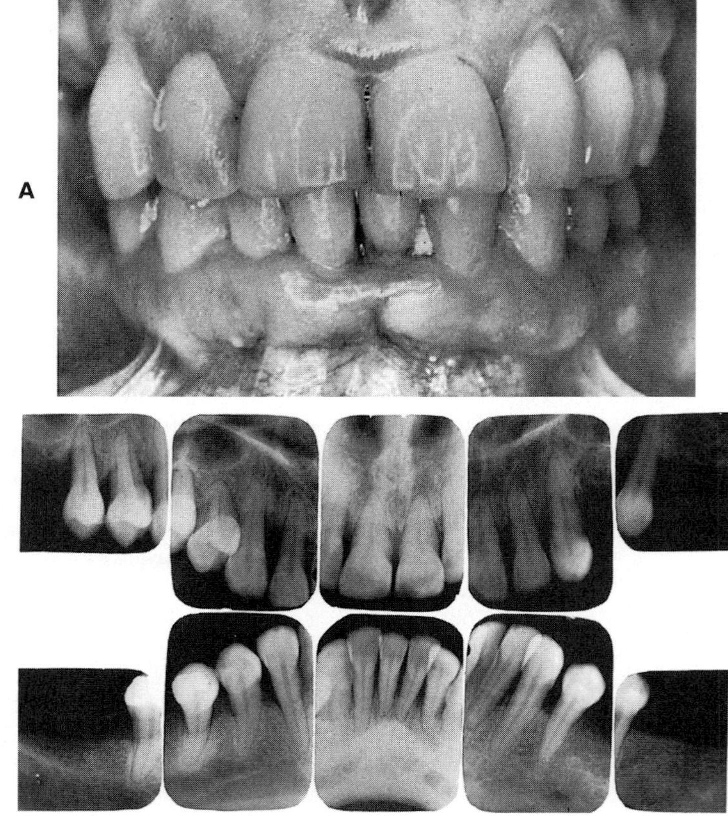

Fig. 12-1 Diabetic patient. **A,** Gingival inflammation and periodontal pockets in a 34-year-old patient with diabetes of long duration. **B,** Extensive generalized bone loss in the patient shown in **A**. Failure to replace posterior teeth adds to the occlusal burden of the remaining dentition.

progression of periodontal disease as well. Poor glycemic control and increased AGEs render the periodontal tissues more susceptible to destruction.[177] Cellular migration through cross-linked collagen is impeded and perhaps more importantly, tissue integrity is impaired as a result of damaged collagen remaining in the tissues for longer periods.

The cumulative effects of altered cellular response to local factors, impaired tissue integrity and altered collagen metabolism undoubtedly play a significant role in the susceptibility of individuals with diabetes to infections and destructive periodontal disease.

A study of risk indicators for a group of 1426 patients, ages 25 to 74, revealed that individuals who are age 45 or older, have diabetes, and smoke are at 20 times greater risk of periodontal disease than patients who do not have these indicators. If they are also infected subgingivally with *Bacteroides forsythus* or *P. gingivalis,* the risk increases to 30 to 50 times.[86]

Hyperparathyroidism

Parathyroid hypersecretion produces generalized demineralization of the skeleton, increased osteoclasis with proliferation of the connective tissue in the enlarged marrow spaces, and formation of bone cysts and giant cell tumors.[207] The disease is called **osteitis fibrosa cystica** or von Recklinghausen's bone disease.

Oral changes include malocclusion and tooth mobility, radiographic evidence of alveolar osteoporosis with closely meshed trabeculae, widening of the periodontal ligament space, absence of the lamina dura, and radiolucent cystlike spaces (Figs. 12-2 and 12-3). Bone cysts become filled with fibrous tissue with abundant hemosiderin-laden macrophages and giant cells. They have been called *brown tumors,* although they are not really tumors but reparative giant cell granulomas.

Loss of the lamina dura and giant cell tumors in the jaws are late signs of hyperparathyroid bone disease, which in itself is uncommon. Complete loss of the lamina dura does not occur often, and there is a danger of attaching too much diagnostic significance to it. Other diseases in which it may occur are Paget's disease, fibrous dysplasia, and osteomalacia.

Different investigators report that 25%, 45%, and 50% of patients with hyperparathyroidism have associated oral changes.[170,188,192] A relationship has been suggested between periodontal disease in dogs and hyperparathyroidism secondary to calcium deficiency in the diet.[90] This has not been confirmed by other studies.[194]

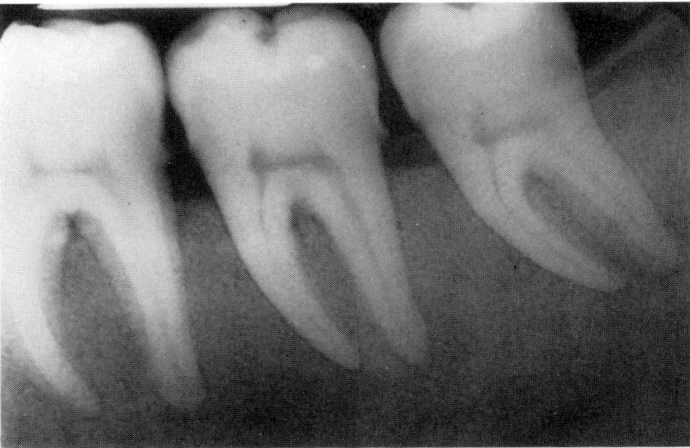

Fig. 12-2 Secondary hyperparathyroidism in a 35-year-old woman with advanced kidney disease. This periapical radiograph shows ground-glass appearance of bone and loss of lamina dura. (Courtesy Dr. L. Roy Eversole, San Francisco, Calif.)

Sex Hormones

There are several types of gingival disease in which modification of the sex hormones is considered to be either the initiating or complicating factor; these types of gingival alterations are associated with physiologic hormonal changes and are characterized by nonspecific inflammatory changes with a predominant vascular component leading clinically to a marked hemorrhagic tendency.

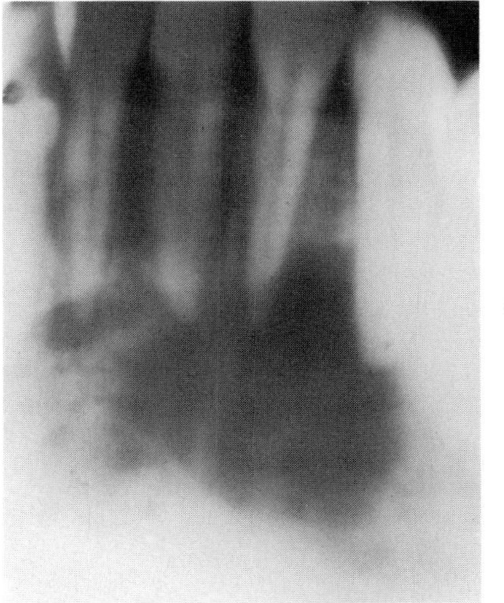

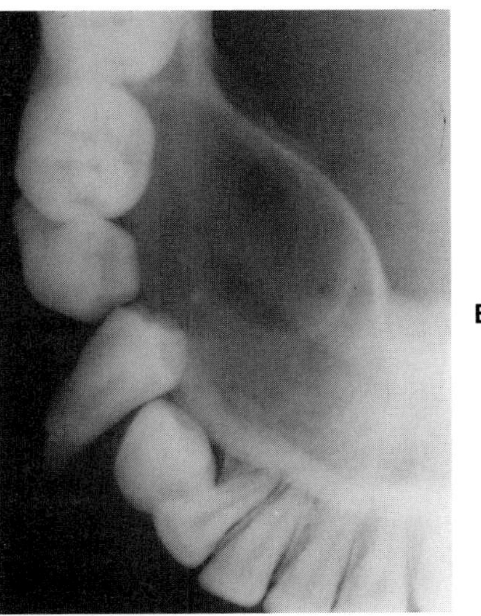

Fig. 12-3 A, Periapical and **B,** occlusal radiographic views of brown tumors in a patient with hyperparathyroidism. (Courtesy Dr. L. Roy Eversole, San Francisco, Calif.)

Experimental Studies. **Progesterone** administration to female dogs produces dilation and increased permeability of the gingival microvasculature, which increases susceptibility to injury and exudation, but it does not affect the morphology of the gingival epithelium.[96]

Repeated injections of **estrogen** in female rats cause increased endosteal bone formation in the jaws and decreased polymerization of mucopolysaccharide protein complexes in the bone ground substance.[21,148,187] Estrogen injections also counteract tendencies toward hyperkeratosis of the gingival epithelium and fibrosis of the vessel walls in ovariectomized female animals. They also stimulate bone formation and fibroplasia, which compensate for destructive changes in the periodontium induced by the systemic administration of cortisone.[76] Locally applied progesterone, estrogen, and gonadotropin appear to reduce the acute inflammatory response to chemical irritation.[122]

Elevated levels of estrogen and progesterone increase gingival exudation in female dogs with and without gingivitis, most likely because of hormone-induced increased permeability of the gingival vessels.[119]

Ovariectomy results in osteoporosis of alveolar bone, reduced cementum formation, and reduced fiber density and cellularity of the periodontal ligament in young adult mice, but not in older animals.[75,159] The gingival epithelium is atrophic in estrogen-deficient animals.[217]

Systemic administration of testosterone retards the downgrowth of sulcular epithelium over the cementum; stimulates osteoblastic activity in alveolar bone; increases the cellularity of the periodontal ligament; and restores osteoblastic activity, which is depressed by hypophysectomy.[171,184,185] The healing of oral wounds is accelerated by castration in males and is unaffected by ovariectomy in females.[34]

The Gingiva in Puberty

Puberty is often accompanied by an exaggerated response of the gingiva to local irritation.[193] Pronounced inflammation, bluish-red discoloration, edema, and enlargement result from local factors that would ordinarily elicit a comparatively mild gingival response (Fig. 12-4).

As adulthood is approached, the severity of the gingival reaction diminishes, even when local factors persist. However, complete return to normal requires removal of these factors. Although the prevalence and severity of gingival disease are increased in puberty, gingivitis is not a universal occurrence during this period; with good oral hygiene, it can be prevented (see Chapter 20).

Gingival Changes Associated with the Menstrual Cycle

As a general rule, the menstrual cycle is not accompanied by notable gingival changes, but occasional problems do occur. Gingival changes associated with menstruation have been attributed to hormonal imbalances and in some instances may be accompanied by a history of ovarian dysfunction.

During the menstrual period, the prevalence of gingivitis increases. Some patients may complain of bleeding gums or a bloated, tense feeling in the gums in the days preceding menstrual flow. The exudate from inflamed gingiva is increased during menstruation, suggesting that existent gingivitis is aggravated by menstruation, but the crevicular fluid of normal gingiva is unaffected.[95] Tooth mobility does not change significantly during the menstrual cycle.[65] The salivary bacterial count is increased during menstruation and at ovulation to 14 days earlier.[27,160]

Gingival Disease in Pregnancy

Gingival changes in pregnancy were described as early as 1898, even before any knowledge about hormonal changes in pregnancy was available.[24]

Pregnancy itself does not cause gingivitis. Gingivitis in pregnancy is caused by bacterial plaque, just as it is in nonpregnant individuals. Pregnancy accentuates the gingival response to plaque and modifies the resultant clinical picture (Figs. 12-5 to 12-7). No notable changes occur in the gingiva during pregnancy in the absence of local factors.

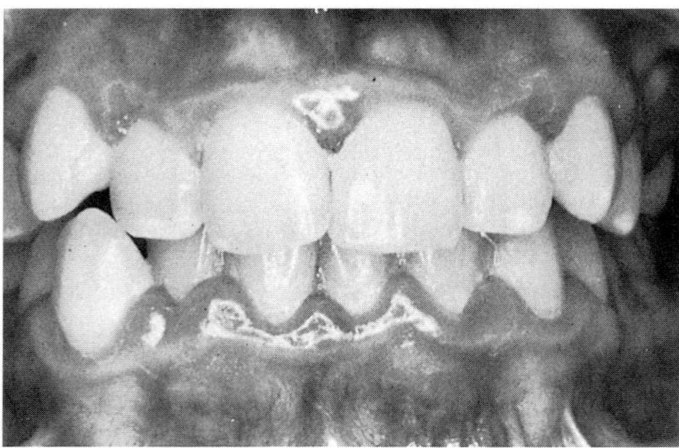

Fig. 12-4 Gingivitis in puberty, with edema, discoloration, and enlargement.

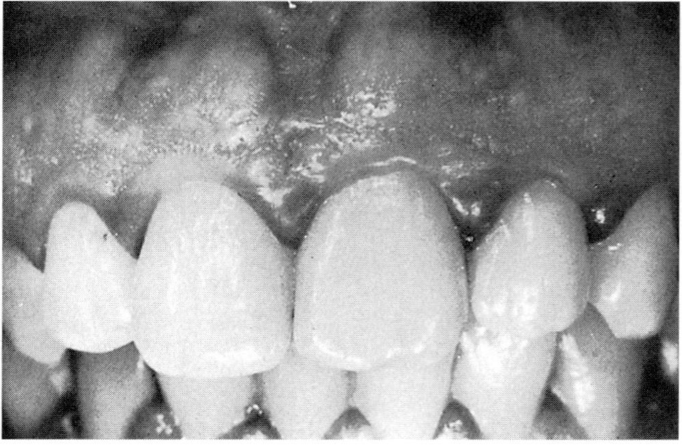

Fig. 12-5 Early changes in the interdental papillae in pregnancy.

The severity of gingivitis is increased during pregnancy beginning in the second or third month. Patients with slight chronic gingivitis that attracted no particular attention before the pregnancy become aware of the gingiva because previously inflamed areas become enlarged, edematous, and more notably discolored. Patients with a slight amount of gingival bleeding before pregnancy become concerned about an increased tendency to bleed (see Color Fig. 12-1, *G*).

Gingivitis becomes more severe by the eighth month and decreases during the ninth; plaque accumulation follows a similar pattern.[124] Some investigators report the greatest severity as being between the second and third trimesters.[47] The correlation between gingivitis and the quantity of plaque is greater after parturition than during pregnancy, which suggests that pregnancy introduces other factors that aggravate the gingival response to local factors.[111]

The reported incidence of gingivitis in pregnancy in well-conducted studies varies from around 50% to 100%.[124,128] Pregnancy affects the severity of previously inflamed areas; it does not alter healthy gingiva. Impressions of increased incidence may be created by the aggravation of previously inflamed but unnoticed areas.[167] Tooth mobility,[164] pocket depth, and gingival fluid[96,118] are also increased in pregnancy.

Partial reduction in the severity of gingivitis occurs by 2 months postpartum, and after 1 year the condition of the gingiva is comparable to that of patients who have not been pregnant.[47] However, the gingiva does not return to normal as long as local factors are present. Also reduced after pregnancy is tooth mobility, pocket depth, and gingival fluid. In a longitudinal investigation of the periodontal changes during pregnancy and for 15 months postpartum, no significant loss of attachment was observed.[47]

Pronounced ease of bleeding is the most striking clinical feature. The gingiva is inflamed and varies in color from a bright red to bluish red.[216,218] The marginal and interdental gingivae are edematous, pit on pressure, appear smooth and shiny, are soft and pliable, and sometimes present a raspberry-like appearance. The extreme redness results from marked vascularity, and there is an increased tendency to bleed (see Color Fig. 12-1, *G*). The gingival changes are usually painless unless complicated by acute infection. In some cases the inflamed gingiva forms discrete "tumorlike" masses, referred to as **pregnancy tumors** (see Color Fig. 12-1, *G*; see Chapter 18).

The microscopic picture of gingival disease in pregnancy is one of nonspecific, vascularizing, proliferative inflammation.[128,218] Marked inflammatory cellular infiltration with edema and degeneration of the gingival epithelium and connective tissue occurs. The epithelium is hyperplastic, with accentuated rete pegs, reduced surface keratinization, and various degrees of intracellular and extracellular edema and infiltration by leukocytes.[200] Newly formed engorged capillaries are present in abundance.

The possibility that bacterial-hormonal interactions may change the composition of plaque and lead to gingival inflammation has not been extensively explored. Kornman and Loesche have reported that the subgingival flora changes to a more anaerobic flora as pregnancy progresses; the only microorganism that increases significantly during pregnancy is *P. intermedia*.[112] This increase appears to be associated with elevations in systemic levels of estradiol and progesterone and to coincide with the peak in gingival bleeding.[112] It has also been suggested that during pregnancy a depression of the maternal T-lymphocyte response may be a factor in the altered tissue response to plaque.[150]

The aggravation of gingivitis in pregnancy has been attributed principally to the increased levels of progesterone, which produce dilation and tortuosity of the gingival microvasculature, circulatory stasis, and increased susceptibility to mechanical irritation, all of which favor leakage of fluid into the perivascular tissues.[142,149] A marked increase in estrogen and progesterone occurs during pregnancy, with a reduction after parturition. The severity of gingivitis varies with the hormonal levels in pregnancy.[96]

The gingiva is a target organ for female sex hormones.

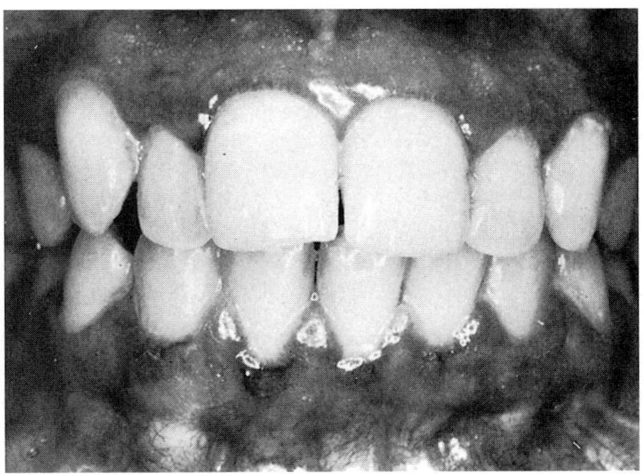

Fig. 12-6 Gingiva in pregnancy, showing edema, discoloration, and bleeding.

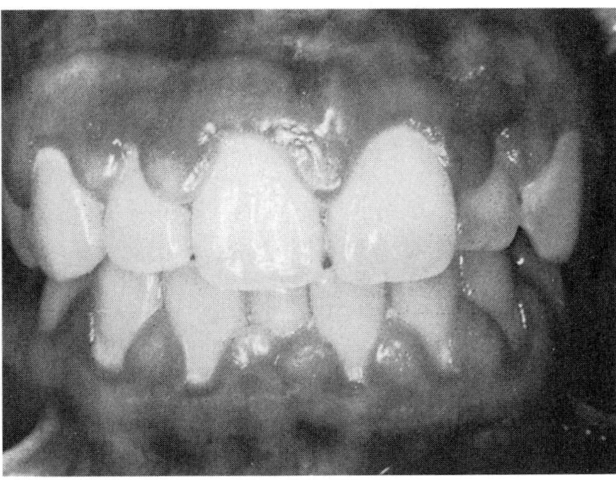

Fig. 12-7 Gingiva in pregnancy, showing edema, discoloration, and enlargement.

Formicola and colleagues have shown that radioactive estradiol injected into female rats appears not only in the genital tract but also in the gingiva.[62]

It has also been suggested that the accentuation of gingivitis in pregnancy occurs in two peaks: during the first trimester, when there is overproduction of gonadotropins, and during the third trimester, when estrogen and progesterone levels are highest.[124] Destruction of gingival mast cells by the increased sex hormones and the resultant release of histamine and proteolytic enzymes may also contribute to the exaggerated inflammatory response to local factors.[121]

Hormonal Contraceptives and the Gingiva

Hormonal contraceptives aggravate the gingival response to local factors in a manner similar to that seen in pregnancy and, when taken for a period of more than 1.5 years, increase periodontal destruction.[56,110,120]

Although some brands of oral contraceptives produce more dramatic changes than others, no correlation has been found to exist on the basis of differences in progesterone or estrogen content in various brands.[128,157] Cumulative exposure to oral contraceptives apparently has no effect on gingival inflammation or oral Debris Index scores.[101]

Menopausal Gingivostomatitis (Senile Atrophic Gingivitis)

This condition occurs during menopause or in the postmenopausal period. Mild signs and symptoms sometimes appear, associated with the earliest menopausal changes. Menopausal gingivostomatitis is not a common condition. The term used for its designation has led to the erroneous impression that it invariably occurs associated with menopause, whereas the opposite is true. Oral disturbances are not a common feature of menopause.[210]

The gingiva and remaining oral mucosa are dry and shiny, vary in color from abnormal paleness to redness, and bleed easily. Fissuring occurs in the mucobuccal fold in some cases, and comparable changes may occur in the vaginal mucosa.[166] The patient complains of a dry, burning sensation throughout the oral cavity, associated with extreme sensitivity to thermal changes; abnormal taste sensations described as "salty," "peppery," or "sour"; and difficulty with removable partial prostheses.[135]

Microscopically, the gingiva exhibits atrophy of the germinal and prickle cell layers of the epithelium and, in some instances, areas of ulceration.

The signs and symptoms of menopausal gingivostomatitis are in some degree comparable to those of chronic desquamative gingivitis (see Chapter 39). Signs and symptoms similar to those of menopausal gingivostomatitis occasionally occur after ovariectomy or sterilization by radiation in the treatment of malignant neoplasms.

Corticosteroid Hormones

In humans, systemic administration of cortisone and adrenocorticotropic hormone (ACTH) appears to have no effect on the incidence and severity of gingival and periodontal disease.[115] However, renal transplant patients who are receiving immunosuppressive therapy (prednisone or methylprednisone and azathioprine or cyclophosphamide) have significantly less gingival inflammation than control subjects with similar amounts of plaque.[16,103,151,198]

The systemic administration of cortisone in experimental animals results in osteoporosis of alveolar bone; capillary dilation and engorgement, with hemorrhage in the periodontal ligament and gingival connective tissue; degeneration and reduction in the number of collagen fibers of the periodontal ligament; and increased destruction of the periodontal tissues associated with inflammation caused by local irritation.[78]

HEMATOLOGIC DISORDERS

All blood cells play a role in the maintenance of a healthy periodontium. White blood cells (WBCs) are involved in peripheral and inflammatory reactions. Red blood cells (RBCs) are responsible for gas exchange and nutrient supply to the periodontal tissues and platelets and are required for normal hemostasis. Disorders of the blood or blood-forming organs can have a profound effect on the periodontium. Certain oral changes such as hemorrhage may suggest the existence of a blood disturbance; specific diagnosis, however, requires a complete physical examination and a thorough hematologic study. Comparable oral changes occur in more than one form of blood dyscrasia, and secondary inflammatory changes produce a wide range of variation in the oral signs.

Gingival and periodontal disturbances associated with blood dyscrasias must be thought of in terms of fundamental interrelationships between the oral tissues and the blood and blood-forming organs rather than in terms of a simple association of dramatic oral changes with hematologic disease. Ecchymosis and petechiae observed most often in the soft palate area is a sign of an underlying bleeding disorder (Figs. 12-8 and 12-9). Abnormal bleeding from the gingiva or other areas of the oral mucosa that is difficult to control is an important clinical sign suggesting a hematologic disorder. Hemorrhagic tendencies occur when the normal hemostatic mechanisms are disturbed.

Leukemia

The leukemias are "malignant neoplasias of WBC precursors, characterized by (1) diffuse replacement of the bone marrow with proliferating leukemic cells; (2) abnormal numbers and forms of immature WBCs in the circulating blood; and (3) widespread infiltrates in the liver, spleen, lymph nodes, and other sites throughout the body."[168]

According to the type of WBC involved, leukemias are classified as *lymphocytic* or *myelocytic;* a subgroup of the myelocytic leukemias is monocytic leukemia. According to their evolution, leukemias can be *acute,* which is rapidly fatal; *subacute;* or *chronic*. In acute leukemia, the primitive "blast" cells are released into the peripheral circulation, whereas in chronic leukemia, the abnormal cells tend to be more mature with normal morphologic characteristics when released into the circulation.

In all leukemias, the replacement of the bone marrow elements by leukemic cells reduces normal production of

RBCs, WBCs, and platelets, leading to anemia, a reduction in the number of nonmalignant WBCs, and thrombocytopenia. Anemia results in poorer tissue oxygenation, making tissues more friable and susceptible to breakdown. A reduction of normal WBCs in the circulation leads to an increased susceptibility to infections. Thrombocytopenia (low platelet counts) leads to bleeding tendency, which can occur in any tissue but has a propensity to occur in the mouth, especially the gingival sulcus (Fig. 12-10). Some patients may have normal blood counts while leukemic cells are present in the bone marrow; this type of disease is called *aleukemic leukemia.*[80]

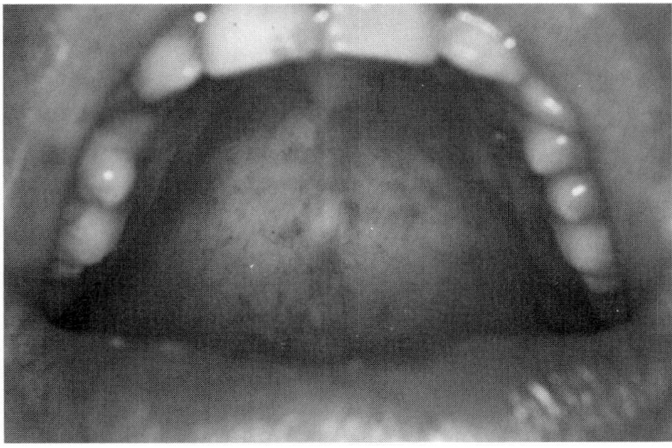

Fig. 12-8 Petechiae evident on the soft palate of patient with underlying bleeding disorder.

The Periodontium in Leukemic Patients

Oral and periodontal manifestations of leukemia consist of leukemic infiltration, bleeding, oral ulcerations, and infections.

Leukemic Infiltration of the Periodontium. Leukemic cells can infiltrate the gingiva and, less frequently, the alveolar bone. Gingival infiltration often results in **leukemic gingival enlargement** (see Chapter 18).

A study of 1076 adult patients with leukemia showed that 3.6% of the patients with teeth had leukemic gingival proliferative lesions, with the highest incidence in patients with acute monocytic leukemia (66.7%), followed by acute myelocytic-monocytic leukemia (18.7%) and acute myelocytic leukemia (3.7%).[54] It should be pointed out, however, that monocytic leukemia is an extremely rare form of the disease. Leukemic gingival enlargement is not found in edentulous patients or in patients with chronic leukemia. Leukemic gingival enlargement consists of a basic infiltration of the gingival corium by leukemic cells that creates gingival pockets where bacterial plaque accumulates, initiating a secondary inflammatory lesion that contributes also to the enlargement of the gingiva.

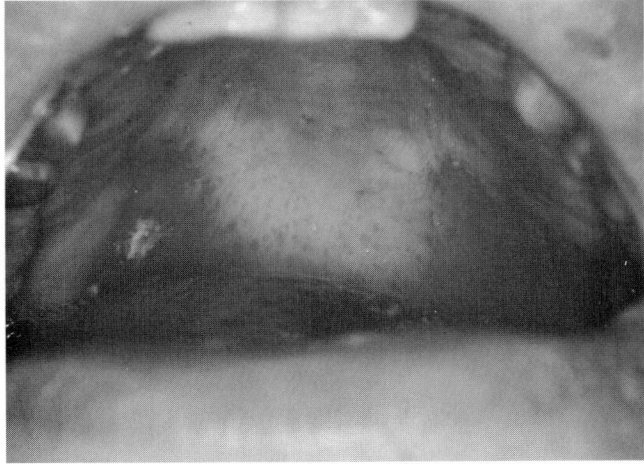

Fig. 12-9 Ecchymosis evident on the lateral aspects of the soft palate and tonsillar pillars of patient with chemotherapy induced thrombocytopenia.

Clinically, the gingiva appears initially bluish red and cyanotic, with a rounding and tenseness of the gingival margin; then it increases in size, most often in the interdental papilla and partially covering the crowns of the teeth (Figs. 12-11, 12-12, and 12-13).

Microscopically, the gingiva exhibits a dense, diffuse infiltration of predominantly immature leukocytes in the attached and marginal gingiva. Occasional mitotic figures indicative of ectopic hematopoiesis may be seen. The normal connective tissue components of the gingiva are displaced by the leukemic cells (Fig. 12-14, *A*). The nature of the cells depends on the type of leukemia. The cellular accumulation is denser in the entire reticular connective tissue layer. In almost all cases, the papillary layer contains comparatively few leukocytes. The blood vessels are distended and contain predominantly leukemic cells, and the RBCs are reduced in number. The epithelium presents a variety of changes. It may be thinned or hyperplastic. Common findings include degeneration associated with intercellular and intracellular edema and leukocytic infiltration with diminished surface keratinization.

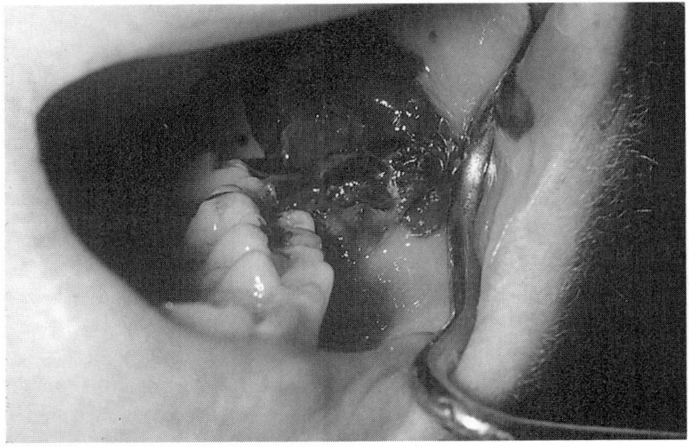

Fig. 12-10 Spontaneous bleeding from the gingival sulcus in a patient with thrombocytopenia. Normal coagulation is evident by the large clot that forms in the mouth. However, platelets are inadequate to establish hemostasis.

The microscopic picture of the marginal gingiva differs from that of the remainder of the gingiva in that it usually exhibits a notable inflammatory component, in

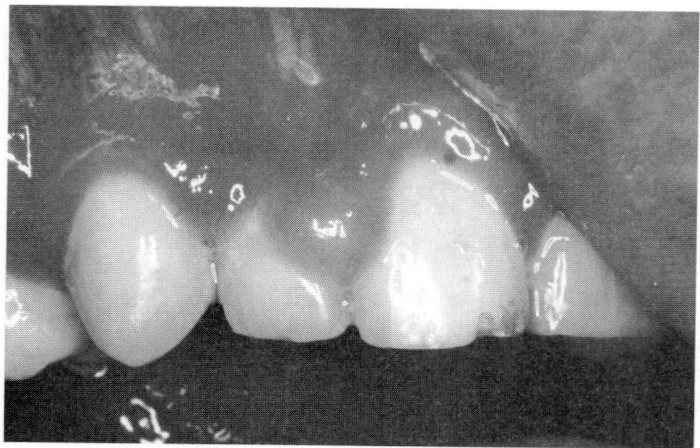

Fig. 12-11 Leukemic infiltration causing localized gingival swelling of the interdental papilla.

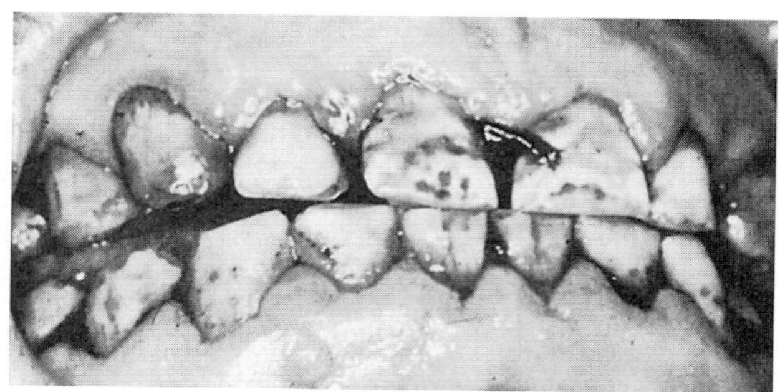

Fig. 12-12 Acute lymphocytic leukemia. The gingiva is inflamed, edematous, and discolored and bleeds spontaneously.

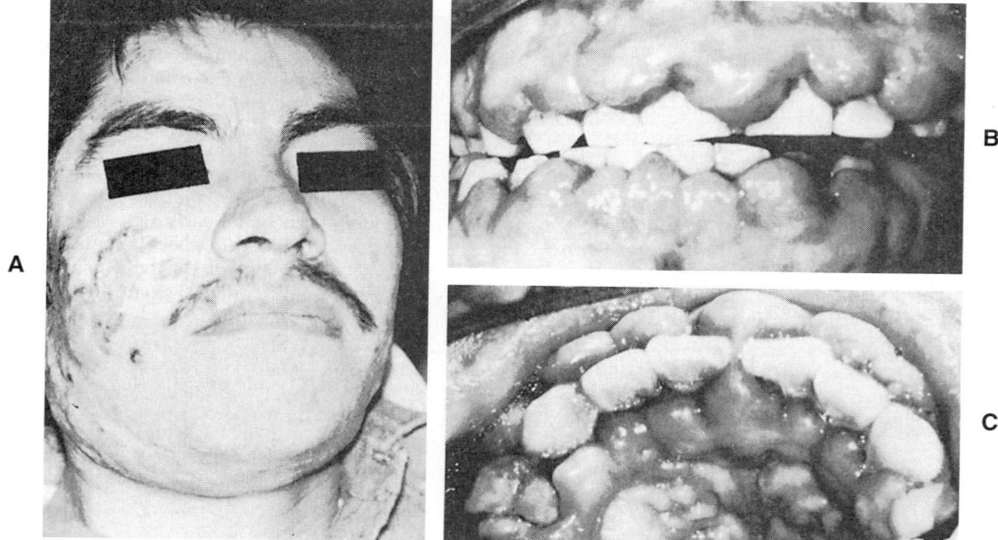

Fig. 12-13 Acute myelocytic leukemia. **A,** View of patient's face. Note the elevated flat macules and papules (leukemia cutis) on the right cheek. **B,** Intraoral view showing the pronounced gingival enlargement. **C,** Occlusal view of upper anterior teeth. Note the marked enlargement in both the facial and the palatal aspects. (Courtesy Dr. Spencer Woolfe, Dublin, Ireland.)

addition to the leukemic cells. Scattered foci of plasma cells and lymphocytes with edema and degeneration are common findings. The inner aspect of the marginal gingiva is usually ulcerated, and marginal necrosis with pseudomembrane formation may also be seen.

The periodontal ligament and alveolar bone may also be involved in acute and subacute leukemia (see Fig. 12-14, *B*). The periodontal ligament may be infiltrated with mature and immature leukocytes. The marrow of the alveolar bone exhibits a variety of changes, such as localized areas of necrosis, thrombosis of the blood vessels, infiltration with mature and immature leukocytes, occasional RBCs, and replacement of the fatty marrow by fibrous tissue.

In leukemic mice, the presence of infiltrate in marrow spaces and the periodontal ligament results in osteoporosis of the alveolar bone with destruction of the supporting bone and disappearance of the periodontal fibers (Fig. 12-15).[30,40]

The abnormal accumulation of leukemic cells in the dermal and subcutaneous connective tissue is called *leukemia cutis* and forms elevated flat macules and papules (see Fig. 12-13, *A*).[54,168]

Bleeding. Gingival hemorrhage is a common finding in leukemic patients (see Fig. 12-10), even in the absence of clinically detectable gingivitis. Bleeding gingiva can be an early sign of leukemia.[180] It is due to the thrombocytopenia that results from replacement of the bone marrow cells by leukemic cells and also from the inhibition of normal stem cell function by leukemic cells or their products.[168]

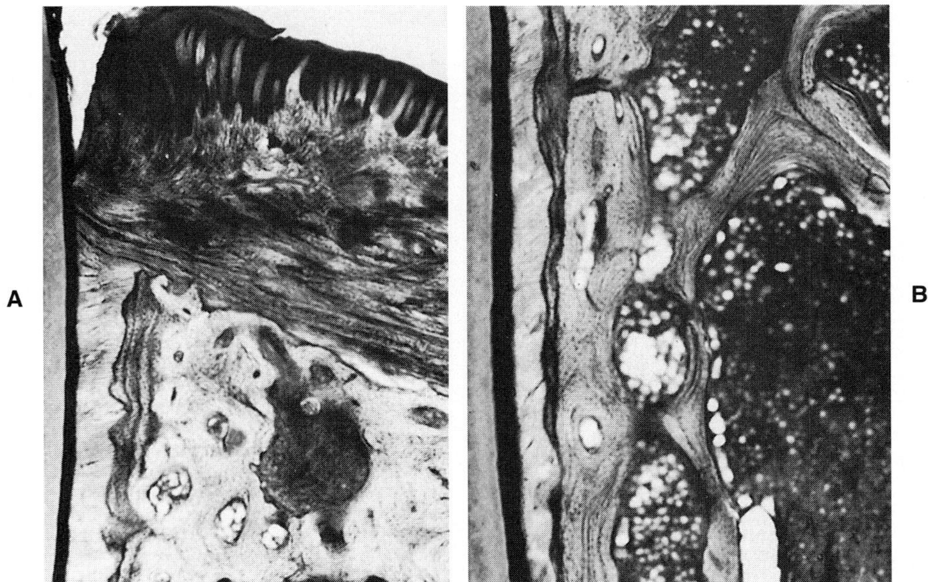

Fig. 12-14 A, Leukemic infiltrate in gingiva and bone in a human autopsy specimen. **B,** Same case as in **A.** Note the dense infiltrate in marrow spaces and the lack of extension to the periodontal ligament.

This bleeding tendency can also manifest itself in the skin and throughout the oral mucosa, where petechiae are often found, with or without leukemic infiltrates. Oral bleeding has been reported as a presenting sign in 17.7% of patients with acute leukemia and in 4.4% of patients with chronic leukemia.[125] This symptom can also result from the chemotherapeutic agents used.

Oral Ulceration and Infection. The granulocytopenia resulting from the replacement of bone marrow cells by leukemic cells reduces the tissue resistance to opportunistic microorganisms and leads to ulcerations and infections. Discrete, punched-out ulcers penetrating deeply into the submucosa and covered by a firmly attached white slough can be found in the oral mucosa.[11] These lesions occur in sites of trauma such as the buccal mucosa in relation to the line of occlusion or the palate. Patients with past history of herpes infection may develop herpetic oral ulcers, often in multiple sites and large atypical forms and after chemotherapy is instituted[85] (Fig. 12-16).

Gingival bacterial infection in leukemic patients can be a primary bacterial infection or result from an increased severity of existing gingival or periodontal disease. Acute gingivitis and lesions of necrotizing ulcerative gingivitis are more frequent and severe in terminal cases of acute leukemia[19] (Figs. 12-17 and 12-18).

In leukemia, the response to irritation is altered so that the cellular component of the inflammatory exudate differs both quantitatively and qualitatively from that which occurs in nonleukemic individuals. There is pronounced infiltration of immature leukemic cells in addition to the usual inflammatory cells.

The inflamed gingiva differs clinically from inflamed gingiva in nonleukemic individuals. It is a peculiar bluish red, is markedly spongelike and friable, and bleeds persistently on the slightest provocation or even spontaneously. This markedly altered and degenerated tissue is extremely susceptible to bacterial infection, which can be so severe as to cause acute gingival necrosis and pseudomembrane formation (Figs. 12-19 and 12-20). These are secondary oral changes superimposed on the

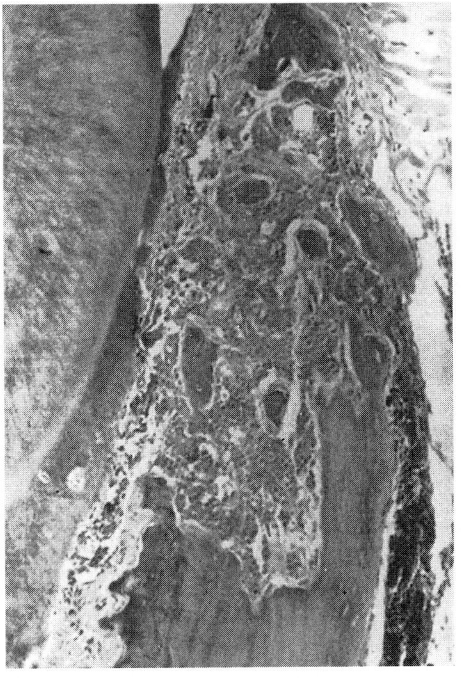

Fig. 12-15 Leukemic infiltrate in alveolar bone in leukemic mouse. Note the leukemic infiltrate producing destruction of bone and loss of periodontal ligament.

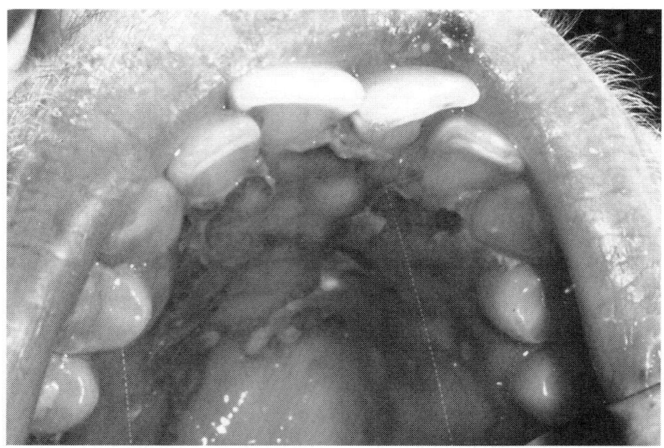

Fig. 12-16 Large ulcerations on the palate of patient with granulocytopenia secondary to leukemia. These atypical ulcerations are caused by herpes virus opportunistic infection. Notice the smaller, discrete round ulcerations that have coalesced into the larger lesion.

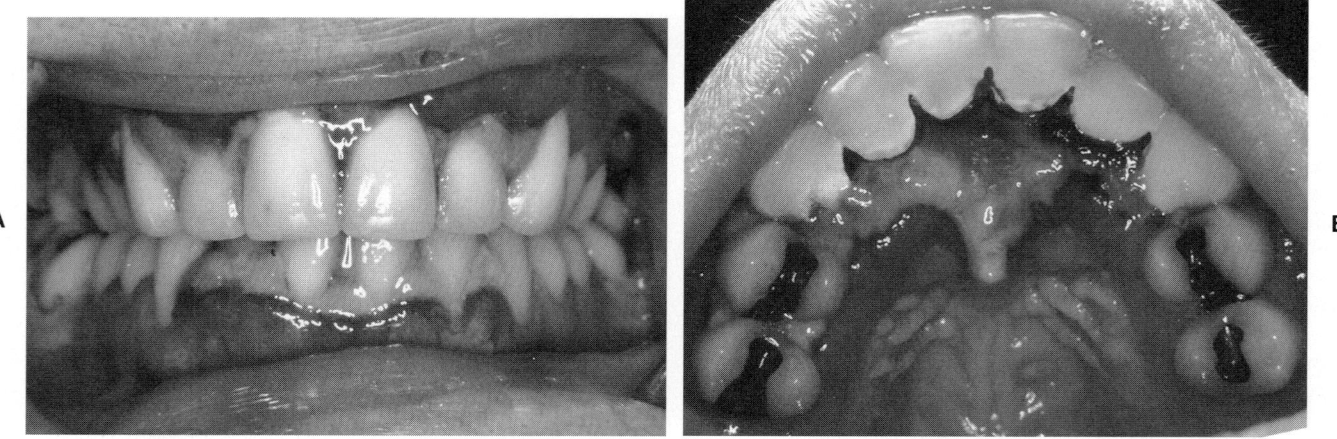

Fig. 12-17 **A,** Anterior view of patient with acute myelocytic leukemia. Interdental papilla are necrotic with a highly inflamed and swollen base. **B,** Palatal view demonstrating extensive necrosis of interdental and palatal tissue.

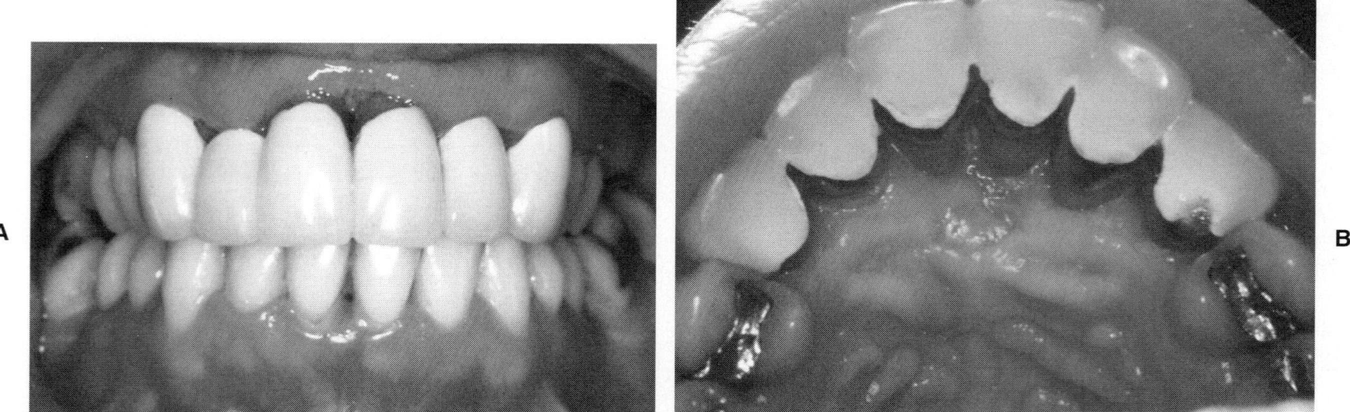

Fig. 12-18 Same patient as in Fig. 12-17 following chemotherapy and initial induction of remission. **A,** Anterior view reveals that although the tissue health has dramatically improved, the interdental papilla have been lost. **B,** Palatal view shows extensive loss of gingival tissue around maxillary incisors.

oral tissues altered by the blood disturbance. They produce associated disturbances that may be a source of considerable difficulty to the patient, such as systemic toxic effects, loss of appetite, nausea, blood loss from persistent gingival bleeding, and constant gnawing pain. By eliminating local factors, it is possible to alleviate severe oral changes in leukemia.

Chronic Leukemia

In chronic leukemia, clinical oral changes suggesting a hematologic disturbance are very rare. The microscopic changes in chronic leukemia may consist of replacing the normal fatty marrow of the jaws with islands of mature lymphocytes or lymphocytic infiltration of the marginal gingiva without dramatic clinical manifestations.

The existence of leukemia is sometimes revealed by a gingival biopsy performed to clarify the nature of a troublesome gingival condition. In such cases, the gingival findings must be corroborated by medical examination and hematologic study. The absence of leukemic involvement in a gingival biopsy specimen does not rule out the possibility of leukemia. In chronic leukemia, the gingiva may simply present inflammatory changes, with no suggestion of a hematologic disturbance. In patients with recognized leukemia, the gingival biopsy indicates the extent to which leukemic infiltration is responsible for the altered clinical appearance of the gingiva. *Although such findings are of interest, their benefit to the patient is insufficient to warrant routine gingival biopsy studies in patients with leukemia.*

Anemia

Anemia is a deficiency in the quantity or quality of the blood as manifested by a reduction in the number of erythrocytes and in the amount of hemoglobin. Anemia may be the result of blood loss, defective blood formation, or increased blood destruction.

Anemias are classified according to cellular morphology and hemoglobin content as 1) macrocytic hyperchromic anemia (pernicious anemia); 2) microcytic hypochromic anemia (iron deficiency anemia); 3) sickle cell anemia; or 4) normocytic-normochromic anemia (hemolytic or aplastic anemia).

Pernicious anemia results in tongue changes in 75% of cases. The tongue appears red, smooth, and shiny, owing to atrophy of the papillae. There is also marked pallor of the gingiva (Figs. 12-21 and 12-22).

Iron deficiency anemia induces similar tongue and gingival changes. A syndrome consisting of glossitis and ulceration of the oral mucosa and oropharynx, inducing dysphagia (Plummer-Vinson syndrome), has been described in patients with iron deficiency anemia.

Sickle cell anemia is a hereditary form of chronic hemolytic anemia that occurs almost exclusively in blacks. It is characterized by pallor, jaundice, weakness, rheumatoid manifestations, and leg ulcers. Oral changes include generalized osteoporosis of the jaws, with a peculiar stepladder alignment of the trabeculae of the interdental septa, along with pallor and yellowish discoloration of the oral mucosa. Periodontal infections may precipitate sickle cell crisis.[162]

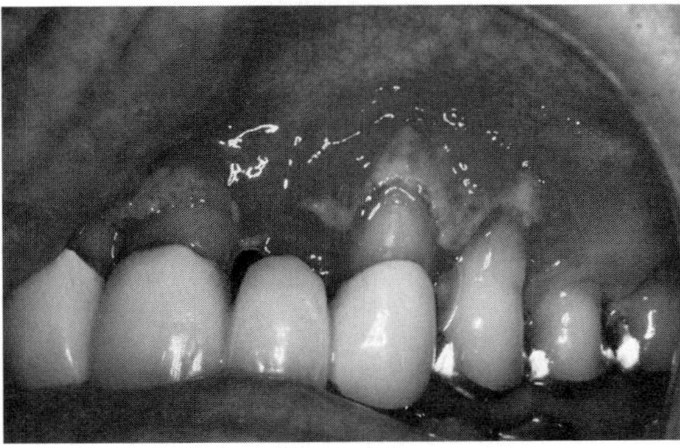

Fig. 12-20 The opportunistic bacterial infection in this immunosuppressed patient caused complete destruction of the gingiva exposing the underlying alveolar bone.

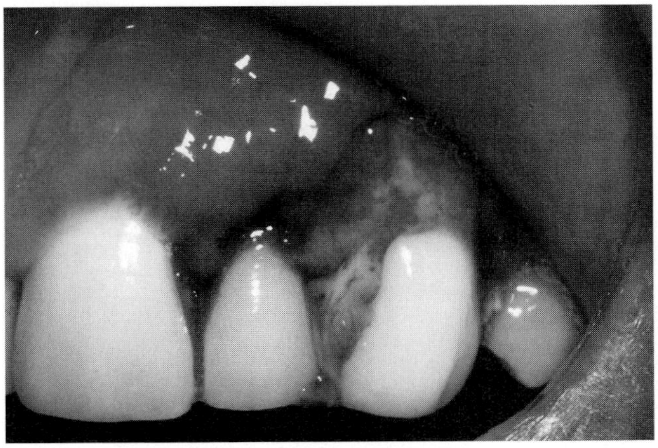

Fig. 12-19 Opportunistic bacterial infection of the gingiva in a patient with leukemia. Gingival tissue is highly inflamed, bleeding and necrotic with pseudomembrane formation.

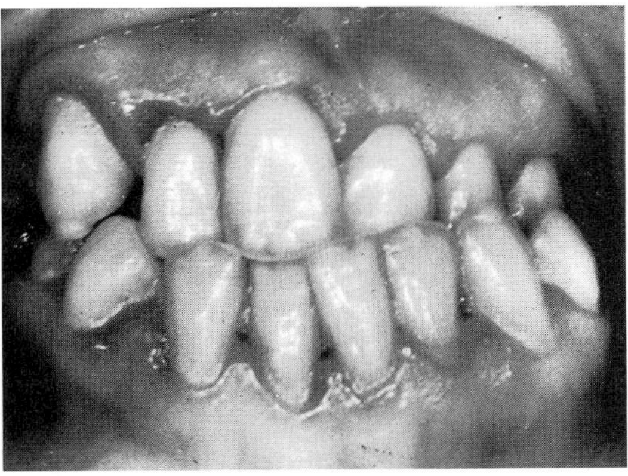

Fig. 12-21 Diffuse pallor of the gingiva in a patient with anemia. The discolored, inflamed gingival margin stands out in sharp contrast to the adjacent pale, attached gingiva.

Aplastic anemias result from a failure of the bone marrow to produce erythrocytes. Their etiology is usually the effect of toxic drugs on the marrow. Oral changes include pale discoloration of the oral mucosa and increased susceptibility to infection, owing to the concomitant neutropenia.

Thrombocytopenia

Thrombocytopenic purpura may be idiopathic (i.e., of unknown etiology, as in Werlhof's disease), or it may occur secondary to some known etiologic factor responsible for a reduction in the amount of functioning marrow and a resultant reduction in the number of circulating platelets. Such etiologic factors include aplasia of the marrow; crowding out of the megakaryocytes in the marrow, as in leukemia; replacement of the marrow by tumor; and destruction of the marrow by irradiation or radium or by drugs such as benzene, aminopyrine, and arsenical agents.

Thrombocytopenic purpura is characterized by a low platelet count, a prolonged clot retraction and bleeding time, and a normal or slightly prolonged clotting time. There is spontaneous bleeding into the skin or from mucous membranes. Petechiae and hemorrhagic vesicles occur in the oral cavity, particularly in the palate, tonsillar pillars, and the buccal mucosa (see Figs. 12-8 and 12-9). *The gingivae are swollen, soft, and friable. Bleeding occurs spontaneously or on the slightest provocation and is difficult to control. Gingival changes represent an abnormal response to local irritation;* the severity of the gingival condition is dramatically alleviated by removal of the local factors (Fig. 12-23).

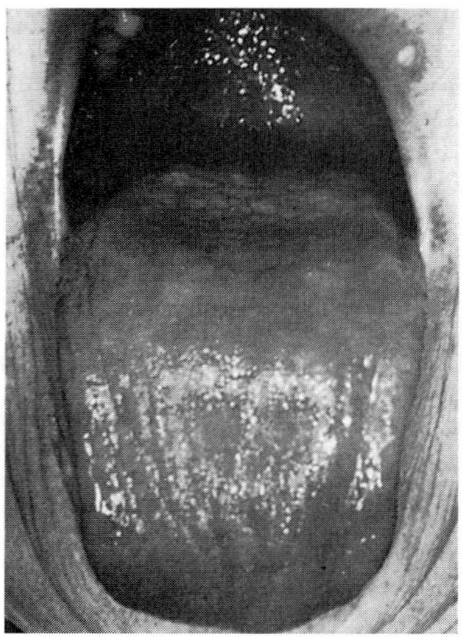

Fig. 12-22 Smooth tongue in a patient with pernicious anemia.

IMMUNODEFICIENCY DISORDERS

Deficiencies in host defense mechanisms may lead to severely destructive periodontal lesions. These deficiencies may be primary, or inherited; or secondary, caused by immunosuppressive drug therapy or pathologic destruction of the lymphoid system. Leukemia, Hodgkin's disease, lymphomas, and multiple myeloma all may result in secondary immunodeficiency disorders.

Leukocyte Disorders

Disorders that affect production or function of leukocytes may result in severe periodontal destruction (see also Chapters 8 and 10).

Agranulocytosis. *Agranulocytosis is characterized by a reduction in the number of circulating granulocytes and results in severe infections, including ulcerative necrotizing lesions of the oral mucosa, skin, and gastrointestinal and genitourinary tracts.* Less severe forms of the disease are called *neutropenia* or *granulocytopenia.*

Drug idiosyncrasy is the most common cause of agranulocytosis, but in some instances, its cause cannot be explained. Agranulocytosis has been reported after the administration of drugs such as aminopyrine, barbiturates and their derivatives, benzene ring derivatives, sulfonamides, gold salts, or arsenical agents.[113,127,139,163] It generally occurs as an acute disease, but it sometimes reappears in cyclic episodes (cyclic neutropenia). It may be periodic with recurring neutropenic cycles.[196]

The onset of the disease is accompanied by fever, malaise, general weakness, and sore throat. Ulceration in

A

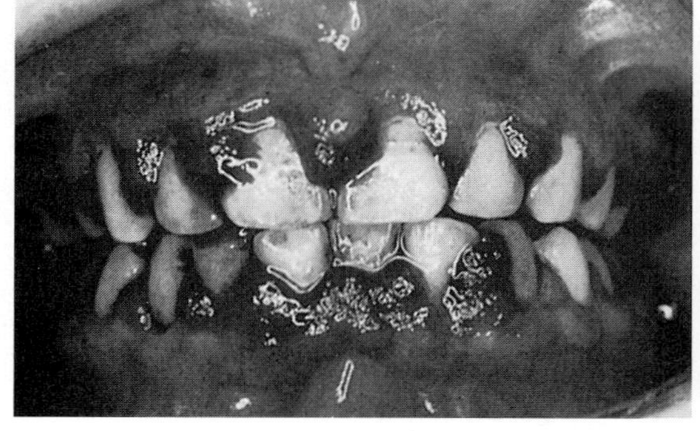

B

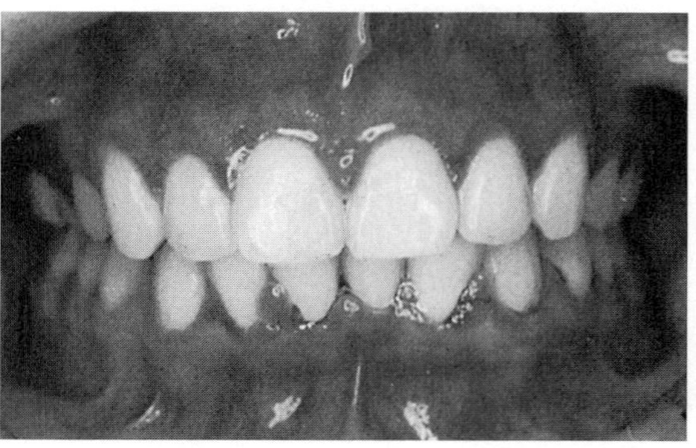

Fig. 12-23 Thrombocytopenic purpura. **A,** Hemorrhagic gingivitis in patient with thrombocytopenic purpura. **B,** Marked reduction in severity of gingival disease after removal of surface debris and careful scaling.

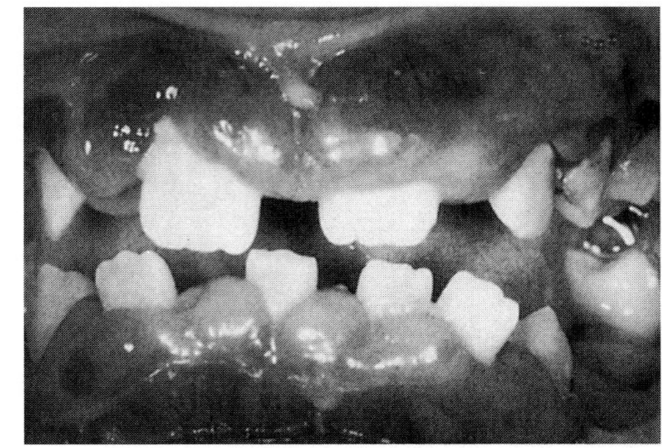

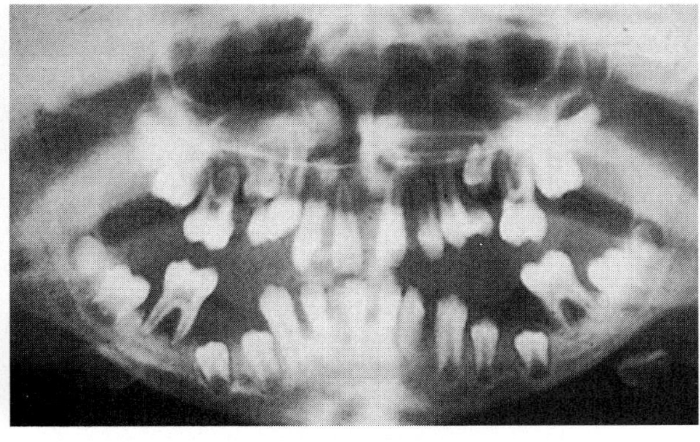

Fig. 12-24 Prepubertal periodontitis **(A),** clinical picture and panoramic radiograph **(B).** The patient is a 10-year-old boy with cyclic neutropenia and agammaglobulinemia.

the oral cavity, oropharynx, and throat is characteristic. The mucosa exhibits isolated necrotic patches that are black and gray and are sharply demarcated from the adjacent uninvolved areas.[104,132] *The absence of a notable inflammatory reaction due to lack of granulocytes is a striking feature.* The gingival margin may or may not be involved. Gingival hemorrhage, necrosis, increased salivation, and fetid odor are accompanying clinical features. The occurrence of rapidly destructive periodontitis has been described in cyclic neutropenia (Fig. 12-24).[181]

The following microscopic changes have been described in the periodontium[13]:

- Hemorrhage into the periodontal ligament with destruction of the principal fibers
- Osteoporosis of the cancellous bone with osteoclastic resorption
- Small fragments of necrotic bone in the hemorrhagic periodontal ligament
- Hemorrhage in the marrow adjacent to the teeth, areas in which the periodontal ligament is widened and consists of dense fibrous tissue with fibers parallel to the tooth surface
- Formation of new bony trabeculae

In cyclic neutropenia the gingival changes recur with recurrent exacerbation of the disease.[46]

Experimentally, neutropenia has been produced in dogs with heterologous antineutrophil serum. Neutrophilic granulocytes disappeared from the tissues, but ulcerative lesions and bacterial invasion were not observed, probably owing to the short duration of the experiment (4 days).[173]

Because infection is a common feature of agranulocytosis, differential diagnosis involves consideration of such conditions as acute necrotizing ulcerative gingivitis, diphtheria, noma, and acute necrotizing inflammation of the tonsils. Definitive diagnosis depends on the hematologic findings of pronounced leukopenia and almost complete absence of neutrophils.

Chédiak-Higashi Syndrome. Chédiak-Higashi syndrome is a rare disease that affects the production of organelles found in almost every cell. It affects mostly the melanocytes, platelets, and phagocytes and produces partial albinism, mild bleeding disorders, and recurrent bacterial infections, including rapidly destructive periodontitis. It has been described as a genetically transmitted disease in ranch-raised mink (see Chapter 10).[8,154]

Antibody Deficiency Disorders

Agammaglobulinemia. Agammaglobulinemia results from a deficiency in B cells; T-cell function remains normal. It can be congenital (X-linked or Bruton's agammaglobulinemia) or acquired. The disease is characterized by recurrent infections, including destructive periodontitis in children (see Fig. 12-24).

Acquired Immunodeficiency Syndrome. Acquired immunodeficiency syndrome (AIDS) is caused by the human immunodeficiency virus (HIV) and is characterized by destruction of lymphocytes, rendering the patient susceptible to opportunistic infections, including destructive periodontal lesions and malignancies (see Chapter 29).

CARDIOVASCULAR DISEASES

Arteriosclerosis

In aged individuals, arteriosclerotic changes characterized by intimal thickening, narrowing of the lumen, thickening of the media, and hyalinization of the media and adventitia, with or without calcification, are common in vessels throughout the jaws, as well as in areas of periodontal inflammation (Fig. 12-25).[84,161,211] Both periodontal disease and arteriosclerosis increase with age, and it has been hypothesized that the circulatory impairment induced by vascular changes may increase the patient's susceptibility to periodontal disease.[11,20,22] Conversely, there is recent evidence to suggest that individuals with periodontal disease may be at greater risk for heart disease as a result of chronic periodontal infections and inflammation. See Chapter 13 for a detailed discussion of the relationship between periodontal inflammatory disease and the risk for systemic diseases.

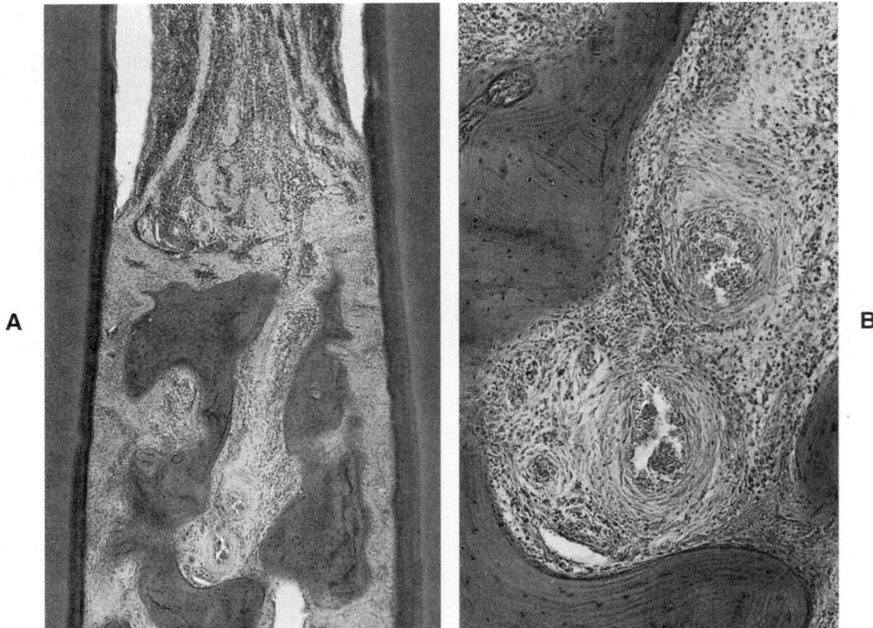

Fig. 12-25 Vascular changes in an aged individual with periodontal disease. **A,** periodontitis, showing inflammation extending from the gingiva into the interdental septum. **B,** Detailed view, showing arterioles with thickened walls in the marrow space of the interdental septum.

In experimental animals, partial ischemia of more than 10 hours' duration created by arteriolar occlusion produces changes in the oxidative enzymes and acid phosphatase activity and in the glycogen and lipid content of the gingival epithelium.[98] Focal necrosis, followed by ulceration, occurs in the epithelium, with the junctional epithelium least affected.[105] DNA duplication is depressed. Changes typical of periodontal disease do not occur. Ischemia is followed by hyperemia, which is accompanied by metabolic changes and increased DNA synthesis in the epithelium. The gingival response to arteriolar occlusion is epithelial proliferation and thickening.

Congenital Heart Disease

Gingival disease and other oral symptoms may occur in children with congenital heart disease.[26,102] In cases of **tetralogy of Fallot,** which is characterized by pulmonary stenosis, right ventricular enlargement, a defect in the interventricular septum, and malposition of the aorta to the right, the oral changes include a purplish-red discoloration of the lips and gingiva and sometimes severe marginal gingivitis and periodontal destruction (Figs. 12-26 and 12-27). The discoloration of the lips and gingivae corresponds to the general degree of cyanosis and returns to normal after corrective heart surgery. The tongue appears coated, fissured, and edematous, and there is extreme reddening of the fungiform and filiform papillae. The number of subepithelial capillaries is increased but will return to normal after heart surgery.[63]

In cases of **tetralogy of Eisenmenger,** there is pulmonary insufficiency and a diastolic murmur; the lips, cheeks, and buccal mucous membranes are cyanotic, but markedly less so than in tetralogy of Fallot. Severe generalized marginal gingivitis may be found. In cases in which there is *transposition of the aorta and superior vena cava,* cyanotic discoloration and marginal gingivitis of a lesser degree are noted. In coarctation of the aorta, there is narrowing of the vessel in the region where it is joined by the ductus arteriosus. Patients with this problem show marked inflammation of the gingiva in the anterior part of the mouth.

OTHER SYSTEMIC CONDITIONS

Metal Intoxication

The ingestion of metals such as mercury, lead, and bismuth in medicinal compounds and through industrial contact may result in oral manifestations owing to either intoxication or absorption without evidence of toxicity.

Bismuth Intoxication. Chronic bismuth intoxication is characterized by gastrointestinal disturbances, nausea, vomiting, and jaundice, as well as by an ulcerative gingivostomatitis, generally with pigmentation and accompanied by a metallic taste and burning sensation of the oral mucosa. The tongue may be sore and inflamed. Urticaria, exanthematous eruptions of different types, bullous and purpuric lesions, and herpes zoster-like eruptions and pigmentation of the skin and mucous membranes are among the dermatologic lesions attributed to bismuth intoxication. Acute bismuth intoxication, which is less commonly seen, is accompanied by methemoglobin formation, cyanosis, and dyspnea.[91]

Bismuth pigmentation in the oral cavity usually appears

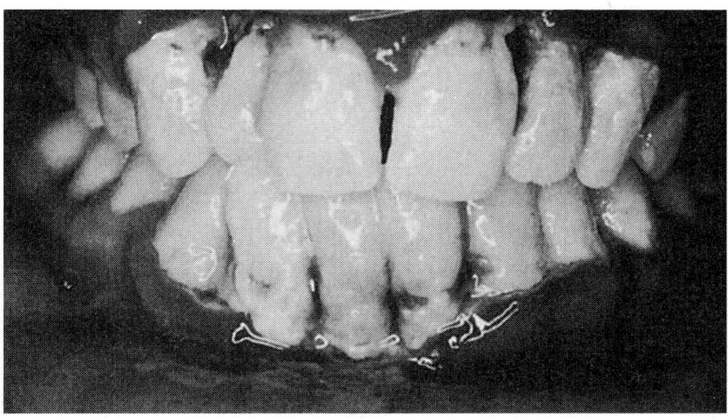

Fig. 12-26 Extensive marginal inflammation with ulceronecrotic lesions and periodontal destruction in an adolescent with tetralogy of Fallot.

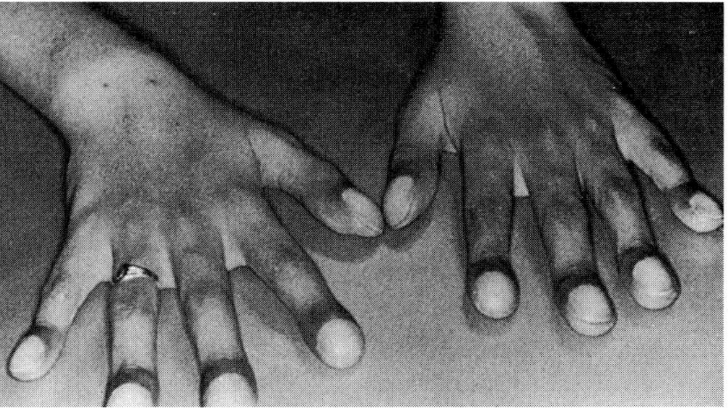

Fig. 12-27 Characteristic clubbing of the fingers in the patient shown in Fig. 12-26, consistent with untreated congenital cyanotic heart disease.

as a narrow, bluish-black discoloration of the gingival margin in areas of preexistent gingival inflammation (see Chapter 17 and Fig. 17-11). Such pigmentation results from the precipitation of particles of bismuth sulfide associated with vascular changes in inflammation. It is not evidence of intoxication but simply indicates the presence of bismuth in the bloodstream. Bismuth pigmentation in the oral cavity also occurs in cases of intoxication. It assumes a linear form if the marginal gingiva is inflamed.

Lead Intoxication. Lead is slowly absorbed, and toxic symptoms are not particularly definitive when they do occur.[100] There is pallor of the face and lips and gastrointestinal symptoms consisting of nausea, vomiting, loss of appetite, and abdominal colic. Peripheral neuritis, psychologic disorders, and encephalitis have been reported. Among the oral signs are salivation, coated tongue, a peculiar sweetish taste, gingival pigmentation, and ulceration. *The pigmentation of the gingiva is linear (burtonian line), steel gray, and associated with local irritation. Oral signs may occur without toxic symptoms.*

Mercury Intoxication. Mercury intoxication is characterized by headache, insomnia, cardiovascular symptoms, pronounced salivation (ptyalism), and a metallic taste.[4] *Gingival pigmentation in linear form results from the deposition of mercuric sulfide. The chemical also acts as an irritant, which accentuates the preexistent inflammation and commonly leads to notable ulceration of the gingiva and adjacent mucosa and destruction of the underlying bone.* Mercurial pigmentation of the gingiva also occurs in areas of local irritation in patients without symptoms of intoxication.

Other Chemicals. Other chemicals, such as phosphorus, arsenic, and chromium, may cause necrosis of the alveolar bone with loosening and exfoliation of the teeth.[117,179] Inflammation and ulceration of the gingiva are usually associated with destruction of the underlying tissues. Benzene intoxication is accompanied by gingival bleeding and ulceration with destruction of the underlying bone.[179]

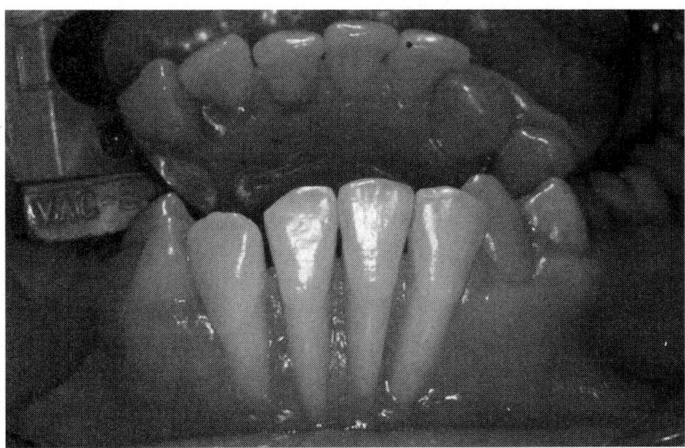

Fig. 12-28 Severe gingival recession of all lower incisors, which was discovered under general anesthetic in an uncooperative, institutionalized adult with mental disorders. The patient was known to habitually pace around the home with all four fingers inside his lower lip.

PSYCHOSOMATIC DISORDERS

Harmful effects that result from psychic influences on the organic control of tissues are known as **psychosomatic disorders.**[87] The two ways in which psychosomatic disorders may be induced in the oral cavity are 1) through the development of habits that are injurious to the periodontium and 2) by the direct effect of the autonomic nervous system on the physiologic tissue balance.

Psychologically, the oral cavity is related directly or symbolically to the major human instincts and passions. In the infant, many oral drives find direct expression as oral receptive and aggressive trends and oral eroticism.[176] In the adult, most of the instinctive drives are normally suppressed by education and are satisfied in substitutive ways, or are taken over by organs more appropriate than the mouth. *However, under conditions of mental and emotional duress, the mouth may subconsciously become an outlet for the gratification of basic drives in the adult.*

Gratification may be derived from neurotic habits, such as grinding or clenching the teeth; nibbling on foreign objects (e.g., pencils or pipes); nail biting; or excessive use of tobacco, which are all potentially injurious to the periodontium.[32,66,176] Self-inflicted gingival injuries such as gingival recession have been described in both children and adults. Correlation between psychiatric and anxiety states and the occurrence of periodontal disease have been reported, but these reports have been questioned by some investigators.[9,18,129,141] Psychologic factors in the cause of necrotizing ulcerative gingivitis are discussed in Chapter 19.

REFERENCES

1. Adler P, Wegner H, Bohatka A: Influence of age and duration of diabetes on dental development in diabetic children. J Dent Res 1973; 52:535, 1973.
2. Afonsky D: Oral lesions in niacin, riboflavin, pyridoxine, folic acid and pantothenic acid deficiencies in adult dogs. Oral Surg 1955; 8:207, 315, 867.
3. Ainamo J, Lahtinen A, Vitto VJ: Rapid periodontal destruction in adult humans with poorly controlled diabetes. A report of two cases. J Clin Periodontol 1990; 17:22.
4. Akers LH: Ulcerative stomatitis following therapeutic use of mercury and bismuth. J Am Dent Assoc 1936; 23:781.
5. Alfano MC: Controversies, perspectives and clinical implications of nutrition in periodontal disease. Dent Clin North Am 1976; 20:519.
6. Alfano MC, Miller SA, Drummond JF: Effect of ascorbic acid deficiency on the permeability and collagen biosynthesis of oral mucosal epithelium. Ann NY Acad Sci 1975; 258:253.
7. Alvares O, Siegel I: Permeability of gingival sulcular epithelium in the development of scorbutic gingivitis. J Oral Pathol 1981; 10:40.
8. Babior BM: Disorders of neutrophil function. In: Wyngaarden JB, Smith LHJ (eds): Cecil Textbook of Medicine, ed 18. Philadephia, Saunders, 1988.
9. Baker EG, Crook GH, Schwabacher (eds): Personality correlates of periodontal disease. J Dent Res 1961; 40:396.
10. Barnett ML, Baker RL, Yancey JM, et al: Absence of periodontitis in a population of insulin-dependent diabetes mellitus (IDDM) patients. J Periodontol 1984; 55:402.
11. Barrett P: Gingival lesions in leukemia. A classification. J Periodontol 1984; 55:585.
12. Bartolucci EG, Parkes RB: Accelerated periodontal breakdown in uncontrolled diabetes. Pathogenesis and treatment. Oral Surg Oral Med Oral Pathol 1981; 52:387.
13. Bauer WH: Agranulocytosis and the supporting dental tissues. J Dent Res 1946; 25:501.
14. Becks H, Collins DA, Freytog RM: Changes in oral structures of the dog persisting after chronic overdoses of vitamin D. Am J Orthod 1946; 32:463.
15. Becks H, Wainwright WW, Morgan AF: Comparative study of oral changes in dogs due to deficiencies of pantothenic acid, nicotinic acid and unknowns of B vitamin complex. Am J Orthod 1943; 29:183.
16. Been V, Engel D: The effects of immunosuppressive drugs on periodontal inflammation in human renal allograft patients. J Periodontol 1982; 53:245.
17. Behbehani MJ, Jordan HV: Comparative colonization of human Actinomyces species in hamsters under different dietary conditions. J Periodont Res 1980; 15:395.
18. Belting CM, Gupta OP: The influence of psychiatric disturbances on the severity of periodontal disease. J Periodontol 1961; 32:219.
19. Bergmann OJ, Ellegaard B, Dahl M, et al: Gingival status during chemical plaque control with or without prior mechanical plaque removal in patients with acute myeloid leukemia. J Clin Periodontol 1992; 19:169.
20. Bernick S: Age changes in the blood supply to human teeth. J Dent Res 1967; 46:544.
21. Bernick S, Ershoff BH: Histochemical study of bone in estrogen-treated rats. J Dent Res 1963; 42:981.
22. Bernick S, Levy BM, Patek PR: Studies on the biology of the periodontium of marmosets. VI. Arteriosclerotic changes in the blood vessels of the periodontium. J Periodontol 1969; 40:355.
23. Bernick SM, Cohen DW, Baker L, et al: Dental disease in children with diabetes mellitus. J Periodontol 1975; 46:241.
24. Biro S: Studies regarding the influence of pregnancy upon caries. Vierteljahrschr Zahnheilk 1898; 14:371.
25. Bissada NF, Schaffer EM, Laarow A: Effect of alloxan diabetes and local irritating factors on the periodontal structures of the rat. Periodontics 1966; 4:233.
26. Blitzer B, Sznajder N, Carranza FA Jr: Hallazgos clinicos periodontales en ninos con cardiopatias congenitas. Rev Assoc Odont Argent 1975; 63:169.
27. Borghelli RF, Devoto FCH, Foglia V, et al: Periodontal changes and dental caries in experimental prediabetes. Diabetes 1967; 16:804.
28. Boyle PE: Effect of vitamin A deficiency on the periodontal tissues. Am J Orthod 1947; 33:744.
29. Boyle PE, Bessey OA: The effect of acute vitamin A deficiency on the molar teeth and paradontal tissues, with a comment on deformed incisor-teeth in this deficiency. J Dent Res 1941; 20:236.
30. Brown LR, Roth GD, Hoover D, et al: Alveolar bone loss in leukemic and nonleukemic mice. J Periodontol 1969; 40:725.
31. Brownlee M: Glycation and diabetic complications. Diabetes 1994; 43:836.
32. Burstoen MS: The psychosomatic aspects of dental problems. J Am Dent Assoc 1946; 33:862.
33. Burwasser P, Hill TJ: The effect of hard and soft diets on the gingival tissues of dogs. J Dent Res 1939; 18:389.
34. Butcher EO, Klingsberg J: Age, gonadectomy and wound healing in the palatal mucosa. J Dent Res 1961; 40:694.
35. Buzina R, Brodarec A, Jušić M, et al: Epidemiology of angular stomatitis and bleeding gums. Int J Vitam Nutr Res 1973; 43:401.
36. Cabrini RL, Carranza FA Jr: Adenosine triphosphatase in normal and scorbutic wounds. Nature 1963; 200:1113.
37. Campbell MJA: Epidemiology of periodontal disease in the diabetic and the nondiabetic. Aust Dent J 1972; 17:274.
38. Cannon P: Some Pathologic Consequences of Protein and Amino Acid Deficiencies. Springfield, IL, Charles C. Thomas, 1948.
39. Carranza FA Jr, Cabrini RL, Lopez Otero R, et al: Histometric analysis of interradicular bone in protein deficient animals. J Periodont Res 1969; 4:292.
40. Carranza FA Jr, Gravina O, Cabrini RL: Periodontal and pulpal pathosis in leukemic mice. Oral Surg 1965; 20:374.
41. Chapman OD, Harris AE: Oral lesions associated with dietary deficiencies in monkeys. J Infect Dis 1941; 69:7.
42. Charbeneau TD, Hurt WC: Gingival findings in spontaneous scurvy. A case report. J Periodontol 1983; 54:694.
43. Chawla TN, Glickman I: Protein deprivation and the periodontal structures of the albino rat. Oral Surg 1951; 4:578.
44. Cianciola LJ, Park BH, Bruck E, et al: Prevalence of periodontal disease in insulin-dependent diabetes mellitus (juvenile diabetes). J Am Dent Assoc 1982; 104:653.
45. Cohen DW, Friedman LA, Shapiro J, et al: Diabetes mellitus and periodontal disease: Two year longitudinal observations. Part I. J Periodontol 1970; 41:709.

46. Cohen DW, Morris AL: Periodontal manifestations of cyclic neutropenia. J Periodontol 1961; 32:159.
47. Cohen DW, Shapiro J, Friedman L, et al: A longitudinal investigation of the periodontal changes during pregnancy and fifteen months postpartum. J Periodontol 1971; 42:653.
48. Cotran RS, Kumar V, Robbins SR: Robbins' Pathologic Basis of Disease, ed 4. Philadelphia, Saunders, 1989.
49. Crandon JH, Lund CC, Dill DB: Experimental human scurvy. N Engl J Med 1940; 223:353.
50. Denton J: A study of tissue changes in experimental black tongue of dogs compared with similar changes in pellagra. Am J Pathol 1928; 4:341.
51. Diabetes and oral health. J Am Dent Assoc 1987; 115:741.
52. Dreizen S: Oral manifestations of human nutritional anemias. Arch Environ Health 1962; 5:66.
53. Dreizen S, Levy BM, Bernick S, et al: Studies of the biology of the periodontium of marmosets. III. Periodontal bone changes in marmosets with osteomalacia and hyperparathyroidism. Isr J Med Sci 1967; 3:731.
54. Dreizen S, McCredie KB, Keating MJ, et al: Malignant gingival and skin infiltrates in adult leukemia. Oral Surg 1983; 55:572.
55. Egelberg J: Local effect of diet on plaque formation and development of gingivitis in dogs. I. Effect of hard and soft diets. Odont Revy 1965; 16:31.
56. El-Ashiry GM, El-Kafrawy AH, Nasr MF, et al: Comparative study of the influence of pregnancy and oral contraceptives on the gingivae. Oral Surg 1970; 30:472.
57. Emrich LJ, Shlossman M, Genco RJ: Periodontal disease in non–insulin-dependent diabetes mellitus. J Periodontol 1991; 62:123.
58. Enwonwu CO, Edozien JC: Epidemiology of periodontal disease in western Nigerians in relation to socioeconomic status. Arch Oral Biol 1970; 15:1231.
59. Falk H, Hugoson A, Thorstensson H: Number of teeth, prevalence of caries and periapical lesions in insulin-dependent diabetics. Scand J Dent Res 1989; 97:198.
60. Ficara AI, Levin MP, Grover MF, et al: A comparison of the glucose and protein content of gingival fluid from diabetics and nondiabetics. J Periodont Res 1975; 10:171.
61. Follis RH: The pathology of nutritional disease. Springfield, IL, Charles C. Thomas, 1948.
62. Formicola AJ, Weatherford T, Grupe H Jr: The uptake of H3-estradiol by the oral tissues in rats. J Periodont Res 1970; 5:269.
63. Forsslund G: Occurrence of subepithelial gingival blood vessels in patients with morbus caeruleus (tetralogy of Fallot). Acta Odontol Scand 1962; 20:301.
64. Frandsen AM: Periodontal tissue changes in vitamin A deficient young rats. Acta Odontol Scand 1963; 21:19.
65. Friedman LA: Horizontal tooth mobility and the menstrual cycle. J Periodont Res 1972; 7:125.
66. Frohman BS: Occlusal neuroses. Psychoanal Rev 1932; 19:297.
67. Galea H, Aganovic I, Anganovic M: The dental caries and periodontal disease experience of patients with early-onset insulin-dependent diabetes. Int Dent J 1986; 36:219.
68. Genco RJ, Shlossman M, Zambon JJ: Immunologic studies of periodontitis patients with type II diabetes (abstract). J Dent Res 1987; 66:257.
69. Gillman CF, Berstein JM, Van Oss C: Increased phagocytosis associated with increased surface hydrophobicity of neutrophils of children with chronic infections (abstract). Fed Proc 1976; 35:227.
70. Glavind L, Lund B, Löe H: The relationship between periodontal state and diabetes duration, insulin dosage and retinal changes. J Periodontol 1968; 39:341.
71. Glickman I: The periodontal structures in experimental diabetes. NY J Dent 1946; 16:226.
72. Glickman I: Acute vitamin C deficiency and periodontal disease. I. The periodontal tissues of the guinea pig in acute vitamin C deficiency. J Dent Res 1948; 27:9.
73. Glickman I: Acute vitamin C deficiency and the periodontal tissues. II. The effect of acute vitamin C deficiency upon the response of the periodontal tissues of the guinea pig to artificially induced inflammation. J Dent Res 1948; 27:201.
74. Glickman I, Morse A, Robinson L: The systemic influence upon bone in periodontoclasia. J Am Dent Assoc 1944; 31:1435.
75. Glickman I, Quintarelli G: Further observations regarding the effect of ovariectomy upon the tissues of the periodontium. J Periodontol 1960; 31:31.
76. Glickman I, Shklar G: The steroid hormones and the tissues of the periodontium. Oral Surg 1955; 8:1179.
77. Glickman I, Stoller M: The periodontal tissues of the albino rat in vitamin A deficiency. J Dent Res 1948; 27:758.
78. Glickman I, Stone IC, Chawla TN: The effect of cortisone acetate upon the periodontium of white mice. J Periodontol 1953; 24:161.
79. Goetzl EJ: Enhancement of random migration and chemotactic response of human leukocytes by ascorbic acid. J Clin Invest 1974; 53:813.
80. Goldman HM: Acute aleukemic leukemia. Am J Orthod 1940; 26:89.
81. Goodman MH: Perlèche: A consideration of its etiology and pathology. Bull Johns Hopkins Hosp 1943; 51:263.
82. Gottsegen R: Dental and oral considerations in diabetes mellitus. NY J Med 1962; 62:389.
83. Govier WM, Grieg ME: Prevention of oral lesions in B1 avitaminotic dogs. Science 1943; 98:216.
84. Grant D, Bernick S: Arteriosclerosis in periodontal vessels of aging humans. J Periodontol 1970; 41:170.
85. Greenberg MS, Cohen SB, Boosz B, et al: Oral herpes infections in patients with leukemia. J Am Dent Assoc 1987; 114:483.
86. Grossi SG, Zambon JJ, Norderyd OM, et al: Microbiological risk indicators for periodontal disease. Abstract 818. J Dent Res 1993; 72:206.
87. Gupta OP: Psychosomatic factors in periodontal disease. Dent Clin North Am 1966; 10:11.
88. Gusberti F, Grossman N, Loesche W: Puberty gingivitis in insulin-dependent diabetes. Abstract 199. J Dent Res (special issue) 1982; 61:201.
89. Hayden P, Buckley LA: Diabetes mellitus and periodontal disease in an Irish population. J Periodont Res 1989; 24:298.
90. Henrikson PA: Periodontal disease and calcium deficiency in the dog. Acta Odont Scand 1968; 26(suppl 50):1.
91. Higgins WH: Systemic poisoning with bismuth. JAMA 1916; 66:648.
92. Hirschfeld I: Periodontal symptoms associated with diabetes. J Periodontol 1934; 5:37.
93. Hodges RE, Baker EM, Hood J, et al: Experimental scurvy in man. Am J Clin Nutr 1969; 22:535.
94. Hojer JA: Studies in scurvy. Acta Paediatr 1924; 3(suppl):119.
95. Holm-Pederson P, Löe H: Flow of gingival exudate as related to menstruation and pregnancy. J Periodont Res 1967; 2:13.
96. Hugoson A: Gingival inflammation and female sex hormones. J Periodontol Res 5(suppl):1970.
97. Ismail AI, Burt BA, Eklund SA: Relation between ascorbic acid intake and periodontal disease in the United States. J Am Dent Assoc 1983; 107:927.
98. Itoiz ME, Litwack D, Kennedy JE, et al: Experimental ischemia in monkeys. III. Histochemical analysis of gingival epithelium. J Dent Res 1969; 48:895.

99. Jeghers H: Riboflavin deficiency. IV. Oral changes. In: Advances in Internal Medicine I. New York, Interscience Publishers, 1942.
100. Jones RR: Symptoms in early stages of industrial plumbism. JAMA 1935; 104:195.
101. Kalkwarf KL: Effect of oral contraceptive therapy on gingival inflammation in humans. J Periodontol 1978; 49:560.
102. Kaner A, Losch P, Green M: Oral manifestations of congenital heart disease. J Pediatr 1946; 29:269.
103. Kardachi BJR, Newcomb GM: A clinical study of gingival inflammation in renal transplant patients taking immunosuppressive drugs. J Periodontol 1978; 49:307.
104. Kastlin G: Agranulocytic angina. Am J Med Sci 1927; 173:799.
105. Kennedy JE, Zander HA: Experimental ischemia in monkeys. I. Effect of ischemia on gingival epithelium. J Dent Res 1969; 48:696.
106. Keys A, Brozek J, Henschel A, et al. In: The Biology of Human Starvation, vol 1. Minneapolis, University of Minnesota Press, 1950.
107. Kim JE, Shklar G: The effect of vitamin E on the healing of gingival wounds in rats. J Periodontol 1983; 54:305.
108. King JD: Vincent's disease treated with nicotinic acid. Lancet 1940; 2:32.
109. King JD, Glover NE: The relative effects of dietary constituents and other factors upon calculus formation and gingival disease in the ferret. J Pathol Bacteriol 1945; 57:353.
110. Knight GM, Wade AB: The effects of hormonal contraceptives on the human periodontium. J Periodont Res 1974; 9:18.
111. Kolodzinski E, Munoa N, Malatesta E: Clinical study of gingival tissue in pregnant women. Abstract. J Dent Res 1974; 53:693.
112. Kornman KS, Loesche WJ: The subgingival microbial flora during pregnancy. J Periodont Res 1980; 15:111.
113. Kracke RR: Granulopenia as associated with amidopyrine administration. Report made at the Annual Session of the AMA 1934.
114. Krasse B, Brill N: Effect of consistency of diet on bacteria in gingival pockets in dogs. Odont Rev 1960; 11:152.
115. Krohn S: The effect of the administration of steroid hormones on the gingival tissues. J Periodontol 1958; 29:300.
116. Lee RE, Lee NZ: The peripheral vascular system and its reactions in scurvy: An experimental study. Am J Physiol 1947; 149:465.
117. Liberman H: Chrome ulcerations of the nose and throat. N Engl J Med 1941; 225:132.
118. Lindhe J, Attstrom R: Gingival exudation during the menstrual cycle. J Periodont Res 1967; 2:194.
119. Lindhe J, Attstrom R, Bjorn A: Influence of sex hormones on gingival exudation in gingivitis-free female dogs. J Periodont Res 1968; 3:272.
120. Lindhe J, Bjorn AL: Influence of hormonal contraceptives on the gingiva of women. J Periodont Res 1967; 2:64.
121. Lindhe J, Branemark PI: Changes in microcirculation after local application of sex hormones. J Periodont Res 1967; 2:185.
122. Lindhe J, Sonesson B: The effect of sex hormones on inflammation. II. Progestogen, oestrogen and chorionic gonadotropin. J Periodont Res 1967; 2:7.
123. Lindhe J, Wicen PO: The effects on the gingivae of chewing fibrous foods. J Periodont Res 1969; 4:193.
124. Löe H: Periodontal changes in pregnancy. J Periodontol 1965; 36:209.
125. Lynch MA, Ship I: Initial oral manifestations of leukemia. J Am Dent Assoc 1967; 75:932.
126. MacKenzie RS, Millard HO: Interrelated effects of diabetes, arteriosclerosis and calculus on alveolar bone loss. J Am Dent Assoc 1963; 66:191.
127. Madison FW, Squier TL: Primary granulocytopenia after administration of benzene chain derivatives. JAMA 1934; 102:755.
128. Maier AW, Orban B: Gingivitis in pregnancy. Oral Surg 1949; 2:234.
129. Manhold JH: Report of a study on the relationship of personality variables to periodontal conditions. J Periodontol 1953; 24:248.
130. Mann AW, Spies TD, Springer M: Oral manifestations of vitamin B complex deficiencies. J Dent Res 1941; 20:269.
131. Manson-Bahr P, Ransford ON: Stomatitis of vitamin B2 deficiency treated with nicotinic acid. Lancet 1938; 2:426.
132. Mark HA: Agranulocytic angina. Its oral manifestations. J Am Dent Assoc 1934; 21:119.
133. Mascola B: The oral manifestations of diabetes mellitus: A review. NY Dent J 1970; 36:139.
134. Mashimo P, Yamamoto Y, Slots J, et al: The periodontal microflora of juvenile diabetes—Culture, immunofluorescence and serum antibody studies. J Periodontol 1983; 54:420.
135. Massler M, Henry J: Oral manifestations during the female climacteric. Alpha Omegan September, 1950; 105.
136. McCarthy P, Shklar G: Diseases of the Oral Mucosa, ed 2. Philadelphia, Lea & Febiger, 1980.
137. McMullen JA, VanDyke TE, Horozewicz HU, et al: Neutrophil chemotaxis in individuals with advanced periodontal disease and a genetic predisposition to diabetes mellitus. J Periodontol 1981; 52:167.
138. Mealey BL: Influence of periodontal infections on systemic health. Periodontology 2000 1999; 21:197.
139. Meyer A: Agranulocytosis. Report of a case caused by sulfadiazine. Calif West Med J 1944; 61:54.
140. Miller SC, Stahl SS, Goldsmith (eds): The effects of vertical occlusal trauma on the periodontium of protein deprived young adult rats. J Periodontol 1957; 28:87.
141. Miller SC, Thaller JL, Soberman A: The use of the Minnesota Multiphasic Personality Inventory as a diagnostic aid in periodontal disease. A preliminary report. J Periodontol 1956; 27:44.
142. Mohammed AH, Waterhouse JP, Friederici HH: The microvasculature of the rat gingiva as affected by progesterone: An ultrastructural study. J Periodontol 1974; 45:50.
143. National Diabetes Data Group: Diabetes in America, ed 2. Bethesda, MD, National Institutes of Health, NIH No. 95-1468, 1995.
144. Nelson MA, Chaudhry AP: Effects of tocopherol (vitamin E) deficient diet on some oral//para-oral and hematopoietic tissues of the rat. J Dent Res 1966; 45:1072.
145. Nichols C, Laster AA, Bodak Gyovai LZ: Diabetes mellitus and periodontal disease. J Periodontol 1978; 49:85.
146. Nishida M, Grossi SG, Dunford RG, et al: Dietary vitamin C and the risk for periodontal disease. J Periodontol 2000; 71(8):1215.
147. Novaes AB Jr, Pereira ALA, Moraes N, et al: Manifestations of insulin-dependent diabetes mellitus in the periodontium of young Brazilian patients. J Periodontol 1991; 62:116.
148. Nutlay AG, Bhaskar SN, Weinmann JP, et al: The effect of estrogen on the gingiva and alveolar bone in rats and mice. J Dent Res 1954; 33:115.
149. O'Leary TM, Shannon I, Prigmore JR: Clinical and systemic findings in periodontal disease. J Periodontol 1962; 32:243.
150. O'Neil TCA: Maternal T-lymphocyte response and gingivitis in pregnancy. J Periodontol 1979; 50:178.

151. Oshrain HI, Mender S, Mandel ID: Periodontal status of patients with reduced immunocapacity. J Periodontol 1979; 50:185.
152. Pack A, Thomson M: Effects of topical and systemic folic acid supplementation on gingivitis in pregnancy. J Clin Periodontol 1980; 7:402.
153. Page RC: The pathobiology of periodontal diseases may affect systemic diseases: inversion of a paradigm. Ann Periodontol 1998; 3:108.
154. Page RC, Schroeder HE: Periodontitis in Man and Other Animals. A Comparative Review. Basel, S. Karger, 1982.
155. Parrish JH Jr, DeMarco TJ, Bissada NF: Vitamin E and periodontitis in the rat. 1977; 44(2):210.
156. Pelzer R: A study of the local oral effect of diet on the periodontal tissues and the gingival capillary structure. J Am Dent Assoc 1940; 27:13.
157. Perry DA: Oral contraceptives and periodontal health. J West Soc Periodontol 1981; 29:72.
158. Phair J: Neutrophil dysfunction in diabetes mellitus. J Lab Clin Med 1975; 85:26.
159. Piroshaw N, Glickman I: The effect of ovariectomy upon the tissues of the periodontium and skeletal bones. Oral Surg 1957; 10:133.
160. Prout RES, Hopps RM: A relationship between human oral bacteria and the menstrual cycle. J Periodontol 1970; 41:98.
161. Quintarelli G: Histopathology of the human mandibular artery and arterioles in periodontal disease. Oral Surg 1957; 10:1047.
162. Rada RE, Bronny AT, Hasiakos PS: Sickle cell crisis precipitated by periodontal infection. J Am Dent Assoc 1987; 11:799.
163. Randall CL: Granulocytopenia following barbiturates and amidopyrine. JAMA 1934; 102:1137.
164. Rateitschak KH: Tooth mobility changes in pregnancy. J Periodont Res 1967; 2:199.
165. Restarski JS, Pijoan M: Gingivitis and vitamin C. J Am Dent Assoc 1944; 31:1323.
166. Richman JJ, Abarbanel AR: Effects of estradiol, testosterone, diethylstilbestrol and several of their derivatives upon the human mucous membrane. J Am Dent Assoc 1943; 30:913.
167. Ringsdorf WM, Powell BJ, Knight LA, et al: Periodontal status and pregnancy. Am J Obstet Gynecol 1962; 83:258.
168. Robbins SL, Cotran RS, Kumar V: Pathologic Basis of Disease, ed 4. Philadephia, Saunders, 1989.
169. Robertson HD, Polk HC Jr: The mechanism of infection in patients with diabetes mellitus. A review of leukocyte malfunction. Surgery 1974; 75:123.
170. Rosenberg EH, Guralnick WC: Hyperparathyroidism. Oral Surg 1962; 15(suppl 2):84.
171. Rushton MA: Epithelial downgrowth: Effect of methyl testosterone. Br Dent J 1952; 93:27.
172. Russell AL: International nutrition surveys: A summary of preliminary dental findings. J Dent Res 1963; 42:233.
173. Rylander H, Attstrom R, Lindhe J: Influence of experimental neutropenia in dogs with chronic gingivitis. J Periodont Res 1975; 10:315.
174. Safkan-Seppala B, Ainamo J: Periodontal conditions in insulin-dependent diabetes mellitus. J Clin Periodontol 1992; 19:24.
175. Sastrowijoto SH, Hillemans P, van Steenbergen TJM, et al: Periodontal condition and microbiology of healthy and diseased periodontal pockets in type I diabetes mellitus patients. J Clin Periodontol 1989; 16:316.
176. Saul LJ: A note on the psychogenesis of organic symptoms. Psychoanal 1935; 4:476.
177. Schmidt AM, Weidman E, Lalla E: Advanced glycation endproducts (AGEs) induce oxidant stress in the gingiva: A potential mechanism underlying accelerated periodontal disease associated with diabetes. J Periodontol Res 1996; 31:508.
178. Schneir M, Imberman M, Ramamurthy N, et al: Streptozotocin-induced diabetes and the rat periodontium: Decreased relative collagen production. Coll Relat Res 1988; 8:221.
179. Schour I, Sarnat BG: Oral manifestations of occupational origin. JAMA 1942; 120:1197.
180. Scopp IW: Healthy periodontium in chronically ill patients. J Periodontol 1957; 28:147.
181. Scully CE, MacFayden A, Campbell A: Oral manifestations in cyclic neutropenia. Br J Oral Surg 1982; 20:96.
182. Shaw JH: The relation of nutrition to periodontal disease. J Dent Res 1962; 41(suppl 1):264.
183. Shilotri PG, Bhat KS: Effect of megadoses of vitamin C on bacterial activity of leukocytes. Am J Clin Nutr 1977; 30:1077.
184. Shklar G, Chauncey H, Peluso D: The effect of testosterone on the periodontium of the male albino rat. IADR Abstracts 1962; vol 68.
185. Shklar G, Chauncey H, Shapiro S: The effect of testosterone on the periodontium of normal and hypophysectomy rats. J Periodontol 1967; 38:203.
186. Shklar G, Cohen MM, Yerganian G: Periodontal disease in the Chinese hamster with hereditary diabetes. J Periodontol 1962; 33:14.
187. Shklar G, Glickman I: The effect of estrogenic hormone on the periodontium of white mice. J Periodontol 1956; 27:16.
188. Silverman S, Gordon G, Grant T, et al: The dental structures in primary hyperparathyroidism. Oral Surg 1962; 15:426.
189. Squire CF, Costley JM: Gingival status during prolonged fasting for weight loss. J Periodontol 1957; 28:87.
190. Stahl SS: The effect of a protein-free diet on the healing of gingival wounds in rats. Arch Oral Biol 1962; 7:551.
191. Stahl SS, Sandler HC, Cahn L: The effects of protein deprivation upon the oral tissues of the rat and particularly upon the periodontal structures under irritation. Oral Surg 1955; 8:760.
192. Strock MS: The mouth in hyperparathyroidism. N Engl J Med 1945; 224:1019.
193. Sutcliffe P: A longitudinal study of gingivitis and puberty. J Periodont Res 1972; 7:52.
194. Svanberg G, Lindhe J, Hugoson A, et al: Effect of nutritional hyperparathyroidism on experimental periodontitis in the dog. Scand J Dent Res 1973; 81:155.
195. Sznajder N, Carraro JJ, Rugna S, et al: Periodontal findings in diabetic and nondiabetic patients. J Periodontol 1978; 49:445.
196. Telsey B, Beube FE, Zegarelli EV, et al: Oral manifestations of cyclical neutropenia associated with hypergammaglobulinemia. Oral Surg 1962; 15:540.
197. Tervonen T, Knuuttila M, Pohjamo L, et al: Immediate response to non-surgical periodontal treatment in subjects with diabetes mellitus. J Clin Periodontol 1991; 18:65.
198. Tollefsen T, Saltvedt E, Koppang HS: The effect of immunosuppressive agents on periodontal disease in man. J Periodont Res 1978; 13:240.
199. Topping NH, Fraser HF: Mouth lesions associated with dietary deficiencies in monkeys. Public Health Rep 1939; 54:416.
200. Turesky S, Fisher B, Glickman I: A histochemical study of the attached gingiva in pregnancy. J Dent Res 1958; 37:1115.

201. Vogel, R: Relationship of folic acid to phenytoin-induced gingival overgrowth. In: Hassell TM, Johnson M, Dudley K (eds): Phenytoin-Induced Teratology and Gingival Pathology. New York, Raven Press, 1980.
202. Vogel R, Deasy M, Alfano M, et al: The effect of folic acid on gingival health of women taking oral contraceptives. J Prev Dent 1980; 6:221.
203. Vogel R, Fink R, Frank O, et al: The effect of topical application of folic acid on gingival health. J Oral Med 1978; 33:20.
204. Vogel R, Fink R, Schneider L, et al: The effect of folic acid on gingival health. J Periodontol 1976; 47:667.
205. Waerhaug J: Effect of C-avitaminosis on the supporting structures of the teeth. J Periodontol 1958; 29:87.
206. Waerhaug J: Epidemiology of periodontal disease. Review of the literature. In: World Workshop in Periodontics. Ann Arbor, MI, American Academy of Periodontology and the University of Michigan Press, 1966.
207. Weinmann JP, Schour I: The effect of parathyroid hormone on the alveolar bone and teeth of the normal and rachitic rat. Am J Pathol 1945; 21:857.
208. Weinmann JP, Schour I: Experimental studies in calcification. Am J Pathol 1945; 21:821, 1047.
209. Willershausen B, Barth S, Preac-Mursic V, et al: Parodontalbefund und Mikroflora bei insulin-abhangigen (Typ I)-Diabetikern. Schweiz Monatsschr Zahnmed 1991; 101:1399.
210. Wingrove FA, Rubright WC, Kerber PE: Influence of ovarian hormone situation on atrophy, hypertrophy, and/or desquamation of human gingiva in premenopausal and postmenopausal women. J Periodontol 1979; 50:445.
211. Wirthlin MR Jr, Ratcliff PA: Arteries, atherosclerosis and periodontics. J Periodontol 40:341.
212. Wolbach SB, Bessey OA: Tissue changes in vitamin deficiencies. Physiol Rev 1942; 22:233.
213. Woolfe SN, Hume WR, Kenney EB: Ascorbic acid and periodontal disease: A review of the literature. J West Soc Periodontol 1980; 28:44.
214. Woolfe SN, Kenney EB, Hume WR, et al: Relationship of ascorbic acid levels of blood and gingival tissue with response to periodontal therapy. J Clin Periodontol 1984; 11:159.
215. Zambon JJ, Reynolds H, Fisher JB, et al: Microbiological and immunological studies of adult periodontitis in patients with non–insulin-dependent diabetes mellitus. J Periodontol 1988; 59:23.
216. Ziskin DE, Blackberg SN: A study of the gingivae during pregnancy. J Dent Res 1933; 13:253.
217. Ziskin DE, Blackberg SN: The effect of castration and hypophysectomy on the gingiva and oral mucous membranes of Rhesus monkeys. J Dent Res 1940; 19:381.
218. Ziskin DE, Blackberg SN, Stout A: The gingivae during pregnancy: An experimental study and a histopathological interpretation. Surg Gynecol Obstet 1933; 57:719.

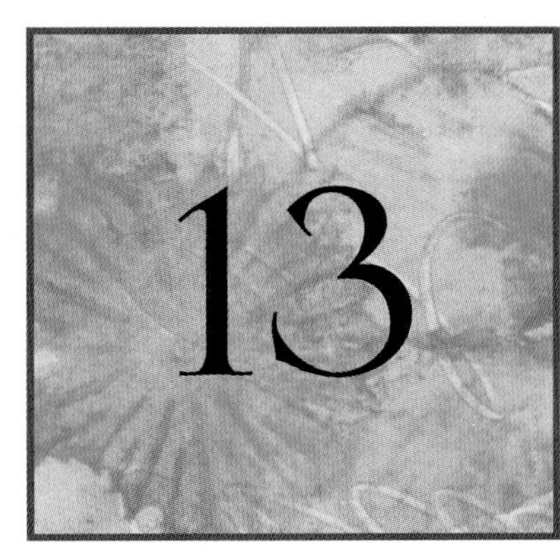

CHAPTER

Periodontal Medicine

Brian L. Mealey and Perry R. Klokkevold

CHAPTER OUTLINE

Advances in science and technology over the last century have greatly expanded our knowledge of the pathogenesis of periodontal diseases. Periodontal disease is an infectious disease. However, environmental, physical, social, and host stresses may affect and modify disease expression. It is clear that certain systemic conditions may affect the initiation and progression of gingivitis and periodontitis. Many of these are discussed in Chapters 10 and 12. Systemic disorders affecting neutrophil, monocyte/macrophage, and lymphocyte function result in altered production or activity of host inflammatory mediators.[53] These alterations may manifest clinically as early onset of periodontal destruction or a more rapid rate of destruction than would occur in the absence of such disorders.

Evidence emerging in the last decade has shed light on the converse side of the relationship between systemic health and oral health—that is, the potential effects of periodontal disease on a wide range of organ systems. This field of periodontal medicine addresses the important questions: Can bacterial infection of the periodontium, commonly known as *periodontitis,* have an effect remote from the oral cavity? Is periodontal infection a risk factor for systemic diseases or conditions that affect human health?

PATHOBIOLOGY OF PERIODONTITIS

Our understanding of the pathogenesis of periodontitis has changed remarkably over the last 30 years.[57] Nonspecific accumulation of bacterial plaque was once thought to be the cause of periodontal destruction, but it is now

BOX 13-1

Organ Systems and Conditions Possibly Influenced by Periodontal Infection

Cardiovascular/Cerebrovascular System
Atherosclerosis
Coronary heart disease
Angina
Myocardial infarction
Cerebrovascular accident (Stroke)

Endocrine System
Diabetes mellitus

Reproductive System
Preterm low birth-weight babies

Respiratory System
Chronic obstructive pulmonary disease
Acute bacterial pneumonia

recognized that periodontitis is an infectious disease associated with a small number of predominantly gram-negative microorganisms. Furthermore, the importance of the host in disease initiation and progression is clearly recognized. Although pathogenic bacteria are necessary for periodontal disease, they are not in and of themselves sufficient to cause the disease. A susceptible host is also imperative. In a host who is not susceptible to disease, pathogenic bacteria may have no clinical effect. Conversely, the susceptible host experiences clinical signs of periodontitis in the presence of pathogenic bacteria.

Recognition of the importance of host susceptibility opens a door to understanding the differences in the onset, natural history, and progression of periodontitis seen throughout the scientific literature. Due to differences in host susceptibility, not all individuals are equally vulnerable to the destructive effects of periodontal pathogens. Thus patients may not necessarily have similar disease expression in spite of the presence of similar bacteria. Likewise, the response to periodontal treatment may vary depending on the wound healing capacity and susceptibility of the host to further disease progression. The importance of host susceptibility is clearly evident in the medical literature. For example, respiratory tract pathogens may have minimal effect on many individuals; yet, in a susceptible host such as an elderly patient, these same pathogens may cause life-threatening respiratory tract illnesses.

Many of the systemic conditions discussed in Chapters 10 and 12 serve to modify the susceptibility of the host to periodontitis. For example, patients with immune suppression may not be able to mount an effective host response to subgingival microorganisms, resulting in more rapid and severe periodontal destruction. Although the potential impact of many systemic disorders on the periodontium is well-documented, recent evidence suggests that periodontal infection may significantly enhance the risk for certain systemic diseases or alter the natural course of systemic conditions.[46] Conditions in which the influences of periodontal infection are documented include coronary heart disease (CHD) and CHD-related events such as angina and infarction, atherosclerosis, stroke, diabetes mellitus, preterm labor, low birth-weight delivery, and respiratory conditions such as chronic obstructive pulmonary disease (COPD) (Box 13-1).[46,58]

FOCAL INFECTION THEORY REVISITED

Recent research in the area of periodontal medicine marks a resurgence in the concept of focal infection. In 1900, William Hunter, a British physician, first developed the idea that oral microorganisms were responsible for a wide range of systemic conditions that were not easily recognized as being infectious in nature[16,51] and claimed that restoration of carious teeth rather than extraction resulted in trapping of infectious agents under restorations. In addition to caries, pulpal necrosis, and periapical abscesses, Hunter also identified gingivitis and periodontitis as foci of infection. He advocated extraction of teeth with these conditions to eliminate the source of sepsis. Hunter believed that teeth were liable to septic infection primarily due to their structure and their relationship to alveolar bone. He stated that the degree of systemic effect produced by oral sepsis depended on the virulence of the oral infection and the degree of resistance of the individual. He also felt that oral organisms had specific actions on different tissues and that these organisms acted by producing toxins, resulting in low-grade "subinfection," which produced systemic effects over prolonged periods. Finally, Hunter believed that the connection between oral sepsis and resulting systemic conditions could be shown by removal of the causative sepsis via tooth extraction and observation of the improvement in systemic health. Since it explained a wide range of disorders for which there was no known explanation at the time, Hunter's theory became widely accepted in Britain and eventually the United States, leading to wholesale extraction of teeth.

The focal infection theory fell into disrepute in the 1940s and 1950s when widespread extraction, often of the entire dentition, failed to reduce or eliminate the systemic conditions to which the supposedly infected dentition had been linked. The theory, while offering a possible explanation for perplexing systemic disorders, had been based on very little, if any, scientific evidence. Hunter and other advocates of the theory were unable to explain how focal oral sepsis produced these systemic maladies. They were unable to elucidate possible interactive mechanisms between oral and systemic health. Furthermore, the suggested intervention of tooth extraction often had no effect on the systemic conditions for which patients sought relief. However, Hunter's ideas did encourage extensive research in microbiology and immunology.

EVIDENCE-BASED CLINICAL PRACTICE

Many of the precepts of the focal infection theory are being revived today in light of recent research demonstrating links between oral and systemic health. Yet, in order for the "hypothesis not to fall into disrepute for a second time, there must be no unsubstantiated attributions, no theories without evidence."[51] Today's era of evidence-based medicine and dentistry provides an excellent environment in which to examine the possible relationships between oral infection and systemic disorders.[17]

To establish a relationship between conditions A and B, different levels of evidence must be examined. All scientific evidence is not given the same weight.[32,52] The stronger the evidence, the more likely it is that a true relationship exists between the conditions. Table 13-1 describes these various levels of evidence.

For example, in examining the relationship between elevated cholesterol levels and CHD-related events, the literature might initially consist entirely of case reports or similar anecdotal information in which individual patients with recent myocardial infarction are found to have elevated cholesterol levels. These anecdotal reports suggest a possible relationship between elevated cholesterol and myocardial infarction, but the evidence is weak. These case reports may lead to cross-sectional studies in which a large subject population is examined to determine whether those individual who have had a myocardial infarction have higher cholesterol levels than other individuals (control subjects) who have not had an infarction. Ideally, these cross-sectional studies are controlled for other potential causes or factors associated with myocardial infarction such as age, gender, and smoking history. In other words, the subjects who had a previous myocardial infarction would be retrospectively "matched" with subjects of similar age, gender, and smoking history. Then their cholesterol levels would be examined for similarities or differences. Significantly higher cholesterol levels in those subjects with a previous infarction compared with those without infarction offers stronger evidence than case reports and further substantiates a possible link between elevated cholesterol and myocardial infarction.

Even stronger evidence is provided by longitudinal studies in which subject populations are examined over time. For example, a group of subjects might periodically have cholesterol levels evaluated over several years. If those individuals with elevated cholesterol levels have a significantly higher rate of myocardial infarction over time compared with those subjects with normal cholesterol levels, even stronger evidence is available to substantiate the link between cholesterol and infarction. Finally, intervention trials may be designed to alter the potentially causative condition and to determine the effect of this change on the resultant condition. For example, patients with elevated cholesterol may be divided into two groups: a group that uses a cholesterol-lowering drug or diet and a control group that has no intervention. These two groups might also be compared with a third group with normal cholesterol levels. Over time, the rate of myocardial infarction in each group would be determined. If the group on the cholesterol-lowering regimen has a significantly lower rate of infarction than the group with continued elevations in cholesterol, strong evidence of a link between cholesterol and myocardial infarction would be established.

At each level of evidence, it is important to determine whether there is a biologically plausible link between conditions A and B. For example, if case reports, cross-sectional studies, longitudinal studies, and intervention trials all support the link between cholesterol levels and

TABLE 13-1

Evaluation of Evidence

Type of Study	Strength of Evidence	Comments
Case report	+/−	• Provides relatively weak retrospective anecdotal evidence • May suggest further study needed
Cross-sectional study	+	• Compares groups of subjects at a single point in time • Stronger than case report • Fairly easy to conduct • Relatively inexpensive to conduct
Longitudinal study	++	• Follows groups of subjects over time • Stronger than cross-sectional study • Studies with control group much stronger than studies without controls • More difficult and expensive to conduct
Intervention trial	+++	• Examines effects of some intervention • Studies with control group (i.e., placebo) much stronger than studies without controls • Strongest form of evidence is randomized controlled intervention trial • Difficult and expensive to conduct

myocardial infarction, the following question remains: How is cholesterol related to infarction? What are the mechanisms by which cholesterol affects the cardiovascular system and thus increases the risk for myocardial infarction? These studies provide explanatory data that further substantiate the link between the two conditions.

The focal infection theory, as proposed and defended in the early part of the 20th century, was based on almost no evidence. Only the occasional case report and other anecdotes were available to substantiate the theory. Although explanatory mechanisms were proposed, none were validated with scientific research. Unfortunately, this theory predated current concepts of evidence-based clinical practice, leading to unnecessary extraction of millions of teeth. Today, in reexamining the potential associations between oral infections and systemic conditions, it is important to determine what evidence is available, is still needed to substantiate the associations, and validates the possible mechanisms of association. This chapter reviews current knowledge relating periodontal infection to overall systemic health.

THE SUBGINGIVAL ENVIRONMENT AS A RESERVOIR OF BACTERIA

The subgingival microbiota in patients with periodontitis provides a significant and persistent gram-negative bacterial challenge to the host (see Chapters 6 and 8). These organisms and their products, such as lipopolysaccharide (LPS), have ready access to the periodontal tissues and to the circulation via the sulcular epithelium, which is frequently ulcerated and discontinuous. Even with treatment, complete eradication of these organisms is difficult, and their reemergence is often rapid. The total surface area of pocket epithelium in contact with subgingival bacteria and their products in a patient with generalized moderate periodontitis has been estimated to be approximately the size of the palm of an adult hand, with even larger areas of exposure in cases of more advanced periodontal destruction.[57] Bacteremias are common after mechanical periodontal therapy and also occur frequently during normal daily function and oral hygiene procedures.[25,45,74] Just as the periodontal tissues mount an immunoinflammatory response to bacteria and their products, systemic challenge with these agents also induces a major vascular response. This host response may offer explanatory mechanisms for the interactions between periodontal infection and a variety of systemic disorders.

PERIODONTAL DISEASE AND MORTALITY

The ultimate medical outcome measure is mortality. In the 1960s a prospective study known as the Normative Aging Study was begun. The study enrolled 2280 healthy men, each of whom received baseline clinical, radiographic, laboratory, and electrocardiographic examinations. Subjects have been seen every 3 years for the past 30 years, and received their medical and dental care in the private sector. The Veterans Affairs (VA) Dental Longitudinal Study began in 1968, using a subset of patients from the Normative Aging Study to examine age-related changes in the oral cavity and to identify risk factors for oral disease.[18] Clinical examinations were performed and alveolar bone level measurements were determined from full-mouth radiographs. The mean percentage of alveolar bone loss and the mean probing depth were determined for each subject. A recent study of data from this subject population sought to determine whether periodontal disease status was a significant predictor of mortality independent of other baseline characteristics within the population.[19] From the original sample of 804 dentate, medically healthy subjects, a total of 166 died during the study. Periodontal status at the baseline examination was a significant predictor of mortality independent of other factors such as smoking, alcohol use, cholesterol levels, blood pressure, family history of heart disease, education level, and body mass. For those subjects with the most alveolar bone loss, having an average of greater than 21% alveolar bone loss at baseline, the risk of dying during the follow-up period was 70% higher than for all other subjects. Interestingly, alveolar bone loss increased the risk of mortality to a greater extent than smoking (52% increased risk), a well-known risk factor for mortality.

In the study described above, periodontitis preceded and increased the risk of mortality. Yet this only establishes an association, not causation. It is possible that periodontal disease reflects other health behaviors not evaluated in this study, rather than acting as a specific cause of mortality. In other words, patients with poor periodontal health may also have other risk factors that increase mortality rate (e.g., smoking).

In examining research that suggests oral health status as a possible risk factor for systemic conditions, it is important to recognize when other known risk factors for those systemic conditions have been accounted for in the analysis. Host susceptibility factors that place individuals at risk for periodontitis may also place them at risk for systemic diseases such as cardiovascular disease. In that case, the association may actually be between the risk factors, rather than between the diseases themselves. For example, periodontitis and cardiovascular disease share risk factors like smoking, age, race, male gender, and stress. Genetic risk factors may also be shared.[57] In the VA Dental Longitudinal Study, smoking was an independent risk factor for mortality. When examining the data to determine if periodontal status was a risk factor, smoking status and other known risk factors for mortality were removed from the equation to allow independent evaluation of periodontal status.

PERIODONTAL DISEASE AND CORONARY HEART DISEASE/ATHEROSCLEROSIS

To further explore the periodontal disease and coronary heart disease/atherosclerosis association, investigators have studied specific systemic disorders and medical outcomes to determine their relationship to periodontal status. CHD-related events are a major cause of death. Myocardial infarction has been associated with acute systemic bacterial and viral infections, and infarction is sometimes preceded by influenza-like symptoms.[38,67] Is it possible that oral infection is similarly related to myocardial infarction? Traditional risk factors such as smoking, dyslipidemia, hypertension, and diabetes mellitus do not explain the presence of coronary atherosclerosis in a large number of patients. Localized infection resulting in a chronic inflammatory reaction has been suggested as a mechanism underlying coronary heart disease in these individuals.[48]

In cross-sectional studies of patients with acute myocardial infarction or confirmed CHD compared with age- and gender-matched control patients, myocardial infarction patients had significantly worse dental health (periodontitis, periapical lesions, caries, and pericoronitis) than did controls.[39,40] This association between poor dental health and myocardial infarction was independent of known risk factors for heart disease such as age, cholesterol levels, hypertension, diabetes, and smoking. Because atherosclerosis is a major determinant of CHD-related events, dental health has also been related to coronary atheromatosis. Mattila and colleagues performed oral radiographic examinations and diagnostic coronary angiography on men with known CHD.[41] There was a significant correlation between the severity of dental disease and the degree of coronary atheromatosis. This relationship remained significant after accounting for other known risk factors for coronary artery disease. Cross-sectional studies thus suggest a link between oral health and CHD; however, such studies cannot determine causality in this relationship. Rather, dental diseases may be indicators of general health practices. For example, periodontal disease and CHD are both related to lifestyle and share numerous risk factors such as smoking, diabetes, and low socioeconomic status. Bacterial infections have significant effects on endothelial cells, blood coagulation, lipid metabolism, and monocytes/macrophages. The research of Mattila and colleagues showed that dental infections were the only factors, other than the classic and well-recognized coronary risk factors, that were associated independently with the severity of coronary atherosclerosis.

Longitudinal studies provide compelling data on this relationship. In a 7-year follow-up study of the patients from the study of Mattila and colleagues, dental disease was significantly related to the incidence of new fatal and nonfatal coronary events, as well as to overall mortality.[42] In a prospective study of a national sample of adults, 9760 subjects were followed for 14 years following baseline dental and medical evaluation.[14] The main outcome measures were incidence of mortality or hospital admission due to CHD. Subjects with periodontitis had a 25% increase in the risk for CHD compared with those with no or minimal periodontal disease after adjusting for other known risk factors. Among younger males (ages 25 to 49), periodontitis increased the risk of CHD by 70%. The level of oral hygiene was also associated with heart disease. Patients with poor oral hygiene, as indicated by higher debris and calculus scores, had a two-fold increased risk for coronary heart disease.

In another large prospective study, 1147 men were followed for 18 years.[5] During that time, 207 men (18%) developed CHD. When periodontal status at baseline was related to the presence or absence of CHD-related events during follow-up, a significant relationship was found. Subjects with greater than 20% mean bone loss had a 50% increased risk of CHD compared with those with 0 to 20% bone loss. The extent of sites with probing depth greater than 3 mm was strongly related to the incidence of CHD. Subjects with probing depths greater than 3 mm on at least half of their teeth had a two-fold increased risk, whereas those with probing depths greater than 3 mm on all teeth had more than a three-fold increased risk on CHD. **This study and others in which the periodontal condition is known to have preceded the CHD-related events, support the concept that periodontal disease is a risk factor for CHD, independent of other classic risk factors.**

The Effect of Periodontal Infection

Periodontal infection may affect the onset or progression of atherosclerosis and CHD through certain mechanisms. Periodontitis and atherosclerosis both have complex etiologic factors, combining genetic and environmental influences. The diseases share many risk factors and have distinct similarities in basic pathogenic mechanisms.

Ischemic Heart Disease. Ischemic heart disease is associated with the processes of atherogenesis and thrombogenesis (Fig. 13-1). Increased viscosity of blood may promote major ischemic heart disease and stroke by increasing the risk of thrombus formation.[36] Fibrinogen is probably the most important factor in promoting this hypercoagulable state. Fibrinogen is the precursor to fibrin, and increased fibrinogen levels increase blood viscosity. Increased plasma fibrinogen is a recognized risk factor for cardiovascular events and peripheral vascular

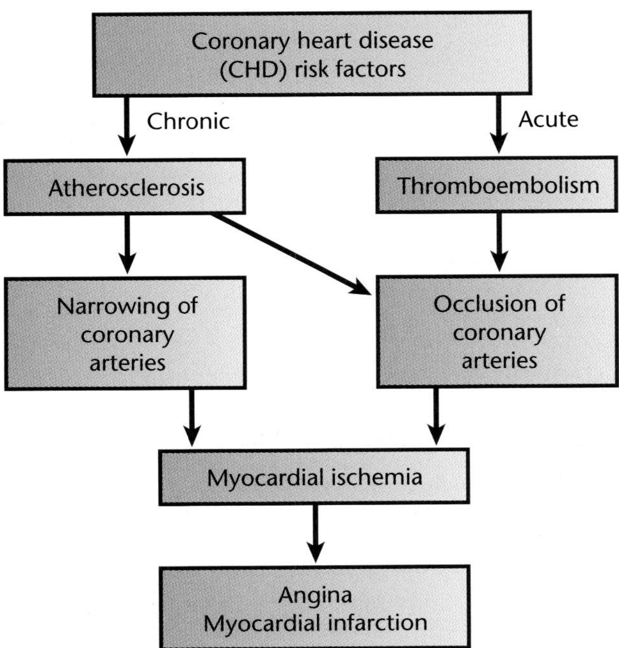

Fig. 13-1 Acute and chronic pathways to ischemic heart disease. CHD-related events such as angina or myocardial infarction may be precipitated by either one or both pathways.

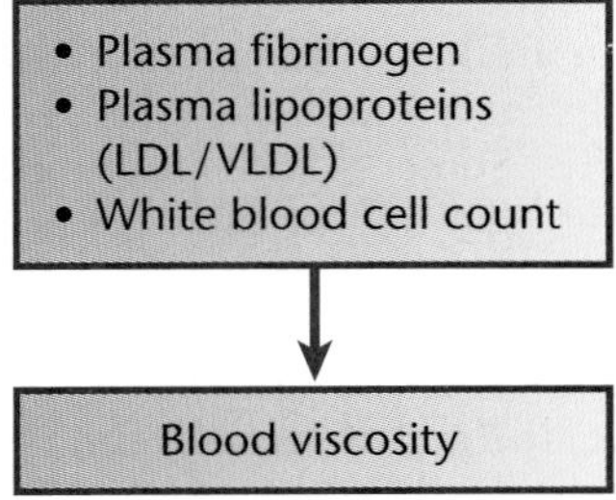

Fig. 13-2 Factors affecting blood viscosity in health

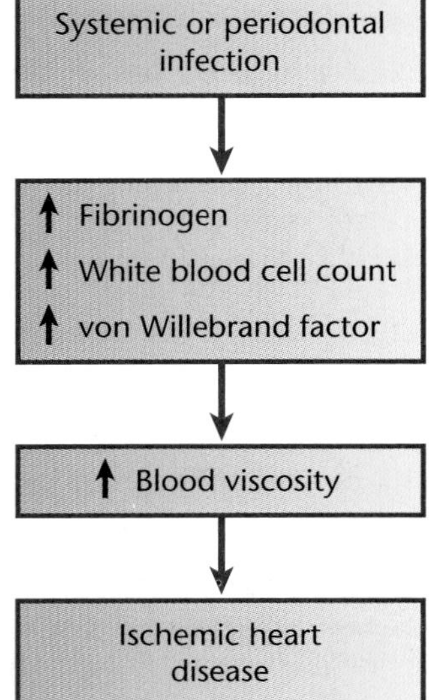

Fig. 13-3 Effect of infection on blood viscosity. Increased plasma fibrinogen and von Willebrand factor cause hypercoagulability. When combined with increased WBC count, blood viscosity increases, increasing the risk of coronary ischemia.

disease (Fig. 13-2).[37] Elevated white blood cell (WBC) count is also a predictor of heart disease and stroke, and circulating leukocytes may promote occlusion of blood vessels. The coagulation factor VIII: von Willebrand factor has likewise been associated with the risk of ischemic heart disease.[61]

Systemic Infections. Systemic infections are known to induce a hypercoagulable state and to increase blood viscosity (Fig. 13-3). Fibrinogen levels and WBC counts are often increased in patients with periodontal disease.[34] Individuals with poor oral health may also have significant elevations in coagulation factor VIII: von Willebrand factor antigen, increasing the risk of thrombus formation. Thus periodontal infection may also promote increased blood viscosity and thrombogenesis, leading to an increased risk for central and peripheral vascular disease.

Daily Activity. Routine daily activities such as mastication and oral hygiene procedures result in frequent bacteremia with oral organisms. The exposure time to bacteremias from routine daily chewing and tooth brushing is much greater than from dental procedures.[25] Periodontal disease may predispose the patient to an increased incidence of bacteremia, including the presence of virulent gram-negative organisms associated with periodontitis. It has been estimated that about 8% of all cases of infective endocarditis are associated with periodontal or dental disease without any preceding dental procedure.[15] Recognition of this fact is implicit in the American Heart Association recommendations on prevention of bacterial endocarditis, which stress the importance of establishing and maintaining "the best possible oral health to reduce potential sources of bacterial seeding."[12]

Thrombogenesis. Platelet aggregation plays a major role in thrombogenesis, and most cases of acute myocardial infarction are precipitated by thromboembolism. Oral organisms may be involved in coronary thrombogenesis. Platelets selectively bind some strains of *Streptococcus sanguis,* a common component of supragingival plaque, and *Porphyromonas gingivalis,* a pathogen closely associated with periodontitis.[28] Aggregation of platelets is induced by the platelet aggregation-associated protein (PAAP) expressed on some strains of these bacteria.[27] In animal models, intravenous infusion of PAAP-positive bacterial strains resulted in alterations of heart rate, blood pressure, cardiac contractility, and electrocardiogram (ECG) consistent with myocardial infarction. Platelet accumulation also occurred in the lungs, leading to tachypnea. No such changes were seen with infusion of PAAP-negative strains. PAAP-positive bacteria caused aggregation of circulating platelets, resulting in formation of thromboemboli and the resultant cardiac and pulmonary changes. Thus it is possible that periodontitis-associated bacteremia with certain strains of *S. sanguis* and *P. gingivalis* may promote acute thromboembolic events via interaction with circulating platelets.

Atherosclerosis. Atherosclerosis is a focal thickening of the arterial intima, the innermost layer lining the vessel lumen, and the media, the thick layer under the intima consisting of smooth muscle, collagen, and elastic fibers (Fig. 13-4). Early in the formation of atherosclerotic plaques, circulating monocytes adhere to the vascular endothelium. This adherence is mediated through several adhesion molecules on the endothelial cell surface, including intercellular adhesion molecule-1 (ICAM-1), endothelial leukocyte adhesion molecule-1 (ELAM-1), and vascular cell adhesion molecule-1 (VCAM-1).[33] These adhesion molecules are up-regulated by a number of factors including bacterial LPS, prostaglandins and pro-inflammatory cytokines. After binding to the endothelial cell lining, monocytes penetrate the endothelium and migrate under the arterial intima. The monocytes ingest circulating low-density lipoprotein (LDL) in its oxidized state and become engorged, forming foam cells characteristic of atheromatous plaques.

Once within the arterial media, monocytes may also transform to macrophages. A host of pro-inflammatory cytokines such as interleukin-1 (IL-1), tumor necrosis factor-alpha (TNF-α), and prostaglandin E2 (PGE_2) are then produced, which propagate the atheromatous lesion. Mitogenic factors such as fibroblast growth factor and platelet-derived growth factor stimulate smooth muscle and collagen proliferation within the media, thickening the arterial wall.[37] Atheromatous plaque formation and thickening of the vessel wall narrow the lumen and dramatically decrease blood flow through the vessel. Arterial thrombosis often occurs after an atheromatous plaque ruptures. Plaque rupture exposes circulating blood to arterial collagen and tissue factor from monocytes/macrophages that activate platelets and the coagulation pathway. Platelet and fibrin accumulation forms a thrombus that may occlude the vessel, resulting in ischemic events such as angina or myocardial infarction. The thrombus may separate from the vessel wall and form an embolus, which may also occlude vessels, again leading to acute events such as myocardial or cerebral infarction (stroke).

The Role of Periodontal Disease in Myocardial or Cerebral Infarction

In animal models, gram-negative bacteria and the associated LPS cause infiltration of inflammatory cells into the arterial wall, proliferation of arterial smooth muscle, and intravascular coagulation. These changes are identical to those seen in naturally occurring atheromatosis. In a study of eight atheromas obtained from humans during endarterectomy, three contained periodonta pathogens.[77] Periodontal diseases result in chronic systemic exposure to products of these organisms. Low-level bacteremia may initiate host responses that alter coagulability, endothelial and vessel wall integrity, and platelet function, resulting in atherogenic changes and possible thromboembolic events (Fig. 13-5).

Research has clearly shown a wide variation in host response to bacterial challenge between patients. Some individuals with heavy plaque accumulation and high proportions of pathogenic organisms appear relatively resistant to bone and attachment loss. Others develop extensive periodontal destruction in the presence of small amounts of plaque and low proportions of putative pathogens. Those patients with abnormally exuberant inflammatory responses often have a hyperinflammatory monocyte/macrophage phenotype ($M\O^+$). Monocytes/macrophages from these individuals secrete significantly increased levels of pro-inflammatory mediators like IL-1, TNF-α, and PGE_2 in response to bacterial LPS than do monocytes/macrophages from patients with a normal monocyte/macrophage phenotype. Patients with aggressive periodontitis, refractory periodontitis, and type 1 diabetes mellitus often possess the $M\O^+$ phenotype.[7]

This monocyte/macrophage phenotype appears to be under both genetic and environmental control.[7] The monocyte/macrophage cell line is intimately involved in the pathogenesis of both periodontal disease and atherosclerosis. Diet-induced elevations in serum LDL levels

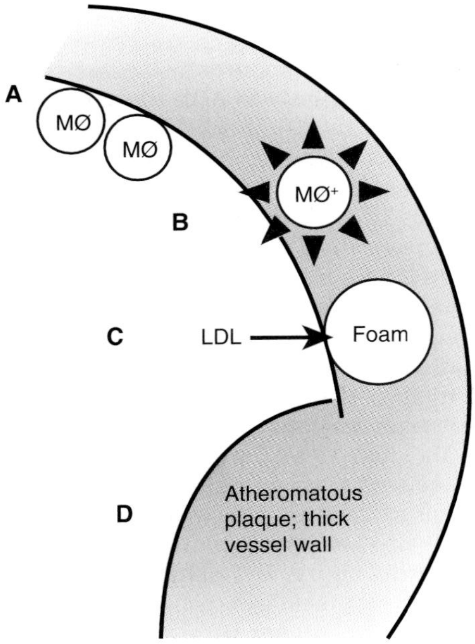

Fig. 13-4 Pathogenesis of atherosclerosis. **A,** Monocytes/macrophages adhere to vascular endothelium. **B,** Monocytes/macrophages penetrate into arterial media, producing pro-inflammatory cytokines and growth factors. **C,** Ingestion of oxidized LDL enlarges monocytes to form foam cells. **D,** Smooth muscle proliferation and plaque formation thicken vessel wall and narrow lumen.

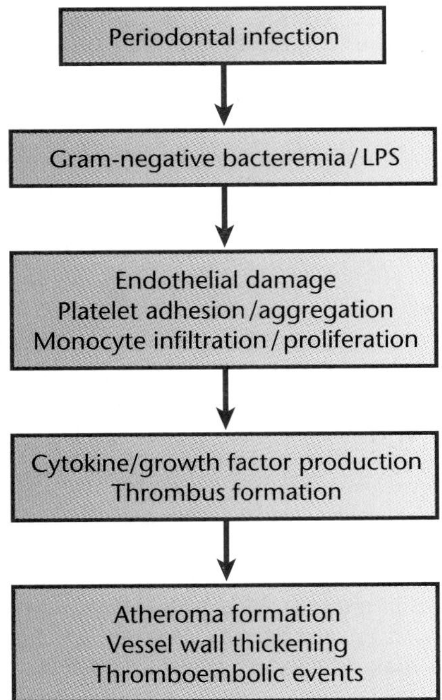

Fig. 13-5 Influence of periodontal infection on atherosclerosis. Periodontal pathogens and their products result in damage to vascular endothelium. Monocytes/macrophages enter vessel wall, producing cytokines that further increase inflammatory response and propagate the atheromatous lesion. Growth factor production leads to smooth muscle proliferation in the vessel wall. Damaged endothelium also activates platelets, resulting in platelet aggregation, and potentiating thromboembolic events.

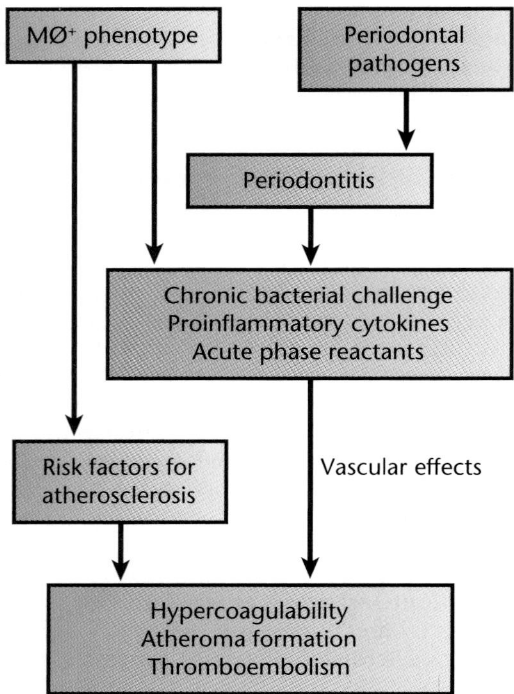

Fig. 13-6 Cardiovascular and periodontal consequences of hyperresponsive monocyte/macrophage phenotype. In combination with other risk factors, the MØ$^+$ phenotype predisposes to both atherosclerosis and periodontitis. Bacterial products and inflammatory mediators associated with periodontitis affect vascular endothelium, monocytes/macrophages, platelets, and smooth muscle; and, may increase blood coagulability. This may further atherosclerosis and result in thromboembolism and ischemic events.

up-regulate monocyte/macrophage responsiveness to bacterial LPS. Thus elevated LDL levels, a known risk factor for atherosclerosis and CHD, may increase secretion of destructive and inflammatory cytokines by monocytes/macrophages. This may result not only in propagation of atheromatous lesions, but also in enhanced periodontal destruction in the presence of pathogenic organisms. This is one example of a potential shared mechanism in the pathogenesis of cardiovascular and periodontal diseases. The presence of a MØ$^+$ phenotype may place patients at risk for both CHD and periodontitis (Fig. 13-6). Periodontal infections may contribute to atherosclerosis and thromboembolic events by repeatedly challenging the vascular endothelium and arterial wall with bacterial LPS and proinflammatory cytokines. Vascularmonocytes/macrophages in patients with a MØ$^+$ phenotype meet this challenge with an abnormally elevated inflammatory response that may directly contribute to atherosclerosis and may precipitate thromboembolic events.[46]

PERIODONTAL DISEASE AND STROKE

Ischemic cerebral infarction, or stroke, is often preceded by systemic bacterial or viral infection.[69] In one study, patients with cerebral ischemia were five times more likely to have had a systemic infection within 1 week before the ischemic event than were nonischemic control subjects. Recent infection was a significant risk factor for cerebral ischemia and was independent of other known risk factors such as hypertension, history of a previous stroke, diabetes, smoking and coronary heart disease.[20] Interestingly, the presence of systemic infection before the stroke resulted in significantly greater ischemia and a more severe post-ischemic neurologic defect than did stroke that was not preceded by infection.[21] Stroke patients with a preceding infection had slightly higher levels of plasma fibrinogen and significantly higher levels of C-reactive protein than did those without infection. C-reactive protein is an acute phase reactant that increases rapidly in inflammatory conditions and infection. C-reactive protein induces monocytes/macrophages to produce tissue factor, which stimulates the coagulation pathway and increases blood coagulability. Increased fibrinogen levels may contribute to this process.

Periodontal Infection Associated with Stroke

In case-control studies, poor dental health was a significant risk factor for cerebrovascular ischemia. In one study, bleeding on probing, suppuration, subgingival calculus, and the number of periodontal or periapical lesions were significantly greater in male stroke patients than in controls.[70] Overall, 25% of all stroke patients had significant dental infections compared with only 2.5% of controls. This study supports an association between poor oral health and stroke in men under age 50. In the other study, men and women age 50 and older who had a stroke had significantly more severe periodontitis and more periapical lesions than did nonstroke control subjects.[22] Poor dental health was an independent risk factor for stroke. In a longitudinal study over 18 years, subjects with greater than 20% mean radiographic bone loss at baseline were almost three times as likely to have a stroke than were subjects with less than 20% bone loss. Periodontitis was a greater risk factor for stroke than was smoking and was independent of other known risk factors.

Most cases of stroke are caused by thromboembolic events, whereas others are related to cerebrovascular atherosclerosis. As discussed in the previous section, periodontal infection may contribute to the pathogenesis of atherosclerosis by providing a persistent bacterial challenge to arterial endothelium, contributing to the monocyte/macrophage-driven inflammatory process that results in atheromatosis and narrowing of the vessel lumen (see Figs. 13-5 and 13-6). Furthermore, periodontal infection is associated with increased plasma fibrinogen and C-reactive protein levels, which contribute to hypercoagulability. Finally, bacteremia with PAAP-positive bacterial strains from the supra- and subgingival plaque can increase platelet aggregation, contributing to thrombus formation and subsequent thromboembolism, the leading cause of stroke.[46]

PERIODONTAL DISEASE AND DIABETES MELLITUS

The relationship between diabetes mellitus and periodontal disease has been extensively examined. It is clear from epidemiologic research that diabetes increases the risk for and severity of periodontal diseases.[59] The biologic mechanisms through which diabetes influences the periodontium are discussed in Chapter 12. The increased prevalence and severity of periodontitis commonly seen in patients with diabetes, especially those with poor metabolic control, led to the designation of periodontal disease as the "sixth complication of diabetes."[35] In addition to the five "classic" complications of diabetes (Box 13-2), the American Diabetes Association has officially recognized that periodontal disease is common in patients with diabetes, and its Standards of Care include taking a history of current or past dental infections as part of the physician's examination.[2,3]

Although many studies have examined the effects of diabetes on the periodontium, fewer have endeavored to examine the effect of periodontal infection on control of diabetes. The following questions remain:

- Does the presence or severity of periodontal disease affect the metabolic state in diabetic patients?
- Does periodontal treatment aimed at reducing the bacterial challenge and minimizing inflammation have a measurable effect on glycemic (blood glucose) control?

In a longitudinal study of patients with type 2 (non-insulin-dependent) diabetes, severe periodontitis was associated with significant worsening of glycemic control over time.[71] Individuals with severe periodontitis at the baseline examination had a greater incidence of worsening glycemic control over a 2- to 4-year period than did those without periodontitis at baseline. In this study, periodontitis is known to have preceded the worsening of glycemic control. Periodontitis has also been associated with the classic complications of diabetes. Diabetic adults with severe periodontitis at baseline had a significantly greater incidence of kidney and macrovascular complications over the subsequent 1 to 11 years than did diabetic adults with only gingivitis or mild periodontitis.[72] This was true despite the fact that both groups had similar glycemic control. One or more cardiovascular complications occurred in 82% of patients with severe periodontitis compared with only 21% of patients without severe periodontitis. Again, severe periodontitis preceded the onset of clinical diabetic complications in these subjects.

BOX 13-2

Complications of Diabetes Mellitus

Retinopathy
Nephropathy
Neuropathy
Macrovascular disease
Altered wound healing
Periodontal disease

Loë H: Periodontal disease: The sixth complication of diabetes mellitus. Diabetes Care 1993; 16(suppl 1):329.

In diabetic patients with periodontitis, periodontal therapy may have beneficial effects on glycemic control.[46,47] This may be especially true for patients with relatively poor glycemic control and more advanced periodontal destruction prior to treatment.[24] Forty years ago, the potential benefits of periodontal therapy were first described in young adults with diabetes and severe periodontitis.[75] Treatment with mechanical debridement, surgery, selected tooth extraction, and systemic antibiotics resulted in decreased insulin demand. In a more recent evaluation of scaling and root planing combined with systemic doxycycline therapy for 2 weeks, type 1 (insulin-dependent) diabetic patients with improved periodontal health also had significant improvement in glycemic control (Fig. 13-7).[49] Conversely, those individuals who demonstrated little beneficial clinical effect from periodontal treatment had no change in glycemic control.

In a placebo-controlled study of poorly controlled individuals with type 2 diabetes and severe periodontitis, nonsurgical mechanical debridement combined with systemic doxycycline for 14 days was compared with similar mechanical treatment combined with systemic placebo.[23] All patient groups had significant improvements in periodontal status, with reduced probing depths and bleeding on probing. Those treated with doxycycline had a greater reduction in the prevalence of *P. gingivalis,* which was more sustained over time. The

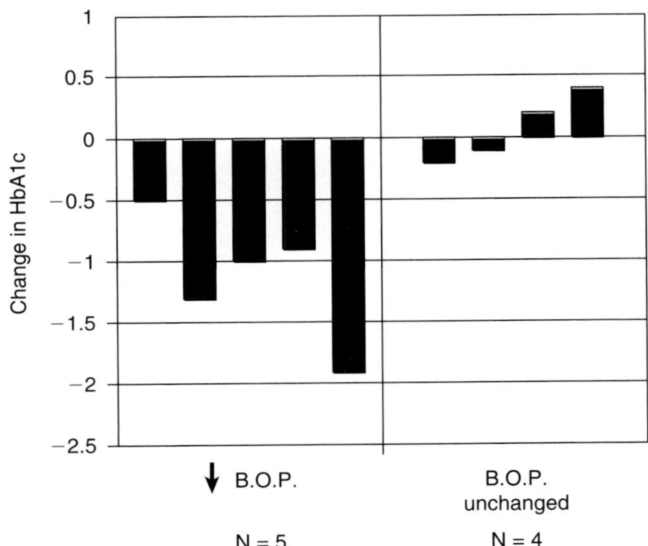

Fig. 13-7 Periodontal treatment: effects on glycemic control. In five patients, reductions in periodontal inflammation after mechanical therapy combined with systemic doxycycline antibiotic were accompanied by improved glycemic control (decreased glycated hemoglobin values HbA1c). In four patients with no improvement in periodontal health, no improvement in glycemic control occurred. (From Miller LS, Manwell MA, Newbold D, et al: The relationship between reduction in periodontal inflammation and diabetes control: A report of 9 cases. J Periodontol 1992; 63:843.)

doxycycline-treated patients also demonstrated significant improvement in glycemic control 3 months after treatment, which gradually reverted to baseline levels at 6 months. Placebo-treated subjects had no significant improvement in glycemic control. These studies suggest that the combination of subgingival mechanical debridement and systemic doxycycline may result in short-term improvement in glycemia in diabetic patients with severe periodontitis and poor metabolic control.

Conversely, moderately or well-controlled individuals with diabetes and periodontitis who are treated by mechanical therapy alone may demonstrate no significant changes in glycemic control, despite improvement in their periodontal condition. In studies of subjects treated by mechanical therapy without adjunctive use of antibiotics, significant changes in glycemic control are less common.[1,8,23,66] Many of the patients in these studies had relatively good glycemic control before treatment, so less benefit on metabolic control might be expected. Although routine use of systemic antibiotics in treatment of chronic periodontitis is not justified, patients with poorly controlled diabetes and severe periodontitis may constitute one patient group for whom such therapy is appropriate. Of course, antibiotics remain an adjunct to the necessary mechanical removal of plaque and calculus.

The mechanisms by which adjunctive antibiotics may induce positive changes in glycemic control when combined with mechanical debridement are unknown at this time. Systemic antibiotics may eliminate residual bacteria following scaling and root planing, further decreasing the bacterial challenge to the host. Tetracyclines are also known to suppress glycation of proteins and to decrease activity of tissue-degrading enzymes such as matrix metalloproteinases. These changes may contribute to improvement in metabolic control of diabetes.

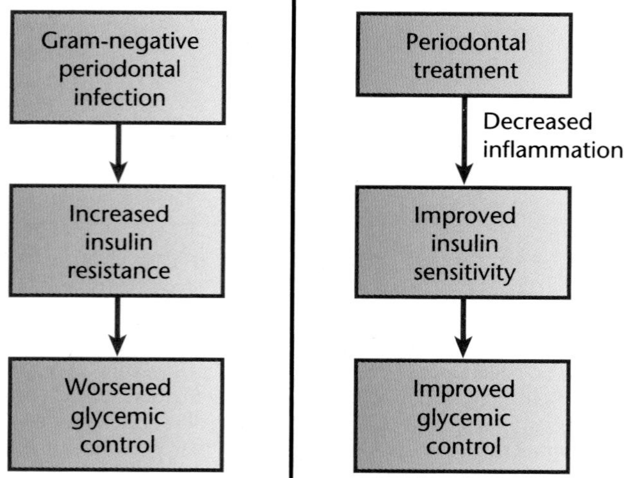

Fig. 13-8 Potential effects of periodontal infection and periodontal therapy on glycemia in patients with diabetes.

Periodontal Infection Associated with Glycemic Control in Diabetes

An understanding of the effects of other infections is useful in delineating the mechanisms by which periodontal infection influences glycemia. Acute bacterial and viral infections have been shown to increase insulin resistance and aggravate glycemic control.[62,76] This occurs in individuals with diabetes and without. Systemic infections increase tissue resistance to insulin, preventing glucose from entering target cells, causing elevated blood glucose levels, and requiring increased pancreatic insulin production to maintain normoglycemia. Insulin resistance may persist for weeks or even months after the patient has recovered clinically from their illness. In the individual with type 2 diabetes, who already has significant insulin resistance, further tissue resistance to insulin induced by infection may considerably exacerbate poor glycemic control. In type 1 patients, normal insulin doses may be inadequate to maintain good glycemic control in the presence of infection-induced tissue resistance. It is possible that chronic gram-negative periodontal infections may also result in increased insulin resistance and poor glycemic control.[24] In patients with periodontitis, persistent systemic challenge with periodontopathic bacteria and their products may act in a way similar to well-recognized systemic infections (Fig. 13-8). This mechanism would explain the worsening of glycemic control associated with severe periodontitis. Periodontal treatment designed to decrease the bacterial insult and reduce inflammation might restore insulin sensitivity over time, resulting in improved metabolic control. The improved glycemic control seen in several studies of periodontal therapy would support such a hypothesis.

PERIODONTAL DISEASE AND PREGNANCY OUTCOME

Low-birth-weight (LBW) infants (those weighing less than 2500 g at birth) are 40 times more likely to die in the neonatal period than normal-birth-weight (NBW) infants.[43] Although about 7% of all infants weigh less than 2500 g at birth, they account for two thirds of neonatal deaths. LBW infants who survive the neonatal period are at increased risk for congenital anomalies, respiratory disorders and neurodevelopmental disabilities. The social and financial costs of LBW infants are enormous, and an emphasis on prevention of low-weight births is preferred to the high-cost intensive care often required to allow survival of LBW infants.

The primary cause of LBW infant deliveries is preterm labor or premature rupture of membranes. Factors such as smoking, alcohol or drug use during pregnancy, inadequate prenatal care, race, low socioeconomic status, hypertension, high or low maternal age, diabetes, and genitourinary tract infections increase the risk of preterm LBW. However, these risk factors are not present in approximately one fourth of preterm LBW cases, leading to a continued search for other causes.[55]

Research has examined the relationship between maternal infection and preterm labor, premature rupture of membranes, and LBW delivery. The true extent of this relationship is difficult to determine, since the majority of maternal infections may be subclinical. Genitourinary tract infections have been associated with adverse pregnancy outcomes. Women with bacteriuria have increased rates of preterm delivery, and antibiotic treatment of bacteriuria has resulted in a significant decrease in preterm delivery rates compared with placebo treatment.[31,55] Vaginal colonization with group-B streptococci or *Bacteroides* species increases the risk of premature rupture of membranes, preterm delivery, and LBW.[44]

Bacterial Vaginosis

Bacterial vaginosis is the most common vaginal disorder in women of reproductive age. It is caused by changes in the vaginal microflora in which normally predominant facultative lactobacilli are replaced by *Gardnerella vaginalis;* anaerobic organisms, including species of the genera *Prevotella, Bacteroides, Peptostreptococcus, Porphyromonas, Mobiluncus;* and others.[29] Bacterial vaginosis is a known risk factor for preterm labor, premature rupture of membranes, and LBW.[31] In fact, treatment of bacterial vaginosis with metronidazole in pregnant women resulted in decreased preterm birth rates compared with placebo treatment.[50]

The exact mechanism by which vaginal colonization or genitourinary tract infection may cause premature rupture of membranes and preterm labor is not known. The primary mechanism has traditionally been thought to be ascending infection from the vagina and endocervix. Endotoxin (LPS) and bioactive enzymes produced by many organisms associated with vaginosis may directly injure tissue, as well as induce release of proinflammatory cytokines and prostaglandins. Throughout normal gestation, amniotic prostaglandin levels rise steadily until a sufficient threshold is reached that induces labor and delivery. Maternal infection may cause increased prostaglandin production and may result in labor-inducing levels being achieved before full gestation. In addition to prostaglandins, various pro-inflammatory cytokines such as IL-1, IL-6, and TNF have been found in the amniotic fluid of women with preterm labor.

Women with preterm labor often have culture-positive amniotic fluid, even in the absence of clinical infection. Of culture-positive patients, the most commonly isolated species is *Fusobacterium nucleatum.*[31] Although *F. nucleatum* is occasionally isolated from the vaginal flora in bacterial vaginosis, its prevalence in women with preterm labor is much greater than in vaginosis. *F. nucleatum* is even less frequently isolated from the vaginal flora of women without bacterial vaginosis. This organism is certainly not the only one isolated from amniotic fluid in women with preterm labor. Many of the isolated species are those commonly found in bacterial vaginosis. Thus an ascending route of infection is supported by the presence of these bacterial vaginosis-associated species. However, the frequency of *F. nucleatum* detection suggests other possible routes of infection. Some investigators have suggested the possibility of infection via a hematogenous route from a location in which the organism is commonly detected.[31] *F. nucleatum* is a common oral species and is highly prevalent in patients with periodontitis. It is possible that this organism reaches the amniotic fluid by hematogenous spread from the oral cavity. This route is also suggested by the occasional isolation of *Capnocytophaga* species in the amniotic fluid of women with preterm labor, an organism rarely isolated from the vagina but common in the oral cavity. Hill found that the species and subspecies of *F. nucleatum* isolated from amniotic fluid cultures in women with preterm labor more closely matched those found in subgingival plaque than strains identified from the lower genital tract.[30] In addition to hematogenous spread, another possible route of infection is by oral-genital contact, with transfer of oral organisms to the vagina.[31]

Although direct effects of microorganisms may play an important role in many cases of preterm labor, premature rupture of membranes, and LBW, indirect mechanisms may also be operative.[46,55] Bacterial infection of the chorioamnion, or extraplacental membrane, may lead to chorioamnionitis, a condition strongly associated with premature membrane rupture and preterm delivery. However, many cases of histologic chorioamnionitis demonstrate negative bacterial cultures, indicating that infection is not the sole cause of this condition.

How might this occur? It is likely that an indirect mechanism may be active in which the cascade of host products produced in response to infection is often responsible for preterm labor. Maternal infection may lead to the presence of amnionic bacterial products, such as LPS from gram-negative organisms, which stimulate production of host-derived cytokines in the amnion and decidua (Fig. 13-9). These cytokines, including IL-1, TNF-α, and IL-6 stimulate increased prostaglandin production

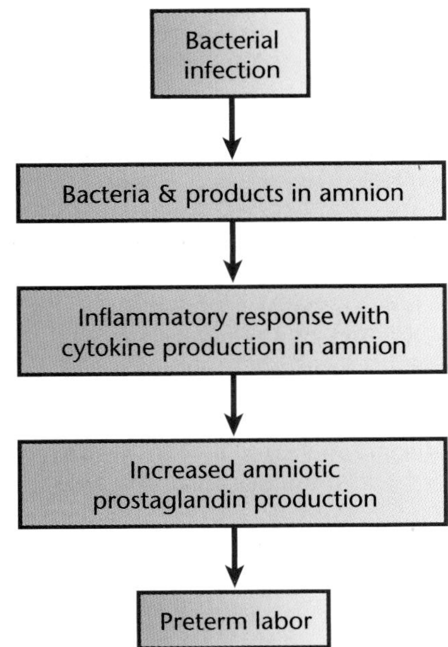

Fig. 13-9 Mechanisms by which infection may induce preterm labor.

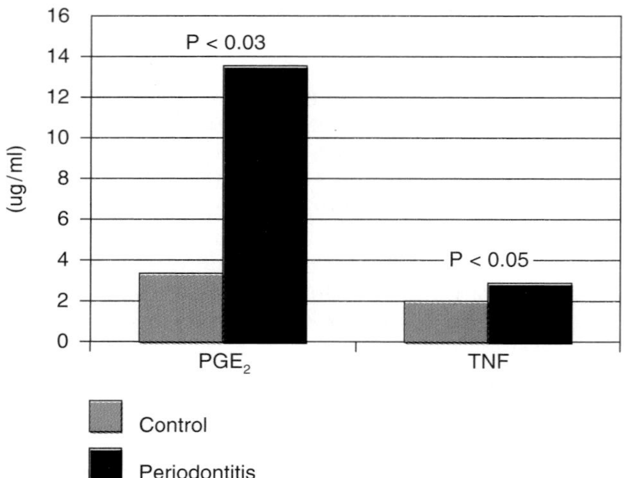

Fig. 13-10 Amniotic fluid levels in experimental periodontitis. Experimental periodontitis resulted in increased amniotic fluid levels of TNF-α and PGE in the pregnant hamster model, providing evidence that periodontal infection can affect the fetal environment. (From Offenbacher S, Jarad HL, O'Reilly PG, et al: Potential pathogenic mechanisms of periodontitis-associated pregnancy complications. Ann Periodontol 1998; 3:233.)

from the amnion and decidua, leading to onset of preterm labor. A premature rise in PGE_2 and $PGF_{2\alpha}$ is characteristic of preterm labor, regardless of whether clinical or subclinical maternal genitourinary tract infection is detected. The question then arises as to what stimulates the increased cytokine levels and resultant increased prostaglandin levels seen in preterm delivery in patients with no evidence of genitourinary infection. Some have suggested that many cases of preterm LBW are a result of infections of unknown origin—that is, infections originating in areas other than the genitourinary tract.

The Role of Periodontitis in Pregnancy Outcome

Periodontitis is a remote gram-negative infection that may play a role in LBW. As discussed previously, periodontopathic organisms and their products may have wide-ranging effects, most likely mediated through stimulation of host cytokine production in target tissues. Animal studies suggest that remote reservoirs of gram-negative organisms and their products may have a negative impact on pregnancy outcome. *P. gingivalis* implanted in subcutaneous chambers during gestation caused significant increases in TNF-α and PGE_2 levels.[9] This localized subcutaneous infection resulted in a significant increase in fetal death and a decrease in fetal birth weight for those that remained viable, when compared with control animals that were not inoculated. There was a significant correlation between both TNF-α and PGE_2 levels, as well as fetal death and growth retardation. These data suggest that a remote, nondisseminated infection with *P. gingivalis* may result in abnormal pregnancy outcomes in this model.

Decreased fetal birth-weight and increased fetal death were also seen after intravenous injections with LPS derived from *P. gingivalis.*[10] This effect was greatly increased when *P. gingivalis* LPS was administered before mating and during gestation, indicating that repeated immunization with *P. gingivalis* LPS does not provide protection during pregnancy, but potentiates the negative effects of LPS exposure during gestation. *P. gingivalis*–induced experimental periodontitis in animal models resulted in decreased fetal birth-weight and increased amniotic fluid levels of TNF-α and PGE_2 (Fig. 13-10).[55] This provides direct evidence that periodontal infection can affect the fetal environment and pregnancy outcome.

These animal studies have led to examination of the potential effects of periodontitis on pregnancy outcome in humans. In a case control study of 124 women (93 cases with at least one LBW delivery and 31 controls with at least one normal birth weight delivery), Offenbacher and coworkers found that women having LBW infants had greater clinical attachment loss than women having NBW infants.[54] After adjusting for known risk factors for LBW, women with periodontitis resulting in greater than 3 mm of attachment loss in at least 60% of sites had a 7.5-fold increased risk of having a LBW infant. In fact, periodontitis contributed to more preterm LBW cases than did smoking or alcohol use during pregnancy. This study indicated a strong association between periodontal infection and adverse pregnancy outcomes. Other studies have demonstrated significantly fewer periodontally healthy sextants and greater gingival bleeding in women having LBW infants.[13]

In a cross-sectional study, women having LBW infants had significantly higher levels of *Actinobacillus actinomycetemcomitans, Bacteroides forsythus, P. gingivalis,* and *Treponema denticola* in their subgingival plaque than did the control women having NBW infants.[55] Women having LBW infants also had higher levels of gingival crevicular fluid PGE_2 and IL-1. In primiparous women (those experiencing a first birth), the gingival crevicular fluid levels of PGE_2 were inversely related to their infants' birth-weight. Women with higher PGE_2 levels in the gingival crevicular fluid had smaller and more premature infants. Gingival crevicular fluid levels of IL-1 and PGE_2 have been shown to correlate highly with intraamniotic IL-1 and PGE_2 levels. In fact, measuring crevicular fluid levels of these inflammatory mediators has been suggested as a less invasive means of screening expectant mothers for elevated amniotic IL-1 and PGE_2 levels than amniocentesis.[55] Thus women having LBW infants have a higher prevalence and severity of periodontitis, more gingival inflammation, higher levels of putative periodontal pathogens, and an elevated subgingival inflammatory response compared with women having NBW infants. When combined with animal studies showing adverse effects of experimental periodontitis on the fetus and data supporting biologically plausible interactive mechanisms, the evidence strongly suggests that periodontal infection may have significant negative impact on pregnancy outcome in some women. To date, however, no longitudinal human studies or intervention trials have been published that examine the potential effects of periodontal treatment or lack of treatment on pregnancy outcome in women with periodontitis.

PERIODONTAL DISEASE AND CHRONIC OBSTRUCTIVE PULMONARY DISEASE

COPD is a disease state characterized by airflow obstruction due to chronic bronchitis or emphysema. Bronchial mucous glands enlarge, and an inflammatory process occurs in which neutrophils and mononuclear inflammatory cells accumulate within the lung tissue.[26,73] About 14 million Americans have COPD, and tobacco smoking is the primary risk factor.

COPD shares similar pathogenic mechanisms with periodontal disease. In both diseases, a host inflammatory response is mounted in response to chronic challenge: by bacteria in periodontal disease and by factors such as cigarette smoke in COPD. The resulting neutrophil influx leads to release of oxidative and hydrolytic enzymes that cause tissue destruction directly. Recruitment of monocytes and macrophages leads to further release of pro-inflammatory mediators.

Less is known about the clinical relationship between periodontal disease and COPD compared with CHD and other systemic conditions. In analyzing data from a longitudinal study of more than 1100 men, alveolar bone loss was associated with the risk for COPD.[26] Over a 25-year period, 23% of subjects were diagnosed with COPD. Subjects with more severe bone loss at the baseline dental examination had a significantly increased risk of subsequently developing COPD compared with subjects with less bone loss. The increase in risk was independent of age, smoking status, and other known risk factors for COPD. Individuals with poor oral hygiene have also been found to be at increased risk for chronic respiratory diseases such as bronchitis and emphysema.[64] These associations remain to be confirmed by further research.

PERIODONTAL DISEASE AND ACUTE RESPIRATORY INFECTIONS

The upper respiratory passages are often contaminated with organisms derived from the oral, nasal, and pharyngeal regions. Conversely, the lower airways in which gas exchange occurs are generally maintained free of microorganisms by a combination of host immune factors and mechanical clearance through the cough reflex, ciliary transport of aspirated contaminants, and movement of secretions from the lower airways into the trachea.[46] Pneumonia is an infection of the lungs caused by bacteria, viruses, fungi, or mycoplasma and is broadly categorized as either community-acquired or hospital-acquired. A wide variety of bacteria may cause pneumonia, and the spectrum of offending organisms differs markedly between community-acquired and hospital-acquired infections.

Community-acquired bacterial pneumonia is caused primarily by inhalation of infectious aerosols or by aspiration of oropharyngeal organisms. *S. pneumoniae* and *Haemophilus influenzae* are most common, although numerous other species may occur, including anaerobic bacteria.[56] Antibiotic therapy is highly successful in resolution of most cases of community-acquired bacterial pneumonia. To date, no associations have been found between oral hygiene or periodontal disease and the risk for acute respiratory conditions such as pneumonia in community-dwelling individuals.[64]

The same cannot be said for individuals in the hospital setting. **Hospital-acquired (nosocomial) bacterial pneumonia** has a very high morbidity and mortality rate. Approximately 20% to 50% of patients with nosocomial pneumonia die.[11] The incidence of nosocomial pneumonia is highest in severely ill patients such as those in intensive care units or on ventilatory support. More than half of patients on mechanical ventilation for several days or more acquire pneumonia. Although nosocomial pneumonia is most commonly caused by gram-negative aerobic organisms, many cases are the result of infection by anaerobic bacteria, including those commonly found in the subgingival environment.

Hospital-acquired pneumonia is usually caused by aspiration of oropharyngeal contents. Oropharyngeal colonization with potential respiratory pathogens (PRPs) increases during hospitalization, and the longer the hospital stay the greater the prevalence of PRPs.[46] PRPs are found predominantly in the gastrointestinal tract and may be passed through esophageal reflux into the oropharynx where they colonize. Subsequent aspiration may lead to pneumonia. Patients whose posterior oropharynx becomes colonized with PRPs have a significantly increased risk of developing nosocomial pneumonia compared with those without oropharyngeal colonization by PRPs.

Selective decontamination is a technique that combines systemic antibiotics with orally administered nonabsorbable antibiotics in an attempt to eradicate PRPs from the digestive tract and oropharynx and to thereby minimize the risk of nosocomial respiratory infections. The technique is used primarily in patients who are intubated and on mechanical ventilators. Selective decontamination significantly decreases the incidence of nosocomial pneumonia.[65] Decontamination of only the digestive tract does not reduce the incidence of pneumonia, but decontamination of the oropharynx alone does.[60,68] This provides further evidence that the oropharynx is the primary site of PRP colonization, with subsequent aspiration of causative organisms leading to pneumonia.

PRPs may also originate in the oral cavity, with dental plaque serving as a reservoir of these organisms. Poor oral hygiene is common in the hospital and nursing home settings, especially in severely ill patients.[6] PRPs are more commonly isolated from supragingival plaque and buccal mucosa of patients in intensive care units than in outpatient settings.[63] Thus organisms that are not routinely found in dental plaque become plaque colonizers after prolonged hospitalization. Subgingival plaque may also harbor PRPs, and putative periodontal pathogens have been associated with nosocomial pneumonia. Furthermore, anaerobic organisms from periodontal pockets may serve as the primary inoculum for suppurative respiratory diseases such as pulmonary abscesses that have significant morbidity and mortality.[4] Although considerable circumstantial evidence suggests that periodontal pathogens may cause acute nosocomial pulmonary infections, currently no published studies specifically demonstrate an increased risk of such infections in patients with periodontal disease. Likewise, there is no research evaluating the effects of periodontal treatment on the incidence of bacterial pneumonia.

PERIODONTAL MEDICINE IN CLINICAL PRACTICE

The concept of periodontal diseases as localized entities affecting only the teeth and supporting apparatus is over simplified and in need of revision. Rather than being confined to the periodontium, periodontal diseases may have wide-ranging systemic effects. In most persons, these effects may be relatively inconsequential or at least not clinically evident. However, in susceptible individuals, periodontal infection may act as an independent risk factor for systemic disease and may be involved in the basic pathogenic mechanisms of these conditions. Furthermore, periodontal infection may exacerbate existing systemic disorders.

Periodontal Disease and Systemic Health in the Clinical Practice of Dentistry

Proper use of the knowledge of potential relationships between periodontal disease and systemic health requires the dental professional to expand his or her horizons, to step back from the technically demanding aspects of the dental art, and to recognize the oral cavity as one of many interrelated organ systems. An infection the size of one's palm on the leg of a pregnant woman would be a major concern to the patient and her health care provider, given the potential negative consequences of this localized infection on fetal and maternal health. A similar suppurating infection on the foot of a person with diabetes would be cause for immediate evaluation and aggressive treatment, knowing the effects of such infections on metabolic control of diabetes. Periodontal infection must be viewed in a similar fashion. Periodontitis is a gram-negative infection resulting in severe inflammation, with potential intravascular dissemination of microorganisms and their products throughout the body. However, periodontitis tends to be a "silent" disease, until destruction results in acute symptoms. Most patients, and many medical professionals, do not recognize the potential infection that may exist within the oral cavity.

Patient Education

Patient education is a priority. Only 30 years ago, the factors involved in CHD were unclear. Yet today, it would be difficult to find an individual who was unfamiliar with the link between cholesterol and heart disease. This change was precipitated by research clearly demonstrating the increased risk for heart disease in individuals with high cholesterol levels, followed by intensive education efforts to spread the message from the scientific community to the wider citizenry. It is important to recognize that high cholesterol levels have not been shown to cause heart disease in all individuals, but rather to significantly increase the risk of disease. Cholesterol has also been demonstrated to have a biologically plausible role in the pathogenesis of CHD. Similarly, patient education efforts in the realm of periodontal medicine must emphasize the nature of periodontal infections, the increased risk for systemic disease associated with the infection, and the biologically plausible role periodontal infection may play in systemic disease. Few individuals had their cholesterol levels evaluated until the knowledge of the link between cholesterol and heart disease became widespread. Likewise, increased appreciation of the potential effects of periodontal infection on systemic health may result in increased patient demand for periodontal evaluation.

Enhanced community awareness may be derived from newspapers, magazines, and other lay sources. However, the most reliable origin of information should be the dental and medical professions through daily contact with patients. The pregnant woman usually knows that infections may adversely affect her pregnancy. Persons with diabetes generally know that infections make glycemic control worse. However, many of these patients do not know that occult periodontal infections can have the same effect as more clinically evident infections. It is up to the dentist to diagnose periodontal infections, provide appropriate treatment, and prevent disease recurrence or progression. Since many medical professionals are unfamiliar with the oral cavity and oral health research, dentists must reach out to the medical community in an effort to improve patient care through education and communication. Likewise, patients must be educated in disease prevention. Just as patients know that lowering cholesterol levels may decrease their risk for heart disease, prevention of periodontal infection should be emphasized. A physician would be remiss if he or she did not provide education on decreasing cholesterol, losing weight, and ceasing a smoking habit to a patient at risk for CHD. Likewise, controlling the risk factor of periodontal infection requires the dentist to emphasize personal and professional preventive measures focused on thorough oral hygiene and regular recall.

Periodontal Disease, CHD, COPD, and Pregnancy

Does periodontal disease cause coronary heart disease, COPD, or adverse pregnancy outcomes? The question may only be answered based on the evidence available today, with the full knowledge that conclusions may change as future evidence dictates. Periodontal disease may increase the risk for many systemic disorders. Biologically plausible mechanisms support the role of periodontal infection in these conditions, but periodontal infection should not be presented as the cause of such systemic diseases any more than cholesterol is said to cause heart disease. Periodontal infection is one of many potential risk factors for a number of systemic conditions. Fortunately, it is a readily modifiable risk factor, unlike age, gender, and genetic influences.

The focal infection theory of the early 20th century was widely and appropriately discredited when treatment based on the theory, namely tooth extraction, had no effect on the underlying diseases that oral sepsis supposedly caused. Similarly, the clinical utility of our current knowledge base is only now evolving. Future research will further delineate the role of periodontal infection in systemic health. It is possible that the associations between periodontal infection and conditions such as LBW delivery, diabetes, cardiovascular and cerebrovascular diseases, and respiratory diseases will be further substantiated. Longitudinal studies and intervention trials are needed before any causative role can be assigned.

The emerging field of periodontal medicine offers new insights into the concept of the oral cavity as one system interconnected with the whole of the human body. For many years, the dental profession has recognized the effects of systemic conditions on the oral cavity. Only now are we coming to more fully understand the impact of the periodontium on systemic health.

REFERENCES

1. Aldridge JP, Lester V, Watts TLP, et al: Single-blind studies of the effects of improved periodontal health on metabolic control in type 1 diabetes mellitus. J Clin Periodontol 1995; 22:271.
2. American Diabetes Association: Report of the expert committee on the diagnosis and classification of diabetes mellitus. Diabetes Care 1997; 20:1183.
3. American Diabetes Association: Standards of medical care for patients with diabetes mellitus. Diabetes Care 1998; 21(suppl 1):523.
4. Bartlett JG: Anaerobic infections of the lung. Chest 1987; 91:901.
5. Beck JD, Garcia RG, Heiss G, et al: Periodontal disease and cardiovascular disease. J Periodontol 1996; 67:1123.
6. Beck JD: Periodontal implications: Older adults. Ann Periodontol 1996; 1:322.
7. Beck JD, Offenbacher S, Williams R, et al: Periodontitis: A risk factor for coronary heart disease? Ann Periodontol 1998; 3:127.
8. Christgau M, Pallitzsch KD, Schmalz G, et al: Healing response to non-surgical periodontal therapy in patients with diabetes mellitus: clinical, microbiological and immunological results. J Clin Periodontol 1998; 25:112.
9. Collins JG, Windley III HW, Arnold RR, et al: Effects of a *Porpyhromonas gingivalis* infection on inflammatory mediator response and pregnancy outcome in hamsters. Infect Immun 1994; 62:4356.
10. Collins JG, Smith MA, Arnold RR, et al: Effects of a *Escherichia coli* and Porpyhromonas gingivalis lipopolysaccharide on pregnancy outcome in the golden hamster. Infect Immun 1994; 62:4652.
11. Craven DE, Steger KE, Barber TW: Preventing nosocomial pneumonia: State of the art and perspectives for the 1990s. Am J Med 1991; 91(suppl 3B):s44.
12. Dajani AS, Taubert KA, Wilson W, et al: Prevention of bacterial endocarditis. Recommendations by the American Heart Association. JAMA 1997; 277:1794.
13. Dasanayake AP: Poor periodontal health of the pregnant woman as a risk factor for low birth weight. Ann Periodontol 1998; 3:202.
14. DeStefano F, Andra RF, Kahn HS, et al: Dental disease and risk of coronary heart disease and mortality. Br Med J 1993; 306:688.
15. Drangsholt MT: A new causal model of dental diseases associated with endocarditis. Ann Periodontol 1998; 3:184.
16. Dussault G, Shieham A: Medical theories and professional development. The theory of focal sepsis and dentistry in early twentieth century Britain. Soc Sci Med 1982; 16:1405.
17. Evidence-Based Medicine Working Group: Evidence-based medicine. A new approach to teaching the practice of medicine. JAMA 1992; 268:2420.
18. Garcia RI, Chauncey HH: Longitudinal studies of aging and oral health. J Dent Res 1991; 70:865.
19. Garcia RI, Krall EA, Vokonas PS: Periodontal disease and mortality from all causes in the VA Dental Longitudinal Study. Ann Periodontol 1998; 3:339.
20. Grau AJ, Buggle F, Heindl S, et al: Recent infection as a risk factor for cerebrovascular ischemia. Stroke 1995; 26:373.
21. Grau AJ, Buggle F, Steichen-Wiehn C, et al: Clinical and biochemical analysis in infection-associated stroke. Stroke 1995; 26:1520.
22. Grau AJ, Buggle F, Ziegler C, et al: Association between acute cerebrovascular ischemia and chronic and recurrent infection. Stroke 1997; 28:1724.
23. Grossi SG, Skrepcinski FB, DeCaro T, et al: Treatment of periodontal disease in diabetics reduces glycated hemoglobin. J Periodontol 1997; 68:713.
24. Grossi SG, Genco RJ: Periodontal disease and diabetes mellitus: A two-way relationship. Ann Periodontol 1998; 3:51.
25. Guntheroth WG: How important are dental procedures as a cause of infective endocarditis? Am J Cardiol 1984; 54:797.
26. Hayes C, Sparrow D, Cohen M, et al: The association between alveolar bone loss and pulmonary function: The VA dental longitudinal study. Ann Periodontol 1998; 3:257.
27. Herzberg MC, Meyer MW: Effects of oral flora on platelets: Possible consequences in cardiovascular disease. J Periodontol 1996; 67:1138.
28. Herzberg MC, Meyer MW: Dental plaque, platelets and cardiovascular diseases. Ann Periodontol 1998; 3:151.
29. Hill GB: The microbiology of bacterial vaginosis. Am J Obstet Gynecol 1993; 169:450.
30. Hill GB: Investigating the source of amniotic fluid isolates of fusobacteria. Clin Infect Dis 1993; 16(suppl 4):s423.
31. Hill GB: Preterm birth: associations with genital and possibly oral microflora. Ann Periodontol 1998; 3:222.
32. Jeffcoat MK, McGuire M, Newman MG: Evidence-based periodontal treatment. Highlights from the 1996 World Workshop in Periodontics. J Am Dent Assoc 1997; 128:713.
33. Kinane DF: Periodontal disease's contributions to cardiovascular disease: An overview of potential mechanisms. Ann Periodontol 1998; 3:142.
34. Kweider M, Lowe GDO, Murray GD, et al: Dental disease, fibrinogen and white cell counts: Links with myocardial infarction? Scott Med J 1993; 38:73.
35. Löe H: Periodontal disease: The sixth complication of diabetes mellitus. Diabetes Care 1993; 16(suppl 1):329.
36. Lowe GDO, Lee AJ, Rumley A, et al: Blood viscosity and risk of cardiovascular events: The Edinburg Artery Study. Br J Haematol 1997; 96:168.
37. Lowe GDO: Etiopathogenesis of cardiovascular disease: Hemostasis, thrombosis, and vascular medicine. Ann Periodontol 1998; 3:121.
38. Mattila KJ: Viral and bacterial infections in patients with acute myocardial infarction. J Intern Med 1989; 225:293.
39. Mattila KJ, Nieminen MS, Valtonen VV, et al: Association between dental health and acute myocardial infarction. Br Med J 1989; 298:779.
40. Mattila KJ: Dental infections as a risk factor for acute myocardial infarction. Eur Heart J 1993; 14:51.
41. Mattila KJ, Valle MS, Nieminen MS, et al: Dental infections and coronary atherosclerosis. Atherosclerosis 1993; 103:205.
42. Mattila KJ, Valtonen VV, Nieminen M, et al: Dental infection and the risk of new coronary events: Prospective study

of patients with documented coronary artery disease. Clin Infect Dis 1995; 20:588.
43. McCormick MC: The contribution of low birth weight to infant mortality and childhood morbidity. N Engl J Med 1985; 312:82.
44. McDonald HM, O'Loughlin JA, Jolley P, et al: Vaginal infections and preterm labour. Br J Obstet Gynecol 1991; 98:427.
45. Mealey BL: Periodontal implications: Medically compromised patients. Ann Periodontol 1996; 1:256.
46. Mealey BL: Influence of periodontal infections on systemic health. Periodontology 2000 1999; 21:197.
47. Mealey BL: Diabetes mellitus. In: Rose LF, Genco RJ, Mealey BL, et al (eds): Periodontal Medicine. Toronto, BC Decker, 2000.
48. Mehta JL, Saldeen TGP, Rand K: Interactive role of infection, inflammation and traditional risk factors in atherosclerosis and coronary artery disease. J Am Coll Cardiol 1998; 31:1217.
49. Miller LS, Manwell MA, Newbold D, et al: The relationship between reduction in periodontal inflammation and diabetes control: A report of 9 cases. J Periodontol 1992; 63:843.
50. Morales WJ, Schorr S, Albritton J: Effect of metronidazole in patients with preterm birth in preceding pregnancy and bacterial vaginosis: A placebo-controlled double-blind study. Am J Obstet Gynecol 1994; 171:345.
51. Newman HN: Focal infection. J Dent Res 1996; 75:1912.
52. Newman MG: Improved clinical decision making using the evidence-based approach. Ann Periodontol 1996; 1:i.
53. Offenbacher S: Periodontal diseases: pathogenesis. Ann Periodontol 1996; 1:821.
54. Offenbacher S, Katz V, Fertik G, et al: Periodontal disease as a possible risk factor for preterm low birth weight. J Periodontol 1996; 67:1103.
55. Offenbacher S, Jarad HL, O'Reilly PG, et al: Potential pathogenic mechanisms of periodontitis-associated pregnancy complications. Ann Periodontol 1998; 3:233.
56. Ostergaard L, Anderson PL: Etiology of community-acquired pneumonia. Evaluation by transtracheal aspiration, blood culture, or serology. Chest 1993; 104:1400.
57. Page RC: The pathobiology of periodontal diseases may affect systemic diseases: inversion of a paradigm. Ann Periodontol 1998; 3:108.
58. Page RC, Beck JD: Risk assessment for periodontal diseases. Int Dent J 1997; 47:61.
59. Papapanou PN: Periodontal diseases: Epidemiology. Ann Periodontol 1996; 1:1.
60. Pugin J, Auckenthaler R, Lew DP, et al: Oropharyngeal decontamination decreases incidence of ventilator-associated pneumonia. A randomized, placebo-controlled, double-blind clinical trial. JAMA 1991; 265:2704.
61. Ridker PM: Fibrinolytic and inflammatory markers for arterial occlusion: the evolving epidemiology of thrombosis and hemostasis. Thromb Haemost 1997; 78:53.
62. Sammalkorpi K: Glucose intolerance in acute infections. J Intern Med 1989; 225:15.
63. Scannapieco FA, Mylotte JM: Relationships between periodontal disease and bacterial pneumonia. J Periodontol 1996; 67:1114.
64. Scannapieco FA, Papandonatos GD, Dunford RG: Associations between oral conditions and respiratory disease in a national sample survey population. Ann Periodontol 1998; 3:251.
65. Selective Decontamination of the Digestive Tract Trialist's Collaborative Group: Meta-analysis of randomised controlled trials of selective decontamination of the digestive tract. Br Med J 1993; 307:525.
66. Smith GT, Greenbaum CJ, Johnson BD, et al: Short-term responses to periodontal therapy in insulin-dependent diabetic patients. J Periodontol 1996; 67:794.
67. Spodick DH, Flessas AP, Johnson MM: Association of acute respiratory symptoms with onset of acute myocardial infarction: Prospective investigation of 150 consecutive patients and matched control patients. Am J Cardiol 1984; 53:481.
68. Stoutenbeek CP, van Saene HKF, Miranda DR, et al: The effect of oropharyngeal decontamination using topical nonabsorbable antibiotics on the incidence of nosocomial respiratory tract infections in multiple trauma patients. J Trauma 1987; 27:357.
69. Syrjanen J, Valtonen VV, Iivanainen M, et al: Preceding infection as an important risk factor for ischemic brain infarction in young and middle aged patients. Br Med J 1988; 296:1156.
70. Syrjanen J, Peltola J, Valtonen V, et al: Dental infections in association with cerebral infarction in young and middle-aged men. J Intern Med 1989; 225:179.
71. Taylor GW, Burt BA, Becker MP, et al: Severe periodontitis and risk for poor glycemic control in patients with non-insulin-dependent diabetes mellitus. J Periodontol 1996; 67:1085.
72. Thorstensson H, Kuylensteirna J, Hugoson A: Medical status and complications in relation to periodontal disease experience in insulin-dependent diabetics. J Clin Periodontol 1996; 23:194.
73. Travis J, Pike R, Imamura T, et al: The role of proteolytic enzymes in the development of pulmonary emphysema and periodontal disease. Am J Respir Crit Care Med 1994; 150:143.
74. Wahl MJ: Myths of dental-induced endocarditis. Arch Intern Med 1994; 154:137.
75. Williams RC, Mahan CJ: Periodontal disease and diabetes in young adults. JAMA 1960; 172:776.
76. Yki-Jarvinen H, Sammalkorpi K, Koivisto VA, et al: Severity, duration and mechanism of insulin resistance during acute infections. J Clin Endocrinol Metab 1989; 69:317.
77. Zambon JJ, Haraszthy VI, Grossi S, et al: Identification of periodontal pathogens in atheromatous plaques. J Dent Res 1997; 76(special issue):408(Abstr 3159).

Smoking and Periodontal Disease

M. John Novak and Karen F. Novak

CHAPTER

CHAPTER OUTLINE

An estimated 27.9% of dentate U.S. adults are current smokers and 23.3% are former smokers. The prevalence of smoking is higher in individuals older than 34 years of age when compared with older age groups and in males (30.9%) compared with females (25.1%), with the highest prevalence seen in non-Hispanic black men (38.6%). Current smoking is more common among low-income adults (37.1%) compared with medium or high-income earners and increases with decreasing years of education.[69] Increasing evidence points to smoking as a major risk factor for periodontitis, affecting the prevalence, extent, and severity of disease. In addition, smoking may influence the clinical outcome of nonsurgical and surgical therapy as well as the long-term success of implant placement. With 41.9% of periodontitis cases in the U.S. being associated with smoking, it has become increasingly important to understand its impact on the initiation, progression, and management of the disease in patients who smoke. This chapter discusses the effects of smoking on the prevalence, severity, etiology, and pathogenesis of periodontal disease as well as the impact on treatment. The reader is referred to several excellent reviews on the topic for the detailed results of studies.[34,49,50,53,71]

EFFECTS OF SMOKING ON THE PREVALENCE AND SEVERITY OF PERIODONTAL DISEASE

Gingivitis

Controlled clinical studies have demonstrated that in human models of experimental gingivitis, the development of inflammation in response to plaque accumulation is reduced in smokers compared with nonsmokers (Table 14-1).[6,16] In addition, cross-sectional studies have consistently demonstrated that smokers present with less gingival inflammation than nonsmokers.[5,8,9,54,55] These data suggest that smokers have a decreased expression of clinical inflammation in the presence of plaque accumulation when compared with nonsmokers. The microbiologic, immunologic, and physiologic factors that might account for this observation are discussed in detail later.

Periodontitis

Although gingival inflammation in smokers appears to be reduced in response to plaque accumulation when compared with nonsmokers, an overwhelming body of data

TABLE 14-1

Effects of Smoking on the Prevalence and Severity of Periodontal Disease

Periodontal Disease	Impact of Smoking
Gingivitis	↓ Gingival inflammation and bleeding on probing
Periodontitis	↑ Prevalence and severity of periodontal destruction
	↑ Pocket depth, attachment loss, and bone loss
	↑ Rate of periodontal destruction
	↑ Prevalence of severe periodontitis
	↑ Tooth loss
	↑ Prevalence with increased number of cigarettes smoked per day
	↓ Prevalence and severity with smoking cessation

↓, Decreased; ↑, increased.

points to smoking as a major risk factor for increasing the prevalence and severity of periodontal destruction. Multiple cross-sectional and longitudinal studies have demonstrated that pocket depth, attachment loss, and alveolar bone loss are more prevalent and severe in patients who smoke compared with nonsmokers.[34,49,50,53,71] An assessment of the relationship between cigarette smoking and periodontitis was performed in more than 12,000 dentate individuals over the age of 18 years as part of the National Health and Nutrition Examination Survey (NHANES III).[69] Periodontitis was defined as ≥1 site with clinical attachment loss of ≥4 mm and pocket depth of ≥4 mm. Using criteria established by the Centers for Disease Control and Prevention (CDC), current smokers were defined as those that had smoked ≥100 cigarettes over their lifetime and smoked at the time of the interview; former smokers had smoked ≥100 cigarettes in their lifetime but were not currently smoking, and nonsmokers had not smoked ≥100 cigarettes in their lifetime. Of the 12,000 individuals studied, 9.2% had periodontitis. This represented approximately 15 million cases of periodontitis in the U.S. On average, smokers were 4 times as likely to have periodontitis as persons who had never smoked after adjusting for age, gender, race/ethnicity, education, and income/poverty ratio. Former smokers were 1.68 times more likely to have periodontitis than persons who had never smoked. This study also demonstrated a dose-response relationship between cigarettes smoked per day and the odds of having periodontitis. In subjects smoking ≤9 cigarettes per day, the odds for having periodontitis was 2.79 whereas subjects smoking ≥31 cigarettes per day were nearly 6 times more likely to have periodontitis. With former smokers, the odds of having periodontitis declined with the number of years since quitting. These data indicated that approximately 42% of periodontitis cases (6.4 million cases) in the U.S. adult population were attributable to current smoking and approximately 11% (1.7 million cases) were attributable to former smoking.

These data are consistent with the findings of other cross-sectional studies performed in the U.S. and Europe. The odds ratio for periodontitis in current smokers has been estimated to range from as low as 1.5 to as high as 7.3, depending on the observed severity of periodontitis.[50] A metaanalysis of data from six such studies involving 2361 subjects indicated that current smokers were nearly 3 times more likely to have severe periodontitis than nonsmokers.[49] The detrimental impact of long-term smoking on the periodontal and dentate status of older adults has been clearly demonstrated. Older-adult smokers are approximately 3 times more likely to have severe periodontal disease,[4,44] and the number of years of tobacco use is a significant factor in tooth loss, coronal root caries, and periodontal disease.[32,33] Smoking also has been shown to affect periodontal disease severity in younger individuals. Cigarette smoking is associated with increased severity of generalized aggressive periodontitis (formerly termed "early onset periodontitis") in young adults,[64] and young adults between the ages of 19 to 30 years who smoke are 3.8 times more likely to have periodontitis than nonsmokers.[26] Longitudinal studies have demonstrated that young individuals smoking more than 15 cigarettes per day showed the highest risk for tooth loss[30] and smokers are greater than 6 times more likely than nonsmokers to demonstrate continued attachment loss.[31] Over a 10-year period, bone loss has been reported to be twice as rapid in smokers when compared with nonsmokers[11] and proceeds more rapidly even in the presence of excellent plaque control.[10]

Less information is available on the effects of cigar and pipe smoking, but it appears that effects similar to cigarette smoking may be observed with this form of tobacco use.[2,20,21,42] The prevalence of moderate and severe periodontitis and the percentage of teeth with ≥5 mm of attachment loss was most severe in current cigarette smokers, but cigar and pipe smokers showed a severity of disease intermediate between the current cigarette smokers and nonsmokers.[2] Tooth loss is also increased in cigar and pipe smokers when compared with nonsmokers.[42]

Smokeless tobacco use has been associated with oral leukoplakia and carcinoma.[15,75] However, there do not appear to be any generalized effects on periodontal disease progression, other than localized attachment loss and recession at the site of tobacco product placement.[60]

Of great interest is the observation that former smokers have less risk for periodontitis than current smokers but more risk than nonsmokers and that the risk for periodontitis decreases with the increasing number of years since quitting smoking.[69] This suggests that the effects of smoking on periodontal disease progression are reversible with smoking cessation and that smoking cessation programs should be an integral component of periodontal education and therapy.

EFFECTS OF SMOKING ON THE ETIOLOGY AND PATHOGENESIS OF PERIODONTAL DISEASE

The increased prevalence and severity of periodontal destruction associated with smoking suggests that the host-bacterial interactions normally seen in chronic periodontitis are altered, resulting in more aggressive periodontal breakdown (see Chapters 6–8) (Table 14-2). This imbalance between bacterial challenge and host response may be due to changes in the composition of the subgingival plaque, with increases in the numbers and/or virulence of pathogenic organisms; changes in the host response to the bacterial challenge; or a combination of both. Recent evidence on the effects of smoking on the microbiology, immunology, and physiology of periodontitis are discussed below.

Microbiology

Studies have failed to demonstrate a difference in the rate of plaque accumulation of smokers compared with nonsmokers, suggesting that if an alteration in the microbial challenge in smokers exists, it is due to a qualitative rather than quantitative alteration in the plaque.[8] Several studies have explored the changes that may occur in subgingival plaque as a result of smoking with conflicting and inconclusive results. In a study of 142 patients with chronic periodontitis, plaque samples from deep pockets (≥6 mm) showed no differences in the counts of *Actinobacillus actinomycetemcomitans, Porphyromonas gingivalis,* and *Prevotella intermedia.*[57] In a similar study of 615 patients, the prevalence of *A. actinomycetemcomitans, P. gingivalis, P. intermedia,* and *Eikenella corrodens* was not found to be significantly different between smokers and nonsmokers using immunoassay.[67] In contrast, other studies have shown differences in the microbial composition of subgingival plaque between smokers and nonsmokers. In a study of 798 subjects with different smoking histories, it was found that smokers had significantly higher levels of *Bacteroides forsythus* and that smokers were 2.3 times more likely to harbor *B. forsythus* than nonsmokers and former smokers.[76] Of particular interest was the observation that smokers do not respond to mechanical therapy as well as nonsmokers and that this is associated with increased levels of *B. forsythus, A. actinomycetemcomitans,* and *P. gingivalis* remaining in the pockets after therapy in the smoking group when compared with nonsmokers.[23,24,27,59] Many discrepancies between the findings of microbiologic studies are a function of the methodology involved, including bacterial counts versus proportions or prevalence of bacteria, number of sites sampled and the pocket depths selected, the sampling technique, the disease status of the subject, and the methods of bacterial enumeration and data analysis.[28] In an attempt to overcome some of these problems, a recent study sampled subgingival plaque from all teeth with the exception of third molars in 272 adult subjects, including 50 current smokers, 98 past smokers, and 124 nonsmokers.[28] Using checkerboard DNA–DNA hybridization technology to screen for 29 different subgingival species, it was found that members of the orange and red complexes (see Chapter 6) including *Eikenella nodatum, Fusobacterium nucleatum* ss. *vincentii, P. intermedia, Peptostreptococcus micros, Prevotella nigrescens, B. forsythus, P. gingivalis, and Treponema denticola* were significantly more prevalent in current smokers than in nonsmokers and former smokers. Of interest was that the increased prevalence of these periodontal pathogens was due to an increased colonization of shallow sites (pocket depth <4 mm) with no differences between smokers, former smokers, and nonsmokers in pockets ≥4 mm. In addition, these pathogenic bacteria were more prevalent in the maxilla than the mandible. These data suggest that smokers have a greater extent of colonization by periodontal pathogens than nonsmokers or former smokers and that this colonization may lead to an increased prevalence of periodontal breakdown.

TABLE 14-2

Effects of Smoking on the Etiology and Pathogenesis of Periodontal Disease

Etiologic Factor	Impact of Smoking
Microbiology	No effect on the rate of plaque accumulation ↑ Colonization of shallow periodontal pockets by periodontal pathogens ↑ Levels of periodontal pathogens in deep periodontal pockets
Immunology	Altered neutrophil chemotaxis, phagocytosis, and oxidative burst ↑ TNF-α, and PGE_2 in GCF ↑ Neutrophil collagenase and elastase in GCF ↑ Production of PGE_2 by monocytes in response to LPS
Physiology	↓ Gingival blood vessels with ↑ inflammation ↓ GCF flow and bleeding on probing with ↑ inflammation ↓ Subgingival temperature ↑ Time needed to recover from local anaesthesia

↓, Decreased; ↑, increased. See text for description of other abbreviations.

Immunology

The immune response of the host to plaque accumulation is essentially protective. In periodontal health and gingivitis, a balance exists between the bacterial challenge of plaque and the immune response from within the gingival tissues, with no resulting loss of periodontal support. In contrast, periodontitis appears to be associated with an alteration in the host-bacterial balance that may be initiated by changes in the bacterial composition of subgingival plaque, changes in the immune response, or a combination of both elements (see Chapters 6–8). Smoking exerts a major effect on the protective elements of the immune response, resulting in an increase in the extent and severity of periodontal destruction. The deleterious effects of smoking appear to be due in part to a down regulation of the immune response to bacterial challenge. The neutrophil is an important component of the host response to bacterial infection, and alterations in neutrophil number or function may result in localized and/or systemic infections. Critical functions of neutrophils include chemotaxis (directed locomotion from the blood stream to the site of infection), phagocytosis (internalization of foreign particles such as bacteria), and killing using oxidative and nonoxidative mechanisms. Neutrophils, obtained from the peripheral blood or saliva of smokers or exposed in vitro to whole tobacco smoke or nicotine, have been shown to demonstrate functional alterations in chemotaxis, phagocytosis, and the oxidative burst. Smoking has been shown to impair the chemotaxis and phagocytosis of neutrophils obtained from the oral cavity,[19,38] and in vitro studies of the effects of tobacco products on neutrophils have shown detrimental effects on cell movement and the oxidative burst.[14,37,43,62,65] In addition, the production of antibody essential for phagocytosis and killing of bacteria, specifically IgG2 levels to periodontal pathogens, has been reported to be reduced in smokers versus nonsmokers with periodontitis,[13,25,58,68] suggesting that smokers may have reduced protection against periodontal infection. In contrast, elevated levels of TNF-α have been demonstrated in the gingival crevicular fluid of smokers[12] as well as elevated levels of PGE_2, neutrophil elastase, and matrix metalloproteinase-8.[66] In vitro studies also have demonstrated that exposure to nicotine increases the secretion of PGE_2 by monocytes in response to LPS.[51]

These data suggest that smoking may impair the response of neutrophils to periodontal infection but may also increase the release of tissue-destructive enzymes. The exact changes in the immunologic mechanisms involved in the rapid tissue destruction seen in smokers are currently unclear. Further studies are needed to define the effects of tobacco use on the immune response and tissue destruction in periodontitis.

Physiology

Previous studies have shown that the clinical signs of inflammation are less pronounced in smokers when compared with nonsmokers.[6,16] These observations may be due to alterations in the inflammatory response in smokers, as outlined previously, or due to alterations in the vascular response of the gingival tissues. Although no significant differences in the vascular density of healthy gingiva have been observed between smokers and nonsmokers,[52] the response of the microcirculation to plaque accumulation appears to be altered in smokers when compared with nonsmokers. With developing inflammation, increases in gingival crevicular fluid flow,[6] bleeding on probing,[6] and gingival blood vessels[7] were less in smokers when compared with nonsmokers. In addition, the oxygen concentration in healthy gingival tissues appears to be less in smokers than nonsmokers, although this condition is reversed in the presence of moderate inflammation.[29] Subgingival temperatures are lower in smokers than nonsmokers,[18] and recovery from the vasoconstriction caused by local anaesthetic administration takes longer in smokers.[39,72] These cumulative data suggest the presence of significant alterations in the gingival microvasculature of smokers when compared with nonsmokers and that these changes lead to decreased blood flow and decreased clinical signs of inflammation.

EFFECTS OF SMOKING ON THE RESPONSE TO PERIODONTAL THERAPY

Nonsurgical Therapy

Numerous studies have indicated that current smokers do not respond as well to periodontal therapy as nonsmokers or former smokers (Table 14-3). The majority of clinical research supports the observation that pocket depth reduction is more effective in nonsmokers than in smokers using nonsurgical periodontal therapy (Phase I therapy) including oral hygiene instruction, scaling, and root planing.[1,23,24,27,36,56,59] In addition, gains in clinical attachment as a result of scaling and root planing are less pronounced in smokers than in nonsmokers. In a study of patients with previously untreated advanced periodontal disease, scaling and root planing plus oral hygiene resulted in significantly greater average reductions in pocket depth and bleeding on probing in nonsmokers than in smokers when evaluated 6 months after completion of therapy.[59] Average pocket reductions of 2.5 mm for nonsmokers and 1.9 mm for smokers were observed in pockets that averaged 7 mm before treatment, even though plaque scores were less than favorable. In another study, the nonsurgical management of pockets ≥5 mm showed that smokers had less pocket depth reduction than nonsmokers after 3 months (1.29 versus 1.76 mm) as well as fewer gains in clinical attachment levels.[23] When a higher level of plaque control can be achieved as part of nonsurgical care, the differences in the resolution of 4- to 6-mm pockets between nonsmokers and smokers become clinically less significant.[56] When pockets persist in smokers and nonsmokers after therapy, adjunctive topical antimicrobial therapy can be used to try to resolve the remaining pocket depths (see Chapter 50). When scaling and root planing is used in combination with either topical subgingivally placed tetracycline fibers, subgingival minocycline gel, or subgingival metronidazole gel, smokers continue to show less pocket reduction than nonsmokers.[40] It can be concluded that smokers respond less well to nonsurgical therapy than nonsmokers. However, in the presence of excellent plaque control, these differences may be minimized. When comparing current smokers with former smokers and nonsmokers, the former and nonsmoking subjects appear to respond equally well to nonsurgical care,[23] reinforcing the need for patients to be informed of the benefits of smoking cessation.

Surgical Therapy and Implants

The less favorable response of the periodontal tissues to nonsurgical therapy that is observed in current smokers also appears to apply to surgical therapy. In a longitudinal comparative study of the effects of four different treatment modalities including coronal scaling, root planing, modified Widman flap surgery, and osseous resection surgery, smokers (*heavy* defined as ≥20 cigarettes/day; *light* defined as ≤19 cigarettes/day) consistently showed less pocket reduction and less gain in clinical attachment levels than nonsmokers or former smokers.[36] These differences began immediately after the completion of therapy and continued throughout 7 years of supportive peri-

TABLE 14-3

Effects of Smoking on the Response to Periodontal Therapy

Therapy	Effects of Smoking
Nonsurgical	↓ Clinical response to scaling and root planing
	↓ Reduction in pocket depth
	↓ Gain in clinical attachment levels
	↓ Negative impact of smoking with ↑ level of plaque control
Surgery and implants	↓ Pocket depth reduction postsurgery
	↑ Deterioration of furcations postsurgery
	↓ Gain in clinical attachment levels, ↓ bone fill, ↑ recession, and ↑ membrane exposure following GTR
	↓ Pocket depth reduction after DFDBA allografts
	↓ Pocket depth reduction and gain in clinical attachment levels after open flap debridement
	Conflicting data on the impact of smoking on implant success
	Smoking cessation should be recommended prior to implants
Maintenance	↑ Pocket depth during maintenance
	↓ Gain in clinical attachment levels
Recurrent (refractory) disease	↑ Recurrent/refractory disease in smokers
	↑ Need for retreatment in smokers
	↑ Need for antibiotics in smokers to control the negative effects of periodontal infection on surgical outcomes
	↑ Tooth loss in smokers after surgical therapy

↓, Decreased; ↑, increased. See text for description of other abbreviations.

odontal therapy. During the 7 years, deterioration of furcation areas was greater in heavy and light smokers when compared with former and nonsmokers.

Smoking also has been shown to have a negative impact on the outcomes of guided tissue regeneration (GTR)[70,73] and the treatment of intrabony defects by bone allografts.[61] By 12 months after GTR therapy for deep intrabony defects, smokers gained less than half as much clinical attachment as nonsmokers (2.1 versus 5.2 mm).[70] **In a second study, 73 smokers also showed less gain in clinical attachment (1.2 versus 3.2 mm), more gingival recession, and less gain in bone fill of the defect. In addition, the GTR membranes were exposed in all the smokers and approximately half of the nonsmokers (Table 14-4).**

Similarly, after the use of decalcified freeze dried bone allograft (DFDBA) for the treatment of intrabony defects, smokers showed less percentage reduction in presurgical pocket depth than nonsmokers (41.9% reduction for smokers versus 48.3% for nonsmokers).[61]

Open flap debridement surgery without regenerative or grafting procedures is the most common surgical procedure used for accessing the root and osseous surfaces. By 6 months after this procedure, smokers showed significantly less reduction of deep pockets (≥7 mm) than nonsmokers (3 mm for smokers versus 4 mm for nonsmokers) and significantly less gain in clinical attachment (1.8 versus 2.8 mm), even though the patients received supportive periodontal therapy every month for 6 months.[63] Of increased significance was the observation that only 16% of deep pockets in smokers returned to ≤3 mm 6 months after surgery, whereas 47% of the deep pockets in nonsmokers were ≤3 mm after completion of therapy.

TABLE 14-4

Postsurgery Changes in Clinical Parameters of the Healing Response in Smoker and Nonsmoker Patients

	Smokers	Nonsmokers	P-Value
CAL gain	1.2 ± 1.3 mm	3.2 ± 2.0 mm	<0.007
GR increase	2.8 ± 1.2 mm	1.3 ± 1.3 mm	<0.008
PBL gain	0.5 ± 1.5 mm	3.7 ± 2.2 mm	<0.000
ME	10/10	15/28	<0.008

CAL, Clinical attachment level; *GR,* gingival recession; *ME,* prevalence of membrane exposure at removal; *PBL,* probing bone level. Adapted from Trombelli M, Kim CK, Zimmerman GJ, et al: Retrospective analysis of factors related to clinical outcome of guided tissue regeneration procedures in intrabony defects. J Clin Periodontol 1997; 24:366.

The impact of smoking on implant success is unclear at present. Several studies have shown that implant success rates are reduced in smokers[3,17,22,35] while other studies have shown no effect.[48,74] Since numerous factors can influence implant success (see Chapters 68–73), further controlled clinical trials are needed to address the role of smoking as an independent variable in implant failure. However, with existing evidence supporting a negative effect of smoking on long-term implant success, patients should be informed and advised of the benefits of smoking cessation and the potential risks of smoking for implant failure.

Maintenance Therapy

The detrimental effects of smoking on treatment outcomes appears to be long lasting, and independent of the frequency of maintenance therapy. After four different modalities of therapy including scaling, scaling and root planing, modified Widman flap surgery, and osseous surgery, maintenance therapy was performed by an hygienist every 3 months for 7 years.[36] Smokers consistently had deeper pockets than nonsmokers and less gain in attachment when evaluated each year for the 7-year period. Heavy smokers (≥20 cigarettes/day) had more plaque than light smokers, former smokers, and nonsmokers. Even with more intensive maintenance therapy given every month for 6 months after flap surgery,[63] smokers had deeper and more residual pockets than nonsmokers, even though no significant differences in plaque or bleeding on probing scores were found. These data suggest that the effects of smoking on the quality of subgingival plaque, the host response, and the healing characteristics of the periodontal tissues may have a long-term effect on pocket resolution in smokers that may not be managed by conventional periodontal therapy. More studies are needed to examine the effects of antimicrobial agents combined with host-modulating agents in an attempt to control periodontal disease in smokers.

Recurrent (Refractory) Disease

Because of the difficulty in controlling periodontal disease in smokers, many smokers become refractory to traditional periodontal treatment and tend to show more periodontal breakdown than nonsmokers after therapy.[45,47] The question has been raised as to whether patients are truly refractive to therapy or whether the therapy administered was insufficient to control the disease process.[41,47] It is now thought that patients formerly considered refractive to therapy actually undergo continuous or recurrent disease; for this reason, the diagnosis of refractory periodontitis has been removed as a distinct classification (see Chapter 4). The complex effects of smoking on the subgingival microflora and host response provide a model for studying new modalities of therapy for controlling periodontitis. In studies of patients who failed to respond to conventional therapy including different combinations of oral hygiene instruction, scaling and root planing, surgery, and antibiotics, approximately 90% of these so-called "refractory" patients were smokers.[45,46] In one study, the mean age of the refractory patients was 42 years and 28 of the 31 refractory patients were smokers.[45] Of the 31 patients, 19% had been retreated once surgically for pocket elimination, 10% had been retreated twice surgically, and the patients had received an average of four episodes of adjunctive antibiotics. During the course of treatment, 36% of patients had lost an average of 3 teeth (range 1–10).

It is clear from these studies that smokers may present with periodontal disease at an early age, may be difficult to treat with conventional therapy, and may continue to have progressive or recurrent periodontitis leading to tooth loss. Further studies are needed to determine the level and type of therapy required to provide long-term maintenance of periodontal health in individuals who wish to continue smoking.

REFERENCES

1. Ah MKB, Johnson GK, Kaldahl WB, et al: The effect of smoking on the response to periodontal therapy. J Clin Periodontol 1994; 21:91.
2. Albandar JM, Streckfus CF, Adesanya MR, et al: Cigar, pipe, and cigarette smoking as risk factors for periodontal disease and tooth loss. J Periodontol 2000; 71:1874.
3. Bain CA, Moy PK: The association between the failure of dental implants and cigarette smoking. Int J Oral Maxillofac Implants 1993; 8:609.
4. Beck JD, Koch GG, Rozier RG, et al: Prevalence and risk indicators for periodontal attachment loss in a population of older community-dwelling blacks and whites. J Periodontol 1990; 61:521.
5. Bergstrom J, Floderus-Myrhed B: Co-twin control study of the relationship between smoking and some periodontal disease factors. Community Dent Oral Epidemiol 1983; 11:113.
6. Bergstrom J, Preber H: The influence of cigarette smoking on the development of experimental gingivitis. J Periodont Res 1986; 21:668.
7. Bergstrom J, Persson L, Preber H: Influence of cigarette smoking on vascular reaction during experimental gingivitis. Scand J Dent Res 1988; 96:34.
8. Bergstrom J: Cigarette smoking as a risk factor in chronic periodontal disease. Community Dent Oral Epidemiol 1989; 17:245.
9. Bergstrom J: Oral hygiene compliance and gingivitis expression in cigarette smokers. Scand J Dent Res 1990; 98:497.
10. Bergstrom J, Eliasson S, Dock J: A 10-year prospective study of tobacco smoking and periodontal health. J Periodontol 2000; 71:1338.
11. Bolin A, Eklund G, Frithiof L, et al: The effect of changed smoking habits on marginal alveolar bone loss: a longitudinal study. Swed Dent J 1993; 17:211.
12. Bostrum L, Linder LE, Bergstrom J: Clinical expression of TNF-α in smoking-associated periodontal disease. J Clin Periodontol 1998; 25:767.
13. Califano JV, Schifferle RE, Gunsolley JC, et al: Anibody reactive with *Porphyromnas gingivalis* serotypes K1–6 in adult and generalized early-onset periodontitis. J Periodontol 1999; 70:730.
14. Codd EE, Swim AT, Bridges RB: Tobacco smokers' neutrophils are desensitized to chemotactic peptide-stimulated oxygen uptake. J Lab Clin Med 1987; 110:648.
15. Creath CJ, Cutter G, Bradley DH, et al: Oral leukoplakia and adolescent smokeless tobacco use. Oral Surg Oral Med Oral Pathol 1991; 72:35.
16. Danielsen B, Manji F, Nagelkerke N, et al: Effect of cigarette smoking on the transition dynamics in experimental gingivitis. J Clin Periodontol 1990; 17:159.
17. De Bruyn H, Collaert B: The effect of smoking on early implant failure. Clin Oral Implants Res 1994; 5:260.
18. Dinsdale CR, Rawlinson A, Walsh TF: Subgingival temperature in smokers and nonsmokers with periodontal disease. J Clin Periodontol 1997; 24:761.

19. Eichel B, Sharik HA: Tobacco smoke toxicity: Loss of human oral leukocyte function and fluid cell metabolism. Science 1969; 166:1424.
20. Feldman RS, Bravacos JS, Close CL: Associations between smoking different tobacco products and periodontal disease indexes. J Periodontol 1983; 54:481.
21. Feldman RS, Alman JE, Chauncey HH: Periodontal disease indexes and tobacco smoking in healthy aging men. Gerodontics 1987; 3:43.
22. Gorman LM, Lambert PM, Morris HF, et al: The effect of smoking on implant survival at second stage surgery: DICRG interim report #5. Dental implant clinical research group. Implant Dent 1994; 3:165.
23. Grossi SG, Skrepcinski FB, DeCaro T, et al: Response to periodontal therapy in diabetics and smokers. J Periodontol 1996; 67:1094.
24. Grossi SG, Zambon J, Machtei EE, et al: Effects of smoking and smoking cessation on healing after mechanical therapy. J Am Dent Assoc 1997; 128:599.
25. Gunsolley JC, Pandey JP, Quinn SM, et al: The effect of race, smoking and immunoglobulin allotypes on IgG subclass concentrations. J Perio Res 1997; 32:380.
26. Haber J, Wattles J, Crowley M, et al: Evidence for cigarette smoking as a major risk factor for periodontitis. J Periodontol 1993; 64:16.
27. Haffajee AD, Cugini MA, Dibart S, et al: The effects of scaling and root planing on the clinical and microbiologic parameters of periodontal diseases. J Clin Periodontol 1997; 24:324.
28. Haffajee AD, Socransky SS: Relationship of cigarette smoking to the subgingival microbiota. J Clin Periodontol 2001; 28:377.
29. Hanioka T, Tanaka M, Ojima M, et al: Oxygen sufficiency in the gingiva of smokers and nonsmokers with periodontal disease. J Periodontol 2000; 71:1846.
30. Holm G: Smoking as an additional risk for tooth loss. J Periodontol 1994; 65:996.
31. Ismail AI, Morrison EC, Burt BA, et al: Natural history of periodontal disease in adults: findings from the Tecumseh Periodontal Disease Study. J Dent Res 1990; 69:430.
32. Jette AM, Feldman HA, Tennstedt SL: Tobacco use: A modifiable risk factor for dental disease among the elderly. Am J Public Health 1993; 83:1271.
33. Jette AM, Feldman HA, Douglass C: Oral disease and physical disability in community dwelling older persons. J Am Geriatr Soc 1993; 41:1102.
34. Johnson GK, Slach NA: Impact of tobacco use on periodontal status. J Dent Educ 2001; 65:313.
35. Jones JK, Triplett RG: The relationship of cigarette smoking to impaired intraoral wound healing: a review of evidence and implications for patient care. J Oral Maxillofac Surg 1992; 50:237.
36. Kaldahl WB, Johnson GK, Patil KD, et al: Levels of cigarette consumption and response to periodontal therapy. J Periodontol 1996; 67:675.
37. Kalra J, Chandhary AK, Prasad K: Increased production of oxygen free radicals in cigarette smokers. Int J Exp Pathol 1991; 72:1.
38. Kenney EB, Kraal JH, Saxe SR, et al: The effect of cigarette smoke on human oral polymorphonuclear leukocytes. J Periodont Res 1977; 12:227.
39. Ketabi M, Hirsch RS: The effects of local anesthetic containing adrenaline on gingival blood flow in smokers and nonsmokers. J Clin Periodontol 1997; 24:888.
40. Kinane DF, Radvar M: The effect of smoking on mechanical and antimicrobial periodontal therapy. J Periodontol 1997; 68:467.
41. Kornman KS: Refractory periodontitis: Critical questions in clinical management. J Clin Periodontol 1996; 23:293.
42. Krall EA, Garvey AJ, Garcia RI: Alveolar bone loss and tooth loss in male cigar and pipe smokers. J Am Dent Assoc 1999; 130:57.
43. Lannan S, McLean A, Drost E, et al: Changes in neutrophil morphology and morphometry following exposure to cigarette smoke. Int J Exp Pathol 1992; 73:183.
44. Locker D, Leake JL: Risk indicators and risk markers for periodontal disease experience in older adults living independently in Ontario, Canada. J Dent Res 1993; 72:9.
45. MacFarlane GD, Herzberg MC, Wolff LF, et al: Refractory periodontitis associated with abnormal polymorphonuclear leukocyte phagocytosis and cigarette smoking. J Periodontol 1992; 63:908.
46. Magnussen I, Low S, McArthur WP, et al: Treatment of subjects with refractory periodontal disease. J Clin Periodontol 1994; 21:628.
47. Magnussen I, Walker CB: Refractory periodontitis or recurrent disease. J Clin Periodontol 1996; 23:289.
48. Minsk L, Polson AM, Weisgold A, et al: Outcome failures of endosseous implants from a clinical training center. Compend Continuing Educ Dent 1996; 17:848.
49. Papapanou PN: Periodontal diseases: Epidemiology. Ann Periodontol 1996; 1:1.
50. Papapanou PN: Risk assessments in the diagnosis and treatment of periodontal diseases. J Dent Educ 1998; 62:822.
51. Payne JB, Johnson GK, Reinhardt RA, et al: Nicotine effects on PGE2 and IL-1ß release by LPS-treated human monocytes. J Periodont Res 1996; 31:99.
52. Persson L, Bergstrom J: Smoking and vascular density of healthy marginal gingival. Eur J Oral Sci 1998; 106:953.
53. Position paper: Tobacco use and the periodontal patient. J Periodontol 1999; 70:1419.
54. Preber H, Bergstrom J: Occurrence of gingival bleeding in smoker and nonsmoker patients. Acta Odontol Scand 1985; 43:315.
55. Preber H, Bergstrom J: Cigarette smoking in patients referred for periodontal treatment. Scad J Dent Res 1986; 94:102.
56. Preber H, Bergstrom J: The effect of non-surgical treatment on periodontal pockets in smokers and nonsmokers. J Clin Periodontol 1986; 13:319.
57. Preber H, Bergstrom J, Linder LE: Occurrence of periopathogens in smoker and nonsmoker patients. J Clin Periodontol 1992; 19:667.
58. Quinn SM, Zhang JB, Gunsolley JC, et al: The influence of smoking and race on adult periodontitis and serum IgG_2 levels. J Periodontol 1998; 69:171.
59. Renvert S, Dahlen G, Wikstrom M: The clinical and microbiologic effects of non-surgical periodontal therapy in smokers and nonsmokers. J Clin Periodontol 1998; 25:153.
60. Robertson PB, Walsh M, Greene J, et al: Periodontal effects associated with the use of smokeless tobacco. J Periodontol 1990; 61:438.
61. Rosen PS, Marks MH, Reynolds MA: Influence of smoking on long-term clinical results of intrabony defects treated with regenerative therapy. J Periodontal 1996; 67:1159.
62. Ryder MI, Fujitaki R, Johnson G, et al: Alterations of neutrophil oxidative burst by in vitro smoke exposure: implications for oral and systemic diseases. Ann Periodontol 1998; 3:76.
63. Scabbia A, Cho K-S, Sigurdsson TJ, et al: Cigarette smoking negatively affects healing response following flap debridement surgery. J Periodontol 2001; 72:43.
64. Schenkein HA, Gunsolley JC, Koertge TE, et al: Smoking and its effects on early-onset periodontitis. J Am Dent Assoc 1995; 126:1107.

65. Selby C, Drost E, Brown D, et al: Inhibition of neutrophil adherence and movement by acute cigarette smoke exposure. Exp Lung Res 1992; 18:813.
66. Soder B: Neutrophil elastase activity, levels of prostaglandin E2, and matrix metalloproteinase-8 in refractory periodontitis sites in smokers and nonsmokers. Acta Odont Scandinavica 1999; 57:77.
67. Stoltenberg JL, Osborn JB, Pihlstrom BL, et al: Association between cigarette smoking, bacterial pathogens and periodontal status. J Periodontol 1993; 64:1225.
68. Tangada SD, Califano JV, Nakashima K, et al: The effect of smoking on serum IgG_2 reactive with *Actinobacillus actinomycetemcomitans* in early-onset periodontitis. J Periodontol 1997; 68:842.
69. Tomar SL, Asma S: Smoking-attributable periodontitis in the United States: findings from NHANES III. J Periodontol 2000; 71:743.
70. Tonetti MS, Pino-Prato G, Cortellini P: Effect of cigarette smoking on periodontal healing following GTR in infrabony defects. J Clin Periodontal 1995; 22:229.
71. Tonetti MS: Cigarette smoking and periodontal diseases: etiology and management of disease. Ann Periodontol 1998; 3:88.
72. Trikilis N, Rawlinson A, Walsh TF: Periodontal probing depth and subgingival temperature in smokers and nonsmokers. J Clin Periodontol 1999; 26:38.
73. Trombelli M, Kim CK, Zimmerman GJ, et al: Retrospective analysis of factors related to clinical outcome of guided tissue regeneration procedures in intrabony defects. J Clin Periodontol 1997; 24:366.
74. Weyant RJ: Characteristics associated with the loss and peri-implant tissue health of endosseous dental implants. Int J Oral Maxillofac Implants 1994; 9:95.
75. Wray A, McGuirt WF: Smokeless tobacco usage associated with oral carcinoma, Incidence, treatment, outcome. Arch Otolaryngol Head Neck Surg 1993; 119:929.
76. Zambon JJ, Grossi SG, Machtei EE, et al: Cigarette smoking increases the risk for subgingival infection with periodontal pathogens. J Periodontol 1996; 67:1050.

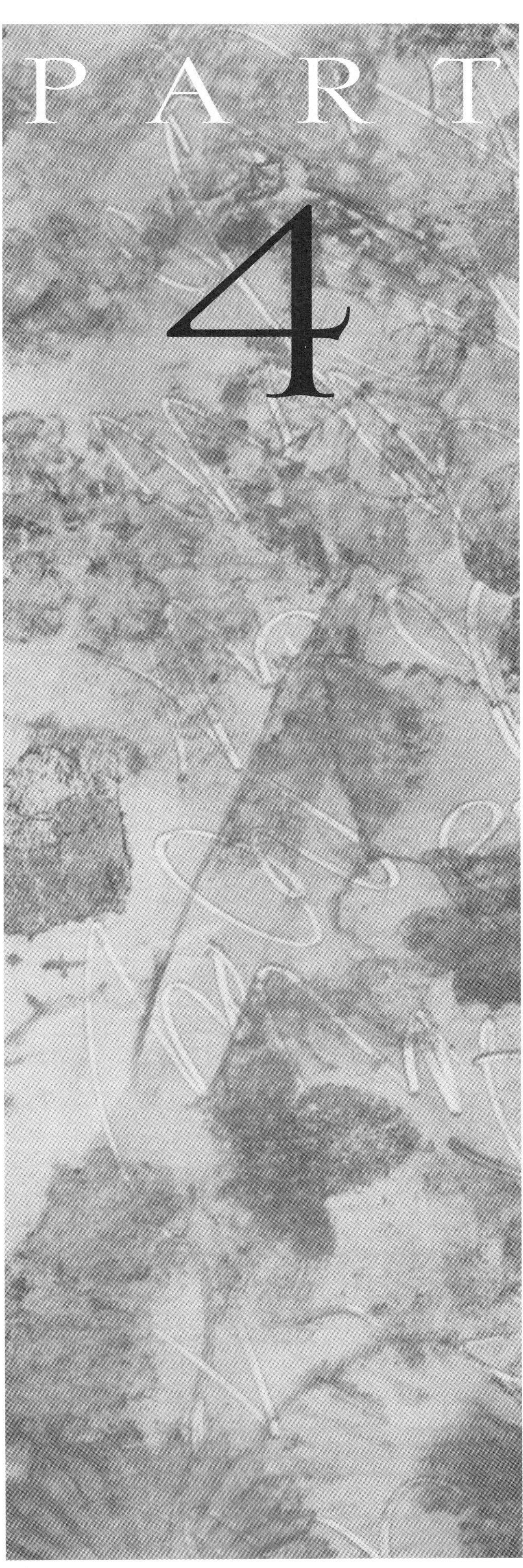

Periodontal Pathology

Michael G. Newman and Fermin A. Carranza

The thorough knowledge of the microscopic tissue changes in disease provides a sound basis for the understanding and interpretation of the clinical and radiographic findings encountered in our patients. This information is essential to comprehend the biologic nature of the periodontal responses to injury and healing.

This part provides information of the gingival diseases (Section One) and periodontal diseases (Section Two). The latter section also presents chapters with detailed descriptions of the different diseases that can affect the periodontium.

SECTION I

Gingival Disease

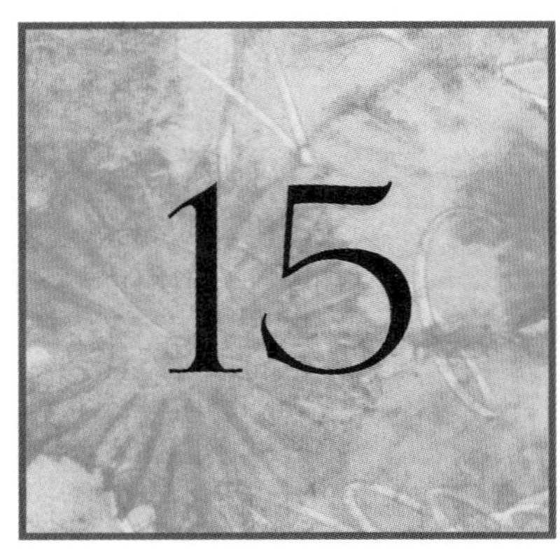

CHAPTER

Defense Mechanisms of the Gingiva

Jaime Bulkacz and Fermin A. Carranza

CHAPTER OUTLINE

The gingival tissue is constantly subjected to mechanical and bacterial aggressions. The saliva, the epithelial surface, and the initial stages of the inflammatory response provide resistance to these actions. The role of the epithelium, through its degree of keratinization and turnover rate, were reviewed in Chapter 1. The permeability of the junctional and sulcular epithelia and the role of sulcular fluid, leukocytes, and saliva is described here.

SULCULAR FLUID

The presence of sulcular fluid or gingival crevicular fluid (GCF) has been known since the nineteenth century, but its composition and possible role in oral defense mechanisms were elucidated by the pioneering work of Waerhaug[128] and Brill and Krasse[14] in the 1950s. The latter investigators introduced filter paper into the gingival sulci of dogs that had previously been injected intramuscularly with fluorescein; within 3 minutes the fluorescent material was recovered on the paper strips. This indicated a passage of fluid from the bloodstream through the tissues and exiting via the gingival sulcus.

In subsequent studies, Brill[11,12] confirmed the presence of GCF in humans and considered it a transudate. However, others[74,129] demonstrated that GCF is an inflammatory exudate, not a continuous transudate. In a strictly normal gingiva, little or no fluid can be collected.

More recently, interest in the development of tests for the detection or prediction of periodontal disease has resulted in numerous research papers dealing with the components, origin, and function of GCF.

Methods of Collection

The most difficult hurdle to overcome when collecting GCF is the scarcity of material that can be obtained from the sulcus. Many collection methods have been tried.[10,13,59,63,64,74,76,104,124,125] These methods include the use of absorbing paper strips, twisted threads placed around and into the sulcus, micropipettes, and intracrevicular washings.

The absorbing paper strips are placed within the sulcus (intrasulcular method) or at its entrance (extrasulcular method) (Fig. 15-1). The placement of the filter paper strip in relation to the sulcus or pocket is important. The Brill technique places it into the pocket until resistance is encountered (see Fig. 15-1, *A*). This method introduces a degree of irritation of the sulcular epithelium that can, by itself, trigger the flow of fluid.

To minimize this irritation, Löe and Holm-Pedersen[74] placed the filter paper strip just at the entrance of the pocket or over the pocket entrance (see Fig. 15-1, *B, C*). In this way, fluid seeping out is picked up by the strip, but the sulcular epithelium is not in contact with the paper.

Preweighed twisted threads were used by Weinstein et al.[129] The threads were placed in the gingival crevice around the tooth, and the amount of fluid collected was estimated by weighing the sample thread.

The use of micropipettes permits the collection of fluid by capillarity. Capillary tubes of standardized length and diameter are placed in the pocket, and their content is later centrifuged and analyzed.[10,12,13]

Crevicular washings can be used to study GCF from clinically normal gingiva. One method uses an appliance consisting of a hard acrylic plate covering the maxilla with soft borders and a groove following the gingival margins; it is connected to four collection tubes. The washings are obtained by rinsing the crevicular areas from one side to the other, using a peristaltic pump.[21]

A modification of the method uses two injection needles fitted one within the other such that during sampling the inside, or ejection, needle is at the bottom of the pocket and the outside, or collecting, one is at the gingival margin. The collection needle is drained into a sample tube by continuous suction.[104]

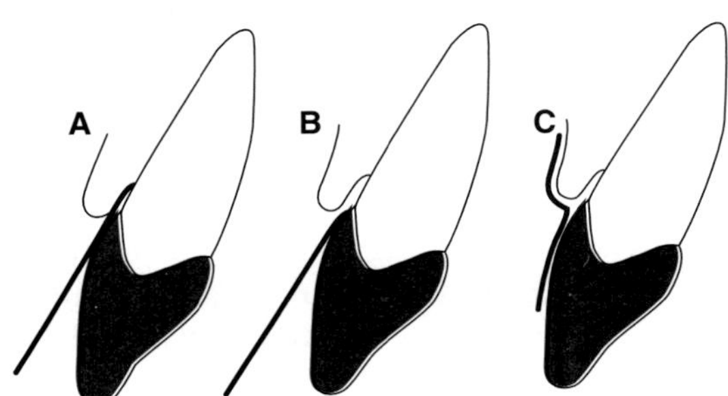

Fig. 15-1 Placement of filter strip in gingival sulcus for collection of fluid. **A,** Intrasulcular method. **B and C,** Extrasulcular methods.

Permeability of Junctional and Sulcular Epithelia

The initial studies by Brill and Krasse[14] with fluorescein were later confirmed with substances such as India ink[97] and saccharated iron oxide.[21] Substances that have been shown to penetrate the sulcular epithelium include albumin,[96,125] endotoxin,[95,100,101,109] thymidine,[49] histamine,[28] phenytoin,[120] and horseradish peroxidase.[80,81] These findings indicate permeability to substances with a molecular weight of up to 1 million.[110]

Squier and Johnson[119] reviewed the mechanisms of penetration through an intact epithelium. Intercellular movement of molecules and ions along intercellular spaces appears to be a possible mechanism. Substances taking this route do not traverse the cell membranes.

Amount

The amount of GCF collected on a paper strip can be evaluated in a variety of ways. The wetted area can be made more visible by staining with ninhydrin; it is then measured planimetrically on an enlarged photograph or with the help of a magnifying glass or a microscope.

An electronic method has been devised for measuring the fluid collected on a "blotter" (Periopaper), employing an electronic transducer (Periotron, Harco Electronics, Winnipeg, Manitoba, Canada) (Fig. 15-2). The wetness of the paper strip affects the flow of an electronic current and gives a digital readout. A comparison of the ninhydrin-staining method and the electronic method performed in vitro revealed no significant differences between the two techniques.[122]

The amount of GCF collected is extremely small. Measurements performed by Cimasoni[21] showed that a strip of paper 1.5-mm wide inserted 1 mm within the gingival sulcus of a slightly inflamed gingiva absorbs about 0.1 mg of GCF in 3 minutes. Challacombe[19] used an isotope dilution method to measure the amount of

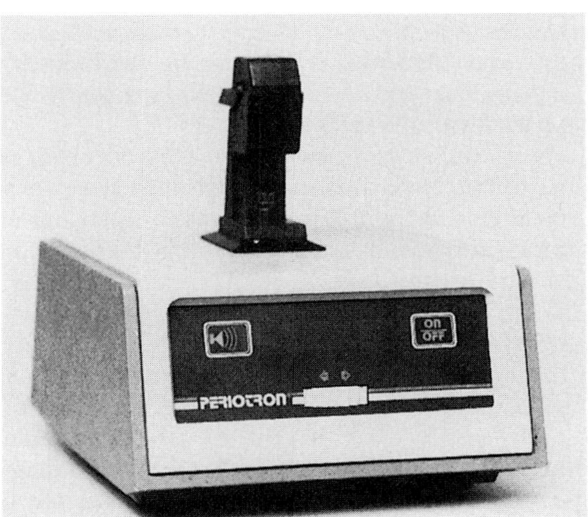

Fig. 15-2 Electronic machine for measuring the amount of fluid collected on filter paper.

BOX 15-1

Enzymes and Other Compounds Reported in Gingival Crevicular Fluid

Compound

Acid phosphatase[40]
Alkaline phosphatase[23]
α1-antitrypsin[2]
α2-macroglobulins[2]
Aryl sulfatase[29]
Aspartate aminotransferase[28]
β-glucuronidase[3,29]
Chrondroitin sulfatase[43]
Citric acid[33]
Cytokines[12,15,34]
  IL-1α
  IL-1β
  IL-6 and -8
IgG, IgA, IgG4, IgM
Cystatins[22]
Endopeptidases:
  Cathepsin D[24]
  Cathepsin B/L[14]
  Cathepsin G[13,14]
  Elastase[13,14]
  Plasminogen activator[20]
  Collagenase[16,32]
  Tryptase-like[14]
  Trypsin-like[14]
Dipeptydilpeptidase IV-like[14]
Elastase-α1 proteinase inhibitor[21]
Exopeptidases[39]
Fibrin[42]
Fibronectin[42]
Glycosidases[4]
  α1-fucosidase
  Sialidase
  B-N-acetylglucosaminidase
  B-galactosidase
  B-mannosidase
Hyaluronidase[44]
Immunoglobulins[18]
Lactate dehydrogenase[29]
Lactoferrin[41]
Lactic acid[30]
Lysozyme[5,41]
Medullasin[27]
Myeloperoxidase[24,25,41]
PGE_2[27,36]
Transferrin[2]
Tromboxane[27,36]

α, alpha; β, beta; *IL,* interleukin; *Ig,* immunoglobulin; *IV,* intravenous; PGE_2, prostaglandin E_2.
References for Box 15-1 are listed at the end of the chapter.

GCF present in a particular space at any given time. His calculations in human volunteers with a mean gingival index of less than 1 showed that the mean GCF volume in proximal spaces from molar teeth ranged from 0.43 to 1.56 μl.

Composition

The components of GCF can be characterized according to individual proteins,[76,87,106] specific antibodies, antigens,[35,94] and enzymes of several specificities.[15] The GCF also contains cellular elements.[28,31,131]

Many research efforts have attempted to use GCF components to detect or diagnose active disease or to predict patients at risk for periodontal disease.[2] So far, more than 40 compounds found in GCF have been analyzed,[91] but their origin is not known with certainty. These compounds can be host derived or produced by the bacteria in the gingival crevice, but their source can be hard to elucidate. Examples of this are X-β-glucuronidase, a lysosomal enzyme and lactic acid dehydrogenase, a cytoplasmic enzyme. The source for collagenases can be fibroblasts or polymorphonuclear neutrophils (PMNs),[89] or collagenases can be secreted by bacteria.[35] Phospholipases are lysosomal and cytoplasmic enzymes but are also produced by microorganisms.[15] The majority of GCF elements detected thus far have been enzymes, but there are nonenzymatic substances as well (Box 15-1).

BOX 15-2

Compounds and Enzymes of Possible Bacterial Origin Detected in Gingival Crevicular Fluid

Product

Acid phosphatase[37,38]
Alkaline phosphatase[15]
Aminopeptidases[31]
β lactamase[37,38]
Chondroitin-sulfatase[45]
Chymotrypsin-like[46]
Collagenase[17,31]
Dipeptidyl-aminopeptidase IV-like[1]
DNase[37]
Fibrinolysin[14,35]
Glucosidases[37]
Hemolysin[11]
Hyaluronidase[44]
Iminopeptidases[5]
Immunoglobulinases[19,26]
Lysophospholipase[6,7]
Phospholipase A[6]
Phospholipase C[8,9]
Prostaglandin-like[10]
Trypsinlike enzyme[37,39]

References for Box 15-2 are listed at the end of the chapter.

Cellular Elements. Cellular elements found in GCF include bacteria, desquamated epithelial cells, and leukocytes (PMNs, lymphocytes, and monocytes/macrophages), which migrate through the sulcular epithelium.[28,31]

Electrolytes. Potassium, sodium, and calcium have been studied in GCF. Most studies have shown a positive correlation of calcium and sodium concentrations and the sodium-to-potassium ratio with inflammation.[56–58,63] (For further information, see references 12 and 13 and Box 15-2.)

Organic Compounds. Both carbohydrates and proteins have been investigated. Glucose hexosamine and hexuronic acid are two of the compounds found in GCF.[47] Blood glucose levels do not correlate with GCF glucose levels; glucose concentration in GCF is three to four times greater than that in serum.[47] This is interpreted not only as a result of metabolic activity of adjacent tissues, but also as a function of the local microbial flora.

The total protein content of GCF is much less than that of serum.[13,14] No significant correlations have been found between the concentration of proteins in GCF and the severity of gingivitis, pocket depth, or extent of bone loss.[7]

Metabolic and bacterial products identified in GCF include lactic acid,[48] urea,[42] hydroxyproline,[93] endotoxins,[114,115] cytotoxic substances, hydrogen sulphide,[118] and antibacterial factors.[27] Many enzymes have also been identified (see Boxes 15-1 and 15-2).

The methodology used for the analysis of GCF components is as varied as the diversity of those components. A few examples suffice, such as fluorometry for the detection of metalloproteases[28]; enzyme-linked immunoabsorbent assay (ELISA) tests to detect enzyme levels and interleukin-1beta (IL-1β)[69]; radio-immunoassays to detect cyclooxygenase derivatives[88] and procollagen III[123]; timidazole detected by high-pressure liquid chromatography (HPLC)[68]; acute phase proteins detected by direct and indirect immunodots[113]; and others.

Cellular and Humoral Activity in Gingival Crevicular Fluid

Monitoring periodontal disease is a complicated task, because there are very few noninvasive procedures that can follow the initiation and progress of the disease. Analysis of GCF constituents in health and disease may be extremely useful because of GCF's simplicity and the fact that it can be obtained with noninvasive methods.

Analysis of GCF has identified cell and humoral responses in both healthy individuals and those with periodontal disease.[66] The cellular immune response includes the appearance in GCF of cytokines (see Box 15-1), but there is no clear evidence of a relationship between them and disease. However, interleukin-1alpha (IL-1α) and IL-1β are known to increase the binding of PMNs and monocytes/macrophages to endothelial cells, stimulate the production of prostaglandin (PGE_2) and release of lysosomal enzymes, and stimulate bone resorption.[69] There is also preliminary evidence of the presence of interferon-α in GCF,[66] which may have a protective role in periodontal disease because of its ability to inhibit the bone resorption activity of IL-1β.[44]

Because the amount of fluid recoverable from gingival crevices is small, only the use of very sensitive immunoassays permits the analysis of the specificity of antibodies.[27] A study comparing antibodies in different crevices with serum antibodies directed at specific microorganisms did not provide any conclusive evidence about the significance of the antibody presence in GCF in periodontal disease.[66]

Even though the role of antibodies in the gingival defense mechanisms is hard to ascertain, there is a consensus indicating that in a patient with periodontal disease, (1) a reduction in antibody response is detrimental and (2) an antibody response plays a protective role in periodontal disease.[65]

Clinical Significance

As mentioned previously, GCF is an inflammatory exudate.[74] Its presence in clinically normal sulci can be explained by the fact that gingiva that appears clinically normal invariably exhibits inflammation when examined microscopically.

The amount of GCF is greater when inflammation is present[34,111] and is sometimes proportional to the severity of inflammation.[90] GCF production is not increased by trauma from occlusion[79] but is increased by mastication of coarse foods, toothbrushing and gingival massage, ovulation,[71] hormonal contraceptives,[72] and smoking.[82] Other factors that influence the amount of GCF are circadian periodicity and periodontal therapy.

Circadian Periodicity. There is a gradual increase in GCF amount from 6 AM to 10 PM and a decrease afterward.[9]

Sex Hormones. Female sex hormones increase GCF flow, probably because they enhance vascular permeability.[69] Pregnancy, ovulation,[68] and hormonal contraceptives[70] all increase gingival fluid production.

Mechanical Stimulation. Chewing[12] and vigorous gingival brushing stimulate the flow of GCF. Even the minor stimuli represented by intrasulcular placement of paper strips increases the production of fluid.

Smoking. Smoking produces an immediate transient but marked increase in GCF flow.[82]

Periodontal Therapy. There is an increase in GCF production during the healing period after periodontal surgery.[3]

Drugs in Gingival Crevicular Fluid

Drugs that are excreted through the GCF may be used advantageously in periodontal therapy. Bader and Goldhaber[6] demonstrated in dogs that tetracyclines are excreted through the GCF; this finding triggered extensive research that demonstrated a concentration of tetracycline's in GCF when compared with serum.[43] Metronidazole is another antibiotic that has been detected in human GCF[32] (see Chapter 50).

LEUKOCYTES IN THE DENTOGINGIVAL AREA

Leukocytes have been found in clinically healthy gingival sulci in humans and experimental animals. The leukocytes found are predominantly PMNs. They appear in small numbers extravascularly in the connective tissue adjacent to the bottom of the sulcus; from there, they travel across the epithelium[18,45] to the gingival sulcus, where they are expelled (Figs. 15-3 and 15-4).

Leukocytes are present in sulci even when histologic sections of adjacent tissue are free of inflammatory infiltrate. Differential counts of leukocytes from clinically

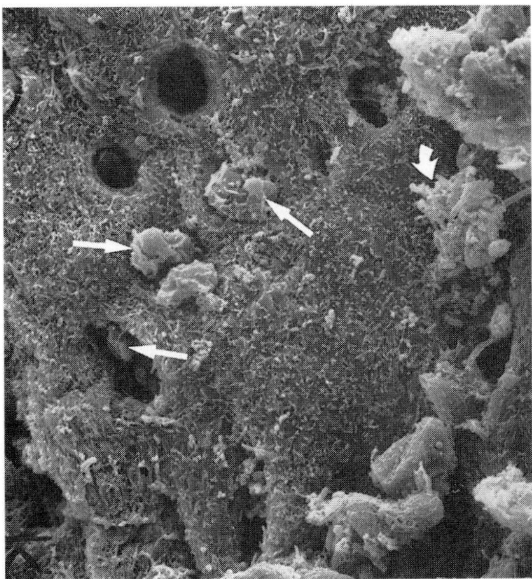

Fig. 15-3 Scanning electron microscope view of periodontal pocket wall. Several leukocytes are emerging *(straight arrows)*, some partially covered by bacteria *(curved arrow)*. Empty holes correspond to tunnels through which leukocytes have emerged.

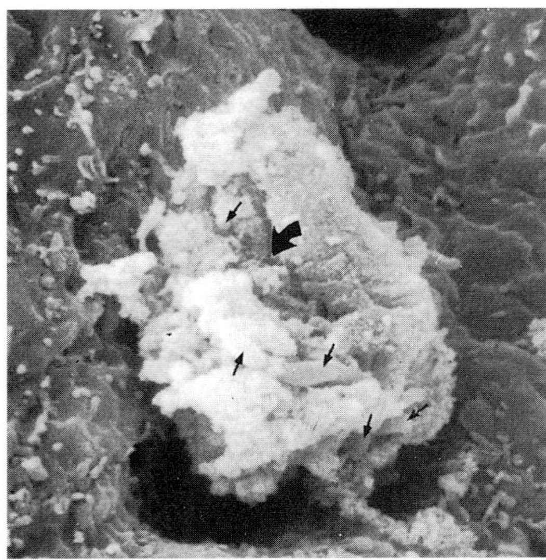

Fig. 15-4 Scanning electron microscope view at higher magnification than Fig. 15-3. A leukocyte emerging from the pocket wall is covered with bacteria *(small arrows)*. The large curved arrow points to a phagosomal vacuole through which bacteria are being engulfed.

healthy human gingival sulci have shown 91.2% to 91.5% PMNs and 8.5% to 8.8% mononuclear cells.[117,131]

Mononuclear cells were identified as 58% B lymphocytes, 24% T lymphocytes, and 18% mononuclear phagocytes. The ratio of T lymphocytes to B lymphocytes was found to be reversed from the normal ratio of about 3:1 found in peripheral blood to about 1:3 in GCF.[131]

Leukocytes are attracted by different plaque bacteria[54,130] but can also be found in the dentogingival region of germ-free adult animals.[75,103] Leukocytes were reported in the gingival sulcus in nonmechanically irritated (resting) healthy gingiva, indicating that their migration may be independent of an increase in vascular permeability.[5,124] The majority of these cells are viable and have been found to have phagocytic and killing capacity.[62,92,98] Therefore they constitute a major protective mechanism against the extension of plaque into the gingival sulcus.

Leukocytes are also found in saliva (see following discussion). The main port of entry of leukocytes into the oral cavity is the gingival sulcus.[107]

SALIVA

Salivary secretions are protective in nature because they maintain the oral tissues in a physiologic state (Table 15-1). Saliva exerts a major influence on plaque by mechanically cleansing the exposed oral surfaces, by buffering acids produced by bacteria, and by controlling bacterial activity.

Antibacterial Factors

Saliva contains numerous inorganic and organic factors that influence bacteria and their products in the oral environment. Inorganic factors include ions and gases, bicarbonate, sodium, potassium, phosphates, calcium, fluorides, ammonium, and carbon dioxide. Organic factors include lysozyme, lactoferrin, myeloperoxidase, lactoperoxidase, and agglutinins such as glycoproteins, mucins, β2-macroglobulins, fibronectins,[123] and antibodies.

Lysozyme is a hydrolytic enzyme that cleaves the linkage between structural components of the glycopeptide muramic acid-containing region of the cell wall of certain bacteria in vitro. Lysozyme works on both gram-negative and gram-positive organisms[50]; *Veillonella* species and *Actinobacillus actinomycetemcomitans* are some of their targets. It probably repels certain transient bacterial invaders of the mouth.[53]

The lactoperoxidase-thiocyanate system in saliva has been shown to be bactericidal to some strains of *Lactobacillus* and *Streptococcus*[84,102] by preventing the accumulation of lysine and glutamic acid, both of which are essential for bacterial growth. Another antibacterial finding includes lactoferrin, which is effective against *Actinobacillus* species.[55]

Myeloperoxidase, an enzyme similar to salivary peroxidase, is released by leukocytes and is bactericidal for *Actinobacillus*[83] but has the added effect of inhibiting the attachment of *Actinomyces* strains to hydroxyapatite.[16]

Salivary Antibodies

Saliva, like GCF, contains antibodies that are reactive with indigenous oral bacterial species. Although immunoglobulins G (IgG) and M (IgM) are present, the preponderant immunoglobulin found in saliva is immunoglobulin A (IgA). However, IgG is more prevalent in GCF.[121] Major and minor salivary glands contribute all the secretory IgA (sIgA) and lesser amounts of IgG and IgM. GCF contributes most of the IgG, complement, and PMN that, in conjunction with IgG or IgM, inactivate or opsonize bacteria.

TABLE 15-1

Role of Saliva in Oral Health

Function	Salivary Components	Probable Mechanism
Lubrication	Glycoproteins, mucoids	Coating similar to gastric mucin
Physical protection	Glycoproteins, mucoids	Coating similar to gastric mucin
Cleansing	Physical flow	Clearance of debris and bacteria
Buffering	Bicarbonate and phosphate	Antacids
Tooth integrity maintenance	Minerals	Maturation, remineralization
	Glycoprotein pellicle	Mechanical protection
Antibacterial action	IgA	Control of bacterial colonization
	Lysozyme	Breaks bacterial cell walls
	Lactoperoxidase	Oxidation of susceptible bacteria

Salivary antibodies appear to be synthesized locally, for they react with strains of bacteria indigenous to the mouth but not with organisms characteristic of the intestinal tract.[36,38] Many bacteria found in saliva have been shown to be coated with IgA, and the bacterial deposits on teeth contain both IgA and IgG in quantities greater than 1% of their dry weight.[37] It has been shown that IgA antibodies present in parotid saliva can inhibit the attachment of oral *Streptococcus* species to epithelial cells.[33,128] Gibbons and colleagues[36–38] suggested that antibodies in secretions may impair the ability of bacteria to attach to mucosal or dental surfaces.

The enzymes normally found in the saliva are derived from the salivary glands, bacteria, leukocytes, oral tissues, and ingested substances; the major enzyme is parotid amylase. Certain salivary enzymes have been reported in increased concentrations in periodontal disease; these are hyaluronidase and lipase,[17] β-glucuronidase and chondroitin sulfatase,[41] amino acid decarboxylases,[41] catalase, peroxidase, and collagenase.[60]

Proteolytic enzymes in the saliva are generated by both the host and oral bacteria. These enzymes have been recognized as contributors to the initiation and progression of periodontal disease.[49,78] To combat these enzymes, saliva contains antiproteases that inhibit cysteine proteases such as cathepsins[51] and antileucoproteases that inhibit elastase.[89] Another antiprotease identified as a tissue inhibitor of matrix metalloproteinase (TIMP) has been shown to inhibit the activity of collagen-degrading enzymes.[26]

High-molecular-weight mucinous glycoproteins in saliva bind specifically to many plaque-forming bacteria. The glycoprotein-bacteria interactions facilitate bacterial accumulation on the exposed tooth surface.[33,36–38,130] The specificity of these interactions has been demonstrated. The interbacterial matrix of human plaque appears to contain polymers similar to salivary glycoproteins that may aid in maintaining the integrity of plaque. In addition, these glycoproteins selectively adsorb to the hydroxyapatite to make up part of the acquired pellicle. Other salivary glycoproteins inhibit the sorption of some bacteria to the tooth surface and to epithelial cells of the oral mucosa. This activity appears to be associated with the glycoproteins that possess blood group reactivity.[1,33,36,38,128] Another effect of mucin is the deletion of bacterial cells from the oral cavity by aggregation with mucin-rich films.

Glycoproteins and a glycolipid present on mammalian cell surfaces appear to serve as receptors for the attachment of some viruses and bacteria. Thus the close similarity between glycoproteins of salivary secretions and components of the epithelial cell surface suggests that the secretions can competitively inhibit antigen sorption and therefore may limit pathologic alterations.

Salivary Buffers and Coagulation Factors

The maintenance of physiologic hydrogen ion concentration (pH) at the mucosal epithelial cell surface and the tooth surface is an important function of salivary buffers. Their primary effect has been studied in relationship to dental caries. In saliva the most important salivary buffer is the bicarbonate-carbonic acid system.[77]

Saliva also contains coagulation factors (factors VIII, IX, and X; plasma thromboplastin antecedent [PTA]; and the Hageman factor) that hasten blood coagulation and protect wounds from bacterial invasion.[67] The presence of an active fibrinolytic enzyme has also been suggested.

Leukocytes

In addition to desquamated epithelial cells, the saliva contains all forms of leukocytes, of which the principal cells are PMNs. The number of PMNs varies from person to person at different times of the day and is increased in gingivitis. PMNs reach the oral cavity by migrating through the lining of the gingival sulcus. Living PMNs in saliva are sometimes referred to as *orogranulocytes,* and their rate of migration into the oral cavity is termed the *orogranulocytic migratory rate.* Some investigators think that the rate of migration is correlated with the severity of gingival inflammation and is therefore a reliable index for assessing gingivitis.[117]

Role in Periodontal Pathology

Saliva exerts a major influence on plaque initiation, maturation, and metabolism. Salivary flow and composition also influence calculus formation, periodontal disease, and caries. The removal of the salivary glands in experimental animals significantly increases the incidence of dental caries[39] and periodontal disease[46] and delays wound healing.[112]

In humans, an increase in inflammatory gingival diseases, dental caries, and rapid tooth destruction associated with cervical or cemental caries is partially a consequence of decreased salivary gland secretion (xerostomia). Xerostomia may result from a variety of factors, among them sialolithiasis, sarcoidosis, Sjogren's syndrome, Mikulicz's disease, irradiation, and surgical removal of the salivary glands (see Chapters 38 and 39).

REFERENCES

1. Adinolfi M, Mollison PL, Polley MJ, et al: A blood group antibodies. J Exp Med 1966; 123:951.
2. Armitage G: Diagnostic tests for periodontal diseases. Curr Opinion Dent 1992; 2:53.
3. Arnold R, Lunstad, G, Bissada, N, et al: Alterations in crevicular fluid flow during healing following gingival surgery. J Periodont Res 1966; 1:303.
4. Attstrom R: Presence of leukocytes in the crevices of healthy and clinically inflamed gingiva. J Periodontol 1970; 5:42.
5. Attstrom R, Egelberg J: Emigration of blood neutrophils and monocytes into the gingival crevices. J Periodont Res 1970; 5:48.
6. Bader HJ, Goldhaber P: The passage of intravenously administered tetracycline in the gingival sulcus of dogs. J Oral Ther 1966; 2:324.
7. Bang J, Cimasoni G: Total protein in human crevicular fluid. J Dent Res 1971; 50:1683.
8. Birkedal-Hansen H, Taylor RE, Zambon JJ, et al: Characterization of collagenolytic activity from strains of Bacteroides gingivalis. J Periodont Res 1988; 23:258.
9. Bissada NF, Schaffer EM, Haus E: Circadian periodicity of human crevicular fluid. J Periodontol 1967; 38:36.
10. Bjorn HL, Koch G, Lindhe J: Evaluation of gingival fluid measurements. Odont Rev 1965; 16:300.
11. Brill N: The gingival pocket fluid. Studies of its occurrence, composition and effect. Acta Odont Scand 1969; 20(suppl 32):159.
12. Brill N: Effect of chewing on flow of tissue fluid into gingival pockets. Acta Odontol Scand 1959; 17:277.
13. Brill N, Bronnestam R: Immunoelectrophoretic study of tissue fluid from gingival pockets. Acta Odontol Scand 1960; 18:95.

14. Brill N, Krasse B: The passage of tissue fluid into the clinically healthy gingival pocket. Acta Odontol Scand 1958; 16:223.
15. Bulkacz J: Enzymatic activities in gingival fluid with special emphasis on phospholipases. J Western Soc Periodont 1986; 36:145.
16. Camargo PM de, Miyasaki KT, Wolinsky LE: Host modulation of adherence: The effect of human neutrophil myeloperoxidase on the attachment of *Actinomyces viscosus* and *naeslundii* to saliva coated hydroxyapatite. J Periodont Res 1988; 23:334.
17. Carlsson J, Egelberg J: Local effect of diet on plaque formation and development of gingivitis in dogs. II. Effect of high carbohydrate versus high protein/fat diets. Odont Rev 1965; 16:42.
18. Cattoni M: Lymphocytes in the epithelium of healthy gingiva. J Dent Res 1951; 30:627.
19. Challacombe SJ: Passage of serum immunoglobulin into the oral cavity. In Lehner, T, Cimasoni, G (eds): Borderland between Caries and Periodontal Disease, vol 2. London, Academic Press, 1980.
20. Cimasoni G: The crevicular fluid. In Myers H (ed): Monographs in Oral Science, vol 3. Basel, S Karger, 1974.
21. Cimasoni G: Crevicular fluid updated. In Myers H (ed): Monographs in Oral Science, vol 12. Basel, S Karger, 1983.
22. Cobb CM, Brown LR: The effects of exudate from the periodontal pocket on cell culture. Periodontics 1967; 5:5.
23. Dawes C: The chemistry and physiology of saliva. In Shaw JH, Sweeney EA, Cappuccino CC, et al (eds): Textbook of Oral Biology. Philadelphia, Saunders, 1978.
24. Dawes C, Jenkins GM, Tonge CH: The nomenclature of the integuments of the enamel surface of teeth. Br Dent J 1963; 115:65.
25. Dinarello CA: Interleukin-1 and its biologically related cytokines. In Cohen S (ed): Lymphokines and the Immune Response. Boca Raton, FL, CRC Press, 1990.
26. Drouin L, Overall CM, Sodek J: Identification of matrix metallo-endoproteinase inhibitor (TIMP) in human parotid and submandibular saliva: partial purification and characterization. J Periodont Res 1988; 23:370.
27. Ebersole JL, Taubman MA, Smith DJ: Gingival crevicular fluid antibody to oral microorganisms. II. Distribution and specificity of local antibody responses. J Periodont Res 1985; 20:349.
28. Egelberg J: Cellular elements in gingival pocket fluid. Acta Odontol Scand 1963; 21:283.
29. Egelberg J: Gingival exudate measurements for evaluation of inflammatory changes of the gingiva. Odont Rev 1964; 15:381.
30. Egelberg J: Permeability of the dentogingival vessels. II. Clinically healthy gingiva. J Periodont Res 1966; 1:276.
31. Egelberg J, Attstrom R: Presence of leukocytes within crevices of healthy and inflamed gingiva and their immigration from the blood. J Periodont Res 1969; (suppl 4):23.
32. Eisenberg L, Suchow R, Coles RS, et al: The effects of metronidazole administration on clinical and microbiologic parameters of periodontal disease. Clin Prevent Dent 1991; 13:28.
33. Ellen RP, Gibbons RJ: Protein associated adherence of Streptococcus pyogenes to epithelial surfaces: Prerequisite for virulence. Infect Immun 1972; 5:826.
34. Garnick JJ, Pearson R, Harrell D: The evaluation of the Periotron. J Periodontol 1979; 50:424.
35. Genco RJ, Zambon JJ, Murray PA: Serum and gingival fluid antibodies as an adjunct in the diagnosis of *Actinobacillus actinomycetemcomitans*–associated periodontal disease. J Periodontol 1985; 56:41.
36. Gibbons RJ, van Houte J: Selective bacterial adherence to oral epithelial surfaces and its role as an ecological determinant. Infect Immun 1971; 3:567.
37. Gibbons RJ, van Houte J: On the formation of dental plaques. J Periodontol 1973; 44:347.
38. Gibbons RJ, van Houte J, Liljemark WF: Some parameters that effect the adherence of S. salivarius to oral epithelial surfaces. J Dent Res 1972; 51:424.
39. Gilda JE, Keyes PH: Increased dental caries activity in the Syrian hamster following desalivation. Proc Soc Exp Biol Med 1947; 66:28.
40. Glas JE, Krasse B: Biophysical studies on dental calculus from germ-free and conventional rats. Acta Odontol Scand 1962; 20:127.
41. Gochman N, Meyer RK, Blackwell RQ, et al: The amino acid decarboxylase of salivary sediment. J Dent Res 1959; 38:998.
42. Golub LM, Borden SM, Kleinberg K: Urea content of gingival crevicular fluid and its relation to periodontal disease in humans. J Periodont Res 1971; 6:243.
43. Gordon JM, Walker CB, Goodson JM, et al: Sensitive assay for measuring tetracycline levels in gingival crevice fluid. Antimicrob Agents Chemother 1980; 17:193.
44. Gowan M, Mundy GR: Actions of recombinant interleukin 1, interleukin 2 and interferon-gamma on bone resorption. In vitro. J Immunol 1986; 136:2478.
45. Grant DA, Orban BJ: Leukocytes in the epithelial attachment. J Periodontol 1960; 31:87.
46. Gupta OH, Blechman H, Stahl SS: The effects of desalivation on periodontal tissues of the Syrian hamster. Oral Surg 1960; 13:470.
47. Hara K, Löe H: Carbohydrate components of the gingival exudate. J Periodont Res 1969; 4:202.
48. Hasegawa K: Biochemical study of gingival fluid. Lactic acid in gingival fluid. Bull Tokyo Med Dent Univ 1967; 14:359.
49. Holt SC, Bramanti TE: Factors in virulence expression and their role on periodontal disease pathogenesis. Crit Rev Oral Biol Med 1991; 2:177.
50. Iacono VC, Bolot PR, Mackay JB, et al: Lytic sensitivity of Actinobacillus actinomycetemcomitans to lysozyme. Infect Immun 1983; 40:773.
51. Isemura S, Ando K, Nakashizoka T, et al: Cystatin S: A cysteinproteinase inhibitor of human saliva. J Biochem 1984; 96:1311.
52. Jensen RL, Folke LEA: The passage of exogenous tritiated thymidine into gingival tissues. J Periodontol 1974; 45:786.
53. Jolles P, Petit JF: Purification and analysis of human saliva lysozyme. Nature 1963; 200:168.
54. Kahnberg KE, Lindhe J, Helden J: Initial gingivitis induced by topical application of plaque extract. A histometric study in dogs with normal gingiva. J Periodont Res 1976; 11:218.
55. Kalmar JP, Arnold RP: Killing of Actinobacillus actin-omycetemcomitans by human lactoferrin. Infect Immun 1988; 56:2552.
56. Kaslick RS, Mandel ID, Chasens AJ, et al: Concentration of inorganic ions in gingival fluid. J Dent Res 1970; 49:887.
57. Kaslick RS, Chasens AI, Mandel ID, et al: Quantitative analysis of sodium, potassium and calcium in gingival fluid from gingiva in varying degrees of inflammation. J Periodontol 1970; 41:93.
58. Kaslick RS, Chasens AI, Mandel ID, et al: Sodium, potassium and calcium in gingival fluid. A study of the relationship of the ions to one another, to circadian rhythms, gingival bleeding, purulence, and to conservative periodontal therapy. J Periodontol 1970; 41:442.
59. Kaslik RS, Chasens AI, Weinstein O, et al: Ultramicromethods for the collection of gingival fluid and quantitative analysis of its sodium content. J Dent Res 1986; 47:1192.
60. King JD: Experimental investigation of periodontal disease in the ferret and in man, with special reference to calculus formation. Dent Pract 1954; 4:157.
61. Kiroshita JJ, Muhlemann HR: Effect of sodium ortho and pyrophosphate on supragingival calculus. Helv Odontol Acta 1966; 10:46.
62. Kowolik MJ, Raeburn JA: Functional integrity of gingival crevicular neutrophil polymorphonuclear leukocytes as demonstrated by nitroblue tetrazolium reduction. J Periodont Res 1980; 15:483.
63. Krasse B, Egelberg J: The relative proportions of sodium, potassium and calcium in gingival pocket fluid. Acta Odontol Scand 1962; 20:143.
64. Krekeler G: Quantitative determination of the gingival sulcus fluid by means of microcapillaries. Dtsch Zahnaertzl Z 1975; 30:544.
65. Lamster IB, Celenti R, Ebersole J: The relationship of serum IgG antibody titers to periodontal pathogens to indicators of the host response in gingival crevicular fluid. J Clin Periodontol 1990; 17:419.
66. Lamster IB, Novak MJ: Host mediators in gingival crevicular fluid: Implications for the pathogenesis of periodontal disease. Crit Rev Oral Biol Med 1992; 3:31.
67. Leung SW, Jensen AT: Factors controlling the deposition of calculus. Int Dent J 1958; 8:613.
68. Liew V, Mack G, Tseng P, et al: Single-dose concentrations of timidazole in gingival crevicular fluid, serum and gingival tissue in adults with periodontitis. J Dent Res 1991; 70:910.
69. Life JS, Johnson NW, Powell JR, et al: Interleukin-1 beta (IL-1b) levels in gingival crevicular fluid from adults without previous evidence of destructive periodontitis. A cross sectional study. J Clin Periodontol 1992; 19:53.

70. Lindhe J, Attstrom R: Gingival exudation during the menstrual cycle. J Periodont Res 1967; 2:194.
71. Lindhe J, Attstrom R, Bjorn AL: Influence of sex hormones on gingival exudate of gingivitis-free female dogs. J Periodont Res 1968; 3:273.
72. Lindhe J, Bjorn AL: Influence of hormonal contraceptives on the gingiva of women. J Periodont Res 1967; 2:1.
73. Lisanti VF: Hydrolytic enzymes in periodontal tissues. Ann NY Acad Sci 1960; 85:461.
74. Löe H, Holm-Pedersen P: Absence and presence of fluid from normal and inflamed gingiva. Periodontics 1965; 3:171.
75. Magnusson B: Mucosal changes at erupting molars in germ-free rats. J Periodont Res 1969; 4:181.
76. Marcus ER, Jooste CP, Driver HS, Hatting J: The quantification of individual proteins in crevicular gingival fluid. J Periodont Res 1985; 20:444.
77. Mandel I: Relation of saliva and plaque to caries. J Dent Res 1974; 53(suppl):246.
78. Mandel ID: Markers of periodontal disease susceptibility and activity derived from saliva. In Johnson NW (ed): Risk Markers of Oral Diseases, vol 3. New York, Cambridge University Press, 1991.
79. Martin LP, Noble WH: Gingival fluid in relation to tooth mobility and occlusal interferences. J Periodontol 1974; 45:444.
80. McDougall WA: Pathways of penetration and effects of horseradish peroxidase in rat molar gingiva. Arch Oral Biol 1970; 15:621.
81. McDougall WA: The effect of topical antigen on the gingiva of sensitized rabbits. J Periodont Res 1974; 9:153.
82. McLaughlin WS, Lovat FM, Macgregor IDM, et al: The immediate effects of smoking on gingival fluid flow. J Clin Periodontol 1993; 20:448.
83. Miyasaki KT, Wilson ME, Genco RJ: Killing of *Actinobacillus actinomycetemcomitans* by the human peroxide chloride system. Infect Immun 1986; 53:161.
84. Muhlemann HR, Schroeder H: Dynamics of supragingival calculus formation. Adv Oral Biol 1964; 1:175.
85. Nagao M: Influence of prosthetic appliances upon the flow of crevicular tissue fluid. I. Relation between crevicular tissue fluid and prosthetic appliances. Bull Tokyo Med Dent Univ 1967; 14:241.
86. Nakamura M, Slots J: Salivary enzymes: origin and relationship to periodontal disease. J Periodont Res 1983; 18:559.
87. Novaes AB Jr, Ruben MP, Kramer GM: Proteins of the gingival exudate: A review and discussion of the literature. J Western Soc Periodontol 1979; 27:12.
88. Offenbacher S, Williams RC, Jeffcoat MK, et al: Effects of NAIDS on beagle crevicular cyclo-oxygenase metabolites and periodontal bone loss. J Periodont Res 1992; 27:207.
89. Ohlsson M, Rosengreen M, Tegner H, et al: Quantification of granulocyte elastase inhibitor in human mixed saliva and in pure parotid secretion. Phys Chem 1983; 364:1323.
90. Orban JE, Stallard RE: Gingival crevicular fluid: A reliable predictor of gingival health? J Periodontol 1969; 40:231.
91. Page RC: Host response tests designed for diagnosing periodontal disease. J Periodontol 1992; 63:356.
92. Passo SA, Tsai CC, McArthur WP, et al: Interaction of inflammatory cells and oral microorganisms. IX. The bacterial effect of human PMN leukocytes on isolated plaque microorganisms. J Periodont Res 1980; 15:470.
93. Paunio K: On the hydroxyproline-containing components in the gingival exudate. J Periodont Res 1971; 6:115.
94. Pollock JJ, Andors L, Gulumoglu A: Direct measurement of hepatitis B virus antibody and antigen markers in gingival crevicular fluid. Oral Surg, Oral Med, Oral Pathol 1984; 57:499.
95. Ranney RR, Montgomery EH: Vascular leakage resulting from topical application of endotoxin to the gingiva of the beagle dog. Arch Oral Biol 1973; 18:963.
96. Ranney RR, Zander HA: Allergic periodontal disease in sensitized squirrel monkeys. J Periodontol 1970; 41:12.
97. Ratcliff P: Permeability of healthy gingival epithelium by microscopically observable particles. J Periodontol 1966; 37:291.
98. Renggli HH: Phagocytosis and killing by crevicular neutrophils. In Lehner T (ed): The Borderland between Caries and Periodontal Disease. New York, Grune and Stratton, 1977.
99. Renggli HH, Regolatti B: Intracrevicular sampling of leukocytes using plastic strips. Helv Odont Acta 1972; 16:93.
100. Rizzo AA: Absorption of bacterial endotoxin into rabbit gingival pocket tissue. Periodontics 1968; 6:65.
101. Rizzo AA: Histologic and immunologic evaluation of antigen penetration with oral tissues after topical application. Periodontics 1970; 41:210.
102. Rosebury R, Karshan M: Salivary Calculus: Dental Science and Dental Art. Philadelphia, Lea & Febiger, 1938.
103. Rovin S, Costich ER, Gordon HA: The influence of bacteria and irritation in the initiation of periodontal disease in germfree and conventional rats. J Periodont Res 1966; 1:193.
104. Salonen JI, Paunio KU: An intracrevicular washing method for collection of intracrevicular contents. Scand J Dent Res 1961; 99:406.
105. Sandalli P, Wade AB: Alterations in crevicular fluid flow during healing following gingivectomy and flap procedures. J Periodont Res 1969; 4:314.
106. Sano K, Nakao M, Shiba A, et al: An ultra-micro assay for proteins in biological fluids other than blood using a combination of agarose gel isoelectric focusing and silver staining. Clin Chim Acta 1984; 137:115.
107. Schiott CR, Löe H: The origin and variation in the number of leukocytes in the human saliva. J Periodont Res 1969; (suppl 4):24.
108. Schultz-Haudt S, Bibby BG, Bruce MA: Tissue destructive products of gingival bacteria from nonspecific gingivitis. J Dent Res 1954; 33:624.
109. Schwartz J, Stinson FL, Parker RB: The passage of tritiated bacterial endotoxin across intact gingival crevicular epithelium. J Periodontol 1972; 43:270.
110. Selvig K: Structure and metabolism of the normal periodontium. Position paper. International Conference on Research in the Biology of Periodontal Disease, Chicago, June 12–15, 1977.
111. Shapiro L, Goldman H, Bloom A: Sulcular exudate flow in gingival inflammation. J Periodontol 1979; 50:301.
112. Shen LS, Ghavamzadeh G, Shklar G: Gingival healing in sialadenectomized rats. J Periodontol 1979; 50:533.
113. Sibraa PD, Reinhardt AA, Dyer JK, et al: Acute-phase protein detection and quantification in gingival crevicular fluid by direct and indirect immuno-dot. J Clin Periodont 1991; 18:101.
114. Simon B, Goldman HM, Ruben MP, et al: The role of endotoxin in periodontal disease. II. Correlation of the amount of endotoxin in human gingival exudate with the clinical degree of inflammation. J Periodontol 1970; 42:81.
115. Simon B, Goldman HM, Ruben MP, et al: The role of endotoxin in periodontal disease. III. Correlation of the amount of endotoxin with the histologic degree of inflammation. J Periodontol 1971; 42:210.
116. Skapski H, Lehner T: A crevicular washing method for investigating immune components of crevicular fluid in man. J Periodont Res 1976; 11:19.
117. Skougaard MR, Bay I, Kilnkhammer JM: Correlation between gingivitis and orogranulocytic migratory rate. J Dent Res 1994; 48:716.
118. Solis Gaffar MC, Rustogi KN, Gaffar A: Hydrogen sulfide production from gingival crevicular fluid. J Periodontol 1980; 51:603.
119. Squier CA, Johnson NW: Permeability of oral mucosa. Br Med Bull 1975; 31:169.
120. Steinberg AD, Steinberg J, Allen P, et al: The effect of alteration in the sulcular environment upon the movement of 14C-diphenylhydantoin through rabbit sulcular tissues. J Periodont Res 1976; 11:47.
121. Sueda T, Bang J, Cimasoni G: Collection of gingival fluid for quantitative analysis. J Dent Res 1969; 48:159.
122. Suppipat W, Suppipat N: Evaluation of an electronic device for gingival fluid quantitation. J Periodontol 1977; 48:388.
123. Talonopoika JT, Hamalainen MM: Collagen III aminoterminal propeptide in gingival crevicular fluid before and after periodontal disease. Scand J Dent Res 1992; 100:107.
124. Theilade J, Egelberg J, Attstrom R: Vascular permeability to colloidal carbon in clinically inflamed gingiva. J Periodont Res 1971; 6:100.
125. Tolo K: Transport across stratified nonkeratinized epithelium. J Periodont Res 1971; 6:237.
126. Tomasi TB, Bienenstock J: Secretory immunoglobulins. Adv Immunol 1968; 9:1.
127. Vogel JJ, Amdur BH: Inorganic pyrophosphate in parotid saliva. Arch Oral Biol 1967; 12:159.

128. Waerhaug J: The gingival pocket. Anatomy, pathology deepening and elimination. Odont Tidskaift 1952; 60(suppl 1):1.
129. Weinstein E, Mandel ID, Salkind A, et al: Studies of gingival fluid. Periodontics 1967, 5:161.
130. Williams RW, Gibbons RG: Inhibition of bacterial adherence by secretory immunoglobulin A: A mechanism of antigen disposal. Science 1972; 177:697.
131. Wilton JMA, Renggli HH, Lehner T: The isolation and identification of mononuclear cells from the gingival crevice in man. J Periodont Res 1976; 11:243.
132. Winkelhoff AJ van, Steenberger TJM van, de Graaff J: The role of black-pigmented Bacteroides in human oral infections. J Clin Periodontol 1988; 15:145.

REFERENCES FOR BOXES 15-1 AND 15-2

1. Abiko Y, Hayakawa M, Murai S, et al: Glycylpropyl dipeptidyl amino-peptidase from *Bacteroides gingivalis.* J Clin Periodontal 1985; 64:106.
2. Adonogianaki E, Mooney J, Kinane DF: The ability of acute gingival crevicular fluid phase proteins to distinguish gingivitis and periodontitis sites. J Clin Periodontol 1992; 19:98.
3. Bang J, Cimasoni G, Held A: Beta glucuronidase correlated with inflammation in the exudate from human gingiva. Arch Oral Biol 1970; 15:45.
4. Beighton D, Radford JR, Naylor MN: Glycosidase activity in gingival crevicular fluid in subjects with adult periodontitis or gingivitis. Arch Oral Biol 1992; 37:43.
5. Brandtzaeg P, Mann WA: A comparative study of the lysozyme activity of human gingival pocket fluid, serum and saliva. Acta Odont Scand 1964; 29:441.
6. Bulkacz J: Enzymatic activities in gingival fluid with special emphasis on phospholipases. J Western Soc Perio 1986; 36:145.
7. Bulkacz J, Erbland JF, MacGregor: Phospholipase activity in supernatants from cultures of *Bacteroides melaninogenicus.* Biochem Biophys Acta 1981; 664:148.
8. Bulkacz J, Erbland JF: Exocellular phospholipase activity from a strain of *Propionibacterium acnes* isolated from a periodontal pocket. J Periodontol 1997; 68:369.
9. Bulkacz J, Garnick J, Barclay JE: Detection of phospholipase activity in crevicular fluid. J Dent Res 1981; 60:abstract #1187.
10. Bulkacz J, Grenett H: Synthesis of prostaglandin-like substances by oral Gram negative rods. J Dent Res 1981; 60:abstract #421.
11. Chu L, Bramanti TE, Holt SC, et al: Hemolytic activity in the periodontopathogen *Porphyromonas gingivalis:* kinectics of enzyme formation and localization. Infec Immun 1991; 59:1932.
12. Chung RM, Grbic JT, Lamster IB: Interleukin-8 and beta- glucuronidase in gingival crevicular fluid. J Clin Periodontol 1997; 24:146.
13. Cimasoni G: Crevicular fluid updated. In Myers H (ed): Monographs in Oral Science, vol 12. Basel, S Karger, 1983.
14. Eley BM, Cox SW: Cathepsin B/L-, elastase-, tryptase-, trypsin- and dipeptidyl peptidase IV-like activities in gingival crevicular fluid: a comparison of levels before and after periodontal surgery in chronic periodontitis patients. J Periodontol 1992; 63:412.
15. Figueiredo CM, Riberio MS, Fischer RG, et al: Increased interleukin-1 beta concentration in gingival crevicular fluid as a characteristic of periodontitis. J Periodontol 1999; 70:1457.
16. Fullmer, HM, Gibson WA: Collagenolytic activity in gingiva in man. Nature 1966; 209:728.
17. Gibbons RJ, MacDonald JB: Degradation of collagenous substrates by *Bacteroides melaninogenicus.* J Bacteriol 1964; 81:614.
18. Grbic JT, Singer RE, Jans HH, et al: Immunoglobulin isotypes in gingival crevicular fluid: possible protective role of IgA. J Periodontol 1995; 66:55.
19. Gregory, RL, Kim DE, Kindel JC, et al: Immunoglobulin-degrading enzymes in localized juvenile periodontitis. J Perio Res 1992; 27:176.
20. Gustaffson GT, Nilsson IM: Fibrinolytic activity in fluid from gingival crevice. Proc Soc Expt Biol Med 1961; 106:277.
21. Huynk C, Roch-Arveiller M, Meyer J, et al: Gingival crevicular fluid of patients with gingivitis or periodontal disease: evaluation of elastase-alpha 1 proteinase inhibitor complexs. J Clin Periodontol 1992; 19:187.
22. Ichimaru E, Imura K, Hara Y, et al: Cystatin activity in gingival crevicular fluid from periodontal disease patients, measured by a new quantitative analysis method. J Perio Res 1992; 27:119.
23. Ishikawa I, Cimasoni G: Alkaline phosphatase in human gingival fluid and its relation to periodontitis. Arch Oral Biol 1970; 15:1401.
24. Ishikawa I, Cimasoni G, Ahmad-Zadeh C: Possible roles of lysosomal enzymes in the pathogenesis of periodontitis: a study in cathepsin D in human gingival fluid. Arch Oral Biol 1972; 17:111.
25. Karhuvaara L, Tenovuo J, Sievers G: Crevicular fluid myeloperoxidase- an indicator of acute gingival inflammation. Proc Finish Dent Soc 1990; 86:3.
26. Killian M: Degradation of immunoglobulins A1, A2, and G by suspected principal peridontal pathogens. Infec Immun 1981; 34:757.
27. Kunamitsu K, Ichimaru E, Kato I, et al: Granulocite medullasin levels in gingival crevicular fluid from chronic adult periodontitis patients and experimental gingivitis subjects. J Perio Res 1990; 25:352.
28. Kuru B, Vilmaz S, Novan U, et al: Microbiological features and crevicular fluid aspartate aminotransferase enzyme activity in early onset periodontitis. J Clin Periodontol 1999; 26:19.
29. Lamster IB, Vogel RI, Hartley LJ, et al: Lactate dehydrogenase, beta-glucuronidase, and arylsulfatase activity in gingival crevicular fluid associated with experimental gingivitis in man. J Periodontol 1985, 56:139.
30. Life JS, Johnson NW, Powell JR, et al; Interleukin-1 beta (IL-1B) levels in gingival crevicular fluid from adults without previous evidence of destructive periodontitis. A cross sectional study. J Clin Periodontol 1992; 19:53.
31. Makinen KK, Syed SA, Löesche WJ, et al: Proteolytic profile of Treponema vincentii ATCC 35580 with special reference to collagenolytic and arginine aminopeptidase activity. Oral Microbiol Immunol 1988; 3:121.
32. Mancini S, Romanelli R, Laschinger CA, et al: Assessment of a novel screening test for neutrophil collagenase activity in the diagnosis of periodontal disease. J Periodontol 1999;70:1292.
33. Miyajima K, Ohmo Y, Iwata T, et al: The lactic lacid and citric acid content in the gingival fluid of orthodontic patients. Aichi-Gakuin Dental Science 1991; 4:75.
34. Mogi M, Otogoto J, Ota N, et al: Interleukin 1 beta, interleukin 6, beta 2-microglobulin, and transforming growth factor-alpha in gingival crevicular fluid from human periodontal disease. Arch Oral Biol 1999; 44:535.
35. Nitzan D, Sperry JF, Wilkins TD: Fibrinolytic activity of oral anaerobic bacteria. Arch Oral Biol 1978; 23:465.
36. Page RC: Host response tests designed for diagnosing periodontal diseases. J Periodontol 1992; 63:356.
37. Slots J: Enzymatic characterization of some oral and non-oral Gram-negative bacteria with the API ZYM system. J Clin Microbiol 1981; 14:288.
38. Slots J, Dahlen G: Subgingival microorganisms and bacterial virulence factors in periodontitis. Scand J Dent Res 1985; 93:119.
39. Smalley J, Birss AJ, Kay HM, et al: The distribution of trypsin-like enzyme activity in cultures of a virulent and an avirulent strain of *Bacteroides gingivalis* W50. Oral Microbiol Immunol 1989; 4:178.
40. Sueda T, Cimasoni G, Held AJ: High levels of acid phosphatase in human crevicular fluid. Arch Oral Biol 1967; 12:1205.
41. Suomalainen K, Saxen L, Vilja P, et al: Peroxidases, lactoferrin and lysozyme in peripheral blood neutrophiles, gingival crevicular fluid and whole saliva in patients with localized juvenile periodontitis. Oral Dis 1996; 2:129.
42. Talonopoika J: Characterization of fibrin(ogen) fragments in gingival crevicular fluid. Scand J Perio Res 1991; 99:40.
43. Tipler LS, Emberg G: Glycosaminoglycan depolimerizing enzymes form oral microorganisms. Arch Oral Biol 1985; 30:391.
44. Tynelius-Brathall G: Hyaluronidase activity in gingival crevicular fluid and in peritoneal exudate leukocytes in dogs. J Perio Res 1972; 7:307.
45. Uito VJ, Degradation of basement membrane collagen by praoteinases from human gingiva, leukocytes and bacterial plaque. J Perio 1983; 54:740.
46. Uito VJ, Grenier D, Chan ECS, et al: Isolation of a chymotrypsin-like enzyme from Treponema denticola. Infec Immun 1988; 56:2717.

Gingival Inflammation

Fermin A. Carranza, John W. Rapley, and Susan Kinder Haake

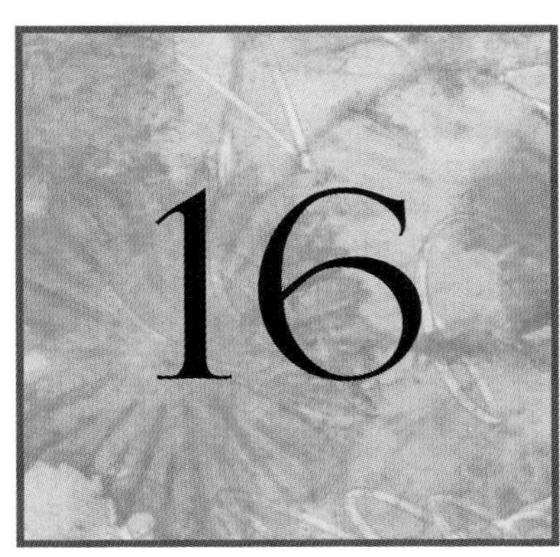

CHAPTER

CHAPTER OUTLINE

Pathologic changes in gingivitis are associated with the presence of oral microorganisms in the gingival sulcus (see Chapter 8). These organisms are capable of synthesizing products (e.g., collagenase, hyaluronidase, protease, chondroitin sulfatase, or endotoxin) that cause damage to epithelial and connective tissue cells, as well as to intercellular constituents, such as collagen, ground substance, and glycocalyx (cell coat). The resultant widening of the spaces between the junctional epithelial cells during early gingivitis may permit injurious agents derived from bacteria, or bacteria themselves, to gain access to the connective tissue.[10,38,42]

Microbial products activate monocytes and macrophages to produce vasoactive substances such as prostaglandin E_2, interferon, tumor necrosis factor, or interleukin-1.[23,32]

The sequence of events in the development of gingivitis occurs in three different stages (Table 16-1).[34] Obviously, one stage evolves into the next, with no clear-cut dividing lines.

STAGE I GINGIVITIS: THE INITIAL LESION

The first manifestations of gingival inflammation are vascular changes consisting essentially of dilation of capillaries and increased blood flow. These initial inflammatory changes occur in response to microbial activation of resident leukocytes and the subsequent stimulation of endothelial cells. Clinically, this initial response of the gingiva to bacterial plaque (**subclinical gingivitis**[25]) is not apparent.

Microscopically, some classic features of acute inflammation can be seen in the connective tissue beneath the junctional epithelium. Changes in blood vessel morphologic features (e.g., widening of small capillaries or venules) and adherence of neutrophils to vessel walls (margination) occur within 1 week and sometimes as early as 2 days after plaque has been allowed to accumulate[18,35] (Fig. 16-1). Leukocytes, mainly polymorphonuclear neutrophils (PMNs), leave the capillaries by migrating through the walls (diapedesis, emigration)[27,37,46] (Fig. 16-2). They can be seen in increased quantities in the connective tissue, the junctional epithelium, and the gingival sulcus (Figs. 16-3 and 16-4).[2,3,24,31,35,39,40] Exudation of fluid from the gingival sulcus[18] and extravascular proteins are present.[20,21]

Subtle changes can also be detected in the junctional epithelium and perivascular connective tissue at this early stage. Lymphocytes soon begin to accumulate (see Fig. 16-2, *D*). The increase in the migration of leukocytes and their accumulation within the gingival sulcus may be correlated with an increase in the flow of gingival fluid into the sulcus.[4]

The character and intensity of the host response determine whether this initial lesion resolves rapidly, with the restoration of the tissue to a normal state, or evolves into a chronic inflammatory lesion. If the latter occurs, an infiltrate of macrophages and lymphoid cells appears within a few days.

TABLE 16-1

Stages of Gingivitis

Stage	Time (Days)	Blood Vessels	Junctional and Sulcular Epithelium	Predominant Immune Cells	Collagen	Clinical Findings
I. Initial Lesion	2–4	Vascular dilation Vasculitis	Infiltrated by PMNs	PMNs	Perivascular loss	Gingival fluid flow
II. Early Lesion	4–7	Vascular proliferation	Same as Stage I Rete peg formation Atrophic areas	Lymphocytes	Increased loss around infiltrate	Erythema Bleeding on probing
III. Established Lesion	14–21	Same as Stage II, plus blood stasis	Same as Stage II but more advanced	Plasma cells	Continued loss	Changes in color, size, texture, etc.

PMNs, Polymorphonuclear neutrophils.

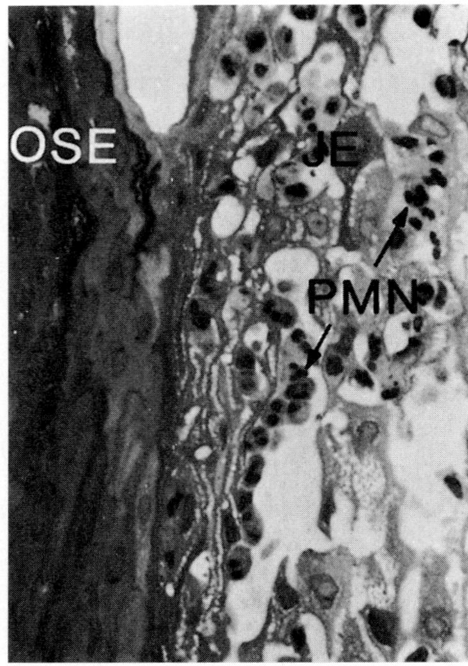

Fig. 16-1 Human biopsy sample, experimental gingivitis. After 4 days of plaque accumulation, the blood vessels immediately adjacent to the junctional epithelium are distended and contain polymorphonuclear neutrophils (PMNs). Neutrophils have also migrated between the cells of the junctional epithelium. *OSE,* oral sulcular epithelium. (Magnification ×500.) (From Payne WA, Page RC, Ogilvie AL, et al: Histopathologic features of the early and initial stages of experimental gingivitis in man. J Periodont Res 1975; 10:51.)

STAGE II GINGIVITIS: THE EARLY LESION

As time goes on, clinical signs of erythema may appear, mainly owing to the proliferation of capillaries and increased formation of capillary loops between rete pegs or ridges. Bleeding on probing may also be evident.[1]

Microscopic examination of the gingiva reveals a leukocyte infiltration in the connective tissue beneath the junctional epithelium, consisting of mainly lymphocytes (75%, with the majority of them T cells)[35,40] but also composed of some migrating neutrophils, as well as macrophages, plasma cells, and mast cells. All the changes seen in the initial lesion continue to intensify.[15,26,29,32,41] The junctional epithelium becomes densely infiltrated with neutrophils, as does the gingival sulcus, and the junctional epithelium may begin to show development of rete pegs or ridges.

There is an increase in the amount of collagen destruction[11,26,41]; 70% of the collagen is destroyed around the cellular infiltrate. The main fiber groups affected appear to be the circular and dentogingival fiber assemblies. Alterations in blood vessel morphologic features and vascular bed patterns have also been described.[18,19]

PMNs that have left the blood vessels in response to chemotactic stimuli from plaque components travel to the epithelium, cross the basement lamina, and are found in the epithelium and are emerging in the pocket area (see Fig. 16-3). PMNs are attracted to bacteria and engulf them in the process of phagocytosis (Fig. 16-5). PMNs release their lysosomes in association with the ingestion of bacteria.[22] Fibroblasts show cytotoxic alterations[34] with a decreased capacity for collagen production.

STAGE III GINGIVITIS: THE ESTABLISHED LESION

In chronic gingivitis (stage III), the blood vessels become engorged and congested, venous return is impaired, and the blood flow becomes sluggish. The result is localized gingival anoxemia, which superimposes a somewhat bluish hue on the reddened gingiva.[17] Extravasation of

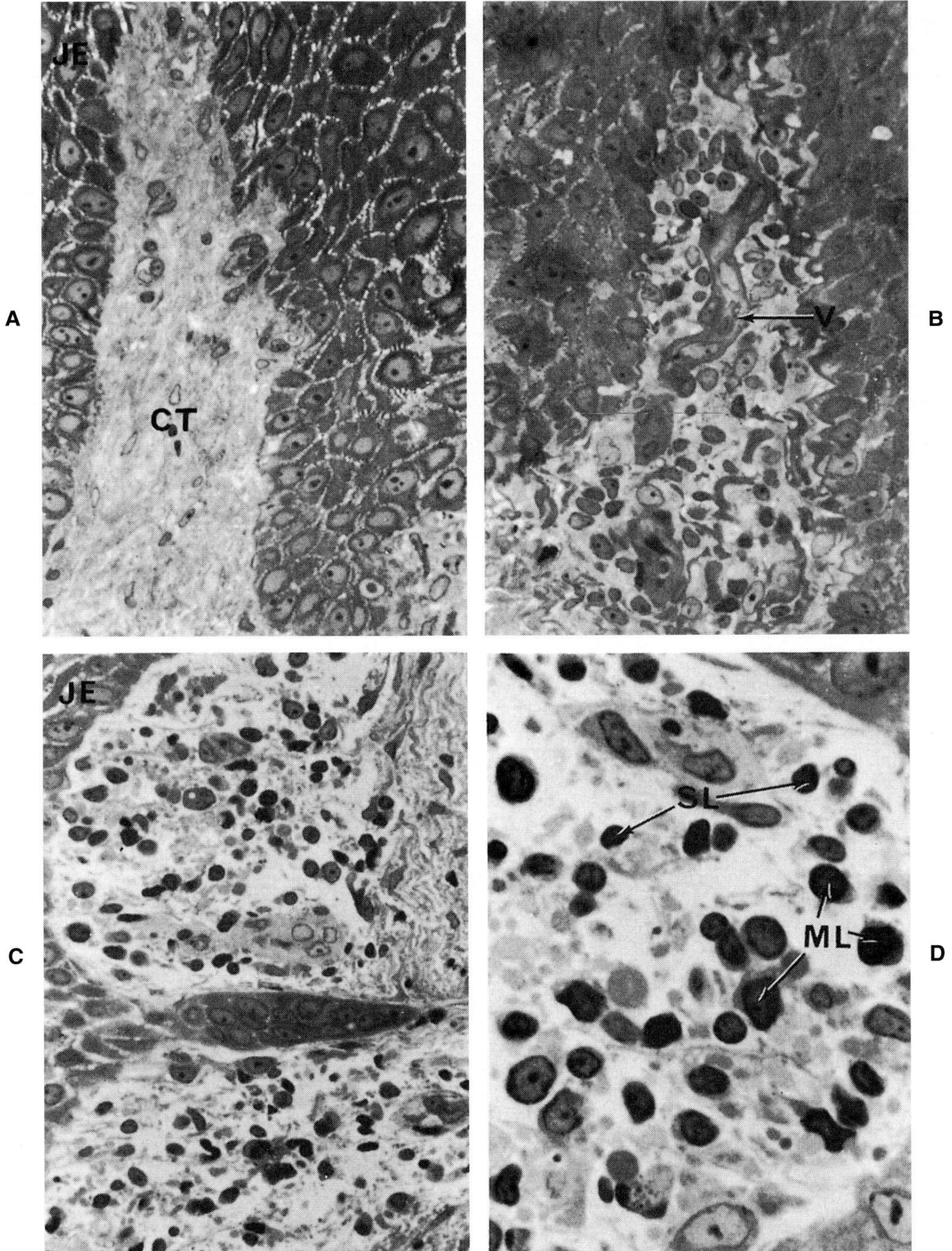

Fig. 16-2 Human biopsy, experimental gingivitis. **A,** Control biopsy specimen from a patient with good oral hygiene and no detectable plaque accumulation. The junctional epithelium is at the left. The connective tissue *(CT)* shows few cells other than fibroblasts, blood vessels, and a dense background of collagen fibers. (Magnification × 500.) **B,** Biopsy specimen taken after 8 days of plaque accumulation. The connective tissue is infiltrated with inflammatory cells, which displace the collagen fibers. A distended blood vessel *(V)* is seen in the center. (Magnification × 500.) **C,** After 8 days of plaque accumulation, the connective tissue next to the junctional epithelium at the base of the sulcus shows a mononuclear cell infiltrate and evidence of collagen degeneration (clear spaces around cellular infiltrate). (Magnification × 500.) **D,** The inflammatory cell infiltrate at higher magnification. After 8 days of plaque accumulation, numerous small- *(SL)* and medium-size *(ML)* lymphocytes are seen within the connective tissue. Most of the collagen fibers around these cells have disappeared, presumably as a result of enzymatic digestion. (Magnification × 1250.) (From Payne WA, Page RC, Ogilvie AL, et al: Histopathologic features of the initial and early stages of experimental gingivitis in man. J Periodont Res 1975; 10:51.)

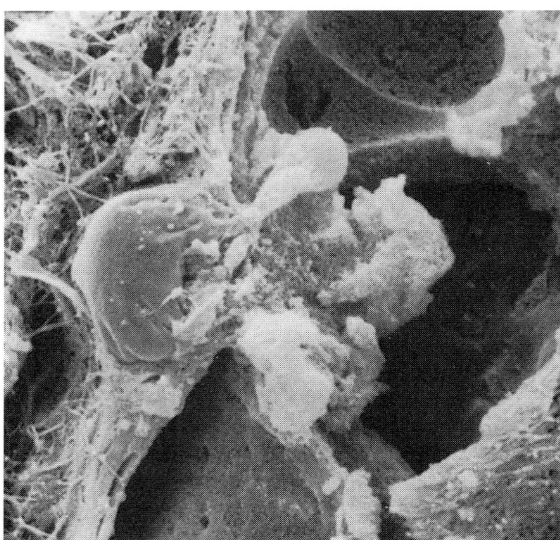

Fig. 16-3 Scanning electron micrograph showing a leukocyte traversing the vessel wall to enter into the gingival connective tissue.

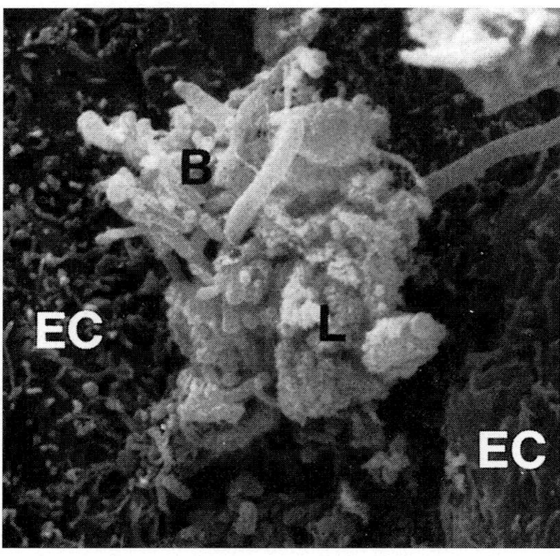

Fig. 16-5 Scanning electron micrograph of leukocyte emerging to pocket wall and covered with bacteria and extracellular lysosomes. *EC,* Epithelial cells.

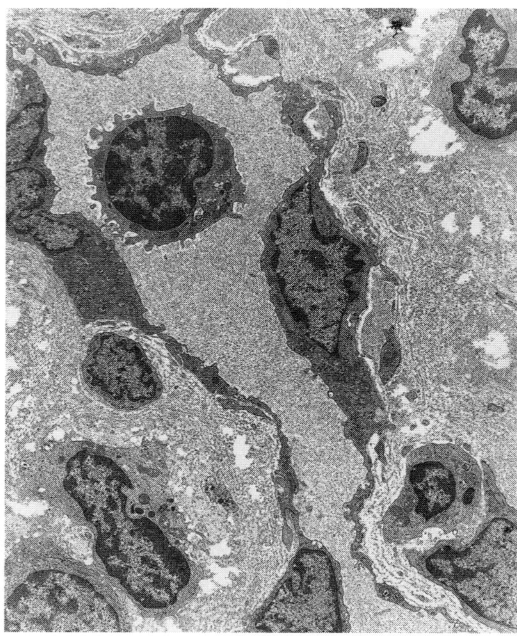

Fig. 16-4 Early human gingivitis lesion. Area of lamina propria subjacent to the crevicular epithelium showing a capillary with several extravascular lymphocytes and one lymphocyte within the lumen. The specimen also exhibits considerable loss of perivascular collagen density. (Magnification ×2500.) (Courtesy Dr. Charles Cobb, Kansas City, Mo.)

red blood cells (RBCs) into the connective tissue and breakdown of hemoglobin into its component pigments can also deepen the color of the chronically inflamed gingiva. The established lesion can be described as moderately to severely inflamed gingiva.

In histologic sections, an intense, chronic inflammatory reaction is observed. Several detailed cytologic studies have been carried out on chronically inflamed gingiva.[12,14,15,33,40,43,45] A key feature that differentiates the established lesion is the increase in the number of plasma cells, which become the preponderant inflammatory cell type. Plasma cells invade the connective tissue not only immediately below the junctional epithelium, but also deep into the connective tissue, around blood vessels, and between bundles of collagen fibers.[6] The junctional epithelium reveals widened intercellular spaces filled with granular cellular debris, including lysosomes derived from disrupted neutrophils, lymphocytes, and monocytes (Fig. 16-6). The lysosomes contain acid hydrolases that can destroy tissue components. The junctional epithelium develops rete pegs or ridges that protrude into the connective tissue, and the basal lamina is destroyed in some areas. In the connective tissue, collagen fibers are destroyed around the infiltrate of intact and disrupted plasma cells, neutrophils, lymphocytes, monocytes, and mast cells (Fig. 16-7).

The predominance of plasma cells is a primary characteristic of the established lesion. However, several studies of human experimental gingivitis have failed to demonstrate plasma cell predominance in the affected connective tissues,[7,8,43] including one study of 6-month duration.[1] Increases in the proportions of plasma cells were evident with long-standing gingivitis,[1] but the time for the development of the classic "established lesion" may exceed 6 months.

An inverse relationship appears to exist between the number of intact collagen bundles and the number of inflammatory cells.[44] Collagenolytic activity is increased

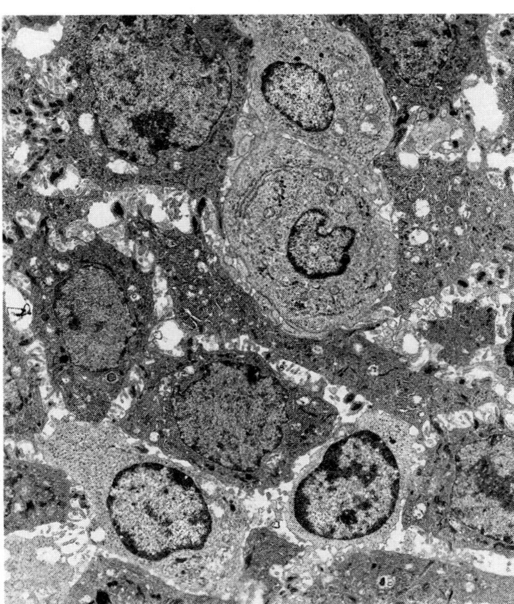

Fig. 16-6 Established gingivitis in a human subject. An area of crevicular epithelium exhibiting enlarged intercellular spaces with numerous microvilli and desmosomal junctions. Several lymphocytes, both small and large, are seen migrating through the epithelial layer. (Magnification ×3000.)

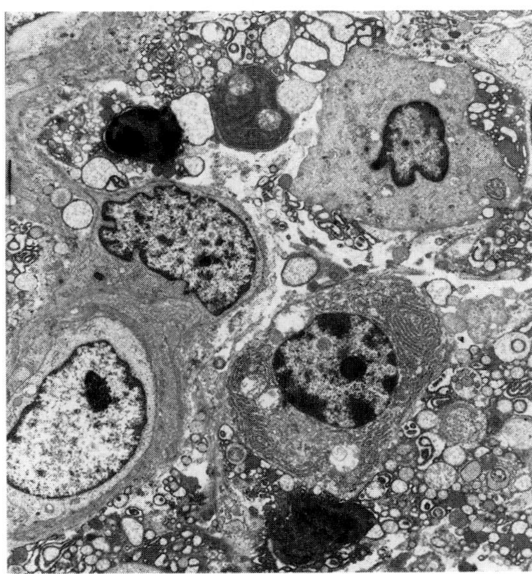

Fig. 16-7 Advanced gingivitis in a human subject. Specimen from the lamina propria exhibiting plasma cell degeneration with abundant cellular debris visible. (Magnification ×3000.) (Courtesy Dr. Charles Cobb, Kansas City, Mo.)

in inflamed gingival tissue[16] by the enzyme collagenase. Collagenase is normally present in gingival tissues[5] and is produced by some oral bacteria and by PMNs.

Enzyme histochemistry studies have shown that chronically inflamed gingiva have elevated levels of acid and alkaline phosphatase,[47] β-glucuronidase, β-glucosidase, β-galactosidase, esterases,[28] aminopeptidase,[30,36] and cytochrome oxidase.[9] Neutral mucopolysaccharide levels are decreased,[45] presumably as a result of degradation of the ground substance.

STAGE IV GINGIVITIS: THE ADVANCED LESION

Extension of the lesion into alveolar bone characterizes a fourth stage known as the *advanced lesion*[33] or *phase of periodontal breakdown*.[26] This is described in detail in Chapters 22 and 23.

REFERENCES

1. Amato R, Caton J, Polson A, Espeland M: Interproximal gingival inflammation related to the conversion of a bleeding to a non-bleeding state. J Periodontol 1986; 57:63.
2. Attström R: Studies on neutrophil polymorphonuclear leukocytes at the dentogingival junction in gingival health and disease. J Periodont Res (Suppl) 1971; 8:6.
3. Attström R: The roles of gingival epithelium and phagocytosing leukocytes in gingival defense. J Clin Periodontol 1975; 2:25.
4. Attström R, Egelberg J: Emigration of blood neutrophils and monocytes into the gingival crevices. J Periodont Res 1970; 5:48.
5. Beutner E H, Triftshauser C, Hazen SP: Collagenase activity of gingival tissue from patients with periodontal disease. Proc Soc Exp Biol Med, 1966; 121:1082.
6. Brecx MC: Histophysiology and histopathology of the gingiva. J West Soc Periodontol 1991; 39:33.
7. Brecx MC, Frohlicher I, Gehr P, et al: Stereological observations on long-term experimental gingivitis in man. J Clin Periodontol 1988; 15:621.
8. Brecx MC, Lehman B, Siegwart CM, et al: Observations on the initial stages of healing following human experimental gingivitis. A clinical and morphological study. J Clin Periodontol 1988; 15:123.
9. Burstone, MS: Histochemical study of cytochrome oxidase in normal and inflamed gingiva. Oral Surg 1960; 13:1501.
10. Caffesse RG, Nasjleti C: Enzymatic penetration through intact sulcular epithelium. J Periodontol 1976; 47:391.
11. Flieder DE, Sun CN: Chemistry of normal and inflamed human gingival tissues. Periodontics 1966; 4:302.
12. Freedman HL, Listgarten MA, Taichman NS: Electron microscopic features of chronically inflamed human gingiva. J Periodont Res 1968; 3:313.
13. Fullmer H, Gibson W: Collagenolytic activity in gingivae of man. Nature 1966; 209:728.
14. Garant PR, Mulvihill JE: The fine structure of gingivitis in the beagle. III. Plasma cell infiltration of the subepithelial connective tissue. J Periodont Res 1971; 7:161.
15. Gavin JR: Ultrastructural features of chronic marginal gingivitis. J Periodont Res 1970; 5:19.
16. Hancock E, Cray R, O'Leary T: The relationship between gingival crevicular inflammation and gingival fluid. A clinical and histologic study. J Periodontol 1979; 50:13.
17. Hanioka T, Shizukuishi S, Tsunemitsu A: Changes in hemoglobin concentration and oxygen saturation in human gingiva with decreasing inflammation. J Periodontol 1991; 62:366.

18. Hock J, Nuki K: A vital microscopy study of the morphology of normal and inflamed gingiva. J Periodont Res 1971; 6:81.
19. Kindlova M: Changes in the vascular bed of the marginal periodontium in periodontitis. J Dent Res 1965; 44:456.
20. Lamster I, Hartley L, Vogel R: Development of a biochemical profile for gingival crevicular fluid. Methodological considerations and evaluation of collagen-degrading and ground substance-degrading enzyme activity during experimental gingivitis. J Periodontol (11 Suppl) 1985; 56:13.
21. Lamster I, Vogel R, Hartley L, et al: Lactate dehydrogenase, β-glucuronidase and arylsulfatase activity in gingival fluid associated with experimental gingivitis in man. J Periodontol 1985; 56:139.
22. Lange D, Schroeder HE: Cytochemistry and ultrastructure of gingival sulcus cells. Helv Odont Acta 15 (Suppl 6) 1971; 65.
23. Lindeman R, Economou J: *Actinobacillus actinomycetemcomitans* and *Bacteroides gingivalis* activate human peripheral monocytes to produce interleukin-1 and tumor necrosis factor. J Periodontol 1988; 59:728.
24. Levy BM, Taylor AC, Bernick S: Relationship between epithelium and connective tissue in gingival inflammation. J Dent Res 1969; 48:625.
25. Lindhe J, Hamp SE, Löe H: Experimental periodontitis in the beagle dog. J Periodont Res 1973; 8:1.
26. Lindhe J, Schroeder HE, Page RC, et al: Clinical and stereologic analysis of the course of early gingivitis in dogs. J Periodont Res 1974; 9:314.
27. Lindhe J, Socransky SS: Chemotaxis and vascular permeability produced by human periodontopathic bacteria. J Periodont Res 1979; 14:138.
28. Lisanti VF: Hydrolytic enzymes in periodontal tissues. Ann NY Acad Sci 1960; 85:461.
29. Listgarten MA, Ellegaard B: Experimental gingivitis in rhesus monkeys. J Periodont Res 1973; 8:199.
30. Mori M, Kishiro A: Histochemical observation of aminopeptidase activity in the normal and inflamed oral epithelium. J Osaka Univ Dent Sch 1961; 1:39.
31. Oliver RC, Holm-Pedersen P, Löe H: The correlation between clinical scoring, exudate measurements, and microscopic evaluation of inflammation of the gingiva. J Periodontol, 1969; 40:201.
32. Page RC: The role of inflammatory mediators in the pathogenesis of periodontal disease. J Periodont Res 1991; 26:230.
33. Page RC, Ammons WF, Simpson DM: Host tissue response in chronic inflammatory periodontal disease. IV. The periodontal and dental status of a group of aged great apes. J Periodontol 1975; 46:144.
34. Page RC, Schroeder, HE: Pathogenic mechanisms. In Schluger S, Youdelis R, Page RC (eds): Periodontal Disease: Basic Phenomena, Clinical Management and Restorative Interrelationships. Philadelphia, Lea & Febiger, 1977.
35. Payne WA, Page RC, Ogilvie AL, et al: Histopathologic features of the initial and early stages of experimental gingivitis in man. J Periodont Res 1975; 10:51.
36. Quintarelli G: Histochemistry of gingiva. III. The distribution of aminopeptidase in normal and inflammatory conditions. Arch Oral Biol 1960; 2:271.
37. Saglie R, Newman MG, Carranza FA Jr: Scanning electron microscopy study of the interaction of leukocytes and bacteria in human periodontitis. J Periodontol 1982; 53:752.
38. Saglie R, Newman MG, Carranza FA Jr, et al: Bacterial invasion of gingiva in advanced periodontitis in humans. J Periodontol 1982; 53:217.
39. Schroeder HE: Transmigration and infiltration of leucocytes in human junctional epithelium. Helv Odontol Acta 1973; 17:6.
40. Schroeder HE, Graf de Beer M, Attström R: Initial gingivitis in dogs. J Periodont Res 1975; 10:128.
41. Schroeder HE, Munzell-Pedrazzoli S, Page RC: Correlated morphological and biochemical analysis of gingival tissue in early chronic gingivitis in man. Arch Oral Biol 1973; 18:899.
42. Schwartz J, Stinson F, Parker R: The passage of bacterial endotoxin across intact gingival crevicular epithelium. J Periodontol 1972; 43:270.
43. Seymour GJ, Powell RN, Aitken RF: Experimental gingivitis in humans. A clinical and histological investigation. J Periodontol 1983; 54:522.
44. Simpson DM, Avery BE: Histopathologic and ultrastructural features of inflamed gingiva in the baboon. J Periodontol 1974; 45:500.
45. Thilander H: Epithelial changes in gingivitis. An electron microscopic study. J Periodont Res 1968; 3:303.
46. Wennstrom J, Heijl L, Lindhe J, et al: Migration of gingival leukocytes mediated by plaque bacteria. J Periodont Res 1980; 15:363.
47. Winer RA, O'Donnell LS, Chauncey HH, et al: Enzyme activity in periodontal disease. J Periodontol 1970; 41:449.

Clinical Features of Gingivitis

Fermin A. Carranza and John W. Rapley

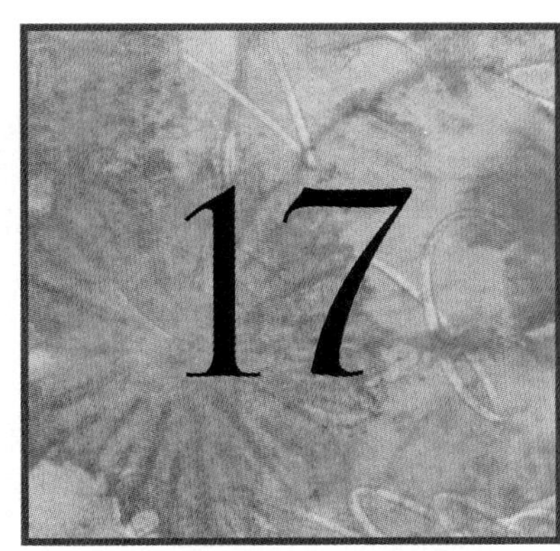

CHAPTER

Chapter Outline

COURSE AND DURATION

Acute gingivitis is of sudden onset and short duration and can be painful. A less severe phase of the acute condition has been termed *subacute.* **Recurrent gingivitis** reappears after having been eliminated by treatment or disappearing spontaneously. **Chronic gingivitis** is slow in onset and of long duration, and is painless, unless complicated by acute or subacute exacerbations. Chronic gingivitis is the type most commonly encountered (Fig. 17-1 and Color Fig. 17-1). Chronic gingivitis is a fluctuating disease in which inflammation persists or resolves and normal areas become inflamed.[14,15]

DISTRIBUTION

Localized gingivitis is confined to the gingiva of a single tooth or group of teeth while **generalized gingivitis** involves the entire mouth. **Marginal gingivitis** involves the gingival margin and may include a portion of the contiguous attached gingiva. **Papillary gingivitis** involves the interdental papillae and often extends into the adjacent portion of the gingival margin. Papillae are involved more frequently than the gingival margin, and the earliest signs of gingivitis often occur in the papillae. **Diffuse gingivitis** affects the gingival margin, the attached gingiva, and the interdental papillae.

The distribution of gingival disease in individual cases is described by combining the preceding terms as follows:

Localized marginal gingivitis is confined to one or more areas of the marginal gingiva (Fig. 17-2).

Localized diffuse gingivitis extends from the margin to the mucobuccal fold but is limited in area (Fig. 17-3; see Color Fig. 17-1, *A*).

Localized papillary gingivitis is confined to one or more interdental spaces in a limited area (Fig. 17-4; see Color Fig. 17-1, *B*).

Generalized marginal gingivitis involves the gingival margins in relation to all the teeth. The interdental papillae are usually affected in generalized marginal gingivitis (Fig. 17-5; see Color Fig. 17-1, *C*).

Generalized diffuse gingivitis involves the entire gingiva. The alveolar mucosa and attached gingiva are affected, so the mucogingival junction is sometimes obliterated (Fig. 17-6; Color Fig. 17-1, *D*). Systemic conditions can be involved in the cause of generalized diffuse gingivitis and should be evaluated if suspected as an etiologic co-factor.

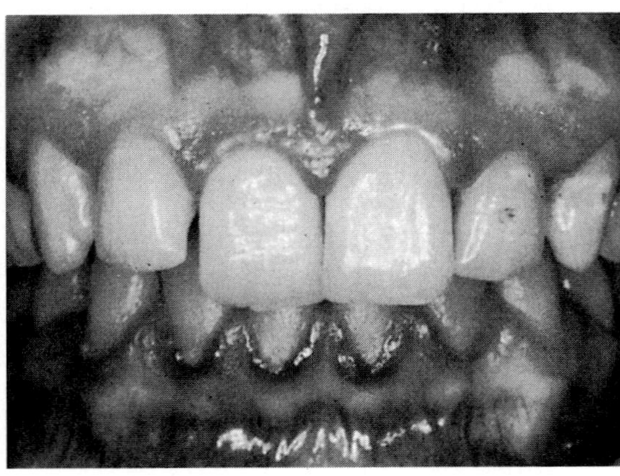

Fig. 17-1 Chronic gingivitis. The marginal and interdental gingivae are smooth, edematous, and discolored.

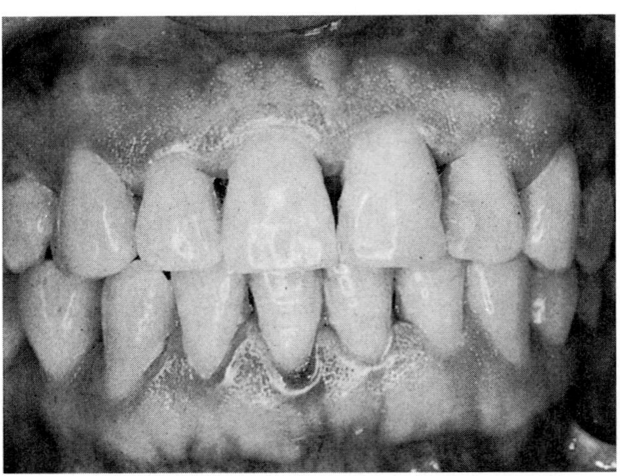

Fig. 17-2 Localized marginal gingivitis in the mandibular anterior region.

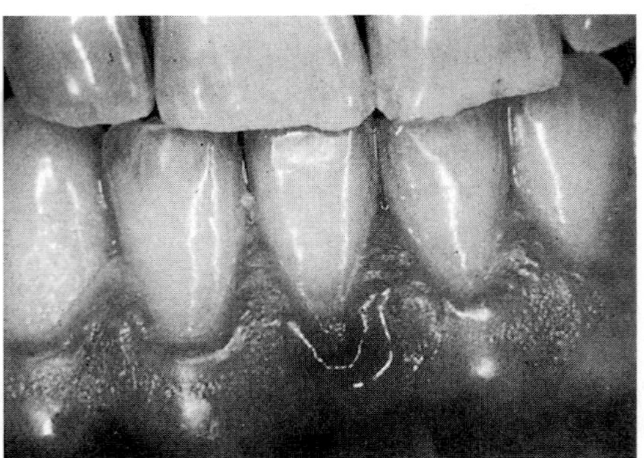

Fig. 17-3 Localized diffuse gingivitis involving both the marginal and the attached gingiva.

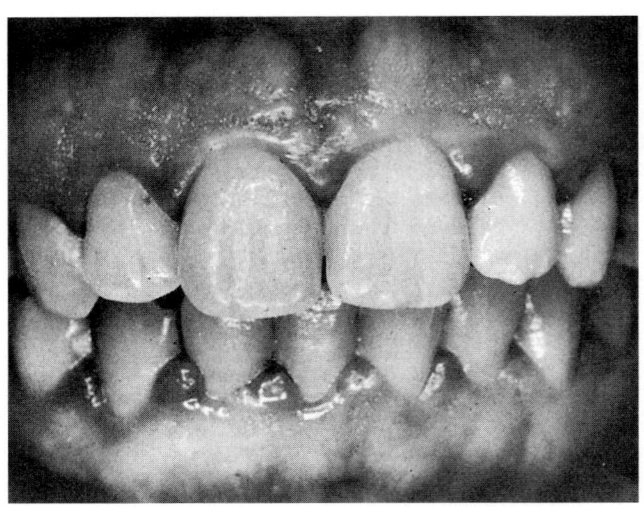

Fig. 17-4 Papillary gingivitis.

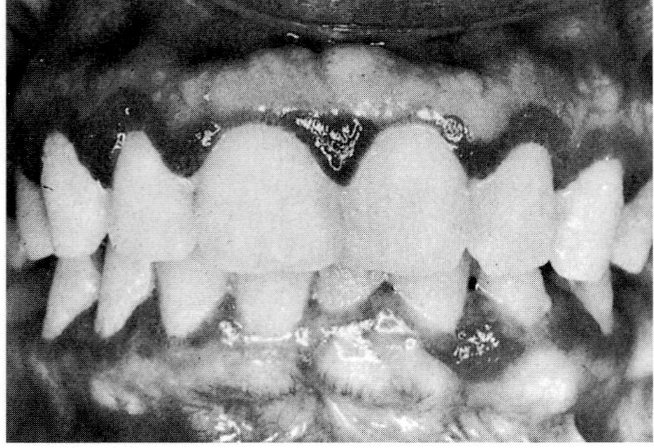

Fig. 17-5 Generalized marginal gingivitis. The interdental papillae are also involved.

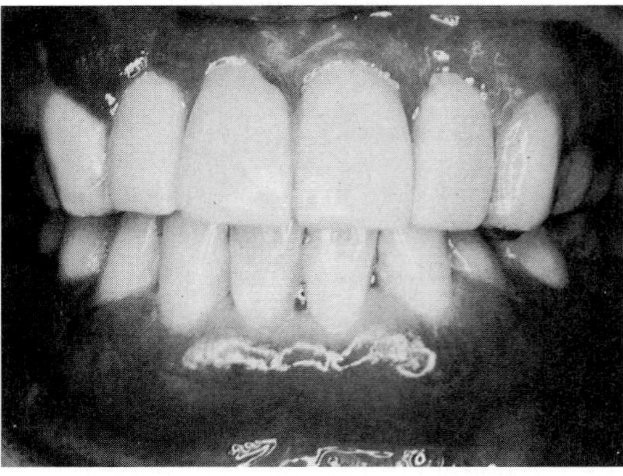

Fig. 17-6 Generalized diffuse gingivitis. The marginal, interdental, and attached gingivae are involved in chronic desquamative gingivitis.

CLINICAL FINDINGS

In evaluating the clinical features of gingivitis, it is necessary to be **systematic.** Attention should be focused on subtle tissue alterations, because these may be of diagnostic significance. A systematic clinical approach requires an orderly examination of the gingiva for color, contour, consistency, position, ease and severity of bleeding, and pain. These clinical characteristics and the microscopic changes responsible for each are discussed in this chapter.

Gingival Bleeding on Probing

The two earliest symptoms of gingival inflammation preceding established gingivitis, are (1) increased gingival crevicular fluid production rate and (2) bleeding from the gingival sulcus on gentle probing (Fig. 17-7; see Color Fig. 17-1, *G,H*). Gingival crevicular fluid is discussed in detail in Chapter 15.

Gingival bleeding varies in severity, duration, and the ease with which it is provoked. *Bleeding on probing is easily detectable clinically and therefore is of value for the early diagnosis and prevention of more advanced gingivitis.* It has been shown that bleeding on probing appears earlier than a change in color or other visual signs of inflammation[15,16,20]; in addition, the use of bleeding rather than color changes to diagnose early gingival inflammation is advantageous in that bleeding is a more objective sign that requires less subjective estimation by the examiner. Several gingival indices based on bleeding have been developed[1,6,26] and are described in Chapter 5. (For further considerations on probing, see Chapter 30.)

A

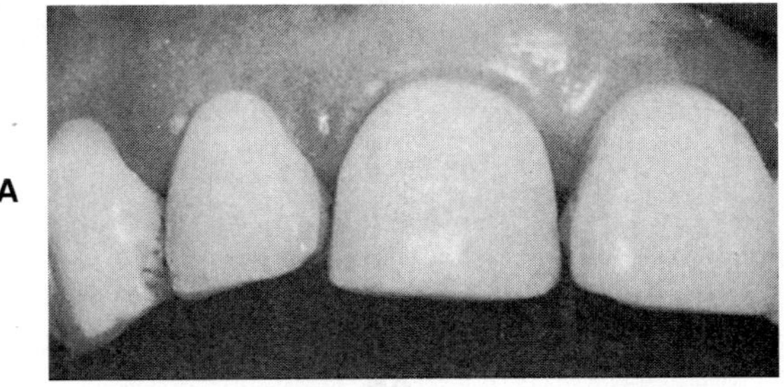

B

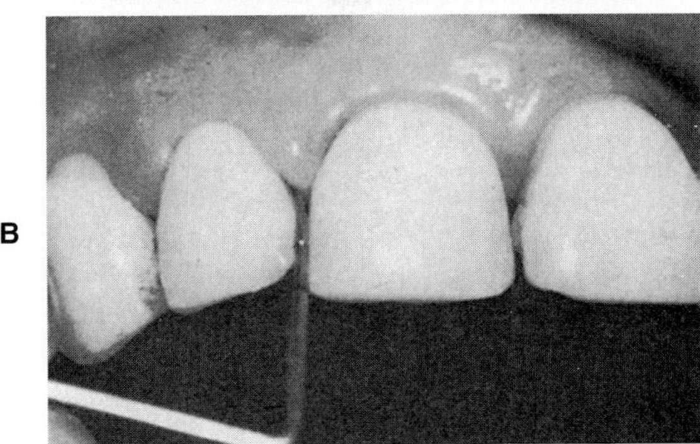

C

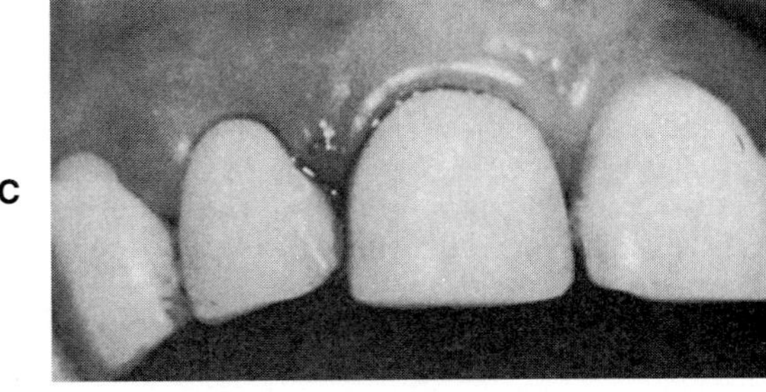

Fig. 17-7 Bleeding on probing. **A,** Mild gingivitis with slight edema. **B,** Introduction of the periodontal probe to the bottom of the gingival sulcus. **C,** Bleeding appears after a few seconds. (Courtesy Dr. Joseph Hsiou, Los Angeles, Calif.)

Gingival Bleeding Caused by Local Factors

Chronic and Recurrent Bleeding. The most common cause of abnormal gingival bleeding on probing is chronic inflammation.[23] The bleeding is chronic or recurrent and is provoked by mechanical trauma (e.g., from toothbrushing, toothpicks, or food impaction) or by biting into solid foods such as apples.

> In gingival inflammation, the following histopathologic alterations result in abnormal gingival bleeding: dilation and engorgement of the capillaries and thinning or ulceration of the sulcular epithelium (Fig. 17-9). Because the capillaries are engorged and closer to the surface and the thinned, degenerated epithelium is less protective, stimuli that are ordinarily innocuous cause rupture of the capillaries and gingival bleeding.

Sites that bleed on probing have a greater area of inflamed connective tissue (i.e., cell-rich, collagen-poor tissue) than do sites that do not bleed. In most cases, the cellular infiltrate of sites that bleed on probing is predominantly lymphocytic (a characteristic of stage II, or early gingivitis).[2,7,10]

The severity of the bleeding and the ease with which it is provoked depend on the intensity of the inflammation. After the vessels are damaged and rupture, a complex of mechanisms induce hemostasis.[35] The vessel walls contract, and blood flow is diminished; blood platelets adhere to the edges of the tissue; and a fibrous clot is formed, which contracts and results in approximation of the edges of the injured area. Bleeding recurs, however, when the area is irritated.

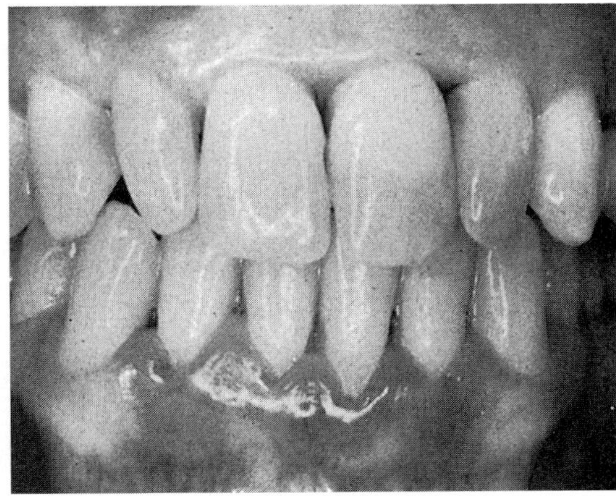

Fig. 17-8 Vertical discoloration of marginal and attached gingivae associated with periodontal pockets.

In cases of moderate or advanced periodontitis, the presence of bleeding on probing is considered a sign of active tissue destruction (see Chapter 22).

Acute Bleeding. Acute episodes of gingival bleeding are caused by injury or occur spontaneously in acute gingival disease. Laceration of the gingiva by toothbrush bristles during aggressive toothbrushing or by sharp pieces of hard food can cause gingival bleeding even in the absence of gingival disease. Gingival burns from hot foods or chemicals increase the ease of gingival bleeding.

Spontaneous bleeding or bleeding on slight provocation can occur in acute necrotizing ulcerative gingivitis. In this condition, engorged blood vessels in the inflamed connective tissue are exposed by ulceration of the necrotic surface epithelium.

Gingival Bleeding Associated with Systemic Changes. In some systemic disorders, gingival hemorrhage occurs spontaneously or after irritation and is excessive and difficult to control. These hemorrhagic diseases represent a wide variety of conditions that vary in etiologic factors and clinical manifestations. Such conditions have the common feature of a hemostatic mechanism failure and result in abnormal bleeding in the skin, internal organs, and other tissues, including the oral mucosa.

The hemorrhagic tendency may be due to failure of one or more of the hemostatic mechanisms.[33] Hemorrhagic disorders in which abnormal gingival bleeding is encountered include vascular abnormalities (vitamin C deficiency or allergy such as Schönlein-Henoch purpura), platelet disorders (thrombocytopenic purpura), hypoprothrombinemia (vitamin K deficiency), other coagulation defects (hemophilia, leukemia, Christmas disease), deficient platelet thromboplastic factor (PF3) resulting from uremia,[21] multiple myeloma,[3] and postrubella purpura.[14] Bleeding may follow the administration of excessive amounts of drugs such as salicylates and the administration of anticoagulants such as dicumarol and heparin. (Periodontal involvement in hematologic disorders is considered in Chapter 12.)

Color Changes in the Gingiva

Color Changes in Chronic Gingivitis. *Change in color is an important clinical sign of gingival disease.* The normal gingival color is "coral pink" and is produced by the tissue's vascularity and modified by the overlying epithelial layers. For this reason, the gingiva becomes more red when there is an increase in vascularization or the degree of epithelial keratinization becomes reduced or disappears. The color becomes more pale when vascularization is reduced (in association with fibrosis of the corium) or epithelial keratinization increases.

Thus chronic inflammation intensifies the red or bluish red color, because of vascular proliferation and reduction of keratinization due to epithelial compression by the inflamed tissue. Additionally, venous stasis will contribute a bluish hue. The gingival color changes with increasing chronicity of the inflammatory process. The changes start in the interdental papillae and gingival margin and spread to the attached gingiva (see Fig. 17-1). Proper diagnosis and treatment require an understanding of the tissue changes that alter the color of the gingiva at the clinical level.

Color Changes in Acute Gingivitis. Color changes in acute gingival inflammation differ in both nature and distribution from those in chronic gingivitis. The color changes may be marginal, diffuse, or patchlike, depending on the underlying acute condition. In acute

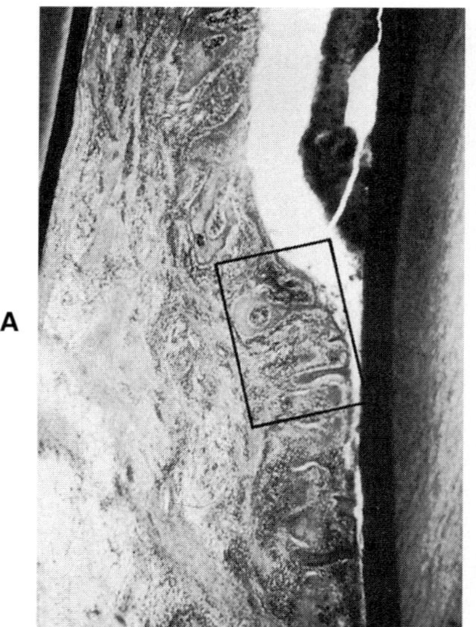

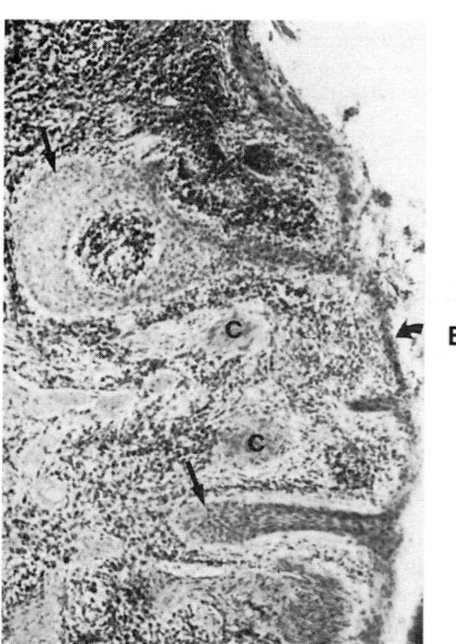

Fig. 17-9 **A,** Microscopic view of interdental space in a human autopsy specimen. **B,** Higher magnification of the area within the rectangle in **A.** Note the dense inflammatory infiltrate, the thinned epithelium (curved arrow), the extension of rete pegs (straight arrows), and the remnants of collagen fibers *(C).*

necrotizing ulcerative gingivitis the involvement is marginal; in herpetic gingivostomatitis, it is diffuse; and in acute reactions to chemical irritation, it is patchlike or diffuse.

Color changes vary with the intensity of the inflammation. Initially, there is an increasingly red erythema. If the condition does not worsen, this is the only color change until the gingiva reverts to normal. In severe acute inflammation, the red color gradually becomes a dull, whitish gray. The gray discoloration produced by tissue necrosis is demarcated from the adjacent gingiva by a thin, sharply defined erythematous zone. Detailed descriptions of the clinical and pathologic features of the various forms of acute gingivitis are found in Chapter 19.

Metallic Pigmentation. Heavy metals (bismuth, arsenic, mercury, lead, silver) absorbed systemically from therapeutic use or occupational or household environments may discolor the gingiva and other areas of the oral mucosa.[19] These changes are rare but still should be ruled out in suspected cases.

Typically, they produce a black or bluish line in the gingiva that follows the contour of the margin (Fig. 17-10). The pigmentation may also appear as isolated black blotches involving the interdental marginal and attached gingiva. This is different from tattooing produced by the accidental embedding of amalgam or other metal fragments[5] (Fig. 17-11).

Gingival pigmentation from systemically absorbed metals results from perivascular precipitation of metallic sulfides in the subepithelial connective tissue. Gingival pigmentation is not a result of systemic toxicity. It occurs only in areas of inflammation, where the increased permeability of irritated blood vessels permits seepage of the metal into the surrounding tissue. In addition to inflamed gingiva, mucosal areas irritated by biting or abnormal chewing habits (e.g., the inner surface of the lips, the cheek at the level of the occlusal line, and the lateral border of the tongue) are common pigmentation sites. Pigmentation can be eliminated by treating the inflammatory changes without necessarily discontinuing the metal-containing medication.

A

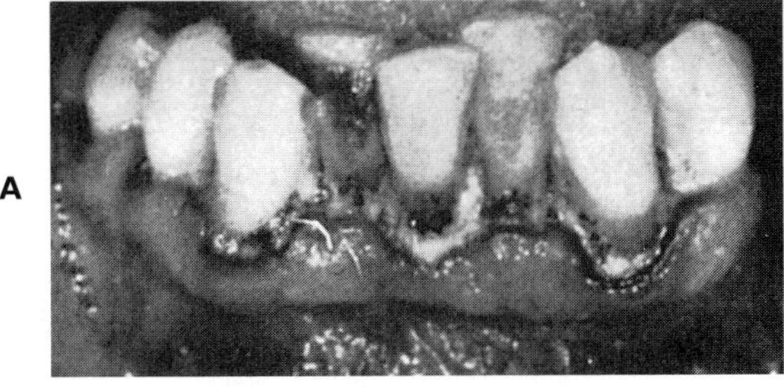

B

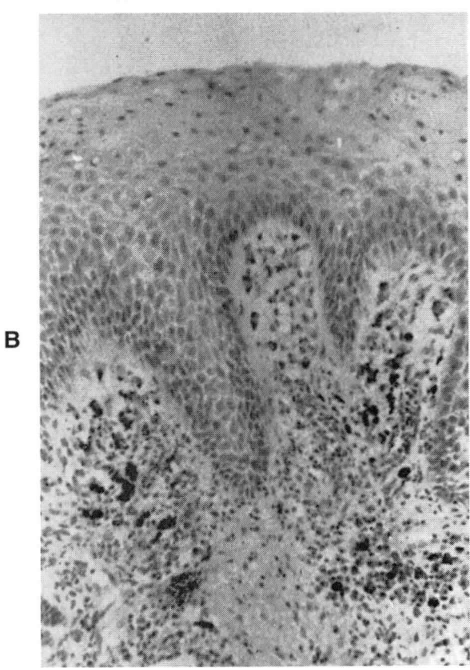

Fig. 17-10 Bismuth line. **A,** Linear discoloration of the gingiva in relation to local irritation in a patient receiving bismuth therapy. **B,** Biopsy specimen showing bismuth particles engulfed by monocytes/macrophages.

Color Changes Associated with Systemic Factors

Many systemic diseases may cause color changes in the oral mucosa, including the gingiva.[8] In general, these abnormal pigmentations are nonspecific in nature and should stimulate further diagnostic efforts or referral to the appropriate specialist.[32]

Endogenous oral pigmentations can be due to melanin, bilirubin, or iron.[19] **Melanin** oral pigmentations can be normal physiologic pigmentations and are commonly found in highly pigmented ethnic groups (see Chapter 1). Diseases that increase melanin pigmentation include the following:

Addison's disease: caused by adrenal dysfunction and produces isolated patches of discoloration varying from bluish black to brown

Peutz-Jeghers syndrome: produces intestinal polyposis and melanin pigmentation in the oral mucosa and lips

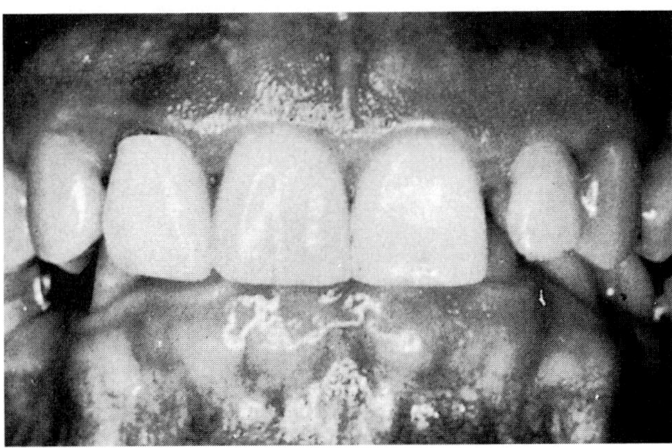

Fig. 17-11 Discoloration of the gingiva over the lateral incisor caused by embedded metal particles.

Albright's syndrome (polyostotic fibrous dysplasia) and von Recklinghausen's disease (neurofibromatosis: produce areas of oral melanin pigmentation

Skin and mucous membranes can also be stained by **bile pigments.** Jaundice is best detected by examination of the sclera, but the oral mucosa may also acquire a yellowish color. The deposition of **iron** in hemochromatosis may produce a blue-gray pigmentation of the oral mucosa. Several endocrine and metabolic disturbances, including diabetes and pregnancy, may result in color changes. Blood dyscrasias such as anemia, polycythemia, and leukemia may also induce color changes.

Exogenous factors capable of producing color changes in the gingiva include atmospheric irritants such as coal and metal dust and coloring agents in food or lozenges. Tobacco causes hyperkeratosis of the gingiva and also may induce a significant increase in melanin pigmentation of the oral mucosa.[27] Localized bluish black areas of pigment are commonly due to amalgam implanted in the mucosa (see Fig. 17-11).

Changes in the Consistency of the Gingiva

Both chronic and acute inflammation produce changes in the normal firm, resilient consistency of the gingiva. As noted in the preceding discussion, in chronic gingivitis, both destructive (edematous) and reparative (fibrotic) changes coexist, and the consistency of the gingiva is determined by their relative predominance (Figs. 17-12 and 17-13). Table 17-1 summarizes the clinical alterations in the consistency of the gingiva and the microscopic changes that produce them.

Calcified Masses in the Gingiva. Calcified microscopic masses may be found in the gingiva.[4,25] They can occur alone or in groups and vary in size, location, shape, and structure. Such masses may be calcified material removed from the tooth and traumatically displaced into the gingiva during scaling,[25] root remnants, cementum fragments, or cementicles (Fig. 17-14). Chronic inflammation and fibrosis and occasionally foreign body giant cell activity occur in relation to these masses. They are sometimes enclosed in an osteoid-like matrix. Crystalline foreign bodies have also been described in the gingiva, but their origin has not been determined.[30]

Changes in the Surface Texture of the Gingiva

Loss of surface stippling is an early sign of gingivitis. In chronic inflammation the surface is either smooth and shiny or firm and nodular, depending on whether the dominant changes are exudative or fibrotic. Smooth surface texture is also produced by epithelial atrophy in atrophic gingivitis, and peeling of the surface occurs in chronic desquamative gingivitis. Hyperkeratosis results in a leathery texture, and drug-induced gingival overgrowth produces a nodular surface.

TABLE 17-1

Clinical and Histopathologic Changes in Gingival Consistency

Clinical Changes	Underlying Microscopic Features
Chronic Gingivitis	
1. Soggy puffiness that pits on pressure.	1. Infiltration by fluid and cells of inflammatory exudate.
2. Marked softness and friability, with ready fragmentation on exploration with probe and pinpoint surface areas of redness and desquamation.	2. Degeneration of connective tissue and epithelium associated with injurious substances that provoke the inflammation and inflammatory exudate; change in connective tissue–epithelium relationship, with the inflamed, engorged connective tissue expanding to within a few epithelial cells of surface; thinning of epithelium and degeneration associated with edema and leukocytic invasion, separated by areas in which rete pegs are elongated to connective tissue.
3. Firm, leathery consistency.	3. Fibrosis and epithelial proliferation associated with longstanding chronic inflammation.
Acute Gingivitis	
1. Diffuse puffiness and softening.	1. Diffuse edema of acute inflammatory origin; fatty infiltration in xanthomatosis.
2. Sloughing with grayish, flake-like particles of debris adhering to eroded surface.	2. Necrosis with formation of a pseudomembrane composed of bacteria, PMNs, and degenerated epithelial cells in a fibrinous meshwork.
3. Vesicle formation.	3. Inter- and intracellular edema with degeneration of nucleus and cytoplasm and rupture of cell wall.

PMN, Polymorphonuclear neutrophils.

Changes in the Position of the Gingiva

Actual and Apparent Positions of the Gingiva. **Recession** is exposure of the root surface by an apical shift in the position of the gingiva. To understand what is meant by recession, one must distinguish between the actual and apparent positions of the gingiva. The **actual position** is the level of the epithelial attachment on the tooth (Fig. 17-15), whereas the **apparent position** is the level of the crest of the gingival margin. *The severity of recession is determined by the actual position of the gingiva, not its apparent position.*

The two types of recession are visible, which is clinically observable, and hidden, which is covered by gingiva and can be measured only by inserting a probe to the level of epithelial attachment (see Fig. 17-15). For example, in periodontal disease, the inflamed pocket wall covers part of the denuded root; thus some of the recession is hidden, and some may be visible. The total amount of recession is the sum of the two.

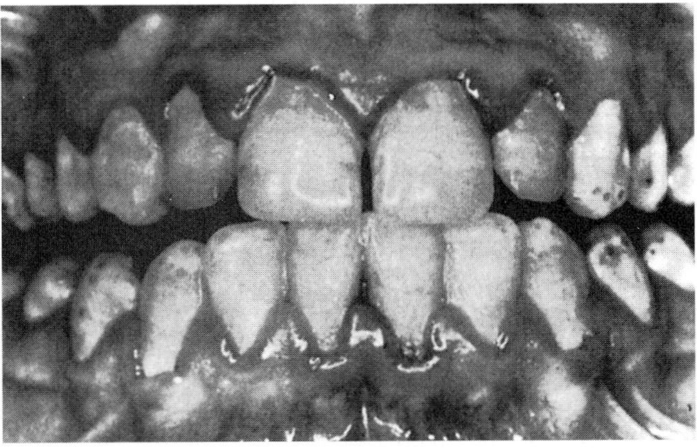

Fig. 17-12 Chronic gingivitis, showing swelling and discoloration produced when inflammatory exudate and tissue degeneration are the predominant microscopic changes. The gingiva is soft and friable and bleeds easily. Note the mottled teeth.

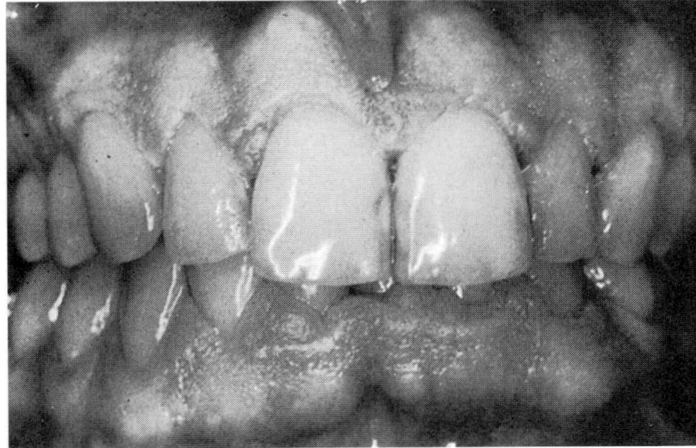

Fig. 17-13 Chronic gingivitis, showing a firm gingiva with a minutely nodular surface produced when fibrosis predominates in the inflammatory process.

Recession refers to the location of the gingiva, not its condition. Receded gingiva can be inflamed (Figs. 17-16 and 17-17) but may be normal except for their position (Fig. 17-18). Recession may be localized to one tooth (Fig. 17-19) or a group of teeth, or it may be generalized throughout the mouth (Fig. 17-20; see also Color Fig. 17-1, *F*).

ETIOLOGIC FACTORS OF RECESSION. Gingival recession increases with age; the incidence varies from 8% in children to 100% after the age of 50 years.[39] This has led some investigators to assume that recession may be a physiologic process related to aging. However, convincing evidence for a physiologic shift of the gingival

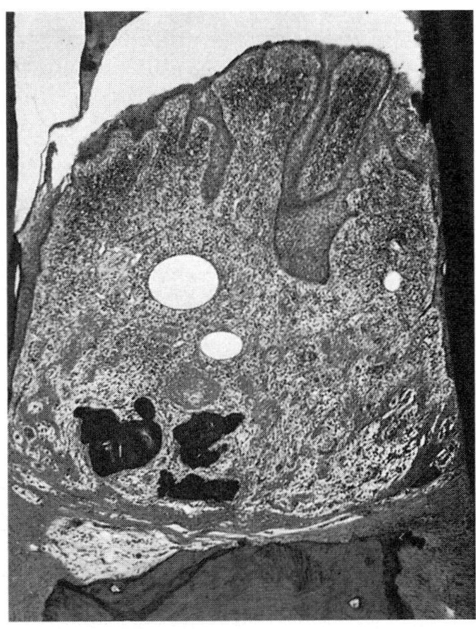

Fig. 17-14 Cementicles in the gingiva.

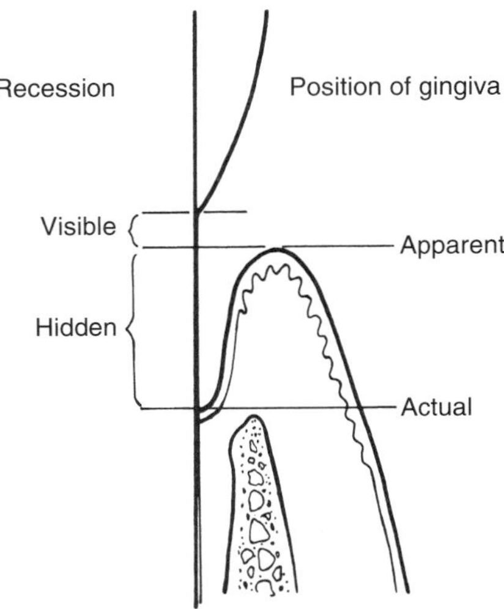

Fig. 17-15 Diagram illustrating the apparent and actual positions of the gingiva and visible and hidden recession.

attachment has never been presented.[17] The gradual apical shift is most probably the result of the cumulative effect of minor pathologic involvement and/or repeated minor direct trauma to the gingiva, but in some populations without access to dental care, recession may be the result of increasing periodontal disease.[13,18]

The following etiologic factors have been implicated in gingival recession: faulty toothbrushing technique (gingival abrasion), tooth malposition, friction from soft tissues (gingival ablation),[34] gingival inflammation, and abnormal frenum attachment. Trauma from occlusion has been suggested in the past, but its mechanism of action has never been demonstrated. Orthodontic movement in a labial direction in monkeys has been shown to result in loss of marginal bone and connective tissue attachment, as well as in gingival recession.[36]

Although toothbrushing is important for gingival health, faulty toothbrushing technique or brushing with hard bristles may cause gingival recession. Recession tends to be more frequent and severe in patients with comparatively healthy gingiva, little bacterial plaque, and good oral hygiene.[9,28,29]

Susceptibility to recession is influenced by the position of teeth in the arch,[38] the root-bone angle, and the mesiodistal curvature of the tooth surface.[24] On rotated, tilted, or facially displaced teeth, the bony plate is thinned or reduced in height. Pressure from mastication or moderate toothbrushing damages the unsupported gingiva and produces recession. The effect of the angle of the root in the bone on recession is often observed in the maxillary molar area (Fig. 17-21). If the lingual inclination of the palatal root is prominent or the buccal roots flare outward, then the bone in the cervical area is thinned or shortened, and recession results from repeated trauma of the thin marginal gingiva.

It has been noted that there may be a relationship between smoking and recession (see Chapter 14). The

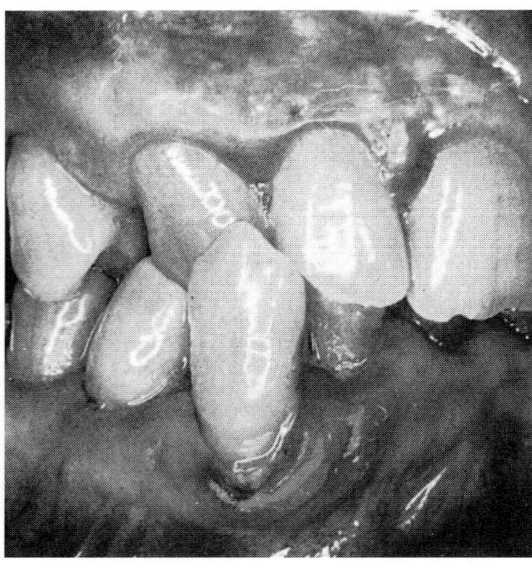

Fig. 17-16 Recession on prominent canine. Note the severe inflammatory reaction to local irritation.

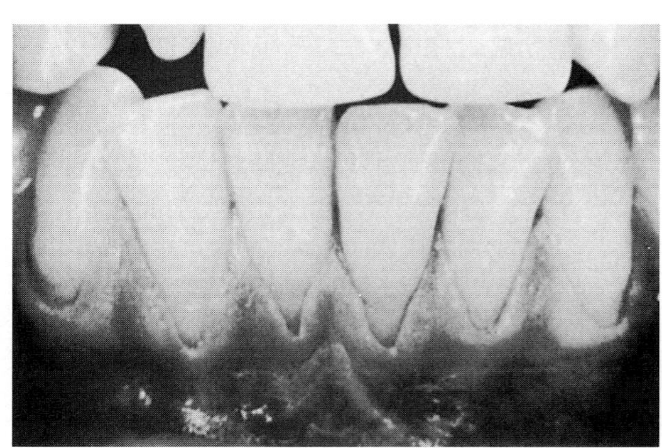

Fig. 17-18 Gingival recession. Note the excellent condition of the gingiva.

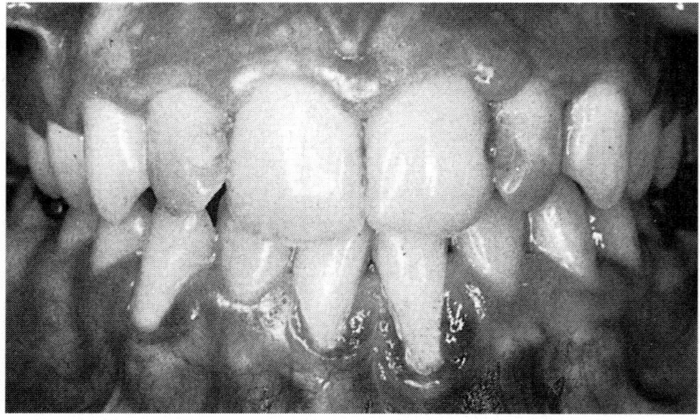

Fig. 17-17 Recession around malposed anterior teeth. The gingiva is markedly inflamed.

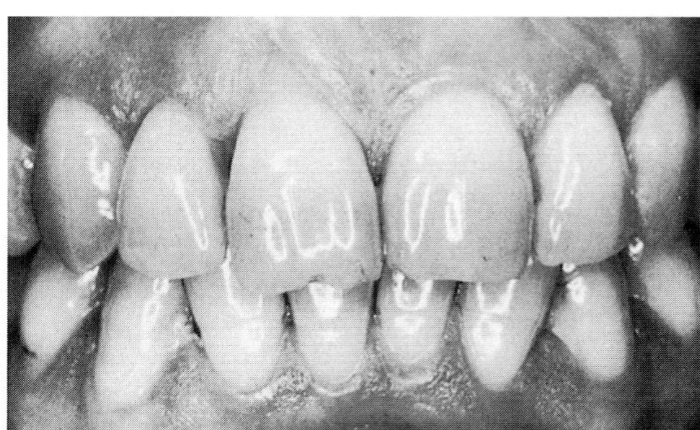

Fig. 17-19 Localized recession on the maxillary central incisor associated with aggressive toothbrushing.

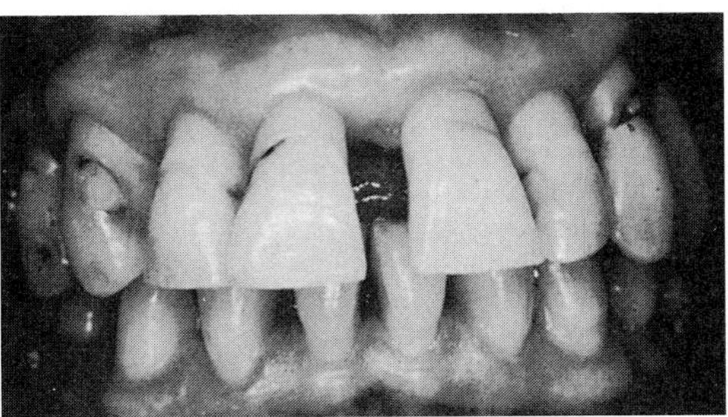

Fig. 17-20 Generalized recession resulting from chronic periodontal disease.

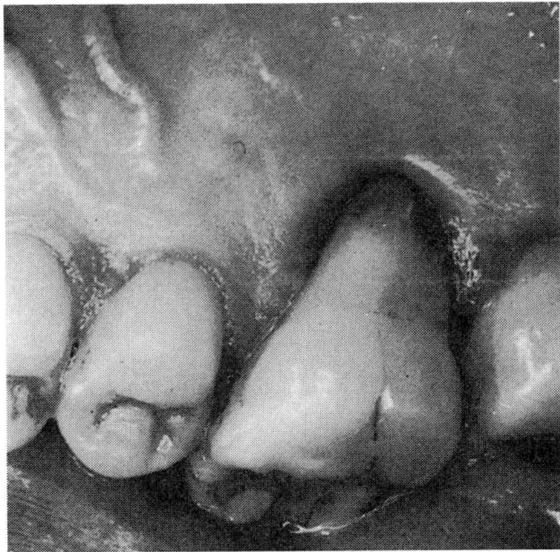

Fig. 17-21 Accentuated recession on a maxillary first molar aggravated by the angulation of the prominent palatal root in the bone.

mechanisms are multifactorial and may include reduction in gingival blood flow and alterations in the immune response but are not, as yet, conclusive.[11,31]

CLINICAL SIGNIFICANCE. Several aspects of gingival recession make it clinically significant. Exposed root surfaces are susceptible to caries. Abrasion or erosion of the cementum exposed by recession leaves an underlying dentinal surface that can be sensitive. Hyperemia of the pulp and associated symptoms may also result from excessive exposure of the root surface.[22] Interproximal recession creates oral hygiene problems and resulting plaque accumulation.

Changes in Gingival Contour

Changes in gingival contour are for the most part associated with gingival enlargement (see Chapter 18), but such changes may also occur in other conditions.

Of historical interest are the descriptions of indentations of the gingival margin referred to as *Stillman's clefts* (Fig. 17-22),[37] and the so-called McCall festoons (life preserver–shaped enlargement of the margin). They were attributed to trauma from occlusion, but this association

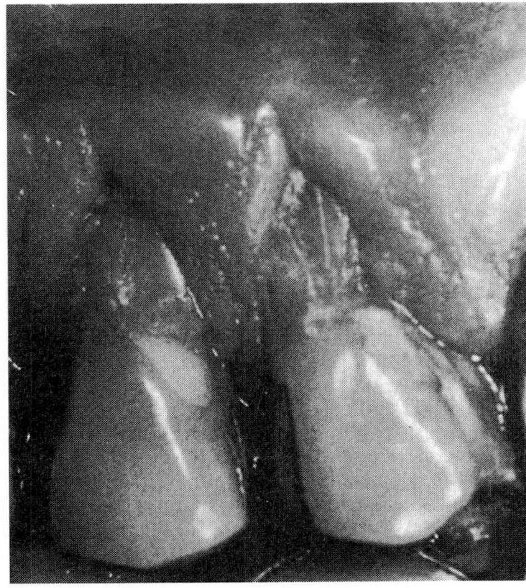

Fig. 17-22 Stillman's clefts in the gingiva.

was never proven; they represent peculiar inflammatory changes of the marginal gingiva.[4]

REFERENCES

1. Ainamo J, Bay I:. Problems and proposals for recording gingivitis and plaque. Int Dent J 1975; 25:229.
2. Amato R, Caton JG, Polson AM, et al: Interproximal gingival inflammation related to the conversion of a bleeding to a nonbleeding state. J Periodontol 1986; 57:63.
3. Bennett JH, Shankar S: Gingival bleeding as the presenting feature of multiple myeloma. Br Dent J 1984; 157:101.
4. Box HK: Gingival clefts and associated tracts. NY State Dent J 1950; 16:3.
5. Buchner A, Hansen LA: Amalgam pigmentation (amalgam tattoo) of the oral mucosa. A clinicopathologic study of 268 cases. Oral Surg 1980; 49:139.
6. Carter HG, Barnes GP: The gingival bleeding index. J Periodontol 1974; 45:801.
7. Cooper PG, Caton JG, Polson AM: Cell populations associated with gingival bleeding. J Periodontol 1983; 54:497.
8. Dummett CO: Oral tissue color changes. Ala J Med Sci 1979; 16:274.
9. Gorman WJ: Prevalence and etiology of gingival recession. J Periodontol 1967; 38:316.
10. Greenstein PG, Caton JG, Polson AM: Histologic characteristics associated with bleeding after probing and ritual signs of inflammation. J Periodontol 1981; 52:420.
11. Gunsolley JC, Quinn SM, Gooss CM, et al: The effect of smoking on individuals with minimal periodontal destruction. J Periodontol 1998; 69:165.
12. Haeb HP: Postrubella thrombocytopenic purpura. A report of cases with discussion of hemorrhagic manifestations of rubella. Clin Pediatr (Phila) 1968; 7:350.
13. Hirschfeld I: A study of skulls in the American Museum of Natural History in relation to periodontal disease. J Dent Res 1923; 5:241.
14. Hoover DR, Lefkowitz W: Fluctuation in marginal gingivitis. J Periodontol 1965; 36:310.
15. Larato D, Stahl SS, Brown R Jr, et al: The effect of a prescribed method of toothbrushing on the fluctuation of marginal gingivitis. J Periodontol 1969; 40:142.

16. Lenox JA, Kopczyk RA: A clinical system for scoring a patient's oral hygiene performance. J Am Dent Assoc 1973; 86:849.
17. Löe H: The structure and physiology of the dentogingival junction. In: Miles AE (ed): Structural and Chemical Organization of Teeth, vol 2. New York, Academic Press, 1967.
18. Löe H, Anerud A, Boysen H: The natural history of periodontal disease in man: Prevalence, severity and extent of gingival recession. J Periodontol 1992; 63:498.
19. McCarthy FP, Shklar G: Diseases of the Oral Mucosa. New York, McGraw-Hill, 1964.
20. Meitner SW, Zander H, Iker HP, et al: Identification of inflamed gingival surfaces. J Clin Periodontol 1979; 6:93.
21. Merril A, Peterson LJ: Gingival hemorrhage secondary to uremia. Review and report of a case. Oral Surg 1970; 29:530.
22. Merritt AA: Hyperemia of the dental pulp caused by gingival recession. J Periodontol 1933; 4:30.
23. Milne AM: Gingival bleeding in 848 army recruits. An assessment. Br Dent J 1967; 122:111.
24. Morris ML: The position of the margin of the gingiva. Oral Surg 1958; 11:969.
25. Moskow BS: Calcified material in human gingival tissues. J Dent Res 1961; 40:644.
26. Muhlemann HR, Son S: Gingival sulcus bleeding, a leading symptom in initial gingivitis. Helv Odontol Acta 1971; 15:107.
27. Neville BW, Damm DD, Allen CM, et al: Oral and Maxillofacial Pathology. Philadelphia, Saunders, 1995.
28. O'Leary TJ, Drake RV, Crump P, et al: The incidence of recession in young males: A further study. J Periodontol 1971; 42:264.
29. O'Leary TJ, Drake RV, Jividen GJ, et al: The incidence of recession in young males: relationship to gingival and plaque scores. USAF School of Aerospace Medicine. November 1967; SAM-TR-67–97:1.
30. Orban B: Gingival inclusions. J Periodontol 1945; 16:16.
31. Preber H, Bergstrom J: Occurrence of gingival bleeding in smokers and non-smoker patients. Acta Odontol Scand 1985; 43:315.
32. Shklar G, McCarthy PL: The Oral Manifestations of Systemic Disease. Boston, Butterworth, 1976.
33. Sodeman WA Jr, Sodeman WA: Pathologic Physiology: Mechanisms of Disease, ed 7. Philadelphia, Saunders, 1985.
34. Sognnaes RF: Periodontal significance of intraoral frictional ablation. J West Soc Periodontol 1977; 25:112.
35. Stefanini M, Dameshek W: The Hemorrhagic Disorders, ed 2. New York, Grune & Stratton, 1962.
36. Steiner GG, Pearson JK, Ainamo J: Changes of the marginal periodontium as a result of labial tooth movement in monkeys. J Periodontol 1981; 52:314.
37. Stillman PR: Early clinical evidence of disease in the gingiva and pericementum. J Dent Res 1921; 3:25.
38. Trott JR, Love B: An analysis of localized gingival recession in 766 Winnipeg high school students. Dent Pract Dent Rec 1966; 16:209.
39. Woofter C: The prevalence and etiology of gingival recession. Periodont Abstr 1969; 17:45.

Gingival Enlargement

Fermin A. Carranza and Eva L. Hogan

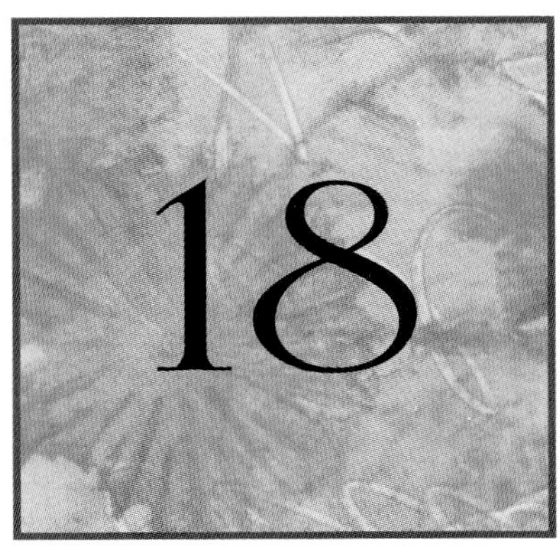

CHAPTER

CHAPTER OUTLINE

Increase in size of the gingiva is a common feature of gingival disease (Color Fig. 18-1). Accepted current terminology for this condition is gingival enlargement and gingival overgrowth. These are strictly clinical descriptive terms and avoid the erroneous pathologic connotations of terms used in the past such as hypertrophic gingivitis or gingival hyperplasia.

The many types of gingival enlargement can be classified according to etiologic factors and pathologic changes as follows:

I. Inflammatory enlargement
  A. Chronic
  B. Acute
II. Drug-induced enlargement
III. Enlargements associated with systemic diseases
  A. Conditioned enlargement
    1. Pregnancy
    2. Puberty
    3. Vitamin C deficiency
    4. Plasma cell gingivitis
    5. Nonspecific conditioned enlargement (granuloma pyogenicum)
  B. Systemic diseases causing gingival enlargement
    1. Leukemia
    2. Granulomatous diseases (Wegener's granulomatosis, sarcoidosis, and so on)
IV. Neoplastic enlargement (gingival tumors)
  A. Benign tumors
  B. Malignant tumors
V. False enlargement

Using the criteria of location and distribution, gingival enlargement is designated as follows:

Localized: Limited to the gingiva adjacent to a single tooth or group of teeth
Generalized: Involving the gingiva throughout the mouth
Marginal: Confined to the marginal gingiva
Papillary: Confined to the interdental papilla
Diffuse: Involving the marginal and attached gingivae and papillae
Discrete: An isolated sessile or pedunculated tumorlike enlargement

The degree of gingival enlargement can be scored as follows[16]:

Grade 0: No signs of gingival enlargement
Grade I: Enlargement confined to interdental papilla
Grade II: Enlargement involves papilla and marginal gingiva
Grade III: Enlargement covers three quarters or more of the crown

INFLAMMATORY ENLARGEMENT

Gingival enlargement may result from chronic or acute inflammatory changes. The former is by far the more common. In addition, inflammatory enlargements commonly are a secondary complication to any of the other types of enlargement, creating a combined gingival enlargement. In these cases it is important to understand the double etiology and treat them adequately.

Chronic Inflammatory Enlargement

Clinical Features. Chronic inflammatory gingival enlargement originates as a slight ballooning of the interdental papilla and/or the marginal gingiva. In the early stages it produces a life preserver-shaped bulge around the involved teeth. This bulge can increase in size until it covers part of the crowns. The enlargement may be localized (Fig. 18-1) or generalized (Fig. 18-2) and progresses slowly and painlessly, unless it is complicated by acute infection or trauma.

Occasionally, chronic inflammatory gingival enlargement occurs as a discrete sessile or pedunculated mass resembling a tumor. It may be interproximal or on the marginal or attached gingiva (see Color Fig. 18-1, *A*). The lesions are slow growing and usually painless. They may undergo spontaneous reduction in size, followed by exacerbation and continued enlargement. Painful ulceration sometimes occurs in the fold between the mass and the adjacent gingiva.

Histopathology. Chronic inflammatory gingival enlargements show the exudative and proliferative features of chronic inflammation (Fig. 18-3). Lesions that are clinically deep red or bluish red are soft and friable with a smooth, shiny surface, and they bleed easily. They also have a preponderance of inflammatory cells and fluid with vascular engorgement, new capillary formation, and associated degenerative changes. Lesions that are relatively firm, resilient, and pink have a greater fibrotic component with an abundance of fibroblasts and collagen fibers.

Etiology. Chronic inflammatory gingival enlargement is caused by prolonged exposure to dental plaque. Factors that favor plaque accumulation and retention[54] include poor oral hygiene (Fig. 18-4), as well as irritation by anatomic abnormalities and improper restorative and orthodontic appliances.

Gingival Changes Associated with Mouth Breathing. Gingivitis and gingival enlargement are often seen in mouth breathers.[74] The gingiva appears red and edematous with a diffuse surface shininess of the exposed area. The maxillary anterior region is the common site of such involvement. In many cases the altered gingiva is clearly demarcated from the adjacent unexposed normal gingiva (Fig. 18-5; see Color Fig. 18-1, *B*). The exact manner in which mouth breathing affects gingival changes has not been demonstrated. Its harmful effect is generally attributed to irritation from surface dehydration. However, comparable changes could not be produced by air drying the gingiva of experimental animals.[67]

Acute Inflammatory Enlargement

Gingival Abscess. A gingival abscess is a localized, painful, rapidly expanding lesion that is usually of sudden onset. It is generally limited to the marginal gingiva or interdental papilla. In its early stages it appears as a red swelling with a smooth, shiny surface. Within 24 to 48 hours, the lesion usually becomes fluctuant and pointed with a surface orifice from which a purulent exudate may be expressed. The adjacent teeth are often sensitive to percussion. If permitted to progress, the lesion generally ruptures spontaneously.

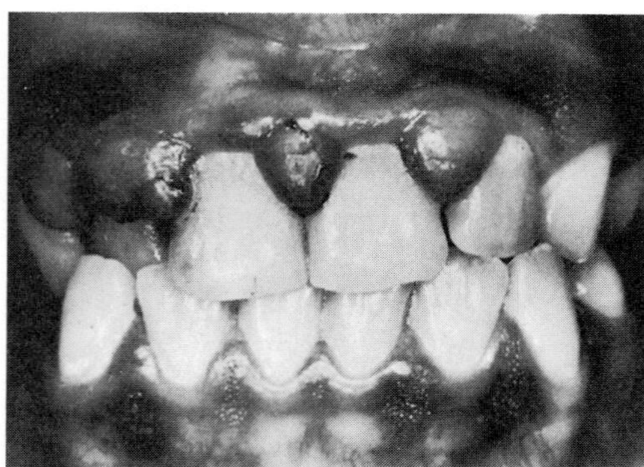

Fig. 18-1 Chronic inflammatory gingival enlargement localized to the anterior region.

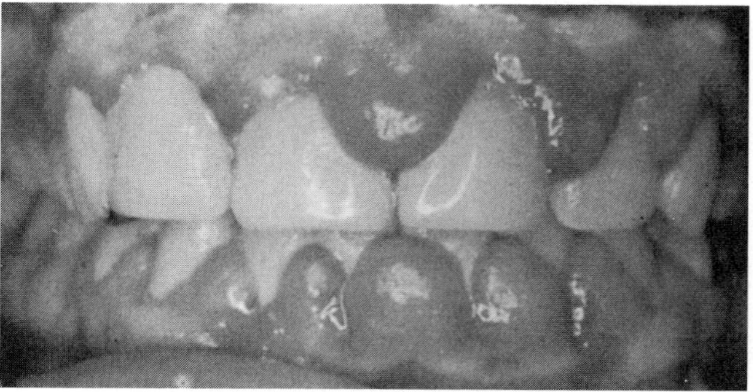

Fig. 18-2 Chronic inflammatory gingival enlargement.

HISTOPATHOLOGY. The gingival abscess consists of a purulent focus in the connective tissue, surrounded by a diffuse infiltration of polymorphonuclear leukocytes, edematous tissue, and vascular engorgement. The surface epithelium has varying degrees of intra- and extracellular edema, invasion by leukocytes, and sometimes ulceration.

ETIOLOGY. Acute inflammatory gingival enlargement results from bacteria carried deep into the tissues when a foreign substance such as a toothbrush bristle, a piece of apple core, or a lobster shell fragment is forcefully embedded into the gingiva. The lesion is confined to the gingiva and should not be confused with periodontal or lateral abscesses.

Periodontal (Lateral) Abscess. Periodontal abscesses generally produce enlargement of the gingiva, but they also involve the supporting periodontal tissues. For a detailed description of periodontal abscesses, see Chapter 22.

DRUG-INDUCED GINGIVAL ENLARGEMENT

Gingival enlargement is a well-known consequence of the administration of some anticonvulsants, immunosuppressants, and calcium channel blockers and may create speech, mastication, tooth eruption, and aesthetic problems.

Clinical and microscopic features of the enlargements caused by the different drugs are similar.[23,108] These are presented first, followed by a description of the particular features of each drug.

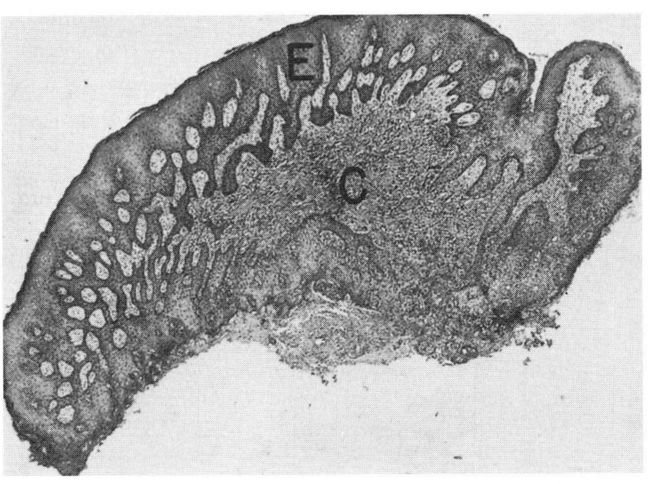

Fig. 18-3 Survey section of chronic inflammatory gingival enlargement showing the central connective tissue core (C) and thickened epithelium at the periphery (E). Note the ulceration of the epithelial surface at the lower border of the mass that was adjacent to the tooth surface.

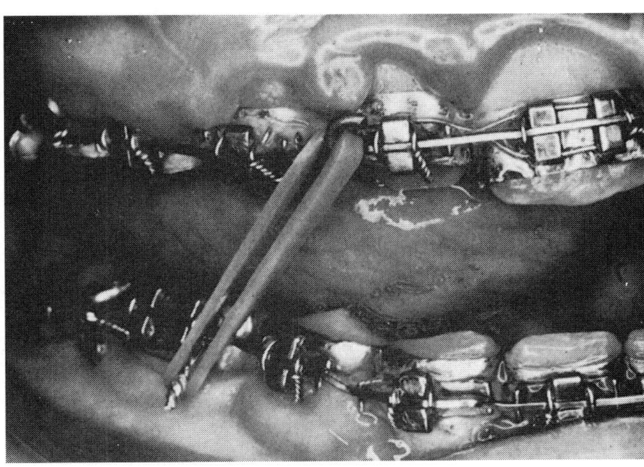

Fig. 18-4 Chronic inflammatory gingival enlargement associated with plaque accumulation around an orthodontic appliance.

A

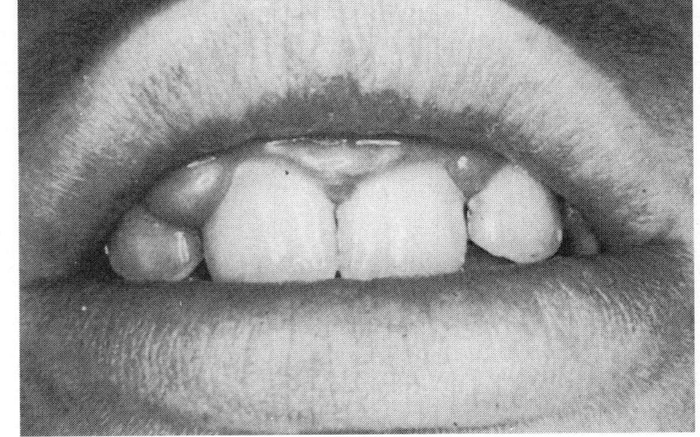

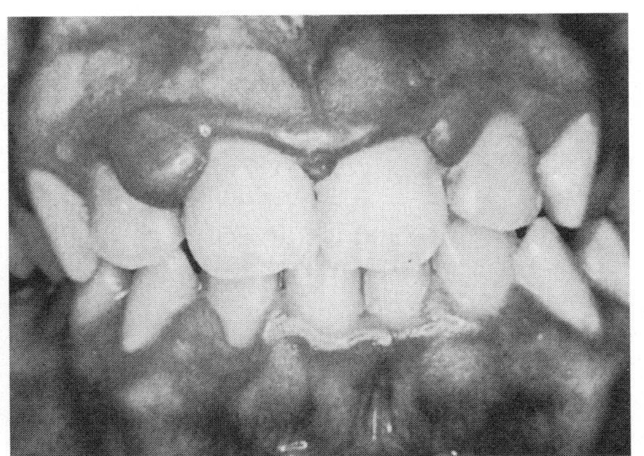

B

Fig. 18-5 Gingivitis in a mouth breather. **A,** High lip line in a mouth breather. **B,** Gingivitis and inflammatory gingival enlargement in the exposed area of the gingiva.

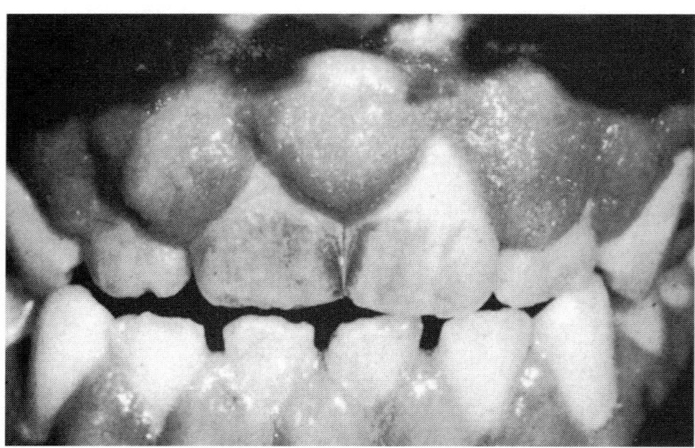

Fig. 18-6 Gingival enlargement associated with phenytoin therapy. Note the prominent papillary lesions and the firm, nodular surface. Black patches in attached gingiva are melanin-pigmented areas.

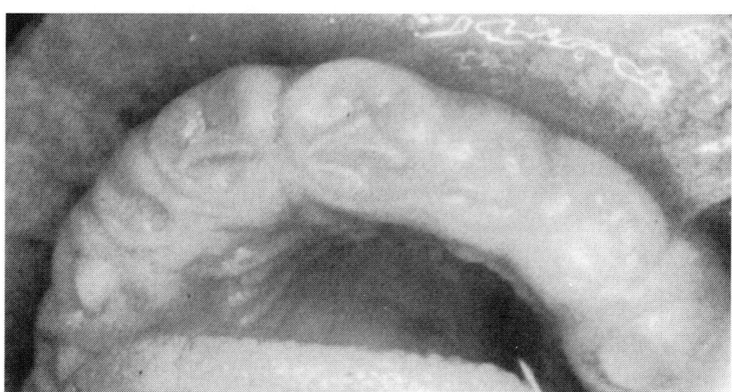

Fig. 18-7 Massive phenytoin-associated gingival enlargement in a 5-year-old patient. The teeth are almost completely covered by firm, dense tissue.

General Information

Clinical Features. The growth starts as a painless, beadlike enlargement of the interdental papilla and extends to the facial and lingual gingival margins (Fig. 18-6). As the condition progresses, the marginal and papillary enlargements unite; they may develop into a massive tissue fold covering a considerable portion of the crowns, and they may interfere with occlusion (Figs. 18-7, 18-8; Color Fig. 18-1, *C, D, E*). When uncomplicated by inflammation, the lesion is mulberry shaped, firm, pale pink, and resilient, with a minutely lobulated surface and no tendency to bleed. The enlargement characteristically appears to project from beneath the gingival margin, from which it is separated by a linear groove.

The enlargement is usually generalized throughout the mouth but is more severe in the maxillary and mandibular anterior regions. It occurs in areas in which teeth are present, not in edentulous spaces, and the enlargement disappears in areas from which teeth are extracted. Hyperplasia of the mucosa in edentulous mouths has been reported but is rare.[32,33]

Some investigators believe that inflammation is a prerequisite for development of the enlargement, which therefore could be prevented by plaque removal and fastidious oral hygiene.[26,44,66,91,114] However, oral hygiene by means of toothbrushing[34] or the use of a chlorhexidine toothpaste[102] reduces the inflammation but does not lessen or prevent the overgrowth. Hassell and coworkers[52] have hypothesized that in noninflamed gingiva, fibroblasts are less active or even quiescent and do not respond to circulating phenytoin, whereas fibroblasts within inflamed tissue are in an active state as a result of the inflammatory mediators and the endogenous growth factors present.

A genetic predisposition is a suspected factor[50,96] in determining whether a person treated with phenytoin will develop gingival enlargement or not.

The enlargement is chronic and slowly increases in size. When surgically removed, it recurs. Spontaneous disappearance occurs within a few months after discontinuation of the drug (see Chapter 59).

Drug-induced enlargement may occur in mouths with little or no plaque and may be absent in mouths with abundant deposits. However, the presence of the enlargement makes plaque control difficult, often resulting in a secondary inflammatory process that complicates the gingival overgrowth caused by the drug. The resultant enlargement becomes then a combination of the increase in size caused by the drug and the complicating inflammation caused by bacteria. Secondary inflammatory changes not only add to the size of the lesion caused by the drug but also produce a red or bluish-red discoloration, obliterate the lobulated surface demarcations, and result in an increased tendency toward bleeding (see Fig. 18-12).

Histopathology. The enlargement consists of a pronounced hyperplasia of the connective tissue and epithelium (Fig. 18-9). There is acanthosis of the epithelium, and elongated rete pegs extend deep into the connective tissue, which exhibits densely arranged collagen bundles with an increase in the number of fibroblasts and new blood vessels. An abundance of amorphous ground substance has also been reported.[78] Structural changes in the outer epithelial cell surface have been reported in cyclosporine enlargements.[4]

The enlargement begins as a hyperplasia of the connective tissue core of the marginal gingiva and increases by its proliferation and expansion beyond the crest of the gingival margin. Sometimes, particularly in cyclosporine enlargements, the connective tissue appears more highly vascularized and with foci of chronic inflammatory cells,[87] particularly plasma cells.[75]

The "mature" phenytoin enlargement has a fibroblast-to-collagen ratio equal to that of normal gingiva from normal individuals, suggesting that at some point in the development of the lesion there must have been an abnormally high fibroblastic proliferation.[51] Oxytalan fibers are numerous beneath the ep-

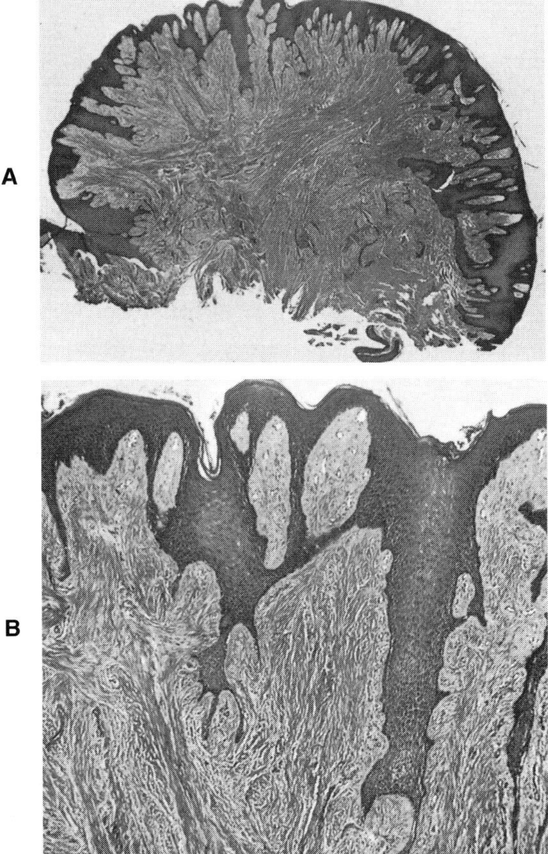

Fig. 18-8 Gingival enlargement associated with phenytoin therapy. **A,** Survey section showing bulbous gingival enlargement. **B,** Detailed view showing hyperplasia and acanthosis of the epithelium with extension of deep rete pegs into the connective tissue. The connective tissue is densely collagenous. There is little evidence of inflammation.

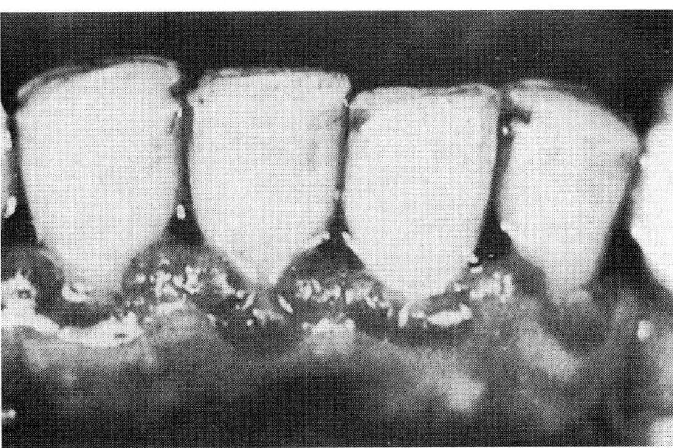

Fig. 18-9 Early recurrence after surgical removal of enlarged gingiva in a patient receiving phenytoin therapy.

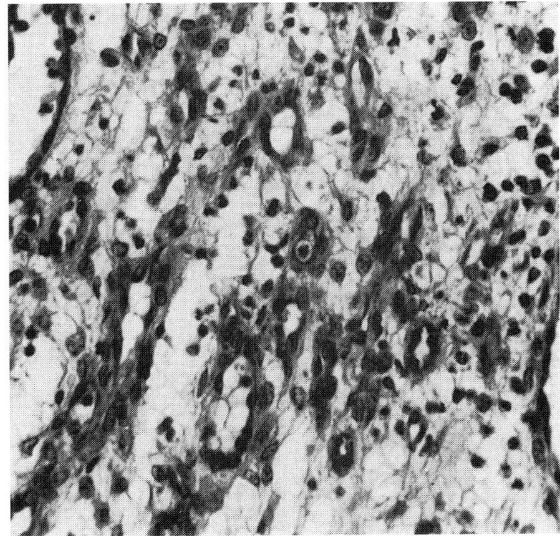

Fig. 18-10 Biopsy specimen of the recurrent gingival enlargement shown in Fig. 18-9. Note the abundance of new blood vessels.

ithelium and in areas of inflammation.[9] Inflammation is common along the sulcular surfaces of the gingiva.

Recurring enlargements appear as granulation tissue composed of numerous young capillaries and fibroblasts and irregularly arranged collagen fibrils with occasional lymphocytes (Figs. 18-10 and 18-11).

Anticonvulsants

The first drug-induced gingival enlargements reported were those produced by phenytoin (Dilantin). Dilantin is a hydantoin, introduced by Merritt and Putnam[80] in 1938 for the treatment of all forms of epilepsy, except petit mal. Shortly thereafter, its relationship with gingival enlargement was reported.[41,65] Other hydantoins known to induce gingival enlargement are ethotoin (Paganone), and mephenytoin (Mesantoin).[45] Other anticonvulsants that have the same side effect are the succinimides (ethosuximide [Zerontin], methsuxinimide [Celontin]), and valproic acid (Depakene).[45]

Gingival enlargement occurs in about 50% of patients receiving the drug,[108] although different authors have reported incidences from 3% to 84.5%.[3,41,92] It occurs more often in younger patients.[6] Its occurrence and severity are not necessarily related to the dosage after a threshold level has been exceeded.[108] Phenytoin appears in the saliva. There is no consensus, however, on whether the severity of the overgrowth is related to the levels of phenytoin in plasma or saliva.[3,6,7,131] Some reports indicate a relation between the drug dosage and the degree of gingival overgrowth.[60,66]

Tissue culture experiments indicate that phenytoin stimulates proliferation of fibroblast-like cells[109] and epithelium.[110] Two analogues of phenytoin (1-allyl-5-phenylhydantoinate and 5-methyl-5-phenylhydantoinate) have a similar effect on fibroblast-like cells.[110] Fibroblasts from a phenytoin-induced gingival overgrowth show increased synthesis of sulfated glycosaminoglycans in vitro.[59] Phenytoin may induce a decrease in collagen degradation as a result of the production of an inactive fibroblastic collagenase[49] (Fig. 18-12).

Experimental attempts to induce gingival enlargement with phenytoin administration in laboratory animals have been successful only in the cat,[56] the ferret, and the *Macaca speciosa monkey.*[116] In experimental animals, phenytoin causes gingival enlargement that is independent of local inflammation.

In cats, one of the metabolic products of phenytoin is 5-(parahydroxyphenyl)-5-phenylhydantoin; administration of this metabolite to cats also induces gingival enlargement in some cases.[51] This led Hassell and Page[51] to hypothesize that gingival enlargement may result from the genetically determined ability or inability of the host to deal effectively with prolonged administration of phenytoin.

Systemic administration of phenytoin accelerates the healing of gingival wounds in nonepileptic humans[112] and increases the tensile strength of healing abdominal wounds in rats.[31,111] The administration of phenytoin may precipitate a megaloblastic anemia[76] and a folic-acid deficiency.[117]

In conclusion, the pathogenesis of gingival enlargement induced by phenytoin is not known, but there is some evidence to link it to a direct effect on specific genetically predetermined subpopulations of fibroblasts, inactivation of collagenase, and plaque-induced inflammation.

Immunosuppressants

Cyclosporine is a potent immunosuppressive agent used to prevent organ transplant rejection and to treat several diseases of autoimmune origin.[24] Its exact mechanism of action is not well known, but it appears to selectively and reversibly inhibit helper T cells, which play a role in cellular and humoral immune responses. Cyclosporine A (Sandimmune, Neoral) is administered intravenously or by mouth, and dosages greater than 500 mg/day have been reported to induce gingival overgrowth.[29]

Cyclosporine-induced gingival enlargement is more vascularized than the phenytoin enlargement, occurs in approximately 30% of patients receiving the drug, is more frequent in children, and its magnitude appears to be related more to the plasma concentration than to the patient's periodontal status.[107] Gingival enlargement is greater in patients who are medicated with both cyclosporine and calcium channel–blocking drugs.[114,125,126]

The microscopic finding of many plasma cells plus the presence of an abundant amorphous extracellular substance has suggested that the enlargement is a hypersensitivity response to the cyclosporine.[78]

It has been reported that in experimental animals (rats) oral administration of cyclosporine also induces abundant formation of new cementum.[5]

In addition to gingival enlargement, cyclosporine induces other major side effects such as nephrotoxicity, hypertension, and hyperthricosis. Another immunosuppressive drug called *tacrolimus* has been used effectively and is also nephrotoxic, but it results in much less severe hypertension, hyperthricosis, and gingival overgrowth.[8,82,115]

A

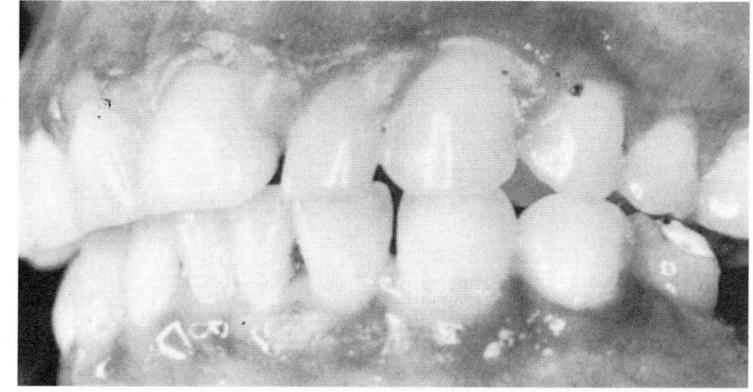

B

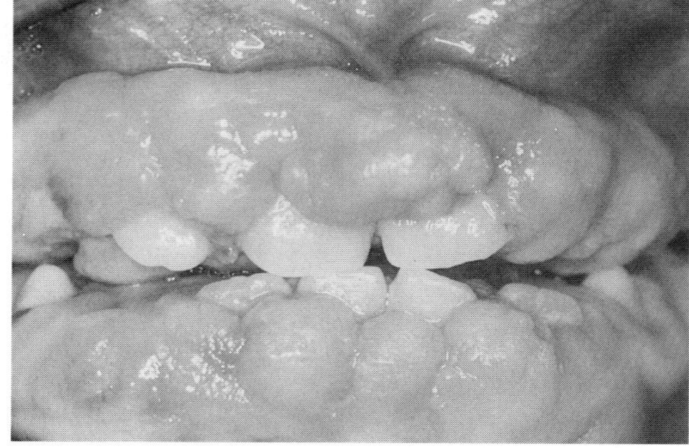

C

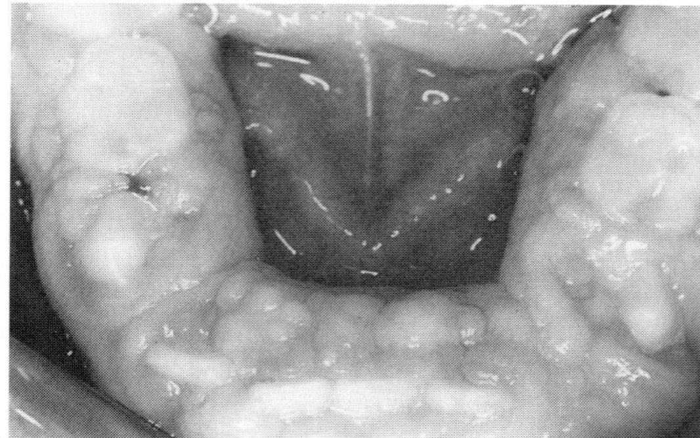

Fig. 18-11 Cyclosporine-associated gingival enlargement. **A,** Mild involvement located particularly on papillae between teeth No. 9 and 10, and 10 and 11. **B,** Advanced enlargement covering most of the crowns of the teeth. **C,** Occlusal view of case shown in **B.**

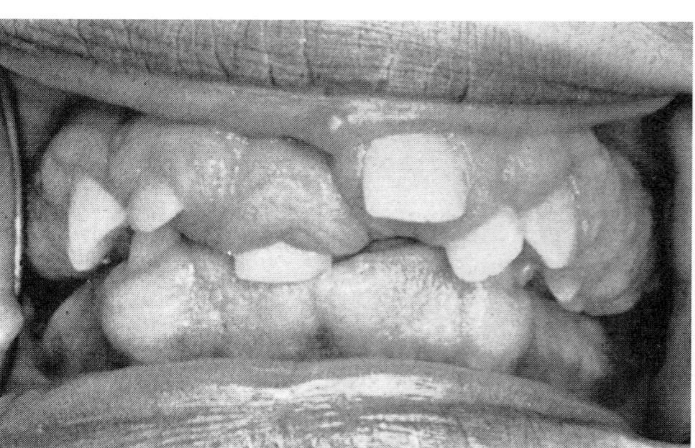

Fig. 18-12 Combined gingival enlargement in a patient receiving phenytoin therapy. The basic overgrowth is complicated by secondary inflammatory involvement. Note the edema and discoloration produced by the inflammation.

Calcium Channel Blockers

Calcium channel blockers are drugs developed for the treatment of cardiovascular conditions such as hypertension, angina pectoris, coronary artery spasms, and cardiac arrythmias.* They inhibit calcium ion influx across the cell membrane of heart and smooth muscle cells, blocking intracellular mobilization of calcium. This induces direct dilation of the coronary arteries and arterioles, improving oxygen supply to the heart muscle; it also reduces hypertension by dilating the peripheral vasculature.

Some of these drugs can induce gingival enlargement. Nifedipine, one of the most commonly used,[73,75,89] induces gingival enlargement in 20% of the cases.[10] Diltiazem, felodipine, nitrendipine, and verapamil also induce gingival enlargement.[17,30] The dihydropyridine derivative isradipidine can in some cases replace nifedipine and does not induce gingival overgrowth.[130]

Nifedipine is also used with cyclosporine in kidney transplant recipients, and the combined use of both drugs induces larger overgrowths.[16] Nifedipine gingival enlargement has been induced experimentally in rats, where it appears to be dose dependent[38]; in humans, however, this dose dependency is not clear.

Idiopathic Gingival Enlargement

Idiopathic gingival fibromatosis is a rare condition of undetermined cause. It has been designated by such terms as *gingivomatosis, elephantiasis, idiopathic fibromatosis, hereditary gingival hyperplasia,* and *congenital familial fibromatosis.*

* These drugs are[45] the *dihydroxypiridine derivatives* (amlodipine [Lotrel, Norvasc], felodipine [Plendil], nicardipine [Cardene], Nifedipine [Adalat, Procardia]); the *benzothiazine derivatives* (diltiazem [Cardizem, Dilacor XR, Tlazac]); and the *phenylalkylamine derivatives* (verapamil [Calan, Isoptin, Verelan, Covera HS]) induced experimentally in rats where it appears to be dose dependent[38]; in humans, however, the dose dependency is not clear.

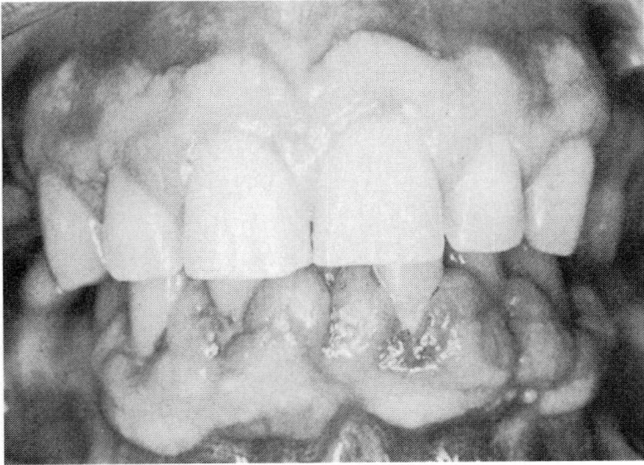

Fig. 18-13 Idiopathic hyperplastic gingival enlargement. The gingiva is firm, with a nodular, pebbled surface. The hyperplastic gingiva deflects the erupting teeth from proper alignment. (Courtesy Dr. E. I. Ball.)

Clinical Features. The enlargement affects the attached gingiva, as well as the gingival margin and interdental papillae, in contrast to phenytoin-induced overgrowth, which is often limited to the gingival margin and interdental papillae. The facial and lingual surfaces of the mandible and maxilla are generally affected, but the involvement may be limited to either jaw. The enlarged gingiva is pink, firm, and almost leathery in consistency and has a characteristic minutely pebbled surface (Fig. 18-12). In severe cases the teeth are almost completely covered, and the enlargement projects into the oral vestibule (see Color Fig. 18-1, *F*). The jaws appear distorted because of the bulbous enlargement of the gingiva. Secondary inflammatory changes are common at the gingival margin.

Histopathology. There is a bulbous increase in the amount of connective tissue that is relatively avascular and consists of densely arranged collagen bundles and numerous fibroblasts. The surface epithelium is thickened and acanthotic with elongated rete pegs.

Etiology. The cause is unknown, and thus the condition is designated as idiopathic. Some cases have a hereditary basis,[35,134,136] but the genetic mechanisms involved are not well understood. A study of several families found the mode of inheritance to be autosomal recessive in some cases and autosomal dominant in others.[58,96] In some families the gingival enlargement may be linked to retardation of physical development.[64] The enlargement usually begins with the eruption of the primary or secondary dentition and may regress after extraction, suggesting the possibility that the teeth (or the plaque attached to them) may be initiating factors. The presence of bacterial plaque is a complicating factor. Gingival enlargement has been described in tuberous sclerosis, which is an inherited condition characterized by a triad of epilepsy, mental deficiency, and cutaneous angiofibromas.[119,124]

ENLARGEMENTS ASSOCIATED WITH SYSTEMIC DISEASES

Many systemic diseases can develop oral manifestations that may include gingival enlargement. These diseases and/or conditions can affect the periodontium by two different mechanisms:

1. Magnification of an existing inflammation initiated by dental plaque. This group of diseases, discussed below under "Conditioned Enlargements," includes some hormonal conditions (e.g., pregnancy and puberty), nutritional diseases such as vitamin C deficiency, and some cases in which the systemic influence is not identified (nonspecific conditioned enlargement).
2. Manifestation of the systemic disease independently of the inflammatory status of the gingiva. This group will be described under "Systemic Diseases Causing Gingival Enlargement" and "Neoplastic Enlargement (Gingival Tumors)."

Conditioned Enlargement

Conditioned enlargement occurs when the systemic condition of the patient exaggerates or distorts the usual gingival response to dental plaque. The specific manner in which the clinical picture of conditioned gingival enlargement differs from that of chronic gingivitis depends on the nature of the modifying systemic influence. *Bacterial plaque is necessary for the initiation of this type of enlargement.* However, plaque is not the sole determinant of the nature of the clinical features.

The three types of conditioned gingival enlargement are hormonal (pregnancy, puberty), nutritional (associated with vitamin C deficiency), and allergic. Nonspecific conditioned enlargement is also seen.

Enlargement in Pregnancy. Pregnancy gingival enlargement may be marginal and generalized or may occur as single or multiple tumor-like masses (see Chapters 12 and 37).

During pregnancy there is an increase in levels of both progesterone and estrogen, which, by the end of the third trimester, reach levels 10 and 30 times the levels during the menstrual cycle, respectively.[2] These hormonal changes induce changes in vascular permeability leading to gingival edema and an increased inflammatory response to dental plaque. The subgingival microbiota may also undergo changes, including an increase in *Prevotella intermedia*.[69,95]

MARGINAL ENLARGEMENT. Marginal gingival enlargement during pregnancy results from the aggravation of previous inflammation, and its incidence has been reported as 10%[23] and 70%.[135] The gingival enlargement does not occur without the presence of bacterial plaque.

Clinical Features. The clinical picture varies considerably. The enlargement is usually generalized and tends to be more prominent interproximally than on the facial and lingual surfaces. The enlarged gingiva is bright red or magenta, soft, and friable and has a smooth, shiny surface. Bleeding occurs spontaneously or on slight provocation.

TUMORLIKE GINGIVAL ENLARGEMENT. The so-called pregnancy tumor is not a neoplasm; it is an inflammatory response to bacterial plaque and is modified by the patient's condition. It usually appears after the third month of pregnancy but may occur earlier. The reported incidence is 1.8% to 5%.[77]

Clinical Features. The lesion appears as a discrete, mushroomlike, flattened spherical mass that protrudes from the gingival margin or more commonly from the interproximal space and is attached by a sessile or pedunculated base (Fig. 18-14). It tends to expand laterally, and pressure from the tongue and the cheek perpetuates its flattened appearance. Generally dusky red or magenta, it has a smooth, glistening surface that often exhibits numerous deep red, pinpoint markings. It is a superficial lesion and ordinarily does not invade the underlying bone. The consistency varies; the mass is usually semifirm, but it may have various degrees of softness and friability. It is usually painless unless its size and shape foster accumulation of debris under its margin or interfere with occlusion, in which case, painful ulceration may occur.

HISTOPATHOLOGY. Gingival enlargement in pregnancy is called *angiogranuloma*. Both marginal and tumorlike enlargements consist of a central mass of connective tissue, with numerous diffusely arranged, newly formed, and engorged capillaries lined by cuboid endothelial cells (Fig. 18-15) and a moderately fibrous stroma with varying degrees of edema and chronic inflammatory infiltrate. The stratified squamous epithelium is thickened, with prominent rete pegs and some degree of intracellular and extracellular edema, prominent intercellular bridges, and leukocytic infiltration.

Although the microscopic findings are characteristic of gingival enlargement in pregnancy, they are not pathognomonic because they cannot be used to differentiate pregnant and nonpregnant patients.[77]

Most gingival disease during pregnancy can be prevented by the removal of plaque and calculus, as well as the institution of fastidious oral hygiene at the outset. In pregnancy, treatment of the gingiva that is limited to the removal of tissue without complete elimination of local irritants is followed by recurrence of gingival enlarge-

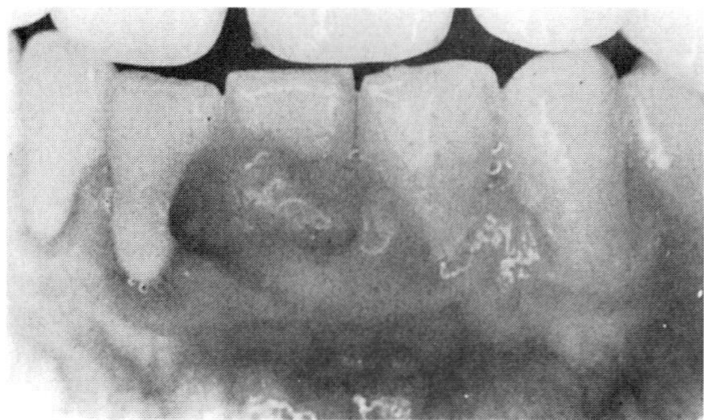

Fig. 18-14 Conditioned gingival enlargement in pregnancy.

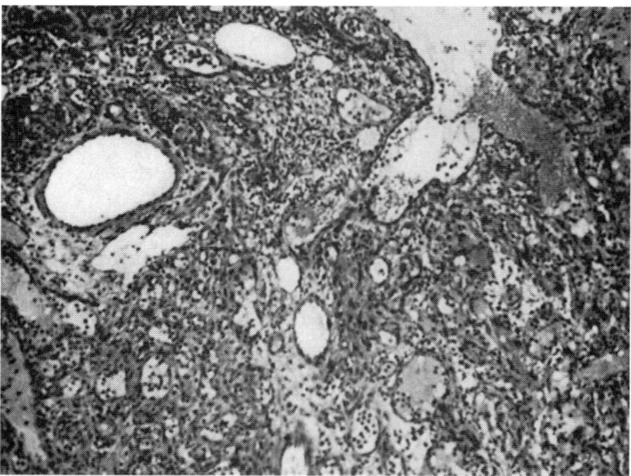

Fig. 18-15 Microscopic view of gingival enlargement in pregnancy showing an abundance of blood vessels and interspersed inflammatory cells.

ment. Although spontaneous reduction in the size of gingival enlargement commonly follows the termination of pregnancy, complete elimination of the residual inflammatory lesion requires the removal of all plaque deposits and factors that favor its accumulation.

Enlargement in Puberty. Enlargement of the gingiva is sometimes seen during puberty (see Chapters 12 and 37). It occurs in both male and female adolescents and appears in areas of plaque accumulation.

CLINICAL FEATURES. The size of the gingival enlargement far exceeds that usually seen in association with comparable local factors. It is marginal and interdental and is characterized by prominent bulbous interproximal papillae (Fig. 18-16). Often only the facial gingivae are enlarged, and the lingual surfaces are relatively unaltered. This is because the mechanical action of the tongue and the excursion of food prevent a heavy accumulation of local irritants on the lingual surface.

Gingival enlargement during puberty has all the clinical features generally associated with chronic inflammatory gingival disease. It is the degree of enlargement and the tendency to develop massive recurrence in the presence of relatively scant plaque deposits that distinguish pubertal gingival enlargement from uncomplicated chronic inflammatory gingival enlargement. After puberty, the enlargement undergoes spontaneous reduction but does not disappear until plaque and calculus are removed.

A longitudinal study of 127 children 11 to 17 years of age showed a high initial prevalence of gingival enlargement that tended to decline with age.[120] When the mean number of inflamed gingival sites per child was determined and correlated with the time at which the maximum number of inflamed sites was observed and the oral hygiene index at that time, it could be clearly seen that a pubertal peak in gingival inflammation that was unrelated to oral hygiene factors occurred. A longitudinal study of subgingival microbiota of children between the ages of 11 and 14 and their association with clinical parameters has implicated *Capnocytophaga* sp. in the initiation of pubertal gingivitis.[83] Other studies have reported that hormonal changes coincide with an increase in the proportion of *Prevotella intermedia* and *Prevotella nigrescens*.[85,132]

HISTOPATHOLOGY. The microscopic picture is that of chronic inflammation with prominent edema and associated degenerative changes.

Enlargement in Vitamin C Deficiency. Enlargement of the gingiva is generally included in classic descriptions of scurvy. It is important to recognize that such enlargement is essentially a conditioned response to bacterial plaque. Acute vitamin C deficiency does not of itself cause gingival inflammation, but it does cause hemorrhage, collagen degeneration, and edema of the gingival connective tissue. These changes modify the response of the gingiva to plaque to the extent that the normal defensive delimiting reaction is inhibited, and the extent of the inflammation is exaggerated.[39,40] The combined effect of acute vitamin C deficiency and inflammation produces the massive gingival enlargement in scurvy (Fig. 18-17) (see Chapter 12).

CLINICAL FEATURES. Gingival enlargement in vitamin C deficiency is marginal; the gingiva is bluish red, soft, and friable and has a smooth, shiny surface. Hemorrhage, occurring either spontaneously or on slight provocation, and surface necrosis with pseudomembrane formation are common features.

HISTOPATHOLOGY. The gingiva has a chronic inflammatory cellular infiltration with a superficial acute response. There are scattered areas of hemorrhage, with engorged capillaries. Marked diffuse edema, collagen degeneration, and scarcity of collagen fibrils or fibroblasts are striking findings.

Plasma Cell Gingivitis. Plasma cell gingivitis is also referred to as *atypical gingivitis* and *plasma cell gingivostomatitis* and often consists of a mild marginal gingival enlargement that extends to the attached gingiva. A localized lesion, referred to as *plasma cell granuloma,* has also been described.[15]

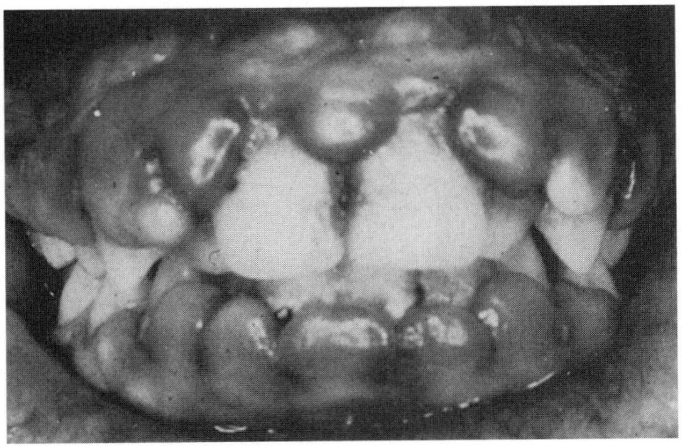

Fig. 18-16 Conditioned gingival enlargement in puberty in a 13-year-old boy.

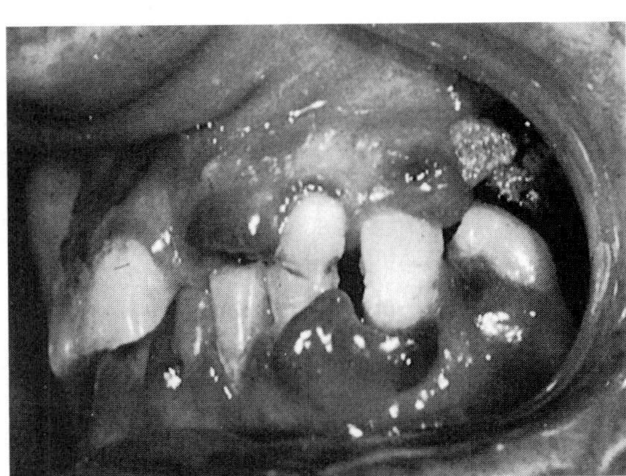

Fig. 18-17 Gingival enlargement in vitamin C deficiency. Note the prominent hemorrhagic areas.

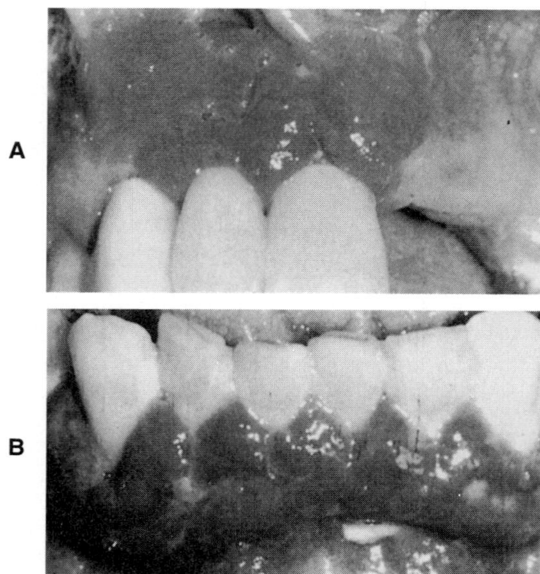

Fig. 18-18 Plasma cell granuloma of the gingiva. **A,** Diffuse lesions on the facial surface of the anterior maxilla. **B,** Mandibular lesions. (Courtesy Dr. Kim D. Zussman, Thousand Oaks, Calif.)

CLINICAL FEATURES. The gingiva appears red, friable, and sometimes granular and bleeds easily; usually it does not induce a loss of attachment (Fig. 18-18). This lesion is located in the oral aspect of the attached gingiva and therefore differs from plaque-induced gingivitis.

HISTOPATHOLOGY. The oral epithelium shows spongiosis and infiltration with inflammatory cells; ultrastructurally there are signs of damage in the lower spinous layers and the basal layers. The underlying connective tissue contains a dense infiltrate of plasma cells that also extends to the oral epithelium, inducing a dissecting type of injury.[88]

An associated cheilitis and glossitis have been reported.[63,104] Plasma cell gingivitis is thought to be allergic in origin, possibly related to components of chewing gum, dentifrices, or various diet components. Cessation of exposure to the allergen brings resolution of the lesion.

In rare instances, marked inflammatory gingival enlargements with a predominance of plasma cells can appear associated with rapidly progressive periodontitis.[90]

Nonspecific Conditioned Enlargement (Pyogenic Granuloma). Pyogenic granuloma is a tumorlike gingival enlargement that is considered an exaggerated conditioned response to minor trauma (Fig. 18-19). The exact nature of the systemic conditioning factor has not been identified.[62]

CLINICAL FEATURES. The lesion varies from a discrete spherical, tumorlike mass with a pedunculated attachment to a flattened, keloidlike enlargement with a broad base. It is bright red or purple and either friable or firm, depending on its duration; in the majority of cases it presents with surface ulceration and purulent exudation. The lesion tends to involute spontaneously to become a fibroepithelial papilloma or persists relatively unchanged for years.

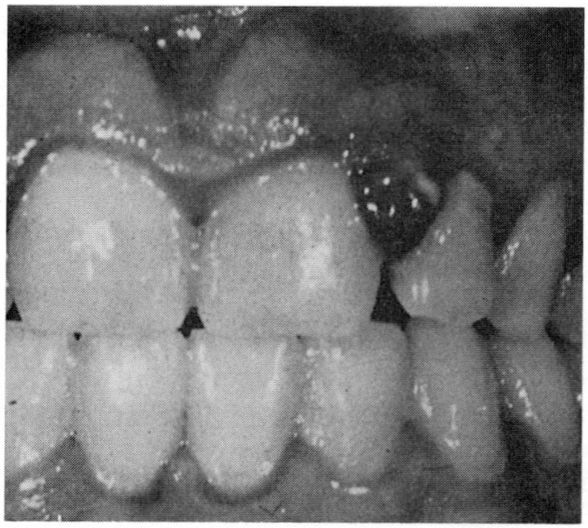

Fig. 18-19 Pyogenic granuloma in a young woman.

HISTOPATHOLOGY. Pyogenic granuloma appears as a mass of granulation tissue with chronic inflammatory cellular infiltration. Endothelial proliferation and the formation of numerous vascular spaces are the prominent features. The surface epithelium is atrophic in some areas and hyperplastic in others. Surface ulceration and exudation are common features.

Treatment consists of removal of the lesions plus the elimination of irritating local factors. The recurrence rate is about 15%.[14] Pyogenic granuloma is similar in clinical and microscopic appearance to the conditioned gingival enlargement seen in pregnancy. Differential diagnosis depends on the patient's history.

Systemic Diseases Causing Gingival Enlargement

Several systemic diseases may, by different mechanisms, result in gingival enlargement. These are uncommon cases and will be only briefly discussed.

Leukemia

CLINICAL FEATURES. Leukemic enlargement may be diffuse or marginal, localized or generalized (see Chapter 12). It may appear as a diffuse enlargement of the gingival mucosa (Fig. 18-20), an oversized extension of the marginal gingiva, or a discrete tumorlike interproximal mass. In leukemic enlargement the gingiva is generally bluish red and has a shiny surface. The consistency is moderately firm, but there is a tendency toward friability and hemorrhage, occurring either spontaneously or on slight irritation. Acute painful necrotizing ulcerative inflammatory involvement sometimes occurs in the crevice formed at the junction of the enlarged gingiva and the contiguous tooth surfaces.

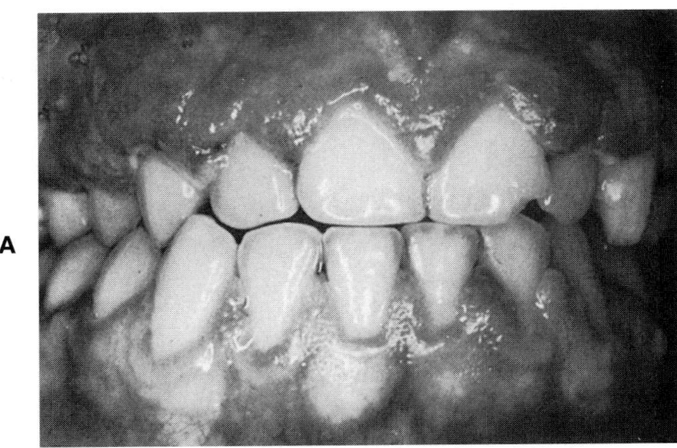

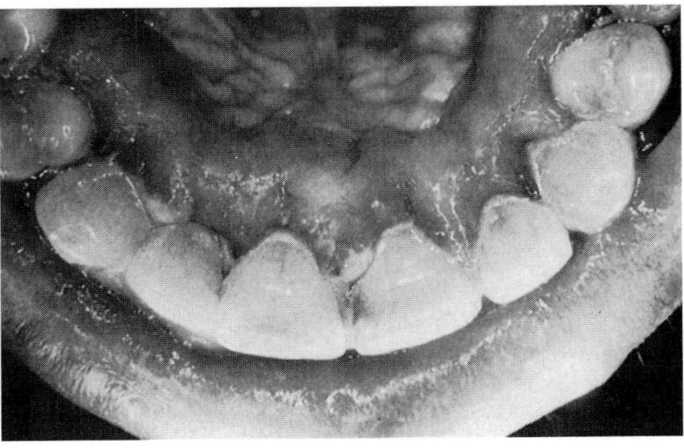

Fig. 18-20 Leukemic gingival enlargement. **A,** Leukemic gingival enlargement in a patient with acute myelocytic leukemia. Note that the enlargement is more prominent in the maxilla and is associated with greater plaque accumulation. **B,** Lingual view of gingival enlargement in a patient with subacute monocytic leukemia, showing a bulbous increase in size with discoloration and a smooth, shiny surface. Note the difference between the enlarged gingiva and the adjacent palatal mucosa.

Patients with leukemia may also have a simple chronic inflammation without the involvement of leukemic cells and may present with the same clinical and microscopic features seen in patients without the disease. Most cases reveal features of both simple chronic inflammation and a leukemic infiltrate.

True leukemic enlargement occurs commonly in acute leukemia but may also be seen in subacute leukemia. It seldom occurs in chronic leukemia.

HISTOPATHOLOGY. Gingival enlargements in leukemic patients show various degrees of chronic inflammation with mature leukocytes and areas of connective tissue infiltrated with a dense mass of immature and proliferating leukocytes, the specific nature of which varies with the type of leukemia. Engorged capillaries, edematous and degenerated connective tissue, and epithelium with various degrees of leukocytic infiltration and edema are found. Isolated surface areas of acute necrotizing inflammation with a pseudomembranous meshwork of fibrin, necrotic epithelial cells, polymorphonuclear neutrophils (PMNs), and bacteria are often seen.

Granulomatous Diseases

WEGENER'S GRANULOMATOSIS. Wegener's granulomatosis is a rare disease characterized by acute granulomatous necrotizing lesions of the respiratory tract, including nasal and oral defects. Renal lesions develop, and acute necrotizing vasculitis affects the blood vessels. The initial manifestations of Wegener's granulomatosis may involve the orofacial region and include oral mucosal ulceration, gingival enlargement, abnormal tooth mobility, exfoliation of teeth, and delayed healing response.[20]

Clinical Features. The granulomatous papillary enlargement is reddish purple and bleeds easily on stimulation.

Histopathology. Chronic inflammation occurs, with scattered giant cells and foci of acute inflammation and microabscesses covered by a thin acanthotic epithelium. Vascular changes have not been described, probably owing to the small size of the gingival blood vessels.[57]

The cause of Wegener's granulomatosis is unknown, but the condition is considered an immunologically mediated tissue injury.[27] At one time the usual outcome was death from kidney failure within a few months, but more recently the use of immunosuppressive drugs has produced prolonged remissions in more than 90% of cases.[68]

Sarcoidosis. Sarcoidosis is a granulomatous disease of unknown etiology. It starts in individuals in their twenties or thirties, affects predominantly blacks and can involve almost any organ, including the gingiva, where a red, smooth, painless enlargement may appear (Fig. 18-21).

HISTOPATHOLOGY. Sarcoid granulomas consist of discrete, noncaseating whorls of epithelioid cells and multinucleated foreign-body–type giant cells with peripheral mononuclear cells.[99]

NEOPLASTIC ENLARGEMENT (GINGIVAL TUMORS)

Only a brief description of some of the most common neoplastic and pseudoneoplastic lesions of the gingiva will be given. The reader is referred to texts on oral pathology for a more comprehensive coverage.[87,99]

Benign Tumors of the Gingiva

Epulis is a generic term used clinically to designate all discrete tumors and tumorlike masses of the gingiva. It

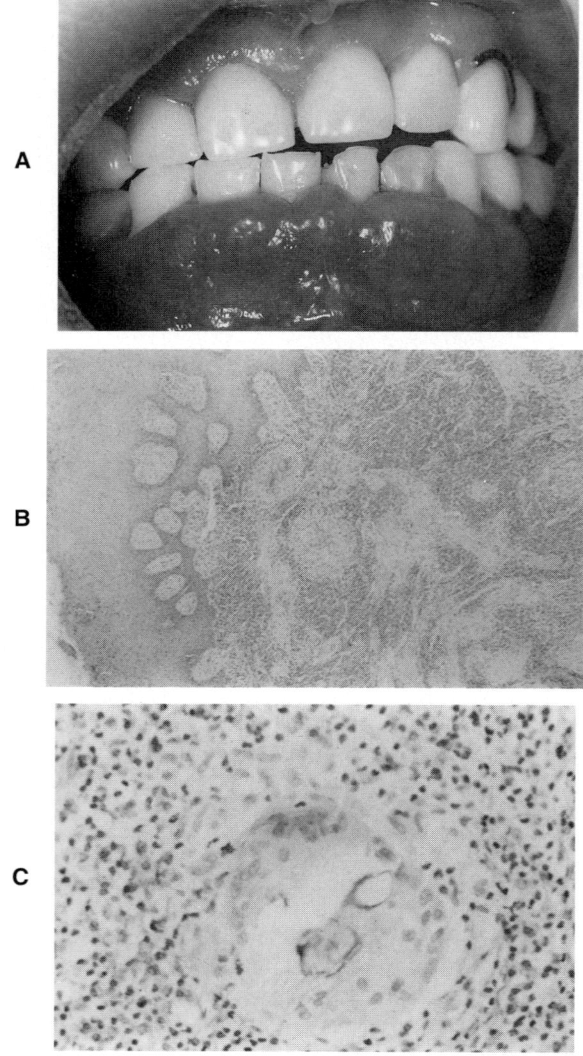

Fig. 18-21 **A,** Gingival enlargement in a case of sarcoidosis. Low power **(B)** and high-power **(C)** microscopic view of sarcoid granuloma. (Courtesy Dr. Silvia Oreamuno, San José, Costa Rica.)

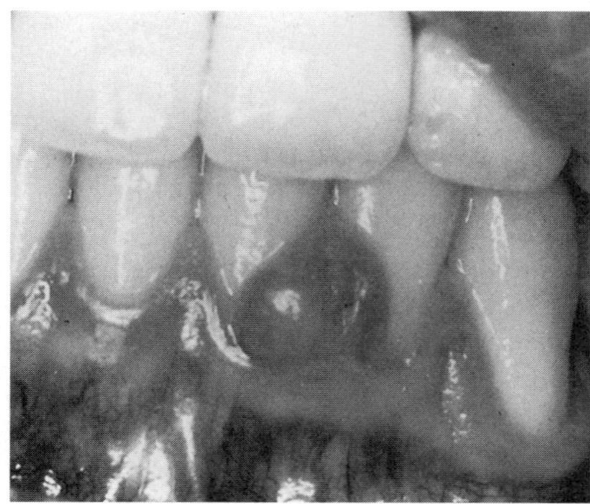

Fig. 18-22 Papilloma of the gingiva in a 26-year-old man.

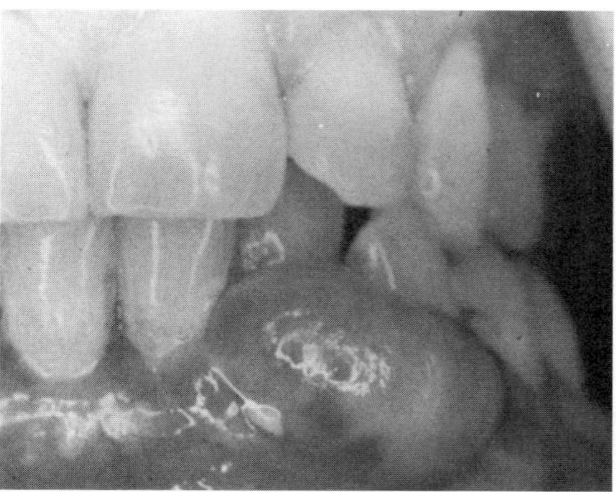

Fig. 18-23 Gingival giant cell granuloma.

serves to locate the tumor but not to describe it. Most lesions referred to as *epulis* are inflammatory rather than neoplastic.

Neoplasms account for a comparatively small proportion of gingival enlargements and make up a small percentage of the total number of oral neoplasms. In a survey of 257 oral tumors,[81] approximately 8% occurred on the gingiva. In another study[12] of 868 growths of the gingiva and palate, of which 57% were neoplastic and the remainder inflammatory, the following incidence of tumors was noted: carcinoma, 11.0%; fibroma, 9.3%; giant cell tumor, 8.4%; papilloma, 7.3%; leukoplakia, 4.9%; mixed tumor (salivary gland type), 2.5%; angioma, 1.5%; osteofibroma, 1.3%; sarcoma, 0.5%; melanoma, 0.5%; myxoma, 0.45%; fibropapilloma, 0.4%; adenoma, 0.4%; and lipoma, 0.3%.

Fibroma. Fibromas of the gingiva arise from the gingival connective tissue or from the periodontal ligament. They are slow-growing, spherical tumors that tend to be firm and nodular but may be soft and vascular. Fibromas are usually pedunculated. Hard fibromas of the gingiva are rare; most of the lesions diagnosed clinically as fibromas are inflammatory enlargements.[103]

HISTOPATHOLOGY. Fibromas are composed of bundles of well-formed collagen fibers with a scattering of fibrocytes and a variable vascularity.

A so-called giant-cell fibroma contains multinucleated fibroblasts. In another variant mineralized tissue (bone, cementum-like material, dystrophic calcifications) may be found; this type of fibroma is called *peripheral ossifying fibroma.*

Papilloma. Papillomas are benign proliferations of surface epithelium associated with the human papillomavirus (HPV). Viral subtypes HPV-6 and HPV-11 have been found in most cases of oral papillomas. Gingival papillomas appear as solitary, wartlike or "cauliflower"-like protuberances (Fig. 18-22) and may be small and discrete or broad, hard elevations with minutely irregular surfaces.

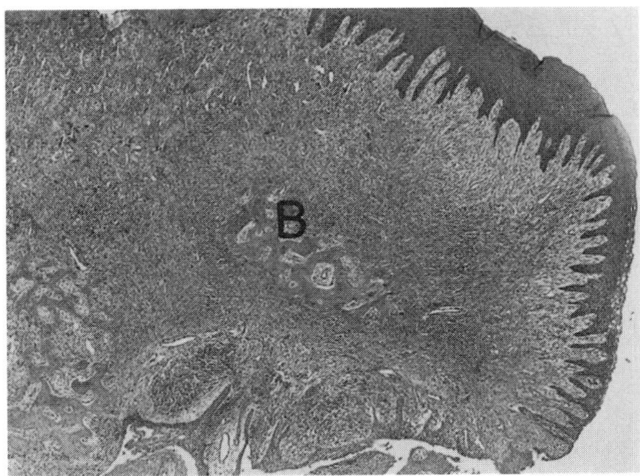

Fig. 18-24 Microscopic survey of peripheral giant cell reparative granuloma. Trabeculae of newly formed bone (B) are contained within the mass.

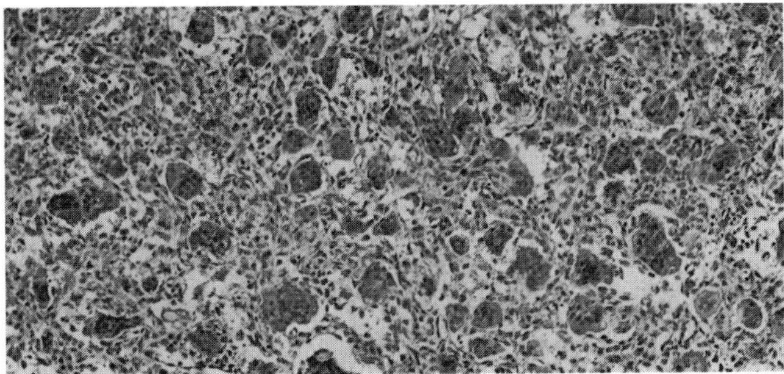

Fig. 18-25 High-power study of the lesion shown in Fig. 18-24 demonstrating the giant cells and intervening stroma that make up the major portion of the mass.

HISTOPATHOLOGY. The lesion consists of fingerlike projections of stratified squamous epithelium, often hyperkeratotic, with a central core of fibrovascular connective tissue.

Peripheral Giant Cell Granuloma. Giant cell lesions of the gingiva arise interdentally or from the gingival margin, occur most frequently on the labial surface, and may be sessile or pedunculated. They vary in appearance from smooth, regularly outlined masses to irregularly shaped, multilobulated protuberances with surface indentations (Fig. 18-23). Ulceration of the margin is occasionally seen. The lesions are painless, vary in size, and may cover several teeth. They may be firm or spongy, and the color varies from pink to deep red or purplish blue. There are no pathognomonic clinical features whereby these lesions can be differentiated from other forms of gingival enlargement. Microscopic examination is required for definitive diagnosis (Figs. 18-24 and 18-25).

In the past, giant cell lesions of the gingiva have been referred to as *peripheral reparative giant cell tumors*. These lesions, however, are essentially responses to local injury and not neoplasms; and their reparative nature has not been proven. Therefore they are now referred to as *peripheral giant cell granulomas*. The prefix peripheral is needed to differentiate them from comparable lesions that originate within the jawbone (central giant cell granulomas).

In some instances, the giant cell granuloma of the gingiva is locally invasive and causes destruction of the underlying bone (Fig. 18-26). Complete removal leads to uneventful recovery.

HISTOPATHOLOGY. The giant cell granuloma has numerous foci of multinuclear giant cells and hemosiderin particles in a connective tissue stroma. Areas of chronic inflammation are scattered throughout the lesion, with acute involvement occurring at the surface. The overlying epithelium is usually hyperplastic, with ulceration at the base. Bone formation occasionally occurs within the lesion (see Figs. 18-24 and 18-25).

Central Giant Cell Granuloma. These lesions arise within the jaws and produce central cavitation. They occasionally create a deformity of the jaw that makes the gingiva appear enlarged.

Mixed tumors, salivary gland type tumors, and plasmacytomas of the gingiva have also been described but are not often seen.

Leukoplakia. *Leukoplakia* is a strictly clinical term defined by the World Health Organization as a white patch or plaque that does not rub off and cannot be diagnosed as any other disease. The cause of leukoplakia remains obscure, although it is associated to the use of tobacco (smoke or smokeless). Other probable factors are *Candida albicans,* HPV-16 and HPV-18, and trauma. Leukoplakia of the gingiva varies in appearance from a grayish white, flattened, scaly lesion to a thick, irregularly shaped keratinous plaque (Fig. 18-27).

Most leukoplakias (80%) are benign, the remaining 20% are malignant or premalignant, and only 3% of these are invasive carcinomas.[37] Biopsy of all leukoplakias, selecting the most suspicious area, is necessary to arrive at a correct diagnosis and institute proper therapy.[37,87]

HISTOPATHOLOGY. Leukoplakia exhibits hyperkeratosis and acanthosis. Premalignant and malignant cases have a variable degree of atypical epithelial changes that may be mild, moderate, or severe, depending on the extent of involvement of the epithelial layers. When dysplastic changes involve all layers, it is diagnosed as a *carcinoma in situ,* and this may become invasive carcinoma when the basement membrane is breached.[37] Inflammatory involvement of the underlying connective tissue is a commonly associated finding.

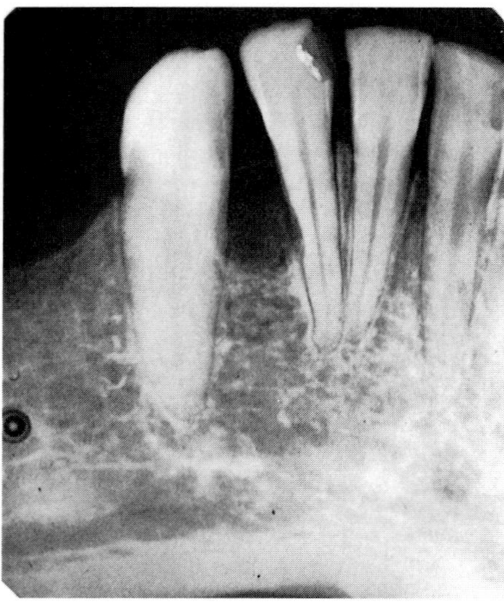

Fig. 18-26 Bone destruction in the interproximal space between the canine and lateral incisor caused by the extension of a peripheral giant cell reparative granuloma of the gingiva. (Courtesy Dr. Sam Toll.)

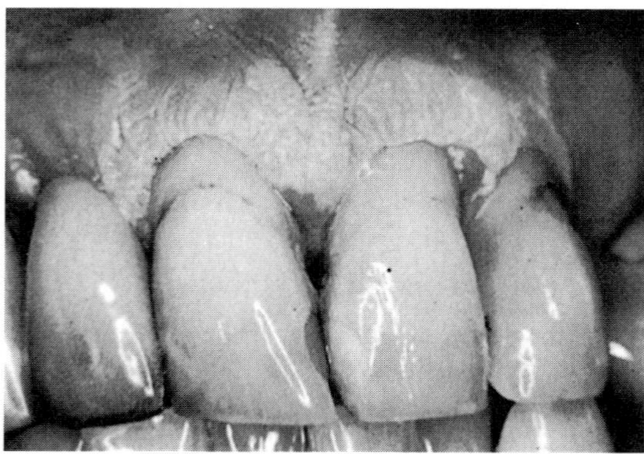

Fig. 18-27 Leukoplakia of the gingiva.

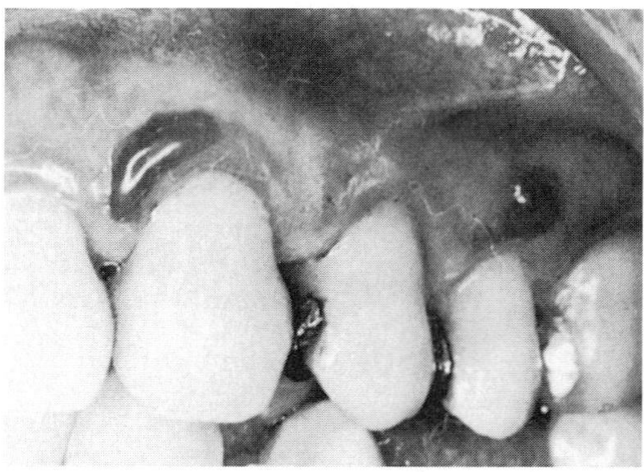

Fig. 18-28 Hematomas produced by trauma.

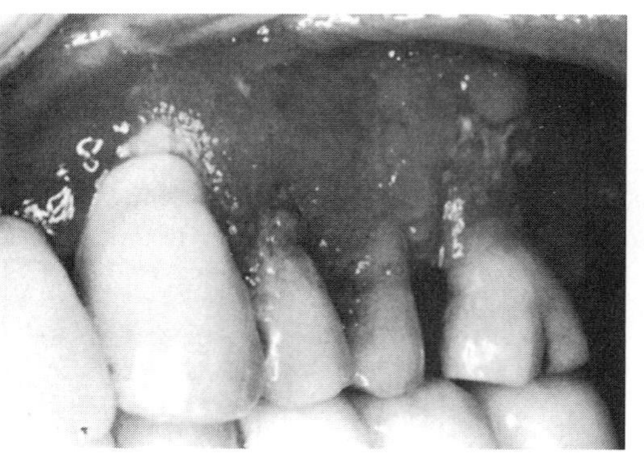

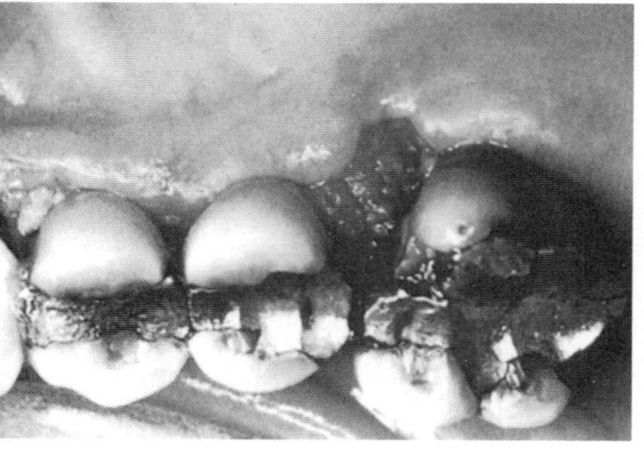

Fig. 18-29 Squamous cell carcinoma of the gingiva. **A,** Facial view. Note the extensive verrucous involvement. **B,** Palatal view. Note the mulberry-like tissue emerging between the second premolar and the first molar.

Gingival Cyst. Gingival cysts of microscopic proportions are common, but they seldom reach a clinically significant size.[84] When they do, they appear as localized enlargements that may involve the marginal and attached gingiva. They occur in the mandibular canine and premolar areas, most often on the lingual surface. They are painless, but with expansion, they may cause erosion of the surface of the alveolar bone. However, it should be differentiated from the lateral periodontal cyst (see Chapter 22), which arises within the alveolar bone, adjacent to the root, and is developmental in origin. The cysts develop from odontogenic epithelium or from surface or sulcular epithelium traumatically implanted in the area. Removal is followed by uneventful recovery.

Microscopically, a cyst cavity is lined by a thin, flattened epithelium with or without localized areas of thickening. Less frequently, the following types of epithelium can be found: unkeratinized stratified squamous epithelium, keratinized stratified squamous epithelium, and parakeratinized epithelium with palisading basal cells.[19]

Other benign tumors have also been described as rare or infrequent findings in the gingiva. They include nevus,[13] myoblastoma,[43,61] hemangioma (Fig. 18-28),[12,121] neurilemoma,[37] neurofibroma,[94] mucus-secreting cysts (mucoceles),[127] and ameloblastoma.[118]

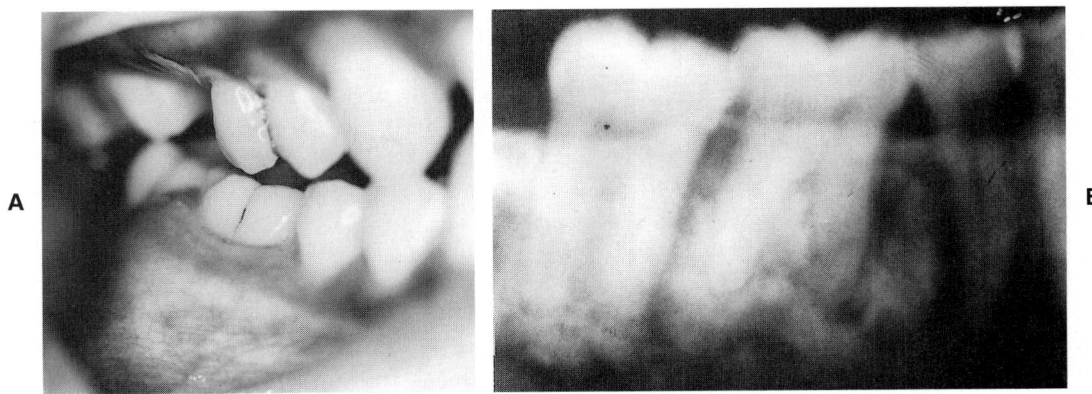

Fig. 18-30 **A,** Apparent gingival enlargement associated with bone augmentation in a case of fibrous dysplasia. **B,** Radiograph of the case shown in **A,** depicting a ground-glass, mottled radiographic pattern.

Malignant Tumors of the Gingiva

Carcinoma. Oral cancer accounts for less than 3% of all malignant tumors in the body but is the sixth most common cancer in males and the twelfth in females.[87] The gingiva is not a frequent site of oral malignancy (6% of oral cancers[70]).

Squamous cell carcinoma is the most common malignant tumor of the gingiva. It may be exophytic, presenting as an irregular outgrowth, or ulcerative, which appear as flat, erosive lesions. It is often symptom free, often going unnoticed until complicated by inflammatory changes that may mask the neoplasm but cause pain; sometimes it becomes evident after tooth extraction. They are locally invasive, involving the underlying bone and periodontal ligament of adjoining teeth and the adjacent mucosa (Fig. 18-29). Metastasis is usually confined to the region above the clavicle; however, more extensive involvement may include the lung, liver, or bone.

Malignant Melanoma. Malignant melanoma is a rare oral tumor that tends to occur in the hard palate and maxillary gingiva of older persons.[87] It is usually darkly pigmented and is often preceded by the occurrence of localized pigmentation.[25] It may be flat or nodular and is characterized by rapid growth and early metastasis. It arises from melanoblasts in the gingiva, cheek, or palate. Infiltration into the underlying bone and metastasis to cervical and axillary lymph nodes are common.

SARCOMA. Fibrosarcoma, lymphosarcoma, and reticulum cell sarcoma of the gingiva are rare; only isolated cases have been described in the literature.[42,47,123] Kaposi's sarcoma often occurs in the oral cavity of patients with acquired immunodeficiency syndrome (AIDS), particularly in the palate and the gingiva (see Chapter 29).

METASTASIS. Tumor metastasis to the gingiva is not common. Such metastasis has been reported with various tumors, including adenocarcinoma of the colon,[55] lung carcinoma, primary hepatocellular carcinoma,[125] renal cell carcinoma,[18] hypernephroma,[93] chondrosarcoma,[122] and testicular tumor.[36]

The low incidence of oral malignancy should not mislead the clinician. *Ulcerations that do not respond to therapy in the usual manner, as well as all gingival tumors and tumorlike lesions must be biopsied and submitted for microscopic diagnosis* (see Chapter 30).

The reader is referred to oral pathology textbooks[87] for more complete information on benign and malignant tumors of the gingiva.

FALSE ENLARGEMENT

False enlargements are not true enlargements of the gingival tissues but may appear as such as a result of increases in size of the underlying osseous or dental tissues. The gingiva usually presents with no abnormal clinical features except the massive increase in size of the area.

Underlying Osseous Lesions

Enlargement of the bone subjacent to the gingival area occurs most commonly in tori and exostoses, but it can also occur in Paget's disease, fibrous dysplasia, cherubism, central giant cell granuloma, ameloblastoma, osteoma, and osteosarcoma. One example of this type of enlargement is shown in Fig. 18-30. In this case a fibrous dysplasia (florid type) in a 38-year-old black female induced an osseous enlargement in the mandibular molar area that appeared as a gingival enlargement. The gingival tissue can appear normal or may have unrelated inflammatory changes.

Underlying Dental Tissues

During the various stages of eruption, particularly of the primary dentition, the labial gingiva may show a bulbous marginal distortion caused by superimposition of the bulk of the gingiva on the normal prominence of the enamel in the gingival half of the crown. This enlargement has been termed *developmental enlargement* and often persists until the junctional epithelium has migrated from the enamel to the cementoenamel junction.

In a strict sense, developmental gingival enlargements are physiologic and ordinarily present no problems. However, when such enlargement is complicated by mar-

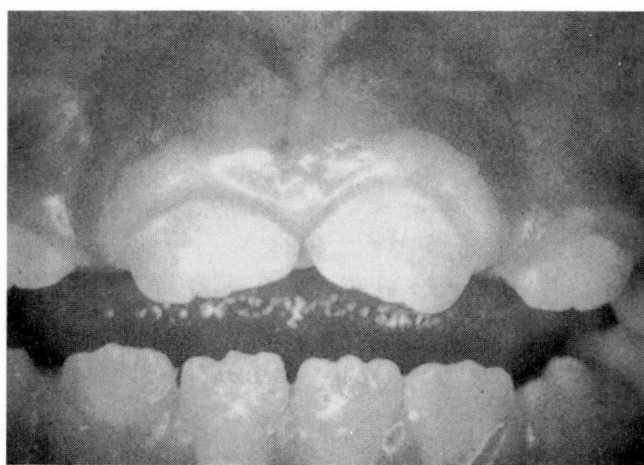

Fig. 18-31 Developmental gingival enlargement. The normal bulbous contour of the gingiva around the incompletely erupted anterior teeth is accentuated by chronic inflammation.

ginal inflammation, the composite picture gives the impression of extensive gingival enlargement (Fig. 18-31). Treatment to alleviate the marginal inflammation, rather than resection of the enlargement, is sufficient in these cases.

REFERENCES

1. Aas E: Hyperplasia Gingivae Diphenylhydantoinea. Oslo, Universitetsforlaget, 1963.
2. Amar S, Chung KM: Influence of hormonal variation on the periodontium in women. Periodontology 2000, 1994; 6:79.
3. Angelopoulos AP, Goaz PW: Incidence of diphenylhydantoin gingival hyperplasia. Oral Surg 1972; 34:898.
4. Ashrafi SH, Slaski K, Thu K, et al: Scanning electron microscopy of cyclosporine-induced gingival overgrowth. Scanning Microscopy 1996; 10:219.
5. Ayanoglou, CM, Lesty C: New cementum formation induced bt cyclosporin A: a histological, ultrastructural and histomorphometric study in the rat. J Periodont 1997; 32:543.
6. Babcock JR: Incidence of gingival hyperplasia associated with dilantin therapy in a hospital population. J Am Dent Assoc 1965; 71:1447.
7. Babcock JR, Nelson GH: Gingival hyperplasia and Dilantin content of saliva. J Am Dent Assoc 1964; 68:195.
8. Bader G, Lejeune S, Messner M: Reduction of cyclosporine-induced gingival overgrowth following a change to tacrolimus. A case history involving a liver transplant patient. J Periodontol 1988; 69:729.
9. Baratieri A: The oxytalan connective tissue fibers in gingival hyperplasia in patients treated with sodium diphenylhydantoin. J Periodont Res 1967; 2:106.
10. Barclay S, Thomason JM, Idle JR, et al: The incidence and severity of nifedipine-induced gingival overgrowth. J Clin Periodontol 1992; 19:311.
11. Bellinger DH: Blood and lymph vessel tumors involving the mouth. J Oral Surg 1944; 2:141.
12. Bernick S: Growth of the gingiva and palate. II. Connective tissue tumors. Oral Surg 1948; 1:1098.
13. Bernier JL, Tiecke RW: Nevus of the gingiva. J Oral Surg 1950; 8:165.
14. Bhaskar SN, Jacoway JR: Pyogenic granuloma: Clinical features, incidence, histology and result of treatment. J Oral Surg 1966; 24:391.
15. Bhaskar SN, Levin MP, Frisch J: Plasma cell granuloma of periodontal tissues. Report of 45 cases. Periodontics 1988; 6:272.
16. Bökenkamp A, Bohnhorst B, Beier C, et al: Nifedipine aggravates cyclosporine A-induced hyperplasia. Pediatr Nephrol 1994; 8:181.
17. Brown RS, Sein P, Corio R, et al: Nitrendipine-induced gingival hyperplasia. Oral Surg 1990; 70:593.
18. Buchner A, Begleiter A: Metastatic renal cell carcinoma in the gingiva mimicking a hyperplastic lesion. J Periodontol 1980; 51:413.
19. Buchner A, Hansen AS: The histomorphologic spectrum of the gingival cyst in the adult. Oral Surg 1979; 48:532.
20. Buckley DJ, Barrett AP, Bilous AM, et al: Wegener's granulomatosis—are gingival lesions pathognomonic? J Oral Med 1987; 42:169.
21. Buckner HJ: Diffuse fibroma of the gums. J Am Dent Assoc 1937; 24:2003.
22. Burket LW: Oral Medicine. Philadelphia, JB Lippincott, 1946.
23. Butler RT, Kalkwarf KL, Kaldhal WB: Drug-induced gingival hyperplasia: Phenytoin, cyclosporine and nifedipine. J Am Dent Assoc 1987; 114:56.
24. Calne R, Rolles K, White DJ, et al: Cyclosporin-A initially as the only immunosuppressant in 34 recipients of cadaveric organs: 32 kidneys, 2 pancreas and 2 livers. Lancet 1979; 2:1033.
25. Chaudry AP, Hampel A, Gorlin RJ: Primary malignant melanoma of the oral cavity: A review of 105 cases. Cancer 1958; 11:923.
26. Ciancio SG, Yaffe SJ, Catz CC: Gingival hyperplasia and diphenylhydantoin. J Periodontol 1972; 43:411.
27. Cotran RS, Kumar V, Robbins SL: Robbins' Pathologic Basis of Disease, 4th ed. Philadelphia, WB Saunders, 1989.
28. Daley TD, Nartey NO, Wysocki GP: Pregnancy tumor: An analysis. Oral Surg 1991; 72:196.
29. Daley TD, Wysocki GP, Day C: Clinical and pharmacologic correlations in cyclosporine-induced gingival hyperplasia. Oral Surg 1986; 62:417.
30. Heijl L, Sundin Y: Nitrendipine-induced gingival overgrowth in dogs. J Periodontol 1989; 60:104.
31. DaCosta ML, Regan MC, al Sader M, et al: Diphenyl hydantoin sodium promotes early and marked angiogenesis and results in increased collagen deposition and tensile strength in healing wounds. Surgery 1988; 123:287.
32. Dallas BM: Hyperplasia of the oral mucosa in an edentulous epileptic. NZ Dent J 1963; 59:54.
33. Dreyer WP, Thomas CJ: DPH-induced hyperplasia of the masticatory mucosa in an edentulous epileptic patient. Oral Surg 1978; 45:701.
34. Elzay RP, Swenson HM: Effect of an electric toothbrush on Dilantin sodium induced gingival hyperplasia. NY J Dent 1964; 34:13.
35. Emerson TG: Hereditary gingival hyperplasia. A family pedigree of four generations. Oral Surg 1965; 19:1.
36. Fantasia JE, Chen A: A testicular tumor with gingival metastasis. Oral Surg 1979; 48:64.
37. Fowler CB: Benign and malignant neoplasms of the periodontium. Periodontology 2000 1999; 21:33.
38. Fu E, Nieh S, Hiao CT, et al: Nifedipine-induced gingival overgrowth in rats: brief review and experimental study. J Periodontol 1988; 69:765.
39. Glickman I: The periodontal tissues of the guinea pig in vitamin C deficiency. J Dent Res 1948; 27:9.
40. Glickman I: The effect of acute vitamin C deficiency upon the response of the periodontal tissues of the guinea pig to artificially induced inflammation. J Dent Res 1948; 27:201.
41. Glickman I, Lewitus M: Hyperplasia of the gingiva associ-

ated with Dilantin (sodium diphenyl hydantoinate) therapy. J Am Dent Assoc 1941; 28:1991.
42. Goldman HM: Sarcoma. Am J Orthod 1944; 30:311.
43. Hagen JD, Soule EH, Gores RJ: Granular cell myoblastoma of the oral cavity. Oral Surg 1961; 14:454.
44. Hall WB: Dilantin hyperplasia: A preventable lesion. J Periodont Res (Suppl) 1969; 4:36.
45. Hallmon WW, Rossmann JA: The role of drugs in the pathogenesis of gingival overgrowth. Periodontology 2000 1999; 21:176.
46. Hancock RH, Swan RH: Nifedipine-induced gingival overgrowth. J Clin Periodontol 1992; 19:12.
47. Hardman FG: Secondary sarcoma presenting clinical appearance of fibrous epulis. Br Dent J 1949; 86:109.
48. Hassell TM: Epilepsy and the Oral Manifestations of Phenytoin Therapy. Monographs in Oral Science, Vol 9. New York, S Karger, 1981.
49. Hassell TM: Evidence for production of an inactive collagenase by fibroblasts from phenytoin-enlarged human gingiva. J Oral Pathol 1982; 11:310.
50. Hassell TM, Burtner AP, McNeal D, et al: Oral problems and genetic aspects of individuals with epilepsy. Periodontology 2000 1994; 6:68.
51. Hassell TM, Page RC: The major metabolite of phenytoin (Dilantin) induces gingival overgrowth in cats. J Periodont Res 1978; 13:280.
52. Hassell TM, Page RC, Lindhe J: Histologic evidence of impaired growth control in diphenylhydantoin gingival overgrowth in man. Arch Oral Biol 1978; 23:381.
53. Henefer EP, Kay LA: Congenital idiopathic gingival fibromatosis in the deciduous dentition. Oral Surg 1967; 24:65.
54. Hirschfeld I: Hypertrophic gingivitis; its clinical aspect. J Am Dent Assoc 1932; 19:799.
55. Humphrey AA, Amos NH: Metastatic gingival adenocarcinoma from primary lesion of colon. Am J Cancer 1936; 28:128.
56. Ishikawa J, Glickman I: Gingival response to the systemic administration of sodium diphenyl hydantoinate (Dilantin) in cats. J Periodontol 1961; 32:149.
57. Israelson H, Binnie WH, Hurt WC: The hyperplastic gingivitis of Wegener's granulomatosis. J Periodontol 1981; 52:81.
58. Jorgenson RJ, Cocker ME: Variation in the inheritance and expression of gingival fibromatosis. J Periodontol 1974; 45:472.
59. Kantor ML, Hassell TM: Increased accumulation of sulfated glycosaminoglycans in cultures of human fibroblasts from phenytoin-induced gingival overgrowth. J Dent Res 1983; 62:383.
60. Kapur RN, Grigis S, Little TM, et al: Diphenylhydantoin induced gingival hyperplasia: Its relation to dose and serum level. Dev Med Child Neurol 1973; 15:483.
61. Kerr DA: Myoblastic myoma. Oral Surg 1949; 2:41.
62. Kerr DA: Granuloma pyogenicum. Oral Surg 1951; 4:155.
63. Kerr DA, McClatchey KD, Regezi JA: Allergic gingivostomatitis (due to gum chewing). J Periodontol 1971; 42:709.
64. Kilpinen E, Raeste AM, Collan Y: Hereditary gingival hyperplasia and physical maturation. Scand J Dent Res 1978; 86:118.
65. Kimball O: The treatment of epilepsy with sodium diphenylhydantoinate. JAMA 1939; 112:1244.
66. Klar LA: Gingival hyperplasia during Dilantin therapy: A survey of 312 patients. J Public Health Dent 1973; 33:180.
67. Klingsberg J, Cancellaro LA, Butcher EO: Effects of air drying in rodent oral mucous membrane. A histologic study of simulated mouth breathing. J Periodontol 1961; 32:38.
68. Kornblut AD, Wolff SM, de Fries HE, et al: Wegener's granulomatosis. Laryngoscope 1980; 90:1453.
69. Kornman KS, Loesche WJ: The subgingival microbial flora during pregnancy. J Periodont Res 1980; 15:111.
70. Krolls SO, Hoffman S: Squamous cell carcinomas of the oral soft tissues: A statistical analysis of 14,253 cases by age, sex and race of patients. J Am Dent Assoc 1976; 92:571.
71. Lamborghini Deliliers G, Santoro F, Polli N, et al: Light and electron microscopic study of cyclosporin-A induced gingival hyperplasia. J Periodontol 1986; 57:771.
72. Larmas LA, Mackinen KK, Paunio KU: A histochemical study of amylaminopeptidase in hydantoin-induced hyperplastic, healthy and inflamed human gingiva. J Periodont Res 1973; 8:21.
73. Lederman D, Lummerman H, Reuben S, et al: Gingival hyperplasia associated with nifedipine therapy. Oral Surg 1984; 57:620.
74. Lite T, Dimaio DJ, Burman LR: Gingival patterns in mouth breathers. A clinical and histopathologic study and a method of treatment. Oral Surg 1955; 8:382.
75. Lucas RM, Howell LP, Wall RA: Nifedipine-induced gingival hyperplasia. A histochemical and ultrastructural study. J Periodontol 1985; 56:211.
76. Lustberg A, Goldman D, Dreskin OH: Megaloblastic anemia due to Dilantin therapy. Ann Intern Med 1961; 54:153.
77. Maier AW, Orban B: Gingivitis in pregnancy. Oral Surg 1949; 2:334.
78. Mariani G, Calastrini C, Carinci F, et al: Ultrastructural features of cyclosporine A-induced gingival hyperplasia. J Periodontol 1993; 64:1092.
79. Mealy BL: Periodontal implications: medically compromised patients. Annals Periodontol 1996; 1:256.
80. Merritt H, Putnam T: Sodium diphenylhydantoinate in the treatment of convulsive disorders. JAMA 1938; 111:1068.
81. McCarthy FP: A clinical and pathological study of oral disease. JAMA 1941; 116:16.
82. Mihatsch MJ, Kyo M, Morozumi K, et al: The side-effects of cyclosporine-A and tacrolimus. Clin Nephrol 1988; 49:356.
83. Mombelli A, Lang NP, Burgin WB, et al: Microbial changes associated with the development of puberty gingivitis. J Periodont Res 1990; 25:331.
84. Moskow BS: The pathogenesis of the gingival cyst. Periodontics 1966; 4:23.
85. Nakagawa S, Fujii H, Machida Y, et al: A longitudinal study from prepuberty to puberty of gingivitis. Correlation between the occurrence of Prevotella intermedia and sex hormones. J Periodontol 1994; 21:658.
86. Nease WJ: Effect of sodium diphenylhydantoinate on tissue cultures of human gingiva. J Periodontol 1965; 36:22.
87. Neville BW, Damm DD, Allen CM, et al: Oral and Maxillofacial Pathology. Philadelphia, WB Saunders, 1995.
88. Newcomb GM, Seymour GJ, Adkins KF: An unusual form of chronic gingivitis: An ultrastructural, histochemical and immunologic investigation. Oral Surg 1982; 53:488.
89. Nishikawa S, Tada H, Hamasaki A, et al: Nifedipine-induced gingival hyperplasia: A clinical and in vitro study. J Periodontol 1991; 62:30.
90. Nitta H, Kameyama Y, Ishikawa I: Unusual gingival enlargement with rapidly progressive periodontitis. Report of a case. J Periodontol 1993; 64:1008.
91. Nuki K, Cooper SH: The role of inflammation in the pathogenesis of gingival enlargement during the administration of diphenylhydantoin sodium in cats. J Periodont Res 1972; 7:91.
92. Panuska HJ, Gorlin RJ, Bearman JE, et al: The effect of anticonvulsant drugs upon the gingiva. A series of 1048 patients. II. J Periodontol 1961; 32:15.
93. Persson PA, Wallenino K: Metastatic renal carcinoma (hypernephroma) in the gingiva of the lower jaw. Acta Odontol Scand 1961; 19:289.

94. Pollack RP: Neurofibroma of the palatal mucosa. A case report. J Periodontol 1990; 61:456.
95. Raber-Durlacher JE, van Steenbergen TJM, van der Velde U, et al: Experimental gingivitis during pregnancy and postpartum: Clinical, endocrinological and microbiological aspects. J Clin Periodontol 1994; 21:549.
96. Raeste AM, Collan Y, Kilpinen E: Hereditary fibrous hyperplasia of the gingiva with varying penetrance and expressivity. Scand J Dent Res 1978; 86:357.
97. Rateitschak-Pluss EM, Hefti A, Lortscher R, et al: Initial observation that cyclosporin A induces gingival enlargement in man. J Clin Periodontol 1983; 10:237.
98. Rees TD: Drugs and oral disorders. Periodontology 2000 1998; 18:21.
99. Rees TD (ed): Disorders affecting the periodontium. Periodontology 2000 1999; 21:145.
100. Rostock MH, Fry HR, Turner JE: Severe gingival overgrowth associated with cyclosporine therapy. J Periodontol 1986; 57:294.
101. Rushton MA: Hereditary or idiopathic hyperplasia of the gums. Dent Pract 1957; 7:136.
102. Russell BJ, Bay LM: Oral use of chlorhexidine gluconate toothpaste in epileptic children. Scand J Dent Res 1978; 86:52.
103. Schneider LC, Weisinger E: The true gingival fibroma; an analysis of 129 fibrous gingival lesions. J Periodontol 1978; 49:423.
104. Serio FG, Siegel MA, Slade BE: Plasma cell gingivitis of unusual origin. A case report. J Periodontol 1978; 49:423.
105. Setia AP: Severe bleeding from a pregnancy tumor. Oral Surg 1973; 36:192.
106. Seymour RA, Jacobs DJ: Cyclosporine and the gingival tissues. J Clin Periodontol 1992; 19:1.
107. Seymour RA, Smith DG, Rogers SR: The comparative effects of azathioprine and cyclosporine on some gingival health parameters of renal transplant patients. J Clin Periodontol 1987; 14:610.
108. Seymour RA, Thomason JM, Ellis JS: The pathogenesis of drug-induced gingival overgrowth. J Clin Periodontol 1996; 23:165.
109. Shafer WG: Effect of Dilantin sodium analogues on cell proliferation in tissue culture. Proc Soc Exp Biol Med 1960; 106:205.
110. Shafer WG: Effect of Dilantin sodium on various cell lines in tissue culture. Proc Soc Exp Biol Med 1961; 108:694.
111. Shafer WG, Beatty RE, Davis WB: Effect of Dilantin sodium on tensile strength of healing wounds. Proc Soc Exp Biol Med 1958; 98:348.
112. Shapiro M: Acceleration of gingival wound healing in nonepileptic patients receiving diphenylhydantoin sodium. Exp Med Surg 1958; 16:41.
113. Silverman S Jr, Lozada F: An epilogue to plasma cell gingivostomatitis (allergic gingivostomatitis). Oral Surg 1977; 43:211.
114. Slavin J, Taylor J: Cyclosporine, nifedipine and gingival hyperplasia. Lancet 1987; ii:739.
115. Spencer CM, Goa KL, Gillis JC: Tacrolimus. An update of its pharmacology and drug efficacy in the management of organ transplantation. Drugs 1997; 54:925.
116. Staple PH, Reed MJ, Mashimo PA: Diphenylhydantoin gingival hyperplasia in Macaca arctoides: A new human model. J Periodontol 1977; 48:325.
117. Stein GM, Lewis H: Oral changes in a folic acid deficient patient precipitated by anticonvulsant drug therapy. J Periodontol 1973; 44:645.
118. Stevenson ARL, Austin BW: A case of ameloblastoma presenting as an exophytic gingival lesion. J Periodontol 1990; 61:378.
119. Stirrups D, Inglis J: Tuberous sclerosis with nonhydantoin gingival hyperplasia. Report of a case. Oral Surg 1980; 49:211.
120. Sutcliffe P: A longitudinal study of gingivitis and puberty. J Periodont Res 1972; 7:52.
121. Sznajder N, Dominguez FV, Carraro JJ, Lis G: Hemorrhagic hemangioma of the gingiva: Report of a case. J Periodontol 1973; 44:579.
122. Taicher S, Mazar A, Hirschberg A, et al: Metastatic chondrosarcoma of the gingiva mimicking a reactive exophytic lesion: A case report. J Periodontol 1991; 623:223.
123. Thoma KH, Holland DJ, Woodbury HW, et al: Malignant lymphoma of the gingiva. Oral Surg 1948; 1:57.
124. Thomas D, Rapley J, Strathman R, et al: Tuberous sclerosis with gingival overgrowth. J Periodontol 1992; 63:713.
125. Thomason JM, Seymour RA, Rice N: The prevalence and severity of cyclosporine and nifedipine-induced gingival overgrowth. J Clin Periodontol 1993; 20:37.
126. Thomason JM, Seymour RA, Ellis JS, et al: Determinants of gingival overgrowth severity in organ transplant patients. J Clin Periodontol 1996; 23:628.
127. Traeger KA: Cyst of the gingiva (mucocele): Report of a case. Oral Surg 1961; 14:243.
128. Varga E, Lennon MA, Mair LH: Pre-transplant gingival hyperplasia predicts severe cyclosporin-induced gingival overgrowth in renal transplant patients. J Clin Periodontol 1988; 25:225.
129. Wedgwood D, Rusen D, Balk S: Gingival metastases from primary hepatocellular carcinoma. Oral Surg 1979; 47:263.
130. Westbrook P, Bednarczyk EM, Carlson M, et al: Regression of nifedipine-induced gingival hyperplasia following switch to a same class calcium channel blocker, isradipine. J Periodontol 1997; 68:645.
131. Westphal P: Salivary secretion and gingival hyperplasia in diphenylhydantoin-treated guinea pigs. Sven Tandlak Tidskr 1969; 62:505.
132. Wojcicki CJ, Harper DS, Robinson PJ: Differences in periodontal-disease associated microorganisms in prepubertal, pubertal and postpubertal children. J Periodontol 1987; 58:219.
133. Wysocki G, Gretsinger HA, Laupacis A, et al: Fibrous hyperplasia of the gingiva: A side effect of cyclosporin A therapy. Oral Surg 1983; 55:274.
134. Zackin SJ, Weisberger D: Hereditary gingival fibromatosis. Oral Surg 1961; 14:828.
135. Ziskin DE, Blackberg SM, Stout AP: The gingivae during pregnancy. Surg Gynecol Obstet 1933; 57:719.
136. Ziskin DE, Zegarelli E: Idiopathic fibromatosis of the gingivae. Ann Dent 1943; 2:50.

Acute Gingival Infections

Fermin A. Carranza and Perry R. Klokkevold

CHAPTER

CHAPTER OUTLINE

NECROTIZING ULCERATIVE GINGIVITIS

Necrotizing ulcerative gingivitis (NUG) is an inflammatory destructive disease of the gingiva, which presents characteristic signs and symptoms.

Clinical Features

Classification. NUG most often occurs as an **acute** disease. NUG often undergoes a diminution in severity, leading to a **subacute** stage with milder clinical symptoms. The disease may sometimes subside spontaneously without treatment. Such patients generally have a history of repeated remissions and exacerbations. Recurrence of the condition in previously treated patients is also frequent. Involvement may be limited to a single tooth or group of teeth (Fig. 19-1) or may be widespread throughout the mouth.

NUG can cause tissue destruction involving the supporting structures. When bone loss occurs the condition is called **necrotizing ulcerative periodontitis (NUP)** (see Chapter 27).

History. NUG is characterized by sudden onset, sometimes following an episode of debilitating disease or acute respiratory tract infection. A change in living habits, protracted work without adequate rest, and psychologic stress are frequent features of the patient's history.

Oral Signs. *Characteristic lesions are punched out, craterlike depressions at the crest of the interdental papillae,* subsequently extending to the marginal gingiva and rarely to the attached gingiva and oral mucosa. The surface of the gingival craters is covered by a *gray, pseudomembranous slough, demarcated from the remainder of the gingival mucosa by a pronounced linear erythema* (Color Fig. 19-1, *A*). In some instances, the lesions are denuded of the surface pseudomembrane, exposing the gingival margin, which is red, shiny, and hemorrhagic. The characteristic lesions may progressively destroy the gingiva and underlying periodontal tissues (Color Fig. 19-1, *B*).

Spontaneous gingival hemorrhage or pronounced bleeding on the slightest stimulation are additional characteristic

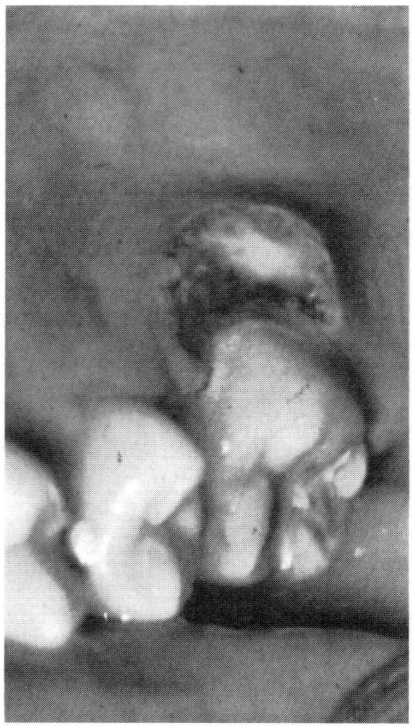

Fig. 19-1 Localized zone of necrotizing ulcerative gingivitis.

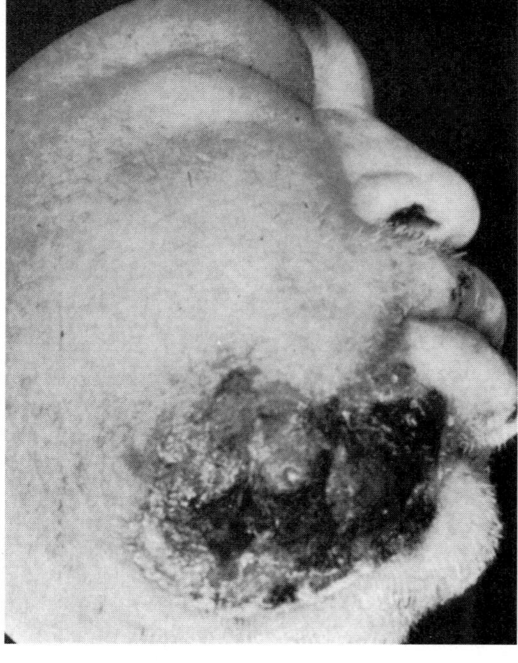

Fig. 19-2 Noma following necrotizing ulcerative gingivitis in a 50-year-old male with severe anemia.

clinical signs (Color Fig. 19-1, *C*). Other signs often found are fetid odor and increased salivation.

NUG can occur in otherwise disease-free mouths or can be superimposed on chronic gingivitis (Color Fig. 19-1, *D*) *or periodontal pockets.* However, it does not usually lead to periodontal pocket formation because the necrotic changes involve the junctional epithelium; a viable junctional epithelium is needed for pocket deepening (see Chapter 22). It is rare in edentulous mouths, but isolated spherical lesions occasionally occur on the soft palate.

Oral Symptoms. The lesions are *extremely sensitive to touch,* and the patient often complains of a *constant radiating, gnawing pain* that is intensified by eating spicy or hot foods and chewing. There is a metallic foul taste, and the patient is conscious of an excessive amount of "pasty" saliva.

Extraoral and Systemic Signs and Symptoms. Patients are usually ambulatory and have a minimum of systemic complications. Local lymphadenopathy and a slight elevation in temperature are common features of the mild and moderate stages of the disease. In severe cases there may be marked systemic complications such as high fever, increased pulse rate, leukocytosis, loss of appetite, and general lassitude. Systemic reactions are more severe in children. Insomnia, constipation, gastrointestinal disorders, headache, and mental depression sometimes accompany the condition.

In very rare cases, severe sequelae such as noma or gangrenous stomatitis[2,3,19] (Fig. 19-2) have been described.

Clinical Course. The clinical course is indefinite. If untreated, NUG may lead to NUP with a progressive destruction of the periodontium and denudation of the roots, accompanied by an increase in the severity of toxic systemic complications.

Pindborg and colleagues[53] have described the following stages in the progress of NUG: (1) only the tip of the interdental papilla is affected; (2) the lesion extends to marginal gingiva and causes punched-out papilla; (3) the attached gingiva is also affected; and (4) bone is exposed.

Horning and Cohen[33] extended the staging of these oral necrotizing diseases as follows:

Stage 1: Necrosis of the tip of the interdental papilla (93%)*
Stage 2: Necrosis of the entire papilla (19%)
Stage 3: Necrosis extending to the gingival margin (21%)
Stage 4: Necrosis extending also to the attached gingiva (1%)
Stage 5: Necrosis extending into buccal or labial mucosa (6%)
Stage 6: Necrosis exposing alveolar bone (1%)
Stage 7: Necrosis perforating skin of cheek (0%)

According to Horning and Cohen, stage 1 is NUG, stage 2 may be either NUG or NUP because attachment loss may have occurred, stages 3 and 4 are NUP, stages 5 and 6 are necrotizing stomatitis, and stage 7 is noma.

* Percent of cases found in Horning and Cohen series.

Histopathology. Microscopically, the lesion is a nonspecific acute necrotizing inflammation of the gingival margin, involving both the stratified squamous epithelium and the underlying connective tissue. The surface epithelium is destroyed and is replaced by a meshwork of fibrin, necrotic epithelial cells, polymorphonuclear neutrophils (PMNs), and various types of microorganisms (Fig. 19-3). This is the zone that appears clinically as the surface pseudomembrane. At the immediate border of the necrotic pseudomembrane, the epithelium is edematous, and the individual cells exhibit varying degrees of hydropic degeneration. In addition, there is an infiltration of PMNs in the intercellular spaces.

The underlying connective tissue is markedly hyperemic, with numerous engorged capillaries and a dense infiltration of PMNs. This acutely inflamed zone appears clinically as the linear erythema beneath the surface pseudomembrane. Numerous plasma cells may appear in the periphery of the infiltrate; this is interpreted as an area of established chronic gingivitis on which the acute lesion became superimposed.[32]

The epithelium and connective tissue alterations decrease as the distance from the necrotic gingival margin increases, blending gradually with the uninvolved gingiva.

It is noteworthy that the microscopic appearance of NUG is nonspecific. Comparable changes result from trauma, chemical irritation, or the application of caustic medications.

Relation of Bacteria to the Characteristic Lesion

The light microscope and the electron microscope have been used to study the relationship of bacteria to the characteristic lesion of NUG. With the former, it appears that the exudate on the surface of the necrotic lesion contains microorganisms that morphologically resemble cocci, fusiform bacilli, and spirochetes.[74] The layer between the necrotic and the living tissue contains enormous numbers of fusiform bacilli and spirochetes, in addition to leukocytes and fibrin. Spirochetes and other bacteria[5,12,17,38] invade the underlying living tissue.

Listgarten[37] described the following four zones, which blend with each other and may not all be present in every case:

Zone 1: Bacterial zone, the most superficial, consists of varied bacteria, including a few spirochetes of the small, medium, and large types.

Zone 2: Neutrophil-rich zone contains numerous leukocytes, preponderantly neutrophils, with bacteria, including many spirochetes of various types, between the leukocytes.

Zone 3: Necrotic zone consists of disintegrated tissue cells, fibrillar material, remnants of collagen fibers, and numerous spirochetes of the medium and large types, with few other organisms.

Zone 4: Zone of spirochetal infiltration consists of well-preserved tissue infiltrated with medium and large spirochetes, without other organisms.

Spirochetes have been found as deep as 300 microns from the surface. The majority of spirochetes in the deeper zones are morphologically different from cultivated strains of *Treponema microdentium.* They occur in nonnecrotic tissue before other types of bacteria and may be present in high concentrations intercellularly in the epithelium adjacent to the ulcerated lesion and in the connective tissue.[37]

Bacterial Flora

Smears from the lesions (Fig. 19-4) present scattered bacteria, predominantly spirochetes and fusiform bacilli, desquamated epithelial cells, and occasional PMNs. A smear containing only spirochetes and fusiform bacilli is rarely seen. Usually these two organisms are seen with other oral spirochetes, vibrios, streptococci, and filamentous organisms. The spirochetal organisms form a light-staining, conspicuous, interlacing network throughout the microscopic field.

Electron microscopic studies indicate that the spirochetes may be classified into three morphologic groups: small (7% to 39% of the total spirochetes present); medium (43.9% to 90%); and large (0% to 20%).[38] It was also suggested that medium-size spirochetes are present in greater numbers in pooled scrapings from lesions of NUG and are found in greater percentages in deeper portions of the lesions.

Diagnosis

Diagnosis is based on clinical findings of gingival pain, ulceration, and bleeding. A bacterial smear is not necessary or definitive because the bacterial picture is not appreciably different from that in marginal gingivitis, periodontal pockets, pericoronitis, or primary herpetic gingivostomatitis.[59] Bacterial studies are useful, however, in the differential diagnosis of NUG and specific infections of the oral cavity such as diphtheria, thrush, actinomycosis, and streptococcal stomatitis.

Microscopic examination of a biopsy specimen is not sufficiently specific to be diagnostic. It can be used to differentiate NUG from specific infections such as tuberculosis or from neoplastic disease, but it does not differentiate between NUG and other necrotizing conditions of nonspecific origin, such as those produced by trauma or caustic medications.

Differential Diagnosis

NUG should be differentiated from other conditions that resemble it in some respects, such as herpetic gingivostomatitis (Table 19-1); chronic periodontitis; desquamative gingivitis (Table 19-2); streptococcal gingivostomatitis; aphthous stomatitis; gonococcal gingivostomatitis; diphtheritic and syphilitic lesions (Table 19-3); tuberculous gingival lesion; candidiasis, agranulocytosis, dermatoses (pemphigus, erythema multiforme, and lichen planus); and stomatitis venenata. See Chapter 21 for a description of most of these conditions.

Streptococcal gingivostomatitis[43] is a rare condition characterized by a diffuse erythema of the gingiva and other areas of the oral mucosa. In some instances it is confined as a marginal erythema with marginal hemorrhage. Necrosis of the gingival margin is not a feature of this disease, and there is no notably fetid odor. Bacterial smears show a preponderance of streptococcal forms, which were identified as *Streptococcus viridans,* but more recent studies report it to be group A beta-hemolytic *streptococcus.*[39]

Agranulocytosis is characterized by a marked decrease in the number of circulating PMNs, lesions of the throat, and other mucous membranes, as well as ulceration and necrosis of the gingiva, which may resemble that of NUG. The oral condition in agranulocytosis is primarily necrotizing. Because of the diminished innate defense mechanisms in agranulocytosis, the clinical picture is not marked by the severe inflammatory reaction seen in NUG. Blood studies serve to differentiate between NUG and the gingival necrosis in agranulocytosis.

Vincent's angina is a fusospirochetal infection of the oropharynx and throat, as distinguished from NUG, which affects the marginal gingiva. In Vincent's angina, there is a painful membranous ulceration of the throat, with edema and hyperemic patches breaking down to form ulcers covered with pseudomembranous material. The process may extend to the larynx and middle ear.

TABLE 19-1

Differentiation between Necrotizing Ulcerative Gingivitis and Primary Herpetic Gingivostomatitis

Necrotizing Ulcerative Gingivitis	Primary Herpetic Gingivostomatitis
Etiology: Interaction between host and bacteria, most probably fusospirochetes	Specific viral etiology
Necrotizing condition	Diffuse erythema and vesicular eruption
Punched out gingival margin; pseudomembrane that peels off, leaving raw areas. Marginal gingiva affected; other oral tissues rarely affected	Vesicles rupture and leave slightly depressed oval or spherical ulcer Diffuse involvement of gingiva, may include buccal mucosa and lips
Uncommon in children	Occurs more frequently in children
No definite duration	Duration of 7 to 10 days
No demonstrated immunity	An acute episode results in some degree of immunity
Contagion not demonstrated	Contagious

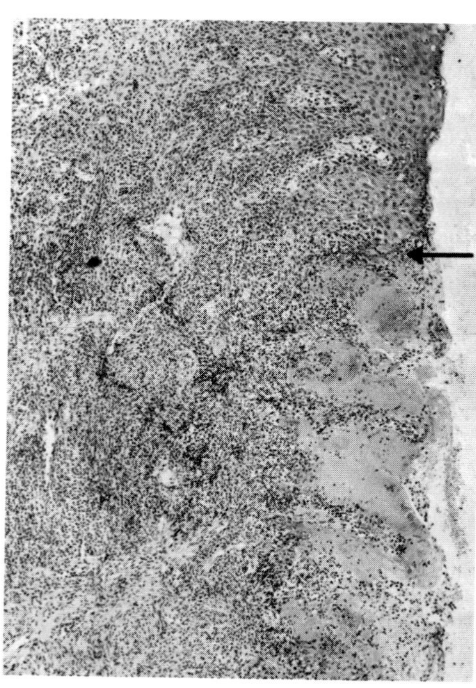

Fig. 19-3 Survey section of the gingiva in necrotizing ulcerative gingivitis. The portion of the section below the arrow shows ulceration and accumulation of leukocytes, fibrin, and necrotic tissue that form the gray marginal pseudomembrane.

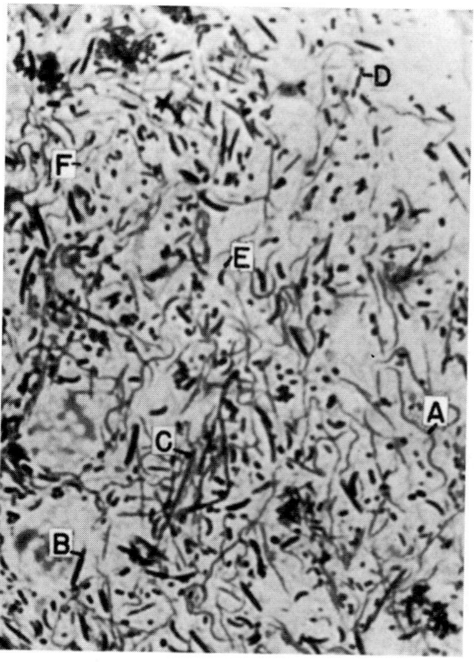

Fig. 19-4 Bacterial smear from lesion in necrotizing ulcerative gingivitis. *A,* Spirochete; *B, Bacillus fusiformis; C,* filamentous organism *(Actinomyces* or *Leptotrichia); D, Streptococcus; E, Vibrio; F, Treponema microdentium.*

TABLE 19-2

Differentiation among Necrotizing Ulcerative Gingivitis, Chronic Desquamative Gingivitis, and Chronic Periodontal Disease

Necrotizing Ulcerative Gingivitis	Desquamative Gingivitis	Chronic Destructive Periodontal Disease
Bacterial smears show fusospirochetal complex	Bacterial smears reveal numerous epithelial cells, few bacterial forms	Bacterial smears are variable
Marginal gingiva affected	Diffuse involvement of marginal and attached gingivae and other areas of oral mucosa	Marginal gingiva affected
Acute history	Chronic history	Chronic history
Painful	May or may not be painful	Painless if uncomplicated
Pseudomembrane	Patchy desquamation of gingival epithelium	No desquamation generally but purulent material may appear from pockets
Papillary and marginal necrotic lesions	Papillae do not undergo necrosis	Papillae do not undergo notable necrosis
Affects adults of both genders, occasionally children	Affects adults, most often women	Generally in adults, occasionally in children
Characteristic fetid odor	None	Some odor present but not strikingly fetid

TABLE 19-3

Differentiation among Necrotizing Ulcerative Gingivitis, Diphtheria, and Secondary Stage of Syphilis

Necrotizing Ulcerative Gingivitis	Diphtheria	Secondary Stage of Syphilis (Mucous Patch)
Etiology: interaction between host and bacteria, possibly fusospirochetes	Specific bacterial etiology: *Corynebacterium diphtheriae*	Specific bacterial etiology: *Treponema pallidum*
Affects marginal gingiva	Rarely affects marginal gingiva	Rarely affects marginal gingiva
Membrane removal easy	Membrane removal difficult	Membrane not detachable
Painful condition	Less painful	Minimal pain
Marginal gingiva affected	Throat, fauces, tonsils affected	Any part of mouth affected
Serologic findings normal	Serologic findings normal	Serologic findings abnormal (Wassermann, Kahn, Venereal Disease Research Laboratory [VDRL])
Immunity not conferred	Immunity conferred by an attack	Immunity not conferred
Doubtful contagiousness	Contagious	Only direct contact will communicate disease
Antibiotic therapy relieves symptoms	Antibiotic treatment has little effect	Antibiotic therapy has excellent results

NUG in leukemia is not produced by leukemia per se but may be the result of a reduction in host defense mechanisms seen with leukemia. However, NUG may be superimposed on gingival tissue alterations caused by leukemia. The differential diagnosis consists not in distinguishing between NUG and leukemic gingival changes, but rather in determining whether leukemia is a predisposing factor in a mouth with NUG. For example, if a patient with necrotizing involvement of the gingival margin also has generalized diffuse discoloration and edema of the attached gingiva, the possibility of an underlying, systemically induced gingival change should be considered. Leukemia is one of the conditions that would have to be ruled out (see Chapter 12).

NUG in acquired immunodeficiency syndrome (AIDS) has the same clinical features, although it follows a very destructive course leading to NUP with the loss of soft tissue, bone, and the formation of bony sequestra[29] (see Chapter 29).

Etiology

The Role of Bacteria. Plaut[54] and Vincent,[77] in 1894 and 1896, respectively, introduced the concept that NUG is caused by specific bacteria, namely a fusiform bacillus and a spirochetal organism.

Opinions still differ regarding whether bacteria are the primary causative factors in NUG. Several observations support this concept, including the fact that spirochetal organisms and fusiform bacilli are always found in the disease, with other organisms also involved. Rosebury and colleagues[59] described a fusospirochetal complex consisting of *T. microdentium,* intermediate spirochetes, vibrios, fusiform bacilli, and filamentous organisms, in addition to several *Borrelia* species.

Loesche and colleagues[40] described a predominant constant flora and a variable flora associated with NUG. The constant flora is composed of *prevotella intermedia,* in addition to the *fusobacteria, treponema,* and *selenomonas* species. The variable flora consists of a heterogeneous array of bacterial types.

Treatment with metronidazole results in a significant reduction of *Treponema* species, *prevotella intermedia,* and *fusobacteria* with resolution of the clinical symptoms.[16,40] Given the antibacterial spectrum of this drug, the anaerobic members of the flora mentioned are thought to be responsible for the symptoms.

These bacteriologic findings have been supported by immunologic data from Chung and colleagues.[9] These investigators reported increased immunoglobulin (IgG and IgM) antibody titers for medium-size spirochetes and *prevotella intermedia* in NUG patients compared with titers in those with chronic gingivitis and healthy controls. Cogen and colleagues[10] described a depression in host defense mechanisms, particularly in PMN chemotaxis and phagocytosis, in NUG patients. For further details on the host-bacteria interactions in NUG, see Chapters 6, 8, and 9.

NUG has not been produced experimentally in humans or animals by inoculation of bacterial exudates from the lesions. Exudates from NUG produce fusospirochetal abscesses when inoculated subcutaneously in experimental animals, and the infection is freely transmissible in series.[58] Local intracutaneous injection of a hyaluronidase- and chondroitinase-containing cell-free filtrate of oral microaerophilic diphtheroid bacilli aggravated spirochetal lesions that were produced by oral treponemes.[31] Only in one animal experiment has the transmission of lesions comparable with those seen in humans been reported.[2]

The specific cause of NUG has not been established. The prevalent opinion is that it is produced by a complex of bacterial organisms but requires underlying tissue changes to facilitate the pathogenic activity of the bacteria.

Local Predisposing Factors. Preexisting gingivitis, injury to the gingiva, and smoking are important predisposing factors. Although NUG may appear in an otherwise disease-free mouth, it most often occurs superimposed on preexisting chronic gingival disease and periodontal pockets. Deep periodontal pockets and pericoronal flaps are particularly vulnerable areas because they offer a favorable environment for the proliferation of anaerobic fusiform bacilli and spirochetes. Areas of the gingiva traumatized by opposing teeth in malocclusion, such as the palatal surface behind the maxillary incisors and the labial gingival surface of the mandibular incisors, are frequent sites of NUG.

The *relationship between NUG and smoking* has often been mentioned in the literature. Pindborg[52] reported that 98% of his patients with NUG were smokers and that the frequency of this disease increases with an increasing exposure to tobacco smoke. The effect of smoking on periodontal disease in general has been the subject of numerous studies in the past two decades, and it has been established that it is a high risk factor for this disease. For an in-depth consideration of this important topic see Chapter 14.

Systemic Predisposing Factors. NUG is often superimposed on gingival alterations caused by severe systemic disease.

NUTRITIONAL DEFICIENCY. Necrotizing gingivitis has been produced by giving animals nutritionally deficient diets.[7,36,46,73,76] Several researchers found an increase in the fusospirochetal flora in the mouths of the experimental animals, but the bacteria were regarded as opportunists, proliferating only when the tissues were altered by the deficiency. A poor diet has been mentioned as a predisposing factor in NUG and its sequelae in developing African countries, although the effects appear to be primarily in diminishing the effectiveness of the immune response.[19,20,33]

Nutritional deficiencies (e.g., vitamin C, vitamin B_2) accentuate the severity of the pathologic changes induced when the fusospirochetal bacterial complex is injected into animals.[68]

DEBILITATING DISEASE. Debilitating systemic disease may predispose the development of NUG. Included among such systemic disturbances are chronic diseases such as syphilis and cancer, severe gastrointestinal disorders such as ulcerative colitis, blood dyscrasias such as the leukemias and anemia, and acquired immunodeficiency syndrome (AIDS). Nutritional deficiency resulting from debilitating disease may be an additional predisposing factor. Experimentally induced leukopenia in animals may produce ulcerative gangrenous stomatitis.[46,71,72,75] Ulceronecrotic lesions appear in the gingival margins of hamsters exposed to total body irradiation[41]; these lesions can be prevented with systemic antibiotics.[42]

Psychosomatic Factors. Psychologic factors appear to be important in the etiology of NUG. The disease often occurs in association with stress situations (induction into the armed forces or school examinations).[26] Psychological disturbances,[27] as well as increased adrenocortical secretion,[64] are common in patients with the disease.

Significant correlation between disease incidence and two personality traits, dominance and abasement, suggests the presence of an NUG-prone personality.[23] The mechanisms whereby psychologic factors create or predispose to gingival damage have not been established, but alterations in digital and gingival capillary responses suggestive of increased autonomic nervous activity have been demonstrated in patients with NUG.[25]

Cohen-Cole and colleagues[11] suggested that a psychiatric disturbance (e.g., trait anxiety, depression, and psychopathic deviance) and the impact of negative life events (stress) may lead to activation of the hypothalamic-pituitary-adrenal axis. This results in elevation of serum and urine cortisol levels, which is associated with a depression of lymphocyte and PMN function that may predispose to NUG.

It can be concluded that opportunistic bacteria are the primary etiologic agents of NUG in patients that demonstrate immunosuppression. Stress, smoking and preexisting gingivitis are common predisposing factors.

Epidemiology and Prevalence

NUG often occurs in groups in an epidemic pattern. At one time, it was considered contagious, but this has not been substantiated.[61]

The prevalence of NUG appears to have been rather low in the United States and Europe before 1914. During World Wars I and II, numerous "epidemics" broke out among the Allied troops, but German soldiers did not seem to have been similarly affected. Similar epidemic-like outbreaks have occurred among civilian populations. In a study conducted at a dental clinic in Prague, Czech Republic, the following incidence of NUG was reported: 0.08% in patients between ages 15 and 19, 0.05% in those between ages 20 and 24, and 0.02% in those between ages 25 and 29.[67]

NUG occurs at all ages,[13] with the highest incidence reported between ages 20 and 30[14,69] and ages 15 and 20 years.[67] It is not common in children in the United States, Canada, and Europe, but it has been reported in children from low socioeconomic groups in underdeveloped countries.[35] In India, 54%[52] and 58%[53] of the patients in two studies were under age 10. In a random school population in Nigeria, NUG occurred in 11.3% of children between the ages of 2 and 6 years,[65] and in a Nigerian hospital population, it was present in 23% of children under age 10.[18] It has been reported in several members of the same family in low socioeconomic groups. NUG is more common in children with Down syndrome than in other children with mental deficiencies.[4]

Opinions differ as to whether it is more common during the winter,[50] summer, or fall,[67] or whether there is a peak seasonal incidence.[15]

Communicability

A distinction must be made between communicability and transmissibility when referring to the characteristics of disease. The term *transmissible* denotes a capacity for the maintenance of an infectious agent in successive passages through a susceptible animal host.[57] The term *communicable* signifies a capacity for the maintenance of infection by natural modes of spread such as direct contact through drinking water, food, and eating utensils; via the airborne route; or by means of arthropod vectors. A disease that is communicable is described as *contagious*. It has been demonstrated that disease associated with the fusospirochetal bacterial complex is transmissible; *however, it has not been shown to be communicable or contagious.*

Attempts have been made to spread NUG from human to human, without success.[62] King[36] traumatized an area in his gingiva and introduced debris from a patient with a severe case of NUG. There was no response until he happened to fall ill shortly thereafter; subsequent to his illness, he observed the characteristic lesion in the experimental area. It may be inferred with reservation from this experiment that systemic debility is a prerequisite for the contagion of NUG.

It is a common impression that, because NUG often occurs in groups using the same kitchen facilities, the disease is spread by bacteria on eating utensils. Growth of fusospirochetal organisms requires carefully controlled conditions and an anaerobic environment; they do not ordinarily survive on eating utensils.[31]

The occurrence of the disease in epidemic-like outbreaks does not necessarily mean that it is contagious. The affected groups may be afflicted by the disease because of common predisposing factors rather than because of its spread from person to person. In all likelihood, both a predisposed immunocompromised host and the presence of appropriate bacteria are necessary for the production of this disease.

PRIMARY HERPETIC GINGIVOSTOMATITIS

Primary herpetic gingivostomatitis is an infection of the oral cavity caused by the herpes simplex virus type 1 (HSV-1).[15,44] It occurs most often in infants and children younger than 6 years of age,[6,63] but it is also seen in adolescents and adults. It occurs with equal frequency in male and female patients. In most persons, however, the primary infection is asymptomatic.

After the primary infection, the virus ascends through sensory and autonomic nerves and persists in neuronal ganglia that innervate the site as latent HSV. In approximately one third of the world's population, secondary manifestations occur as a result of various stimuli such as sunlight, trauma, fever, or stress. These secondary manifestations include herpes labialis (Fig. 19-5), herpes genitalis, ocular herpes, and herpetic encephalitis.

Clinical Features

Oral Signs. The condition appears as a diffuse, erythematous, shiny involvement of the gingiva and the adjacent oral mucosa, with varying degrees of edema and gingival bleeding (see Color Fig. 19-1, *E*). In its initial stage, it is characterized by the presence of discrete, spherical gray vesicles (see Color Fig. 19-1, *F*), which may occur on the gingiva, labial and buccal mucosae,

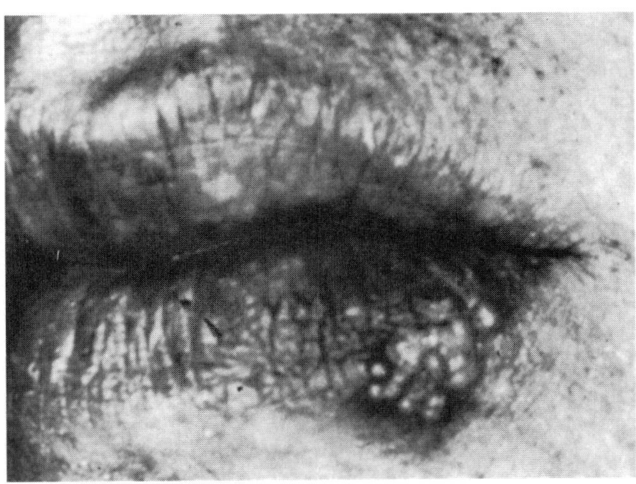

Fig. 19-5 Cluster of herpetic vesicles (cold sores).

soft palate, pharynx, sublingual mucosa, and tongue (Fig. 19-6). After approximately 24 hours the vesicles rupture and form painful, small ulcers with a red, elevated, halolike margin and a depressed, yellowish- or grayish-white central portion. These occur either in widely separated areas or in clusters where confluence occurs (Figs. 19-7 and 19-8).

Occasionally, primary herpetic gingivitis may occur without overt vesiculation. Diffuse, erythematous, shiny discoloration and edematous enlargement of the gingivae with a tendency toward bleeding make up the clinical picture.

The course of the disease is limited to 7 to 10 days. The diffuse gingival erythema and edema that appear early in the disease persist for several days after the ulcerative lesions have healed. Scarring does not occur in the areas of healed ulcerations.

Oral Symptoms. The disease is accompanied by generalized "soreness" of the oral cavity, which interferes with eating and drinking. The ruptured vesicles are the focal sites of pain and are particularly sensitive to touch, thermal changes, foods such as condiments and fruit juices, and the action of coarse foods. In infants the disease is marked by irritability and refusal to take food.

Extraoral and Systemic Signs and Symptoms. Cervical adenitis, fever as high as 101° F to 105° F (38.3° C to 40.6° C), and generalized malaise are common.

History. Recent acute infection is a common feature of the history of patients with primary herpetic gingivostomatitis. The condition often occurs during and immediately after an episode of such febrile diseases as pneumonia, meningitis, influenza, and typhoid. It also tends to occur during periods of anxiety, strain, or exhaustion, as well as during menstruation. A history of exposure to patients with herpetic infection of the oral cavity or lips may also be elicited. Primary herpetic gingivostomatitis often occurs in the early stage of infectious mononucleosis.[47]

Histopathology. The virus targets the epithelial cells, which show "ballooning degeneration" consisting of acantholysis, nuclear clearing and nuclear enlargement. These cells are called *Tzanck cells*. Infected cells fuse, forming multinucleated cells, and intercellular edema leads to formation of an intraepithelial vesicles that rupture and develop a secondary inflammatory response with a fibropurulent exudate.[48] Discrete ulcerations resulting from rupture of the vesicles have a central portion of acute inflammation, with varying degrees of purulent exudate, surrounded by a zone rich in engorged blood vessels.

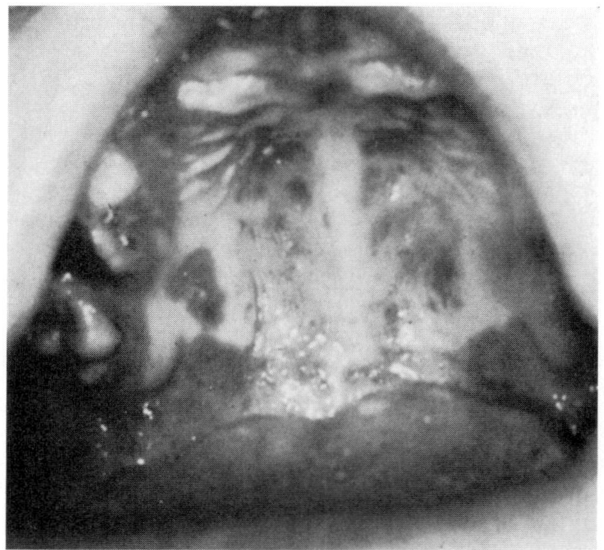

Fig. 19-7 Involvement of the palate in primary herpetic gingivostomatitis.

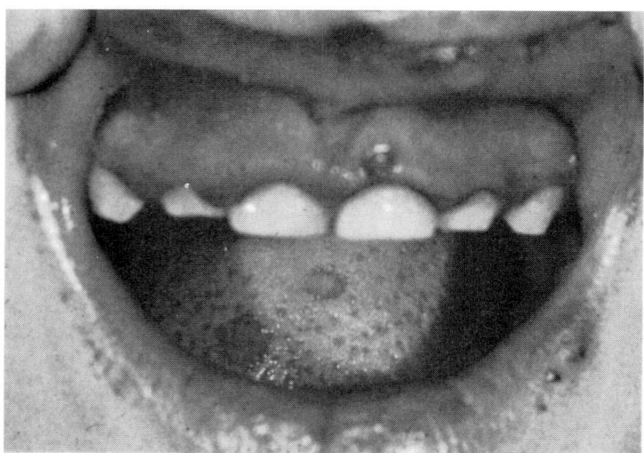

Fig. 19-6 Vesicles on the tongue in primary herpetic gingivostomatitis.

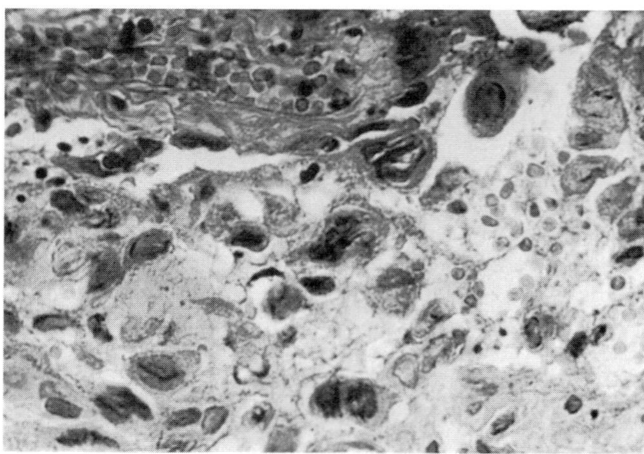

Fig. 19-8 Biopsy showing giant cells at base of herpetic lesion.

Diagnosis

The diagnosis is usually established from the patient's history and the clinical findings. Material may be obtained from the lesions and submitted to the laboratory for confirmatory tests, including virus culture and immunologic tests using monoclonal antibodies or DNA hybridization techniques.[6,24,55]

Differential Diagnosis

Primary herpetic gingivostomatitis should be differentiated from the following conditions. *NUG* can be differentiated in different ways (see Table 19-1).

Erythema multiforme can be differentiated because the vesicles in erythema multiforme are generally more extensive than those in primary herpetic gingivostomatitis and on rupture demonstrate a tendency toward pseudomembrane formation. In addition, in the former condition the tongue is usually markedly involved, with infection of the ruptured vesicles resulting in varying degrees of ulceration. Oral involvement in erythema multiforme may be accompanied by skin lesions. The duration of erythema multiforme may be comparable with that of primary herpetic gingivostomatitis, but prolonged involvement for a period of weeks is not uncommon.

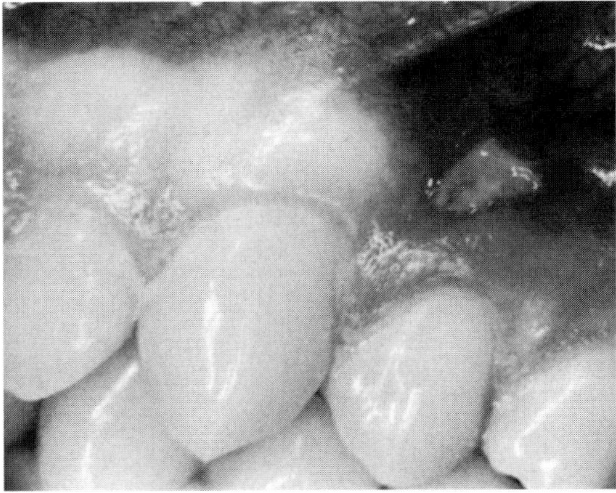

Fig. 19-9 Aphthous lesion in the mucobuccal fold. The depressed gray center is surrounded by an elevated red border.

Stevens-Johnson syndrome is a comparatively rare form of erythema multiforme, characterized by vesicular hemorrhagic lesions in the oral cavity, hemorrhagic ocular lesions, and bullous skin lesions.

Bullous lichen planus is a very rare and painful condition. It is characterized by large blisters on the tongue and cheek that rupture and undergo ulceration; it runs a prolonged, indefinite course. Patches of linear, gray, lace-like lesions of lichen planus are often interspersed among the bullous eruptions. Lichen planus involvement of the skin may coexist with the oral lesions and facilitate differential diagnosis.

Desquamative gingivitis is characterized by diffuse involvement of the gingiva, with varying degrees of "peeling" of the epithelial surface and exposure of the underlying tissue. It is a chronic condition (see Chapter 21).

Lesions of *recurrent aphthous stomatitis (RAS)*[21] Fig. 19-9) range from occasional small (0.5 to 1 cm in diameter), well-defined, round or ovoid, shallow ulcers with a yellowish-gray central area surrounded by an erythematous halo, which heal in 7 to 10 days without scarring, to larger (1 to 3 cm in diameter) oval or irregular ulcers, which persist for weeks and heal with scarring. The cause is unknown, although immunopathologic mecanisms appear to play a role. RAS is a different clinical entity from primary herpetic gingivostomatitis. The ulcerations may look the same in the two conditions, but diffuse erythematous involvement of the gingiva and acute toxic systemic symptoms do not occur in RAS.

Communicability

Primary herpetic gingivostomatitis is contagious.[8,39] Most adults have developed immunity to HSV as the result of infection during childhood, which in most instances is subclinical. For this reason acute herpetic gingivostomatitis usually occurs in infants and children. Although recurrent herpetic gingivostomatitis has been

A

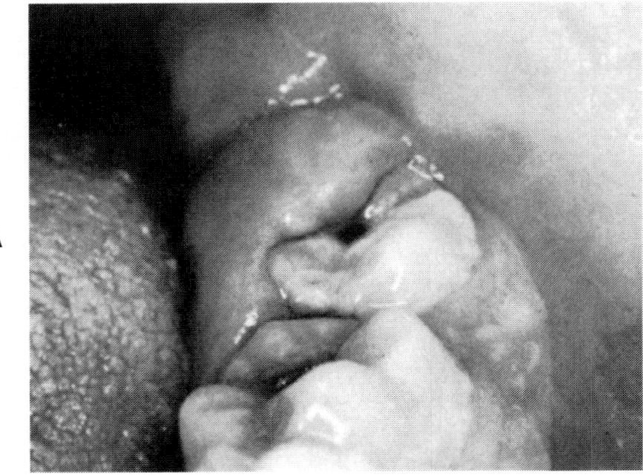

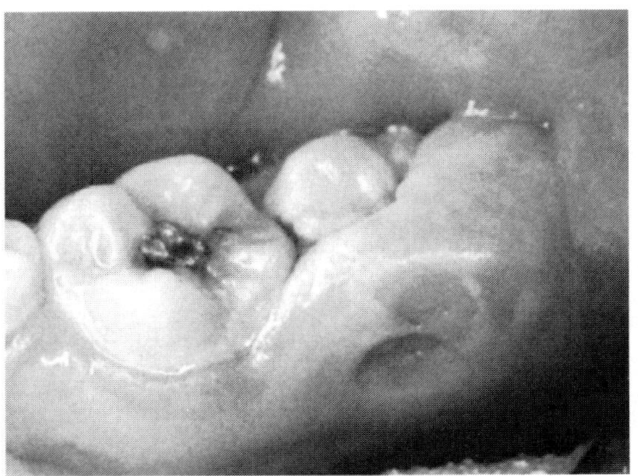

B

Fig. 19-10 Pericoronitis. **A,** Third molar partially covered by infected flap. **B,** Lingual view showing sinus draining from infected flap.

reported,[30] it does not ordinarily recur unless immunity is destroyed by debilitating systemic disease. Secondary herpetic infection of the skin, such as herpes labialis, does recur.[66]

PERICORONITIS

The term *pericoronitis* refers to inflammation of the gingiva in relation to the crown of an incompletely erupted tooth (Fig. 19-10). It occurs most often in the mandibular third molar area. Pericoronitis may be acute, subacute, or chronic.

Clinical Features

The partially erupted or impacted mandibular third molar is the most common site of pericoronitis. The space between the crown of the tooth and the overlying gingival flap is an ideal area for the accumulation of food debris and bacterial growth. Even in patients with no clinical signs or symptoms, the gingival flap is often chronically inflamed and infected and has varying degrees of ulceration along its inner surface. Acute inflammatory involvement is a constant possibility.

Acute pericoronitis is identified by varying degrees of inflammatory involvement of the pericoronal flap and adjacent structures as well as systemic complications. The inflammatory fluid and cellular exudate increase the bulk of the flap, which then may interfere with complete closure of the jaws, and can be traumatized by contact with the opposing jaw, aggravating the inflammatory involvement.

The resultant clinical picture is that of a markedly red, swollen, suppurating lesion that is exquisitely tender, with radiating pains to the ear, throat, and floor of the mouth. The patient is extremely uncomfortable because of a foul taste and an inability to close the jaws, in addition to the pain. Swelling of the cheek in the region of the angle of the jaw and lymphadenitis are common findings. The patient may also have toxic systemic complications such as fever, leukocytosis, and malaise.

Complications

The involvement may become localized in the form of a pericoronal abscess. It may spread posteriorly into the oropharyngeal area and medially to the base of the tongue, making it difficult for the patient to swallow. Depending on the severity and extent of the infection, there is involvement of the submaxillary, posterior cervical, deep cervical, and retropharyngeal lymph nodes.[34,51] Peritonsillar abscess formation, cellulitis, and Ludwig's angina are infrequent but potential sequelae of acute pericoronitis.

REFERENCES

1. Barnes GP, Bowles WF III, Carter HG: Acute necrotizing ulcerative gingivitis. A survey of 218 cases. J Periodontol 1973; 44:35.
2. Berke JD: Experimental study of acute ulcerative stomatitis. J Am Dent Assoc 1961; 63:86.
3. Box HK: Necrotic Gingivitis. Toronto, University of Toronto Press, 1930.
4. Brown RH: Necrotizing ulcerative gingivitis in mongoloid and nonmongoloid retarded individuals. J Periodont Res 1973; 8:290.
5. Cahn LR: The penetration of the tissue by Vincent's organisms. A report of a case. J Dent Res 1929; 9:695.
6. Cawson RA: Infections of the oral mucous membrane. In Cohen B, Kramer IRH (eds): Scientific Foundations of Dentistry. Chicago, Year–Book Medical Publishers, 1976.
7. Chapman OD, Harris AE: Oral lesions associated with dietary deficiencies in monkeys. J Infect Dis 1941; 69:7.
8. Chilton NW: Herpetic stomatitis. Am J Orthod Oral Surg 1944; 30:335.
9. Chung CP, Nisengard RJ, Slots J, et al: Bacterial IgG and IgM antibody titers in acute necrotizing ulcerative gingivitis. J Periodontol 1983; 54:557.
10. Cogen RB, Stevens AW Jr, Cohen-Cole SA, et al: Leukocyte function in the etiology of acute necrotizing ulcerative gingivitis. J Periodontol, 54:402, 1983.
11. Cohen-Cole SA, et al: Psychiatric, psychosocial and endocrine correlates of acute necrotizing ulcerative gingivitis (trench mouth): a preliminary report. Psychiatr Med 1:215, 1983.
12. Curtois GJ III, Cobb CM, Killoy WJ: Acute necrotizing ulcerative gingivitis. A transmission electron microscope study. J Periodontol 1983; 54:671.
13. Daley FH: Studies of Vincent's infection at the clinic of Tufts College Dental School from October 1926 to February 1928. J Dent Res 1928; 8:408.
14. Dean HT, Singleton JE Jr: Vincent's infection—a wartime disease. Am J Pub Health 1945; 35:433.
15. Dodd, K, Johnston LM, Budding GJ: Herpetic stomatitis. J Pediatr 1938; 12:95.
16. Duckworth R, Waterhouse JP, Britton DG, et al: Acute ulcerative gingivitis. A double blind controlled clinical trial with metronidazole. Br Dent J 1966; 120:599.
17. Ellerman V: Vincent's organisms in tissue. Z Hyg Infekt Pr 1907; 56:453.
18. Emslie RD: Cancrum oris. Dent Pract, 13:481, 1963.
19. Enwonwu CO: Epidemiological and biochemical studies of necrotizing ulcerative gingivitis and noma (cancrum oris) in Nigerian children. Arch Oral Biol 1972; 17:1357, 1972.
20. Enwonwu CO: Cellular and molecular effects of malnutrition and their relevance to periodontal diseases. J Clin Periodontol 1994; 21:643.
21. Eversole LR: Diseases of the oral mucous membranes. Review of the literature. In Millard HD, Mason DK (eds): World Workshop on Oral Medicine. Chicago, Year–Book Medical Publishers, 1989.
22. Falkler WA Jr, Martin SA, Vincent JW, et al: A clinical, demographic and microbiologic study of NUG patients in an urban dental school. J Clin Periodontol 1987; 14:307.
23. Formicola AJ, Witte ET, Curran PM: A study of personality traits and acute necrotizing ulcerative gingivitis. J Periodontol 1970; 41:36.
24. Gardner PS, McQuillin J, Black MM, et al: Rapid diagnosis of herpesvirus hominis infections in superficial lesions by immunofluorescent antibody techniques. Br Med J 1968; 4:89.
25. Giddon DB: Psychophysiology of the oral cavity. J Dent Res (Suppl 6) 1966; 45:1627.
26. Giddon DB, Zackin SJ, Goldhaber P: Acute necrotizing gingivitis in college students. J Am Dent Assoc 1964; 68:381.
27. Goldhaber P, Giddon DB: Present concepts concerning the etiology and treatment of acute necrotizing ulcerative gingivitis. Int Dent J 1964; 14:468.
28. Greenberg MS, Brightman VJ, Ship II: Clinical and laboratory differentiation of recurrent intraoral herpes simplex virus infections following fever. J Dent Res 1969; 48:385.
29. Greenspan D, Pindborg JJ, Greenspan JS, et al: AIDS and the Dental Team. Copenhagen, Munksgaard, 1986.

30. Griffin JW: Recurrent intraoral herpes simplex virus infection. Oral Surg 1965; 19:209.
31. Hampp EG, Mergenhagen SE: Experimental infection with oral spirochetes. J Infect Dis 1961; 109:43.
32. Hooper PA, Seymour GJ: The histopathogenesis of acute ulcerative gingivitis. J Periodontol 1979; 50:419.
33. Horning GM, Cohen ME: Necrotizing ulcerative gingivitis, periodontitis and stomatitis: clinical staging and predisposing factors. J Periodontol 1995; 66:990.
34. Jacobs MH: Pericoronal and Vincent's infections: bacteriology and treatment. J Am Dent Assoc 1953; 30:392.
35. Jimenez M, Baer PN: Necrotizing ulcerative gingivitis in children: a 9-year clinical study. J Periodontol 1975; 46:715.
36. King JD: Nutritional and other factors in trench mouth with special reference to the nicotinic acid component of vitamin B complex. Br Dent J 1943; 74:113.
37. Listgarten MA: Electron microscopic observations on the bacterial flora of acute necrotizing ulcerative gingivitis. J Periodontol 1965; 36:328.
38. Listgarten MA, Lewis DW: The distribution of spirochetes in the lesion of acute necrotizing ulcerative gingivitis: an electron microscopic and statistical survey. J Periodontol 1967; 38:379.
39. Littner MM, Dayan D, Kaffe I, et al: Acute streptococcal gingivostomatitis. Report of five cases. Oral Surg Oral Med Oral Pathol Oral Radiol Endod 1982; 53:144.
40. Loesche WJ, Syed SA, Langhorn BE, Stoll J: The bacteriology of acute necrotizing ulcerative gingivitis. J Periodontol 1982; 53:223.
41. Mayo J, Carranza FA Jr, Cabrini RL: Comparative study of the effect of antibiotics, bone marrow and cysteamine on oral lesions produced in hamsters by total body irradiation. Experientia 1964; 20:403.
42. Mayo J, Carranza FA Jr, Epper CE, et al: The effect of total-body irradiation on the oral tissues of the Syrian hamster. Oral Surg 1962; 15:739.
43. McCarthy PL, Shklar G: Diseases of the Oral Mucosa, 2nd ed. Philadelphia, Lea & Febiger, 1980.
44. McNair ST: Herpetic stomatitis. J Dent Res 1950; 29:647.
45. Miglani DC, Sharma OP: Incidence of acute necrotizing gingivitis and periodontosis among cases seen at the government hospital, Madras. J All India Dent Assoc 1965; 37:183.
46. Miller DK, Rhoads CP: The experimental production in dogs of acute stomatitis associated with leukopenia and a maturation defect of the myeloid elements of the bone marrow. J Exp Med 1935; 61:173.
47. Nathanson I, Morin GE: Herpetic stomatitis. An aid in the early diagnosis of infectious mononucleosis. Oral Surg 1953; 6:1284.
48. Neville BW, Damm DD, Allen CM, et al: Oral and Maxillofacial Pathology. Philadelphia, Saunders, 1995.
49. Park NH: Virology. In: Newman MG, Nisengard R (eds.): Oral Microbiology and Immunology. Philadelphia, Saunders, 1988.
50. Pedler JA, Radden BG: Seasonal influence of acute ulcerative gingivitis. Dent Pract 1957; 8:23, 1957.
51. Perkins AE: Acute infections around erupting mandibular third molar. Br Dent J 1944; 76:199.
52. Pindborg JJ: Gingivitis in military personnel with special reference to ulceromembranous gingivitis. Odontol Tidskr 1951; 59:407.
53. Pindborg JJ, Bhat M, Devanath KR, et al: Occurrence of acute necrotizing gingivitis in South Indian children. J Periodontol 1966; 37:14.
54. Plaut HC: Studienzur bakterielle Diagnostik der Diphtheriae un der Aginen. Dtsch Med Wochenschr 1894; 20:920.
55. Regezi JA, Sciubba JJ: Oral Pathology. Clinico-Pathologic Correlations. Philadelphia, Saunders, 1989.
56. Rivera-Hidalgo F, Stanford TW: Oral mucosal lesions caused by infective microorganisms. I. Virus and bacteria. Periodontology 2000 1999; 21:106.
57. Rosebury T: Is Vincent's infection a communicable disease? J Am Dent Assoc 1942; 29:823.
58. Rosebury T, Foley G: Experimental Vincent's infection. J Am Dent Assoc 1939; 26:1978.
59. Rosebury T, MacDonald JB, Clark A: A bacteriologic survey of gingival scrapings from periodontal infections by direct examination, guinea pig inoculation and anaerobic cultivation. J Dent Res 1950; 29:718.
60. Roy S, Wolman L: Electron microscopic observations on the virus particles in herpes simplex encephalitis. J Clin Pathol 1969; 22:51.
61. Schluger S: Necrotizing ulcerative gingivitis in the army. Incidence, communicability, and treatment. J Am Dent Assoc 1949; 38:174.
62. Schwartzman J, Grossman L: Vincent's ulceromembranous gingivostomatitis. Arch Pediatr 1941; 58:515.
63. Scott TFM, Steigman AS, Convey JH: Acute infectious gingivostomatitis. Etiology, epidemiology, and clinical picture of common disorders caused by virus of herpes simplex. JAMA 1941; 117:999.
64. Shannon IL, Kilgore WG, Leary TJ: Stress as a predisposing factor in necrotizing ulcerative gingivitis. J Periodontol 1969; 40:240.
65. Sheiham A: An epidemiological study of oral disease in Nigerians. J Dent Res 1965; 44:1184.
66. Ship II, Brightman VJ, Laster LL: The patient with recurrent aphthous ulcers and the patient with recurrent herpes labialis. A study of two population samples. J Am Dent Assoc 1967; 75:645.
67. Skach M, Zabrodsky S, Mrklas L: A study of the effect of age and season on the incidence of ulcerative gingivitis. J Periodont Res 1970; 5:187.
68. Smith DT: Spirochetes and related organisms in fusospirochetal disease. Baltimore, Williams & Wilkins, 1932.
69. Stammers AF: Vincent's infection. Br Dent J 1944; 76:171.
70. Stevens AWJ, Cogen RB, Cohen-Cole SA, et al: Demographic and clinical data associated with acute necrotizing ulcerative gingivitis in a dental school population. J Clin Periodontol 1984; 11:487.
71. Swenson HM: Induced Vincent's infection in dogs. J Dent Res 1944; 23:190.
72. Swenson HM, Muhler, JC: Induced fusospirochetal infection in dogs. J Dent Res 1947; 26:161.
73. Topping NH, Fraser HF: Mouth lesions associated with dietary deficiencies in monkeys. US Pub Health Rep 1939; 54:431.
74. Tunnicliff R, Fink EB, Hammond C: Significance of fusiform bacilli and spirilla in gingival tissue. J Am Dent Assoc 1936; 23:1959.
75. Tunnicliff R, Hammond C: Abscess production by fusiform bacilli in rabbits and mice by the use of scillaren-B or mucin. J Dent Res 1937; 16:479.
76. Underhill FP, Mendel LB: Further experiments on the pellagra-like syndrome in dogs. Am J Physiol 1928; 83:589.
77. Vincent H: Sur l'etiologie et sur les lesions anatomopathologiques de la pourritute d'hopital. Ann de l'Inst Pasteur 1896; 10:448.
78. Wilton JMA, Ivanyi A, Lehner T: Cell-mediated immunity and humoral antibodies in acute ulcerative gingivitis. J Periodont Res 1971; 6:9.

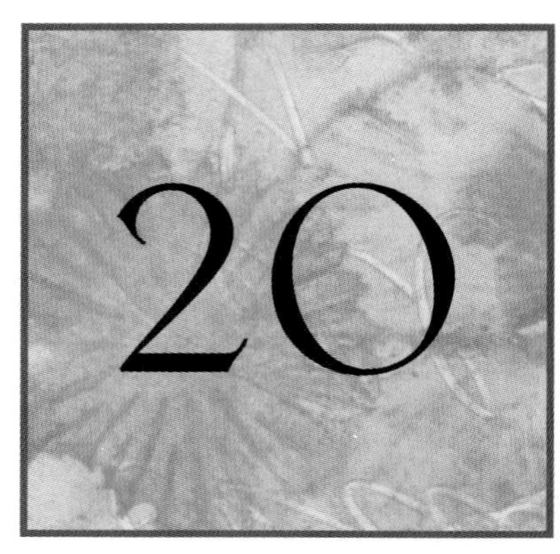

CHAPTER 20

Gingival Disease in Childhood

Fermin A. Carranza

Chapter Outline

The effects of periodontal disease observed in adults have their inception earlier in life. Gingival disease in the child may progress to jeopardize the periodontium of the adult.

The developing dentition and certain systemic metabolic patterns are peculiar to childhood. There are also gingival and periodontal disturbances that occur more often in childhood and are therefore identified with this period. Consequently, some degree of coherence is provided by considering gingival and periodontal problems in childhood and in adolescence separately. This chapter will cover gingival diseases; juvenile forms of periodontitis are covered in Chapter 28.

THE PERIODONTIUM OF THE DECIDUOUS DENTITION

The gingiva of the deciduous dentition is pale pink and firm and may be either smooth or stippled (stippling is found in 35% of children between ages 5 and 13 years)[26] (Fig. 20-1). The interdental gingiva is broad faciolingually and tends to be relatively narrow mesiodistally, in conformity with the contour of the approximal tooth surfaces. Its structure is comparable to that of the adult in that it consists of a facial papilla and a lingual papilla with an intervening depression, or col.

The mean gingival sulcus depth for the primary dentition is 2.1 mm ± 0.2 mm.[24] The width of the attached gingiva is greater in the incisor area, decreases over the cuspids, and increases again over premolars (primary molars) and permanent molars.[27] The attached gingiva increases in width with age.

Microscopically, the stratified squamous epithelium of the gingiva presents well-differentiated rete pegs with a parakeratinized (Fig. 20-2) or keratinized surface, the latter correlated with stippling. The connective tissue is predominantly fibrillar, but the well-differentiated collagen bundles seen in the adult are not present in childhood. The epithelium covering the col is a few cells thick and nonkeratinized.

The periodontal ligament of the deciduous teeth is wider than that of the permanent dentition. During eruption the principal fibers are parallel to the long axis of the teeth; the bundle arrangement seen in the adult dentition occurs when the teeth encounter their functional antagonists.

Radiographically, the alveolar bone in relation to the deciduous dentition shows a prominent lamina dura, both in the crypt stage and during eruption. The trabeculae of the alveolar bone are fewer but thicker than in the adult, and the marrow spaces tend to be larger. The crests of the interdental septa are flat.[6]

Oral flora and dental plaque in childhood are discussed in Chapter 6.

PHYSIOLOGIC GINGIVAL CHANGES ASSOCIATED WITH TOOTH ERUPTION

During the transition period in the development of the dentition, changes associated with eruption of the permanent teeth occur in the gingiva. It is important to recognize these physiologic changes and to differentiate them from the gingival disease that often accompanies tooth eruption.

Preeruption Bulge

Before the crown appears in the oral cavity, the gingiva presents a bulge that is firm, may be slightly blanched, and conforms to the contour of the underlying crown.

Formation of the Gingival Margin

The marginal gingiva and sulcus develop as the crown penetrates the oral mucosa. In the course of eruption the gingival margin is usually edematous, rounded, and slightly reddened (Fig. 20-3).

Normal Prominence of the Gingival Margin

During the period of mixed dentition, it is normal for the marginal gingiva around the permanent teeth to be quite prominent, particularly in the maxillary anterior region. At this stage in tooth eruption the gingiva is still attached to the crown, and it appears prominent when superimposed on the bulk of the underlying enamel (Fig. 20-4).

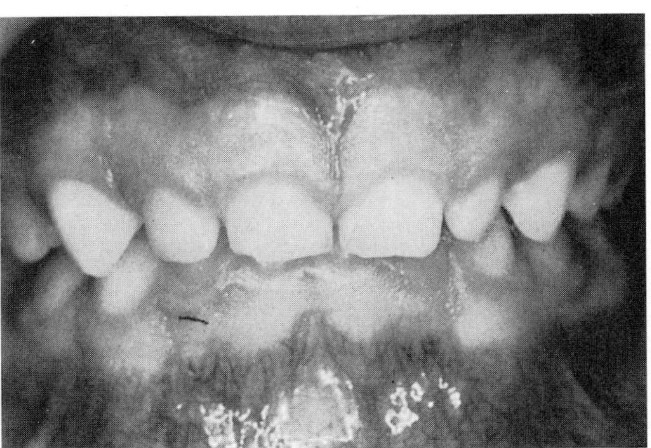

Fig. 20-1 Deciduous dentition with stippled gingiva.

TYPES OF GINGIVAL DISEASE

Chronic Marginal Gingivitis

Chronic marginal gingivitis is the most prevalent type of gingival change in childhood. The gingiva exhibits all the changes in color, size, consistency, and surface texture characteristic of chronic inflammation. A fiery red

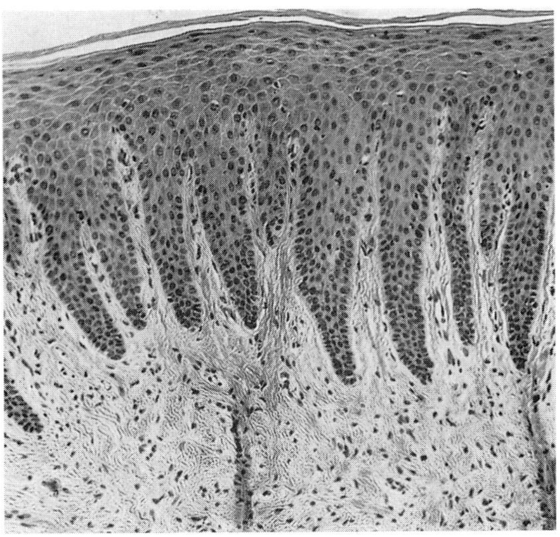

Fig. 20-2 Normal gingiva in a 4-year-old patient showing stratified squamous epithelium with rete pegs and surface keratinization. The papillary arrangement of the underlying connective tissue can also be seen.

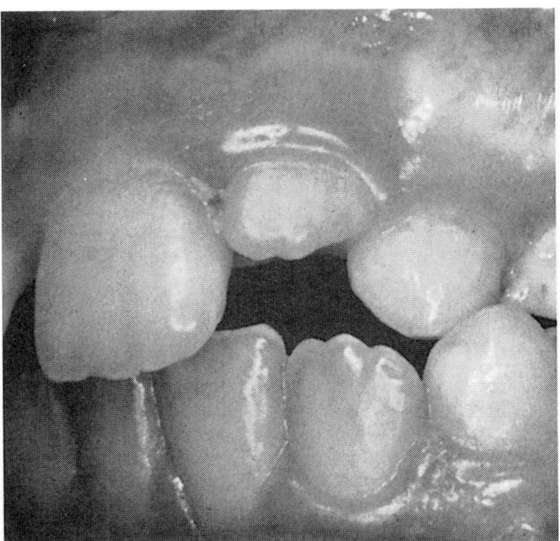

Fig. 20-3 Gingivitis associated with tooth eruption. Note the prominent rolled gingival margin, which is slightly inflamed and edematous around the erupting maxillary lateral incisor.

surface discoloration is often superimposed on underlying chronic changes. Gingival color change and swelling appear to be more common expressions of gingivitis in children than are bleeding and increased pocket depth.[5]

Etiology. In children, as in adults, the cause of gingivitis is plaque; local conditions such as *materia alba* and poor oral hygiene favor its accumulation (Fig. 20-5). In preschool children, however, the gingival response to bacterial plaque has been found to be markedly less than that in adults.[16,17] Dental plaque appears to form more rapidly in children age 8 to 12 years than in adults.

Calculus is uncommon in infants; it occurs in approximately 9% of children ages 4 to 6, in 18% of those ages 7 to 9, and in 33% to 43% of those ages 10 to 15. In children with cystic fibrosis, calculus formation is more common (occurring in 77% of those ages 7 to 9 and in 90% of those ages 10 to 15) and more severe; this is probably related to increased concentrations of phosphate, calcium, and protein in the saliva.[20]

Gingivitis associated with tooth eruption is frequent and has given rise to the term eruption gingivitis. However, tooth eruption per se does not cause gingivitis. The inflammation results from plaque accumulation around erupting teeth. The initiation of gingivitis appears to be related to plaque accumulation rather than to tissue remodeling associated with eruption.[10] Plaque retention around deciduous teeth facilitates plaque formation around juxtaposed permanent teeth.[10] The inflammatory changes accentuate the normal prominence of the gingival margin and may create the impression of a marked gingival enlargement (Fig. 20-6).

Partially exfoliated, loose deciduous teeth often cause gingivitis. The eroded margin of partially resorbed teeth favors plaque accumulation, which causes gingival changes varying from slight discoloration and edema to abscess formation with suppuration. Other factors favoring plaque buildup are food impaction and *materia alba* accumulation around teeth partially destroyed by caries. Children often develop unilateral chewing habits to avoid loose or carious teeth, aggravating the accumulation of plaque on the nonchewing side.

Gingivitis occurs more often and with greater severity around **malposed teeth** because of their increased tendency to accumulate plaque and *materia alba*. Severe changes include gingival enlargement, bluish-red discoloration, ulceration (Fig. 20-7), and the formation of deep pockets from which pus can be expressed. Gingival health and contour are restored by correction of the malposition (Figs. 20-8 and 20-9); plaque elimination; and, when necessary, surgical removal of the enlarged gingiva.

Gingivitis is increased in children with *excessive overbite* and *overjet, nasal obstruction,* and *mouth-breathing habit.*

According to Maynard and Wilson,[18] mucogingival problems start in the primary dentition as a consequence of developmental aberrations in eruption and deficiencies in the thickness of the periodontium. If there is also inadequate plaque control or excessive toothbrushing trauma, a mucogingival problem develops. However, the width of the attached gingiva increases with age, and these problems may resolve.

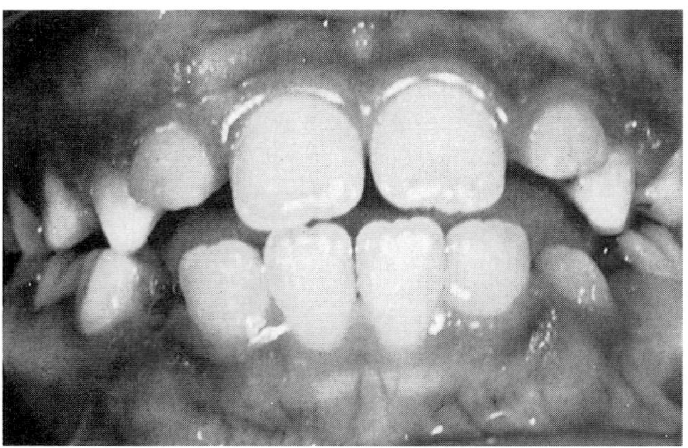

Fig. 20-4 Prominent marginal gingiva on the cervical third of partially erupted maxillary anterior teeth.

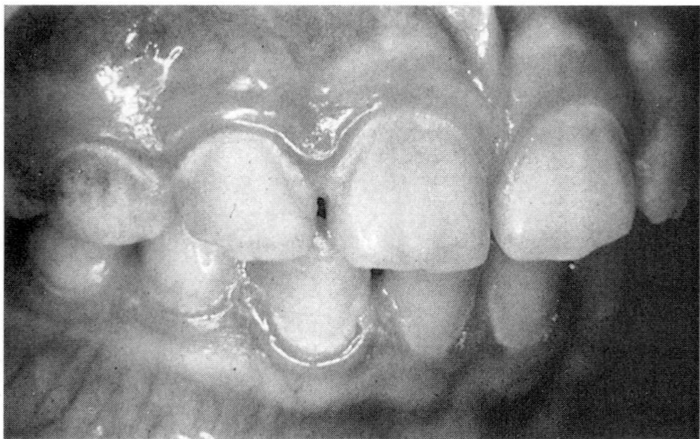

Fig. 20-5 Chronic marginal gingivitis associated with plaque and *materia alba.*

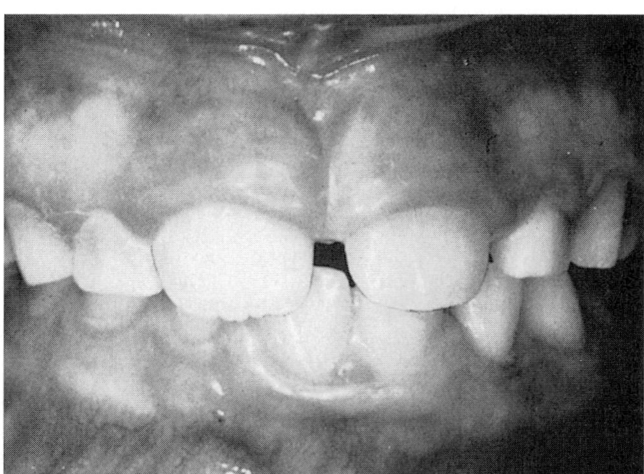

Fig. 20-6 Developmental gingival enlargement caused by inflammation superimposed on the normal prominence of the teeth at this stage of tooth eruption.

Histopathology. Chronic gingivitis in children[13,14] is characterized by loss of collagen in the area around the junctional epithelium, an important vascular component, and an infiltrate consisting mostly of lymphocytes and small numbers of polymorphonuclear leukocytes, plasma cells, monocytes, mast cells, fibroblasts, and endothelial cells.

The composition of the inflammatory infiltrate in gingivitis in children has given rise to controversy. According to Gillett and colleagues,[8] the inflammatory infiltrate is composed mostly of untransformed B lymphocytes, and the resulting clinical lesions are nondestructive and nonprogressive. This may also characterize the composition of the infiltrate in quiescent lesions in adults. According to Longhurst et al[13,14] and Seymour et al,[25] the infiltrate is predominantly composed of T cells that shift to B cells (plasma cells) when the lesion becomes destructive.

A higher prevalence and severity of gingivitis and gingival enlargement is found in the circumpubertal period; this form of gingivitis has been termed **pubertal gingivitis.** The most frequent manifestation is a significant increase in bleeding interdental sites.[19] This inflammatory lesion may include a gingival enlargement as a result of hormonal changes that magnify the tissue response to dental plaque. It occurs in males and females and resolves partially after puberty (see Chapter 18).

Localized Gingival Recession

Gingival recession around individual teeth or groups of teeth is a common source of concern. The gingiva may be inflamed or free of disease, depending on the presence or absence of local irritants. There are many causes of gingival recession (see Chapter 17), but in children the position of the tooth in the arch is the most important.[22] Gingival recession occurs on teeth in labial version (Fig. 20-10) and on those that are tilted or rotated so that the roots project labially. Anterior open bite increases the prevalence of gingival recession.[15] The recession may be a transitional phase in tooth eruption and may correct itself when the teeth attain proper alignment, or it may be necessary to realign the teeth orthodontically.[3]

Acute Gingival Infections

Primary Herpetic Gingivostomatitis. This is the most common type of acute gingival infection in childhood and often occurs as a sequela of upper respiratory tract infection (see Chapter 19).

Candidiasis. This is a mycotic infection of the oral cavity caused by the fungus *Candida albicans*. For a complete discussion, see Chapter 21.

Necrotizing Ulcerative Gingivitis. The incidence of necrotizing ulcerative gingivitis (NUG) in childhood is low (see Chapter 19). In children living in areas

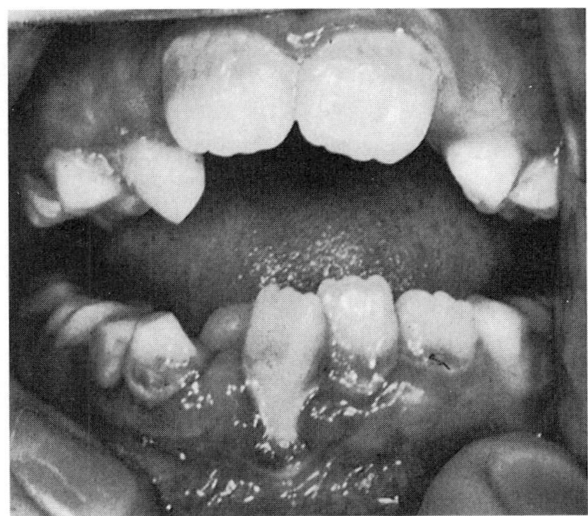

Fig. 20-7 Severe gingivitis associated with accumulation of plaque around malposed teeth.

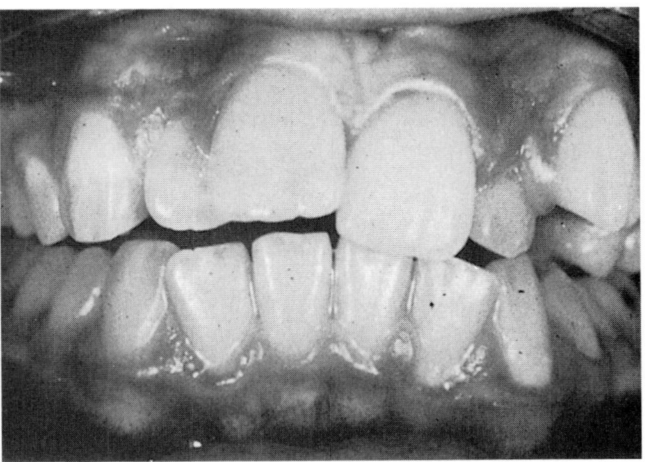

Fig. 20-8 Gingival enlargement in relation to malposed maxillary lateral and canine teeth (left side).

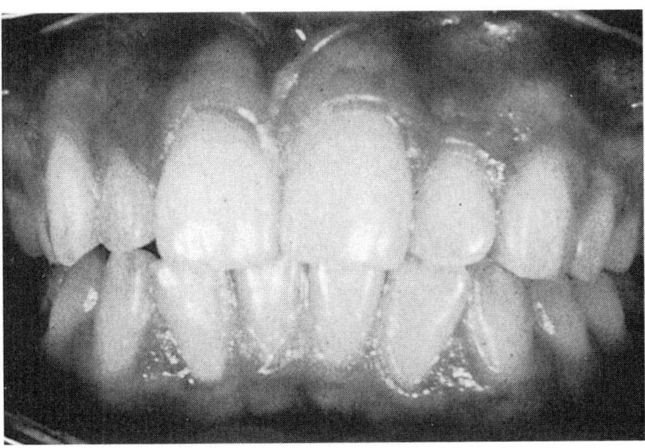

Fig. 20-9 Disappearance of the gingival enlargement shown in Fig. 20-8 after orthodontic correction of the malposed teeth.

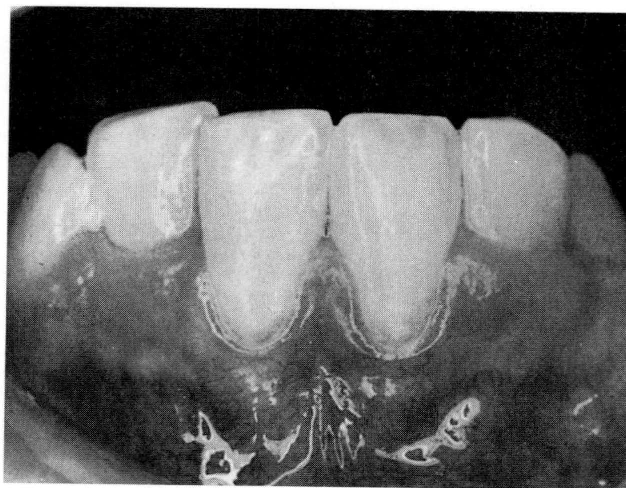

Fig. 20-10 Gingival recession on labially positioned mandibular central incisors.

where chronic malnutrition is common and in children with Down syndrome, the incidence and severity of NUG are increased.[11,23] Primary herpetic gingivostomatitis, which is more common in childhood, is occasionally erroneously diagnosed as NUG.

TRAUMATIC CHANGES IN THE PERIODONTIUM

Traumatic changes may occur in the periodontal tissues of deciduous teeth under several conditions. In the process of shedding deciduous teeth, resorption of teeth and bone weakens the periodontal support so that the existing functional forces are injurious to the remaining supporting tissues.[4] Excessive occlusal forces may be produced by malalignment, mutilation, loss or extraction of teeth, or dental restorations. In the mixed dentition stage, the periodontium of the permanent teeth may be traumatized, because the permanent teeth bear an increased occlusal load when the adjacent deciduous teeth are shed. The periodontal ligament of an erupting permanent tooth may be injured by occlusal forces transmitted through the deciduous tooth it is replacing.[9]

Microscopically,[12,21] the least severe traumatic changes involve compression, ischemia, and hyalinization of the periodontal ligament. With severe injury there is crushing and necrosis of the periodontal ligament (see Chapter 24).

In most instances the injuries are repaired, and tooth loss does not result. However, traumatized teeth may be sore or loose. Repair may result in ankylosis of the tooth to the bone, fixing the tooth in situ. When the permanent dentition erupts, ankylosed deciduous teeth appear to be submerged.

THE ORAL MUCOUS MEMBRANE IN CHILDHOOD DISEASES

Some childhood diseases present specific alterations in the oral mucosa, including the gingival tissues. Among these are the communicable diseases, such as varicella (chickenpox), rubeola (measles), scarlatina (scarlet fever), and diphtheria. For a more thorough discussion of this topic, the reader is referred to books in oral and pediatric pathology.

REFERENCES

1. Alcoforado GA, Kristoffersen T, Johannessen AC, et al: The composition of gingival inflammatory cell infiltrates in children studied by enzyme histochemistry. J Clin Periodontol 1990; 17:335.
2. Andlin-Sobocki A, Marcusson A, Persson M: 3-year observations on gingival recession in mandibular incisors in children. J Clin Periodontol 1991; 18:155.
3. Baer PN, Benjamin SD: Periodontal Disease in Children and Adolescents. Philadelphia, JB Lippincott, 1974.
4. Bernick S, Freedman N: Microscopic studies of the periodontium of the primary dentitions of monkeys. II. Posterior teeth during the mixed dentitional period. Oral Surg Oral Med Oral Pathol 1954; 7:322.
5. Bimstein E, Lustmann J, Soskolne WA: A clinical and histometric study of gingivitis associated with the human deciduous dentition. J Periodontol 1985; 56:293.
6. Brauer JC, Highley LB, Massler M, et al: Dentistry for Children. 2nd ed. Philadelphia, Blakiston, 1947.
7. Everett FG, Tuchler H, Lu KH: Occurrence of calculus in grade school children in Portland, Oregon. J Periodontol 1963; 34:54.
8. Gillett R, Cruckley A, Johnson NW: The nature of the inflammatory infiltrates in childhood gingivitis, juvenile periodontitis and adult periodontitis: Immunocytochemical studies using a monoclonal antibody to HLA Dr. J Clin Periodontol 1986; 13:281.
9. Grimmer EA: Trauma in an erupting premolar. J Dent Res 1939; 18:267.
10. Hock J: A clinical study of gingivitis of deciduous and succedaneous permanent teeth in dogs. J Periodont Res 1978; 13:68.
11. Jimenez M, Ramos J, Garrington G, et al: The familial occurrence of acute necrotizing gingivitis in Colombia. J Periodontol 1969; 40:414.
12. Kronfeld R, Weinmann J: Traumatic changes in the periodontal tissues of deciduous teeth. J Dent Res 1940; 19:441.
13. Longhurst P, Gillett R, Johnson NW: Electron microscope quantitation of inflammatory infiltrates in childhood gingivitis. J Periodont Res 1980; 15:255.
14. Longhurst P, Johnson NW, Hopps RM: Differences in lymphocyte and plasma cell densities in inflamed gingiva from adults and young children. J Periodontol 1977; 48:705.
15. Machtei EE, Zubery Y, Bimstein E, et al: Anterior open bite and gingival recession in children and adolescents. Int Dent J 1990; 40:369.
16. Mackler SB, Crawford JJ: Plaque development in the primary dentition. J Periodontol 1973; 44:18.
17. Mattson L: Development of gingivitis in preschool children and young adults. A comparative experimental study. J Clin Periodontol 1978; 5:24.
18. Maynard JG, Wilson RD: Diagnosis and management of mucogingival problems in children. Dent Clin North Am 1980; 24:683.

19. Mombelli R, Gusberti FR, van Oosten MA, et al: Gingival health and gingivitis development during puberty. A 4-year longitudinal study. J Clin Periodontol 1989; 16:451.
20. Notman S, Mandel ID, Mercadante J: Calculus in normal children and children with cystic fibrosis. International Association for Dental Research Program and Abstracts, 48th General Meeting, 1970.
21. Orban B, Weinmann J: Signs of traumatic occlusion in average human jaws. J Dent Res 1933; 13:216.
22. Parfitt GJ, Mjor IA: A clinical evaluation of local gingival recession in children. J Dent Child 1964; 31:257.
23. Pindborg JJ, Bhat M, Devanath KR, et al: Occurrence of acute necrotizing gingivitis in South India children. J Periodontol 1966; 37:14.
24. Rosenblum FN: Clinical study of the depth of the gingival sulcus in the primary dentition. J Dent Child 1966; 5:289.
25. Seymour GJ, Crouch MS, Powell RN, et al: The identification of lymphoid cell subpopulations in sections of human lymphoid tissue and gingivitis in children using monoclonal antibodies. J Periodont Res 1982; 17:247.
26. Soni NN, Silberkweit M, Hayes RL: Histological characteristics of stippling in children. J Periodontol 1963; 34:31.
27. Srivastava B, Chandra S, Jaiswal JS, et al: Cross-sectional study to evaluate variations in attached gingiva and gingival sulcus in the three periods of dentition. J Clin Pediatr Dent 1990; 15:17.

Desquamative Gingivitis

Alfredo Aguirre, Mirdza E. Neiders, and Russell J. Nisengard

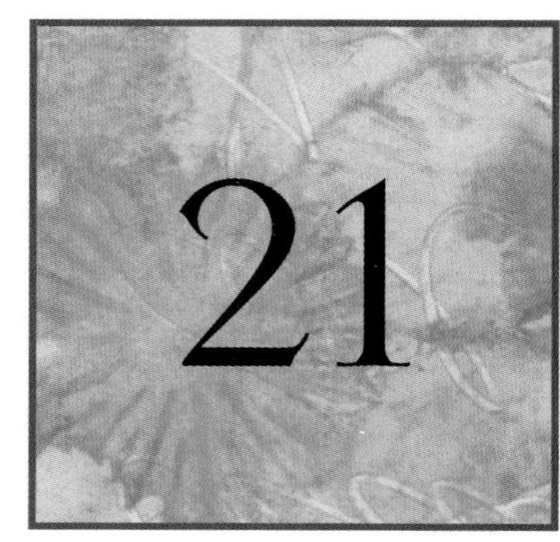

CHAPTER

CHAPTER OUTLINE

CHRONIC DESQUAMATIVE GINGIVITIS

Although first recognized and reported in 1894,[118] the term *chronic desquamative gingivitis* was coined in 1932 by Prinz[92] to describe a peculiar condition characterized by intense erythema, desquamation, and ulceration of the free and attached gingiva (Fig. 21-1). Patients may be asymptomatic, however, when symptomatic, their complaints range from a mild burning sensation to an intense pain. Approximately 50% of desquamative gingivitis cases are localized to the gingiva, although involvement of the gingiva plus other intraoral and even extraoral sites is not uncommon.[85] Initially, the cause of this condition was unclear with a variety of possibilities suggested. Because most cases were diagnosed in women in the fourth to fifth decades of life (although desquamative gingivitis may occur as early as puberty or as late as the seventh or eighth decades), a hormonal derangement was suspected.* However, in 1960 McCarthy and colleagues[72] suggested that *desquamative gingivitis was not a specific disease entity, but a gingival response associated with a variety of conditions.* This concept has been further supported by numerous immunopathologic studies.[57,86,97,113]

Use of clinical and laboratory parameters have revealed that approximately 75% of desquamative gingivitis cases have a dermatologic genesis. Cicatricial pemphigoid and lichen planus account for over 95% of the dermatologic cases.[85] However, many other mucocutaneous autoimmune conditions such as bullous pemphigoid, pemphigus vulgaris, linear immunoglobulin A (IgA), dermatitis herpetiformis, lupus erythematosus, and chronic ulcerative stomatitis can clinically manifest as desquamative gingivitis.[103]

Other conditions that must be considered in the differential diagnosis of desquamative gingivitis include chronic bacterial, fungal, and viral infections, as well as reactions to medications, mouthwashes, and chewing gum. Although less common, Crohn's disease, sarcoidosis, some leukemias, and even factitious lesions have also been reported to clinically present as desquamative gingivitis.[103,122]

* See references 37, 42, 75, 92, 114, 124, and 125.

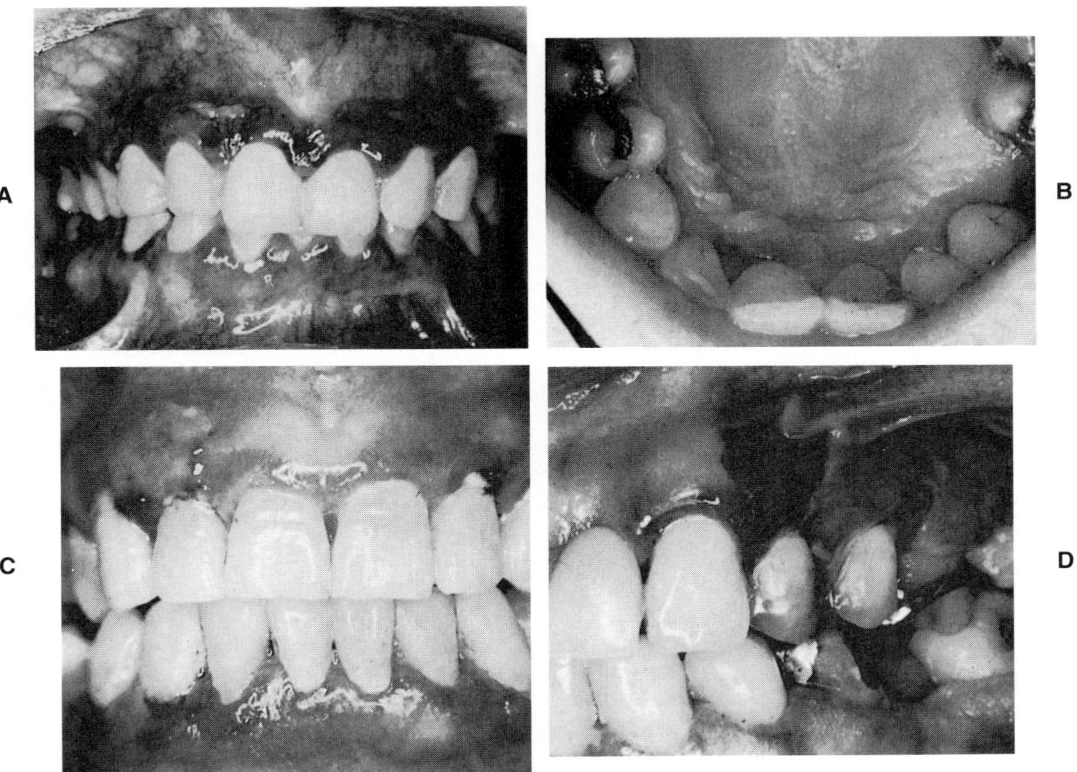

Fig. 21-1 Chronic desquamative gingivitis of varied severity. **A,** Moderate, with generalized edema and erythema associated with inflammation and exposure of underlying connective tissue. **B,** Lingual view of patient shown in **A.** Aside from slight marginal erythema, there is little evidence of change in the gingiva and adjacent mucosa. **C,** Severe, with scattered, irregularly shaped, denuded areas producing a mosaic appearance. Note the ulceration between the right maxillary lateral and canine teeth. **D,** Severe, with complete denudation of the epithelium and exposure of underlying erythematous inflamed connective tissue. (Courtesy Dr. Gerald Shklar, Boston, Mass.)

Therefore it is of paramount importance to ascertain the identity of the disease responsible for desquamative gingivitis to establish the appropriate therapeutic approach and management. To achieve this goal, the clinical examination has to be coupled with a thorough history, and routine histologic and immunofluorescent studies.[122] It should be mentioned, however, that despite this diagnostic approach, the cause of desquamative gingivitis cannot be elucidated in up to one third of the cases.[93]

DIAGNOSIS OF DESQUAMATIVE GINGIVITIS: A SYSTEMATIC APPROACH

The previous sections have made clear that *desquamative gingivitis* is only a clinical term that describes a peculiar clinical picture. This term is not a diagnosis per se and once it is rendered, a series of laboratory procedures should be used to arrive to a final diagnosis. Thus the success of any given therapeutic approach resides on the establishment of an accurate final diagnosis. The following represents a systematic approach to elucidate the disease triggering desquamative gingivitis. This approach is also illustrated in Fig 21-2.

Clinical History. A thorough clinical history is mandatory to begin the assessment of desquamative gingivitis. Data regarding the symptomatology associated with this condition, as well as its historical aspects (i.e., when did the lesion start, has it gotten worse, is there a habit that exacerbates the condition, etc.), provide the foundation for a thorough examination. Information regarding previous therapy that has been directed to alleviate the condition should also be documented.

Clinical Examination. Recognition of the pattern of distribution of the lesions (i.e., focal or multifocal, with or without confinement to the gingival tissues) provides leading information to begin the formulation of a differential diagnosis. In addition, a simple clinical maneuver such as Nikolsky's sign offers insight into the plausibility of the presence of a vesiculobullous disorder.

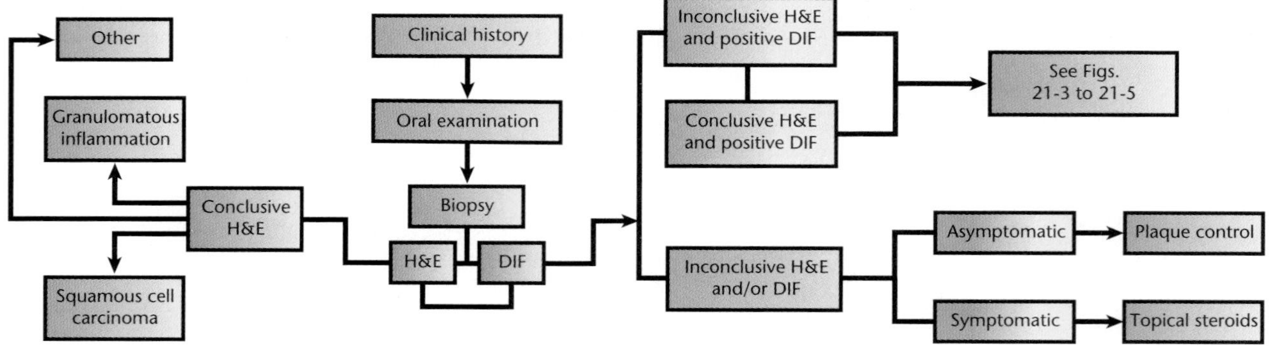

Fig. 21-2 Diagnostic approach for desquamative gingivitis.

Biopsy. Given the extent and number of lesions that may be present in a given individual, an incisional biopsy is the best alternative to begin the microscopic and immunological evaluation. An important consideration is selection of the biopsy site. A perilesional incisional biopsy should avoid areas of ulceration because necrosis and epithelial denudation severely hamper the diagnostic process. Once the tissue is excised from the oral cavity, the specimen can be bisected and then submitted for microscopic examination. Buffered formalin (10%) should be used to fix the tissue for conventional hematoxylin and eosin (H&E) evaluation. Michell's buffer (ammonium sulfate buffer, pH 7.0) is used as transport solution for immunofluorescent assessment. In general, an incisional biopsy of uninvolved (normal) mucosa will show the same immunofluorescent findings as the biopsy of the perilesional tissue. However, there are notable exceptions such as in lichen planus and subacute lupus erythematosus (Table 21-1) where only the lesional tissue will exhibit the corresponding immunologic markers.

Microscopic Examination. Approximately 5-μm sections of formalin-fixed, paraffin embedded, tissue stained with conventional H&E are obtained for light microscopy examination.

Immunofluorescence. For direct immunofluorescence, unfixed frozen sections are incubated with a variety of fluorescein-labeled, anti-human serum (anti-IgG, anti-IgA, anti-IgM, anti-fibrin and anti-C3). With indirect immunofluorescence, unfixed frozen sections of oral or esophageal mucosa from an animal such as a monkey are first incubated with the patient's serum to allow attachment of any serum antibodies to the mucosal tissue. The tissue is then incubated with fluorescein-labeled anti-human serum (anti-IgG, anti-IgA, anti-IgM, anti-fibrin, and anti-C3). Immunofluorescence tests are positive if a fluorescent signal is observed either in the epithelium, its associated basement membrane or in the underlying connective tissue.

Management. Once the diagnosis is established, the dentist has to choose the optimum management for the patient. This is accomplished according to the following three factors: 1) practitioner's experience, 2) systemic impact of the disease, and 3) systemic complications of the medications.

A detailed consideration of these three factors dictates three different scenarios (Figs. 21-3 to 21-5). In the first one, the dental practitioner takes direct and exclusive responsibility for the treatment of the patient. Such is the case in erosive lichen planus that is responsive to topical steroids. In the second scenario, the dentist collaborates with another health care provider to concurrently evaluate and/or treat a patient. The classic example is seen in cicatricial pemphigoid where dentists and ophthalmologists work together. Although the dentist addresses the oral lesions, the ophthalmologist monitors the integrity of the ocular conjunctiva. The third and final scenario is when the patient is immediately referred to a dermatologist for further evaluation and treatment. This occurs in conditions where the systemic impact of the disease transcends the boundaries of the oral cavity and results in significant morbidity and even mortality. Pemphigus vulgaris is a clear example of a condition that once diagnosed by the dentist requires immediate referral to a dermatologist. In addition, the complications of chronically administered systemic medications that are indicated for the management of diseases such as pemphigus vulgaris or nonresponsive mucous membrane pemphigoid (e.g., diabetes mellitus, osteoporosis, methemoglobinemia, etc.) warrant the referral to a dermatologist or a specialist in internal medicine.

When oral treatment is provided, periodic evaluation is needed to monitor the response of the patient to the selected therapy. Initially, the patient should be evaluated at 2 to 4 weeks after beginning treatment to ensure that the condition is under control. This observation should continue until the patient is free of discomfort. Appointments every 3 to 6 months would then be appropriate. Adjustment to the doses of medication(s) used is expected to occur during this interval. Table 21-2 summarizes suggested contemporary therapeutic approaches commonly used to treat selected conditions that clinically present as desquamative gingivitis. It is clear that dentists play an important role in the diagnosis and management of desquamative gingivitis. The importance

TABLE 21-1

Histopathologic, Direct, and Indirect Immunofluorescence Findings in Selected Conditions That May Present Clinically as Desquamative Gingivitis

		Direct Immunofluorescence		Indirect Immunofluorescence
Disease	**Histopathology**	**Biopsy Perilesional Mucosa**	**Biopsy Uninvolved Mucosa**	**Serum**
Pemphigus	Intraepithelial clefting above the basal cell layer. The basal cells have a characteristic "tombstone" appearance. Acantholysis is present.	Intercellular deposits in epithelium; IgG in all cases, C3 in most cases.	Same as perilesional mucosa.	Intercellular (IgG) antibodies in ≥90% of cases.
Cicatricial pemphigoid	Subepithelial clefting with epithelial separation from the underlying lamina propria, leaving an intact basal layer.	Linear deposits of C3, with or without IgG at the basement membrane zone in almost all cases.	Same as perilesional mucosa.	Basement membrane zone (IgG) antibodies in 10% of cases.
Bullous pemphigoid	Subepithelial clefting with epithelial separation from the underlying lamina propria, leaving an intact basal layer.	Linear deposits of C3, with or without IgG at the basement membrane zone in almost all cases.	Same as perilesional mucosa.	Basement membrane zone (IgG) antibodies in 40% to 70% of cases.
Epidermolysis bullosa acquisita	Similar to bullous and cicatricial pemphigoid.	Linear deposits of IgG and C3 at the basement membrane zone in almost all cases.	Same as perilesional mucosa.	Basement membrane zone (IgG) antibodies in 25% of cases.
Lichen planus	Hyperkeratosis, hydropic degeneration of the basal layer, "saw-toothed" rete pegs. The lamina propria exhibits a dense, band-like infiltrate primarily of T lymphocytes. Colloid bodies are present.	Fibrilar deposits of fibrin at the dermal-epidermal junction.	Negative.	Negative.
Chronic ulcerative stomatitis	Similar to erosive lichen planus (hyperkeratosis, acanthosis, basal cell layer liquefaction, subepithelial clefting, and lympho-histiocytic chronic infiltrate in a bandlike configuration.	IgG deposits in nuclei of basal layer epithelial cells.	Same as perilesional mucosa.	ANA specific for basal cells of stratified squamous epithelium.
Linear IgA disease	Similar to erosive lichen planus.	Linear deposits of IgA at the basement membrane zone.	Same as perilesional mucosa.	IgA basement membrane zone (IgA) antibodies in 30% of cases.
Dermatitis herpetiformis	Collection of neutrophils, eosinophils, and fibrin in connective tissue papillae.	IgA deposits in dermal papillae in 85% of cases.	IgA deposits in dermal papillae in 100% of cases.	IgA endomysial antibodies in 70% of cases, gliadin antibodies in 30% of cases.

Continued

TABLE 21-1

Histopathologic, Direct, and Indirect Immunofluorescence Findings in Selected Conditions That May Present Clinically as Desquamative Gingivitis—cont'd

		Direct Immunofluorescence		Indirect Immunofluorescence
Disease	**Histopathology**	**Biopsy Perilesional Mucosa**	**Biopsy Uninvolved Mucosa**	**Serum**
Systemic lupus erythematosus	Hyperkeratosis, basal cell degeneration, epithelial atrophy, and perivascular inflammation.	Ig (G or M), with or without C3 deposits at dermal-epidermal junction.	Same as perilesional mucosa.	ANA in more than 95% of cases, DNA and ENA antibodies in more than 50% of cases.
Chronic cutaneous lupus erythematosus	Hyperkeratosis, basal cell degeneration, epithelial atrophy, and perivascular inflammation.	Ig (G or M), with or without C3 deposits at dermal-epidermal junction.	Negative.	Usually negative.
Subacute lupus erythematosus	Less inflammatory cell infiltrate than systemic and chronic cutaneous lupus erythematosus but with similar microscopic features.	Ig (G or M), with or without C3 deposits at dermal-epidermal junction in 60% of cases; granular IgG deposits in basal cell cytoplasm in 30% of cases.	Same as perilesional mucosa.	ANA in 60% to 90%, SS-A (Ro) in 80%, RF in 30%, and RNP in 10% of cases.

Modified from Rinaggio J, Neiders ME, Aguirre A, et al: Using immunofluorescence in the diagnosis of chronic ulcerative lesions of the oral mucosa. Compend 1999; 20:943.

of being able to recognize and properly diagnose this condition is accentuated by the fact that a serious and life-threatening disease may initially manifest as desquamative gingivitis. The following is a discussion of the most common conditions presenting clinically as desquamative gingivitis.

DISEASES CLINICALLY PRESENTING AS DESQUAMATIVE GINGIVITIS

Lichen Planus

Lichen planus is a relatively common, chronic, dermatosis characterized by the presence of cutaneous violaceous papules that may coalesce to form plaques. The current evidence suggests that lichen planus is an immunologically mediated mucocutaneous disorder where host T lymphocytes play a central role.[7,48,70] Although the oral cavity may present lichen planus lesions with a distinct clinical configuration and distribution, the clinical presentation sometimes may simulate other mucocutaneous disorders. Therefore a clinical diagnosis of oral lichen planus should be accompanied by a broad differential diagnosis. Numerous epidemiologic studies have shown that oral lichen planus presents in 0.1% to 4% of the population.[100] The majority of patients with oral lichen planus are middle-aged and older females with a 2:1 ratio of females to males. Although possible, children are rarely affected. In a dental setting, cutaneous lichen planus is observed in about one third of the patients diagnosed with oral lichen planus.[67] In contrast, two thirds of patients seen in dermatologic clinics exhibit oral lichen planus.[102]

Oral Lesions. Although there are several clinical forms of oral lichen planus (reticular, patch, atrophic, erosive and bullous), the most common are the reticular and erosive subtypes. The typical reticular lesions are asymptomatic, bilateral, and consist of interlacing white lines on the posterior region of the buccal mucosa. The lateral border and dorsum of the tongue, hard palate, alveolar ridge, and gingiva may also be affected. In addition, it is not unusual for the reticular lesions to have an erythematous background, a feature that is associated with the coexistence of candidiasis. Oral lichen planus lesions follow a chronic course and have alternating, unpredictable periods of quiescence and flares.

The erosive subtype of lichen planus is often associated with pain and clinically manifests as atrophic, erythematous areas. Fine white radiating striations are observed bordering the atrophic zones. These areas may be sensitive to heat, acid, and spicy foods (Color Fig. 21-1).

Gingival Lesions. Up to 10% of patients with oral lichen planus have lesions restricted to the gingival

Text continued on page 320

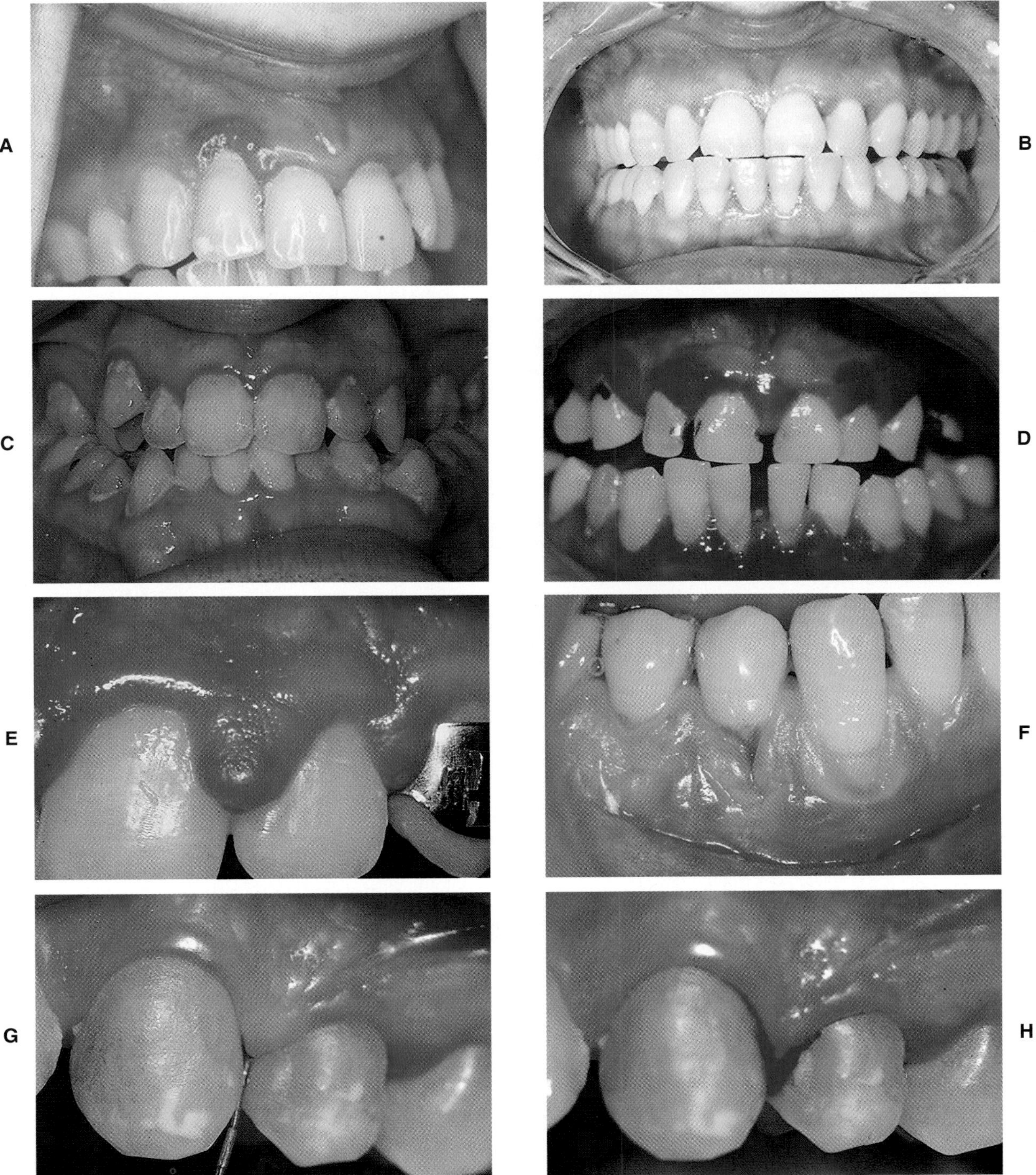

Color Fig. 17-1 Gingivitis: clinical features. **A,** Localized, diffuse, intensely red area facial of tooth #7 and dark pink marginal changes in the remaining anterior teeth. **B,** Generalized papillary gingivitis. **C,** Generalized marginal inflammatory lesion. **D,** Generalized diffuse inflammatory lesion. **E,** Papillary gingival enlargement. **F,** Different degrees of recession. Recession is slight in teeth #26 and 29 and marked in #27 and 28. Note the irregular contours of the gingiva in #28 and the lack of attached gingiva in #27. **G,** Insertion of a probe into the gingival sulcus. Note the lack of stippling, the slightly rolled margins, and the dark red color. **H,** Bleeding appears about 30 seconds after probing.

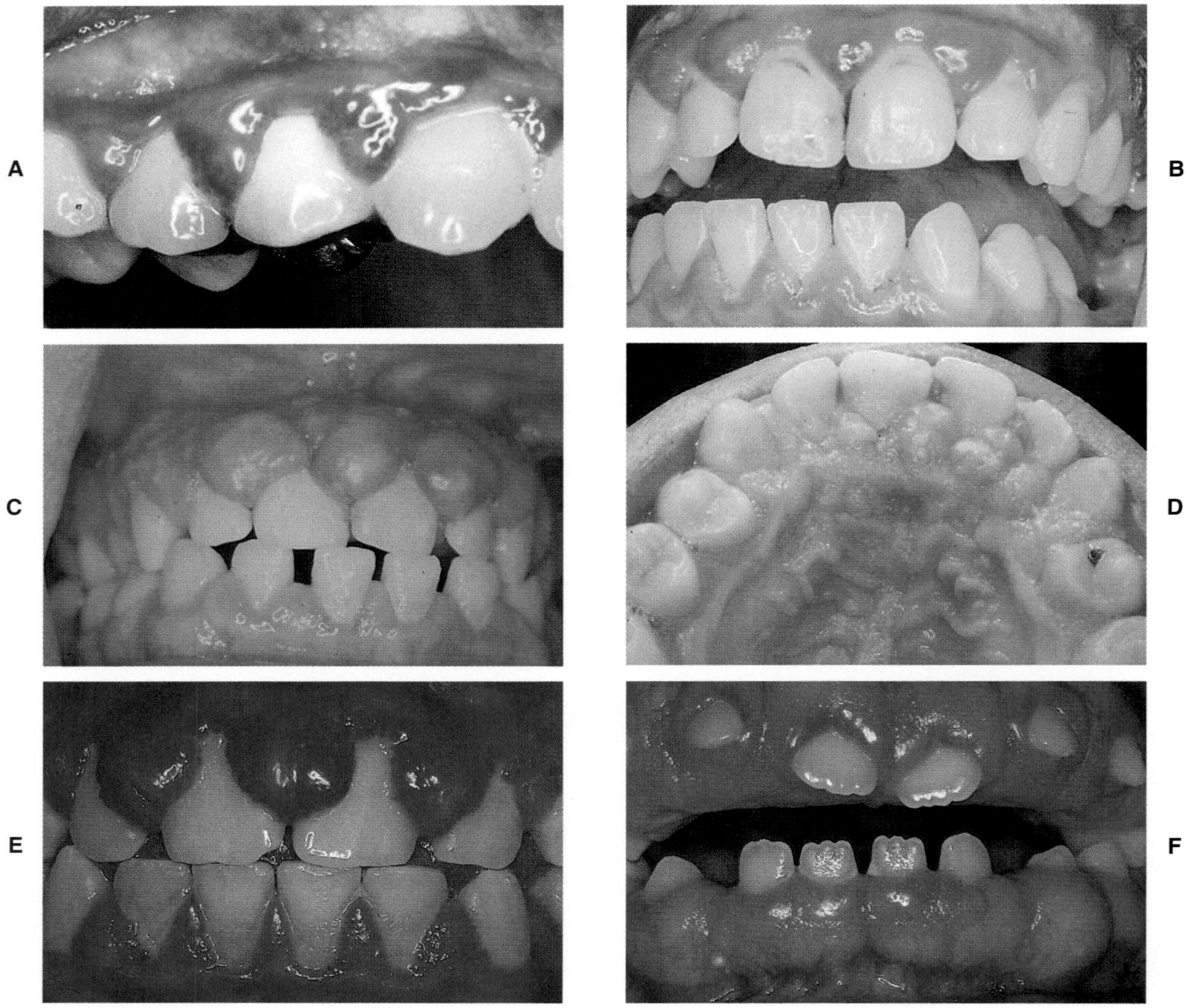

Color Fig. 18-1 Gingival enlargements. **A,** Chronic inflammatory gingival enlargement in a 27-year-old woman. Note the papillary enlargement and the red, smooth surfaces. **B,** Gingival enlargement associated with mouth breathing, typically localized to the marginal and papillary areas of teeth #6–11, in an 18-year-old man. **C,** Phenytoin-associated gingival enlargement in a 21-year-old man. In the maxilla, note the bulbous papillary enlargement, leaving a trough between enlarged papillae, and the pink, stippled surface. **D,** Occlusal view of the same case shown in **C. E,** Cyclosporine-associated gingival enlargement in a 14-year-old boy. Note the enlarged papillae and margin, the deep red color, and the smooth surface. **F,** Gingival fibromatosis in a 16-year-old boy. Dense fibrotic enlargement partially covers the crowns of the teeth, and the pink, stippled surface shows minor marginal inflammatory changes.

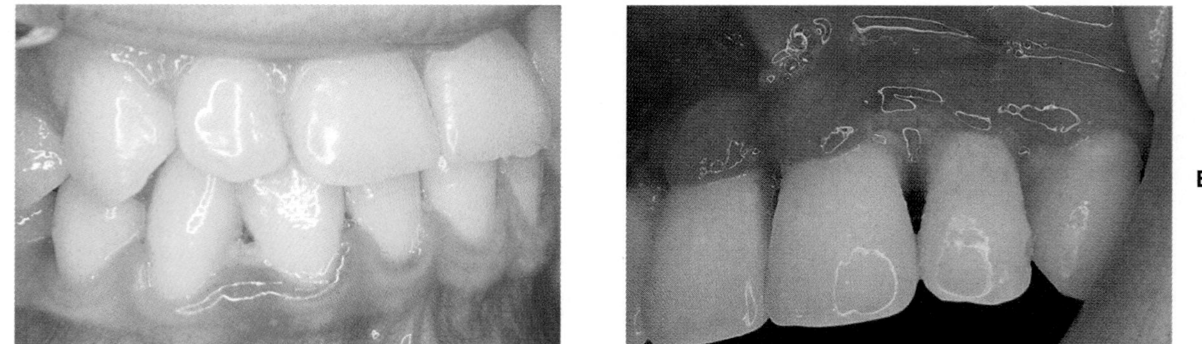

Color Fig. 19-1 **A,** *Necrotizing ulcerative gingivitis*: typical punched out interdental papilla between mandibular canine and lateral incisor. **B,** *Necrotizing ulcerative gingivitis:* typical lesions with progressive tissue destruction.

Continued

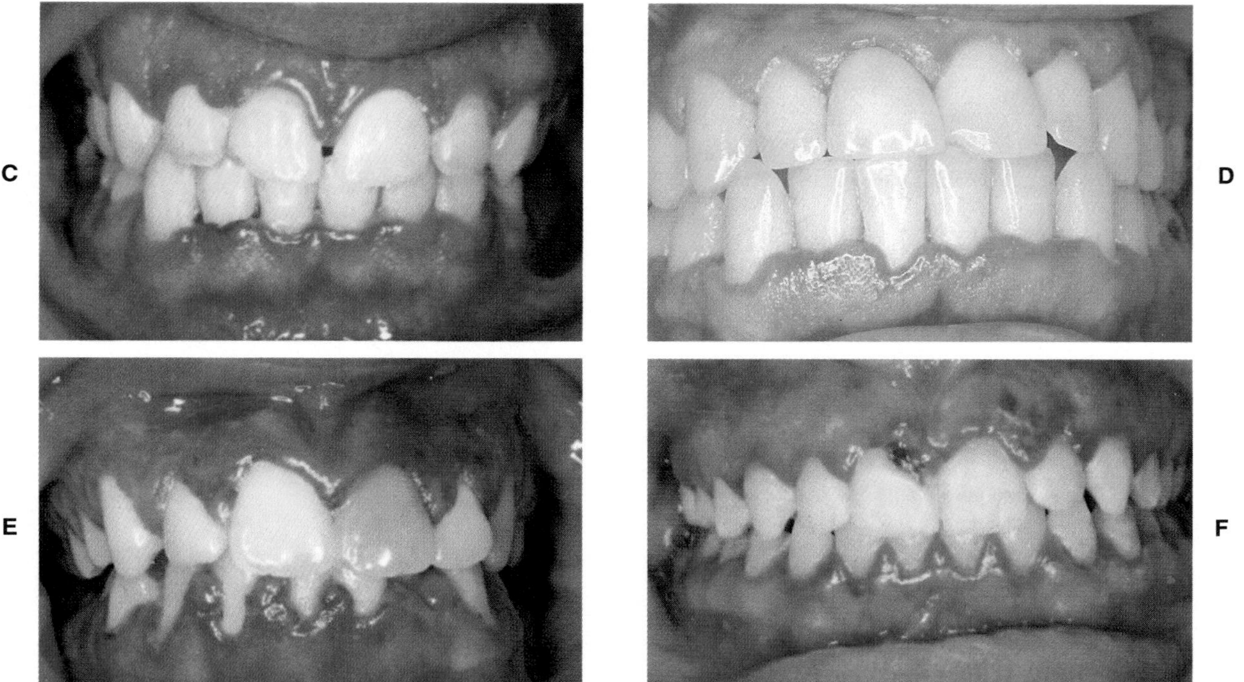

Color Fig. 19-1 cont'd C, *Necrotizing ulcerative gingivitis*: typical lesions with spontaneous hemorrhage. **D,** *Necrotizing ulcerative gingivitis*: typical lesions producing irregular gingival contour. **E,** *Primary herpetic gingivostomatitis*: typical diffuse erythema. **F,** *Primary herpetic gingivostomatitis*: vesicles on the gingiva.

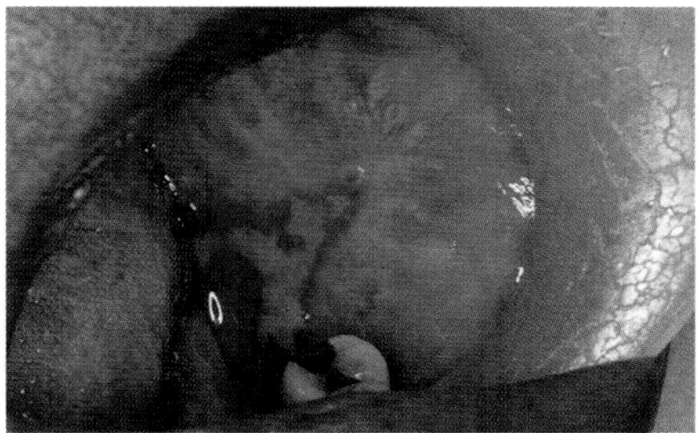

Color Fig. 21-1 Erosive lichen planus. Large ulcerative lesion on the left buccal mucosa exhibiting bordering erythema. The typical white striations of lichen planus are evident in the periphery of the ulcer.

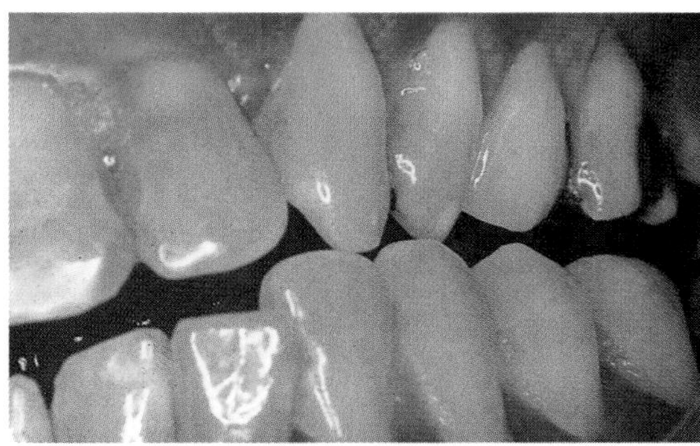

Color Fig. 21-2 Erosive lichen planus presenting as desquamative gingivitis. The gingival tissues are erythematous, ulcerated, and painful.

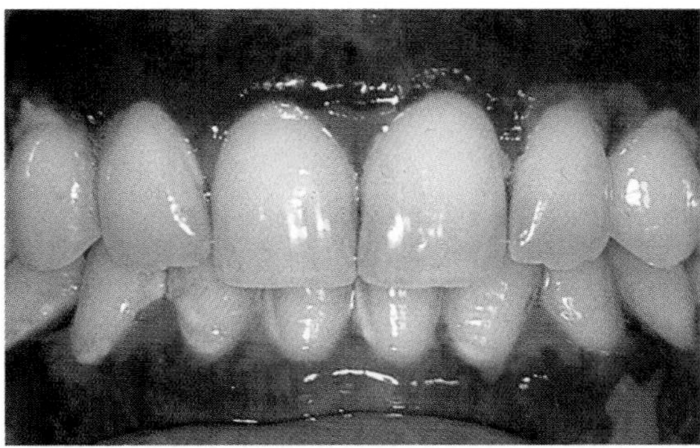

Color Fig. 21-3 Gingival mucous membrane pemphigoid. Lesions of cicatricial pemphigoid confined to the gingival tissues, producing a typical desquamative gingivitis appearance. (Courtesy Dr. Stuart L. Fischman, State University of New York at Buffalo, Buffalo, N.Y.).

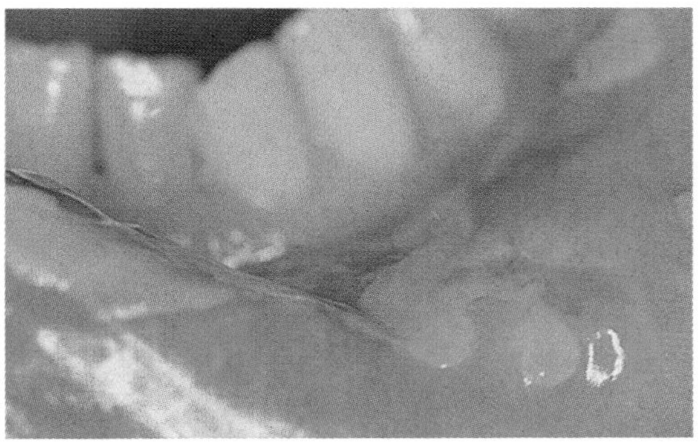

Color Fig. 21-4 Pemphigus vulgaris of the oral cavity. Multiple and coalescent areas of ulceration covered by necrotic epithelium. This patient presented with large ulcers in the labial mucosa, tongue, and soft palate.

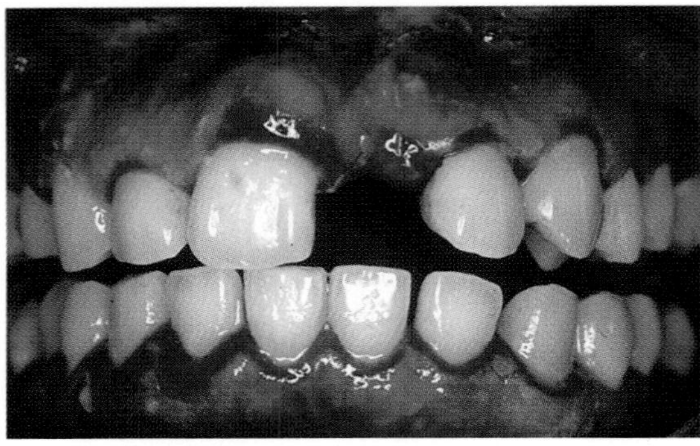

Color Fig. 21-5 Pemphigus vulgaris of the gingiva. Clinical appearance of a patient with pemphigus vulgaris presenting oral lesions confined to the gingiva. The clinical diagnosis was consistent with desquamative gingivitis. (Courtesy Dr. Beatriz Aldape, National Autonomous University of Mexico, Mexico City, Mexico).

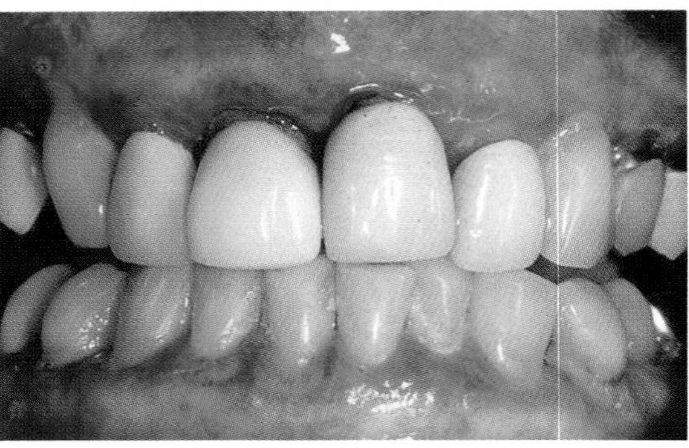

Color Fig. 21-6 Chronic ulcerative stomatitis. Erythema and ulceration of the gingiva consistent with a clinical diagnosis of desquamative gingivitis. (Courtesy Dr. Douglas Damm, University of Kentucky, Lexington, Ky.).

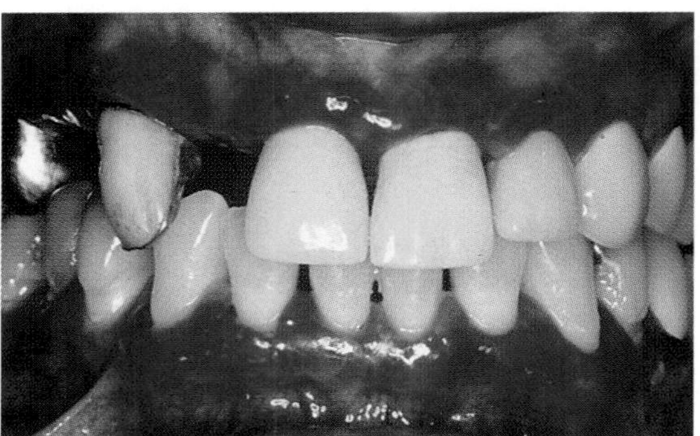

Color Fig. 21-7 Linear IgA. Intense erythema and ulceration of the gingiva consistent with desquamative gingivitis.

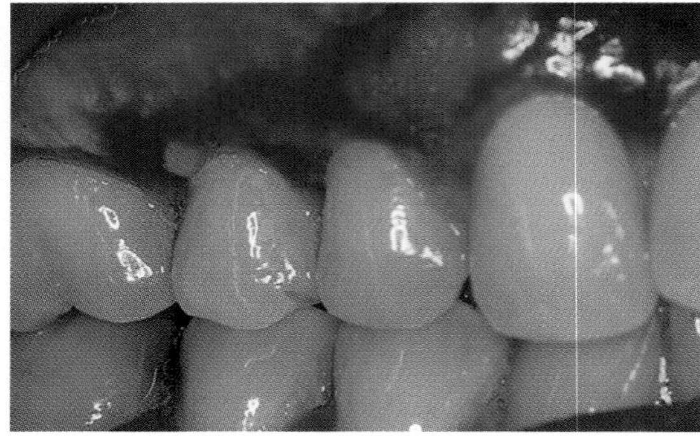

Color Fig. 21-8 Lupus erythematosus of the oral cavity presenting as desquamative gingivitis. Intense erythema with ulceration bordered by white radial lines (Courtesy Dr. Stuart Fischman, Buffalo, N.Y.)

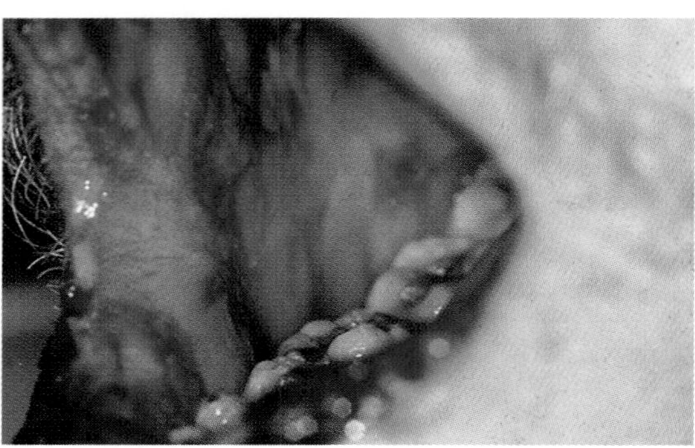

Color Fig. 21-9 Erythema multiforme. Large, shallow, and painful ulcers involving the labial and buccal mucosae. Hemorrhagic crusting of the mandibular vermilion border of the lips is observed. (Courtesy Dr. Stuart Fischman, Buffalo, N.Y.)

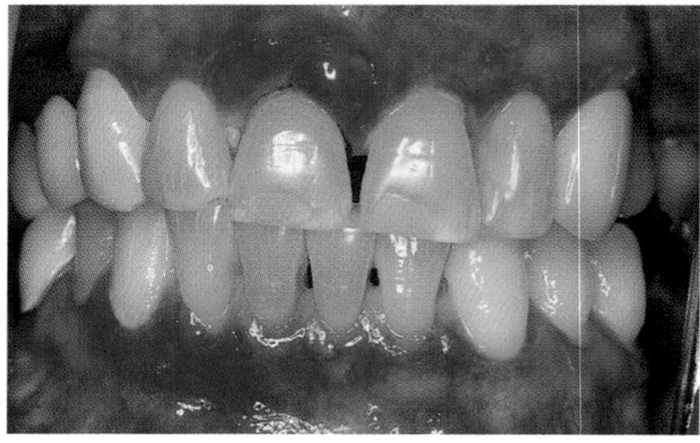

Color Fig. 21-10 Plasma cell gingivitis. The gingiva presents a band of moderate to severe inflammation reminiscent of desquamative gingivitis.

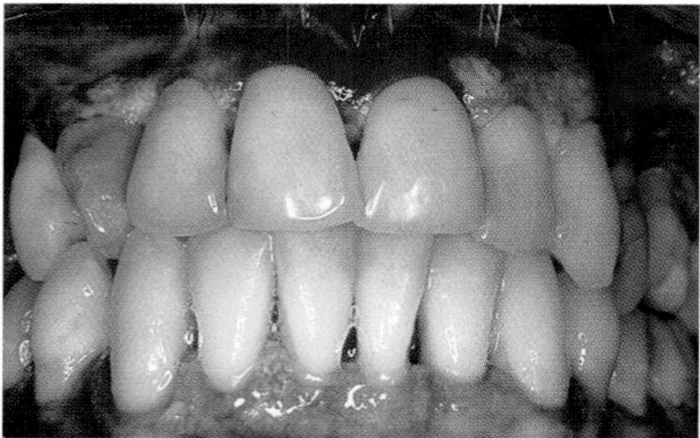

Color Fig. 21-11 Graft versus host disease in a recipient of an allogenic bone marrow transplant. The maxillary gingiva exhibits features consistent with desquamative gingivitis. (Courtesy Dr. Linda Lee, University of Toronto, Toronto, Ontario.)

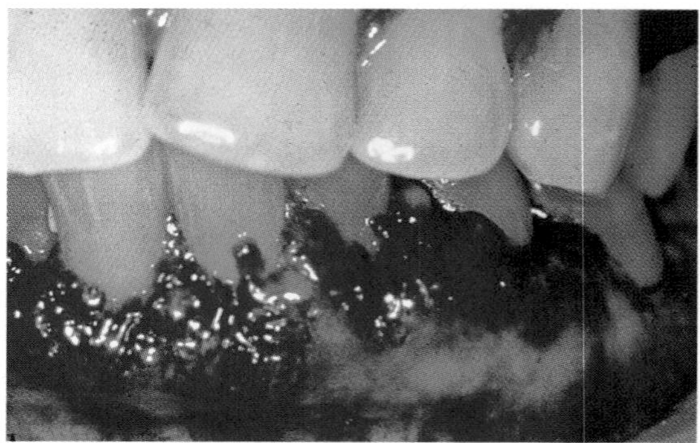

Color Fig. 21-12 Wegener's granulomatosis affecting the gingival tissues. The classic "strawberry gums" appearance of the mandibular gingiva is seen in this patient. A slight resemblance with desquamative gingivitis is evident.

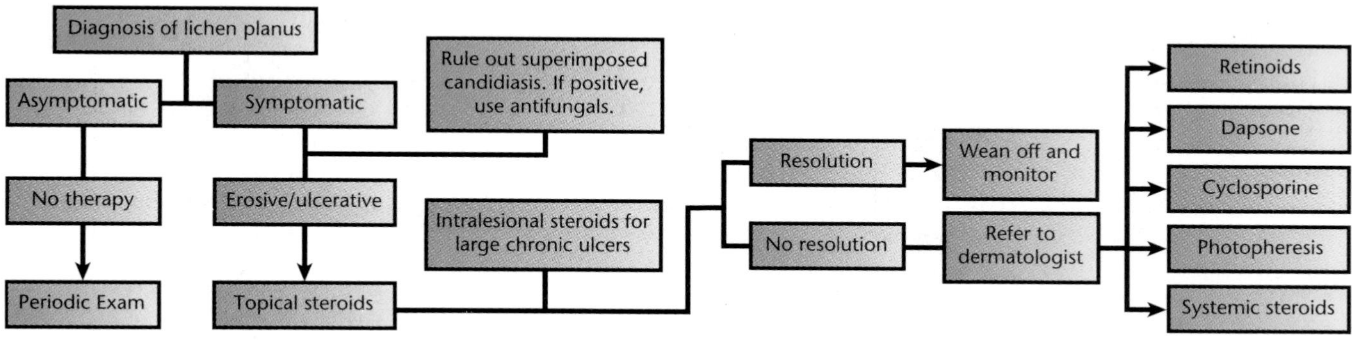

Fig. 21-3 Treatment of lichen planus.

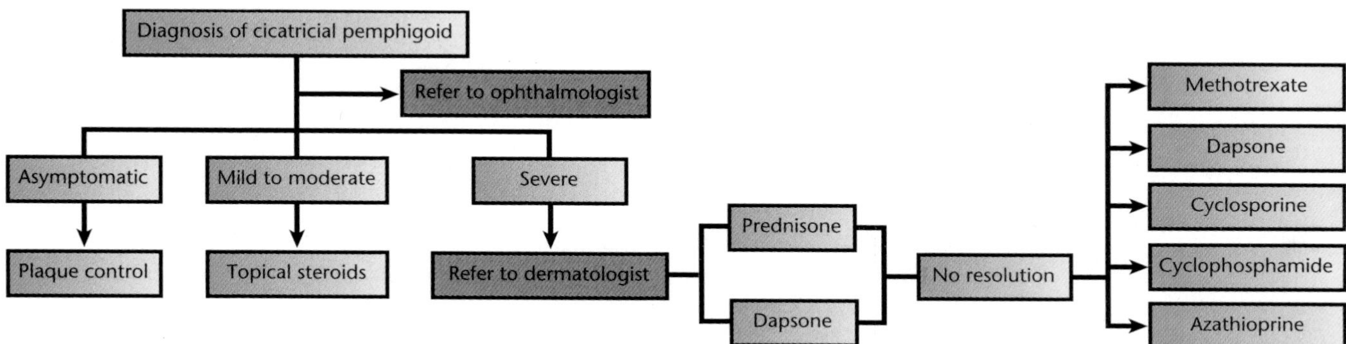

Fig. 21-4 Treatment of cicatricial pemphigoid.

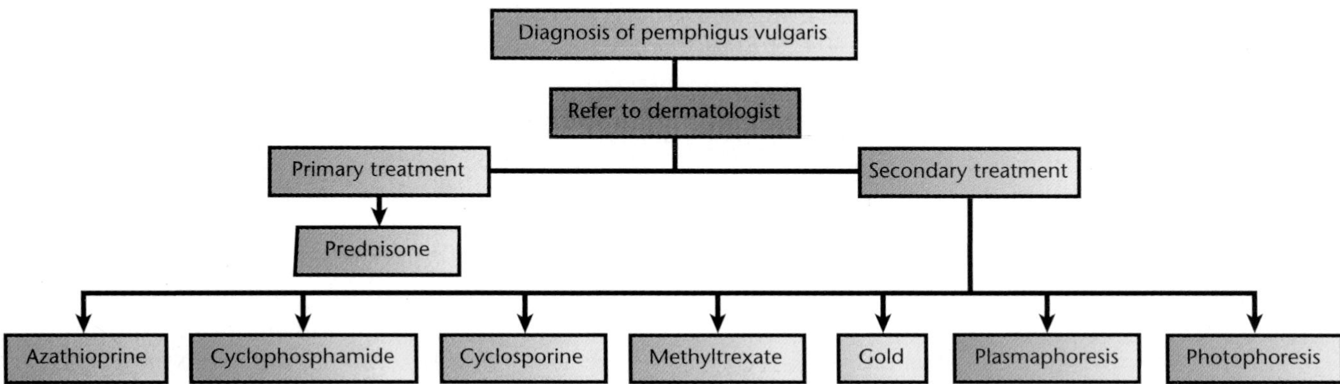

Fig. 21-5 Treatment of pemphigus vulgaris.

TABLE 21-2

Accepted Contemporary Therapeutic Approaches Used to Treat Selected Conditions That Clinically Present as Desquamative Gingivitis

Disease	Therapy
Erosive Lichen Planus	Mild cases: Delivery of the therapeutic agent can be enhanced with the use of vacuum-formed custom trays. **Rx.:** Lidex (0.05% fluocinonide) gel **Disp.:** One tube 15 gm **Sig.:** Apply to affected area p.c. and h.s. Monitoring the oral cavity of the patient is warranted because candidiasis may develop after few weeks of use of topical steroids. Therefore concomitant use of an antifungal may be necessary. **Rx.:** Nystatin oral pastilles (100,000 IU) **Disp.:** 60 pastilles **Sig.:** Dissolve in mouth b.i.d. and then expectorate for 30 consecutive days Severe or refractory cases: Refer to dermatologist for management with systemic corticosteroids.
Cicatricial Pemphigoid	Mild cases: **Rx.:** Lidex (0.05% fluocinonide) gel **Disp.:** One tube 15 gm **Sig.:** Apply to affected area p.c. and h.s. **Rx.:** Temovate (0.05% clobetasol propionate) **Disp.:** One tube 15 gm **Sig.:** Apply to affected areas q.i.d. Severe or refractory cases: Refer to a dermatologist for management with prednisone (20–30 mg/day). Concomitant use of azathioprine may be needed. Dapsone, sulfonamide, and tetracycline are other alternatives.
Pemphigus	Refer to dermatologist for management with prednisone (20–30 mg/day). Concomitant use of azathioprine may be needed.
Chronic Ulcerative Stomatitis	Mild cases: **Rx.:** Lidex (0.05% fluocinonide) gel **Disp.:** One tube 15 gm **Sig.:** Apply to affected areas q.i.d. **Rx.:** Temovate (0.05% clobetasol propionate) **Disp.:** One tube 15 gm **Sig.:** Apply to affected areas q.i.d. Severe or refractory cases: Refer to dermatologist for management with hydroxychloroquinine sulfate (200–400 mg/day) and/or systemic corticosteroids.

tissue[102] that may occur as one or more types of four distinctive patterns:

1. *Keratotic lesions.* These raised white lesions may present as groups of individual papules, linear or reticulate lesions, or plaquelike configurations (Fig. 21-6).
2. *Erosive or ulcerative lesions.* These extensive erythematous areas with a patchy distribution may present as focal or diffuse hemorrhagic areas. These lesions are exacerbated by slight trauma (e.g., toothbrushing) (Color Fig. 21-2).
3. *Vesicular or bullous lesions.* These raised, fluid-filled lesions are uncommon and short lived on the gingiva, quickly rupturing and leaving an ulceration.
4. *Atrophic lesions.* Atrophy of the gingival tissues with ensuing epithelial thinning results in erythema confined to the gingiva.

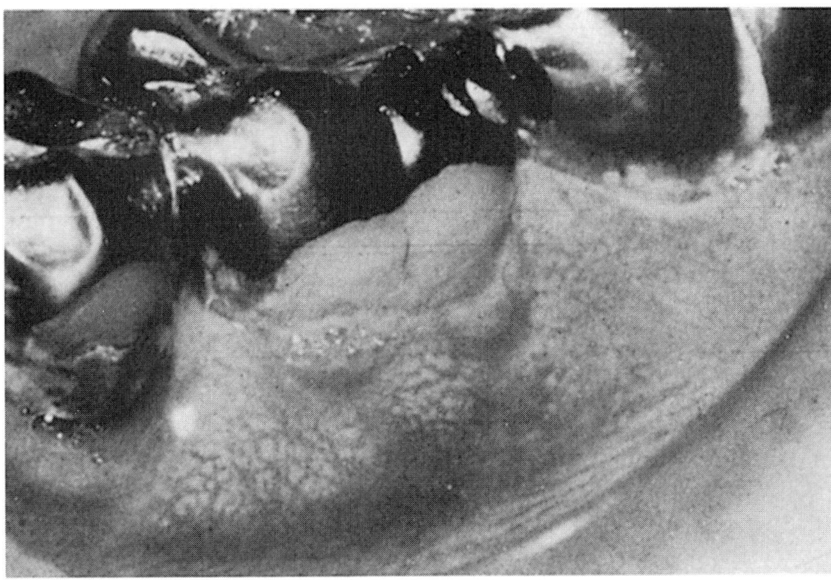

Fig. 21-6 Lichen planus. Unusual papular appearance of lichen planus on the gingiva.

Histopathology. Microscopically, three main features characterize oral lichen planus: (1) hyperkeratosis or parakeratosis, (2) hydropic degeneration of the basal layer, and (3) a dense, bandlike infiltrate primarily of T lymphocytes in the lamina propria (Fig. 21-7). Classically, the epithelial rete ridges have a "saw-tooth" configuration. Hydropic degeneration of the basal layer of the epithelium may be sufficiently extensive that the epithelium becomes thin and atrophic or detaches off the underlying connective tissue and produces either a subepithelial vesicle or an ulcer. Colloid bodies (Civatte bodies) are often seen at the epithelium-connective tissue interface. A microscopic diagnosis of oral lichen planus is straightforward in the keratotic lesions, and biopsy specimens should be obtained from these areas if possible. However, these classic histologic features may be obscured in the areas of ulceration, making a conclusive diagnosis of oral lichen planus difficult based solely on conventional microscopy.

Electron microscopic studies indicate that lichen planus can be divided into three stages: (1) degeneration of the cytoplasm of the epithelial cells, (2) loss of collagen fibers in the superficial lamina propria, and (3) degeneration and necrosis of the basal and parabasal layers of the epithelium. The superficial lamina propria is also degenerated and necrotic, and the basement lamina is no longer visible. Separation of the basal lamina from the basal cell layer is an early manifestation of lichen planus.[106]

It is noteworthy that oral lesions of lichen planus may change in pattern, and in certain unusual cases, a second or even a third biopsy may be necessary to arrive at a definitive diagnosis. More importantly, controversy exists about the malignant potential of oral lichen planus. In some studies, it has been estimated that oral cancer emerges in 0.4 to 5.6% of patients with oral lichen planus.[46,47,112] In contrast, other researchers reject or question the connection between oral lichen planus and oral cancer.[32,65] In spite of this controversy, biopsy and close follow-up are warranted in these patients.

Immunopathology. Direct immunofluorescence of both lesional and perilesional oral lichen planus biopsy specimens reveal linear-fibrilar deposits of fibrin in the basement membrane zone (Fig. 21-8), along with scattered immunoglobulin-staining cytoid bodies in the upper areas of the lamina propria (Fig. 21-9). Serum tests using indirect immunofluorescence are negative in lichen planus.

Differential Diagnosis. The classic clinical presentation of oral lichen planus can be simulated by other conditions mainly, lichenoid mucositis. When an erosive component is present, lupus erythematosus and chronic ulcerative stomatitis should be included in the differential diagnosis. In the event that oral lichen planus is confined to the gingival tissues (erosive oral lichen planus), the identification of fine white radiating striations bordering the erosive areas support a clinical diagnosis of oral lichen planus. If the white striations are absent, the differential diagnosis should primarily include cicatricial pemphigoid and pemphigus vulgaris. Other less common possibilities encompass linear IgA and chronic ulcerative stomatitis.

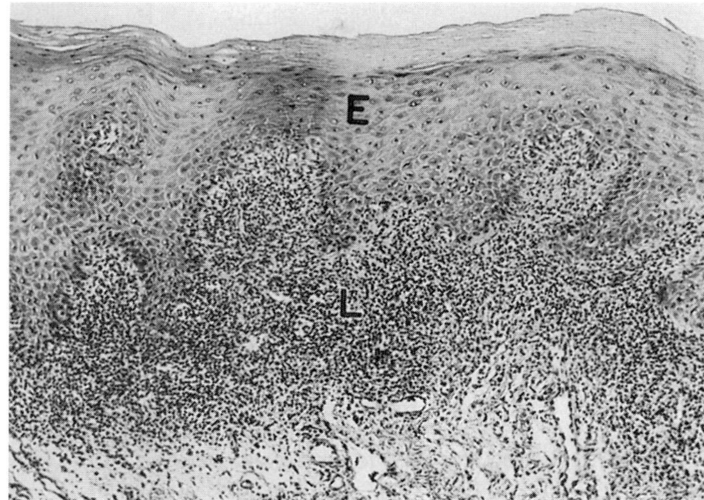

Fig. 21-7 Microscopic appearance of lichen planus. Biopsy specimen from a gingival lesion showing hyperkeratosis and acanthosis of the epithelium *(E),* as well as extension of rete pegs. There is dense, bandlike lymphocytic infiltrate in the lamina propria (*L*) confined to a broad zone immediately beneath the epithelium.

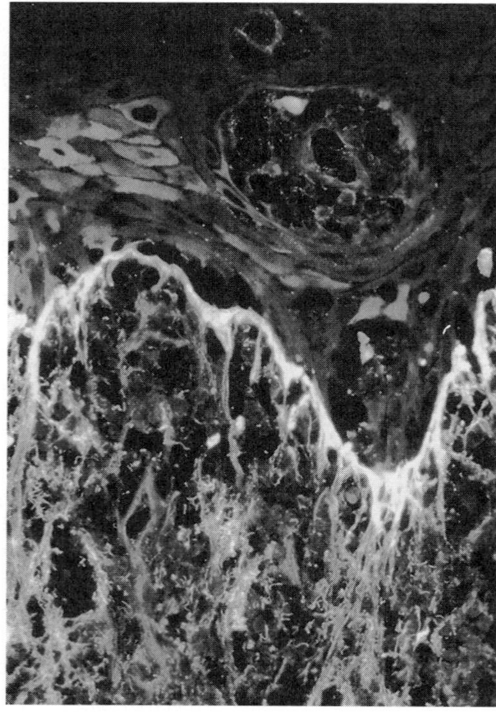

Fig. 21-8 Direct immunofluorescence of lichen planus. Fibrin deposits along the basement membrane of the epithelium.

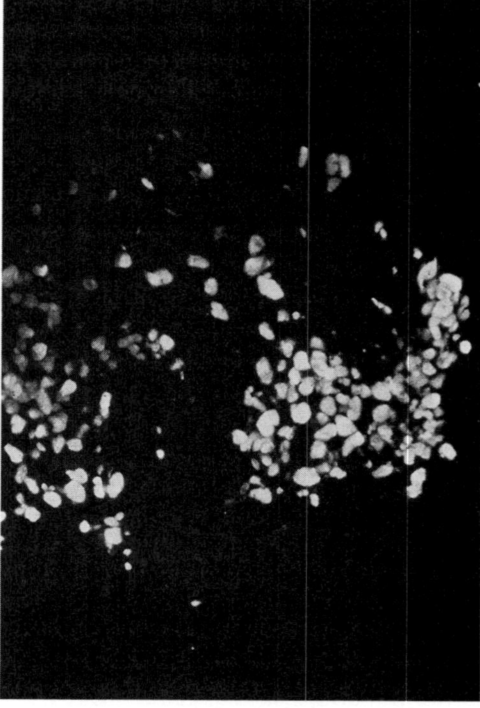

Fig. 21-9 Direct immunofluorescence of lichen planus. Clusters of cytoid bodies exhibiting IgM deposits in the lamina propria.

Therapy. The keratotic lesions of oral lichen planus are asymptomatic and do not require treatment once the microscopic diagnosis is established. However, follow-up of the patient every 6 to 12 months is warranted to monitor suspicious clinical changes and the emergence of an erosive component.

In contrast, the erosive, bullous, or ulcerative lesions of oral lichen planus are treated with high-potency topical steroid such as 0.05% fluocinonide ointment (Lidex, three times daily). Lidex can also be mixed 1:1 with carboxymethyl cellulose (Orabase) paste or other adhesive ointment. Intralesional injections of triamcinolone acetonide (10 to 20 mg) or short-term regimens of 40 mg prednisone daily for 5 days followed by 10 to 20 mg daily for an additional 2 weeks have also been employed in more severe cases.[85] Because of the potential side effects, administration of systemic steroids should be prescribed and monitored by a dermatologist. Other treatment modalities (e.g., retinoids, hydroxychloroquine, cyclosporine, and free gingival grafts) have also been used.[85] Because candidiasis is often associated with symptomatic oral lichen planus, antifungal therapy should be considered.[14,39]

Pemphigoid

The term *pemphigoid* applies to a number of cutaneous, immune-mediated, subepithelial bullous diseases that are characterized by a separation of the basement membrane zone (bullous pemphigoid, mucous membrane pemphigoid and pemphigoid [herpes] gestationis).[89,101] Among these conditions, bullous pemphigoid and mucous membrane pemphigoid (also known as *benign mucous membrane pemphigoid* and *cicatricial pemphigoid*) have received considerable attention. Current molecular findings on these two diseases have made clear that they are separate entities.[101] However, there is considerable histologic and immunopathologic overlap between them to the point that their differentiation may be impossible on these two criteria.[89] In many occasions, the clinical findings are probably the best cognitive element to discriminate them. Accordingly, the term *bullous pemphigoid* is preferred when the disease is nonscarring and mainly affects the skin. The term *cicatricial pemphigoid* is favored when scarring occurs and the disease is mainly confined to mucous membranes (although scarring may be absent in some subtypes of mucous membrane pemphigoid).[119] Until more research allows better understanding of this family of diseases, bullous pemphigoid and mucous membrane pemphigoid will be discussed separately.

Bullous Pemphigoid. Bullous pemphigoid is a chronic, autoimmune, subepidermal, bullous disease with tense bullae that rupture and become flaccid in the skin. Oral involvement occurs in about a third of the patients.[110] Although the skin lesions clinically resemble those of pemphigus, the microscopic picture is quite distinct. There is no evidence of acantholysis, and the developing vesicles are subepithelial rather than intraepithelial. The epithelium separates from the underlying connective tissue at the basement membrane zone. Electron microscopic studies show an actual horizontal splitting or replication of the basal lamina. The separating epithelium remains relatively intact, and the basal layer is present and appears to be regular. The two major antigenic determinants for bullous pemphigoid are the 230-kDa protein plaque known as *BP1* and the 180-kDa collagen-like transmembrane protein BP2.[79,98]

IMMUNOFLUORESCENCE. Immunologically, bullous pemphigoid is characterized by IgG and C3 immune deposits along epithelial basement membranes and circulating IgG antibodies to the epithelial basement membrane.[52,82] Direct immunofluoresence is positive in 90% to 100% of these patients, whereas indirect immunofluorescence is positive in 40% to 70% of affected patients.[83]

ORAL LESIONS. Oral lesions have been reported to occur secondarily in up to 40% of the cases. There is an erosive or desquamative gingivitis presentation and occasional vesicular or bullous lesions.[110]

THERAPY. Because its etiologic factors are unknown, treatment of bullous pemphigoid is designed to control its signs and symptoms.[52,82] The primary treatment is a moderate dose of systemic prednisone. Steroid-sparing strategies (prednisone plus other immunomodulator drugs) are used when high doses of steroids are needed or the steroid alone fails to control the disease.[29] For localized lesions of bullous pemphigoid, high-potency topical steroids or tetracycline with or without nicotinamide can be effective.[84]

Mucous Membrane Pemphigoid (Cicatricial Pemphigoid). Mucous membrane pemphigoid, also known as *cicatricial pemphigoid,* is a chronic, vesiculobullous autoimmune disorder of unknown cause that predominantly affects women in the fifth decade of life. Although rare, it has been reported in young children.[101] Cicatricial pemphigoid involves the oral cavity, conjunctiva, and the mucosa of the nose, vagina, rectum, esophagus, and urethra. However, in about 20% of cases, the skin may also be involved. Recent investigations have suggested that cicatricial pemphigoid encompasses a group of heterogeneous conditions with distinct clinical and molecular features.[26,76,99] An elaborate cascade of events is involved in the pathogenesis of cicatricial pemphigoid. Initially, antigen/antibody complexing occurs at the basement membrane zone and is followed by complement activation and subsequent leukocyte recruitment. Next, proteolytic enzymes are released and dissolve or cleave the basement membrane zone, usually at the level of the lamina lucida.[34] The two major antigenic determinants for cicatricial pemphigoid are bullous pemphigoid 1 and 2 (BP1 and BP2). Most cases of cicatricial pemphigoid are the result of an immune response directed against BP2 and less commonly against BP1 and epiligrin (laminin-5, a lamina lucida protein in the basement membrane of the stratified epithelium).[5,26] Current research strongly suggests that there are at least five subtypes of cicatricial pemphigoid (oral pemphigoid, anti-epiligrin pemphigoid, anti-BP antigen mucosal pemphigoid, ocular pemphigoid and multiple antigens pemphigoid).[101]

OCULAR LESIONS. In cases presenting first to the dentist (mainly desquamative gingivitis), the eyes are affected in approximately 25% of the patients.[83] In contrast, in cases presenting first to the dermatologist, 66% of the patients present conjunctival lesions, where in ophthalmic studies, 100% of the patients have ocular involvement.[38,61,77] The initial lesion is characterized by unilateral conjunctivitis that becomes bilateral within 2 years. Subsequently, there may be adhesions of eyelid to eyeball (symblepharon) (Fig. 21-10). Adhesions at the edges of the eyelids (ankyloblepharon) may lead to a narrowing of the palpebral fissure. Small vesicular lesions may develop on the conjunctiva, which may eventually produce scarring, corneal damage, and blindness.

ORAL LESIONS. The most characteristic feature of oral involvement is the presence of desquamative gingivitis (Color Fig. 21-3) with typical areas of erythema, desquamation, ulceration, and vesiculation, of the attached gingiva.[40,109] Vesiculobullous lesions may occur elsewhere in the mouth.[40] The bullae tend to have a relatively thick roof and rupture in 2 to 3 days, leaving irregularly shaped areas of ulceration. Healing of the lesions may take up to 3 weeks or longer.

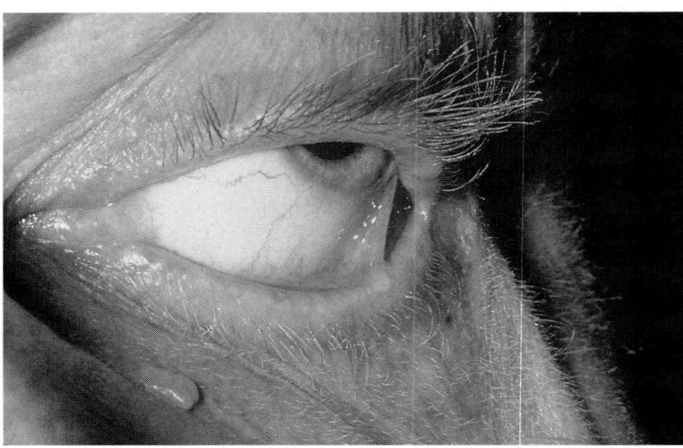

Fig. 21-10 Mucous membrane pemphigoid. Characteristic ocular lesion (symblepharon) in a patient presenting with cicatricial pemphigoid. (Courtesy Dr. Carl Allen; Ohio State University, Columbus, Ohio)

HISTOPATHOLOGY. The microscopic appearance of the oral lesions, although not completely diagnostic for mucous membrane pemphigoid, is sufficiently distinctive that a tentative diagnosis can be considered. A striking subepithelial vesiculation with the epithelium separated from the underlying lamina propria leaves an intact basal layer (Fig. 21-11). The separation of the epithelium and the connective tissue occurs at the basement membrane zone. Electron microscopic studies demonstrate a split in the basal lamina.[116] A mixed inflammatory infiltrate (lymphocytes, plasma cells, neutrophils, and scarce eosinophils) is observed in the underlying fibrous connective tissue.

IMMUNOFLUORESCENCE. Positive immunofluorescence findings along the basement membrane area has been reported by both direct and indirect immunofluorescence.[27,51,56] In biopsy tests by direct immunofluorescence, the main immunoreactants are IgG and C3, which are confined to the basement membrane (Fig. 21-12). Recent studies indicate that a positive indirect immunofluorescence is rare in these patients (<25%).[84] The lack of indirect immunofluorescence findings may be due to an earlier diagnosis of mucous membrane pemphigoid that results in the identification of patients with less extensive disease.[1,59] In any event, circulating autoantibodies do not appear to play a role in the pathogenesis of the disease.

DIFFERENTIAL DIAGNOSIS. Several disease entities present with similar clinical and histologic (subepithelial bulla) features.[31] These include bullous pemphigoid, bullous lichen planus, dermatitis herpetiformis, linear IgA, erythema multiforme, herpes gestationis, and epidermolysis bullosa acquisita.

Pemphigus may be confined to the oral cavity in its early stage, and the vesicular and ulcerative lesions may resemble those of mucous membrane pemphigoid. An erosive or desquamative gingivitis may also be seen in pemphigus as a rare manifestation. Biopsy studies can quickly rule out pemphigus by revealing the absence or presence of acantholytic changes. In erythema multiforme, there are obvious vesiculobullous lesions, but the onset is usually acute rather than chronic, labial involvement is severe, and the gingivae are usually not affected. Desquamative gingivitis is an unusual finding in erythema multiforme, although occasional vesicular lesions may develop. A biopsy study of an oral lesion reveals an unusual degeneration of the upper stratum spinosum, characteristically seen in oral erythema multiforme lesions.

Cicatricial pemphigoid must be differentiated from epidermolysis bullosa acquisita, which can present with similar histopathology and immunopathology. When the biopsy is treated with salt to separate the dermis from the epidermis, basement membrane immunodeposits occur on the epidermal side in pemphigoid and the dermal side in epidermolysis bullosa acquisita.[33]

THERAPY. Topical steroids are the mainstay of treatment for mucous membrane pemphigoid, in particular when localized lesions are present. Fluocinonide (0.05%) and clobetasol propionate (0.05%) in an adhesive vehicle can be used three times a day for up to 6 months.[101] When the oral lesions of mucous membrane pemphigoids are confined to the gingival tissues, topical corticosteroids are effectively delivered with vacuum-formed custom trays or veneers.[101] Optimal oral hygiene is essential because local irritants on the tooth surface result in an exaggerated gingival inflammatory response. Gingival irritation from any dental prosthesis should also be minimized. If the disease is not severe and symptoms are mild, systemic corticosteroids may be omitted. If ocular involvement exists, systemic corticosteroids are indicated.

When lesions do not respond to steroids, systemic Dapsone (4-4′diaminodiphenylsulfone) has proven to be effective.[22,36,76,81] Because of the systemic side effects to

A

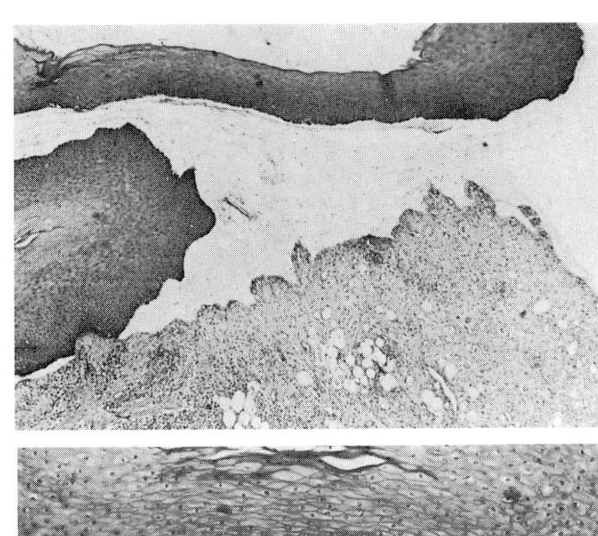

B

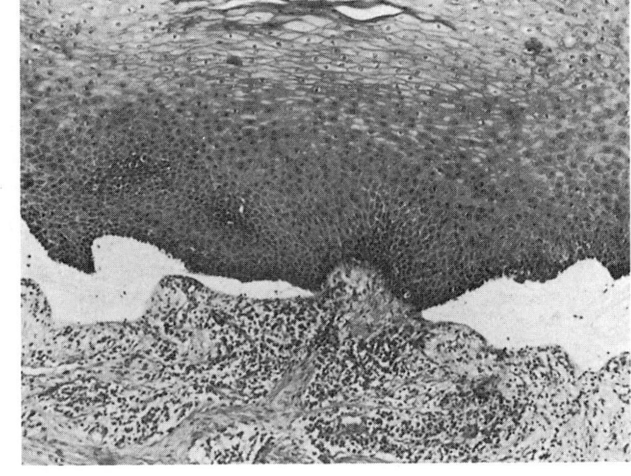

Fig. 21-11 Microscopic features of oral mucous membrane pemphigoid. **A,** A low-power view shows clean separation of the epithelium from the underlying connective tissue. **B,** A high-power view shows an intact basal layer as the epithelium separates from the connective tissue at the basement membrane zone. Foci of inflammatory cells are also present. (Courtesy of Dr. Gerald Shklar, Boston, Mass.)

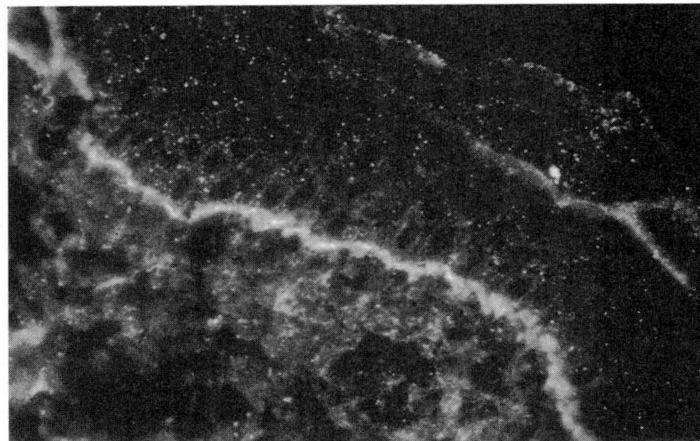

Fig. 21-12 Direct immunofluorescence of mucous membrane pemphigoid. C3 deposits confined along the basement membrane.

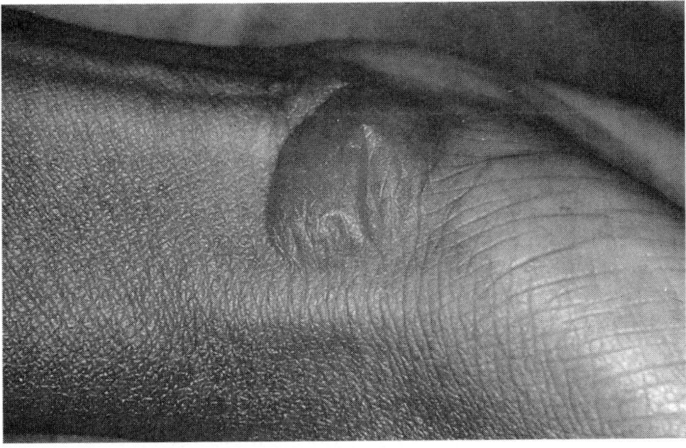

Fig. 21-13 Pemphigus vulgaris. Cutaneous lesion of a patient with pemphigus vulgaris. A large bulla is present on the flexor surface of the wrist.

this drug including hemolysis and methemaglobulinemia, particularly in patients with glucose-6-phosphate dehydrogenase deficiency, referral to a dermatologist is often indicated.[87] Some authors have also advocated sulfonamides and tetracycline; surgery, although not a treatment for mucous membrane pemphigoid, is used in some cases to prevent blindness as well as esophageal and upper airways stenosis.[101]

Pemphigus Vulgaris

The pemphigus diseases are a group of autoimmune bullous disorders that produce cutaneous and/or mucous membranes blisters (Fig. 21-13). Pemphigus vulgaris is the most common of the pemphigus diseases (pemphigus vulgaris, pemphigus foliaceous, pemphigus vegetants, and pemphigus erythematosus).[96] Pemphigus vulgaris is a potentially lethal chronic condition (10% mortality rate) with a worldwide incidence of 0.1 to 0.5 cases per year per 100,000 individuals.[9,96] A predilection in women, usually after the fourth decade of life, has been observed.[96] However, pemphigus vulgaris has also been reported in unusually young children and even in newborns.[20,96,120] The epidermal and/or mucous membrane blisters occur when the cell to cell adhesion structures are damaged by the action of circulating and *in vivo* binding of autoantibodies to the pemphigus vulgaris antigen, a cell surface glycoprotein present in keratinocytes. This pemphigus vulgaris glycoprotein is a member of the desmoglein (DSG) subfamily of the cadherin superfamily of cell to cell adhesion molecules, which is present in desmosomes.[58] Recent evidence suggests that DSG3, the gene coding for pemphigus vulgaris is located in chromosome 18. Most cases of pemphigus vulgaris are idiopathic; however, medications such as penicillamine and captopril can produce drug-induced pemphigus, which is usually reversible on withdrawal of the causative drug. Paraneoplastic pemphigus is antigenically distinct from pemphigus vulgaris and is associated with underlying malignancies.[80]

In approximately 60% of patients with pemphigus vulgaris, the oral lesions are the first sign of the disease and may herald the dermatologic involvement by a year or more.[111]

Oral Lesions. Oral lesions of pemphigus range from small vesicles to large bullae. When the bullae rupture, they leave extensive areas of ulceration (Color Fig. 21-4). Virtually, any region of the oral cavity can be involved, but multiple lesions often develop at sites of irritation or trauma. The soft palate is more often involved (80%), followed by the buccal mucosa (46%), ventral aspect or dorsum of tongue (20%), and lower labial mucosa (10%). Oral lesions of pemphigus vulgaris are confined less often to the gingival tissues.[55] In these cases a clinical diagnosis of erosive gingivitis or desquamative gingivitis is seen as the sole manifestation of oral pemphigus (Color Fig. 21-5).

Histopathology. Lesions of pemphigus demonstrate a characteristic intraepithelial separation, which occurs above the basal cell layer. The intraepithelial vesiculation begins as a microscopic alteration (Fig. 21-14) and gradually results in a grossly visible, fluid-filled bulla. Occasionally, the entire superficial layers of epithelium are lost, leaving only the basal cells attached to the underlying lamina propria, conferring a characteristic "tombstone" appearance to the epithelial cells. Acantholysis, a separation of the epithelial cells of the lower stratum spinosum, takes place and is characterized by the presence of round rather than polyhedral epithelial cells. The intercellular bridges are lost, and the nuclei are large and hyperchromatic.[25,60,123] The underlying connective tissue usually presents as a mild to moderate chronic inflammatory cell infiltrate. As the vesicle or bulla ruptures, the ulcerated lesion becomes infiltrated with polymorphonuclear leukocytes, and the surface may show suppuration.

Cytology. Cytologic smears of oral pemphigus lesions represent a preliminary test and should not replace the histologic and immunopathologic examinations. Cytologic examination may be used as corroborating evidence for a definitive diagnosis. A positive smear reveals large numbers of rounded acantholytic cells with serrated borders and large, hyperchromatic nuclei.[12,104]

Electron Microscopy. Electron microscopic studies indicate that breakdown of the epithelial intercellular cement substance is the first stage in the development of acantholysis. Other investigations suggest that the destruction starts in the tonofilaments[45] or in the desmosomes[107] (Fig. 21-15).

Immunofluorescence. The presence of autoantibodies can be demonstrated in the oral mucosa of patients with oral pemphigus by the use of immunofluorescent techniques. For direct immunofluorescence, perilesional unfixed frozen sections are incubated with fluorescein-labeled human anti-IgG. In indirect immunofluorescence, unfixed frozen sections of oral or esophageal mucosa from an animal such as a monkey is first incubated with the patient's serum to allow attachment of any serum antibodies to the mucosal tissue. The tissue is then incubated with fluorescein-labeled, antihuman IgG serum. The test is positive if immunofluorescence is observed in the intercellular spaces of the stratified squamous epithelium of the mucosa (Fig. 21-16). The indirect technique is less sensitive than the direct technique and may be negative in early stages of the disease, particularly in localized forms. However, in most cases, the indirect immunofluorescence titers are valuable to monitor disease activity and are of prognostic value.

Differential Diagnosis. The oral lesions of pemphigus vulgaris may be similar to those seen in erythema multiforme. In erythema multiforme however, recurrent active episodes of comparatively short duration are followed by long intervals free of skin or oral lesions. Erythema multiforme affects the lips with consid-

A
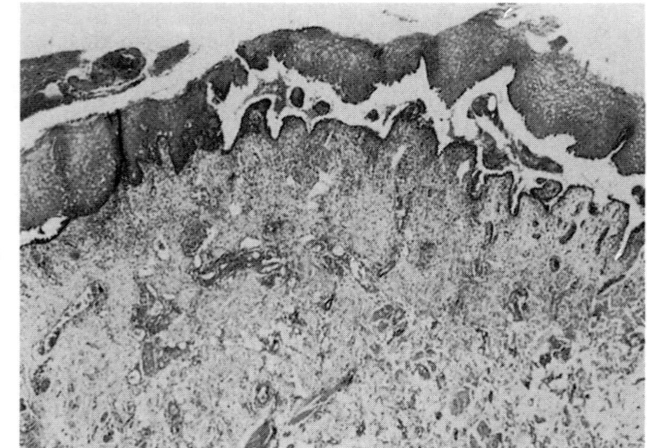
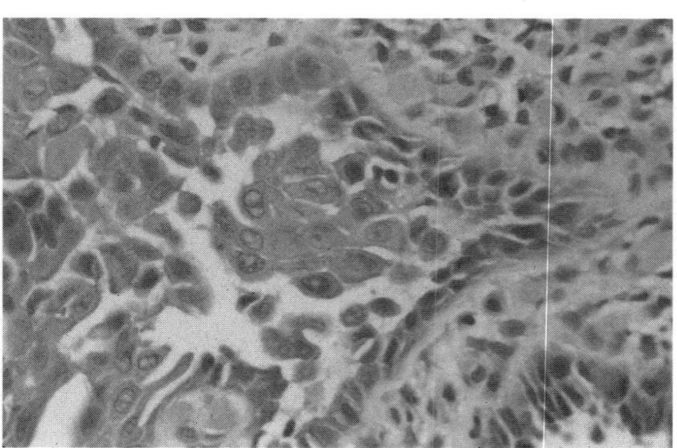
B

Fig. 21-14 Microscopic features of pemphigus vulgaris. **A,** Oral mucosa showing acantholysis and an intraepithelial vesicle. **B,** Detailed view of an intraepithelial vesicle in pemphigus vulgaris.

erable severity. Microscopic examination with conventional H&E and direct immunofluorescence can discriminate oral lesions of pemphigus from those of erythema multiforme. Pemphigus vulgaris will show characteristic intraepithelial clefting at the basal-spinous cell layers interface with acantholysis, whereas erythema multiforme shows microvesiculation of the superficial epithelial layers and numerous necrotic keratinocytes. Pemphigus vulgaris shows an intercellular and intraepithelial signal with direct immunofluorescence. In contrast, erythema multiforme exhibits negative immunofluorescence.

Pemphigoid may clinically resemble pemphigus when it is confined to the mouth. Microscopic examination and direct immunofluorescence studies are needed to establish a correct diagnosis. Bullous pemphigoid and mucous membrane pemphigoid exhibit detachment of the epithelium from the underlying connective tissue ("lifting off"), instead of the acantholytic lesion characteristic of pemphigus.

Bullous lichen planus must also be considered in the differential diagnosis. The primary lesion of pemphigus may be of a bullous character, followed by erosion with associated pain and discomfort. In lichen planus, however, the characteristic reticular lesions are invariably found associated with the bullae. Microscopic examination and direct immunofluorescence studies are necessary to differentiate this condition from pemphigus. Bullous lichen planus shows separation of the epithelium form the underlying fibrous connective tissue, "sawtooth" rete pegs and a bandlike chronic inflammatory infiltrate in the lamina propria. Direct immunofluorescence reveals linear fibrilar deposits of fibrin in the basement membrane of bullous lichen planus, whereas pemphigus vulgaris has intercellular immunoglobulin deposition within the epithelium.

If the oral lesions of pemphigus vulgaris are restricted to the gingival tissues, erosive lichen planus, pemphigoid, linear IgA, and chronic ulcerative stomatitis should be ruled out.

Therapy. The main therapy for pemphigus vulgaris is systemic corticosteroid therapy with or without the addition of other immunosuppressive agents.[111] Initially, when only steroids were employed, high initial and maintenance doses of steroids were necessary to control the disease.[62] Currently, if the patient responds well to corticosteroids, the dosage can be gradually reduced, but a low-maintenance dosage is usually necessary to prevent or minimize the recurrence of lesions. Many dermatologists monitor the dose of steroids by periodic indirect immunofluorescence for changes in titer. Increasing titers are often associated with an impending exacerbation and warrant an increase of the steroid dose. A decrease in the indirect immunofluorescence titer justifies a reduction of the steroid dose.[83] In patients not responsive to corticosteroids or who gradually adapt to them, "steroid-sparing" therapies are used. They consist of combinations of steroids plus other medications such as azathioprine, cyclophosphamide, cyclosporine, dapsone, gold, methotrexate, photoplasmaphoresis, and plasmaphoresis.[84]

The maintenance phase aims to control the disease with the lowest dose of medication. To minimize the risk of morbidity associated with the long-term use of steroids, alternate-day steroid therapy, steroid-sparing drugs, and topical steroids can be combined. Since topical steroids may promote the development of candidiasis, topical antifungal medication may be also needed.[68]

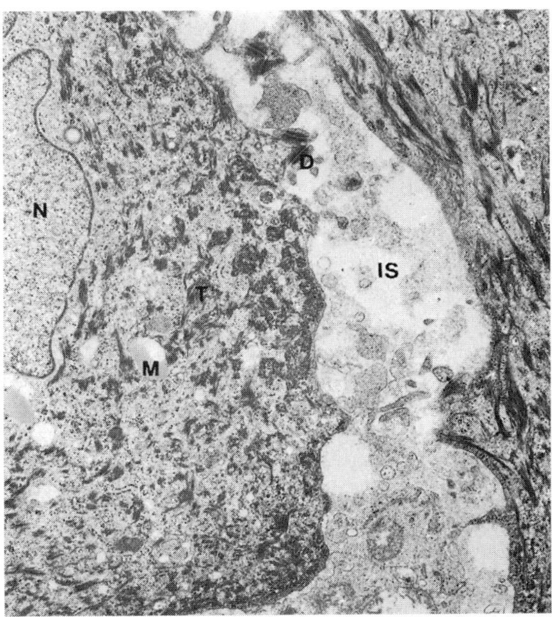

Fig. 21-15 Oral pemphigus. Electron micrograph of acantholytic cells showing the disappearance of desmosomes *(D)* and the separation of cells by widening of the intercellular space *(IS)*. Tonofibrils *(T)* show clumping, and mitochondria *(M)* are degenerating. The nucleus *(N)* demonstrates on intact membrane.

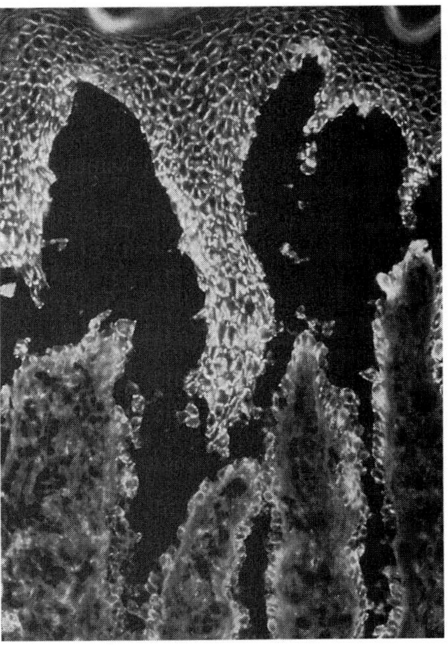

Fig. 21-16 Direct immunofluorescence of oral pemphigus. A positive intercellualr signal for IgG deposition is seen in the entire keratinized stratified epithelium.

Minimization of oral irritation is important in patients with oral pemphigus vulgaris. Optimal oral hygiene is essential, because there is usually widespread involvement of the marginal and attached gingivae in pemphigus vulgaris, as well as other areas of the mouth, which can be exacerbated by plaque-associated gingivitis and periodontitis. Periodontal care is an important issue of the overall management of patients with pemphigus vulgaris. To prevent flare-ups, patients in the maintenance phase should receive prednisone before professional oral prophylaxis and periodontal surgery.[96] In addition, attention should be given to the fit and design of removable prosthetic appliances, as even slight irritation from these prostheses can cause severe inflammation with vesiculation and ulceration.

Chronic Ulcerative Stomatitis

Chronic ulcerative stomatitis was first reported in 1990.[49] Clinically, this condition presents with chronic oral ulcerations and has a predilection for women in their fourth decade of life. The erosions and ulcerations present predominantly in the oral cavity, with only few cases exhibiting cutaneous lesions.[19,63,121]

Oral Lesions. Painful, solitary small blisters and erosions with surrounding erythema are present mainly on the gingiva and the lateral border of the tongue. Because of the magnitude and clinic features of the gingival lesions, a diagnosis of desquamative gingivitis is considered (Color Fig. 21-6). The hard palate may also present similar lesions.

Histopathology. The microscopic features of chronic ulcerative stomatitis are similar to those observed in erosive lichen planus. Hyperkeratosis, acanthosis, and liquefaction of the basal cell layer with areas of subepithelial clefting are prominent features of the epithelium. The underlying lamina propria exhibits a lymphohistiocytic chronic infiltrate in a band-like configuration.

Immunofluorescence. Direct immunofluorescence of normal and perilesional tissues reveal typical stratified epithelium-specific antinuclear antibodies (SES-ANA). These are nuclear deposits of IgG with a speckled pattern, mainly in the basal cell layer of the normal epithelium (Fig. 21-17). In addition, fibrin deposits are visualized at the epithelial-connective tissue interface. Indirect immunofluorescence studies also reveal the presence of SES-ANA.

Differential Diagnosis. Chronic ulcerative stomatitis is clinically similar to erosive lichen. Pemphigus vulgaris, cicatricial pemphigoid, linear IgA, bullous pemphigoid, and lupus erythematosus have to be included in the clinical differential diagnosis. Microscopic examination usually reduces the number of possibilities to chronic ulcerative stomatitis, linear IgA dermatosis, and erosive lichen planus. Direct and indirect immunofluorescence are needed to arrive at the correct diagnosis.

Treatment. For mild cases, topical steroids (fluocinonide, clobetasol propionate) and topical tetracycline may produce clinical improvement; however, recurrences are common.[64] For severe cases, a high dose of systemic corticosteroids is needed to achieve remission. Unfortunately, reduction of the corticosteroids doses results in relapse of the lesions. Hydroxychloroquinine sulfate at a dosage of 200 to 400 mg per day seems to be the treatment of choice to produce complete, long-lasting remission.[10,21,49] However, a recent long-term follow-up study demonstrated that a combined therapy (small doses of corticosteroids and chloroquine) may be required, as the initial good response to chloroquine ceases after several months or even years of treatment.[19]

Linear IgA Disease (Linear IgA Dermatosis)

Linear IgA disease (LAD), also known as *linear IgA dermatosis,* is an uncommon mucocutaneous disorder with predilection in women. It clinically presents as a pruritic vesiculobullous rash usually during middle to late age, although younger individuals may be affected. Characteristic plaques or crops with an annular presentation surrounded by a peripheral rim of blisters affect the skin of the upper and lower trunk, shoulders, groin, and lower limbs. The face and perineum may also be affected. Mucosal involvement, including the oral mucosa, ranges from 50% to 100% of the cases published.[23,50]

LAD may mimic lichen planus both clinically and histologically. Immunofluorescent studies are needed to establish the correct diagnosis.

Oral Lesions. Oral manifestations of LAD consist of vesicles, painful ulcerations or erosions, and erosive gingivitis/cheilitis. The hard and soft palates are more commonly affected. Tonsillar pillars, buccal mucosa, tongue, and gingiva follow in frequency. Rarely, oral lesions may be the only manifestation of LAD for several years before the presentation of cutaneous lesions.[17] In addition, oral lesions of LAD have been clinically reported as desquamative gingivitis (Color Fig. 21-7).[90,91]

Histopathology. The microscopic features of LAD are similar to those observed in erosive lichen planus.

Immunofluorescence. Linear deposits of IgA are observed at the epithelial-connective tissue interface. They differ from the granular pattern observed in dermatitis herpetiformis.

Differential Diagnosis. The differential diagnosis of LAD includes erosive lichen planus, chronic ulcerative stomatitis, pemphigus vulgaris, bullous pemphigoid, and lupus erythematosus. Microscopic examination and immunofluorescence studies are necessary to establish the correct diagnosis.

Treatment. The primary treatment for LAD is a combination of sulfones and dapsone. Small amounts of prednisone (10 to 30 mg per day) can be added if the initial response is inadequate.[18] Alternatively, tetracycline (2 g per day) combined with nicotinamide (1.5 g per day) have shown promising results.[88]

Dermatitis Herpetiformis

Dermatitis herpetiformis is a chronic condition that usually develops in young adults (ages 20 to 30 years) and has a slight predilection for males.[30] Although its cause is still unclear, all patients have gluten enteropathy, which can be severe in about two thirds of the individuals affected and mild or subclinical in the remaining third. In severe cases, patients may complain of dysphagia, weakness, diarrhea, and weight loss.[71] Clinically, dermatitis herpetiformis presents with bilateral and symmetric pruritic papules or vesicles predominantly restricted to the extensor surfaces of the extremities. The sacrum, buttocks, and occasionally the face, as well as the oral cavity may be also affected.[13,30] The name "herpetic" derives from the initial presentation of this disease, where clusters of vesicles or papules arise on the skin. These vesicles or papules eventually resolve and are followed by hyperpigmentation of the skin, which ultimately wanes. The oral lesions of dermatitis herpetiformis are characterized by the presence of painful ulcerations preceded by the collapse of ephemeral vesicles or bullae.

Microscopic examination of the initial lesions of dermatitis herpetiformis reveals focal aggregates of neutrophils and eosinophils amidst deposits of fibrin at the apices of the dermal pegs.[126] Direct immunofluorescence show that IgA and C3 are present at the dermal papillary apices. These findings are present in perilesional and normal, uninvolved tissue. In contrast, biopsies taken from lesional sites may fail to exhibit IgA or C3, resulting in false negatives.[126] Although no circulating autoantibodies to epithelial basement membrane are present in dermatitis herpetiformis, close to 80% of the individuals affected have anti-endomysial and gliadin antibodies.[11]

Lupus Erythematosus

Lupus erythematosus is an autoimmune disease with three different clinical presentations: systemic, chronic cutaneous, and subacute cutaneous.

Systemic Lupus Erythematosus. Systemic lupus erythematosus (SLE) is a severe disease with predilection for females (10:1) that affects vital organs such as kidneys and heart, as well as the skin and mucosa. Its diagnosis is usually hampered by an insidious presentation during the early stages of the disease. However, fever, weight loss, and arthritis are common. The classic cutaneous lesions are characterized by the presence of a rash on the malar area with a butterfly distribution (Fig. 21-18). The oral lesions of SLE are usually ulcerative or lichen planus–like. Oral ulcerations present in 36% of SLE patients. In about 4% of these patients, hyperkeratotic plaques reminiscent of lichen planus appear on the buccal mucosa and palate.[15] In extremely rare instances, lupus erythematosus may occur on the oral mucous membrane without skin lesions. Direct immunofluorescence of the perilesional and normal tissue reveals immunoglobulins and C3 deposits at the dermal-epidermal interface. Antinuclear antibodies (ANA) are present in more than 95% of cases, whereas deoxyribonucleic acid (DNA) and extractable nuclear antigen (ENA) antibodies are present in more than 50% of the cases.

Chronic Cutaneous Lupus Erythematosus. Chronic cutaneous lupus erythematosus (CCLE) usually has no systemic signs or symptoms, with lesions being limited to skin or mucosal surfaces. The skin lesions are referred to as *discoid lupus erythematosus (DLE)*. It is im-

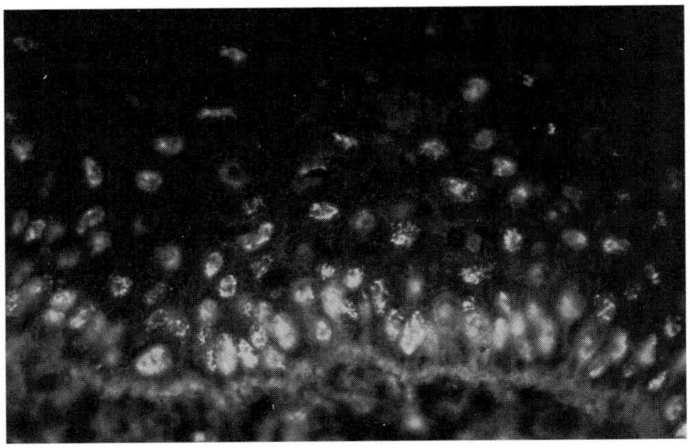

Fig. 21-17 Immunofluorescence of chronic ulcerative stomatitis. Nuclear deposits of IgG are prominent in the basal cell layer and fade towards the superficial epithelial layers. (Courtesy Dr. Douglas Damm; University of Kentucky, Lexington, Ky.).

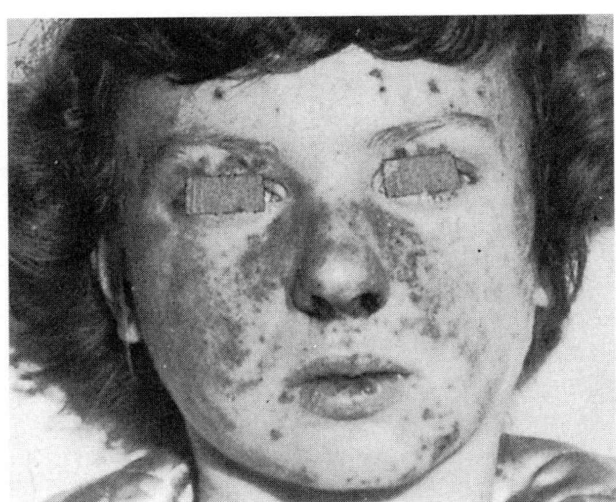

Fig. 21-18 Lupus erythematosus showing "butterfly" distribution of lesions on the face and crusting of the lips.

portant to recognize that the term DLE refers to a specific skin lesion, not a subset of SLE. The term DLE merely describes the chronic scarring, atrophy-producing lesion that may develop hyperpigmentation or hypopigmentation of the healing area. In contrast, the subacute cutaneous lupus erythematosus skin lesions do not produce scarring and/or atrophy.[16]

In the oral cavity, about 9% of patients with CCLE present lichen planus–like plaques on the palate and buccal mucosa.[4,15] The lesions are usually localized and at their borders, numerous dilated blood vessels in a radial arrangement may extend into the surrounding tissue, coupled with whitish, pinhead papules. In the early stages the center of the lesion is slightly depressed and eroded and is covered with a bluish-red epithelial surface showing scarring. In older lesions the erythematous border becomes less elevated and is transformed into a whitish or bluish-white peripheral zone of thickened epithelium. White lines with the same diverging radial arrangement replace the dilated vessels. On the tongue the disease occurs as circumscribed, smooth, reddened areas in which the papillae are lost or as patches with a whitish sheen resembling leukoplakia.

On the lip the lesions are somewhat similar to those in the mouth, and in most cases the lip is involved by direct extension from perioral skin lesions. Localized patches may be present, or the entire lip may be involved. Early in the disease the lip is swollen, bluish-red, and often everted. The lip lesions may be covered with adherent scales and crusts, which remain localized and are rarely diffuse. At the margins of the patches, dilated capillaries or fine, branching radial lines may be seen. The lip is tender and sensitive, and on removal of the adherent scales, bleeding from the raw surface is noted. Depressed scars may follow healing of the deeper lesions. The gingiva may be affected and clinically present as desquamative gingivitis (Color Fig. 21-8).

Periods of activity and quiescence occur. The lesions enlarge by peripheral extension and are accompanied by fresh erosions and superficial ulcerations, followed by atrophic changes. Some burning sensation occurs in the erosions and deeper ulcerations.

Histopathology. The histopathology of the oral lesions consists of hyperkeratosis or parakeratosis, alternated acanthosis and atrophy, and hydropic degeneration of the basal layer of the epithelium. In addition, the lamina propria exhibits a chronic inflammatory cell infiltrate similar to that observed in lichen planus. However, a more diffuse, and deeper inflammatory infiltrate with a perivascular pattern is observed.[108]

Direct immunofluorescence of lesional tissue reveals immunoglobulins and C3 deposits at the dermal-epidermal junction of the lesional or perilesional tissue but not in normal tissue. This seems to differentiate SLE from DLE. Indirect immunofluorescence reveals the presence of ANAs in more than 95% of these patients, whereas DNA- and ENA-circulating antibodies are present in more than 50% of cases.

Subacute Cutaneous Lupus Erythematosus. Subacute cutaneous lupus erythematosus (SCLE) has been used to describe a group of patients who have a characteristic cutaneous lesion that has similarities to DLE but lacks the development of scarring and atrophy.[16] In addition, arthritis/arthralgia, low-grade fever, malaise and myalgia may present in up to 50% of SCLE patients.[16,117] Direct immunofluorescence reveals immunoglobulins and C3 deposits at the dermal-epidermal junction in 60% of cases, and granular IgG deposits in the cytoplasm of basal cells in 30% of cases. About 80% of patients with SCLE have Ro (SSA) antibodies to nuclear antigens, whereas 25% to 30% have La (SSB) antibodies to nuclear antigens. Rheumatoid factor is positive in about 30% of these patients, ANA is positive in 60% to 90%, and 10% of cases have anti-ribonucleoprotein (anti-RNP) antibodies to nuclear antigens.

Differential Diagnosis. Diagnosis usually depends on the identification of the accompanying skin lesions. The diagnosis of DLE confined to the oral cavity is very difficult to make, but microscopic studies may suggest the characteristic histopathology.[3] Erosive lichen planus, erythema multiforme, and pemphigus vulgaris may sometimes simulate the lesions observed in lupus erythematosus. Biopsy studies (H&E and direct immunofluorescence) aid in differentiating between lupus erythematosus and other erosive diseases.

Treatment. The therapy for SLE is dependent on the severity and extent of the disease. Cutaneous rashes are treated with topical steroids, sunscreens, and hydroxychloroquinine. For arthritis and mild pleuritis, nonsteroidal antiinflamatory agents or hydroxychloroquinine are used. For severe systemic organ involvement, moderate-to-high doses of prednisone are effective. For severe cases of SLE or when side effects to prednisone develop, immunosuppressive drugs such as cytotoxic drugs (cyclophosphamide and azathioprine) and plasmaphoresis alone or in conjunction with steroids are useful.[84] For CCLE, topical steroids are effective to manage the cutaneous and oral lesions. For cases resistant to topical therapy, systemic antimalarial drugs may be used with good results.[83]

Erythema Multiforme

Erythema multiforme is an acute bullous and/or macular inflammatory mucocutaneous disease where a series of immunopathologic mechanisms occur.[34] It is believed that the genesis of ulcerative lesions affecting the skin and mucosa resides in the development of immune complex vasculitis. This is followed by complement fixation leading to leukocytoclastic destruction of vascular walls and small vessel occlusion. The culmination of these events produces ischemic necrosis of the epithelium and underlying connective tissue.[34] Target or "iris" lesions with central clearing, are the "hallmark" of erythema multiforme. It may be a mild condition (erythema multiforme minor), or it may be a severe, possibly life-threatening condition (erythema multiforme major or Stevens-Johnson syndrome). Erythema multiforme minor lasts approximately 4 weeks and exhibits a moderate cutaneous and mucosal involvement. Stevens-Johnson syndrome may last a month or longer and involves the skin, conjunctiva, oral mucosa, and genitalia, requiring a more aggressive therapy. Toxic epidermal necrolysis is considered by some researchers as the most severe form of erythema multiforme; however, other investigators feel that they are unrelated entities.[6] The three most common etiologic factors for the development of erythema multiforme are (1) herpes simplex infection, (2) mycoplasma infection, and (3) drug reactions. The most common causative drugs are sulfonamides, penicillins, phenylbutazone, and phenytoin.[115]

Oral lesions in erythema multiforme are common and present in more than 70% of patients with skin involvement.[35,66,73] However, in rare instances, erythema multiforme may be confined to the mouth.[69,103]

Oral Lesions. The oral lesions consist of multiple, large, shallow, painful ulcers with an erythematous border. They may affect the entire oral mucosa in approximately 20% of erythema multiforme patients. The lesions are so painful that chewing and swallowing are impaired (Color Fig. 21-9). The buccal mucosa and tongue are the most commonly affected sites, followed by the labial mucosa. Less commonly affected are the floor of the mouth, hard and soft palate, and the gingiva.[35] There are rare instances in which erythema multiforme may be confined exclusively to the gingival tissues, resulting in a clinical diagnosis of desquamative gingivitis.[8] Hemorrhagic crusting of the vermilion border of the lips is not uncommon. The presence of hemorrhagic crusting of the lips is helpful in arriving at a clinical diagnosis of erythema multiforme.

Histopathology. A wide spectrum of tissue changes occur in erythema multiforme. In several cases, the value of the microscopic examination is to rule out other conditions. Some of the most common microscopic findings of erythema multiforme include liquefaction degeneration of the upper epithelium and the development of intraepithelial microvesicles, but without the acantholysis that occurs in pemphigus.[105] In addition, acanthosis, pseudoepitheliomatous hyperplasia, and necrotic keratinocytes are observed in the epithelium. Degenerative changes also occur in the basement membrane. In some cases, the junction between the epithelium and the lamina propria is indistinct due to a dense inflammatory cell infiltrate. Edema of the lamina propria, vascular dilation, and congestion are also present. Deeper layers of the connective tissue stroma exhibit a perivascular chronic inflammatory cell infiltrate. Nonetheless, neutrophils and esosinophils may also be present.

Immunofluorescence. Immunofluorescence examination is negative in erythema multiforme. Its value resides in ruling out other vesiculo-bullous and ulcerative disorders.

Treatment. There is no specific treatment for erythema multiforme. Some cases may even resolve spontaneously, and erythematous lesions may require no treatment. In contrast, patients exhibiting bullous or ulcerative lesions require intervention. For mild symptoms, systemic and local antihistamines coupled to topical anesthetics and débridement of lesions with an oxygenating agent is adequate. In patients with severe symptoms, corticosteroids are considered the drug of choice although, its use is controversial and not completely accepted.[85]

DRUG ERUPTIONS

An increase in the incidence of skin and oral manifestations of hypersensitivity to drugs has been noted since the advent of the sulfonamides, barbiturates, and various antibiotics. The eruptive skin and oral lesions are attributed to the fact that the drug acts as an allergen, either alone or in combination, sensitizing the tissues and then causing the allergic reaction.

Eruptions in the oral cavity resulting from sensitivity to drugs that have been taken by mouth or parenterally are termed *stomatitis medicamentosa.* The local reaction from the use of a medicament in the oral cavity (e.g., an aspirin burn or the stomatitis resulting from topical penicillin) is referred to as *stomatitis venenata* or *contact stomatitis.* Such changes may result either from the irritating local action of the drug or from drug sensitivity. In many cases, skin eruptions may accompany the oral lesions.

In general, drug eruptions in the oral cavity are multiform. Vesicular and bullous lesions occur most commonly, but pigmented or nonpigmented macular lesions are also often observed. Erosions, often followed by deep ulceration with purpuric lesions, may also occur. The lesions are seen in different areas of the oral cavity, with the gingiva often affected.[41]

The development of gingival lesions due to contact allergy to mercurial compounds present in dental amalgam has been clearly documented.[53] Because of financial considerations, biopsy and patch testing may be indicated before the indiscriminate replacement of dental amalgam restorations. Similarly, desquamative gingivitis has been reported with the use of tartar control toothpaste. Pyrophosphates and flavoring agents have been identified as the main causative agents of this unusual condition.[28] Oral reactions to cinnamon compounds (cinnamon oil, cinnamic acid and cinnamic aldehyde) used to mask the taste of pyrophosphates in tartar control toothpaste, include an intense erythema of the attached gingival tissues characteristic of plasma cell gingivitis (Color Fig. 21-10).[2,54] A thorough clinical history usually discloses the source of the gingival disturbance. Elimination of the offending agent (e.g., tartar control toothpaste) leads to resolution of the gingival lesions within a week. Challenge with the offending agent leads to recurrence of the oral lesions.

MISCELLANEOUS

Another group of heterogeneous conditions may masquerade as desquamative gingivitis. Factitious lesions, candidiasis, graft vs. host disease, Wegener's granulomatosis, foreign body gingivitis, Kindler syndrome, and even squamous cell carcinoma can divert the attention of the clinician and result in a diagnostic challenge. Factitious lesions are consciously and intentionally produced injuries without a clear motive, although, guilt, seeking sympathy, or monetary compensation may be the driving forces behind this abnormal behavior. Factitious desquamative gingivitis has been reported in the literature and may be very difficult to diagnose and become apparent only after extensive and costly laboratory tests fail to reveal the genesis of the lesions.[74] Rarely, candidiasis may be limited to the gingival tissues and may simulate desquamative gingivitis (Fig. 21-19). Graft vs. host disease may occur in recipients of allogenic bone marrow transplants where oral lesions may occasionally resemble desquamative gingivitis (Color Fig. 21-11). Wegener's granulomatosis is a systemic disease that may initially present with striking alterations that are confined to the gingival tissues. Classically, the gingival tissues exhibit erythema and enlargement and are typically described as "strawberry gums" (Color Fig. 21-12).[24] Foreign body gingivitis is clinically characterized by red or red and white chronic lesions that may be painful and are reminiscent of desquamative gingivitis. This condition does not have a gingival site predilection and is more common in women approaching the fifth decade of life. Microscopic analysis reveals small (<5 μm in diameter) foreign bodies associated with a chronic inflammatory cell response that may exhibit granulomatous and lichenoid characteristics. Energy dispersive x-ray microanalysis has revealed that in this condition, most foreign bodies are of dental material origin (more specifically abrasives and restorative material).[43,44] Kindler syndrome (cutaneous neonatal bullae, poikiloderma, photosensitivity, and acral atrophy) may also present with oral lesions that are clinically consistent with desquamative gingivitis.[94] Failure to properly and systematically evaluate a patient with a clinical condition that is consistent with desquamative gingivitis can lead to unpleasant outcomes. This is particularly true when therapy for a putative desquamative gingivitis is established before a biopsy of the lesional tissue is obtained. Every year we see in our laboratory at least two examples of clinically diagnosed desquamative gingivitis where microscopic and immunofluorescence studies were not performed to rule out the genesis of the gingival lesions. In those cases, the patients have been either "carefully" followed-up or placed on topical steroids for several months (Fig. 21-20). The lack of response of the gingival tissues impels the clinician to obtain a biopsy, which reveals that the gingival lesions are bona fide squamous cell carcinomas. Thus the clinician should be alert to the possibility of squamous cell carcinoma of the gingival tissues presenting initially as desquamative gingivitis.

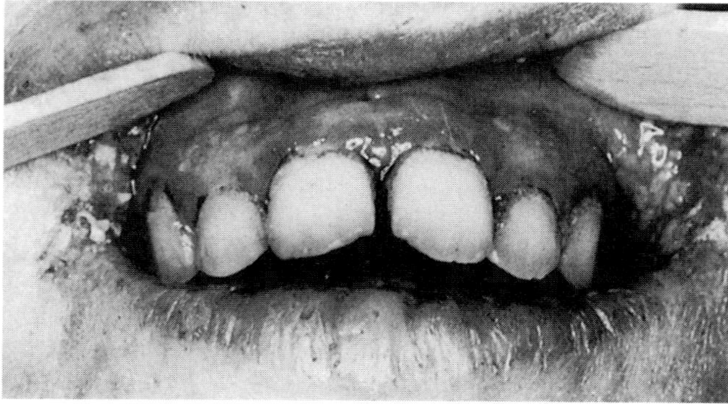

Fig. 21-19 Chronic candidiasis involving the gingiva in an 18-year-old woman.

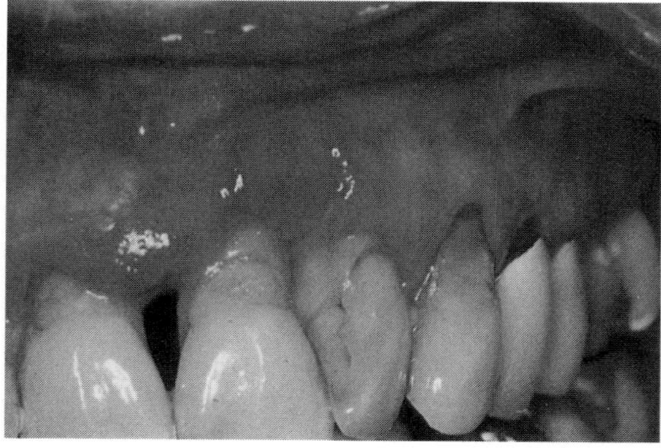

Fig. 21-20 Squamous cell carcinoma masquerading as desquamative gingivitis.

REFERENCES

1. Ahmed AR, Kurgis BS, Rogers RS: Cicatricial pemphigoid. J Am Acad Dermatol 1991; 24:987.
2. Allen CM, Blozis GG: Oral mucosal reactions to cinnamon-flavores chewing gum. JADA 1988; 116:664.
3. Andreasen JO, Poulsen HE: Oral manifestations in discoid and systemic lupus erythematosus. Histologic investigation. Acta Odontol Scand 1964; 22:389.
4. Archard HO, Roebuck NF, Stanley HR: Oral manifestations of chronic discoid lupus erythematosus. Oral Surg 1963; 16:696.
5. Balding SD, Prost C, Diaz LA: Cicatricial pemphigoid autoantibodies react with multiple sites on the BP 180 extracellular domain. J Invest Dermatol 1996; 106:141.
6. Bastuji-Garin S, Rzany B, Stern RS, et al: Clinical classification of cases of toxic epidermal necrolysis, Stevens-Johnson syndrome, and erythema multiforme. Arch Dermatol 1993; 129:92.
7. Baudet-Pommel M, Janin-Mercier A, Souteyrand P: Sequential immunopathologic study of oral lichen planus treated with tretinoin and etretinate. 1991; Oral Surg 71:197.
8. Barrett AW, Scully C, Eveson JW: Erythema multiforme involving gingiva. J Periodontol 1993; 64:910.
9. Becker BA, Gaspari AA: Pemphigus vulgaris and vegetants. Dermatol Clin 1993; 11:453.
10. Beutner EH, Chorzelski TP, Parodi A, et al: Ten cases of chronic ulcerative stomatitis with stratified epithelium-specific antinuclear antibody. J Am Acad Dermatol 1991; 24:781.

11. Beutner EH, Chorzelski TP, Reunala TL, et al: Immunopathology of dermatitis herpetiformis. Clin Dermatol 1992; 9:295.
12. Blank H, Burgoon CF: Abnormal cytology of epithelial cells in pemphigus vulgaris: A diagnostic aid. J Invest Dermatol 1952; 18:213.
13. Boh EE, Milikan LE: Vesiculobullous diseases with prominent immunologic features. JAMA 1992; 268:2893.
14. Brown RS, Bottomley WK, Puente E, et al: A retrospective evaluation of 193 patients with oral lichen planus. J Oral Pathol Med 1993; 22:69.
15. Burge SM, Frith PA, Juniper RP, et al: Mucosal involvement in systemic and chronic cutaneous lupus erythematosus. Brit J Dermatol 1989; 121:727.
16. Callen JP, Kulick KB, Stelzer G, et al: Subacute cutaneous lupus erythematosus: Clinical, serologic, and immunogenetic studies on 49 patients seen in a non-referral setting. J Am Acad Dermatol 1986; 15:1227.
17. Chan LS, Regezi JA, Cooper KD: Oral manifestations of linear IgA disease. J Am Acad Dermatol 1990; 22:362.
18. Chorzelski TP, Jablonska S, Maciejowska E: Linear IgA bullous dermatosis of adults. Clin Dermatol 1992; 9:383.
19. Chorzelski TF, Olszewska M, Jarzabek-Chorzelska M, et al: Is chronic ulcerative stomatitis an entity? Clinical and immunological findings in 18 cases. Euro J Dermatol 1998; 8:261.
20. Chowdhury MM, Natarajan S: Neonatal pemphigus vulgaris associated with mild oral pemphigus vulgaris in the mother during pregnancy. Br J Dermatol 139:500, 1998.
21. Church LF Jr, Schosser RH: Chronic ulcerative stomatitis associated with stratified epithelial specific antinuclear antibodies. A case report of a newly described disease entity. Oral Surg Oral Med Oral Pathol 1992; 73:579.
22. Ciarrocca KN, Greenberg MS: A retrospective study of the management of oral mucous membrane pemphigoid with dapsone. Oral Surg Oral Med Oral Pathol Oral Radiol Endod 1999; 88:159.
23. Cohen DM, Bhattacharyya I, Zunt SL, et al: Linear IgA disease histopathologically and clinically masquerading as lichen planus. Oral Surg Oral Med Oral Pathol Oral Radiol Endod 1999; 88:196.
24. Cohen RE, Cardoza TT, Drinnan AJ, et al: Gingival manifestations of Wegener's granulomatosis. J Periodontol 1990; 61:705.
25. Combes FL, Canizares O: Pemphigus vulgaris, a clinicopathological study of one hundred cases. Arch Dermatol Syph 1950; 62:786.
26. Dabelsteen E: Molecular biological aspects of acquired bullous diseases. Crit Rev Oral Biol Med 1998; 9:162.
27. Dabelsteen E, Ullman S, Thomson K, et al: Demonstration of basement membrane autoantibodies in patients with benign mucous membrane pemphigoid. Acta Dermatol Venereol (Stockh) 1974; 54:189.
28. DeLattre V: Factors contributing to adverse soft tissue reactions due to the use of tartar control toothpastes: Report of a case and literature review. Periodontol 1999; 70:803.
29. De Vita S, Neri R, Bombardieri S: Cyclophosphamide pulses in the treatment of rheumatic diseases: an update. Clin Exp Rheumatol 1991; 9:179.
30. Economopoulou P, Laskaris G: Dermatitis herpetiformis: Oral lesions as an early manifestation. Oral Surg Oral Med Oral Pathol 1986; 62:77.
31. Eisen D, Ellis CN, Duell GA, et al: Effect of topical cyclosporin rinse on oral lichen planus. N Engl J Med 1990; 323:290.
32. Eisenberg E, Krutchkoff DJ: Lichenoid lesions of oral mucosa. Diagnostic criteria and their importance in the alleged relationship to oral cancer. Oral Surg Oral Med Oral Pathol 1992; 73:699.
33. Engel M, Ray HG, Orban B: The pathogenesis of desquamative gingivitis. J Dent Res 1950; 29:410.
34. Eversole LR: Immunopathology of oral mucosal ulcerative, desquamative and bullous diseases. Oral Surg Oral Med Oral Pathol 1994; 77:55.
35. Farthing PM, Margou P, Coates M, et al: Characteristics of the oral lesions in patients with cutaneous recurrent erythema multiforme. J Oral Pathol Med 1995; 24:9.
36. Fine JD: Management of acquired bullous diseases. New Engl J Med 1995; 5:33.
37. Foss CL, Grupe HE, Orban B: Gingivosis. J Periodontol 1953; 24:207.
38. Foster CS: Cicatricial pemphigoid. Trans Am Ophthalmol Soc 1986; 84:527.
39. Fotos PG, Vincent SD, Hellstein JW: Oral candidosis: Clinical, historical and therapeutic features of 100 cases. Oral Surg 1992; 74:41.
40. Gallagher G, Shklar G: Oral involvement in mucous membrane pemphigoid. Clin Dermatol 1987; 5:19.
41. Gallagher GT: Oral mucous membrane reactions to drugs and chemicals. Curr Opin Dent 1991; 1:777.
42. Goadby K: Diseases of the Gums and Oral Mucous Membrane. London, Henry Froude and Hodder and Staughton, 1923.
43. Gordon SC, Daley TD: Foreign body gingivitis. Clinical and microscopic features of 61 cases. Oral Surg Oral Med Oral Pathol Oral Radiol Endod 1997; 83:562.
44. Gordon SC, Daley TD: Foreign body gingivitis. Identification of the foreign material by energy-dispersive x-ray microanalysis. Oral Surg Oral Med Oral Pathol Oral Radiol Endod 1997; 83:571.
45. Hashimoto K, Dibella R, Shklar G, et al: Electron microscopic studies of oral lichen planus. G Ital Dermatol 1966; 107:765.
46. Holmstrup P: The controversy of a premalignant potential of lichen planus is over. Oral Surg Oral Med Oral Pathol 1992; 73:704.
47. Eisenberg E. Lichen planus and oral cancer: Is there a connection between the two? JADA 1992; 123:104.
48. Ishii T: Immunohistochemical demonstration of T cell subsets and accessory cells in oral lichen planus. J Oral Pathol 1987; 15:268.
49. Jaremko WM, Beutner EH, Kumar V, et al: Chronic ulcerative stomatitis associated with a specific immunologic marker. J Am Acad Dermatol 1990; 22:215.
50. Kelly SE, Frith PA, Millard PR, et al: A clinicopathological study of mucosal involvement in linear IgA disease. Br J Dermatol 1988; 119:161.
51. Komori A, Welton NA, Kelln EE: The behavior of the basement membrane of skin and oral lesions in patients with lichen planus, erythema multiforme, lupus erythematosus, pemphigus vulgaris, pemphigoid and epidermolysis bullosa. Oral Surg 1966; 22:752.
52. Korman NJ: Bullous pemphigoid. Dermatol Clin 1993; 11:483.
53. Laine J, Kalimo K, Happonen R: Contact allergy to dental restorative materials in patients with oral lichenoid lesions. Cont Derm 1997; 36:141.
54. Lamey PJ, Lewis MAO, Ress TD, et al: Sensitivity reaction to the cinnamonaldehyde component of toothpaste. Br Dent J 1990; 168:115.
55. Lamey PJ, Rees TD, Binnie WH, et al: Oral presentation of pemphigus vulgaris and its response to systemic steroid therapy. Oral Surg Oral Med Oral Pathol 1992; 74:54.
56. Laskaris G, Angelopoulos A: Cicatricial pemphigoid: Direct and indirect immunofluorescent studies. Oral Surg 1981; 51:48.

57. Laskaris G, Demetrou N, Angelopoulos A: Immunofluorescent studies in desquamative gingivitis. J Oral Pathol 1981; 10:398.
58. Lenz P, Amagai M, Volc-Platzer B, et al: Desmoglein 3-ELISA: a pemphigus vulgaris specific diagnostic tool. Arch dermatol 1999; 135:142.
59. Leonard J: Immunofluorescent studies in ocular cicatricial pemphigoid. Br J Dermatol 1988; 118:209.
60. Lever WF: Pemphigus. Medicine 1953; 32:1.
61. Lever WF. Pemphigus and pemphigoid: A review of the advances made since 1964. J Am Acad Derm 1979; 1:2.
62. Lever WF, Schaumburg-Lever G: Immunosuppressants and prednisone in pemphigus vulgaris. Arch Dermatol 1977; 113:1236.
63. Lewis JE, Beutner EH, Rostami R, et al: Chronic ulcerative stomatitis with stratified epithelium-specific antinuclear antibodies. Int Jour Dermatol 1996; 35:272.
64. Lorenzana ER, Rees TD, Glass M, et al: Chronic ulcerative stomatitis: A case report. J Periodontol 2000; 71:104.
65. Lozada-Nur F: Oral lichen planus and oral cancer: Is there enough epidemiologic evidence? Oral Surg Oral Med Oral Pathol Oral Radiol Endod 2000; 89:265.
66. Lozada-Nur F, Gorsky M, Silverman S Jr: Oral erythema multiforme: clinical observations and treatment of 95 patients. Oral Surg Oral Med Oral Pathol 1989; 67:36.
67. Lozada-Nur F, Miranda C: Oral lichen planus: Epidemiology, clinical characteristics, and associated diseases. Sem Cutan Med Surg 1997; 16:273.
68. Lozada-Nur F, Miranda C, Maliski R: Double-blind clinical trial of 0.05% clobetasole propionate ointment in orabase and 0.05% fluocinonide ointment in orabase in the treatment of patients with vesiculoerosive diseases. Oral Surg Oral Med Oral Pathol 1994; 77:598.
69. Lozada F, Silverman S: Erythema multiforme: Clinical characteristics and natural history in fifty patients. Oral Surg 1978; 46:628.
70. Malmstrom M, Kontinnen YT, Jungell P, et al: Lymphocyte activation in oral lichen planus in situ. Am J Clin Pathol 1988; 89:329.
71. Marsh MN: The natural history of gluten sensitivity: Defining, refining and re-defining. Q J Med 1995; 85:9.
72. McCarthy FP, McCarthy PL, Shklar G: Chronic desquamative gingivitis: A reconsideration. Oral Surg 1960; 13:1300.
73. McCarthy PL, Shklar G: Diseases of the Oral Mucosa, ed 2. Philadelphia, Lea & Febiger, 1980.
74. McGrath KG, Pick R, leboff-Ries E, Patterson R: Factitious desquamative gingivitis simulating a possible immunologic disease. J Allergy Clin Immunol 1985; 75:44.
75. Merritt AH: Chronic desquamative gingivitis. J Periodontol 1933; 4:30.
76. Mobini N, Nagarwalla N, Ahmed AR: Oral pemphigoid: Subset of cicatricial pemphigoid? Oral Surg Oral Med Oral Pathol Oral Radiol Endod 1998; 85:37.
77. Mondino BJ, Brown SI: Ocular cicatricial pemphigoid. Ophthalmology 1981; 99:95.
78. Mondino BJ, Linstone FA: Ocular pemphigoid. Clin Dermatol 1987; 5:28.
79. Muller S, Klaus-Kovtun V, Stanley JR: A 230-kD basic protein is the major bullous pemphigoid antigen. J Invest Dermatol 1989; 92:33.
80. Mutasim DF, Pelc DJ, Anhalt GJ: Paraneoplastic pemphigus. Dermatol Clin 1993; 11:473.
81. Mutasim DF, Pelc NJ, Anhalt GJ: Cicatricial pemphigoid. Dermatol Clin 1993; 11:499.
82. Nemeth AJ, Klein AD, Gould EW, et al: Childhood bullous pemphigoid: Clinical and immunologic features, treatment, and prognosis. Arch Dermatol 1991; 127:378.
83. Neville BW, Damm DD, Allen C, et al: Dermatologic disease. In Neville BW, Damm DD, Allen C, Bouquot JE (eds): Oral and Maxillofacial Pathology. Philadelphia, Saunders, 1995.
84. Nisengard R: Periodontal implications: Mucocutaneous disorders. Ann Periodontol 1996; 1:401.
85. Nisengard R, Levine R: Diagnosis and management of desquamative gingivitis. Periodontal Insights 1995; 2:4.
86. Nisengard RJ, Neiders M: Desquamative lesions of the gingiva. J Periodontol 1981; 52:500.
87. Nisengard RJ, Rogers RS III: The treatment of desquamative gingival lesions. J Periodontol 1987; 58:167.
88. Peoples D, Fivenson DP: Linear IgA bullous dermatosis: Successful treatment with tetracycline and nicotinamide. J Am Acad Dermatol 1992; 26:498.
89. Pleyer U, Bruckner-Tuderman L, Friedmann A, et al: The immunology of bullous oculo-muco-cutaneous disorders. Imm Today 1996; 17:111.
90. Porter SR, Bain SE, Scully CM: Linear IgA disease manifesting as recalcitrant desquamative gingivitis. Oral Surg Oral Med Oral Pathol 1992; 74:179.
91. Porter SR, Scully C, Midda M, et al: Adult linear immunoglobulin A: A disease manifesting as desquamative gingivitis. Oral Surg Oral Med Oral Pathol 1990; 70:450.
92. Prinz H: Chronic diffuse desquamative gingivitis. Dent Cosmos 1932; 74:331.
93. Rees TD: Adjunctive therapy. Proceedings of the World Workshop in Clinical Periodontics. Chicago. The American Academy of Periodontology, 1989, X1–X31.
94. Ricketts DNJ, Morgan CL, McGregor JM, et al: Kindler syndrome. A rare cause of desquamative lesions of the gingiva. Oral Surg Oral Med Oral Pathol Oral Radiol Endod 1997; 84:488.
95. Rinaggio J, Neiders ME, Aguirre A, et al: Using immunofluorescence in the diagnosis of chronic ulcerative lesions of the oral mucosa. Compendium 1999; 20:943.
96. Robinson JC, Lozada-Nur F, Frieden I: Oral pemphigus vulgaris: a review of the literature and a report on the management of 12 cases. Oral Surg Oral Med Oral Pathol Oral Radiol Endod 1997; 84:349.
97. Rogers RS, Sheridan PJ, Jordon RC: Desquamative gingivitis: Clinical, histopathologic and immunopathologic investigations. Oral Surg 1976; 42:316.
98. Robledo MA, Soo-Chan K, Korman NJ, et al: Studies of the relationship of the 230-kD and 180-kD bullous pemphigoid antigens. J Invest Dermatol 1990; 94:793.
99. Sciubba JJ: Autoimmune aspects of pemphigus vulgaris and mucosal pemphigoid. Advances Dent Res 1996; 10:52.
100. Scully C, Beyli M, Ferreiro MC, et al: Update on oral lichen planus: Etiopathogenesis and management. Crit Rev Oral Biol Med 1998; 9:86.
101. Scully C, Carrozzo M, Gandolfo S, et al: Update on mucous membrane pemphigoid. A heterogeneous immune-mediated subepithelial blistering entity. Oral Surg Oral Med Oral Pathol Oral Radiol Endod 1999; 88:56.
102. Scully C, El-Kom M: Lichen planus: Review and update on pathogenesis. J Oral Pathol 1985; 14:431.
103. Scully C, Porter SR: The clinical spectrum of desquamative gingivitis. Sem Cutan Med and Surg 1997; 16:308.
104. Shklar G, Cataldo E: Histopathology and cytology of oral pemphigus vulgaris. Arch Dermatol 1970; 101:36.
105. Shklar G: Oral lesions of erythema multiforme: Histologic and histochemical observations. Arch Dermatol 1965; 92:495.
106. Shklar G, Flynn E, Szabo G: Basement membrane changes in oral lichen planus. J Invest Dermatol 1978; 70:45.
107. Shklar G, Frim S, Flynn E: Gingival lesions of pemphigus. J Periodontol 1978; 49:428.

108. Shklar G, McCarthy PL: Histopathology of oral lesions of chronic discoid lupus erythematous. Arch Dermatol 1978; 114:1031.
109. Shklar G, McCarthy PL: The oral lesions of mucous membrane pemphigoid. A study of 85 cases. Arch Otolaryngol 1971; 93:354.
110. Shklar G, Meyer I, Zacarian S: Oral lesions in bullous pemphigoid. Arch Dermatol 1969; 99:663.
111. Siegel MA, Balciunas BA: Oral presentation and management of vesiculobullous disorders. Sem Dermatol 13:78–86, 1994.
112. Silverman S, Shachi B: Oral lichen planus update: Clinical characteristics, treatment responses, and malignant transformation. Am J Dent 1997; 10:259.
113. Sklavounou A, Laskaris G: Frequency of desquamative gingivitis in skin disease. Oral Surg Oral Med Oral Pathol 1983; 56:141.
114. Sorrin S: Chronic desquamative gingivitis. J Am Dent Assoc 1940; 27:250.
115. Stampien TM, Schwartz RA: Erythema multiforme. Am Fam Phys 1992; 46:1171.
116. Susi FR, Shklar G: Histochemistry and fine structure of oral lesions of mucous membrane pemphigoid. Arch Dermatol 1971; 104:244.
117. Tan EM, Cohen AS, Fries JR, et al: The 1982 revised criteria for the classification of systemic lupus erythematosus. Arthritis Rheum 1982; 25:1271.
118. Tomes J, Tomes G: Dental Surgery, ed 4. London, Churchill, 1894.
119. Venning VA, Frith PA, Bron AJ, et al: Mucosal involvement in bullous and cicatricial pemphigoid. A clinical and immunopathological study. Brit J Dermatol 1988; 118:7.
120. Weston WL, Morelli JG, Huff JC: Misdiagnosis, treatments and outcomes in the immunobullous diseases in children. Pediatr Dermatol 1997; 14:164.
121. Worle B, Wollenberg A, Schaller M, et al: Chronic ulcerative stomatitis. Brit J Dermatol 1997; 137:262.
122. Yih WY, Maier T, Kratochvil FJ, et al: Analysis of desquamative gingivitis using direct immunofluorescence in conjunction with histology. J Periodontol 1998; 69:678.
123. Zegarelli DJ, Zegarelli EV: Intraoral pemphigus vulgaris. Oral Surg 1977; 44:384.
124. Ziskin D, Silvers HF: Report of a case of desquamative gingivitis and lichen planus. J Periodontol 1945; 16:7.
125. Ziskin D, Zegarelli EV: Chronic desquamative gingivitis. Am J Orthod 1947; 33:756.
126. Zone JJ, Meyer LJ, Petersen MJ: Deposition of granular IgA relative to clinical lesions in dermatitis herpetiformis. Arch Dermatol 1996; 132:912.

SECTION II Periodontal Disease

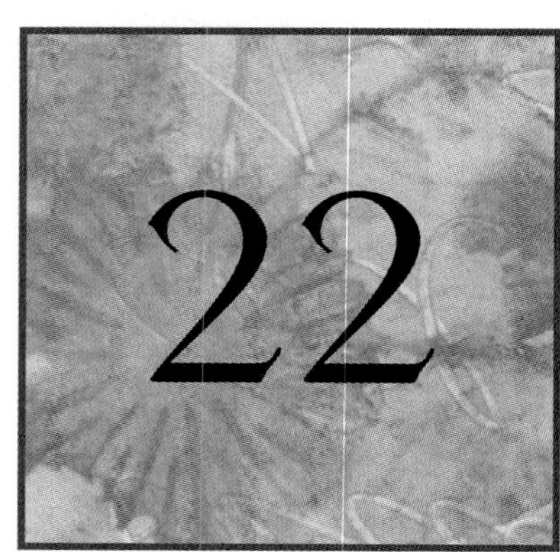

CHAPTER 22

The Periodontal Pocket

Fermin A. Carranza and Paulo M. Camargo

CHAPTER OUTLINE

The periodontal pocket, defined as a pathologically deepened gingival sulcus, is one of the most important clinical features of periodontal disease. All different types of periodontitis, outlined in Chapter 4, share histopathologic features such as tissue changes in the periodontal pocket, mechanisms of tissue destruction, and healing mechanisms. They differ, however, in their etiology, natural history, progression, and response to therapy.[36]

CLASSIFICATION

Deepening of the gingival sulcus may occur by coronal movement of the gingival margin, apical displacement of the gingival attachment, or a combination of the two processes (Fig. 22-1). Pockets can be classified as follows:

Gingival pocket (pseudo pocket): This type of pocket is formed by gingival enlargement without destruction of the underlying periodontal tissues. The sulcus is deepened because of the increased bulk of the gingiva (Fig. 22-2, *A*).

Periodontal pocket: This type of pocket occurs with destruction of the supporting periodontal tissues. Progressive pocket deepening leads to destruction of the supporting periodontal tissues and loosening and exfoliation of the teeth. The remainder of this chapter refers to this type of pocket.

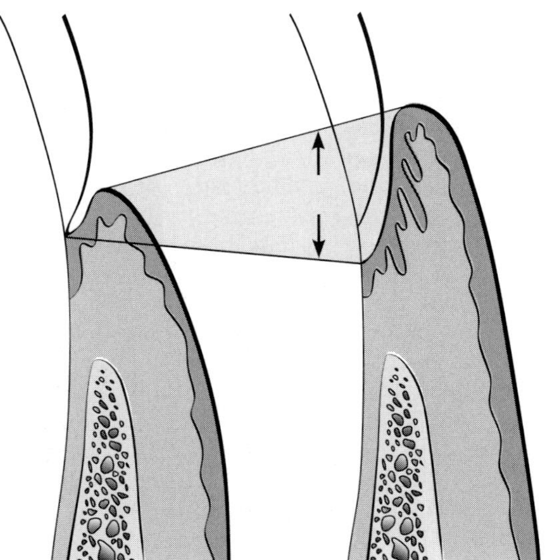

Fig. 22-1 Illustration of pocket formation indicating expansion in two directions *(arrows)* from the normal gingival sulcus (left) to the periodontal pocket (right).

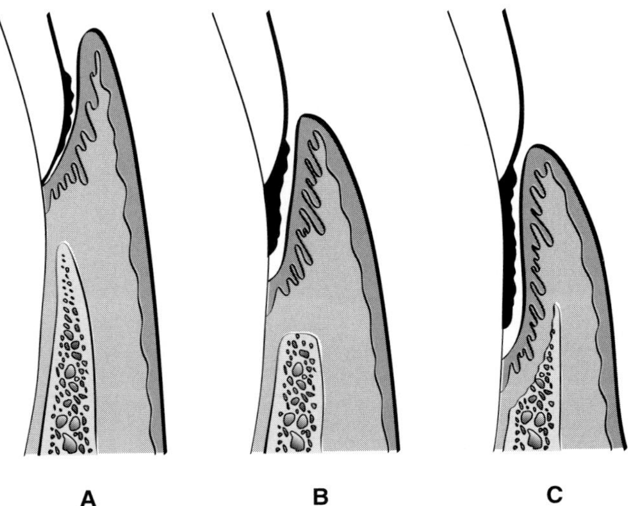

Fig. 22-2 Different types of periodontal pockets. **A,** Gingival pocket. There is no destruction of the supporting periodontal tissues. **B,** Suprabony pocket. The base of the pocket is coronal to the level of the underlying bone. Bone loss is horizontal. **C,** Intrabony pocket. The base of the pocket is apical to the level of the adjacent bone. Bone loss is vertical.

Two types of periodontal pockets exist:

Suprabony (supracrestal or supraalveolar), in which the bottom of the pocket is coronal to the underlying alveolar bone (Fig. 22-2, *B*).

Intrabony (infrabony, subcrestal or intraalveolar), in which the bottom of the pocket is apical to the level of the adjacent alveolar bone. In this second type, the lateral pocket wall lies between the tooth surface and the alveolar bone (Fig. 22-2, *C*).

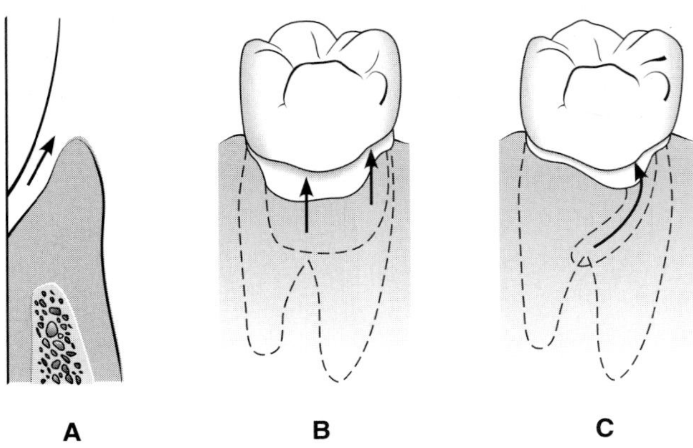

Fig. 22-3 Classification of pockets according to involved tooth surfaces. **A,** Simple pocket. **B,** Compound pocket. **C,** Complex pocket.

Pockets can involve one, two, or more tooth surfaces and can be of different depths and types on different surfaces of the same tooth and on approximating surfaces of the same interdental space.[32,42] Pockets can also be spiral (i.e., originating on one tooth surface and twisting around the tooth to involve one or more additional surfaces) (Fig. 22-3). These types of pockets are most common in furcation areas.

CLINICAL FEATURES

Clinical signs such as bluish-red, thickened marginal gingiva; a bluish-red vertical zone from the gingival margin to the alveolar mucosa; gingival bleeding, suppuration, or both; tooth mobility; and diastema formation and symptoms such as localized pain or pain "deep in the bone" are suggestive of the presence of periodontal pockets. The only reliable method of locating periodontal pockets and determining their extent is careful probing of the gingival margin along each tooth surface (Fig. 22-4 and Table 22-1). On the basis of depth alone, however, it is sometimes difficult to differentiate between a deep normal sulcus and a shallow periodontal pocket. In such borderline cases, pathologic changes in the gingiva distinguish the two conditions.

For a more detailed discussion of the clinical aspects of periodontal pockets, see Chapter 30.

PATHOGENESIS

The initial lesion in the development of periodontitis is the inflammation of the gingiva in response to a bacterial challenge. Changes involved in the transition from the normal gingival sulcus to the pathologic periodontal pocket are associated with different proportions of bacterial cells in dental plaque. Healthy gingiva is associated with few microorganisms, mostly coccoid cells and straight rods. Diseased gingiva is associated with increased numbers of spirochetes and motile rods.[44,45,47] However, the microbiota of diseased sites cannot be used as a predictor of future attachment or bone loss because their presence alone is not sufficient for disease to start or progress.[39]

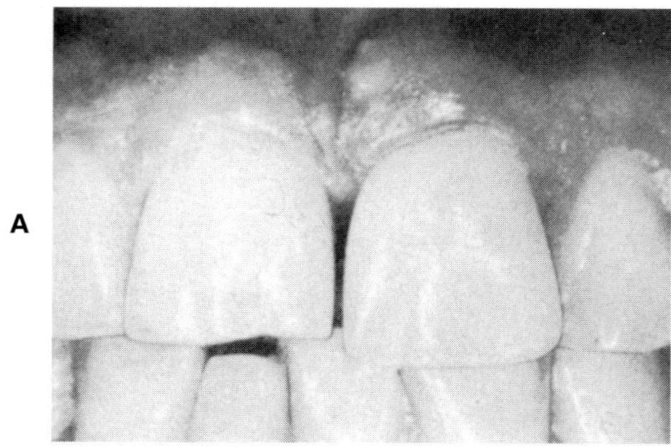

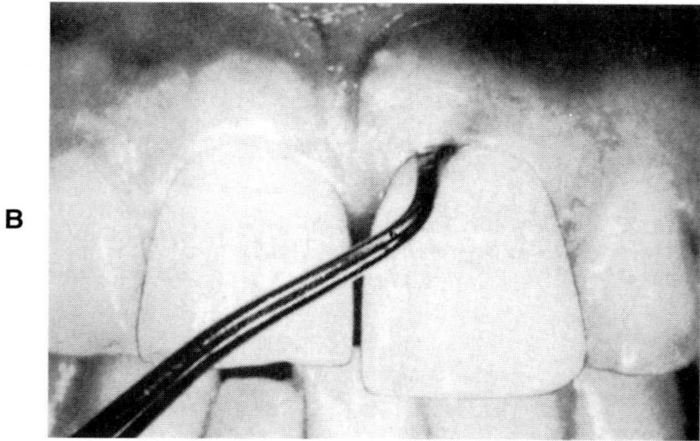

Fig. 22-4 A, Extrusion of the central incisor and diastema associated with the periodontal pocket. **B,** The entire length of the periodontal probe inserted to the base of the periodontal pocket in the central incisor.

Pocket formation starts as an inflammatory change in the connective tissue wall of the gingival sulcus. The cellular and fluid inflammatory exudate causes degeneration of the surrounding connective tissue, including the gingival fibers. Just apical to the junctional epithelium, collagen fibers are destroyed[21,65] and the area becomes occupied by inflammatory cells and edema.

Two mechanisms are considered to be associated with collagen loss: (1) collagenases and other enzymes secreted by various cells in healthy and inflamed tissue such as fibroblasts,[78] polymorphonuclear leukocytes,[77] and macrophages[57] become extracellular and destroy collagen; these enzymes that degrade collagen and other matrix macromolecules into small peptides are called *matrix metalloproteinases*[79]; (2) fibroblasts phagocytize collagen fibers by extending cytoplasmic processes to the ligament-cementum interface and degrade the inserted collagen fibrils and the fibrils of the cementum matrix.[21,22]

As a consequence of the loss of collagen, the apical cells of the junctional epithelium proliferate along the root, extending fingerlike projections two or three cells in thickness.

The coronal portion of the junctional epithelium detaches from the root as the apical portion migrates. As a result of inflammation, polymorphonuclear neutrophils (PMNs) invade the coronal end of the junctional epithelium in increasing numbers. The PMNs are not joined to one another or to the remaining

Continued

TABLE 22-1

Correlation of Clinical and Histopathologic Features of the Periodontal Pocket

Clinical Features	Histopathologic Features
1. The gingival wall of the periodontal pocket presents various degrees of bluish-red discoloration; flaccidity; a smooth, shiny surface; and pitting on pressure.	1. The discoloration is caused by circulatory stagnation; the flaccidity, by destruction of the gingival fibers and surrounding tissues; the smooth, shiny surface, by the atrophy of the epithelium and edema; the pitting on pressure, by edema and degeneration.
2. Less frequently, the gingival wall may be pink and firm.	2. In such cases, fibrotic changes predominate over exudation and degeneration, particularly in relation to the outer surface of the pocket wall. However, despite the external appearance of health, the inner wall of the pocket invariably presents some degeneration and is often ulcerated (see Fig. 22-13).
3. Bleeding is elicited by gently probing the soft tissue wall of the pocket.	3. Ease of bleeding results from increased vascularity, thinning and degeneration of the epithelium, and the proximity of the engorged vessels to the inner surface.
4. When explored with a probe, the inner aspect of the periodontal pocket is generally painful.	4. Pain on tactile stimulation is due to ulceration of the inner aspect of the pocket wall.
5. In many cases, pus may be expressed by applying digital pressure.	5. Pus occurs in pockets with suppurative inflammation of the inner wall.

epithelial cells by desmosomes. When the relative volume of PMNs reaches approximately 60% or more of the junctional epithelium, the tissue loses cohesiveness and detaches from the tooth surface. Thus the sulcus bottom shifts apically, and the oral sulcular epithelium occupies a gradually increasing portion of the sulcular (pocket) lining.[66]

The initial deepening of the pocket has been described as occurring between the junctional epithelium and the tooth[33,34,65] or by an intraepithelial cleavage within the junctional epithelium.[10,24,46,78]

Extension of the junctional epithelium along the root requires the presence of healthy epithelial cells. Marked degeneration or necrosis of the junctional epithelium retards rather than accelerates pocket formation. Degenerative changes seen in the junctional epithelium at the base of periodontal pockets are usually less severe than those in the epithelium of the lateral pocket wall. Because migration of the junctional epithelium requires healthy, viable cells, it is reasonable to assume that the degenerative changes seen in this area occur after the junctional epithelium reaches its position on the cementum.

The degree of leukocyte infiltration of the junctional epithelium is independent of the volume of inflamed connective tissue, and thus this process may occur in gingiva with only slight signs of clinical inflammation.[65]

With continued inflammation, the gingiva increases in bulk, and the crest of the gingival margin extends coronally. The junctional epithelium continues to migrate along the root and separate from it. The epithelium of the lateral wall of the pocket proliferates to form bulbous, cordlike extensions into the inflamed connective tissue. Leukocytes and edema from the inflamed connective tissue infiltrate the epithelium lining the pocket, resulting in various degrees of degeneration and necrosis.

The transformation of a gingival sulcus into a periodontal pocket creates an area where plaque removal becomes impossible, and the following feedback mechanism is established:

Plaque → Gingival inflammation → Pocket formation →
→ More plaque formation

The rationale for pocket reduction is based on the need to eliminate areas of plaque accumulation.

HISTOPATHOLOGY

Changes occurring in the initial stages of gingival inflammation are presented in Chapter 16. Once the pocket is formed, several microscopic features are present, as discussed in the following sections.

Soft Tissue Wall

The connective tissue is edematous and densely infiltrated with plasma cells (approximately 80%),[86] lymphocytes, and a scattering of PMNs. The blood vessels are increased in number, dilated, and engorged, particularly in the subepithelial connective tissue layer.[11] The connective tissue exhibits varying degrees of degeneration. Single or multiple necrotic foci are occasionally present.[56] In addition to exudative and degenerative changes, the connective tissue shows proliferation of the endothelial cells, with newly formed capillaries, fibroblasts, and collagen fibers (Fig. 22-5).

The junctional epithelium at the base of the pocket is usually much shorter than that of a normal sulcus. Although marked variations are found as to length, width, and condition of the epithelial cells, usually the coronoapical length of the junctional epithelium is reduced to only 50 to 100 μm.[15] The cells may be well formed and in good condition or may exhibit slight to marked degeneration (Fig. 22-6).

The most severe degenerative changes in the periodontal pocket occur along the lateral wall (Fig. 22-7). The epithelium of the lateral wall of the pocket presents striking proliferative and degenerative changes. Epithelial buds or interlacing cords of epithelial cells project from the lateral wall into the adjacent inflamed connective tissue and may extend farther apically than the junctional epithelium. These epithelial projections, as well as the remainder of the lateral epithelium, are densely infiltrated by leukocytes and edema from the inflamed connective tissue. The cells undergo vacuolar degeneration and rupture to form vesicles. Progressive degeneration and necrosis of the epithelium lead to ulceration of the lateral wall, exposure of the underlying inflamed connective tissue, and suppuration. In some cases, acute inflammation is superimposed on the underlying chronic changes.

A comparative study of gingival histopathologic changes in rapidly progressive (aggressive) and adult periodontitis (chronic)[39] revealed more pronounced degenerative changes in the epithelium of aggressive cases with more open intercellular spaces, with microclefts and necrotic areas.

The severity of the degenerative changes is not necessarily related to pocket depth. Ulceration of the lateral wall may occur in shallow pockets, and deep pockets are occasionally observed in which the lateral epithelium is relatively intact or shows only slight degeneration.

The epithelium at the gingival crest of a periodontal pocket is generally intact and thickened, with prominent rete pegs.

A detailed electron microscopic study of the pocket epithelium in experimentally induced pockets in dogs has been performed by Müller-Glauser and Schröder.[53]

Bacterial Invasion. Bacterial invasion of the apical and lateral areas of the pocket wall has been described in

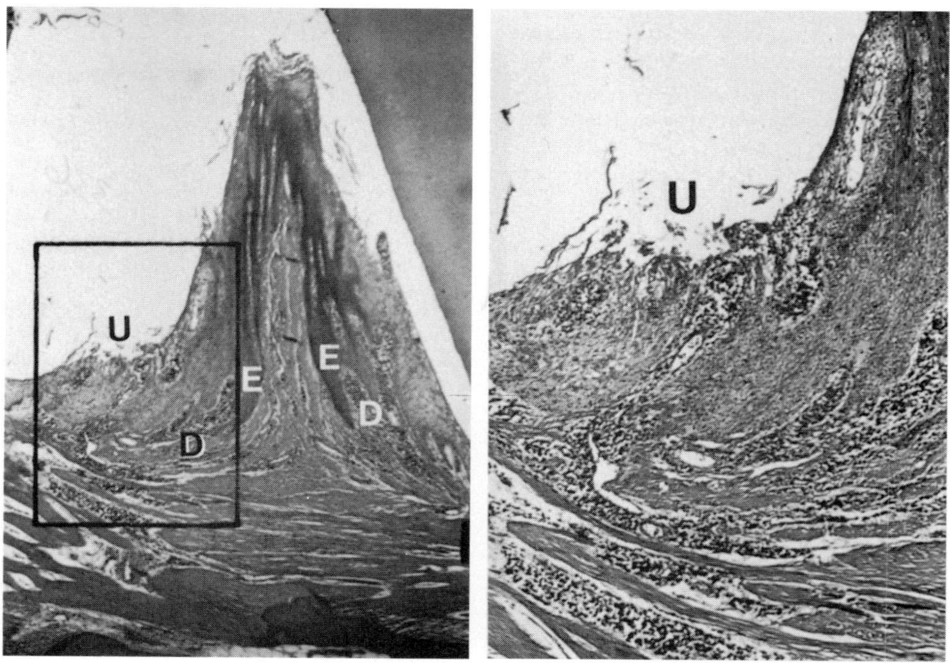

Fig. 22-5 *Left,* Interdental papilla with suprabony pockets on proximal tooth surfaces. *D,* Densely inflamed connective tissue; *E,* proliferating pocket epithelium; *U,* ulcerated pocket epithelium. *Right,* Magnification of the rectangular area on the left. Note the ulcerated area *(U)* and the infiltrate between the collagen fibers.

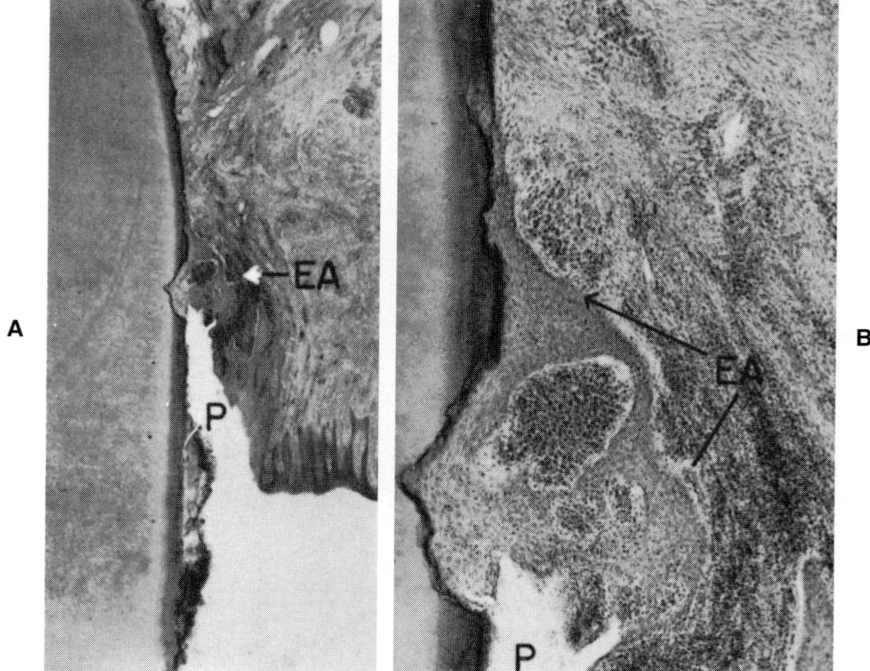

Fig. 22-6 **A,** Low-power section of periodontal pocket *(P).* The location of the junctional epithelium is indicated by the arrow *(EA).* The lateral epithelial wall is ulcerated. **B,** Detailed study of junctional epithelium *(EA)* at the base of the pocket *(P).* Note the extension of well-formed epithelial cells *(arrow)* along the resorbed root surface. There is a dense accumulation of leukocytes enclosed within the epithelium.

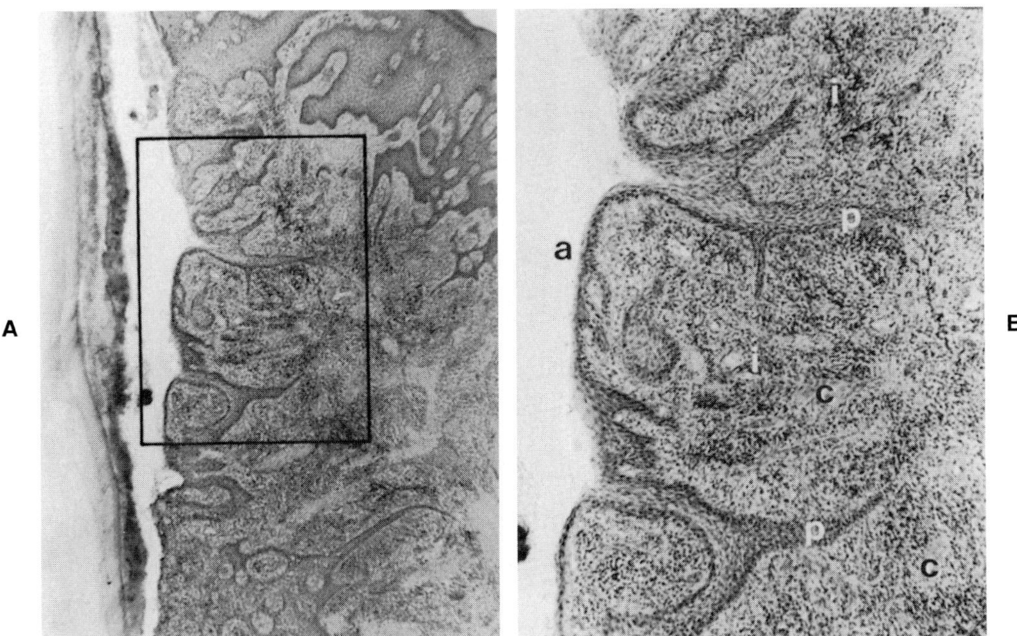

Fig. 22-7 **A,** Low-power view of the lateral wall of a periodontal pocket. Note the dense inflammatory infiltrate and the proliferating epithelium. **B,** High-power view of the rectangular area in **A.** Note the areas of atrophic epithelium *(a)* and epithelial proliferation *(p)*. The connective tissue is densely infiltrated *(i)*; some remnants of collagen fibers *(c)* can be seen.

human chronic periodontitis. Filaments, rods, and coccoid organisms with predominant gram-negative cell walls have been found in intercellular spaces of the epithelium.[27,28] Hillmann et al[39] have reported the presence of *Porphyromonas gingivalis* and *Prevotella intermedia* in the gingiva of aggressive periodontitis cases. *Actinobacillus actinomycetemcomitans* has also been found in the tissues.[17,51,63]

Bacteria may invade the intercellular space under exfoliating epithelial cells, but they are also found between deeper epithelial cells and accumulating on the basement lamina. Some bacteria traverse the basement lamina and invade the subepithelial connective tissue[64] (Figs. 22-8 and 22-9).

The presence of bacteria in the gingival tissues has been interpreted by different investigators as bacterial invasion or as passive translocation of plaque bacteria. This important point has significant clinicopathologic implications and has not yet been clarified.[18,43,47]

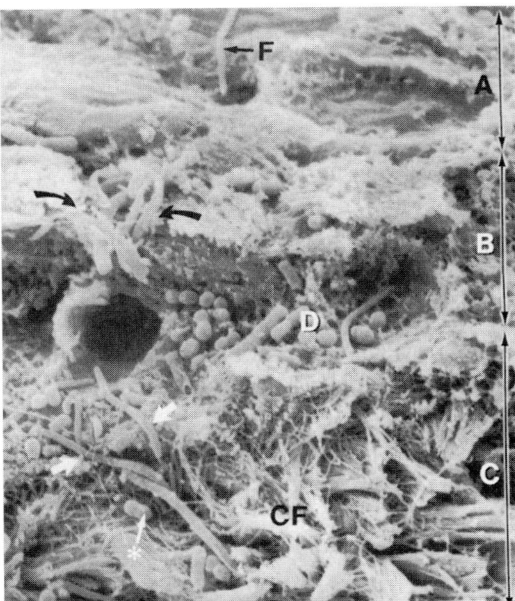

Fig. 22-8 Electron micrograph of a section of pocket wall in advanced periodontitis in a human specimen, showing bacterial penetration into the epithelium and connective tissue. Scanning electron microscope view of surface of pocket wall *(A)*, sectioned epithelium *(B)*, and sectioned connective tissue *(C)*. Curved arrows point to areas of bacterial penetration into the epithelium. Thick white arrows point to bacterial penetration into the connective tissue through a break in the continuity of the basal lamina. *CF,* Connective tissue fibers; *D,* accumulation of bacteria (rods, cocci, filaments) on basal lamina; *F,* filamentous organism on surface of epithelium. Asterisk points to coccobacillus in connective tissue.

Microtopography of the Gingival Wall of the Pocket

Scanning electron microscopy has permitted the description of several areas in the soft tissue wall of the pocket where different types of activity take place.[60] These areas are irregularly oval or elongated and adjacent to one another and measure about 50 to 200 μm. These findings suggest that the pocket wall is constantly changing as a

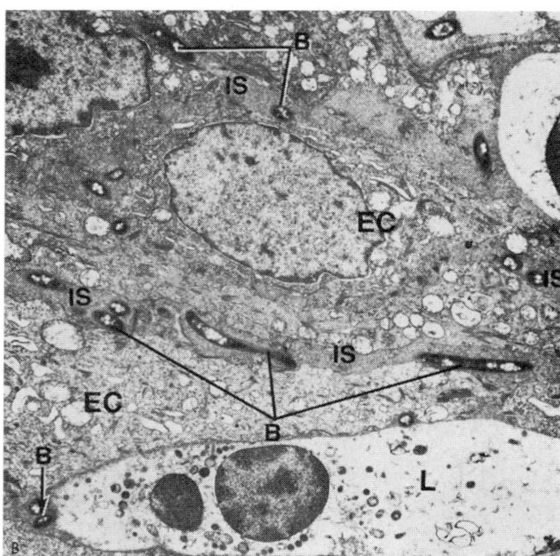

Fig. 22-9 Transmission electron micrograph of the epithelium in the periodontal pocket wall showing bacteria in the intercellular spaces. *B,* Bacteria; *EC,* epithelial cell; *IS,* intercellular space; *L,* leukocyte about to engulf bacteria. Magnification ×8000.

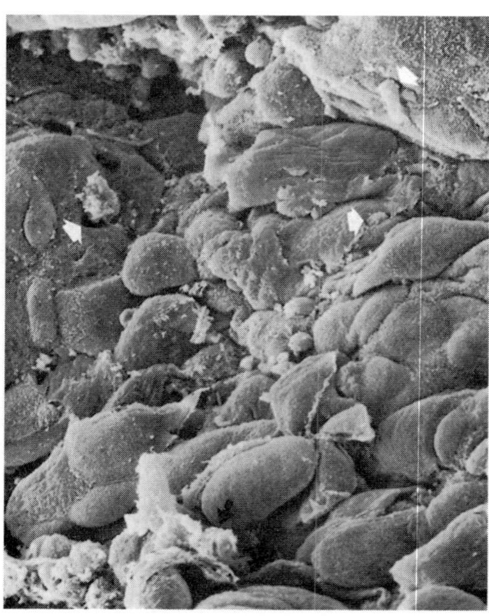

Fig. 22-11 Scanning electron micrograph of the periodontal pocket wall, frontal view, in a case of advanced periodontitis in a human. Note the desquamating epithelial cells and leukocytes *(white arrows)* emerging onto the pocket space. Scattered bacteria can also be seen *(black arrow).* Magnification ×1500.

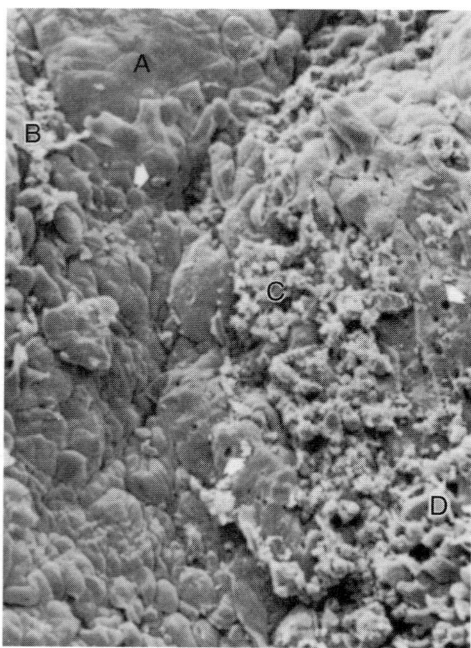

Fig. 22-10 Scanning electron frontal micrograph of the periodontal pocket wall. Different areas can be seen in the pocket wall surface. *A,* Area of quiescence; *B,* bacterial accumulation; *C,* bacterial-leukocyte interaction; *D,* intense cellular desquamation. Arrows point to emerging leukocytes and holes left by them in the pocket wall. Magnification ×800.

result of the interaction between the host and the bacteria. The following areas have been noted:

1. *Areas of relative quiescence,* showing a relatively flat surface with minor depressions and mounds and occasional shedding of cells (Fig. 22-10, *A*).
2. *Areas of bacterial accumulation,* which appear as depressions on the epithelial surface, with abundant debris and bacterial clumps penetrating into the enlarged intercellular spaces. These bacteria are mainly cocci, rods, and filaments, with a few spirochetes (see Fig. 22-10, *B*).
3. *Areas of emergence of leukocytes,* where leukocytes appear in the pocket wall through holes located in the intercellular spaces (Fig. 22-11).
4. *Areas of leukocyte-bacteria interaction,* where numerous leukocytes are present and covered with bacteria in an apparent process of phagocytosis. Bacterial plaque associated with the epithelium is seen either as an organized matrix covered by a fibrin-like material in contact with the surface of cells or as bacteria penetrating into the intercellular spaces (see Fig. 22-10, *C*).
5. *Areas of intense epithelial desquamation,* which consist of semi-attached and folded epithelial squames, sometimes partially covered with bacteria (Fig. 22-10, *D*).
6. *Areas of ulceration,* with exposed connective tissue (Fig. 22-12).
7. *Areas of hemorrhage,* with numerous erythrocytes.

The transition from one area to another could be postulated as follows: bacteria accumulate in previously quiescent areas, triggering the emergence of leukocytes and

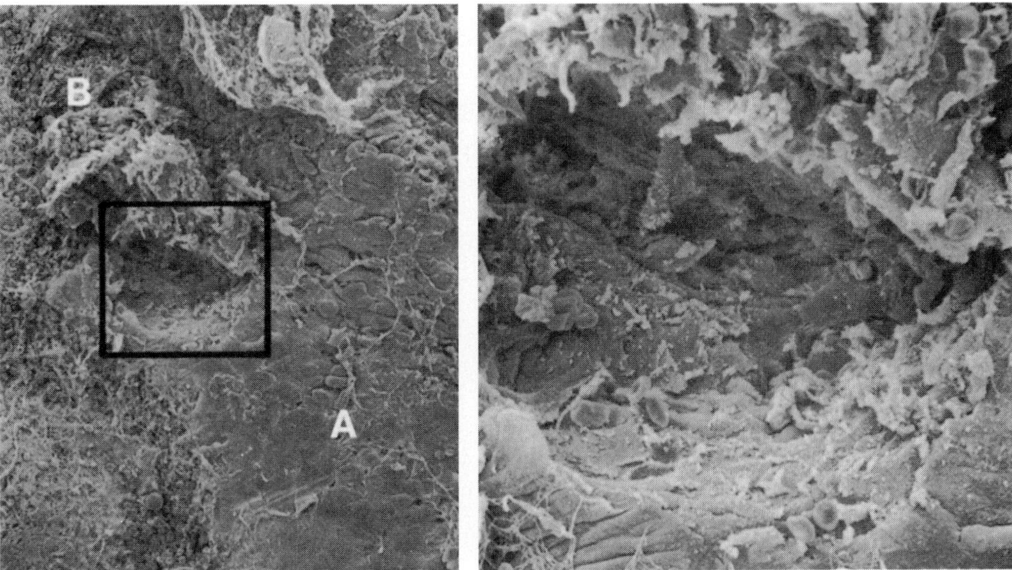

Fig. 22-12 *Left,* Area of ulceration in the lateral wall of a deep periodontal pocket in a human specimen. *A,* Surface of pocket epithelium in a quiescent state; *B,* area of hemorrhage. Magnification ×800. *Right,* Magnification of the square area on the left. Connective tissue fibers and cells can be seen in the bottom of the ulcer. Scanning electron microscopy. Magnification ×3000.

the leukocyte-bacteria interaction. This would lead to intense epithelial desquamation and finally to ulceration and hemorrhage.

Periodontal Pockets as Healing Lesions

Periodontal pockets are chronic inflammatory lesions and as such are constantly undergoing repair. Complete healing does not occur because of the persistence of the bacterial attack, which continues to stimulate an inflammatory response, causing degeneration of the new tissue elements formed in the continuous effort at repair.

The condition of the soft tissue wall of the periodontal pocket results from the interplay of the destructive and constructive tissue changes. Their balance determines clinical features such as color, consistency, and surface texture of the pocket wall. If the inflammatory fluid and cellular exudate predominate, the pocket wall is bluish-red, soft, spongy, and friable, with a smooth, shiny surface. If there is a relative predominance of newly formed connective tissue cells and fibers, the pocket wall is more firm and pink. At the clinical level, the former condition is generally referred to as an *edematous pocket wall* and the latter as a *fibrotic pocket wall* (see Chapter 30).

Edematous and fibrotic pockets represent opposite extremes of the same pathologic process, not different disease entities. They are subject to constant modification, depending on the relative predominance of exudative and constructive changes.

Fibrotic pocket walls may be misleading because they do not necessarily reflect what is taking place throughout the pocket wall. The most severe degenerative changes in periodontal tissues occur adjacent to the tooth surface and subgingival plaque. In some cases, inflammation and ulceration on the inside of the pocket are walled off by fibrous tissue on the outer aspect (Fig. 22-13). Outwardly the pocket appears pink and fibrotic, despite the inflammatory changes occurring within.

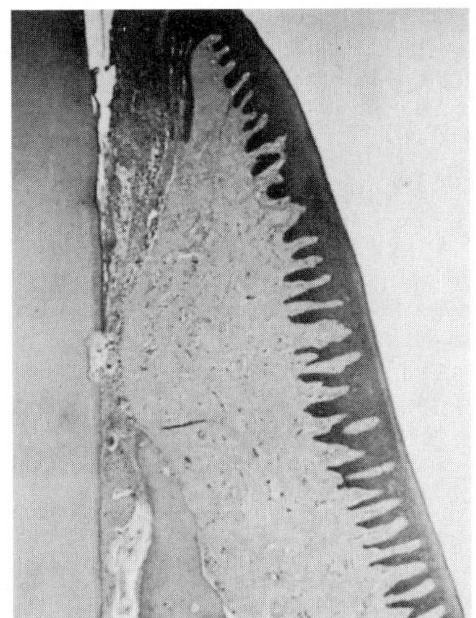

Fig. 22-13 Periodontal pocket wall. The inner half is inflamed and ulcerated; the outer half is densely collagenous.

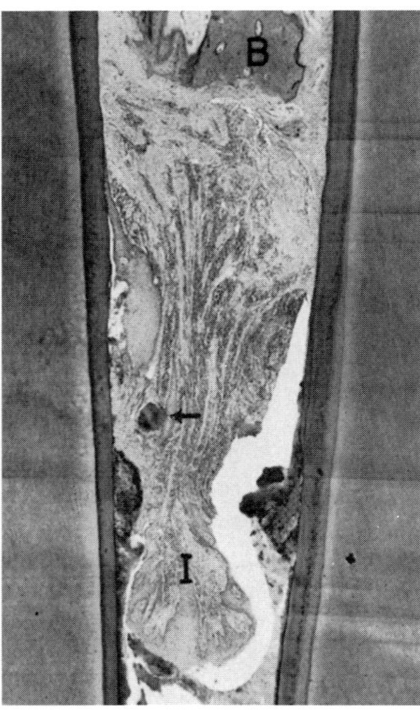

Fig. 22-14 Interdental papilla *(I)* with ulcerated suprabony periodontal pockets on its mesial and distal aspects. Calculus is present on the approximal tooth surfaces and within the gingiva *(arrow)*. The bone is shown at *B*.

Pocket Contents

Periodontal pockets contain debris consisting principally of microorganisms and their products (enzymes, endotoxins, and other metabolic products), gingival fluid, food remnants, salivary mucin, desquamated epithelial cells, and leukocytes. Plaque-covered calculus usually projects from the tooth surface (Fig. 22-14). Purulent exudate, if present, consists of living, degenerated, and necrotic leukocytes; living and dead bacteria; serum; and a scant amount of fibrin.[50] The contents of periodontal pockets filtered free of organisms and debris have been demonstrated to be toxic when injected subcutaneously into experimental animals.[35]

Significance of Pus Formation. There is a tendency to overemphasize the importance of the purulent exudate and to equate it with severity of periodontal disease. Because it is a dramatic clinical finding, early observers assumed that it was responsible for the loosening and exfoliation of the teeth. *Pus is a common feature of periodontal disease, but it is only a secondary sign.* The presence of pus or the ease with which it can be expressed from the pocket merely reflects the nature of the inflammatory changes in the pocket wall. It is not an indication of the depth of the pocket or the severity of the destruction of the supporting tissues. Extensive pus formation may occur in shallow pockets, whereas deep pockets may exhibit little or no pus.

Localized accumulation of pus constitutes an abscess, which is discussed later in this chapter.

Root Surface Wall

The root surface wall of periodontal pockets often undergoes changes that are significant because they may perpetuate the periodontal infection, cause pain, and complicate periodontal treatment.

As the pocket deepens, collagen fibers embedded in the cementum are destroyed and cementum becomes exposed to the oral environment. Collagenous remnants of Sharpey's fibers in the cementum undergo degeneration, creating an environment favorable to the penetration of bacteria. Viable bacteria have been found in the roots of 87% of periodontally diseased noncarious teeth.[1] Bacterial penetration into the cementum can be found as deep as the cementodentinal junction[2,19] and may also enter the dentinal tubules (Fig. 22-15).[31]

Pathologic granules[9] have been observed with optical and electron microscopy[6,7] and may represent areas of collagen degeneration or areas where collagen fibrils have not been fully mineralized initially.

Penetration and growth of bacteria leads to fragmentation and breakdown of the cementum surface and result in areas of necrotic cementum, separated from the tooth by masses of bacteria (Fig. 22-16).

In addition, bacterial products such as endotoxins[4,5] have also been detected in the cementum wall of periodontal pockets. When root fragments from teeth with periodontal disease are placed in tissue culture, they induce irreversible morphologic changes in the cells of the culture. Such changes are not produced by normal roots.[37] Diseased root fragments also prevent the in vitro attachment of human gingival fibroblasts, whereas normal root surfaces allow the cells to attach freely.[3] When reimplanted in the oral mucosa of the patient, diseased root fragments induce an inflammatory response even if they are autoclaved.[48]

These changes are manifested clinically by softening of the cementum surface, which is usually asymptomatic but painful when a probe or explorer penetrates the area. They also constitute a possible reservoir for reinfection of the area after treatment. In the course of treatment, these necrotic areas are removed by root planing until a hard smooth surface is reached. Cementum is very thin in the cervical areas, and scaling and root planing often removes it entirely, exposing the underlying dentin. Sensitivity to cold may result until secondary dentin is formed by the pulp tissue.

The following changes may also occur in the root surface wall of periodontal pockets:

Decalcification and Remineralization of Cementum. Areas of *increased mineralization*[69] are probably

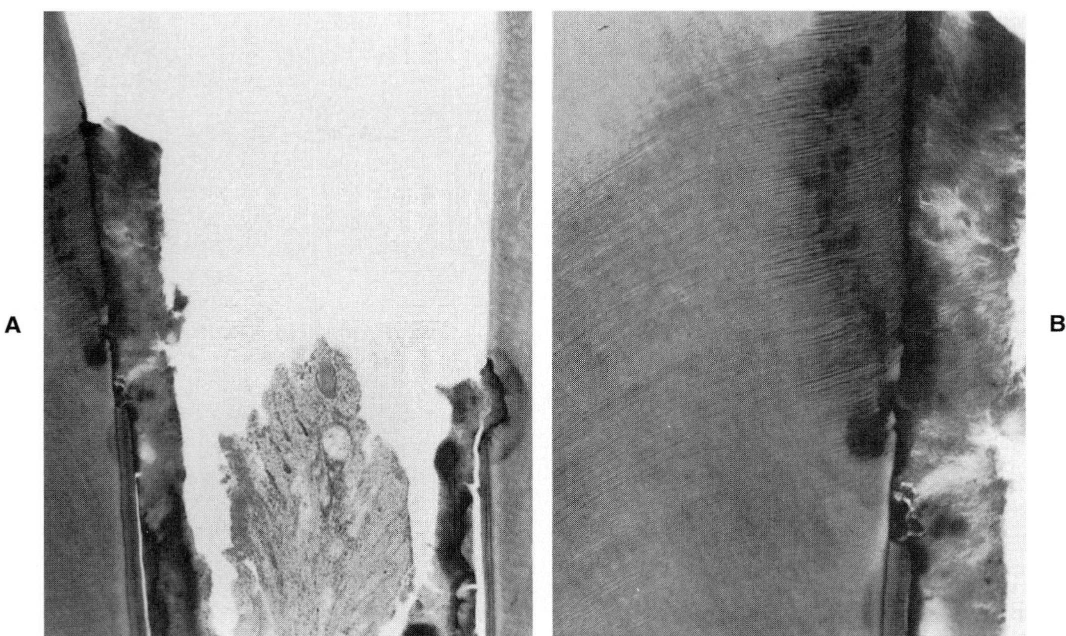

Fig. 22-15 Caries on root surfaces exposed by periodontal disease. **A,** Interdental space, showing inflamed gingiva and caries on proximal tooth surfaces. **B,** Caries of cementum and dentin, showing bacterial invasion of dentinal tubules. Note the filamentous structure of the dental plaque and darker staining of calculus adherent to the root.

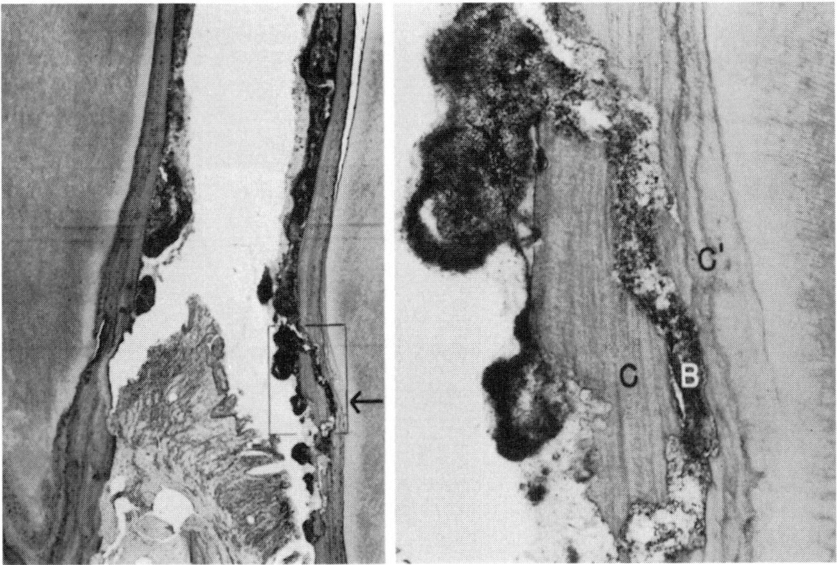

Fig. 22-16 *Left,* Mesiodistal section through an interdental space in a patient with extensive periodontal destruction. An area of cementum necrosis is enclosed within the rectangle designated by the arrow. *Right,* Detailed section of the rectangular area showing a necrotic fragment of cementum *(C)* separated from lamellated cementum *(C')* by clumps of bacteria *(B).*

a result of an exchange, on exposure to the oral cavity, of minerals and organic components at the cementum-saliva interface. The mineral content of exposed cementum increases.[68] The following minerals are increased in diseased root surfaces: calcium,[71] magnesium,[54,71] phosphorus,[54] and fluoride.[54] Microhardness, however, remains unchanged.[59,85] The development of a highly mineralized superficial layer may increase the tooth resistance to decay.[3]

The hypermineralized zones are detectable by electron microscopy and are associated with increased perfection of the crystal structure and organic changes suggestive of a subsurface cuticle.[68,69] These zones have also been seen in microradiographic studies[70] as a layer 10 to 20 μm thick, with areas as thick as 50 μm. No decrease in mineralization was found in deeper areas, thereby indicating that increased mineralization does not come from adjacent areas. A loss of, or reduction in, the cross-banding of collagen near the cementum surface[29,30] and a subsurface condensation of organic material of exogenous origin[68] have also been reported.

Areas of demineralization are commonly related to **root caries.** Exposure to oral fluid and bacterial plaque results in proteolysis of the embedded remnants of Sharpey's fibers; the cementum may be softened and may undergo fragmentation and cavitation.[38] Unlike enamel caries, root surface caries tend to progress around rather than into the tooth.[52] Active root caries lesions appear as well-defined yellowish or light-brown areas, are frequently covered by plaque, and have a softened or leathery consistency on probing.[26] Inactive lesions are well-defined darker lesions with a smooth surface and a harder consistency on probing.[26]

The dominant microorganism in root surface caries is *Actinomyces viscosus,*[76] although its specific responsibility in the development of the lesion has not been established.[26] Other bacteria such as *Actinomyces naeslundii, Streptococcus mutans, Streptococcus salivarius, Streptococcus sanguis,* and *Bacillus cereus* have been found to produce root caries in animal models. Quirynen et al[58] reported that when plaque levels and pocket depths fall after periodontal therapy (both conservative and surgical), a shift in oral bacteria occurs, leading to a reduction in periodontal pathogens and an increase in *S. mutans* and the development of root caries.

A prevalence rate study of root caries in 20- to 64-year-old individuals revealed that 42% had one or more root caries lesions and that these lesions tended to increase with age.[41]

The tooth may not be painful, but exploration of the root surface reveals the presence of a defect, and penetration of the involved area with a probe causes pain. Caries of the root, however, may lead to pulpitis, sensitivity to sweets and thermal changes, or severe pain. Pathologic exposure of the pulp occurs in severe cases. Root caries may be the cause of toothache in patients with periodontal disease and no evidence of coronal decay.

Caries of the cementum requires special attention when the pocket is treated. The necrotic cementum must be removed by scaling and root planing until firm tooth surface is reached, even if this entails extension into the dentin.

Areas of cellular resorption of cementum and dentin are common in roots unexposed by periodontal disease (see Figs. 2-16 and 22-16).[72] These areas are of no particular significance because they are symptom free, and as long as the root is covered by the periodontal ligament, they are apt to undergo repair. However, if the root is exposed by progressive pocket formation before repair of such areas occurs, these appear as isolated cavitations that penetrate into the dentin. These areas can be differentiated from caries of the cementum by their clear-cut outline and hard surface. They may be sources of considerable pain, requiring the placement of a restoration.

Surface Morphology of the Tooth Wall of Periodontal Pockets. This topic has been studied by several authors.[8,13,40,61,62,82] The following zones can be found in the bottom of a periodontal pocket (Fig. 22-17):

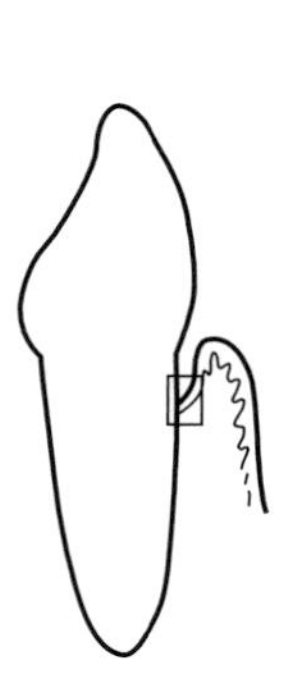

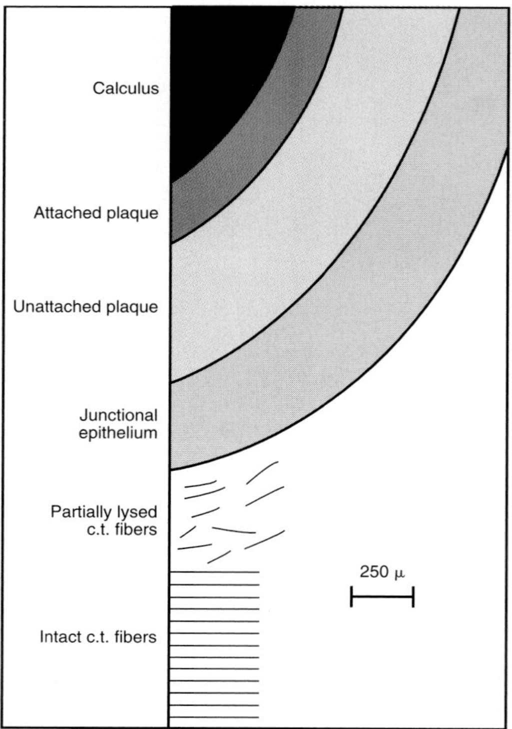

Fig. 22-17 Diagram of the area at the bottom of a pocket.

1. *Cementum covered by calculus,* where all the changes described in the preceding paragraphs can be found.
2. *Attached plaque,* which covers calculus and extends apically from it to a variable degree, probably 100 to 500 μm.
3. *The zone of unattached plaque* that surrounds attached plaque and extends apically to it.
4. The zone where the *junctional epithelium is attached to the tooth.* The extension of this zone, which in normal sulci is more than 500 μm, is usually reduced in periodontal pockets to less than 100 μm.
5. Apical to the junctional epithelium, there may be *a zone of semidestroyed connective tissue fibers* (see "Pathogenesis").

Areas 3, 4, and 5 compose the so-called *plaque-free zone* seen in extracted teeth. The total width of the plaque-free zone varies according to the type of tooth (it is wider in molars than in incisors) and the depth of the pocket (it is narrower in deeper pockets).[61] It is important to remember that the term *plaque-free zone* refers only to attached plaque because unattached plaque contains a variety of gram-positive cocci and various gram-negative morphotypes including cocci, rods, filaments, fusiforms, and spirochetes. The most apical zone contain predominantly gram-negative rods and cocci.[80]

PERIODONTAL DISEASE ACTIVITY

For many years the loss of attachment produced by periodontal disease was thought to be a slow but continuously progressive phenomenon. More recently, as a result of studies on the specificity of plaque bacteria, the concept of periodontal disease activity has evolved.

According to this concept, periodontal pockets go through periods of exacerbation and quiescence, resulting from episodic bursts of activity followed by periods of remission. *Periods of quiescence* are characterized by a reduced inflammatory response and little or no loss of bone and connective tissue attachment. A buildup of unattached plaque, with its gram-negative, motile, and anaerobic bacteria (see Chapter 6), starts a *period of exacerbation* in which bone and connective tissue attachment are lost and the pocket deepens. This period may last for days, weeks, or months and is eventually followed by a period of remission or quiescence in which gram-positive bacteria proliferate and a more stable condition is established. Based on a study of I_{125} absorptiometry, McHenry and colleagues have confirmed that bone loss in untreated periodontal disease occurs in an episodic manner.[49]

These periods of quiescence and exacerbation are also known as *periods of activity* and *inactivity.* Clinically, active periods show bleeding, either spontaneously or with probing, and greater amounts of gingival exudate. Histologically, the pocket epithelium appears thin and ulcerated, and an infiltrate composed predominantly of plasma cells,[20] polymorphonuclear leukocytes,[57] or both are seen. Bacterial samples from the pocket lumen, analyzed with darkfield microscopy, show high proportions of motile organisms and spirochetes.[47] Over time, loss of bone should be detected radiographically.

Methods to detect periods of activity or inactivity are currently being investigated (see Chapter 34).

SITE SPECIFICITY

Periodontal destruction does not occur in all parts of the mouth at the same time but rather on a few teeth at a time or even only some aspects of some teeth at any given time. This is referred to as the *site specificity* of periodontal disease. It is very common to find sites of periodontal destruction next to sites with little or no destruction. Therefore the severity of periodontitis increases by the development of new disease sites, the increased breakdown of existing sites, or both.

PULP CHANGES ASSOCIATED WITH PERIODONTAL POCKETS

The spread of infection from periodontal pockets may cause pathologic changes in the pulp. Such changes may give rise to painful symptoms or adversely affect the response of the pulp to restorative procedures. Involvement of the pulp in periodontal disease occurs through either the apical foramen or the lateral canals in the root after infection spreads from the pocket through the periodontal ligament. Atrophic and inflammatory pulpal changes occur in such cases (see also Chapters 64 and 65).

RELATION OF ATTACHMENT LOSS AND BONE LOSS TO POCKET DEPTH

Pocket formation causes loss of attachment of the gingiva and denudation of the root surface. The severity of the attachment loss is generally, but not always, correlated with the depth of the pocket. This is because the degree of attachment loss depends on the location of the base of the pocket on the root surface, whereas the pocket depth is the distance between the base of the pocket and the crest of the gingival margin. Pockets of the same depth may be associated with different degrees of attachment loss (Fig. 22-18), and pockets of different depths may be associated with the same amount of attachment loss (Fig. 22-19).

Severity of bone loss is generally, but not always, correlated with pocket depth. Extensive attachment and bone loss may be associated with shallow pockets if the

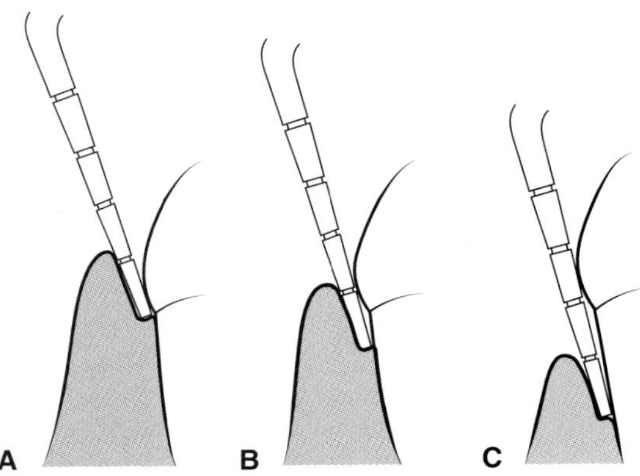

Fig. 22-18 Same pocket depth with different amounts of recession. **A,** Gingival pocket with no recession. **B,** Periodontal pocket of similar depth as in **A,** but with some degree of recession. **C,** Pocket depth same as in **A** and **B,** but with still more recession.

attachment loss is accompanied by recession of the gingival margin, and slight bone loss can occur with deep pockets.

AREA BETWEEN THE BASE OF THE POCKET AND THE ALVEOLAR BONE

Normally, the distance between the apical end of the junctional epithelium and the alveolar bone is relatively constant. The distance between the apical extent of calculus and the alveolar crest in human periodontal pockets is most constant, having a mean length of 1.97 mm ± 33.16%.[75,81]

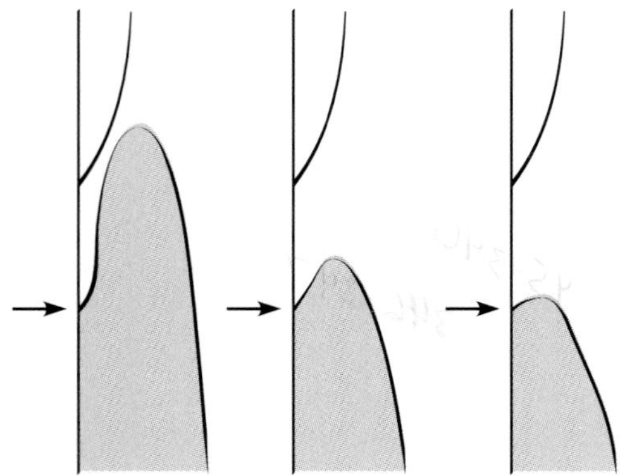

Fig. 22-19 Different pocket depths with the same amount of attachment loss. Arrows point to bottom of the pocket. The distance between the arrow and the cementoenamel junctions remains the same despite different pocket depths.

The distance from attached plaque to bone is never less than 0.5 mm and never more than 2.7 mm.[81,82] These findings suggest that the bone-resorbing activity induced by the bacteria is exerted within these distances. However, the finding of isolated bacteria, clumps of bacteria, or both in the connective tissue[64] and on the bone surface[28] may modify these considerations.

RELATIONSHIP OF THE PERIODONTAL POCKET TO BONE

In intrabony pockets, the base of the pocket is apical to the crest of the alveolar bone, and the pocket wall lies between the tooth and the bone. Intrabony pockets most often occur interproximally but may be located on the facial and lingual tooth surfaces. Most often the pocket spreads from the surface on which it originated to one or more contiguous surfaces. The suprabony pocket has its base coronal to the crest of the bone.

The inflammatory, proliferative, and degenerative changes in intrabony and suprabony pockets are the same, and both lead to destruction of the supporting periodontal tissues.

Differences between Intrabony and Suprabony Pockets

The principal differences between intrabony and suprabony pockets are the relationship of the soft tissue wall of the pocket to the alveolar bone, the pattern of bone destruction, and the direction of the transseptal fibers of the periodontal ligament[16] (Figs. 22-20 to 22-22).

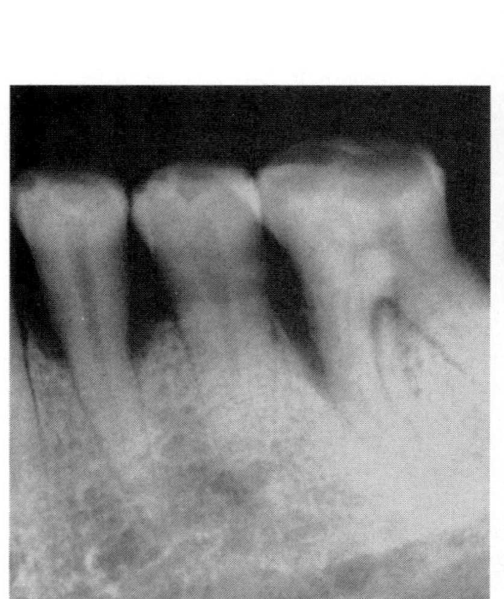

A

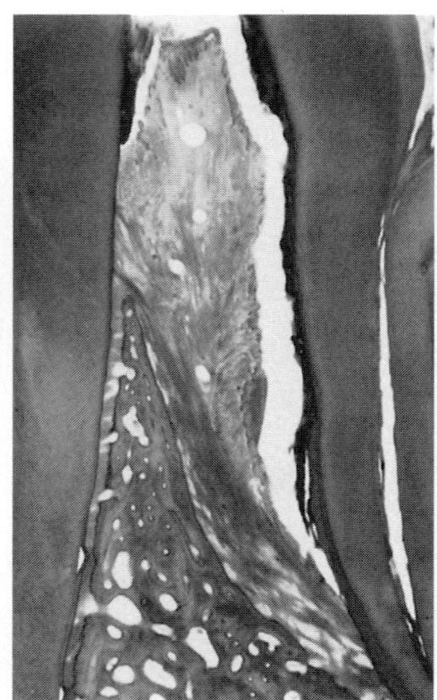

B

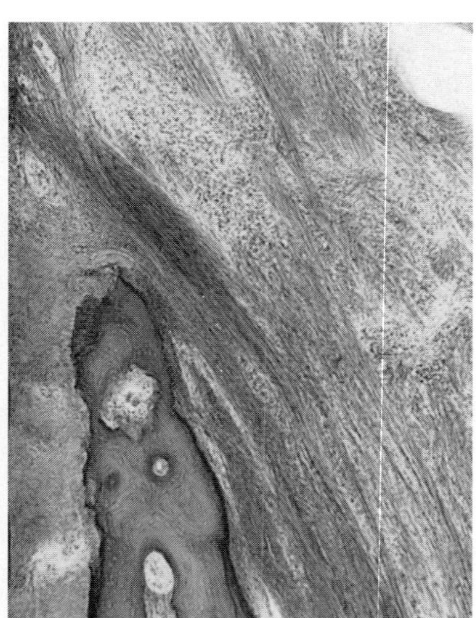

C

Fig. 22-20 Intrabony pocket on the mesial surface of a molar. **A,** Radiograph showing a deep angular defect on the mesial surface of the first molar. The bifurcation is also involved. Note the calculus on the mesial surface of the molar. **B,** Interdental space between the second premolar with a suprabony pocket *(left)* and the first molar with an intrabony pocket. Note the transseptal fibers that extend from the base of the intrabony pocket along the bone to the root of the premolar, the relationship of the epithelial lining of the pocket to the transseptal fibers, and the calculus on the root. **C,** Transseptal fibers extending from the distal surface of the premolar over the crest of the bone into the infrabony pocket. Note the leukocytic infiltration of the transseptal fibers.

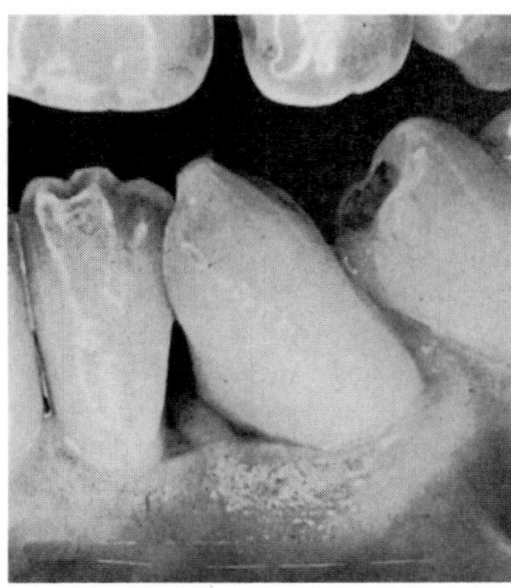

A

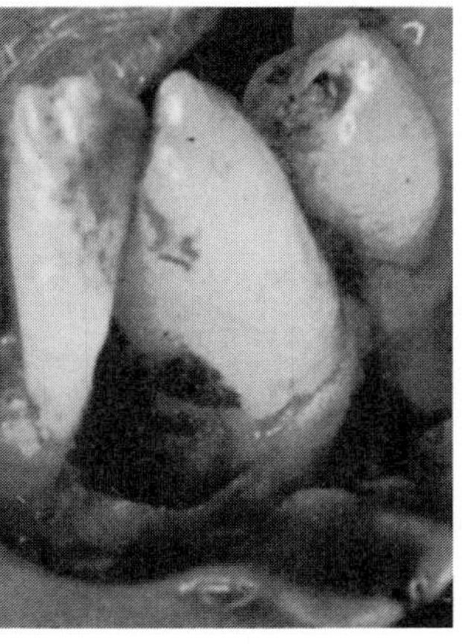

B

Fig. 22-21 Intrabony pocket on the mesial surface of the mandibular canine. **A,** Rolled gingival margin and space between gingiva and canine suggest the presence of a periodontal pocket. **B,** Flap reflected to show calculus on the root and a three-wall bone defect.

When loss of attachment and bone occur as a result of suprabony pockets, the alveolar crest and the periodontal ligament gradually attain a more apical position in relation to the tooth but retain their general morphology and architecture. This is usually associated with a horizontal pattern of bone loss. In intrabony pockets, the morphology of the alveolar crest changes completely with the formation of angular bony defects as a result of vertical bone loss. This may affect the function of the area.[14]

The distinguishing features of suprabony and intrabony pockets are summarized in Table 22-2. The morphologic features of the intrabony pocket are important because they necessitate modification in treatment techniques (see Chapters 62 and 63). The classification of intrabony pockets is discussed in Chapter 23.

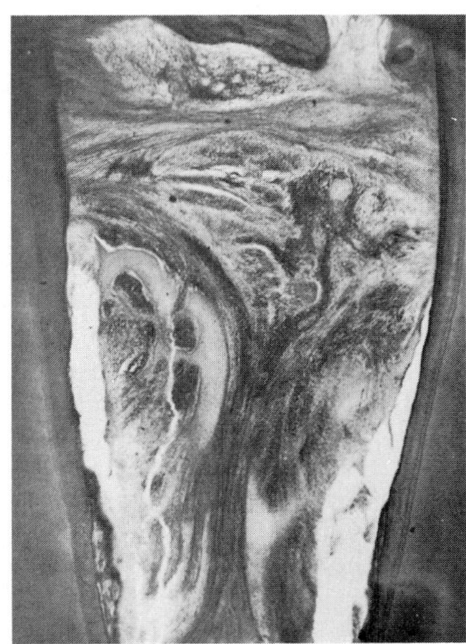

Fig. 22-22 Two suprabony pockets in an interdental space between the maxillary cuspid and the lateral incisor. Note the normal horizontal arrangement of the transseptal fibers.

PERIODONTAL ABSCESS

A periodontal abscess is a localized purulent inflammation in the periodontal tissues (Fig. 22-23). It is also known as a *lateral* or *parietal abscess.* Abscesses localized in the gingiva, caused by injury to the outer surface of the gingiva, and not involving the supporting structures are called *gingival abscesses.* They may occur in the presence or absence of a periodontal pocket (see Chapter 18).

Periodontal abscess formation may occur in the following ways:

1. Extension of infection from a periodontal pocket deeply into the supporting periodontal tissues and localization of the suppurative inflammatory process along the lateral aspect of the root.
2. Lateral extension of inflammation from the inner surface of a periodontal pocket into the connective tissue of the pocket wall. Localization of the abscess results when drainage into the pocket space is impaired (Fig. 22-24).
3. In a pocket that describes a tortuous course around the root, a periodontal abscess may form in the cul-de-sac, the deep end of which is shut off from the surface.
4. Incomplete removal of calculus during treatment of a periodontal pocket. In this instance, the gingival wall shrinks, occluding the pocket orifice, and a periodontal abscess occurs in the sealed-off portion of the pocket.
5. A periodontal abscess may occur in the absence of periodontal disease after trauma to the tooth or perforation of the lateral wall of the root in endodontic therapy.

Periodontal abscesses are classified according to location as follows:

1. *Abscess in the supporting periodontal tissues* along the lateral aspect of the root. In this condition, a sinus generally occurs in the bone that extends laterally from the abscess to the external surface.
2. *Abscess in the soft tissue wall of a deep periodontal pocket.*

TABLE 22-2

Distinguishing Features of the Suprabony and Intrabony Pockets

Suprabony Pocket	Intrabony Pocket
1. The base of the pocket is coronal to the level of the alveolar bone.	1. The base of the pocket is apical to the crest of the alveolar bone so that the bone is adjacent to the soft tissue wall (see Fig. 22-2).
2. The pattern of destruction of the underlying bone is horizontal.	2. The bone destructive pattern is vertical (angular) (see Figs. 22-20 and 22-21).
3. Interproximally, the transseptal fibers that are restored during progressive periodontal disease are arranged horizontally in the space between the base of the pocket and the alveolar bone (see Fig. 22-22).	3. Interproximally, the transseptal fibers are oblique rather than horizontal. They extend from the cementum beneath the base of the pocket along the bone and over the crest to the cementum of the adjacent tooth (see Fig. 22-20).
4. On the facial and lingual surfaces, the periodontal ligament fibers beneath the pocket follow their normal horizontal-oblique course between the tooth and the bone.	4. On the facial and lingual surfaces, the periodontal ligament fibers follow the angular pattern of the adjacent bone. They extend from the cementum beneath the base of the pocket along the bone and over the crest to join with the outer periosteum.

Microscopically, an abscess is a localized accumulation of viable and nonviable PMNs within the periodontal pocket wall. The PMNs liberate enzymes that digest the cells and other tissue structures, forming the liquid product known as *pus,* which constitutes the center of the abscess. An acute inflammatory reaction surrounds the purulent area, and the overlying epithelium exhibits intracellular and extracellular edema and invasion of leukocytes (Fig. 22-25).

The localized acute abscess becomes a chronic abscess when its purulent content drains through a fistula into the outer gingival surface or into the periodontal pocket and the infection causing the abscess is not resolved.

Bacterial invasion of tissues has been reported in abscesses; the invading organisms were identified as gram-negative cocci, diplococci, fusiforms, and spirochetes.[23] Invasive fungi were also found and were interpreted as being opportunistic invaders.[23] Microorganisms that colonize the periodontal abscess have been reported to be primarily gram-negative anaerobic rods.[55]

PERIODONTAL CYST

The periodontal cyst is an uncommon lesion that produces localized destruction of the periodontal tissues along a lateral root surface, most often in the mandibular canine–premolar area.[25,73]

The following possible etiologies have been suggested:

1. Odontogenic cyst caused by proliferation of the epithelial rests of Malassez; the stimulus initiating the cellular activity is not known.
2. Lateral dentigerous cyst retained in the jaw after tooth eruption.
3. Primordial cyst of supernumerary tooth germ.
4. Stimulation of epithelial rests of the periodontal ligament by infection from a periodontal abscess or the pulp through an accessory root canal.

A periodontal cyst is usually asymptomatic and without grossly detectable changes, but it may present as a localized tender swelling. Radiographically, an interproximal periodontal cyst appears on the side of the root as a radiolucent area bordered by a radiopaque line. Its radiographic appearance cannot be differentiated from that of a periodontal abscess.

Microscopically, the cystic lining may be (1) a loosely arranged, nonkeratinized, thickened, proliferating epithelium; (2) a thin, nonkeratinized epithelium; or (3) an odontogenic keratocyst.[25]

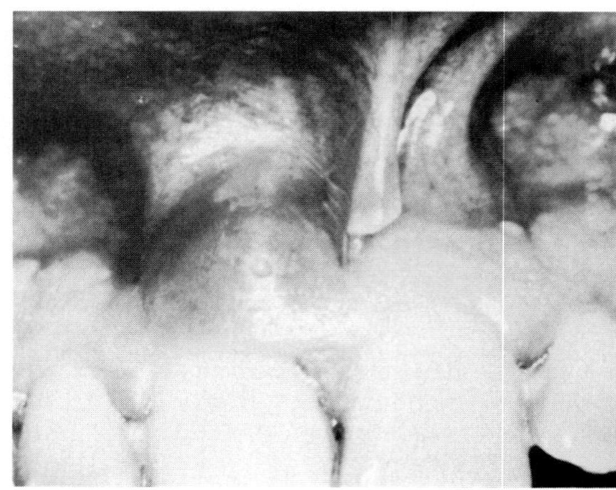

Fig. 22-23 Periodontal abscess on an upper central incisor.

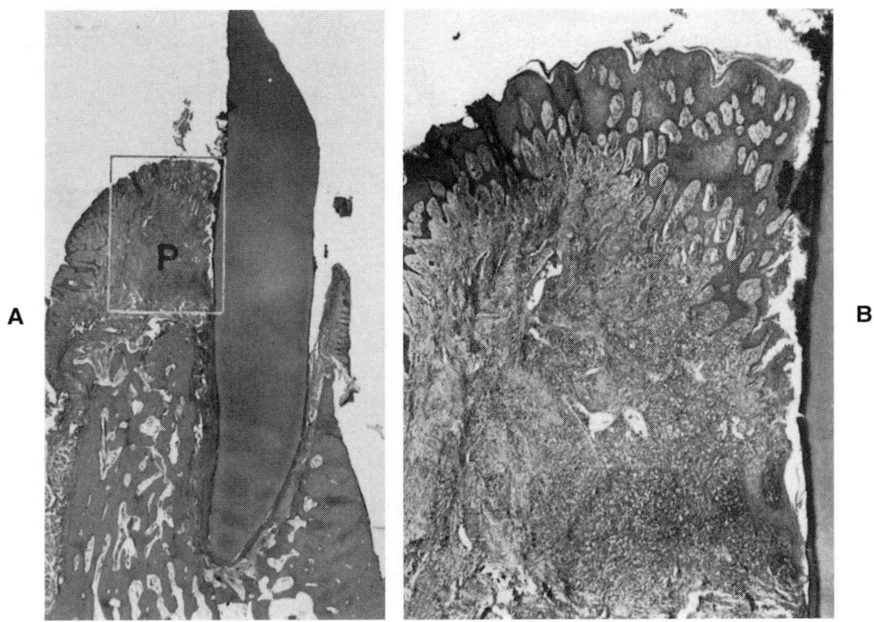

Fig. 22-24 **A,** Periodontal abscess (*P,* enclosed in rectangle) on the lingual surface of the mandibular incisor. **B,** Detailed view of a periodontal abscess showing dense leukocytic infiltration and suppuration.

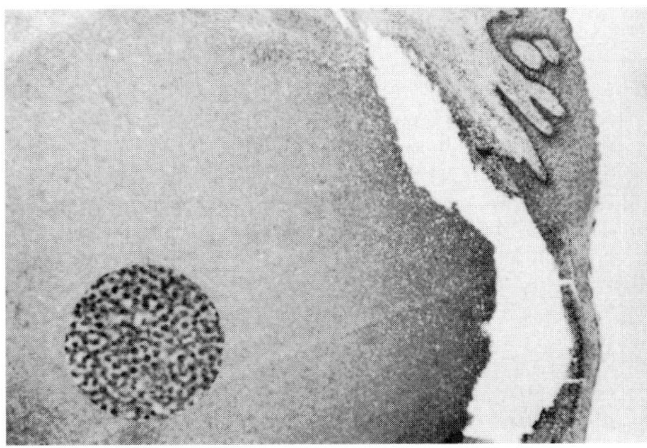

Fig. 22-25 Microscopic view of a periodontal abscess showing dense accumulation of polymorphonuclear neutrophils covered by stratified squamous epithelium. Inset, Magnification of PMNs. Bone loss and patterns of bone destruction.

REFERENCES

1. Adriaens PA, DeBoever JA, Loesche WJ: Bacterial invasion in root cementum and radicular dentin of periodontally diseased teeth in humans. A reservoir of periodontopathic bacteria. J Periodontol 1988; 59:222.
2. Adriaens, PA, DeBoever JA: Ultrastructural study of bacterial invasion in roots of periodontally diseased, caries-free human teeth. J Dent Res 1986; 65:770.
3. Aleo JJ, DeRenzis FA, Farber PA: In vitro attachment of human gingival fibroblasts to root surfaces. J Periodontol 1975; 46:639.
4. Aleo JJ, Vandersall DC: Cementum. Recent concepts related to periodontal disease therapy. Dent Clin North Am 1980; 24:627.
5. Aleo JJ, DeRenzis FA, Farber PA, et al: The presence and biologic activity of cementum-bound endotoxin. J Periodontol 1974; 45:672.
6. Armitage GC, Christie TM: Structural changes in exposed cementum. I. Light microscopic observations. J Periodont Res 1973; 8:343.
7. Armitage GC, Christie TM: Structural changes in exposed cementum. II. Electronmicroscopic observations. J Periodont Res 1973; 8:356.
8. Bass CC: A demonstrable line on extracted teeth indicating the location of the outer border of the epithelial attachment. J Dent Res 1946; 25:401.
9. Bass CC: A previously undescribed demonstrable pathologic condition in exposed cementum and the underlying dentine. Oral Surg 1951; 4:641.
10. Becks H: Normal and pathologic pocket formation. J Am Dent Assoc 1929; 16:2167.
11. Bonakdar MPS, Barber PM, Newman HN: The vasculature in chronic adult periodontitis: a qualitative and quantitative study. J Periodontol 1997; 68:50.
12. Bosshardt DD, Selvig KA: Dental cementum: the dynamic tissue covering the root. Periodontology 2000 1997; 13:41.
13. Brady JM: A plaque-free zone on human teeth: Scanning and transmission electron microscopy. J Periodontol 1973; 44:416.
14. Carranza FA, Carranza FA Jr: The management of alveolar bone in the treatment of the periodontal pocket. J Periodontol 1956; 27:29.
15. Carranza FA Jr: Histometric evaluation of periodontal pathology. A review of recent studies. J Periodontol 1967; 38:741.
16. Carranza FA Jr, Glickman I: Some observations on the microscopic features of the infrabony pockets. J Periodontol 1957; 28:33.
17. Christersson LA, Albini B, Zambon JJ, et al: Tissue localization of *Actinobacillus actinomycetemcomitans* in human periodontitis. I. Light, immunofluorescence and electronmicroscopic studies. J Periodontol 1987; 58:529.
18. Coons DB, Charbeneau TD, Rivera-Hidalgo F: Quantification of bacterial penetration in spontaneous periodontal disease in beagle dogs. J Periodontol 1989; 60:23.

19. Daly CG, Seymour GJ, Kieser JB, et al: Histological assessment of periodontally involved cementum. J Clin Periodontol 1982; 9:266.
20. Davenport RH Jr, Simpson DM, Hassell TM: Histometric comparison of active and inactive lesions of advanced periodontitis. J Periodontol 1982; 53:285.
21. Deporter DA, Brown DJ: Fine structural observations on the mechanisms of loss of attachment during experimental periodontal disease in the rat. J Periodont Res 1980; 15:304.
22. Deporter DA, Ten Cate AR: Collagen resorption by periodontal ligament fibroblasts at the hard tissue–ligament interfaces of the mouse molar periodontium. J Periodontol 1980; 51:429.
23. DeWitt GV, Cobb CM, Killoy WJ: The acute periodontal abscess: Microbial penetration of the soft tissue wall. Int J Periodont Restor Dent 1985; 5:39.
24. Euler H: Der Epithelansatz in neuere Beleuchtung. Vjschr Zahnheilk 1923; 29:103.
25. Fantasia JE: Lateral periodontal cyst. An analysis of 46 cases. Oral Surg Oral Med Oral Pathol 1979; 48:237.
26. Fejerskov O, Nyvad B: Pathology and treatment of dental caries in the aging individual. In: Holm-Pedersen P, Loe H (eds): Geriatric Dentistry. Copenhagen, Munksgaard, 1986.
27. Frank RM: Bacterial penetration in the apical wall of advanced human periodontitis. J Periodont Res 1980; 15:563.
28. Frank RM, Voegel RC: Bacterial bone resorption in advanced cases of human periodontitis. J Periodont Res 1978; 13:251.
29. Furseth R: Further observations on the fine structure of orally exposed carious human dental cementum. Arch Oral Biol 1971; 16:71.
30. Furseth R, Johanson E: The mineral phase of sound and carious human dental cementum studies by electron microscopy. Acta Odontol Scand 1970; 28:305.
31. Giuliana G, Ammatuna P, Pizzo G, et al: Occurrence of invading bacteria in radicular dentin of periodontally diseased teeth: microbiological findings. J Clin Periodontol 1997; 24:478.
32. Glickman I, Smulow JB: Periodontal disease: clinical, radiographic and histopathologic features. Philadelphia, Saunders, 1974.
33. Gottlieb B: Der Epithelansatz am Zahne. Dtsch Monatsschr Zahnheilk 1921; 39:142.
34. Gottlieb B: Biology of the cementum. J Periodontol 1942; 13:13.
35. Graham JW: Toxicity of sterile filtrate from parodontal pockets. Proc R Soc Med 1937; 30:1165.
36. Greenstein G, Lamster I: Changing periodontal paradigms: Therapeutic Implications. Int J Periodontics Restorative Dent 2000; 20:337.
37. Hatfield CG, Baumhammers A: Cytotoxic effects of periodontally involved surfaces of human teeth. Arch Oral Biol 1971; 16:465.
38. Herting HC: Electron microscope studies of the cementum surface structures of periodontally healthy and diseased teeth. J Dent Res 1967; 46(suppl):127.
39. Hillmann G, Dogan S, Gewrtsen W: Histopathological investigation of gingival tissue from patients with rapidly progressive periodontitis. J Periodontol 1998; 69:195.
40. Hoffman ID, Gold W: Distances between plaque and remnants of attached periodontal tissues on extracted teeth. J Periodontol 1971; 42:29.
41. Katz RV, Hazen SP, Chilton NW, et al: Prevalence and intraoral distribution of root caries in an adult population. Caries Res 1982; 16:265.
42. Krayer JW, Rees TD: Histologic observations on the topography of a human periodontal pocket viewed in transverse step-serial sections. J Periodontol 1993; 64:585.
43. Liakoni H, Barber P, Newman HN: Bacterial penetration of pocket soft tissues in chronic adult and juvenile periodontitis cases. An ultrastructural study. J Clin Periodontol 1987; 14:22.
44. Lindhe J, Liljenberg B, Listgarten MA: Some microbiological and histopathological features of periodontal disease in man. J Periodontol 1980; 52:264.
45. Listgarten MA: Structure of the microbial flora associated with periodontal health and disease in man. J Periodontol 1976; 47:1.
46. Listgarten MA: Pathogenesis of periodontitis. J Clin Periodontol 1986; 13:418.
47. Listgarten MA, Hellden L: Relative distributions of bacteria at clinically healthy and periodontally diseased sites in humans. J Clin Periodontol 1978; 5:665.
48. Lopez NJ, Belvederessi M, de la Sotta R: Inflammatory effects of periodontally diseased cementum studied by autogenous dental root implants in humans. J Periodontol 1980; 51:582.
49. McHenry KR, Hausman E, Genco RJ, et al: 125I absorptiometry: Alveolar bone mass measurements in untreated periodontal disease. Abstract. J Dent Res 1981; 60(suppl A):387.
50. McMillan L, Burrill DY, Fosdick LS: An electron microscope study of particulates in periodontal exudate. Abstract. J Dent Res 1958; 37:51.
51. Meyer DH, Screenivasan PK, Fives-Taylor PM: Evidence for the invasion of a human oral cell line by *Actinobacillus actinomycetemcomitans*. Infect Immun 1991; 59:2719.
52. Mount GJ: Root surface caries: A recurrent dilemma. Austr Dent J 1986; 31:288.
53. Müller-Glauser W, Schröder HE: The pocket epithelium: A light and electron microscopic study. J Periodontol 1982; 53:133.
54. Nakata T, Stepnick R, Zipkin I: Chemistry of human dental cementum. The effect of age and exposure on the concentration of F, Ca, P and Mg. J Periodontol 1972; 43:115.
55. Newman MG, Sims TN: The predominant cultivable microbiota of the periodontal abscess. J Periodontol 1979; 50:350.
56. Orban B, Ray AG: Deep necrotic foci in the gingiva. J Periodontol 1948; 19:91.
57. Page RC, Schroeder HH: Structure and pathogenesis. In: Schluger S, Youdelis R, Page R (eds): Periodontal Disease. Philadelphia, Lea & Febiger, 1977.
58. Quirynen M, Gizani S, Mongardini C, et al: The effect of periodontal therapy on the number of cariogenic bacteria in different intraoral niches. J Clin Periodontol 1999; 26:322.
59. Rautiola CA, Craig RG: The micro hardness of cementum and underlying dentin of normal teeth and teeth exposed to periodontal disease. J Periodontol 1961;32:113.
60. Saglie FR, Carranza FA Jr, Newman MG, et al: Scanning electron microscopy of the gingival wall of deep periodontal pockets in humans. J Periodont Res 1982j; 17:284.
61. Saglie FR, Johansen JR, Flotra L: The zone of completely and partially destroyed periodontal fibers in pathologic pockets. J Clin Periodontol 1975; 2:198.
62. Saglie FR, Johansen JR, Tollefsen T: Plaque-free zones on human teeth in periodontitis. J Clin Periodontol 1975; 2:190.
63. Saglie FR, Marfany A, Camargo P: Intragingival occurrence of *Actinobacillus actinomycetemcomitans* and *Bacteroides gingivalis* in active destructive periodontal lesions. J Periodontol 1988; 59:259.
64. Saglie FR, Newman MG, Carranza FA Jr, et al: Bacterial invasion of gingiva in advanced periodontitis in humans. J Periodontol 1982; 53:217.
65. Schroeder HE: Quantitative parameters of early human gingival inflammation. Arch Oral Biol 1970; 15:383.
66. Schroeder HE, Attstrom R: The Borderland between Caries and Periodontal Disease, vol 2. London, Grune & Stratton, 1980.

67. Schroeder HE, Listgarten MA: Fine Structure of the Developing Epithelial Attachment of Human Teeth. Monographs in Developmental Biology, vol 2. Basel, S Karger, 1977.
68. Selvig KA: Ultrastructural changes in cementum and adjacent connective tissue in periodontal disease. Acta Odontol Scand 1966; 24:459.
69. Selvig KA: Biological changes at the tooth-saliva interface in periodontal disease. J Dent Res 1969; 48(suppl):846.
70. Selvig KA, Hals E: Periodontally diseased cementum studied by correlated microradiography, electron probe analysis and electron microscopy. J Periodont Res 1977; 12:419.
71. Selvig KA, Zander HA: Chemical analysis and microradiography of cementum and dentin from periodontally diseased human teeth. J Periodontol 1962; 33:303.
72. Sottosanti JS: A possible relationship between occlusion, root resorption, and the progression of periodontal disease. J West Soc Periodontol 1977; 25:69.
73. Spouge JD: A new look at the rests of Malassez. A review of their embryological origin, anatomy, and possible role in periodontal health and disease. J Periodontol 1980; 51:437.
74. Standish SN, Shafer WG: The lateral periodontal cyst. J Periodontol 1958; 29:27.
75. Stanley HR: The cyclic phenomenon of periodontitis. Oral Surg Oral Med Oral Pathol 1955; 8:598.
76. Syed SA, Loesche WJ, Pape HL, et al: Predominant cultivable flora isolated from human root surface caries plaque. Infect Immunol 1975; 11:727.
77. Taichman N: Potential mechanisms of tissue destruction in periodontal disease. J Dent Res 1968; 47:928.
78. Takada T, Donath K: The mechanism of pocket formation. A light microscopic study of undecalcified human material. J Periodontol 1988; 59:215.
79. Ten Cate AR: Fibroblasts and their products. In: Ten Cate JR (ed): Oral Histology—Development, Structure and Function, ed 4. St Louis, Mosby, 1994.
80. Vrahopoulos TP, Barber PM, Newman HN: The apical border plaque in severe periodontitis. An ultrastructural study. J Periodontol 1995; 66:113.
81. Wade AB: The relation between the pocket base, the epithelial attachment and the alveolar process. In: Les Parodontopathies. 16th ARPA Congress, Vienna, 1960.
82. Waerhaug J: The gingival pocket. Odont Tidsk 1952; 60(suppl 1).
83. Waerhaug J: The angular bone defect and its relationship to trauma from occlusion and downgrowth of subgingival plaque. J Clin Periodontol 1979; 6:61.
84. Waerhaug J: The infrabony pocket and its relationship to trauma from occlusion and subgingival plaque. J Periodontol 1979; 50:355.
85. Warren EB, Hanse NM, Swartz ML, et al: Effects of periodontal disease and of calculus solvents on microhardness of cementum. J Periodontol 1964; 35:505.
86. Wittwer JW, Dickler EH, Toto PDL Comparative frequencies of plasma cells and lymphocytes in gingivitis. J Periodontol 1969; 40:274.
87. Zander HA: The attachment of calculus to root surfaces. J Periodontol 1953; 24:16.

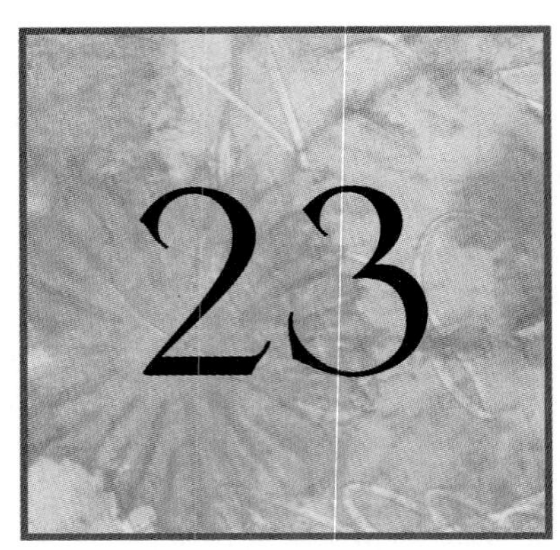

CHAPTER

Bone Loss and Patterns of Bone Destruction

Fermin A. Carranza

CHAPTER OUTLINE

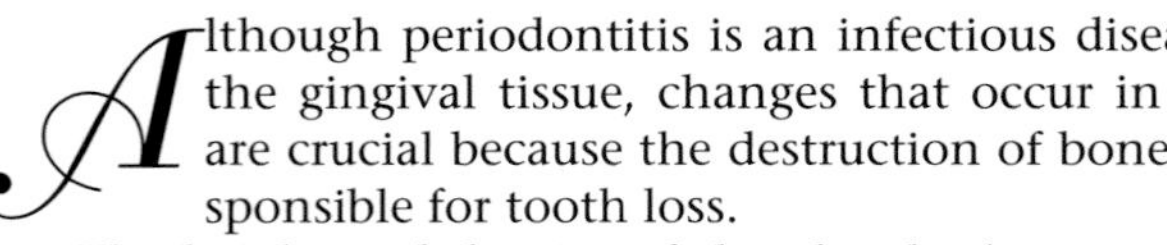

Although periodontitis is an infectious disease of the gingival tissue, changes that occur in bone are crucial because the destruction of bone is responsible for tooth loss.

The height and density of the alveolar bone are normally maintained by an equilibrium, regulated by local and systemic influences[12,16] between bone formation and bone resorption. When resorption exceeds formation, bone height, density, or both are reduced.

The level of bone is the consequence of past pathologic experiences, whereas changes in the soft tissue of the pocket wall reflect the present inflammatory condition. Therefore the degree of bone loss is not necessarily correlated with the depth of periodontal pockets, severity of ulceration of the pocket wall, or presence or absence of pus.

BONE DESTRUCTION CAUSED BY EXTENSION OF GINGIVAL INFLAMMATION

The most common cause of bone destruction in periodontal disease is the extension of inflammation from the marginal gingiva into the supporting periodontal tissues. The inflammatory invasion of the bone surface and the initial bone loss that follows mark the transition from gingivitis to periodontitis.

Periodontitis is always preceded by gingivitis, but not all gingivitis progresses to periodontitis. Some cases of gingivitis apparently never become periodontitis, and others go through a brief gingivitis phase and rapidly develop into periodontitis. The factors that are responsible for the extension of inflammation to the supporting structures and bring about the conversion of gingivitis to periodontitis are not known at this time.

The transition from gingivitis to periodontitis is associated with changes in the composition of bacterial plaque. In advanced stages of disease, the number of motile organisms and spirochetes increases whereas the number of coccoid rods and straight rods decreases.[36]

The cellular composition of the infiltrated connective tissue also changes with increasing severity of the lesion (see Chapter 16). Fibroblasts and lymphocytes predominate in stage I gingivitis, whereas the number of plasma cells and blast cells increases gradually as the disease progresses. Seymour and associates[66,67] have postulated a stage of "contained" gingivitis in which T lymphocytes are preponderant; they believe that as the lesion becomes a B-lymphocyte lesion, it becomes progressively destructive.

Heijl and co-workers[24] were able to convert a confined, naturally occurring chronic gingivitis into a progressive periodontitis in experimental animals by placing a silk ligature into the sulcus and tying it around the neck of the tooth. This induced ulceration of the sulcular epithelium, a shift in the connective tissue population from predominantly plasma cells to predominantly polymorphonuclear leukocytes, and osteoclastic resorption of the alveolar crest. The recurrence of episodes of acute destruction over time may be one mechanism leading to progressive bone loss in marginal periodontitis.

The extension of inflammation to the supporting structures of a tooth may be modified by the pathogenic potential of plaque or the resistance of the host. The latter includes immunologic activity and other tissue-related mechanisms, such as the degree of fibrosis of the gingiva, probably the width of the attached gingiva, and the reactive fibrogenesis and osteogenesis that occur peripheral to the inflammatory lesion. A fibrin-fibrinolytic system has been mentioned as "walling off" the advancing lesion.[59] The pathway of the spread of inflammation is critical because it affects the pattern of bone destruction in periodontal disease. Considerable controversy exists about the possible changes in the pathway of gingival inflammation caused by trauma from occlusion. The suggested change in the pathway of inflammation, going toward the periodontal ligament rather than to the bone,[13,39] has not been confirmed.[8,68]

Histopathology

Gingival inflammation extends along the collagen fiber bundles and follows the course of the blood vessels through the loosely arranged tissues around them into the alveolar bone[77] (Fig. 23-1). Although the inflammatory infiltrate is concentrated in the marginal periodontium, the reaction is a much more diffuse one, often reaching the bone and eliciting a response before evidence of crestal resorption or loss of attachment exists.[45] In the upper molar region, inflammation can extend to the maxillary sinus, resulting in thickening of the sinus mucosa.[44]

Interproximally, inflammation spreads to the loose connective tissue around the blood vessels, through the fibers, and then into the bone through vessel channels that perforate the crest of the interdental septum at the center of the crest (Fig. 23-2), toward the side of the crest (Fig. 23-3), or at the angle of the septum, and it may enter the bone through more than one channel. Less frequently, the inflammation spreads from the gingiva directly into the periodontal ligament and from there into the interdental septum (Fig. 23-4).[1]

Continued

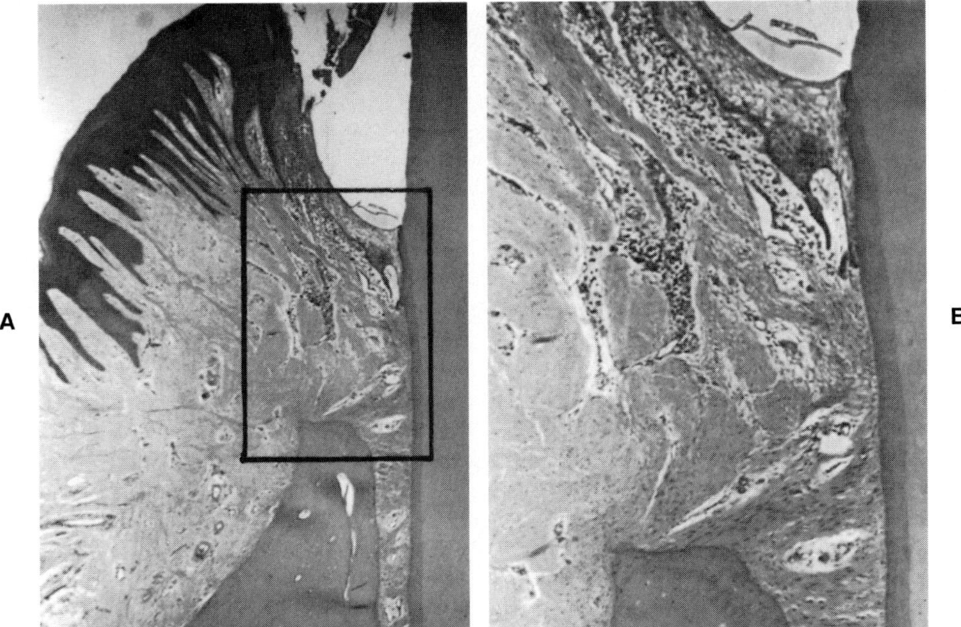

Fig. 23-1 **A,** Area of inflammation extending from the gingiva into the suprabony area. **B,** Detailed view of rectangular area in **A,** showing extension of inflammation along blood vessels in between collagen bundles.

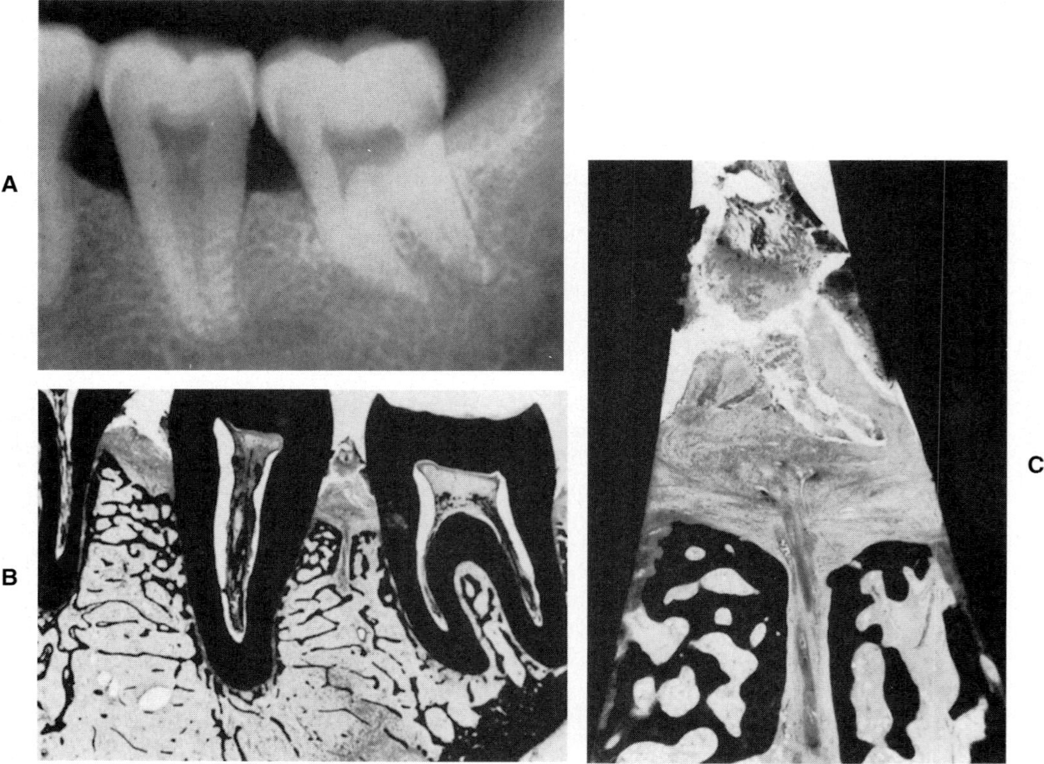

Fig. 23-2 Extension of inflammation into the center of the interdental septum. **A,** Molar region showing periodontal bone loss. **B,** Survey section of the second and third molars. **C,** Inflammation from the gingiva penetrates the transseptal fibers and enters the bone around blood vessel in the center of the septum.

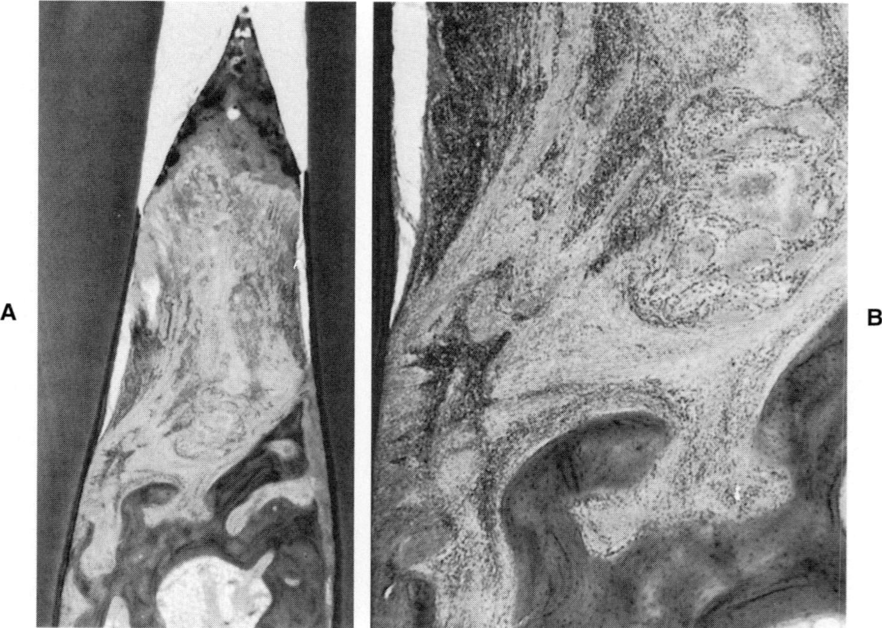

Fig. 23-3 Inflammation enters the interdental septum at the center of the crest and near the crestal angle. **A,** Interdental periodontal pockets with inflammation extending into the bone. **B,** Inflammation enters the crest of the interdental bone at two areas. Note the granular necrosis of the collagen fibers in the inflamed area above the bone.

Histopathology—cont'd

Facially and lingually, inflammation from the gingiva spreads along the outer periosteal surface of the bone (see Fig. 23-4) and penetrates into the marrow spaces through vessel channels in the outer cortex.

Along its course from the gingiva to the bone, the inflammation destroys the gingival and transseptal fibers, reducing them to disorganized granular fragments interspersed among the inflammatory cells and edema (Fig. 23-5).[49] However, there is a continuous tendency to recreate transseptal fibers across the crest of the interdental septum farther along the root as the bone destruction progresses. As a result, transseptal fibers are present, even in cases of extreme periodontal bone loss (Fig. 23-6).

The dense transseptal fibers are of clinical importance when surgical procedures are used to eradicate periodontal pockets. They form a firm covering over the bone, which is encountered after the superficial granulation tissue is removed.[54]

After inflammation reaches the bone by extension from the gingiva, it spreads into the marrow spaces and replaces the marrow with a leukocytic and fluid exudate, new blood vessels, and proliferating fibroblasts (Fig. 23-7). Multinuclear osteoclasts and mononuclear phagocytes increase in number, and the bone surfaces appear, lined with Howship's lacunae (Fig. 23-8).

In the marrow spaces, resorption proceeds from within, causing a thinning of the surrounding bony trabeculae and enlargement of the marrow spaces, followed by destruction of the bone and a reduction in bone height. Normally fatty bone marrow is partially or totally replaced by a fibrous type of marrow in the vicinity of the resorption.

Bone destruction in periodontal disease is not a process of bone necrosis.[29] It involves the activity of living cells along viable bone. When tissue necrosis and pus are present in periodontal disease, they occur in the soft tissue walls of periodontal pockets, not along the resorbing margin of the underlying bone.

The amount of inflammatory infiltrate correlates with the degree of bone loss but not with the number of osteoclasts. However, the distance from the apical border of the inflammatory infiltrate to the alveolar bone crest correlates with both the number of osteoclasts on the alveolar crest and the total number of osteoclasts.[58] Similar findings have been reported in experimentally induced periodontitis in animals.[34]

Radius of Action

Garant and Cho[11] suggested that locally produced bone resorption factors may have to be present in the proximity of the bone surface to be able to exert their action. Page and Schroeder,[53] on the basis of Waerhaug's measurements made on human autopsy specimens,[74,76] postulated a range of effectiveness of about 1.5 to 2.5 mm within which bacterial plaque can induce loss of bone.

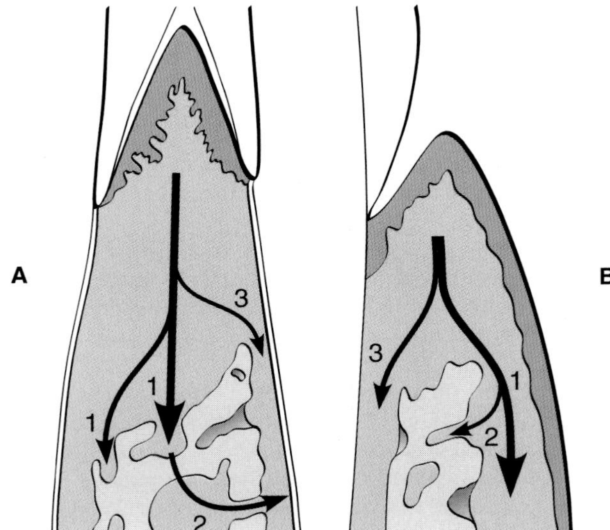

Fig. 23-4 Pathways of inflammation from the gingiva into the supporting periodontal tissues in periodontitis. **A,** Interproximally, from the gingiva into the bone *(1)*, from the bone into the periodontal ligament *(2)*, and from the gingiva into the periodontal ligament *(3)*. **B,** Facially and lingually, from the gingiva along the outer periosteum *(1)*, from the periosteum into the bone *(2)*, and from the gingiva into the periodontal ligament *(3)*.

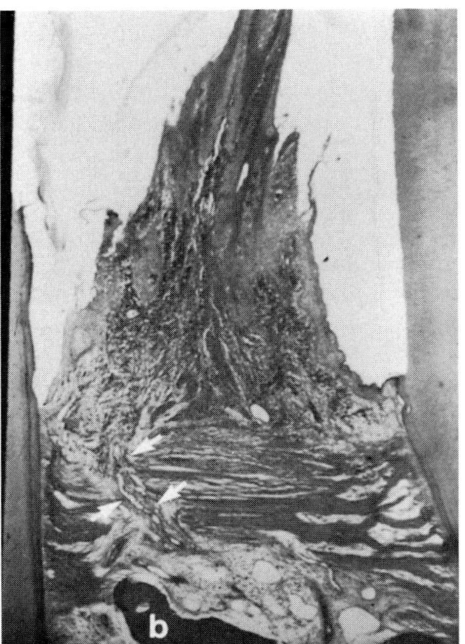

Fig. 23-5 Interruption, destruction, or both of transseptal fibers *(arrows)* as inflammation extends to the bone *(b)* around blood vessels.

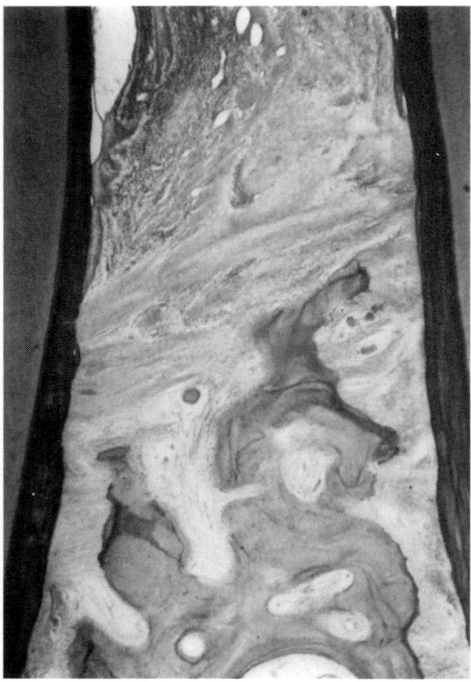

Fig. 23-6 Reformation of transseptal fibers. Mesiodistal section through interdental septum showing gingival inflammation and bone loss. Recreated transseptal fibers can be seen above the bone margin, partially infiltrated by the inflammatory process.

Beyond 2.5 mm there is no effect; interproximal angular defects can appear only in spaces that are wider than 2.5 mm because narrower spaces would be destroyed entirely. Tal[70] corroborated this with measurements in human patients.

Large defects far exceeding a distance of 2.5 mm from the tooth surface (as described in aggressive types of periodontitis) may be caused by the presence of bacteria in the tissues.[6,10,62]

Rate of Bone Loss

In a study of Sri Lankan tea laborers with no oral hygiene and no dental care, Löe and associates found the rate of bone loss to average about 0.2 mm a year for facial surfaces and about 0.3 mm a year for proximal surfaces when periodontal disease was allowed to progress untreated.[37] However, the rate of bone loss may vary, depending on the type of disease present. Löe and co-workers[38] identified three subgroups of patients with periodontal disease based on interproximal loss of attachment* and tooth mortality:

1. Approximately 8% of persons had rapid progression of periodontal disease, characterized by a yearly loss of attachment of 0.1 to 1 mm.
2. Approximately 81% of individuals had moderately progressive periodontal disease, with a yearly loss of attachment of 0.05 to 0.5 mm.
3. The remaining 11% of persons had minimal or no progression of destructive disease (0.05 to 0.09 mm yearly).

*Loss of attachment can be equated with loss of bone, although the former precedes the latter by about 6 to 8 months.[21]

Periods of Destruction

Periodontal destruction occurs in an episodic, intermittent fashion, with periods of inactivity or quiescence. The destructive periods result in loss of collagen and alveolar bone with deepening of the periodontal pocket. The reasons for the onset of destructive periods have not been totally elucidated, although the following theories have been offered:

1. Bursts of destructive activity are associated with subgingival ulceration and an acute inflammatory reaction, resulting in rapid loss of alveolar bone.[53,63]
2. Bursts of destructive activity coincide with the conversion of a predominately T-lymphocyte lesion to one with a predominance of B-lymphocyte–plasma cell infiltrate.[67]
3. Periods of exacerbation are associated with an increase of the loose, unattached, motile, gram-negative, anaerobic pocket flora, and periods of remission coincide with the formation of a dense, unattached, nonmotile, gram-positive flora with a tendency to mineralize.[47]
4. Tissue invasion by one or several bacterial species is followed by an advanced local host defense that controls the attack.[61]

Mechanisms of Bone Destruction

The factors involved in bone destruction in periodontal disease are bacterial and host mediated. Bacterial plaque products induce the differentiation of bone progenitor cells into osteoclasts and stimulate gingival cells to release mediators that have the same effect.[23,65] Plaque products and inflammatory mediators can also act directly on osteoblasts or their progenitors, inhibiting their action and reducing their numbers.

In addition, in rapidly progressing diseases such as localized juvenile periodontitis, bacterial microcolonies or single bacterial cells may be present between collagen fibers and over the bone surface, suggesting a direct effect.[6,65]

Several host factors released by inflammatory cells are capable of inducing bone resorption in vitro and can play a role in periodontal disease. These include host-produced prostaglandins and their precursors, interleukin 1-α and -β, and tumor necrosis factor (TNF)-α.

When injected intradermally, prostaglandin E_2 induces the vascular changes seen in inflammation; when injected over a bone surface, it induces bone resorption in the absence of inflammatory cells and with few multinucleated osteoclasts.[18,28] In addition, nonsteroidal anti-inflammatory drugs, such as flurbiprofen or ibuprofen, inhibit prostaglandin E_2 production, slowing bone loss in naturally occurring periodontal disease in beagle dogs and humans. This effect occurs without changes in gingival inflammation and rebounds 6 months after cessation of administration of the drug.[27,78] (See also Chapters 6 to 9.)

Bone Formation in Periodontal Disease

Areas of bone formation are also found immediately adjacent to sites of active bone resorption (Fig. 23-9) and along trabecular surfaces at a distance from the inflammation in an apparent effort to reinforce the remaining bone (buttressing bone formation). This osteogenic response is clearly found in experimentally produced periodontal bone loss in animals.[7] In humans, it is less obvious but has been confirmed by histometric[4,5] and histologic studies.[14]

The response of alveolar bone to inflammation includes bone formation and resorption; thus bone loss in periodontal disease is not simply a destructive process but results from the predominance of resorption over formation. New bone formation retards the rate of bone loss, compensating in some degree for the bone destroyed by inflammation.

Autopsy specimens from individuals with untreated disease occasionally show areas where bone resorption has ceased and new bone is being formed on previously eroded bone margins. This confirms the intermittent character of bone resorption in periodontal disease and is consistent with the varied rates of progression observed clinically in untreated periodontal disease.

These periods of remission and exacerbation (or inactivity and activity, respectively) appear to coincide with the quiescence or exacerbation of gingival inflammation, manifested by changes in the extent of bleeding, amount of exudate, and composition of bacterial plaque (see Chapter 22).

The presence of bone formation in response to inflammation, even in active periodontal disease, has a bearing on the outcome of treatment. The basic aim of periodontal therapy is the elimination of inflammation to remove the stimulus for bone resorption and therefore allow the inherent constructive tendencies to predominate.

BONE DESTRUCTION CAUSED BY TRAUMA FROM OCCLUSION

Another cause of periodontal destruction is trauma from occlusion. Trauma from occlusion can produce bone destruction in the absence or presence of inflammation (see also Chapter 24).

In the absence of inflammation, the changes caused by trauma from occlusion vary from increased compression and tension of the periodontal ligament and increased osteoclasis of alveolar bone to necrosis of the periodontal ligament and bone and resorption of bone and tooth structure. These changes are reversible in that they can be repaired if the offending forces are removed. However, persistent trauma from occlusion results in funnel-shaped widening of the crestal portion of the periodontal ligament, with resorption of the adjacent bone.[35] These changes, which may cause the bony crest to have an angular shape, represent adaptation of the periodontal tissues aimed at "cushioning" increased occlusal forces, but the modified bone shape may weaken tooth support and cause tooth mobility.

When combined with inflammation, trauma from occlusion aggravates the bone destruction caused by the inflammation[35] and causes bizarre bone patterns.

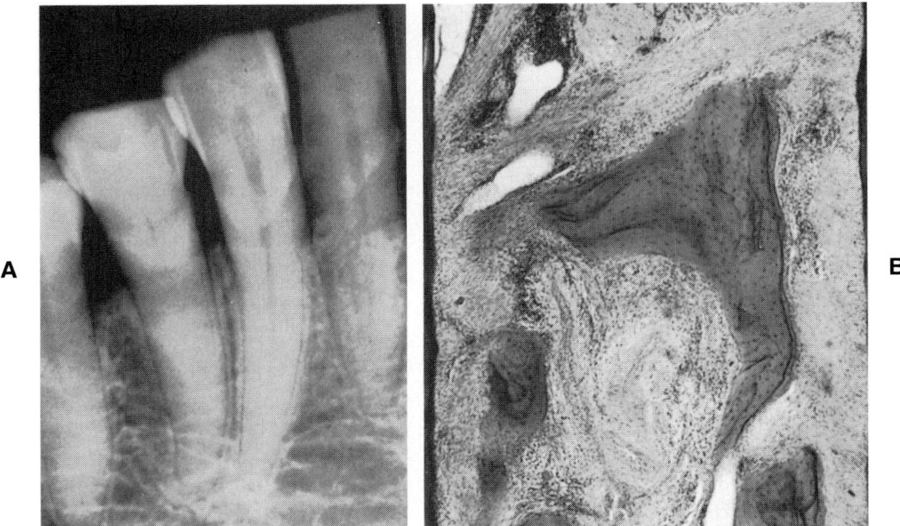

Fig. 23-7 Early periodontal bone destruction. **A,** Early bone loss in the canine and premolar areas. **B,** Interdental septum beneath the periodontal pockets between the canine and first premolar. The inflammation has invaded the marrow space, and lacunar resorption of the surrounding bone surface is evident. Note the inflammation in the periodontal ligament in the right side.

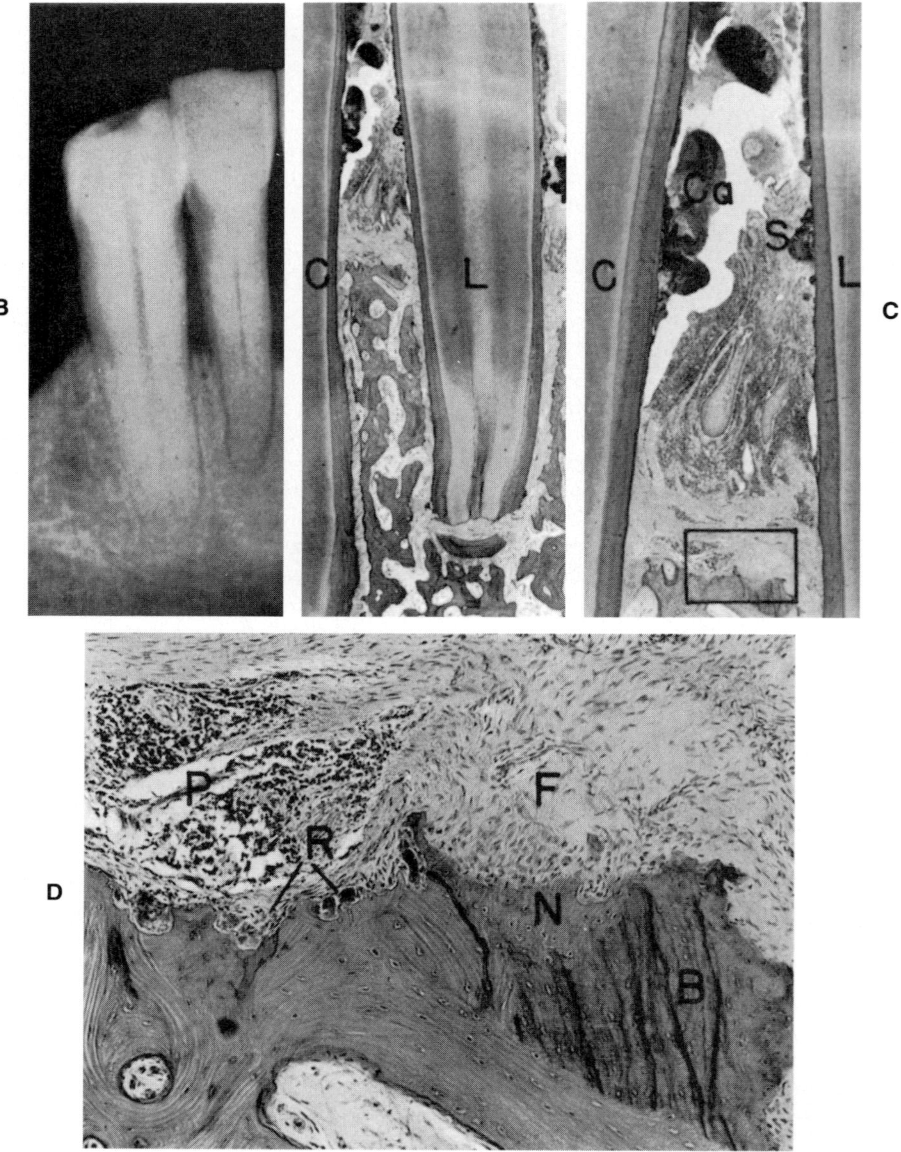

Fig. 23-8 Bone resorption and formation in periodontal disease. **A,** Lateral incisor and canine with bone loss. **B,** Survey section of lateral incisor *(L)* and canine *(C)*. **C,** Interdental space between lateral incisor *(L)* and canine *(C)*, showing calculus *(Ca)* and periodontal pockets with suppuration *(S)*. **D,** A detailed view of the bone margin within the rectangle showing bone margin beneath the periodontal pockets. Note the osteoclastic resorption *(R)* beneath the inflammation *(P)* and newly formed bone *(N)* with a thin surface layer of osteoid and osteoblasts adjacent to the resorption. The new bone is separated from the lamellated bone *(B)* by an irregular resorption line. An area of fibrosis is shown at *F.*

BONE DESTRUCTION CAUSED BY SYSTEMIC DISORDERS

Local and systemic factors regulate the physiologic equilibrium of bone. When a generalized tendency toward bone resorption exists, bone loss initiated by local inflammatory processes may be magnified. This systemic influence on the response of alveolar bone has been termed the *bone factor in periodontal disease.*[12]

The *bone factor concept,* developed by Irving Glickman[12] in the early 1950s, envisioned a systemic component in all cases of periodontal disease. In addition to the amount and virulence of plaque bacteria, the nature of the systemic component, not its presence or absence, influences the severity of periodontal destruction. Although the term *bone factor* is not in current use, the concept of a role played by systemic defense mechanisms has been validated, particularly by studies of immune deficiencies in severely destructive types of periodontitis, such as the juvenile forms of the disease.

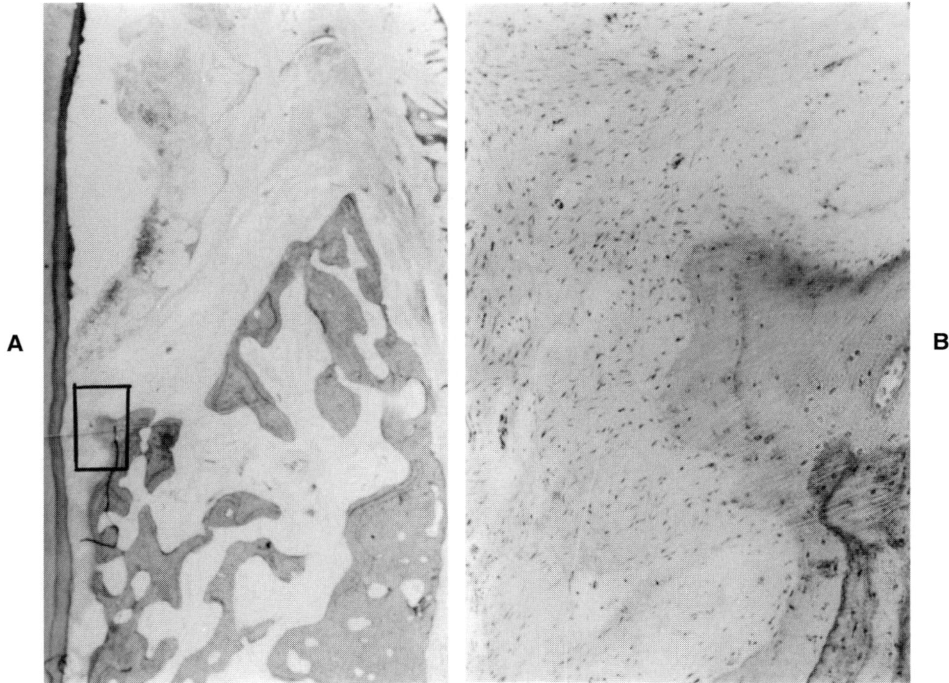

Fig. 23-9 Bone formation in untreated periodontal disease. **A,** Section showing an infrabony pocket with deep angular bone loss. **B,** Magnification of the rectangular area in **A,** showing newly formed bone at bottom of defect.

In recent years, interest has increased in the possible relationship between periodontal bone loss and osteoporosis. **Osteoporosis** is a physiologic condition of postmenopausal women, resulting in loss of bone mineral content and structural bone changes. Periodontitis and osteoporosis share a number of risk factors (e.g., aging, smoking, diseases, and medications that interfere with healing). Few studies on the relationship between periodontitis and osteoporosis are available, and some show relationships between skeletal density and oral bone density and between crestal height and residual ridge resorption. In 1968, Groen et al[20] reported relationships between osteopenia and periodontal disease, tooth mobility and tooth loss. Several more recent studies have indicated that such an association may exist, but final proof is lacking.[25,26,62,73]

Periodontal bone loss may also occur in generalized skeletal disturbances (e.g., hyperparathyroidism, leukemia, or Langerhans' cell histiocytosis) by mechanisms that may be totally unrelated to the usual periodontal problem.

FACTORS DETERMINING BONE MORPHOLOGY IN PERIODONTAL DISEASE

Normal Variation in Alveolar Bone

Considerable normal variation in the morphologic features of alveolar bone exists (see Chapter 2), which affects the osseous contours produced by periodontal disease. The anatomic features that substantially affect the bone destructive pattern in periodontal disease include the following:

- The thickness, width, and crestal angulation of the interdental septa
- The thickness of the facial and lingual alveolar plates
- The presence of fenestrations, dehiscences, or both
- The alignment of the teeth
- Root and root trunk anatomy
- Root position within the alveolar process
- Proximity with another tooth surface

For example, angular osseous defects cannot form in thin facial or lingual alveolar plates, which have little or no cancellous bone between the outer and inner cortical layers. In such instances the entire crest of the plate is destroyed, and the height of the bone is reduced (Fig. 23-10).

Exostoses

Exostoses are outgrowths of bone of varied size and shape. Palatal exostoses have been found in 40% of human skulls.[46] They can occur as small nodules, large nodules, sharp ridges, spike-like projections, or any combination of these (see Fig. 23-20). Exostoses have been described in rare cases as developing after the placement of free gingival grafts.[50]

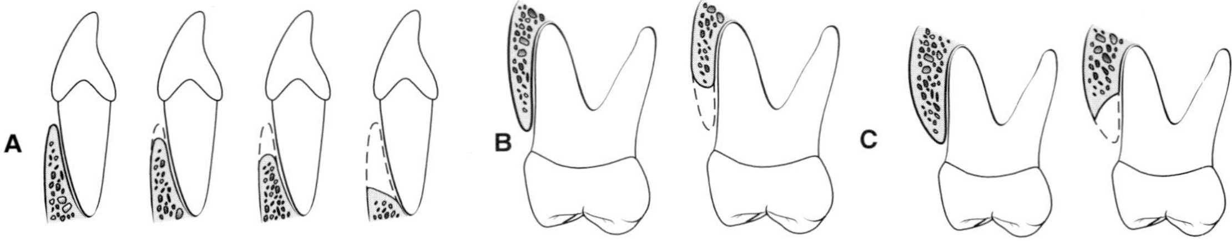

Fig. 23-10 **A,** A lower incisor with thin labial bone. Bone loss can become vertical only when it reaches thicker bone in apical areas. **B,** Upper molars with thin facial bone, where only horizontal bone loss can occur. **C,** Upper molar with a thick facial bone, allowing for vertical bone loss.

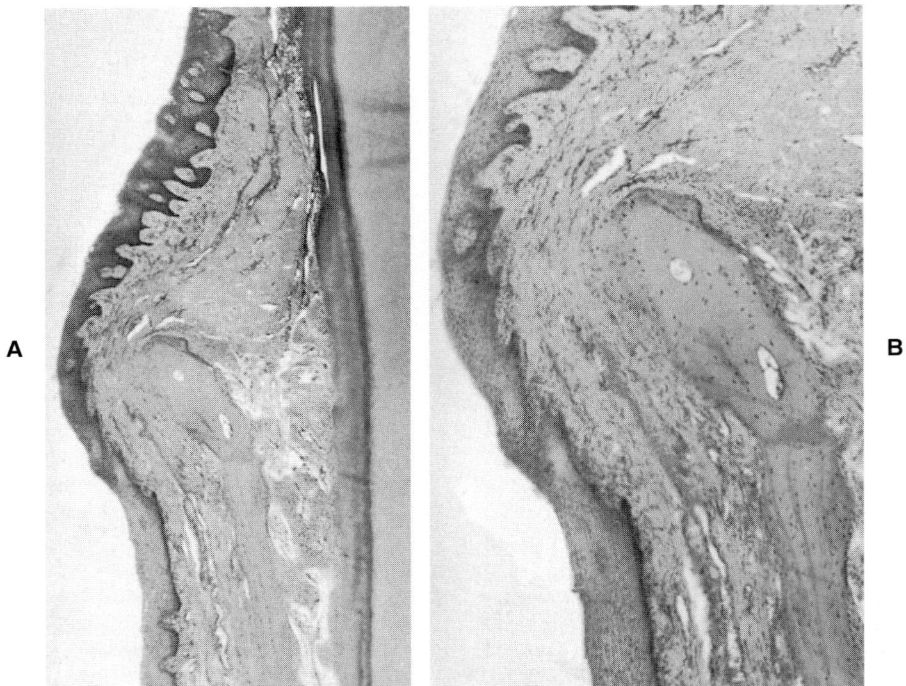

Fig. 23-11 Lipping of facial bone. **A,** Peripheral buttressing bone formation along the external surface of the facial bony plate and at the crest. Note the deformity in the bone produced by the buttressing bone formation and the bulging of the mucosa. **B,** Detailed view showing lipping and deformity produced by buttressing bone formation.

Trauma from Occlusion

Trauma from occlusion may be a factor in determining the dimension and shape of bone deformities. It may cause a thickening of the cervical margin of alveolar bone or a change in the morphology of the bone (e.g., angular defects and buttressing bone [see following discussion]) on which inflammatory changes will later be superimposed.

Buttressing Bone Formation (Lipping)

Bone formation sometimes occurs in an attempt to buttress bony trabeculae weakened by resorption. When it occurs within the jaw, it is termed *central buttressing bone formation.* When it occurs on the external surface, it is referred to as *peripheral buttressing bone formation.*[14] The latter may cause bulging of the bone contour, termed *lipping,* which sometimes accompanies the production of osseous craters and angular defects (Fig. 23-11).

Food Impaction

Interdental bone defects often occur where proximal contact is abnormal or absent. Pressure and irritation from food impaction contribute to the inverted bone architecture. In some instances the poor proximal relationship may be the result of a shift in tooth position because of extensive bone destruction preceding food

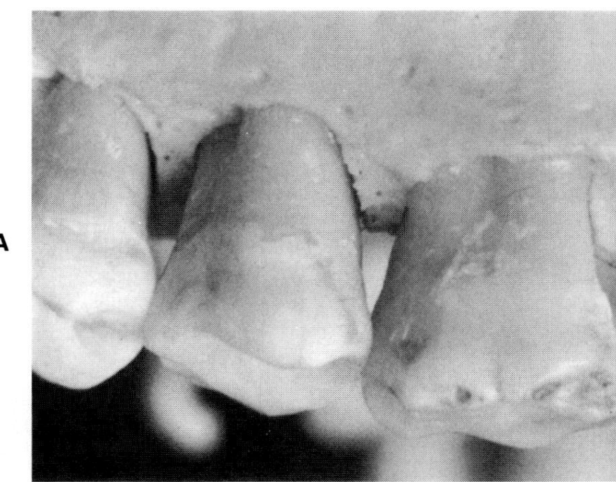
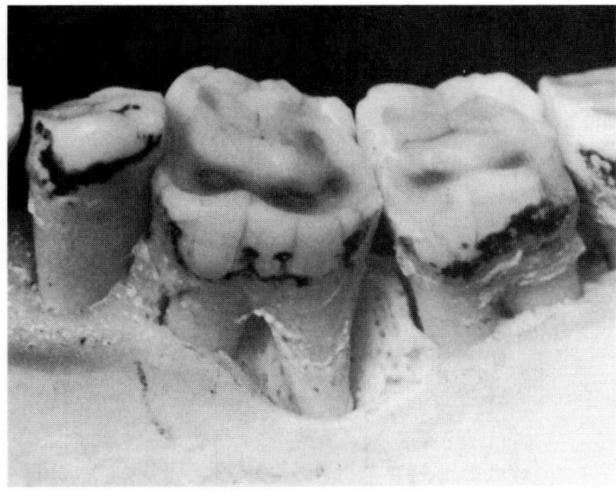

Fig. 23-12 A, Horizontal bone loss. Note the reduction in height of the marginal bone, exposing cancellous bone and reaching the furca of the second molar. **B,** Vertical (angular) bone loss on the distal root of the first molar.

impaction. In such cases, food impaction is a complicating factor rather than the cause of the bone defect.

Juvenile Periodontitis

A vertical or angular pattern of alveolar bone destruction is found around the first molars in juvenile periodontitis. The cause of the localized bone destruction in this type of periodontal disease is unknown (see Chapter 28).

BONE DESTRUCTION PATTERNS IN PERIODONTAL DISEASE

Periodontal disease alters the morphologic features of the bone in addition to reducing bone height. An understanding of the nature and pathogenesis of these alterations is essential for effective diagnosis and treatment.

Horizontal Bone Loss

Horizontal bone loss is the most common pattern of bone loss in periodontal disease. The bone is reduced in height, but the bone margin remains roughly perpendicular to the tooth surface. The interdental septa and facial and lingual plates are affected, but not necessarily to an equal degree around the same tooth (Fig. 23-12, *A*).

Bone Deformities (Osseous Defects)

Different types of bone deformities can result from periodontal disease. These usually occur in adults and have been reported in human skulls with deciduous dentitions.[30] Their presence may be suggested on radiographs, but careful probing and surgical exposure of the areas is required to determine their exact conformation and dimensions.

Vertical or Angular Defects

Vertical or angular defects are those that occur in an oblique direction, leaving a hollowed-out trough in the bone alongside the root; the base of the defect is located apical to the surrounding bone (see Figs. 23-12, *B*; 23-13; and 23-14). In most instances, angular defects have accompanying infrabony pockets; such pockets always have an underlying angular defect.

Angular defects are classified on the basis of the number of osseous walls.[17] Angular defects may have one, two, or three walls (Figs. 23-15 to 23-17). The number of walls in the apical portion of the defect may be greater than that in its occlusal portion, in which case the term *combined osseous defect* is used (Fig. 23-18).

Vertical defects occurring interdentally can generally be seen on the radiograph, although thick, bony plates sometimes may obscure them. Angular defects can also appear on facial and lingual or palatal surfaces, but these defects are not seen on radiographs. Surgical exposure is the only sure way to determine the presence and configuration of vertical osseous defects.

Vertical defects increase with age.[48,52,79] Approximately 60% of persons with interdental angular defects have only a single defect.[48] Vertical defects detected radiographically have been reported to appear most commonly on the distal surfaces[48] and mesial surfaces.[52,79] However, three-wall defects are more frequently found on the mesial surfaces of upper and lower molars.[31]

The three-wall vertical defect was originally called an *intrabony defect.** This defect appears most frequently on the mesial aspects of second and third maxillary and mandibular molars. The one-wall vertical defect is also called a *hemiseptum.*

* The term *intrabony* was later expanded to designate all vertical defects.

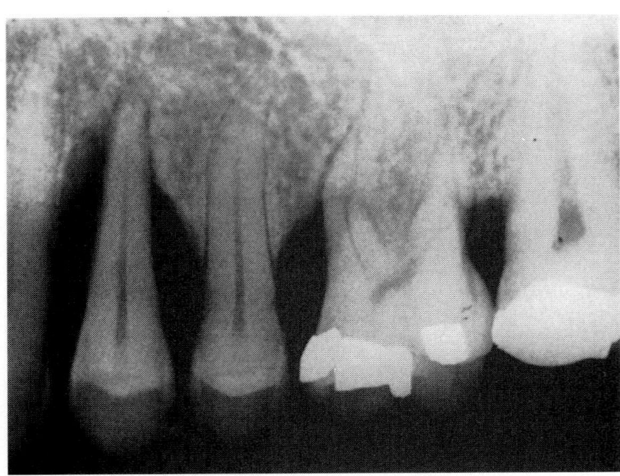

Fig. 23-13 Angular (vertical) defects of different depths.

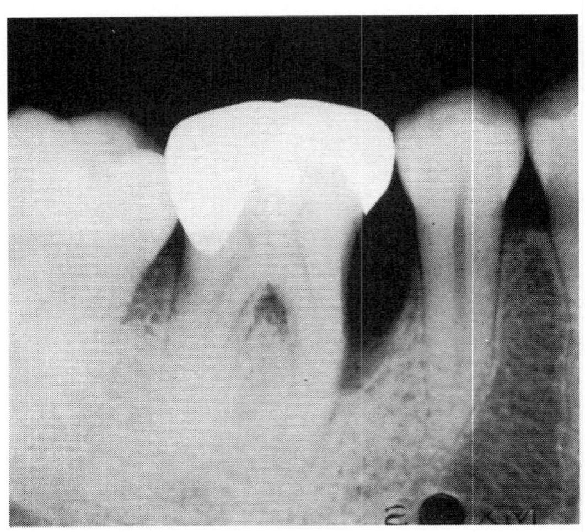

Fig. 23-14 Angular defect on the mesial surface of the first molar. Note also the furcation involvement.

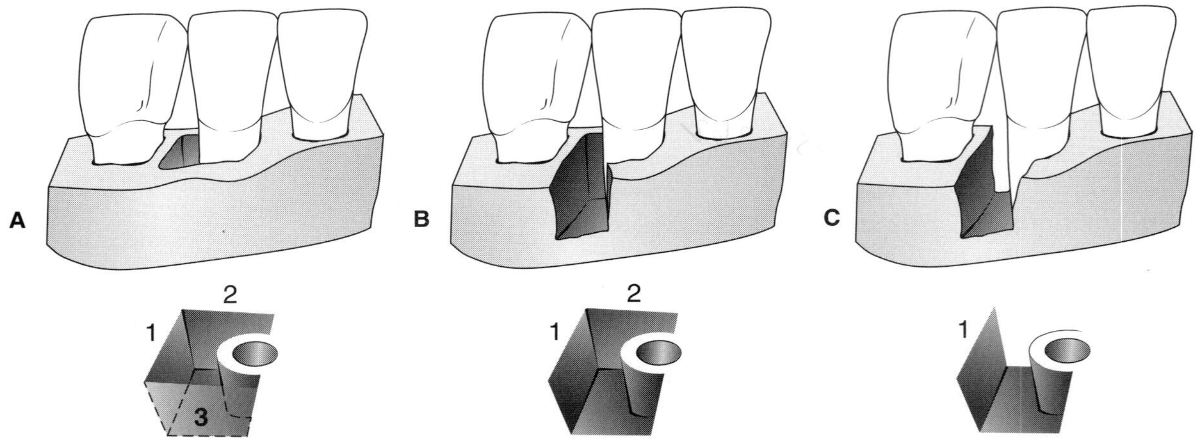

Fig. 23-15 One-, two-, and three-walled vertical defects on right lateral incisor. **A,** Three bony walls: distal *(1)*, lingual *(2)*, and facial *(3)*. **B,** Two-wall defect: distal *(1)* and lingual *(2)*. **C,** One-wall defect: distal wall only *(1)*.

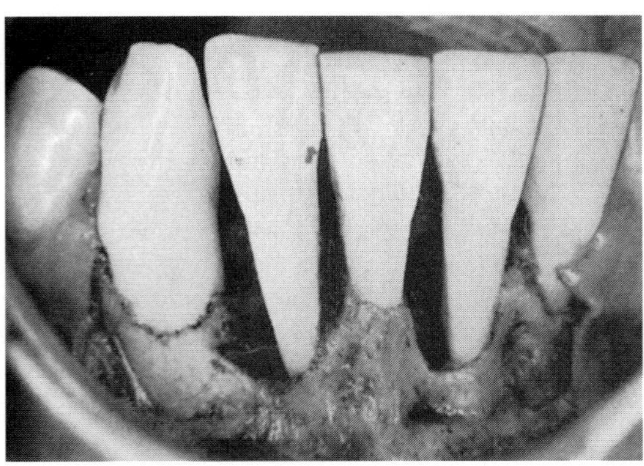

Fig. 23-16 One-wall vertical defect on the mesial surface of the left lateral incisor and $1\frac{1}{2}$-wall defect (distal wall and half of the labial wall) on the distal surface of the right lateral incisor.

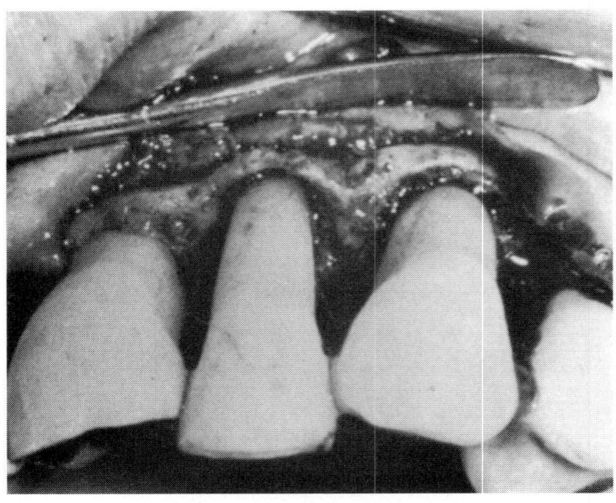

Fig. 23-17 Circumferential vertical defect in relation to the upper lateral incisor and canine.

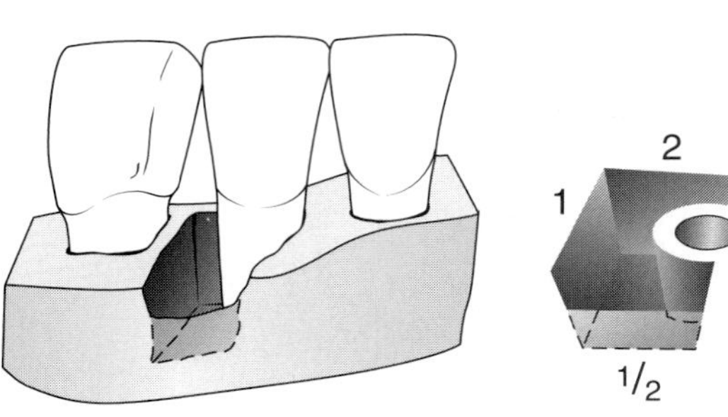

Fig. 23-18 Combined type of osseous defect. Because the facial wall is half the height of the distal *(1)* and lingual *(2)* walls, this is an osseous defect with three walls in its apical half and two walls in the occlusal half.

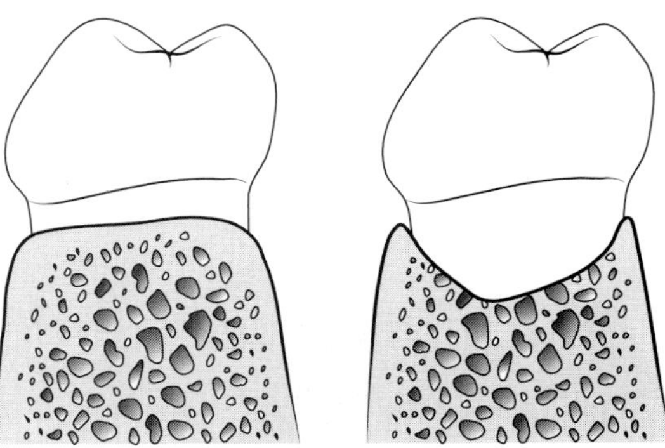

Fig. 23-19 Diagrammatic representation of an osseous crater in a faciolingual section between two lower molars. *Left,* Normal bone contour. *Right,* Osseous crater.

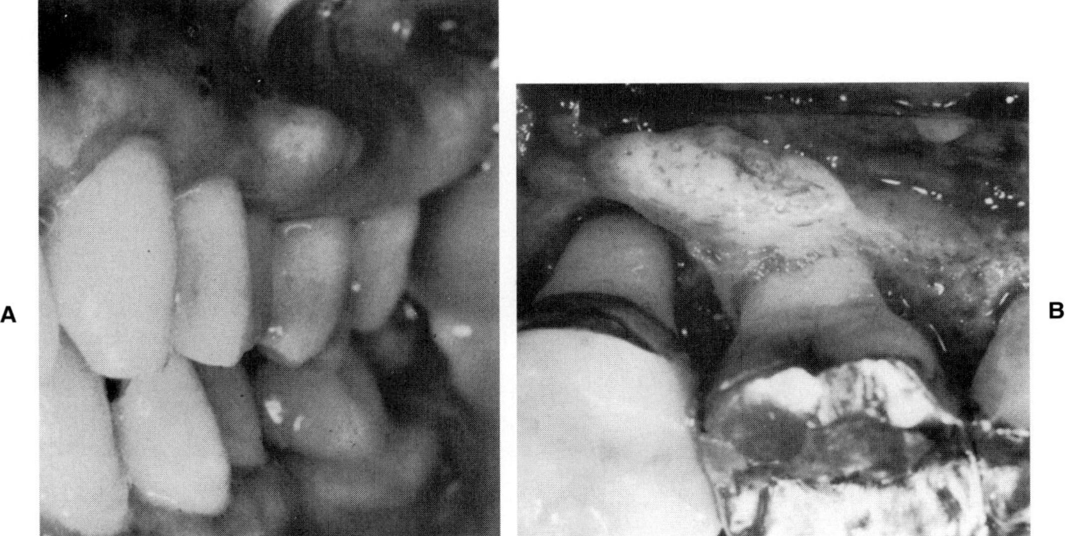

Fig. 23-20 **A,** Exostosis in the facial aspect. **B,** Exostosis in the palatal aspect. Note also the circumferential defect in the second molar.

Osseous Craters

Osseous craters are concavities in the crest of the interdental bone confined within the facial and lingual walls (Fig. 23-19). Craters have been found to make up about one third (35.2%) of all defects and about two thirds (62%) of all mandibular defects. They are twice as common in posterior segments as in anterior segments.[42,43]

The heights of the facial and lingual crests of a crater have been found to be identical in 85% of cases, with the remaining 15% being nearly equally divided between higher facial crests and higher lingual crests.[60] The following reasons for the high frequency of interdental craters have been suggested:

- The interdental area collects plaque and is difficult to clean.
- The normal flat or even concave faciolingual shape of the interdental septum in lower molars may favor crater formation.
- Vascular patterns from the gingiva to the center of the crest may provide a pathway for inflammation.[40,41,60]

Bulbous Bone Contours

Bulbous bone contours are bony enlargements caused by exostoses, adaptation to function, or buttressing bone formation (Fig. 23-20). They are found more frequently in the maxilla than in the mandible.

Reversed Architecture

Reversed architecture defects are produced by loss of interdental bone, including the facial plates, lingual plates,

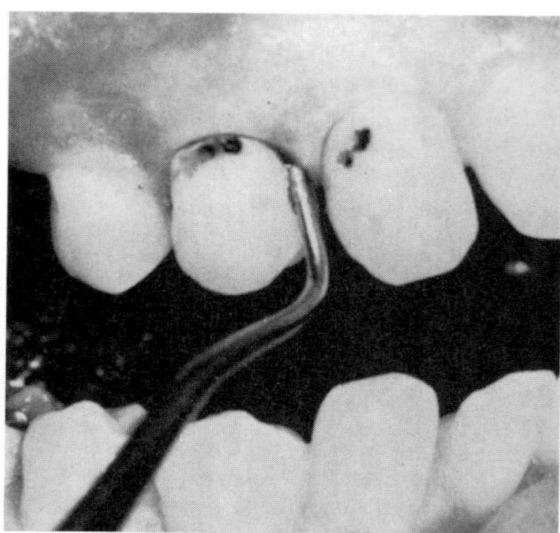

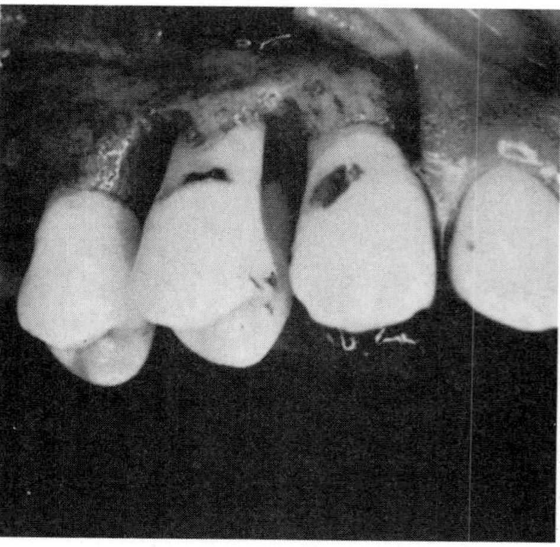

Fig. 23-21 Reversed architecture. *Left,* Probe in the deep infrabony pocket on the mesial surface of the maxillary premolar. *Right,* Elevated flap shows irregular bone margin with notching of interdental bone.

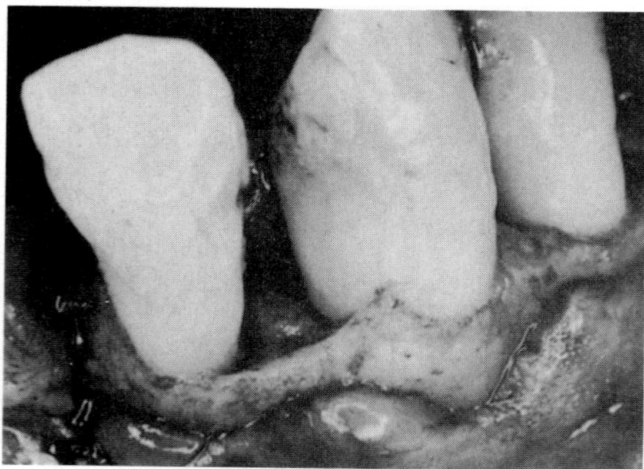

Fig. 23-22 Labial ledge produced by interproximal resorption.

or both, without concomitant loss of radicular bone, thereby reversing the normal architecture (Fig. 23-21). Such defects are more common in the maxilla.[48]

Ledges

Ledges are plateau-like bone margins caused by resorption of thickened bony plates (Fig. 23-22).

Furcation Involvements

The term *furcation involvement* refers to the invasion of the bifurcation and trifurcation of multirooted teeth by periodontal disease. The prevalence of furcation-involved molars is not clear.[9,51] Whereas some reports[32] indicate that the mandibular first molars are the most common sites and the maxillary premolars are the least common, others[70] have found higher prevalence in upper molars. The number of furcation involvements increases with age.[32,33]

The denuded furcation may be visible clinically or covered by the wall of the pocket. The extent of involvement is determined by exploration with a blunt probe, along with a simultaneous blast of warm air to facilitate visualization (Figs. 23-23 and 23-24).

Furcation involvements have been classified as grades I, II, III, and IV according to the amount of tissue destruction. Grade I is incipient bone loss, grade II is partial bone loss (cul-de-sac), and grade III is total bone loss with through-and-through opening of the furcation. Grade IV is similar to grade III, but with gingival recession exposing the furcation to view.

Microscopically, furcation involvement presents no unique pathologic features. It is simply a phase in the rootward extension of the periodontal pocket. In its early stages, a widening of the periodontal space occurs, with cellular and fluid inflammatory exudation (Fig. 23-25), followed by epithelial proliferation into the furcation area from an adjoining periodontal pocket (Fig. 23-26). Extension of the inflammation into the bone leads to resorption and reduction in bone height (Fig. 23-27). The bone destructive pattern may produce horizontal loss, or angular osseous defects associated with infrabony pockets may exist (Figs. 23-28 and 23-29). Plaque, calculus, and bacterial debris occupy the denuded furcation space.

The destructive pattern in a furcation involvement varies in different cases and with the degree of involvement. Bone loss around each individual root may be horizontal or angular, and very frequently a crater develops in the interradicular area. Probing to determine the presence of these destructive patterns must be done horizontally and vertically around each involved root and in the crater area to establish the depth of the vertical component.

Furcation involvement is a stage of progressive periodontal disease and has its same etiology. The difficulty, and sometimes the impossibility,[2,3] of controlling plaque in furcations are responsible for the presence of extensive lesions in this area.[75]

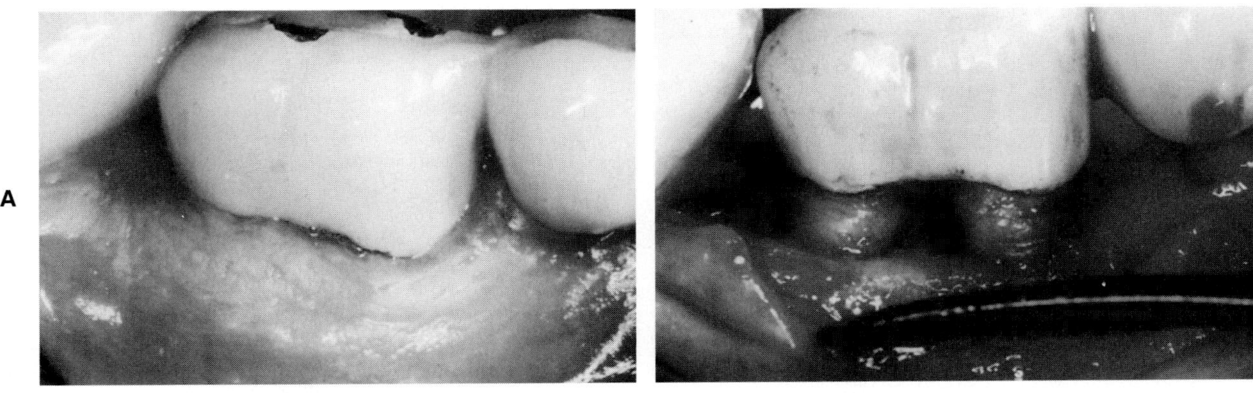

Fig. 23-23 **A,** Partially stippled gingiva covering the furcation area of the lower first molar. **B,** Flap elevation reveals furcation involvement.

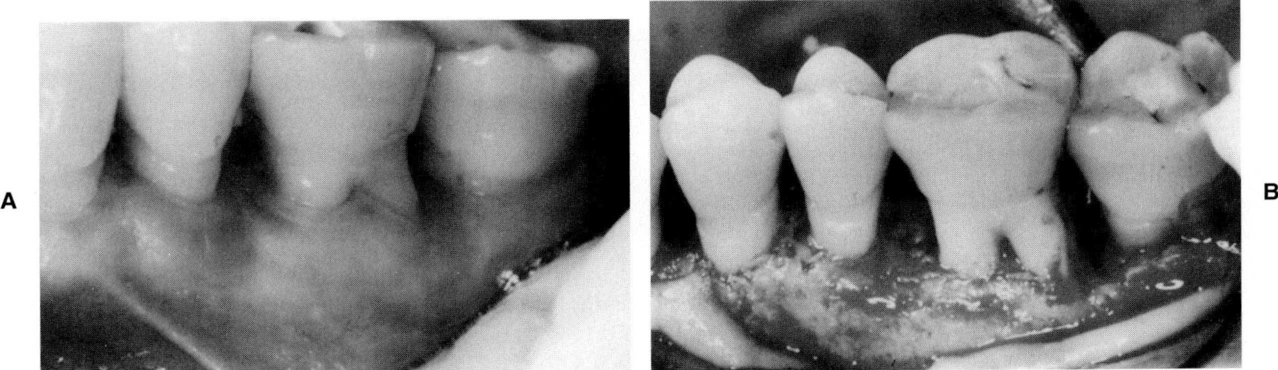

Fig. 23-24 **A,** Furcation area barely covered by gingival tissue. **B,** Flap elevation reveals partial furcation involvement.

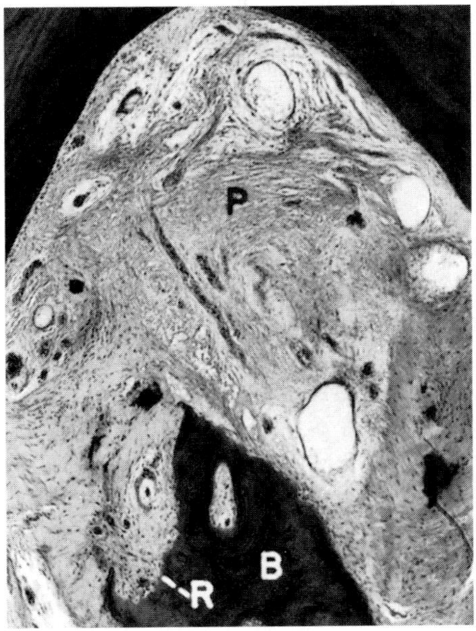

Fig. 23-25 Furcation area in a mandibular molar. The periodontal space is widened. There is edema, slight leukocytic infiltration of the periodontal ligament *(P)*, and an area of resorption *(R)* at the margin of the bone *(B)*.

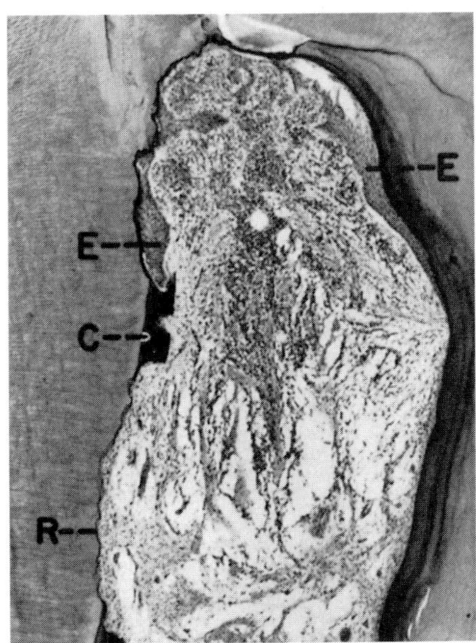

Fig. 23-26 Furcation area showing proliferation of epithelium *(E)*, edema and degeneration of connective tissue, bone loss, and destruction of cementum *(C)* and dentin with irregularly hollowed-out lacunae along the dentinal surface *(R)*.

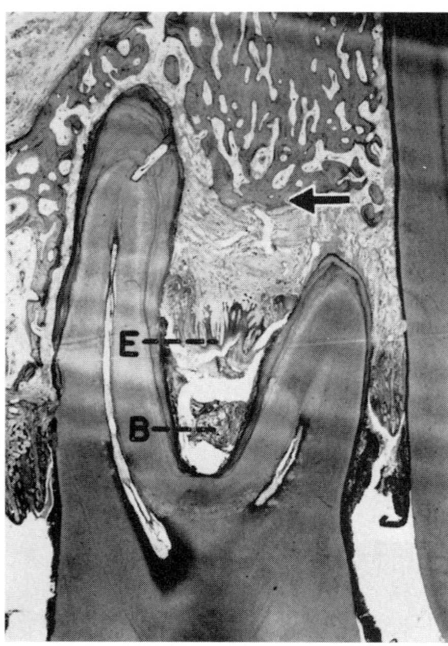

Fig. 23-27 Furcation involvement. Maxillary first molar showing pronounced bone loss, inflammation, and epithelial proliferation *(E)*. Bacterial debris is shown at *B*. Note the different height of bone between the mesial surface *(left)* and the furcation area *(arrow)*.

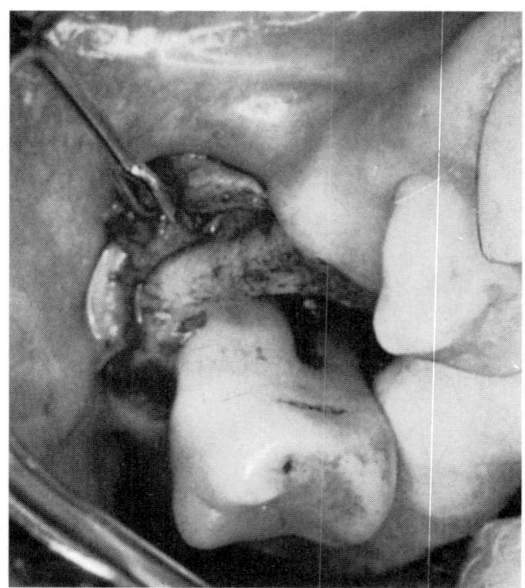

Fig. 23-29 Crater-like osseous defect in trifurcation of a molar.

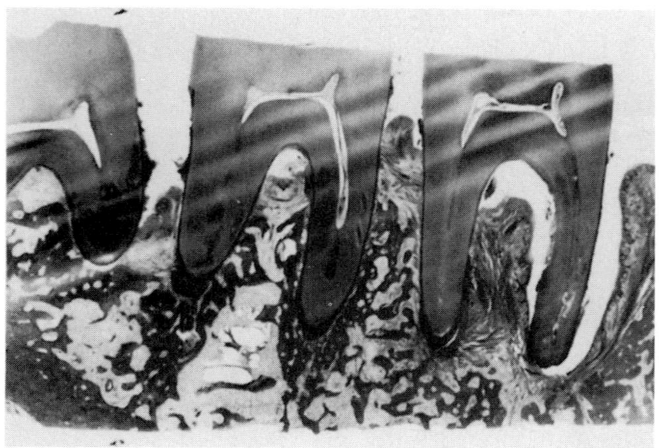

Fig. 23-28 Different degrees of furcation involvement in a human autopsy specimen. Moderate involvement is found in the third molar; a more advanced lesion in the second molar; and a very severe lesion in the first molar, exposing almost the entire mesial root.

The role of trauma from occlusion in the etiology of furcation lesions is controversial. Some assign a key role to trauma, believing that furcation areas are most sensitive to injury from excessive occlusal forces.[15] Others deny the initiating effect of trauma and consider that inflammation and edema caused by plaque in the furcation area tend to extrude the tooth, which then becomes traumatized and sensitive.[75]

Trauma from occlusion has been suspected as a contributing etiologic factor in cases of furcation involvement with craterlike or angular deformities in the bone and especially when bone destruction is localized to one of the roots.

Other factors that may play a role are the presence of enamel projections into the furcation,[42] which occurs in about 13% of multirooted teeth, and the proximity of the furcation to the cementoenamel junction, which occurs in about 75% of cases of furcation involvement.[33]

The presence of accessory pulpal canals in the furcation area may extend pulpal inflammation to the furcation[21]; this possibility should be carefully explored, particularly when mesial and distal bone retain their normal height. Accessory canals connecting the pulp chamber floor to the furcation have been found in 36% of maxillary first molars, 12% of maxillary second molars, 32% of mandibular first molars, and 24% of mandibular second molars.[72]

The diagnosis of furcation involvement is made by clinical examination and careful probing with one of the specially designed probes (see Chapter 30). Radiographic examination of the area is helpful, but lesions can be obscured by angulation of the beam and the radiopacity of neighboring structures (see Chapter 31).

For more detailed clinical considerations in the diagnosis and treatment of furcation involvements, see Chapters 30 and 64.

REFERENCES

1. Akiyoshi M, Mori K: Marginal periodontitis: A histological study of the incipient stage. J Periodontol 1967; 38:45.
2. Bower RC: Furcation morphology relative to periodontal treatment. Furcation entrance architecture. J Periodontol 1979; 50:23.

3. Bower RC: Furcation morphology relative to periodontal treatment. Furcation root surface anatomy. J Periodontol 1979; 50:366.
4. Carranza FA Jr: Histometric evaluation of periodontal pathology. A review of recent studies. J Periodontol 1967; 38:741.
5. Carranza FA Jr, Cabrini RL: Histometric studies of periodontal tissues. Periodontics 1967; 5:308.
6. Carranza FA Jr, Saglie R, Newman MG: Scanning and transmission electron microscopy study of tissue invading microorganisms in juvenile periodontitis. J Periodontol 1983; 54:598.
7. Carranza FA Jr, Simes RJ, Mayo J, et al: Histometric evaluation of periodontal bone loss in rats. J Periodont Res 1971; 6:65.
8. Comar MD, Kollar JD, Gargiulo AW: Local irritation and occlusal trauma as cofactors in the periodontal disease process. J Periodontol 1969; 40:193.
9. Easley JR, Drennan GA: Morphological classification of the furca. J Can Dent Assoc 1969; 35:104.
10. Frank RM, Voegel JC: Bacterial bone resorption in advanced cases of human periodontitis. J Periodont Res 1978; 13:251.
11. Garant PR, Cho MJ: Histopathogenesis of spontaneous periodontal disease in conventional rats. I. Histometric and histologic study. J Periodont Res 1979; 14:297.
12. Glickman I: The experimental basis for the "bone factor" concept in periodontal disease. J Periodontol 1951; 20:7.
13. Glickman I, Smulow JB: Alterations in the pathway of gingival inflammation into the underlying tissues induced by excessive occlusal forces. J Periodontol 1962; 33:7.
14. Glickman I, Smulow J: Buttressing bone formation in the periodontium. J Periodontol 1965; 36:365.
15. Glickman I, Stein RS, Smulow JB: The effects of increased functional forces upon the periodontium of splinted and nonsplinted teeth. J Periodontol 1961; 32:290.
16. Glickman I, Wood H: Bone histology in periodontal disease. J Dent Res 1942; 21:35.
17. Goldman HM, Cohen DW: The intrabony pocket: classification and treatment. J Periodontol 1958; 29:272.
18. Goodson JM, Haffajee AD, Socransky SS: The relationship between attachment level loss and alveolar bone loss. J Clin Periodontol 1984; 11:348.
19. Goodson JM, McClatchy K, Revell C: Prostaglandin-induced resorption of the adult calvarium. J Dent Res 1974; 53:670.
20. Groen JJ, Menczel J, Shapiro S: Chronic destructive periodontal disease in patients with presenile osteoporosis. J Periodontol 1968; 39:19.
21. Gutman JL: Prevalence, location and patency of accessory canals in the furcation region of permanent molars. J Periodontol 1978; 49:21.
22. Hausmann E: Potential pathways for bone resorption in human periodontal disease. J Periodontol 1974; 45:338.
23. Hausmann E, Raisz LG, Miller WA: Endotoxin: Stimulation of bone resorption in tissue culture. Science 1970; 168:793.
24. Heijl L, Rifkin BR, Zander HA: Conversion of chronic gingivitis to periodontitis in squirrel monkeys. J Periodontol 1976; 47:710.
25. Jeffcoat MK: Osteoporosis: a possible modifying factor in oral bone loss. Ann. Periodontol 1998; 3:312.
26. Jeffcoat MK, Lewis CE, Reddy MS, et al: Post-menopausal bone loss and its relationship to oral bone loss. Periodontology 2000 2000; 23:94.
27. Jeffcoat MK, Williams RC, Wachter WJ, et al: Flurbiprofen treatment of periodontal disease in beagles. J Periodont Res 1986; 21:624.
28. Klein DC, Raisz LG: Prostaglandins: Stimulation of bone resorption in tissue culture. Endocrinology 1970; 86:1436.
29. Kronfeld R: Condition of alveolar bone underlying periodontal pockets. J Periodontol 1935; 6:22.
30. Larato DC: Periodontal bone defects in the juvenile skull. J Periodontol 1970; 41:473.
31. Larato DC: Intrabony defects in the dry human skull. J Periodontol 1970; 41:496.
32. Larato DC: Furcation involvements: Incidence of distribution. J Periodontol 1970; 41:499.
33. Larato DC: Some anatomical factors related to furcation involvements. J Periodontol 1975; 46:608.
34. Lindhe J, Ericsson I: Effect of ligature placement and dental plaque on periodontal tissue breakdown in the dog. J Periodontol 1978; 49:343.
35. Lindhe J, Svanberg G: Influence of trauma from occlusion on progression of experimental periodontitis in beagle dogs. J Clin Periodontol 1974; 1:3.
36. Lindhe J, Liljenberg B, Listgarten MA: Some microbiological and histopathological features of periodontal disease in man. J Periodontol 1980; 51:264.
37. Löe H, Anerud A, Boysen H, et al: Natural history of periodontal disease in man. Rapid, moderate and no loss of attachment in Sri Lankan laborers 14 to 46 years of age. J Clin Periodontol 1986; 13:431.
38. Löe H, Anerud A, Boysen H, et al: The natural history of periodontal disease in man. The rate of periodontal destruction before 40 years of age. J Periodontol 1978; 49:607.
39. Macapanpan LC, Weinmann JP: The influence of injury to the periodontal membrane on the spread of gingival inflammation. J Dent Res 1954; 33:263.
40. Manson JD, Nicholson K: The distribution of bone defects in chronic periodontitis. J Periodontol 1974; 45:88.
41. Manson JD: Bone morphology and bone loss in periodontal disease. J Clin Periodontol 1976; 3:14.
42. Masters DH, Hoskins SW: Projection of cervical enamel into molar furcations. J Periodontol 1963; 35:49.
43. Melcher AH, Eastoe JE: Biology of the Periodontium. New York, Academic Press, 1969.
44. Moskow BS: A histomorphologic study of the effects of periodontal inflammation on the maxillary sinus mucosa. J Periodontol 1992; 63:674.
45. Moskow BS, Polson AM: Histologic studies on the extension of the inflammatory infiltrate in human periodontitis. J Clin Periodontol 1991; 18:534.
46. Nery EB, Corn H, Eisenstein IL: Palatal exostoses in the molar region. J Periodontol 1977; 48:663.
47. Newman MG: The role of *Bacteroides melaninogenicus* and other anaerobes in periodontal infections. Rev Infect Dis 1979; 1:313.
48. Nielsen JI, Glavind L, Karring T: Interproximal periodontal intrabony defects. Prevalence, localization and etiological factors. J Clin Periodontol 1980; 7:187.
49. Ooya K, Yamamoto H: A scanning electron microscopic study of the destruction of human alveolar crest in periodontal disease. J Periodont Res 1978; 13:498.
50. Pack ARC, Gaudie WM, Jennings AM: Bony exostosis as a sequela to free gingival grafting: Two case reports. J Periodontol 1991; 62:269.
51. Papapanou PN, Tonetti MS: Diagnosis and epidemiology of periodontal osseous lesions. Periodontology 2000 2000; 22:8.
52. Papapanou PN, Wennström JL, Grondahl K: Periodontal status in relation to age and tooth type. A cross-sectional radiographic study. J Clin Periodontol 1988; 15:469.
53. Page RC, Schroeder HE: Periodontitis in Man and Other Animals. A Comparative Review. Basel, Karger, 1982.
54. Prichard JF: Periodontal Surgery, Practical Dental Monographs. Chicago, Year Book Medical, 1961.
55. Raisz LG, Sandberg AL, Goodson JM, et al: Complement-dependent stimulation of prostaglandin synthesis and bone resorption. Science 1974; 185:789.
56. Rifkin BR, Heijl L: The occurrence of mononuclear cells at sites of osteoclastic bone resorption in experimental periodontitis. J Periodontol 1979; 50:636.

57. Rizzo AA, Mergenhagen SE: Histopathologic effects of endotoxin injected into rabbit oral mucosa. Arch Oral Biol 1964; 9:659.
58. Rowe DJ, Bradley LS: Quantitative analyses of osteoclasts, bone loss and inflammation in human periodontal disease. J Periodont Res 1981; 16:13.
59. Ruben M, Cooper SJ: Tissue factors modifying the spread of periodontal inflammation: A perspective. Contin Educ Dent 1981; 2:387.
60. Saari JT, Hurt WC, Briggs NL: Periodontal bony defects on the dry skull. J Periodontol 1968; 39:278.
61. Saglie RF, Rezende M, Pertuiset J, et al: Bacterial invasion during disease activity as determined by significant loss of attachment. Abstract. J Periodontol 1987; 58:336.
62. Salvi GE, Lawrence HP, Offenbacher S, et al: Sequence of risk factors on the pathogenesis of periodontitis. Periodontology 2000 1997; 14:173.
63. Schroeder HE, Lindhe J: Conditions and pathological features of rapidly destructive experimental periodontitis in dogs. J Periodontol 1980; 51:6.
64. Schroeder HE: Discussion: Pathogenesis of periodontitis. J Clin Periodontol 1986; 13:426.
65. Schwartz Z, Goultschin J, Dean DD, et al: Mechanisms of alveolar bone destruction in periodontitis. Periodontology 2000 1997; 14:158.
66. Seymour GJ, Dockrell HM, Greenspan JS: Enzyme differentiation of lymphocyte subpopulations in sections of human lymph nodes, tonsils, and periodontal disease. Clin Exp Immunol 1978; 32:169.
67. Seymour GJ, Powell RN, Davies WJR: Conversion of a stable T cell lesion to a progressive B cell lesion in the pathogenesis of chronic inflammatory periodontal disease: A hypothesis. J Clin Periodontol 1979; 6:267.
68. Stahl SS: The response of the periodontium to combined gingival inflammation and occlusofunctional stresses in four surgical specimens. Periodontics 1968; 6:14.
69. Svärdström G, Wennström JL: Prevalence of furcation involvements in patients referred for periodontal treatment. J Clin Periodontol 1996; 23:1093.
70. Tal H: Relationship between interproximal distance of roots and the prevalence of intrabony pockets. J Periodontol 1984; 55:604.
71. Ubios AM, Costa OR, Cabrini RL: Early steps in bone resorption in experimental periodontitis. A histomorphometric study. Acta Odont Lat-Am 1993; 7:45.
72. Vertucci FJ, Anthony RL: An SEM investigation of accessory foramina in the furcation and pulp chamber floor of molar teeth. Oral Surg 1986; 62:319.
73. Wactawski-Wende J, Grossi SG, Trevisan M, et al: The role of osteopenia in oral bone loss and periodontal disease. J Periodontol 1996; 67:1076.
74. Waerhaug J: The angular bone defect and its relationship to trauma from occlusion and downgrowth of subgingival plaque. J Clin Periodontol 1979; 6:61.
75. Waerhaug J: The furcation problem. Etiology, pathogenesis, diagnosis, therapy and prognosis. J Clin Periodontol 1980; 7:73.
76. Waerhaug J: The infrabony pocket and its relationship to trauma from occlusion and subgingival plaque. J Periodontol 1979; 50:355.
77. Weinmann JP: Progress of gingival inflammation into the supporting structures of the teeth. J Periodontol 1941; 12:71.
78. Williams RC, Jeffcoat MK, Kaplan ML, et al: Flurbiprofen: A potent inhibitor of alveolar bone resorption in beagles. Science 1985; 227:640.
79. Wouters FR, Salonen LE, Helldén LB, et al: Prevalence of interproximal periodontal infrabony defects in an adult population in Sweden. A radiographic study. J Clin Periodontol 1989; 16:144.

Periodontal Response to External Forces

Fermin A. Carranza and Paulo M. Camargo

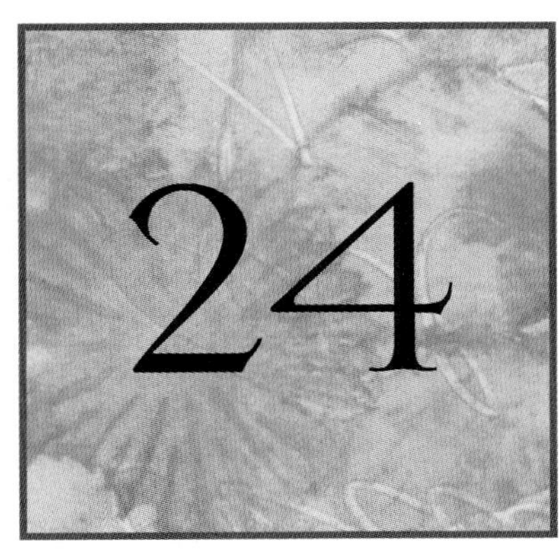

CHAPTER

CHAPTER OUTLINE

ADAPTIVE CAPACITY OF THE PERIODONTIUM TO OCCLUSAL FORCES

The periodontium tries to accommodate to the forces exerted on the crown. This adaptive capacity varies in different persons and in the same person at different times. The effect of occlusal forces on the periodontium is influenced by the magnitude, direction, duration, and frequency of the forces.

When the **magnitude** of occlusal forces is increased, the periodontium responds with a widening of the periodontal ligament space, an increase in the number and width of periodontal ligament fibers, and an increase in the density of alveolar bone.

Changing the **direction** of occlusal forces causes a reorientation of the stresses and strains within the periodontium[24] (Fig. 24-1). The principal fibers of the periodontal ligament are arranged so that they best accommodate occlusal forces along the long axis of the tooth. Lateral (horizontal) forces and torque (rotational) forces are more likely to injure the periodontium.

The response of alveolar bone is also affected by the **duration** and **frequency** of occlusal forces. Constant pressure on the bone is more injurious than intermittent forces. The more frequent the application of an intermittent force, the more injurious the force to the periodontium.

TRAUMA FROM OCCLUSION

An inherent "margin of safety" common to all tissues permits some variation in occlusion without adversely affecting the periodontium. However, *when occlusal forces exceed the adaptive capacity of the tissues, tissue injury results.*[13,35,53,54] The resultant injury is termed *trauma from occlusion.**

Thus *trauma from occlusion refers to the tissue injury, not the occlusal force.* An occlusion that produces such injury is called a *traumatic occlusion.*[2] Excessive occlusal forces may also disrupt the function of the masticatory musculature and cause painful spasms, injure the temporomandibular joints, or produce excessive tooth wear, but the term *trauma from occlusion* is generally used in connection with injury in the periodontium.

* The term is used throughout this text to designate periodontal tissue injury produced by occlusal forces. It is also known as *traumatism* and *occlusal trauma.*

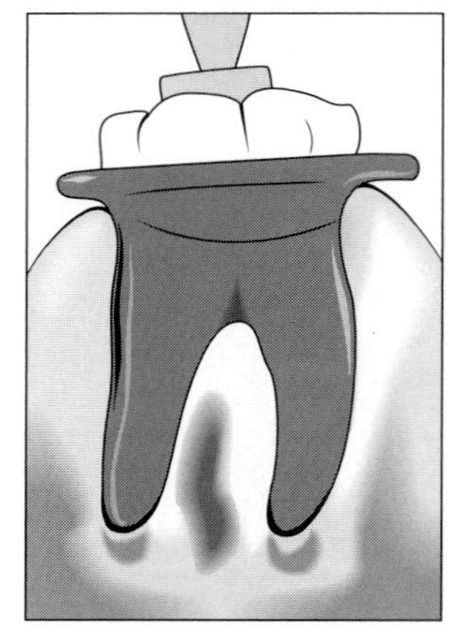
A

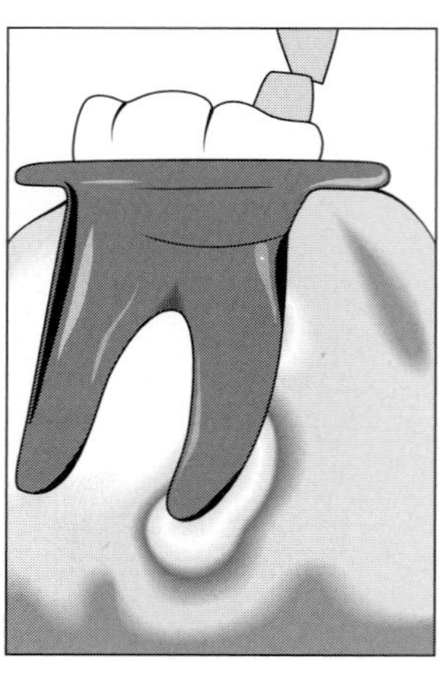
B

Fig. 24-1 Stress patterns around the roots changed by shifting the direction of occlusal forces (experimental model using photoelastic analysis). **A,** Buccal view of an ivorine molar subjected to an axial force. The shaded fringes indicate that the internal stresses are at the root apices. **B,** Buccal view of ivorine molar subjected to a mesial tilting force. The shaded fringes indicate that the internal stresses are along the mesial surface and at the apex of the mesial root. (From Glickman I, Roeber F, Brion M, et al: Photoelastic analysis of internal stresses in the periodontium created by occlusal forces. J Periodontol 1970; 41:30.)

Acute and Chronic Trauma

Trauma from occlusion may be acute or chronic. *Acute trauma from occlusion* results from an abrupt occlusal impact, such as that produced by biting on a hard object (e.g., an olive pit). In addition, restorations or prosthetic appliances that interfere with or alter the direction of occlusal forces on the teeth may induce acute trauma. The results are tooth pain, sensitivity to percussion, and increased tooth mobility. If the force is dissipated by a shift in the position of the tooth or by wearing away or correction of the restoration, the injury heals and the symptoms subside. Otherwise, periodontal injury may worsen and develop into necrosis accompanied by periodontal abscess formation or persist as a symptom-free chronic condition. Acute trauma can also produce cementum tears (see Chapter 2).

Chronic trauma from occlusion is more common than the acute form and is of greater clinical significance. It most often develops from gradual changes in occlusion produced by tooth wear, drifting movement, and extrusion of teeth, combined with parafunctional habits such as bruxism and clenching, rather than as a sequela of acute periodontal trauma (see Chapters 25 and 51). The features of chronic trauma from occlusion and their significance are discussed in the following text.

The criterion that determines whether an occlusion is traumatic is whether it produces periodontal injury, not how the teeth occlude. Any occlusion that produces periodontal injury is traumatic. Malocclusion is not necessary to produce trauma; periodontal injury may occur when the occlusion appears normal. The dentition may be anatomically and aesthetically acceptable but functionally injurious. Similarly, not all malocclusions are necessarily injurious to the periodontium. Traumatic occlusal relationships are referred to by such terms as *occlusal disharmony, functional imbalance,* and *occlusal dystrophy.* These terms refer to the occlusion's effect on the periodontium, not to the position of the teeth. Because *trauma from occlusion* refers to the tissue injury rather than the occlusion, an increased occlusal force is not traumatic if the periodontium can accommodate it.

Primary and Secondary Trauma from Occlusion

Trauma from occlusion may be caused by alterations in occlusal forces, reduced capacity of the periodontium to withstand occlusal forces, or both. When trauma from occlusion is the result of alterations in occlusal forces, it is called *primary trauma from occlusion.* When it results from reduced ability of the tissues to resist the occlusal forces, it is known as *secondary trauma from occlusion.*

Primary trauma from occlusion occurs if trauma from occlusion is considered the primary etiologic factor in periodontal destruction and if the only local alteration to which a tooth is subjected is from occlusion. Examples include periodontal injury produced around teeth with a previously healthy periodontium following 1) the insertion of a "high filling," 2) the insertion of a prosthetic replacement that creates excessive forces on abutment and antagonistic teeth, 3) the drifting movement or extrusion of teeth into spaces created by unreplaced missing teeth, or 4) the orthodontic movement of teeth into functionally unacceptable positions. Most studies on experimental animals of the effect of trauma from occlusion have examined the primary type of trauma. Changes produced by primary trauma do not alter the level of connective tissue attachment and do not initiate pocket formation. This is probably because the supracrestal gingival fibers are not affected and therefore prevent apical migration of the junctional epithelium.[57]

Secondary trauma from occlusion occurs when the adaptive capacity of the tissues to withstand occlusal forces is impaired by bone loss resulting from marginal inflammation. This reduces the periodontal attachment area and alters the leverage on the remaining tissues. The periodontium becomes more vulnerable to injury, and previously well-tolerated occlusal forces become traumatic.

Fig. 24-2 depicts three different situations on which excessive occlusal forces can be superimposed:

1. Normal periodontium with normal height of bone
2. Normal periodontium with reduced height of bone
3. Marginal periodontitis with reduced height of bone

The first case is an example of primary trauma from occlusion, whereas the last two represent secondary trauma from occlusion. The effects of trauma from occlusion in these different situations are analyzed in the following discussion.

It has been found in experimental animals that systemic disorders can reduce tissue resistance and that previously tolerable forces may become excessive.[30,61,72] This could theoretically represent another mechanism by which tissue resistance to increased forces is lowered, resulting in secondary trauma from occlusion.

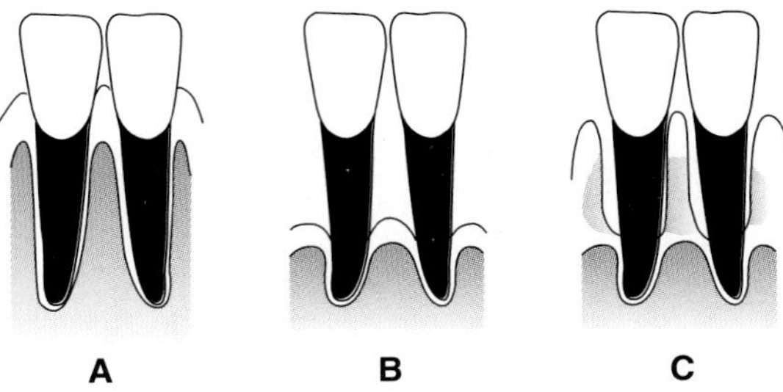

Fig. 24-2 Traumatic forces can occur on **A**, normal periodontium with normal height of bone; **B**, normal periodontium with reduced height of bone; or **C**, marginal periodontitis with reduced height of bone.

TISSUE RESPONSE TO INCREASED OCCLUSAL FORCES

Stages of Tissue Response

Tissue response occurs in three stages[9,16]: injury, repair, and adaptive remodeling of the periodontium.

Stage I: Injury. Tissue injury is produced by excessive occlusal forces. The body then attempts to repair the injury and restore the periodontium. This can occur if the forces are diminished or if the tooth drifts away from them. However, if the offending force is chronic, the periodontium is remodeled to cushion its impact. The ligament is widened at the expense of the bone, resulting in angular bone defects without periodontal pockets, and the tooth becomes loose.

Under the forces of occlusion, a tooth rotates around a fulcrum or axis of rotation, which in single-rooted teeth is located in the junction between the middle third and the apical third of the clinical root (see Fig. 2-12). This creates areas of pressure and tension on opposite sides of the fulcrum. Different lesions are produced by different degrees of pressure and tension. If jiggling forces are exerted, these different lesions may coexist in the same area.

Slightly excessive pressure stimulates resorption of the alveolar bone, with a resultant widening of the periodontal ligament space. Slightly excessive tension causes elongation of the periodontal ligament fibers and apposition of alveolar bone. In areas of increased pressure, the blood vessels are numerous and reduced in size; in areas of increased tension, they are enlarged.[79]

Greater pressure produces a gradation of changes in the periodontal ligament, starting with compression of the fibers, which produces areas of hyalinization.[64-66] Subsequent injury to the fibroblasts and other connective tissue cells leads to necrosis of areas of the ligament.[62,66] Vascular changes are also produced: within 30 minutes, retardation and stasis of blood flow occur; at 2 to 3 hours, blood vessels appear to be packed with erythrocytes, which start to fragment; and between 1 and 7 days, disintegration of the blood vessel walls and release of the contents into the surrounding tissue occur.[63] In addition, increased resorption of alveolar bone and resorption of the tooth surface occur[39,44] (Figs. 24-3 and 24-4).

Severe tension causes widening of the periodontal ligament, thrombosis, hemorrhage, tearing of the periodontal ligament, and resorption of alveolar bone.

Pressure severe enough to force the root against bone causes necrosis of the periodontal ligament and bone. The bone is resorbed from viable periodontal ligament adjacent to necrotic areas and from marrow spaces, a process called *undermining resorption.*[34,53]

The areas of the periodontium most susceptible to injury from excessive occlusal forces are the furcations.[31]

Injury to the periodontium produces a temporary depression in mitotic activity and the rate of proliferation and differentiation of fibroblasts,[73] in collagen formation, and in bone formation.[39,71,73] These return to normal levels after dissipation of the forces.

Stage II: Repair. Repair is constantly occurring in the normal periodontium, and trauma from occlusion stimulates increased reparative activity.

The damaged tissues are removed, and new connective tissue cells and fibers, bone, and cementum are formed in an attempt to restore the injured periodontium (Fig. 24-5). Forces remain traumatic only as long as the damage produced exceeds the reparative capacity of the tissues.

When bone is resorbed by excessive occlusal forces, the body attempts to reinforce the thinned bony trabeculae with new bone (Fig. 24-6). This attempt to compensate for lost bone is called *buttressing bone formation* and is an important feature of the reparative process associated with trauma from occlusion.[28] It also occurs when bone is destroyed by inflammation or osteolytic tumors.

Buttressing bone formation occurs within the jaw (central buttressing) and on the bone surface (peripheral buttressing). In central buttressing, the endosteal cells deposit new bone, which restores the bony trabeculae and reduces the size of the marrow spaces (see Fig. 24-6). Peripheral buttressing occurs on the facial and lingual surfaces of the alveolar plate. Depending on its severity, peripheral buttressing may produce a shelf-like thickening of the alveolar margin, referred to as lipping (Fig. 24-7; see also Fig. 24-3), or a pronounced bulge in the contour of the facial and lingual bone[16,26] (see Chapter 23).

Cartilage-like material sometimes develops in the periodontal ligament space as an aftermath of the trauma.[21] Formation of crystals from erythrocytes has also been shown.[67]

Stage III: Adaptive Remodeling of the Periodontium. If the repair process cannot keep pace with the destruction caused by the occlusion, the periodontium is remodeled in an effort to create a structural

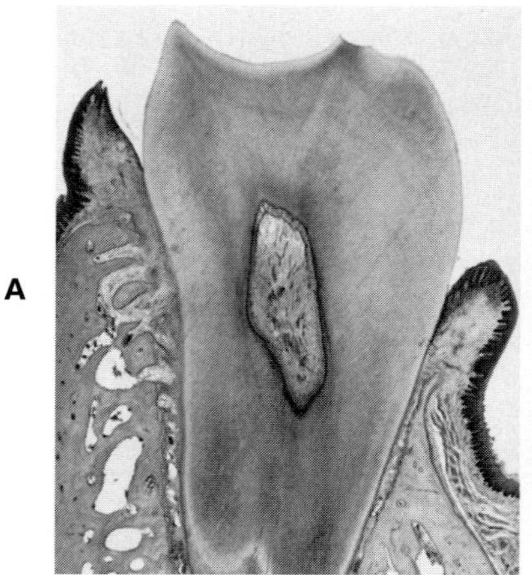

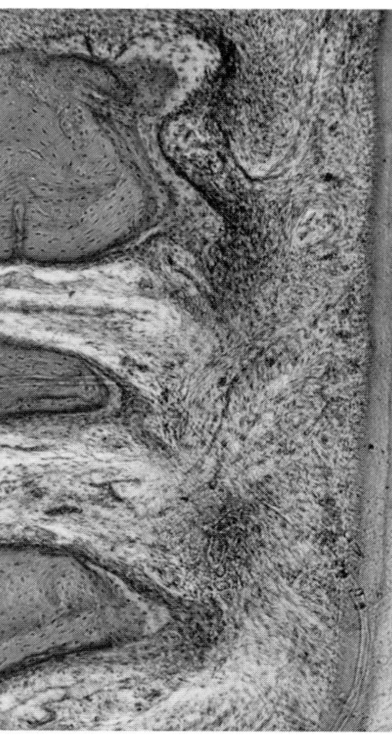

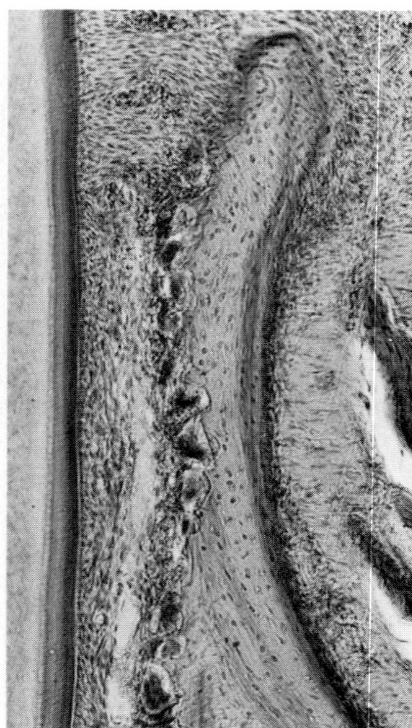

Fig. 24-3 Periodontal accommodation to lateral forces. **A,** Mandibular premolar. **B,** Lingual surface, showing new bone formation in response to tension on the periodontal ligament. Note the pale-staining osteoid bordered by osteoblasts and the incremental lines indicative of previous additions to the bone. **C,** Facial surface shows compression of the periodontal ligament and osteoclastic resorption of the bony plate. Note the new bone formed on the external surface. This is peripheral buttressing bone, which reinforces the resorbing facial plate. Note also that the buttressing bone has produced a bulge in the bony contour.

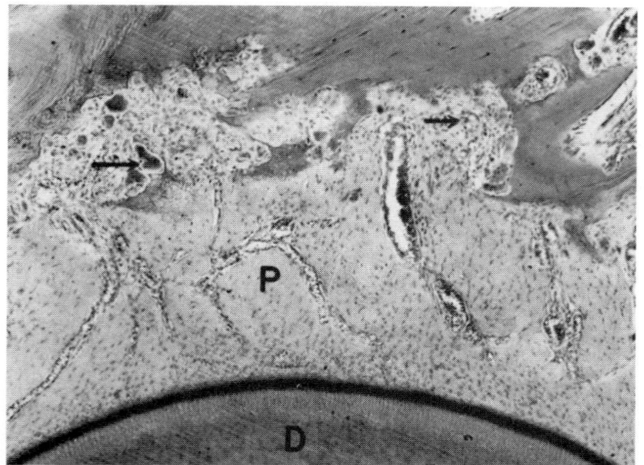

Fig. 24-4 Trauma from occlusion at the root apex. Note bone resorption with prominent osteoclasts *(arrows).* The periodontal ligament *(P)* is widened as the result of bone resorption, and the blood vessels are engorged. The root is shown at *D.*

relationship in which the forces are no longer injurious to the tissues. *This results in a thickened periodontal ligament, which is funnel shaped at the crest, and angular defects in the bone, with no pocket formation. The involved teeth become loose.*[78] *Increased vascularization has also been reported.*[15]

The three stages in the evolution of traumatic lesions have been differentiated histometrically by means of the relative amounts of periodontal bone surface undergoing resorption or formation[10,16] (Fig. 24-8). The injury phase shows an increase in areas of resorption and a decrease in bone formation, whereas the repair phase demonstrates decreased resorption and increased bone formation. After adaptive remodeling of the periodontium, resorption and formation return to normal.

EFFECTS OF INSUFFICIENT OCCLUSAL FORCE

Insufficient occlusal force may also be injurious to the supporting periodontal tissues.[11,46] Insufficient stimulation causes thinning of the periodontal ligament, atrophy of the fibers, osteoporosis of the alveolar bone, and reduction in bone height. Hypofunction can result from an open-bite relationship, an absence of functional antagonists, or unilateral chewing habits that neglect one side of the mouth.

REVERSIBILITY OF TRAUMATIC LESIONS

Trauma from occlusion is reversible. When trauma is artificially induced in experimental animals, the teeth move away or intrude into the jaw. When the impact of the artificially created force is relieved, the tissues undergo

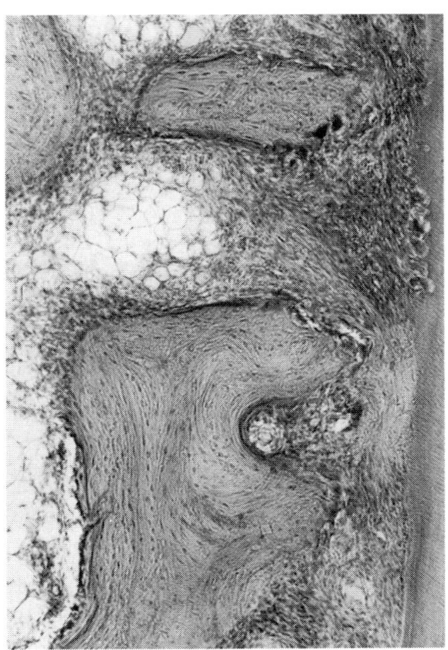

Fig. 24-5 Trauma from occlusion. Injury is more severe than that shown in Fig. 24-4. The cementum *(right)* is undergoing resorption, the periodontal ligament is compressed and necrotic, and the bone is undergoing resorption. Note the osteoblasts and new bone (central buttressing bone formation) on the trabecular margins adjacent to the marrow.

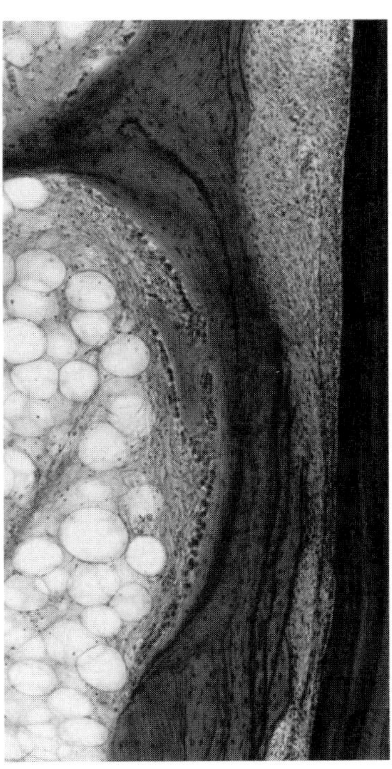

Fig. 24-6 Central buttressing bone. Note the new bone formation on the marrow side of alveolar bone that is undergoing resorption on the side of the periodontal ligament.

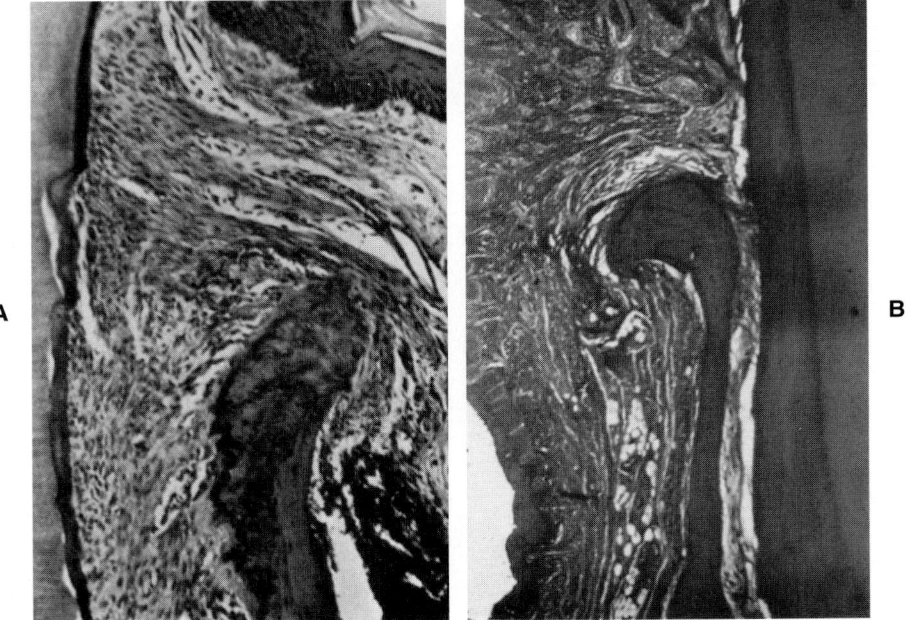

Fig. 24-7 **A,** Widening of the periodontal ligament space in cervical area and a change in the shape of marginal alveolar bone as a result of chronic prolonged trauma from occlusion in rats. **B,** A comparable change in shape of marginal bone found in a human autopsy case.

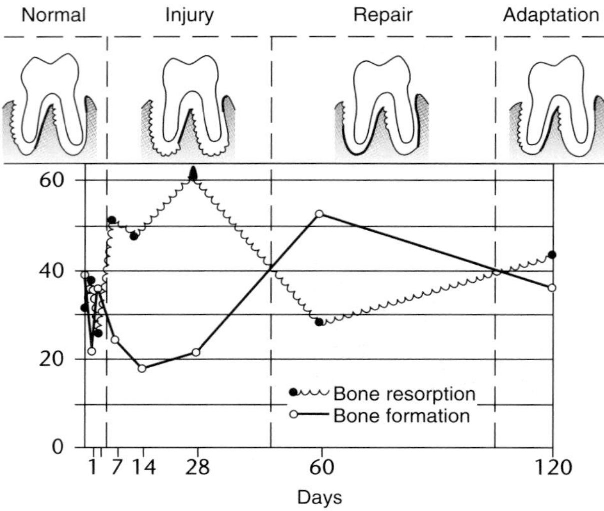

Fig. 24-8 Evolution of traumatic lesions as depicted experimentally in rats by variations in relative amounts of areas of bone formation and bone resorption in periodontal bone surfaces. *Horizontal axis:* days after initiation of traumatic interference. *Vertical axis:* percentage of bone surface undergoing resorption or formation. The stages in the evolution of the lesions are represented in the top drawings, which show the average amount of bone activity for each group. See references 9, 16, and 39.

repair. Although trauma from occlusion is reversible under such conditions, it does not always correct itself, nor is it therefore always temporary and of limited clinical significance. The injurious force must be relieved for repair to occur.[31,58] If conditions in humans do not permit the teeth to escape from or adapt to excessive occlusal force, periodontal damage persists and worsens.

The presence of inflammation in the periodontium as a result of plaque accumulation may impair the reversibility of traumatic lesions.[40,58]

EFFECTS OF EXCESSIVE OCCLUSAL FORCES ON DENTAL PULP

The effects of excessive occlusal forces on the dental pulp have not been established. Some clinicians report the disappearance of pulpal symptoms after correction of excessive occlusal forces. Pulpal reactions have been noted in animals subjected to increased occlusal forces[14,45] but did not occur when the forces were minimal and occurred over short periods.[45]

INFLUENCE OF TRAUMA FROM OCCLUSION ON PROGRESSION OF MARGINAL PERIODONTITIS

The clinical impressions of early investigators and clinicians assigned an important role to trauma from occlusion in the etiology of periodontal lesions. Numerous studies have since been performed attempting to determine the mechanisms by which trauma from occlusion may affect periodontal disease.

Initial studies involved the placement of high crowns or restorations on the teeth of dogs or monkeys, resulting in a continuous or intermittent force in one direction.[2,32] These investigations provided an orthodontic type of force and gave clear descriptions of changes occurring in pressure zones and tension zones. These procedures usually resulted in tooth displacement and consolidation in a new, nontraumatized position.

Trauma from occlusion in humans, however, occurs as a result of forces that act alternatively in opposing directions. These were analyzed in experimental animals with jiggling forces, usually produced by means of a high crown combined with an orthodontic appliance that would bring the traumatized tooth back to its original position when the force was dissipated by separating the teeth. In another method, the teeth were separated by wooden or elastic material wedged interproximally to displace a tooth toward the opposite proximal side. After 48 hours the wedge was removed, and the procedure was repeated on the opposite side.

These studies resulted in a combination of changes produced by pressure and tension on both sides of the tooth, with an increase in the width of the ligament and increased tooth mobility. None of these methods caused gingival inflammation or pocket formation, and the results essentially represented different degrees of functional adaptation to increased forces.[57,79]

To more closely mimic the problem in humans, studies were then conducted on the effect produced by jiggling trauma and simultaneous plaque-induced gingival inflammation.

The accumulation of bacterial plaque that initiates gingivitis and results in periodontal pocket formation affects the marginal gingiva, but trauma from occlusion occurs in the supporting tissues and does not affect the gingiva (Fig. 24-9). The marginal gingiva is unaffected by trauma from occlusion because its blood supply is sufficient to maintain it, even when the vessels of the periodontal ligament are obliterated by excessive occlusal forces.[33] It has been repeatedly proven that *trauma from occlusion does not cause pockets or gingivitis,*[2,32,39,60,77,78,80*] nor does it increase gingival fluid flow.[37,43,51] Furthermore, experimental trauma in dogs does not influence bacterial repopulation of pockets after scaling and root planing.[41] However, mobile teeth in humans harbor significantly higher proportions of *Campylobacter rectus* and *Peptostreptococcus micros* than nonmobile teeth.

As long as inflammation is confined to the gingiva, the inflammatory process is not affected by occlusal forces.[42] When inflammation extends from the gingiva into the supporting periodontal tissues (i.e., when gingivitis becomes periodontitis), plaque-induced inflammation enters the zone influenced by occlusion, which Glickman has called the *zone of co-destruction.*[23,25,27]

* Of historical interest are references 5 and 74, which describe periodontal pocket formation in animals as a result of trauma from occlusion.

Two groups have studied this topic extensively with conflicting results, probably owing to the different methods used. The Eastman Dental Center group in Rochester, NY, used squirrel monkeys, produced trauma by repetitive interdental wedging, and added mild to moderate gingival inflammation; experimental times were up to 10 weeks. They reported that the presence of trauma did not increase the loss of attachment induced by periodontitis.[52,55,56,59] The University of Gothenburg group in Sweden used beagle dogs, produced trauma by placing cap splints and orthodontic appliances, and induced severe gingival inflammation; experimental times were up to 1 year. This group found that occlusal stresses increase the periodontal destruction induced by periodontitis.[18,19,49]

When trauma from occlusion is eliminated, a substantial reversal of bone loss occurs, except in the presence of periodontitis. This indicates that inflammation inhibits the potential for bone regeneration.[40,48,57,58] *Thus it is important to eliminate the marginal inflammatory component in cases of trauma from occlusion because the presence of inflammation affects bone regeneration after the removal of the traumatizing contacts.*[40] It also has been shown in experimental animals that trauma from occlusion does not induce progressive destruction of the periodontal tissues in regions kept healthy after the elimination of preexistent periodontitis.[18]

Trauma from occlusion also tends to change the shape of the alveolar crest. The change in shape consists of a widening of the marginal periodontal ligament space, a narrowing of the interproximal alveolar bone, and a shelf-like thickening of the alveolar margin.[16,49,52] Therefore although trauma from occlusion does not alter the inflammatory process, it changes the architecture of the area around the inflamed site.[16,49] *Thus in the absence of inflammation, the response to trauma from occlusion is limited to adaptation to the increased forces. However, in the presence of inflammation, the changes in the shape of the alveolar crest may be conducive to angular bone loss, and existing pockets may become intrabony.*

Other theories that have been proposed to explain the interaction of trauma and inflammation include the following:

1. Trauma from occlusion may alter the pathway of extension of gingival inflammation to the underlying tissues. This may be favored by the reduced collagen density and increased number of leukocytes, osteoclasts, and blood vessels in the coronal portion of increasingly mobile teeth.[3] Inflammation then may proceed to the periodontal ligament rather than to the bone. Resulting bone loss would be angular, and pockets could become intrabony.[1,23,25,27,29,50]
2. Trauma-induced areas of root resorption uncovered by apical migration of the inflamed gingival attachment may offer a favorable environment for the formation and attachment of plaque and calculus and therefore may be responsible for the development of deeper lesions.[69]
3. Supragingival plaque can become subgingival if the tooth is tilted orthodontically or migrates into an edentulous area, resulting in the transformation of a suprabony pocket into an intrabony pocket.[17,20]
4. Increased mobility of traumatically loosened teeth may have a pumping effect on plaque metabolites, increasing their diffusion.[76]

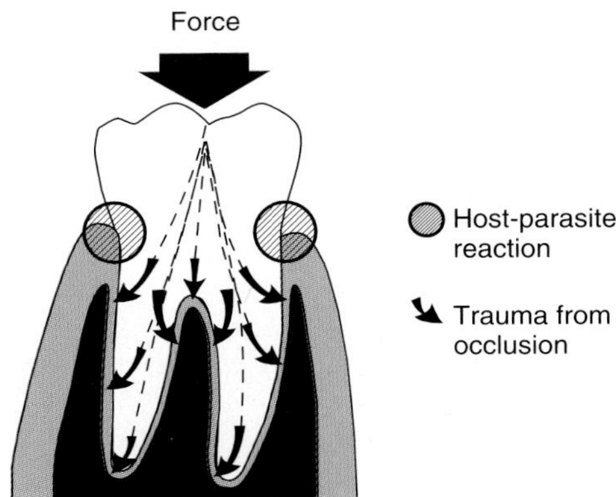

Fig. 24-9 The reaction between dental plaque and the host takes place in the gingival sulcus region. Trauma from occlusion appears in the tissues supporting the tooth.

Clinical and Radiographic Signs of Trauma from Occlusion Alone

The most common clinical sign of trauma to the periodontium is increased tooth mobility. In the injury stage of trauma from occlusion, destruction of periodontal fibers occurs, which increases the mobility of the tooth. In the final stage, the accommodation of the periodontium to increased forces entails a widening of the periodontal ligament, which also leads to increased tooth mobility. Although this tooth mobility is greater than the so-called normal mobility, it cannot be considered pathologic because it is an adaptation and not a disease process. When it becomes progressively worse, it can be considered pathologic.

Other causes of increased tooth mobility include advanced bone loss, inflammation of the periodontal ligament that is of periodontal or periapical origin, and some systemic causes (e.g., pregnancy). The destruction of surrounding alveolar bone, such as occurs in osteomyelitis or jaw tumors, may also increase tooth mobility (see Chapter 30).

Radiographic signs of trauma from occlusion may include the following:

1. Increased width of the periodontal space, often with thickening of the lamina dura along the lateral aspect of the root, in the apical region, and in bifurcation areas. These changes do not *necessarily* indicate destructive changes because they may result from thickening and strengthening of the periodontal ligament and alveolar bone, constituting a favorable response to increased occlusal forces (Fig. 24-10).
2. A "vertical" rather than "horizontal" destruction of the interdental septum.

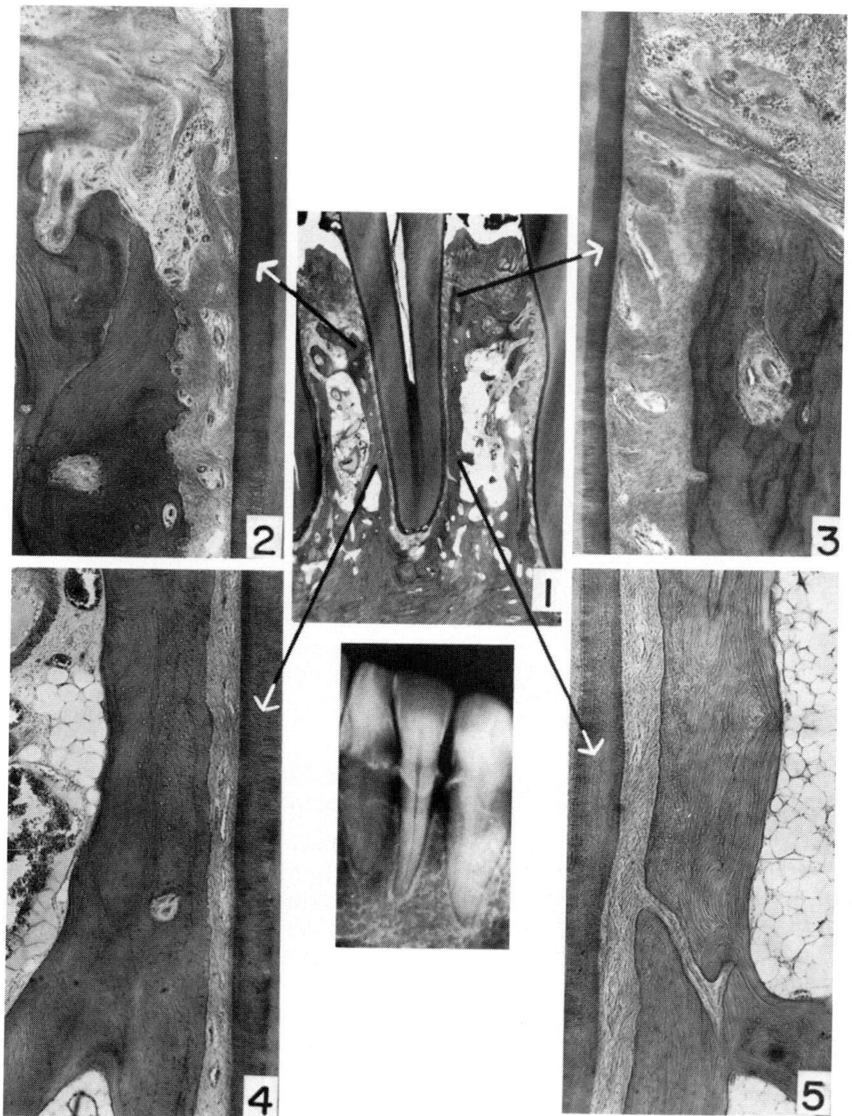

Fig. 24-10 Widened periodontal space produced by two types of tissue response to increased occlusal forces. Radiograph shows thickening of periodontal space and lamina dura around the lateral incisor. *1,* Survey microscopic section of the lateral incisor. *2,* Mesial surface widening of the periodontal space has resulted from resorption of alveolar bone associated with pressure. *3,* Distal surface widening of the periodontal space has resulted from thickening of the periodontal ligament, which is a favorable response to increased tension. *4* and *5,* Thinned periodontal ligament at axis of rotation, one third the distance from the apex.

3. Radiolucence and condensation of the alveolar bone.
4. Root resorption (see Chapter 22).

In summary, trauma from occlusion does not initiate gingivitis or periodontal pockets, but it may constitute an additional risk factor for the progression and severity of the disease. An understanding of the effect of trauma from occlusion on the periodontium is useful in the clinical management of periodontal problems.

PATHOLOGIC TOOTH MIGRATION

Pathologic migration refers to tooth displacement that results when the balance among the factors that maintain physiologic tooth position is disturbed by periodontal disease. Pathologic migration is relatively common and may be an early sign of disease, or it may occur in association with gingival inflammation and pocket formation as the disease progresses.

Pathologic migration occurs most frequently in the anterior region, but posterior teeth may also be affected. The teeth may move in any direction, and the migration is usually accompanied by mobility and rotation. Pathologic migration in the occlusal or incisal direction is termed *extrusion*. All degrees of pathologic migration are encountered, and one or more teeth may be affected (Fig. 24-11). It is important to detect it in its early stages and prevent more serious involvement by eliminating the causative factors. Even in the early stage, some degree of bone loss occurs.

Pathogenesis

Two major factors play a role in maintaining the normal position of the teeth: the health and normal height of the periodontium and the forces exerted on the teeth. The latter includes the forces of occlusion and pressure from the lips, cheeks, and tongue. The following factors are important in relation to the forces of occlusion: tooth morphologic features and cuspal inclination; the presence of a full complement of teeth; a physiologic tendency toward mesial migration; the nature and location of contact point relationships; proximal, incisal, and occlusal attrition; and the axial inclination of the teeth. Alterations in any of these factors start an interrelated sequence of changes in the environment of a single tooth or group of teeth that results in pathologic migration. Thus pathologic migration occurs under conditions that weaken the periodontal support, increase or modify the forces exerted on the teeth, or both.

Weakened Periodontal Support. The inflammatory destruction of the periodontium in periodontitis creates an imbalance between the forces maintaining the tooth in position and the occlusal and muscular forces on which it is ordinarily called to bear. The tooth with weakened support is unable to maintain its normal position in the arch and moves away from the opposing force unless it is restrained by proximal contact. The force that moves the weakly supported tooth may be created by factors such as occlusal contacts or pressure from the tongue.

It is important to understand that the abnormality in pathologic migration rests with the weakened periodontium. The force itself need not be abnormal. Forces that are acceptable to an intact periodontium become injurious when periodontal support is reduced. An example of this is the tooth with abnormal proximal contacts. Abnormally located proximal contacts convert the normal anterior component of force to a wedging force that moves the tooth occlusally or incisally. The wedging

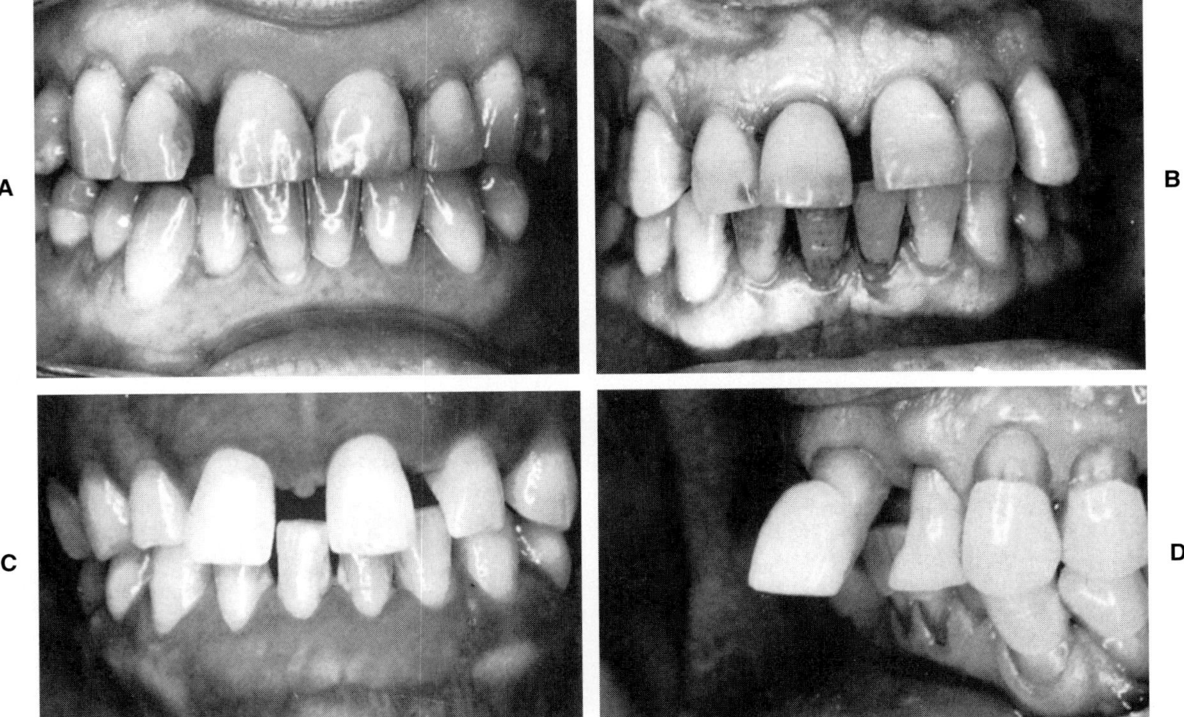

Fig. 24-11 Stages in pathologic migration. **A,** Migration of the right maxillary lateral incisor. **B,** Labial migration of maxillary central incisors and left canine, and mesial migration of the right lateral incisor. **C,** Migration and extrusion of maxillary and mandibular incisors. **D,** Severe migration of the maxillary central incisor.

force, which can be withstood by the intact periodontium, causes the tooth to extrude when the periodontal support is weakened by disease. *As its position changes, the tooth is subjected to abnormal occlusal forces, which aggravate the periodontal destruction and the tooth migration.*

Pathologic migration may continue after a tooth no longer contacts its antagonist. Pressures from the tongue, the food bolus during mastication, and proliferating granulation tissue provide the force.

Pathologic migration is also an early sign of localized aggressive periodontitis. Weakened by loss of periodontal support, the maxillary and mandibular anterior incisors drift labially and extrude, creating diastemata between the teeth (see Chapter 28).

Changes in the Forces Exerted on the Teeth. Changes in the magnitude, direction, or frequency of the forces exerted on the teeth can induce pathologic migration of a tooth or group of teeth. These forces do not have to be abnormal to cause migration if the periodontium is sufficiently weakened. Changes in the forces may occur as a result of unreplaced missing teeth, failure to replace first molars, or other causes.

UNREPLACED MISSING TEETH. Drifting of teeth into the spaces created by unreplaced missing teeth often occurs. Drifting differs from pathologic migration in that it does not result from destruction of the periodontal tissues. However, it usually creates conditions that lead to periodontal disease, and thus the initial tooth movement is aggravated by loss of periodontal support (Fig. 24-12).

Drifting generally occurs in a mesial direction, combined with tilting or extrusion beyond the occlusal plane. The premolars frequently drift distally (Fig. 24-13). Although drifting is a common sequela when missing teeth are not replaced, it does not always occur (Fig. 24-14).

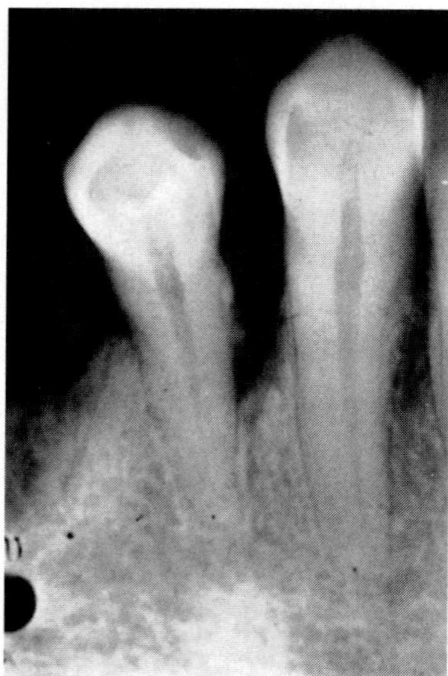

Fig. 24-12 Calculus and bone loss on the mesial surface of a canine that has drifted distally.

FAILURE TO REPLACE FIRST MOLARS. The pattern of changes that may follow failure to replace missing first molars is characteristic. In extreme cases it consists of the following:

1. The second and third molars tilt, resulting in a decrease in vertical dimension (Fig. 24-15).
2. The premolars move distally, and the mandibular incisors tilt or drift lingually. While drifting distally, the mandibular premolars lose their intercuspating relationship with the maxillary teeth and may tilt distally.
3. Anterior overbite is increased. The mandibular incisors strike the maxillary incisors near the gingiva or traumatize the gingiva.
4. The maxillary incisors are pushed labially and laterally (Fig. 24-16).
5. The anterior teeth extrude because the incisal apposition has largely disappeared.
6. Diastemata are created by the separation of the anterior teeth (see Fig. 24-15).

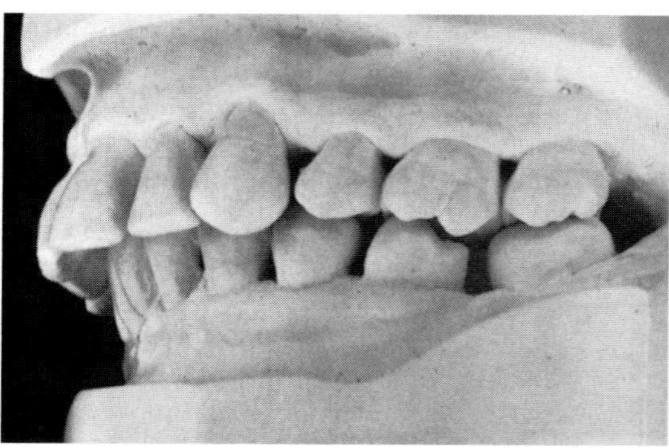

Fig. 24-13 Maxillary first molar tilted and extruded into the space created by a missing mandibular tooth.

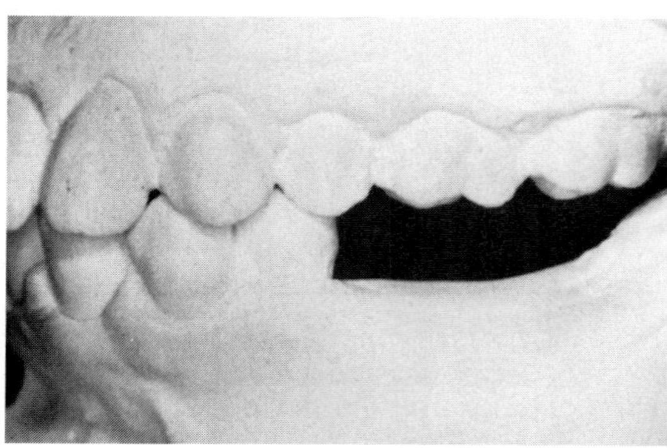

Fig. 24-14 No drifting or extrusion despite 4 years' absence of mandibular teeth.

The disturbed proximal contact relationships lead to food impaction, gingival inflammation, and pocket formation, followed by bone loss and tooth mobility. Occlusal disharmonies created by the altered tooth positions traumatize the supporting tissues of the periodontium and aggravate the destruction caused by the inflammation. Reduction in periodontal support leads to further migration of the teeth and mutilation of the occlusion.

OTHER CAUSES. *Trauma from occlusion* may cause a shift in tooth position either by itself or in combination with inflammatory periodontal disease. The direction of movement depends on the occlusal force.

Pressure from the tongue may cause drifting of the teeth in the absence of periodontal disease or may contribute to pathologic migration of teeth with reduced periodontal support (Fig. 24-17).

In tooth support weakened by periodontal destruction, *pressure from the granulation tissue of periodontal pockets* has been mentioned as contributing to pathologic migration.[38] The teeth may return to their original positions after the pockets are eliminated, but if more destruction has occurred on one side of a tooth than the other, the healing tissues tend to pull in the direction of the lesser destruction.

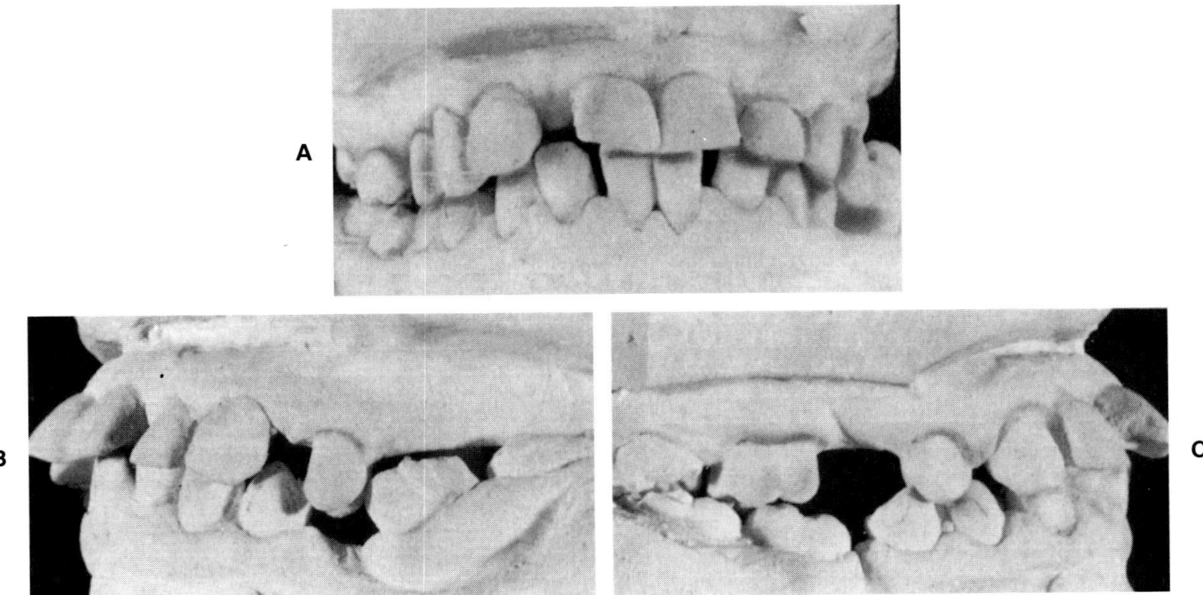

Fig. 24-15 A–C, Mutilation of occlusion associated with unreplaced missing teeth. Note pronounced pathologic migration, disturbed proximal contacts, and functional relationships with closing of the bite.

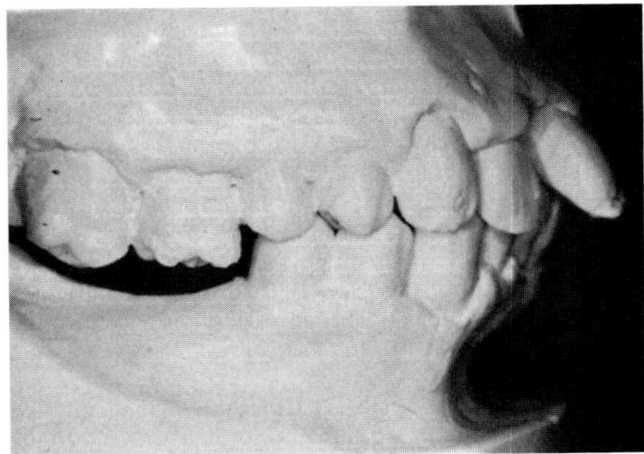

Fig. 24-16 Maxillary incisors pushed labially in patient with bilateral unreplaced mandibular molars. Note extrusion of the maxillary molars.

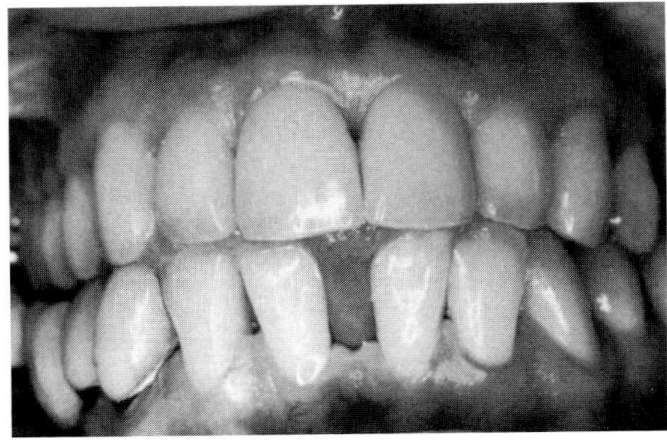

Fig. 24-17 Pathologic migration associated with tongue pressure.

REFERENCES

1. Ballbe R, Carranza FA, Erausquin R: Los paradencios del caso ocho. Rev Odont (Buenos Aires) 1938; 26:606.
2. Bhaskar SN, Orban B: Experimental occlusal trauma. J Periodontol 1955; 26:270.
3. Biancu S, Ericsson I, Lindhe J: Periodontal ligament tissue reactions to trauma and gingival inflammation. An experimental study in the beagle dog. J Clin Periodontol 1995; 22:772.
4. Box HK: Traumatic occlusion and traumatogenic occlusion. Oral Health 1930; 20:642.
5. Box HK: Experimental traumatogenic occlusion in sheep. Oral Health 1935; 25:9.
6. Box HK: Twelve Periodontal Studies. Toronto, University of Toronto Press, 1940.
7. Budtz-Jorgensen E: Bruxism and trauma from occlusion. J Clin Periodontol 1980; 7:149.
8. Burgett FG: Trauma from occlusion. Periodontal concerns. D Clin N Amer 1995; 39(2):301.
9. Carranza FA Jr: Histometric evaluation of periodontal pathology. J Periodontol 1970; 38:741.
10. Carranza FA Jr, Cabrini RL: Histometric studies of periodontal tissues. Periodontics 1967; 5:308.
11. Cohn SA: Disuse atrophy of the periodontium in molar teeth of mice. J Dent Res 1961; 40:707.
12. Comar MD, Kollar JA, Gargiulo AW: Local irritation and occlusal trauma as cofactors in the periodontal disease process. J Periodontol 1969; 40:193.
13. Coolidge ED: Traumatic and functional injuries occurring in the supporting tissues on human teeth. J Am Dent Assoc 1938; 25:343.
14. Cooper MB, Landay MA, Seltzer S: The effects of excessive occlusal forces on the pulp. II. Heavier and longer term forces. J Periodontol 1971; 42:353.
15. Dotto CA, Carranza FA Jr, Cabrini RL, et al: Vascular changes in experimental trauma from occlusion. J Periodontol 1967; 38:183.
16. Dotto CA, Carranza FA Jr, Itoiz ME: Efectos mediatos del trauma experimental en ratas. Rev Asoc Odontol Argent 1966; 54:48.
17. Ericsson I: The combined effects of plaque and physical stress on periodontal tissues. J Clin Periodontol 1986; 13:918.
18. Ericsson I, Lindhe J: Lack of effect of trauma from occlusion on the recurrence of experimental periodontitis. J Clin Periodontol 1977; 4:115.
19. Ericsson I, Lindhe J: Effect of longstanding jiggling on experimental marginal periodontitis in the beagle dog. J Clin Periodontol 1982; 9:497.
20. Ericsson I, Thilander B, Lindhe J, et al: The effect of orthodontic tilting movements on the periodontal tissues of infected and noninfected dentitions in dogs. J Clin Periodontol 1977; 4:278.
21. Everett FG, Bruckner RJ: Cartilage in the periodontal ligament space. J Periodontol 1970; 41:165.
22. Gher ME: Changing concepts. The effects of occlusion on periodontitis. D Clin N Amer 1998; 42(2):285.
23. Glickman I: Occlusion and the periodontium. J Dent Res 1967; 46(suppl 53):53.
24. Glickman I, Roeber F, Brion M, et al: Photoelastic analysis of internal stresses in the periodontium created by occlusal forces. J Periodontol 1970; 41:30.
25. Glickman I, Smulow JB: Alterations in the pathway of gingival inflammation into the underlying tissues induced by excessive occlusal forces. J Periodontol 1962; 33:7.
26. Glickman I, Smulow JB: Buttressing bone formation in the periodontium. J Periodontol 1965; 36:365.
27. Glickman I, Smulow JB: Effect of excessive occlusal forces upon the pathway of gingival inflammation in humans. J Periodontol 1965; 36:141.
28. Glickman I, Smulow JB: Adaptive alterations in the periodontium of the rhesus monkey in chronic trauma from occlusion. J Periodontol 1968; 39:101.
29. Glickman I, Smulow JB: The combined effects of inflammation and trauma from occlusion to periodontitis. Int Dent J 1969; 19:393.
30. Glickman I, Smulow JB, Moreau J: Effect of alloxan diabetes upon the periodontal response to excessive occlusal forces. J Periodontol 1966; 37:146.
31. Glickman I, Stein RS, Smulow JB: The effects of increased functional forces upon the periodontium of splinted and nonsplinted teeth. J Periodontol 1961; 32:290.
32. Glickman I, Weiss L: Role of trauma from occlusion in initiation of periodontal pocket formation in experimental animals. J Periodontol 1955; 26:14.
33. Goldman H: Gingival vascular supply in induced occlusal traumatism. Oral Surg Oral Med Oral Pathol 1956; 9:939.
34. Gottlieb B, Orban B: Changes in the Tissue due to Excessive Force upon the Teeth. Leipzig, G Thieme, 1931.
35. Gottlieb B, Orban B: Tissue changes in experimental traumatic occlusion with special reference to age and constitution. J Dent Res 1931; 11:505.
36. Grant DA, Grant DA, Flynn MJ, et al: Periodontal microbiota of mobile and nonmobile teeth. J Periodontol 1985; 66:386.
37. Hakkarainen K: Relative influence of scaling and root influence and occlusal adjustment on sulcular fluid flow. J Periodontol 1986; 57:681.
38. Hirschfeld I: The dynamic relationship between pathologically migrating teeth and inflammatory tissue in periodontal pockets: A clinical study. J Periodontol 1933; 4:35.
39. Itoiz ME, Carranza FA Jr, Cabrini RL: Histologic and histometric study of experimental occlusal trauma in rats. J Periodontol 1963; 34:305.
40. Kantor M, Polson AN, Zander HA: Alveolar bone regeneration after removal of inflammatory and traumatic factors. J Periodontol 1976; 46:687.
41. Kaufman H, Carranza FA Jr, Enders B, et al: The influence of trauma from occlusion on the bacterial repopulation of periodontal pockets in dogs. J Periodontol 1984; 55:86.
42. Kenney EB: A histopathologic study of incisal dysfunction and gingival inflammation in the rhesus monkey. J Periodontol 1971; 42:3.
43. Kobayashi K, Kobayashi K, Soeda W, et al: Gingival crevicular pH in experimental gingivitis and occlusal trauma in man. J Periodontol 1998; 69:1036.
44. Kvam E: Scanning electron microscopy of tissue changes on the pressure surface of human premolars following tooth movement. Scand J Dent Res 1972; 80:357.
45. Landay MA, Nazimov H, Seltzer S: The effects of excessive occlusal forces on the pulp. J Periodontol 1970; 41:3.
46. Levy G, Mailland ML: Etude quantitative des effets de l'hypofonction occlusale sur la largeur desmodontale et la resorption osteoclastique alveolaire chez le rat. J Biol Buccale 1980; 8:17.
47. Lindhe J, Ericsson I: The influence of trauma from occlusion on reduced but healthy periodontal tissues in dogs. J Clin Periodontol 1976; 3:110.
48. Lindhe J, Ericsson I: The effect of elimination of jiggling forces on periodontally exposed teeth in the dog. J Periodontol 1982; 53:562.
49. Lindhe J, Svanberg G: Influence of trauma from occlusion on progression of experimental periodontitis in the beagle dog. J Clin Periodontol 1974; 1:3.

50. Macapanpan LC, Weinmann JP: The influence of injury to the periodontal membrane on the spread of gingival inflammation. J Dent Res 1954; 33:263.
51. Martin LP, Noble WH: Gingival fluid in relation to tooth mobility and occlusal interferences. J Periodontol 1974; 45:444.
52. Meitner S: Co-destructive factors of marginal periodontitis and repetitive mechanical injury. J Dent Res 1975; 54:C78.
53. Orban B: Tissue changes in traumatic occlusion. J Am Dent Assoc 1928; 15:2090.
54. Orban B, Weinmann JP: Signs of traumatic occlusion in average human jaws. J Dent Res 1933; 13:216.
55. Polson AM: Trauma and progression of marginal periodontitis in squirrel monkeys. II. Codestructive factors of periodontitis and mechanically produced injury. J Periodont Res 1974; 9:108.
56. Polson AM: The relative importance of plaque and occlusion in periodontal disease. J Clin Periodontol 1986; 13:923.
57. Polson AM, Meitner SW, Zander HA: Trauma and progression of marginal periodontitis in squirrel monkeys. III. Adaption of interproximal alveolar bone to repetitive injury. J Periodont Res 1976; 11:279.
58. Polson AM, Meitner SW, Zander HA: Trauma and progression of marginal periodontitis in squirrel monkeys. IV. Reversibility of bone loss due to trauma alone and trauma superimposed upon periodontitis. J Periodont Res 1976; 11:290.
59. Polson AM, Zander HA: Effect of periodontal trauma upon intrabony pockets. J Periodontol 1983; 54:586.
60. Ramfjord SP, Kohler CA: Periodontal reaction to functional occlusal stress. J Periodontol 1959; 30:95.
61. Rothblatt JM, Waldo CM: Tissue response to tooth movement in normal and abnormal metabolic states. J Dent Res 1953; 32:678.
62. Rygh P: Ultrastructural cellular reactions in pressure zones of rat molar periodontium incident to orthodontic movement. Acta Odontol Scand 1972; 30:575.
63. Rygh P: Ultrastructural vascular changes in pressure zones of rat molar periodontium incident to orthodontic movement. Scand J Dent Res 1972; 80:307.
64. Rygh P: Ultrastructural changes in pressure zones of human periodontium incident to orthodontic tooth movement. Acta Odontol Scand 1973; 31:109.
65. Rygh P: Ultrastructural changes of the periodontal fibers and their attachment in rat molar periodontium incident to orthodontic tooth movement. Scand J Dent Res 1973; 81:467.
66. Rygh P: Elimination of hyalinized periodontal tissues associated with orthodontic tooth movement. Scand J Dent Res 1974; 82:57.
67. Rygh P, Selvig KA: Erythrocytic crystallization in rat molar periodontium incident to tooth movement. Scand J Dent Res 1973; 81:62.
68. Solt CW, Glickman I: A histologic and radioautographic study of healing following wedging interdental injury in mice. J Periodontol 1968; 39:249.
69. Sottosanti JS: A possible relationship between occlusion, root resorption and the progression of periodontal disease. J West Soc Periodontol 1977; 25:69.
70. Stahl SS: The responses of the periodontium to combined gingival inflammation and occlusofunctional stresses in four human surgical specimens. Periodontics 1968; 6:14.
71. Stahl SS: Accommodation of the periodontium to occlusal trauma and inflammatory periodontal disease. Dent Clin North Am 1975; 19:531.
72. Stahl SS, Miller SC, Goldsmith ED: The effects of vertical occlusal trauma on the periodontium of protein deprived young adult rats. J Periodontol 1957; 28:87.
73. Stallard RE: The effect of occlusal alterations on collagen formation within the periodontium. Periodontics 1964; 2:49.
74. Stones HH: An experimental investigation into the association of traumatic occlusion with paradontal disease. Proc Soc Med 1938; 31:479.
75. Svanberg G, Lindhe J: Vascular reactions to the periodontal ligament incident to trauma from occlusion. J Clin Periodontol 1974; 1:58.
76. Vollmer WH, Rateitschak KH: Influence of occlusal adjustment by grinding on gingivitis and mobility of traumatized teeth. J Clin Periodontol 1975; 2:113.
77. Waerhaug J, Hansen ER: Periodontal changes incidental to prolonged occlusal overload in monkeys. Acta Odontol Scand 1966; 24:91.
78. Wentz FM, Jarabak J, Orban B: Experimental occlusal trauma imitating cuspal interferences. J Periodontol 1958; 29:117.
79. Zaki AE, Van Huysen G: Histology of the periodontium following tooth movement. J Dent Res 1963; 42:1373.
80. Zander HA, Muhlemann HR: The effect of stresses on the periodontal structures. Oral Surg Oral Med Oral Pathol 1956; 9:380.

Masticatory System Disorders

*Michael J. McDevitt**

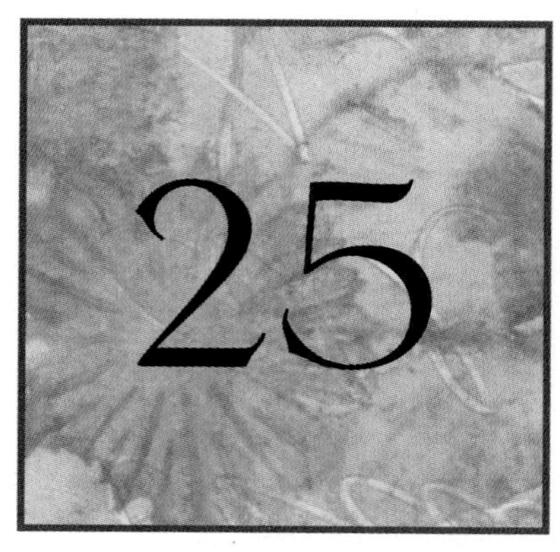

CHAPTER

CHAPTER OUTLINE

The masticatory system consists of the temporomandibular joints (TMJs), masticatory muscles, teeth in occlusion, and neurologic and vascular supplies supporting all these structures.

Research suggests that masticatory system disorders include many varied conditions with multiple possible contributing factors rather than different manifestations of a single disease or syndrome.[2,73,111] The ability to understand the anatomy and function of the masticatory system and correctly interpret relevant diagnostic information is a prerequisite to fulfilling comprehensive standards of care. Our diagnostic process must be broad based and inclusive enough to determine the most appropriate cause of masticatory dysfunction.[119]

* I would like to acknowledge the incredible efforts of Dr. David K. Warfield in helping me compile the numerous references reviewed during the development of this chapter. His encouragement, along with that of Drs. Peter Dawson and Henry Gremillion, was very meaningful and often timely. Drs. Dawson, Gremillion, Parker Mahan, and Okeson provided invaluable foundations through their publications, texts, and lectures. Although there are many others from whom I have learned much, these four exceptional dentists certainly deserve my public appreciation. I would especially like to acknowledge my precious wife, Martha-Anne, whose patience and support was priceless, as always.

THE TEMPOROMANDIBULAR JOINT

Harmonious function of the TMJs is a product of the coordination of the muscles of mastication by intricate mechanisms of neurologic control. Understanding the dynamics and the relationship of the TMJ to the associated muscles and nerves provides the working knowledge required for effective assessment and diagnosis.

The TMJ is one of the most complex joints in the human body. It is capable of providing both hinging (rotation) and gliding (translation) movements and sustaining incredible forces of mastication. The TMJ is formed by the head of the condyle of the mandible as it fits into the articular fossa of the temporal bone (Fig. 25-1). The body of the mandible effectively connects both condyles so that neither condyle functions independently of the other. Interposed between the head of the condyle and the articular surface of the temporal bone is the articular disc, consisting of dense connective tissue, resulting in a compound joint with two joint cavities (see Figs. 25-1 and 25-2). The articulating surfaces of the osseous structures are essentially convex in a healthy situation, so the biconcave configuration of the articular disc compensates for the opposing convexities (see Fig. 25-1). The articular surfaces of the condyles and temporal bones consist of fibrous connective tissue, rendering them resistant to breakdown and capable of repair. Deep to the superficial connective tissue layer, articular cartilage provides the cellular and structural basis for response to the functional loading and movement of the TMJs.[73,119,164] The discal ligaments and attachments to the capsule along with the disc itself become the means of separating the joint into superior and inferior joint spaces (see Figs. 25-1 and 25-2). Synovial lubrication of the articular surfaces is a function of synovial fluid production by endothelial cells along the borders of each joint cavity and at the anterior extent of the retrodiscal tissues.*

MUSCLES AND NERVES OF THE MASTICATORY SYSTEM

The muscles and nerves of the masticatory system are extensively reviewed elsewhere and are only briefly discussed here for the purpose of understanding the mechanisms involved. Appropriate references are provided for further reading.

The muscles of mastication consist principally of two groups: the elevator muscles and depressor muscles. The muscles responsible for elevating the mandible are the masseter, internal pterygoid, and much of the temporal muscle. The posteriorly oriented fibers of the temporal muscle also retrude the mandible. The superficial muscle bundle of the masseter muscle may also assist in protruding the mandible, while the deeper bundle serves to stabilize the condylar head against the articular eminence. Juxtaposed with the masseter muscle, the medial pterygoid forms a muscular support for the mandible at its angle. Although the primary function of this muscle is elevation of the mandible, it is also active during protrusion.[73,119] The lateral pterygoid muscle is now known to function as two distinct muscles, the inferior and superior lateral pterygoid muscles, having independent and nearly opposite functions.[6,14] The inferior lateral pterygoid muscle depresses and protrudes the mandible. The superior lateral pterygoid muscle does not contract during depression of the mandible but rather contracts along with the elevator muscles, bracing the condyle anteromedially.[99,107,117,119,139]

Physiologic mandibular posture and movement are products of harmonious muscular contraction among masticatory and supportive muscles. The neurologic input to produce synergy of complementary and antagonistic muscles is extremely complex. Motor and sensory innervation of the TMJs and the rest of the masticatory system are provided by structures of the trigeminal nerve. Mechanoreceptors in the skin, muscle, and ligamentous structures, especially the periodontal ligament, discern pressure differences at sensitive degrees of discrimination. Painful stimuli are perceived by nociceptors and result in both pain perception and reflex responses. The innervation of both the capsular ligaments and discal ligaments provide essential proprioceptive input with regard to joint position. Efferent or motor neurons cause muscle contraction in response to central cortical stimulation and in response to afferent stimuli in reflex activity.[38,119,164]

*See references 38, 73, 119, 159, 161, and 164.

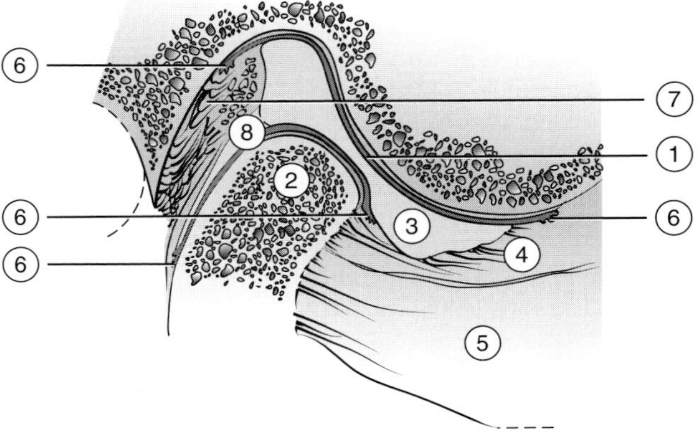

Fig. 25-1 Lateral view of cross-section through the temporomandibular joint. *1,* Posterior slope of the articular eminence of the temporal bone; *2,* head of the condyle; *3,* disc (note biconcave shape); *4,* superior lateral pterygoid muscle (note attachment to both the head of the condyle and disc); *5,* inferior lateral pterygoid muscle; *6,* synovial tissue; *7,* retrodiscal tissue; *8,* discal ligament attachment to the posterior surface of the head of the condyle. (Modified from Dawson PE: Evaluation, Diagnosis, and Treatment of Occlusal Problems, ed 2. St Louis, Mosby, 1989.)

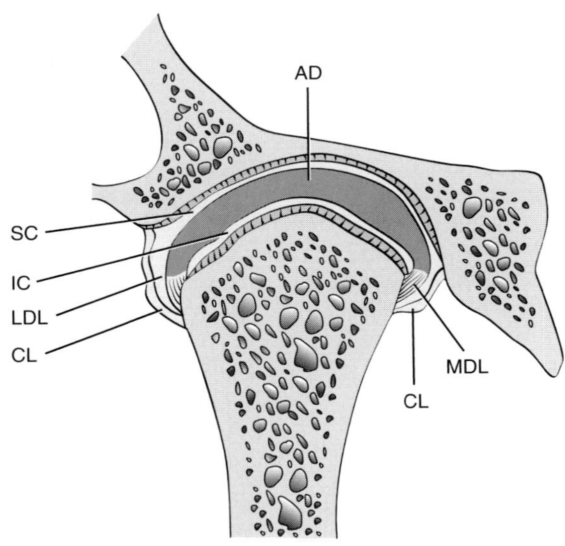

Fig. 25-2 Temporomandibular joint (anterior view), showing collateral ligaments. The following are identified: *AD,* articular disc; *CL,* capsular ligament; *IC,* inferior joint cavity; *LDL,* lateral discal ligament; *MDL,* medial discal ligament; *SC,* superior joint cavity. (From Okeson JP: Management of Temporomandibular Joint Disorders and Occlusion, ed 4. St Louis, Mosby, 1998.)

Sensory input from the periodontal ligament (PDL) offers the potential to be an important component of the complex neurologic management of the masticatory system. Currently, little evidence of the existence of proprioceptive sensory organs within the neuroanatomy of the PDL is available, although it was once considered likely. Pain perception causes the nociceptive reflex to rapidly open the mouth through contraction of depressor muscles and suppression of elevator muscles, consistent with other protective reflexes within the musculoskeletal system.[119] Protective reflexes may be suppressed in individuals experiencing chronic occlusal parafunction (clenching or grinding of their teeth).[23,46] Pressure perception is a function of the numerous mechanoreceptors within the PDL of teeth in contact. Discrimination within the dentition based on specific teeth in contact, direction of force, and intensity of force and their influence on muscle activity have been demonstrated in human study populations and animal studies.[22,35,90,98,142] Both research and clinical observations suggest that elevator muscle contraction is suppressed when anterior teeth promote disclusion or separation of posterior teeth during excursive mandibular movements.[160] Implicit in the experience of loss of attachment due to periodontitis is the loss of some mechanoreceptors. Patients with significant bone loss, significant inflammatory disruption of the integrity of the PDL, or chronic occlusal parafunction may experience compromised regulation of muscle activity.*

CENTRIC RELATION

The mandible is suspended from the cranial base by ligaments and muscles. Understanding mandibular movement begins from an initial reference point for each condyle, commonly referred to as *centric relation*. In this clinically determined relationship of the mandible to the maxilla, occurring when both condyle-disc assemblies are positioned in their most superior position in the maxillary (or glenoid) fossa and against the slope of the articular eminence of the temporal bone. Verification of centric relation is obtained by loading the TMJs bilaterally with the teeth apart, using the bimanual mandibular manipulation technique advocated by Dawson and others.[38,39,152] When both condyles are in this relationship, rotation or hinging action occurs around an axis defined by the medial poles of each condyle (Fig. 25-3). The term *centric relation* is limited to the rotation axis through both condyles while they are seated in their respective glenoid fossa. The only occlusal consideration relative to centric relation occurs when rotation of the mandible brings about initial contact of opposing occlusal surfaces. The term *retruded contact position,* as used in the chapters of this text dealing with occlusion, can be used to define this relationship. Should the contraction of elevator muscles occur at the point of initial occlusal contact, resulting in the distraction of one or both condyle-disc assemblies from their seated relationship, then centric relation is no longer occurring.[38,39]

For TMJs to maintain orthopedic stability, the condyles must remain fully seated in their respective fossa when the teeth occlude in maximal intercuspation. Orthopedic instability occurs when the occlusal relationships are such that contraction of elevator muscles is required to achieve stable occlusion in maximal intercuspal position, resulting in the unseating of one or both condyles from their respective fossa (Fig. 25-4). The strain on the discal ligaments caused by a loaded joint being displaced from the fossa can lead to internal derangement of that joint, as is described later. Postural and parafunctional stress can also be a source of orthopedic instability of a TMJ. An individual's susceptibility to masticatory system disorders determines whether that person adapts with minimal consequence or suffers dysfunction or degeneration.[24,38,119,152]

*See references 2, 23, 46, 70, 73, 111, 119, and 137.

BIOMECHANICS OF THE MASTICATORY SYSTEM

Biomechanics of mandibular movement are a function of neurologic input from cortical and stomatognathic sources acting to initiate or restrict muscular contraction. Muscular action either stabilizes the condyle against the articular eminence or directs its rotational and/or translational movement relative to each respective temporal bone. The position and functional movement of one condyle is always dependent on the status or activity of the other. Because the maxillary teeth have a fixed relationship to the cranial base, just as mandibular teeth have a fixed relationship to the condyle, contact of their respective occlusal surfaces may directly influence condylar position or movement.[38,119]

The mandible can move within a range of motion that is limited by skeletal, muscular, and ligamentous structures. Pure rotation of up to approximately 25 mm can occur before translation of the condyle is required to continue toward maximal opening of the jaw. Movement of the condyle is relative to the disc, so rotation effectively occurs within the inferior joint space (Fig. 25-5, *A*). Strict translation protrudes the mandible while the condyle-disc assembly moves anterior and inferior toward the articular eminence of the temporal bone. The disc moves relative to the temporal bone, and movement occurs within the upper joint space (see Fig. 25-5, *B*). In combination translation/rotation movement of the condyle, the axis of rotation for each condyle changes as the condyle translates down the articular eminence to a position inferior to its respective fossa (see Fig. 25-5, *C*). Harmonious muscle function and ligament attachments keep the condyle-disc assembly properly related so that the articular disc remains loaded in its concave, avascular central portion between the condyle and the articular surface of the temporal bone. The elasticity and vascularity of the retrodiscal tissues permit anterior movement of the disc during translation of each respective condyle. Rotation and translation of the condyle can occur in the absence of any tooth-to-tooth contact because the condyle-disc assembly can be supported by the muscles of mastication against the articular eminence during rotation, translation, and combination movements. When the teeth are in contact, their ability to influence both the position and the direction of movement of condyle-disc assemblies is defined by the intensity of muscle activity and the steepness of the inclines of those teeth.[38,67,77,93,119]

DYSFUNCTION AND DETERIORATION

Ideally, function never exceeds the integrity or adaptive limits of the structural elements of the masticatory system. In clinical experience, the tolerance of the components of the masticatory system can be exceeded by both acute trauma and chronic trauma.

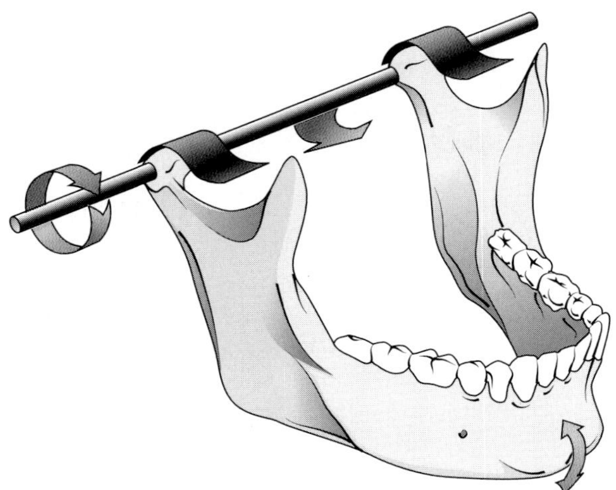

Fig. 25-3 In centric relation, the condyles can rotate on a fixed axis. As long as the rotational axis stays fixed at the most superior position against the eminentiae, the mandible can open or close and still be in centric relation. If the condyle axis moves forward, it is no longer in centric relation. (From Dawson PE: Evaluation, Diagnosis, and Treatment of Occlusal Problems, ed 2. St Louis, Mosby, 1989.)

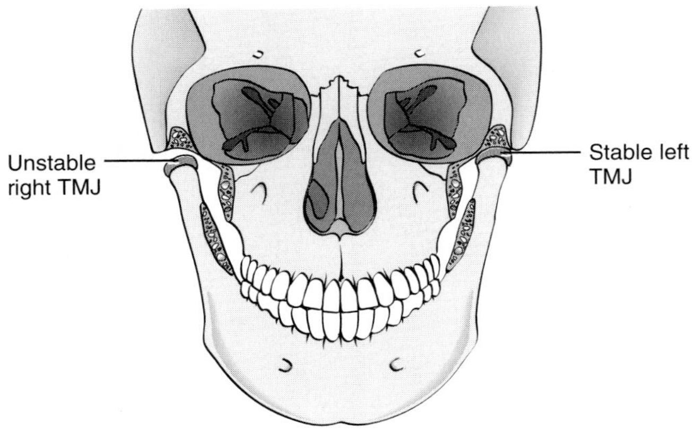

Fig. 25-4 An example of orthopedic instability. Note that with the teeth in their stable position (maximal intercuspation), the left temporomandibular joint is in a stable relationship with the fossa. The right temporomandibular joint, however, is not in a stable position in the fossa. When the elevator muscles contract, the right condyle moves superiorly, seeking a more stable relationship with the disc and fossa (the musculoskeletally stable position). This type of loading can lead to an intracapusular disorder. (From Okeson JP: Management of Temporomandibular Joint Disorders and Occlusion, ed 4. St Louis, Mosby, 1998.)

Acute trauma to the head and neck region can range from a distinct event, such as an accident or a blow to the face, to a sustained overuse experience, such as a long dental appointment. Acute trauma can serve as an initiating event leading toward a chronic condition, so accurate documentation and careful monitoring may prove extremely valuable should symptoms or dysfunction persist.[12,19,41]

Chronic trauma is defined as any experience that repeatedly exceeds the tolerances of the affected masticatory system structure. Postural stresses and parafunctional occlusal habits, with or without occlusal discrepancies, may produce musculoskeletal disharmony and orthopedic instability of the TMJ. Occlusal relationships that disrupt the condyle during physiologic movement of rotation or translation require muscular and TMJ compensation. The extent to which the repeated loading of the teeth and/or the condyles during function and parafunction exceeds the tolerance of an individual determine whether structural or muscular compromise occurs.[119] In the absence of prospective research, it is somewhat difficult to associate defined occlusal patterns with specific muscle or joint disorders; however, retrospective studies and clinical experience still offer valuable perspectives. When correlation of TMJ dysfunction could be made with specific occlusal relationships, the trend was to recognize that when inclines of posterior teeth dominated occlusal function, masticatory system harmony was disrupted.* Other researchers have found that various occlusal interferences and relationships are common among individuals with and without masticatory system disorders. They could not distinguish a particular occlusal feature as a specific etiologic or predisposing factor to the development of masticatory system disorders, although some found that several factors occurring together encouraged dysfunction.[33,66,127,129,151] There seems to be less correlation between static references, such as class of malocclusion, and masticatory system disorders than when functional or extrafunctional occlusal force exceed the tolerance of the TMJ and masticatory musculature.[119,141]

The general terms for occlusal parafunction to be used in this text include *bruxism,* or grinding of the teeth, and *clenching,* where a person holds the teeth firmly together with significant force. Bruxism is commonly confirmed by observing excessive tooth wear. Clenching type of parafunction can be distinguished from grinding the teeth and seems to be more commonly associated with masticatory system disorders than does bruxism.* Discrimination between occlusal function or parafunction-related masticatory system disorders and those with other etiology requires exacting standards of occlusal evaluation. Should there be sufficient evidence to suspect that the occlusal relationships in function or parafunction may have exceeded the tolerances of that individual's masticatory system, then responsible intervention or monitoring can be initiated.[39,57,122,127]

Disruption of the relationship or alignment of the condyle, disc, and articular surface of the temporal bone is commonly called an *intracapsular disorder* or *internal derangement* of the TMJ. The articular disc can be displaced as a result of an acute blow to the jaw, the effect of chronic trauma, and/or the result of uncoordinated

*See references 1, 27, 39, 62, 66, 71, 110, 119, 158, and 160.

*See references 28, 53, 55, 72, 122, and 128.

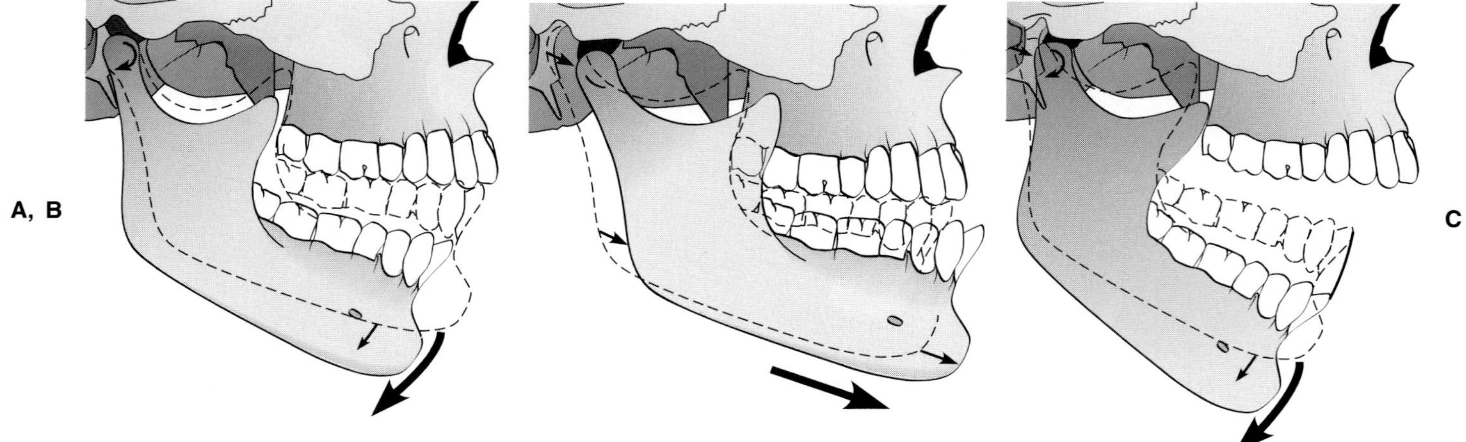

Fig. 25-5 **A,** Rotational movement of the mandible with the condyles in centric relation. This pure rotational opening can occur until the anterior teeth are about 20 to 25 mm apart. **B,** Translational movement of the condyle-disc assembly during protrusion of the mandible. **C,** Second stage of rotational movement during opening. Note the dual activity relative to the disc. *1,* Rotation of the condylar head, relative to the disc, occurs in the inferior space. *2,* Movement of the disc anteriorly and inferiorly along the articular surface of the temporal bone. The disc moves anteriorly and inferiorly with the head of the condyle, which continues to rotate against the disc. Translation occurs in the superior joint space and rotation in the inferior joint space. (From Okeson JP: Management of Temporomandibular Joint Disorders and Occlusion, ed 4. St Louis, Mosby, 1998.)

contraction of the lateral pterygoid muscle. When the disc cannot return to its normal relationship to the condyle on full closure of the mouth, it is considered to be *displaced* or *dislocated.* Progressive disc displacement most commonly occurs in an anterior and medial direction due to the insertion of muscle fibers into the anteromedial aspect of the disc and the reported variability in resistance of the attachment of the lateral aspect of the disc.[11,143] Stretching of the retrodiscal tissues and collateral ligaments permits the disc to be displaced and function to be limited because of pain due to compressive forces on retrodiscal tissues. At some stage of opening, the remaining elasticity of the retrodiscal tissues and tension of the capsular ligaments can pull the disc onto the head of the condyle, often with a discernible sound. Closing then results in the disc again becoming dislocated anteriorly, with a commonly occurring joint sound often referred to as a *reciprocal click* (Fig. 25-6).*

When the disc remains anterior to the head of the condyle during rotation and the limited range of translation possible, the condition is called *closed lock* or *disc displacement (dislocation) without reduction* (Fig. 25-7). The entire disc need not be locked anterior to the head of the condyle for this condition to limit function, cause pain, or both. The lateral aspect of the disc would be more likely than the medial aspect to be displaced anteriorly if a *partial anterior disc displacement without reduction* were to occur. A history of joint sounds is commonly reported, although this state of the condyle-disc assembly may not result in currently discernible sounds.[38,119]

*See references 9, 38, 39, 119, 130, and 154.

The vascular portion of the retrodiscal tissues being loaded (between the condyle and the articular surface of the eminentia) accounts for most current or history of pain originating within the TMJ. Adaptation of the retrodiscal tissues to completely nonvascular fibrous tissue or perforation of the disc may account for cessation of those painful symptoms.[123]

The presence of abnormal anatomic features of the condyle and fossa results in deviation in shape of the affected articular surface to which the disc then must adapt its normal anatomy, resulting in a deviation in form and function. If this type of functional limitation or irregularity is observed at a consistently occurring point in jaw opening and/or closing, it is often within the compensation mechanisms of the patient and should be distinguished from the disc derangements described previously.[119]

When the intensity and duration of the functional and dysfunctional loading of the TMJs result in injury, molecular agents appear to be active in the degeneration of joints. Free radicals, various catabolic enzymes, neuropeptides, estrogen, cytokines, and prostaglandins are implicated in inflammatory reactions that have an impact on the articular surfaces, synovial fluid, or both.* Loss of the ability of the synovial fluid to lubricate articular surfaces can result in adherence of the disc. Limitation of rotation occurs with adherence between the disc and the condyle, whereas fixation of the disc against the fossa permits rotation but does not allow the disc to move forward during translation.[119]

*See references 50, 60, 81, 84, 86, 108, 109, 115, 133, and 145.

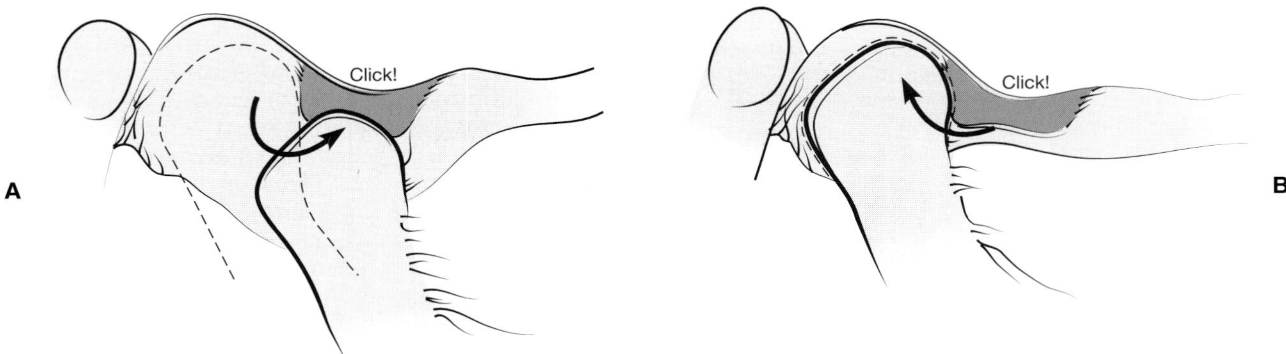

Fig. 25-6 Reciprocal click. **A,** Reciprocal click occurs when the condyle moves onto the disc from a position behind the posterior band of the disc and then clicks off the disc **(B)** when the condyle moves back. This occurs as the condyle translates forward and back in the opening and closing movements. (From Dawson PE: Evaluation, Diagnosis, and Treatment of Occlusal Problems, ed 2. St Louis, Mosby, 1989.)

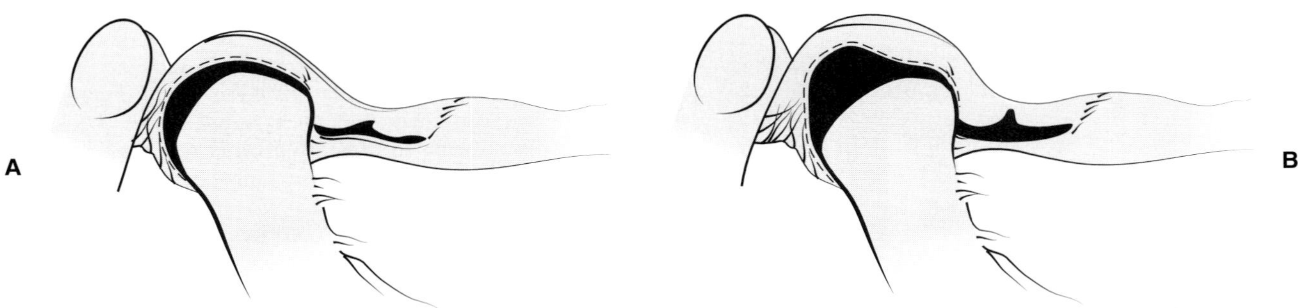

Fig. 25-7 Anterior disc displacement without reduction. **A,** Condyle positioned in the fossa on retrodiscal tissues with the disc remaining anterior to head of condyle. **B,** During translation, the disc is further misshaped, restricting full opening of the mandible.

Hypermobility (subluxation) of the TMJ can permit the condyle to translate beyond the eminentia with both the disc and the condyle beyond its prominence. The combination of anatomic features, which predispose individuals to subluxation, often allows for self-reduction of the condyles. When condyles translate beyond the eminentia but the discs are trapped posteriorly, the combined steepness of the disc and the eminentia prevents reduction of each condyle so that the mandible is locked open.[119]

OROFACIAL PAIN

Discomfort associated with masticatory system disorders falls under the larger umbrella of orofacial pain. Pain associated with TMJ dysfunction is most frequently muscular in origin.[38] Working knowledge of even the uncommon sources of pain perceived in the region of the masticatory system is essential to providing comprehensive diagnosis and treatment. Sources of dental or periodontal pain should be identified by clinical, radiographic, and/or historical information. Nondental sources of pain include TMJ structures, muscles, cervical structures, neuropathies, vascular inflammation, all types of headache, sleep disorders, systemic disorders, and psychoimmune neurologic sources.[118] A survey of 45,700 American households revealed that 22% of respondents had experienced some type of orofacial pain in the previous 6 months, establishing a meaningful probability that the periodontal patient's list of symptoms includes pain.[94] The current list of possible sources of orofacial pain, prepared by the American Academy of Orofacial Pain, is depicted in Box 25-1.[118]

Headache pain is perceived primarily within the trigeminal nerve pathways, although other cranial and cervical nerves may offer painful sensory input.[73,118] Pain originating in masticatory system structures, which are also innervated by the trigeminal nerve, requires diagnostic differentiation from headache pain.[141] Headache can present in a myriad of forms and can influence perception of pain and diagnosis of origin of pain.[73,118] Pain of dental and periodontal origin must be clearly defined and differentiated from heart attack, sinus pain or myofascial pain.[118,119] Pain originating in pulpal or periodontal nociceptors would be differentiated within a comprehensive clinical and radiographic

BOX 25-1

Differential Diagnosis of Orofacial Pain

Intracranial Pain Disorders[65,73,118,124]
Neoplasm, aneurysm, abscess, hemorrhage, hematoma, edema

Primary Headaches Disorders (Neurovascular Disorders)[87,119]
Migraine, migraine variants, cluster headache, paroxysmal hemicrania, cranial arteritis, carotidynia, tension-type headache[80,118,119,140]

Neurogenic Pain Disorders
Paroxysmal neuralgias: Trigeminal, glossopharyngeal, nervus intermedius and superior laryngeal neuralgias[156]
Continuous pain disorders: Deafferentation pain syndromes (peripheral neuritis, postherpetic neuritis, posttraumatic and postsurgical neuralgia, neuralgia–inducing cavitation osteonecrosis[16,17])
Sympathetically maintained pain

Intraoral Pain Disorders
Dental pulp, periodontium, mucogingival tissues, tongue[13,105]

Temporomandibular Disorders
Masticatory muscle, temporomandibular joint, associated structures

Associated Structures[118,119]
Ears, eyes, nose, paranasal sinuses, throat, lymph nodes, salivary glands, neck

Axis II, Mental Disorders
Somatoform disorders
Pain syndromes of psychogenic origin

evaluation. Orofacial pain originating in the TMJs and/or the muscles of mastication can occur as a product of neoplasm, macrotrauma, repeated microtrauma, systemic disease, or anatomic predisposition. Within the joint structures, inflammation and/or compression of vascularized components are the direct source of pain. Synovitis or capsulitis, with or without osteoarthritis, and the polyarthritides are characterized by local pain, which increases with function while limiting range of motion of the affected TMJ. In addition to the potential for pain, symptoms of arthritis can include limited mandibular opening, disruption of other jaw mechanics, and joint sounds characteristic of degenerative change to and/or direct contact between articular surfaces.* Orofacial pain originating in the muscles of mastication may be perceived in that region or may be referred to other structures such as individual teeth. Similarly, pain referral to the region of certain muscles requires definition of origin. Because local provocation at the origin of pain should produce symptoms at the site of perception of pain, movement of the jaw would be expected to elicit pain in painful muscles of mastication. Cranial nerves experience referral on the same side, whereas skeletal nerve referral can occur to the opposite side; both sources generally refer pain centrally or superiorly.[73,119,146] The muscles of mastication can be subject to a variety of disorders and dysfunction, many of which can be painful. The American Academy of Orofacial Pain designates myofascial pain, myositis, myospasm, local myalgia, and myofibrotic contracture as major categories of these conditions. Muscle palpation that reveals a taut band of muscle or fascia and that results in pain, which is also frequently referred, is virtually diagnostic for myofascial pain. Myostitis of masticatory muscles arises from direct trauma or infection in close proximity to muscle. Associated pain increases with mandibular movement, thereby limiting range of motion. Muscle spasm is the sustained involuntary contraction resulting in pain and dramatic shortening of the affected muscle. Myospasm of masticatory muscles greatly limits mandibular movement and can change occlusion suddenly due to its rapid onset. Local myalgia, pain specific to individual muscles, may result from ischemia or fatigue and may present as delayed-onset muscle soreness and/or protective co-contraction. Occlusal parafunction, extended dental appointments, metabolic imbalances, and sympathetic nervous system influences have been associated with this painful muscular reaction. An extended period of limited range of mandibular movement can result in fibrosis of the muscle and related attachments, creating a painless condition called *myofibrotic contracture*.[118]

Otolaryngologic symptoms associated with masticatory system disorders have been reported and include degrees of deafness, tinnitus, and vertigo.* Trauma and postural stress in the cervical spine can be responsible for both the perception and origin of pain within the masticatory system.[12,19,73,119]

Determination of a specific origin or source of pain can be made more difficult by both pain referral and modulation of painful experiences by the central nervous system. Sensitization of peripheral nocioceptors by higher neural centers and inflammation at the site of origin of pain can alter pain perception. Persistent inflammation therefore may be a contributing factor to chronic pain.[74,101,144] Systemic conditions that may contribute to or predispose an individual to compromised pain regulation include sleep disorders, fibromyalgia, chronic depression, chronic fatigue syndrome, hypothyroidism, insufficient thyroid receptor activity, prolactin feedback disorder, epinephrine sensitivity related to mitral valve prolapse, premenstrual syndrome, androgen excess in women, and posttraumatic stress disorder. Although some of these situations exhibit gender bias due to hor-

*See references 42, 45, 56, 58, 68, 82, 83, 97, 100, 102, 118, and 165.

*See references 15, 21, 25, 26, 34, 36, 52, 76, 113, 119, 121, 135, 136, and 163.

monal factors, the influence of stress on pain experiences and the effect of variable coping skills are reported for both genders.*

COMPREHENSIVE EVALUATION

Patient History and Interview

The written history and personal interview should be designed to invite open-ended response and reflection by the patient on past experiences and current condition. Standard dental or medical history forms may require modification to include questions regarding any history of limited or painful jaw movement, noise in either joint, and masticatory muscle symptoms (Box 25-2). These issues should be documented with regard to timing, duration, frequency, and relationship to any history of trauma.[118]

Clinical Examination

The clinical examination continues the interview process through codiscovery of the patient's masticatory system status. The dentist leads the patient to understand the meaning of signs and symptoms of dysfunction or deterioration, seeking opportunities to expand responses to questions asked of the patient. The physical examination actually begins during the interview when asymmetries in facial form, head posture, and mandibular movement patterns can be observed. Clinical evaluation of the various structures of the masticatory system, although individual to each practitioner, should include the following[9,38,119]:

1. Observation and measurement of full range motion of the mandible
2. Auscultation and light palpation of each TMJ in its full range of motion
3. Load testing of each TMJ
4. Palpitation of each muscle of mastication and related head and neck muscles
5. Evaluation of all the soft tissues of the face, oral cavity, and oropharynx
6. Periodontal and dental examinations
7. Complete occlusal analysis, including accurately mounted diagnostic models

Evaluation of the TMJ begins with range-of-motion analysis. Observation of departure from a straight path of opening and closing the mandible suggests an intracapsular disorder or masticatory muscle incoordination.[38,119] An average maximal opening of 50 mm is common; findings of less than 40 mm of opening suggest limited opening due to a masticatory system disorder. The range of right and left lateral excursions is usually about 9 mm, and protrusion of mandible is commonly 7 mm. Limitation in range of motion may be normal for some patients, but for most, these observations are of diagnostic value.[9,44,64,119,147] Auscultation of the joint by listening with a stethoscope or Doppler instrument, which amplifies joint sound for both the patient and the dentist, can reveal noises diagnostic for numerous conditions. The intensity and nature of any sounds, clicks, pops, and/or crepitus (grinding, grating, or rubbing sounds) should be recorded accurately. Any sound detected as part of the initial evaluation should be tracked consistently to detect any change. Diagnostic interpretation and management based on specific sounds correlated with status of the TMJ can be found in other references.[7,9,38,119,157]

Firm palpation of the TMJ with the mouth closed can be uncomfortable to the patient with inflammation in joint structures or superficial muscles. Palpation while opening may become more uncomfortable if retrodiscal tissues are also inflamed. Load testing of the TMJ is essentially a means to palpate the head of the condyle, surface of the glenoid fossa, and tissue interposed between

BOX 25-2

Examples of Questions or Subjects to Be Included in Patient History

Are you now experiencing or have you ever experienced any of the following?

1. Pain in either jaw joint or pain when opening or closing your mouth[8]
2. Acute or direct trauma to the face, jaw, head, or neck such as during an accident
3. Any locking or restricted movement of either jaw joint[44,147]
4. Inability to bite or close teeth together completely without discomfort of one or both jaw joints
5. Earache without infection, especially if it is recurring
6. Ringing or rushing sounds in either ear
7. Any type of neuralgia, especially with trigger points
8. Tooth pain without diagnosed dental problem or following tooth removal[103,104,162]
9. Fibromyalgia[37,126,131]
10. Sleep apnea or any sleep disturbance
11. Any sounds (clicks, pops, etc.) in either jaw joint, especially when opening or while eating
12. Chronic or frequently recurring headaches, especially migraine or cluster type of headache[4]
13. Shingles or any painful infection of face or neck
14. Having to "adjust" the jaw or manipulate jaw joint with your hand to be able to open or close your mouth
15. An occupation or activity that requires regular stressful posture such as cradling a telephone between head and shoulder, working at a computer, playing a musical instrument, or scuba diving[150,166]
16. Awareness of frequently keeping your teeth together, maintaining a clenched jaw, or holding your jaw in an assumed position such as holding a pipe
17. Lyme disease[61]
18. Neck muscles that are commonly tired or sore
19. Sleep position or posture that maintains pressure on your lower jaw

*See references 5, 20, 51, 92, 116, 118, 138, and 149.

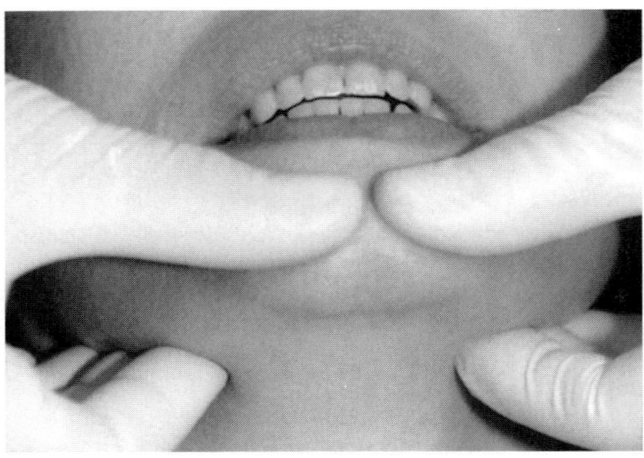

Fig. 25-8 Bimanual manipulation load testing in centric relation with the teeth apart.

them, except in the case of bone-to-bone contact. With bimanual mandibular manipulation, the dentist loads the joints equally and may detect resistance or tension on either side. The patient is in a supine position in the dental chair to minimize postural influence on muscle activity. The patient's head is braced by the support of the chair and by being cradled against the dentist's arm and/or abdomen. The dentist's middle fingers locate the notch in the mandible just anterior to the angle, and the thumbs are placed near the midline in the mental region of the mandible (Fig. 25-8). Initially, the dentist provides very gentle guidance to the hinging action of the mandible, with a slight lifting force applied by the fingers and slight depressing force applied with the thumbs. Should the patient remain comfortable, then increasing force can be applied at both points, ultimately with enough pressure to load test the joints (see Fig. 25-8). With the avascular fibrous discs interposed, the condyles are in centric relation and the loading of both joints is comfortable. Discomfort may occur with muscle incoordination or bracing or with an anterior displaced disc and attempted loading of vascular retrodiscal tissues of either TMJ. When performed properly, the patient can bite firmly as part of guided loading of the TMJs and report the nature or absence of pain or tension.[9,38,59,119]

Muscle palpation is also a learned technique that requires both experience and expertise to derive the most reliable information. Too little pressure is not diagnostic of modest muscle pain or spasm, while too much pressure can hurt even when normal musculature is palpated.[54] Externally, the muscles palpated include the anterior, middle, and posterior temporalis; superficial masseter; anterior and posterior digastric; sternocleidomastoid; trapezeius; posterior cervical muscles; and insertion of the medial pterygoid muscle. Intraorally, the deep masseter is tested with moderate squeezing pressure and the medial pterygoid muscle is palpated directly in the general region of the insertion point for mandibular block local anesthesia. The lateral pterygoid is difficult to palpate due to the dominance of the medial pterygoid in the same region. Its palpation superior and distal to the palpation point for the medial pterygoid can be attempted distal to the maxillary tuberosity. Offering manual resistance to the patient's efforts to protrude the mandible is also a test of the lateral pterygoid muscle. Neither method of evaluation of the possible soreness of the lateral pterygoid muscle is completely reliable, although some insight into muscle status is obtained.*

During any of the muscle palpation portion of the clinical examination, it may be possible for the dentist to detect a particularly taut and uncomfortable band of muscle fibers. This condition represents regional myofascial pain or trigger point myalgia, which can be responsible for referral of pain to the teeth and other orofacial regions. Diagnostic injection of local anesthesia can be very effective in identifying trigger point pain and pain referral patterns but is beyond the scope of this text.[119,146]

The occlusal analysis is a logical extension of the evaluation of the teeth and periodontium. Tooth mobility is assessed in both static and dynamic modes. Pressure applied to a tooth with a firm object allows detection of movement with both visual and tactile evaluation possible. Asking the patient to move in excursions of the mandible while maintaining firm contact of opposing teeth also permits visual and tactile assessment. Sources of tooth mobility include inadequate periodontal support, inflammation of the periodontium, and excessive occlusal loading of the teeth with adequate periodontium, resulting in adaptive mobility. The physical evaluation of the teeth and any restorations can reflect history of trauma or wear. Visual observation, registration with marking paper or wax, and electronic assessment of tooth contacts as the patient moves in all excursions may reveal disharmonies sufficient to cause orthopedic instability of either TMJ. If the teeth are found to be relatively firm, then the relationship of the maxillary and mandibular teeth may influence the direction of condylar movement as soon as tooth-to-tooth contact is made. While maintaining centric relation, the physical examination continues by positioning the condyles in a fully seated relationship without tooth-to-tooth contact using bimanual manipulation or a leaf gauge technique. The mandible is manually guided to close until the first tooth-to-tooth contact is made. If that position is also maximal intercuspation, then optimal seating of the condyles is maintained. If the initial tooth-to-tooth contact is not maximal intercuspation, then the condyles will be directed from a fully seated position to an inferior position relative to their respective fossae, resulting in an orthopedic instability. The direction and extent of the accommodation of the mandible should be carefully measured and recorded at the initial evaluation and consistently evaluated at subsequent appointments so that any trend may be discovered.**

To increase the reliability of this evaluation, a muscle deprogramming effort may be employed. The simplest approach is to use cotton rolls placed between the anterior teeth for 5 to 15 minutes to allow possible muscle relaxation through avoidance of proprioceptive or

* See references 3, 9, 38, 47, 49, 73, 119, and 148.

** See references 9, 29, 30, 38–40, 48, 69, 71, 78, 79, 85, 95, 96, 119, 120, 132, 134, 141, and 155.

pressure neurologic input. A prefabricated or directly fabricated acrylic or composite bite stop for anterior teeth will offer the same advantage.[9,10,119] A more complex means of confirming the seating of the condyles in centric relation is achieved with a maxillary or mandibular muscle relaxation occlusal appliance. These appliances provide full coverage for the respective arch and occlusal contact for at least one cusp or incisal edge of the opposing teeth so that teeth are protected from spontaneous shifting. The occlusal design provides immediate disclusion of all the posterior teeth in every protrusive or lateral excursion. This allows for the progressive deprogramming of muscles through the advantage of reduced muscle contractions and limited noxious neurologic input.[39,88,160]

Models of the dentition must be accurately mounted to be diagnostic. The facebow transfer relates the maxillary cast to the axis of rotation of the articulator as the maxillary teeth relate to the cranial case. With careful bimanual manipulation or the use of an anterior bite stop, a transfer wafer is generated with the condyles fully seated in their glenoid fossa. The maxillary and mandibular teeth of each diagnostic model then relate to one another in centric relation as determined by condylar position, and they may reveal an occlusal discrepancy in centric relation, which would require compensation by the patient.[9,38]

Imaging

When the clinical evaluation and the history of the patient indicate the possibility of structural masticatory system disorders or the possible presence of pathology, especially neoplasm, then appropriate imaging of the TMJ is warranted. The current state of the art technique for imaging of soft tissue, especially the articular disc, is magnetic resonance (MR) imaging. The current highest standard for imaging for hard tissue, such as the condyle or the temporal bone, is computed tomography (CT). Both techniques are usually reserved for more difficult or strategic diagnosis, such as when joint surgery is being considered. Their interpretation usually requires specialized training for the clinician or access to a radiologist. Though arthrography is still being used for certain diagnostic situations, such as suspected perforation of the articular disc, CT and MR imaging are experiencing greater utilization.[9,18,75,89,125] Although plain film tomography is occasionally a feature of some of the newer radiographic equipment, the technique most readily available to a majority of practitioners is panoramic radiography. The image produced depicts only general relationships and gross anatomy, so the information provided should be regarded for screening purposes only. When pathology or marked deformation is suggested by a panoramic radiograph, further diagnostic imaging and procedures may be warranted.[18,73]

DIAGNOSTIC DECISION MAKING

Complete evaluation of every patient's periodontal status must include the diagnostic components required to reveal any form of masticatory system disorder. The existence of factors responsible for historical, current, or potential impairment of masticatory system function can be integrated into a comprehensive treatment plan. Patients who require substantial periodontal therapy or have suffered the effects of advanced periodontal disease may be at increased risk to develop masticatory system disorders, so diagnostic processes must remain consistently thorough and inclusive for all patients.[23,137] For the patient presenting with symptomatic masticatory system disorder, the diagnostic strategy would logically begin with the inclusion of all potential sources of pain or dysfunction followed by the systematic exclusion of possible causative or contributing factors, beginning with the least likely. When no symptoms are reported, the history and clinical examination would need to be just as thorough due to the tendency for a number of patients to tolerate modest dysfunction or mild transient discomfort. The diagnostic strategy for the patient presenting minimal or no signs and symptoms of masticatory system disorders would be to attempt to confirm a stable condition while identifying risk factors. Careful and complete documentation of the indication of past or current trauma and disharmony would provide the basis for trend analysis and anticipation of possible future problems.*

Consistent professional maintenance care has been clearly demonstrated to be a key ingredient in successful management of a patient's periodontal condition.[63,106] Complementing any treatment sequence, these appointments afford dentists the opportunity at every stage of comprehensive care to provide continuing evaluation of the status of the entire masticatory system and to provide timely and appropriate intervention when needed.

REFERENCES

1. Al-Hadi LA: Prevalence of temporomandibular disorders in relation to some occlusal parameters. J Prosthet Dent 1993; 70:345.
2. Allen EP, Bayne SC, Becker IM, et al: Annual review of selected dental literature: Report of the Committee of Scientific Investigation of the American Academy of Restorative Dentistry. J Prosthet Dent 1999; 82:39.
3. Atwood MJ, Dixon DC, Talcott GW, et al: Comparison of two scales in the assessment of muscle and joint palpation tenderness in chronic temporomandibular disorders. J Orofacial Pain 1993; 7:403.
4. Austin DG: Special considerations in orofacial pain and headache. Dent Clin North Am 1997; 41:325.
5. Auvenshine RC: Psychoneuroimmunology and its relationship to the differential diagnosis of temporomandibular disorders. Dent Clin North Am 1997; 41:279.
6. Aziz MA, Cowie RJ, Skinner CE, et al: Are the two heads of the human lateral pterygoid separate muscles? A perspective based on their nerve supply. J Orofacial Pain 1998; 12:226.
7. Bade DM, Lovasko JH, Dimitroff M, et al: Clinical comparison of temporomandibular joint sound auscultation and emission imaging studies. J Orofacial Pain 1994; 8:55.
8. Bates RE, Gremillion HA, Stewart CM: Degenerative joint disease, part II: Symptoms and examination findings. J Craniomandib Pract 1994; 12:88.

*See references 31, 32, 43, 54, 91, 111, 112, 114, and 153.

9. Becker IM, Tarantola GJ: Parameters of Care: Temporomandibular Disorders. Key Biscayne, FL, L.D. Pankey Institute of Advanced Dental Education, 1994.
10. Becker I, Tarantola G, Zambrano J, et al: Effect of a prefabricated anterior bite stop on electromyographic activity of masticatory muscles. J Prosthet Dent 1999; 82:22.
11. Ben Amor F, Carpentier P, Foucart JM, et al: Anatomic and mechanical properties of the lateral disc attachment of the temporomandibular joint. J Oral Maxillofac Surg 1998; 56:1164.
12. Benoliel R, Eliav E, Elishoov H, et al: Diagnosis and treatment of persistent pain after trauma to the head and neck. J Oral Maxillofac Surg 1994; 52:1138.
13. Bergdahl J, Anneroth G, Anneroth I: Clinical study of patients with burning mouth. Scand J Dent Res 1994; 102:229.
14. Bertilsson O, Ström D: A literature survey of a hundred years of anatomic and functional lateral pterygoid muscle research. J Orofacial Pain 1995; 9:17.
15. Bjorne A, Agerberg G: Craniomandibular disorders in patients with Ménière's disease: A controlled study. J Orofacial Pain 1996; 10:28.
16. Bouquot JE, Roberts AM, Person P, et al: NICO (neuralgia-inducing cavitational osteonecrosis): osteomyelitis in 224 jawbone samples from patients with facial neuralgias. Oral Surg 1992; 73:307.
17. Bouquot J, Roberts A: NICO (neuralgia-inducing cavitational osteonecrosis): radiographic appearance of the "invisible" osteomyelitis. Oral Surg 1992; 74:600.
18. Brooks SL, Brand JW, Gibbs SJ, et al: Imaging of the temporomandibular joint: A position paper of the American Academy of Oral and Maxillofacial Radiology. Oral Surg Oral Med Oral Pathol Oral Radiol Endod 1997; 83:609.
19. Burgess JA, Kolbinson DA, Lee PT, et al: Motor vehicle accidents and TMDs: Assessing the relationship. JADA 1996; 127:1767.
20. Bush FM, Harkins SW: Pain-related limitation in activities of daily living in patients with chronic orofacial pain: Psychometric properties of a disability index. J Orofacial Pain 1995; 9:57.
21. Bush FM, Harkins SW, Harrington WG: Otalgis and aversive symptoms in temporomandibular disorders. Ann Otol Rhino Laryngol 1999; 108:884.
22. Byers MR, Dong WK: Comparison of trigeminal receptor location and structure in the periodontal ligament of different types of teeth from the rat, cat, and monkey. J Comp Neurol 1989; 279:117.
23. Cathelineau G, Yardin M: The relationship between tooth vibratory sensation and periodontal disease. J Periodontol 1982; 53:704.
24. Carranza FA, Newman MG: Clinical Periodontology, ed 8. Philadelphia, Saunders, 1996.
25. Chan SWY, Reade PC: Tinnitus and temporomandibular pain-dysfunction disorder. Clin Otolaryngol 1994; 19:370.
26. Chole RA, Parker WS: Tinnitus and vertigo in patients with temporomandibular disorder. Arch Otolaryngol Head Neck Surg 1992; 118:817.
27. Christensen GJ: Abnormal occlusal conditions: A forgotten part of dentistry. JADA 1995; 126:1667.
28. Christensen GJ: Treating bruxism and clenching. JADA 2000; 131:233.
29. Christensen LV, Rassouli NM: Experimental occlusal interferences. Part I. A review. J Oral Rehabil 1995; 22:515.
30. Christensen LV, Rassouli NM: Experimental occlusal interferences. Part V. Mandibular rotations versus hemimandibular translations. J Oral Rehabil 1995; 22:865.
31. Christensen LV, McKay DC: TMD diagnostic decision-making and probability theory. Part I. J Craniomandib Pract 1996; 14:240.
32. Christensen LV, McKay DC: TMD diagnostic decision-making and probability theory. Part II. J Craniomandib Pract 1996; 14:312.
33. Clark GT, Tsukiyama Y, Baba K, et al: Sixty-eight years of experimental occlusal interference studies: What have we learned? J Prosthet Dent 1999; 82:704.
34. Ciancaglini R, Loreti P, Radaelli G: Ear, nose, and throat symptoms in patients with TMD: The association of symptoms according to severity of arthropathy. J Orofacial Pain 1994; 8:293.
35. Coffey JP, Williams WN, Turner GE, et al: Human bite force discrimination using specific maxillary and mandibular teeth. J Oral Rehabil 1989; 16:529.
36. Cooper BC, Cooper DL: Recognizing otolaryngologic symptoms in patients with temporomandibular disorders. J Craniomandib Pract 1993; 11:260.
37. Dao TTT, Reynolds WJ, Tenenbaum HC: Comorbidity between myofascial pain of the masticatory muscle and fibromyalgia. J Orofacial Pain 1997; 11:232.
38. Dawson PE: Evaluation, Diagnosis, and Treatment of Occlusal Problems, ed 2. St Louis, Mosby, 1989.
39. Dawson PE: New definition for relating occlusion to varying conditions of the temporomandibular joint. J Prosthet Dent 1995; 74:619.
40. Dawson PE: A classification system that relates maximal intercuspation to the position and condition of the temporomandibular joint. J Prosthet Dent 1996; 75:60.
41. De Boever JA, Keersmaeker K: Trauma in patients with temporomandibular disorders: Frequency and treatment outcomes. J Oral Rehabil 1996; 23:91.
42. de Bont LGM, Stengenga B: Pathology of temporomandibular joint internal derangement and osteoarthrosis. Int J Oral Maxillofac Surg 1993; 22:71.
43. De Wijer A, Lobbezoo-Scholte AM, Steenks MH, et al: Reliability of clinical findings in temporomandibular disorders. J Orofacial Pain 1995; 9:181.
44. Dimitroulis G, Dolwick MF, Gremillion HA: Temporomandibular disorders. 1. Clinical evaluation. Aus Dent J 1995; 40:301.
45. Donaldson KW: Rheumatoid diseases and the temporomandibular joint: A review. J Craniomandib Pract 1995; 13:264.
46. Dong WK, Shiwaku T, Kawakami Y, et al: Static and dynamic responses of periodontal ligament mechanoreceptors and intradental mechanoreceptors. J Neurophysiol 1993; 69:1567.
47. Ehrlich R, Garlick D, Ninio M: The effect of jaw clenching on the electromyographic activities of 2 neck and 2 trunk muscles. J Orofacial Pain 1999; 13:115.
48. Ferrario VF, Sforza C, Sigurta D, et al: Temporomandibular joint dysfunction and flat lateral guidances: A clinical association. J Prosthet Dent 1996; 75:534.
49. Ferrario VF, Sforza C, Colombo A, et al: An electromyographic investigation of masticatory muscle symmetry in normo-occlusion subjects. J Oral Rehabil 2000; 27:33.
50. Fu K, Ma X, Zhang Z, et al: Interleukin-6 in synovial fluid and HLA-DR expression in synovium from patients with temporomandibular disorders. J Orofacial Pain 1995; 9:131.
52. Gelb H, Gelb ML, Wagner ML: The relationship of tinnitus to craniocervical mandibular disorders. J Craniomandib Pract 1997; 15:136.
53. Glaros AG, Baharloo L, Glass EG: Effect of parafunctional clenching and estrogen on temporomandibular disorder pain. J Craniomandib Pract 1998; 16:78.
54. Glaros AG, Glass EG, Williams KB: Clinical examination findings of temporomandibular disorder patients: A factor analytic study. J Orofacial Pain 1998; 12:193.

55. Glaros AG, Tabacchi KN, Glass EG: Effect of parafunctional clenching on TMD pain. J Orofacial Pain 1998; 12:145.
56. Goupille P, FouQuet B, Goga D, et al: The temporomandibular joint in rheumatoid arthritis: Correlations between clinical and tomographic features. J Dent 1993; 21:141.
57. Gremillion HA: TMD and maladaptive occlusion: Does a link exist? J Craniomandib Pract 1995; 13:205.
58. Gynther GW, Holmlund AB, Reinholt FP, et al: Temporomandibular joint involvement in generalized osteoarthritis and rheumatoid arthritis: A clinical, arthroscopic, histologic, and immunohistochemical study. Int J Oral Maxillofac Surg 1997; 26:10.
59. Harper RP, Schneiderman E: Condylar movement and centric relation in patients with internal derangement of the temporomandibular joint. J Prosthet Dent 1996; 75:67.
60. Haskin CL, Milam SB, Cameron IL: Pathogenesis of degenerative joint disease in the human temporomandibular joint. Crit Rev Oral Biol Med 1995; 6:248.
61. Heir GM: Differentiation of orofacial pain related to Lyme disease from other dental and facial pain disorders. Dent Clin North Am 1997; 41:243.
62. Hickman DM, Cramer R: The effect of different condylar positions on masticatory muscle electromyography activity in humans. Oral Surg Oral Med Oral Pathol Radiol Endod 1998; 85:18.
63. Hirschfield L, Wasserman B: A long-term survey of tooth loss in 600 treated periodontal patients. J Periodontol 1978; 49:225.
64. Hochstedler JL, Allen JD, Follmar MA: Temporomandibular joint range of motion: A ratio of interincisal opening to excursive movement in a healthy population. J Craniomandib Pract 1996; 14:296.
65. Huntley TA, Wiesenfeld D: Delayed diagnosis of the cause of facial pain in patients with neoplastic disease: A report of eight cases. J Oral Maxillofac Surg 1994; 52:81.
66. Ingervall B, Hähner R, Kessi S: Pattern of tooth contacts in eccentric mandibular positions in young adults. J Prosthet Dent 1991; 66:169.
67. Isberg A, Westesson P-L: Steepness of articular eminence and movement of the condyle and disk in asymptomatic temporomandibular joints. Oral Surg Oral Med Oral Pathol Oral Radiol Endod 1998; 86:152.
68. Israel HA, Diamond B, Saed-Nejad F, et al: Osteoarthritis and synovitis as major pathoses of the temporomandibular joint: Comparison of clinical diagnosis with arthroscopic morphology. J Oral Maxillofac Surg 1998; 56:1023.
69. Ito T, Gibbs CH, Marguelles-Bonnet R, et al: Loading on the temporomandibular joints with five occlusal conditions. J Prosthet Dent 1986; 56:478.
70. Jacobs R, van Steenberghe D: Role of periodontal ligament receptors in the tactile function of teeth: A review. J Periodont Res 1994; 29:153.
71. Kahn J, Tallents RH, Katzberg RW, et al: Association between dental occlusal variables and intraarticular temporomandibular joint disorders: Horizontal and vertical overlap. J Prosthet Dent 1998; 79:658.
72. Kampe T, Tagdae T, Bader G, et al: Reported symptoms and clinical findings in a group of subjects with longstanding bruxing behavior. J Oral Rehabil 1997; 24:581.
73. Kaplan AS, Assaed LA: Temporomandibular Disorders: Diagnosis and Treatment. Philadelphia, Saunders, 1991.
74. Katz MA: Approach to the management of nonmalignant pain. A J Med 1996; 101(suppl 1A):54S.
75. Katzberg RW, Westesson P: Diagnosis of the Temporomandibular Joint. Philadelphia, Saunders, 1993.
76. Keersmaeker K, De Boever JA, Van Den Berghe L: Otalgia in patients with temporomandibular joint disorders. J Prosthet Dent 1996; 75:72.
77. Kenworthy CR, Morrish RB, Mohn C, et al: Bilateral condylar movement patterns in adult subjects. J Orofacial Pain 1997; 11:328.
78. Kerstein RB: Disclusion time measurement studies: A comparison of disclusion time between chronic myofascial pain dysfunction patients and nonpatients: A population analysis. J Prosthet Dent 1994; 72:473.
79. Kerstein R: Disclusion time measurement studies: Stability of disclusion time: A 1-year follow up. J Prosthet Dent 1994; 72:164.
80. Kleinegger CL, Lilly GE: Cranial arteritis: A medical emergency with orofacial manifestations. J Am Dent Assoc 1999; 130:1203.
81. Kelmetti E, Vainio P, Kroger H: Craniomandibular disorders and skeletal mineral status. J Craniomandib Pract 1995; 13:89.
82. Koh ET, Yap AU-J, Koh CKH, et al: Temporomandibular disorders in rheumatoid arthritis. J Rheumatol 1999; 26:1918.
83. Könönen M, Wenneberg B, Kallenberg A: Craniomandibular disorders in rheumatoid arthritis, psoriatic arthritis, and ankylosing spondylitis: A clinical study. Acta Odontol Scand 1992; 50:281.
84. Kopp S: The influence of neuropeptides, serotonin, and interleukin 1B on temporomandibular joint pain and inflammation. J Oral Maxillofac Surg 1998; 56:189.
85. Kuboki T, Azuma Y, Orsini MG, et al: Effects of sustained unilateral molar clenching on the temporomandibular joint space. Oral Surg Oral Med Oral Pathol Oral Radiol Endod 1996; 82:616.
86. Kubota E, Kubota T, Matsumoto J, et al: Synovial fluid cytokines and proteinases as markers of temporomandibular joint disease. J Oral Maxillofac Surg 1998; 56:192.
87. Kumar KL, Cooney TG: Headaches. Med Clin North Am 1995; 79:261.
88. Kurita H, Ikeda K, Kurashina K: Evaluation of the effect of a stabilization splint on occlusal force in patient occlusions with masticatory muscle disorders. J Oral Rehabil 2000; 27:79.
89. Larheim TA: Current trends in temporomandibular joint imaging. Oral Surg Oral Med Oral Pathol Oral Radiol Endod 1995; 80:555.
90. Lavigne G, Kim JS, Valiquette C, et al: Evidence that periodontal pressoreceptors provide positive feedback to jaw closing muscles during mastication. J Neurophysiol 1987; 58:342.
91. Levitt SR, McKinney MW: Appropriate use of predictive values in clinical decision making and evaluating diagnostic tests for TMD. J Orofacial Pain 1994; 8:298.
92. Levitt SR, McKinney MW: Validating the TMJ scale in the national sample of 10,000 patients: Demographic and epidemiologic characteristics. J Orofacial Pain 1994; 8:25.
93. Lindauer SJ, Sabol G, Isaccson RJ, et al: Condylar movement and mandibular rotation during jaw opening. Am J Orthod Dentofac Orthop 1995; 107:573.
94. Lipton JA, Ship JA, Larach-Robinson D: Estimated prevalence and distribution of reported orofacial pain in the United States. J Am Dent Assoc 1993; 124:115.
95. Liu ZJ, Yamagata K, Kashara Y, et al: Electromyographic examination of jaw muscles in relation to symptoms and occlusion of patients with temporomandibular joint disorders. J Oral Rehabil 1999; 26:33.
96. Lobbezoo F, Lavigne GJ: Do bruxism and temporomandibular disorders have a cause-and-effect relationship? J Orofacial Pain 1997; 11:15.
97. Locher MC, Felder M, Sailer HF: Involvement of the temporomandibular joints in ankylosing spondylitis (Bechterew's disease). J Cranio-Maxillofac Surg 1996; 24:205.

98. Louca C, Cadden SW, Linden RWA: The roles of periodontal ligament mechanoreceptors in the reflex control of human jaw-closing muscles. Brain Res 1996; 731:63.
99. Loughner BA, Gremillion HA, Larkin LH, et al: Muscle attachment to the lateral aspect of the articular disc of the human temporomandibular joint. Oral Surg Oral Med Oral Pathol Oral Radiol Endod 1996; 82:139.
100. Lyssy KJ, Escalante A: Perioperative management of rheumatoid arthritis: Areas of concern for primary care physicians. Postgraduate Medicine: Rheumatoid Arthritis 1996; 99:191.
101. Maixner W, Fillingham R, Kincaid S, et al: Relationship between pain sensitivity and resting arterial blood pressure in patients with painful temporomandibular disorders. Psychosomatic Med 1997; 59:503.
102. Major P, Ramos-Remus C, Suarez-Almazor ME, et al: Magnetic resonance imaging and clinical assessment of temporomandibular joint pathology in ankylosing spondylitis. J Rheumatol 1999; 26:616.
103. Marbach JL: Is phantom tooth pain a deafferentation (neuropathic) syndrome? Oral Surg Oral Med Oral Pathol 1993; 75:225.
104. Marbach JL: Orofacial phantom pain: Theory and phenomenology. JADA 1996; 127:221.
105. Marbach JJ: Medically unexplained chronic orofacial pain: Temporomandibular pain and dysfunction syndrome, orofacial phantom pain, burning mouth syndrome, and trigeminal neuralgia. Med Clinics North Am 1999; 83:691.
106. McGuire MK, Nunn ME: Prognosis versus actual outcome: A long-term survey of 100 treated periodontal patients under maintenance care. J Periodontol 1991; 62:51.
107. Merida-Velasco JR, Rodriguez-Vazquez JF, Jimenez-Collado J: The relationships between the temporomandibular joint disc and related masticatory muscles in humans. J Oral Maxillofac Surg 1993; 51:390.
108. Milam SB, Schmitz JP: Molecular biology of temporomandibular joint disorders: Proposed mechanisms of disease. J Oral Maxillofac Surg 1995; 53:1448.
109. Milam SB, Zardeneta G, Schmitz JP: Oxidative stress and degenerative temporomandibular joint disease: A proposed hypothesis. J Oral Maxillofac Surg 1998; 56:214.
110. Minagi S, Ohtsuki H, Sato T, et al: Effect of balancing-side occlusion on the ipsilateral TMJ dynamics under clenching. J Oral Rehabil 1997; 24:57.
111. Mohl ND, Ohrbach R: Clinical decision making for temporomandibular disorders. J Dent Educ 1992; 56:823.
112. Mohl ND: Reliability and validity of diagnostic modalities for temporomandibular disorders. Adv Dent Res 1993; 7:113.
113. Morgan DH, Goode RL, Christiansen RL, et al: The TMJ-ear connection. J Craniomandib Pract 1995; 13:42.
114. Moses AJ: Scientific methodology in temporomandibular disorders, Part I: Epidemiology. J Craniomandib Pract 1994; 12:114.
115. Murakami K, Kubota E, Maeda H, et al: Intraarticular levels of prostoglandin E_2, hyaluronic acid, and chrondroitin-4 and -6 sulfates in the temporomandibular joint synovial fluid of patients with internal derangements. J Oral Maxillofac Surg 1998; 56:199.
116. Murray H, Locker D, Mock D, et al: Pain and the quality of life in patients referred to a craniofacial pain unit. J Orofacial Pain 1996; 10:316.
117. Neff PA: TMJ Occlusion and Function. Georgetown, Georgetown University School of Dentistry, 1975.
118. Okeson JP: Orofacial Pain: Guidelines for Assessment, Diagnosis, and Management. Carol Stream, IL, Quintessence, 1996.
119. Okeson JP: Management of Temporomandibular Joint Disorders and Occlusion, ed 4. St. Louis, Mosby, 1998.
120. Parker MW: The significance of occlusion in restorative dentistry. Dent Clinics North Am 1993; 37:341.
121. Parker WS, Chole RA: Tinnitus, vertigo, and temporomandibular disorders. Am J Orthod Dentofac Orthop 1995; 107:153.
122. Pavone BW: Bruxism and its effect on the natural teeth. J Prosthet Dent 1985; 53:692.
123. Pereira FL, Lundh H, Eriksson L, et al: Microscopic changes in the retrodiscal tissues of painful temporomandibular joints. J Oral Maxillofac Surg 1996; 54:461.
124. Pertes RA: Differential diagnosis of orofacial pain. Mount Sinai J Med 1998; 65:348.
125. Pharoah MJ: The prescription of diagnostic images for temporomandibular joint disorders. J Orofacial Pain 1999; 13:251.
126. Pleash O, Wolfe F, Lane N: The relationship between fibromyalgia and temporomandibular disorders: Prevalence and symptom severity. J Rheumatol 1996; 23:1948.
127. Pullinger AG, Seligman DA, Gornbein JA: A multiple logistic regression analysis of the risk and relative odds of temporomandibular disorders as a function of common occlusal features. J Dent Res 1993; 72:968.
128. Pullinger AG, Seligman DA: The degree to which attrition characterizes differentiated patient groups of temporomandibular disorders. J Orofacial Pain 1993; 7:196.
129. Pullinger AG, Seligman DA: Quantification and validation of predictive values of occlusal variables in temporomandibular disorders using multifactorial analysis. J Prosthet Dent 2000; 83:66.
130. Rammelsberg P, Pospiech PR, Jäger L, et al: Variability of disc position in asymptomatic volunteers and patients with internal derangements of the TMJ. Oral Surg Oral Med Oral Pathol Oral Radiol Endod 1997; 83:393.
131. Raphael KG, Marbach JJ, Klausner J: Myofascial face pain: Clinical characteristics of those with regional versus widespread pain. JADA 2000; 131:161.
132. Rassouli NM, Christensen LV: Experimental occlusal interferences. Part III. Mandibular rotations induced by a rigid interference. J Oral Rehabil 1995; 22:781.
133. Ratcliffe A, Israel H, Saed-Nejad F, et al: Proteoglycans in the synovial fluid of the temporomandibular joint as an indicator of changes in cartilage metabolism during primary and secondary osteoarthritis. J Oral Maxillofac Surg 1998; 56:204.
134. Raustia AM, Pirttiniemi PM, Pyhtinen J: Correlation of occlusal factors and condyle position asymmetry with signs and symptoms of temporomandibular disorders in young adults. J Craniomandib Pract 1995; 13:152.
135. Ren Y, Isberg A: Tinnitus in patients with temporomandibular joint internal derangement. J Craniomandib Pract 1995; 13:75.
136. Rodriguez-Vazquez JF, Merida-Velasco JR, Merida-Velasco JA, et al: Anatomical considerations on the discomalleolar ligament. J Anat 1998; 192:617.
137. Rosenbaum RS: The possible effects of periodontal disease on occlusal function. Curr Opin Periodont 1993; 163.
138. Ruf S, Cecere F, Kupfer J, et al: Stress-induced changes in the functional electromyographic activity of the masticatory muscles. Acta Odontol Scand 1997; 55:44.
139. Sarnat BG, Laskin DM: The Temporomandibular Joint: Biologic Basis for Clinical Practice, ed 4. Philadelphia, Saunders, 1992.
140. Schiffman E, Haley D, Baker C, et al: Diagnostic criteria for screening headache patients for temporomandibular disorders. Headache 1995; 35:121.

141. Schiffman EL, Fricton JR, Haley D: The relationship of occlusion, parafunctional habits and recent life events to mandibular dysfunction in a nonpatient population. J Oral Rehabil 1992; 19:201.
142. Schindler JH, Stengel E, Spiess WEL: Feedback control during mastication of solid food textures: A clinical-experimental study. J Prosthet Dent 1998; 80:330.
143. Schmolke C: The relationship between the temporomandibular joint capsule, articular disc, and jaw muscles. J Anat 1994; 184:335.
144. Sessle BJ: The neural basis of the temporomandibular joint and masticatory muscle pain. J Orofacial Pain 1999; 13:238.
145. Shibata T, Murakami K, Kubota E, et al: Glycosaminoglycan components in temporomandibular joint synovial fluid as markers of joint pathology. J Oral Maxillofac Surg 1998; 56:209.
146. Simons DG, Travell JG, Simons LS: Myofascial Pain and Dysfunction: The Trigger Point Manual. Baltimore, Williams & Wilkins, 1999.
147. Stegenga B, de Bont LGM, de Leeuw R, et al: Assessment of mandibular function impairment associated with temporomandibular joint osteoarthrosis and internal derangement. J Orofacial Pain 1993; 7:183.
148. Stratmann U, Mokyrs K, Meyer U, et al: Clinical anatomy and palpability of the inferior lateral pterygoid muscle. J Prosthet Dent 2000; 83:548.
149. Suvinen TI, Reade PC: Temporomandibular disorders: A critical review of the nature of pain and its assessment. J Orofacial Pain 1995; 9:317.
150. Taddey JJ: Musicians and temporomandibular disorders: Prevalence and occupational etiologic considerations. J Craniomandib Pract 1992; 10:241.
151. Tanne K, Tanaka E, Sakuda M: Association between malocclusion and temporomandibular disorders in orthodontic patients before treatment. J Orofacial Pain 1993; 7:156.
152. Tarantola GJ, Becker IM, Gremillion H: The reproducibility of centric relation: A clinical approach. JADA 1997; 128:1245.
153. Tasaki MM, Westesson P, Isberg AM, et al: Classification and prevalence of temporomandibular joint disc displacement in patients and symptom-free volunteers. Am J Orthod Dentofac Orthop 1996; 109:249.
154. Tenenbaum HC, Freeman BV, Psutka DJ, et al: Temporomandibular disorders: Disc displacements. J Orofacial Pain 1999; 13:285.
155. Tsolka P, Walter JD, Wilson RF, et al: Occlusal variables, bruxism and temporomandibular disorders: A clinical and kinesiographic assessment. J Oral Rehabil 1995; 22:849.
156. Turp JG, Gobetti JP: Trigeminal neuralgia: An update. Compend 2000; 21:279.
157. Wabeke KB, Spruijt RJ, van der Zaag J: The reliability of clinical methods for recording temporomandibular joint sounds. J Dent Res 1994; 73:1157.
158. Watanabe EK, Yatani H, Kuboki T, et al: The relationship between signs and symptoms of temporomandibular disorders and bilateral occlusal contact patterns in lateral excursions. J Oral Rehabil 1998; 25:409.
159. Wilkinson TM, Crowley CM: A histologic study of retrodiscal tissues of the human temporomandibular joint in the open and closed position. J Orofacial Pain 1994; 8:7.
160. Williamson EH, Ludquist DO: Anterior guidance: Its effect on electromyographic activity of the temporal and masseter muscles. J Prosthet Dent 1983; 49:816.
161. Wish-Baratz S, Ring GD, Hiss J, et al: The microscopic structure and function of the vascular retrodiscal pad of the human temporomandibular joint. Arch Oral Biol 1993; 38:265.
162. Wright EF, Bifano SL: Tinnitus improvement through TMD therapy. JADA 1997; 128:1424.
163. Wright EF, Gullickson DC: Identifying acute pulpalgia as a factor in TMD pain. JADA 1996; 127:773.
164. Zarb GA, Carlsson GE, Sessle BJ, et al: Temporomandibular Joint and Masticatory Muscle Disorders. St Louis, Mosby, 1994.
165. Zarb GA, Carlsson GE: Temporomandibular disorders: Osteoarthritis. J Orofacial Pain 1999; 13:295.
166. Zimers PL, Gobetti JP: Head and neck lesions commonly found in musicians. JADA 1994; 125:1487.

Chronic Periodontitis

Richard J. Nagy and M. John Novak

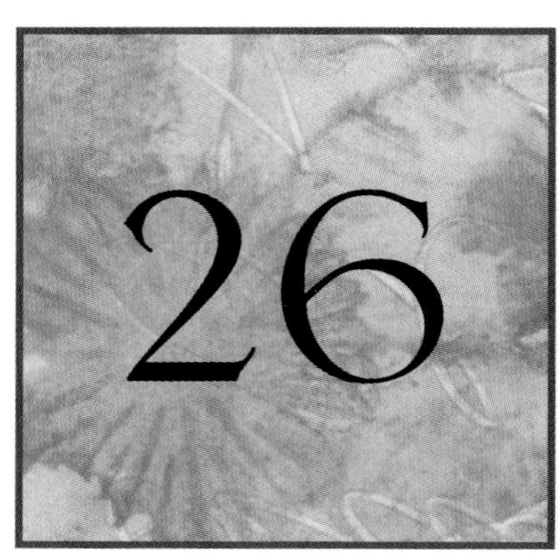

CHAPTER

CHAPTER OUTLINE

Chronic periodontitis, formerly known as "adult periodontitis" or "chronic adult periodontitis," is the most prevalent form of periodontitis. It is generally considered to be a slowly progressing disease. However, in the presence of systemic or environmental factors that may modify the host response to plaque accumulation, such as diabetes, smoking, or stress, disease progression may become more aggressive. Although chronic periodontitis is most frequently observed in adults, it can occur in children and adolescents in response to chronic plaque and calculus accumulation. This observation underlies the recent name change from "adult" periodontitis, which suggests that chronic, plaque-induced periodontitis is only observed in adults, to a more universal description of "chronic" periodontitis that can occur at any age (reviewed in Chapter 4).

Chronic periodontitis has recently been defined as "an infectious disease resulting in inflammation within the supporting tissues of the teeth, progressive attachment loss, and bone loss."[2] This definition outlines the major clinical and etiologic characteristics of the disease: microbial plaque formation, periodontal inflammation, and loss of attachment and alveolar bone. Periodontal pocket formation is usually a sequela of the disease process unless gingival recession accompanies attachment loss, in which case pocket depths may remain shallow even in the presence of ongoing attachment and bone loss.

CLINICAL FEATURES

General Characteristics

Characteristic clinical findings in patients with chronic periodontitis include supragingival and subgingival plaque accumulation that is frequently associated with calculus formation, gingival inflammation, pocket formation, loss of periodontal attachment and loss of alveolar bone (Fig. 26-1). The gingiva ordinarily is slightly to moderately swollen and exhibits alterations in color ranging from pale red to magenta. Loss of gingival stippling and changes in the surface topography may include blunted or rolled gingival margins and flattened or cratered papillae. In many patients, the changes in color, contour, and consistency that are frequently associated with gingival inflammation may not be visible on inspection, and inflammation may be detected only as bleeding of the gingiva in response to examination of the periodontal pocket with a periodontal probe. Gingival bleeding, either spontaneous or in response to probing, is frequent, and inflammation-related exudates of crevicular fluid and suppuration from the pocket also

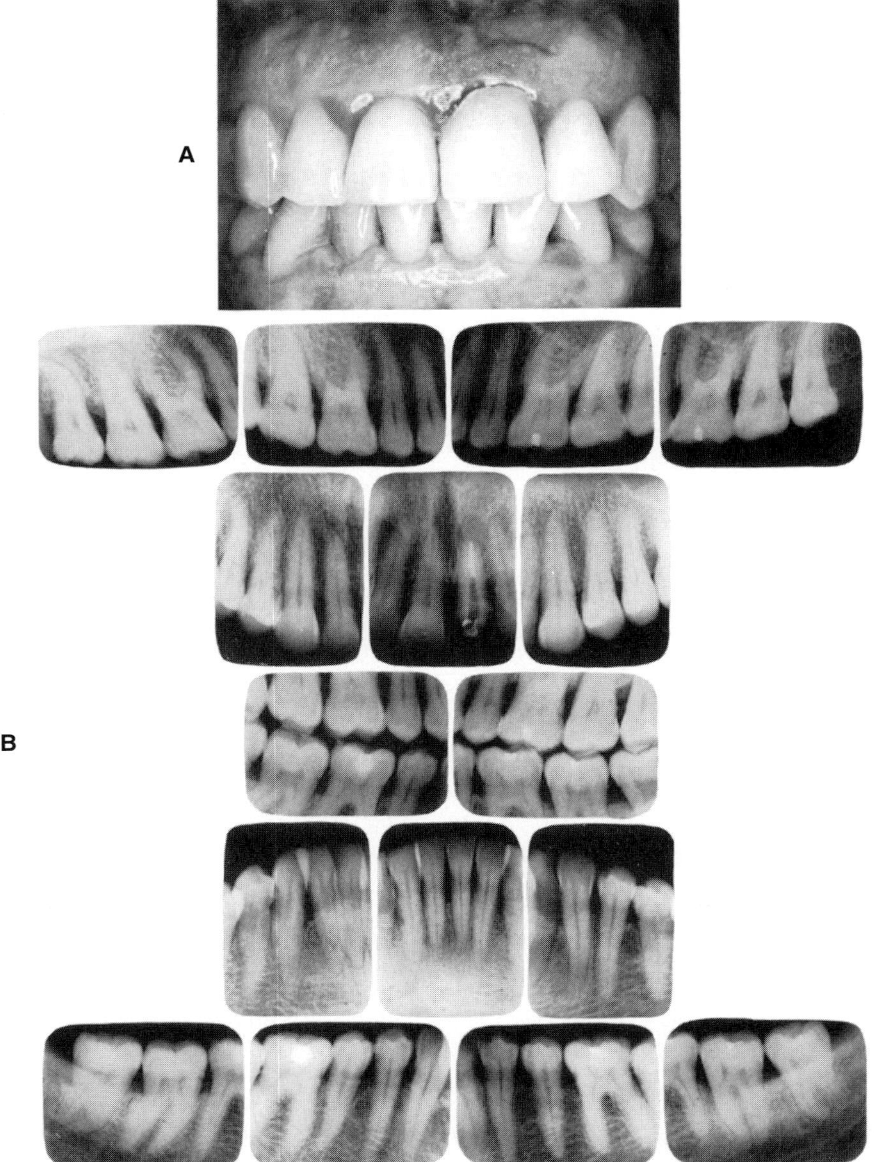

Fig. 26-1 Chronic periodontitis in a 47-year-old female. **A,** Clinical view showing generalized gingival inflammation and periodontal pocket formation. **B,** Radiographs showing generalized horizontal bone loss that varies in severity in different areas.

may be found. In some cases, probably as a result of long standing, low-grade inflammation, thickened, fibrotic marginal tissues may obscure the underlying inflammatory changes. Pocket depths are variable, and both horizontal and vertical bone loss can be found. Tooth mobility often appears in advanced cases when bone loss has been considerable.

Chronic periodontitis can be clinically diagnosed by the detection of chronic inflammatory changes in the marginal gingiva, presence of periodontal pockets, and loss of clinical attachment. It is diagnosed radiographically by evidence of bone loss. These findings may be similar to those seen in aggressive disease. A differential diagnosis is based on the age of the patient, rate of disease progression over time, familial nature of aggressive disease, and relative absence of local factors in aggressive disease compared with the presence of abundant plaque and calculus in chronic periodontitis.

Disease Distribution

Chronic periodontitis is considered a *site-specific* disease. The clinical signs of chronic periodontitis—namely inflammation, pocket formation, attachment loss, and bone loss—are considered to be due to the direct, site-specific effects of subgingival plaque accumulation. As a result of this local effect, pocketing, attachment, and bone loss may occur on one surface of a tooth while other surfaces maintain normal attachment levels. For example, a proximal surface with chronic plaque accumulation may have loss of attachment, whereas the plaque-free facial surface of the same tooth may be free of disease. In addition to being site specific, chronic periodontitis may be described as being *localized* when few sites demonstrate attachment and bone loss or *generalized* when many sites around the mouth are affected (see Chapter 4).

Localized periodontitis: Periodontitis is considered localized when <30% of the sites assessed in the mouth demonstrate attachment loss and bone loss.

Generalized periodontitis: Periodontitis is considered generalized when >30% of the sites assessed in the mouth demonstrate attachment loss and bone loss.

The pattern of bone loss observed in chronic periodontitis may be vertical, when attachment and bone loss on one tooth surface is greater than that occurring on an adjacent surface, or horizontal, when attachment and bone loss proceeds at a uniform rate on the majority of tooth surfaces. Vertical bone loss is usually associated with angular bony defects and intrabony pocket formation. Horizontal bone loss is usually associated with suprabony pockets (see Chapters 24 and 25).

Disease Severity

The severity of destruction of the periodontium that occurs as a result of chronic periodontitis is generally considered a function of time. With increasing age, attachment loss and bone loss becomes more prevalent and more severe due to an accumulation of destruction (see Chapter 5). Disease severity may be described as being *slight (mild), moderate,* or *severe* (see Chapter 4). These terms may be used to describe the disease severity of the entire mouth, a part of the mouth such as a quadrant or sextant, or the disease status of an individual tooth.

Slight (mild) periodontitis: Periodontal destruction is generally considered slight when no more than 1 to 2 mm of clinical attachment loss has occurred.

Moderate periodontitis: Periodontal destruction is generally considered moderate when 3 to 4 mm of clinical attachment loss has occurred.

Severe periodontitis: Periodontal destruction is considered severe when 5 mm or more of clinical attachment loss has occurred.

Symptoms

Because chronic periodontitis is usually painless, patients may be less likely to seek treatment and accept treatment recommendations. In addition, a negative response to questions such as "Are you in pain?" is not sufficient to eliminate suspicion of periodontitis. Occasionally, pain may be present in the absence of caries due to exposed roots that are sensitive to heat, cold, or both. Areas of localized dull pain, sometimes radiating deep into the jaw, have been associated with periodontitis. The presence of areas of food impaction may add to the patient's discomfort. Gingival tenderness or "itchiness" can also be found.

Disease Progression

Patients appear to have the same susceptibility to plaque-induced chronic periodontitis throughout their lives. The rate of disease progression is usually slow but may be modified by systemic and/or environmental and behavioral factors. Onset of chronic periodontitis can occur at any time, and the first signs may be detected during adolescence in the presence of chronic plaque and calculus accumulation. However, because of its slow rate of progression, chronic periodontitis usually becomes clinically significant in the mid-30s or later.

Chronic periodontitis does not progress at an equal rate in all affected sites throughout the mouth. Some involved areas may remain static for long periods of time,[4] whereas others may progress more rapidly. More rapidly progressive lesions occur most frequently in interproximal areas[5] and are usually associated with areas of greater plaque accumulation and inaccessibility to plaque control measures (e.g., furcation areas, overhanging margins, sites of malposed teeth, or areas of food impaction). Several models have been proposed to describe the rate of disease progression.[8] In these models, progression is measured by determining the amount of attachment loss during a given time. The *continuous model,* the *random* or *episodic burst model,* and the *asynchronous multiple burst model* of disease progression are described in Chapter 9.

Prevalence

Chronic periodontitis increases in prevalence and severity with age, generally affecting both sexes equally. Periodontitis is an age-associated, not age-related, disease. In other words, it is not the age of the individual that causes the increase in disease prevalence, but rather the length of time that the periodontal tissues are challenged by chronic plaque accumulation. The incidence and prevalence of chronic periodontitis are discussed in detail in Chapter 5.

RISK FACTORS FOR DISEASE

Prior History of Periodontitis

Although not a true risk factor for disease but rather a disease predictor, a prior history of periodontitis puts patients at greater risk for developing further loss of attachment and bone, given a challenge from bacterial plaque accumulation.[7] This means that a patient who presents with pocketing and attachment and bone loss will continue to lose periodontal support if not successfully treated. In addition, a chronic periodontitis patient that has been successfully treated will develop continuing disease if plaque is allowed to accumulate. This stresses the need for continuous monitoring and maintenance of periodontitis patients to prevent a reoccurrence of the disease. The risk factors that contribute to patient susceptibility are discussed in the following sections.

Local Factors

Plaque accumulation on tooth and gingival surfaces at the dentogingival junction is considered the primary initiating agent in the etiology of chronic periodontitis. Attachment and bone loss are associated with an increase in the proportion of gram-negative organisms in the subgingival plaque biofilm, with specific increases in organisms known to be exceptionally pathogenic and virulent. *Bacteroides gingivalis, Bacteroides forsythus,* and *Treponema denticola,* otherwise known as the "red complex," are frequently associated with ongoing attachment and bone loss in chronic periodontitis. These microorganims and their virulence factors are described in detail in Chapters 6 and 8. The identification and characterization of these and other pathogenic microorganisms and their association with attachment and bone loss has led to the specific plaque hypothesis for the development of chronic periodontitis. This hypothesis implies that although a general increase occurs in the proportion of gram-negative microorganisms in the subgingival plaque in periodontitis, it is the presence of increased proportions of members of the red complex and perhaps other microorganisms that precipitates attachment and bone loss. The mechanisms by which this occurs have not been clearly delineated, but these bacteria may impart a local effect on the cells of the inflammatory response and the cells and tissues of the host, resulting in a local, site-specific disease process. The interactions between pathogenic bacteria and the host and their potential effects on disease progression are discussed in detail in Chapter 8.

Because plaque accumulation is the primary initiating agent in periodontal destruction, anything that facilitates plaque accumulation or prevents plaque removal by oral hygiene procedures can be detrimental to the patient. *Plaque retentive factors* are important in the development and progression of chronic periodontitis because they retain plaque microorganisms in close proximity to the periodontal tissues, providing an ecologic niche for plaque growth and maturation. Calculus is considered the most important plaque retentive factor because of its ability to retain and harbor plaque bacteria on its rough surface. As a result, calculus removal is essential for the maintenance of a healthy periodontium. Other factors that are known to retain plaque or prevent its removal are subgingival and/or overhanging margins of restorations; carious lesions that extend subgingivally; furcations exposed by loss of attachment and bone; crowded and malaligned teeth; and root grooves and concavities. These potential risk factors for periodontitis are discussed further in Chapter 32, and their impact on the prognosis of periodontal treatment is discussed in Chapter 33.

Systemic Factors

The rate of progression of plaque-induced chronic periodontitis is generally considered to be slow. However, when chronic periodontitis occurs in a patient who also suffers from a systemic disease that influences the effectiveness of the host response, the rate of periodontal destruction may be significantly increased. Diabetes is a systemic condition that can increase the severity and extent of periodontal disease in an affected patient. Type II or non–insulin-dependent diabetes mellitus (NIDDM) is the most prevalent form of diabetes and accounts for 90% of diabetics.[1] In addition, Type II diabetes is most likely to develop in an adult population at the same time as chronic periodontitis. The synergistic effect of plaque accumulation and modulation of an effective host response through the effects of diabetes can lead to severe and extensive periodontal destruction that may be difficult to manage with standard clinical techniques without controlling the systemic condition. An increase in Type II diabetes in teenagers and young adults has been observed and may be associated with an increase in juvenile obesity. In addition, Type I or insulin-dependent diabetes (IDDM) is observed in children, teenagers, and young adults and may lead to increased periodontal destruction when it is uncontrolled. It is likely that chronic periodontitis, aggravated by the complications of Type I and/or Type II diabetes may increase in prevalence in the near future and will provide therapeutic challenges to the clinician.

Environmental and Behavioral Factors

Smoking has been shown to increase the severity and extent of periodontal disease. When combined with plaque-induced chronic periodontitis, an increase in the rate of periodontal destruction may be observed in nonsmoking patients who have chronic periodontitis. As a result, smokers with chronic periodontitis have more attachment and bone loss, more furcation involvements, and deeper pockets. In addition, they appear to form more supragingival and less subgingival calculus and demonstrate less bleeding on probing than nonsmokers. The reasons for this effect are receiving considerable attention at present. Initial evidence points to changes in the subgingival microflora between smokers and nonsmokers in addition to the effects of smoking on the host response. The clinical, microbiologic, and immunologic effects of smoking also appear to have an influence on the response to therapy and the frequency of recurrent disease. The effects of smoking are reviewed further in Chapter 14.

Emotional stress has previously been associated with necrotizing ulcerative disease, perhaps because of the effects of stress on immune function. Increasing evidence suggests that emotional stress also may influence the extent and severity of chronic periodontitis, probably through the same mechanisms.

Genetic Factors

Periodontitis is considered to be a multifactorial disease in which the normal balance between microbial plaque and host response is disrupted. This disruption, as described previously, can occur through changes in the plaque composition, changes in the host response, or environmental and behavioral influences that can affect both plaque response and host response. In addition, periodontal destruction is frequently seen among family members and across different generations within a family, suggesting the possibility of a genetic basis to the susceptibility to periodontal disease. Recent studies have demonstrated a familial aggregation of localized and generalized aggressive periodontitis (reviewed in Chapters 10 and 27). In addition, studies of monozygotic twins suggest a genetic component to chronic periodontitis, but the influences of bacterial transmission among family members and environmental effects make it difficult to interpret a complex interaction. These studies are discussed in detail in Chapter 10.

Although no clear genetic determinants have been described for patients with chronic periodontitis, a genetic predisposition to more aggressive periodontal breakdown in response to plaque and calculus accumulation may exist. Recent data indicate that a genetic variation or polymorphism in the genes encoding interleukin 1-α and interleukin 1-β is associated with an increased susceptibility to a more aggressive form of chronic periodontitis in subjects of Northern European origin.[3] In addition, smokers demonstrating the composite IL-1 genotype are at even greater risk for severe disease. A recent study suggested that patients with the IL-1 genotype increased the risk for tooth loss by 2.7 times; those who were heavy smokers and IL-1 genotype negative increased the risk for tooth loss by 2.9 times. The combined effect of the IL-1 genotype and smoking increased the risk of tooth loss by 7.7 times.[6] With increased characterization of genetic polymorphisms that may exist in other target genes, a complex genotype is likely to be identified for many different clinical forms of periodontitis.

REFERENCES

1. Diagnosis and Classification. In: Raskin P (ed): Medical Management of Non-Insulin-Dependent (Type II) Diabetes, ed 3. Alexandria, VA, American Diabetes Association, 1994.
2. Flemmig TF: Periodontitis. Ann Periodontol 1999; 4:32.
3. Kornman KS, di Giovine FS: Genetic variations in cytokine expression: a risk factor for severity of adult periodontitis. Ann Periodontol 1998; 3:327.
4. Lindhe J, Okamoto H, Yoneyama T, et al: Longitudinal changes in periodontal disease in untreated subjects. J Clin Periodontol 1989; 16:662.
5. Lindhe J, Okamoto H, Yoneyama T, et al: Periodontal loser sites in untreated adult subjects. J Clin Periodontol 1989; 16:671.
6. McGuire MK, Nunn ME: Prognosis versus actual outcome. IV. The effectiveness of clinical parameters and IL-1 genotype in accurately predicting prognoses and tooth survival. J Periodontol 1999; 70:49.
7. Papapanou PN: Risk assessment in the diagnosis and treatment of periodontal diseases. J Dent Ed 1998; 62:822.
8. Socransky SS, Haffajee AD, Goodson JM, et al: New concepts of destructive periodontal disease. J Clin Periodontol 1984; 11:21.

Necrotizing Ulcerative Periodontitis, Refractory Periodontitis, and Periodontitis as a Manifestation of Systemic Diseases

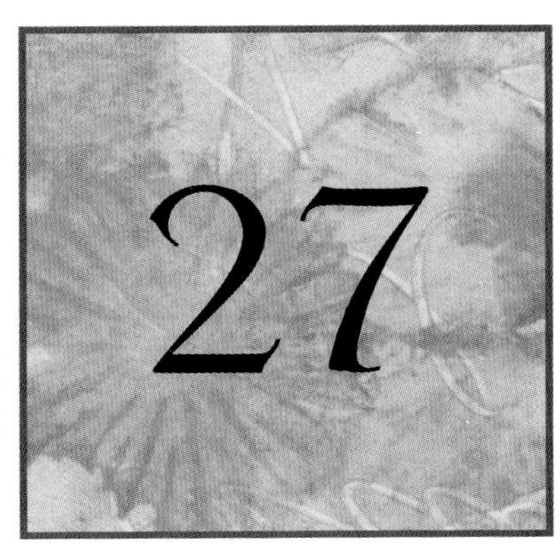

CHAPTER 27

Richard J. Nagy, Fermin A. Carranza, and Michael G. Newman

CHAPTER OUTLINE

Unusual and severe forms of periodontitis can be more frequently seen in certain severe combined and acquired immunodeficiency diseases and in some patients who were treated yet continue to show periodontal deterioration. This chapter reviews the following aggressive periodontal diseases: necrotizing ulcerative periodontitis (NUP), the refractory forms of periodontitis, and periodontitis as a manifestation of systemic diseases.

NECROTIZING ULCERATIVE PERIODONTITIS

NUP is an extension of necrotizing ulcerative gingivitis (NUG) into the periodontal structures, leading to attachment and bone loss. NUP may include combinations of the following signs and symptoms: necrosis and ulceration of the coronal portion of the interdental papillae and/or gingival margin; painful, bright-red marginal gingiva that bleeds on even slight manipulation; mouth malodor (halitosis); and systemic manifestations including fever, malaise, and lymphadenopathy. In addition, increased levels of stress, heavy smoking, and poor nutrition have been shown to be contributing factors to NUP.

Two types of NUP have been described according to their relationship with acquired immunodeficiency syndrome (AIDS).

NON-AIDS TYPE NECROTIZING ULCERATIVE PERIODONTITIS

Clinical Features

This type of periodontitis occurs after repeated long-term episodes of NUG. NUG is characterized by areas of ulceration and necrosis of the gingival margin that become covered by a whitish-yellowish soft material known as a *pseudomembrane*. The ulcerated margin is surrounded by an erythematous halo. The lesions are painful and bleed often, giving rise to localized lymphadenopathy and even fever and malaise. Microscopically, NUG lesions are the result of nonspecific necrotizing inflammation presenting a predominantly polymorphonuclear neutrophil (PMN) infiltrate in the ulcerated areas with an abundant chronic component (lymphocytes and plasma cells) in the peripheral and deeper areas.[38]

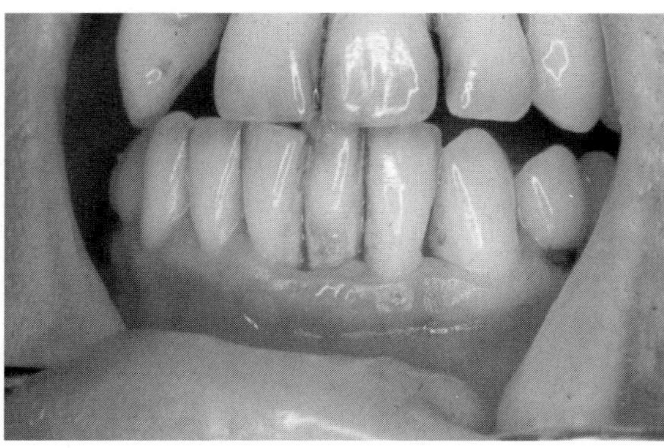

Fig. 27-1 Necrotizing ulcerative periodontitis in a 42-year-old, HIV-negative, white male.

The inflammatory infiltrate in lesions of NUG, especially in long-standing cases, can extend to the underlying bone, resulting in deep, crater-like osseous lesions, most often located in interdental areas. These cases are diagnosed as NUP.

Lesions resembling this description and progressing to become *gangrenous stomatitis,* or *noma,* have been described in children with severe malnutrition in underdeveloped countries. Jimenez and Baer[18] described NUG in children and adolescents aged 2 to 14 with malnutrition in Colombia; in advanced stages, NUG extended from the gingiva to other areas of the oral cavity, becoming gangrenous stomatitis or noma and causing exposure, necrosis, and sequestration of the alveolar bone. Experimentally, noma-like lesions have been produced in rats by administering cortisone and causing mechanical injury to the gingiva[34] and in hamsters by total body irradiation.[25]

NUP is characterized by deep interdental osseous craters (Fig. 27-1; Color Fig. 27-1, *A–C*), but deep "conventional" pockets are not found because the ulcerative and necrotizing character of the gingival lesion destroys the marginal epithelium, resulting in recession. Lesions of NUP can lead to advanced bone loss, tooth mobility, and tooth loss.

Etiology

The etiologic agents of NUP have not been studied, but they can be assumed to be similar to those present in NUG, which has been extensively investigated. However, this similarity has not been established. The mechanisms by which cases of NUG may become NUP have also not been investigated. Cutler et al[9] have described impaired bactericidal activity of PMNs in two children with NUP.

AIDS-ASSOCIATED NECROTIZING ULCERATIVE PERIODONTITIS

Clinical Features

Typical changes of inflammatory periodontal diseases can arise in the course of infection by the human immunodeficiency virus (HIV). The prevalence of these illnesses may be up to 5%.[9] The HIV-associated periodontal diseases include linear gingival erythema (LGE), NUG, and NUP.[30] The necrotizing forms appear particularly in severe or advanced immunosuppression. Gingival and periodontal lesions are frequently found in patients with AIDS. These gingival and periodontal lesions in HIV-positive patients appear to be similar to those seen in NUP in HIV-negative patients but frequently result in complications that are extremely rare in non-AIDS patients. These complications consist of large areas of soft tissue necrosis with exposure of bone and sequestration of bone fragments, which sometimes extend to the vestibular area and/or the palate and become necrotizing stomatitis.

Progression

Bone loss associated with HIV-positive NUP may be extremely rapid. Winkler and colleagues[40] mention cases in which 10 mm of bone were lost in 3 months.

Etiology

AIDS favors the occurrence of opportunistic infections leading to NUG, atypical gingivitis (an aggressive form of chronic periodontitis), and NUP. Murray and co-workers[27] have reported that cases of NUP in AIDS patients demonstrate greater numbers of the opportunistic fungus *Candida albicans* and higher prevalence of *Actinobacillus actinomycetemcomitans, Prevotella intermedia, Porphyromonas gingivalis, Fusobacterium nucleatum,* and *Campylobacter* spp. They also observed that the destructive periodontal lesions seen in AIDS patients differ substantially from NUG lesions; particularly noteworthy is the low or variable level of spirochetes, which is inconsistent with the NUG flora. The flora found in NUP in AIDS patients is more in line with that of chronic periodontitis.

For a more detailed description of these diseases, see Chapters 15 and 19; treatment is discussed in Chapters 39 and 45.

REFRACTORY PERIODONTITIS

Refractory periodontitis has been defined by the American Academy of Periodontology as "those patients who are unresponsive to any treatment provided, whatever the thoroughness or frequency." Refractory periodontitis should be distinguished from recurrent disease, in which a complete remission occurs after therapy, followed by recurrence of the disease as a result of reformation of plaque, and calculus. To classify cases as refractory (unresponsive), the clinician must clearly differentiate them from incompletely treated cases. In such patients the irritants may not have been completely removed, and the disease may temporarily have become less severe but never completely resolved.

Because of the lack of clear guidelines and parameters for the diagnosis and classification of patients as having refractory periodontitis, two different opinions have been expressed in the literature:

1. Refractory periodontitis is a distinct entity, different from other types of periodontitis.[6,10] Refractory peri-

odontitis results from different bacterial agents, specific alterations of the host response, or a combination of these factors. According to this view, multiple categories or subtypes of refractory patients may exist. Until more information is known, these patients should be grouped together into the default designation of refractory periodontitis.

2. Refractory periodontitis is not a distinct entity, and all cases of refractory periodontitis can fall into some of the other categories of periodontitis.[1] Refractory cases are most often seen during the management of aggressive forms of periodontitis, periodontitis as a manifestation of a systemic disease that cannot be resolved, and chronic periodontitis exacerbated by smoking or uncontrolled systemic conditions such as diabetes and AIDS

The incorporation of refractory periodontitis into the classification of periodontal diseases may have been a reflection of our ignorance with respect to the factors that result in unresponsiveness to therapy. As a result, the term *refractory periodontitis* has been removed as a single disease entity (see Chapter 4), even though it is appreciated that any of the forms of periodontitis may be unresponsive to conventional therapy due to inadequate or inappropriate therapy or to factors as yet undefined.

Clinical Features

Pretreatment clinical findings and severity are not diagnostic of refractory periodontitis. After the initial treatment, Magnusson et al reported no difference in the amount of plaque in sites that were gaining or losing attachment, but losing sites had persistent bleeding on probing and suppuration.[23]

Deterioration in cases of refractory periodontitis occurs either by new involvement of additional teeth or by increased bone and attachment loss in previously treated areas.

Etiology

Refractory periodontitis may be due to an abnormal host response, an unusually pathogenic and virulent microflora, failure to eliminate plaque-retentive factors, or a combination of any of these factors. Plaque accumulation and smoking have been consistently associated with the lack of clinical responsiveness.

A high proportion of *A. actinomycetemcomitans*[11] and *P. intermedia* has been reported in refractory periodontitis cases.[32] Rodenburg et al noted that the total number of bacteria in the pockets of refractory patients was lower than that in untreated patients, but *A. actinomycetemcomitans* comprised a larger proportion of the subgingival microflora than in untreated patients.[32] This has been explained (1) by the assumption that *A. actinomycetemcomitans* is more difficult to eradicate from the subgingival area than are other bacteria because of its invasive capability and (2) by reinfection from other sites of the mouth.[31]

Slots and Rams[35] have noted the following microorganisms and their incidence in refractory chronic periodontitis: *F. nucleatum* (75% of patients/sites), *P. intermedia* (40%), *A. actinomycetemcomitans* (30%), *Peptostreptococcus micros* (30%), *Staphylococcus* sp. (30%), *Bacteroides forsythus* (25%), *Campylobacter rectus* (25%), *P. gingivalis* (15%), *Candida* sp. (15%), and *Enterobacteriaceae* or *Pseudomonadacea* spp. (10%).

Haffajee et al[14] identified three major microbial complexes in patients with refractory periodontitis: (1) *B. forsythus, F. nucleatum,* and *C. rectus;* (2) *Streptococcus intermedius, B. gingivalis,* and *Peptostreptococcus micros;* and (3) *S. intermedius* and *F. nucleatum.*

Walker et al[39] have indicated that at least two patterns or rates of attachment loss may be associated with refractory periodontitis; each pattern may be indicative of a different flora. The pattern associated with a relatively rapid loss of attachment was characterized by a gram-negative flora that contained spirochetes, *P. intermedia,* and *Fusobacterium* species. A slow, continuous rate was associated with a predominantly gram-negative flora containing a high proportion of *S. intermedius* or *S. intermedius*-like organisms. However, Colombo et al[8] reported that elevated levels of *Streptococcus constellatus* was more related to refractory disease in test subjects compared to control subjects with similar levels of the known putative periodontopathogens found in each group. This shows the wide variation in microbial species known to be related to refractory disease. Thus refractory periodontal disease may not be related to the persistence of microbial species alone.

MacFarlane et al[22] have described impaired PMN phagocytosis in cases of refractory periodontitis and reduction of PMN chemotaxis. They also found a high percentage of smokers in the group of refractory cases. Hernichel-Gorbach et al[15] have evaluated the host responses of patients with generalized refractory periodontitis and reported that a majority of these patients may have some alteration in the mononuclear cell–cytokine system.

Frequency

Cases of refractory periodontitis may be similar to cases identified by Hirschfeld and Wasserman[16] as "extreme downhill," which constituted 4.2% of the 600 patients studied and followed for 22 years. In McFall's study of 100 patients followed for 19 years, 8% were identified as "extreme downhill."[26]

PERIODONTITIS AS A MANIFESTATION OF SYSTEMIC DISEASES

Many systemic conditions associated with or predisposing to periodontal attachment loss have defective numbers of neutrophils or defective neutrophil function as a common finding. This underscores the importance of the neutrophil in the protection of the periodontium against infection. Severe periodontitis has been observed in individuals with primary neutrophil disorders including agranulocytosis, neutropenia, Chediak-Higashi syndrome, and lazy leukocyte syndrome. In addition, more frequent and severe periodontitis has been observed in

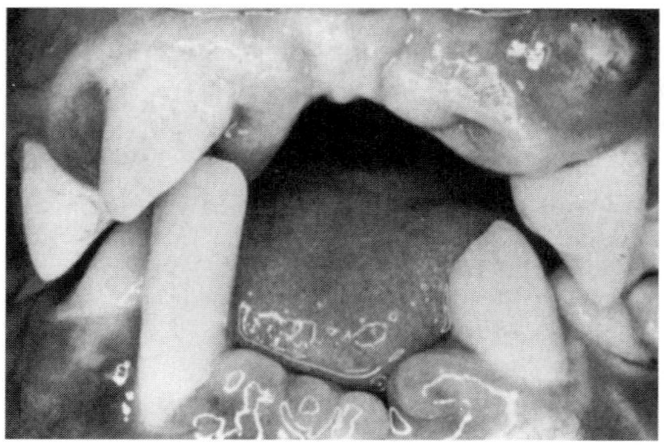

Fig. 27-2 Dentition of a 17-year-old boy with Papillon-Lefèvre syndrome. The missing teeth were exfoliated.

A

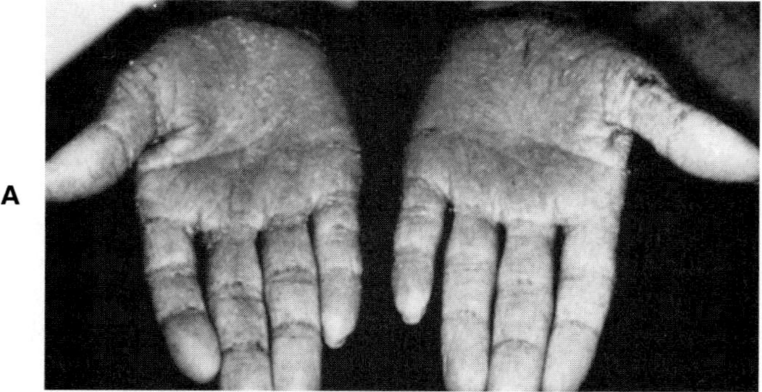

B

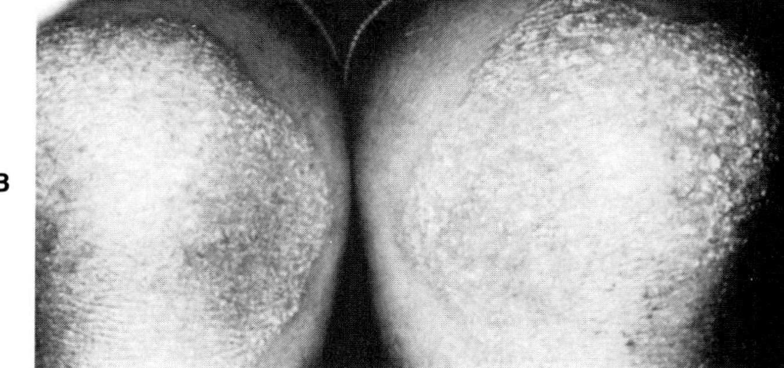

Fig. 27-3 Palms **(A)** and knees **(B)** of the patient in Fig. 27-1. Note the hyperkeratotic scaly lesions.

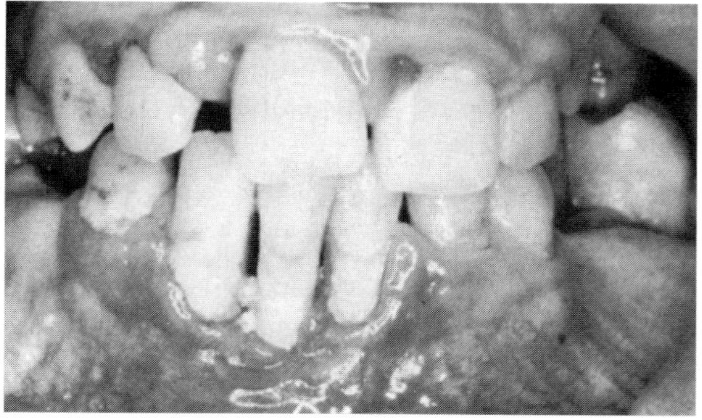

Fig. 27-4 A 14-year-old patient with Down syndrome and severe periodontal destruction.

individuals who exhibit secondary neutrophil impairment as seen in Down syndrome, Papillon-Lefèvre syndrome, and inflammatory bowel disease. The remainder of this chapter discusses some of these entities.

Papillon-Lefèvre Syndrome

Papillon-Lefèvre syndrome is characterized by hyperkeratotic skin lesions, severe destruction of the periodontium, and in some cases, calcification of the dura.[4,12] The cutaneous and periodontal changes usually appear together before the age of 4 years. The skin lesions consist of hyperkeratosis and ichthyosis of localized areas on palms, soles, knees, and elbows (Figs. 27-2 and 27-3).

Periodontal involvement consists of early inflammatory changes that lead to bone loss and exfoliation of teeth. Primary teeth are lost by 5 or 6 years of age. The permanent dentition then erupts normally, but within a few years the permanent teeth are lost owing to destructive periodontal disease. By the age of 15 years, patients are usually edentulous except for the third molars. These also are lost a few years after they erupt. Tooth extraction sites heal uneventfully.[13] The microscopic changes reported include marked chronic inflammation of the lateral wall of the pocket with a predominantly plasma cell infiltrate, considerable osteoclastic activity and apparent lack of osteoblastic activity, and an extremely thin cementum.[24] Bacterial flora studies of plaque in a case of Papillon-Lefèvre syndrome revealed a similarity to bacterial flora in chronic periodontitis.[21] Spirochete-rich zones in the apical portion of the pockets, as well as spirochete adherence to the cementum and microcolony formation of *Mycoplasma* spp., have been reported in Papillon-Lefèvre syndrome.[20] Gram-negative cocci and rods appear at the apical border of plaque.[37] No significant alterations have been found in peripheral blood lymphocytes and polymorphonuclear neutrophils (PMNs).[33]

Papillon-Lefèvre syndrome is inherited and appears to follow an autosomal recessive pattern. Parents are not affected, and both must carry the autosomal genes for the syndrome to appear in the offspring. It may occur in siblings; males and females are equally affected. The estimated frequency is 1 to 4 cases per 1 million individuals. Rare cases of adult onset of this syndrome, albeit with mild periodontal lesions, have also been described.[3]

Down Syndrome

Down syndrome (mongolism, trisomy 21) is a congenital disease caused by a chromosomal abnormality and characterized by mental deficiency and growth retardation. The prevalence of periodontal disease in Down syndrome is high (occurring in almost 100% of patients younger than 30 years). Although plaque, calculus, and local irritants (e.g., diastemata, crowding of teeth, high frenum attachments, and malocclusion) are present and oral hygiene is poor, the severity of periodontal destruction exceeds that explainable by local factors alone.[5,7,36]

Periodontal disease in Down syndrome is characterized by formation of deep periodontal pockets associated with substantial plaque accumulation and moderate gingivitis (Fig. 27-4). These findings are usually generalized, although they tend to be more severe in the lower anterior region; marked recession is also sometimes seen in this region, apparently associated with high frenum attachment. The disease progresses rapidly. Acute necrotizing lesions are a frequent finding.

Two factors have been proposed to explain the high prevalence and increased severity of periodontal destruction associated with Down syndrome: a reduced resistance to infections because of poor circulation, especially in areas of terminal vascularization such as the gingival tissue,[9,10] and a defect in T-cell maturation and polymorphonuclear leukocyte chemotaxis.[17] Increased numbers of *P. intermedia* have been reported in the mouths of children with Down syndrome.[19]

Neutropenia

Destructive generalized periodontal lesions have been described in children with neutropenia. For further information, see Chapter 14.

Chediak-Higashi Syndrome

Chediak-Higashi syndrome is rare and is characterized by recurrent bacterial infections including rapidly destructive periodontitis. It is discussed in Chapters 10 and 14.

Hypophosphatasia

Hypophosphatasia is a rare familial skeletal disease characterized by rickets, poor cranial bone formation, craneostenosis, and premature loss of primary teeth, particularly the incisors. Patients have a low level of serum alkaline phosphatase, and phosphoethanolamine is present in serum and urine.

Teeth are lost with no clinical evidence of gingival inflammation and show reduced cementum formation.[2] In patients with minimal bone abnormalities, premature loss of deciduous teeth may be the only symptom of hypophosphatasia. In adolescents, this disease resembles localized *juvenile periodontitis*.[41]

Leukocyte Adhesion Deficiency

Cases of leukocyte adhesion deficiency (LAD) are rare and begin during or immediately after eruption of the primary teeth. Extremely acute inflammation and proliferation of the gingival tissues with rapid destruction of bone are found. Profound defects in peripheral blood neutrophils and monocytes and an absence of neutrophils in the gingival tissues have been noted in patients with LAD[28,29]; these patients also have frequent respiratory tract infections and sometimes otitis media. All primary teeth are affected, but the permanent dentition may not be affected.[29]

REFERENCES

1. Adams DF: Diagnosis and treatment of refractory periodontitis. Curr Opin Dent 1992; 2:33.
2. Beumer J III, Trowbridge HO, Silverman S Jr, et al: Childhood hypophosphatasia and the premature loss of teeth. Oral Surg Oral Med Oral Pathol 1973; 35:631.
3. Bullon P, Pascual A, Fernandez-Novoa MC, et al: Late onset Papillon-Lefèvre syndrome? J Clin Periodontol 1993; 20:662.
4. Carvel RI: Palmar-plantar hyperkeratosis and premature periodontal destruction. J Oral Med 1969; 24:73.
5. Cichon P, Crawford L, Grimm WD: Early-onset periodontitis associated with Down's syndrome—clinical interventional study. Ann Periodontol 1998; 3:370.
6. Cram S, Rasheed A, Meador H, et al: Objective parameters of refractory periodontitis. Abstract 1428. J Dent Res 1989; 68(special issue):360.
7. Cohen MM, Winer RA, Schwartz S, et al: Oral aspects of mongolism. Part I. Periodontal disease in mongolism. Oral Surg Oral Med Oral Pathol 1961; 14:92.
8. Colombo AP, Haffajee AD, Dewhirst FE, et al: Clinical and microbiological features of refractory periodontitis subjects. J Clin Periodontol 1998; 25:169.
9. Cutler CW, Wasfy MO, Ghaffar K, et al: Impaired bactericidal activity of PMN from two brothers with necrotizing ulcerative gingivo-periodontitis. J Periodontol 1994;*65*:357.
10. Dow RS. Preliminary study of periodontoclasia in mongoloid children at Polk State School. Am J Ment Defic 1951; 55:535.
11. Eggert FM, Flowerdew G, McLeod MH, et al: Diagnostic utility of specific microbiological markers for periodontal diseases. J Periodontol 1998; 69:1373.
12. Fardal O, Drangsholt E, Olsen I: Palmar plantar keratosis and unusual periodontal findings. Observations from a family of 4 members. J Clin Periodontol 1998; 25:181.
13. Farzim I, Edalat M: Periodontitis with hyperkeratosis palmaris et plantaris (Papillon-Lefèvre syndrome). J Periodontol 1974; 45:316.
14. Haffajee AD, Socransky SS, Dzink JL, et al: Clinical, microbiological and immunological features of subjects with refractory periodontal diseases. J Clin Periodontol 1988; 15:390.
15. Hernichel-Gorbach E, Kornman KS, Holt SC, et al: Host responses in patients with generalized refractory periodontitis. J Periodontol 1994; 65:8.
16. Hirschfeld L, Wasserman B: A long-term survey of tooth loss in 600 treated periodontal patients. J Periodontol 1978; 49:225.
17. Izumi Y, Sugiyama S, Shinozuka O, et al: Defective neutrophil chemotaxis in Down's syndrome patients and its relationship to periodontal disease. J Periodontol 1989; 60:238.
18. Jimenez M, Baer PN: Necrotizing ulcerative gingivitis in children: A 9 year clinical study. J Periodontol 1975; 46:715.
19. Loesche WJ, Hockett RN, Syed SA: The predominant cultivable flora of tooth surface plaque removed from institutionalized subjects. Arch Oral Biol 1972; 17:1311.
20. Jung JR, Carranza FA Jr, Newman MG: Scanning electronmicroscopy of plaque in Papillon-Lefèvre syndrome. J Periodontol 1981; 52:442.
21. Lundgren T, Renvert S, Papapanou PN, et al: Subgingival microbial profile of Papillon-Lefèvre patients assessed by DNA probes. J Clin Periodontol 1998; 25:624.
22. MacFarlane GD, Herzberg MC, Wolff LF, et al: Refractory periodontitis associated with abnormal PMN leukocyte phagocytosis and cigarette smoking. J Periodontol 1993; 63:908.
23. Magnusson I, Marks RG, Clark WB, et al: Clinical, microbiological and immunological characteristics of subjects with "refractory" periodontal disease. J Clin Periodontol 1991; 18:291.
24. Martinez Lalis RR, Lopez Otero R, Carranza FA Jr: A case of Papillon-Lefèvre syndrome. Periodontics 1965; 3:292.
25. Mayo J, Carranza FA Jr, Epper CE, et al: The effect of total body irradiation on the oral tissues of the Syrian hamster. Oral Surg Med Pathol 1962; 15:739.

26. McFall WT, Jr: Tooth loss in 100 treated patients with periodontal disease. A long-term study. J Periodontol 1982; 53:539.
27. Murray PA, Holt SC: Microbiology of HIV-associated gingivitis and periodontitis. In Robertson PB, Greenspan JS (eds): Perspectives on Oral Manifestations of AIDS. Littleton, MA, PSG Publishing, 1988.
28. Page RC, Bowen T, Altman L, et al: Prepubertal periodontitis. I. Definition of a clinical disease entity. J Periodontol 1983; 54:257.
29. Page RC, Schroeder HE: Periodontitis in Man and Other Animals. Basel, S Karger, 1982.
30. Pistorius A, Willershausen B: Cases of HIV-associated characteristic periodontal diseases. Eur J Med Res 1999; 4:121.
31. Renvert S, Wikström M, Dahlen G, et al: On the inability of root debridement and periodontal surgery to eliminate *Actinobacillus actinomycetemcomitans* from periodontal pockets. J Clin Periodontol 1990; 17:351.
32. Rodenburg JP, Winkelhoff AJ, Winkel EG, et al: Occurrence of *Bacteroides gingivalis, Bacteroides intermedius* and *Actinobacillus actinomycetemcomitans* in severe periodontitis in relation to age and treatment history. J Clin Periodontol 1990; 17:392.
33. Schroeder HE, Seger RA, Keller HU, et al: Behavior of neutrophilic granulocytes in a case of Papillon-Lefèvre syndrome. J Clin Periodontol 1983; 10:618.
34. Selye H: Effect of cortisone and somatotrophic hormone upon the development of a noma-like condition in the rat. Oral Surg Med Pathol 1953; 6:557.
35. Slots J, Rams T: New views on periodontal microbiota in special patient categories. J Clin Periodontol 1991; 18:411.
36. Sznajder N, Carraro JJ, Otero E, Carranza FA, Jr: Clinical periodontal finding in trisomy 21 (mongolism). J Periodont Res 1968; 3:1.
37. Vrahopoulos TP, Barber P, Liakoni H, et al: Ultrastructure of the periodontal lesion in a case of Papillon-Lefèvre syndrome (PLS). J Clin Periodontol 1988; 15:17.
38. Wade DN, Kerns DG: Acute necrotizing ulcerative gingivitis-periodontitis: a literature review. Mil Med 1998; 16:337.
39. Walker CB, Gordon JM, Magnusson I, et al: A role for antibiotics in the treatment of refractory periodontitis. J Periodontol 1993; 64:772.
40. Winkler JR, Grassi M, Murray PA: Clinical description and etiology of HIV-associated periodontal diseases. In Robertson PB, Greenspan JS (eds): Perspectives on Oral Manifestations of AIDS. Littleton, MA, PSG Publishing, 1988.
41. Yendt ER: The parathyroids and calcium metabolism. In Volpe R (ed): Clinical Medicine. Vol 8: Endocrinology. Philadelphia, Harper & Row, 1986.

Aggressive Periodontitis

Richard J. Nagy and Karen F. Novak

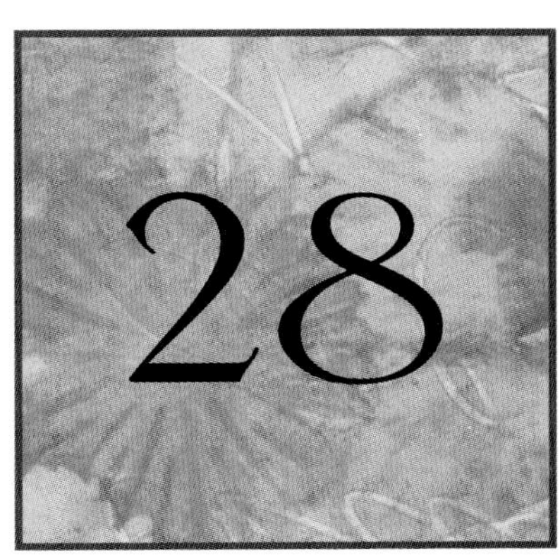

CHAPTER

CHAPTER OUTLINE

Aggressive periodontitis generally affects systemically healthy individuals less than 30 years old, although patients may be older. Aggressive periodontitis may be universally distinguished from chronic periodontitis by the age of onset, the rapid rate of disease progression, the nature and composition of the associated subgingival microflora, alterations in the host's immune response, and a familial aggregation of diseased individuals.[18] In addition, a strong racial influence is observed in the United States; the disease is more prevalent among African-Americans.[27] Aggressive periodontitis describes three of the diseases formerly classified as early onset periodontitis. Localized aggressive periodontitis was formerly classified as localized juvenile periodontitis (LJP). Generalized aggressive periodontitis encompasses the diseases previously classified as generalized juvenile periodontitis (GJP) and rapidly progressive periodontitis (RPP) (see Chapter 4).

LOCALIZED AGGRESSIVE PERIODONTITIS

Historical Background

In 1923, Gottlieb[13] reported a patient with a fatal case of epidemic influenza and a disease that he called *diffuse atrophy of the alveolar bone.* This disease was characterized by a loss of collagen fibers in the periodontal ligament and their replacement by loose connective tissue and extensive bone resorption, resulting in a widened periodontal ligament space. The gingiva apparently was not involved. In 1928, Gottlieb[14] attributed this condition to the inhibition of continuous cementum formation, which he considered essential for maintenance of the periodontal ligament fibers. He then termed the disease *deep cementopathia.* Gottlieb hypothesized that deep cementopathia was a "disease of eruption" and that cementum initiated a foreign body response. As a result, it was postulated that the host attempted to exfoliate the tooth, resulting in the observed bone resorption and pocket formation.[14]

In 1938, Wannenmacher[49] described incisor-first molar involvement and called the disease *parodontitis marginalis progressiva.* Several explanations evolved for the etiology and pathogenesis of this type of disease. Many individuals considered this to be a degenerative, noninflammatory disease process[12,34,45] and therefore gave it the name *periodontosis.* Other investigators denied the existence of a degenerative type of periodontal disease and attributed the changes observed to trauma from occlusion.[6] Ultimately, in 1966 the World Workshop in Periodontics[38] concluded that the concept of periodontosis as a degenerative entity was unsubstantiated and that the term should be eliminated from periodontal nomenclature. The committee did recognize that a clinical entity different from adult periodontitis might occur among adolescents and young adults.

The term *juvenile periodontitis* was introduced by Chaput and colleagues in 1967 and by Butler[4] in 1969. In 1971, Baer[2] defined it as "a disease of the periodontium occurring in an otherwise healthy adolescent which is characterized by a rapid loss of alveolar bone about more than one tooth of the permanent dentition. The amount of destruction manifested is not commensurate with the amount of local irritants." In 1989 the World Workshop in Clinical Periodontics[8] categorized this disease as localized juvenile periodontitis (LJP), a subset of the broad classification of early onset periodontitis (EOP). Under this classification system, age of onset and distribution of lesions were of primary importance when making a diagnosis of LJP. Most recently, disease with the characteristics of LJP has been renamed *localized aggressive periodontitis.*

Clinical Characteristics

Localized aggressive periodontitis usually has an age of onset around puberty.[22] Clinically, it is characterized as having "localized first molar/incisor presentation with interproximal attachment loss on at least two permanent teeth, one of which is a first molar, and involving no more than two teeth other than first molars and incisors" (Color Fig. 28-1, *A–D*). The localized distribution of lesions in localized aggressive periodontitis is characteristic but as yet unexplained. The following possible reasons for the limitation of periodontal destruction to certain teeth have been suggested:

1. After initial colonization of the first permanent teeth to erupt (the first molars and incisors), *Actinobacillus actinomycetemcomitans* evades the host defenses by different mechanisms, including production of polymorphonuclear leukocyte chemotaxis-inhibiting factors, endotoxin, collagenases, leukotoxin, and other factors that allow the bacteria to colonize the pocket and initiate the destruction of the periodontal tissues. After this initial attack, adequate immune defenses are stimulated to produce opsonic antibodies to enhance the clearance and phagocytosis of invading bacteria and neutralize leukotoxic activity. In this manner, colonization of other sites may be prevented.[51] A strong antibody response to infecting agents is one characteristic of localized aggressive periodontitis.[22]
2. Bacteria antagonistic to *A. actinomycetemcomitans* may colonize the periodontal tissues and inhibit *A. actinomycetemcomitans* from further colonization of periodontal sites in the mouth. This would localize *A. actinomycetemcomitans* infection and tissue destruction.[19]
3. *A. actinomycetemcomitans* may lose its leukotoxin-producing ability for unknown reasons.[44] If this happens, the progression of the disease may become arrested or retarded and colonization of new periodontal sites averted.
4. The possibility that a defect in cementum formation may be responsible for the localization of the lesions has been suggested.[25,35] Root surfaces of teeth extracted from patients with localized aggressive periodontitis have been found to have hypoplastic or aplastic cementum. This was true not only of root surfaces exposed to periodontal pockets but also of roots still surrounded by their periodontium.

A striking feature of localized aggressive periodontitis is the lack of clinical inflammation despite the presence of deep periodontal pockets (see Color Fig. 28-1, *E* and *F*). Furthermore, in many cases the amount of plaque on the affected teeth is minimal, which seems inconsistent with the amount of periodontal destruction present.[22] The plaque that is present forms a thin biofilm on the teeth and rarely mineralizes to form calculus.[48] Although the quantity of plaque may be limited, it often contains elevated levels of *A. actinomycetemcomitans,* and in some patients, *Porphyromonas gingivalis*. The potential significance of the qualitative composition of the microbial flora in localized aggressive periodontitis is discussed later in this chapter (Risk Factors for Aggressive Periodontitis: Microbiologic Factors).

As the name suggests, localized aggressive periodontitis progresses rapidly. Evidence suggests that the rate of bone loss is about three to four times faster than in chronic periodontitis.[2] Other clinical features of localized aggressive periodontitis may include distolabial migration of the maxillary incisors with concomitant diastema formation (see Color Fig. 28-1, *B*), increasing mobility of the first molars, sensitivity of denuded root surfaces to thermal and tactile stimuli, and deep, dull, radiating pain during mastication, probably because of irritation of the supporting structures by mobile teeth and impacted food. Periodontal abscesses may form at this stage, and regional lymph node enlargement may occur.[30]

It should be noted that not all cases of localized aggressive periodontitis progress to the degree described previously. In some patients, the progression of attachment loss and bone loss may be self-arresting.[22]

Radiographic Findings

Vertical loss of alveolar bone around the first molars and incisors, beginning around puberty in otherwise healthy teenagers, is a classic diagnostic sign of localized aggressive periodontitis. Radiographic findings may include an "arc-shaped loss of alveolar bone extending from the distal surface of the second premolar to the mesial surface of the second molar"[33] (see Color Fig. 28-1, *D*).

Prevalence and Distribution by Age and Sex

The prevalence of localized aggressive periodontitis in geographically diverse adolescent populations is estimated to be below 1%. Most reports suggest a low prevalence, about 0.2%.[27] Two independent radiographic studies of 16-year-old adolescents, one in Finland[41] and the other in Switzerland,[21] followed the strict diagnostic criteria delineated by Baer[2] and reported a prevalence rate of 0.1%. A clinical and radiographic study of 7266 English adolescents 15 to 19 years old also showed a prevalence rate of 0.1%.[40] In the U.S., a national survey of adolescents age 14 to 17 reported that 0.53% had localized aggressive periodontitis.[27] Blacks were at much higher risk for localized aggressive periodontitis, and black males were 2.9 times more likely to have the disease than black females. In contrast, white females were more likely to have localized aggressive periodontitis than white males. Several other studies have found the highest prevalence of localized aggressive periodontitis among black males,[5,32,40] followed in descending order by black females, white females, and white males.[32]

Localized aggressive periodontitis affects both males and females and is seen most frequently in the period between puberty and 20 years of age. Some studies have suggested a predilection for female patients, particularly in the youngest age groups,[20] whereas others report no male-female differences in incidence when studies are designed to correct for ascertainment bias.[17] (For additional epidemiologic data on localized aggressive periodontitis, see Chapter 5.)

GENERALIZED AGGRESSIVE PERIODONTITIS

Clinical Characteristics

Generalized aggressive periodontitis usually affects individuals under the age of 30, but older patients also may be affected.[22] In contrast to localized aggressive periodontitis, evidence suggests that individuals affected with generalized aggressive periodontitis produce a poor antibody response to the pathogens present. Clinically, generalized aggressive periodontitis is characterized by "generalized interproximal attachment loss affecting at least three permanent teeth other than first molars and incisors" (Figs. 28-1, *A* and *B*, and 28-2, *A* and *B*). The destruction appears to occur episodically with periods of advanced destruction followed by stages of quiescence of variable length (weeks to months or years). Radiographs often show bone loss that has progressed since the previous evaluation (see Fig. 28-2, *B* and *C*).

As seen in localized aggressive periodontitis, patients with generalized aggressive periodontitis often have small amounts of bacterial plaque associated with the affected teeth.[22] Quantitatively, the amount of plaque seems inconsistent with the amount of periodontal destruction. Qualitatively, *P. gingivalis, A. actinomycetemcomitans,* and *Bacteriodes forsythus* frequently are detected in the plaque that is present.[46]

Two gingival tissue responses can be found in cases of generalized aggressive periodontitis. One is a severe, acutely inflamed tissue, often proliferating, ulcerated, and fiery red (see Fig. 28-1, *A*). Bleeding may occur spontaneously or with slight stimulation. Suppuration may be an important feature. This tissue response is considered to occur in the destructive stage, in which attachment and bone are actively lost. In other cases, the gingival tissues may appear pink, free of inflammation, and occasionally with some degree of stippling, although the last feature may be absent (see Fig. 28-2, *A*). However, despite the apparently mild clinical appearance, deep pockets can be demonstrated by probing. This tissue response has been considered by Page and Schroeder[37] to coincide with periods of quiescence in which the bone level remains stationary. Some patients with generalized aggressive periodontitis may have systemic manifestations such as weight loss, mental depression, and general malaise.[36] Patients with a presumptive diagnosis of generalized aggressive periodontitis must have their medical histories updated and reviewed. These patients should receive medical evaluations to rule out possible systemic involvement. As seen with localized aggressive periodontitis, cases of generalized aggressive periodontitis may be arrested spontaneously or after therapy, whereas others may continue to progress inexorably to tooth loss despite intervention with conventional treatment.

Radiographic Findings

The radiographic picture in generalized aggressive periodontitis can range from severe bone loss associated with the minimal number of teeth, as described previously, to advanced bone loss affecting the majority of teeth in the dentition (see Fig. 28-1, *B*). A comparison of radiographs taken at different times illustrates the aggressive nature of this disease (see Fig. 28-2, *B* and *C*). Page and co-workers[36] described sites in generalized aggressive periodontitis (formerly RPP) patients that demonstrated osseous destruction of 25% to 60% during a 9-week period. Despite this extreme loss, other sites in the same patient showed no bone loss.

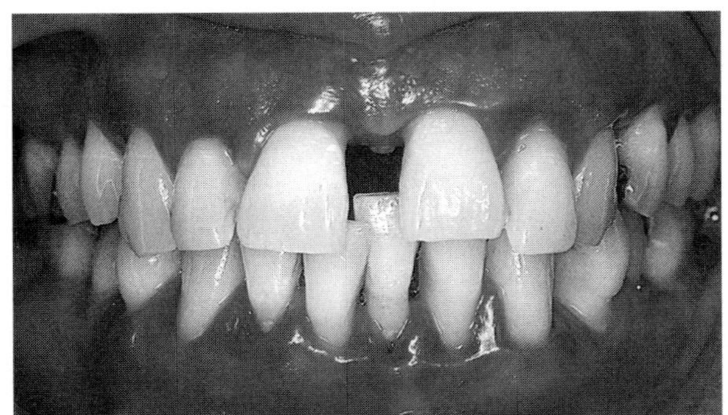

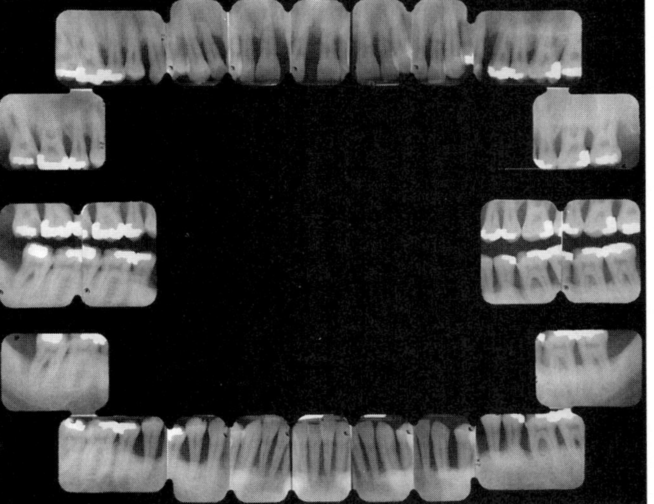

Fig. 28-1 A, Generalized aggressive periodontitis in a 30-year-old white patient. Note the generalized discoloration and smooth surface of the gingival tissues. **B,** Radiographs of this same patient, showing advanced generalized bone loss. (Courtesy Dr. Philip Melnick, Los Angeles, Calif.)

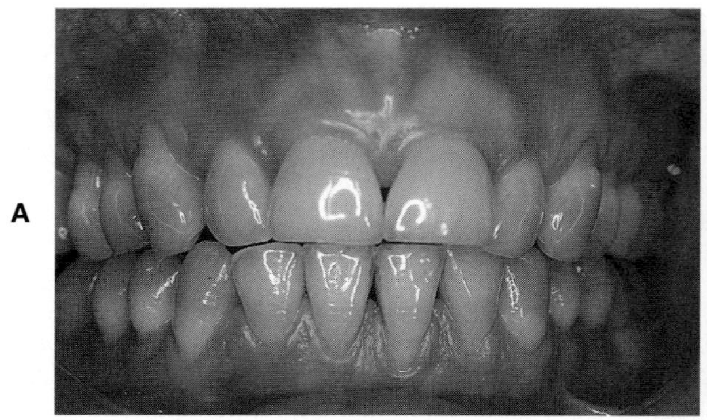

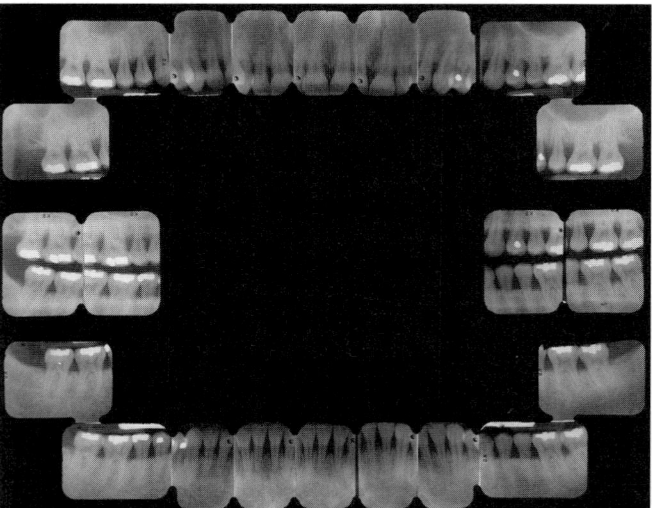

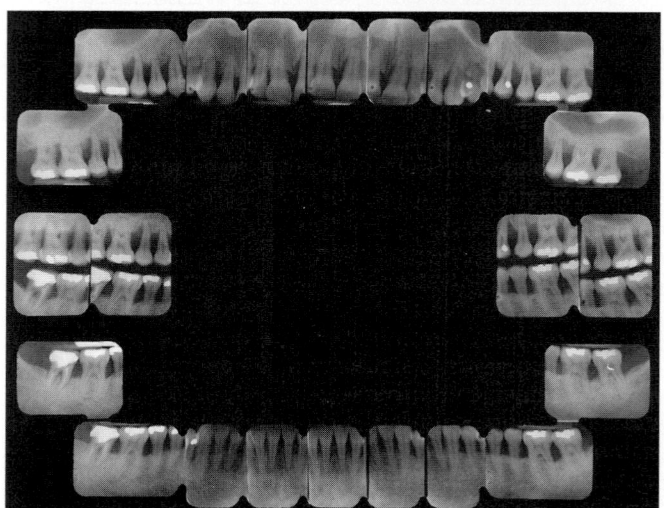

Fig. 28-2 A, Generalized aggressive periodontitis in a 32-year-old white female. Note the apparently normal color and surface texture of the gingival tissues. **B,** Radiographs of this patient taken in 1988, showing advanced generalized bone loss. Despite repeated aggressive treatment, the patient's condition continued to deteriorate. **C,** Radiographs taken in 1992, showing progressive bone loss. Clinical pictures were taken at the later date. (Courtesy Dr. Philip Melnick, Los Angeles, Calif.)

Prevalence and Distribution by Age and Sex

In a study of untreated periodontal disease conducted in Sri Lanka by Löe and colleagues,[26] 8% of the population had rapid progression of periodontal disease characterized by a yearly loss of attachment of 0.1 to 1.0 mm. In the U.S., a national survey of adolescents aged 14 to 17 reported that 0.13% had generalized aggressive periodontitis.[27] In addition, blacks were at much higher risk than whites for all forms of aggressive periodontitis and males were more likely to have generalized aggressive periodontitis than females. (For additional epidemiologic data on aggressive periodontitis, see Chapter 5.)

RISK FACTORS FOR AGGRESSIVE PERIODONTITIS

Microbiologic Factors

Although several specific microorganisms frequently are detected in patients with localized aggressive periodontitis (*A. actinomycetemcomitans, Capnocytophaga* sp., *Eikenella corrodens, Prevotella intermedia,* and *Campylobacter rectus*), *A. actinomycetemcomitans* has been implicated as the primary pathogen associated with this disease. As summarized by Tonetti and Mombelli,[46] this link is based on the following evidence: (1) *A. actinomycetemcomitans* is found in high frequency (approximately 90%) in lesions characteristic of localized aggressive periodontitis, (2) sites with evidence of disease progression often show elevated levels of *A. actinomycetemcomitans,* (3) many patients with the clinical manifestations of localized aggressive periodontitis have significantly elevated serum antibody titers to *A. actinomycetemcomitans,* (4) clinical studies show a correlation between reduction in the subgingival load of *A. actinomycetemcomitans* during treatment and a successful clinical response, and (5) *A. actinomycetemcomitans* produces a number of virulence factors that may contribute to the disease process (see also Chapter 6).

It should be noted that not all reports support the association of *A. actinomycetemcomitans* and localized aggressive periodontitis. In some studies, *A. actinomycetemcomitans* either could not be detected in patients with this form of disease or could not be detected at the previously reported frequencies. Another study found elevated levels of *P. gingivalis, P. intermedia, Fusobacterium nucleatum, C. rectus,* and *Treponema denticola* in patients with either localized or generalized aggressive disease, but no significant association was found between the presence of aggressive disease and *A. actinomycetemcomitans*. In addition, *A. actinomycetemcomitans* often can be detected in periodontally healthy subjects, suggesting that this microorganism may be part of the normal flora in many individuals.

Electron microscopic studies of localized aggressive periodontitis have revealed bacterial invasion of connective tissue[9,11] that reaches the bone surface.[7] The invading flora has been described as morphologically mixed but composed mainly of gram-negative bacteria, including cocci, rods, filaments, and spirochetes.[11] Using different methods, including immunocytochemistry and electromicroscopy, several tissue-invading microorganisms have been identified as *A. actinomycetemcomitans, Capnocytophaga sputigena, Mycoplasma* spp., and spirochetes.[39]

Immunologic Factors

Some immune defects have been implicated in the pathogenesis of aggressive periodontitis. The human leukocyte antigens (HLA), which regulate immune responses, have been evaluated as candidate markers for aggressive periodontitis. Although the findings with many HLA antigens have been inconsistent, HLA-A9 and B15 antigens are consistently associated with aggressive periodontitis (see Chapter 10).

Several investigators[10,23,24] have shown that patients with aggressive periodontitis display functional defects of polymorphonuclear leukocytes (PMNs), monocytes, or both. These defects can impair either the chemotactic attraction of PMN to the site of infection or their ability to phagocytose and kill microorganisms. Current studies have also demonstrated a hyperresponsiveness of monocytes from localized aggressive periodontitis patients with respect to their production of PGE_2 in response to lipopolysaccharide (LPS).[43] This hyperresponsive phenotype could lead to increased connective tissue or bone loss due to excessive production of these catabolic factors. Additionally, poorly functional inherited forms of monocyte FcγRII, the receptor for human IgG2 antibodies, have been shown to be disproportionately present in patients with localized aggressive periodontitis.[50] These PMN and monocyte defects may be induced by the bacterial infection or may be genetic in origin. Further studies are needed to characterize the origin of these cellular alterations.

Autoimmunity has been considered to have a role in generalized aggressive periodontitis according to Anusaksathien and Dolby,[1] who found host antibodies to collagen, DNA, and immunoglobulin G (IgG). Possible immune mechanisms include an increase in the expression of type II major histocompatibility complex (MHC) molecules, HLA DR4[3], altered helper or suppressor T-cell function, polyclonal activation of B cells by microbial plaque, and genetic predisposition. (For additional information on the immunology of aggressive periodontitis, see Part Three.)

Genetic Factors

Results from several studies support the concept that all individuals are not equally susceptible to aggressive periodontitis.[46] Specifically, several authors have described a familial pattern of alveolar bone loss and have implicated genetic factors in aggressive periodontitis.[4,28,29,31] Currently, specific genes have not been identified that are responsible for these diseases. However, segregational analyses and linkage analyses of families with a genetic predisposition for localized aggressive periodontitis suggest that a major gene plays a role in this disease, which is transmitted through an autosomal dominant mode of inheritance in U.S. populations[31] (see Chapter 10). It should be noted that most of the segregational studies were conducted in African-American populations and therefore other modes of inheritance may exist in different populations.

Evidence suggests that some immunologic defects associated with aggressive periodontitis may be inherited. For example, Van Dyke et al[47] reported a familial clustering of the neutrophil abnormalities seen in localized aggressive periodontitis. This clustering suggests that the defect(s) may be inherited.[46] Studies also have demonstrated that the antibody response to periodontal pathogens, particularly *A. actinomycetemcomitans,* is under genetic control and that the ability to mount high titers of specific, protective antibody (primarily IgG2) against *A. actinomycetemcomitans* may be race dependent.[15]

In summary, data support the idea that a gene of major effect exists for aggressive periodontitis. Data also support a genetic basis for some of the immunologic defects seen in patients with aggressive periodontitis. However, it is unlikely that all patients affected with aggressive periodontitis have the same genetic defect. As summarized by Tonetti and Mombelli,[46] "It seems that specific genes may be different in various populations and/or ethnic groups and therefore true heterogeneity in disease susceptibility may be present. The role of specific genes remains to be elucidated." (For additional information on genetic factors, see Chapter 10.)

Environmental Factors

The amount and duration of smoking are important variables that can influence the extent of destruction seen in young adults.[46] Patients with generalized aggressive periodontitis who smoke have more affected teeth and more loss of clinical attachment than nonsmoking patients with generalized aggressive periodontitis.[16] However, smoking may not have the same impact on attachment levels in younger patients with localized aggressive periodontitis.[42] (For additional information on smoking and periodontal disease, see Chapter 14.)

REFERENCES

1. Anusaksathien O, Dolby AE: Autoimmunity in periodontal disease. J Oral Pathol Med 1991; 20:101.
2. Baer PN: The case for periodontosis as a clinical entity. J Periodontol 1971; 42:516.
3. Bonfil JJ, Dillier FL, Mercier P: A "case control" study on the role of HLA DR4 in severe periodontitis and rapidly progressive periodontitis. Identification of types and subtypes using molecular biology. J Clin Periodontol 1999; 26:77.
4. Butler JH: A familial pattern of juvenile periodontitis (periodontosis). J Periodontol 1969; 40:115.

5. Burmeister JA, Best AM, Palcanis KG, et al: Localized juvenile periodontitis and generalized severe periodontitis: Clinical findings. J Clin Periodontol 1984; 11:181.
6. Carranza FA Sr, Carranza FA Jr: A suggested classification of common periodontal disease. J Periodontol 1959; 30:140.
7. Carranza FA Jr, Saglie R, Newman MG: Scanning and transmission electron microscopy study of tissue invading microorganisms in localized juvenile periodontitis. J Periodontol 1983; 54:598.
8. Caton J. Consensus Report: Periodontal diagnosis and diagnostic aids. In: Proceedings of the World Workshop in Clinical Periodontics. The American Academy of Periodontology. Chicago. 1989.
9. Christersson LA, Albini B, Zambon J, et al: Demonstration of *Actinobacillus actinomycetemcomitans* in gingiva in localized juvenile periodontitis in humans. Abstract. J Dent Res 1983; 62:255.
10. Clark RA, Page RC, Wilde G: Defective neutrophil chemotaxis in juvenile periodontitis. Infect Immun 1977; 18:694.
11. Gillett R, Johnson NW: Bacterial invasion of the periodontium in a case of juvenile periodontitis. J Clin Periodontol 1982; 9:93.
12. Goldman HM: Similar condition to periodontosis in two spider monkeys. Am J Orthod 1947; 33:749.
13. Gottlieb B: Die diffuse Atrophy des Alveolarknochens. Z Stomatol 1923; 21:195.
14. Gottlieb B: The formation of the pocket: Diffuse atrophy of alveolar bone. J Am Dent Assoc 1928; 15:462.
15. Gunsolley JC, Tew JG, Gooss CM, et al: Effects of race, smoking and immunoglobulin allotypes on IgG subclass concentrations. J Periodont Res 1997: 32:381.
16. Haber J, Wattles J, Crowley M, et al: Evidence for cigarette smoking as a major risk factor for periodontitis. J Periodontol 1993; 64:16.
17. Hart TC, Marazita ML, Schenkein HA, et al: No female preponderance in juvenile periodontitis after correction of ascertainment bias. J Periodontol 1991; 62:745.
18. Hart TC: Genetic risk factors for early-onset periodontitis. J Periodontol 1996; 67:355.
19. Hillman JD, Socransky SS: Bacterial interference in the oral ecology of *Actinobacillus actinomycetemcomitans* and its relationship to human periodontosis. Arch Oral Biol 1982; 27:75.
20. Hormand J, Frandsen A: Juvenile periodontitis. Localization of bone loss in relation to age, sex, and teeth. J Clin Periodontol 1979; 6:407.
21. Kronauer E, Borsa G, Lang NP: Prevalence of incipient juvenile periodontitis at age 16 years in Switzerland. J Clin Periodontol 1986; 13:103.
22. Lang N, Bartold PM, Cullinan M, et al: Consensus Report: Aggressive periodontitis. Ann Periodontol 1999; 4:53.
23. Lavine WS, Maderazo EG, Stolman J, et al: Impaired neutrophil chemotaxis in patients with juvenile and rapidly progressing periodontitis. J Periodont Res 1979; 14:10.
24. Leino L, Hurttia H: A potential role of an intracellular signaling defect in neutrophil functional abnormalities and promotion of tissue damage in patients with localized juvenile periodontitis. Clin Chem Lab Med 1999; 37:215.
25. Lindskog S, Blomlof L: Cementum hypoplasia in teeth affected by juvenile periodontitis. J Clin Periodontol 1983; 10:443.
26. Löe H, Anerud A, Boysen H, et al: Natural history of periodontal disease in man. Rapid, moderate and no loss of attachment in Sri Lankan laborers 14 to 46 years of age. J Clin Periodontol 1986; 13:431.
27. Löe H, Brown LJ: Early-onset periodontitis in the United States of America. J. Periodontol 1991; 62:608.
28. Long JC, Nance WE, Waring P, et al: Early onset periodontitis: A comparison and evaluation of two modes of inheritance. Genet Epidemiol 1987; 4:13.
29. Lopez NJ: Clinical, laboratory and immunological studies of a family with a high prevalence of generalized prepubertal and juvenile periodontitis. J Periodontol 1992; 63:457.
30. Manson JD, Lehner T: Clinical features of juvenile periodontitis (periodontosis). J Periodontol 1974; 45:636.
31. Marazita ML, Burmeister JA, Gunsolley JC, et al: Evidence for autosomal dominant inheritance and race-specific heterogeneity in early-onset periodontitis. J Periodontol 1994; 65:623.
32. Melvin WL, Sandifer JB, Gray JL: The prevalence and sex ratio of juvenile periodontitis in a young racially mixed population. J Periodontol 1991; 62:330.
33. Miller SC: Precocious advanced alveolar atrophy. J Periodontol 1948; 19:146.
34. Orban B, Weinmann JP: Diffuse atrophy of alveolar bone. J Periodontol 1942; 13:31.
35. Page RC, Baab DA: A new look at the etiology and pathogenesis of early-onset periodontitis. Cementopathia revisited. J Periodontol 1985; 56:748.
36. Page RC, Altman LC, Ebersole JL, et al: Rapidly progressive periodontitis. A distinct clinical condition. J Periodontol 1983; 54:197.
37. Page RC, Schroeder HE: Periodontitis in Man and Other Animals. A Comparative Review. Basel, Karger, 1982.
38. Ramfjord SP, Ash MM, Kerr DA (eds): World Workshop in Periodontics. Ann Arbor, University of Michigan, 1966.
39. Saglie FR, Carranza FA Jr, Newman MG, et al: Identification of tissue invading bacteria in juvenile periodontitis. J Periodont Res 1982; 17:452.
40. Saxby MS: Juvenile periodontitis: An epidemiologic study in the West Midlands of the United Kingdom. J Clin Periodontol 1987; 14:594.
41. Saxen L: Prevalence of juvenile periodontitis in Finland. J Clin Periodontol 1980; 7:177
42. Schenkein JA, Gunsolley JC, Koertge TE, et al: Smoking and its effects on early-onset periodontitis. J Am Dent Assoc 1995; 126:1107.
43. Shapira L, Soskolone WA, Van Dyke TE, et al: Prostaglandin E_2 secretion, cell maturation, and CD 14 expression by monocyte-derived macrophages from localized juvenile periodontitis patients. J Periodontol 1996; 67:224.
44. Slots J, Zambon JJ, Rosling BC, et al: *Actinobacillus actinomycetemcomitans* in human periodontal disease. Association, serology, leukotoxicity, and treatment. J Periodont Res 1982; 17:447.
45. Thoma KH, Goldman HM: Wandering and elongation of the teeth and pocket formation in paradontosis. J Am Dent Assoc 1940; 27:335.
46. Tonetti MS, Mombelli A: Early-onset periodontitis. Ann Periodontol 1999: 4:39.
47. Van Dyke TE, Schweinebraten M, Cinaciola LJ, et al: Neutrophil chemotaxis in families with localized juvenile periodontitis. J Periodont Res 1985: 20:503.
48. Waerhaug J: Subgingival plaque and loss of attachment in periodontosis as well as observed in autopsy material. J Periodontol 1976; 47:636.
49. Wannenmacher E: Ursachen auf dem Gebiet der Paradentopathien. Zbl Gesant Zahn Mund Kieferheilk 1938; 3:81.
50. Wilson ME, Kalmar JR: FcγRIIa (CD32): A potential marker defining susceptibility to localized juvenile periodontitis. J Periodontol 1996; 67:323.
51. Zambon JJ, Christersson LA, Slots J: *Actinobacillus actinomycetemcomitans* in human periodontal disease. Prevalence in patient groups and distribution of biotypes and serotypes within families. J Periodontol 1983; 54:707.

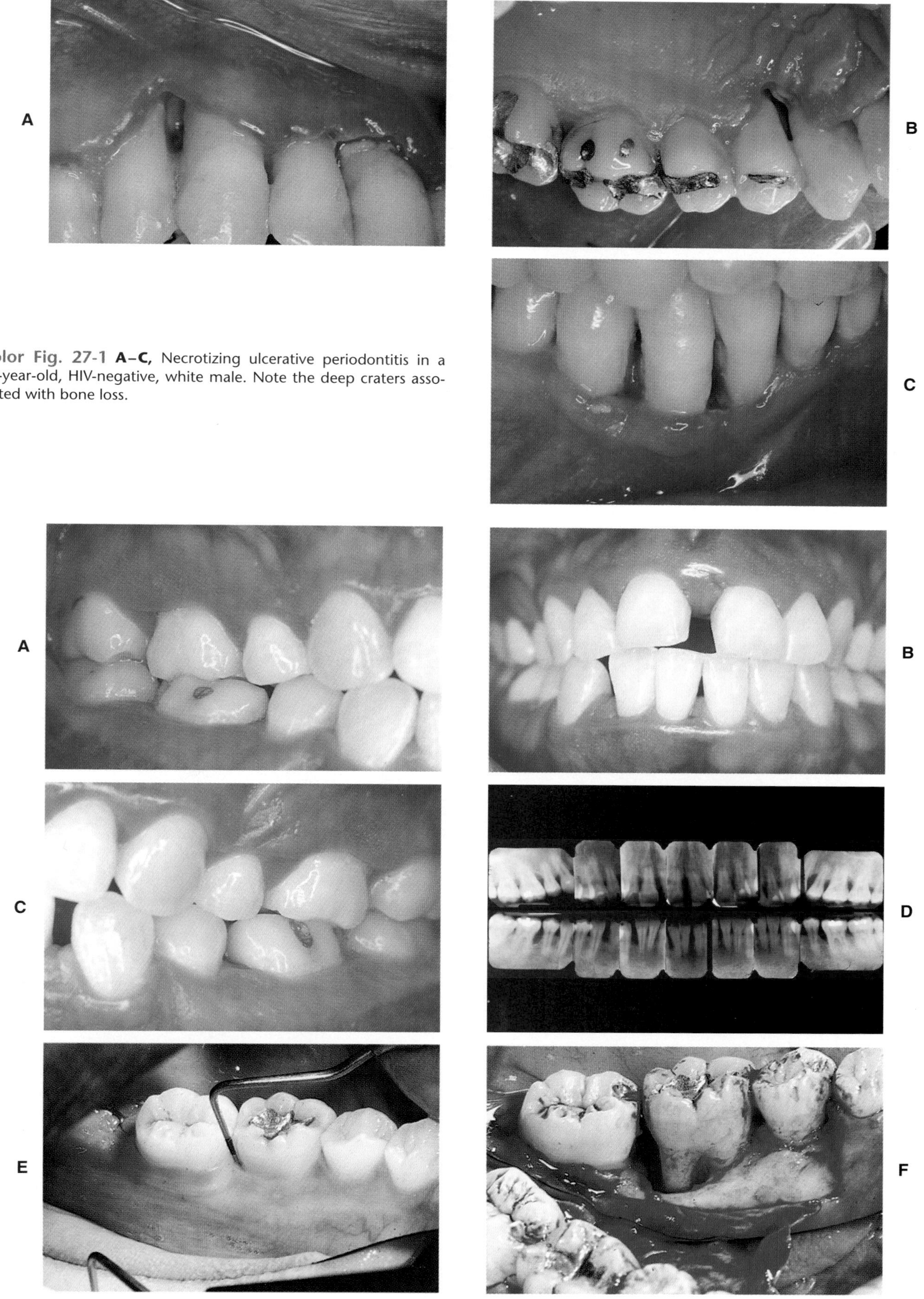

Color Fig. 27-1 **A–C,** Necrotizing ulcerative periodontitis in a 45-year-old, HIV-negative, white male. Note the deep craters associated with bone loss.

Color Fig. 28-1 Localized aggressive periodontitis. **A–C,** Clinical views of a case of localized aggressive periodontitis in a 19-year-old female. Note the migration of the maxillary anterior teeth, lack of calculus, and scant clinical inflammation. **D,** Radiographs of the same case, showing typical molar-incisor lesions. **E,** Lingual view of the left mandibular molar area in a patient with localized aggressive periodontitis. Note the apparently normal gingival tissue and the presence of a deep pocket, as denoted by the probe. **F,** The same area after the elevation of a mucoperiosteal flap. Note the advanced bone loss localized to the first molar. (**D,** Courtesy Dr. Philip Melnick, Los Angeles, Calif.; **F,** courtesy Dr. Terry Fiori, Palo Alto, Calif.)

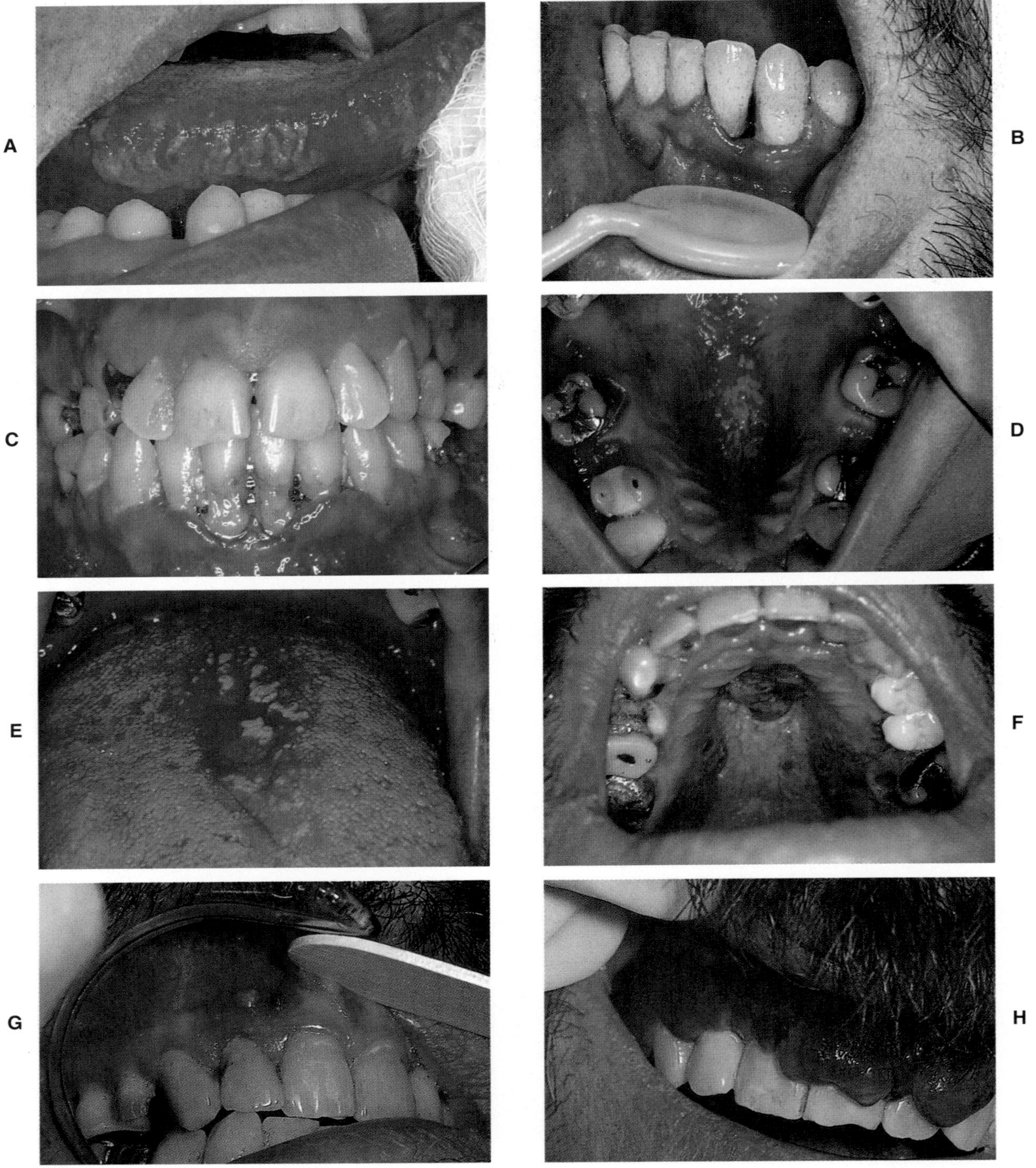

Color Fig. 29-1 AIDS and the periodontium. **A,** Hairy leukoplakia on the lateral margin of the tongue, causing a corrugated appearance. **B,** Painless ANUG-like lesion of several months' duration. The patient had a second ANUG-like lesion that was painful. **C–E,** ANUG-like lesion and candidiasis of the palate and tongue in a 29-year-old woman. **F,** Kaposi's sarcoma involving the anterior hard palate and right and left palatal mucosa. Candidiasis is also noted on the hard palate. **G,** Same patient as in **F,** with Kaposi's sarcoma of the labial gingiva presenting as a small purple nodule next to a parulis. **H,** Kaposi's sarcoma involving the anterior facial gingiva and producing a gingival enlargement. (Courtesy Dr. Frank Lucatorto.)

AIDS and the Periodontium

Terry D. Rees

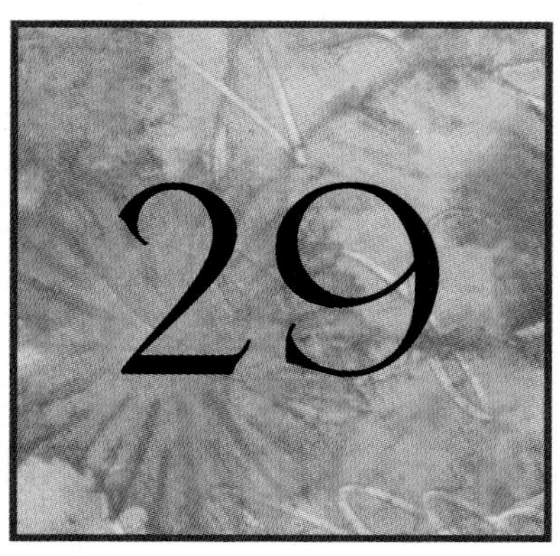

CHAPTER

Chapter Outline

Acquired immunodeficiency syndrome (AIDS) is characterized by profound impairment of the immune system. The condition was first reported in 1981, and a viral pathogen, the human immunodeficiency virus (HIV), was identified in 1984.[111]

HIV has a strong affinity for cells of the immune system, most specifically those that carry the CD4 cell surface receptor molecule. Thus helper T lymphocytes are most profoundly affected, but monocytes, macrophages, Langerhans cells, and some neuronal and glial brain cells may also be involved.[27] Viral replication occurs continuously in the lymphoreticular tissues of lymph nodes, spleen, gut-associated lymphoid cells, and macrophages.[141] In recent years, combined therapeutic regimens consisting of antiretroviral agents and protease-inhibiting drugs have resulted in marked improvement in the health status of HIV-infected individuals and occasionally a reduction in viral plasma bioloads below detectable levels, although the infection is still transmissible.[31,50,55,146] Current evidence indicates that the virus is never completely eradicated; rather, it is sequestered at low levels in resting CD4 cells even in individuals with no detectable plasma virus.[15,30] These findings suggest that effective combination drug therapy may be necessary for the lifetime of infected individuals. Long-term control of the infection may be difficult because the antiviral agents currently used have many adverse side effects and readily develop drug-resistant varient strains.[141] In untreated or inadequately treated HIV infection, the overall effect is to gradually impair the immune system by interference with helper T lymphocytes and other immune cell functions.[142]

B lymphocytes are not infected, but the altered function of infected T lymphocytes secondarily results in B-cell dysregulation and altered neutrophil function.[76] This may place the HIV-positive individual at increased risk for malignancy and disseminated infections with microorganisms such as viruses, mycobacterioses, and mycoses.[49,100,106,117] HIV-positive individuals are also at increased risk for adverse drug reactions owing to altered antigenic regulation.

HIV has been detected in most body fluids, although it is found in high quantities only in blood, semen, and cerebrospinal fluid. Transmission occurs almost exclusively by sexual contact, illicit use of injectable drugs, or exposure to blood or blood products. Transmission following a human bite has been reported, although the risk is extremely low.[139]

BOX 29-1

1993 CDC AIDS Surveillance Case Definition Conditions

- Candidiasis of bronchi, trachea, or lungs
- Candidiasis, esophageal
- Cervical cancer, invasive
- Coccidioidomycosis, disseminated or extrapulmonary
- Cryptococcosis, extrapulmonary
- Cryptosporidiosis, chronic intestinal (>1 month's duration)
- Cytomegalovirus disease (other than liver, spleen, or nodes)
- Cytomegalovirus retinitis (with loss of vision)
- Encephalopathy, HIV-related
- Herpes simplex: chronic ulcer(s) (>1 month's duration) or bronchitis, pneumonitis, or esophagitis
- Histoplasmosis, disseminated or extrapulmonary
- Isosporiasis, chronic intestinal (1 month's duration)
- Kaposi's sarcoma
- Lymphoma, Burkitt's (or equivalent term)
- Lymphoma, immunoblastic (or equivalent term)
- Lymphoma, primary, of brain
- *Mycobacterium avium* complex or *Mycobacterium kansasii,* disseminated or extrapulmonary
- *Mycobacterium tuberculosis,* any site (pulmonary or extrapulmonary)
- *Mycobacterium,* other species or unidentified species, disseminated or extrapulmonary
- *Pneumocystis carinii* pneumonia
- Pneumonia, recurrent
- Progressive multifocal leukoencephalopathy
- *Salmonella* septicemia, recurrent
- Toxoplasmosis of brain
- Wasting syndrome owing to HIV

From Centers for Disease Control: 1993 Revised classification system for HIV infection and expanded surveillance case definition for AIDS among adolescents and adults. MMWR 1993; 41:RR-17.

The high-risk population includes homosexual and bisexual men; users of illegal, injectable drugs; hemophiliacs or others with coagulation disorders; recipients of blood transfusions before April 1985; infants of HIV-infected mothers (in whom transmission occurs by fetal transmission, at delivery, or by breast feeding); promiscuous heterosexuals; and individuals who engage in unprotected sex with HIV-positive cohorts. Heterosexual transmission is a common cause of AIDS in the world population and is increasing significantly in the United States.[12,97] Transmission is more likely to occur through contact with HIV-infected individuals with a high plasma bioload of the virus.[97,112] HIV transmission has also been reported to occur through organ transplantation and artificial insemination.[14]

EPIDEMIOLOGY AND DEMOGRAPHICS

As of December 31,1998, 688,200 AIDS cases had been reported in the U.S.[12] The increase in numbers of patients with AIDS in the U.S. and other developed countries is due in part to prolonged survival since the advent of multidrug anti-HIV therapy.[7,31,54,98,138] The World Health Organization (WHO) estimates that as many as 21 million individuals worldwide are infected with one of the 10 known subtypes of HIV.[127] This number may increase to more than 40 million people early in the 21st century.[101,127]

AIDS affects individuals of all ages, but more than 98% of cases occur among adults and adolescents over the age of 12. The majority of adult victims in the U.S. are men, 54% of whom are homosexuals or bisexuals. Approximately 6% of this group also use illicit injectable drugs. An additional 26% contract the infection exclusively through injectable drug use, and 10% of all patients with AIDS have contracted the infection through heterosexual contact.[12] The majority of women who contract AIDS are those who have sex with intravenous drug users or bisexual males.[12,96] Others were born in countries such as Haiti or one of several high-incidence African nations where heterosexual contact is the major mode of transmission. Only 1% of individuals contracted AIDS from blood products or blood transfusions in the U.S. because of stringent blood bank controls. A disproportionately high number of African-American and Hispanic male homosexuals, male and female heterosexuals, and children suffer from HIV infection. The major risk factor for this disparity appears to be a more frequent history of use of injectable drugs and needle sharing and unprotected sexual activity in these groups.[12,18,76,78,86,88]

Transmission from health care workers to patients has been documented on rare occasions (6 from 1 dentist, 1 from an orthopedic surgeon).[73] Conversely, 94 health care workers have had documented seroconversion following occupational injury, especially from patients with high plasma viral loads. The majority of these incidences involved nurses, and no documented seroconversion has been reported among dental health care workers.[11,60]

CLASSIFICATION AND STAGING

In 1982 the Centers for Disease Control (CDC) developed a surveillance case definition for AIDS based on the presence of opportunistic illnesses or malignancies secondary to defective cell-mediated immunity in HIV-positive individuals.[9] This definition was further expanded in 1985, 1987, and 1993.[10] The 1993 revision added invasive cervical cancer in women, bacillary tuberculosis, and recurrent pneumonia into the AIDS designation. Currently, any of 25 specific clinical conditions found in HIV-positive individuals can establish the diagnosis of AIDS (Box 29-1). The most significant change in the most recent CDC case definition was the inclusion of severe immunodeficiency (CD4-T4 lymphocyte count of less than 200/mm^3 or a T4 lymphocyte percentage of less than 14% of total lymphocytes) as definitive for AIDS. This change was based on recognition that severe immunodeficiency results in increased risk for opportunistic life-threatening conditions. Many HIV-positive individuals have been designated as patients with AIDS due solely to low CD4-T4 cell counts or percentages even in the absence of life-threatening conditions. New combined drug therapy for HIV, however, has resulted in a rise of CD4 levels, often reaching or exceeding 200/mm³.[51,70] Such individuals are still considered to have AIDS although their CD4 cells may even reach normal levels. These individuals may continue to be susceptible to opportunistic infections although the risk of secondary disease generally is diminished in those who are responsive to AIDS therapy.[23]

A few weeks to a few months after initial exposure, some HIV-infected individuals may experience acute symptoms (e.g., sudden onset of an acute mononucleosis-like illness characterized by malaise, fatigue, fever, myalgia, erythematous cutaneous eruption, oral candidiasis, oral ulcerations, and thrombocytopenia).[32,71,135] This acute phase may last for up to 2 weeks, with seroconversion occurring 3 to 8 weeks later.[72,136] However, antigenic viremia may sometimes be present for an extended period of time before seroconversion occurs.[58,72,86] Some individuals experience asymptomatic HIV infection, whereas others may become asymptomatic after the initial acute infection. In any event, infected individuals eventually become seropositive for HIV antibody, but the mean time from infection until development of AIDS is estimated to be up to 12 or more years.[138]

CDC Surveillance Case Classification

AIDS patients have been grouped as follows, according to the CDC Surveillance Case Classification (1993)[10]:

Category A includes patients with acute symptoms or asymptomatic diseases, along with individuals with persistent generalized lymphadenopathy, with or without malaise, fatigue, or low-grade fever.

Category B patients have symptomatic conditions such as oropharyngeal or vulvovaginal candidiasis; herpes zoster; oral hairy leukoplakia; idiopathic thrombocytopenia; or constitutional symptoms of fever, diarrhea, and weight loss.

Category C patients are those with outright AIDS as manifested by life-threatening conditions identified by $CD4^+$ T lymphocyte levels of less than 200 per cubic millimeter.

These staging categories reflect progressive immunologic dysfunction, but patients do not necessarily progress serially through the three stages, and the predictive value of these categories is not known.

ORAL AND PERIODONTAL MANIFESTATIONS OF HIV INFECTION

Oral lesions are very common in HIV-infected patients, although geographic and environmental variables may exist.* Previous reports indicate that most AIDS patients have head and neck lesions,[112] while oral lesions are quite common in HIV positive individuals who do not yet have AIDS.[35,74,83] Several reports have identified a strong correlation between HIV infection and oral candidiasis, oral hairy leukoplakia, atypical periodontal diseases, oral Kaposi's sarcoma, and oral non-Hodgkin's lymphoma.[22,47,77,94,120,133]

*See references 24, 29, 34, 35, 53, 68, 77, 92, 94, 103, and 134.

Oral lesions less strongly associated with HIV infection include melanotic hyperpigmentation, mycobacterial infections, necrotizing ulcerative stomatitis, miscellaneous oral ulcerations, and viral infections (e.g., herpes simplex virus, herpes zoster, condyloma acuminatum). Lesions seen in HIV-infected individuals but of undetermined frequency include less-common viral infections (e.g., cytomegalovirus, molluscum contagiosum); recurrent aphthous stomatitis; and bacillary angiomatosis (epithelioid angiomatosis).[22]

Oral Hairy Leukoplakia

Oral hairy leukoplakia (OHL) primarily occurs in persons with HIV infection.[43,45] Found on the lateral borders of the tongue, it frequently has a bilateral distribution and may extend to the ventrum. This lesion is characterized by an asymptomatic, poorly demarcated keratotic area ranging in size from a few millimeters to several centimeters (Fig. 29-1). Often, characteristic vertical striations, imparting a corrugated appearance, are present, or the surface may be shaggy and may appear "hairy" when dried (Color Fig. 29-1, *A*). The lesion does not rub off and may resemble other keratotic oral lesions.

Microscopically, the lesion shows a hyperparakeratotic surface with projections that often resemble hairs. Beneath the parakeratotic surface are acanthosis and some characteristic balloon cells resembling koilocytes (Fig. 29-2). It has been demonstrated that these cells contain virus particles of the human herpesvirus group; these particles have been interpreted as the Epstein-Barr virus (EBV).[43,46] Epithelial dysplasia is not a feature, and in most lesions, little or no inflammatory infiltrate in the underlying connective tissue is present.[118]

OHL is found almost exclusively on the lateral borders of the tongue, although it has been reported on the dorsum of the tongue, buccal mucosa, floor of the mouth, retromolar area, and soft palate.[26,43,64] In addition, most of these lesions reveal surface colonization by *Candida* organisms, which are secondary invaders and not the cause of the lesion.

OHL was originally believed to be caused by the human papilloma virus, but subsequent evidence suggests that this condition is associated with EBV.[43,46] In the late 1980s a so-called pseudo-hairy leukoplakia was described in HIV- and EBV-negative individuals who manifested

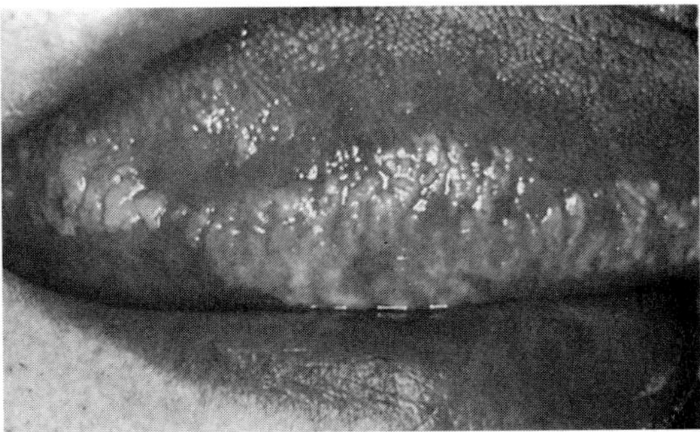

Fig. 29-1 Hyperkeratotic areas in the lateral border of the tongue in a patient with AIDS.

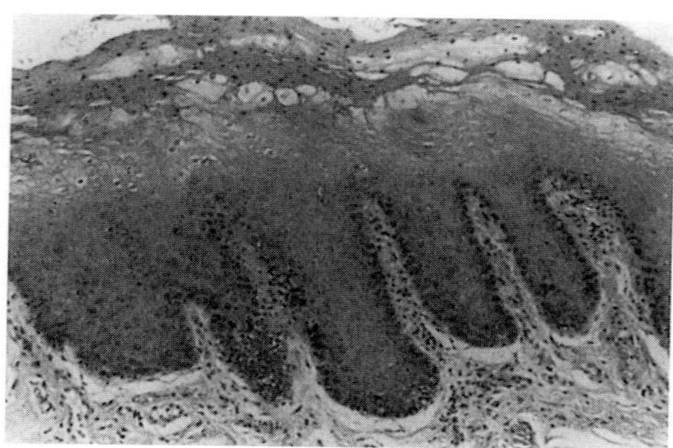

Fig. 29-2 Microscopic view of hairy leukoplakia.

with lesions clinically identical to OHL. In addition, several case reports have described OHL in EBV-infected but HIV-negative individuals suffering from a variety of immunosuppressed conditions (e.g., acute myelogenous leukemia) or who are immunosuppressed as a result of organ transplantation or extensive systemic corticosteroid therapy.[44,129] Regardless, biopsy identification of a lesion suggestive of OHL should dictate that HIV testing be performed.

The differential diagnosis of OHL must consider white lesions of the mucosa, which include dysplasia, carcinoma, frictional and idiopathic keratosis, lichen planus, tobacco-related leukoplakia, psoriasiform lesions (e.g., geographic tongue), and hyperplastic candidiasis. The microscopic confirmation of OHL of the tongue in a high-risk patient is considered to be a specific early sign of HIV infection and a strong indicator that the patient will develop AIDS.[45] However, earlier diagnosis and treatment of HIV infection appears to have resulted in a marked reduction in occurrence of OHL, although incidence studies have not been performed. Prior to the advent of effective therapy for HIV, survival analysis indicated that 83% of HIV-infected patients with hairy leukoplakia would develop AIDS within 31 months,[44] and the number of patients with hairy leukoplakia who eventually developed AIDS approached 100%.[47]

It should be emphasized that the severity of the lesion is not correlated with the likelihood of developing AIDS. Thus small lesions are as diagnostically significant as extensive lesions.[118]

Oral Candidiasis

Candida, a fungus found in normal oral flora, proliferates on the surface of the oral mucosa under certain conditions. A major factor associated with overgrowth of *Candida* is diminished host resistance, as seen in debilitated patients or in patients receiving immunosuppressive therapy. The incidence of candidal infection has been demonstrated to progressively increase in relationship to diminishing immune competency.[1,28,59,80,81] Most oral candidal infections (85% to 95%) are associated with *Candida albicans,* but other species of *Candida* may be involved.[53] Currently, at least 11 strains of *Candida* have been identified, and non-*C. albicans* infections are more common among immunocompromised individuals already receiving antifungal therapy for *C. albicans.*[4,119]

Candidiasis is the most common oral lesion in HIV diseases and has been found in approximately 90% of AIDS patients.[102] It usually has one of four clinical presentations: pseudomembranous, erythematous, or hyperplastic candidiasis or angular cheilitis.[94]

Pseudomembranous candidiasis (thrush) presents as painless or slightly sensitive white lesions that can be readily scraped and separated from the surface of the oral mucosa. This type is most common on the hard and soft palate and the buccal or labial mucosa.

Erythematous candidiasis may be present as a component of the pseudomembranous type, appearing as red patches on the buccal or palatal mucosa, or it may be associated with depapillation of the tongue (Fig. 29-3).

Hyperplastic candidiasis is the least common form and may be seen in the buccal mucosa and tongue. It is more resistant to removal than the other types (Fig. 29-4).

In **angular cheilitis,** the commissures appear erythematous with surface crusting and fissuring.

Diagnosis of candidiasis is made by microscopic examination of a tissue sample or smear of material scraped from the lesion, which shows hyphae and yeast forms of the organisms. When oral candidiasis appears in patients with no apparent predisposing causes, the clinician should be alerted to the possibility of HIV infection.[1] Many patients at risk for HIV infection who present with oral candidiasis also have esophageal candidiasis, a diagnostic sign of AIDS.[131]

Although candidiasis in HIV-infected patients may respond to antifungal therapy, it is often refractory or recurrent. Traditionally, 30% of AIDS related candidiasis relapse within 4 weeks of treatment and 60% to 80% within 3 months. This relapse may result from decreasing immunocompetency or development of antifungal resistant candidial strains. As many as 10% of candidial organisms become resistant to long-term fluconazole therapy, and cross-resistance to other antifungal agents may develop to include itraconazole, amphotericin B oral suspension, and intravenous amphotericin B.[65,95,99] Resistant candidiasis is more common in individuals who have low CD4 counts at baseline.[56]

Recent reports indicate that the administration of effective combined antiretroviral and protease-inhibiting drugs in HIV infections has resulted in a significant decrease in incidence of oropharyngeal candidiasis and oral candidal carriage and has reduced the rate of fluconazole resistance.[19,79]

Kaposi's Sarcoma

Kaposi's sarcoma (KS) is a rare, multifocal, vascular neoplasm; it was originally described in 1872 as occurring in the skin of the lower extremities of older men of Mediterranean origin. Its cause is unknown, although sexually transmitted viral infection has been suspected. Recently, a new strain of herpes virus has been identified

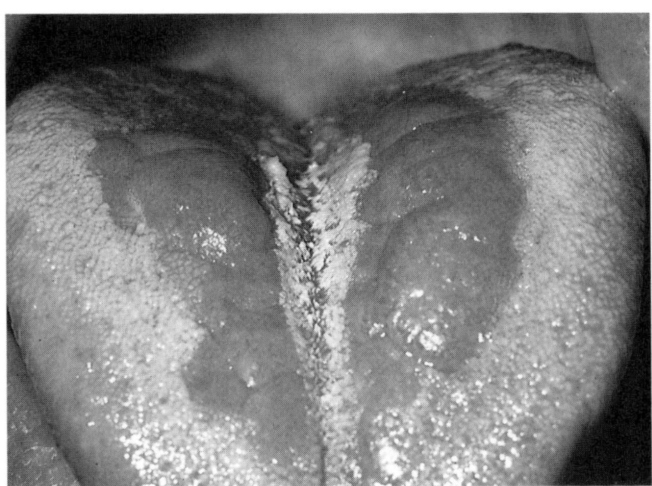

Fig. 29-3 Depapillation of the tongue. A smear obtained from the tongue was positive for *Candida* sp.

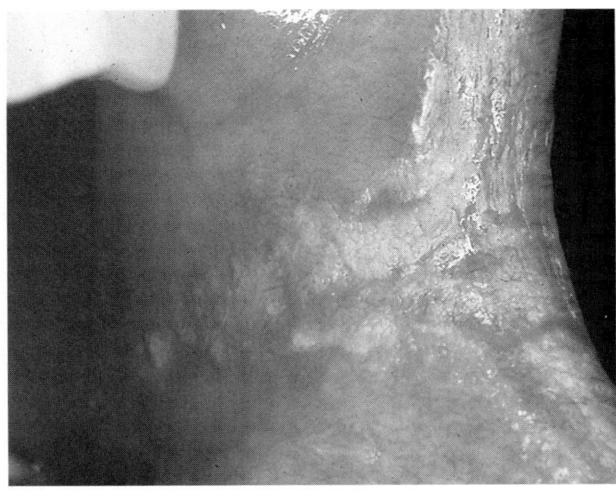

Fig. 29-4 Large area of mucosal necrosis extending from the lingual gingival tissue onto the floor of the mouth in a 28-year-old patient with AIDS.

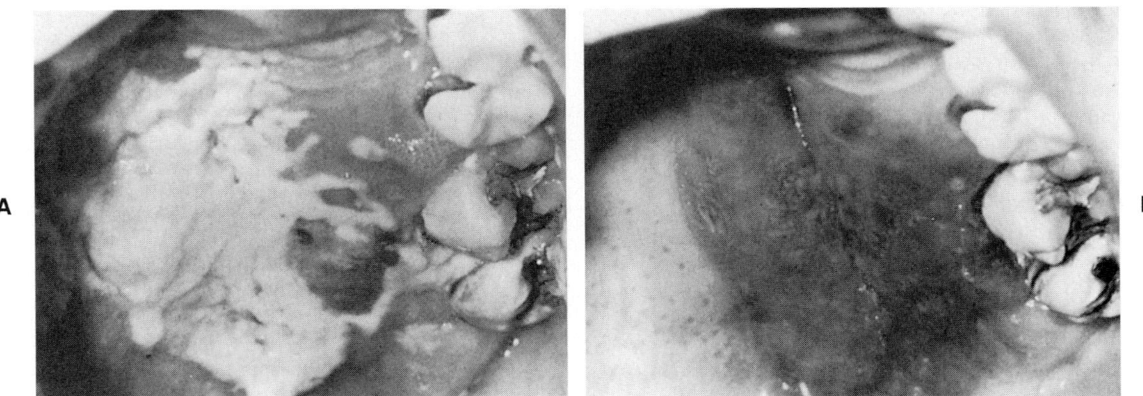

Fig. 29-5 **A,** Kaposi's sarcoma of the palate and gingiva covered with *Candida* sp. **B,** After antifungal therapy, the candidiasis has disappeared and the underlying sarcoma is more apparent. (Courtesy Dr. Frank Lucatorto, Los Angeles, Calif.)

as closely associated with KS. This virus was originally named the *KS-herpes virus* but has now been designated *as human herpes virus-8 (HHV-8)*. HHV-8 has been associated both with AIDS-related and non–AIDS-related KS.[114] However, HIV-infected individuals are 7000-fold more likely to develop KS.[63] Despite this strong association, an etiologic association between HHV-8 and KS has not been established.[62,63] The virus has been isolated from 29% of American adults and 8% of children in the non-AIDS general population. It has also been isolated from lesions of non-Hodgkin's lymphoma, Castleman's disease, other lymphoproliferative disorders, and a variety of additional abnormalities, although these findings may coincide with those of the healthy general population.[39,62,125] In contrast, one study identified HHV-8 in 53 of 54 AIDS-related KS lesions.[114] Thus it appears that decreasing immunocompetence results in activation of latent HHV-8. Although the virus may be sexually transmitted, it may also be transmitted from infected mothers to children.[126]

Although KS is a malignant tumor, in its classic form it is a localized and slowly growing lesion. The KS that occurs in HIV-infected patients presents different clinical features (Figs. 29-5 to 29-7; see Color Fig. 29-1, *E*). In these individuals, it is a much more aggressive lesion and the majority (71%) develop lesions of the oral mucosa, particularly the palate and gingiva (see Color Fig. 29-1, *H*).[63] The oral cavity may often be the first or only site of the lesion.[5]

In the early stages, the oral lesions are painless, reddish-purple macules of the mucosa. As the lesions progress, they frequently become nodular and can easily be con-

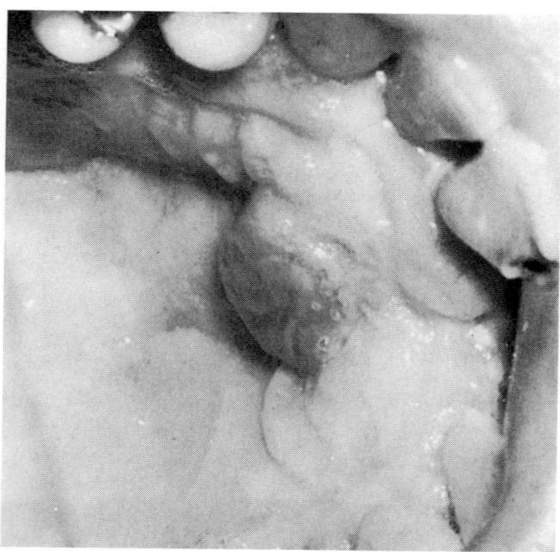

Fig. 29-6 Kaposi's sarcoma of the palate extending to the gingiva. (Courtesy Dr. Frank Lucatorto, Los Angeles, Calif.)

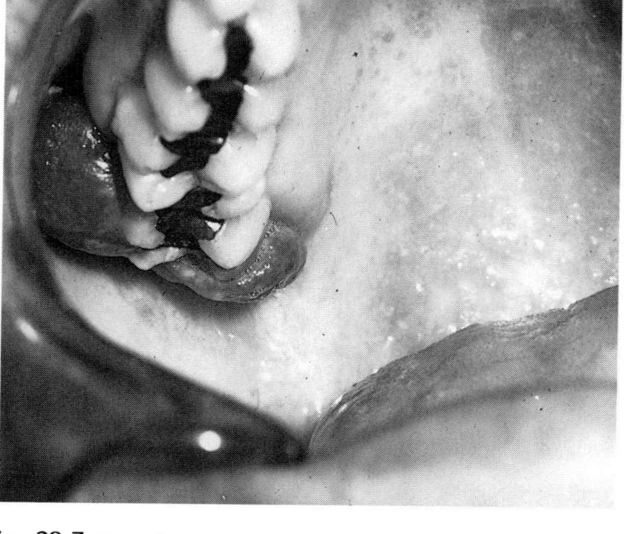

Fig. 29-7 Kaposi's sarcoma of the gingiva in a 26-year-old man.

fused with other oral vascular entities such as hemangioma, hematoma, varicosity, or pyogenic granuloma (when occurring in the gingiva).[121]

Lesions manifest as nodules, papules, or nonelevated macules that are usually brown, blue, or purple in color. On occasion, however, lesions may display normal pigmentation. Diagnosis is based on histologic findings.[67,109]

Microscopically, KS consists of four components: endothelial cell proliferation with the formation of atypical vascular channels; extravascular hemorrhage with hemosiderin deposition; spindle cell proliferation in association with atypical vessels; and a mononuclear inflammatory infiltrate consisting mainly of plasma cells[42] (Fig. 29-8).

Regional and gender differences are apparent; oral KS is more common in the U.S. than in Europe and the male-to-female ratio is 20:1.[108,132] The condition has also been reported in patients with lupus erythematosus who are receiving immunosuppressant therapy and in renal transplant patients and other individuals receiving corticosteroid or cyclosporin therapy. Case reports describe gingival KS in HIV-negative patients experiencing cyclosporin-induced gingival enlargement.[105,131] In an HIV-positive individual, the presence of KS signifies transition to outright AIDS. Before the advent of combined drug therapy for AIDS, the median survival time after onset of KS ranged from 7 to 31 months.[15,16]

The differential diagnosis of oral KS includes pyogenic granuloma, hemangioma, atypical hyperpigmentation, sarcoidosis, bacillary angiomatosis, angiosarcoma, pigmented nevi, and cat-scratch disease (skin).[109]

Bacillary (Epithelioid) Angiomatosis

Bacillary (epithelioid) angiomatosis (BA) is an infectious vascular proliferative disease with clinical and histologic features very similar to those of KS. BA is believed to be caused by rickettsia-like organisms, *Bartonellaciae henselia, quintana,* or others.[22,29,85,93,104,143] Skin lesions are similar to those seen in KS or cat-scratch disease. Gingival BA manifests as red, purple, or blue edematous soft tissue lesions that may cause destruction of periodontal ligament and bone (Fig. 29-9).[33] The condition is more prevalent in HIV-positive individuals with low CD4 levels.[85]

Differentiation of BA from KS is based on biopsy, which reveals an "epithelioid" proliferation of angiogenic cells accompanied by an acute inflammatory cell infiltrate. The causative organism in the biopsy specimen sometimes reacts with Warthen-Starry silver stain.

Oral Hyperpigmentation

An increased incidence of oral hyperpigmentation has been described in HIV-infected individuals.[69] Oral pigmented areas often appear as spots or striations on the buccal mucosa, palate, gingiva, or tongue (Figs. 29-10 and 29-11). In some instances, the pigmentation may relate to prolonged use of drugs such as zidovudine, ketoconazole, or clofazimine.[147] Zidovudine is also associated with excessive pigmentation of the skin and nails. On occasion, oral pigmentation may be the result of adrenocorticoid insufficiency induced in an HIV-positive individual by prolonged use of ketoconazole or by *Pneumocystis carinii* infection or cytomegalovirus or other viral infections (see Fig. 29-11).

Atypical Ulcers and Delayed Healing

Nonspecific oral ulcerations in HIV-infected individuals may have multiple etiologies to include neoplasms such as lymphoma, KS, and squamous cell carcinoma. Recent case reports suggest that HIV-associated neutropenia may also feature oral ulcerations. Neutropenia has been successfully treated using recombinant human granulocyte

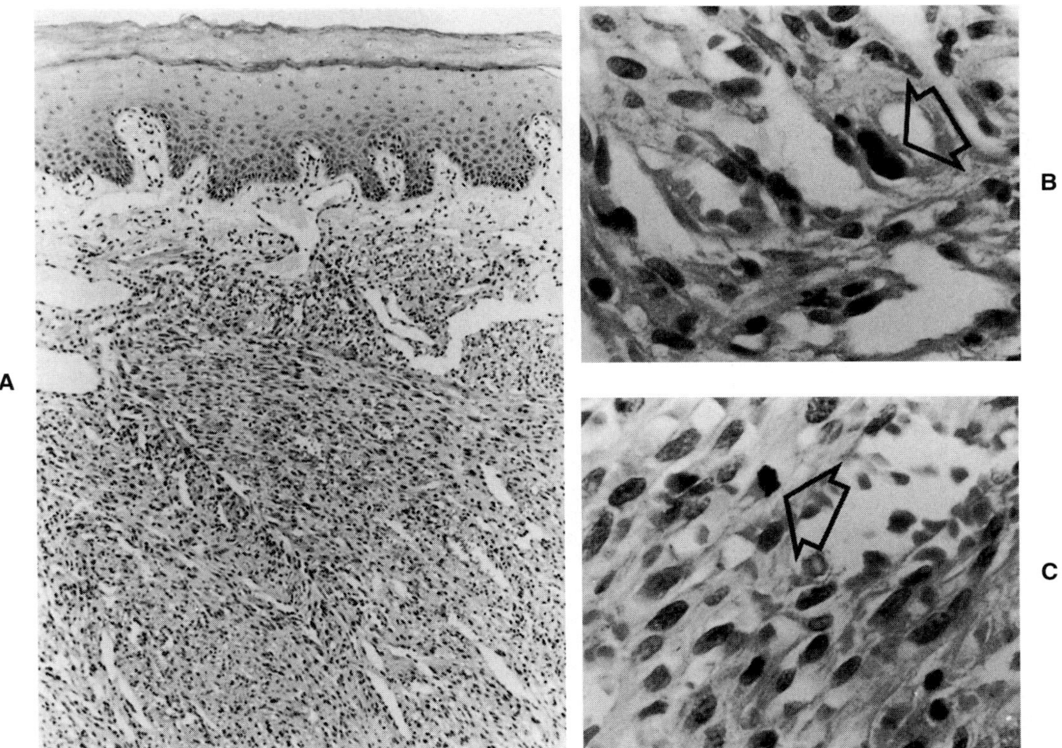

Fig. 29-8 Kaposi's sarcoma of the palate in a patient with AIDS. **A,** Low-power view of hyperkeratotic epithelium overlying large vascular spaces and a dense tumoral mass. **B,** High-power view showing small blood vessels with occasional large hyperchromatic cells (*arrow*). **C,** High-power view showing dense endothelial cells with occasional mitotic figures (*arrow*). (Courtesy Dr. Gerald Shklar, Boston, Mass.)

colony-stimulating factor with resultant resolution of oral ulcers.[76] Severe, prolonged oral ulcers have been successfully managed using prednisone or thalidomide, a drug that inhibits tissue necrosis factor alpha (TNF-α). Recurrence is likely, however, if either drug is discontinued.[20,36,40,61,144]

HIV-infected patients have a higher incidence of recurrent herpetic lesions and aphthous stomatitis (Figs. 29-12 and 29-13). Approximately 10% of HIV-infected patients have herpes infection,[102,124] and multiple episodes are common. Aphthae and aphthae-like lesions are common when patients are followed throughout the course of their immunosuppression.[37]

In healthy patients, herpetic and aphthous lesions are self-limiting and relatively easy to diagnose by their characteristic clinical features (i.e., herpes on the keratinizing mucosa, aphthae on the nonkeratinizing surfaces). In HIV-infected patients, the clinical presentation and course of these lesions may be altered. Herpes may involve all mucosal surfaces and extend to the skin and may persist for months.[25] Currently the CDC includes mucocutaneous herpes present for more than 1 month as a sign of AIDS.[10]

Atypical large, persistent, nonspecific, painful ulcers are common in immunocompromised individuals. If healing is delayed, these lesions are secondarily infected and may become indistinguishable from persistent herpetic or aphthous lesions.[110] A wide variety of bacterial and viral infections may produce severe oral ulcerations in HIV-infected individuals. Essentially, immunocompromised individuals are at risk from infectious agents

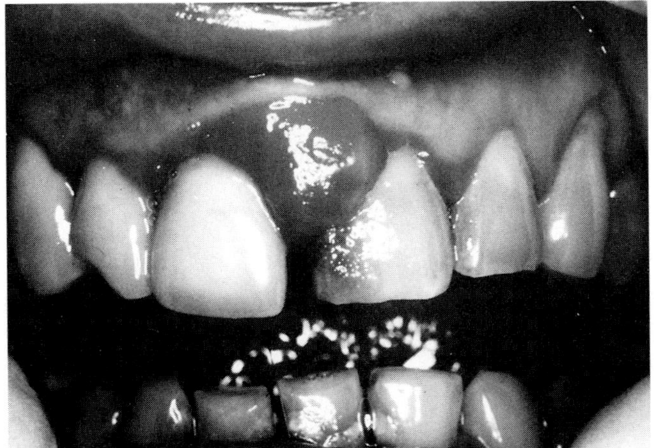

Fig. 29-9 Bacillary angiomatosis in a 30-year-old, HIV-positive man.

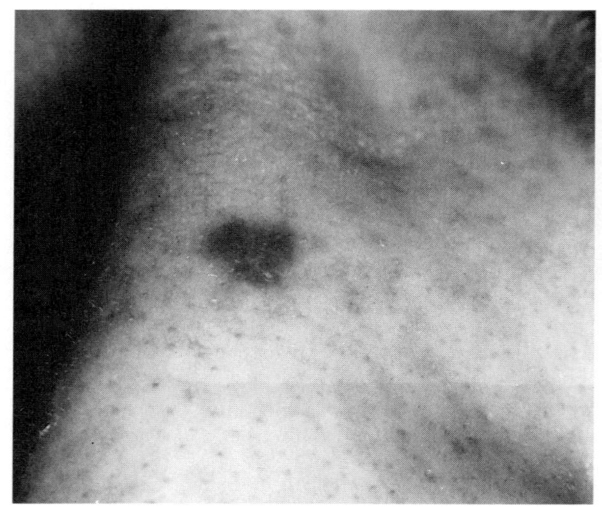

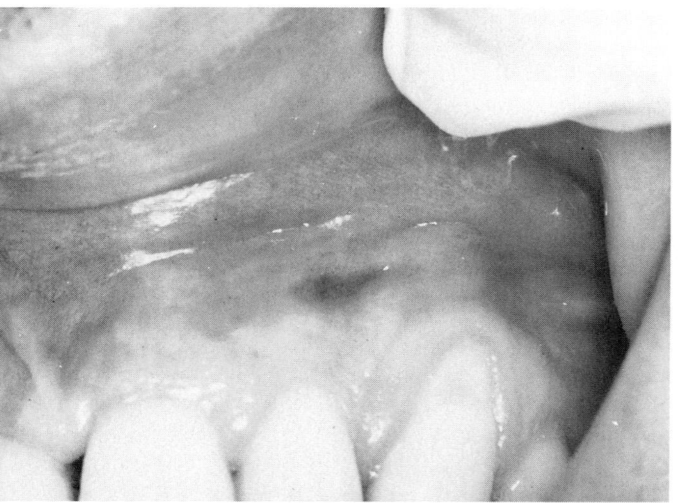

Fig. 29-10 Oral hyperpigmentation in a 32-year-old AIDS patient with Kaposi's sarcoma of the skin. **A,** Kaposi's sarcoma of the bridge of the nose. **B,** Pigmented lesion of the alveolar mucosa. A biopsy specimen was negative for Kaposi's sarcoma.

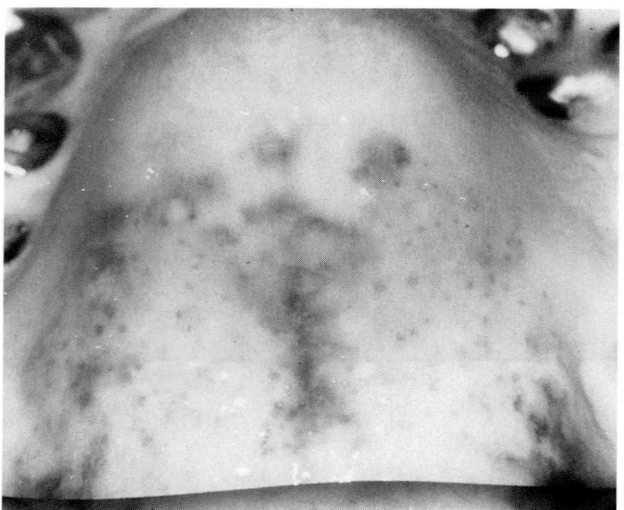

Fig. 29-11 Palatal hyperpigmentation in a patient with drug-induced adrenocortical insufficiency.

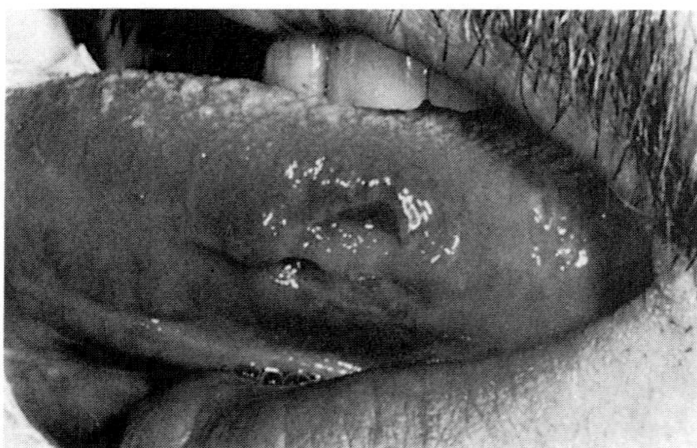

Fig. 29-12 Ulcerous lesion in the tongue of a patient with AIDS.

endemic to the patient's geographic location. Atypical or nonhealing ulcers may require biopsy, microbial cultures, or both to determine the etiology. Oral ulcerations have been described in association with enterobacterial organisms such as *Klebsiella pneumoniae, Enterobacter cloacae,* and *Escherichia coli.*[110] Such infections are rare and are usually associated with systemic involvement. Specific antibiotic therapy is indicated, and close coordination of oral therapy with the patient's physician is usually necessary.

Herpes simplex virus (HSV), varicella-zoster virus (VZV), Epstein-Barr virus (EBV), or cytomegalovirus (CMV) are frequently retrieved from nonspecific oral ulcers, indicating a possible etiologic role.[130] Recently, atypical ulcers were found to be co-infected with HSV and CMV or with EBV and CMV.[108,129] These ulcers may be more common in individuals who are neutropenic in conjunction with their HIV infection. Neutropenia may also be induced by drugs such as zidovodine, trimethoprim-sulfamethoxazole, or gancyclovir.[76] Atypical ulcers may be more severe and persistent in individuals with low CD4 cell counts, and the presence of oral CMV-induced ulcers may be indicative of systemic CMV infection.[37]

Recurrent aphthous stomatitis (RAS) has been described in HIV-infected individuals, but the overall incidence may be no greater than that in the general population.[22] RAS may occur, however, as a component of the initial acute illness of HIV seroconversion.[82] The incidence of major aphthae may be increased, and the oropharynx, esophagus, or other areas of the gastrointestinal tract may be involved.[2,3]

Adverse Drug Effects

A number of adverse drug-induced effects have been reported in HIV-positive patients and the dentist may be the first to recognize an oral drug reaction. Foscarnet, interferon, and 2′–3′-dideoxycytidine (DDC) occasionally

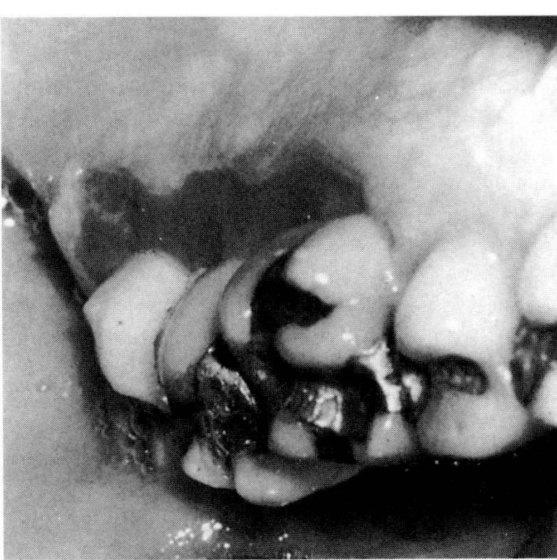

Fig. 29-13 Nonhealing ulcer in the palatal gingiva of 6 weeks' duration. Biopsy revealed Kaposi's sarcoma. (Courtesy Dr. Frank Lucatorto, Los Angeles, Calif.)

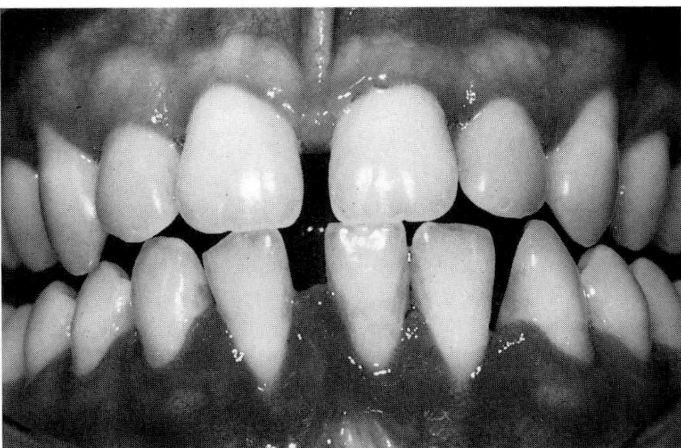

Fig. 29-14 Marginal gingival erythema of the maxillary gingiva and diffuse erythema of the mandibular attached gingiva in a 28-year-old man. Early necrosis of some of the interdental papillae is seen.

induce oral ulcerations, and erythema multiforme has been reported with use of didanosine (DDI).[17] Zidovudine and ganciclovir may induce leukopenia, resulting in oral ulcers.[84] Xerostomia and altered taste sensation have been described in conjunction with diethyldithiocarbamate (Dithiocarb). HIV-positive patients are believed to be generally more susceptible to drug-induced mucositis and lichenoid drug reactions than the general population.[6,17,52,122] In some instances, mouth ulcers and mucositis resolve if drug therapy is continued beyond 2 to 3 weeks, but when drug effects are severe or persistent, alternative therapy with different drugs should be used.

The advent of protease-inhibiting drugs used in double or triple drug therapy has been associated with a variety of generalized adverse reactions. These may include nausea, development of kidney stones, lypodystrophy (possibly including hyperlipidemia), an increase in abdominal fat mass, enlarged breast size, and development of the classic "buffalo hump" usually associated with administration of systemic corticosteroids.[8,127] Impaired glucose tolerance or diabetes mellitus may occur, apparently resulting from increased insulin resistance.[8,140] Combined drug therapy may also induce more severe liver cirrhosis in individuals with hepatitis C/HIV co-infections.[148] The dentist should remain alert for general signs and symptoms of adverse drug effects, some of which can affect oral tissues (e.g., nausea and vomiting, diabetes mellitus).

PERIODONTAL DISEASE

Considerable interest has been directed toward the nature and incidence of dental and periodontal diseases in HIV-infected individuals. Available evidence indicates that those diseases are more common among HIV-infected intravenous (IV) drug users. This appears to relate to poor oral hygiene and lack of dental care rather than decreased CD4 cell counts.[48,68,107]

Linear Gingival Erythema

A persistent, linear, easily bleeding, erythematous gingivitis (LGE) has been described in some HIV-positive patients. This may or may not serve as a precursor to rapidly progressive necrotizing ulcerative periodontitis (NUP)[35,41,83] (see Color Fig. 29-1, *B* and *C,* and Fig. 29-14). The microflora of LGE may closely mimic that of periodontitis rather than gingivitis.[41] Linear gingivitis lesions may be localized or generalized in nature. The erythematous gingivitis may (1) be limited to marginal tissue, (2) extend into attached gingiva in a punctate or a diffuse erythema, or (3) extend into the alveolar mucosa.

LGE is often unresponsive to corrective therapy, yet such lesions may undergo spontaneous remission.[89] Concomitant oral candidiasis and LGE lesions have been identified, suggesting a possible etiologic role for candidial species in LGE.[68] Recently, direct microscopic cultures from LGE lesions implicated *Candida dubliniensis* in four patients, all of whom experienced complete or partial remission after systemic antifungal therapy.[137] It is not yet known whether candidial infections are etiologic in all LGE cases.

Necrotizing Ulcerative Gingivitis

Some reports have described an increased incidence of necrotizing ulcerative gingivitis (NUG) (Fig. 29-15) among HIV-infected individuals, although this has not been substantiated by other studies.[21,38,57,116,128]

Necrotizing Ulcerative Stomatitis

A severely destructive, acutely painful necrotizing ulcerative stomatitis (NUS) has occasionally been reported in HIV-positive patients. NUS is characterized by necrosis of significant areas of oral soft tissue and underlying bone. It may occur separately or as an extension of NUP[21] and is commonly associated with severe depression of CD4

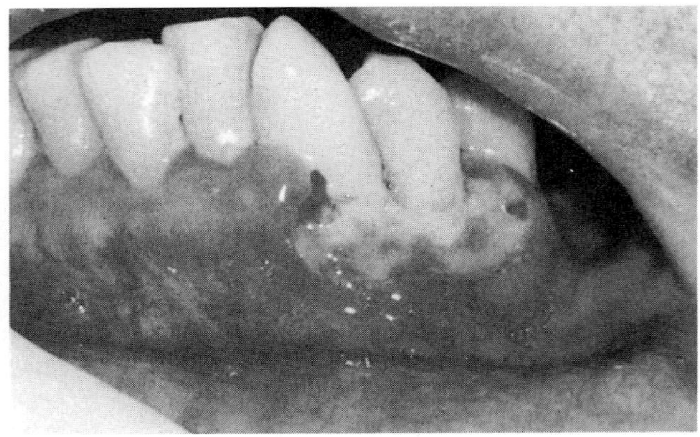

Fig. 29-15 Acute necrotizing ulcerative gingivitis (ANUG)-like lesion and ulcer involving the facial gingiva. (Courtesy Dr. Frank Lucatorto, Los Angeles, Calif.)

immune cells. The condition appears to be identical to cancrum oris (noma), a rare destructive process occasionally reported in nutritionally deprived individuals, especially those in Africa. NUS may be associated with severe immunodeficiency regardless of the cause of onset.[114]

Necrotizing Ulcerative Periodontitis

A necrotizing, ulcerative, rapidly progressive form of periodontitis occurs more frequently among HIV-positive individuals, although such lesions were described long before the onset of the AIDS epidemic. NUP may represent an extension of NUG in which bone loss and periodontal attachment loss occurs.

NUP is characterized by soft tissue necrosis, rapid periodontal destruction, and interproximal bone loss[35] (Figs. 29-16 and 29-17). Lesions may occur anywhere in the dental arches and are usually localized to a few teeth, although generalized NUP is sometimes present after marked $CD4^+$ cell depletion. Bone is often exposed, resulting in necrosis and subsequent sequestration. NUP is severely painful at onset, and immediate treatment is necessary. On occasion, however, patients undergo spontaneous resolution of the necrotizing lesions, leaving painless, deep interproximal craters that are difficult to clean and may lead to conventional periodontitis.[35]

Some evidence suggests slight differences between the microbial flora found in NUP lesions and that found in chronic periodontitis,[87] but the bulk of data implicate a similar microbial component in both diseases.[38,90,91,115] The periodontal health of HIV-infected individuals is subject to wide variations.[113,145] Riley and associates[113] examined 200 HIV-positive patients and found that 85 were periodontally healthy; none had NUG; 59 were suffering from gingivitis; 54 were experiencing mild, moderate, or advanced periodontitis; and only 2 had NUP. Using a different approach, Rowland and associates[116] studied 20 patients with NUG and found that 7 were HIV positive, 2 of whom had $CD4^+$ lymphocyte depression ($<400/mm^3$). They concluded that dentists should recognize NUG as a possible early marker for HIV infection. In contrast, Drinkard and associates[21] found no evidence of NUG in 106 HIV-positive individuals; 97 were asymptomatic, and 9 exhibited Category B symptoms.

Klein and associates[66] evaluated 181 heterosexuals with AIDS and found a larger percentage of women (91%) than men (73%) with gingivitis or periodontitis. Overall, most heterosexuals with AIDS had only gingivitis (70%) while others had moderate (27%) to severe periodontitis (27%). This study suggests that periodontal diseases are no more frequent in heterosexuals with AIDS than the general population. The finding of more frequent disease in women may reflect the fact that more women with AIDS have used illicit injectable drugs.

Swango and associates[128] reported early findings among 230 HIV-positive patients with relatively high $CD4^+$ counts. They found no correlation between linear gingival erythema and $CD4^+$ T-cell levels in these patients, although 6% experienced NUG-like papillary destruction. Others have reported a relationship between NUP and decreased $CD4^+$ lymphocytes.[75,133] Glick and associates[38] reported the incidence of periodontal diseases in 700 HIV-positive individuals. They found NUP in only 6.3% but concluded that NUP is a predictive marker for severe immune deficiency because patients with NUP were 20.8 times as likely to have $CD4^+$ lymphocyte counts $<200/mm^3$.

It can be concluded from these studies that periodontal diseases can occur among HIV-infected individuals in all categories, but susceptibility to periodontal infections increases as the immune system becomes more compromised. Lamster and associates compared frequency of oral lesions and periodontal diseases between HIV-positive and HIV-negative individuals, some of whom were injectable drug users (IDUs). They concluded that the lifestyle associated with IDU may play a larger role in oral disease than the individual's HIV status. They also found tongue lesions consistent with hairy leukoplakia to be most common among seropositive homosexual males, whereas oral candidiasis and LGE were most common among injectable drug users.[68] The majority of HIV-positive individuals experience periodontal disease in a manner similar to the general population. Under some circumstances, however, immunocompromised individuals experience less common types of severe gingival or periodontal destruction. With proper home care and appropriate periodontal treatment and maintenance, HIV-positive individuals can anticipate reasonably good periodontal health throughout the course of their disease. The median period between initial HIV infection and outright AIDS is approximately 12 years, and the life expectancy of persons living with AIDS has been significantly prolonged with current anti-HIV drug therapy.[12] This indicates that HIV-infected patients are potential candidates for conventional periodontal treatment procedures to include periodontal surgery and implant placement. Treatment decisions should be based on the overall health status of the patient, the degree of periodontal involvement, and the motivation and ability of the patient to perform effective oral hygiene procedures. (Chapter 51 describes in detail the periodontal management of AIDS patients.)

A

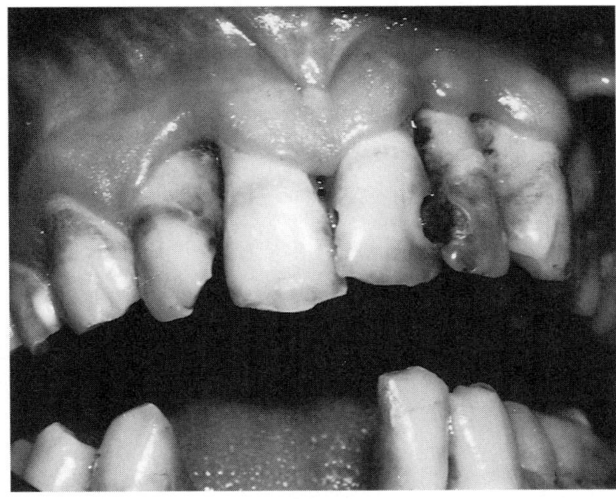

B

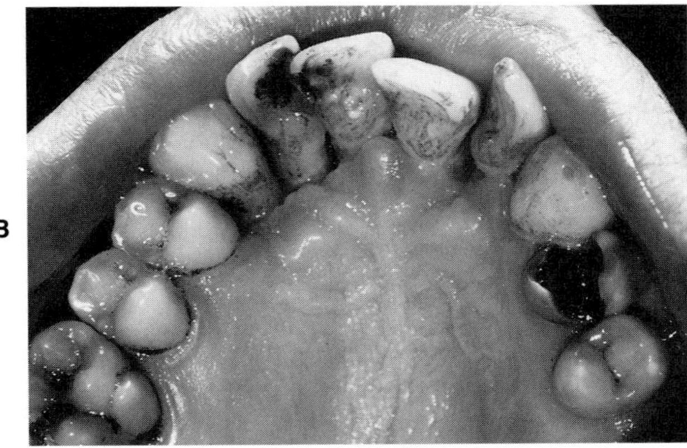

Fig. 29-16 Necrotizing ulcerative periodontitis in an HIV-negative patient. **A,** Facial view. **B,** Lingual view.

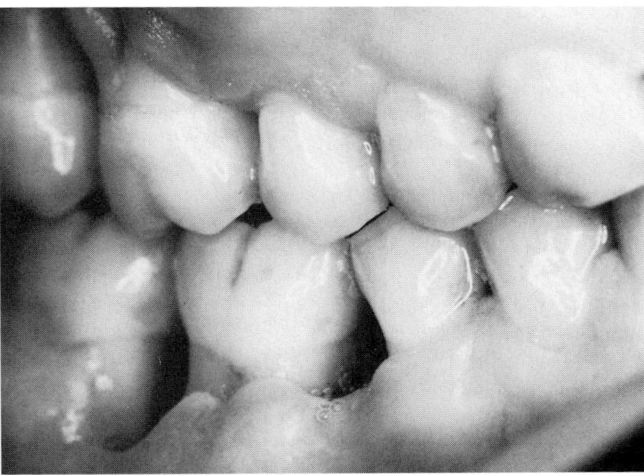

A

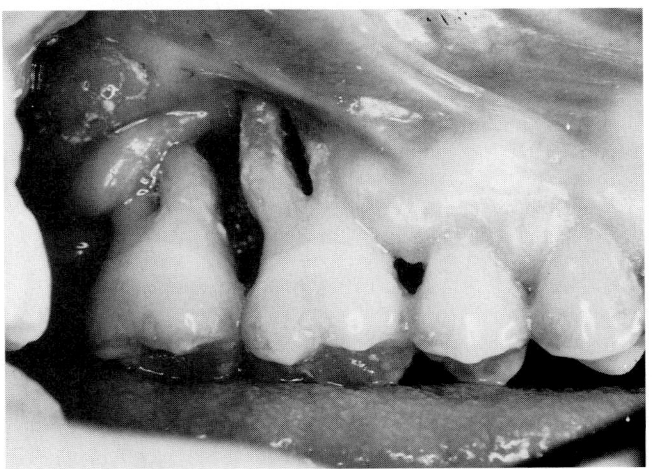

B

Fig. 29-17 Necrotizing ulcerative periodontitis in a 30-year-old, HIV-positive man. **A,** Mandibular/maxillary posterior facial view. **B,** Facial view of maxillary molars.

REFERENCES

1. Aly R, Berger T: Common superficial fungal infections in patients with AIDS. Clinical Infectious Diseases 1996; 22(Suppl 2):S128.
2. Bach MC, Howell DA, Valenti AJ, et al: Aphthous ulceration of the gastrointestinal tract in patients with the acquired immunodeficiency syndrome (AIDS). Ann Intern Med 1990; 112:465.
3. Bach MC, Valenti AJ, Howell DA, et al: Odynophagia from aphthous ulcers of the pharynx and oesophagus in the acquired immunodeficiency syndrome (AIDS). Ann Intern Med 1988; 108:338.
4. Baily GG, Moore CB, Essayag SM, et al: *Candida inconspicua,* a fluconazole-resistant pathogen in patients infected with human immunodeficiency virus. Clin Infect Dis 1997; 25:161.
5. Barrett AP, Bilous AM, Buckley DJ, et al: Clinicopathological presentations of oral Kaposi's sarcoma in AIDS. Aust Dent J 1988; 33(5):395.
6. Bayard PJ, Berger TG, Jacobson MA: Drug hypersensitivity reactions and human immunodeficiency virus disease. J Acq Immune Defic Syn 1992; 5(12):1237.
7. Buve A, Rogers MF: Epidemiology. AIDS 1998; 12(suppl A):S53.
8. Carr A, Samaras K, Thorisdottir A, et al: Diagnosis, prediction, and natural course of HIV-1 protease-inhibitor-associated lipodystrophy, hyperlipidaemia, and diabetes mellitus: a cohort study. Lancet 1999; 353:2093.
9. Centers for Disease Control: Update on AIDS—United States. MMWR 1982; 31:507.
10. Centers for Disease Control: 1993 Revised classification system for HIV infection and expanded surveillance case definition for AIDS among adolescents and adults. MMWR 1993; 41:RR-17.
11. Centers for Disease Control: Case-control study of HIV seroconversion in health-care workers after percutaneous exposure to HIV-infected blood—France, United Kingdom, and United States, January 1988–August 1994. MMWR 1995; 44:929.
12. Centers for Disease Control and Prevention: HIV surveillance report. US HIV and AIDS cases reported through December 1998. HIV Surveillance Report 1998; 10(2):1.
13. Chachoua A, Krigel R, Lafleur F, et al: Prognostic factors and staging classification of Kaposi's sarcoma. J Clin Oncol 1989; 7:774.

14. Chiasson MA, Stoneburner RL, Joseph SC: Human immunodeficiency virus transmission through artificial insemination. J Acq Immune Defic Syn 1990; 3:69.
15. Chun T-W, Carruth L, Finzi D, et al: Quantification of latent tissue reservoirs and total body viral load in HIV-1 infection. Nature 1997; 387:183.
16. Conant MA, Opp KM, Paretz D, et al: Reduction on Kaposi's sarcoma lesions following treatment of AIDS with ritonovir. AIDS 1997; 11:1300.
17. Coopman SA, Stern RS: Cutaneous drug reactions in human immunodeficiency virus infection. Arch Dermatol 1991; 127:714.
18. DeRienzo B, Mongairdo N, Pellegrino F, et al: Heterosexual transmission of the human immunodeficiency virus: A seroepidemiological study. Arch Dermatol Res 1989; 281:369.
19. Diz Dios P, Ocampo A, Miralles C, et al: Frequency of oropharyngeal candidiasis in HIV-infected patients on protease inhibitor therapy. Oral Surg Oral Med Oral Pathol Oral Radiol Endod 1999; 87:437.
20. Domingo P, Ris J, Lopez-Conteras J: Esophageal ulcers in AIDS. Ann Int Med 1996; 124:928.
21. Drinkard CR, Decher L, Little JW, et al: Periodontal status of individuals in early stages of human immunodeficiency virus infection. Commun Dent Oral Epidemiol 1991; 19:281.
22. EC-Clearinghouse on Oral Problems Related to HIV Infection and WHO Collaborating Centre on Oral Manifestations of the Immunodeficiency Virus: Classification and diagnostic criteria for oral lesions in HIV infection. J Oral Pathol Med 1993; 22:289.
23. Enger C, Graham N, Peng Y, et al: Survival from early, intermediate and late stages of HIV infection. J Am Med Assoc 1996; 275:1329.
24. Epstein JB, Silverman S: Head and neck malignancies associated with HIV infection. Oral Surg Oral Med Oral Pathol 1992; 73:193.
25. Eversole LR: Viral infections of the head and neck among HIV-seropositive patients. Oral Surg Oral Med Oral Pathol 1992; 73:155.
26. Eversole LR, Jacobsen P, Stone CE, et al: Oral condyloma planus (hairy leukoplakia) among homosexual men. A clinico-pathologic study of thirty-six cases. Oral Surg 1986; 61:249.
27. Fauci AS, Schnittman SM, Poli G, et al: Immunopathogenic mechanisms in human immunodeficiency virus (HIV) infection. Ann Intern Med 1993; 114:678.
28. Fetter A, Partisani M, Koenig H, et al: Asymptomatic oral *Candida albicans* carriage in HIV-infection: Frequency and predisposing factors. J Oral Pathol Med 1993; 22:57.
29. Ficarra G, Berson AM, Silverman S Jr, et al: Kaposi's sarcoma of the oral cavity: A study of 134 patients with a review of the pathogenesis, epidemiology, clinical aspects and treatment. Oral Surg Oral Med Oral Pathol 1988; 66:543.
30. Finzi D, Blankson J, Siliciano JD, et al: Latent infection of CD+4 T cells provides a mechanism for lifelong persistence of HIV-1, even in patients on effective combination therapy. Nature Med 1999; 5:512.
31. Fleming PL, Ward JW, Karon JM, et al: Declines in AIDS incidence and deaths in the USA: a signal change in the epidemic. AIDS 1998; 12(suppl A):S55.
32. Gaines H, Von Sydow M, Pehrson PO, et al: Clinical picture of primary HIV infection presenting as a glandular-fever-like illness. Br Med J 1988; 97:1363.
33. Glick M, Cleveland DB: Oral mucosal bacillary epithelioid angiomatosis in a patient with AIDS associated with rapid alveolar bone loss: A case report. J Oral Pathol Med 1993; 22:235.
34. Glick M, Garfunkel AA: Common oral findings in two different diseases—leukemia and AIDS: Part 1. Compend Contin Educ Dent 1992; XIII(6):432.
35. Glick M, Holmstrup P: HIV infection and periodontal diseases. In: Genco R, Mealey B, Rose L (eds): Periodontal Medicine. Hamilton, Canada, BC Decker, 2000.
36. Glick M, Muzyka BC: Alternative therapies for major aphthous ulcers in AIDS patients. J Am Dent Assoc 1992; 123:61.
37. Glick M, Muzyka BC, Lurie D, et al: Oral manifestations associated with HIV disease as markers for immune suppression and AIDS. Oral Surg Oral Med Oral Pathol 1994; 77:344.
38. Glick M, Muzyka BC, Salkin LM, et al: Necrotizing ulcerative periodontitis: A marker for immune deterioration and a predictor for the diagnosis of AIDS. J Periodontol 1994; 65:393.
39. Gompels UA, Kasolo FC: HHV-8 serology and Kaposi's sarcoma. Lancet 1996; 348:1587.
40. Gorin I, Vilette B, Gehanno P, et al: Thalidomide in hyperalgic pharyngeal ulceration of AIDS. Lancet 1990; 335:1343.
41. Gornitsky M, Clark DC, Siboo R, et al: Clinical documentation and occurrence of putative periodontopathic bacteria in human immunodeficiency virus-associated periodontal disease. J Periodontol 1991; 62:576.
42. Green TS, Beckstead JH, Lozada-Nur F, et al: Histopathologic spectrum of oral Kaposi's sarcoma. Oral Surg 1984; 58:306.
43. Greenspan D, Conant M, Silverman S Jr, et al: Oral hairy leukoplakia in male homosexuals. Evidence of association with both papilloma virus and a herpes-group virus. Lancet 1984; 2:831.
44. Greenspan D, Greenspan JS, de Souza Y, et al: Oral hairy leukoplakia in an HIV-negative renal transplant recipient. J Oral Pathol Med 1989; 18:32.
45. Greenspan D, Greenspan JS, Hearst NG, et al: Relations of oral hairy leukoplakia with HIV and the risk of developing AIDS. J Infect Dis 1987; 155:475.
46. Greenspan JS, Greenspan D, Lennette ET, et al: Replication of Epstein-Barr virus within the epithelial cells of oral hairy leukoplakia, and AIDS associated lesion. N Engl J Med 1985; 313:1564.
47. Greenspan D, Pindborg JJ, Greenspan JS, et al: AIDS and the Mouth. Copenhagen, Munksgaard, 1990.
48. Guarinos J, Bagan JV, Martinez-Canut P: Dental health in patients infected by human immunodeficiency virus (HIV). A study of 94 cases. Bull Group Int Rech Sci Stomatol et Odontol 1996; 39:119.
49. Gupta G: Viral pathogenesis and opportunistic infections. CDA J 1993; 21(9):29.
50. Haase AT, Schacker TW: Potential for the transmission of HIV-1 despite highly active antiretroviral therapy. N Engl J Med Dec 1998; 17:339:1846.
51. Hammer SM: Advances in antiretroviral therapy and viral load monitoring. AIDS 1996; 10(suppl 3):S1.
52. Harb GE, Alldredge BK, Coleman R, et al: Pharmacoepidemiology of adverse drug reactions in hospitalized patients with human immunodeficiency virus disease. J Acq Immune Defic Syn 1993; 6:919.
53. Hauman CHJ, Thompson IOC, Theunissen F, et al: Oral carriage of *Candida* in healthy and HIV-seropositive persons. Oral Surg Oral Med Oral Pathol 1993; 76:570.
54. Hicks JM: Assessing survival in HIV-seropositive individuals with extremely low CD4 counts. DAAC Forum 1997; March:10.
55. Ho DD, Neumann AU, Perelson AS, et al: Rapid turnover of plasma virions and CD4 lymphocytes in HIV-1 infection. Nature 1995; 373:123.

56. Hood SV, Hollis S, Percy M, et al: Assessment of therapeutic response of oropharyngeal and esophageal candidiasis in AIDS with use of a new clinical scoring system: studies with D0870. Clinical Infectious Diseases 1999; 28:587.
57. Horning GM, Cohen ME: Necrotizing ulcerative gingivitis, periodontitis and stomatitis: clinical staging and predisposing factors. J Periodontol 1995; 66:990.
58. Imagawa DT, Lee MH, Wolinsky SM, et al: Human immunodeficiency virus type 1 infection in homosexual men who remain seronegative for prolonged periods. N Engl J Med 1989; 320:1458.
59. Imam N, Carpenter CCJ, Mayer KH, et al: Hierarchical pattern of mucosal candida infections in HIV-seropositive women. Am J Med 1990; 89:142.
60. Ippolito G, Puro V, Heptonstall J, et al: Occupational human immunodeficiency virus infection in health care workers: worldwide cases through September 1997. Clin Infect Dis 1999; 28:365.
61. Jacobson JM, Greenspan JS, Spritzler J, et al: Thalidomide for the treatment of oral aphthous ulcers in patients with human immunodeficiency virus infection. N Engl J Med 1997; 336:1487.
62. Jaffe HW, Pellett PE: Human Herpesvirus 8 and Kaposi's sarcoma—some answers, more questions. New Engl J Med 1999; 340:1912.
63. Jin Y-T, Tsai S-T, Yan J-J, et al: Presence of human herpesvirus-like DNA sequence in oral Kaposi's sarcoma. Oral Surg Oral Med Oral Pathol Oral Radiol Endod 1996; 81:442.
64. Kabani S, Greenspan D, DeSouza YD, et al: Oral hairy leukoplakia with extensive oral mucosal involvement: Report of two cases. Oral Surg Oral Med Oral Pathol 1989; 67:411.
65. Kelly SL, Lamb DC, Kelly DE, et al: Resistance to fluconazole and amphotericin in *Candida albicans* from AIDS patients. Lancet 1996; 348:1523.
66. Klein RS, Quart AM, Small CB: Periodontal disease in heterosexuals with acquired immunodeficiency syndrome. J Periodontol 1991; 62:535
67. Kuntz AA, Gelderblum HR, Reichart PA: Ultrastructural findings on oral Kaposi's sarcoma (AIDS). J Oral Pathol 1987; 16:372.
68. Lamster IB, Begg MD, Mitchell-Lewis D, et al: Oral manifestations of HIV infection in homosexual men and intravenous drug users. Oral Surg Oral Med Oral Pathol 1994; 78:163.
69. Langford A, Pohle HD, Gelderblum HR, et al: Oral hyperpigmentation in HIV-infected patients. Oral Surg Oral Med Oral Pathol 1989; 67:301.
70. Law MG, de Winter L, McDonald A, et al: AIDS diagnoses at higher CD4 counts in Australia following the introduction of highly active antiretroviral treatment. AIDS 1999; 13:263.
71. Leaf AN, Laubenstein LJ, Raphael B, et al: Thrombotic thrombocytopenic purpura associated with human immunodeficiency virus type I (HIV-1) infection. Ann Intern Med 1988; 109:194.
72. Lindhardt BO, Ulrich K, Sindrup JH, et al: Seroconversion to human immunodeficiency virus (HIV) in persons attending an STD clinic in Copenhagen. Acta Derm Venereol (Stockh) 1998; 68:250.
73. Lot F, Seguier J-C, Fegueux S, et al: Probable transmission of HIV from an orthopedic surgeon to a patient in France. Ann Intern Med 1999; 130:1.
74. Lozada-Nur F, Silverman S Jr, Migliorati C, et al: The diagnosis of AIDS and AIDS related complex in the dental office, findings in 171 homosexual males. Calif Dent Assoc J 1984; 12:21.
75. Lucht E, Helmdahl A, Nord CE: Periodontal disease in HIV-infected patients in relation to lymphocyte subsets and specific micro-organisms. J Clin Periodontol 1991; 18:252.
76. Luzzi GA, Jones BJ: Treatment of neutropenic oral ulceration in human immunodeficiency virus infection with G-CSF. Oral Surg Oral Med Oral Pathol Oral Radiol Endod 1996; 81:53.
77. Margiotta V, Campisi G, Mancuso S, et al: HIV infection: oral lesions, CD4+ cell count and viral load in an Italian study population. J Oral Pathol Med 1999; 28:173.
78. Marmor M, Krasinski K, Sanchez M, et al: Sex, drugs, and HIV infection in a New York city hospital outpatient population. J Acq Immune Defic Syn 1990; 3:307.
79. Martins MD, Lozano-Chiu M, Rex JH: Declining rates of oropharyngeal candidiasis and carriage of *Candida albicans* associated with trends toward reduced rates of carriage of fluconazole-resistant *C. albicans* in human immunodeficiency virus-infected patients. Clin Infect Dis 1998; 27:1291.
80. McCarthy GM: Host factors associated with HIV-related oral candidiasis. Oral Surg Oral Med Oral Pathol 1992; 73:181.
81. McCarthy GM, Mackie ID, Koval J, et al: Factors associated with increased frequency of HIV-related oral candidiasis. J Oral Pathol Med 1991; 20:332.
82. McLeod AW: Dermatologic manifestations of AIDS. Med (North Am) 1986; 32:4448.
83. Mealey BL: Periodontal implications: medically compromised patients. Ann Periodontol 1996; 1:256.
84. Medical Letter: Drugs for AIDS and associated infections. Med Lett 1993; 35:79.
85. Michael NL, Brown AD, Voigt RF, et al: Rapid disease progression without seroconversion following primary human immunodeficiency virus type 1 infection—Evidence for highly susceptible human hosts. J Infect Dis 1997; 175: 1352.
86. Mohle-Boetani JC, Koehler JE, Berger TG, et al: Bacillary angiomatosis and bacillary peliosis in patients infected with human immunodeficiency virus: clinical characteristics in a case-control study. Clin Inf Dis 1996; 22:794.
87. Moore LVH, Moore WEC, Riley C, et al: Periodontal microflora of HIV-positive subjects with gingivitis or adult periodontitis. J Periodontol 1993; 64(1):48.
88. Mulligan R. The changing profile of the HIV/AIDS epidemic. CDA J 1993; 21(9):23.
89. Murray PA: Periodontal diseases in patients infected by human immunodeficiency virus. Periodontol 2000 1994; 6:50.
90. Murray PA, Grassi M, Winkler JR: The microbiology of HIV-associated periodontal lesions. J Clin Periodontol 1989; 16:636.
91. Murray PA, Winkler JR, Peros WJ, et al: DNA probe detection of periodontal pathogens in HIV-associated periodontal lesions. Oral Microbial Immunol 1991; 6:34.
92. Navazesh M, Lucatorto F: Common oral lesions associated with HIV infection. CDA J 1993; 21(9):37.
93. Newell AM, Francis N, Nelson MR: Nephrotic syndrome associated with bacillary angiomatosis in a patient with AIDS. Clin Infect Dis 1997; 25:750.
94. Nicolatou O, Theodoridou M, Mostrou G, et al: Oral lesions in children with perinatally acquired human immunodeficiency virus infection. J Oral Pathol Med 1999; 28:49.
95. Nguyen M-T, Weiss PJ, LaBarre RC, et al: Orally administered amphotericin B in the treatment of oral candidiasis in HIV-infected patients caused by azole-resistant *Candida albicans*. AIDS 1996; 10:1745.
96. Padian NS, Shiboski SC, Glass SO, et al: Heterosexual transmission of human immunodeficiency virus in northern

California: Results from a ten-year study. Am J Epidemiol 1997; 146:350.
97. Pedraza M-A, del Romero J, Roldan F, et al: Heterosexual transmission of HIV-1 is associated with high plasma viral load levels and a positive viral isolation in the infected partner. J AIDS 1999; 21:120.
98. Pezzotti P, Napoli PA, Acciai S, et al: Increasing survival time after AIDS in Italy: the role of new combination antiretroviral therapies. AIDS 1999; 13:249.
99. Phillips P. Refractory mucosal candidiasis in patients with human immunodeficiency virus infection. Clin Infect Dis 1999; 28:407.
100. Piliero PJ: HIV and hepatitis coinfection. AIDS Clin Care 1993; 5:93, 102.
101. Pindborg JJ: Global aspects of the AIDS epidemic. Oral Surg Oral Med Oral Pathol 1992; 73:138.
102. Phelan JA, Saltzman BR, Friedland GH, et al: Oral findings in patients with acquired immunodeficiency syndrome. Oral Surg 1987; 64:50.
103. Porter SR, Luker J, Scully C, et al: Orofacial manifestions of a group of British patients infected with HIV-1. J Oral Pathol Med 1989; 18:47.
104. Price DA, Birtles RJ, Levine TS, et al: Bacillary angiomatosis: a role for Phyllobacterium? AIDS 1997; 11:1186.
105. Qunibi WY, Akhtar M, Ginn E, et al: Kaposi's sarcoma in cyclosporine-induced gingival hyperplasia. Am J Kidney Dis 1988; 11:349.
106. Rahman MA, Kingsley LA, Breinig MK, et al: Enhanced antibody responses to Epstein-Barr virus in HIV-infected homosexual men. J Infect Dis 1989; 159:472.
107. Rees TD: Oral effects of drug abuse. Crit Rev Oral Biol Med 1992; 3:163.
108. Regezi JA, Eversole LR, Barker BF, et al: Herpes simplex and cytomegalovirus coinfected oral ulcers in HIV-positive patients. Oral Surg Oral Med Oral Pathol Oral Radiol Endod 1996; 81:55.
109. Regezi JA, MacPhail LA, Daniels TE, et al: Oral Kaposi's sarcoma: A 10-year retrospective histopathologic study. J Oral Pathol Med 1993; 22:292.
110. Reichart PA: Oral ulceration and iatrogenic disease in HIV infection. Oral Surg Oral Med Oral Pathol 1992; 73:212.
111. Relman AS: Pathogenic human retroviruses. N Engl J Med 1988; 318:243.
112. Richards JM: Notes on AIDS. Br Dent J 1985; 158:199.
113. Riley C, London JP, Burmeister JA: Periodontal health in 200 HIV-positive patients. J Oral Pathol Med 1992; 21:124.
114. Rivera-Hidalgo F, Stanford T: Oral mucosal lesions caused by infective microorganisms 1. Lesions caused by viruses and bacteria. Periodontal 2000 1999; 21:125.
115. Robinson P: Periodontal diseases and HIV infection. J Clin Periodontol 1992; 19:609.
116. Rowland RW, Escobar MR, Friedman RB, et al: Painful gingivitis may be an early sign of infection with the human immunodeficiency virus. Clin Infect Dis 1993; 16(2):233.
117. Safai B, Diaz B, Schwartz J: Malignant neoplasms associated with human immunodeficiency virus infection. AIDS Patient Care 1993; October:262.
118. Schiodt M, Greenspan D, Daniels TE, et al: Clinical and histologic spectrum of oral hairy leukoplakia. Oral Surg Oral Med Oral Pathol 1987; 64:716.
119. Schuman P, Sobel JD, Ohmit SE, et al: Mucosal candidal colonization and candidiasis in women with or without risk for human immunodeficiency virus infection. Clin Inf Dis 1998; 27:1161.
120. Schulten EAJM, ten Kate RW, van der Waal I: Oral manifestations of HIV infection in 75 Dutch patients. J Oral Pathol Med 1989; 18:42.
121. Sciubba JJ: Recognizing the oral manifestations of AIDS. Oncology 1992; 6:64.
122. Scully C, McCarthy G: Management of oral health in persons with HIV infection. Oral Surg Oral Med Oral Pathol 1992; 73:215.
123. Siegal B, Levinton-Kriss S, Schiffer A, et al: Kaposi's sarcoma in immunosuppression. Possibly the result of a dual viral infection. Cancer 1990; 65:492.
124. Silverman S: Color Atlas of Oral Manifestations of AIDS. Toronto, Decker, 1989.
125. Sitas F, Carrara H, Beral V, et al: Antibodies against human herpesvirus 8 in black South African patients with cancer. New Eng J Med 1999; 340:1863.
126. Sitas F, Newton R, Boshoff C: Increasing probability of mother-to-child transmission of HHV-8 with increasing maternal antibody titer for HHV-8. New Eng J Med 1999; 340:1923.
127. Slavkin HC: An update on HIV/AIDS. J Am Dent Assoc 1996; 127:1401.
128. Swango PA, Kleinman DV, Konzelman JL: HIV and periodontal health. A study of military personnel with HIV. J Am Dent Assoc 1991; 122:49.
129. Syrjanen S, Laine P, Niemela M, et al: Oral hairy leukoplakia is not a specific sign of HIV-infection but related to immunosuppression in general. J Oral Pathol Med 1989; 18:28.
130. Syrjanen S, Leimola-Virtanen R, Schmidt-Westhausen A, et al: Oral ulcers in AIDS patients frequently associated with cytomegalovirus (CMV) and Epstein-Barr virus (EBV) infection. J Oral Pathol Med 1999; 28:204
131. Tavitian A, Raufman J-P, Rosenthal LE: Oral candidiasis as a marker for esophageal candidiasis in the acquired immunodeficiency syndrome. Ann Intern Med 1986; 104:54.
132. Tomlinson DR, Coker RJ, Fisher M: Management and treatment of Kaposi's sarcoma in AIDS. Int J STD and AIDS 1996; 7:466.
133. Thompson SH, Charles GA, Craig DB: Correlation of oral disease with the Walter Reed staging scheme for HIV-1-seropositive patients. Oral Surg Oral Med Oral Pathol 1992; 73:289.
134. Tsang PCS, Samaranayake LP: Oral manifestations of HIV infection in a group of predominantly ethnic Chinese. J Oral Pathol Med 1999; 28:122.
135. Vanhems P, Allard R, Toma E, et al: Prognostic value of the CD4-T cell count for HIV-1 infected patients with advanced immunosuppression. Int J STD and AIDS 1996; 7:495.
136. Vanhems P, Dassa C, Lambert J, et al: Comprehensive classification of symptoms and signs reported among 218 patients with acute HIV-1 infection. J AIDS 1999; 21:99.
137. Velegraki A, Nicolatou O, Theodoridou M, et al: Paediatric AIDS-related linear gingival erythema; a form of erythematous candiasis? J Oral Path Med 1999; 28:178.
138. Veugelers PJ, Cornelisse PGA, Craib KJP, et al: Models of survival in HIV infection and their use in the quantification of treatment benefits. Am J Epidemiol 1998; 148:487.
139. Vidmar L, Poljak M, Tomazic J, et al: Transmission of HIV-1 by human bite. Lancet 1996; 347:1762.
140. Walli R, Goebel FD: Impaired glucose tolerance and protease inhibitors. Ann Int Med 1998; 129:837.
141. Wei X, Ghosh SK, Taylor ME, et al: Dynamics in human immunodeficiency virus type 1 infection. Nature 1995; 12:117.
142. Weisman Z, Kalinkovich A, Borkow G, et al: Infection by different HIV-1 subtypes (B and C) resuts in a similar immune activation profile despite distinct immune backgrounds. J AIDS 1999; 21:157.

143. Welch DF, Pickett DA, Slater LN, et al: Rochalimaea henselae sp. nov., a cause of septicemia, bacillary angiomatosis and parenchymal bacillary peliosis. J Clin Microbiol 1992; 30:275.
144. Wilcox CM: Esophageal ulcers in AIDS: In response. Ann Int Med 1996; 124:928.
145. Yeung SCH, Stewart GJ, Cooper DA, et al: Progression of periodontal disease in HIV seropositive patients. J Periodontol 1993; 64(7):651.
146. Zhang H, Dornadula G, Beumont M, et al: Human immunodeficiency virus type 1 in the semen of men receiving highly active antiretroviral therapy. New Engl J Med 1998; 17:339.
147. Zhang X, Langford A, Gelderblom H, et al: Ultrastructural findings in oral hyperpigmentation of HIV-infected patients. J Oral Pathol Med 1989; 18:471.
148. Zylberberg H, Pialoux G, Carnot F, et al: Rapidly evolving hepatitis C cirrhosis in a human immunodeficiency virus-infected patient receiving triple antiretroviral therapy. Clin Inf Dis 1998; 27:1255.

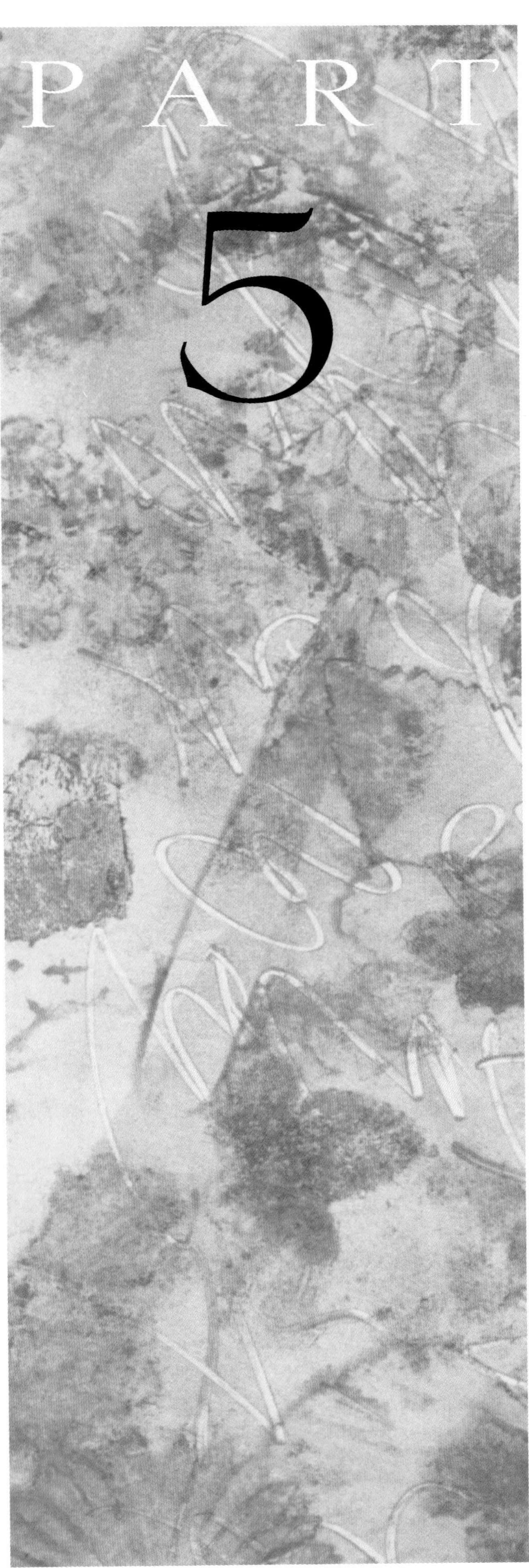

Treatment of Periodontal Disease

Michael G. Newman

Periodontal treatment requires an interrelationship between the care of the periodontium and other phases of dentistry. The concept of total treatment is based on the elimination of gingival inflammation and the factors that lead to it (e.g., plaque accumulation favored by calculus and pocket formation, inadequate restorations, and areas of food impaction).

Total treatment requires consideration of systemic aspects, including the possibility of interaction of periodontal disease with other diseases, systemic adjuncts to local treatment, and special precautions in patient management necessitated by systemic conditions. It may also entail consideration of functional aspects for the establishment of optimal occlusal relationships for the entire dentition.

All these aspects are embodied in a master plan, which consists of a rational sequence of dental procedures that includes periodontal and other measures necessary to create a well-functioning dentition in a healthy periodontal environment.

SECTION I

Diagnosis, Prognosis, and Treatment Plan

Michael G. Newman and Henry H. Takei

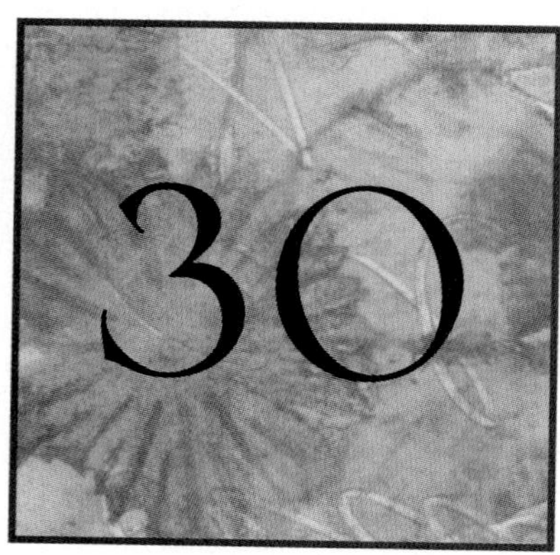

CHAPTER

Clinical Diagnosis

Fermin A. Carranza

Chapter Outline

Proper diagnosis is essential to intelligent treatment. Periodontal diagnosis should first determine whether disease is present; then identify its type, extent, distribution, and severity; and finally provide an understanding of the underlying pathologic processes and its cause. Chapters 26 to 29 provide a detailed description of the different diseases that can afflict the periodontium. In general, they fall into three broad categories.

1. The gingival diseases (Box 30-1)
2. The various types of periodontitis (Table 30-1)
3. The periodontal manifestations of systemic diseases

Periodontal diagnosis is determined after careful analysis of the case history and evaluation of the clinical signs and symptoms, as well as the results of various tests (e.g., probing mobility assessment, radiographs, blood tests, and biopsies).

The interest should be in the patient who has the disease and not simply in the disease itself. Diagnosis must therefore include a general evaluation of the patient and consideration of the oral cavity.

Diagnostic procedures must be systematic and organized for specific purposes. It is not enough to assemble facts. The findings must be pieced together so that they provide a meaningful explanation of the patient's periodontal problem.

The following is a recommended sequence of procedures for the diagnosis of periodontal diseases.

BOX 30-1

Gingival Diseases

Chronic marginal gingivitis
Acute necrotizing ulcerative gingivitis
Acute herpetic gingivostomatitis
Allergic gingivitis
Gingivitis associated with skin diseases
Gingivitis associated with endocrine-metabolic disturbances
Gingivitis associated with hematologic-immunologic disturbances
Gingival enlargement associated with medications
Gingival tumors

FIRST VISIT

Overall Appraisal of the Patient

From the first meeting, the clinician should attempt an overall appraisal of the patient. This includes consideration of the patient's mental and emotional status, temperament, attitude, and physiologic age.

Medical History

Most of the medical history is obtained at the first visit and can be supplemented by pertinent questioning at subsequent visits. The health history can be obtained verbally by questioning the patient and recording his or her responses on a blank piece of paper or by means of a printed questionnaire the patient completes.

The importance of the medical history should be explained to the patient because patients often omit information that they cannot relate to their dental problems. The patient should be made aware of (1) the possible role that some systemic diseases, conditions or behavioral factors may play in the cause of periodontal disease; and (2) oral infection may have a powerful influence on the occurrence and severity of a variety of systemic diseases and conditions (see Chapters 12 and 13).

The medical history aids the clinician in the diagnosis of oral manifestations of systemic disease and in the detection of systemic conditions that may be affecting the periodontal tissue response to local factors or that require special precautions and/or modifications in treatment procedures. For a detailed discussion of conditions requiring special precautions, see Chapters 37 to 39.

The medical history should include reference to:

1. Is the patient under the care of a physician and, if so, what is the nature and duration of the problem and the therapy? The name, address, and telephone number of the physician should be recorded, since direct communication with him or her may be necessary.
2. Details on hospitalization and operations, including diagnosis, kind of operation, and untoward events such as anesthetic, hemorrhagic, or infectious complications, should be provided.
3. A list should be supplied of all medications being taken and whether they were prescribed or obtained over the counter. All the possible effects of these medications should be carefully analyzed to determine their effect, if any, on the oral tissues and also to avoid administering medications that would interact adversely with them. Special inquiry should be made regarding the dosage and duration of therapy with anticoagulants and corticosteroids.
4. History should be taken of all medical problems (cardiovascular, hematologic, endocrine, etc.), including infectious diseases, sexually transmitted diseases, and high-risk behavior for human immunodeficiency virus (HIV) infection.
5. Any possibility of occupational disease should be noted.
6. Abnormal bleeding tendencies such as nosebleeds, prolonged bleeding from minor cuts, spontaneous ecchymoses, tendency toward excessive bruising, and excessive menstrual bleeding should be cited.
7. History of allergy should be taken, including hay fever, asthma, sensitivity to foods, or sensitivity to drugs such as aspirin, codeine, barbiturates, sulfonamides, antibiotics, procaine, and laxatives, to dental materials such as eugenol or acrylic resins.
8. Information is needed regarding the onset of puberty and, for females, menopause, menstrual disorders, hysterectomy, pregnancies, and miscarriages.
9. Family medical history should be taken, including bleeding disorders and diabetes.

Dental History

Current Illness. Some patients may be unaware of any problems but many may report bleeding gums; loose teeth; spreading of the teeth with the appearance of spaces where none existed before; foul taste in the mouth; and an itchy feeling in the gums, relieved by digging with a toothpick. There may also be pain of varied types and duration, including constant, dull, gnawing pain; dull pain after eating; deep, radiating pains in the jaws; acute throbbing pain; sensitivity when chewing; sensitivity to heat and cold; burning sensation in the gums; and extreme sensitivity to inhaled air.

A preliminary oral examination is done to explore the source of the patient's chief complaint and to determine whether immediate emergency care is required. If this is the case, the problem is addressed after consideration of the medical history (see Chapters 45 and 46).

The dental history should include reference to:

1. A list of visits to the dentist should be supplied, including frequency; date of the most recent visit; nature of the treatment; and oral prophylaxis or cleaning by a dentist or hygienist, including frequency and date of most recent cleaning.
2. The patient's oral hygiene regimen should be noted, including toothbrushing frequency, time of day, method, type of toothbrush and dentifrice, and interval at which brushes are replaced. Other methods for mouth care, such as mouthwashes, finger massage,

TABLE 30-1

Features of Types of Periodontitis

Parameter	CP	AP	PPP	LJP	NUP
Age (years)	35+	20–35	<11	11–19	15–35
Calculus	Moderate to abundant	Scanty to moderate	Scanty	Moderate	Scanty
Disease progression	Slow	Rapid	Rapid	Rapid	Rapid
Distribution	Generalized; associated with etiologic factors	Generalized; no consistent pattern	Primary molars and incisors	First molar and incisors, and no more than two other teeth	?
Prevalence	US: >50% Sri Lanka: 81%	US: 4–5% (?) Sri Lanka: 11%	?	<0.50%	?
Racial predilection	No	No	No	More common in blacks	No
Familial tendency	No	?	Yes	Yes	?
Sex distribution	More severe in males	?	?	?	?
PMN/macrophage defects	No	Yes	Yes	Yes	Yes
Association with systemic problems	No	Some cases	Yes	Yes	Yes
Response to therapy	Very good	Variable	Poor	Good	Variable

AP, Aggressive periodontitis; *CP,* chronic periodontitis; *LJP,* localized juvenile periodontitis; *NUP,* necrotizing ulcerative periodontitis; *PPP,* prepubertal periodontitis.
Prevalence in adolescents 14–17 years of age in the United States.

interdental stimulation, water irrigation, and dental floss.

3. Any orthodontic treatment, including duration and approximate date of termination, should be noted.
4. If the patient is experiencing pain in the teeth or in the gums, the manner in which the pain is provoked, its nature and duration, and the manner in which it is relieved should all be noted.
5. Bleeding gums should be cited, including when first noted; whether it occurs spontaneously, on brushing or eating, at night, or with regular periodicity; whether it is associated with the menstrual period or other specific factors; and the duration of the bleeding and the manner in which it is stopped.
6. A bad taste in the mouth and areas of food impaction should be recorded.
7. Do the teeth feel "loose" or insecure? Is there difficulty in chewing? Any tooth mobility should be recorded.
8. What are the patient's general dental habits? If there is any grinding or clenching of the teeth during the day or at night, it should be noted. Do the teeth or jaw muscles feel "sore" in the morning? Are there other habits, such as tobacco smoking or chewing, nail biting, or biting on foreign objects?
9. History of previous periodontal problems should be noted, including the nature of the condition and, if previously treated, the type of treatment received (surgical or nonsurgical) and approximate period of termination of previous treatment. If, in the opinion of the patient, the present problem is a recurrence of previous disease, what does he or she think caused it?

Intraoral Radiographic Survey

The radiographic survey should consist of a minimum of 14 intraoral films and four posterior bite-wing films (Fig. 30-1).

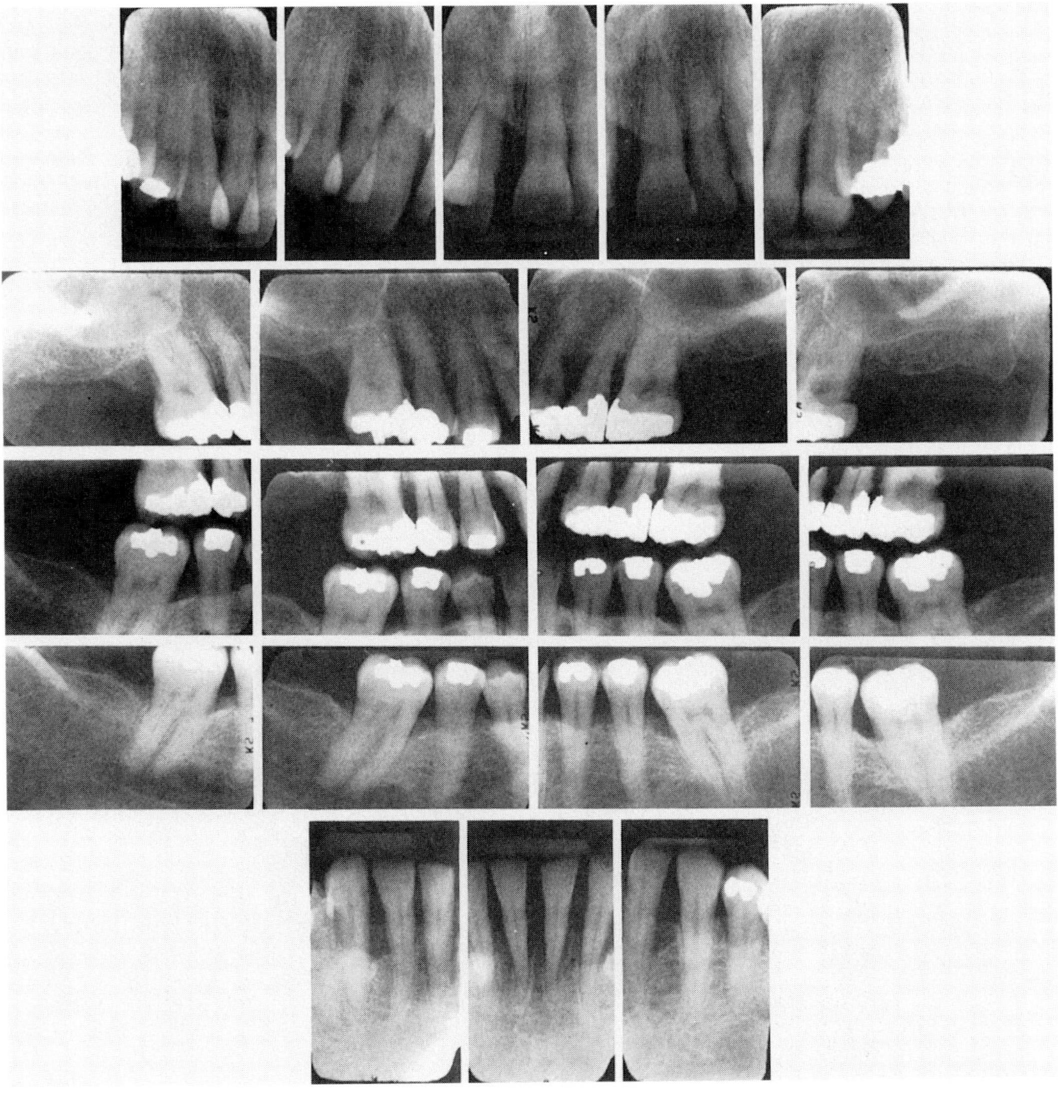

Fig. 30-1 Full-mouth intraoral radiographic series (16 periapical films and four bite-wing films) used as an adjunct in periodontal diagnosis.

Panoramic radiographs are a simple and convenient method of obtaining a survey view of the dental arch and surrounding structures (see Fig. 30-1). They are helpful for the detection of developmental anomalies, pathologic lesions of the teeth and jaws, and fractures (Fig. 30-2), as well as dental screening examinations of large groups. They provide an informative overall radiographic picture of the distribution and severity of bone destruction in periodontal disease, but *a complete intraoral series is required for periodontal diagnosis and treatment planning.* Chapter 31 gives a detailed description of radiographic interpretation in periodontics.

Casts

Casts from dental impressions are extremely useful adjuncts in the oral examination. They indicate the position of the gingival margins and the position and inclination of the teeth, proximal contact relationships, and food impaction areas. In addition, they provide a view of lingual-cuspal relationships. They are important records of the dentition before it is altered by treatment. Finally, casts also serve as visual aids in discussions with the patient and are useful for pre- and post-treatment comparisons, as well as for reference at checkup visits.

Clinical Photographs

Color photographs are not essential, but they are useful for recording the appearance of the tissue before and after treatment. Photographs cannot always be relied on for comparing subtle color changes in the gingiva, but they do depict gingival morphologic changes.

Review of the Initial Examination

If no emergency care is required, the patient is dismissed and instructed as to when to report for the second visit. Before this visit, a correlated examination is made of the radiographs and casts to relate the radiographic changes to unfavorable conditions represented on the casts. The casts are checked for evidence of abnormal wear, plunger cusps, uneven marginal ridges, malposed or extruded teeth, crossbite relationships, or other conditions that could cause occlusal disharmony or food impaction. Such areas are marked on the casts to serve as a reference during the detailed examination of the oral cavity. The radiographs and casts are valuable diagnostic aids; however, it is *the clinical findings in the oral cavity that constitute the basis for diagnosis.*

SECOND VISIT

Oral Examination

Oral Hygiene. The cleanliness of the oral cavity is appraised in terms of the extent of accumulated food debris, plaque, materia alba, and tooth surface stains (Fig. 30-3). Disclosing solution may be used to detect plaque that would otherwise be unnoticed. The amount of plaque detected, however, is not necessarily related to the severity of the disease present. For example, aggressive periodontitis is a destructive type of periodontitis in which plaque is scanty. Qualitative assessments of plaque are more meaningful, and their value in diagnosis is discussed in Chapter 34.

Mouth Odors. Halitosis, also termed *fetor ex ore, fetor oris,* and *oral malodor,* is foul or offensive odor emanating from the oral cavity. Mouth odors may be of diagnostic significance, and their origin may be either oral or extraoral (remote).

Halitosis is caused primarily by volatile sulfur compounds, specifically, hydrogen sulfyde and methyl mercaptan, which result from the bacterial putrefaction of proteins containing sulfur aminoacids. These products

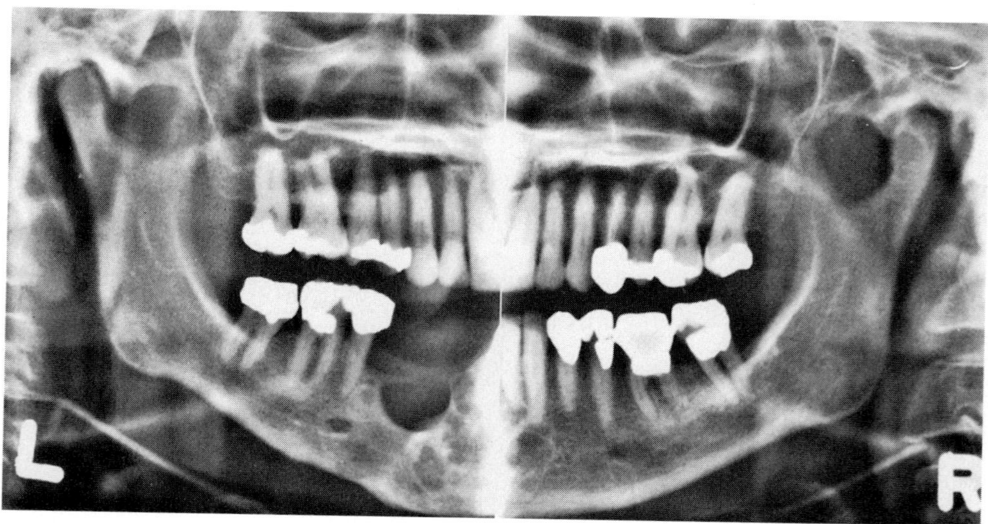

Fig. 30-2 Panoramic radiograph showing temporomandibular joints and "cystic" spaces in the jaw. Areas of periodontal bone loss are not seen in detail. (Compare with Fig. 30-1.)

could be involved in the transition from health to gingivitis and then to periodontitis.[47]

Local sources of mouth odors are mainly the tongue and the gingival sulcus[49] and include retention of odoriferous food particles on and between the teeth, coated tongue, necrotizing ulcerative gingivitis (NUG), dehydration states, caries, artificial dentures, smoker's breath, and healing surgical or extraction wounds. The fetid odor that is a characteristic of NUG is easily identified. Chronic periodontitis with pocket formation may also cause unpleasant mouth odor from any accumulated debris and the increased rate of putrefaction of the saliva.[9]

Extraoral sources of mouth odors include various infections or lesions of the respiratory tract (bronchitis, pneumonia, bronchiectasis, or others) and odors that are excreted through the lungs from aromatic substances in the bloodstream, such as metabolites from ingested foods or excretory products of cell metabolism. Alcoholic breath, the acetone odor of diabetes, and the uremic breath that accompanies kidney dysfunction are examples of the last group.

Examination of the Oral Cavity. The entire oral cavity should be carefully examined. The examination should include the lips, floor of the mouth, tongue, palate, and oropharyngeal region, as well as the quality and quantity of saliva. Although findings may not be related to the periodontal problem, they should enable the dentist to detect any pathologic changes present in the mouth. Textbooks in oral medicine and oral diagnosis cover these topics in detail.

Examination of Lymph Nodes. Because periodontal, periapical, and other oral diseases may result in lymph node changes, the diagnostician should routinely examine and evaluate head and neck lymph nodes. Lymph nodes can become enlarged and/or indurated as a result of an infectious episode, malignant metastases, or residual fibrotic changes.

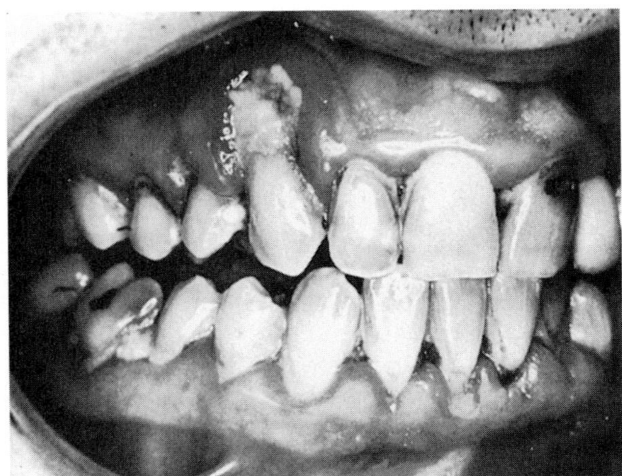

Fig. 30-3 Poor oral hygiene. Gingival inflammation associated with plaque, materia alba, and calculus in a patient with hemophilia.

Inflammatory nodes become enlarged, palpable, tender, and fairly immobile. The overlying skin may be red and warm. Patients are often aware of the presence of "swollen glands." Primary herpetic gingivostomatitis, NUG, and acute periodontal abscesses may produce lymph node enlargement. After successful therapy, lymph nodes return to normal in a matter of days or a few weeks.

Examination of the Teeth

The teeth are examined for caries, developmental defects, anomalies of tooth form, wasting, hypersensitivity, and proximal contact relationships.

Wasting Disease of the Teeth. *Wasting is defined as any gradual loss of tooth substance characterized by the formation of smooth, polished surfaces, without regard to the possible mechanism of this loss.* The forms of wasting are erosion, abrasion, and attrition.

Erosion (cuneiform defect) is a sharply defined wedge-shaped depression in the cervical area of the facial tooth surface.[48] The long axis of the eroded area is perpendicular to the vertical axis of the tooth (Fig. 30-4). The surfaces are smooth, hard, and polished. Erosion generally affects a group of teeth. In the early stages, it may be confined to the enamel, but it generally extends to involve the underlying dentin as well as the cementum.

The cause of erosion is not known. Decalcification by acid beverages[31] or citrus fruits, along with the combined effect of acid salivary secretion and friction,[33] are suggested causes. Sognnaes[53] refers to these lesions as *dentoalveolar ablations* and attributes them to forceful frictional actions between the oral soft tissues and the adjacent hard tissues. In patients with erosion, the salivary pH, buffering capacity, and calcium and phosphorus content have been reported as normal, with the mucin level elevated.[30]

Abrasion refers to the loss of tooth substance induced by mechanical wear other than that of mastication. Abrasion results in saucer-shaped or wedge-shaped indentations with a smooth, shiny surface. Abrasion starts on exposed cementum surfaces rather than on the enamel and extends to involve the dentin of the root. A sharp "ditching" around the cementoenamel junction appears due to the softer cemental surface, as compared with the much harder enamel surface.

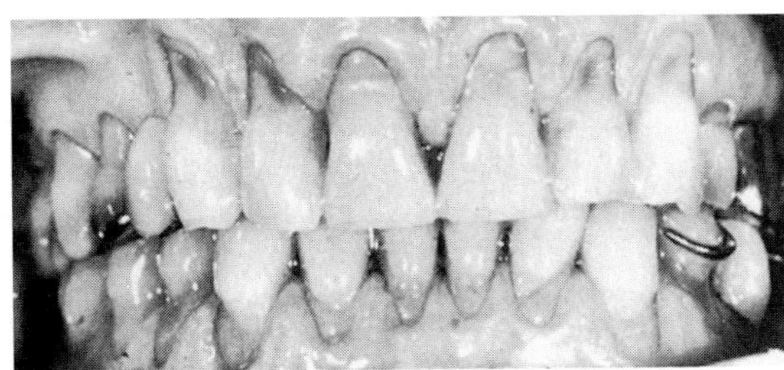

Fig. 30-4 Erosion involving the enamel, cementum, and dentin.

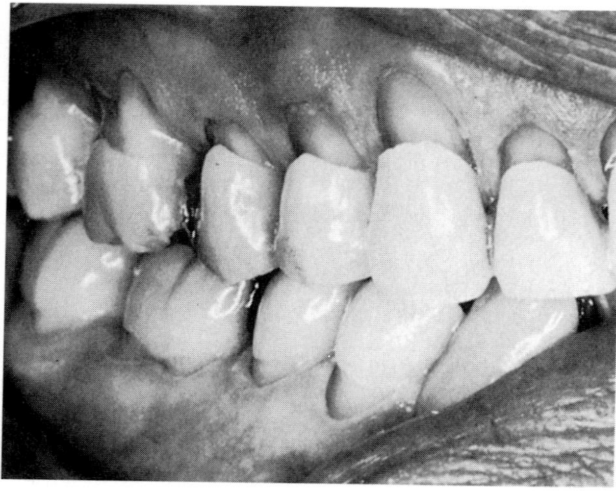

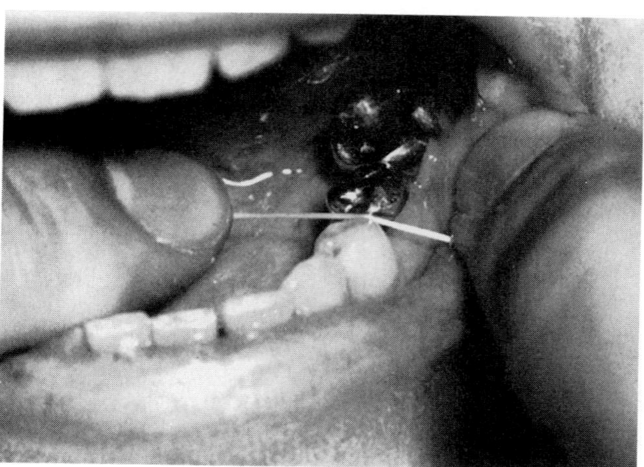

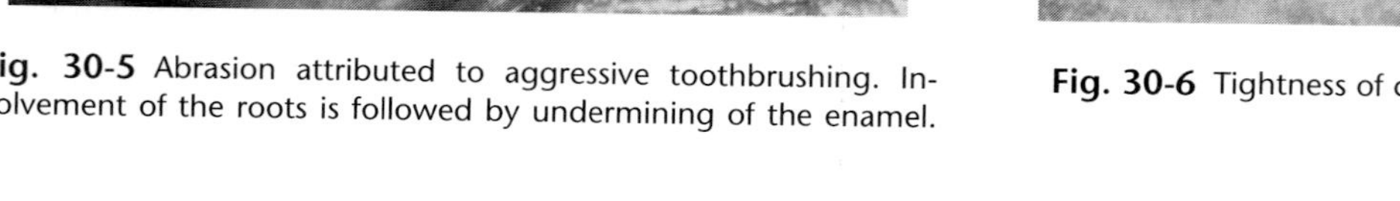

Fig. 30-5 Abrasion attributed to aggressive toothbrushing. Involvement of the roots is followed by undermining of the enamel.

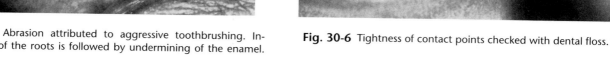

Fig. 30-6 Tightness of contact points checked with dental floss.

Continued exposure to the abrasive agent, combined with decalcification of the enamel by locally formed acids, may result in loss of enamel, followed by loss of the dentin of the crown (Fig. 30-5).

Toothbrushing[21] with an abrasive dentifrice and the action of clasps are common causes of abrasion; the former is by far the more prevalent. The degree of tooth wear from toothbrushing depends on the abrasive effect of the dentifrice and the angle of brushing.[28,29] Horizontal brushing at right angles to the vertical axis of the teeth results in the severest loss of tooth substance. Occasionally, abrasion of the incisal edges occurs as a result of habits such as holding objects (e.g., a bobby pin or tacks) between the teeth.

Attrition is occlusal wear resulting from functional contacts with opposing teeth.

Dental Stains. These are pigmented deposits on the teeth. They should be carefully examined to determine their origin (see Chapter 11).

Hypersensitivity. Root surfaces exposed by gingival recession may be hypersensitive to thermal changes or tactile stimulation. Patients often direct the operator to the sensitive areas. These may be located by gentle exploration with a probe or cold air.

Proximal Contact Relations. Slightly open contacts permit food impaction. The tightness of contacts should be checked by means of clinical observation and with dental floss (Fig. 30-6). Abnormal contact relationships may also initiate occlusal changes such as a shift in the median line between the central incisors, labial version of the maxillary canine, buccal or lingual displacement of the posterior teeth, and an uneven relationship of the marginal ridges.

Tooth Mobility. All teeth have a slight degree of physiologic mobility, which varies for different teeth and at different times of the day.[37] It is greatest on arising in the morning and progressively decreases. The increased mobility in the morning is attributed to slight extrusion of the tooth because of limited occlusal contact during sleep. During the waking hours, mobility is reduced by chewing and swallowing forces, which intrude the teeth in the sockets. These 24-hour variations are less marked in persons with a healthy periodontium than in those with occlusal habits such as bruxism and clenching.

Single-rooted teeth have more mobility than multirooted teeth, with incisors having the most. Mobility is principally in a horizontal direction, although some axial mobility occurs, to a much lesser degree.[39]

Tooth mobility occurs in two stages:

1. The initial or intrasocket stage is where the tooth moves within the confines of the periodontal ligament. This is associated with viscoelastic distortion of the ligament and redistribution of the periodontal fluids, interbundle content, and fibers.[23] This initial movement occurs with forces of about 100 lb and is of the order of 0.05 to 0.10 mm (50 to 100 microns).[34]
2. The secondary stage, which occurs gradually and entails elastic deformation of the alveolar bone in response to increased horizontal forces.[36] When a force of 500 lbs is applied to the crown, the resulting displacement is about 100 to 200 microns for incisors, 50 to 90 microns for canines, 8 to 10 microns for premolars, and 40 to 80 microns for molars.[34]

When a force such as that applied to teeth in occlusion is discontinued, the teeth return to their original position in two stages: the first is an immediate, springlike elastic recoil; the second is a slow, asymptomatic recovery movement. The recovery movement is pulsating and is apparently associated with the normal pulsation of the periodontal vessels, which occurs in synchrony with the cardiac cycle.[35]

Many attempts have been made to develop mechanical or electronic devices for the precise measurement of tooth mobility.[35,38,40,51] Even though standardization of the grading of mobility would be helpful in diagnosing periodontal disease and in evaluating the outcome of treatment, these devices are not widely used. As a general rule, mobility is graded clinically with a simple method such as the following: the tooth is held firmly between the handles of two metallic instruments or with one metallic instrument and one finger (Fig. 30-7), and an effort is made to move it in all directions; abnormal mobility most often occurs faciolingually. Mobility is graded according to the ease and extent of tooth movement as follows:

Normal mobility
Grade I: Slightly more than normal.
Grade II: Moderately more than normal.
Grade III: Severe mobility faciolingually and/or mesiodistally, combined with vertical displacement.

Mobility beyond the physiologic range is termed *abnormal* or *pathologic*. It is pathologic in that it exceeds the limits of normal mobility values; the periodontium is not necessarily diseased at the time of examination.

Increased mobility is caused by one or more of the following factors:

1. *Loss of tooth support (bone loss)* can result in mobility. The amount of mobility depends on the severity and distribution of bone loss at individual root surfaces, the length and shape of the roots, and the root size compared with that of the crown.[42] A tooth with short, tapered roots is more likely to loosen than one with normal-size or bulbous roots with the same amount of bone loss. Because bone loss usually results from a combination of factors and does not occur as an isolated finding, the severity of tooth mobility does not necessarily correspond to the amount of bone loss.
2. *Trauma from occlusion* (i.e., injury produced by excessive occlusal forces or incurred because of abnormal occlusal habits such as bruxism and clenching) is a common cause of tooth mobility. Mobility is also increased by hypofunction. Mobility produced by trauma from occlusion occurs initially as a result of resorption of the cortical layer of bone, leading to reduced fiber support, and later as an adaptation phenomenon resulting in a widened periodontal space.
3. *Extension of inflammation from the gingiva or from the periapex into the periodontal ligament* results in changes that increase mobility. The spread of inflammation from an acute periapical abscess may increase tooth mobility in the absence of periodontal disease.
4. *Periodontal surgery* temporarily increases tooth mobility for a short period.[43-46]
5. *Tooth mobility is increased in pregnancy and is sometimes associated with the menstrual cycle or the use of hormonal contraceptives.* It occurs in patients with or without periodontal disease, presumably because of physicochemical changes in the periodontal tissues.
5. *Pathologic processes of the jaws that destroy the alveolar bone and/or the roots of the teeth* can also result in mobility. Osteomyelitis and tumors of the jaws belong in this category.

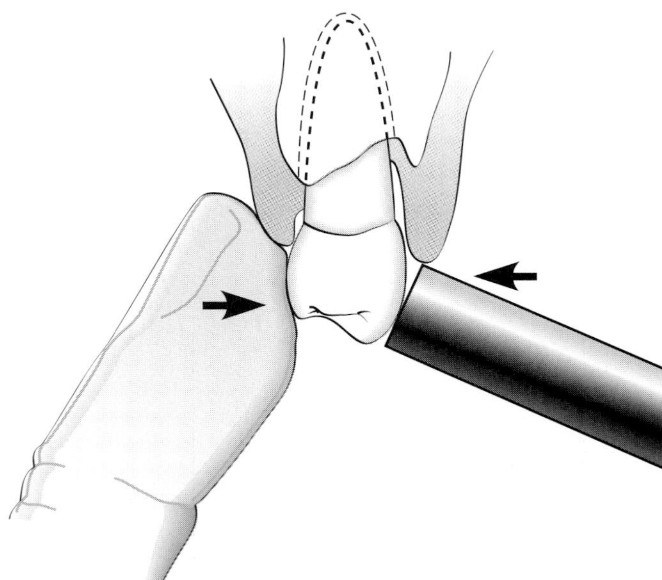

Fig. 30-7 Tooth mobility checked with one metal instrument and one finger.

6. One study[13] has suggested that pockets around mobile teeth harbor higher proportions of *Campylobacter rectus* and *Peptostreptococcus micros,* and possibly of *Porphyromonas gingivalis* than nonmobile teeth. This hypothesis needs further verification.

Trauma from Occlusion. *Trauma from occlusion* refers to tissue injury produced by occlusal forces, not to the occlusal forces themselves (see Chapter 24). The criterion that determines if an occlusal force is injurious is whether it causes damage in the periodontal tissues; therefore the diagnosis of trauma from occlusion is made from the condition of the periodontal tissues. The periodontal findings are then used as a guide for locating the responsible occlusal relationships.

Periodontal findings that suggest the presence of trauma from occlusion include excessive tooth mobility, particularly in teeth showing radiographic evidence of a widened periodontal space (see Chapter 31); vertical or angular bone destruction; infrabony pockets; and pathologic migration, especially of the anterior teeth (see following discussion).

Pathologic Migration of the Teeth. Alterations in tooth position should be carefully noted, particularly with a view toward identifying abnormal forces, a tongue-thrusting habit, or other habits that may be contributing factors (see Chapter 24). Premature tooth contacts in the posterior region that deflect the mandible anteriorly contribute to destruction of the periodontium of the maxillary anterior teeth and to pathologic migration (Fig. 30-8). Pathologic migration of anterior teeth in young persons may be a sign of localized aggressive (juvenile) periodontitis.

Sensitivity to Percussion. Sensitivity to percussion is a feature of acute inflammation of the periodontal ligament. Gentle percussion of a tooth at different angles to the long axis often aids in localizing the site of inflammatory involvement.

Dentition with the Jaws Closed. Examination of the dentition with the jaws closed can detect conditions such as irregularly aligned teeth, extruded teeth, improper proximal contacts, and areas of food impaction, all of which may favor plaque accumulation.

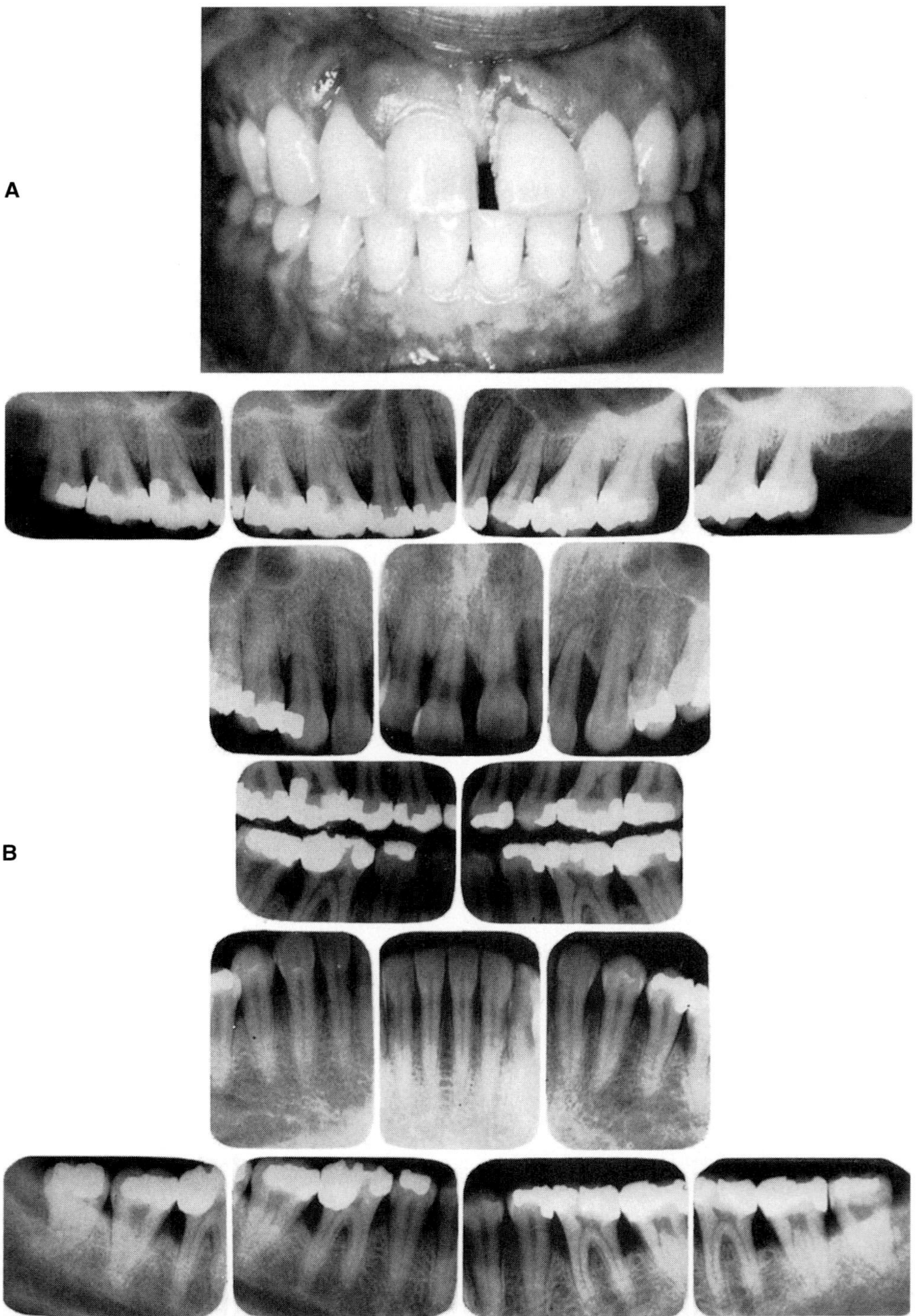

Fig. 30-8 Periodontal disease with pathologic migration of the anterior teeth. **A,** Clinical picture. **B,** Radiographic view.

Excessive overbite, seen most often in the anterior region, may cause impingement of the teeth on the gingiva and food impaction, followed by gingival inflammation, gingival enlargement, and pocket formation. The real significance of excessive overbite for gingival health, however, is controversial.[2]

In *open bite* relationships, abnormal vertical spaces exist between the maxillary and mandibular teeth. The condition occurs most often in the anterior region, although posterior open bite is occasionally seen. Reduced mechanical cleansing by the passage of food may lead to accumulation of debris, calculus formation, and extrusion of teeth.

In *crossbite,* the normal relationship of the mandibular teeth to the maxillary teeth is reversed, with the maxillary teeth being lingual to the mandibular teeth. Crossbite may be bilateral or unilateral, or it may affect only a pair of antagonists. Trauma from occlusion, food impaction, spreading of the mandibular teeth, and associated gingival and periodontal disturbances may be caused by crossbite.

Functional Occlusal Relationships. Examination of functional occlusal relationships is an important part of the diagnostic procedure. Dentitions that appear normal when the jaws are closed may present marked functional abnormalities. Systematic procedures for the detection and correction of functional abnormalities are presented in Chapter 52.

Examination of the Periodontium

The periodontal examination should be systematic, starting in the molar region in either the maxilla or the mandible and proceeding around the arch. This avoids overemphasis of spectacular findings at the expense of other conditions, which, although less striking, may be equally important. It is important to detect the earliest signs of gingival and periodontal disease.

Charts to record the periodontal and associated findings provide a guide for a thorough examination and record of the patient's condition (Fig. 30-9). They are also used for evaluating the response to treatment and for comparison at recall visits. However, excessively complicated mouth charting may lead to identification of a frustrating maze of minutiae rather than clarification of the patient's problem. Computerized dental examination systems using high-resolution graphics and voice-activated technology permit easy retrieval and comparison of data.[8]

A method for periodontal screening and recording (PSR) has been developed jointly by the American Academy of Periodontology and the American Dental Association, with the support of the Procter & Gamble Company.[41] This method is designed for the general dental practitioner, and its purpose is to identify patients requiring periodontal care and to determine, in general terms, the type of care required. This method is presented at the end of this chapter.

Plaque and Calculus. There are many methods for assessing plaque and calculus accumulation.[11] The presence of supragingival plaque and calculus can be directly observed and the amount measured with a calibrated probe. For the detection of subgingival calculus, each tooth surface is carefully checked to the level of the gingival attachment with a sharp no. 17 or no. 3A explorer (Fig. 30-10). Warm air may be used to deflect the gingiva and aid in visualization of the calculus.

Although the radiograph may sometimes reveal heavy calculus deposits interproximally (see Chapter 31) and even on the facial and lingual surfaces, it cannot be relied on for the thorough detection of calculus.

Gingiva. The gingiva must be dried before accurate observations can be made (Fig. 30-11). Light reflection from moist gingiva obscures detail. In addition to visual examination and exploration with instruments, firm but gentle palpation should be used for detecting pathologic alterations in normal resilience, as well as for locating areas of pus formation.

Each of the following features of the gingiva should be considered: color, size, contour, consistency, surface texture, position, ease of bleeding, and pain (see Chapters 17 and 18). No deviation from the norm should be overlooked. The distribution of gingival disease and its acuteness or chronicity should also be noted.

From a clinical point of view, gingival inflammation can produce two basic types of tissue response: edematous and fibrotic. Edematous tissue response is characterized by a smooth, glossy, soft, red gingiva. In the fibrotic tissue response, some of the characteristics of normalcy persist; the gingiva is more firm, stippled, and opaque, although it is usually thicker, and its margin appears rounded (Color Fig. 30-1).

Use of Clinical Indices in Dental Practice. There has been a tendency to extend the use of indices originally designed for epidemiologic studies into dental practice. A detailed description of these indices can be found in Chapter 5. Of all the indices that have been proposed, the Gingival Index and the Sulcus Bleeding Index appear to be the most useful and most easily transferred to clinical practice.

The *Gingival Index* (Löe and Silness) provides an assessment of gingival inflammatory status that can be used in practice to compare gingival health before and after Phase I therapy or before and after surgical therapy. It can also be used to compare gingival status at recall visits. Attaining good intra- and interexaminer calibration is imperative in the dental office.

The *Sulcus Bleeding Index* (Mühlemann and Son) provides an objective, easily reproducible assessment of the gingival status. It is extremely useful for detecting early inflammatory changes and the presence of inflammatory lesions located at the base of the periodontal pocket, an area inaccessible to visual examination. Because it is easily understood by the patient, the Sulcus Bleeding Index can be used to enhance the patient's motivation for plaque control.

Periodontal Pockets. Examination for periodontal pockets must include consideration of the following: presence and distribution on each tooth surface, pocket depth, level of attachment on the root, and type of pocket (suprabony or intrabony).

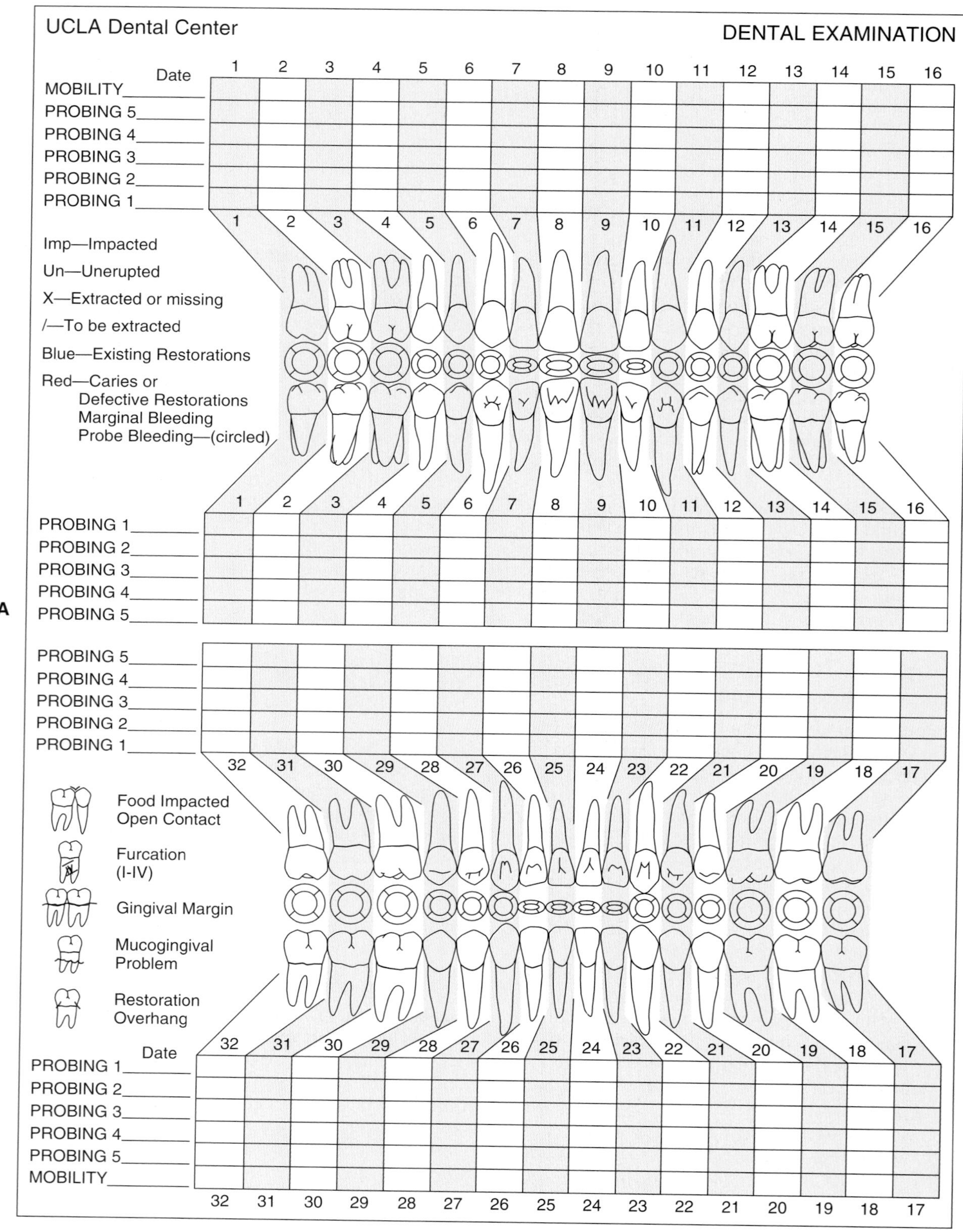

Fig. 30-9 A, UCLA periodontal chart.

Continued

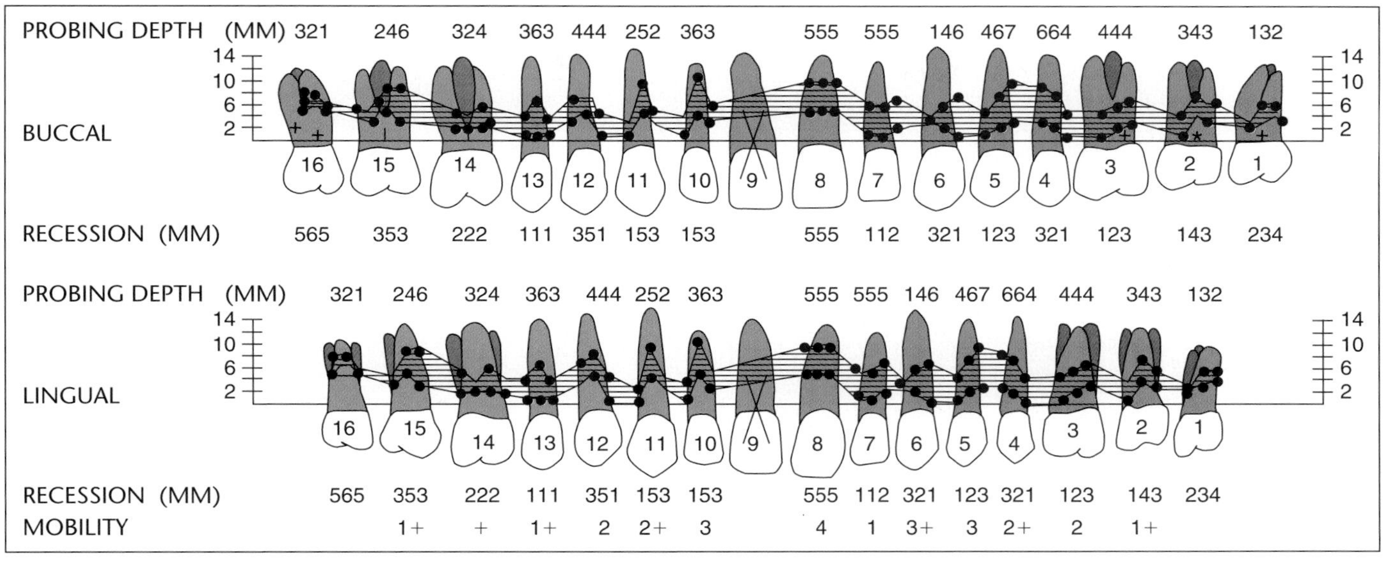

Fig. 30-9, cont'd. B, Computerized diagram showing various periodontal parameters.

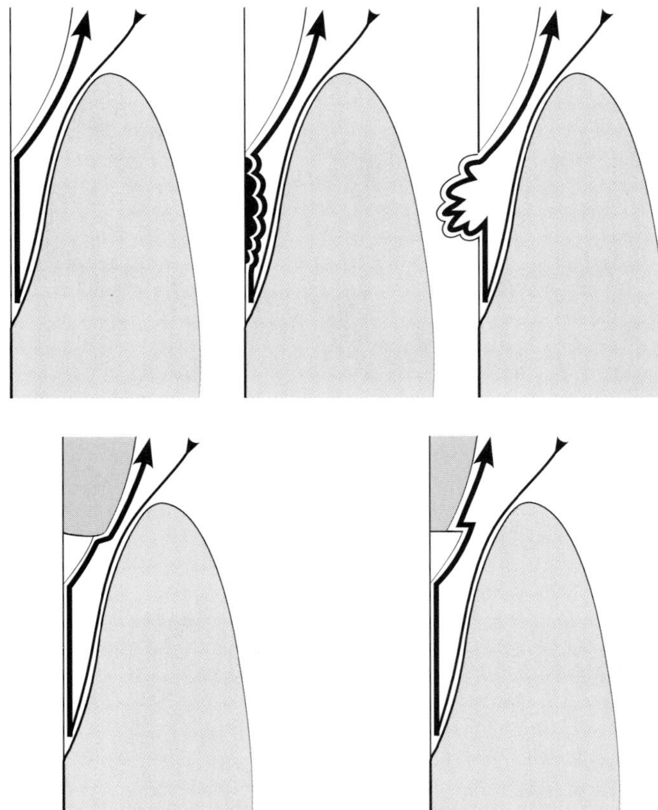

Fig. 30-10 *Top left,* Detection of smoothness or various irregularities on the root surface with outward motion of a probe or explorer. *Top center,* Calculus. *Top right,* Caries. *Bottom left and right,* Irregular margins of restorations.

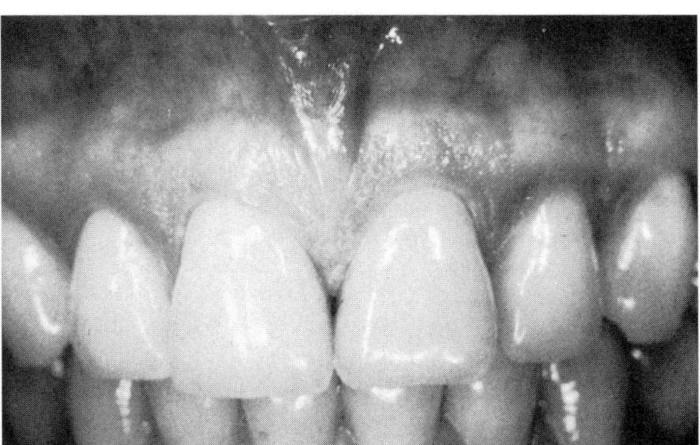

Fig. 30-11 Normal gingiva. Normal surface features are revealed by drying the gingiva.

SIGNS AND SYMPTOMS. Although probing is the only reliable method of detecting pockets, clinical signs such as color changes (bluish-red marginal gingiva or bluish-red vertical zone extending from the gingival margin to the attached gingiva); a "rolled" edge separating the gingival margin from the tooth surface; or an enlarged, edematous gingiva may suggest their presence. The presence of bleeding, suppuration, and loose, extruded teeth may also denote the presence of a pocket (Figs. 30-12 to 30-16 and see Color Fig. 30-1).

Periodontal pockets are generally painless but may give rise to symptoms such as localized or sometimes radiating pain or sensation of pressure after eating, which gradually diminishes. A foul taste in localized areas, sensitivity to hot and cold, and toothache in the absence of caries is also sometimes present.

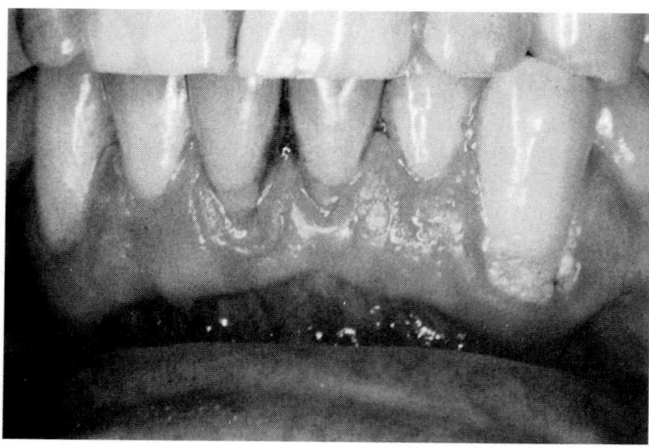

Fig. 30-12 Periodontal pockets around the central incisors and left canine, showing rolled margins and separation from the tooth surface. Note the materia alba on the canine.

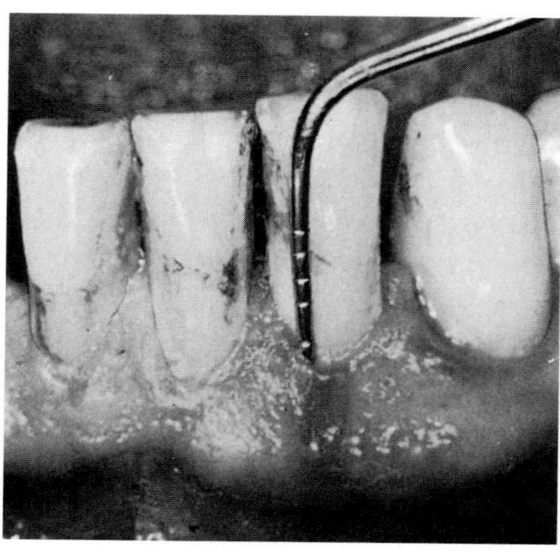

Fig. 30-13 Periodontal pocket with vertical discolored zone extending to the alveolar mucosa.

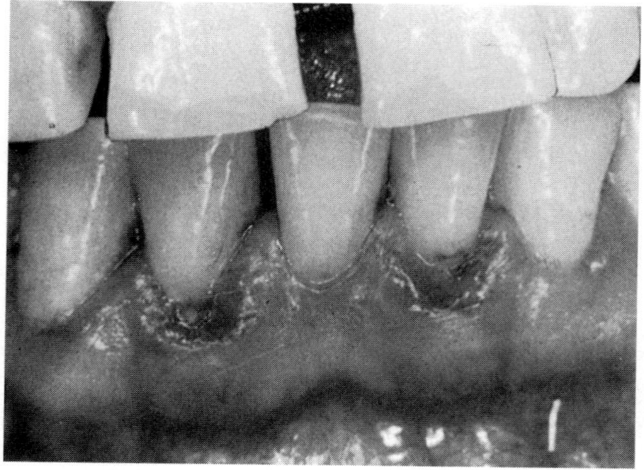

Fig. 30-14 Periodontal pocket with puffy, discolored gingiva and exposed root surfaces.

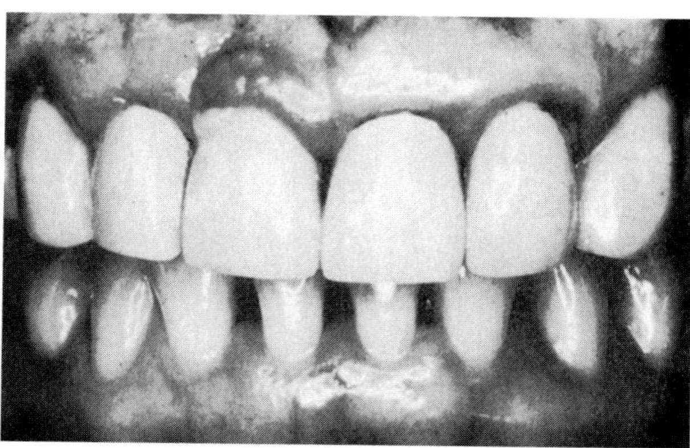

Fig. 30-15 Purulent exudate from the periodontal pocket on the maxillary left central incisor.

A

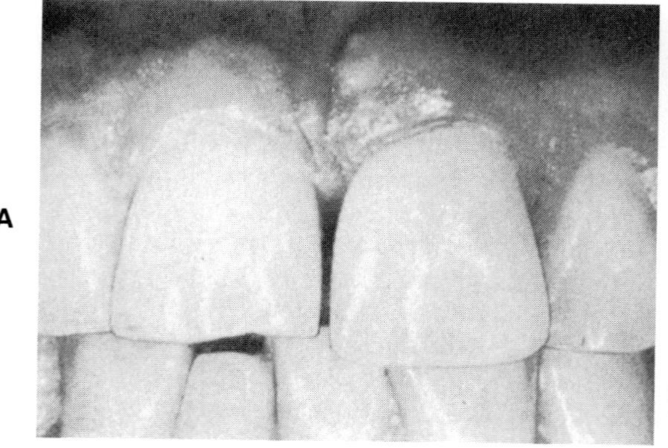

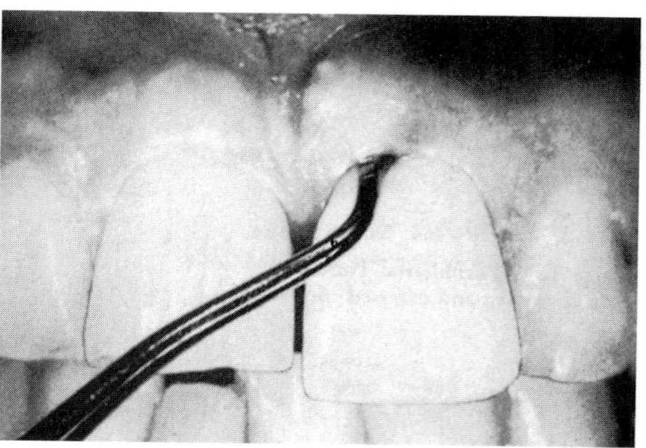

B

Fig. 30-16 A, Extrusion of the maxillary left central incisor and diastema associated with a periodontal pocket. **B,** Deep periodontal pocket revealed by probing. The probe has penetrated to its entire length.

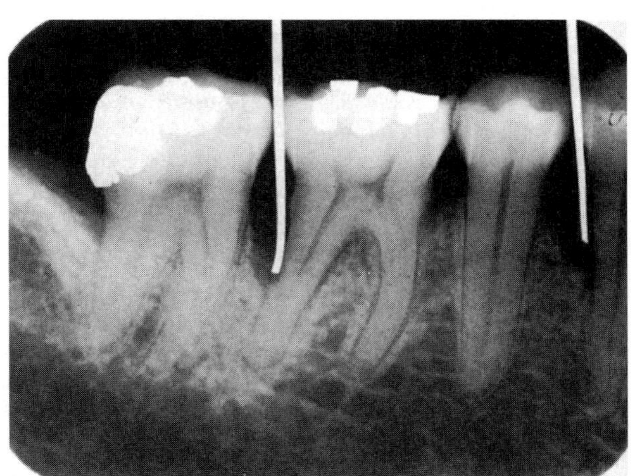

Fig. 30-17 Blunted silver points assist in locating the base of pockets.

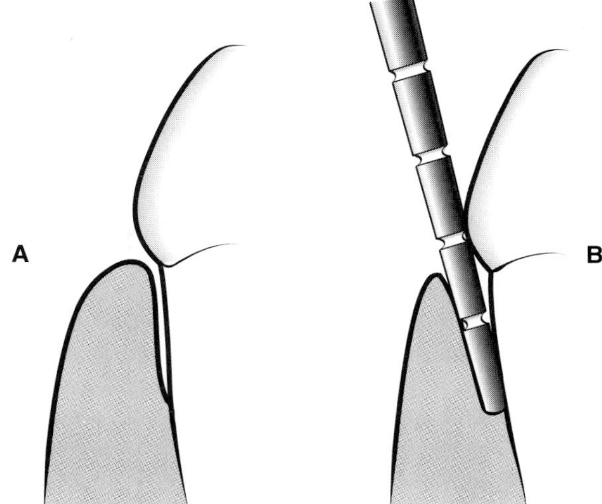

Fig. 30-18 **A,** Biologic or histologic pocket depth. **B,** Probing or clinical pocket depth.

DETECTION OF POCKETS. The only accurate method of detecting and measuring periodontal pockets is careful exploration with a periodontal probe. Pockets are not detected by radiographic examination. The periodontal pocket is a soft tissue change. Radiographs indicate areas of bone loss where pockets may be suspected; they do not show pocket presence or depth, and consequently they show no difference before or after pocket elimination unless bone has been modified.

Gutta percha points or calibrated silver points[19] can be used with the radiograph to assist in determining the level of attachment of periodontal pockets (Fig. 30-17). They may be used effectively for individual pockets or in clinical research, but their routine use throughout the mouth would be rather cumbersome. Clinical examination and probing are more direct and efficient.

POCKET PROBING. The two different pocket depths are (1) biologic or histologic depth and (2) clinical or probing depth[24] (Fig. 30-18) (see Chapter 1).

The **biologic depth** is the distance between the gingival margin and the base of the pocket (the coronal end of the junctional epithelium). This can be measured only in carefully prepared and adequately oriented histologic sections. The **probing depth** is the distance to which an ad hoc instrument (probe) penetrates into the pocket. The depth of penetration of a probe in a pocket depends on factors such as size of the probe, force with which it is introduced, direction of penetration, resistance of the tissues, and convexity of the crown. Probes presently used are described in Chapter 41.

Probe penetration can vary depending on the force of introduction, the shape and size of the probe tip and the degree of tissue inflammation.[4] Several studies have been made to determine the depth of penetration of a probe in a sulcus or pocket. Armitage and colleagues[5] used beagle dogs to evaluate the penetration of a probe using a standardized force of 25 grams. They reported that in healthy specimens, the probe penetrated the epithelium to about two thirds of its length; in gingivitis specimens, it stopped 0.1 mm short of its apical end; and in periodontitis specimens, the probe tip consistently went past the most apical cells of the junctional epithelium (Fig. 30-19).

In humans, the probe tip penetrates to the most coronal intact fibers of the connective tissue attachment.[25,52] The depth of penetration of the probe in the connective tissue apical to the junctional epithelium in a periodontal pocket is about 0.3 mm.[25,50,54] This is important in evaluating differences in probing depth before and after treatment, as the reduction in probe penetration may be a result of reduced inflammatory response rather than gain in attachment.[24,26]

The probing forces have been explored by several investigators[12,57]; forces of 0.75 N have been found to be well tolerated and accurate.[56] Interexaminer error (depth discrepancies between examiners) was reported to be as much as 2.1 mm, with an average of 1.5 mm, in the same areas.[18]

PROBING TECHNIQUE. The probe should be inserted parallel to the vertical axis of the tooth and "walked" circumferentially around each surface of each tooth to detect the areas of deepest penetration (Fig. 30-20).

In addition, special attention should be directed to detecting the presence of interdental craters and furcation involvements. To detect an interdental crater, the probe should be placed obliquely from both the facial and lingual surfaces so as to explore the deepest point of the pocket located beneath the contact point (Fig. 30-21). In multirooted teeth the possibility of furcation involvement should be carefully explored. The use of specially designed probes (e.g., Nabers probe) allows an easier and more accurate exploration of the horizontal component of furcation lesions (Fig. 30-22).

LEVEL OF ATTACHMENT VERSUS POCKET DEPTH. Pocket depth is the distance between the base of the pocket and the gingival margin. It may change from

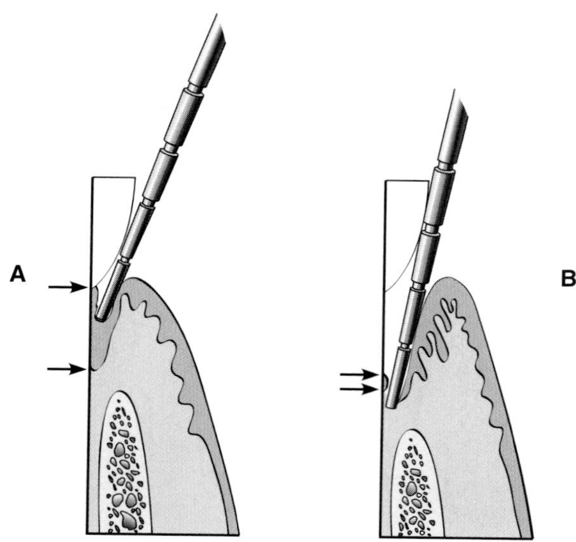

Fig. 30-19 A, In a normal sulcus with a long junctional epithelium (between arrows), the probe penetrates about one third to one half the length of the junctional epithelium. **B,** In a periodontal pocket with a short junctional epithelium (between arrows), the probe penetrates beyond the apical end of the junctional epithelium.

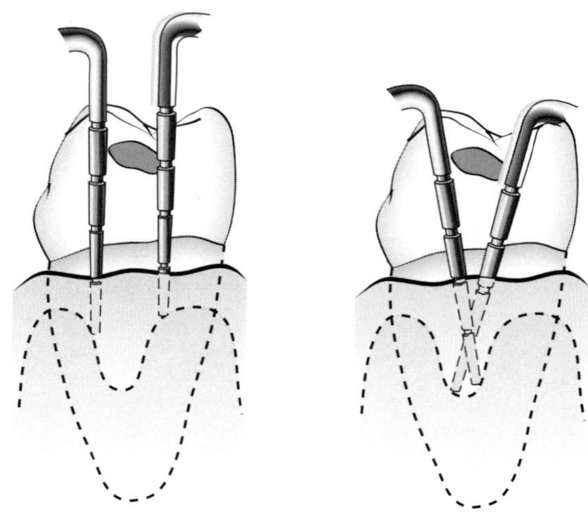

Fig. 30-21 Vertical insertion of the probe (left) may not detect interdental craters; oblique positioning of the probe (right) reaches the depth of the crater.

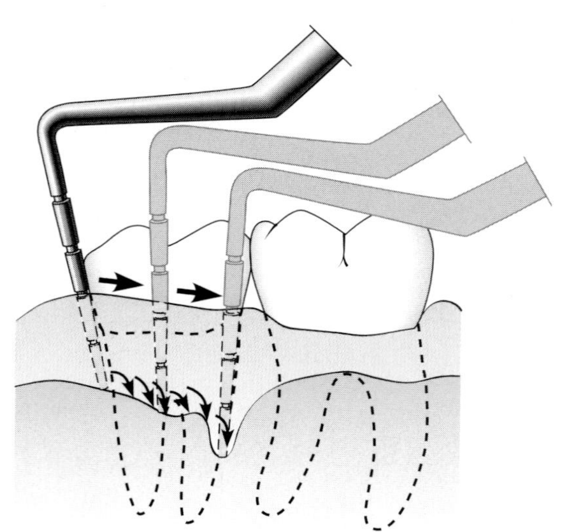

Fig. 30-20 "Walking" the probe to explore the entire pocket.

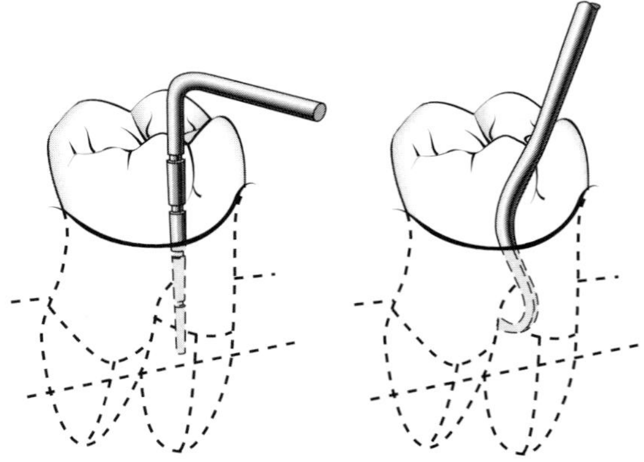

Fig. 30-22 Exploring with a periodontal probe (left) may not detect furcation involvement; specially designed instruments (Nabers probe) (right) can enter the furcation area.

time to time even in untreated periodontal disease owing to changes in the position of the gingival margin, and therefore it may be unrelated to the existing attachment of the tooth.

The level of attachment, on the other hand, is the distance between the base of the pocket and a fixed point on the crown, such as the cementoenamel junction. Changes in the level of attachment can be due only to gain or loss of attachment and afford a better indication of the degree of periodontal destruction. *Shallow pockets attached at the level of the apical third of the root connote more severe destruction than deep pockets attached at the coronal third of the roots* (see Chapter 22 and Figs. 22-19 and 22-20).

DETERMINING THE LEVEL OF ATTACHMENT. When the *gingival margin is located on the anatomic crown,* the level of attachment is determined by subtracting from the depth of the pocket the distance from the gingival margin to the cementoenamel junction. If both are the same, the loss of attachment is zero.

When the *gingival margin coincides with the cementoenamel junction,* the loss of attachment equals the pocket depth.

When the *gingival margin is located apical to the cementoenamel junction,* the loss of attachment is greater than the pocket depth, and therefore the distance between the cementoenamel junction and the gingival margin should be added to the pocket depth. Drawing the gingival margin on the chart where pocket depths are entered helps clarify this important point.

BLEEDING ON PROBING. The insertion of a probe to the bottom of the pocket elicits bleeding if the gingiva is inflamed and the pocket epithelium is atrophic or ulcerated. Noninflamed sites rarely bleed. In most cases, bleeding on probing is an earlier sign of inflammation than gingival color changes[32] (see Chapter 17). However, sometimes color changes are found with no bleeding on probing.[15] Depending on the severity of inflammation, bleeding can vary from a tenuous red line along the gingival sulcus to profuse bleeding.[1] After successful treatment, bleeding on probing ceases.[3]

To test for bleeding after probing, the probe is carefully introduced to the bottom of the pocket and gently moved laterally along the pocket wall. Sometimes bleeding appears immediately after removal of the probe; other times it may be delayed a few seconds. Therefore the clinician should recheck for bleeding 30 to 60 seconds after probing.

As a single test, bleeding on probing is not a good predictor of progressive attachment loss; however its absence is an excellent predictor of periodontal stability.[4] When present in multiple sites of advanced disease, bleeding on probing is a good indicator of progressive attachment loss.[4,17] Armitage analyzed the literature on this subject up to 1996, performing a meta-analysis of the various papers and concluded that the presence of bleeding on probing in a "treated and maintained patient population" is an important risk predictor for increased loss of attachment.[4]

Insertion of a soft wooden interdental stimulator in the interdental space produces a similar bleeding response[3] and can be used by the patient to self-examine the gingiva for the presence of inflammation.[10]

WHEN TO PROBE. Probing of pockets is done at various times for diagnosis, and for monitoring the course of treatment and maintenance. The initial probing of moderate or advanced cases is usually hampered by the presence of heavy inflammation and abundant calculus and cannot be done very accurately. The purpose of this initial probing, together with the clinical and radiographic examination is done, however, with the main purpose of determining whether the tooth can be saved or should be extracted. After the patient has performed an adequate plaque control for some time and calculus has been removed, the major inflammatory changes disappears, and a more accurate probing of the pockets can be performed. This second probing is for the purpose of accurately establishing the level of attachment and degree of involvement of roots and furcations. Data obtained from this probing provides valuable information for treatment decisions.

Further along periodontal treatment probings are done to determine changes in pocket depth and to ascertain healing progress after different procedures.

PROBING AROUND IMPLANTS. Since periimplantitis can create pockets around implants, probing around them becomes part of examination and diagnosis. To prevent scratching of the implant surface, plastic periodontal probes should be used instead of the usual steel probes used for the natural dentition.

Determination of Disease Activity. The determination of pocket depth or attachment levels does not provide information on whether the lesion is in an active or inactive state. Currently there is no sure method to determine activity or inactivity of a lesion. Inactive lesions may show little or no bleeding on probing and minimal amounts of gingival fluid; the bacterial flora, as revealed by dark-field microscopy, consists mostly of coccoid cells. Active lesions bleed more readily on probing and have large amounts of fluid and exudate; their bacterial flora shows a greater number of spirochetes and motile bacteria.[16] In patients with aggressive periodontitis, progressing and nonprogressing sites may show no differences in bleeding on probing.[27]

The precise determination of disease activity has a direct influence on diagnosis, prognosis, and therapy. The goals of therapy may change, depending on the state of the periodontal lesion. Chapter 34 describes in more detail the current state of knowledge in this important area.

Amount of Attached Gingiva. It is important to establish the relation between the bottom of the pocket and the mucogingival line. *The width of the attached gingiva is the distance between the mucogingival junction and the projection on the external surface of the bottom of the gingival sulcus or the periodontal pocket.* It should not be confused with the width of the keratinized gingiva, because the latter also includes the marginal gingiva (Fig. 30-23).

The width of the attached gingiva is determined by subtracting the sulcus or pocket depth from the total width of the gingiva (gingival margin to mucogingival line). This is done by stretching the lip or cheek to demarcate the mucogingival line while the pocket is being probed (Fig. 30-24). The amount of attached gingiva is generally considered to be insufficient when stretching of the lip or cheek induces movement of the free gingival margin.

Other methods used to determine the amount of attached gingiva include pushing the adjacent mucosa coronally with a dull instrument or painting the mucosa with Schiller's potassium iodide solution, which stains keratin.

Degree of Gingival Recession. During periodontal examination, it is necessary to record the data regarding the amount of gingival recession. This measurement is taken with a periodontal probe from the cemento-enamel junction to the gingival crest.

Alveolar Bone Loss. Alveolar bone levels are evaluated by clinical and radiographic examination. Probing is helpful for determining (1) the height and contour of the facial and lingual bones obscured on the radiograph by the dense roots and (2) the architecture of the interdental bone. Transgingival probing, performed after the area is anesthetized, is a more accurate method of evaluation and provides additional information on bone architecture[14,22,55] (see Chapter 62).

Palpation. Palpating the oral mucosa in the lateral and apical areas of the tooth may help locate the origin of radiating pain that the patient cannot localize. Infection deep in the periodontal tissues and the early stages of a periodontal abscess may also be detected by palpation.

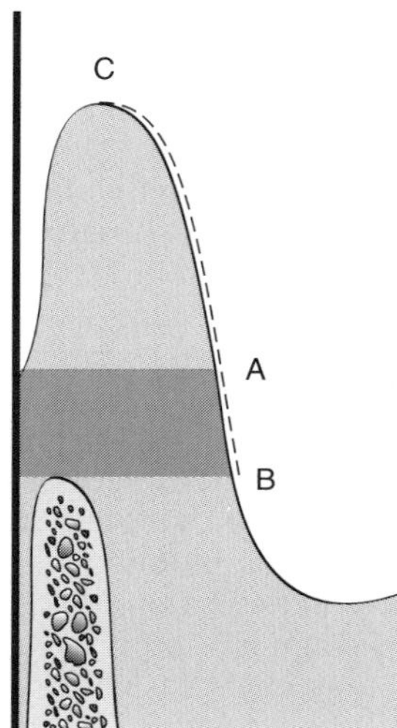

Fig. 30-23 The shaded area shows the attached gingiva, which extends between the projection on the external surface of the bottom of the pocket *(A)* and the mucogingival junction *(B)*. The keratinized gingiva may extend from the mucogingival junction *(B)* to the gingival margin *(C)*.

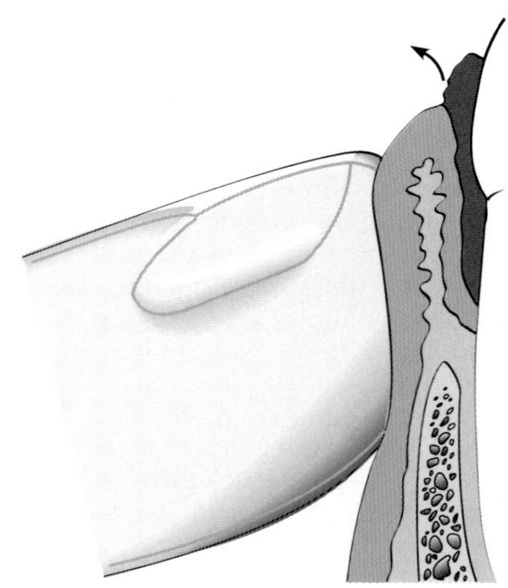

Fig. 30-25 Purulent exudate expressed from a periodontal pocket by digital pressure.

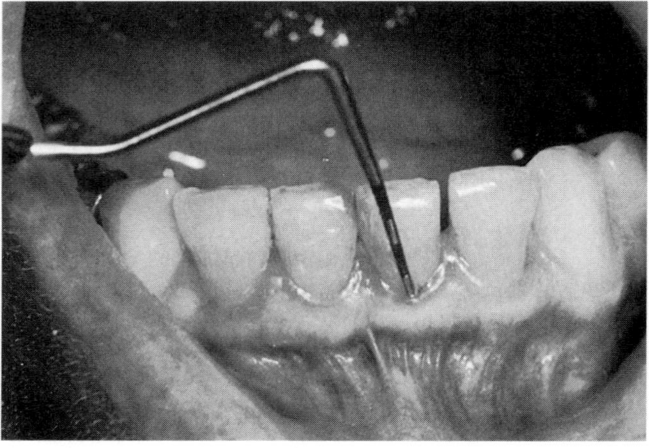

Fig. 30-24 To determine the width of the attached gingiva, the pocket is probed at the same time that the lip (or cheek) is extended to demarcate the mucogingival line.

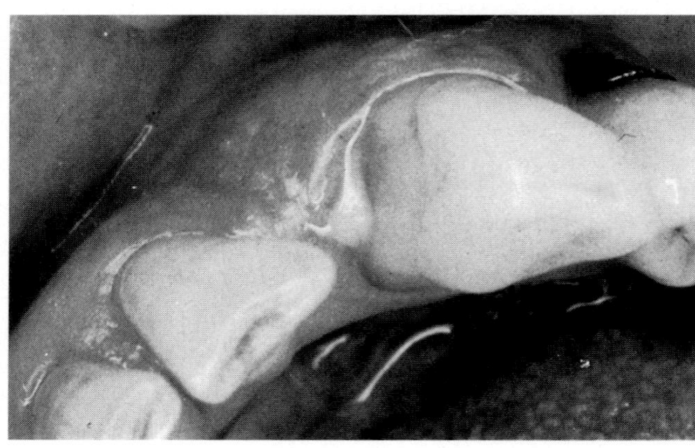

Fig. 30-26 Pus formation on the mesial surface of the mandibular canine.

Suppuration. The presence of an abundant number of neutrophils in the gingival fluid transforms it into a purulent exudate.[4] Several studies[6,7,10,20] have evaluated the association between suppuration and the progression of periodontitis and reported that this sign is present in a very low percentage of sites with the disease (3 to 5%).[4] Therefore it is not by itself a good indicator.

Clinically, the presence of pus in a periodontal pocket is determined by placing the ball of the index finger along the lateral aspect of the marginal gingiva and applying pressure in a rolling motion toward the crown (Fig. 30-25). Visual examination without digital pressure is not enough. The purulent exudate is formed in the inner pocket wall, and therefore the external appearance may give no indication of its presence. Pus formation does not occur in all periodontal pockets, but digital pressure often reveals it in pockets where its presence is not suspected (Fig. 30-26).

Periodontal Abscess. A periodontal abscess is a localized accumulation of pus within the gingival wall of a periodontal pocket (see Chapter 22). Periodontal abscesses may be acute or chronic.

The *acute periodontal abscess* appears as an ovoid elevation of the gingiva along the lateral aspect of the root (Figs. 30-27 to 30-29). The gingiva is edematous and red, with a smooth, shiny surface. The shape and consistency of the elevated area vary; the area may be domelike and

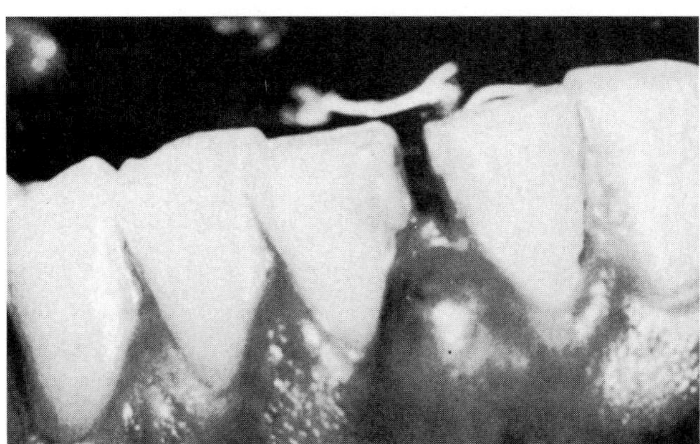

Fig. 30-27 Acute periodontal abscess between the lower central incisors.

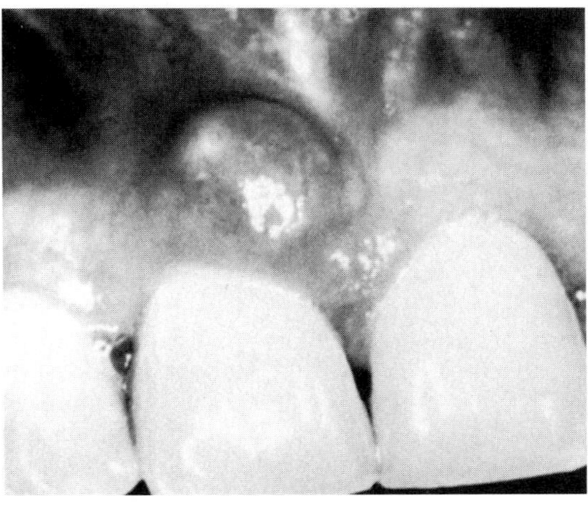

Fig. 30-28 Acute periodontal abscess associated with a deep periodontal pocket facial and mesial of upper central incisor.

relatively firm, or pointed and soft. In most cases, pus may be expressed from the gingival margin with gentle digital pressure.

The acute periodontal abscess is accompanied by symptoms such as throbbing, radiating pain; exquisite tenderness of the gingiva to palpation; sensitivity of the tooth to palpation; tooth mobility; lymphadenitis; and, less frequently, systemic effects such as fever, leukocytosis, and malaise. Occasionally, the patient may have symptoms of an acute periodontal abscess without any notable clinical lesion or radiographic changes.

The *chronic periodontal abscess* usually presents a sinus that opens onto the gingival mucosa somewhere along the length of the root. There may be a history of intermittent exudation. The orifice of the sinus may appear as a difficult-to-detect pinpoint opening, which, when probed, reveals a sinus tract deep in the periodontium (Fig. 30-30). The sinus may be covered by a small, pink, beadlike mass of granulation tissue (Fig. 30-31). The chronic periodontal abscess is usually asymptomatic. However, the patient may report episodes of dull, gnawing pain; slight elevation of the tooth; and a desire to bite down on and grind the tooth. The chronic periodontal abscess often undergoes acute exacerbations, with all the associated symptoms.

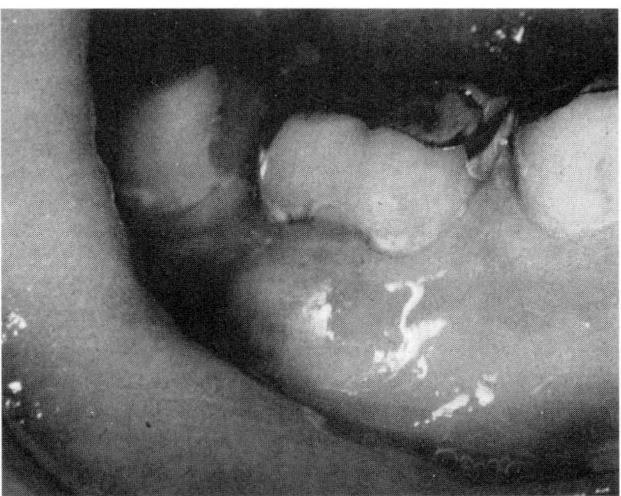

Fig. 30-29 Acute periodontal abscess in the wall of a deep pocket.

Diagnosis of the periodontal abscess requires correlation of the history and clinical and radiographic findings. The suspected area should be probed carefully along the gingival margin in relation to each tooth surface to detect a channel from the marginal area to the deeper periodontal tissues. Continuity of the lesion with the gingival margin is clinical evidence that the abscess is periodontal.

The abscess is not necessarily located on the same surface of the root as the pocket from which it is formed. A pocket at the facial surface may give rise to a periodontal abscess interproximally. It is common for a periodontal abscess to be located at a root surface other than that along which the pocket originated, because drainage is more likely to be impaired when a pocket follows a tortuous course.

In children a sinus orifice along the lateral aspect of a root is usually the result of periapical infection of a deciduous tooth. In the permanent dentition such an orifice may be caused by a periodontal abscess, as well as by apical involvement. The orifice may be patent and draining, or it may be closed and appear as a red, nodular mass (Fig. 30-32). Exploration of such masses with a probe usually reveals a pinpoint orifice that communicates with an underlying sinus.

Periodontal Abscess and Gingival Abscess. The principal differences between the periodontal abscess and the gingival abscess are the location and history

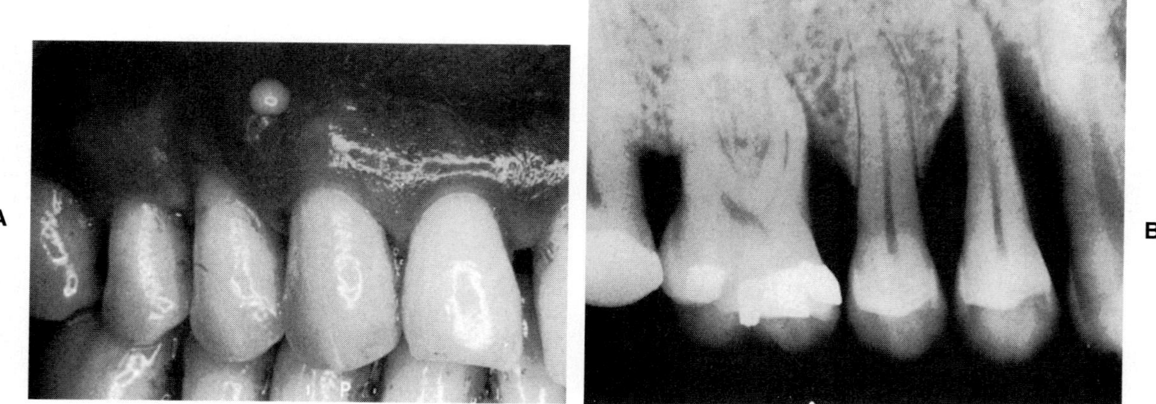

Fig. 30-30 Suppuration from a chronic periodontal abscess. **A,** Suppurative draining sinus between the canine and first premolar. **B,** Radiograph showing extensive bone destruction in the area of the draining sinus.

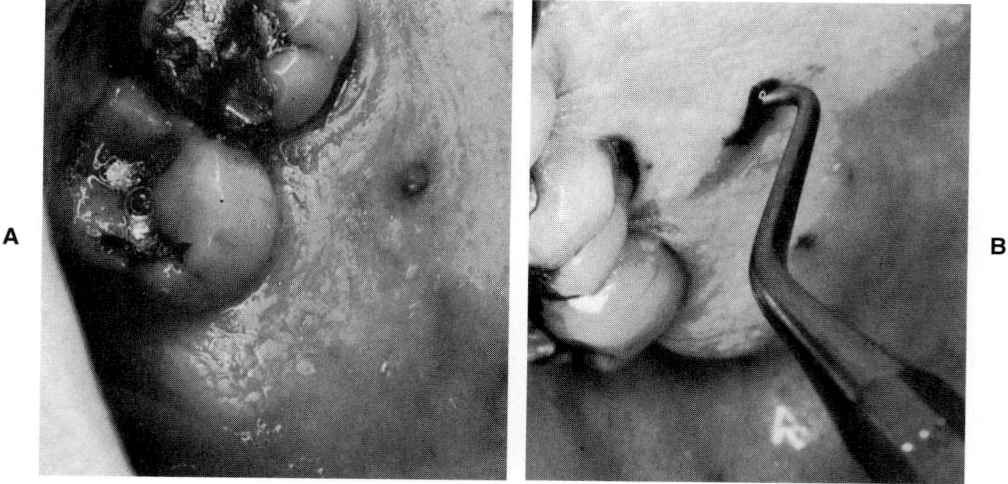

Fig. 30-31 Pinpoint orifice of a sinus from a palatal periodontal abscess. **A,** Pinpoint orifice on the palate indicative of a sinus from a periodontal abscess. **B,** Probe extends into the abscess deep in the periodontium.

(see Chapters 18 and 65). The gingival abscess is confined to the marginal gingiva, and it often occurs in previously disease-free areas (Fig. 30-33). It is usually an acute inflammatory response to forcing of foreign material into the gingiva. The periodontal abscess involves the supporting periodontal structures and generally occurs in the course of chronic destructive periodontitis.

Periodontal Abscess and Periapical Abscess. Several characteristics can be used as guidelines in differentiating a periodontal abscess from a periapical abscess. If the tooth is nonvital, the lesion is most likely periapical. However, a previously nonvital tooth can have a deep periodontal pocket that can abscess. Moreover, a deep periodontal pocket can extend to the apex and cause pulpal involvement and necrosis.

An apical abscess may spread along the lateral aspect of the root to the gingival margin. However, when the apex and lateral surface of a root are involved by a single lesion that can be probed directly from the gingival margin, the lesion is more likely to have originated in a periodontal abscess.

Radiographic findings are sometimes helpful in differentiating between a periodontal and a periapical lesion (see Chapter 31). Early acute periodontal and periapical abscesses present no radiographic changes. Ordinarily, a radiolucent area along the lateral surface of the root suggests the presence of a periodontal abscess, whereas apical rarefaction suggests a periapical abscess. However, acute periodontal abscesses that show no radiographic changes often cause symptoms in teeth with long-standing, radiographically detectable periapical lesions that are not con-

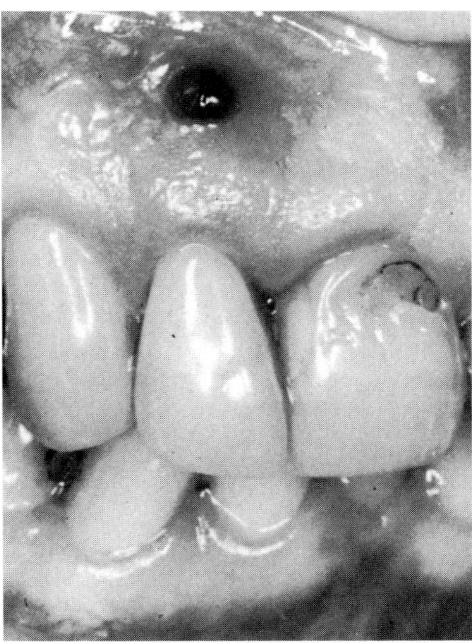

Fig. 30-32 Nodular mass at the orifice of a draining sinus.

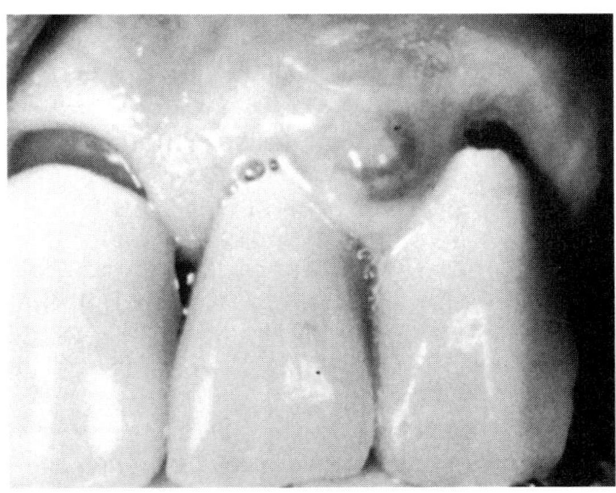

Fig. 30-33 Gingival abscess between upper lateral incisor and canine. The area is essentially free of gingivitis.

tributing to the patient's complaint. Clinical findings, such as the presence of extensive caries, pocket formation, lack of tooth vitality, and the existence of continuity between the gingival margin and the abscess area, often prove to be of greater diagnostic value than radiographic appearance.

A draining sinus on the lateral aspect of the root suggests periodontal rather than apical involvement; a sinus from a periapical lesion is more likely to be located further apically. However, sinus location is not conclusive. In many instances, particularly in children, the sinus from a periapical lesion drains on the side of the root rather than at the apex (see Chapter 65).

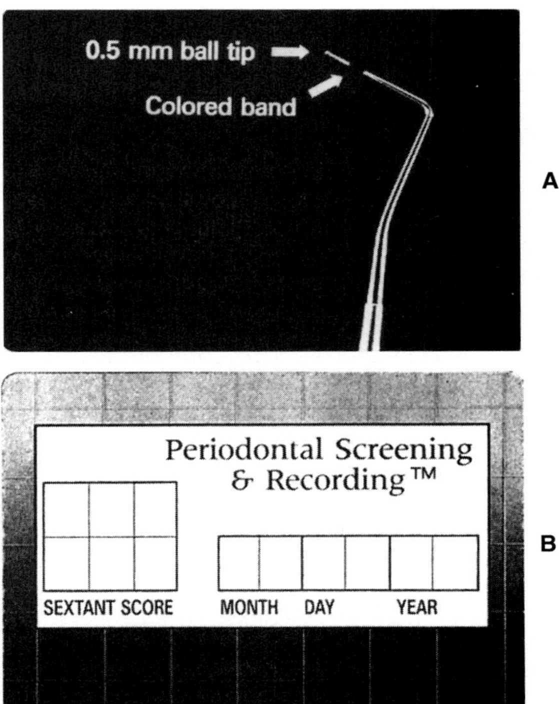

Fig. 30-34 **A,** Periodontal probe especially designed for the PSR system. Note the ball tip and the color coding, 3.5 to 5.5 mm from the probe tip. **B,** Special sticker to be placed in the patient's chart with the code for each sextant. (From the American Dental Association and the American Academy of Periodontology: Periodontal Screening & Recording Training Manual, 1992. Reprinted with permission from the American Dental Association.)

THE PERIODONTAL SCREENING AND RECORDING SYSTEM*

The Periodontal Screening & Recording™ (PSR®) system is designed for easier and faster screening and recording of the periodontal status of a patient by a general practitioner or a dental hygienist.[34] It uses a specially designed probe that has a 0.5-mm ball tip and is color coded from 3.5 to 5.5 mm (Fig. 30-34, *A*).

The patient's mouth is divided into six sextants (maxillary right, anterior, and left; mandibular left, anterior, and right). Each tooth is probed, with the clinician walking the probe around the entire tooth to examine at least six points around each tooth: mesiofacial, midfacial, distofacial, and the corresponding lingual/palatal areas. The deepest finding is recorded in each sextant, along with other findings, according to the following code:

Code 0: In the deepest sulcus of the sextant, the probe's colored band remains completely visible. Gingival tissue is healthy and does not bleed on gentle probing. No calculus or defective margins are found. These patients require only appropriate preventive care.

*Periodontal Screening & Recording™ and PSR® are service marks and trademarks of the American Dental Association.

Code 1: The colored band of the probe remains completely visible in the deepest sulcus of the sextant; no calculus or defective margins are found, but some bleeding after gentle probing is detected. Treatment for these patients consists of subgingival plaque removal and appropriate oral hygiene instructions.

Code 2: The probe's colored band is still completely visible, but there is bleeding on probing, and supragingival or subgingival calculus and/or defective margins are found. Treatment should include plaque and calculus removal, correction of plaque-retentive margins of restorations, and oral hygiene instruction.

Code 3: The colored band is partially submerged. This indicates the need for a comprehensive periodontal examination and charting of the affected sextant to determine the necessary treatment plan. If two or more sextants score Code 3, a comprehensive full-mouth examination and charting is indicated.

Code 4: The colored band completely disappears in the pocket, indicating a depth greater than 5.5 mm. In this case a comprehensive full-mouth periodontal examination, charting, and treatment planning are needed.

*Code *:* When any of the following abnormalities are seen, an asterisk (*) is entered, in addition to the code number: furcation involvement, tooth mobility, mucogingival problem, or gingival recession extending to the colored band of the probe (3.5 mm or greater).

The code finding for each sextant and the date are entered on a sticker (Fig. 30-34, *B*), which is placed on the patient's record.

LABORATORY AIDS TO CLINICAL DIAGNOSIS

When unusual gingival or periodontal problems are present and cannot be explained by local causes, the possibility of contributing systemic factors must be explored. The dentist must understand the oral manifestations of systemic disease so that he or she can question the patient's physician regarding the type of systemic disturbance that may be involved in individual cases.

Numerous laboratory tests aid in the diagnosis of systemic diseases. Descriptions of the manner in which they are performed and the interpretation of findings are provided in standard texts on the subject. Tests pertinent to the diagnosis of disturbances often manifested in the oral cavity are referred to briefly here.

Nutritional Status

If, when examining a patient, it is the dentist's impression that a nutritional deficiency exists, this suspicion must be corroborated by a medical evaluation of the patient's nutritional status. Nutritional therapy in the treatment of periodontal disturbances must be based on a demonstrated need, which is best determined by a nutritionist.

Certain signs and symptoms have been identified with different nutritional deficiencies. However, many patients with nutritional disease do not exhibit classic signs of deficiency disorders, and different types of deficiency produce comparable clinical findings. Clinical findings are suggestive, but definitive diagnosis of nutritional deficiencies and their nature requires the combined information revealed by the history, clinical and laboratory findings, and therapeutic trial. Clinical findings identified with specific nutritional deficiencies and the oral manifestations of nutritional disorders are described in Chapter 12.

Patients on Special Diets for Medical Reasons

Patients on low-residue, nondetergent diets often develop gingivitis because the prescribed foods lack cleansing action and the tendency for plaque and food debris to accumulate on the teeth is increased. Because fibrous foods are contraindicated, special effort is made to compensate for the soft diet by emphasizing the patient's oral hygiene procedures. Patients on salt-free diets should not be given saline mouthwashes, nor should they be treated with saline preparations without consulting their physician. Diabetes, gallbladder disease, and hypertension are examples of conditions in which particular care should be taken to avoid the prescription of contraindicated foodstuffs.

Blood Tests

Analyses of blood smears, red and white blood cell counts, white blood cell differential counts, and erythrocyte sedimentation rates are used to evaluate the presence of blood dyscrasias and generalized infections. Determination of coagulation time, bleeding time, clot retraction time, prothrombin time, capillary fragility test, and bone marrow studies may be required at times. They may be useful aids in the differential diagnosis of certain types of periodontal diseases; the reader is referred to books on hematology for a consideration of this subject.

Chapter 38 describes the use of these tests for the evaluation and management of medically compromised patients.

REFERENCES

1. Abrams K, Caton J, Polson AM: Histologic comparisons of interproximal gingival tissues related to the presence or absence of bleeding. J Periodontol 1984; 55:629.
2. Alexander AG, Tipnis AK: The effect of irregularity of teeth and the degree of overbite and overjet on the gingival health. Br Dent J 1970; 128:539.
3. Amato R, Caton J, Polson A, et al: Interproximal gingival inflammation related to the conversion of a bleeding to a non-bleeding state. J Periodontol 1986; 57:63.
4. Armitage GC: Periodontal diseases: Diagnosis. Ann Periodontol 1996; 1:37.
5. Armitage GC, Svanberg GK, Löe H: Microscopic evaluation of clinical measurements of connective tissue attachment levels. J Clin Periodontol 1977; 4:173.
6. Badersten A, Nilvéus R, Egelberg J: Effect of nonsurgical therapy. VII. Bleeding, suppuration and probing depth in sites with probing attachment loss. J Clin Periodontol 1985; 12:432.

7. Badersten A, Nilvéus R, Egelberg J: Scores of plaque, bleeding, suppuration and probing depth top predict probing attachment loss. Five years of observation following nonsurgical periodontal therapy. J Clin Periodontol 1990; 17:102.
8. Baumgartner HS: A voice-input computerized dental examination system using high resolution graphics. Compend Contin Educ Dent 1988; 9:446.
9. Berg M, Burrill DY, Fosdick LS: Chemical studies in periodontal disease. IV. Putrefactive rate as index of periodontal disease. J Dent Res 1947; 26:67.
10. Caton J, Polson A: The interdental bleeding index: A simplified procedure to monitor gingival health. Compend Contin Educ Dent 1985; 6:89.
11. Fischman SL, Picozzi A: Review of the literature: The methodology of clinical calculus evaluation. J Periodontol 1969; 40:607.
12. Gabathuler H, Hassel TM: A pressure sensitive periodontal probe. Helv Odontol Acta 1971; 15:114.
13. Grant DA, Grant DA, Flynn MJ, et al: Periodontal microbiota of mobile and non-mobile teeth. J Periodontol 1995; 66:386.
14. Greenberg J, Laster L, Listgarten MA: Transgingival probing as a potential estimator of alveolar bone level. J Periodontol 1976; 47:514.
15. Greenstein G: The role of bleeding upon probing in the diagnosis of periodontal disease. A literature review. J Periodontol 1984; 55:684.
16. Greenstein G, Caton J, Polson AM: Histologic characteristics associated with bleeding after probing and visual signs of inflammation. J Periodontol 1981; 52:420.
17. Haffajee, AD, Socransky, SS, Lindhe, J et al: Clinical risk indicators for periodontal attachment loss. J Clin Periodontol 1991; 18:117.
18. Hassel TM, German MA, Saxer UP: Periodontal probing: Interinvestigator discrepancies and correlations between probing force and recorded depth. Helv Odontol Acta 1973; 17:38, 1973.
19. Hirschfeld L: A calibrated silver point for periodontal diagnosis and recording. J Periodontol 1953; 24:94.
20. Kaldahl WB, Kalkwarf KL, Patil KD, et al: Relationship of gingival bleeding, gingival suppuration and supragingival plaque to attachment loss. J Periodontol 1990; 61:347.
21. Kitchen PC: The prevalence of tooth root exposure and the relation of the extent of such exposure to the degree of abrasion in differing age classes. J Dent Res 1941; 20:565.
22. Kim HY, Yi SW, Choi SH, et al: Bone probing measurement as a reliable evaluation of the bone level in periodontal defects. J Periodontol 2000; 71:729.
23. Kurashima K: Viscoelastic properties of periodontal tissue. Bull Tokyo Med Dent Univ 1965; 12:240.
24. Listgarten MA: Periodontal probing: What does it mean? J Clin Periodontol 1980; 7:165.
25. Listgarten MA, Mao R, Robinson PJ: Periodontal probing: The relationship of the probe tip to periodontal tissues. J Periodontol 1976; 47:511.
26. Magnusson I, Listgarten MA: Histological evaluation of probing depth following periodontal treatment. J Clin Periodontol 1980; 7:26.
27. Mandell RL, Ebersole JL, Socransky SS: Clinical, immunologic and microbiologic features of active disease sites in juvenile periodontitis. J Clin Periodontol 1987; 14:534.
28. Manly RS: Abrasion of cementum and dentin by modern dentifrices. J Dent Res 20:583, 1941.
29. Manly RS: Factors influencing tests on the abrasion of dentin by brushing with dentifrices. J Dent Res 1944; 23:59.
30. Mannerberg F: Saliva factors in cases of erosion. Odont Rev 1963; 14:156.
31. McCay CM, Wills L: Erosion of molar teeth by acid beverages. J Nutr 1949; 39:313.
32. Meitner SW, Zander HA, Iker HP, et al: Identification of inflamed gingival surfaces. J Clin Periodontol 1979; 6:93.
33. Miller WD: Experiments and observations on the wasting of tooth tissue variously designated as erosion, abrasion, chemical abrasion, denudation, etc. D Cosmos 1907; 49:1.
34. Mühlemann HR: Ten years of tooth mobility measurements. J Periodontol 1960; 31:110.
35. Mühlemann HR: Tooth mobility: A review of clinical aspects and research findings. J Periodontol 1967; 38:686.
36. Mühlemann HR, Savdir S, Rateitschak KH: Tooth mobility—its causes and significance. J Periodontol 1965; 36:148.
37. O'Leary TJ: Tooth mobility. Dent Clin North Am 1969; 3:567.
38. O'Leary TJ, Rudd KD: An instrument for measuring horizontal mobility. Periodontics 1963; 1:249.
39. Parfitt GJ: Measurement of the physiologic mobility of individual teeth in an axial direction. J Dent Res 1960; 39:608.
40. Parfitt GJ: The dynamics of a tooth in function. J Periodontol 1961; 32:102.
41. Periodontal Screening and Recording, Training Program: From the American Academy of Periodontology and the American Dental Association, sponsored by Procter & Gamble, 1992.
42. Perlitsch MJ: A systematic approach to the interpretation of tooth mobility and clinical implications. Dent Clin North Am 1980; 24:177.
43. Persson R: Assessment of tooth mobility using small loads. II. Effect of oral hygiene procedures. J Clin Periodontol 1980; 7:506.
44. Persson R: Assessment of tooth mobility using small loads. III. Effect of periodontal treatment including a gingivectomy procedure. J Clin Periodontol 1981; 8:4.
45. Persson R: Assessment of tooth mobility using small loads. IV. The effect of periodontal treatment including gingivectomy and flap procedures. J Clin Periodontol 1981; 8:88.
46. Persson R, Svensson A: Assessment of tooth mobility using small loads. I. Technical devices and calculations of tooth mobility in periodontal health and disease. J Clin Periodontol 1980; 7:259.
47. Ratcliff PA, Johnson PW. The relationship between malodor, gingivitis and periodontitis. A review. J Periodontol 1999; 70:485.
48. Robinson HBG: Abrasion, attrition and erosion of teeth. Health Center J Ohio State Univ 1949; 3:21.
49. Rosenberg M: Clinical assessment of bad breath: Current concepts. J Amer Dent Assoc 1966; 127:475.
50. Saglie R, Johanson JR, Flotra L: The zone of completely and partially destructed periodontal fibers in pathological pockets. J Clin Periodontol 1975; 2:198.
51. Schulte W, D'Hoedt B, Scholz F, et al: Periotest-neues Messverfahren der Funktion des Parodontiums. Zahnarztl Mitt 1983; 73:1229.
52. Sivertson JF, Burgett FG: Probing of pockets related to the attachment level. J Periodontol 1976; 47:281.
53. Sognnaes RF: Periodontal significance of intraoral frictional ablation. J West Soc Periodontol 1977; 25:112.
54. Spray JR, Garnick JJ, Doles LR, et al: Microscopic demonstration of the position of periodontal probes. J Periodontol 1978; 49:148.
55. Tibbetts LS: Use of diagnostic probes for detection of periodontal disease. J Am Dent Assoc 78:549, 1969.
56. Van der Velden U: Probing force and the relationship of the probe tip to the periodontal tissues. J Clin Periodontol 1979; 6:106.
57. Van der Velden U, De Vries JH: Introduction of a new periodontal probe. The pressure probe. J Clin Periodontol 1978; 5:188.

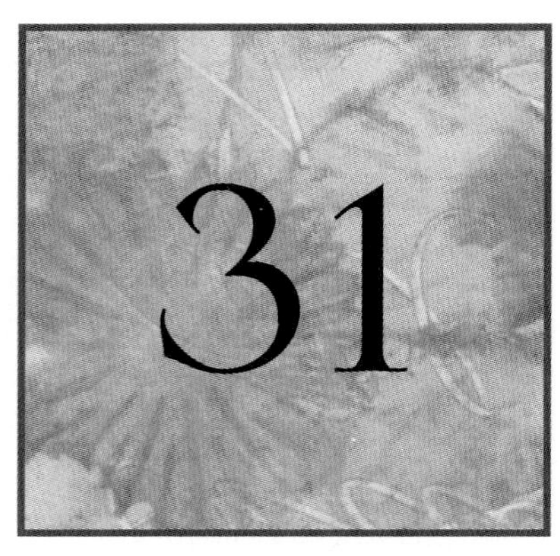

CHAPTER 31

Radiographic Aids in the Diagnosis of Periodontal Disease

Fermin A. Carranza and Henry H. Takei

CHAPTER OUTLINE

RADIOGRAPHS IN THE DIAGNOSIS OF PERIODONTAL DISEASE

The radiograph is a valuable aid in the diagnosis of periodontal disease, determination of the prognosis, and evaluation of the outcome of treatment. However, *it is an adjunct to the clinical examination, not a substitute for it.*

The radiograph reveals alterations in calcified tissue; it does not reveal current cellular activity but shows the effects of past cellular experience on the bone and roots. Special techniques that are not yet in routine clinical usage are required to show changes in the soft tissues of the periodontium.

Normal Interdental Septa

Radiographic evaluation of bone changes in periodontal disease is based mainly on the appearance of the interdental septa, because the relatively dense root structure obscures the facial and lingual bony plates. The interdental septum normally presents a thin radiopaque border, adjacent to the periodontal ligament and at the crest, that is referred to as the *lamina dura* (Fig. 31-1). This appears radiographically as a continuous white line, but in reality it is perforated by numerous small foramina, traversed by blood vessels, lymphatics, and nerves, which pass between the periodontal ligament and the bone. *Because the lamina dura represents the bone surface lining the tooth socket, the shape and position of the root and changes in the angulation of the x-ray beam produce considerable variations in its appearance.*[15]

The width and shape of the interdental septum and the angle of the crest normally vary according to the convexity of the proximal tooth surfaces and the level of the cementoenamel junction of the approximating teeth.[27] The interdental space and therefore the interdental septum between teeth with prominently convex proximal surfaces are wider anteroposteriorly than are those between teeth with relatively flat proximal surfaces. The faciolingual diameter of the bone is related to the width of the proximal root surface. The angulation of the crest of the interdental septum is generally parallel to a line between the cementoenamel junctions of the approximating teeth (see Fig. 31-1). When there is a difference in the levels of the cementoenamel junctions, the crest of the interdental bone appears angulated rather than horizontal.

Distortions Produced by Variations in Radiographic Technique

Variations in technique produce artifacts that limit the diagnostic value of the radiograph. The bone level, pattern of bone destruction, and width of the periodontal ligament space,[31] as well as the radiodensity, trabecular pattern, and marginal contour of the interdental septum are modified by altering the exposure and development time, type of film, and x-ray angulation.[17] Standardized, reproducible techniques are required to obtain reliable radiographs for pretreatment and posttreatment comparisons.[16,22,29] A grid calibrated in millimeters, superimposed on the finished film, is helpful for comparing bone levels in radiographs taken under similar conditions[6] (Fig. 31-2).

The following discussion includes useful facts regarding the effects of angulation. The long cone paralleling technique projects the most realistic image of the level of the alveolar bone[8] (Fig. 31-3). The bisection-of-the-angle technique increases the projection and makes the bone margin appear closer to the crown; the level of the facial bone margin is distorted more than that of the lingual margin (see Fig. 31-3). Shifting the cone mesially or distally without changing the horizontal plane projects the x-rays obliquely and changes the shape of the interdental bone on the radiograph, the radiographic width of the periodontal ligament space, and the appearance of the lamina dura. It may also distort the extent of furcation involvement (Fig. 31-4).[18]

Prichard[21] established the following four criteria to determine adequate angulation of periapical radiographs:

1. The radiograph should show the tips of molar cusps with little or none of the occlusal surface showing.
2. Enamel caps and pulp chambers should be distinct.
3. Interproximal spaces should be open.
4. Proximal contacts should not overlap unless teeth are out of line anatomically.

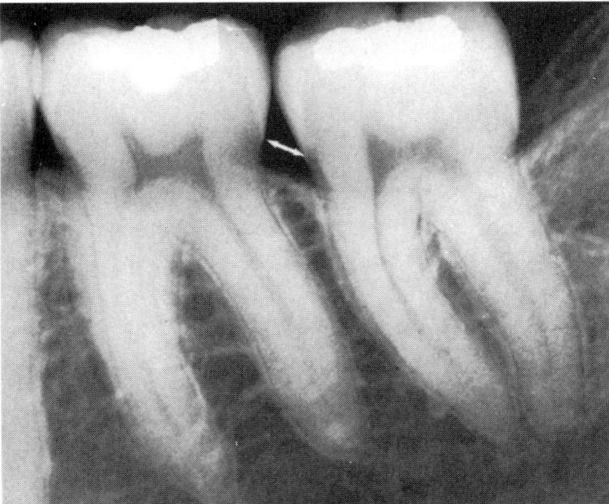

Fig. 31-1 Crest of interdental septum normally parallel to a line drawn between the cementoenamel junction of adjacent teeth *(arrow)*. Note also the radiopaque lamina dura around the roots and interdental septum.

Bone Destruction in Periodontal Disease

The radiograph does not reveal minor destructive changes in bone[3,4,23]; therefore slight radiographic changes in the periodontal tissues mean that the disease has progressed beyond its earliest stages. *The earliest signs of periodontal disease must be detected clinically.*

The radiographic image tends to show less severe bone loss than that actually present.[30] The difference between the alveolar crest height and the radiographic appearance ranges from 0 to 1.6 mm,[25] mostly accounted for by x-ray angulation.

Amount of Bone Loss. The radiograph is an indirect method for determining the amount of bone loss in periodontal disease; it shows the amount of remaining bone rather than the amount lost. The amount of bone lost is estimated to be the difference between the physiologic bone level of the patient and the height of the remaining bone.

The distance from the cementoenamel junction (CEJ) to the alveolar crest has been analyzed by several investigators.[12,14,25] Most studies have been conducted in adolescents and the general consensus seems to be a distance of 2 mm; this distance may be greater in older patients.

Distribution of Bone Loss. The distribution of bone loss is an important diagnostic sign. It points to the location of destructive local factors in different areas of the mouth and in relation to different surfaces of the same tooth.

Pattern of Bone Destruction. *In periodontal disease, the interdental septa undergo changes that affect the*

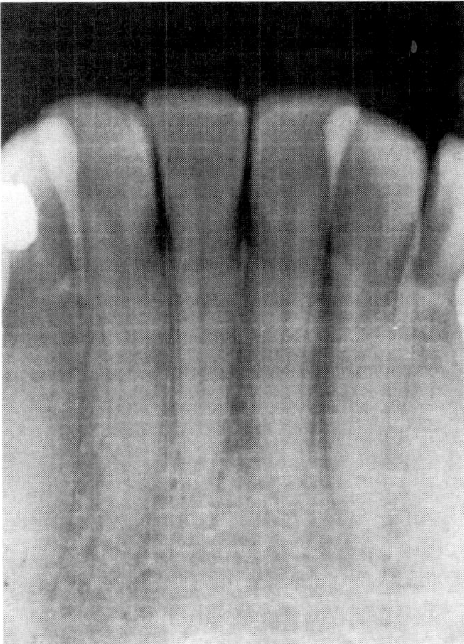

Fig. 31-2 Radiograph with superimposed grid calibrated in millimeters.

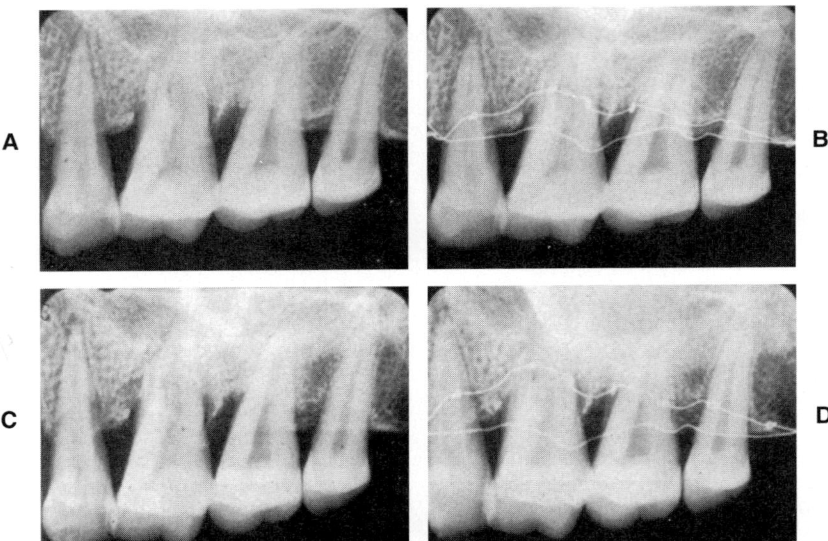

Fig. 31-3 Long cone paralleling technique and bisection of the angle technique compared. **A,** Long cone technique. Radiograph of dried specimen. **B,** Long cone technique. Same specimen. The smooth wire is on the margin of the facial plate and the knotted wire is on the lingual plate to show their relative positions. **C,** Bisection of the angle technique. Same specimen. **D,** Bisection of the angle technique. Same specimen. Both bone margins are shifted toward the crown, the facial margin (smooth wire) more than the lingual margin (knotted wire), creating the illusion that the lingual bone margin has shifted apically. (Courtesy Dr. Benjamin Patur, Hartford, CT.)

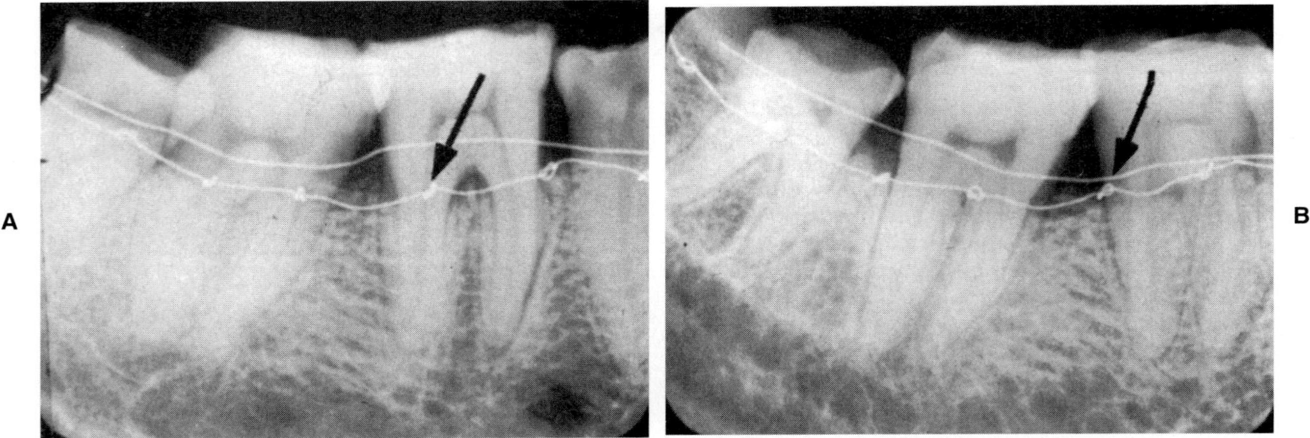

Fig. 31-4 Distortion by oblique projection. **A,** Long cone technique. The smooth wire is on the facial bony plate, the knotted wire on the lingual. Note the knot *(arrow)* near the center of the distal root of the first molar, which shows bifurcation involvement. **B,** Long cone technique. Cone is placed distally, projecting the rays mesially and obliquely. The oblique projection shifts the image of all structures mesially. *The structures closest to the cone shift the most.* This creates the illusion that the knot *(arrow)* has moved distally. Note that the bifurcation involvement shown in **A** is obliterated in **B.** (Courtesy Dr. Benjamin Patur, Hartford, CT.)

lamina dura, crestal radiodensity, size and shape of the medullary spaces, and height and contour of the bone. The interdental septa may be reduced in height, with the crest horizontal and perpendicular to the long axis of the adjacent teeth (Fig. 31-5), or they may have angular or arcuate defects (Fig. 31-6). The former condition is called *horizontal bone loss,* the latter *angular* or *vertical bone loss* (see Chapter 23).

Radiographs do not indicate the internal morphology or depth of the craterlike interdental defects, which appear as angular or vertical defects, nor do they reveal the extent of involvement on the facial and lingual surfaces. There are several reasons for this. Facial and lingual surface bone destruction is obscured by the dense root structure, and bone destruction on the mesial and distal root surfaces may be partially hidden by a dense mylo-

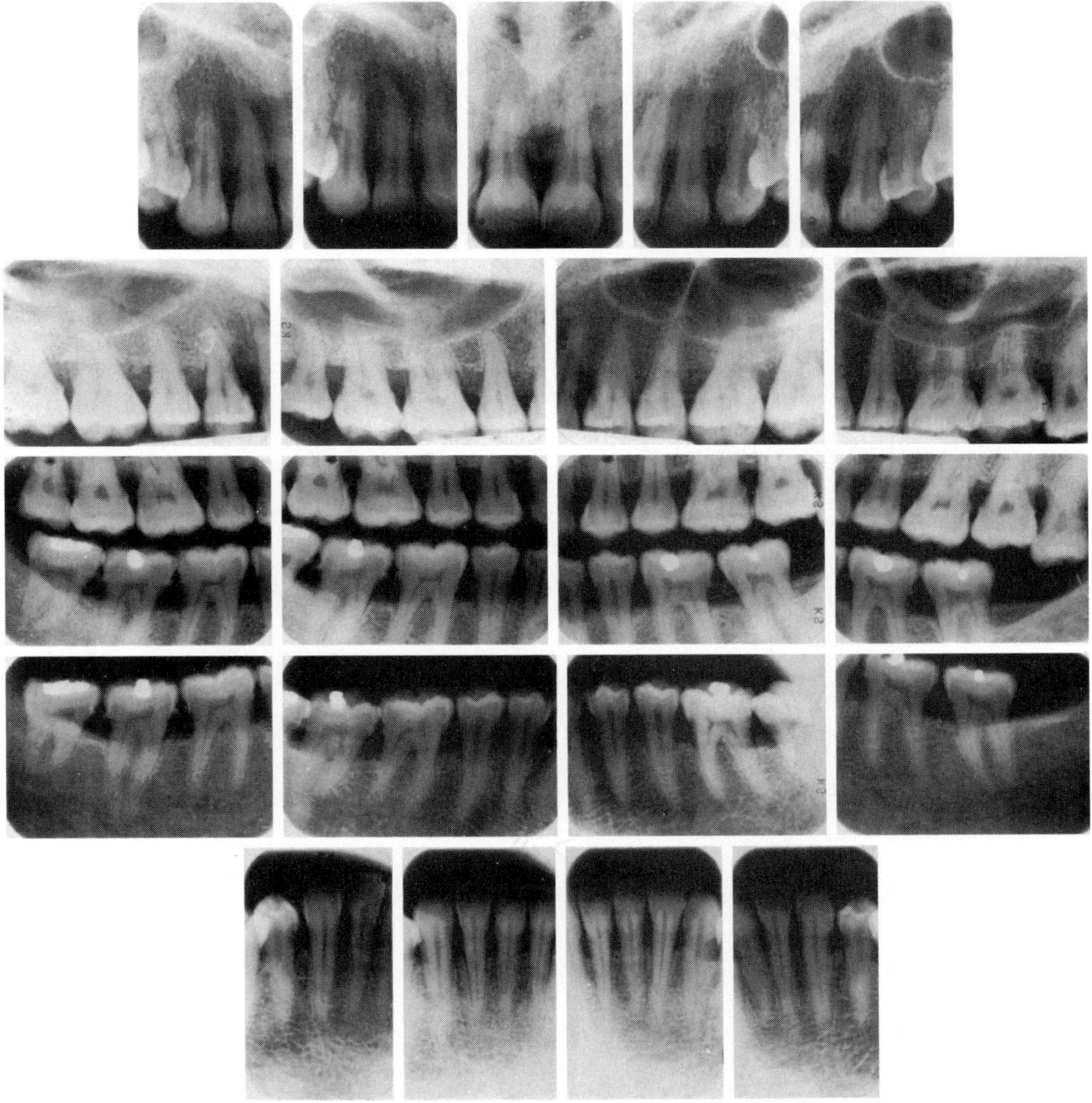

Fig. 31-5 Generalized horizontal bone loss.

hyoid ridge (Fig. 31-7). In most cases it can be assumed that bone losses seen interdentally continue in either the facial or lingual aspects creating a troughlike lesion. The true lesion can only be detected by clinically probing the defect.

Dense cortical plates on the facial and lingual surfaces of the interdental septa obscure destruction that occurs in the intervening cancellous bone. Thus it is possible to have a deep crater in the bone between the facial and lingual plates without radiographic indications of its presence. For destruction of the interproximal cancellous bone to be recorded radiographically, the cortical bone must be involved. A reduction of only 0.5 or 1.0 mm in the thickness of the cortical plate is sufficient to permit radiographic visualization of destruction of the inner cancellous trabeculae.[19]

Interdental vertical lesions in the posterior area with thick facial or lingual bone may not be isolated in the interdental area but may continue facially or lingually or both to form a troughlike defect that cannot be seen radiographically. These lesions may terminate on either the radicular surface or may communicate with the adjacent interdental area to form one continuous lesion (Fig. 31-8).

Fig. 31-9 shows two adjacent interdental lesions connecting on the radicular surface to form one interconnecting osseous lesion. Along with clinical probing of these lesions, the use of a radiopaque pointer placed in these radicular defects will demonstrate the extent of the bone loss.

Gutta percha packed around the teeth increases the usefulness of the radiograph for detecting the morphologic changes of osseous craters and involvement of the facial and lingual surfaces (Fig. 31-10). However, this is a cumbersome technique and is seldom performed. Surgical exposure and visual examination provide the most

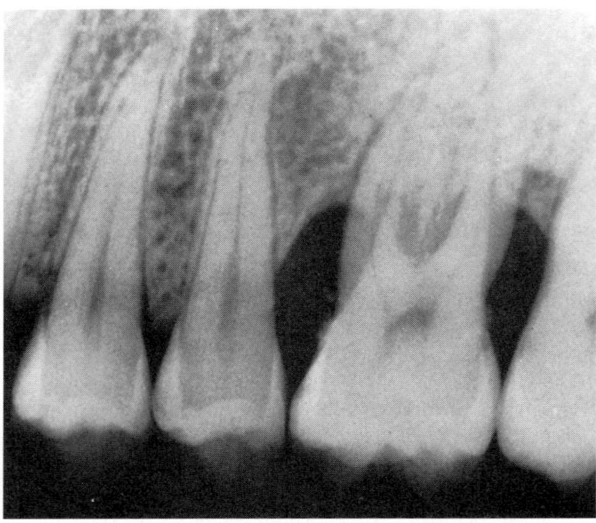

Fig. 31-6 Angular bone loss on first molar with involvement of the furcation.

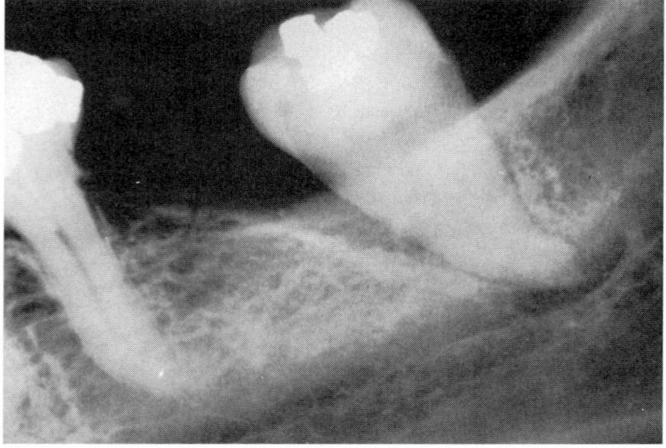

Fig. 31-7 Angular bone loss on mandibular molar partially obscured by dense mylohyoid ridge.

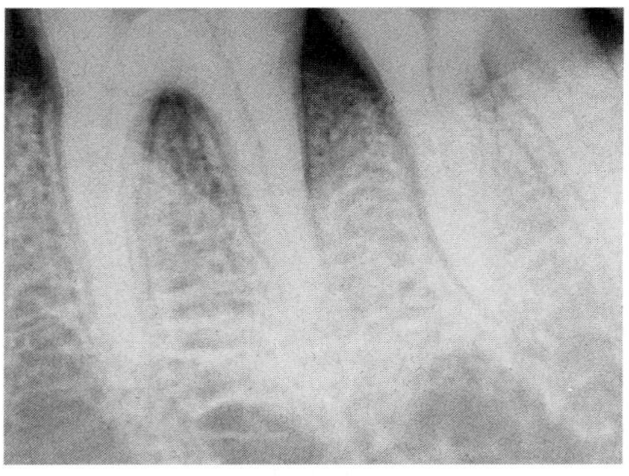

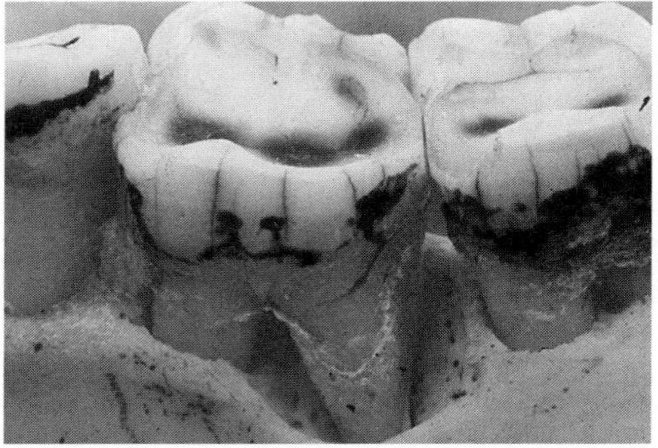

Fig. 31-8 **A and B,** Interdental lesion that extends to the facial or lingual surfaces in a trough-like manner.

definitive information regarding the bone architecture produced by periodontal destruction.[20]

Radiographic Changes in Periodontitis

The following is the sequence of radiographic changes in periodontitis and the tissue changes that produce them:

1. *Fuzziness and a break in the continuity of the lamina dura* at the mesial or distal aspect of the crest of the interdental septum have been considered as the earliest radiographic changes in periodontitis (Fig. 31-11). These result from the extension of gingival inflammation into the bone causing widening of the vessel channels and a reduction in calcified tissue at the septal margin.

   These changes are however highly dependent on the radiographic technique (angulation of the tube, placement of the film) and on anatomical variations (thickness and density of the interdental bone, position of adjoining teeth). No correlation has been found between crestal lamina dura in radiographs and the presence or absence of clinical inflammation, bleeding on probing, periodontal pockets, or loss of attachment.[11,24] Therefore it can be concluded that the presence of an intact crestal lamina dura may be an indicator of periodontal health, whereas its absence lacks diagnostic relevance.[2]
2. A *wedge-shaped radiolucent area* is formed at the mesial or distal aspect of the crest of the septal bone (see Fig. 31-11, *B*). The apex of the area is pointed in the direction of the root. This is produced by resorption of the bone of the lateral aspect of the interdental septum, with an associated widening of the periodontal space.
3. The destructive process extends across the crest of the interdental septum and *the height is reduced.* Fingerlike radiolucent projections extend from the crest into the septum (see Fig. 31-11, *C*). The radiolucent projections into the interdental septum are the result of the deeper extension of the inflammation into the bone. Inflammatory cells and fluid, proliferation of connective tissue cells, and increased osteoclasis cause increased bone resorption along the endosteal margins of the medullary spaces. The radiopaque projections, separating the radiolucent spaces, are the composite images of the partially eroded bony trabeculae.

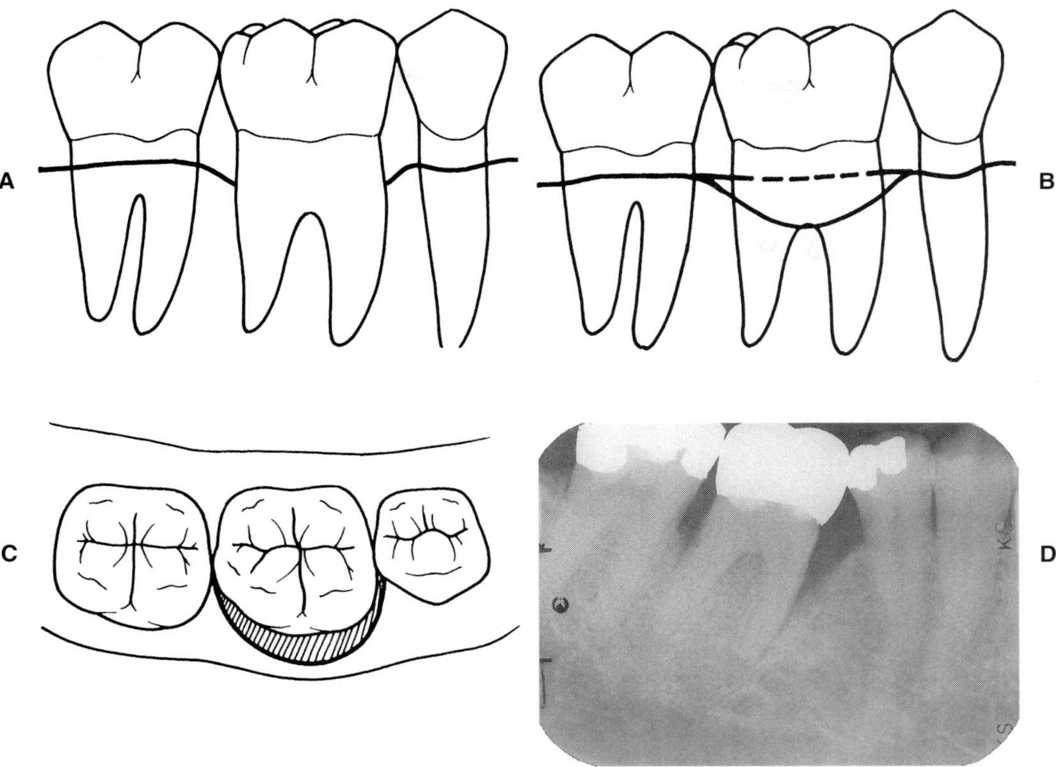

Fig. 31-9 **A,** Interdental mesial and distal lesions. **B,** Facial or lingual outlines of actual lesion. **C,** Occlusal view of lesion. **D,** Actual radiograph of mesial and facial lesions.

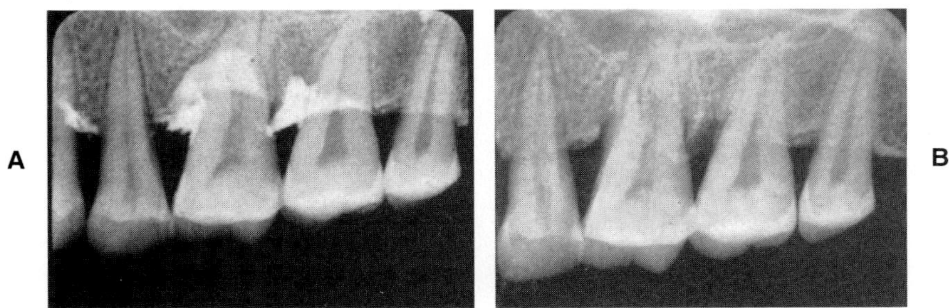

Fig. 31-10 Gutta percha aids in detecting bone defects. **A,** Gutta percha packed around teeth shows interproximal and facial and lingual bone loss. **B,** Same area without gutta percha gives little indication of the extent of bone involvement.

4. The height of the interdental septum (see Fig. 31-11, *D*) is progressively reduced by the extension of inflammation and the resorption of bone.

Radiographic Appearance of Interdental Craters

Interdental craters are seen as irregular areas of reduced radiopacity on the alveolar bone crests[26]; they are generally not sharply demarcated from the rest of the bone, with which they blend gradually. Radiographs do not accurately depict the morphology or depth of interdental craters, which sometimes appear as vertical defects.

Radiographic Appearance of Furcation Involvements

Definitive diagnosis of furcation involvement is made by clinical examination, which includes careful probing with a specially designed probe (Nabers probe). Radiographs are helpful but show artifacts that make it

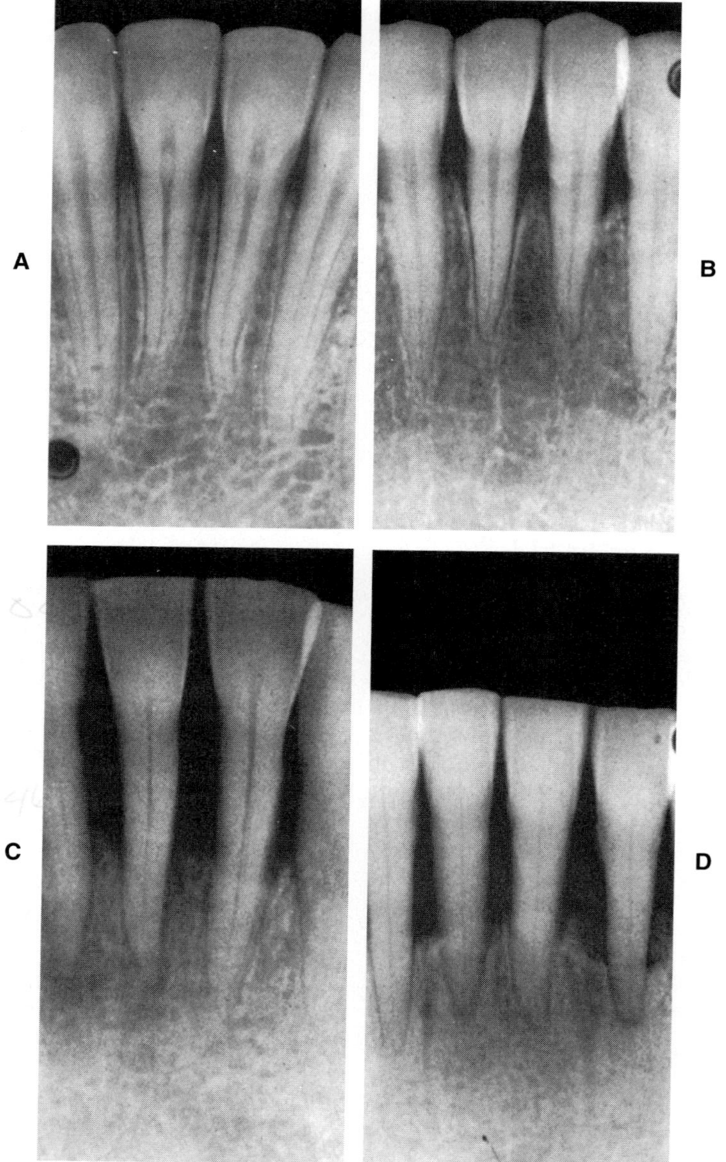

Fig. 31-11 Radiographic changes in periodontitis. **A,** Normal appearance of interdental septa. **B,** Fuzziness and a break in the continuity of the lamina dura at the crest of the bone distal to the central incisor *(left).* There are wedge-shaped radiolucent areas at the crests of the other interdental septa. **C,** Radiolucent projections from the crest into the interdental septum indicate extension of destructive processes. **D,** Severe bone loss.

possible for furcation involvement to be present without detectable radiographic changes.

As a general rule, bone loss is always greater than it appears in the radiograph. Variations in the radiographic technique may obscure the presence and extent of furcation involvement. A tooth may present marked bifurcation involvement in one film (Fig. 31-12, *A*) but appear to be uninvolved in another (see Fig. 31-12, *B*). Radiographs should be taken at different angles to reduce the risk of missing furcation involvement.

The recognition of large, clearly defined radiolucency in the furcation area presents no problem (see Fig. 31-12, *A*), but less clearly defined radiographic changes produced by furcation involvement are often overlooked. To assist in the radiographic detection of furcation involvement, the following diagnostic criteria are suggested:

1. The slightest radiographic change in the furcation area should be investigated clinically, especially if there is bone loss on adjacent roots (Fig. 31-13).
2. Diminished radiodensity in the furcation area in which outlines of bony trabeculae are visible (Fig. 31-14) suggests furcation involvement.
3. Whenever there is marked bone loss in relation to a single molar root, it may be assumed that the furcation is also involved (Figs. 31-15 and 31-16).

A

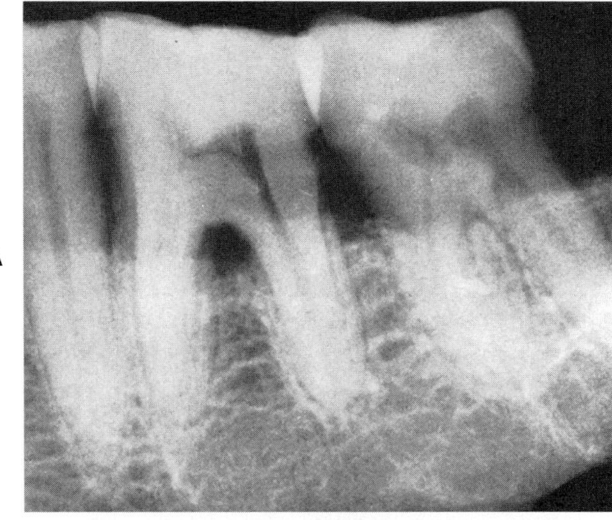

B

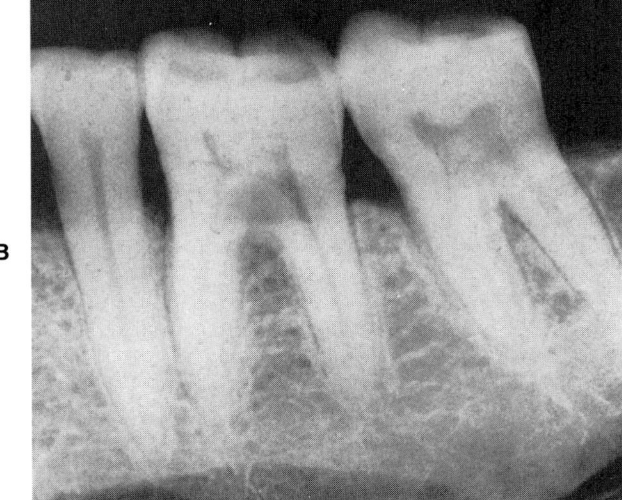

Fig. 31-12 A, Furcation involvement indicated by triangular radiolucency in bifurcation area of mandibular first molar. The second molar presents only a slight thickening of the periodontal space in the bifurcation area. **B,** Same area, different angulation. The triangular radiolucency in the bifurcation of the first molar is obliterated, and involvement of the second molar bifurcation is apparent.

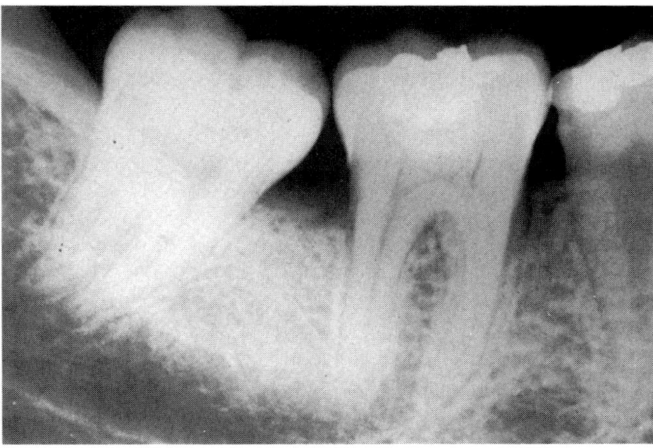

Fig. 31-13 Early furcation involvement suggested by fuzziness in the bifurcation of the mandibular first molar, particularly when associated with bone loss on the roots.

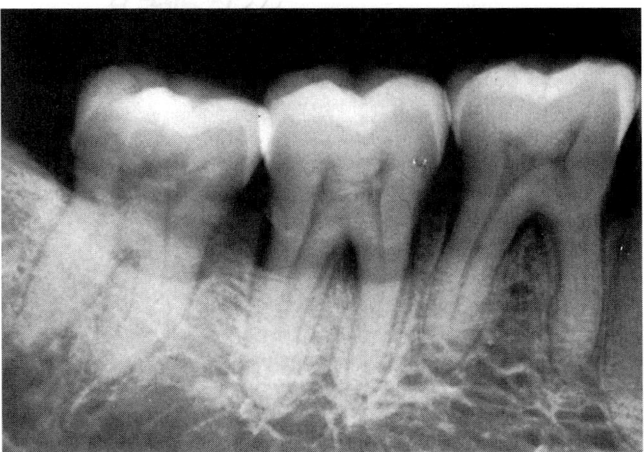

Fig. 31-14 Furcation involvement of mandibular first and second molars indicated by thickening of periodontal space in furcation area. The furcation of the third molar is also involved, but the thickening of the periodontal space is partially obscured by the external oblique line.

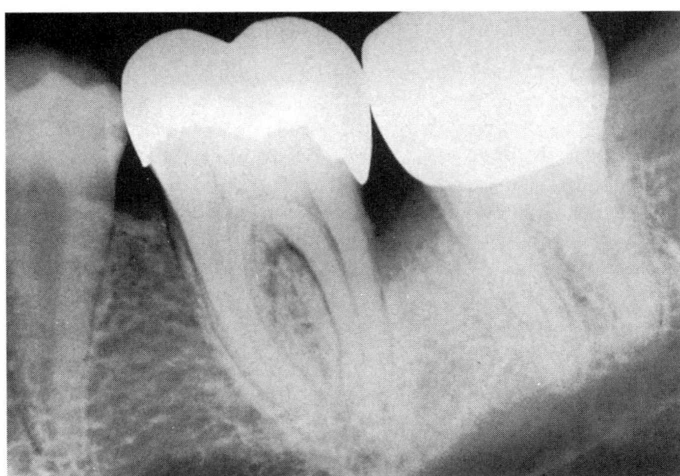

Fig. 31-15 Furcation involvement of the first molar, associated with bone loss on the distal root.

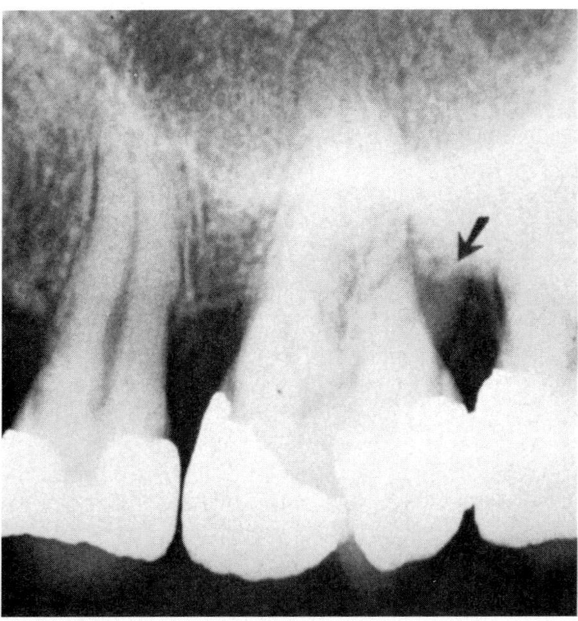

Fig. 31-16 Furcation involvement of the first molar partially obscured by the radiopaque lingual root. The horizontal line across the distobuccal root demarcates the apical portion *(arrow),* which is covered by bone, from the remainder of the root, where the bone has been destroyed.

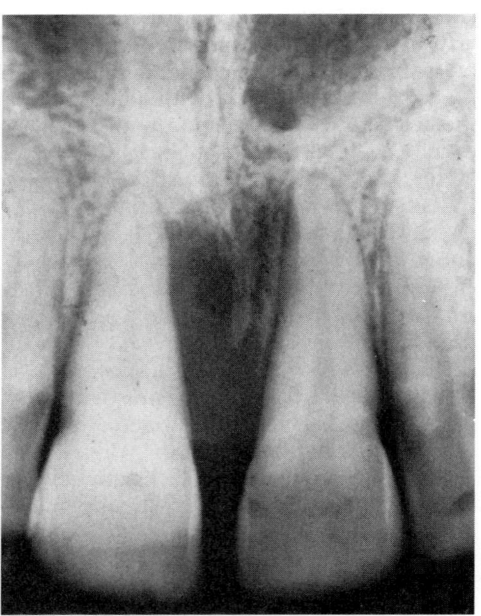

Fig. 31-18 Typical radiographic appearance of periodontal abscess on right central incisor.

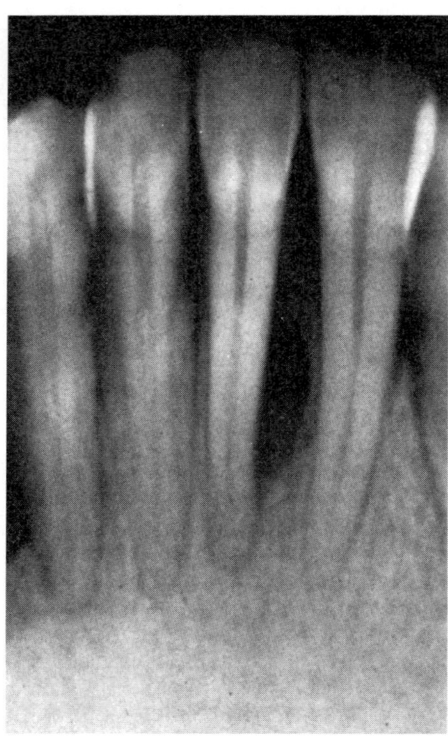

Fig. 31-17 Radiolucent area on the lateral aspect of the root with chronic periodontal abscess.

Radiographic Appearance of the Periodontal Abscess

The typical radiographic appearance of the periodontal abscess is that of a discrete area of radiolucency along the lateral aspect of the root (Figs. 31-17 and 31-18). *However, the radiographic picture is often not typical* (Fig. 31-19) because of many variables such as the following:

1. *The stage of the lesion.* In the early stages the acute periodontal abscess is extremely painful but presents no radiographic changes.
2. *The extent of bone destruction and the morphologic changes of the bone.*
3. *The location of the abscess.* Lesions in the soft tissue wall of a periodontal pocket are less likely to produce radiographic changes than those deep in the supporting tissues. Abscesses on the facial or lingual surface are obscured by the radiopacity of the root; interproximal lesions are more likely to be visualized radiographically.

Therefore *the radiograph alone cannot be relied on for the diagnosis of a periodontal abscess.*

Radiographs and Clinical Probing

Regenerative and resective flap designs and incisions require prior knowledge of the underlying osseous topography. Careful probing of these pocket areas after scaling

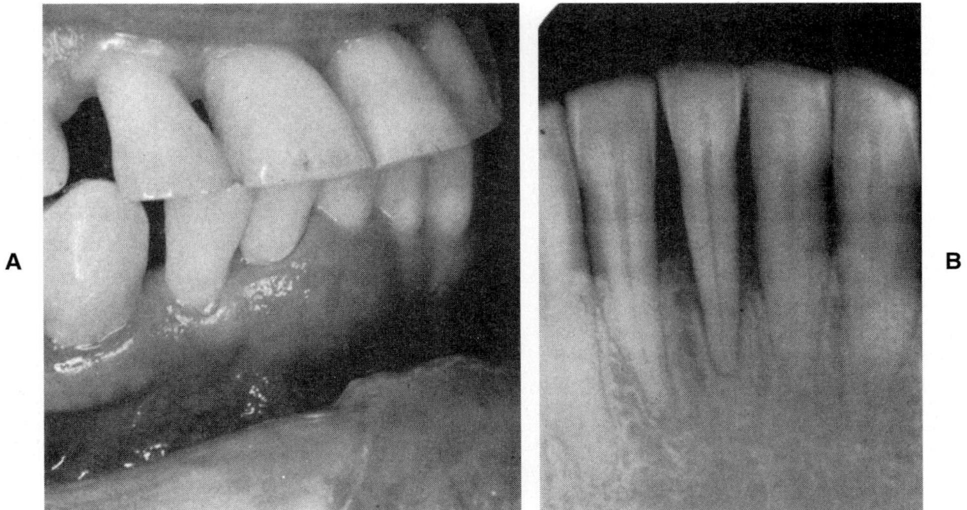

Fig. 31-19 Chronic periodontal abscess. **A,** Periodontal abscess in the right central and lateral incisor area. **B,** Extensive bone destruction and thickening of the periodontal ligament space around the right central incisor.

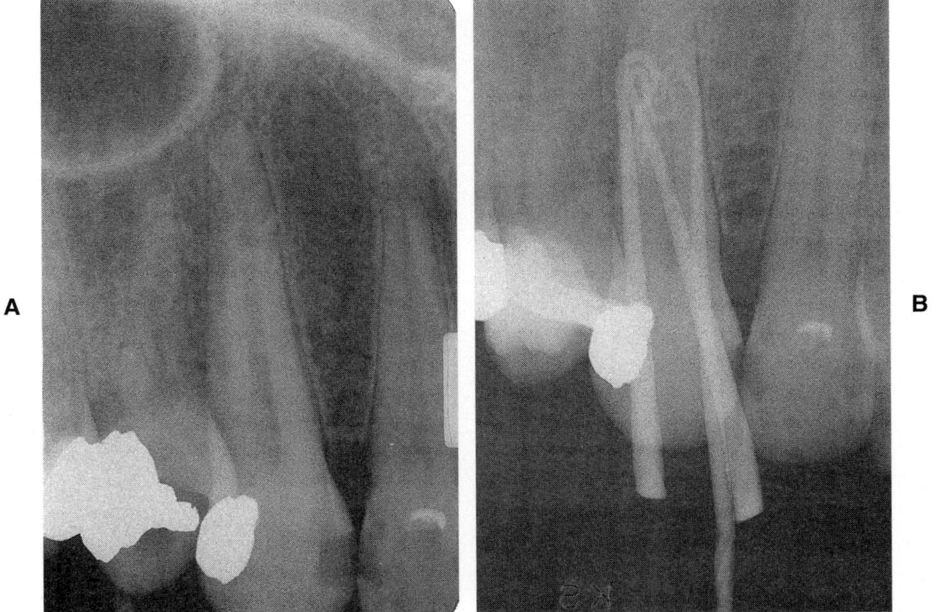

Fig. 31-20 **A,** Radiograph of maxillary cuspid. Does not show facial bone loss. **B,** Radiograph of same maxillary cuspid with gutta percha points placed in the facial pocket to indicate bone loss.

and root planing often require local anesthesia and definitive radiographic evaluation of the osseous lesions. Radiographs taken with periodontal probes or other indicators (e.g., Hirschfeld pointers) placed into the anesthetized pocket show the true extent of the bone lesion. As indicated previously, the attachment level on the radicular surface or interdental lesions with thick facial or lingual bone cannot be visualized in the radiograph. The use of radiopaque indicators is an efficient diagnostic aid for the clinician to better visualize every aspect of the defect. Figs. 31-20, *A* and *B,* are examples of probes placed in pockets to indicate the bone level.

Radiographic Changes in Localized, Aggressive Periodontitis

Juvenile periodontitis is characterized by a combination of the following radiographic features:

1. Bone loss may occur initially in the maxillary and mandibular incisor and/or first molar areas, usually bilaterally, and results in vertical, arclike destructive patterns (Fig. 31-21).
2. Loss of alveolar bone may become generalized as the disease progresses but remains less pronounced in the premolar areas.

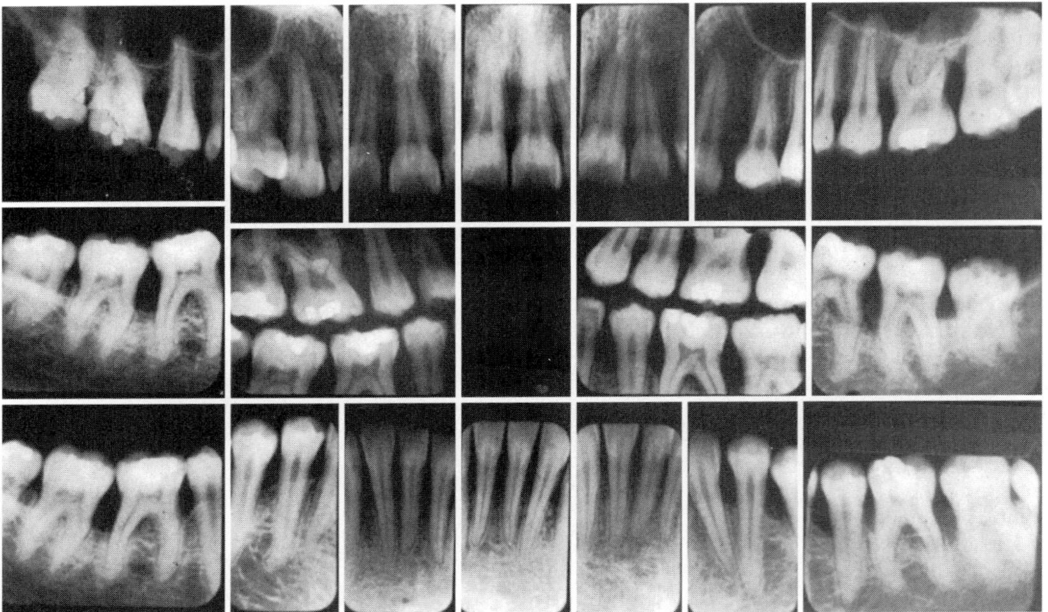

Fig. 31-21 Localized aggressive periodontitis. The accentuated bone destruction in the anterior and first molar areas is considered to be characteristic of this disease.

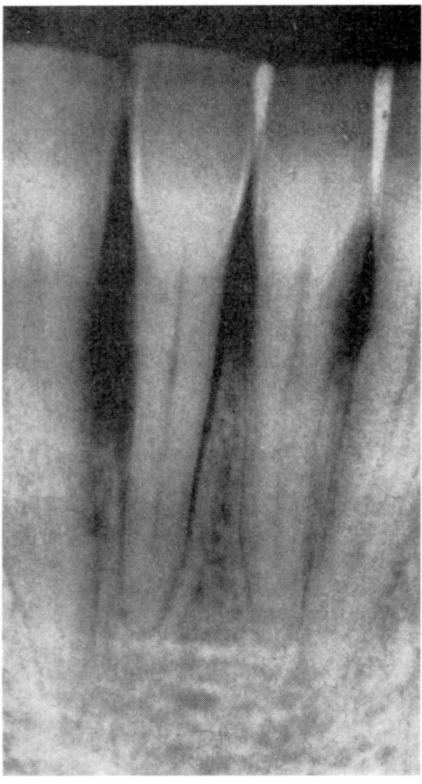

Fig. 31-22 Widened periodontal space caused by trauma from occlusion. Note the increased density of the surrounding bone caused by new bone formation in response to increased occlusal forces.

Radiographic Changes in Trauma from Occlusion

Trauma from occlusion can produce radiographically detectable changes in the lamina dura, morphology of the alveolar crest, width of the periodontal space, and density of the surrounding cancellous bone.

Traumatic lesions manifest themselves more clearly in faciolingual aspects, because mesiodistally, the tooth has the added stability provided by the contact areas with adjacent teeth. Therefore slight variations in the proximal surfaces may indicate greater changes in the facial and lingual aspects. *The radiographic changes listed below are not pathognomonic of trauma from occlusion and have to be interpreted in combination with clinical findings,* particularly tooth mobility, presence of wear facets, pocket depth, and analysis of occlusal contacts and habits.

The *injury phase* of trauma from occlusion produces a loss of the lamina dura that may be noted in apices, furcations, and/or marginal areas. This loss of lamina dura results in widening of the periodontal ligament space (Fig. 31-22). This change, particularly when incipient or circumscribed, may easily be confused with technical variations due to x-ray angulation or malposition of the tooth; it can be diagnosed with certainty only in radiographs of the highest quality.

The *repair phase* of trauma from occlusion results in an attempt to strengthen the periodontal structures to better support the increased loads. Radiographically, this is manifested by a widening of the periodontal ligament space, which may be generalized or localized.

Although microscopic measurements have determined that there are normal variations in the width of the periodontal space in the different regions of the root, these are not generally detected in radiographs. When variations in width between the marginal area and midroot or between the midroot and apex are detected, it means that the tooth is being subjected to increased forces. Successful attempts to reinforce the periodontal structures by widening of the periodontal space is accompanied by increased width of the lamina dura and sometimes by condensation of the perialveolar cancellous bone.

More advanced traumatic lesions may result in deep angular bone loss, which, when combined with marginal inflammation, may lead to intrabony pocket formation. In terminal stages these lesions extend around the root apex, producing a wide radiolucent periapical image (cavernous lesions).

Root resorption may also occur as a result of excessive forces on the periodontium, particularly those caused by orthodontic appliances. Although trauma from occlusion produces many root resorption areas, they are usually of a magnitude insufficient to be detected radiographically.

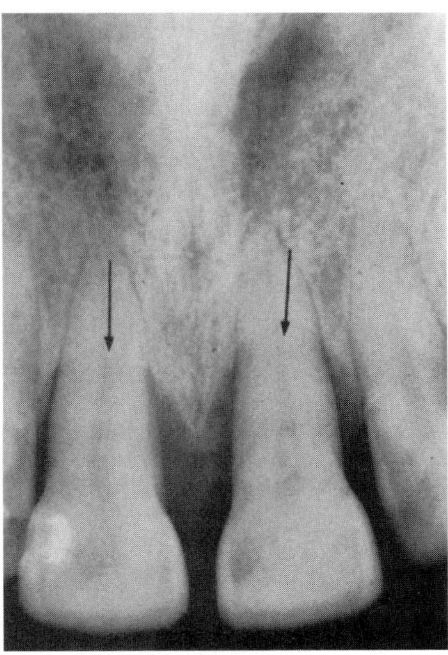

Fig. 31-23 Horizontal lines across the roots of the central incisors *(arrows)*. The area of the roots below the horizontal lines is partially or completely denuded of the facial and/or lingual bony plates.

Additional Radiographic Criteria in the Diagnosis of Periodontal Disease

The following diagnostic criteria can be used to aid in the diagnosis of periodontal disease:

Radiopaque horizontal line across the roots. This line demarcates the portion of the root where the labial and/or lingual bony plate has been partially or completely destroyed from the remaining bone-supported portion (Fig. 31-23).

Vessel canals in the alveolar bone. Hirschfeld[13] described linear and circular radiolucent areas produced by interdental canals and their foramina, respectively (Fig. 31-24). These canals indicate the course of the vascular supply of the bone and are normal radiographic findings. The radiographic image of the canals is often so prominent, particularly in the anterior region of the mandible, that they might be confused with radiolucency resulting from periodontal disease.

Differentiation between treated and untreated periodontal disease. It is sometimes necessary to determine whether the reduced bone level is the result of periodontal disease that is no longer destructive (usually after treatment and proper maintenance) or if destructive periodontal disease is present. Clinical examination is the basic determinant. However, radiographically detectable alterations in the normal clear-cut peripheral outline of the septa are corroborating evidence of destructive periodontal disease.

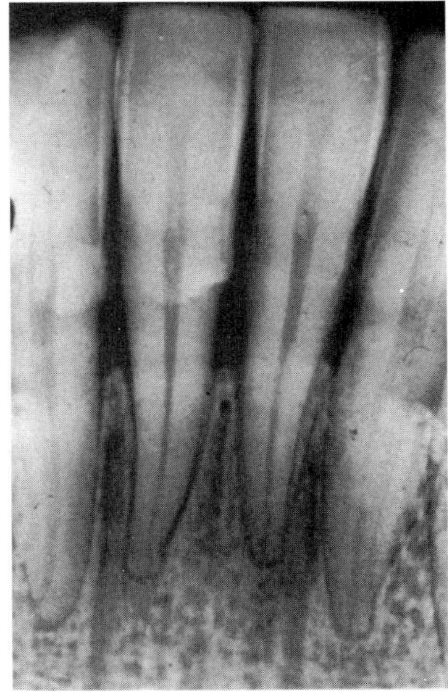

Fig. 31-24 Prominent vessel canals in the mandible.

Skeletal Disturbances Manifested in the Jaws

Skeletal disturbances may produce changes in the jaws that affect the interpretation of radiographs from the periodontal perspective. Destruction of tooth-supporting bone may occur in the following diseases:

Osteitis fibrosa cystica (Recklinghausen's disease of bone) develops in advanced primary or secondary hyperparathyroidism and causes osteoclastic resorption of bone with fibrous replacement and hemorrhage with hemosiderin deposition, creating a mass known as *brown tumor*[5] (see Figs. 12-1 and 12-2). It often appears as a cystic lesion of the jaw. This disease results in a diffuse granular mottling, scattered "cystlike" radiolucent areas throughout the jaws, and a

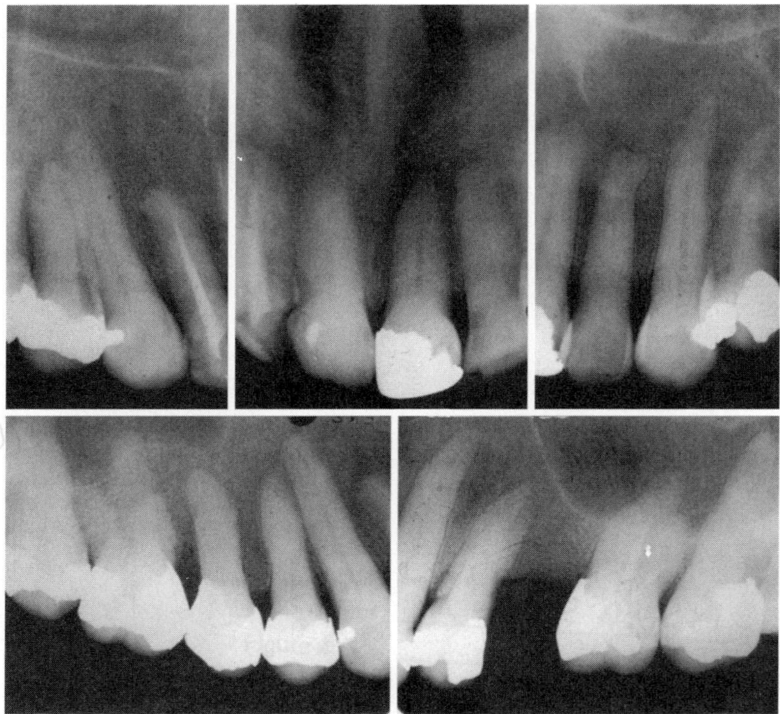

Fig. 31-25 Altered trabecular pattern and diminution in the prominence of the lamina dura in Paget's disease.

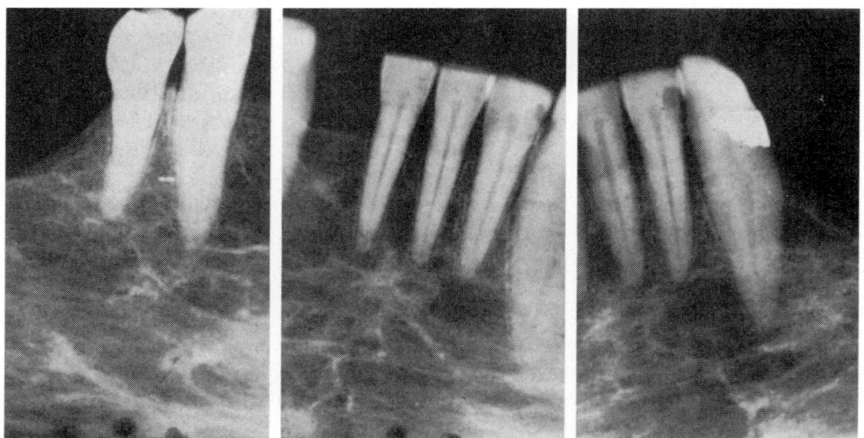

Fig. 31-26 Osteoporosis and altered trabecular arrangement in fibrous dysplasia.

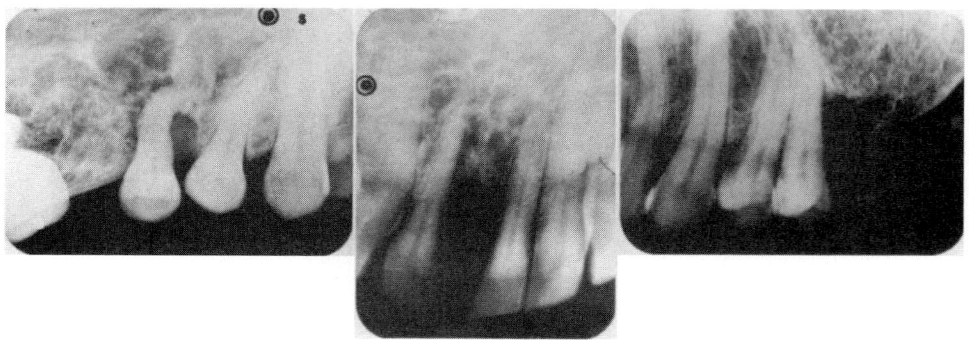

Fig. 31-27 Osteoporosis in Gaucher's disease.

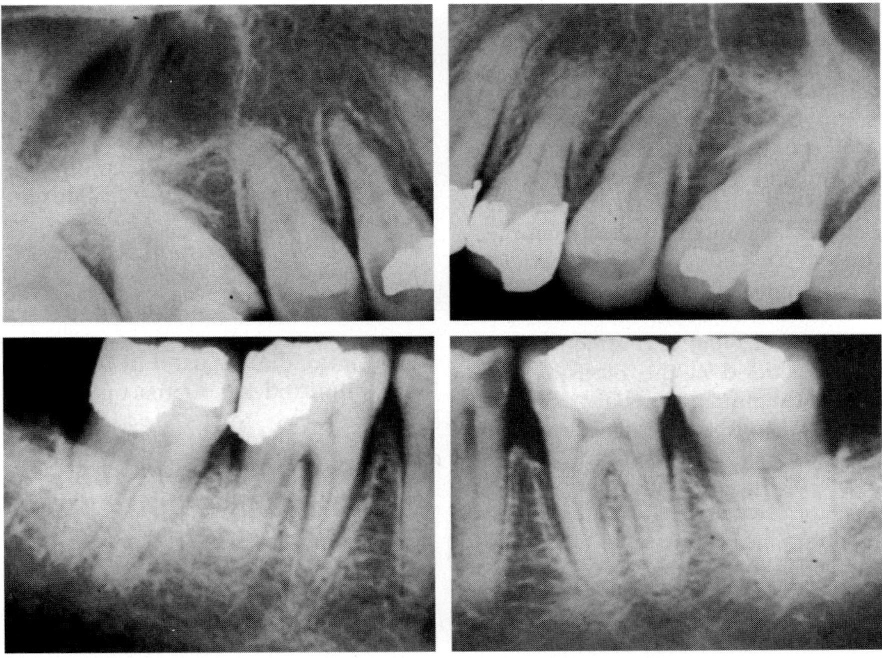

Fig. 31-28 Scleroderma, showing typical uniform widening of the periodontal ligament and thickening of the lamina dura. (Courtesy Drs. David F. Mitchell and Anand P. Chaudhry.)

generalized disappearance of the lamina dura.[28] Correction of the parathyroid hyperfunction usually results in rapid reversion of the bone to normal.

In *Paget's disease,* the normal trabecular pattern is replaced by a hazy, diffuse meshwork of closely knit, fine trabecular markings, with the lamina dura absent (Fig. 31-25), or scattered radiolucent areas may contain irregularly shaped radiopaque zones.[10,32]

Fibrous dysplasia may appear as a small radiolucent area at a root apex or as an extensive radiolucent area with irregularly arranged trabecular markings.[9] There may be enlargement of the cancellous spaces, with distortion of the normal trabecular pattern ("ground glass" appearance) and obliteration of the lamina dura (Fig. 31-26).

Langerhans' cell histiocytosis results from disturbances in immunoregulation, and its different forms comprise the diseases formerly called *Hand-Schüller-Christian disease, Letterer-Siwe disease, Gaucher's disease* and *eosinophilic granuloma.*[5,32] They appear as single or multiple radiolucent areas, which may be unrelated to the teeth or entail destruction of the tooth-supporting bone (Fig. 31-27).

Numerous radiolucent areas occur when the jaws are involved by *multiple myeloma.*

In *osteopetrosis* (marble-bone disease, Albers-Schönberg disease)[7,32] the outlines of the roots may be obscured by diffuse radiopacity of the jaws. In less severe cases the increased density is confined to the bone in relation to the nutrient canals and the lamina dura.

In *scleroderma,* the periodontal ligament is uniformly widened at the expense of the surrounding alveolar bone[1] (Fig. 31-28).

REFERENCES

1. Alexandridis C, White SC: Periodontal ligament changes in patients with progressive systemic sclerosis. Oral Surg 1984; 58:113.
2. Armitage G: Periodontal diseases: Diagnosis. Ann Periodontol 1996; 1:37.
3. Bender IB, Seltzer S: Roentgenographic and direct observation of experimental lesions in bone. I. J Am Dent Assoc 1961; 62:152.
4. Bender IB, Seltzer S: Roentgenographic and direct observation of experimental lesions in bone. II. J Am Dent Assoc 1961; 62:708.
5. Cotran RS, Kumar V, Robbins SL: Robbins Pathologic Basis of Disease, ed 5. Philadelphia. Saunders, 1994.
6. Everett FG, Fixott HC: Use of an incorporated grid in the diagnosis of oral roentgenograms. Oral Surg 1963; 9:1061.
7. Fairbank HAT: Osteopetrosis. J Bone Joint Surg 1948; 30:339.
8. Fitzgerald GM: Dental radiography. IV. The voltage factor (kp). J Am Dent Assoc 1950; 41:19.
9. Glickman I: Fibrous dysplasia in alveolar bone. Oral Surg 1948; 1:895.
10. Glickman I, Glidden S: Paget's disease of the maxillae and mandible. Clinical analysis and case reports. J Am Dent Assoc 1942; 29:2144.
11. Greenstein G, Polson A, Iker H, et al: Associations between crestal lamina dura and periodontal status. J Periodontol 1981; 52:362.
12. Hausmann E, Allen K, Clerehugh V: What alveolar crest level on a bite-wing radiograph represents bone loss? J Periodontol 1991; 62:570.
13. Hirschfeld I: Interdental canals. J Am Dent Assoc 1927; 14:617.
14. Källestål C, Matsson L: Criteria for assessment of interproximal bone loss on bite-wing radiographs in adolescents. J Clin Periodontol 1989; 16:300.

15. Manson JD: The lamina dura. Oral Surg 1963; 16:432.
16. Nicopoulos-Karayianni K, Mombelli A, Lang NO: Diagnostic problems of periodontitis-like lesions caused by eosinophilic granuloma. J Clin Periodontol 1989; 16:505.
17. Parfitt GJ: An investigation of the normal variations in alveolar bone trabeculations. Oral Surg 1962; 15:1453.
18. Patur B, Glickman I: Roentgenographic evaluation of alveolar bone changes in periodontal disease. J Clin N Am 1960; 4:47.
19. Pauls V, Trott JR: A radiological study of experimentally produced lesions in bone. Dent Pract 1966; 16:254, 1966.
20. Prichard JF: Role of the roentgenogram in the diagnosis and prognosis of periodontal disease. Oral Med 1961; 14:182.
21. Prichard JF: Advanced Periodontal Disease: Surgical and Prosthetic Management, ed 2. Philadelphia, Saunders, 1972.
22. Puckett J: A device for comparing roentgenograms of the same mouth. J Periodontol 1968; 39:38.
23. Ramadan ABE, Mitchell DF: A roentgenographic study of experimental bone destruction. Oral Surg 1962; 15:934.
24. Rams TE, Listgarten MA, Slots J: Utility of radiographic crestal lamina dura for predicting periodontal disease activity. J Clin Periodontol 1995; 21:571.
25. Regan JE, Mitchell DF: Roentgenographic and dissection measurements of alveolar crest height. J Am Dent Assoc 1962; 66:356.
26. Rees TD, Biggs NL, Collings CK: Radiographic interpretation of periodontal osseous lesions. Oral Surg Oral Med Oral Pathol 1962; 5:934.
27. Ritchey B, Orban B: The crests of the interdental septa. J Periodontol 1953; 24:75.
28. Rosenberg EH, Guralnick WC: Hyperparathyroidism. Oral Surg 1962; 15(Suppl 2):84.
29. Rosling B, Hollender L, Nyman S, et al: A radiographic method for assessing changes in alveolar bone height following periodontal therapy. J Clin Periodontol 1975; 2:211.
30. Theilade J: An evaluation of the reliability of radiographs in the measurement of bone loss in periodontal disease. J Periodontol 1960; 31:143.
31. Van der Linden, LWJ, Van Aken J: The periodontal ligament in the roentgenogram. J Periodontol 1970; 41:243.
32. Waldron CA: Bone pathology. In: Neville BW, Damm DD, Allen CM, et al: Oral and Maxillofacial Pathology. Philadelphia, Saunders, 1995.

Risk Assessment

Karen F. Novak and M. John Novak

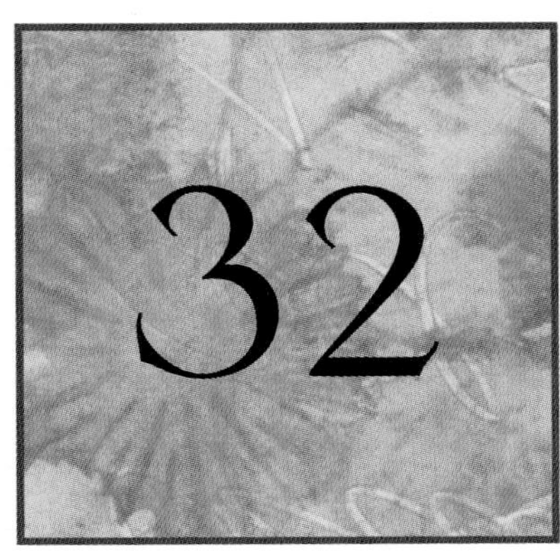

CHAPTER

CHAPTER OUTLINE

DEFINITIONS

Risk assessment is defined by numerous components.[2,27] **Risk** is the probability that an individual will get a specific disease in a given period. The risk of developing the disease will vary from individual to individual. **Risk factors** may be environmental, behavioral, or biologic factors that, when present, increase the likelihood that an individual will get the disease. They are part of the "causal chain" and directly related to disease occurrence. Risk factors are identified through longitudinal studies of patients with the disease of interest. Exposure to a risk factor or factors may occur at a single point in time; over multiple, separate points in time; or continuously. However, to be identified as a risk factor, the exposure must occur prior to disease onset. Interventions often can be identified and, when implemented, can help modify risk factors. The term *risk determinant/background characteristic,* which is sometimes substituted for the term *risk factor,* should be reserved for those risk factors that cannot be modified.

Risk indicators are *probable* or *putative* risk factors that have been identified in cross-sectional studies but not confirmed through longitudinal studies. *Risk predictors/markers,* although associated with increased risk for disease, do not cause the disease. These factors also are identified in cross-sectional and longitudinal studies.

RISK FACTORS FOR PERIODONTAL DISEASE

The following is a discussion on the risk factors for periodontal disease (Table 32-1).

Tobacco Smoking

Tobacco smoking is a well-established risk factor for periodontitis.[2,29] A direct relationship exists between smoking and the prevalence of periodontal disease (see Chapter 5). This association is independent of other factors such as oral hygiene or age.[18] Studies comparing the response to periodontal therapy in smokers, previous

TABLE 32-1

Risk Elements for Periodontal Disease

Risk Factors	Risk Determinants/ Background Characteristics	Risk Indicators	Risk Markers/ Predictors
Tobacco smoking Diabetes Pathogenic bacteria Microbial tooth deposits	Genetic factors Age Gender Socioeconomic status Stress	HIV/AIDS Osteoporosis Infrequent dental visits	Previous history of periodontal disease Bleeding on probing

HIV, human immunodeficiency virus; *AIDS,* acquired immunodeficiency syndrome.

smokers and nonsmokers have shown that smoking has a negative impact on the response to therapy. However, former smokers respond similarly to nonsmokers.[3] These studies demonstrate the impact intervention strategies can have in patients who smoke (see Chapter 14).

Diabetes

Diabetes is a clear risk factor for periodontitis.[2] Epidemiologic data demonstrate that the prevalence and severity of periodontitis is significantly higher in patients with type I and type II diabetes than in those without diabetes and that the level of diabetic control is an important variable in this relationship (see Chapter 5).

Pathogenic Bacteria and Microbial Tooth Deposits

It is well documented that accumulation of bacterial plaque at the gingival margin results in the development of gingivitis and that the gingivitis can be reversed with the implementation of oral hygiene measures.[24] These studies demonstrate a causal relationship between accumulation of bacterial plaque and gingival inflammation. However, a causal relationship between plaque accumulation and periodontitis has been more difficult to establish. Often, patients with severe loss of attachment have minimal levels of bacterial plaque on the affected teeth, indicating that the *quantity* of plaque is not of major importance in the disease process. However, although quantity may not indicate risk, there is evidence that the composition, or *quality,* of the complex plaque biofilm is of importance. In terms of quality of plaque, three specific bacteria have been identified as etiologic agents for periodontitis: *Actinobacillus actinomycetemcomitans, Porphyromonas gingivalis,* and *Bacteroides forsythus.*[12] *P. gingivalis* and *B. forsythus* are often found in chronic periodontitis, whereas *A. actinomycetemcomitans* is often associated with aggressive periodontitis. Cross-sectional and longitudinal studies support the delineation of these three bacteria as risk factors for periodontal disease. Additional evidence that they are causal agents include (1) their elimination or suppression impacts the success of therapy, (2) there is a host reponse to these pathogens, (3) virulence factors are associated with these pathogens and (4) inoculation of these bacteria into animal models induces periodontal disease.[16] Although not completely supported by these criteria for causation, there also is moderate evidence that *Campylobacter rectus, Eubacterium nodatum, Fusobacterium nucleatum, Prevotella intermedia/nigrescens, Peptostreptococcus micros, Streptococcus intermedius* and *Treponema denticola* are etiologic factors in periodontitis.[12] Therefore the quantity of plaque present may not be as important as the quality of the plaque in determining risk for periodontitis.

Anatomic factors such as furcations, root concavities, developmental grooves, cervical enamel projections, enamel pearls, and bifurcation ridges may predispose the periodontium to disease as a result of their potential to harbor bacterial plaque and present a challenge to the clinician during instrumentation. Similarly, the presence of subgingival and/or overhanging margins can result in increased plaque accumulation, increased inflammation, and increased bone loss. Although not clearly defined as risk factors for periodontitis, anatomic and restorative factors that influence plaque accumulation may play a role in disease susceptibility for specific teeth.[8]

The presence of calculus, which serves as a reservoir for bacterial plaque, has been suggested as a risk factor for periodontitis. Although the presence of some calculus in healthy individuals receiving routine dental care does not result in significant loss of attachment, the presence of calculus in other groups of patients, such as those not receiving regular care and patients with poorly controlled diabetes, can have a negative impact on periodontal health.[27]

RISK DETERMINANTS/BACKGROUND CHARACTERISTICS FOR PERIODONTAL DISEASE

Genetic Factors

There is evidence that genetic differences between individuals may explain why some patients develop periodontal disease and others do not. Studies conducted in twins have shown that genetic factors influence clinical measures of gingivitis, probing pocket depth, attachment loss, and interproximal bone height.[25,26] The familial aggregation seen in localized and generalized aggressive periodontitis also is indicative of genetic involvement in these diseases (see Chapter 27). A specific interleukin 1 (IL-1) genotype has been associated with severe chronic periodontitis.[20] Immunologic alterations, such as neutrophil abnormalities,[17] monocytic hyperresponsiveness to lipopolysaccharide stimulation in patients with localized aggressive periodontitis,[34] and alterations in the monocyte/macrophage FcγRII receptor for IgG2 also appear to be under genetic control.[43] In addition, genetics plays a role in regulating the titer of the protective IgG2 antibody response to *A. actinomycetemcomitans* in patients with aggressive periodontitis[15] (see Chapter 10).

Age

Both the prevalence and severity of periodontal disease increases with age.[9,28,29] It is possible that degenerative changes related to aging may increase susceptibility to periodontitis. However, it also is possible that the attachment loss and bone loss seen in older individuals is a result of prolonged exposure to other risk factors over a person's life, creating a cumulative effect over time. In support of this, studies have shown minimal loss of attachment in aging subjects enrolled in preventive programs throughout their lives.[30,31] Therefore it is suggested that periodontal disease is not an inevitable consequence of the aging process and that aging alone does not increase disease susceptibility. However, it remains to be determined whether changes related to the aging process, such as intake of medications, decreased immune function, and altered nutritional status interact with other well-defined risk factors to increase susceptibility to periodontitis.

Evidence of loss of attachment may be of more consequence in younger patients. The younger the patient, the longer they have for exposure to causative factors. In addition, aggressive periodontitis in young individuals often is associated with an unmodifiable risk factor such as a genetic predisposition to disease.[29] Therefore young individuals with periodontal disease may be at greater risk for continued disease as they age.

Gender

Gender plays a role in periodontal disease.[2] United States national surveys conducted since 1960 demonstrate that males have more loss of attachment than females.[38,40,41] In addition, males have poorer oral hygiene than females, as evidenced by higher levels of plaque and calculus.[1,39,41] Therefore it appears that gender differences in prevalence and severity of periodontitis are related to preventive practices rather than any genetic factor.

Socioeconomic Status

Gingivitis and poor oral hygiene can be related to lower socioeconomic status (SES).[2,38,40] This can most likely be attributed to decreased dental awareness and decreased frequency of dental visits when compared with more educated individuals of higher SES. After adjusting for other risk factors such as smoking and poor oral hygiene, lower SES alone does not result in increased risk for periodontitis (see Chapter 5).

Stress

The incidence of necrotizing ulcerative gingivitis increases during periods of emotional and physiologic stress, suggesting a link between the two.[11,35] Emotional stress may interfere with normal immune function[6,36] and may result in increased levels of circulating hormones that can have an impact on the periodontium.[32] Stressful life events such as bereavement and divorce appear to lead to a greater prevalence of periodontal disease,[14] and there is an apparent association between psychosocial factors and risk behaviors such as smoking, poor oral hygiene, and chronic periodontitis.[10] Adult patients with periodontitis who are resistant to therapy are more stressed than those who respond to therapy.[5] Individuals with financial strain, distress, depression, or inadequate coping mechanisms have more severe loss of attachment.[13] Although epidemiologic data on the relationship between stress and periodontal disease is limited, it appears that stress may be a putative risk factor for periodontitis.[29]

RISK INDICATORS FOR PERIODONTAL DISEASE

Human Immunodeficiency Virus/Acquired Immunodeficiency Syndrome

It has been hypothesized that the immune dysfunction associated with human immunodeficiency virus (HIV) infection and acquired immunodeficiency syndrome (AIDS) increases susceptibility to periodontal disease. Early reports on the periodontal status of patients with AIDS or individuals who are HIV seropositive revealed that these patients often had severe periodontal destruction characteristic of necrotizing ulcerative periodontitis.[44] More recent reports, however, have failed to demonstrate significant differences in the periodontal status of individuals with HIV infection and healthy controls.[23,37] The apparent discrepancy in these reports may have been due to the inclusion of patients with AIDS (as opposed to patients who were exclusively HIV seropositive) in some studies.[29] Conflicting results also exist in studies examining the level of immunosuppression and severity of periodontal destruction. In a 20-month study of 114 homosexual and bisexual men, the relative risk of longitudinal attachment loss $\geq$3 mm was 4.8 when CD4 counts were less than 400/mm^3 and increased to 6.16 when CD4 counts were less than 200/mm^3, suggesting a correlation between the severity of periodontal disease and the level of immunosuppression.[7] In contrast, a study of 119 individuals with HIV, 73 patients with AIDS and 156 individuals who were HIV seronegative found no significant differences in bleeding on probing, pocket formation, or attachment loss among the three groups and no significant associations by odds ratio analysis between these clinical parameters and CD4 T-cell counts.[33] Therefore although it seems reasonable to hypothesize that HIV infection and immunosuppression are risk factors for periodontal disease, the evidence is not conclusive.[2,29]

Osteoporosis

Osteoporosis has been suggested as another risk factor for periodontitis. Although studies in animal models indicate that osteoporosis does not initiate periodontitis, there is evidence that the reduced bone mass seen in osteoporosis may aggravate periodontal disease progression.[4,22] However, reports in humans are conflicting. In a study of 12 women with osteoporosis and 14 healthy women, Von Wowern et al[42] reported that the women with osteoporosis had greater loss of attachment than the control subjects. In contrast, Kribbs[21] examined pocket depth, bleeding on probing, and gingival recession in women with and without osteoporosis. Although the two groups had significant differences in bone mass, no differences in periodontal status were noted. However, it appears that a link may exist between osteoporosis and periodontitis, and additional studies may need to be conducted to clearly determine if osteoporosis is a true risk factor for periodontal disease.[19]

Infrequent Dental Visits

Identifying failure to visit the dentist on a regular basis as a risk factor for periodontitis is controversial.[27] One study demonstrated an increased risk for severe periodontitis in patients who had not visited the dentist for three or more years, whereas another demonstrated that there was no more loss of attachment or bone loss in individuals who did not seek dental care when compared with those that did over a 6-year period. However, the ages of the subjects in these two studies were different, which may explain the differences in the results. Additional longitudinal and intervention studies are necessary to determine if infrequency of dental visits is a risk factor for periodontal disease.

RISK MARKERS/PREDICTORS FOR PERIODONTAL DISEASE

Previous History of Periodontal Disease

A history of previous periodontal disease is a good clinical predictor of risk for future disease.[27] Patients with the most severe existing loss of attachment are at the greatest risk for future loss of attachment. Conversely, patients currently free of periodontitis have decreased risk for developing loss of attachment than those who currently have periodontitis (see Chapter 5).

Bleeding on Probing

Bleeding on probing is the best clinical indicator of gingival inflammation.[27] Although bleeding on probing alone does not serve as a predictor for loss of attachment, bleeding on probing coupled with increasing pocket depth may serve as an excellent predictor for future loss of attachment. Lack of bleeding on probing does appear to serve as an excellent indicator of periodontal health.

CLINICAL RISK ASSESSMENT FOR PERIODONTAL DISEASE

Information concerning individual risk for developing periodontal disease is obtained through careful evaluation of the patient's demographic data, medical history, dental history, and clinical examination (Table 32-2). The elements that contribute to increased risk that can be identified through the collection of demographic data include the patient's age, gender, and SES. The medical history may reveal elements such as a history of diabetes, smoking, HIV/AIDS, or osteoporosis, as well as the perceived level of stress. The dental history can reveal a

TABLE 32-2

Clinical Risk Assessment for Periodontal Disease

Demographic Data	Medical History	Dental History	Clinical Examination
Age	Diabetes	Family history of early tooth loss	Plaque accumulation
• Duration of exposure to risk elements	Tobacco smoking	• Genetic predisposition to aggressive disease	• Microbial sampling for putative periodontal pathogens
• Postmenopausal women	HIV/AIDS	Previous history of periodontal disease	Calculus
• Evidence of aggressive disease	Osteoporosis	Frequency of dental care	Bleeding on probing
Gender	Stress		Extent of loss of attachment
• Males			• Aggressive forms of disease
Preventive practices			Tooth examination
Frequency of care			• Plaque retentive areas
SES			• Anatomic factors
• Dental awareness			Restorative factors
• Frequency of care			

AIDS, Acquired immunodeficiency syndrome; *HIV,* human immunodeficiency syndrome; *SES,* socioeconomic status.

family history of early tooth loss (suggestive of a genetic predisposition for aggressive periodontitis), a previous history of periodontal disease, and information concerning the frequency of oral health care in the past. Important elements identified during the clinical examination can include the location and extent of bacterial plaque accumulation, the presence of plaque retentive factors such as overhanging restorations and subgingival margins, the presence of anatomic plaque-retentive areas such as grooves and furcation involvements, the presence of calculus, the extent of attachment loss, and the presence or absence of bleeding on probing.

Once an at-risk patient is identified and a diagnosis is made, their treatment plan may be modified accordingly (Fig. 32-1). For example, a patient with a history of cigarette smoking should be informed of the relationship between smoking and periodontitis. They also should be informed of the impact of smoking on their prognosis and the likelihood of success of their periodontal therapy should they continue to smoke. Part of their recommended treatment plan for initial therapy may include referral to a smoking cessation program, or implementation of self-administered smoking cessation aids. As another example, a patient diagnosed with severe, chronic periodontitis may be encouraged to be tested for the IL-1 positive genotype. If positive, their treatment may involve the administration of systemic antimicrobial agents and/or host modifiers that would not be used in a patient without this genetic marker. If alterations in the host response are identified, the prognosis and treatment plan may be modified. Previously identified risk elements also may need to be reassessed at the reevaluation stage of treatment. This is especially important in patients who do not respond favorably to periodontal therapy (see Fig. 32-1).

In summary, risk assessment involves identifying elements that either may predispose a patient to developing periodontal disease or may influence the progression of disease that already exists. In either case, these patients may require modification of their prognosis and treatment plan. In addition to an evaluation of the factors

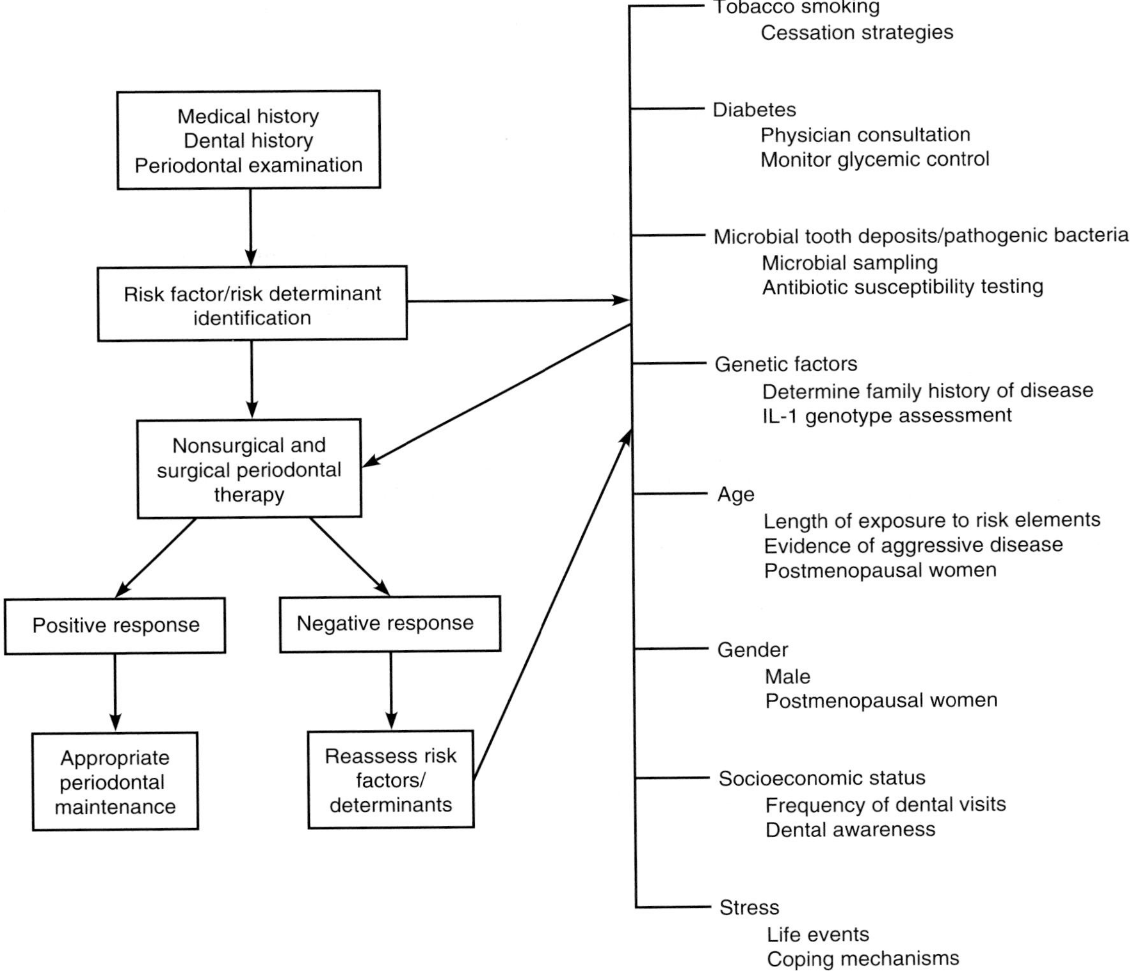

Fig. 32-1 Risk assessment in periodontal therapy. The major risk elements to be considered in the diagnosis and treatment of periodontal disease are indicated. The importance of risk assessment before the initiation of therapy is highlighted, as well as the need for reassessment after a negative response to therapy.

contributing to their risk, these patients should be educated concerning their risk and, when appropriate, suitable intervention strategies implemented.

REFERENCES

1. Abdellatif HM, Burt BA: An epidemiological investigation into the relative importance of age and oral hygiene status as determinants of periodontitis. J Dent Res 1987; 66:13–18.
2. American Academy of Periodontology: Position paper. Epidemiology of periodontal diseases. J Periodontol 1996; 67:935–945.
3. American Academy of Periodontology: Position paper. Tobacco use and the periodontal patient. J Periodontol 1999; 70:1419–1427.
4. Aufdemorte TB, Boyan BD, Fox WC, et al: Diagnostic tools and biologic markers: animal models in the study of osteoporosis and oral bone loss. J Bone Miner Res 1993; 8 (suppl 1):S29034.
5. Axtelius B, Söderfeldt B, Nilsson A, et al: Therapy-resistant periodontitis. Psychosocial characteristics. J Clin Periodontol 1998; 25:482–491.
6. Ballieux RE: Impact of mental stress on the immune response. J Clin Periodontol 1991; 18:427–430.
7. Barr C, Lopez MR, Rua-Dobles A: Periodontal changes by HIV serostatus in a cohort of homosexual and bisexual men. J Clin Periodontol 1992; 19:794–801.
8. Blieden TM: Tooth-related issues. Ann Periodontol 1999; 4:91–96.
9. Burt BA: Periodontitis and aging: reviewing recent evidence. J Am Dent Assoc 1994; 125:273–279.
10. Croucher R, Marcenes WS, Torres MCMB, et al: The relationship between life-events and periodontitis. A case-control study. J Clin Periodontol 1997; 24:39–43.
11. Enwonwu CO: Epidemiological and biochemical studies of necrotizing ulcerative gingivitis and noma (cancrum oris) in Nigerian children. Arch Oral Biol 1972; 17:1357–1371.
12. Genco R, Kornman K, Williams R, et al: Consensus report: Periodontal diseases: Pathogenesis and microbial factors. Ann Periodontol 1996; 1:926–932.
13. Genco RJ, Ho AW, Grossi SG, et al: Relationship of stress, distress, and inadequate coping behaviors to periodontal disease. J Periodontol 1999; 70:711–723.
14. Green LW, Tryon WW, Marks B, et al: Periodontal disease as a function of life events stress. J Stress 1986; 12:32–36.
15. Gunsolley JC, Tew JG, Gooss CM, et al: Effects of race, smoking and immunoglobulin allotypes on IgG subclass concentrations. J Periodont Res 1997; 32:381–387.
16. Haffajee AD, Socransky SS: Microbial etiological agents of destructive periodontal diseases. Periodontol 2000 1994; 5:78–111.
17. Hart TC, Shapira L, Van Dyke TE: Neutrophil defects as risk factors for periodontal diseases. J Periodontol 1994; 65: 521–529.
18. Ismail AI, Burt BA, Eklund SA: Epidemiologic patterns of smoking and periodontal disease in the United States. J Am Dent Assoc 1983; 106:617–621.
19. Kinane DF: Periodontitis modified by systemic factors. Ann Periodontol 1999; 4:55–63.
20. Kornman KS, Crane S, Wang HY, et al: The interleukin-1 genotype as a severity factor in adult periodontal disease. J Clin Periodontol 1997; 24:72–77.
21. Kribbs PJ: Comparison of mandibular bone in normal and osteoporotic women. J Prosthet Dent 1990; 63:218–222.
22. Krook L, Whalen JP, Lesser GV, et al: Experimental studies on osteoporosis. Methods Achiev Exp Pathol 1975; 7:72–108.
23. Lamster IB, Begg MD, Mitchell L, et al: Oral manifestations of HIV infection in homosexual men and intravenous drug users: study design and relationship of epidemiologic, clinical, and immunologic parameter to oral lesions. Oral Surg Oral Med Oral Pathol 1994; 78:163–174.
24. Löe H, Theilade E, Jensen SB: Experimental gingivitis in man. J Periodontol 1965; 36:177–187.
25. Michalowicz BS, Aeppli DP, Kuba RK, et al: A twin study of genetic variation in proportional radiographic alveolar bone height. J Dent Res 1991; 70:1431–1435.
26. Michalowicz BS, Aeppli DP, Virag JG, et al: Risk findings in adult twins. J Periodontol 1991; 62:293–299.
27. Page RC, Beck JD: Risk assessment for periodontal diseases. Int Den J 1997; 47:61–87.
28. Papapanou PN: Epidemiology and natural history of periodontal disease. In: Lang NP, Karring T (eds): Proceeding of the First European Workshop on Periodontology. London, Quintessence, 1994.
29. Papapanou PN: Risk assessments in the diagnosis and treatment of periodontal diseases. J Den Edu 1998; 62:822–839.
30. Papapanou PN, Lindhe J: Preservation of probing attachment and alveolar bone levels in two random population samples. J Clin Periodontol 1992; 19:583–588.
31. Papapanou PN, Lindhe J, Sterrett JD, et al: Considerations on the contribution of aging to loss of periodontal tissue support. J Clin Periodontol 1991; 18:611–615.
32. Rose RM: Endocrine responses to stressful psychological events. Psychiatr Clin N Am 1980; 3:251–276.
33. Scheutz F, Matee MI, Andsager L, et al: Is there an association between periodontal condition and HIV infection? J Clin Periodontol 1997; 24:580–587.
34. Shapira L, Soskolone WA, Van Dyke TE, et al: Prostaglandin E2 secretion, cell maturation, and CD14 expression by monocyte-derived macrophages from localized juvenile periodontitis patients. J Periodontol 1996; 67:224–228.
35. Shields WD: Acute necrotizing ulcerative gingivitis. A study of some of the contributing factors and their validity in an Army population. J Periodontol 1977; 48:346–349.
36. Sternberg EM, Chrousos GP, Wilder RL, et al: The stress response and the regulation of inflammatory disease. Ann Intern Med 1992; 117:854–866.
37. Swango PA, Kleinman DV, Konzelman JL: HIV and periodontal health: a study of military personnel with HIV. J Am Dent Assoc 1991; 122:49–54.
38. U.S. Public Health Service, National Center for Health Statistics: *Periodontal Disease in Adults, United States 1960–1962.* PHS Publ No 1000, Series 11 No 12. Washington, DC, Government Printing Office, 1965.
39. U.S. Public Health Service, National Center for Health Statistics: *Oral Hygiene in Adults, United States 1960–1962.* PHS Publ No 1000, Series 11 No 16. Washington, DC, Government Printing Office, 1966.
40. U.S. Public Health Service, National Center for Health Statistics: *Basic Data on Dental Examination Findings of Persons 1–74 years; United States 1971–1974.* DHEW PHS Publ No 79–1662, Series 11 No. 214. Washington, DC, Government Printing Office, 1979.
41. U.S. Public Health Service, National Institute of Dental Research: *Oral Health of United States Adults; National Findings.* NIH Publ No 87–2868. Bethesda, Md, NIDR, 1987.
42. Van Wowern J, Klausen B, Kollerup G: Osteoporosis: a risk factor in periodontal disease. J Periodontol 1994; 65: 134.
43. Wilson ME, Kalmar JR: FcγIIa (CD32): A potential marker defining susceptibility to localized juvenile periodontitis. J Periodontol 1996; 76:323–331.
44. Winkler JR, Herrera C, Westenhouse J, et al: Periodontal disease in HIV-infected and uninfected homosexual and bisexual men [letter]. AIDS 1992; 6:1041–1043.

Determination of Prognosis

Stephen F. Goodman and Karen F. Novak

CHAPTER

CHAPTER OUTLINE

DEFINITION OF PROGNOSIS

The **prognosis** is a prediction of the probable course, duration, and outcome of a disease based on a general knowledge of the pathogenesis of the disease and the presence of risk factors for the disease. It is established after the diagnosis is made and before the treatment plan is established. The prognosis is based on specific information about the disease and the manner in which it can be treated, but it also can be influenced by the clinician's previous experience with treatment outcomes (successes and failures) as they relate to the particular case.

Prognosis is often confused with the term *risk*. Risk generally deals with the likelihood that an individual will get a disease in a specified period (see Chapter 5). Risk factors are those characteristics of an individual that put them at increased risk for getting a disease. In contrast, prognosis is the prediction of the course or outcome of a disease. Prognostic factors are characteristics that predict the outcome of disease once the disease is present. In some cases, risk factors and prognostic factors are the same (see Chapter 5). For example, patients with diabetes or patients who smoke are more at risk for acquiring periodontal disease, and once they have it, they generally have a worse prognosis.

DETERMINATION OF A PROGNOSIS

The factors often considered when determining the prognosis are listed in Table 33-1. Although some of these factors may be more important than others when assigning a prognosis,[29,30] consideration of each may be beneficial to the clinician. In most cases, careful analysis of these factors allows the clinician to establish one of the following prognoses[28]:

Excellent prognosis: No bone loss, excellent gingival condition, good patient cooperation, no systemic/environmental factors.

Good prognosis: One or more of the following: adequate remaining bone support, adequate possibilities to control etiologic factors and establish a maintainable dentition, adequate patient cooperation, no systemic/environmental factors or if systemic factors are present, they are well controlled.

Fair prognosis: One or more of the following: less-than-adequate remaining bone support, some tooth mobility, grade I furcation involvement, adequate maintenance possible, acceptable patient cooperation, presence of limited systemic/environmental factors.

Poor prognosis: One or more of the following: moderate-to-advanced bone loss, tooth mobility, grade I and II

TABLE 33-1

Factors to be Considered When Determining a Prognosis

Overall Clinical Factors	Systemic/Environmental Factors	Local Factors	Prosthetic/Restorative Factors
Patient age Disease severity Plaque control Patient compliance	Smoking Systemic disease/condition Genetic factors Stress	Plaque/calculus Subgingival restorations Anatomic factors: • Short, tapered roots • Cervical enamel projections • Enamel pearls • Bifurcation ridges • Root concavities • Developmental grooves • Root proximity • Furcation involvement • Tooth mobility	Abutment selection Caries Nonvital teeth Root resorption

furcation involvements, difficult-to-maintain areas and/or doubtful patient cooperation, presence of systemic/environmental factors.

Questionable prognosis: One or more of the following: advanced bone loss, grade II and III furcation involvements, tooth mobility, inaccessible areas, presence of systemic/environmental factors.

Hopeless prognosis: One or more of the following: advanced bone loss, nonmaintainable areas, extraction(s) indicated, presence of uncontrolled systemic/environmental factors.

It should be recognized that excellent, good, and hopeless prognoses are the only prognoses that can be established with a reasonable degree of accuracy. Fair, poor, and even questionable prognoses depend on a large number of factors that can interact in an unpredictable number of ways.[6,11,42] In many of these cases, it may be advisable to establish a provisional prognosis until phase I therapy is completed and evaluated.

The *provisional prognosis* allows the clinician to initiate treatment of teeth that have a doubtful outlook in the hope that a favorable response may tip the balance and allow teeth to be retained. The reevaluation phase in the treatment sequence allows the clinician to examine the tissue response to scaling, oral hygiene, and root planing, as well as to the possible use of chemotherapeutic agents where indicated. The patient's compliance with the proposed treatment plan also can be determined.

Overall versus Individual Tooth Prognosis

Prognosis can be divided into *overall prognosis* and *individual tooth prognosis.* The overall prognosis is concerned with the dentition as a whole. Factors that may influence the overall prognosis include patient age, current severity of disease, systemic factors, smoking, the presence of plaque, calculus and other local factors, patient compliance, and prosthetic possibilities (see Table 33-1). The overall prognosis answers the following questions:

- Should treatment be undertaken?
- Is it likely to succeed?
- When prosthetic replacements are needed, are the remaining teeth able to support the added burden of the prosthesis?

The prognosis for individual teeth is determined after the overall prognosis and is affected by it.[28] For example, in a patient with a poor overall prognosis, the dentist likely would not attempt to retain a tooth that has a questionable prognosis because of local conditions. Many of the factors listed under Local Factors and Prosthetic/Restorative Factors in Table 33-1 have a direct effect on the prognosis for individual teeth in addition to any overall systemic or environmental factors that may be present.

FACTORS TO CONSIDER WHEN DETERMINING A PROGNOSIS

Please refer to Table 33-1 during the following discussion.

Overall Clinical Factors

Patient Age. For two patients with comparable levels of remaining connective tissue attachment and alveolar bone, the prognosis is generally better in the older of the two. For the younger patient, the prognosis is not as good because of the shorter time frame in which the periodontal destruction has occurred. In some cases this may be because the younger patient suffers from an aggressive type of periodontitis or disease progression may have increased due to systemic disease or smoking. In addition, although the younger patient would ordinarily be expected to have a greater reparative capacity, the occurrence of so much destruction in a relatively short period would exceed any naturally occurring periodontal repair.

Disease Severity. Studies have demonstrated that a patient's history of previous periodontal disease may be indicative of their susceptibility for future periodontal breakdown (see Chapter 5). Therefore the following variables should be carefully recorded because they are important for determining the patient's past history of periodontal disease: pocket depth, level of attachment, degree of bone loss, and type of bony defect. They are determined by clinical and radiographic evaluation (see Chapters 30 and 31).

The determination of the level of clinical attachment reveals the approximate extent of root surface that is devoid of periodontal ligament; the radiographic examination shows the amount of root surface still invested in bone. Pocket depth is less important than level of attachment, because it is not necessarily related to bone loss. In general, a tooth with deep pockets and little attachment and bone loss has a better prognosis than one with shallow pockets and severe attachment and bone loss. However, deep pockets are a source of infection and may contribute to progressive disease.

Prognosis is adversely affected if the base of the pocket (level of attachment) is close to the root apex. The presence of apical disease as a result of endodontic involvement also worsen the prognosis. However, surprisingly good apical and lateral bone repair can sometimes be obtained by combining endodontic and periodontal therapy (see Chapter 65).

The prognosis also can be related to the height of remaining bone. Assuming bone destruction can be arrested, is there enough bone remaining to support the teeth? The answer is readily apparent in extreme cases, that is, when there is so little bone loss that tooth support is not in jeopardy (Fig. 33-1) or when bone loss is so severe that the remaining bone is obviously insufficient for proper tooth support (Fig 33-2). Most patients, however, do not fit into these extreme categories. The height of remaining bone is usually somewhere in between, making bone level assessment alone insufficient for determining the overall prognosis.

The type of defect also must be determined. The prognosis for horizontal bone loss depends on the height of the existing bone, because it is unlikely that clinically significant bone height regeneration will be induced by therapy. In the case of angular, intrabony defects, if the contour of the existing bone and the number of osseous walls are favorable, there is an excellent chance that therapy could regenerate bone to approximately the level of the alveolar crest.[40]

When greater bone loss has occurred on one surface of a tooth, the bone height on the less involved surfaces should be taken into consideration when determining the prognosis. Because of the greater height of bone in relation to other surfaces, the center of rotation of the tooth will be nearer the crown (Fig. 33-3). This results in a more favorable distribution of forces to the periodontium and less tooth mobility.[44]

In dealing with a tooth with a questionable prognosis, the chances of successful treatment should be weighed against any benefits that would accrue to the adjacent teeth if the tooth under consideration were extracted. Heroic attempts to retain a hopelessly involved tooth may jeopardize the adjacent teeth. Extraction of the questionable tooth may be followed by partial restoration of the bone support of the adjacent teeth (Fig. 33-4).

Plaque Control. Bacterial plaque is the primary etiologic factor associated with periodontal disease (see Chapter 6). Therefore effective removal of plaque on a daily basis by the patient is critical to the success of periodontal therapy and to the prognosis.

Patient Compliance/Cooperation. The prognosis for patients with gingival and periodontal disease is critically dependent on the patient's attitude, desire to retain the natural teeth, and willingness and ability to maintain good oral hygiene. Without these, treatment cannot succeed. Patients should be clearly informed of the important role they must play for treatment to succeed. If patients are unwilling or unable to perform adequate plaque control and to receive the timely periodic maintenance checkups and treatments deemed necessary by the dentist, then the dentist can (1) refuse to accept the patient for treatment or (2) extract teeth that have a hopeless or poor prognosis and perform scaling and root planing on the remaining teeth. The dentist should make it clear to the patient and in the patient record that further treatment is needed but will not be performed because of a lack of patient cooperation.

Systemic/Environmental Factors

Smoking. Epidemiologic evidence suggests that smoking may be the most important environmental risk factor impacting the development and progression of periodontal disease (see Chapter 5). Therefore it should be made clear to the patient that a direct relationship exists between smoking and the prevalence and incidence of periodontitis. In addition, patients should be informed that smoking affects not only the severity of periodontal destruction, but also the healing potential of the periodontal tissues. As a result, patients who smoke do not respond as well to conventional periodontal therapy as patients who have never smoked.[38,39] Therefore the prognosis in patients who smoke and have slight-to-moderate periodontitis is generally fair to poor. In patients with severe periodontitis, the prognosis may be poor to hopeless.

However, it should be emphasized that smoking cessation can affect the treatment outcome and therefore the prognosis.[3,14] Patients with slight to moderate periodontitis who stop smoking can often be upgraded to a good prognosis, whereas those with severe periodontitis who stop smoking may be upgraded to a fair prognosis.

Systemic Disease/Condition. The patient's systemic background affects overall prognosis in several ways. For example, evidence from epidemiologic studies clearly demonstrates that the prevalence and severity of periodontitis is significantly higher in patients with type I and type II diabetes than in those without diabetes and that the level of control of the diabetes is an important

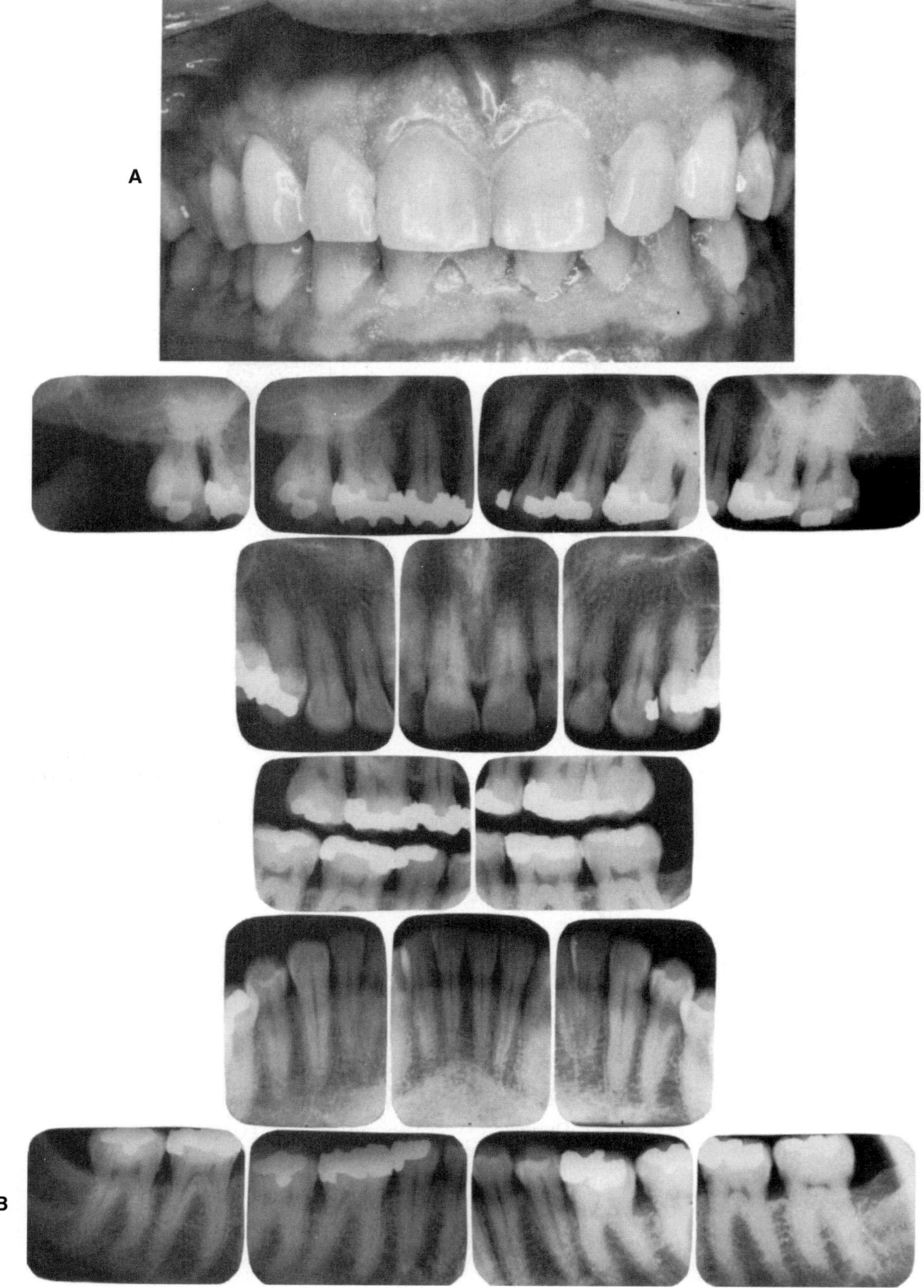

Fig. 33-1 Chronic periodontitis, overall prognosis good. **A,** Gingival inflammation, poor oral hygiene, and pronounced anterior overbite in a systemically healthy, nonsmoking 42-year-old man. **B,** Although local factors are present, the patient presents with adequate remaining bone support and a good prognosis, provided local factors can be controlled.

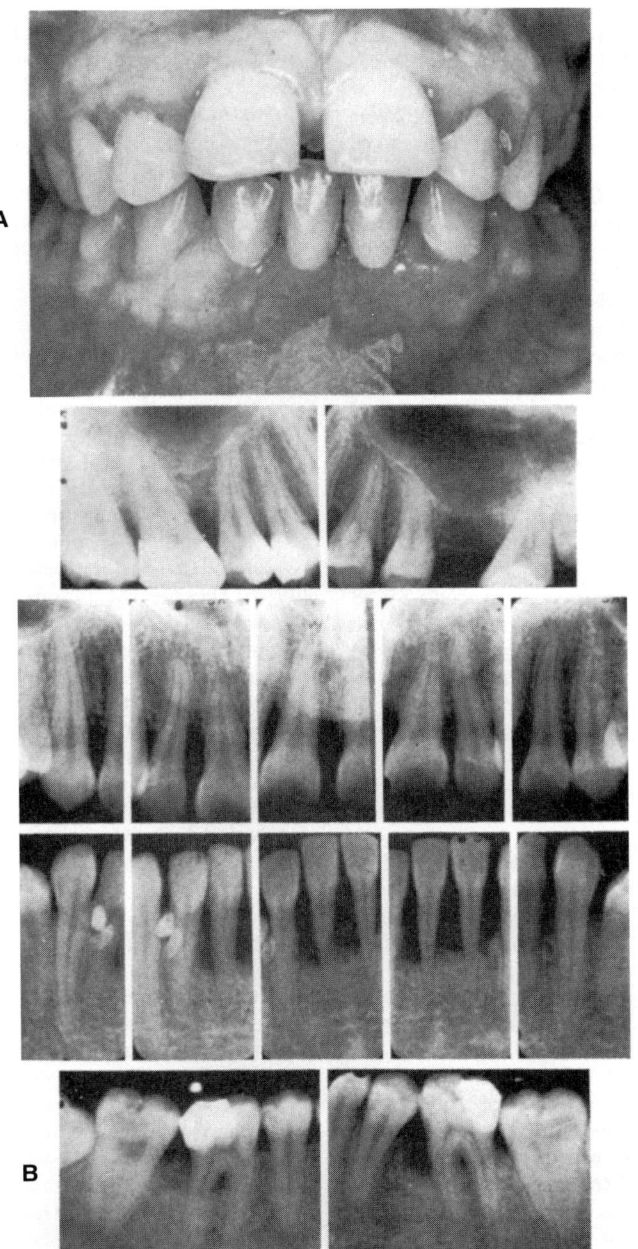

Fig. 33-2 Localized aggressive periodontitis in a 17-year-old girl, overall prognosis fair. **A,** Gingival inflammation, periodontal pockets, and pathologic migration. **B,** Severe bone destruction.

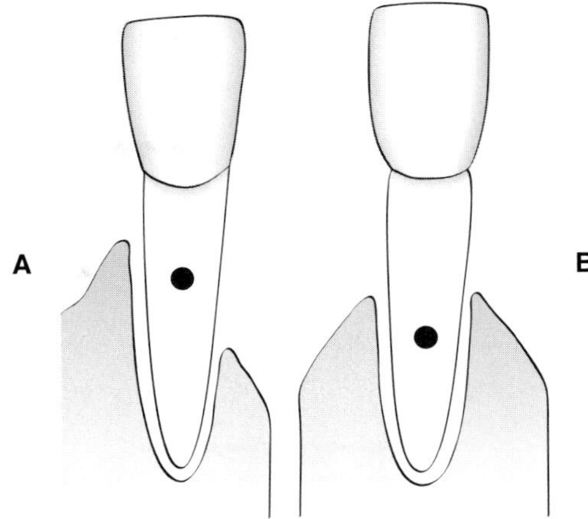

Fig. 33-3 The prognosis of tooth **A** is better than that for tooth **B,** despite the fact that there is less bone on one of the surfaces of **A.** Because the center of rotation of tooth **A** is closer to the crown, the distribution of occlusal forces to the periodontium is more favorable than in **B.**

variable in this relationship (see Chapter 5). Therefore patients at risk for diabetes should be identified as early as possible and informed of the relationship between periodontitis and diabetes. Similarly, patients diagnosed with diabetes must be informed of the impact of diabetic control on the development and progression of periodontitis. It follows that the prognosis in these cases is dependent on patient compliance relative to both their medical and dental status. Well-controlled patients with diabetes with slight-to-moderate periodontitis who comply with their recommended periodontal treatment should have a good prognosis. Similarly, in patients with other systemic disorders that could affect disease progression, prognosis improves with correction of the systemic problem.

The prognosis is questionable when surgical periodontal treatment is required but cannot be provided because of the patient's health (see Chapter 38). Incapacitating conditions that limit the patient's performance of oral procedures (e.g., Parkinson's disease) also adversely affect the prognosis. Newer "automated" oral hygiene devices such as electric toothbrushes may be helpful for these patients and improve their prognosis (see Chapter 49).

Genetic Factors. Periodontal diseases represent a complex interaction between a microbial challenge and the host's response to that challenge, both of which may be influenced by environmental factors such as smoking. In addition to these external factors, there also is evidence that genetic factors may play an important role in determining the nature of the host response.[15] Evidence for this type of genetic influence exists for patients with both chronic and aggressive periodontitis. Genetic polymorphisms in the interleukin-1 (IL-1) genes, resulting in increased production of IL1-β, have been associated with a significant increase in risk for severe, generalized, chronic periodontitis.[20,32] It has been demonstrated that knowledge of the patient's IL-1 genotype and smoking status can aid the clinician in assigning a prognosis.[31] Genetic factors also appear to influence serum IgG2 antibody titers and the expression of Fc-γRII receptors on the neutrophil, both of which may be significant in aggressive periodontitis.[15] Other genetic disorders such as leukocyte adhesion deficiency type I can influence neutrophil function, creating an additional risk factor for aggressive periodontitis.[15] Finally, the familial aggregation that is characteristic of aggressive periodontitis indicates that additional, as yet unidentified, genetic factors may be important in susceptibility to this form of disease (see Chapter 28).

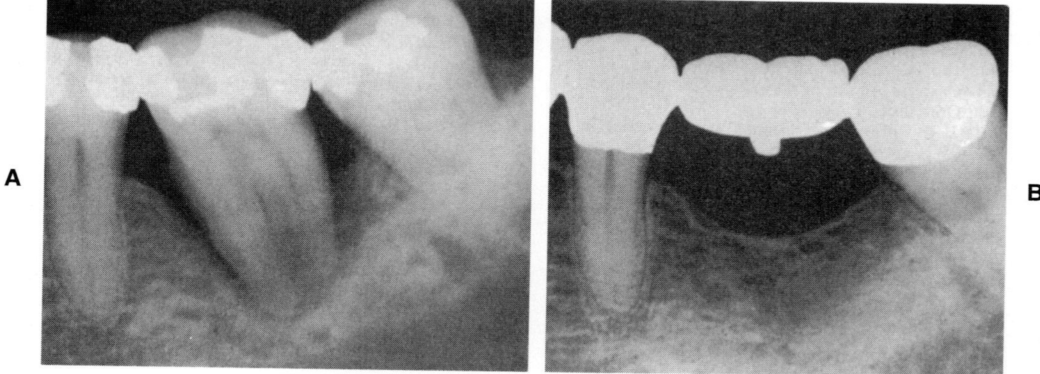

Fig. 33-4 Extraction of severely involved tooth to preserve bone on adjacent teeth. **A,** Extensive bone destruction around the mandibular first molar. **B,** Radiograph made 8.5 years after extraction of the first molar and replacement by a prosthesis. Note the excellent bone support.

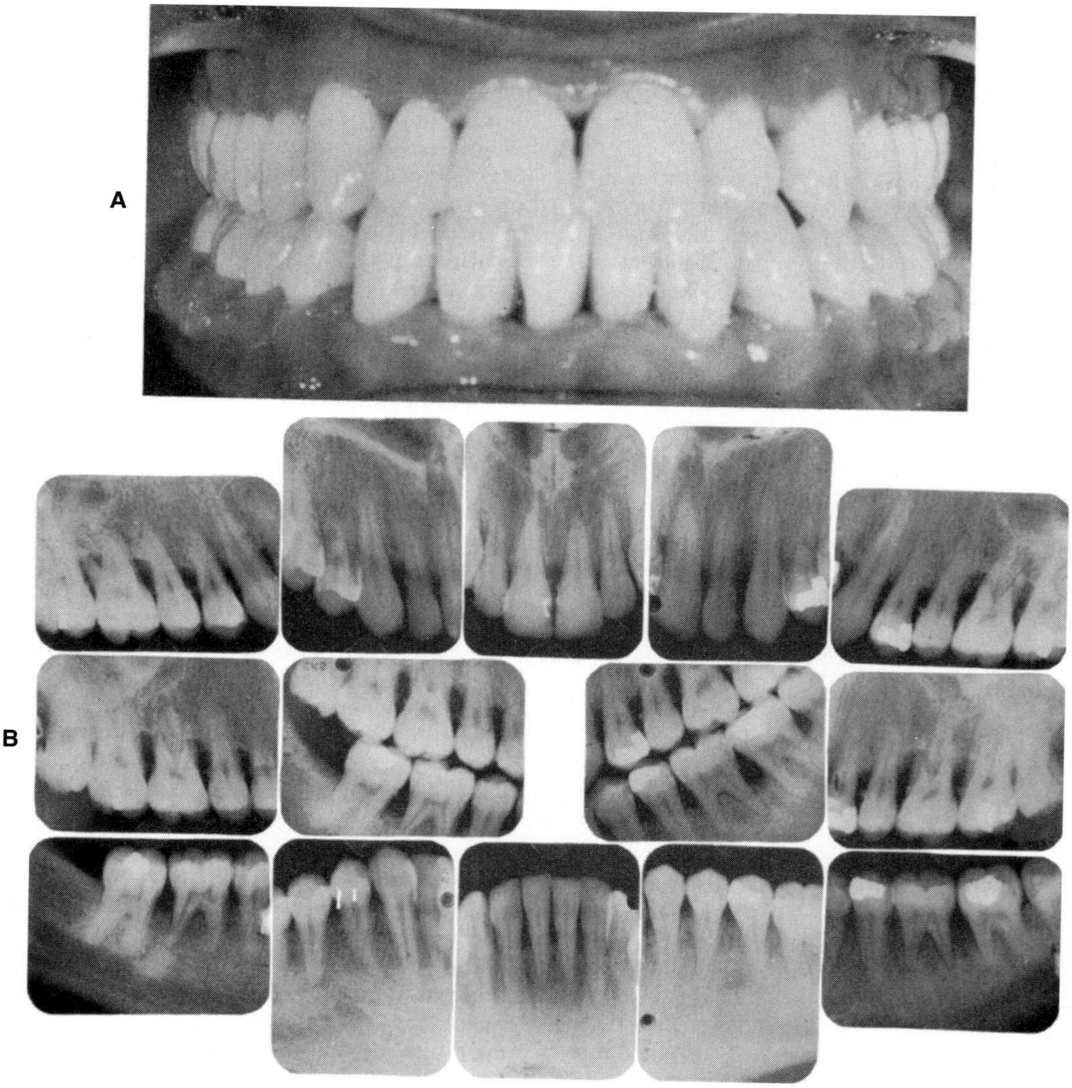

Fig. 33-5 Generalized aggressive periodontitis, poor crown-to-root ratio, overall prognosis poor. **A,** A 24-year-old patient with generalized periodontal attachment loss and pocket formation. **B,** Moderate to advanced bone destruction. The contrast between the well-formed crowns and the relatively short, tapered roots worsens the prognosis.

The influence of genetic factors on prognosis is not simple. Although microbial and environmental factors can be altered through conventional periodontal therapy and patient education, genetic factors currently cannot be altered. However, detection of genetic variations that are linked with periodontal disease can potentially influence the prognosis in several ways. First, early detection of patients at risk due to genetic factors can lead to early implementation of preventive and treatment measures for these patients. Second, identification of genetic risk factors later in the disease and/or during the course of treatment can influence treatment recommendations, such as the use of adjunctive antibiotic therapy or increased frequency of maintenance visits. Finally, identification of young individuals who have not been evaluated for periodontitis, but who are recognized as being at risk because of the familial aggregation seen in aggressive periodontitis, can lead to the development of early intervention strategies. In each of these cases, early diagnosis, intervention and/or alterations in the treatment regimen may lead to an improved prognosis for the patient.

Stress. Physical and emotional stress, as well as substance abuse, may alter the patient's ability to respond to the periodontal treatment performed (see Chapter 5). These factors have to be realistically faced in attempting to establish a prognosis.

Local Factors

Plaque/Calculus. The microbial challenge presented by bacterial plaque and calculus is the most important local factor in periodontal diseases. Therefore in most cases, having a good prognosis is dependent on the ability of the patient and the clinician to remove these etiologic factors (see Chapters 6 and 11).

Subgingival Restorations. Subgingival margins may contribute to increased plaque accumulation, increased inflammation and increased bone loss[2,35,43] when compared with supragingival margins. Furthermore, discrepancies in these margins (e.g., overhangs) can negatively impact the periodontium (see Chapter 11). The size of these discrepancies and amount of time they have been present are important factors in the amount of destruction that occurs. However, in general, a tooth with a discrepancy in its subgingival margins has a poorer prognosis than a tooth with well-contoured, supragingival margins.

Anatomic Factors. Anatomic factors that may predispose the periodontium to disease, and therefore affect the prognosis, include short, tapered roots with large crowns, cervical enamel projections (CEPs) and enamel pearls, intermediate bifurcation ridges, root concavities, and developmental grooves. The clinician must also consider root proximity and the location and anatomy of furcations when developing a prognosis.

Prognosis is poor for teeth with short, tapered roots and relatively large crowns (Fig. 33-5). Because of the disproportionate crown-to-root ratio and the reduced root surface available for periodontal support,[17] the periodontium may be more susceptible to injury by occlusal forces.

CEPs are flat, ectopic extensions of enamel that extend beyond the normal contours of the cementoenamel junction.[27] They extend into the furcation of 28.6% of mandibular molars and 17% of maxillary molars.[27] They are most likely to be found on buccal surfaces of maxillary second molars.[13,45] Enamel pearls are larger, round deposits of enamel that can be located in furcations or other areas on the root surface.[34] Enamel pearls are less frequent (1.1% to 5.7% of permanent molars; 75% appearing in maxillary third molars[34]) than CEPs. An intermediate bifurcation ridge has been described in 73% of mandibular first molars, crossing from the mesial to the distal root at the midpoint of the furcation.[7] The presence of these enamel projections on the root surface interferes with the attachment apparatus and may prevent regenerative procedures from achieving their maximum potential. Therefore their presence may have a negative effect on the prognosis for an individual tooth.

Scaling with root planing is a fundamental procedure in periodontal therapy. Anatomic factors that decrease the efficiency of this procedure can have a negative impact on the prognosis. Therefore the morphology of the tooth root is an important consideration when discussing prognosis. Root concavities exposed through loss of attachment can vary from shallow flutings to deep depressions. They appear more marked on maxillary first premolars, the mesiobuccal root of the maxillary first molar, both roots of mandibular first molars, and the mandibular incisors[4,5] (Figs. 33-6 and 33-7). Any tooth, however, can have a proximal concavity.[10] Although

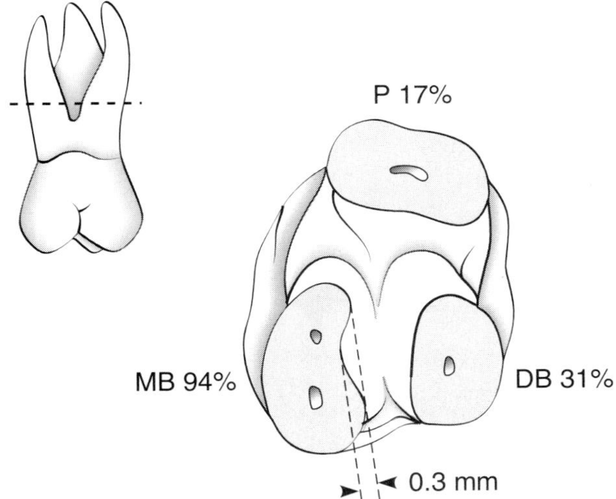

Fig. 33-6 Root concavities in maxillary first molars sectioned 2 mm apical to the furca. The furcal aspect of the root is concave in 94% of the mesiobuccal (MB) roots, 31% of the distobuccal (DB) roots, and 17% of the palatal (P) roots. The deepest concavity is found in the furcal aspects of the mesiobuccal root (mean concavity, 0.3 mm). The furcal aspect of the buccal roots diverges toward the palate in 97% of teeth (mean divergence: 22 degrees). (Redrawn from Bower RC: Furcation morphology relative to periodontal treatment-furcation root surface anatomy. J Periodontol 1979; 50:366.)

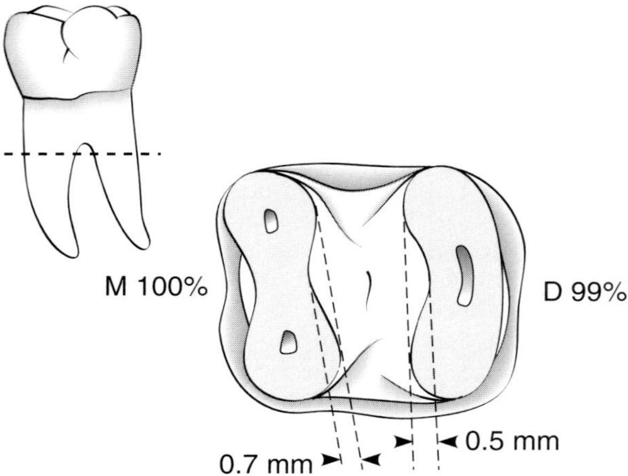

Fig. 33-7 Root concavities in mandibular first molars sectioned 2 mm apical to the furca. Concavity of the furcal aspect was found in 100% of mesial (M) roots and 99% of distal (D) roots. Deeper concavity was found in the mesial roots (mean concavity, 0.7 mm). (Redrawn from Bower RC: Furcation morphology relative to periodontal treatment-furcation root surface anatomy. J Periodontol 1979; 50:366.)

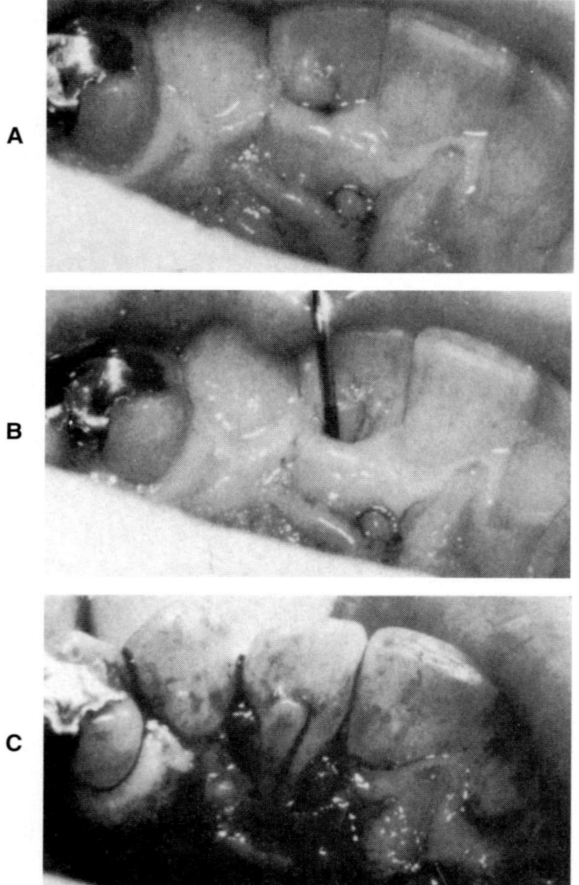

Fig. 33-8 Palatogingival groove. **A,** Gingival inflammation and exudate in an area palatal to the upper lateral incisor. **B,** Probing shows deep pocket. **C,** The area is flapped, and the presence of a palatogingival groove is confirmed. (Courtesy Dr. Robert Merin, Woodland Hills, Calif.)

these concavities increase the attachment area and produce a root shape that may be more resistant to torquing forces, they also create areas that can be difficult for both the dentist and the patient to clean.

Other anatomic considerations that present accessibility problems are developmental grooves, root proximity, and furcation involvements. The presence of any of these can worsen the prognosis. Developmental grooves, which sometimes appear in the maxillary lateral incisors (palatogingival groove)[46] (Fig. 33-8) or in the lower incisors, create an accessibility problem.[8,12] They initiate on enamel and can extend a significant distance on the root surface, providing a plaque-retentive area that is difficult to instrument. These palatogingival grooves are found on 5.6% of maxillary lateral incisors and 3.4% of maxillary central incisors.[19] Similarly, root proximity can result in interproximal areas that are difficult for the clinician and patient to access. Finally, access to the furcation area is usually difficult to obtain. In 58% of maxillary and mandibular first molars, the furcation entrance diameter is narrower than the width of conventional periodontal curettes.[5] (Fig. 33-9) Maxillary first premolars offer the greatest difficulties, and therefore their prognosis is usually unfavorable when the lesion reaches the mesial-distal furcation. Maxillary molars also offer some degree of difficulty; sometimes their prognosis can be improved by resecting one of the buccal roots (see Chapter 64), thereby improving access to the area. When mandibular first molars or buccal furcations of maxillary molars offer good access to the furcation area, their prognosis is usually better.

Tooth Mobility. The principal causes of tooth mobility are loss of alveolar bone, inflammatory changes in the periodontal ligament, and trauma from occlusion. Tooth mobility caused by inflammation and trauma from occlusion may be correctable.[33] However, tooth mobility resulting from loss of alveolar bone is not likely to be corrected. The likelihood of restoring tooth stability is inversely proportional to the extent to which mo-

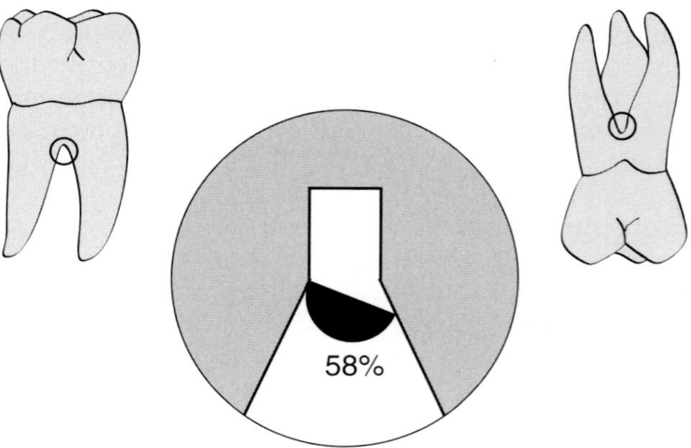

Fig. 33-9 The furcation entrance is narrower than a standard curette in 58% of first molars. (Redrawn from Bower RC: Furcation morphology relative to periodontal treatment-furcation root surface anatomy. J Periodontol 1979; 50:366.)

bility is caused by loss of supporting alveolar bone. A longitudinal study of the response to treatment of teeth with different degrees of mobility revealed that pockets on clinically mobile teeth do not respond as well to periodontal therapy as pockets on nonmobile teeth exhibiting the same initial disease severity.[9] Another study however, in which ideal plaque control was attained, found similar healing in both hypermobile and firm teeth.[40] The stabilization of tooth mobility through the use of splinting may have a beneficial impact on the overall and individual tooth prognosis.

Prosthetic/Restorative Factors

The overall prognosis requires a general consideration of bone levels (evaluated radiographically) and attachment levels (determined clinically) to establish whether enough teeth can be saved either to provide a functional and aesthetic dentition or to serve as abutments for a useful prosthetic replacement of the missing teeth.

At this point, the overall prognosis and the prognosis for individual teeth overlap because the prognosis for key individual teeth may affect the overall prognosis for prosthetic rehabilitation. For example, saving or losing a key tooth may determine whether other teeth are saved or extracted or whether the prosthesis used is fixed or removable (see Fig. 33-4). When few teeth remain, the prosthodontic needs become more important, and sometimes periodontally treatable teeth may have to be extracted if they are not compatible with the design of the prosthesis.

Teeth that serve as abutments are subjected to increased functional demands. More rigid standards are required when evaluating the prognosis of teeth adjacent to edentulous areas. A tooth that has undergone endodontic treatment that has a post is more likely to fracture when serving as a distal abutment supporting a distal removable partial denture. Additionally, special oral hygiene measures must be instituted in these areas.

Caries, Nonvital Teeth, and Root Resorption. For teeth mutilated by extensive caries, the feasibility of adequate restoration and endodontic therapy should be considered before undertaking periodontal treatment. Extensive idiopathic root resorption or root resorption that has occurred as a result of orthodontic therapy, jeopardizes the stability of teeth and adversely affects the response to periodontal treatment. The periodontal prognosis of treated nonvital teeth is not different from that of vital teeth. New attachment can occur to the cementum of both nonvital and vital teeth.

RELATIONSHIP BETWEEN DIAGNOSIS AND PROGNOSIS

Many of the criteria used in the diagnosis and classification of the different forms of periodontal disease[1] (see Chapter 4) are also used in developing a prognosis (see Table 33-1). Factors such as patient age, severity of disease, genetic susceptibility, and presence of systemic disease are important criteria in the diagnosis of the condition. These are also important in developing a prognosis. These common factors suggest that for any given diagnosis, there should be an expected prognosis under ideal conditions. The following section discusses the potential prognoses of the various periodontal diseases outlined in Chapter 4.

Prognosis for Patients with Gingival Disease

Dental Plaque-Induced Gingival Diseases

GINGIVITIS ASSOCIATED WITH DENTAL PLAQUE ONLY. Plaque-induced gingivitis is a reversible disease that occurs when bacterial plaque accumulates at the gingival margin.[24,26] This disease can occur on a periodontium that has experienced no attachment loss, or on a periodontium with nonprogressing attachment loss (see Chapter 4). In either case, the prognosis for patients with gingivitis associated with dental plaque only is good, provided all local irritants are eliminated, other local factors contributing to plaque retention are eliminated, gingival contours conducive to the preservation of health are attained, and the patient cooperates by maintaining good oral hygiene.

PLAQUE-INDUCED GINGIVAL DISEASES MODIFIED BY SYSTEMIC FACTORS. The inflammatory response to bacterial plaque at the gingival margin can be influenced by systemic factors such as endocrine-related changes associated with puberty, menstruation, pregnancy, and diabetes, and the presence of blood dyscrasias. In many instances, the frank signs of gingival inflammation that occur in these patients are seen in the presence of relatively small amounts of bacterial plaque. Therefore the long-term prognosis for these patients depends not only on control of bacterial plaque, but also on control or correction of the systemic factor(s).

PLAQUE-INDUCED GINGIVAL DISEASES MODIFIED BY MEDICATIONS. Gingival diseases associated with medications include drug-influenced gingival enlargement, often seen with phenytoin, cyclosporin, nifedipine, and oral contraceptive-associated gingivitis. In drug-influenced gingival enlargement, it has been shown that reductions in dental plaque can limit the severity of the lesions. However, plaque control alone does not prevent development of the lesions, and surgical intervention is usually necessary to correct the alterations in gingival contour. Continued use of the drug usually results in recurrence of the enlargement, even following surgical intervention (see Chapter 18). Therefore the long-term prognosis is dependent on whether the patient's systemic problem can be treated with an alternative medication that does not have gingival enlargement as a side effect.

In oral contraceptive-associated gingivitis, frank signs of gingival inflammation can be seen in the presence of relatively little plaque. Therefore as seen in plaque-induced gingival diseases modified by systemic factors, the long-term prognosis in these patients is dependent on not only the control of bacterial plaque, but also on the likelihood of continued use of the oral contraceptive.

GINGIVAL DISEASES MODIFIED BY MALNUTRITION. Although malnutrition has been suspected to play a role in the development of gingival diseases, most clinical studies have not shown a relationship between the two. One possible exception is severe vitamin C deficiency. In early experimental vitamin C deficiency, gingival inflammation and bleeding on probing were independent of plaque levels present. The prognosis in these cases may be dependent on the severity and duration of the deficiency and on the likelihood of reversing the deficiency through dietary supplementation.

Non–Plaque-Induced Gingival Lesions

Non–plaque-induced gingivitis can be seen in patients with a variety of bacterial, fungal, and viral infections.[16] Since the gingivitis in these patients is not usually attributed to plaque accumulation, prognosis is dependent on elimination of the source of the infectious agent. Dermatologic disorders such as lichen planus, pemphigoid, pemphigus vulgaris, erythema multiforme, and lupus erythematosus also can manifest in the oral cavity as atypical gingivitis (see Chapter 21). Prognosis for these patients is linked to management of the associated dermatologic disorder. Finally, allergic, toxic, and foreign body reactions, as well as mechanical and thermal trauma can result in gingival lesions. Prognosis for these cases is dependent on elimination of the causative agent.

Prognosis for Patients with Periodontitis

Chronic Periodontitis. Chronic periodontitis is a slowly progressive disease associated with well-known local environmental factors.[22] It can present in a localized or generalized form (see Chapter 26). In cases where the clinical attachment loss and bone loss are not very advanced (slight-to-moderate periodontitis), the prognosis is generally good, provided the inflammation can be controlled through good oral hygiene and the removal of local plaque-retentive factors (see Fig. 33-1). In patients with more severe disease, as evidenced by furcation involvement and increasing clinical mobility, or in patients who are noncompliant with oral hygiene practices, the prognosis may be downgraded to fair to poor.

Aggressive Periodontitis. Aggressive periodontitis can present in a localized or a generalized form.[21] Two common features of both forms are (1) rapid attachment loss and bone destruction in an otherwise clinically healthy patient and (2) a familial aggregation. These patients often present with limited microbial deposits that seem inconsistent with the severity of tissue destruction. However, the deposits that are present often have elevated levels of *Actinobacillus actinomycetemcomitans* or *Porphyromonas gingivalis*. These patients also may present with phagocyte abnormalities and a hyperresponsive monocyte/macrophage phenotype. These clinical, microbiologic and immunologic features would suggest that patients diagnosed with aggressive periodontitis would have a poor prognosis.

However, the clinician should consider additional specific features of the localized form of disease when determining the prognosis (see Fig. 33-2). Localized aggressive periodontitis usually occurs around the age of puberty and is localized to first molars and incisors. The patient often exhibits a strong serum antibody response to the infecting agents, which may contribute to localization of the lesions (see Chapter 27). When diagnosed early, these cases can be treated conservatively with oral hygiene instruction and systemic antibiotic therapy,[37] resulting in an excellent prognosis. When more advanced disease occurs, the prognosis can still be good if the lesions are treated with débridement, local and systemic antibiotics, and regenerative therapy.[25,47]

In contrast, although patients with generalized aggressive periodontitis also are young patients (usually under age 30), they present with generalized interproximal attachment loss and a poor antibody response to infecting agents (see Fig. 33-5). Secondary contributing factors such as cigarette smoking are often present. These factors, coupled with the alterations in host defense seen in many of these patients, may result in a case that does not respond well to conventional periodontal therapy (scaling with root planing, oral hygiene instruction, and surgical intervention). Therefore these patients often have a fair, poor, or questionable prognosis, and the use of systemic antibiotics should be considered to help control the disease (see Chapter 45).

PERIODONTITIS AS A MANIFESTATION OF SYSTEMIC DISEASES. Periodontitis as a manifestation of systemic diseases can be divided into two categories[18,23]: (1) those associated with hematologic disorders such as leukemia and acquired neutropenias and (2) those associated with genetic disorders such as familial and cyclic neutropenia, Down syndrome, Papillon-Lefèvre syndrome, and hypophosphastasia. Although the primary etiologic factor in periodontal diseases is bacterial plaque, systemic diseases that alter the ability of the host to respond to the microbial challenge presented may affect the progression of disease and therefore the prognosis for the case. For example, decreased numbers of circulating neutrophils (as in acquired neutropenias) may contribute to widespread destruction of the periodontium. Unless the neutropenia can be corrected, these patients present with a fair-to-poor prognosis. Similarly, genetic disorders that alter the way the host responds to bacterial plaque (as in leukocyte adhesion deficiency syndrome) also can contribute to the development of periodontitis. Because these disorders generally manifest early in life, the impact on the periodontium may be clinically similar to generalized aggressive periodontitis. The prognosis in these cases will be fair to poor. Other genetic disorders exist that do not affect the host's ability to combat infections, but still have an affect on the development of periodontitis. Examples include hypophosphatasia, where patients have decreased levels of circulating alkaline phosphatase, severe alveolar bone loss, premature loss of deciduous and permanent teeth, and the connective tissue disorder, Ehlers-Danlos syndrome, where patients may present with the clinical characteristics of aggressive periodontitis. In both of these examples, the prognosis will be fair to poor.

Necrotizing Periodontal Diseases. Necrotizing periodontal disease can be divided into necrotic diseases that affect the gingival tissues exclusively (necrotizing ulcerative gingivitis [NUG]) and necrotic diseases that affect deeper tissues of the periodontium, resulting in loss of connective tissue attachment and alveolar bone (necrotizing ulcerative periodontitis [NUP]).[36,41] In NUG, the primary predisposing factor is bacterial plaque. However, this disease is usually complicated by the presence of secondary factors such as acute psychologic stress, tobacco smoking, and poor nutrition, all of which can contribute to immunosuppression. Therefore superimposition of these secondary factors on a preexisting gingivitis can result in the painful, necrotic lesions characteristic of NUG. With control of both the bacterial plaque and the secondary factors, the prognosis for a patient with NUG is good. However, the tissue destruction in these cases is not reversible, and poor control of the secondary factors may make these patients susceptible to recurrence of the disease. With repeated episodes of NUG, the prognosis may be downgraded to fair.

The clinical presentation of NUP is similar to that of NUG, except the necrosis extends from the gingiva into the periodontal ligament and alveolar bone. In systemically healthy patients, this progression may have resulted from multiple episodes of NUG or the necrotizing disease may occur at a site previously affected with periodontitis. In these cases the prognosis is dependent on alleviating the plaque and secondary factors associated with NUG. However, many patients presenting with NUP are immunocompromised through systemic conditions, such as HIV infection. In these cases, the prognosis is dependent on not only reducing local and secondary factors, but also on dealing with the systemic problem (see Chapter 40).

REEVALUATION OF PROGNOSIS AFTER PHASE I THERAPY

A frank reduction in pocket depth and inflammation after phase I therapy points to a favorable response to treatment and may suggest a better prognosis than previously assumed. If the inflammatory changes present cannot be controlled or reduced by phase I therapy, the overall prognosis may be unfavorable. In these cases, the prognosis can be directly related to the severity of inflammation. Given two patients with comparable bone destruction, the prognosis may be better for the patient with the greater degree of inflammation, since a larger component of that patient's bone destruction may be attributable to local irritants. In addition, phase I therapy allows the clinician an opportunity to work with the patient and the patients' physician to control systemic/environmental factors such as diabetes and smoking, which may have a positive effect on prognosis if adequately controlled.

It should be noted that the progression of periodontitis generally occurs in an episodic manner, alternating periods of quiescence with shorter destructive stages (see Chapter 22). There are no methods available at present to accurately determine whether a given lesion is in a stage of remission or exacerbation. Advanced lesions, if active, may progress rapidly to a hopeless stage, whereas similar lesions in a quiescent stage may be maintainable for long periods. Phase I therapy will, at least temporarily, transform an active advanced lesion's prognosis so that it should be reanalyzed after completion of Phase I therapy.

REFERENCES

1. Armitage GC: Development of a classification system for periodontal diseases and conditions. Annals Periodontol 1999; 4:1.
2. Björn A-L, Björn H, Grkovic B: Marginal fit of restorations and its relation to periodontal bone levels. I. Metal fillings. Odontol Rev 1969; 20:311.
3. Bolin A, Eklund G, Frithiof L, et al: The effect of changed smoking habits on marginal alveolar bone loss. A longitudinal study. Swed Dent J 1993; 17:211.
4. Bower RC: Furcation morphology relative to periodontal treatment—furcation entrance architecture. J Periodontol 1979; 50:23.
5. Bower RC: Furcation morphology relative to periodontal treatment-furcation root surface anatomy. J Periodontol 1979; 50:366.
6. Chace R Sr, Low SB: Survival characteristics of periodontally-involved teeth: A 40-year study. J Periodontol 1993; 64:701.
7. Everett FG, Jump EB, Holder TD, et al: The intermediate bifurcational ridge: A study of the morphology of the bifurcation of the lower first molar. J Dent Res 1958; 37:162.
8. Everett FG, Kramer GN: The distolingual groove in the maxillary lateral incisor, a periodontal hazard. J Periodontol 1972; 43:352.
9. Flezar TJ, Knowles JW, Morrison EC, et al: Tooth mobility and periodontal therapy. J Clin Periodontol 1980; 7:495.
10. Fox SC, Bosworth BL: A morphological study of proximal root concavities: A consideration in periodontal therapy. J Am Dent Assoc 1987; 114:811.
11. Ghaia S, Bissada NF: Prognosis and actual treatment outcome of periodontally involved teeth. Periodont Clin Invest 1996; 18:7.
12. Gher, ME, Vernino AR: Root morphology-clinical significance in pathogenesis and treatment of periodontal disease. J Am Dent Assoc 1980; 101:627.
13. Grewe JM, Meskin LH, Miller T: Cervical enamel projections: prevalence, location, and extent; with associated periodontal implications. J Periodontol 1965; 36:460.
14. Grossi SD, Zambon J, Machtei EE, et al: Effects of smoking and smoking cessation on healing after mechanical therapy. J Am Dent Assoc 1997; 128:599.
15. Hart TC, Kornman KS: Genetic factors in the pathogenesis of periodontitis. Periodontol 2000 1997; 14:202.
16. Holmstrup P: Non–plaque-induced gingival lesions. Ann Periodontol 1999; 4:20.
17. Kay S, Forscher BK, Sackett LM: Tooth root length-volume relationships. An aid to periodontal prognosis. I. Anterior teeth. Oral Surg 1954; 7:735.
18. Kinane D: Periodontitis modified by systemic factors. Ann Periodontol 1999; 4:54.
19. Kogan SL: The prevalence, location and conformation of palato-radicular grooves in maxillary incisors. J Periodontol 1986; 57:2312.
20. Kornman KS, di Giovine FS: Genetic variations in cytokine expression: a risk factor for severity of adult periodontitis. Ann Periodontol 1998; 3:327.
21. Lang N, Bartold PM, Cullinan M, et al: Consensus report: aggressive periodontitis. Ann Periodontol 1999; 4:53.
22. Lindhe J, Ranney R, Lamster I, et al: Consensus report: chronic periodontitis. Ann Periodontol 1999; 4:38.
23. Lindhe J, Ranney R, Lamster I, et al: Consensus report: periodontitis as a manifestation of systemic diseases. Ann Periodontol 1999; 4:64.
24. Löe H, Theilade E, Jensen SB: Experimental gingivitis in man. J Periodontol 1965; 36:177.

25. Mabry T, Yukna R, Sepe W: Freeze-dried bone allografts with tetracycline in the treatment of juvenile periodontitis. J Periodontol 1985; 56:74.
26. Mariotti A: Dental plaque-induced gingival disease. Ann Periodontol 1999; 4:7.
27. Masters DH, Hoskins SWP: Projection of cervical enamel into molar furcations. J Periodontol 1964; 35:49.
28. McGuire MK: Prognosis versus actual outcome: a long-term survey of 100 treated periodontal patients under maintenance care. J Periodontol 1991; 62:51.
29. McGuire MK, Nunn ME: Prognosis versus actual outcome. II. The effectiveness of clinical parameters in developing an accurate prognosis. J Periodontol 1996; 67:658.
30. McGuire MK, Nunn ME: Prognosis versus actual outcome. III. The effectiveness of clinical parameters in accurately predicting tooth survival. J Periodontol 1996; 67:666.
31. McGuire MK, Nunn ME: Prognosis versus actual outcome. IV. The effectiveness of clinical parameters and IL-1 genotype in accurately predicting prognoses and tooth survival. J Periodontol 1999; 70:49.
32. Michalowicz BS, Diehl SR, Gunsolley JC, et al: Evidence of a substantial genetic basis for risk of adult periodontitis. J Periodontol 2000; 71:1699.
33. Morris ML: The diagnosis, prognosis and treatment of loose tooth. Oral Surg 1953; 6:1037.
34. Moskow BS, Canut PM: Studies on root enamel (2). Enamel pearls. A review of their morphology, localization, nomenclature, occurrence, classification, histogenesis and incidence. J Clin Periodontol 1990; 17:275.
35. Newcomb GM: The relationship between the location of subgingival crown margins and gingival inflammation. J Periodontol 1974; 45:151.
36. Novak MJ: Necrotizing ulcerative periodontitis. Ann Periodontol 1999; 4:74.
37. Novak MJ, Polson AM, Adair SM: Tetracycline therapy in patients with early juvenile periodontitis. J Periodontol 1988; 59:366.
38. Preber J, Bergström J: The effect of non-surgical treatment on periodontal pockets in smokers and non-smokers. J Clin Periodontol 1986; 13:319.
39. Renvert S, Dahlen G, Wikström M: The clinical and microbiological effects of non-surgical periodontal therapy in smokers and non-smokers. J Clin Periodontol 1998; 25:153.
40. Rosling B, Nyman S, Lindhe J: The effect of systematic plaque control on bone regeneration in infrabony pockets. J Clin Periodontol 1976; 3:38.
41. Rowland RW: Necrotizing ulcerative gingivitis. Ann Periodontol 1999; 4:65.
42. Shapiro N: Retaining periodontally "hopeless" teeth. A case report. J Am Dent Assoc 1994; 125:596.
43. Silness J: Periodontal conditions in patients treated with dental bridges. III. The relationship between the location of the crown margin and the periodontal condition. J Periodont Res 1970; 5:225.
44. Sorrin S, Burman LR: A study of cases not amenable to periodontal therapy. J Am Dent Assoc 1944; 31:204.
45. Tsatsas B, Mandi F, Kerani S: Cervical enamel projections in the molar teeth. J Periodontol 1973; 44:312.
46. Withers JA, Brunsvold MA, Killoy WJ, et al: The relationship of palato-gingival grooves to localized periodontal disease. J Periodontol 1981; 52:41.
47. Yukna R, Sepe W: Clinical evaluation of localized periodontosis defects with freeze-dried bone allografts combined with local and systemic tetracyclines. Internat J Periodont Restor Dent 1982; 5:9.

Advanced Diagnostic Techniques

Mariano Sanz and Michael G. Newman

CHAPTER

CHAPTER OUTLINE

LIMITATIONS OF CONVENTIONAL PERIODONTAL DIAGNOSIS

Periodontal diseases are prevalent human diseases defined by the signs and symptoms of gingival inflammation and/or periodontal tissue destruction. These diseases are conventionally diagnosed by clinical evaluation of the signs of inflammation in the gingiva without periodontal tissue destruction (gingivitis) or by the presence of both inflammation and tissue destruction (periodontitis). A clinical diagnosis of *periodontitis* is made by measuring the loss of connective tissue attachment to the root surface (clinical attachment loss) and loss of alveolar bone (radiographic bone loss) (Fig. 34-1). This information provides evidence of past periodontal destruction, as well as its extent and severity. However this approach does not provide any information on the cause of the condition, on the patient's susceptibility to disease, whether the disease is progressing, whether it is in remission or whether the response to therapy will be positive or negative.

The current view of the natural history of destructive periodontal disease is that disease susceptibility is subject related. This means that a person's susceptibility and host defense mechanisms are generalized. However, the disease process itself is considered to be site specific and has a multifactorial origin where periodontal pathogens, host response, genetic, systemic, and behavioral risk factors interplay to develop the disease process. In light of this information, consideration should be given to including microbiologic, immunologic, systemic, genetic, and behavioral factors, in addition to the traditional clinical and radiographic parameters, when assessing patient status. Considerable advances have been made[51] in the use of these parameters and these advances will be systematically reviewed.

ADVANCES IN CLINICAL DIAGNOSIS

Gingival Bleeding

Clinical evaluation of the degree of gingival inflammation includes assessment of the redness and swelling of

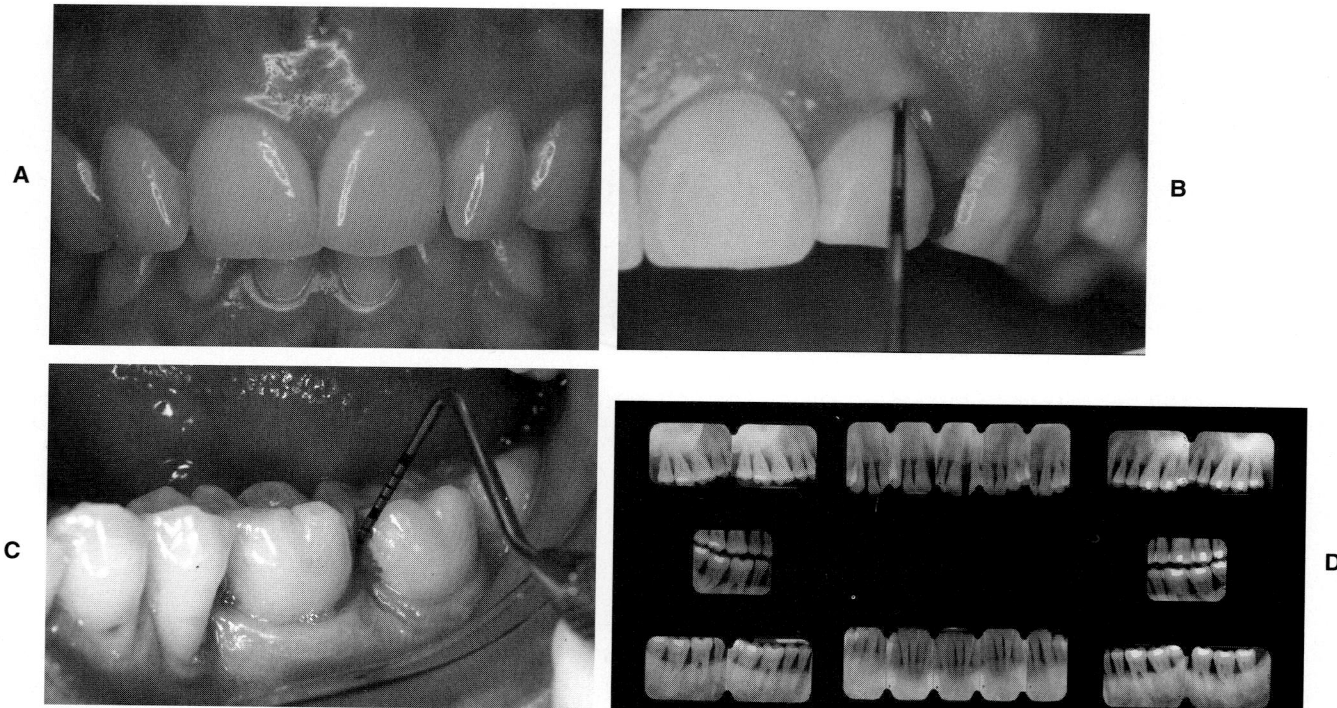

Fig. 34-1 Conventional clinical diagnostic tools. **A,** Visual diagnosis. Changes in color and contour of the gingival tissues are indicative of pathologic changes within the gingiva. **B,** Periodontal probing is used to determine pocket depth and clinical attachment levels. **C,** Bleeding on probing is indicative of periodontal inflammation. An absence of bleeding is associated with a healthy, stable periodontium. **D,** Periapical radiographs. A full mouth series of intraoral periapical radiographs is essential for the diagnosis of changes in the alveolar bone in response to periodontal disease.

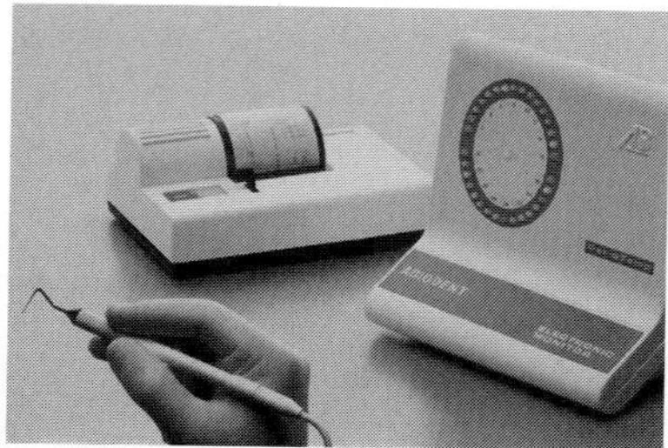

Fig. 34-2 Thermal periodontal probe system. Temperature changes detected within periodontal pockets are associated with inflammation and may be a predictor of future attachment loss. (Courtesy Abiomed, Inc., Danvers, MA.)

the gingiva along with assessment of gingival bleeding. Although the earliest clinical signs of gingivitis consist of color and texture changes, there may be underlying structural alterations without corresponding clinical signs (Fig. 34-1, *A*). Several studies have shown that gingival bleeding is a sensitive clinical indicator of early gingival inflammation.[62] Moreover, the use of gingival bleeding as an indicator of inflammation has the clinical advantage of being more objective, since color changes require a subjective estimation. It has also been shown that gingival bleeding is a good indicator of the presence of an inflammatory lesion in the connective tissue at the base of the sulcus and that the severity of bleeding increases with an increase in size of the inflammatory infiltrate.[26] Therefore there is a tendency to evaluate gingivitis by gingival bleeding alone, either with the use of a periodontal probe or a wooden interdental cleaner, instead of using visual signs of both inflammation and bleeding[2] (Fig. 34-1, *C*). Gingival bleeding has universally been considered an indicator of gingival inflammation and, by some investigators, an indicator of disease activity[73]; *however, its relationship to disease progression is unclear.*

Lang et al,[49] in a retrospective study, reported that sites that bled on probing at several visits had a higher probability of losing attachment than those that bled at one visit or did not bleed. However, well-controlled longitudinal studies[7,31] investigated the predictive values of such clinical signs, trying to correlate them with attachment loss, but failed to demonstrate a significant correlation between bleeding on probing and other clinical signs and subsequent loss of attachment. A further limitation of the use of bleeding as an inflammatory parameter is the possibility that healthy sites may bleed on probing. Lang et al[50] demonstrated that any force greater than 0.25 N may evoke bleeding in healthy sites with an intact periodontium.

A 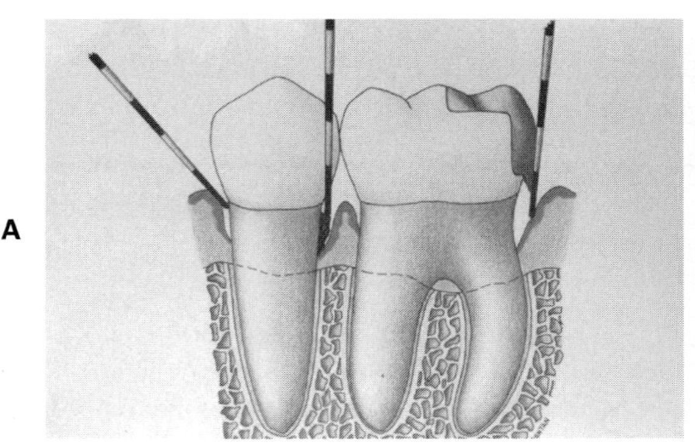 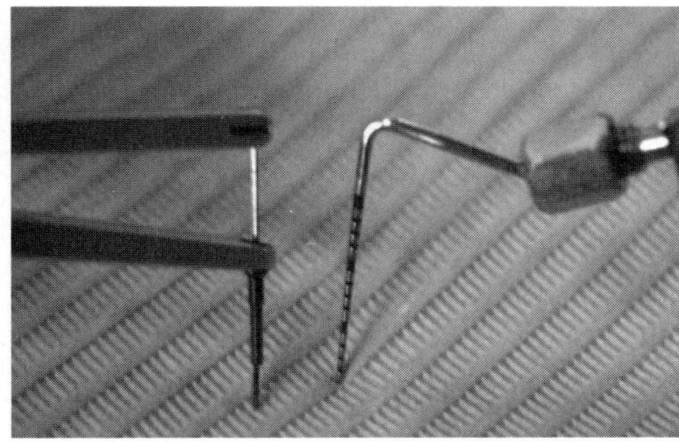 B

Fig. 34-3 Limitations in periodontal probing. **A,** Probing measurements can be affected by the incorrect angulation of the probe, by interference from calculus on the tooth or root surface, and by the presence of overhanging restorations. **B,** Probing measurements can be affected by the amount of pressure applied to the probe. Probes that provide a standardized force may be used to overcome this variable. (**A,** Courtesy Dr. J. Frontan.)

Gingival Temperature

Instruments that measure the temperature in the gingival tissues have been developed; Kung et al[46] claim that these thermal probes are sensitive diagnostic devices for measuring early inflammatory changes in the gingival tissues. Studies demonstrate that suspected active periodontitis lesions can create measurable elevations in sulcular temperature. One commercially available system, the PerioTemp® probe (Abiodent, Inc., Danvers, Mass.) (Fig. 34-2), detects pocket temperature differences of 0.1° C from a referenced subgingival temperature. A naturally occurring temperature gradient exists between maxillary and mandibular teeth and between posterior and anterior teeth. Individual temperature differences are compared with those expected for each tooth, and higher-temperature pockets are signalled with a red-emitting diode. Haffajee et al[33] used this probe to assess its predictability in identifying loss of attachment, concluding that sites with a red (higher) temperature indication had more than twice the risk for future attachment loss than did those with a green indication. However, the influence of pocket depth on temperature is still not clear, and further studies are needed to demonstrate the accuracy of this device and its utility in clinical diagnosis.

Periodontal Probing

The most widely used diagnostic tool for the clinical assessment of connective tissue destruction in periodontitis is the periodontal probe. Increased probing depth and loss of clinical attachment are pathogneumonic for periodontitis. Therefore pocket probing is a crucial and mandatory procedure in diagnosing periodontitis and evaluating periodontal therapy (see Chapter 30). Reduction of pocket depth and gain of clinical attachment are the major clinical outcome measurements used to determine success of treatment (Fig. 34-1, *B*).

However, use of the periodontal probe presents many problems in terms of sensitivity and reproducibility of the measurements. Readings of clinical pocket depth obtained with the periodontal probe do not normally coincide with the histologic pocket depth, since the probe normally penetrates the coronal level of the junctional epithelium,[74] and the precise location of the probe tip depends on the degree of inflammation of the underlying connective tissues. If the tissue is inflamed, it offers less resistance to probe penetration, and the probe tip either coincides with or is apical to the coronal level of connective tissue attachment.[54] Conversely, healed gingiva following subgingival instrumentation demonstrates an increased resistance to periodontal probing.[59]

The disparity between measurements also depends on the probing technique, probing force, size of the probe, angle of insertion of the probe, and precision of the probe calibration[54] (Fig. 34-3, *A*). All of these variables contribute to the large standard deviations (0.5 to 1.3 mm) in clinical probing results, which make detection of small changes difficult.[30]

Since the mid-1980s, different probe prototypes have been developed and tested to overcome these limitations.[86] One of the main problems in reproducibility has been the variation in probing force. Different studies have shown that the penetration of the probe was positively correlated with probing force.[62] This has been solved with the development of pressure-sensitive probes, which have a standardized controlled insertion pressure[85] (Fig. 34-3, *B*). These studies have shown that with forces of up to 30 g, the tip of the probe seems to remain within the junctional epithelium,[4] and forces of up to 50 g are necessary to diagnose periodontal osseous defects.[43] Standardization of probe tips (less than 1 mm) and use of registration stents to maintain reproducible probing angulation have also been used to overcome sources of error.[6] However, fabrication of stents is time consuming and impractical for clinical diagnosis. In addition, current techniques for data readout and storage are inaccurate and time consuming. This has resulted in the development of new periodontal probing systems.

TABLE 34-1

Criteria Defined by the National Institute of Craniofacial Research (NIDCR) for Overcoming the Limitations of Conventional Periodontal Probing

Limitation	Conventional Probing	NIDCR-Criteria
Precision	1 mm	0.1 mm
Range	12 mm	10 mm
Probing force	Nonstandardized	Constant and standardized
Applicability	Noninvasive and easy to use	Noninvasive, light-weight, and easy to use
Reach	Easy to access any location around all teeth	Easy to access any location around all teeth
Angulation	Subjective	A guidance system to ensure proper angulation
Security	Easily sterilized	Complete sterilization of all portions entering the mouth
	Simple stainless steel instrument	No biohazard from material or electric shock
Readout	Depending on voice dictation and recording in writing	Direct electronic reading and digital output

After a National Institute of Craniofacial Research (NIDCR) workshop on the quantitative evaluation of periodontal diseases by physical measurement techniques,[69] there was a proposal to develop and clinically evaluate an improved periodontal pocket depth-attachment level measurement system that would meet the nine criteria shown in Table 34-1.

Following these criteria, the Florida Probe System was developed.[24] This automated probe system consists of a probe hand-piece, digital readout, foot switch, computer interface, and computer (Fig. 34-4). The end of the probe tip is 0.4 mm in diameter. This probe tip reciprocates through a sleeve, and the edge of the sleeve provides a reference by which measurements are made. These measurements are made electronically and transferred automatically to the computer when the foot switch is pressed. Constant probing force is provided by coil springs inside the probe hand-piece and digital readout. This probing method combines the advantages of constant probing force with precise electronic measurement and computer storage of data, thus eliminating the potential errors associated with visual reading and also eliminates the need for an assistant to record the measurements. These automated probes offer many solutions to the problems of conventional probing but also introduce problems of their own. The probing elements lack tactile sensitivity, mostly because of their independent movement, which forces the operator to predetermine an insertion point and angle. In addition, the use of a fixed-force setting throughout the mouth, regardless of the site or inflammatory status, may generate inaccurate measurements or patient discomfort. One common problem reported in different studies where the Florida Probe System has been compared with conventional probing is the underestimation of deep probing depths by the automated probe[70]. In fact, several studies have suggested that the use of this automated probing system does not offer any advantage over conventional probing, rendering a similar level of reproducibility. However, other studies have clearly shown that with the use of trained operators and performing the "double pass" method the measurements taken with the Florida Probe System are significantly less variable (lower standard deviation) than those obtained with a conventional probe.[76,89] Magnusson et al[15,57,58] obtained mean standard deviations (reproducibility) for clinical attachment level measurements of about 0.3 mm, which is clearly superior to an average of 0.82 mm, with a range of 0.52 to 1.30 mm reported by Haffajee et al using manual probing.[32]

Electronic probing systems, such as the Interprobe System® or the Periprobe System®, are also commercially available. They provide constant probing force, computer storage of data, and precise electronic management of the resulting inflammation. However, clinical evaluations of these systems have reported only slightly improved reproducibility when compared with conventional probing, although not clinically significant.[75,85] Other electronic probing systems have been reported in the literature, although they have never been released for general use. One of these systems is the electronic probe described by Jeffcoat et al[39,40] (the Foster-Miller probe), capable of coupling pocket depth measurement with the detection of the cemento-enamel junction from which the clinical attachment level is automatically detected. Researchers at the University of Toronto have also described a probe (the Toronto Automated probe) that, like the Florida probe, uses the occlusal-incisal surface to measure relative clinical attachment levels.[61] The sulcus is probed with a 0.5-mm nickel-titanium wire that is extended under air pressure. It controls angular discrepancies by means of a mercury tilt sensor that limits angulation within ± 30 degrees, but it requires reproducible positioning of the patient's head and cannot easily measure second or third molars.

The measurement of clinical attachment levels has traditionally been used in the diagnosis of periodontitis; however, this measurement only reflects the history of past disease and does not assess current or future disease

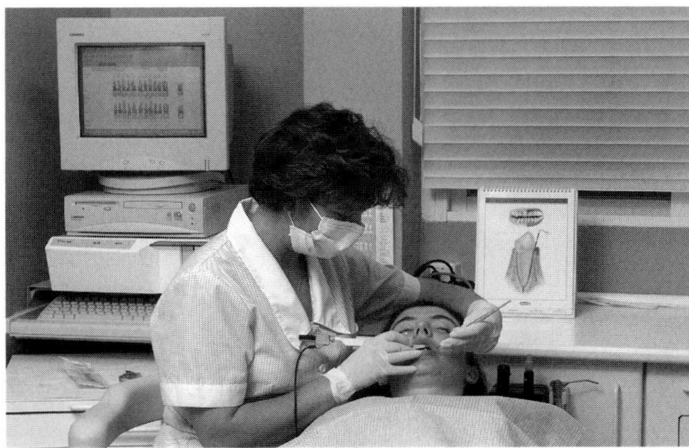

Fig. 34-4 Automated periodontal probes. Probing systems have been developed that allow the integration of direct electronic measurements at a constant probing force with computer storage and on-line data readout. The figure shows the Florida Probe System®.

activity. The most practical method of determining that disease is progressing (active) is the demonstration that a significant loss of attachment has occurred over time. To detect progression of periodontal disease over a short period, the clinician must overcome sources of error introduced by a lack of probing reproducibility. Various methods have been used to overcome these errors; these include regression analysis of measurements over time, running medians, the tolerance method, end-point analysis, and the cumulative sum method.[3,24,42] The development of electronic and automated probes (described in the preceding section) will probably allow more sensitive clinical assessments of disease progression in the near future.

ADVANCES IN RADIOGRAPHIC ASSESSMENT

Dental radiographs are the traditional method used to assess the destruction of alveolar bone associated with periodontitis. Although radiographs cannot accurately reflect the bone morphology buccally and lingually, they provide useful information on interproximal bone levels. Moreover, they provide information on the periodontium that cannot be obtained by any other noninvasive methods (e.g., root length, root proximity, and presence of periapical lesions and estimates of remaining alveolar bone) (Fig. 34-1, *D*). However, it is well known that substantial volumes of alveolar bone must be destroyed before the loss is detectable in radiographs[25]; specifically, more than 30% of the bone mass at the alveolar crest must be lost for a change in bone height to be recognized on radiographs.[66] *Therefore conventional radiographs are very specific, but lack sensitivity.* (See Chapters 32 and 33.)

Numerous cross-sectional and longitudinal epidemiologic studies have used radiographs as the principal method of determining the presence or absence of periodontal destruction. The primary criterion for bone loss in these studies was the distance from the cementoenamel junction (CEJ) to the alveolar crest as measured from bite-wing radiographs. The threshold distance of *bone loss* has varied from 1 mm to 3 mm, although most of the studies have used >2 mm as the criterion for bone loss.[1] This low degree of sensitivity is mainly due to the subjectivity of radiographic assessment and to the inherent sources of variability affecting the conventional radiographic technique, such as (1) variations in projection geometry; (2) variations in contrast and density due to differences in film processing, voltage and exposure time; and (3) masking of osseous changes by other anatomic structures (Fig. 34-5). The variations in projection geometry can be reduced by the use of well-standardized long cone parallel radiographic techniques (Fig. 34-6). To standardize the radiographic assessment, radiographs should be obtained in a constant and reproducible plane, using film holders with a template containing some kind of impression material, which is placed in a constant position on a group of teeth, and an extension arm that can be precisely attached to both the film holder and the x-ray tube[78] (Fig. 34-7). The use of a parallel radiographic technique should be standard to all radiographic assessments for periodontal diagnosis. The use of individualized film holders has been shown to be valid in evaluating bone changes in longitudinal studies and clinical trials.[44]

Digital Radiography

The variations in image quality due to the variables inherent to conventional radiography can be reduced with the use of digital intraoral radiography. Digital radiography enables the use of computerized images, which can be stored, manipulated, and corrected for under- and overexposures. Digital radiography may yield almost equal image properties compared with conventional radiographs, but through digital storage and processing, diagnostic information can be enhanced.[38] Moreover, there is an important dose reduction obtained with this technique (between $\frac{1}{3}$ to $\frac{1}{2}$ of dose reduction compared with conventional radiographs).

Two digital radiography systems rely on the sensor—the *direct* and *indirect* methods. The direct method uses a charge coupled device (CCD) sensor linked with a fiber optic or other wire to the computer system. This direct digital radiography obtains *real-time* imaging, offering both the clinician and the patient an improved visualization of the periodontium by image manipulation and comparison with previously stored images. The main disadvantage of this technique is the limited sensor area, which is only large enough to depict one or two teeth. In addition, the sensor rigidity attached to a wire, which besides sterility issues, makes ideal image projection by using film holders very difficult.

The indirect method (Digora System®) uses a phosphor luminescence plate, which is a flexible filmlike radiation energy sensor placed intraorally and exposed to conventional x-ray tubes. A laser scanner (Fig. 34-8) reads the exposed plates offline and reveals digital image data, which can be enhanced, stored, and compared with previous images. The real advantage of this indirect

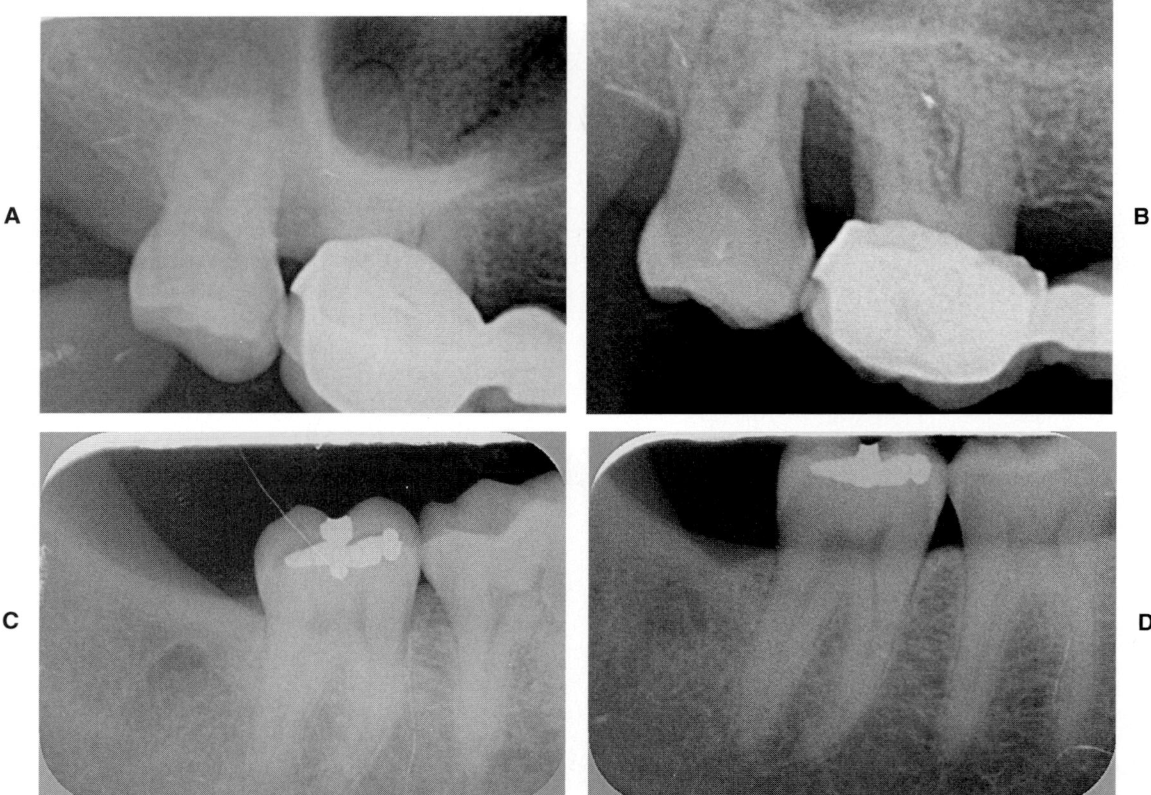

Fig. 34-5 Limitations in conventional periapical radiography. Examples of the importance of image projection in the diagnostic utility of oral periapical raciography. **A,** Radiograph taken without a paralleling technique showing a clear distortion of the root length relative to the crown. The alveolar bone height is and fills the interproximal space. **B,** Image of the same tooth with a proper image projection showing the real alveolar bone height demonstrating severe bone loss in the distal of the upper first molar. **C,** Radiograph taken without a paralleling technique showing a clear distortion of the root length relative to the crown. The alveolar bone height is and fills the interproximal space. **D,** Image of the same tooth with a proper image projection showing the real alveolar bone height and the open interproximal space. (Courtesy Dr. Fredrico Herrero.)

method is due to the plate size and flexibility, which is almost identical to conventional x-ray films. Therefore a paralleling technique with the use of film holders can be easily applied.

Digital intraoral radiography is in a state of rapid development. Sensors, as well as computer hardware and software, are continually modified and improved. Due to the clear advantage of *real or almost real images* that can be improved and to the important educational component of online images presented to the patient, it is expected that digital radiography will soon replace conventional radiography in modern daily practice. However, certain improvements should be expected in order to overcome some of the current limitations.

Subtraction Radiography

Subtraction radiography, a well-established technique in medicine, has been introduced as a technique in periodontal diagnosis.[27] This technique relies on the conversion of serial radiographs into digital images. The serially obtained digital images can then be superimposed and the resultant composite viewed on a video screen. Changes in the density and/or volume of bone can be detected as lighter areas (bone gain) or dark areas (bone loss). Quantitative changes in comparison with the baseline images can be detected using an algorithm for gray-scale levels. This is accomplished by means of a computer **(computer-assisted subtraction radiography)** (Fig. 34-9). This technique requires a parallelization technique to obtain a standardized geometry and accurate superimposable radiographs. Radiographs taken with identical exposure geometry can then be scanned using a microphotometer that determines a gray-scale value for each picture point. After superimposition of two subsequent radiographs, this technique can show differences in relative densities. Studies using this technique have shown (1) a high degree of correlation

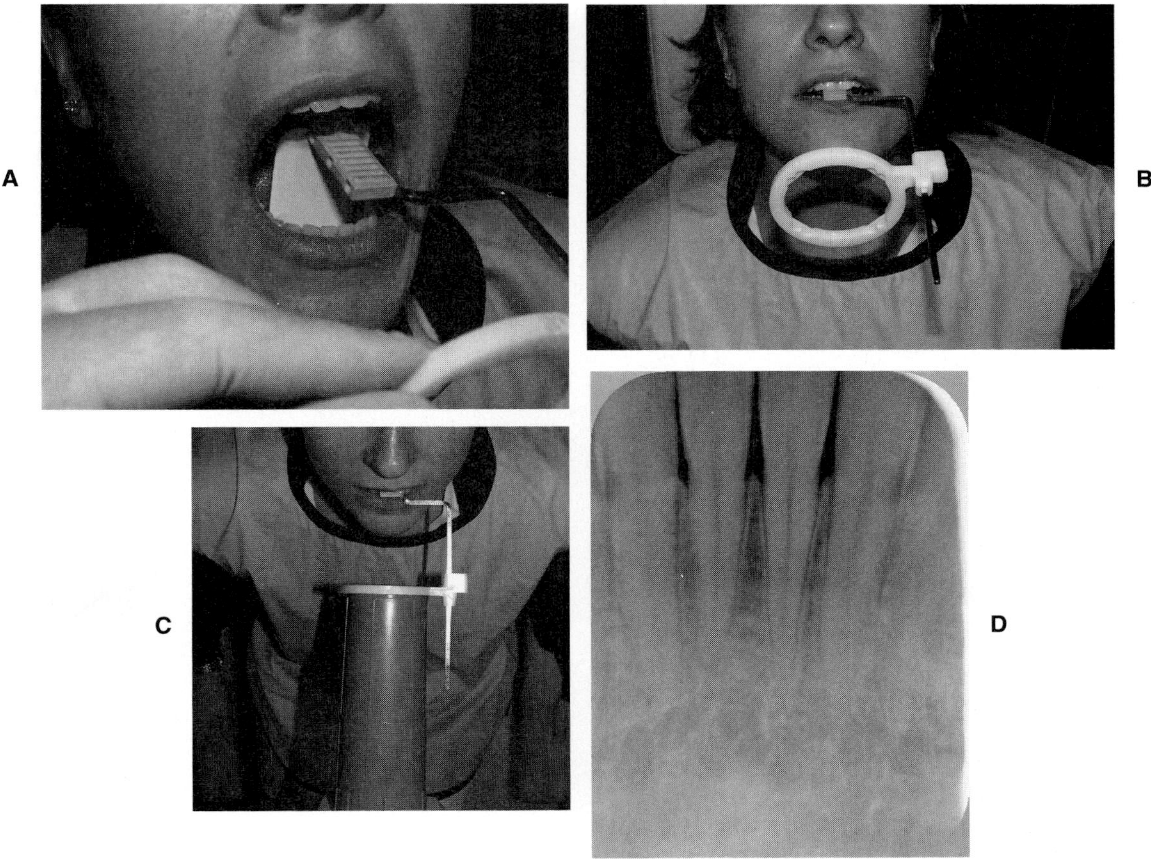

Fig. 34-6 Radiographic paralleling technique. **A,** Position of the film holder relative to the teeth. **B,** Position of the film holder relative to the paralleling device. **C,** Position of the paralleling device to the radiograph long cone tube. **D,** Obtained x-ray with proper image projection. (Courtesy Dr. Fredrico Herrero.)

between changes in alveolar bone determined by subtraction radiography and attachment level changes in periodontal patients after therapy[35] and (2) increased detectability of small osseous lesions compared with the conventional radiographs from which the subtraction images are produced.[77] Grondahl et al,[28] using subtraction analysis, showed nearly perfect accuracy at a lesion depth corresponding to 0.49 mm of compact bone, whereas a lesion must be at least three times larger to be detectable with a conventional radiology technique. Subtraction radiography has also shown a degree of sensitivity similar to that for I^{125} absorptiometry.[36] It can detect a change in bone mass of as little as 5%.[66]

Subtraction radiography has been applied to longitudinal clinical studies. Hausmann et al detected significant differences in crestal bone height of 0.87 mm,[37] and Jeffcoat et al[41] showed a strong relationship between probing attachment loss detected using sequential measurements made with an automated periodontal probe and bone loss detected with digital subtraction radiography. **Subtraction radiography** is a technique that facilitates both qualitative and quantitative visualization of even minor density changes in bone by removing the unchanged anatomic structures from the image. This enhances the detection of bone structures with true density change and significantly improved the sensitivity and accuracy of the evaluation. The main disadvantage of digital subtraction radiography techniques is the need to be close to identical projection alignment during the exposure of the sequential radiographs, which makes this method very impractical in a clinical setting. Recently, new image subtraction methods (diagnostic subtraction radiography [DSR®]) have been introduced combining the use of a positioning device during film exposure with specialized software designed for digital image subtraction using conventional personal computers in dental offices (see Fig. 34-9). This image analysis software system applies an algorithm that corrects for the effects of angular alignment discrepancies and provides some degree of flexibility in the imaging procedure. Recently, the use of the DSR technique has been compared with the conventional subtraction radiography technique and with the conventional intraoral radiography technique yielding statistically significant gains in diagnostic accuracy over conventional radiographs and no differences against the classical subtraction radiography technique.[64]

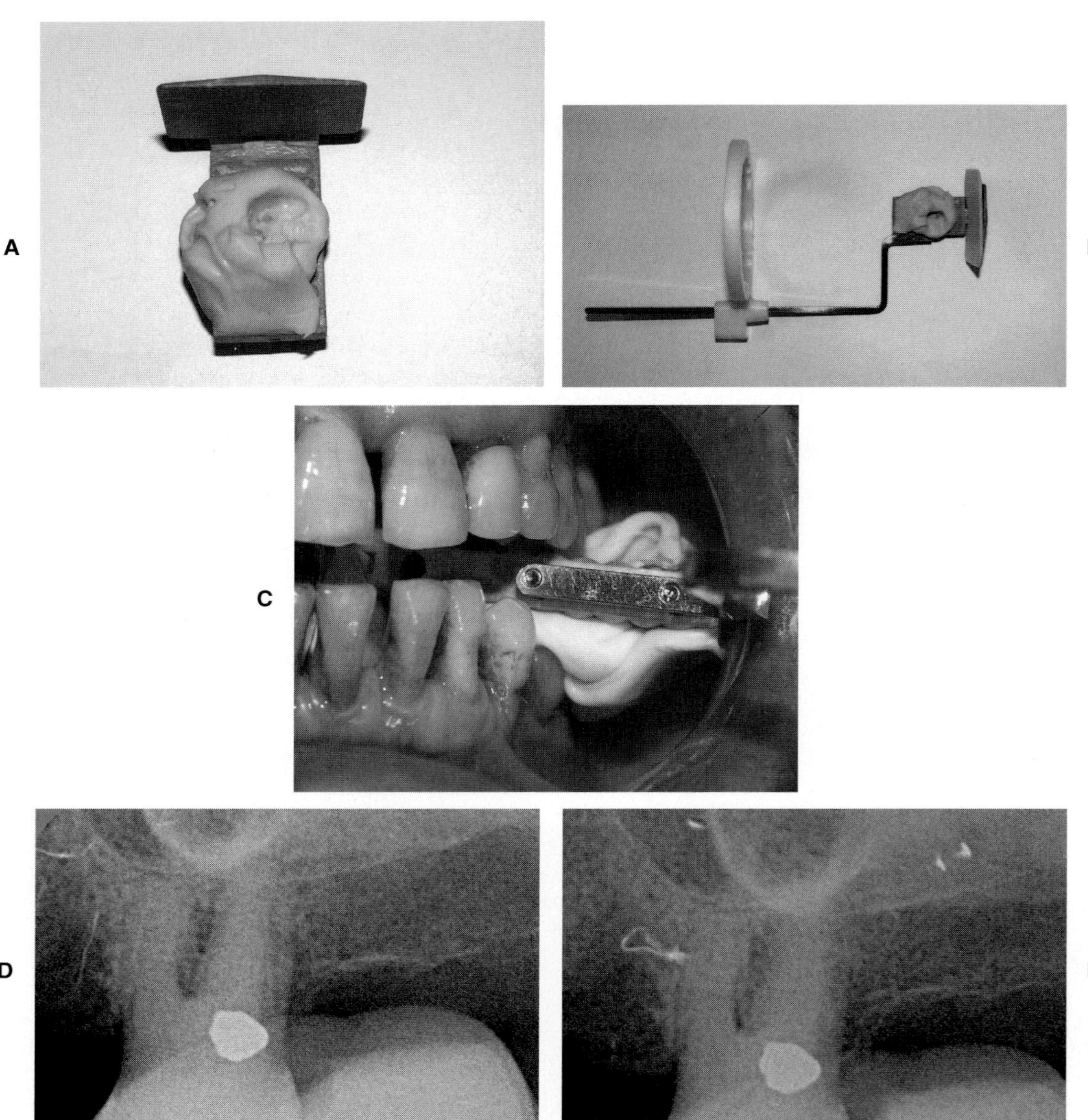

Fig. 34-7 Individualized radiographic paralleling technique for the assessment of alveolar bone changes. **A,** Occlusal imprint in film holder. **B,** Individualized film holder in paralleling device. **C,** Individualized paralleling technique in place intraorally. **D and E,** Two radiographs obtained 6 months apart demonstrating identical projection geometry. (Courtesy Dr. Fredrico Herrero.)

This method has great diagnostic potential, especially in clinical practice, because of the development of personal computers with capability for digitizing and image processing.

Computer-Assisted Densitometric Image Analysis System (CADIA)

Another technique that has been introduced is the video-based **computer-assisted densitometric image analysis system (CADIA).**[11] In this system, a video camera measures the light transmitted through a radiograph, and the signals from the camera are converted into gray-scale images. The camera is interfaced with an image processor and a computer that allow the storage and mathematical manipulation of the images. This system appears to offer an objective method for following alveolar bone density changes quantitatively over time, and, when compared with I^{125} absorptiometry and digital subtraction analysis, it has shown a higher sensitivity and a high degree of reproducibility and accuracy.

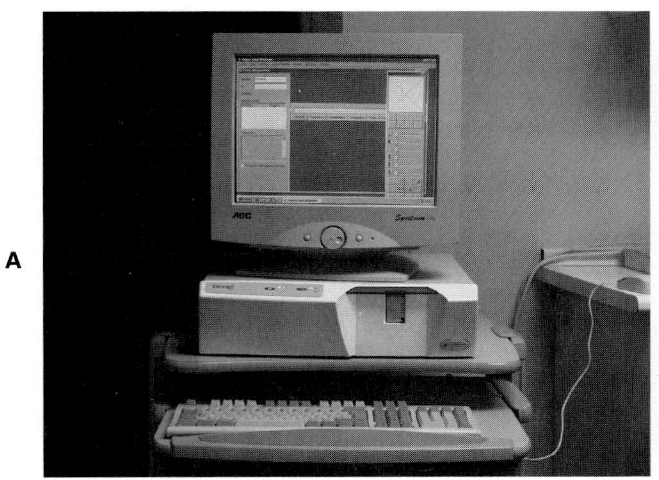

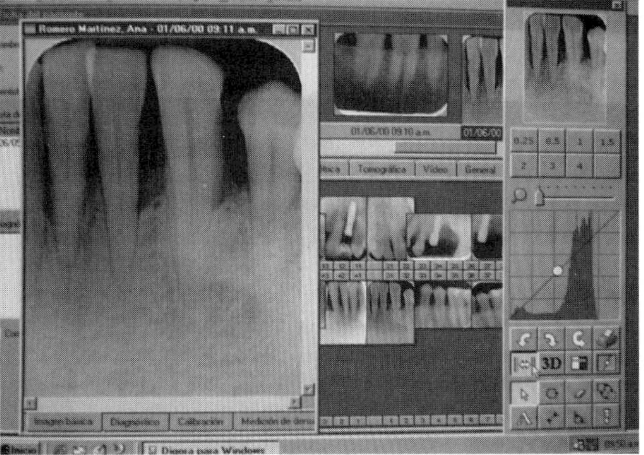

A B

Fig. 34-8 Digital Radiographic System-Digora®. Digitized radiographs can be used for patient education and for demonstrating the effects of therapy.

This technique has also been applied to longitudinal clinical studies. Deas et al,[17] using replicate measurements of clinical attachment levels and CADIA, demonstrated that the prevalence of progressing lesions in periodontitis (38% of sites per patient), as detected by this radiographic method, may be much higher than previously thought.

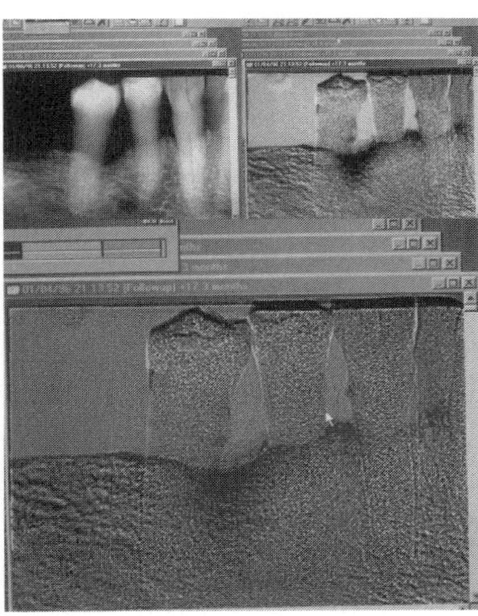

Fig. 34-9 Digital Subtraction Analysis (DSR®). Digital subtraction analysis can be used to evaluate the effects of therapy on bone density and morphology. The effects of surgical therapy on an angular defect are seen, with the new bone formation represented by the dark area.

ADVANCES IN MICROBIOLOGIC ANALYSIS

Since subgingival oral bacteria are the main initiating agents in the development of periodontal disease, it makes sense to look for specific bacteria in the subgingival microflora of patients with disease.[34,81] These microbiologic tests have the potential to support the diagnosis of the various forms of periodontal disease, to serve as indicators of disease initiation and progression (i.e., disease activity), and to determine which periodontal sites are at higher risk for active destruction. Microbial tests can also be used to monitor periodontal therapy directed at the suppression or eradication of periodontopathic microorganisms.[87]

Several methods have been employed for the detection of putative periodontal pathogens in subgingival samples. Some of these methods have been strictly used for research purposes, whereas others have been adapted or modified for clinical use. All of these methods share the common need for an appropriate subgingival plaque sample. Selecting the proper specimen site and collecting an adequate sample are essential elements in periodontal microbiology. These samples may be difficult to obtain in patients infected by organisms that are unevenly distributed in the dentition, Mombelli et al[63] have shown that four individual subgingival specimens, each from the deepest periodontal pocket in each quadrant, should be pooled to be able to detect *Porphyromonas gingivalis*. If a microbial culture is contemplated, the sample must be collected and transported in an anaerobic environment and minimal transport time should be assured to reach the laboratory and to maintain the growth of the microorganisms sampled. Fig. 34-10 shows the standard subgingival sampling technique by means of sterile paper-points inserted into the deepest area of the selected periodontal pocket.

Bacterial Culturing

Historically, culture methods have been widely used in studies aimed at characterizing the composition of the subgingival microflora and are still considered the reference method (gold standard) when determining the

A

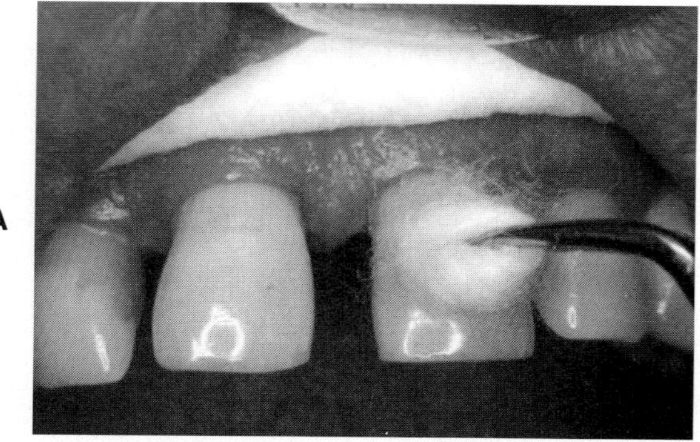

B

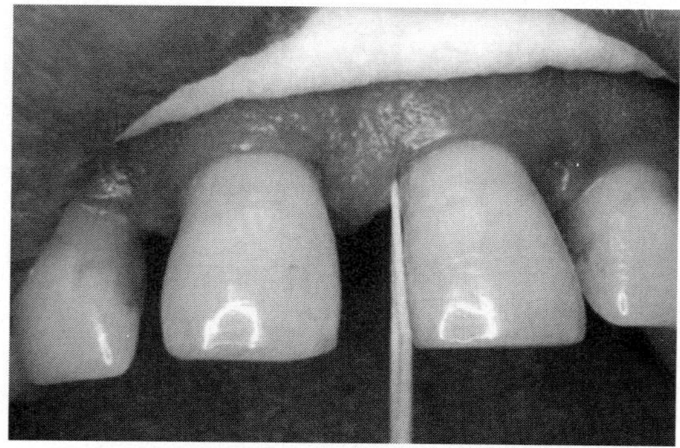

C

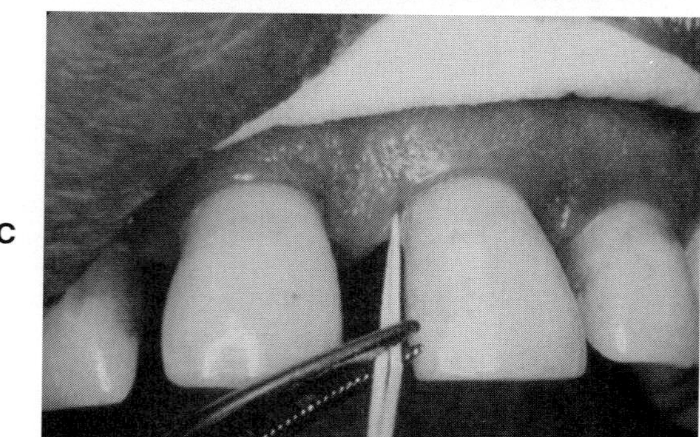

D

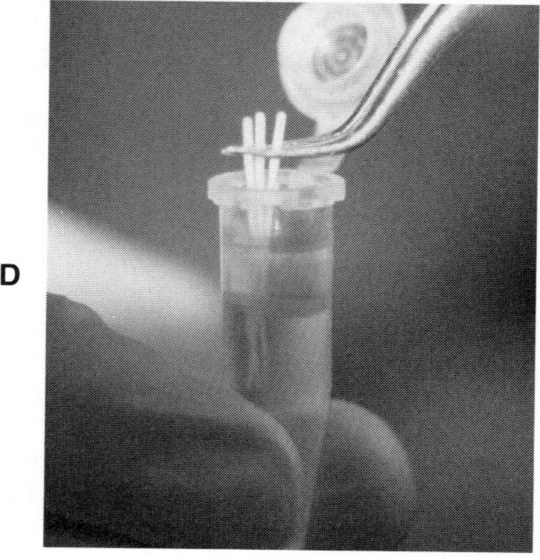

Fig. 34-10 Microbial sampling of the subgingival microflora. **A and B,** The tooth is dried and supragingival plaque is removed from the sampling site. **C,** Three sterile endodontic paper points are placed subgingivally to the base of the pocket. **D,** The paper points are removed and placed in a vial of anaerobic transport media for immediate transport to the laboratory for analysis.

performance of new microbial diagnostic methods. Generally, plaque samples are cultivated anaerobically and by using selective and nonselective media, together with several biochemical and physical tests, the different putative pathogens can be identified. The main advantage of this method is one can obtain relative and absolute counts of the cultured species. Moreover, it is the only in vitro method able to assess for antibiotic susceptibility of the microbes. However, culture techniques have important shortcomings. Culture methods can only grow live bacteria, therefore strict sampling and transport conditions are essential. Moreover, some of the putative pathogens, such as *Treponemas* sp. and *Bacteroides forsythus* are fastidious and difficult to culture. The sensitivity of culture methods is rather low, since the detection limits for selective and nonselective media average 10^3 to 10^4 bacteria and hence low numbers of a specific pathogen in a pocket are undetected. However, the most important drawback is that culture requires sophisticated equipment and experienced personnel and is relatively time-consuming and expensive. Clinicians, when using this method, must be confident that the laboratory has the appropriate technology and expertise in periodontal microbiology to communicate diagnostically and therapeutically useful information to them.

Direct Microscopy

Darkfield or **phase contrast microscopy** has been suggested as an alternative to culture methods[53] on the basis of its ability to directly and rapidly assess the morphology and motility of bacteria in a plaque sample. It has been used to indicate periodontal disease status and to structure maintenance programs. However, most of the main putative periodontopathogens, including *Actinobacillus actinomycetemcomitans, P. gingivalis, B. forsythus, Eikenella corrodens,* and *Eubacterium* species, are nonmotile, and therefore this technique is unable to identify these species. It is also unable to differentiate among the various species of *Treponema*. Therefore darkfield microscopy seems an unlikely candidate as a diagnostic test of destructive periodontal diseases.[55]

Immunodiagnostic Methods

Immunologic assays employ antibodies that recognize specific bacterial antigens to detect target microorganisms. This reaction can be revealed using a variety of procedures, including direct and indirect immunofluorescent microscopy assays (IFA), flow cytometry, enzyme-linked immunoabsorbent assay (ELISA), membrane assay, and latex agglutination.

Direct IFA employs both monoclonal and polyclonal antibodies conjugated to a fluorescein marker that binds with the bacterial antigen to form a fluorescent immune-complex detectable under a microscope. Indirect IFA employs a secondary fluorescein-conjugated antibody that reacts with the primary antigen-antibody complex. Both direct and indirect immunofluorescence assays are able to identify the pathogen and quantify the percentage of the pathogen directly using a plaque smear. IFA has been used mainly to detect *A. actinomycetemcomitans* and *P. gingivalis*. Zambon et al[90] showed that this technique is comparable to bacterial culture in its ability to identify these pathogens in subgingival dental plaque samples. In fact, immune-fluorescence microscopy may be even more likely to detect them in clinical samples because it does not require viable bacterial cells. Comparative studies indicate that the sensitivity of these assays ranges from 82% to 100% for detection of *A. actinomycetemcomitans* and from 91% to 100% for detection of *P. gingivalis,* with specificity values of 88% to 92% and 87% to 89%, respectively.[91]

Cytofluorography or flow cytometry for the rapid identification of oral bacteria involves labelling bacterial cells from a patient plaque sample with both species-specific antibody and a second fluorescein-conjugated antibody. The suspension is then introduced into the flow cytometer, which separates the bacterial cells into an almost single-cell suspension by means of a laminar flow through a narrow tube. The sophistication and cost involved in this procedure precludes its wide usage.

ELISA is similar in principle to other radioimmunoassays, but an enzymatically derived color reaction is substituted as the label in place of the radioisotope. The intensity of the color depends on the concentration of the antigen and is usually read photometrically for optimal quantitation. ELISA has been used primarily to detect serum antibodies to periodontopathogens; however it has also been used in research studies to quantify specific pathogens in subgingival samples using specific monoclonal antibodies.[91]

Latex agglutination is a very simple immunological assay based on the binding of protein to latex. Latex beads are coated with the species-specific antibody, and when these beads come in contact with the microbial cell surface antigens or antigen extracts, cross-linking occurs; its agglutination or clumping is then visible usually in 2 to 5 minutes. Because of their simplicity and rapidity, these assays have great potential for chairside detection of periodontal pathogens. There are two types of latex agglutination tests—the indirect assay and inhibition assay. The **indirect assay** is the most common latex agglutination test for bacteria. The antibody is bound to latex. When a suspension of the plaque sample is mixed with the sensitized latex and gently agitated for 3 to 5 minutes, resulting agglutination or clumping is indicative of a positive result for the bacteria being tested. The **inhibition assay** is based on the principle of inhibiting the expected agglutination reaction between known antigen and known antibody as a result of competition.

A membrane immunoassay has been recently marketed (Evalusite®). It involves linkage between the antigen and a membrane-bound antibody to form an immunocomplex that is later revealed through a colorimetric reaction. Evalusite has been designed to detect *A. actinomycetemcomitans, P. gingivalis,* and *P. intermedia.*[91] Immunological assays for oral bacteria, although extensively used for research purposes, lack the clinical validation since most of them have never been available commercially. Cross reactivity leading to detection of false positives may represent a major problem, mostly when polyclonal antibodies are used. On the other hand the use of monoclonal antibodies may cause the occurrence of false negatives when compared with culture, due to their high specificity. Immunological assays can identify dead target cells, thus not requiring stringent sampling and transport methodology. However, they cannot be used to determine antibiotic susceptibility. Most of these assays provide a quantitative or semiquantitative estimate of target microorganisms; however, these methods generally show poorer detection limits than nucleic acid probes of PCR assays. Snyder et al[80] tested the sensitivity of the Evalusite test, demonstrating a detection limit of 10^5 for *A. actinomycetemcomitans* and 10^6 for *P. gingivalis.*

Enzymatic Methods of Bacterial Identification

B. forsythus, P. gingivalis, the small spirochete *Treponema denticola,* and *Capnocytophaga* species share a common enzymatic profile, since all have in common a trypsin-like enzyme. The activity of this enzyme can be measured with the hydrolysis of the colorless substrate *N*-benzoyl-dl-arginine-2-naphthylamide (BANA). When the hydrolysis takes place, it releases the chromophore *β*-naphthylamide, which turns orange red when a drop of fast garnet is added to the solution. Diagnostic kits has been developed using this reaction for the identification of this bacteria profile in plaque isolates (Perioscan®). Loesche et al[56] proposed the use of this BANA reaction in subgingival plaque samples to detect the presence of any of these periodontal pathogens and thus serve as a marker of disease activity. Using probing depths as a measure of periodontal morbidity, Loesche et al[56] showed that shallow pockets exhibited only 10% positive BANA reactions, whereas deep pockets (7 mm) exhibited 80% to 90% positive BANA reactions. Beck et al[8] used the BANA test as a risk indicator for periodontal attachment loss. Taken collectively, results using this diagnostic method suggest that positive BANA findings are a good indication that *T. denticola, P. gingivalis,* or both are present at sampled sites. One of the potential difficulties of this test is that it may be positive at clinically healthy sites and remains to be proven whether this test can detect sites undergoing periodontal destruction. Besides, since it only detects a very limited number of pathogens, its negative result does not rule out the presence of other important periodontal pathogens.

Deoxyribonucleic Acid Probe Technology

Nucleic Acid Probes. Deoxyribonucleic acid (DNA) probes entail segments of single-stranded nucleic acid, labelled with an enzyme or radioisotope, that can locate and bind to their complementary nucleic acid sequences with low cross-reactivity to nontarget organisms. DNA probe may target whole genomic DNA or individual genes. Whole genomic probes are more likely to cross-react with nontarget microorganisms due to the presence of homologous sequences between different bacterial species. However, specific genes, such as 16S rRNA (ribonucleic acid) genes, contain signature sequences limited to organisms of the same species. These oligonucleotide probes display limited or no cross-reactivity with nontarget microorganisms.[14] To prepare the probe, specific pathogens used as marker organisms are lysed to remove their DNA. Their double helix is denatured, creating single strands that are individually labeled with a radioactive isotope. Subsequently, when a plaque sample is sent for analysis, it undergoes lysis and denaturation. Single strands are chemically treated, attached to a special filter paper, and then exposed to the DNA library. If complementary base pairs hybridize (cross-link), the radiolabeled strands will also be fixed to the filter paper. After the filter is washed to remove any unhybridized strands, it is covered with a radiographic plate. The radioactive labels create spots on the film, which are read with a densitometer. The darkness and size of the spots indicate the concentration of the organisms present in the given plaque sample. The assay can rapidly test for multiple bacteria, including *A. actinomycetemcomitans, P. gingivalis, B. intermedius, C. rectus, E. corrodens, Fusobacterium nucleatum,* and *T. denticola* in multiple clinical plaque samples. The probes are able to detect as few as 10^2 to 10^4 bacteria, and the sensitivity and specificity are not affected by the presence of unrelated bacteria in mixed culture samples.[18,68]

Restriction Endonuclease Analysis. Restriction endonucleases recognize and cleave double-stranded DNA at specific base pair sequences. The DNA fragments generated are separated by electrophoresis, stained with ethidium bromide, and visualized with ultraviolet light. The genetic heterogeneity and homogeneity of strains can then be evaluated by comparing the number and size (electrophoretic pattern) of the DNA fragments obtained. These DNA fragment patterns constitute a specific "fingerprint" to characterize each strain. Restriction endonuclease analysis is thus a powerful tool for determining the distribution of a specific pathogenic strain throughout a population.[22] This technology has also been applied to the molecular genetic analysis of the natural diversity of such oral bacteria as *A. actinomycetemcomitans, P. gingivalis, P. intermedia, E. corrodens, F. nucleatum,* and *T. denticola* and has been very useful in studying the transmission patterns of putative periodontal pathogens among family members.[72]

Polymerase Chain Reaction. Polymerase chain reaction (PCR) involves a reiterate amplification of a region of DNA flanked by a selected primer specific for the target species. The presence of the specific amplification product indicates the presence of the target microorganism. Among the different nucleic acid assays, PCR demonstrates the best detection limits, as few as five to ten cells and shows no cross-reactivity under optimized amplification conditions. Different bacterial species may be detected simultaneously by multiplex PCR in which several distinct primer pairs, each specific for a given target microorganism are employed in a single-tube amplification process.[20,21,88] Most PCR assays have the drawback that relatively small aliquots are used for the amplification process. If this small quantity of the plaque sample does not contain the targeted microorganism, the assay will not detect it. Moreover, subgingival plaque may contain enzymes that can alter the amplification process. Until recently, PCR assays were able just to assess the presence of the target microorganism. Fujise et al[19] have developed a quantitative PCR method. PCR assays have the potential for being an ideal detection method of periodontal microorganisms. It is relatively easy to perform and demonstrates excellent detection limits and little cross-reactivity under optimal conditions.

ADVANCES IN CHARACTERIZING THE HOST RESPONSE

Our understanding of the initiation and progression of periodontal disease and the pathogenic processes involved has expanded enormously in light of advances in clinical and basic science research. Diagnostic tests have been developed that add measures of the inflammatory process to conventional clinical measures. These tests may provide information on the destructive process itself, current activity of the disease, rate of disease progression, patterns of destruction, extent and severity of future breakdown, and likely response to therapy. With this information the clinician would be able to better individualize his therapeutic approach, thus customizing the recommended treatment. Assessment of the host response refers to the study of mediators, by immunologic or biochemical methods, that are recognized as part of the individual's response to the periodontal infection. These mediators are either specifically identified with the infection, such as antibody to a putative pathogen, or represent a less specific reaction like the local release of inflammatory mediators, host-derived enzymes, or tissue breakdown products. The host response in periodontal disease involves aspects of acute and chronic inflammation, humoral and cellular immune responses. Mediators representing each of these systems have been evaluated as diagnostic tests in clinical periodontics from samples that usually involve non-invasive or minimally invasive techniques.[48]

Source of Samples

Potential sample sources include saliva, gingival crevicular fluid (GCF), gingival crevicular cells, blood serum, blood cells, and urine. However, analysis of urine shows little promise except for its use in the differential diagnosis of tooth loss related to hypophosphatasia in young children, in whom the presence of phosphoethanolamine in urine is diagnostic of the disease. Most efforts to date have been based on the use of components of GCF and, to a lesser extent, saliva and blood.[67] Different studies have demonstrated a high correlation between clinical and histologic signs of gingivitis and increased amounts of gingival fluid flow.[16] In addition, more than 40 components of GCF have been studied. They can be divided into three main groups: host-derived enzymes, tissue breakdown products, and inflammatory mediators. For the collection of gingival crevicular fluid (GCF) a number of approaches have been used, which range from the use of paper strips, to microcapillary tubes and micropipettes, to micro-syringes and plastic strips. The method most widely used is the use of paper strips.

These strips are placed in the gingival sulcus for a standard period of time until the filter paper is saturated (Fig. 34-11). The fluid volume collected on the strips can be then quantified in a number of ways. At present the most popular way is using the Periotron® (Fig. 34-11, *B*). This electronic device measures the change in capacitance across the wetted strip, and this change is converted to a digital readout, which can be correlated to the volume of gingival crevicular fluid. Researchers have established that the Periotron 6000 achieves the easiest and quickest measurement and shows high correlation with other clinical gingival indices.[84] Research on GCF has focused on the search for biochemical markers of the progression of periodontitis many of which are discussed below.

Saliva is another fluid that can be easily collected and may contain both locally and systemically derived markers of periodontal disease, which can be evaluated for diagnostic purposes. Saliva can be collected from the parotid, submandibular, or sublingual glands or as "whole saliva" consisting of a mixture of oral fluids, including secretions from the major and minor salivary glands, in addition to constituents of nonsalivary origin (GCF, bacteria and bacterial products, desquamated cells, expectorated bronchial secretions, and so on). In addition, saliva samples can be collected with or without stimulation. The use of saliva for periodontal diagnosis has been the subject of considerable research activity, although no saliva-based diagnostic tests are available to be used in clinical practice. Proposed diagnostic markers in saliva include proteins and enzymes of host origin, phenotypic markers, host cells, hormones (cortisol), bacteria and bacterial products, volatile compounds, and ions.[42]

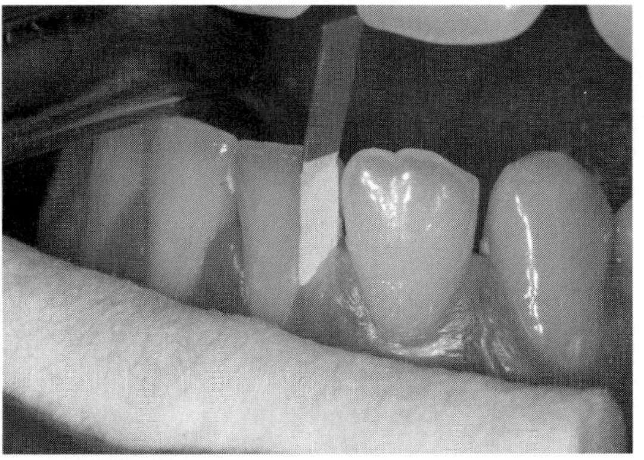

A

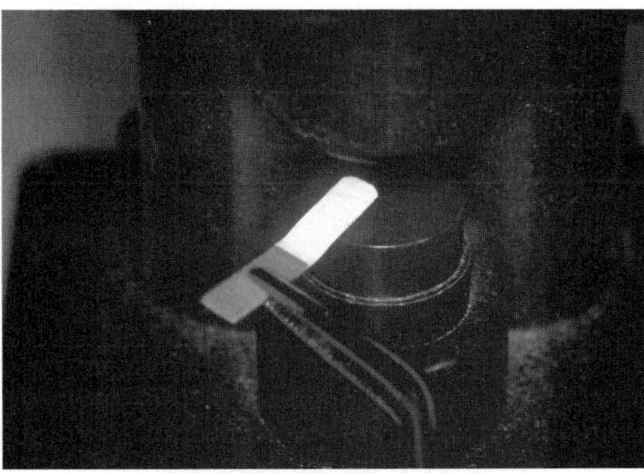

B

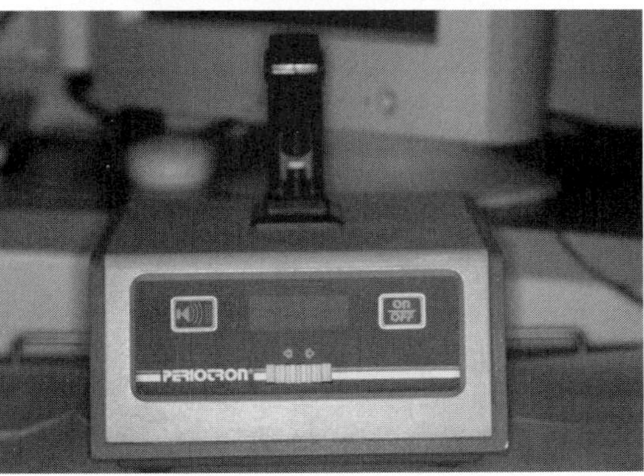

Fig. 34-11 Sampling method for crevicular fluid analysis (Periotron System). **A,** Saliva is removed from the tooth surface with cotton wool prior to placement of a periopaper strip into the pocket to collect GCF. **B,** The moist paper strip is removed and placed between the jaws of the Periotron for the assessment of fluid content.

Inflammatory Mediators and Products

Cytokines are potent local mediators of inflammation that are produced by a variety of cells. Cytokines that are present in GCF and have been investigated as potential diagnostic markers include tumor necrosis factor alpha (TNF-α),[79] interleukin-1 alpha (IL-1α), interleukin-1 beta (IL-1β),[83] interleukin-6 (IL-6), and interleukin 8 (IL-8). IL-1, IL-6, and TNF-α are cytokines produced by a variety of cells at inflamed sites. They are potent immune-regulatory molecules with a variety of biologic effects, including metalloproteinase stimulation and bone resorption; therefore they seem good candidates for markers of disease progression (see Chapter 7). Cross-sectional studies have shown good correlation with disease status and severity,[83] but not disease progression. Prostaglandin E_2 is a product of the cyclooxygenase pathway of the metabolism of arachidonic acid. It is a potent mediator of inflammation and induces bone resorption. In cases of untreated periodontitis, the concentration of prostaglandin E_2 found in GCF increased during active phases of periodontal destruction.[65]

Host-Derived Enzymes

Various enzymes are released from host cells during the initiation and progression of periodontal disease.[10,45] The enzymes that have received the most attention as possible markers of active periodontal destruction are aspartate aminotransferase (AST), akaline phosphatase, β-glucuronidase, elastase, cathepsins, and matrix metalloproteinases. Some of these enzymes are released from dead and dying cells of the periodontium; some come from polymorphonuclear neutrophils; and others are produced by inflammatory, epithelial, and connective tissue cells at affected sites.

AST is an enzyme released from dead cells from a variety of tissues throughout the body, including the heart (after myocardial infarction) and the liver (during hepatitis). Several studies evaluating the association between elevated AST levels in GCF and periodontal disease have demonstrated a marked elevation in AST levels in GCF samples from sites with severe gingival inflammation[12] and sites with a recent history of progressive attachment loss. A rapid chairside test kit for AST has been developed (Periogard®). The test involves collection of GCF with a filter paper strip, which is then placed in tromethamine hydrochloride buffer. A substrate reaction mixture containing L-aspartic and α-ketoglutaric acids are added and allowed to react for 10 minutes. In the presence of AST, the aspartate and α-glutarate are catalyzed to oxalacetate and glutamate. The addition of a dye, such as fast red, results in a color product, the intensity of which is proportional to the AST activity in the GCF sample. A potential problem with the AST test is its inability to discriminate between sites with severe inflammation but with no attachment loss from sites that are losing attachment. It remains to be demonstrated whether this test offers some advantage over existing clinical measures of disease.[60,71]

Alkaline phosphatase (ALP) is an enzyme found in many cells of the periodontium, including osteoblasts, fibroblasts, and neutrophils. Cross-sectional studies show that concentrations of this enzyme in GCF from diseased sites are significantly higher than from healthy sites. Only one longitudinal study has associated whole mouth ALP levels with the progression of periodontitis,[9] but this study has not been reproduced.

β-glucuronidase (βG) is a lysosomal enzyme found in the primary (azurophilic) granules of neutrophils. Cross-sectional data clearly show elevated βG activity in sites with more severe periodontal disease. Two longitudinal studies from the same research group have shown that the concentration of this enzyme may have predictive value in identifying patients at higher risk for losing attachment.[47] Elastase is a serine protease also stored in the primary granules of neutrophils. Cross-sectional studies clearly indicate that GCF samples taken from sites with periodontitis have significantly higher elastase activity than GCF from healthy or gingivitis sites.[29] A rapid chairside test kit (Periocheck®) has been developed to detect neutral proteases in GCF. A limited number of longitudinal studies have evaluated its value as marker of periodontal disease progression.[5] They have shown some predictive value for disease progression in a short-term evaluation of an untreated population, but it remains unclear if its validity can be applied to a treated population in a maintenance program. Similar results have been obtained studying cathepsins. These enzymes are a group of acidic lysosomal enzymes that play an important role in intracellular protein degradation. Although they have shown correlation with disease severity and significant decrease after periodontal therapy, they have not been evaluated longitudinally as markers of disease progression.[13]

Matrix metalloproteinases (MMPs) are members of a large subfamily of zinc- and calcium-dependent proteolytic enzymes (proteinases) responsible for remodeling and degradation of extracellular matrix components. The homeostasis of extracellular matrices is regulated by the release of MMPs by different cells such as fibroblasts and macrophages and the presence of tissue inhibitors of MMPs that are widely distributed in tissues and fluids. Different cross-sectional studies have shown that high MMP levels are associated with periodontitis, as are low levels of tissue inhibitors. Recently Sorsa et al[82] suggested that MMPs be used as a method for detecting destructive periodontitis, especially MMP-8. However, no rapid chairside test kit has been developed for clinical use.

Tissue Breakdown Products

One of the major features of periodontitis is the destruction of collagen and extracellular matrices. Analysis of GCF obtained from sites with periodontitis clearly shows elevated levels of hydroxyproline from collagen breakdown and glycosaminoglycans from matrix degradation.[52] Other bone and connective tissue proteins, including osteocalcin and type 1 collagen peptides, have been correlated with the progression of alveolar bone loss induced in beagle dogs.[23] Both markers gave high positive predictive values and now need to be extended to longitudinal studies in humans.

In conclusion, although there are many potential markers for periodontal disease activity and progression, still numerous features hamper the ability to use them as diagnostic tests of proven utility. There is still a lack of a proven gold standard of disease progression and thus the correlation of these potential markers with proven clinical attachment loss may be a potential confounder in any proposed test. After all these years of intensive research we still lack a proven diagnostic test that has demonstrated high predictive value for disease progression, has a proven impact on disease incidence and prevalence and is simple, safe and cost effective.[54]

REFERENCES

1. Aas AM, Albandar J, Aasenden R, et al: Variation in prevalence of radiographic alveolar bone loss in subgroups of 14-year old schoolchildren in Oslo. J Clin Periodontol 1989; 16:300.
2. Abrams K, Caton J, Polson A: Histologic comparisons of interproximal gingival tissues related to the presence or absence of bleeding. J Periodontol 1984; 55:629.
3. Aeppli DM, Pihlstrom BL: Detection of longitudinal changes in periodontitis. J Periodont Res 1989; 24:329.
4. Armitage GC, Svanberg GK, Löe H: Microscopic evaluation of clinical measurements of connective tissue attachment levels. J Clin Periodontol 1977; 4:173.
5. Armitage GC, Jeffcoat MK, Chadwick DE, et al: Longitudinal evaluation of elastase as a marker for the progression of periodontitis. J Periodontol 1994; 65; 120.
6. Badersten A, Nilveus R, Egelberg J: Reproducibility of probing attachment level measurements. J Clin Periodontol 1984; 11:475.
7. Badersten A, Nilveus R, Egelberg J: Effect of non-surgical periodontal therapy. VII. Bleeding, suppuration and probing depth in sites with probing attachment loss. J Clin Periodontol 1985; 12:432.
8. Beck JD: Issues in assessment of diagnostic tests and risk for periodontal diseases. Periodontol 2000 1995; 7:100.
9. Binder TA, Goodson JM, Socransky SS: Gingival fluid levels of acid and alkaline phosphatase. J Perio Res 1987; 22:14.
10. Bowers JE, Zahradnik M: Evaluation of a chairside gingival protease test for use in periodontal diagnosis. J Clin Dent 1989; 1:106.

11. Brägger U, Pasquali L, Rylander H, et al: Computer assisted densitometric image analysis in periodontal radiography. A methodological study. J Clin Periodontol 1988; 15:27.
12. Chambers DA, Imrey PB, Cohen R, et al: A longitudinal study of aspartate aminotransferase in human gingival crevicular fluid. J Periodont Res 1991; 26:65.
13. Chen HY, Cox SW, Eley BM: Cathepsin B, A-2 macroglobulin and cytastin levels in gingival crevicular fluid from chronic periodontitis patients. J Clin Periodontol 1998; 25:34.
14. Chen C, Slots J: Microbial tests for *Actinobacillus actinomycetemcomitans* and *Porphyromona gingivalis*. Periodontol 2000 1999; 20:53.
15. Clark WB, Yang MCK, Magnusson I: Measuring clinical attachment: Reproducibility and relative measurements with an electronic probe. J Periodontol 1992; 63:831.
16. Daneshmann H, Wade AB: Correlation between gingival fluid measurements and macroscopic and microscopic characteristics of gingival tissue. J Periodont Res 1976; 11:35.
17. Deas D, Pasquali LA, Yuan CH, et al: The relationship between probing attachment loss and computerized radiographic analysis in monitoring the progression of periodontitis. J Periodontol 1991; 62:135.
18. French CK, Savitt ED, Simon SL, et al: DNA detection of periodontal pathogens. Oral Microbiol Immunol 1986; 1:58.
19. Fujise O, Hamachi T, Hirofuchi T, et al: Colorimetric microtiter plate based assay for detection and quantification of amplified *Actinobacillus actinomycetemcomitans* DNA. Oral Microbiol Immunol 1995; 10:372.
20. Gangbar S, Overall CM, McCuloch GAG, et al: Identification of polymorphonuclear leukocyte collagenase and gelatinase activities in mouthrinse samples. Correlation with periodontal disease activity in adult and juvenile periodontitis. J Periodont Res 1990; 25:257.
21. Garcia L, Tercero JC, Legido B et al: Rapid detection of *Actinobacillus actinomycetemcomitans, Prevotella intermedia* and *Porphyromona gingivalis* by multiplex PCR. J Perio Res 1998; 33:59.
22. Genco RJ, Loos BG: The use of genomic DNA fingerprinting in studies of the epidemiology of bacteria in periodontitis. J Clin Periodontol 18:396, 1991.
23. Giannobile WV, Lynch SE, Denmark RG et al: Crevicular fluid osteocalcin and piridoline cross-linked carboxyterminal telopeptide of type I collagen (ICTP) as markers of rapid bone turn over in periodontitis. J Clin Periodontol 1995; 22:903.
24. Gibbs CH, Hirschfeld JW, Lee JG, et al: Description and clinical evaluation of a new computerized periodontal probe—the Florida probe. J Clin Periodontol 1988; 15:137.
25. Goodson JM, Haffajee AD, Socransky SS: The relationship between attachment level loss and alveolar bone loss. J Clin Periodontol 1984; 11:348.
26. Greenstein G, Caton J, Polson AM: Histologic characteristics associated with bleeding after probing and visual signs of inflammation. J Periodontol 1981; 52:420.
27. Grondahl HG, Grondahl K: Subtraction radiography for the diagnosis of periodontal bone lesions. Oral Surg 1983; 55:208.
28. Grondahl K, Kullendorff B, Strid H-G, et al: Detectability of artificial marginal bone lesions as a function of lesion depth. J Clin Periodontol 1988; 15:156.
29. Gustafsson A, Asman B, Bergstrom KG: Granulocyte elastase in gingival crevicular fluid; a possible discriminator between gingivitis and periodontitis. J Clin Periodontol 1992; 19: 535.
30. Haffajee AD, Socransky SS: Attachment level changes in destructive periodontal diseases. J Clin Periodontol 1986; 13:461.
31. Haffajee AD, Socransky SS, Goodson JM: Clinical parameters as predictors of destructive periodontal activity. J Clin Periodontol 1983; 10:257.
32. Haffajee AD, Socransky SS, Goodson JM: Comparisons of different data analysis for detecting changes in attachment level. J Clin Periodontol 1983; 10:298.
33. Haffajee AD, Socransky SS, Goodson JM: Subgingival temperature. Relation to future periodontal attachment loss. J Clin Periodontol 1992; 19:409.
34. Haffajee AD, Socransky SS: Microbial etiologic agents of destructive periodontal diseases. Periodontol 2000 1994; 5:78.
35. Hausmann E, Christersson L, Dunford R, et al: Usefulness of subtraction radiography in the evaluation of periodontal therapy. J Periodontol 1985; 56(suppl 11):4.
36. Hausmann E, McHenry K, Christersson L, et al: Techniques for assessing alveolar bone mass changes in periodontal disease with emphasis on I^{125} absorptiometry. J Clin Periodontol 1983; 10:455.
37. Hausmann E, Allen K, Carpio L, et al: Computerized methodology for detection of alveolar crestal bone loss from serial intraoral radiographs. J Periodontol 1992; 63:657.
38. Hausmann E: Radiographic and digital imaging in periodontal practice. J Periodontol 2000; 71:497.
39. Jeffcoat MK, Jeffcoat RL, Jens SC, et al: A new periodontal probe with automated cemento-enamel junction detection. J Clin Periodontol 1986; 13:276.
40. Jeffcoat MK: Diagnosing periodontal disease: New tools to solve old problems. J Am Dent Assoc 122:54, 1991.
41. Jeffcoat MK. Radiographic methods for the detection of progressive alveolar bone loss. J Periodontol 1992; 63:367.
42. Kaufman E, Lamster IB: Analysis of saliva for periodontal diagnosis. A review. J Clin Periodontol 2000; 27:453.
43. Kalkwarf KL, Kahldal WD, Patil KD: Comparison of manual and pressure controlled periodontal probing. J Periodontol 1986; 57:467.
44. Kelly GP, Cain RJ, Knowles JW, et al: Radiographs in clinical periodontal trials. J Periodontol 1975; 46:381.
45. Kinane D: Host-based chemical agents in diagnosis. In Lang NP, Karring T, Lindhe J (eds): Proceedings of the Second European Workshop on Periodontology. Berlin, Quintessence, 1997.
46. Kung RT, Ochs B, Goodson JM: Temperature as a periodontal diagnostic. J Clin Periodontol 1990; 17:557.
47. Lamster IB, Oshrain RL, Harper CS, et al: Enzyme activity in crevicular fluid for the detection and prediction of clinical attachment loss in patients with chronic adult periodontitis. J Periodontol 1988; 59:516.
48. Lamster IB: Evaluation of components of gingival crevicular fluid as diagnostic tests. Ann Periodontol 1997; 2:123.
49. Lang NP, Joss A, Orsanic T, et al: Bleeding on probing. A predictor for the progression of periodontal disease? J Clin Periodontol 1986; 13:590.
50. Lang NP, Nyman S, Senn C, et al: Bleeding on probing as it relates to probing pressure and gingival health. J Clin Periodontol 1991; 18:257.
51. Lang NP, Brägger U: Periodontal diagnosis in the 1990s. J Clin Periodontol 1991; 18:370.
52. Last KS, Stanbury JB, Embery G: Glycosaminoglycans in human gingival sulcus fluid as indicators of active periodontal disease. Arch Oral Biol 1985; 30:275.
53. Listgarten MA: Direct microscopy of periodontal pathogens. Oral Microbiol Immunol 1986; 1:31.
54. Listgarten MA, Mao R, Robinson PJ: Periodontal probing and the relationship of the probe tip to periodontal tissues. J Periodontol 1976; 47:511.
55. Listgarten MA, Schifter CC, Sullivan P, et al: Failure of a microbial assay to reliably predict disease recurrence in a

treated periodontitis population receiving regularly scheduled prophylaxis. J Clin Periodontol 1987; 13:768.
56. Loesche WJ: The identification of bacteria associated with periodontal disease and dental caries by enzymatic methods. Oral Microbiol Immunol 1986; 1:65.
57. Magnusson I, Clark WB, Marks RG, et al: Attachment level measurements with a constant force electronic probe. J Clin Periodontol 1988; 15:185.
58. Magnusson I, Fuller WW, Heins PJ, et al: Correlation between electronic and visual readings of pocket depths with a newly developed constant force probe. J Clin Periodontol 1988; 15:180.
59. Magnusson I, Listgarten MA: Histological evaluation of probing depth following periodontal treatment. J Clin Periodontol 1980; 7:26.
60. Magnusson I, Persson RG, Page RC et al: A multicenter clinical trial of a new chairside test in distinguishing diseased and healthy periodontal sites. J Periodontol 1995; 67:589.
61. McCulloch CA, Birek P: Automated probe: Futuristic technology for diagnosis of periodontal disease. Univ Toronto Dent J 1991; 4:6.
62. Mombelli A, Graf H: Depth force patterns in periodontal probing. J Clin Periodontol 1986; 13:126.
63. Mombelli A, Mc Nabb H, Lang NP: Black pigmenting gram-negative bacteria in periodontal disease. II. Screening strategies for detection of *Porphyromona gingivalis*. J Periodont Res 1991; 26:308.
64. Nummikoski PV, Steffensen B, Hamilton K, et al: Clinical validation of a new substraction radiographic technique for periodontal bone loss detection. J Periodontol 2000; 71:598.
65. Offenbacher S, Odle BM, Van Dyke TE: The use of crevicular fluid prostaglandin E2 levels as predictor of periodontal attachment loss. J Periodont Res 1986; 21:101.
66. Ortman LF, McHenry K, Hausmann E: Relationship between alveolar bone measured by 125I absorptiometry with analysis of standardized radiographs. J Periodontol 1982; 53:311.
67. Page RC: Host response tests for diagnosing periodontal diseases. J Periodontol 1992; 63:356.
68. Papanou PN, Neiderud AM, Papadimitriou A, et al: Checkerboard assessments of Periodontal Microbiota and serum antibody responses: A case control study. J Periodontol 2000; 71:885.
69. Parakkal PF: Proceedings of the workshop on quantitative evaluation of periodontal diseases by physical measurement techniques. J Dent Res 1979; 58:547.
70. Perry DA, Taggart EJ, Leung A, et al: Comparison of a conventional probe with electronic and manual pressure-regulated probes. J Periodontol 1994; 65:908.
71. Persson GR, Alves MEAF, Chambers DA, et al: A multicenter clinical trial of Periogard in distinguishing between diseased and heathy periodontal sites. J Clin Periodontol 1995; 22:794.
72. Petit MD, van Steenbergen TJ, Timmerman MF, et al: Prevalence of periodontitis and suspected periodontal pathogens in families of adult periodontitis patients. J Clin Periodontol 1994; 21:76.
73. Polson AM, Caton JG: Current status of bleeding in the diagnosis of periodontal diseases. J Periodontol 1985; 56(suppl 11):1.
74. Polson AM, Caton JG, Yeaple RN, et al: Histological determination of probe tip penetration into gingival sulcus of humans using an electronic pressure-sensitive probe. J Clin Periodontol 1980; 7:479.
75. Quirynen M, Callens A, van Steenberghe, et al: Clinical evaluation of a constant force electronic probe. J Periodontol 1993; 64:35.
76. Rams TE, Slots J: Comparison of two pressure-sensitive periodontal probes and a manual periodontal probe in shallow and deep pockets. Int J Periodontics Restorative Dent 1993; 13:521.
77. Rethman M, Ruttimann U, O'Neal R, et al: Diagnosis of bone lesions by subtraction radiography. J Periodontol 1985; 56:324.
78. Rosling B, Hollender L, Nyman S, et al: A radiographic method for assessing changes in alveolar height following periodontal therapy. J Clin Periodontol 1975; 2:211.
79. Rossomando EF, Kennedy JE, Hadjimichael J: Tumor necrosis factor alpha in gingival crevicular fluid as a possible indicator of periodontal disease in humans. Arch Oral Biol 1990; 35:431.
80. Snyder B, Ryersson CG, Corona H, et al: Analytical performance of an immunologic-based periodontal bacterial test for simultaneous detection of Aa, Pg, and Pi. J Periodontol 1996; 67:497.
81. Socransky SS, Haffajee AD, Cugini M, et al: Microbial complexes in subgingival plaque. J Clin Periodontol 1998; 25:134.
82. Sorsa T, Golup LM, Lee HM, et al: The anticollagenolytic effect of low-dose doxycycline regimen in adult human periodontitis from gingival crevicular fluid can be monitored by the immunological test for neutrophil collagenase (MMP-8) J Dent Res 1998; 77:647.
83. Stashenko P, Fujiyoshi P, Obernesser MS, et al: Levels of interleukin 1b in tissue from sites of active periodontal disease. J Clin Periodontol 1991; 18:548.
84. Tsuchida K, Hara K: Clinical significance of gingival fluid measurement by Periotron. J Periodontol 1981; 52:599.
85. Tupta-Veselicky L, Famili P, Ceravolo FJ et al: A clinical study of an electronic constant force periodontal probe. J Periodontol 1994; 65:616.
86. Van der Velden U, de Vries JH: Introduction of a new periodontal probe: The pressure probe. J Clin Periodontol 1978; 5:188.
87. Van Winkelhoff AJ, Rams TE, Slots J: Systemic antibiotic therapy in Periodontics. Periodontol 2000 1996; 10:45.
88. Wahlors J, Meurman JH, Vaiseanen P, et al: Simultaneous detection of Pg and Aa by a rapid PCR method. J Dent Res 1995; 74:1796.
89. Yang MCK, Marks RG, Clark WB, et al: Predictive power of various models for longitudinal attachment level change. J Clin Periodontol 1992; 19:77.
90. Zambon JJ, Bochacki V, Genco RJ: Immunological assays for putative periodontal pathogens. Oral Microbiol Immunol 1986; 1:39.
91. Zambon JJ, Haraszthy VI: The laboratory diagnosis of periodontal infections. Periodontol 2000 1995; 7:69.

The Treatment Plan

Fermin A. Carranza and Henry H. Takei

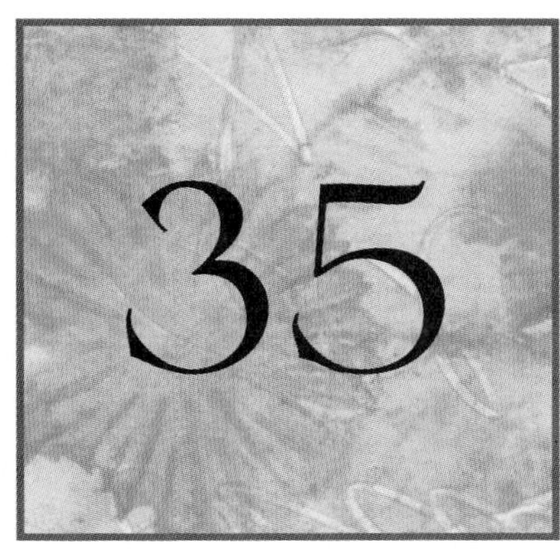

CHAPTER

CHAPTER OUTLINE

After the diagnosis and prognosis have been established, the treatment is planned. *The treatment plan is the blueprint for case management.* It includes all procedures required for the establishment and maintenance of oral health, such as the following decisions:

- Teeth to be retained or extracted
- Pocket therapy, by means of surgical or nonsurgical methods, and the techniques to be used
- The need for occlusal correction, prior, during, or after pocket therapy
- The use of implant therapy
- The need for temporary restorations
- Final restorations that will be needed after therapy and which teeth will be abutments if fixed prosthesis is used
- The need for orthodontic consultation
- Endodontic therapy
- Regarding esthetic considerations in periodontal therapy
- On sequence of therapy

Unforeseen developments during treatment may necessitate modification of the initial treatment plan. However, **except for emergencies, no treatment should be started until the treatment plan has been established.**

THE MASTER PLAN FOR TOTAL TREATMENT

The aim of the treatment plan is **total treatment**—that is, the coordination of all treatment procedures for the purpose of creating a well-functioning dentition in a healthy periodontal environment. The master plan of periodontal treatment encompasses different areas of therapeutic objectives for each patient according to his or her needs. It is based on the diagnosis, disease severity, and other factors outlined in previous chapters and should include a reasoned decision on the possible and desirable therapeutic endpoints and the techniques to be used to reach this objective.

The primary goal is elimination of gingival inflammation and correction of the conditions that cause and/or perpetuate it. This includes not only elimination of root irritants, but also pocket eradication/reduction, establishment of gingival contours and mucogingival relationships conducive to the preservation of periodontal health, restoration of carious areas, and correction of existing restorations.

Extracting or Preserving a Tooth

Periodontal treatment requires long-range planning. Its value to the patient is measured in years of healthy functioning of the entire dentition, not by the number of teeth retained at the time of treatment. **It is directed**

to establishing and maintaining the health of the periodontium throughout the mouth rather than to spectacular efforts to "tighten loose teeth."

The welfare of the dentition should not be jeopardized by a heroic attempt to retain questionable teeth. **The periodontal condition of the teeth to be retained is more important than the number of such teeth.** Teeth that can be retained with minimal doubt and a maximal margin of safety provide the basis for the total treatment plan. Teeth on the borderline of hopelessness do not contribute to the overall usefulness of the dentition, even if they can be saved in a somewhat precarious state. Such teeth become sources of recurrent annoyance to the patient and detract from the value of the greater service rendered by the establishment of periodontal health in the remainder of the oral cavity.

Removal, retention or temporary (interim) retention of one or more teeth is a very important part of the overall treatment plan.

A tooth should be extracted when any of the following occurs:

- It is so mobile that function becomes painful.
- It can cause acute abscesses during therapy.
- There is no use for it in the overall treatment plan.

A tooth can be retained temporarily, postponing the decision to extract it until after treatment, when any of the following occurs:

- It maintains posterior stops; it can be removed after treatment when it can be replaced by a prosthesis.
- It maintains posterior stops and may be functional after implant placement in adjacent areas. When implant is exposed these teeth can be extracted.
- In anterior esthetic areas, a tooth can be retained during periodontal therapy and removed when treatment is completed and a permanent restorative procedure can be performed. This will replace wearing temporary appliances. This can be considered when retention of this tooth will not jeopardize adjacent teeth.
- Removal of hopeless teeth can also be performed during periodontal surgery of neighboring teeth. This would reduce surgical appointments for surgery in the same area.

Teeth will be retained when their prognosis is good to excellent (see Chapter 33).

In the formulation of the treatment plan, in addition to proper function of the dentition, *esthetic considerations* play an increasingly important role in many cases. Different patients value esthetics differently according to their age, gender, profession, social status, and other reasons, and the clinician should carefully evaluate and consider a final outcome of treatment that will be acceptable to the patient without jeopardizing the basic consideration of attaining health.

With the predictable use of implants, questionable teeth should be carefully evaluated as to whether their removal and replacement with an implant may be a better and more satisfactory course of therapy.

In complex cases, the interdisciplinary consultation with other specialty areas is necessary before a final plan can be made. The opinion of orthodontists and prosthodontists is especially important for the final decision in these cases.

Consideration of occlusal relationships may be in order and may necessitate occlusal adjustment, restorative, prosthetic and orthodontic procedures, splinting, and correction of bruxism and clamping and clenching habits.

Systemic conditions should be carefully evaluated, as they may require special precautions during the course of periodontal treatment and may also affect the tissue response to treatment procedures or threaten the preservation of periodontal health after treatment is completed. Such situations should be taken in conjunction with the patient's physician.

Supportive periodontal care is also of paramount importance for case maintenance. Such care entails all procedures for maintaining periodontal health after it has been attained. It consists of instruction in oral hygiene and checkups at regular intervals according to the patient's needs to examine the condition of the periodontium and the status of the restoration as it affects the periodontium.

THERAPEUTIC PROCEDURES

Periodontal therapy is an inseparable part of dental therapy. The list of procedures presented here includes periodontal procedures (in italics) and other procedures not considered to be within the province of the periodontist. They are listed together to emphasize the close relationship of periodontal therapy with other phases of therapy performed by general dentists or other specialists (Box 35-1).

The sequence in which the above phases of therapy are performed may vary to some extent in response to the requirements of the case. However, the preferred sequence, which covers the vast majority of cases, is shown in Box 35-2.

Although the phases of treatment have even been numbered, as mentioned above, their recommended sequence does not follow their numbers. The etiotropic phase, even when successfully performed, stops the progression of dental and periodontal disease. Immediately after completion of Phase I therapy, the patient should be placed on the Maintenance Phase (Phase IV) to preserve the results obtained and prevent any further deterioration and recurrence of disease. While the patient is on the Maintenance Phase, with its periodic checkups and controls, he/she enters into the surgical and reparative phases of treatment (Phases III and IV). This includes periodontal surgery to repair and improve the condition of the periodontal and surrounding tissues and esthetics, rebuild lost structures, place implants, and construct the necessary restorative work.

EXPLAINING THE TREATMENT PLAN TO THE PATIENT

The following discussion includes suggestions for explaining the treatment plan to the patient.

BOX 35-1

Phases of Periodontal Therapy

Preliminary Phase
Treatment of emergencies:

- Dental or periapical
- *Periodontal*
- Other

Extraction of hopeless teeth and provisional replacement if needed (may be postponed to a more convenient time)

Etiotropic Phase (Phase I Therapy)
Plaque control and patient education

- Diet control (in patients with rampant caries)
- *Removal of calculus and root planing*
- *Correction of restorative and prosthetic irritational factors*
- Excavation of caries and restoration (temporary or final, depending on whether a definitive prognosis for the tooth has been arrived at and on the location of caries)
- *Antimicrobial therapy (local or systemic)*
- *Occlusal therapy*
- *Minor orthodontic movement*
- *Provisional splinting and prosthesis*

Evaluation of Response to Etiotropic Phase
Rechecking:

- *Pocket depth and gingival inflammation*
- *Plaque and calculus, caries*

Surgical Phase (Phase II Therapy)
Periodontal therapy, including placement of implants
Endodontic therapy

Restorative Phase (Phase III Therapy)
Final restorations
Fixed and/or removable prosthodontics

Evaluation of Response to Restorative Procedures
Periodontal examination

Maintenance Phase (Phase IV Therapy)
Periodic rechecking:

- *Plaque and calculus*
- *Gingival condition (pockets, inflammation)*
- *Occlusion, tooth mobility*
- Other pathologic changes

BOX 35-2

Preferred Sequence of Periodontal Therapy

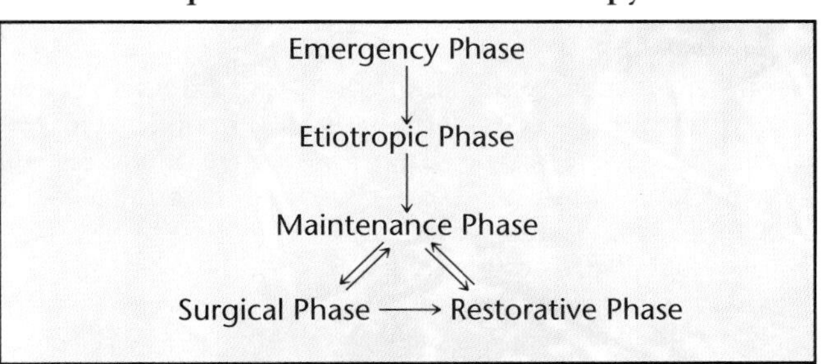

Be specific. Tell your patient: "You have gingivitis," or "You have periodontitis." Then explain exactly what these conditions are, how they are treated, and prognosis for the patient after treatment. *Avoid vague statements* such as: "You have trouble with your gums," or "Something should be done about your gums." Patients do not understand the significance of such statements and disregard them.

Begin your discussion on a positive note. Talk about the teeth that can be retained and the long-term service they can be expected to render. Do not begin your discussion with the statement: "The following teeth have to be extracted." This creates a negative impression, which adds to the erroneous attitude of hopelessness the patient already may have regarding his or her mouth. Make it clear that every effort will be made to retain as many teeth as possible, *but do not dwell on the patient's loose teeth.* Emphasize that the important purpose of the treatment is to prevent the other teeth from becoming as severely diseased as the loose teeth.

Present the entire treatment plan as a unit. Avoid creating the impression that treatment consists of separate procedures, some or all of which may be selected by the patient. *Make it clear that dental restorations and prostheses contribute as much to the health of the gums as does the elimination of inflammation and periodontal pockets.* Do not speak in terms of "having the gums treated and then taking care of the necessary restorations later" as if these were unrelated treatments.

Patients often seek guidance from the dentist with such questions as: "Are my teeth worth treating?" "Would you have them treated if you were me?" or "Why don't I just go along the way I am until the teeth really bother me and then have them all extracted?"

Explain that "doing nothing" or holding onto hopelessly diseased teeth as long as possible is inadvisable for the following reasons:

- Periodontal disease is a microbial infection, and research has clearly shown it to be an important risk factor for severe life-threatening diseases such as stroke, cardiovascular disease, pulmonary disease, and diabetes as well as for premature low birth-weight babies in women of childbearing age. Correcting the periodontal condition eliminates a serious potential risk of systemic disease, which in some cases ranks as high in the danger list as smoking.
- It is not feasible to place restorations or bridges on teeth with untreated periodontal disease because the usefulness of the restoration is limited by the uncertain condition of the supporting structures.

- Failure to eliminate periodontal disease not only results in the loss of teeth already severely involved but also shortens the life span of other teeth that, with proper treatment, could serve as the foundation for a healthy, functioning dentition.
- Therefore the dentist should make it clear to the patient that if the periodontal condition is treatable, the best results are obtained by prompt treatment. If the condition is not treatable, the teeth should also be promptly extracted.

It is the dentist's responsibility to advise the patient of the importance of periodontal treatment. However, if treatment is to be successful, the patient must be sufficiently interested in retaining the natural teeth to maintain the necessary oral hygiene. Individuals who are not particularly perturbed by the thought of losing their teeth are generally not good candidates for periodontal treatment.

Rationale for Periodontal Treatment

Fermin A. Carranza

CHAPTER

CHAPTER OUTLINE

WHAT DOES PERIODONTAL THERAPY ACCOMPLISH?

The effectiveness of periodontal therapy is made possible by the remarkable healing capacity of the periodontal tissues (Fig. 36-1). Periodontal therapy can restore chronically inflamed gingiva so that from a clinical and structural point of view it is almost identical with gingiva that has never been exposed to excessive plaque accumulation[19] (see Chapter 77).

Properly performed, periodontal treatment can be relied on to accomplish the following: eliminate pain, eliminate gingival inflammation[25] and gingival bleeding, reduce periodontal pockets and eliminate infection, stop pus formation, arrest the destruction of soft tissue and bone,[26] reduce abnormal tooth mobility,[6] establish optimal occlusal function, restore tissue destroyed by disease in some instances, reestablish the physiologic gingival contour necessary for the preservation of periodontal health, prevent the recurrence of disease, and reduce tooth loss (Fig. 36-2).[22]

Local Therapy

The cause of periodontitis and gingivitis is bacterial plaque accumulation on the tooth surface in close proximity to the gingival tissue. The accumulation of plaque can be favored by a variety of local factors, such as calculus, overhanging margins of restorations, and food impaction. **The removal of plaque and of all the factors that favor its accumulation is therefore the primary consideration in local therapy.**

Abnormal forces on the tooth increase tooth mobility. The thorough elimination of plaque and the prevention of its new formation, by themselves, maintain periodontal health, even if traumatic forces are allowed to persist.[17,18] However, the elimination of trauma may increase the chances of bone regeneration and gain of attachment.[14] Although this point is not widely accepted,[23] it appears that creating occlusal relations that are more tolerable to the periodontal tissues increases the margin of safety of the periodontium to minor buildup of plaque, in addition to reducing tooth mobility. It should be remembered that total plaque elimination as obtained in experimental studies may not be possible in all human subjects.

Systemic Therapy

Systemic therapy may be employed *as an adjunct to local measures and for specific purposes,* such as the control of systemic complications from acute infections, chemotherapy to prevent harmful effects of posttreatment bacteremia, supportive nutritional therapy, and the control of systemic diseases that aggravate the patient's periodontal

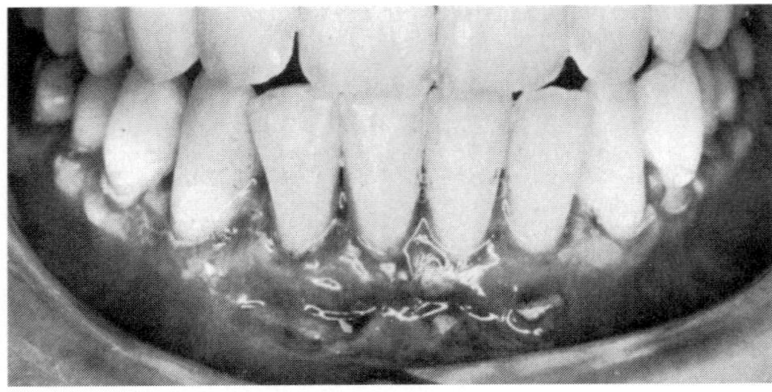

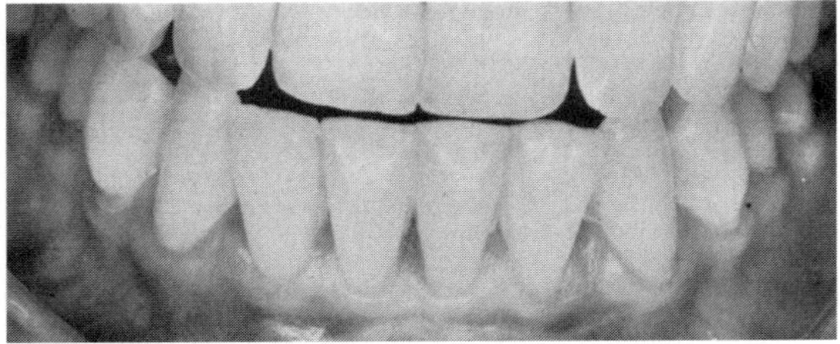

Fig. 36-1 Excellent healing capacity of the periodontium. *Above,* One week following periodontal surgery, after removal of periodontal dressing. *Below,* After 7 months, showing healed tissues and restoration of physiologic gingival contour.

condition or necessitate special precautions during treatment (see Chapter 38).

Systemic therapy *for treatment of the periodontal condition and in conjunction with local therapy* is indicated in localized and generalized aggressive periodontitis. In these diseases, systemic antibiotics are used to completely eliminate the bacteria that invade the gingival tissues and can repopulate the pocket after scaling and root planing (see Chapters 40 and 50).

In addition, *periodontal manifestations of systemic diseases* (see Chapter 12) are treated primarily by other than local measures. However, local therapy may still be indicated to reduce or prevent complications of gingival inflammation.

Evidence has been presented that some *nonsteroidal antiinflammatory drugs* such as flurbiprofen and ibuprofen can slow down the development of experimental gingivitis,[8] as well as the loss of alveolar bone in periodontitis.[10,31-33] These drugs are propionic acid derivatives and act by inhibiting the cyclooxygenase pathway of arachidonic acid metabolism, thereby reducing prostaglandin formation; they can be administered by mouth[12] or applied topically.[31] This type of therapy is still in experimental stages, and protocols for its clinical use have not been established. However, it shows that future treatment modalities may attempt not only to control the bacterial cause of the disease, but also to suppress the self-destructive components of the host inflammatory response.[10]

Another drug that has a strong inhibitory effect on bone resorption is alendronate, a *bisphosphonate,* which is currently used to treat metabolic diseases in humans, such as Paget's disease or hypercalcemia of malignancy, which result in bone resorption. Experimental studies in monkeys have shown that the bisphosphonate alendronate reduced the bone loss associated with periodontitis.[3,30]

FACTORS THAT AFFECT HEALING

In the periodontium, as elsewhere in the body, healing is affected by local and systemic factors.

Local Factors

Systemic conditions that impair healing may reduce the effectiveness of local periodontal treatment and should be corrected before, or along with, local procedures. However, local factors, particularly plaque microorganisms are the most common deterrents to healing following periodontal treatment.

Healing is also delayed by excessive tissue manipulation during treatment, trauma to the tissues, the presence of foreign bodies, and repetitive treatment procedures that disrupt the orderly cellular activity in the healing process. An adequate blood supply is needed for the increased cellular activity during healing; if this is impaired or insufficient, areas of necrosis will develop and delay the healing process.

Healing is improved by débridement (the removal of degenerated and necrotic tissue), immobilization of the healing area, and pressure on the wound. The cellular activity in healing entails an increase in oxygen consumption, but healing of the gingiva is not accelerated by artificially increasing the oxygen supply beyond the normal requirements.[7]

Systemic Factors

The effects of systemic conditions on healing have been extensively documented in animal experiments but are less clearly defined in humans. Healing capacity diminishes with age,[4,9] probably due to atherosclerotic vascular changes, which are common in aging, and result in reduction in blood circulation. Healing is delayed in patients with generalized infections and in those with diabetes and other debilitating diseases.

Healing is retarded by insufficient food intake; bodily conditions that interfere with the use of nutrients; and deficiencies in vitamin C,[1,29] proteins,[28] and other nutrients. However, the nutrient requirements of the healing tissues in minor wounds, such as those created by periodontal surgical procedures, are ordinarily satisfied by a well-balanced diet.

Healing is also affected by hormones. Systemically administered glucocorticoids such as cortisone hinder repair by depressing the inflammatory reaction or by inhibiting the growth of fibroblasts, the production of collagen, and the formation of endothelial cells. Systemic stress,[27] thyroidectomy, testosterone, adrenocorticotropic hormone (ACTH), and large doses of estrogen suppress the formation of granulation tissue and retard healing.[4] Progesterone increases and accelerates the vascularization of immature granulation tissue[16] and appears to increase the susceptibility of the gingiva to mechanical injury by causing dilation of the marginal vessels.[11]

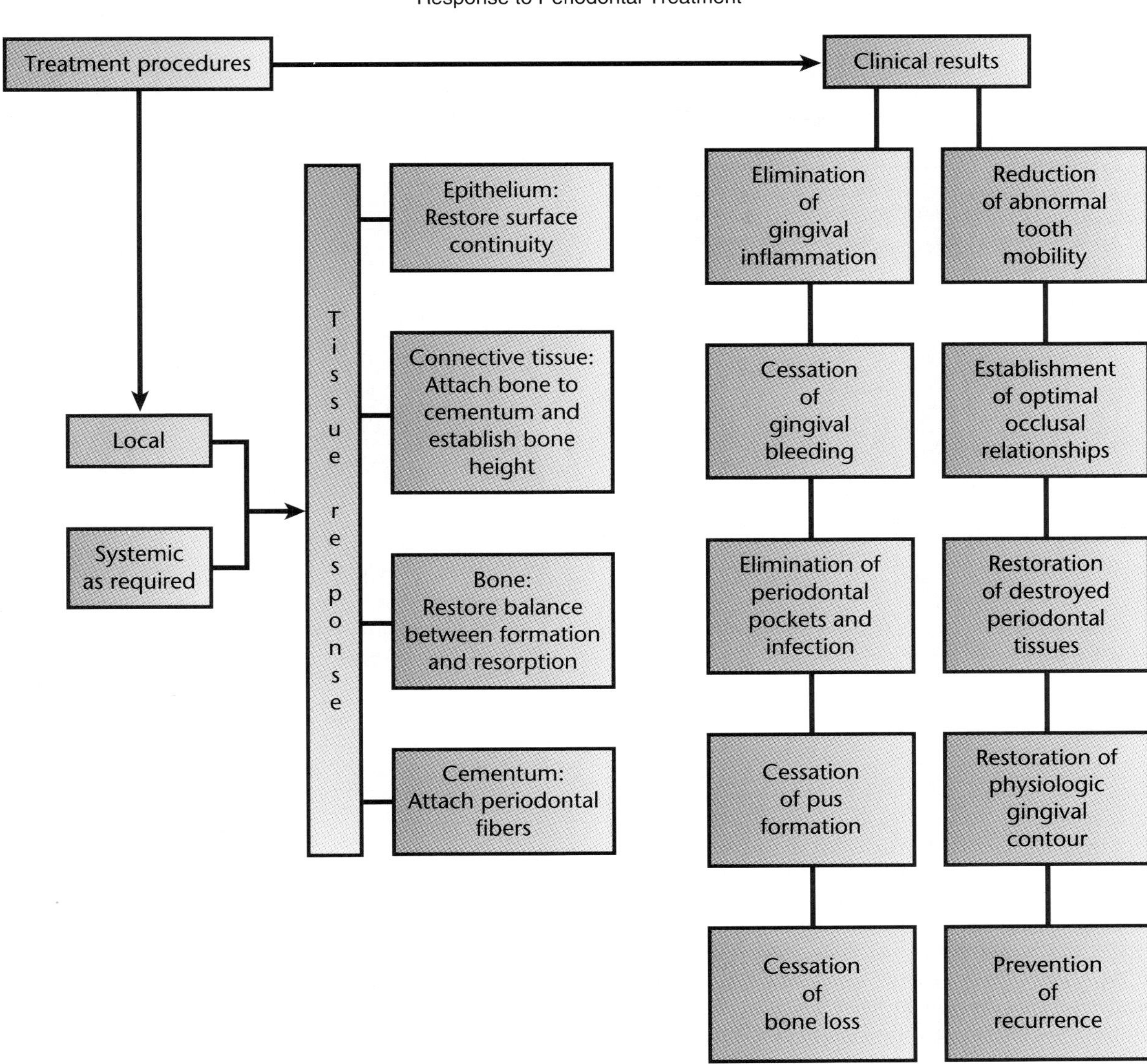

Fig. 36-2 Tissue response and clinical results after periodontal treatment.

HEALING AFTER PERIODONTAL THERAPY

The basic healing processes are the same following all forms of periodontal therapy. They consist of the removal of degenerated tissue debris and the replacement of tissues destroyed by disease. Regeneration, repair, and new attachment are aspects of periodontal healing that have a special bearing on the results obtainable by treatment.

Regeneration

Regeneration is the **growth and differentiation of new cells and intercellular substances to form new tissues or parts.** Regeneration takes place by growth from the same type of tissue that has been destroyed or from its precursor. In the periodontium, gingival epithelium is replaced by epithelium, and the underlying connective tissue and periodontal ligament are derived from connective tissue. Bone and cementum are not replaced by existing bone or cementum but by connective tissue, which is the precursor of both. Undifferentiated connective tissue cells develop into osteoblasts and cementoblasts, which form bone and cementum.

Regeneration of the periodontium is a continuous physiologic process. Under normal conditions new cells and tissues are constantly being formed to replace those that mature and die. This is termed *wear and tear repair.*[15] It is manifested by mitotic activity in the epithelium of the gingiva and the connective tissue of the periodontal ligament, by the formation of new bone, and by the continuous deposition of cementum.

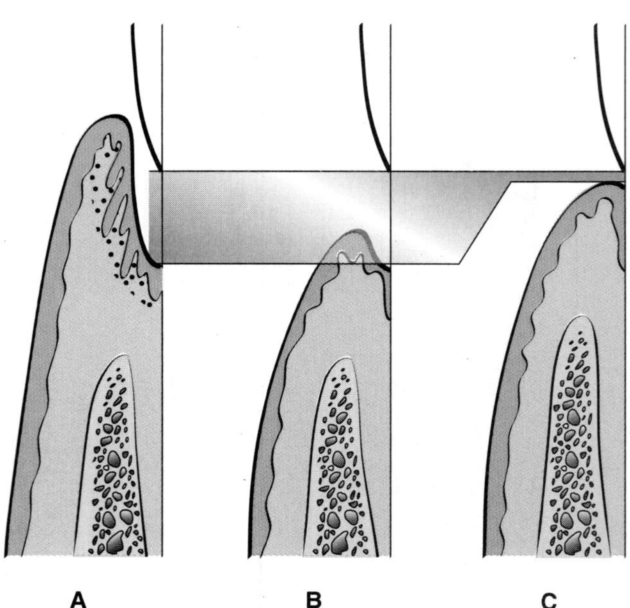

Fig. 36-3 Two possible outcomes of pocket elimination. **A,** Periodontal pocket before treatment. **B,** Normal sulcus reestablished at the level of the base of the pocket. **C,** Periodontium restored on the root surface previously denuded by disease. The latter is called *new attachment.* Shaded areas show denudation caused by periodontal disease.

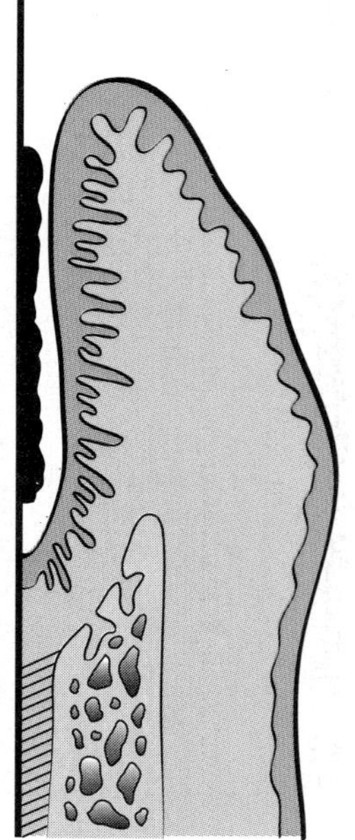

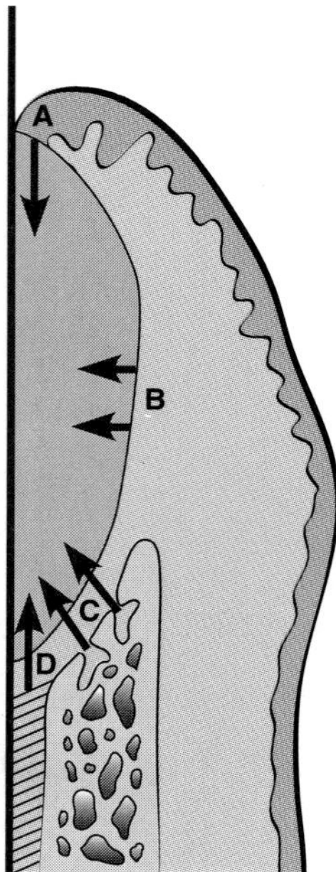

Fig. 36-4 Sources of regenerating cells in the healing stages of a periodontal pocket. *Left,* Intrabony pocket. *Right,* After therapy, the clot formed is invaded by cells from **A,** the marginal epithelium; **B,** the gingival connective tissue; **C,** the bone marrow; and **D,** the periodontal ligament.

Regeneration is also going on during destructive periodontal disease. Most gingival and periodontal diseases are chronic inflammatory processes and, as such, are healing lesions. Regeneration is part of the healing. However, bacteria and bacterial products that perpetuate the disease process and the inflammatory exudate they elicit are injurious to the regenerating cells and tissues and prevent the healing from proceeding to completion.

By removing bacterial plaque and creating the conditions to prevent its new formation, periodontal treatment removes the obstacles to regeneration and enables the patient to benefit from the inherent regenerative capacity of the tissues. There is a brief spurt in regenerative activity immediately following periodontal treatment, but there are no local treatment procedures that promote or accelerate regeneration.

Repair

Repair simply restores the continuity of the diseased marginal gingiva and reestablishes a normal gingival sulcus at the same level on the root as the base of the preexistent periodontal pocket (Fig. 36-3). This process, called *healing by scar,*[24] arrests bone destruction without necessarily increasing bone height. Restoration of the destroyed periodontium involves mobilization of epithelial and connective tissue cells into the damaged area and increased local mitotic divisions to provide sufficient number of cells (Fig. 36-4).

New Attachment

New attachment is the embedding of new periodontal ligament fibers into new cementum and the attachment of the gingival epithelium to a tooth surface previously denuded by disease (see Fig. 36-3). The critical phrase in this definition is "tooth surface previously denuded by disease" (Fig. 36-5). Attachment of the gingiva or the periodontal ligament to areas of the tooth from which they may be removed in the course of treatment or during the preparation of teeth for restorations represents *simple healing* or *reattachment* of the periodontium, not new attachment.[13] The term *reattachment* has been used in the past to refer to the restoration of the marginal periodontium, but because it is not the existing fibers that reattach but new fibers that are formed and attach to new cementum, the term has been replaced by the term *new attachment.* Reattachment is currently used only to refer to repair in areas of the root not previously exposed to the pocket, such as after surgical detachment of the tissues or following traumatic tears in the cementum, tooth fractures, or the treatment of periapical lesions.

Epithelial adaptation differs from new attachment in that it is the close apposition of the gingival epithelium to the tooth surface without complete obliteration of the pocket. The pocket space does not permit passage of a probe (Fig. 36-6). Studies have shown that these deep sulci lined by long, thin epithelium may be as resistant to disease as true connective tissue attachments.[2,20] The absence of bleeding or secretion on probing, the absence of clinically visible inflammation, and

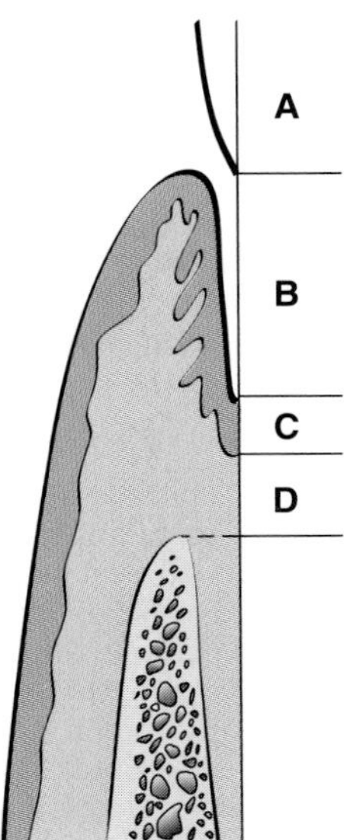

Fig. 36-5 **A,** Enamel surface. **B,** Area of cementum denuded by pocket formation. **C,** Area of cementum covered by junctional epithelium. **D,** Area of cementum apical to the junctional epithelium. The term *new attachment* refers to a new junctional epithelium and attached connective tissue fibers formed on zone B.

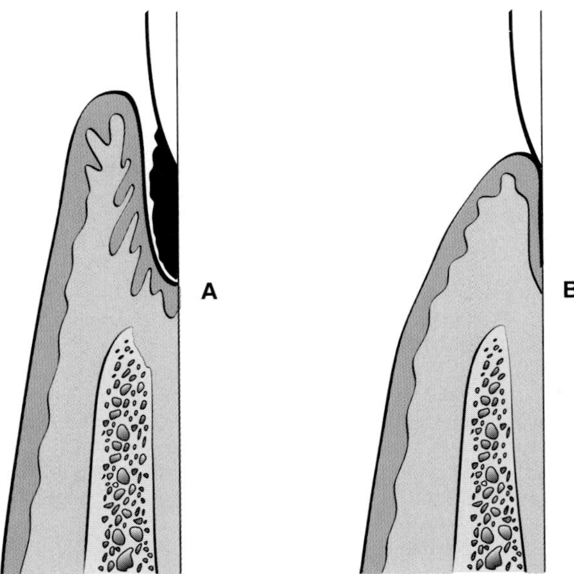

Fig. 36-6 Epithelial adaptation following periodontal treatment. **A,** Periodontal pocket. **B,** After treatment. The pocket epithelium is closely adapted to, but not attached to, the root.

the absence of stainable plaque on the root surface when the pocket wall is deflected from the tooth may indicate that the "deep sulcus" persists in an inactive state, causing no further loss of attachment.[5,34] A post-therapy depth of 4 or even 5 mm may therefore be acceptable in these cases.

New attachment and osseous regeneration have been a constant but elusive goal of periodontal therapy since beginning of this century. Since the 1970s, renewed laboratory and clinical research efforts have resulted in new concepts and techniques that have moved us much closer to attaining this ideal result of therapy. Chapter 63 presents the recommended methods of treatment and their indications and accomplishments.

Melcher pointed out that the regeneration of the periodontal ligament is the key to new attachment because it "provides continuity between the alveolar bone and the cementum and also because it contains cells that can synthesize and remodel the three connective tissues of the alveolar part of the periodontium."[21]

During the healing stages of a periodontal pocket, the area is invaded by cells from four different sources (see Fig. 36-4): oral epithelium, gingival connective tissue, bone, and periodontal ligament.

The final outcome of periodontal pocket healing depends on the sequence of events during the healing stages.[21] If the epithelium proliferates along the tooth surface before the other tissues reach the area, the result will be a long junctional epithelium. If the cells from the gingival connective tissue are the first to populate the area, the result will be fibers parallel to the tooth surface and remodeling of the alveolar bone with no attachment to the cementum. If bone cells arrive first, root resorption and ankylosis may occur. Finally, only when cells from the periodontal ligament proliferate coronally is there new formation of cementum and periodontal ligament.[21]

Several methods have been recommended to improve the likelihood of attaining new attachment. They are presented in Chapter 63.

REFERENCES

1. Barr CE: Oral healing in ascorbic acid deficiency. Periodontics 1965; 3:286.
2. Beaumont RH, O'Leary TJ, Kafrawy AH: Relative resistance of long junctional epithelial adhesions and connective tissue attachments to plaque-induced inflammation. J Periodontol 1984; 55:213.
3. Brunsvold MA, Chaves ES, Kornman KS, et al: Effects of a bisphosphonate on experimental periodontitis in monkeys. J Periodontol 1992; 63:825.
4. Butcher EO, Klingsberg J: Age, gonadectomy, and wound healing in the palatal mucosa. J Dent Res 1961; 40:694.
5. Caffesse RG, Ramfjord SP, Nasjleti CE: Reverse bevel periodontal flaps in monkeys. J Periodontol 1968; 39:219.
6. Ferris RT: Quantitative evaluation of tooth mobility following initial periodontal therapy. J Periodontol 1966; 37:190.
7. Glickman I, Turesky SS, Manhold J: The oxygen consumption of healing gingiva. J Dent Res 1950; 29:429.
8. Heasman PA, Seymour RA: The effect of a systemically-administered non-steroidal anti-inflammatory drug (flurbiprofen) on experimental gingivitis in humans. J Clin Periodontol 1989; 16:551.

9. Holm-Pedersen P, Löe H: Wound healing in the gingiva of young and old individuals. Scand J Dent Res 1971; 79:40.
10. Howell TH, Williams RC: Nonsteroidal antiinflammatory drugs as inhibitors of periodontal disease progression. Crit Rev Oral Biol Med 1993; 4:177.
11. Hugoson A: Gingival inflammation and female sex hormones. J Periodont Res 1970; 5(suppl):1.
12. Jeffcoat MK, Williams RC, Reddy MS, et al: Flurbiprofen treatment of human periodontitis: effect on alveolar bone height and metabolism. J Periodont Res 1988; 23:381.
13. Kalkwarf KL: Periodontal new attachment without the placement of osseous potentiating grafts. Periodont Abs 1974; 22:53.
14. Kantor M, Polson AM, Zander HA: Alveolar bone regeneration after removal of inflammatory and traumatic factors. J Periodontol 1976; 47:687.
15. Leblond CP, Walker BE: Renewal of cell populations. Physiol Rev 1956; 36:255.
16. Lindhe J, Branemark PI.: The effect of sex hormones on vascularization of a granulation tissue. J Periodont Res 1968; 3:6.
17. Lindhe J, Ericsson I: The influence of trauma from occlusion on reduced but healthy periodontal tissues in dogs. J Clin Periodontol 1976; 3:110.
18. Lindhe J, Nyman S: The effect of plaque control and surgical pocket elimination on the establishment and maintenance of periodontal health. A longitudinal study of periodontal therapy in cases of advanced periodontal disease. J Clin Periodontol 1975; 2:67.
19. Lindhe J, Parodi R, Liljenberg B, et al: Clinical and structural alterations characterizing healing gingiva. J Periodont Res 1978; 13:410.
20. Magnusson I, Runstad L, Nyman S, et al: A long junctional epithelium—a locus minoris resistentiae in plaque infection? J Clin Periodontol 1983; 10:33.
21. Melcher AH: On the repair potential of periodontal tissues. J Periodontol 1976; 47:256.
22. Oliver RC: Tooth loss with and without periodontal therapy. Periodont Abst 1969; 17:8.
23. Polson AM: Interrelationship of inflammation and tooth mobility (trauma) in pathogenesis of periodontal disease. J Clin Periodontol 1980; 7:351.
24. Ratcliff PA: An analysis of repair systems in periodontal therapy. Periodont Abst 1966; 14:57.
25. Rateitschak K: The therapeutic effect of local treatment on periodontal disease assessed upon evaluation of different diagnostic criteria. 2. Changes in gingival inflammation. J Periodontol 1964; 35:155.
26. Rateitschak K, Engelberger A, Marthaler TM: The therapeutic effect of local treatment on periodontal disease assessed upon evaluation of different diagnostic criteria. 3. Radiographic changes in appearance of bone. J Periodontol 1964; 35:263.
27. Stahl SS: Healing gingival injury in normal and systemically stressed young adult male rats. J Periodontol 1961; 32:63.
28. Stahl SS: The effect of a protein-free diet on the healing of gingival wounds in rats. Arch Oral Biol 1962; 7:551.
29. Turesky SS, Glickman I: Histochemical evaluation of gingival healing in experimental animals on adequate and vitamin C deficient diets. J Dent Res 1954; 33:273.
30. Weinreb M, Quartuccio H, Seedor JG, et al: Histomorphometrical analysis of the effects of the bisphosphonate alendronate on bone loss caused by experimental periodontitis in monkeys. J Periodont Res 1994; 29:35.
31. Williams RC, Jeffcoat MK, Howell TH, et al.: Topical flurbiprofen treatment of periodontitis in beagles. J Periodont Res 1988; 23:166.
32. Williams RC, Jeffcoat MK, Howell H, et al: Altering the progression of human alveolar bone loss with the non-steroidal anti-inflammatory drug flurbiprofen. J Periodontol 1989; 60:485.
33. Williams RC, Jeffcoat MK, Kaplan ML, et al: Flurbiprofen: A potent inhibitor of alveolar bone resorption in beagles. Science 1985; 227:640.
34. Yukna RA: A clinical and histologic study of healing following the excisional new attachment procedure in rhesus monkeys. J Periodontol 1976; 47:701.

Periodontal Therapy in the Female Patient (Puberty, Menses, Pregnancy, and Menopause)

Joan Otomo-Corgel

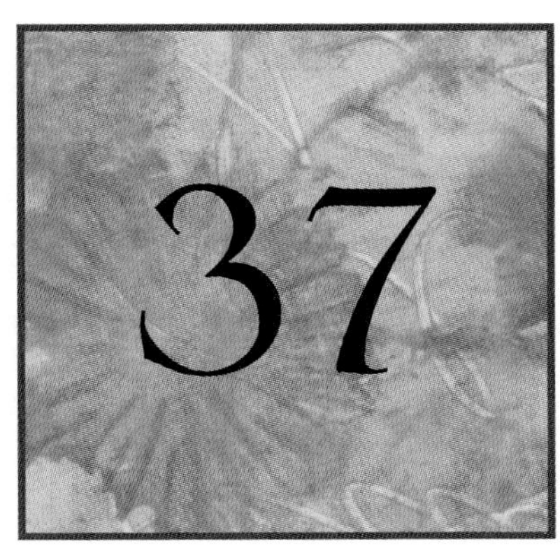

CHAPTER

CHAPTER OUTLINE

Throughout a woman's life cycle, hormonal influences affect therapeutic decision making in periodontics. Historically, therapies have been gender biased. However, the advent of new research has provided keener appreciation of the unique systemic influences on oral, periodontal, and implant tissues. Oral health care professionals have greater awareness and capabilities of dealing with hormonal influences associated with the reproductive process. Periodontal and oral tissue responses may be altered, creating diagnostic and therapeutic dilemmas. Therefore it is imperative that the clinician recognize, customize, and appropriately alter periodontal therapy according to the individual woman's needs based on the stage of her life cycle.

This chapter reviews phases of the female life cycle from puberty through menopause. Periodontal manifestations, systemic effects, and clinical management are presented.

PUBERTY

Puberty occurs between the average ages of 11 to 14 in most women. An increase in the production of sex hormones (estrogen and progesterone) occurs, which then remains relatively constant during the remainder of the reproductive phase.

Also, the prevalence of gingivitis increases without an increase in the amount of plaque. Gram-negative anaerobes, especially *Prevotella intermedia,* have been implicated in association with puberty gingivitis. Kornman and Loesche postulated that this anaerobic organism may use ovarian hormone as a substitute for vitamin K growth factor.[41] Delaney and Kornman suggest levels of black pigmented *Bacteroides,* especially *P. intermedia* (formerly known as *Bacteroides intermedius*), increase with increased levels of gonadotrophic hormones in puberty. *Capnocytophaga* species also increase in incidence as well as in proportion. These organisms have been implicated in the increased bleeding tendency observed during puberty.[32] Recent studies associated with puberty gingivitis indicate proportionately elevated motile rods, spirochetes, and *P. intermedia.*[55] Statistically significant increases in gingival inflammation and in the proportions of *P. intermedia* and *Prevotella nigrescens* were seen in puberty gingivitis.[58]

During puberty, periodontal tissues may have an exaggerated response to local factors. A hyperplastic reaction of the gingiva may occur in areas where food debris, materia alba, plaque, and calculus are deposited. The inflamed tissues become erythematous, lobulated, and retractable. Bleeding may occur easily with mechanical debridement of the gingival tissues. Histologically, the appearance is consistent with inflammatory hyperplasia.

During the reproductive years, women tend to have a more vigorous immune response including higher immunoglobulin concentrations, stronger primary and secondary responses, increased resistance to the induction of immunologic tolerance, and a greater ability to reject tumors and homografts.[81] Allergy sensitivity and asthma is higher in young men, but after puberty, women become more susceptible than their male counterparts.

Management

During puberty, education of the parent or caregiver is part of successful periodontal therapy. Preventive care, including a vigorous program of oral hygiene, is also vital. Milder gingivitis cases respond well to scaling and root planing with frequent oral hygiene reinforcement.[4] Severe cases of gingivitis may require microbial culturing, antimicrobial mouthwashes and local site delivery, or antibiotic therapy. Periodontal maintenance appointments may need to be more frequent when periodontal instability is noted.

The clinician should recognize the intraoral effects of chronic regurgitation of gastric contents on intraoral tissues because this age group also is susceptible to eating disorders, namely bulimia and anorexia nervosa. Perimylosis (smooth erosion of the enamel and dentin), typically on the lingual surfaces of maxillary anterior teeth, varies with the duration and frequency of the behavior.[12] Also, enlargement of the parotid glands (occasionally sublingual glands) has been estimated to occur in 10% to 50% of patients who binge and purge.[52] Therefore a diminished salivary flow rate may also be present, which will increase oral mucous membrane sensitivity, gingival erythema, and caries susceptibility.

MENSES

Periodontal Manifestations

During the reproductive years, the ovarian cycle is controlled by the anterior pituitary gland. Gonadotrophins FSH (follicle stimulating hormone) and LH (luteinizing hormone) are produced from the anterior pituitary gland. The secretion of gonadotrophins is also dependent on the hypothalamus. Ongoing changes in the concentration of the gonadotrophins and ovarian hormones occur during the monthly menstrual cycle (Fig. 37-1). Under the influence of FSH and LH, estrogen and progesterone are steroid hormones produced by the ovaries during the menstrual cycle. During the reproductive cycle, the purpose of estrogen and progesterone is to prepare the uterus for implantation of the egg.

The monthly reproductive cycle has two phases. The first phase is referred to as the *follicular phase.* Levels of FSH are elevated, and estradiol (E_2), the major form of estrogen, is synthesized by the developing follicle and peaks approximately 2 days before ovulation. The effect of estrogen stimulates the egg to move down the fallopian tubules (ovulation) and stimulates proliferation of the stroma cells, blood vessels, and glands of the endometrium.

Phase II is called the *luteal phase.* The developing corpus luteum synthesizes both estradiol and progesterone. Note that estrogen peaks to 0.2 ng/ml and progesterone 10.0 ng/ml to complete the rebuilding of the endometrium for fertilized egg implantation. The corpus luteum involutes, ovarian hormone levels drops, and menstruation ensues.

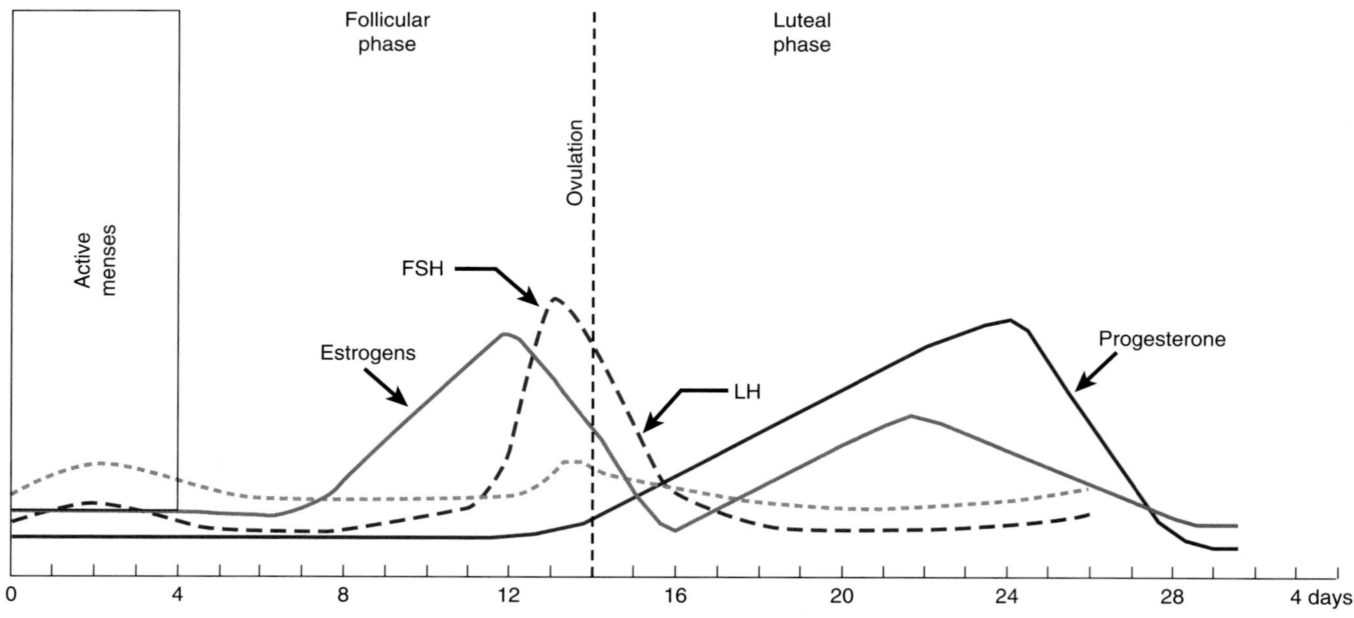

Fig. 37-1 Female reproductive cycle. Note the peak of progesterone and estrogen to FSH and LH.

The concept that ovarian hormones may increase inflammation in gingival tissues and exaggerate the response to local irritants has been postulated by several studies. Gingival inflammation seems to be aggravated by an imbalance and/or increase in sex hormones. Numerous studies have demonstrated in vitro and in vivo that sex hormones affect and modify the actions of cells of the immune system. In addition, evidence suggests that the interaction between estrogen and cells of the immune system can have nonimmune regulatory effects.[5,15]

Progesterone has been associated with increased permeability of the microvasculature, altering the rate and pattern of collagen production in the gingiva,[50] increasing folate metabolism,[66,87] and altering the immune response. During menses, progesterone increases from the second week, peaks at approximately 10 days, and dramatically drops before menstruation. (Note that this is based on a 28-day cycle; individual cycles are variable.) Progesterone plays a role in stimulating the production of prostaglandins that mediate the body's response to inflammation. Prostaglandin E_2 (PGE_2) is one of the major secretory products of monocytes and is higher in inflamed gingiva. Miyagi et al[53] found that the chemotaxis of PMNs was enhanced by progesterone but reduced by estradiol. Testosterone did not have a measurable effect on PMN chemotaxis. The researchers suggested that the altered PMN chemotaxis associated with gingival inflammation may be due to the effects of sex hormones. Physiologic, experimental, and clinical data confirm differences in immune responses between the two sexes.[92]

Gingival tissues have been reported to be more edematous during menses and erythematous preceding the onset of menses in some individuals. In addition, an increase of gingival exudate has been observed during the menstrual period and is sometimes associated with a minor increase in tooth mobility.[30] The incidence of postextraction osteitis has also been reported to be higher during the initiation of menses. No significant hematologic laboratory findings accompany this, other than a slightly reduced platelet count and a slight increase in clotting time.

When progesterone is highest (during the luteal phase of the cycle), intraoral recurrent apthous ulcers,[24] herpes labialis lesions, and candida infections occur in some women as a cyclic pattern. Because the esophageal sphincter is relaxed by progesterone, women may be more susceptible to gastroesophageal reflux disease (GERD) during this time of the cycle as well. Symptoms of GERD include heartburn, regurgitation, and chest pain, and when reflux is severe, some people develop unexplained coughing, hoarseness, sore throat, gingivitis, or asthma.[79]

During the peak level of progesterone (about 7 to 10 days before menstruation), premenstrual syndrome (PMS) may also occur. There appears to be no significant difference in the estrogen and progesterone levels between women who suffer from PMS and those who do not. Yet women with PMS seem to have lower levels of certain neurotransmitters such as enkephalins, endorphins, gamma-aminobutyric acid (GABA), and serotonin. Depression, irritability, mood swings, and difficulty with memory and concentration may be symptoms of neurotransmitter reduction. Patients are more sensitive and less tolerant of procedures, have a heightened gag reflex, and may have an exaggerated response to pain.

Management

Increased gingival bleeding and tenderness associated with the menstrual cycle, requires closer periodontal monitoring. Periodontal maintenance should be titrated to the individual patient's need and, if problematic, 3- to 4-month intervals should be recommended. An antimicrobial mouthrinse before cyclic inflammation may be indicated. Emphasis should be placed on oral hygiene.

For the patient with a history of excessive postoperative hemorrhage or menstrual flow, scheduling surgical visits after cyclic menstruation is prudent. Anemia is common, and appropriate consultation with a physician and recent laboratory tests, where indicated, should be maintained.

During PMS, many women exhibit physical symptoms including fatigue, sweet and salty food cravings, abdominal bloating, swollen hands or feet, headaches, breast tenderness, nausea, and gastrointestinal upset.[92] GERD may make it more uncomfortable for the patient to lay fully supine, especially within hours immediately after consuming a meal, and there may be a more sensitive gag reflex. The clinician should be aware that nonsteroidal antiinflammatory medication, infection, and acidic foods exacerbate GERD. Patients taking over-the counter antacids, H_2-receptor antagonists (cimetidine, famotidine, nizatidine, and ranitidine), prokinetic agents (cisapride and metoclopramide), and proton-pump inhibitors (lansoprazole, omeprazole, pantoprazole, and abeprazole)[78] may be GERD patients. The aforementioned medications have interactions with some antibiotics and antifungal medications, thus review of their pharmacology is necessary. Fluoride rinses and/or trays, frequent periodontal debridement, and avoidance of high-alcohol-content mouthwashes may reduce the associated gingival and caries sequela.

PMS is often treated by antidepressants. Selective serotonin reuptake inhibitors (SSRIs) are generally the first-line choice because they have fewer side effects than other antidepressants, do not require blood monitoring, and are safe in overdoses. The SSRI fluoxetine reported a 70% response rate. It was ranked the 5th most dispensed prescription (new and refills) in the U.S. in 1998. (Sertraline was ranked 12th and is the drug of choice for treatment of PMS).[97] The clinician should be aware that patients on fluoxetine have increased side effects with highly protein-bound drugs (e.g., aspirin) and the half-life of diazepam and other CNS depressants is increased. Additional common selective serotonin reuptake inhibitors are fluvoxamine, paroxetine, and citalopram. Other antidepressants that may be prescribed are the selective serotonin and norepinephrine reuptake inhibitors (SNRIs), tricyclics, trazodone, mirtazapine, nefazodone, or maprotiline.

The PMS patient may be difficult to treat due to emotional and physiologic sensitivity. Treat the gingival and oral mucosal tissues gently. Moisten gauzes or cotton rolls with a lubricant, chlorhexidine rinse, or water before placing them in the apthous prone patient. Careful retraction of the oral mucosa, cheeks, and lips is necessary in both the apthous and herpetic prone patient. Because the hypoglycemic threshold is elevated, advise the patient to have a light snack before her appointment. Note that 70% of menstruating women have PMS symptoms, but only 5% meet the strict diagnostic criteria.

PERIODONTAL MANIFESTATIONS OF PREGNANCY

The link between pregnancy and periodontal inflammation has been known for many years. In 1778, Vermeeren discussed "toothpains" in pregnancy. In 1818, Pitcarin described gingival hyperplasia in pregnancy.[71] Despite awareness regarding pregnancy and its effect on periodontal disease, only recently has evidence indicated an inverse relationship to systemic health. Current research implies periodontal disease may alter the systemic health of the patient and adversely affect the well-being of the fetus by elevating the risk for low-birth-weight, preterm infants.

Periodontal Diseases

In 1877, Pinard[70] recorded the first case of "pregnancy gingivitis." Only recently has periodontal research begun to focus on causative mechanisms. The occurrence of "pregnancy gingivitis" is extremely common, occurring in approximately 30% to 100% of all pregnant women.[33,44,48,80] It is characterized by erythema, edema, hyperplasia, and increased bleeding. Histologically, the description is the same as gingivitis. However, the etiologic factors are different despite clinical and histologic similarities. Cases range from mild to severe inflammation (Fig. 37-2). This can progress to severe hyperplasia, pain, and bleeding (Figs. 37-3 to 37-6). Other growths that resemble pregnancy granulomas must be ruled out, such as central giant cell granulomas or underlying systemic diseases. Periodontal status before pregnancy may influence the progression or severity as the circulating hormones fluctuate. The anterior region of the mouth is more commonly affected, and interproximal sites tend to be most involved.[19] Increased tissue edema may lead to increased pocket depths and relate to a transient tooth mobility.[73] Anterior site inflammation may be exacerbated by increased mouth breathing, primarily in the third trimester from pregnancy rhinitis. The gingiva is the most common site involved (approximately 70% of all cases), followed by the tongue and lips, buccal mucosa, and palate.[8]

Pyogenic granulomas, pregnancy tumors, or pregnancy epulides occur in 0.2% to 9.6% of pregnancies. They are clinically and histologically indistinguishable from pyogenic granulomas occurring in women who are not pregnant or in men. They appear most commonly during the second or third month of pregnancy. Clinically, they bleed easily and become hyperplastic and nodular. When excised, they do not usually leave a large defect. They may be sessile or pedunculated, ulcerated, and ranging in color from purplish red to deep blue, depending on the vascularity of the lesion and degree of venous stasis. The lesion classically occurs in an area of gingivitis and is associated with poor oral hygiene and calculus. Alveolar bone loss is not usually associated with pyogenic granulomas of pregnancy.

Role of Pregnancy Hormones

Subgingival Plaque Composition. Epidemiologic studies indicate a relationship between the level of home care and the severity of gingival inflammation. It appears that the relation between signs of gingival inflammation and the amount of plaque is closer after parturition than during pregnancy. An alteration in the compositions of subgingival plaque occurs during pregnancy. Kornman and Loesche found that during the second trimester, gingivitis and gingival bleeding increased without an increase in plaque levels.[42] Bacterial anaerobic to aerobic ratios increased in addition to *B. melaninogenicus* and *P. intermedia* proportions (2.2% to 10.1%). These authors suggested that estradiol or progesterone can substitute for menadione (vitamin K) as an essential growth factor for *P. intermedia* but not *Porphyromonas gingivalis* or *Bacteroides coherences*. There was also an increase in *P. gingivalis* during the 21st to 27th weeks of gestation, but this was not statistically significant. The relative increase in the numbers of *P. intermedia* may be a

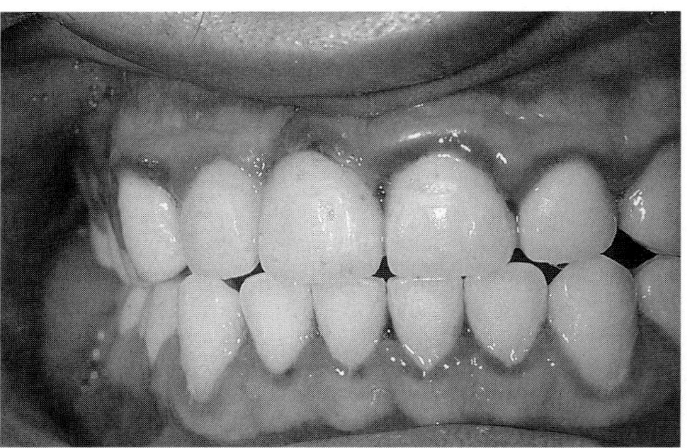

Fig. 37-2 Moderate pregnancy gingivitis.

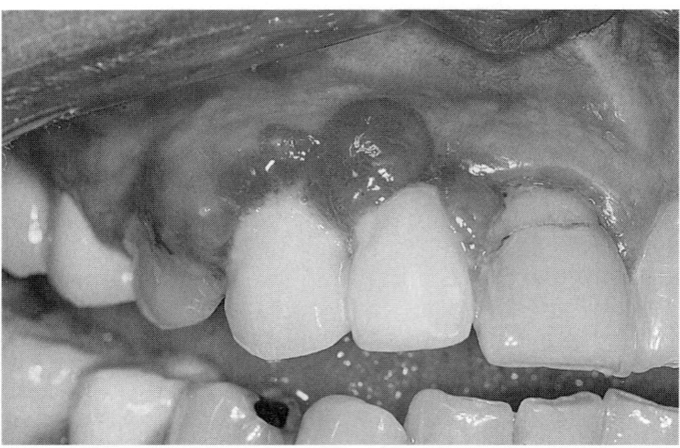

Fig. 37-3 Pregnancy tumor.

more sensitive indicator of an altered systemic hormonal situation than clinical parameters of gingivitis.[83]

Periodontal Disease and Preterm, Low-Birth-Weight Births. Due to the pioneering research by Offenbacher, evidence exists that untreated periodontal disease in pregnant women may be a significant risk factor for preterm (<37 weeks' gestation), low-birth-weight (<2500 g) babies.[62] The relationship between genitourinary tract infection and preterm, low-birth-weight (PLBW) is well documented in human and animal studies. Periodontal researchers, suspecting periodontal disease as another source of infection, found that otherwise low-risk mothers of PLBW infants had significantly more periodontal attachment loss than control mothers having normal-weight infants at birth. The current opinion is that the correlation of periodontal disease to PLBW births occurs as a result of infection and is mediated indirectly, principally by the translocation of bacterial products such as endotoxin (lipopolysaccharide, LPS) and the action of maternally produced inflammatory mediators.[27] Biologically active molecules such as prostaglandin E_2 (PGE_2) and tumor necrosis factor-alpha (TNFα), which are normally involved in normal parturition, are raised to artificially high levels by the infection process, which may foster premature labor.[3] Gram-negative bacteria in periodontal diseases therefore may permit selective overgrowth or invasion of gram-negative bacteria within the genitourinary tract. Recently, gingival crevicular fluid levels of PGE_2 were positively associated with intraamniotic PGE_2 levels ($P = 0.018$), suggesting that gram-negative periodontal infection may present a systemic challenge sufficient to initiate the onset of premature labor as a source of LPS and/or through stimulation of secondary inflammatory mediators such as PGE_2 and interleukin 1 beta (IL-1β).[16] Ongoing research supports the association of periodontal disease and PLBW.[17,18] Offenbacher has recently published data suggesting a dose response relationship for increasing gingival crevicular fluid PGE_2 as a marker of current periodontal disease activity and decreasing birth weight. Four organisms associated with mature plaque and progressing periodontitis (*Bacteroides forsythus, P. gingivalis, Actinobacillus actinomycetemcomitans,* and *Treponema denticola*) were detected at higher levels in PLBW mothers as compared with normal-birth-weight controls[61] (see also Chapter 13).

Maternal Immunoresponse

The maternal immune system is thought to be suppressed during pregnancy. This response may allow the fetus to survive as an allograft. Documentation of immunosuppressive factors in the sera of pregnant women can be noted by marked increase of monocytes (which in large numbers inhibit in vitro proliferative responses to mitogens, allogenic cells, and soluble antigen),[88] and

A

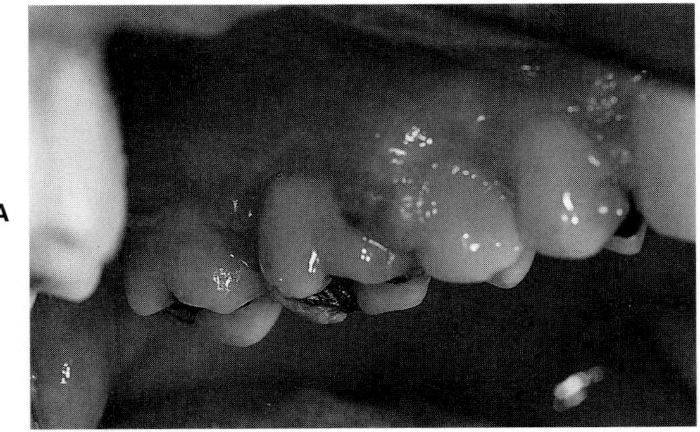

B

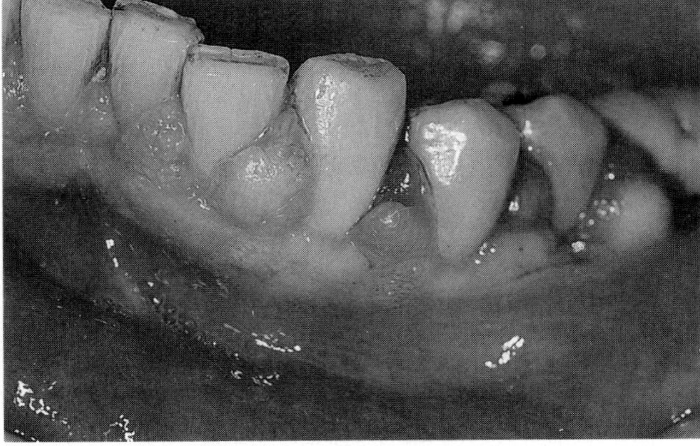

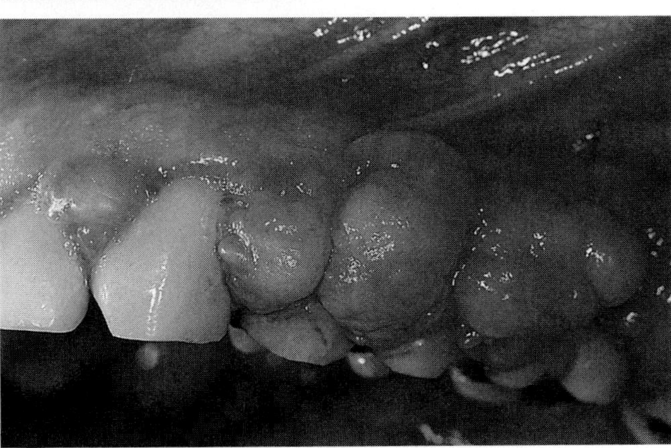

C

Fig. 37-4 Severe pregnancy gingivitis with hyperplasia in a patient with non–insulin-dependent diabetes mellitus in poor control. **A,** Lingual view of the upper jaw. **B,** Lower mandibular incisors and premolars. **C,** Buccal view.

BOX 37-1

Etiology of Gingival Responses to Elevated Estrogen and Progesterone during Pregnancy

Subgingival Plaque Composition

Anaerobic to aerobic ratio increases
Higher concentrations of *Prevotella intermedia* (substitutes sex hormone for Vitamin K–growth factor)
Higher concentrations of *Bacteroides melaninogenicus*
Higher concentrations of *Porphyromonous gingivalis*

Maternal Immunoresponse

Depression of cell-mediated immunity
Decreased neutrophil chemotaxis
Depression of antibody and T cell responses
- Decrease in the ratio of peripheral T helper cells to T suppressor–cytotoxic cells (CD4/CD8 ratio)

Cytotoxicity directed against macrophages and B cells may result in diminished immunoresponsiveness
Decrease in absolute numbers or CD3, CD4, and CD19 positive cells in peripheral blood during pregnancy versus postpartum
Stimulation of the production of prostaglandin

Sex Hormone Concentration

Estrogen
- Increases cellular proliferation in blood vessels (known in the endometrium)
- Decreases keratinization, while increasing epithelial glycogen
- Specific receptors are found in gingival tissues

Progesterone
- Increases vascular dilation, thus increases permeability (result in edema and accumulation of inflammatory cells)
- Increases proliferation of newly formed capillaries in gingival tissues (increased bleeding tendency)
- Alters rate and pattern of collagen production
- Increased metabolic breakdown of folate (a deficiency can inhibit tissue repair)
- Specific receptors are found in gingival tissues
- Decreases plasminogen activator inhibitor factor type 2, thus increases tissue proteolysis

Estrogen and Progesterone
- Effect ground substance of connective tissue by increasing fluidity
- Concentrations increase in saliva and fluid with increased concentrations in serum

pregnancy-specific B-l-glycoproteins contribute to diminished lymphocyte responsiveness to mitogens and antigens.[9] In addition, a decrease in the ratio of peripheral T helper cells to T suppressor cells (CD4/CD8) ratio has been reported to occur throughout pregnancy.[83]

These changes in maternal immunoresponsiveness suggest an increased susceptibility to developing gingival inflammation. In one study, the gingival index was higher but percentages of T3, T4, and B cells appeared to decrease in peripheral blood and gingival tissues during pregnancy as compared with a control group.[1] Other studies report decreased neutrophil chemotaxis, depression of cell-mediated immunity, phagocytosis, and a decreased T cell response with elevated ovarian hormones levels, especially progesterone.[72] A decrease in in vitro responses of peripheral blood lymphocytes to several mitogens and a preparation of *P. intermedia* has been reported,[10,49,60] and evidence suggests a decrease in the absolute numbers of CD4 positive cells in peripheral blood during pregnancy as compared with the number of these cells postpartum.[74,84] Lapp et al suggests that high levels of progesterone during pregnancy affect the development of localized inflammation by down-regulation of IL-6 production, rendering the gingiva less efficient at resisting the inflammatory challenges produced by the bacteria.[43]

Also, ovarian hormone stimulates the production of prostaglandins, in particular PGE_1 and PGE_2, which are potent mediators of the inflammatory response. With the prostaglandin acting as an immunosuppressant, gingival inflammation may increase when the mediator level is high.[20,63] Kinnby et al[39] found that high progesterone levels during pregnancy influenced plasminogen activator inhibitor type 2 (PAI-2) and disturbed the balance of the fibrinolytic system. Because PAI-2 serves as an important inhibitor of tissue proteolysis, the research of Kinnby et al implies that components of the fibrinolytic system may be involved in the development of pregnancy gingivitis.

Sex Hormone Levels

During pregnancy, hormonal levels rise dramatically (Box 37-1). Progesterone reaches levels of 100 ng/mL, 10 times the peak luteal phase of menses. Estradiol in the plasma may reach 30 times higher levels than during the reproductive cycle. In early pregnancy and during the normal ovarian cycle, the corpus luteum is the major source of estrogen and progesterone. During pregnancy, the placenta begins to produce estrogens and progesterone.

Estrogen may regulate cellular proliferation, differentiation, and keratinization, whereas progesterone influences the permeability of the microvasculature,[45,46] alters the rate and pattern of collagen production, and increases the metabolic breakdown of folate (necessary for tissue maintenance).[95] High concentration of sex hormones in gingival tissues, saliva, serum, and crevicular fluid also may exaggerate the response.

Regulation via hormones of most cellular processes occurs by interaction of these products with intracellular receptors. The resulting effects are dependent on the concentration of unbound hormone diffused through the cell membrane. Vittek has demonstrated specific estrogen and progesterone receptors in gingival tissues.[90] This is direct biochemical evidence that this tissue may function as a target organ for sex hormones. Muramatsu and Takaesu found increasing concentration of sex hormones in saliva from the first month and peaking in the ninth month of gestation, along with increasing percentages of *P. intermedia*. Probing depths, increasing numbers of gingival sites with bleeding, and redness increased until 1 month postpartum.[56] Also, evidence of sex hormone concentration in crevicular fluid exists, providing a growth media for periodontal pathogens.

Other Oral Manifestations of Pregnancy

Perimylolysis or acid erosion of teeth may occur if "morning sickness" or esophageal reflux is severe and involves repeated vomiting of the gastric contents. Note that severe reflux may cause scarring of the esophageal sphincter and the patient may become a more likely candidate for GERD later in life.

Xerostomia is a frequent complaint among pregnant women. One study found this persistent dryness in 44% of pregnant participants.[22]

A rare finding in pregnancy is ptyalism or sialorrhea. This excessive secretion of saliva usually begins at 2 to 3 weeks of gestation and may abate at the end of the first trimester. The etiology of ptyalism has not been identified, but it may occur because of the inability of nauseated gravid women to swallow normal amounts of saliva rather than from a true increase in the production of saliva.[14]

Because pregnancy places the woman in an immunocompromised state, the clinician must be aware of the total health of the patient. Gestational diabetes, leukemia, and other medical conditions may appear during pregnancy.

Clinical Management

A thorough medical history is an imperative component of the periodontal examination, especially in the pregnant patient. Due to immunologic alterations, increase in blood volume (ruling out mitral valve prolapse and heart murmurs), and fetal interactions, the clinician must diligently and consistently monitor the patient's medical and periodontal stability. Medical history dialogue should include pregnancy complications, previous miscarriages, recent history of cramping, spotting, or pernicious vomiting. Next, the patient's obstetrician should be contacted to discuss her medical status, periodontal or dental needs, and the proposed treatment plan.

Establishment of a healthy oral environment and optimal oral hygiene levels are primary objectives in the pregnant patient. A preventive periodontal program consisting of nutritional counseling and rigorous plaque control measures in the dental office and at home should be reinforced.

Plaque Control. The heightened tendency for gingival inflammation should be clearly explained to the patient so that acceptable oral hygiene techniques may be taught, reinforced, and monitored throughout pregnancy. Scaling, polishing, and root planing may be performed whenever necessary throughout the pregnancy. Some practitioners avoid the use of high-alcohol-content antimicrobial mouthrinses in pregnant women and prefer to use those that are non–alcohol based.

Prenatal Fluoride. The prescribing of prenatal fluoride supplements has been an area of controversy for quite some time. Although two studies have claimed beneficial results,[28,29] others suggest that the clinical efficacy of prenatal fluoride supplements is uncertain and the mechanism by which prenatal fluorides might impart cariostasis is unclear.[69]

The American Dental Association does not recommend the use of prenatal fluoride because its efficacy has not been demonstrated. The American Academy of Pediatric Dentistry supports this position as well. The American Academy of Pediatrics has no stated position on prescribing prenatal fluorides.

Treatment

Elective Dental Treatment. Other than good plaque control, it is prudent to avoid elective dental care if possible during the first trimester and the last half of the third trimester. The first trimester is the period of organogenesis when the fetus is highly susceptible to environmental influences. In the last half of the third trimester, a hazard of premature delivery exists because the uterus is very sensitive to external stimuli. Prolonged chair time may need to be avoided because the woman is most uncomfortable at this time. Further, supine hypotensive syndrome may possibly occur. In a semi-reclining or supine position, the great vessels, particularly the inferior vena cava, are compressed by the gravid uterus. By interfering with venous return, this compression will cause maternal hypotension, decreased cardiac output, and eventual loss of consciousness. Supine hypotensive syndrome can usually be reversed by turning the patient on her left side, thereby removing pressure on the vena cava and allowing blood to return from the lower extremities and pelvic area. A preventive 6-inch soft wedge (rolled towel) should be placed on the patient's right side when she is reclined for clinical treatment.

The second trimester is the safest period for providing routine dental care. The emphasis at this time is on controlling active disease and eliminating potential problems that could arise in late pregnancy. Major oral or periodontal surgery should be postponed until after delivery. Pregnancy tumors that are painful, interfere with mastication, or continue to bleed or suppurate after mechanical debridement may require excision and biopsy before delivery.

Dental Radiographs. The safety of dental radiography has been well established, provided features such as high-speed film, filtration, collimation, and lead aprons are used. However, it is most desirable not to have any irradiation during pregnancy, especially during the first trimester, because the developing fetus is particularly susceptible to radiation damage.[47] When radiographs are needed for diagnosis, the most important aid for the patient is the protective lead apron. Studies have shown that when an apron is used during contemporary dental radiography, gonadal and fetal radiation is virtually immeasurable.[7]

Even in light of the obvious safety of dental radiography, radiographs should be used selectively during pregnancy and only when necessary and appropriate to aid in diagnosis and treatment. In most instances, only

BOX 37-2

FDA Classification System

The following table represents the five category systems used by the FDA to classify drugs based on their potential for causing birth defects.

A	Controlled studies in women fail to demonstrate a risk to the fetus in the first trimester (there is no evidence of a risk in later trimesters), and the possibility of fetal harm appears remote.
B	Either animal-reproduction studies have not demonstrated a fetal risk but there are no controlled studies in pregnant women, or animal-reproduction studies have shown an adverse effect (other than a decrease in fertility) that was not confirmed in controlled studies in women in the first trimester (and there is no evidence of a risk in later trimesters).
C	Either studies in animals have revealed adverse effects on the fetus (teratogenic or embryocidal, or other) and there are not controlled studies in women or studies in women and animals are not available. Drugs should be given only if the potential benefit justifies the potential risk to the fetus.
D	There is positive evidence of human fetal risk, but the benefits from use in pregnant women may be acceptable despite the risk (e.g., if the drug is needed in a life-threatening situation or for a serious disease for which safer drugs cannot be used or are ineffective).
X	Studies in animals or human beings have demonstrated fetal abnormalities, or there is evidence of fetal risk based on human experience, or both, and the risk of the use of the drug in pregnant women clearly outweighs any possible benefit. The drug contraindicated in women who are or may become pregnant.

bitewing, panoramic, or selected periapical films are indicated.

Medications. Drug therapy in the pregnant patient is controversial because drugs can affect the fetus by diffusion across the placenta. Prescriptions should be only the duration absolutely essential for the pregnant patient's well-being and only after careful consideration of potential side effects. The classification system established by the FDA in 1979 to rate fetal risk levels associated with many prescription drugs provides safety guidelines (Box 37-2). The prudent practitioner should consult references such as Briggs' *Drugs in Pregnancy and Lactation*[11] or Olin's *Drug Facts and Comparisons*[64] for information on the FDA pregnancy risk factor associated with prescription drugs. Ideally, no drug should be administered during pregnancy, especially the first trimester.[47] However, it is sometimes impossible to adhere to this rule. It is therefore fortunate that most commonly used drugs in dental practice can be given during pregnancy with relative safety, although there are a few important exceptions (see Tables 37-1 to 37-3). The table of drugs presented is considered a general guideline.[75] Refer to the tables regarding local anesthetic, antibiotic, and analgesic prescriptions. In particular, antibiotics are often needed in periodontal therapy. Note that the effect of a particular medication on the fetus depends on the type of antimicrobial, dosage, trimester, and duration of the course of therapy. [65] Research regarding subgingival irrigation and local site delivery in relation to the developing fetus is inadequate at this date.

Breast Feeding. Usually, there is a risk that the drug can enter breast milk and be transferred to the nursing infant, in whom exposure could have adverse effects (see Tables 37-4 and 37-5). Unfortunately, there is little conclusive information about drug dosage and effects via breast milk; however, retrospective clinical studies and empiric observations coupled with known pharmacologic pathways allow recommendations to be made.[47] The amount of drug excreted in breast milk is usually not more than 1% to 2% of the maternal dose; therefore it is highly unlikely that most drugs have any pharmacologic significance for the infant.[85,94]

The mother should take prescribed drugs just after breastfeeding and then avoid nursing for 4 hours or more, if possible,[47,85] to markedly decrease the drug concentration in breast milk.

ORAL CONTRACEPTIVES

Oral contraceptives (OC) may have similar responses to those witnessed in pregnant patients. An exaggerated response to local irritants occurs in gingival tissues. Inflammation ranges from mild edema and erythema to severe inflammation with hemorrhagic or hyperplasic gingival tissues. It has been reported more exudate is present in inflamed gingival tissues of OC users versus that of pregnancy.[82,96]

Investigators have reported several mechanisms for the heightened response in gingival tissues. Kalkwarf reported the response may be due to alteration of the microvasculature, increased gingival permeability, and increasing synthesis of prostaglandin.[38] Prostaglandin E appears to rise significantly with increasing sex hormones. Prostaglandin E is a potent mediator of inflammation.[23] Jensen et al found dramatic microbial changes in pregnant and OC groups as compared with a nonpregnant group.[37] A 16-fold increase in *Bacteroides* species was noted in the OC group versus the nonpregnant group, despite no statistically significant clinical differences in gingival index or crevicular fluid flow. Jensen et al stated that the increased female sex hormones substituting for the napthaquinone requirement of certain *Bacteroides* species were most likely responsible for this increase.

TABLE 37-1

Local Anesthetic/Analgesic Administration during Pregnancy

Drug	FDA Category (Prescription Drug)	During Pregnancy
Local Anesthetics*		
Lidocaine	B	Yes
Mepivacaine	C	Use with caution; consult physician
Prilocaine	B	Yes
Bupivacaine	C	Use with caution; consult physician
Etidocaine	B	Yes
Procaine	C	Use with caution; consult physician
Analgesics		
Aspirin	C/D, 3rd trimester	Caution; avoid in 3rd trimester
Acetaminophen	B	Yes
Ibuprofen	B/D, 3rd trimester	Caution; avoid in 3rd trimester
Codeine**	C	Use with caution; consult physician
Hydrocodone**	B	Use with caution; consult physician
Oxycodone**	B	Use with caution; consult physician
Propoxyphene	C	Use with caution; consult physician

* Can use vasoconstrictors if necessary

** Avoid prolonged use

TABLE 37-2

Antibiotic Administration during Pregnancy

Drug	FDA Category (Prescription Drug)	During Pregnancy	Risks
Penicillins	B	Yes	Diarrhea
Erythromycin	B	Yes; avoid estolate form	Intrahepatic jaundice in mother
Clindamycin	B	Yes, with caution	Drug concentrated in fetal bone, spleen, lung, and liver
Cephalosporins	B	Yes	Limited information
Tetracycline	D	Avoid	Depression of bone growth, enamel hypoplasia, gray-brown tooth discoloration
Ciprofloxacin	C	Avoid	Possible developing cartilage erosion
Metronidazole	B	Avoid; controversial	Theoretic carcinogenic data in animals
Gentamicin	C	Caution; consult physician	Limited information ototoxicity
Vanocomycin	C	Caution; consult physician	Limited information
Clarithromycin	D	Avoid; use only if the potential benefit justifies the risk to the fetus	Limited information Adverse effects on pregnancy, outcome, and embryo/fetal development in animals

TABLE 37-3

Sedative-Hypnotic Drug Administration during Pregnancy

Drug	FDA Category	During Pregnancy
Sedative-Hypnotics		
Benzodiazepines	D	Avoid
Barbiturates	D	Avoid
Nitrous oxide	Not assigned	Avoid in 1st trimester; otherwise use with caution; consult physician

TABLE 37-4

Dental Drug Administration during Breastfeeding

Drug	During Breastfeeding
Local Anesthetics	
Lidocaine	Yes
Mepivacaine	Yes
Prilocaine	Yes
Bupivacaine	Yes
Etidocaine	Yes
Procaine	Yes
Analgesics	
Aspirin	Avoid
Acetaminophen	Yes
Ibuprofen	Yes
Codeine	Yes
Hydrocodone	No data
Oxycodone	Yes
Propoxyphene	Yes

The OC-associated gingival inflammation may become chronic (versus that of acute inflammation of pregnancy) due to the extended periods of time that women are exposed to elevated levels of estrogen and progesterone.[40,68] Some have reported that the inflammation increases with prolonged use of OCs. Kalkawarf did not find that duration of use made a significant difference; however, the brand used had different responses. It is apparent that further studies need to be performed in relation to dosage, duration, and type of OC used in association with the periodontium. The concentration of female sex hormones in today's OC is significantly less than that of the 1970s with the same level of contraceptive efficacy.

Salivary composition has a noted change in patients taking OCs in studies conducted in the 1970s. A decrease concentration of protein, sialic, acid, hexosamine fucose, hydrogen ions, and total electrolytes has been reported. Salivary flow rates have been reported to be increased in one report[51] and decreased in 30% of subjects in another report.[21]

TABLE 37-5

Dental Drug Administration during Breastfeeding

Drug	During Breastfeeding
Antibiotics	
Penicillins	Yes
Erythromycin	Yes
Clindamycin	Yes (with caution)
Cephalosporins	Yes
Tetracycline	Avoid
Ciprofloxacin	Avoid
Metronidazole	Avoid
Gentamicin	Avoid
Vancomycin	Avoid
(Note: antibiotics have the risk of diarrhea and sensitization in the mother and infant.)	
Sedative-Hypnotics	
Benzodiazepines	Avoid
Barbiturates	Avoid
Nitrous oxide	Yes

The dental literature reports that women taking OCs experience a twofold to threefold increase in the incidence of localized osteitis following extraction of mandibular third molars.[86] The higher incidence of osteitis is these patients may be attributed to the effects of OCs (estrogens) on clotting factors. However, a number of studies refute these finding.[13] Evidence to this date is inconclusive with regard to osteitis following third molar extractions and use of OCs.

Also, it has been reported in the medical literature that a spotty melanotic pigmentation of the skin may occur with use of oral contraceptives. This suggests a relationship between the use of OCs and the occurrence of gingival melanosis,[34] especially in fair-skinned individuals.

Management

Medical histories should include OCs under the heading of "Medications," and an oral dialogue should include questions regarding OCs in women of childbearing age. The patient should be informed of the oral and periodontal side effects of OCs and the need for meticulous home care and compliance with periodontal maintenance. Treatment of gingival inflammation exaggerated by OCs should include establishing an oral hygiene program and eliminating local predisposing factors. Periodontal surgery may be indicated if resolution after initial therapy (scaling and root planing) is inadequate. It may be advisable to perform extraction of teeth (especially of third molars) on nonestrogenic days (days 23 to 28) of the OC cycle to reduce the risk of a postoperative localized osteitis,[25] but note that evidence of this association is inconclusive and warrants further investigation.

Although the results from animal studies have demonstrated antibiotic interference adversely affecting contraceptive sex hormone levels, several studies involving human subjects have failed to support such an interaction.[6,26,57,59] This issue is controversial, and antibiotics possibly could render OCs ineffective in preventing pregnancies. In 1991 an ADA Health Foundation Report stated that all women of childbearing age should be informed of possible reduced efficacy of steroid OCs during antibiotic therapy and advised to use additional forms of contraception during short-term antibiotic therapy. During long-term antibiotic therapy, they should consult their physician about using high-dose OC preparations.[2] Although research regarding oral manifestations attributed to OCs has been reported in the literature, it can be presumed that the same effects could occur with the use of contraceptive implants. Along the same lines, the remote possibility of reduced efficacy of the contraceptive implant with concurrent antibiotic administration also exists and the same precautions can be adhered to as with OCs.

MENOPAUSE

Female life expectancy is 80+ years, therefore many women will live 40% of their lives in menopause. This cohort represents a large number of the patients that present in clinical practices. Therefore we must be aware of the implications that reduced hormones have on the periodontal tissues as well as the systemic changes that may manifest.

Throughout a woman's lifetime, the number of oocytes steadily diminishes. Menopause is associated with symptoms of estrogen deficiency. Estradiol levels fall gradually in the years before menopause. Levels of the gonadotophins FSH and LH begin to rise, and levels of sex hormones begin to fluctuate. This stage of "perimenopause" is characterized by increasing ovarian unresponsiveness, therefore sporadic ovulation ensues. Anovulatory cycles indicate low estradiol and progesterone because of absent corpus luteum function.

Oral Changes

Important to the clinician is recognition of the effect of hormonal alterations on the oral cavity as well as systemic and psychologic changes. Oral changes in menopause include thinning of the oral mucosa, oral discomfort ("burning mouth"), gingival recession, xerostomia, altered taste sensation, alveolar bone loss, and alveolar ridge resorption.

Fluctuations of sex hormones during menopause have been implicated as factors in inflammatory changes in the human gingiva, hypertrophy, or atrophy. Estrogen affects cellular proliferation, differentiation, and keratinization of the gingival epithelium. Hormone receptors have been identified in basal and spinous layers of the epithelium and connective tissue,[2] implicating gingiva and other oral tissues as targets to manifest hormone deficiencies. Sex steroids are known to have a direct effect on connective tissue, with estrogens increasing the intracellular fluid content. Estrogen deficiency can lead to a reduction in collagen formation in connective tissues, resulting in a decrease in skin thickness.[93] Alterations in collagen affect tissues such as joints, hair, nails, and glands. In 1996, Mohammed et al noted significant increased recession in postmenopausal patients with low bone density.[54]

Osteopenia and osteoporosis have been associated with the menopausal patient. Osteopenia is a reduction in bone mass due to an imbalance between bone resorption and formation, favoring resorption and resulting in demineralization and osteoporosis. Osteoporosis is a disease characterized by low bone mass and fragility and a consequent increase in fracture risk.[91] In most women, peak bone mass occurs between 20 to 30 years of age and declines from this point. Menopause accelerates declining bone mass.[89] It is estimated that 25 million Americans are affected with osteoporosis, of whom 80% are female. Ongoing studies are examining the association of postmenopausal primary osteoporosis with mandibular/maxillary bone mineral density, tooth loss, alveolar ridge atrophy, and clinical periodontal attachment loss. The effects of hormone replacement therapy (HRT) or estrogen replacement therapy (ERT) on the oral bone and tooth loss is under investigation. Much of the latest evidence points to an probable association between osteoporosis and tooth loss as well as alveolar bone loss.[36,67,76,77]

Clinical Management

It is the clinician's responsibility to review the patient's medical history and keep information up to date. Due to possible alterations in oral soft and osseous tissues during perimenopause and postmenopause, appropriate questioning regarding hormone changes should be performed and documented. A myriad of therapies for HRT/ERT are available, from prescriptions to holistic approaches that need to be followed. Many medications may alter clotting times, prolong other medications, and interfere with absorption or effectiveness of prescription medications.

If gingival and mucosal tissue thinning occurs, soft tissue augmentation may be performed. Brushing with an extra-soft toothbrush using the toe or heal of the brush may prevent "scrubbing" the thinning gingiva. Dentifrices with minimal abrasive particles should be used. Rinses should have low alcohol concentrations. During periodontal maintenance, root surfaces should be debrided gently with minimal soft tissue trauma. Oral pain may be from thinning tissues, xerostomia, inadequate nutritional intake, or hormone depletion. It has been noted that when patients with oral symptoms were placed on HRT, symptoms were significantly reduced.

If the patient is osteoporosis susceptible (menopausal, female, Caucasian or Asian, smoker, minimal physical activity, low calcium intake, thin build or low body weight <58 kg, systemic disease associated with predisposition, and genetic history),[35] consult the patient's physician as to the risks versus benefits of HRT/ERT and calcium/vitamin D supplementation for the individual patient. Sodium fluoride, biphosphonates (alendronate),

BOX 37-3

National Institutes of Health (NIH) Consensus Conference Recommendations for Optimal Calcium Intake[31]

Premenopausal women (25–50 years old):	1000 mg/d
Postmenopausal women (estrogen therapy):	1000 mg/d
Postmenopausal women (no estrogen therapy):	1500 mg/d
Men (25–65 years old):	1000 mg/d
Women and men >65 years old:	1500 mg/d

selective estrogen receptor modulators, and parathyroid hormone may be other possible therapies for the osteoporotic patient. Close monitoring of the periodontal stability of the patient, performing titrated periodontal maintenance, informing the patient regarding potential risks of hormone depletion on the oral tissues, and consulting the treating physician is advised. The 1994 NIH Conference on Optimal Calcium Intake recommends 1000 mg of calcium per day for premenopausal women and 1500 mg per day for postmenopausal women (Box 37-3). To date, no data are available regarding success or failure with periodontal regeneration procedures in osteoporotic versus nonosteoporotic individuals. Also, no scientific data are available to contraindicate the use of osseointegrated implants in osteoporotic patients, despite articles stating osteoporosis as a risk factor. Much research is needed to address the increasing number of patients who may present to our periodontal practices with osteoporosis or osteopenia, most of whom will be undiagnosed.

CONCLUSION

Clinical periodontal therapy includes an understanding of our role in the total health and well-being of our patients. We do not treat localized site infections without affecting other systemic systems (and the possible unborn fetus or breastfed infant). Therefore female patients may present with periodontal and systemic considerations that alter conventional therapy.

The cyclic nature of the female sex hormones often reflect in the gingival tissues as the initial signs and symptoms. Our medical histories and dialogues should include thoughtful investigation of the individual patient's problems and needs. Questioning should reflect hormonal stability and medications associated with regulation. Patients should be educated regarding the profound effects the sex hormones may play on periodontal and oral tissues as well as the consistent need for home and office removal of local irritants.

Research regarding female issues and medical/periodontal therapy is in process. In the near future, information regarding specific management and etiology of sex hormone–mediated infections will enhance our ability to provide quality care to our patients.

REFERENCES

1. Aboul-Dahab OM, el-Sherbiny MM, Abdel-Rahman R, et al: Identification of lymphocytes subsets in pregnancy. Egyptian Dental J 1994; 40(1):653.
2. ADA Health Foundation Research Institute, Department of Toxicology: Antibiotic interference with oral contraceptives. JADA 1991; 122:79.
3. American Academy of Periodontology Position Paper: Periodontal disease as a potential risk factor for systemic disease. J Periodontol 1998; 69(7):841.
4. American Dental Association, Council on Access, Prevention, and Interpersonal Relations: Women's Oral Health Issues, Dec. 1995. Chicago, ADA, 1995.
5. Aschkenazi S, Naftolin F, Mor G: Menopause, sex hormones and the immune system. Menopause Mgt 2000; 9:6, 18.
6. Back DJ, Orme M: Pharmacokinetic drug interactions with oral contraceptives. Clin Pharmacokinet 1990; 18(6), 472.
7. Bean, LR Jr, Devore WD: The effects of protective aprons in dental roentgenography. Oral Surg 1969; 28:505.
8. Bhashkar SN, Jacoway JR: Pyogenic granuloma: clinical features, incidence, histology, and results of treatment report of 242 cases. J Oral Surg 1966; 24:391.
9. Bischof P, Lauber K, Girard JP, et al: Circulating levels of pregnancy proteins and depression of lymphoblastogenesis during pregnancy. J Clin Lab Immunol 1983; 12:93.
10. Brabin BJ: Epidemiology of infection in pregnancy. Rev Infect Dis 1985; 7:579.
11. Briggs GG, Freeman RK, Yaffe SJ: Drugs in Pregnancy and Lactation, ed 4. Baltimore, Williams & Wilkins, 1994.
12. Brown S, Bonifaz DZ: An overview of anorexia and bulimia nervosa and the impact of eating disorders on the oral cavity. Compend Contin Educ Dent 1993; 14(12):1594.
13. Cohen ME, Simecek JW: Effects of gender-related factors on the incidence of localized alveolar osteitis. Oral Surg Oral Med Oral Path 1995; 79(4):416.
14. Cruikshank O, Hayes PM: Maternal physiology. In: Gabbe S, Niebyl JR, Simpson JL (eds): Pregnancy in Obstretrics: Normal and Problem Pregnancies. Livingstone, NY, Churchill, 1986.
15. Cutolo M, Sulli A, Seriolo B, et al: Estrogens, the immune response and autoimmunity. Clin Exp Rheumatol 1995; 13:217.
16. Damare SM, Wells S, Offenbacher S: Eicosanoids in periodontal diseases potential for systemic involvement. Adv Experiment Med Bio 1997; 433:23.
17. Dasanayake AP: Poor periodontal health of the pregnant woman as a risk. Ann Periodontol 1998; 3(1):206.
18. Davenport ES, Williams CE, Sterne JA, et al: The East London study of maternal chronic periodontal disease and preterm low birth weight infants: Study design and prevalence. Ann Periodontol 1998; 3(1):213.
19. DeLiefde B: The dental care of pregnant women. NZ Dent J 1984; 80:41.
20. El Attar TMA: Prostaglandins F2 in human gingiva in health and disease and its stimulation by female sex steroids. Prostaglandins 1976; 11:331.
21. El-Ashiry G, El-Kafrawy AH, Nasr MF, et al: Effects of oral contraceptives on the gingiva. J Periodontol 1971; 42:273.
22. El-Ashiry G: Comparative study of the influence of pregnancy and oral contraceptives on the gingivae. Oral Surg 1970; 30:472.
23. El-Attar TMA, Roth GD, Hugoson A: Comparative metabolism of 4-C progesterone in normal and chronically inflamed human gingival tissue. J Periodontol Res 1973; 8:79.
24. Ferguson MM, Carter J, Boyle P: An epidemiological study of factors associated with recurrent apthae in women. J Oral Med 1984; 39(4):212.

25. Fleisher AB, Jr, Resnick SD: The effect of antibiotics in the efficacy of oral contraceptives: Arch Dermatol 1980; 125:1582.
26. Fraser IS, Jansen RPS: Why do inadvertent pregnancies occur in oral contraceptive users? Effectiveness of oral contraceptive regimens and interfering factors. Contraception 1983; 27:531.
27. Gibbs RS, Romero R, Hillier SL, et al: A review of premature birth and subclinical infections. Am J Obstet 1992; 166:1515.
28. Glenn FB, Glenn WD III, Duncan RC: Fluoride tablet supplementation during pregnancy for caries immunity: A study of the offspring produced. Am J Obstet Gynecol 1982; 143:560.
29. Glenn FB: Immunity conveyed by a fluoride supplement during pregnancy. J Dent Child 1977; 44:391.
30. Grant D, Stern J, Listgarten M:. The epidemiology, etiology and public health aspects of periodontal disease. In: Grant D, Stern J, Listegarten M (eds): Periodontics. St Louis, Mosby, 1988.
31. Grossi SG, Jeffcoat MK, Genco RJ: Osteopenia, osteoporosis, and oral disease. In Rose LR, Genco RJ, Cohen DW, et al (eds): Periodontal Medicine. St Louis, BC Decker, 2000.
32. Gusberti FA, Mombelli A, Lang NP, et al: Changes in subgingival microbiota during puberty. J Clin Periodont 1990; 17:685.
33. Hanson L, Sobol SM, Abelson T: The otolaryngologic manifestations of pregnancy. J Fam Pract 1986; 23:151.
34. Hertz RS, Beckstead PC, Brown WJ: Epithelial melanosis of the gingiva possibly resulting from the use of oral contraceptives. JADA 1980; 100(5):173.
35. Jeffcoat MK, Lewis CE, Reddy MS, et al: Postmenopausal bone loss and its relationship to oral bone loss. Periodontol 2000 2000; 23:94.
36. Jeffcoat MK: Osteoporosis: A possible modifiying factor in oral bone loss. Ann Periodontol 1998; 3:312.
37. Jensen J, Lilijmack W, Blookquist C: The effect of female sex hormones on subgingival plaque. J Periodontol 1981; 52(10):599.
38. Kalkwarf KL: Effect of oral contraceptive therapy on gingival inflammation in humans. J Periodontol 1978; 49:560.
39. Kinnby B, Matsson L, Astedt B: Aggravation of gingival inflammatory symptoms during pregnancy associated with the concentration of activator inhibitor type 2 (PAI-2) in gingival fluid. J Periodontol Res 1996; 31(4):271.
40. Knight GM, Wade AB: The effects of oral contraceptives on the human periodontium. J Peridont Res 1974; 9:18.
41. Kornman K, Loseche JF: Direct interaction of estradiol and progesterone with *Bacteroides melaninogenicus*. J Dent Res 1979; 58A:10.
42. Kornman KS, Loesche WJ: The subgingival flora during pregnancy. J Peridontol 1980; 15:111.
43. Lapp CA, Thomas ME, Lewis JB: Modulation by progesterone of interleukin-6 production by gingival fibroblasts. J Periodontol 1995; 66(4):279.
44. Levin RP: Pregnancy gingivitis. Maryland State Dental Association 1987; 30:27.
45. Lindhe J, Branemark P: Changes in microcirculation after local application of sex hormones. J Periodontol Res 1967a; 2:185.
46. Lindhe J, Branemark P: Changes in vascular permeability after local application of sex hormones. J Periodontol Res 1967b; 2:259.
47. Little JW, Falace DA: Dental Management of the Medically Compromised Patient, ed 4. St Louis, Mosby, 1993.
48. Löe H, Silness J: Periodontal disease in pregnancy. 1. Prevalence and severity. Acta Odontol Scan 1984; 21:533.
49. Lopatin DE, Kornman KS, Loesche WJ: Modulation of immunoreactivity to periodontal disease-associated microorganisms during pregnancy. Infect Immun 1980; 28:713.
50. Lundgren D, Magnssen B, Lindhe J: Connective tissue alterations in gingiva of rats treated with estrogens and progesterone. Odontol 1973; 24:49.
51. Magnusson T, Ericson T. Hugoson A: The effect of oral contraceptives on some salivary substance in women. Arch Oral Bio 1975; 20:119.
52. Mandel L, Kaynar A: Bulimia and parotid swelling: A review and case report. J Oral Maxillofac Surg 1992; 50:1122.
53. Miyagi M, Aoyama H, Morishita M, et al: Effects of sex hormones on chemotaxis of polymorphonuclearleukocytes and monocytes. J Periodontol 1992; 63:28.
54. Mohammad AR, Brunsvold M, Bauer R: The strength of association between systemic postmenopausal osteoporosis and periodontal disease. Int J Prosth 1996; 9:479.
55. Mombelli A, Rutar A, Lan NP: Correlation of the periodontal status 6 years after puberty with clinical and microbiological conditions during puberty. J Clin Periodont 1995; 22(4):300.
56. Muramatsu Y, Takaesu Y: Oral health status related to subgingival bacterial flora and sex hormones in saliva during pregnancy. Bull Tokyo Dent College 1994; 35(3):139.
57. Murphy AA, Zacur HA, Charache P, et al: The effect of tetracycline on levels of oral contraceptives. Am J Obstet Gynecol 1991; 164:28.
58. Nakagawa S, Fujii H, Machida Y, et al: A longitudinal study from prepuberty to puberty of gingivitis. Correlation between the occurrence of *Prevotella intermedia* and sex hormones. J Clin Periodont 1994; 21(10):658.
59. Neely JL, Abate M, Swinker M, et al: The effect of doxycycline on serum levels on ethinyl estradiol, norethindrone, and endogenous progesterone. Obstet Gynecol 1991; 77:416.
60. O'Neil TCA: Maternal T-lymphocyte response and gingivitis in pregnancy. J Periodontol 1979; 50:178.
61. Offenbacher S, Jared HL, O'Reilly PG, et al: Potential pathogenic mechanisms of periodontitis associated pregnancy complications. Ann Periodontol 1998; 3(1):233.
62. Offenbacher S, Katz V, Fertik G, et al: Periodontal infection as a possible risk factor for preterm low birthweight. J Periodontol 1996; 67(10 Suppl):1103.
63. Ojanotko-Harri AO, Harri MOP, Hurrita HP, et al: Altered tissue metabolism of progesterone in pregnancy gingivitis and granuloma. J Clin Periodontol 1991; 18:262.
64. Olin BR: Drug Facts and Comparisons. St Louis, Walters Kluwer, 1994.
65. Otomo-Corgel J: Systemic considerations for female patients. In: Antibiotics/Antimicrobial Use in Dental Practice. Tokyo, Quintessence, 1990.
66. Pack ARC, Thomson ME: Effects of topical and systemic folic acid supplementation on gingivitis in pregnancy. J Clin Periodontol 1980; 7:402.
67. Paganini-Hill A: Benefits of estrogen replacement therapy on oral health: the leisure world cohort. Arch Intern Med 1995; 155:2325.
68. Pankhurst CL: The influence of oral contraceptive therapy on the periodontium: Duration of drug therapy. J Periodontol 1981; 52:617.
69. Pediatric Dentistry Special Issue: Reference manual. Pediatr Dent 1994; 16(7).
70. Pinard A: Gingivitis in pregnancy. Dent Register 1877; 31:258–259.
71. Pitcarin J: A case of disease of the gums which occurred during pregnancy. Dubing Hosp Rep 1818; 2:309.
72. Raber-Durlacher JE, Leene W, Palmer-Bouva CCR, et al: Experimental gingivitis during pregnancy and postpartum: Immunohistochemical aspects. J Periodontal 1993; 64:211.
73. Raber-Durlacher JE, van Steenbergen TJM, van der Velden U: Experimental gingivitis during pregnancy and postpartum; clinical endocrinological and microbiological aspects. J Clin Periodontol 1994; 21:549.

74. Raber-Durlacher JE, Zeylemaker WP, Meinesz AAP, et al: CD4 to CD8 ratio and in vitro lymphoproliferative responses during experimental gingivitis in pregnancy and postpartum. J Periodontol 1991; 62:663.
75. Reese RE, Betts RF: Handbook of Antibiotics, ed 2. Boston, Little, Brown, and Co, 1993.
76. Reinhardt RA, Payne JB, Maze C, et al: Gingival fluid IL-beta in postmenopausal females on supportive peridontal therapy. A longitudinal 2-year study. J Clin Periodontol 1998; 25:1029.
77. Reinhardt RA, Payne JB, Maze CA, et al: Influence of estrogen and osteopenia/osteoporosis on clinical periodontitis in postmenopausal women. J Periodontol 1999; 70:823.
78. Robb-Nicholson C: Gastroesophageal reflux disease. Harvard Women's Health Watch 1999; 4(6):4.
79. Robb-Nicholson C: PMS: It's real. Harvard Women's Health Watch 1994; 1(11):2.
80. Samant A, Malik CP, Chabra SK, et al: Gingivitis and periodontal disease in pregnancy. J Periodontol 1976; 47:415.
81. Schuurs A, Verheul H: Effects of gender and sex steroids on the immune response and autoimmune disease. J Steroid Biochem 1990; 35:157.
82. Sooriyamoorthy M, Gower DB: Hormonal influences on gingival tissues: Relationship to periodontal disease. J Clin Periodontol 1989; 16:201.
83. Sridama V, Pacini F, Yang SL, et al: Decreased levels of helper T cells. A possible cause of immunodeficiency in pregnancy. New Engl J Med 1982; 307:352.
84. Sridama V, Pacini F, Yang SL, et al: Decreased levels of helper T cells. A possible cause of immunodeficiency in pregnancy. New Engl J Med 1982; 307:352.
85. Steinberg BJ: Sex hormonal alterations. In: Rose LD, Kay D (eds): Internal Medicine for Dentistry, ed 2. St Louis, Mosby, 1990.
86. Sweet JB, Butler DP: Increased incidence of postoperative localized osteitis in mandibular 3rd molar surgery associated with patients using oral contraceptives. Am J Obset Gynecol 1977; 127:518.
87. Thomson ME, Pack ARC: Effects of extended systemic and topical folate supplementation on gingivitis in pregnancy. J Clin Periodontol 1982; 9:275.
88. Valdimarsson H, Mulholland C, Fridriksdottir V, et al: A longitudinal study of leukocyte blood counts and lymphocyte responses in pregnancy: A marked early increase of monocyte-lymphocyte ratio. Clin Exp Immunol 1983; 53:437.
89. Vinco L, Prallet B, Chappard D, et al: Contributions of chronological age, age at menarche and menopause and of anthropometric parameters to axial and peripheral bone densities. Osteoporosis Int 1992; 2:153.
90. Vittek J, Gordon G, Rappaport C, et al: Specific progesterone receptors in rabbit gingiva. J Perio Res 1982; 17:657.
91. Wactawski-Wende J, Grossi SG, Trevisan M, et al: The role of osteopenia in oral bone loss and periodontal disease. J Periodontol 1996; 67:1076.
92. Whitacre CC, Reingold SC, O'Looney PA: A gender gap in autoimmunity. Science 1999; 283:1277.
93. Whitehear MI, Whitcroft SIJ, Hillard TC: An Atlas of the Menopause. New York, Parthenon, 1993.
94. Wilson JT, Brown RD, Cherek DR, et al: Drug excretion in human breast milk: principles, pharmacokinetics and projects consequences. Clin Pharmacokinet 1980; 5:1.
95. Zachariasen RD: Ovarian hormones and oral health: pregnancy gingivitis. Compend Contin Educ Dent 1989; 10(9):508.
96. Zachariasen RD: The effects of elevated ovarian hormones on periodontal health: oral contraceptives and pregnancy. Women Health 1993; 20(2):21.
97. Zoeller J: The top 200 drugs. American Druggist 1999; p 41.

Periodontal Treatment of Medically Compromised Patients

Brian L. Mealey, Perry R. Klokkevold, and Joan Otomo-Corgel

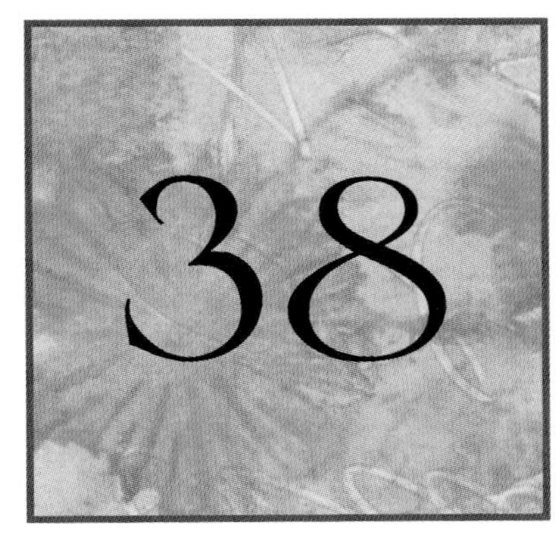

CHAPTER

CHAPTER OUTLINE

Many patients seeking dental care have significant medical conditions that may alter both the course of their oral disease and the therapy provided. The older age of the average periodontal patient increases the likelihood of underlying disease. Therefore the therapeutic responsibility of the clinician includes identification of the patient's medical problems to formulate proper treatment plans. Thorough medical histories are paramount.[52] If significant findings are unveiled, consultation with or referral of the patient to an appropriate physician may be indicated. This ensures correct patient management and provides medicolegal coverage to the clinician.

This chapter covers common medical conditions and associated periodontal management. Review of each topic area is general, and the reader is encouraged to consult other references for more detailed coverage of specific disorders. Understanding these conditions will enable the clinician to treat the total patient, not merely the periodontal reflection of underlying disease.

CARDIOVASCULAR DISEASES

Cardiovascular diseases are the most prevalent category of systemic disease in the U.S. and many other countries, and they are more common with increasing age.[69] Health histories should be closely scrutinized for cardiovascular problems. These conditions include hypertension, angina pectoris, myocardial infarction, previous cardiac bypass surgery, previous cerebrovascular accident, congestive heart failure, presence of cardiac pacemakers or automatic defibrillators, and infective endocarditis.

In most cases the patient's physician should be consulted, especially if stressful or prolonged treatment is anticipated. Short appointments and a calm, relaxing environment help minimize stress and maintain hemodynamic stability.

Hypertension

Hypertension, the most common cardiovascular disease, affects more than 20% of American adults, many of whom are undiagnosed.[34] Hypertension is defined as a systolic blood pressure of 140 mm Hg or greater, or a diastolic blood pressure of 90 mm Hg or greater.[25,29,30,40] Hypertension is not diagnosed on a single elevated blood pressure recording. Rather, classification is based on the average value of three or more blood pressure readings taken at three or more appointments (Table 38-1). The higher value of either the systolic or diastolic blood pressure determines the patient's classification. Patients with hypertension enter the dental practice every day and are particularly common amongst the older population seen in most periodontal practices.

Hypertension is divided into primary and secondary types. Primary (essential) hypertension occurs when no underlying pathologic abnormality can be found to explain the disease. Approximately 95% of all hypertensive patients have primary hypertension. The remaining 5% have secondary hypertension, in which an underlying etiology can be found and often treated. Examples of the conditions responsible for secondary hypertension are renal disease, endocrinologic changes, and neurogenic disorders.

In early hypertension, the patient may be asymptomatic. If not identified and diagnosed, hypertension may persist and increase in severity, leading eventually to coronary artery disease, angina, myocardial infarction, congestive heart failure, cerebrovascular accident, or kidney failure.[35] The dental office can play a vital role in the detection of hypertension and maintenance care of the patient with hypertensive disease. The first dental office visit should include two blood pressure readings spaced at least 10 minutes apart, which are averaged and used as a baseline. Before the clinician refers a patient to a physician because of elevated blood pressure, readings should be taken at a minimum of two appointments, unless the measurements are extremely high (i.e., systolic pressure >180 mm Hg or diastolic pressure >100 mm Hg). The periodontal recall system is an ideal method for hypertension detection and monitoring. Nearly 3 of every 4 adult hypertension patients in the U.S. do not control their blood pressure well enough to attain the goal of systolic pressure <140 mm Hg and diastolic pressure <90 mm Hg.[7] Lack of compliance with antihypertensive therapy is the primary reason for this failure. Dentists can help achieve greater success in managing hypertension by taking blood pressure recordings at each periodontal recall visit.

Periodontal procedures should not be performed until accurate blood pressure measurements and histories have been taken to identify those patients with significant hypertensive disease. The time of day should be recorded along with the blood pressure reading because blood pressure varies significantly throughout the day.[48] Table 38-1 outlines appropriate medical referral or consultation and dental treatment modifications, depending on the patient's stage of hypertension.

Dental treatment for hypertensive patients is generally safe as long as stress is minimized.[35,40] If a patient is currently receiving antihypertensive therapy, consultation with the physician may be warranted regarding the current medical status, medications, periodontal treat-

TABLE 38-1

Classification of Adult Blood Pressure

Classification	Systolic Blood Pressure (mm Hg)	Diastolic Blood Pressure (mm Hg)	Dental Treatment Modifications
Normal	<130	<85	No changes in dental treatment.
High normal	130–139	85–89	No changes in dental treatment.
Hypertension			
Stage 1	140–159	90–99	• Inform patient of findings. • Routine medical consultation/referral. • No changes in dental treatment; minimize stress.
Stage 2	160–179	100–109	• Inform patient. • Routine medical referral. • Selective dental care (routine exam, prophylaxis, restorative, nonsurgical endodontics and periodontics); minimize stress.
Stage 3	≥180	≥110	• Inform patient. • Immediate medical consultation/referral. • Emergency dental care only (to alleviate pain, bleeding, infection)*; minimize stress.

* Risk of providing emergency dental care must outweigh risk of possible hypertensive complications.
See references 25, 29, and 30.

ment plan, and patient management. Many physicians are not knowledgeable about the nature of specific periodontal procedures. The dentist must inform the physician regarding the estimated degree of stress, length of the procedures, and complexity of the individualized treatment plan. Morning dental appointments were once suggested for hypertensive patients. However, recent evidence indicates that blood pressure generally increases around awakening and peaks at mid-morning.[5,48,64] Lower blood pressures occur in the afternoon. Therefore afternoon dental appointments may be preferred.

No routine periodontal treatment should be given to a patient who is hypertensive and not under medical management. For patients with stage 3 hypertension, treatment should be limited to emergency care until hypertension is controlled. Analgesics are prescribed for pain and antibiotics for infection. Acute infections may require surgical incision and drainage, although the surgical field should be limited because excessive bleeding may be seen with elevated blood pressures.

When treating hypertensive patients, the clinician should not use a local anesthetic containing an epinephrine concentration greater than 1:100,000, nor should a vasopressor be used to control local bleeding. Local anesthesia without epinephrine may be used for short procedures (less than 30 minutes). In a patient with hypertensive disease, however, it is important to minimize pain by providing profound local anesthesia to avoid an increase in endogenous epinephrine secretion.[35,40] The benefits of the small doses of epinephrine used in dentistry far outweigh the potential for hemodynamic compromise. The smallest possible dose of epinephrine should be used, and aspiration before injection of local anesthetics is critical. Intraligamentary injection is generally contraindicated because hemodynamic changes are similar to intravascular injection.[63]

β-adrenergic receptor antagonists or β-blockers are commonly used to treat hypertension (Table 38-2). β-blockers are either cardioselective, blocking only β-1 cardiac receptors, or non-selective, blocking both β-1 cardiac receptors and β-2 peripheral receptors. Epinephrine, an α- and β-adrenergic agonist, produces an increase in heart rate via direct stimulation of cardiac β-1 receptors. Epinephrine also stimulates α-adrenergic receptors, producing vasoconstriction of arteries, as well as β-2 receptors, causing vasodilation of skeletal muscle arterioles. Administration of local anesthetics containing epinephrine to patients taking nonselective β-blockers such as propanolol or nadolol may cause elevated blood pressure.[72] Epinephrine-induced α-adrenergic stimulation results in vasoconstriction and an increase in blood pressure. Because the patient's nonselective medication has blocked the β-2 receptors, epinephrine will not stimulate the normal compensatory β-2-induced vasodilation. This may result in dramatically increased blood pressure, which is then followed by a reflex bradycardia mediated by the vagus nerve and carotid baroreceptors. The end result is a patient with severe hypertension and bradycardia, resulting in a dangerous decrease in vascular perfusion and possible death. Because of this potential complication, epinephrine-containing local anesthetics should be used cautiously and only in very small amounts in patients taking nonselective β-blockers, with careful monitoring of vital signs.[35,72]

The clinician should be aware of the many side effects of various antihypertensive medications. Postural hypotension is very common and can be minimized by slow positional changes in the dental chair.[25,35] Depression is a side effect of which many patients are unaware. Nausea, sedation, oral dryness, lichenoid drug reactions, and gingival overgrowth are associated with certain classes of antihypertensive agents.[25,40]

Ischemic Heart Diseases

Ischemic heart disease includes disorders such as angina pectoris and myocardial infarction (Fig. 38-1). Angina occurs when myocardial oxygen demand exceeds supply, resulting in temporary myocardial ischemia.[26] Patients with a history of unstable angina pectoris (angina that occurs irregularly or on multiple occasions without predisposing factors) should be treated for emergencies only and then in consultation with the patient's physician. Patients with stable angina (angina that occurs infrequently, is associated with exertion or stress, and is easily controlled with medication and rest) can undergo elective dental procedures. Because stress often induces an acute anginal attack, stress reduction is important. Profound local anesthesia is vital, and conscious sedation may be indicated for anxious patients. Supplemental oxygen delivered via nasal cannula may also help prevent intraoperative anginal attacks.

Patients who treat acute anginal attacks with nitroglycerine should be instructed to bring their medication to dental appointments. Nitroglycerine should also be kept in the office emergency medical kit. For particularly stressful procedures, the patient may take a nitroglycerine

TABLE 38-2

Nonselective and Selective β-Adrenergic Receptor Antagonists (β-Blockers)

Generic Name	Trade Name
Nonselective	
Carteolol hydrochloride	Cartrol
Nadolol	Corgard
Penbutolol sulfate	Levatol
Pindolol	Visken
Propanolol hydrochloride	Inderal; Inderal LA
Timolol maleate	Blocadren
Selective	
Acebutolol hydrochloride	Sectral
Atenolol	Tenormin
Betaxolol hydrochloride	Kerlone
Bisoprolol fumarate	Zebeta
Metoprolol tartrate	Lopressor
Metoprolol succinate	Toprol-XL

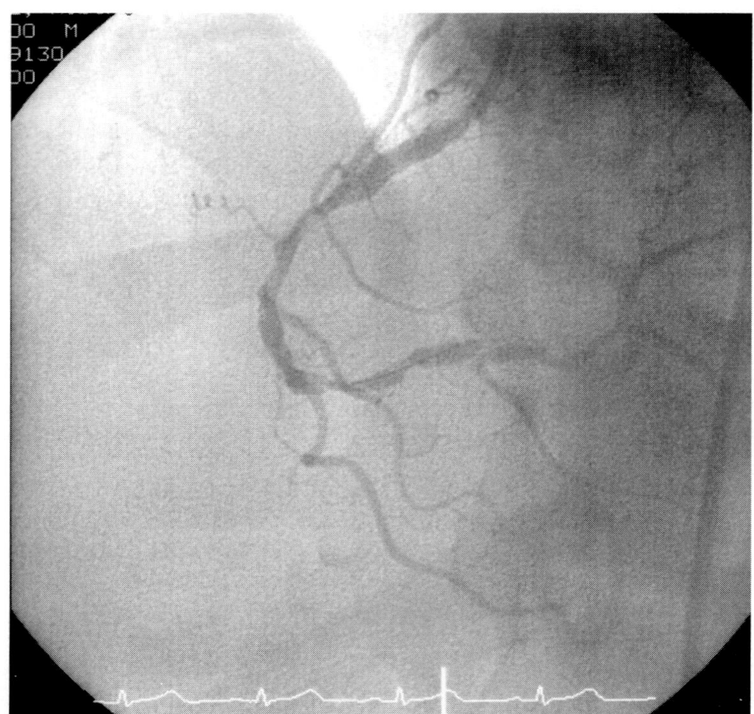

Fig. 38-1 Coronary angiogram. Atherosclerosis can result in narrowing of the coronary arteries and onset of signs and symptoms of ischemic heart disease.

tablet preoperatively to prevent angina, although this is generally not necessary. The patient's nitroglycerin should be readily accessible on the dental tray in case it is needed during treatment. As the shelf life of nitroglycerin is relatively short, the expiration date of the patient's nitroglycerin should be noted, as should the expiration date of the nitroglycerin in the office's emergency medical kit. Also, patients with angina may be taking longer-acting nitroglycerins (in tablet or patch form), β-blockers, or calcium channel blockers (also used in the treatment of hypertension) for prevention of angina. Restrictions on use of local anesthetics containing epinephrine are similar to the patient with hypertension. In addition, intraosseous injection with epinephrine-containing local anesthetics using systems such as the Stabident system (Fairfax Dental Inc.) should be done cautiously in patients with ischemic heart disease, because it results in transient increases in heart rate and myocardial oxygen demand.[50]

If the patient becomes fatigued or uncomfortable or has a sudden change in heart rhythm or rate during a periodontal procedure, the procedure should be discontinued as soon as possible. A patient who has an anginal episode in the dental chair should receive the following emergency medical treatment:

1. Discontinue the periodontal procedure.
2. Administer one tablet (0.3 to 0.6 mg) of nitroglycerin sublingually.
3. Reassure the patient and loosen restrictive garments.
4. Administer oxygen with the patient in a reclined position.
5. If the signs and symptoms cease within 3 minutes, complete the periodontal procedure if possible, making sure that the patient is comfortable. Terminate the procedure at the earliest convenient time.
6. If the anginal signs and symptoms do not resolve with this treatment within 2 to 3 minutes, administer another dose of nitroglycerin, monitor the patient's vital signs, call his or her physician, and be ready to accompany the patient to the emergency department.
7. A third nitroglycerin tablet may be given 3 minutes after the second. Chest pain that is not relieved by 3 tablets of nitroglycerin indicates likely myocardial infarction. The patient should be transported to the nearest emergency medical facility immediately.

Myocardial infarction is the other category of ischemic heart disease frequently encountered in dental practice. Dental treatment is generally deferred for at least 6 months following a myocardial infarction because the peak mortality rate occurs during this time.[20] After 6 months, myocardial infarction patients can usually be treated using techniques similar to the stable angina patient.

Cardiac (aortocoronary) bypass, femoral artery bypass, angioplasty, and endarterectomy have become common surgical procedures in patients with ischemic heart disease. The physician should be consulted before elective dental therapy if one of these procedures was performed recently to determine the degree of heart damage or arterial occlusive disease, the stability of the patient's condition, and the potential for infective endocarditis or graft rejection. Prophylactic antibiotics are not usually necessary for cardiac bypass patients unless recommended by the cardiologist.

Congestive Heart Failure

Congestive heart failure (CHF) is a condition in which the pump function of the heart is unable to supply sufficient amounts of oxygenated blood to meet the body's needs.[20] CHF usually begins with left ventricular failure caused by a disproportion between the hemodynamic load and the capacity to handle that load. It may be due to a chronic increase in workload (as in hypertension or aortic, mitral, pulmonary, or tricuspid valvular disease), direct damage to the myocardium (as in myocardial infarction or rheumatic fever), or an increase in the body's oxygen requirements (as in anemia, thyrotoxicosis, or pregnancy).

Patients with poorly controlled or untreated congestive heart failure are not candidates for elective dental procedures. These individuals are at risk for sudden death, usually from ventricular arrhythmias. For patients with treated congestive heart failure, the clinician should consult with the physician regarding the severity of CHF, underlying etiology, and current medical management. Medical management of CHF may include use of calcium channel blockers, direct vasodilators, diuretics, ACE inhibitors, α-receptor blockers, and cardiotonic agents such as digoxin.[43] Each of these medications has potential side effects that may have an impact on periodontal therapy. Due to the presence of orthopnea (the inability to breathe unless in an upright position) in some CHF patients, the dental chair should be adjusted to a comfortable level for the patient rather than being placed in a supine position. Short appointments, stress reduction with profound local anesthesia and possibly conscious sedation, and use of supplemental oxygen should be considered.[20,35]

Cardiac Pacemakers and Automatic Defibrillators

Some cardiac arrhythmias are treated with implantable pacemakers or automatic defibrillators.[35] Pacemakers are usually implanted in the chest wall and enter the heart transvenously. Automatic defibrillators are more often implanted subcutaneously near the umbilicus and have electrodes passing into the heart transvenously or directly attached to the epicardium. Consultation with the patient's physician allows determination of the underlying cardiac status, the type of pacemaker or automatic defibrillator, and any precautionary measures to be taken. Older pacemakers were unipolar and could be disrupted by dental equipment that generates electromagnetic fields such as ultrasonic and electrocautery units. Newer units are bipolar and are generally not affected by dental equipment. Automatic defibrillators activate without warning when certain arrhythmias occur. This may endanger the patient during dental treatment because such activation often causes sudden patient movement. Stabilization of the operating field during periodontal treatment with bite blocks or other devices can prevent unexpected trauma.

Infective Endocarditis

Infective endocarditis (IE) is a disease in which microorganisms colonize the damaged endocardium or heart valves.[22] Although the incidence of IE is low, it is a serious disease with a poor prognosis, despite modern therapy. The term *infective endocarditis* is preferred to the previous term *bacterial endocarditis* because the disease can also be caused by fungi and viruses. The organisms most commonly encountered in IE are α-hemolytic streptococci (e.g., *Streptococcus viridans*). However, nonstreptococcal organisms often found in the periodontal pocket have been increasingly implicated, including *Eikenella corrodens, Actinobacillus actinomycetemcomitans, Capnocytophaga,* and *Lactobacillus* species.[4]

IE has been divided into acute and subacute forms. The acute form involves virulent organisms, generally nonhemolytic streptococci and strains of staphylococci, which invade normal cardiac tissue, produce septic emboli, and cause infections that run a rapid, generally fatal course. The subacute form, on the other hand, occurs as a result of colony formation on damaged endocardium or heart valves by low-grade pathogenic organisms; the classic example is rheumatic carditis consequent to rheumatic fever.

The risk for IE varies with the underlying disorder (Box 38-1).[14,15] The high-risk category includes patients at high risk of developing IE after dental-induced bacteremia and those in whom the resultant IE is associated with high morbidity and mortality. The moderate-risk category includes patients at higher risk for IE than the general population.

The practice of periodontics is intimately concerned with the prevention of IE. Because dental procedures that involve bleeding may induce a transient bacteremia, the American Heart Association (AHA) recommends antibiotic prophylaxis before procedures "associated with significant bleeding from hard or soft tissues, periodontal surgery, scaling and professional teeth cleaning."[15] However, bacteremia may occur even in the absence of dental procedures, especially in individuals with poor oral hygiene and significant periodontal inflammation. Thus prevention of periodontal inflammation is paramount. The AHA states that patients who are at risk for IE should "establish and maintain the best possible oral health to reduce potential sources of bacterial seeding." To provide adequate preventive measures for IE, the clinician's major concern should be to reduce the microbial population in the oral cavity so as to minimize soft tissue inflammation and bacteremia.

Preventive measures to reduce the risk of IE should consist of the following:

1. *Define the susceptible patient.* A careful medical history will disclose the aforementioned susceptible patients. Health questioning should cover history of all potential categories of risk (see Box 38-1). If any doubt exists, the patient's physician should be consulted.
2. *Provide oral hygiene instruction.* Oral hygiene should be practiced with methods that improve gingival health yet minimize bacteremia. In patients with significant gingival inflammation, oral hygiene should initially be limited to gentle procedures (i.e., oral rinses and

BOX 38-1

Heart Conditions Associated with Infective Endocarditis (IE)*

Endocarditis Prophylaxis Recommended

High-risk patients
- Previous history of IE
- Prosthetic heart valves
- Major congenital heart disease
  - Tetralogy of Fallot
  - Transposition of great arteries
  - Single ventricle states
  - Surgically constructed systemic pulmonary shunts, or conduits

Moderate-risk patients
- Acquired valvular dysfunction (e.g., rheumatic heart disease)
- Most other congenital heart malformations
- Hypertrophic cardiomyopathy
- Mitral valve prolapse with valvular regurgitation, thickened leaflets, or both

Endocarditis Prophylaxis* Not *Recommended (No Greater Risk than General Population)

Mitral valve prolapse without valvular regurgitation
Previous coronary artery bypass graft surgery
Physiologic, functional, or innocent heart murmurs
Previous rheumatic fever without valvular dysfunction
Cardiac pacemakers and implanted defibrillators
Isolated secundum atrial septal defect
Surgically repaired atrial septal defect, ventricular septal defect, or patent ductus arteriosus
Previous Kawasaki disease without valvular dysfunction

* Recommendations by the American Heart Association.[14,15]

gentle toothbrushing with a soft brush) to minimize bleeding. As gingival health improves, more aggressive oral hygiene may be initiated. Oral irrigators are generally not recommended because their use may induce bacteremia.[44] Susceptible patients should be encouraged to maintain the highest level of oral hygiene once soft tissue inflammation is controlled.

3. *During periodontal treatment, currently recommended antibiotic prophylactic regimens should be practiced with all susceptible patients* (Table 38-3). If any doubt regarding susceptibility exists, the patient's physician should be consulted. In patients who have been receiving continuous oral penicillin for secondary prevention of rheumatic fever, penicillin-resistant α-hemolytic streptococci are occasionally found in the oral cavity. It therefore is recommended that an alternate regimen be followed instead. Likewise, if the periodontal patient is taking a systemic antibiotic as part of periodontal therapy, changes in the IE prophylaxis regimen may be indicated. For example, a patient currently taking a penicillin agent after regenerative therapy may be placed on azithromycin before the next periodontal procedure. Patients with early onset forms of periodontitis often have high levels of *Actinobacillus actinomycetemcomitans* in the subgingival plaque. This organism has been associated with IE and is often resistant to penicillins. Therefore in patients with early onset periodontitis who are also at risk for IE, Slots and co-workers have suggested using tetracycline, 250 mg, four times daily for 14 days to eliminate or reduce *A. actinomycetemcomitans,* followed by the conventional prophylaxis protocol at the time of dental treatment.[62]
4. *Periodontal treatment should be designed for susceptible patients to accommodate their particular degree of periodontal involvement.* The nature of periodontal therapy enhances the problems related to the prophylaxis of subacute IE. Patients are faced with long-term therapy, healing periods that extend beyond a 1-day antibiotic regimen, multiple visits, and procedures that easily elicit gingival bleeding. The following guidelines should aid in the development of periodontal treatment plans for patients susceptible to IE:
   - Periodontal disease is an infection with potentially wide-ranging systemic effects. In patients at risk for IE, every effort should be made to eliminate this infection. Teeth with severe periodontitis and a poor prognosis may require extraction. Teeth with less severe involvement in a motivated patient should be retained, treated, and maintained closely.
   - All periodontal treatment procedures (including probing) require antibiotic prophylaxis; gentle oral hygiene methods are excluded. Pretreatment chlorhexidine mouthrinses are recommended before all procedures, including periodontal probing, because they significantly reduce the presence of bacteria on mucosal surfaces.[15]
   - To reduce the number of visits required and thereby minimize the risk of developing resistant bacteria, numerous procedures may be accomplished at each appointment, depending on the patient's needs and ability to tolerate dental treatment.[35]
   - When possible, allow at least 7 days between appointments (preferably 10 to 14 days). If this is not possible, select an alternative antibiotic regimen for appointments within a 7-day time period.
   - Evidence does not support nor refute a need to place patients at risk for IE on extended antibiotic regimens after treatment.[35] Therefore patients who have had periodontal surgery are not generally placed on antibiotics for the first week of healing (unless there are specific indications to do so). If patients are placed on such regimens, the dosages are inadequate to prevent endocarditis during ensuing appointments. Therefore the standard prophylactic antibiotic dose is still needed. For example, if a patient was placed on 250 mg of amoxicillin three times a day for 10 days after periodontal surgery and was returning to the office for more treatment on the seventh day, he or she would still require a full 2.0 g dose of amoxicillin before that treatment. Alternatively, clindamycin or azithromycin could be used at the second appointment.
   - The need for antibiotic prophylaxis before simple suture removal is controversial. Some authors

TABLE 38-3

Recommended Antibiotic Prophylaxis Regimens for Periodontal Procedures in Adults at Risk for Infective Endocarditis

Regimen	Antibiotic	Dosage
Standard oral regimen	Amoxicillin	2.0 g 1 hour before procedure
Alternate regimen for patients allergic to amoxicillin, penicillin, or both	Clindamycin	600 mg 1 hour before procedure
	OR	
	Azithromycin or clarithromycin	500 mg 1 hour before procedure
	OR	
	Cephalexin or cefadroxil*	2.0 g 1 hour before procedure
Patients unable to take oral medications	Ampicillin	2.0 g intramuscularly or intravenously within 30 minutes before procedure
Patients unable to take oral medications and allergic to penicillin	Clindamycin	600 mg intravenously within 30 minutes before procedure (must be diluted and injected slowly)
	OR	
	Cefazolin*	1.0 g intramuscularly or intravenously within 30 minutes before procedure

* Cephalosporins should *not* be used in patients with immediate-type hypersensitivity reactions to penicillins (e.g., urticaria, angioedema, anaphylaxis).
Note: Children's dosages are lower
See References 14 and 15.

suggest it is needed, whereas others suggest it is not. When possible, sutures that resorb in a short period of time, such as chromic gut, may be indicated for patients at risk of IE.

- Regular recall appointments, with an emphasis on oral hygiene reinforcement and maintenance of periodontal health, are extremely important in this population.

Cerebrovascular Accident

A cerebrovascular accident (CVA), or stroke, occurs as a result of ischemic changes (e.g., cerebral thrombosis owing to an embolus) or hemorrhagic phenomena. Hypertension and atherosclerosis are predisposing factors to a CVA and should alert the clinician to evaluate the patient's medical history carefully for the possibility of early cerebrovascular insufficiency and to be aware of symptoms of the disease. A physician's referral should precede periodontal therapy if the signs and symptoms of early cerebrovascular insufficiency are evident.

To prevent a repeat stroke, active infections should be treated aggressively because even minor infection may alter blood coagulation and trigger thrombus formation and ensuing cerebral infarction. The clinician should counsel the patient as to the importance of thorough oral hygiene. Post-stroke weakness of the facial area or paralysis of extremities may make oral hygiene procedures extremely difficult.[42] The clinician may need to modify oral hygiene instruments for ease of use, perhaps in consultation with an occupational therapist. Long-term chlorhexidine rinses may greatly aid in plaque control.

Patients who are seen after a stroke should be treated following these guidelines:

1. No periodontal therapy (unless for an emergency) should be performed for 6 months because of the high risk of recurrence during this period.
2. After 6 months, periodontal therapy may be performed using short appointments with an emphasis on minimizing stress. Profound local anesthesia should be obtained using the minimal effective dose of local anesthetic agents. Concentrations of epinephrine greater than 1:100,000 are contraindicated.
3. Light conscious sedation (inhalation, oral or parenteral) may be used for very anxious patients. Supplemental oxygen is indicated to maintain thorough cerebral oxygenation.
4. Stroke patients are frequently placed on oral anticoagulants. For procedures that entail significant bleeding, such as periodontal surgery or tooth extraction, the anticoagulant regimen often needs adjustment in consultation with the physician.
5. Monitor blood pressure carefully. Recurrence rates for CVAs are high, as are rates of associated functional deficits.

ENDOCRINE DISORDERS

Diabetes

The diabetic patient requires special precautions before periodontal therapy. The two major types of diabetes are type 1 (formerly known as "insulin-dependent diabetes")

BOX 38-2

Diagnostic Criteria for Diabetes Mellitus

Diabetes mellitus may be diagnosed by any 1 of 3 different laboratory methods. Whatever method is used *must be confirmed on a subsequent day* by using any 1 of the 3 methods.

1. *Symptoms of diabetes plus casual (nonfasting) plasma glucose ≥200 mg/dl.* Casual glucose may be drawn at any time of day without regard to time since the last meal. Classic symptoms of diabetes include polyuria, polydipsia, and unexplained weight loss.
2. *Fasting plasma glucose ≥126 mg/dl.* Fasting is defined as no caloric intake for at least 8 hours. (Normal fasting glucose is 70–100 mg/dl.)
3. *2 hour postprandial glucose ≥200 mg/dl during an oral glucose tolerance test.** The test should be performed using a glucose load containing the equivalent of 75 g of anhydrous glucose dissolved in water. (Normal 2 hour postprandial glucose is <140 mg/dl.)

* The third method is *not* recommended for routine clinical use. See reference 3.

BOX 38-3

Laboratory Evaluation of Diabetes Control (American Diabetes Association Guidelines)

Glycated Hemoglobin Assay (HbA1c)	
4% to 6%	Normal
<7%	Good diabetes control
7% to 8%	Moderate diabetes control
>8%	Action suggested to improve diabetes control

BOX 38-4

Signs and Symptoms of Hypoglycemia

Shakiness or tremors
Confusion
Agitation and anxiety
Sweating
Tachycardia
Dizziness
Feeling of "impending doom"
Unconsciousness
Seizures

and type 2 (formerly called "non–insulin-dependent diabetes").[37] Over the last decade, the medical management of diabetes has changed significantly in an effort to minimize the debilitating complications associated with this disease.[17,68] Patients are more tightly managing their blood glucose levels (glycemia) through diet, oral agents, and insulin therapy.[36]

If the clinician detects intraoral signs of undiagnosed or poorly controlled diabetes, a thorough history is indicated. The classic signs of diabetes include polydipsia (excessive thirst), polyuria (excessive urination), and polyphagia (excessive hunger, often with unexplained concurrent weight loss). If the patient has any of these signs or symptoms, or if the clinician's index of suspicion is high, further investigation via laboratory studies and physician consultation is indicated. Periodontal therapy has limited success in the presence of undiagnosed or poorly controlled diabetes.

If a patient is suspected of having undiagnosed diabetes, the following procedures should be performed:

1. Consult the patient's physician.
2. Analyze laboratory tests (Box 38-2): fasting blood glucose, casual glucose, and postprandial blood glucose.[3]
3. Rule out acute orofacial infection or severe dental infection, and provide emergency care only until diagnosis is established.

If a patient is known to have diabetes, it is critical that the level of glycemic control be established before initiating periodontal treatment. The fasting glucose and casual glucose tests provide "snapshots" of the blood glucose concentration at the time the blood was drawn. They reveal nothing about long-term glycemic control. The primary test used to assess glycemic control in a known diabetic individual is the glycosylated or glycated hemoglobin assay (Box 38-3). Two different tests are available, the HbA1 and the HbA1c test; the HbA1c is more commonly used.[36] This assay reflects blood glucose concentrations over the preceding 6 to 8 weeks and may provide an indication of the potential response to periodontal therapy. Patients with relatively well-controlled diabetes (HbA1c < 8%) usually respond to therapy in a manner similar to nondiabetic individuals.[11,66,71] Poorly controlled patients (HbA1c > 10%) often have a poor response to treatment, with more postoperative complications and less favorable long-term results.[37,66]

As discussed in Chapter 13, periodontal infection may worsen glycemic control, and should be managed aggressively. Diabetic patients with periodontitis should received oral hygiene instructions, mechanical debridement to remove local factors, and regular maintenance. When possible, an HbA1c of <10% should be established before surgical treatment is performed. Systemic antibiotics are not needed routinely, although recent evidence indicates that tetracycline antibiotics in combination with scaling and root planing may positively influence glycemic control (see Chapter 13). If the patient has poor glycemic control and surgery is absolutely needed, prophylactic antibiotics may be given. Penicillins are most often used for this purpose. Frequent reevaluation

TABLE 38-4

Oral Agents Used in Management of Diabetes

Agent	Action	Risk of Hypoglycemia
Sulfonylureas (first generation) Chlorpropamide Tolbutamide Tolazamide	Stimulate pancreatic insulin secretion.	++
Sulfonylureas (second generation) Glyburide Glipizide	Stimulate pancreatic insulin secretion.	+++
Sulfonylureas (third generation) Glimepiride	Stimulates pancreatic insulin secretion.	+
Meglitinides: Repaglinide	Stimulates rapid pancreatic insulin secretion.	+
Phenylalanine derivatives: Nateglinide	Stimulates rapid pancreatic insulin secretion.	+
Biguanides Metformin	Blocks production of glucose by liver; improves tissue sensitivity to insulin.	−
Thiazolidinediones Rosiglitazone Pioglitazone	Improves tissue sensitivity to insulin.	−
α-Glucosidase inhibitors Acarbose Miglitol	Slows absorption of some carbohydrates from gut, decreasing postprandial peaks in glycemia.	−

after active therapy is needed to assess treatment response and prevent recurrence of periodontitis.

Many diabetic patients today use glucometers for immediate blood glucose self-monitoring. These devices use capillary blood from a simple finger stick to provide blood glucose readings in a matter of seconds to minutes. Diabetic patients should be asked whether they have glucometers and how often they use them. Because these devices provide an instantaneous assessment of blood glucose, they are highly beneficial in the dental office environment. The following guidelines should be observed:

1. Patients should be asked to bring their glucometer to the dental office at each appointment.
2. Patients should check their blood glucose before any long procedure to get a baseline level. Patients with blood glucose levels at or below the lower end of normal before the procedure may become hypoglycemic intraoperatively. It is advisable to have such a patient consume some carbohydrate before starting treatment. For example, if a 2-hour procedure is planned and the pretreatment glucose level is 70 mg/dl (the lower end of normal range), providing 4 oz of juice preoperatively may help prevent hypoglycemia during treatment. If pretreatment glucose levels are excessively high, the procedure may need to be postponed until better glycemic control is established.
3. After the procedure, the blood glucose can be checked again to assess fluctuations over time.
4. Any time the patient feels symptoms of hypoglycemic, the glucose should be checked immediately. This may prevent onset of severe hypoglycemia, a medical emergency.

The most common dental office complication seen in diabetic patients taking insulin is symptomatic low blood glucose or hypoglycemia (Box 38-4). Hypoglycemia is also associated with the use of numerous oral agents (Table 38-4). In patients receiving conscious sedation, the warning signs of an impending hypoglycemic episode may be masked, making the glucometer one of the best diagnostic aids. Hypoglycemia does not usually occur until blood glucose levels fall below 60 mg/dl. However, in patients with poor glycemic control who have prolonged hyperglycemia (high blood glucose levels), a rapid drop in glucose can precipitate signs and symptoms of hypoglycemia at levels well above 60 mg/dl.

As medical management of diabetes has intensified over the last decade, the incidence of severe hypoglycemia has risen.[18] The clinician should question diabetic patients about past episodes of hypoglycemia. Hypoglycemia is more common in patients with better glycemic control. When planning dental treatment, it is best to schedule appointments before or after periods of peak insulin activity. This requires knowledge of the

TABLE 38-5

Types of Insulin

Insulin Type	Insulin Classification	Onset of Activity	Peak Activity	Duration of Activity
Lispro	Rapid acting	15 min	30 to 90 min	<5 hrs
Regular	Short acting	30 to 60 min	2 to 3 hrs	4 to 12 hrs
NPH	Intermediate acting	2 to 4 hrs	4 to 10 hrs	14 to 18 hrs
Lente	Intermediate acting	3 to 4 hrs	4 to 12 hrs	16 to 20 hrs
Ultralente	Long acting	6 to 10 hrs	12 to 16 hrs	20 to 30 hrs
Glargine	Long acting	6 to 8 hrs	No peak in activity	22 to 28 hrs

pharmacodynamics of the drugs being taken by the diabetic patient. Patients taking insulin are at greatest risk, followed by those on sulfonylurea agents. Metformin and thiazolidinediones generally do not cause hypoglycemia (see Table 38-4).

Insulins are classified as rapid-, short-, intermediate-, or long-acting (Table 38-5). The categories vary in their onset, peak, and duration of activity. It is important that the clinician establish exactly which insulins the diabetic patient takes, the amount, the number of times per day, and the time of the last dose. Periodontal treatment often can be timed to avoid peak insulin activity. Many diabetic patients take multiple injections each day, in which case it is difficult, if not impossible, to avoid peak insulin activity. Checking the pretreatment glucose with the patient's glucometer, checking again during long procedures, and again at the end of the procedure provides a better understanding of the patient's insulin pharmacodynamics and helps prevent hypoglycemia.

If hypoglycemia occurs during dental treatment, therapy should be immediately terminated. If a glucometer is available, the blood glucose level should be checked. Treatment guidelines include the following[36]:

1. Provide approximately 15 g of oral carbohydrate to the patient:
   - 4 to 6 oz of juice or soda
   - 3 or 4 tsp of table sugar
   - Hard candy with 15 g of sugar
2. If the patient is unable to take food or drink by mouth, or if the patient is sedated:
   - Give 25 ml to 30 ml of 50% dextrose intravenously, or
   - Give 1 mg of glucagon intravenously (glucagon results in rapid release of stored glucose from the liver), or
   - Give 1 mg of glucagon intramuscularly (if no IV access)

Emergencies due to hyperglycemia are rare in the dental office. They generally take days to weeks to develop. However, the glucometer may be used to rule out hyperglycemic emergencies such as diabetic ketoacidosis, a life-threatening event.

Because periodontal therapy may render the patient unable to eat for some time, adjustment in insulin or oral agent dosages may be required. It is absolutely critical that patients eat their normal meal before dental treatment. Taking insulin without eating is the primary cause of hypoglycemia. If the patient is restricted from eating before treatment (e.g., for conscious sedation), normal insulin doses will need to be reduced. As a general guideline, well-controlled diabetic patients having routine periodontal treatment may take their normal insulin doses as long as they also eat their normal meal. If the procedures are going to be particularly long, the insulin dose before treatment may need to be reduced. Likewise, if the patient will have dietary restrictions after treatment, insulin or sulfonylurea dosages may need to be reduced. Consultation with the patient's physician is prudent and allows both practitioners to review the proposed treatment plan and determine any modifications needed. When periodontal surgery is indicated, it is usually best to limit the size of the surgical fields so that the patient will be comfortable enough to resume a normal diet immediately.

Thyroid and Parathyroid Disorders

Periodontal therapy requires minimal alterations in the patient with adequately managed thyroid disease.[58] Patients with thyrotoxicosis and those with inadequate medical management should not receive periodontal therapy until their conditions are stabilized. Patients with histories of hyperthyroidism should be carefully evaluated to determine the level of medical management, and they should be treated in a way that limits stress and infection. Hyperthyroidism may cause tachycardia and other arrhythmias, increased cardiac output, and myocardial ischemia. Medications such as epinephrine and other vasopressor amines should be given with caution in patients with treated hyperthyroidism, although the small amounts used in dental anesthetics rarely cause problems.[72] They should not be given to patients with thyrotoxicosis or poorly controlled thyroid disorders. Patients with hypothyroidism require careful administration of sedatives and narcotics due to the potential for excessive sedation.

Routine periodontal therapy may be provided to patients with parathyroid disease once that disorder has been identified and the proper medical treatment given.

BOX 38-5

Manifestations of Acute Adrenal Insufficiency

Mental confusion, fatigue, and weakness
Nausea, vomiting, or both
Hypertension
Syncope
Intense abdominal, lower back, leg pain, or all
Loss of consciousness
Coma

TABLE 38-6

Equilvalent Doses of Corticosteroids

Corticosteroid	Equivalent Dose (mg)
Cortisone	25
Hydrocortisone	20
Prednisone	5
Prednisolone	5
Methylprednisone	5
Methylprednisolone	4
Triamcinolone	4
Dexamethasone	0.75
Betamethasone	0.6

However, patients who have not received medical care may have significant renal disease, uremia, and hypertension. Also, if hypercalcemia or hypocalcemia is present, the patient may be more prone to cardiac arrhythmias.

Adrenal Insufficiency

Acute adrenal insufficiency is associated with significant morbidity and mortality owing to peripheral vascular collapse and cardiac arrest. Therefore the periodontist should be aware of the clinical manifestations (Box 38-5) and ways of preventing acute adrenal insufficiency in patients with histories of primary adrenal insufficiency (Addison's disease) or secondary adrenal insufficiency (most often caused by use of exogenous glucocorticosteroids).

The use of systemic corticosteroids is common in allergic, endocrine, respiratory, joint, intestinal, neurologic, renal, liver, skin, and connective tissue disorders. Significant complications associated with corticosteroid use include alterations in glucose metabolism (steroid-induced diabetes), increased risk of infection, altered wound healing, osteoporosis, skin disorders, cataracts, glaucoma, and suppression of the hypothalamic-pituitary-adrenal (HPA) axis.[24,35] In the normal healthy patient, stress activates the HPA axis, stimulating increased endogenous cortisol production by the adrenal glands. Exogenous steroids may suppress the HPA axis and impair the patient's ability to respond to stress with increased endogenous cortisol production, leading to the potential for acute adrenal crisis (see Table 38-5). The degree of adrenal suppression depends on the drugs used, dose, duration of administration, length of time elapsed since steroid therapy was terminated, and route of administration.

It has been common practice in the past to administer prophylactic systemic steroids before dental treatment for patients who are taking or recently have taken exogenous steroids. A thorough review of the literature and recent clinical evidence suggests such steroid supplementation may not be required for many periodontal procedures.[24] Shapiro et al found that patients taking 5 to 20 mg/day prednisone maintained at least some adrenal reserve after immediate termination of steroid therapy.[57] Higher doses may suppress the adrenal glands to a greater degree. Although exogenous steroids may suppress normal adrenal cortisol secretion for an extended period of time, the ability of the adrenal gland to respond to stress may return quickly after termination of steroid therapy. However, the severe consequences of adrenal crisis suggest caution in patient management. Before treating a patient with a history of recent or current steroid use, physician consultation is indicated to determine whether the patient's periodontal needs and proposed treatment plan suggest a requirement for supplemental steroids. Use of a stress reduction protocol and profound local anesthesia may help minimize the physical and psychologic stress associated with therapy and reduce the risk of acute adrenal crisis. A rapid assay is available to determine the degree of adrenal reserve by measurement of serum cortisol levels 30 and 60 minutes after intravenous administration of synthetic corticotrophin.[57]

There is no set protocol for steroid prophylaxis. Topical corticosteroids generally have minimal to no HPA effect, and steroid supplementation generally is not required for these patients. For the patient currently receiving systemic steroid therapy, the need for corticosteroid prophylaxis depends on the drug used because of the variance in equivalent therapeutic doses (Table 38-6). Glucocorticosteroid coverage regimens vary, but most provide a 2- to 4-fold increase in coverage, depending on the stress produced by the procedure. For patients taking large doses of >20 mg cortisol-equivalent per day and requiring stressful periodontal procedures, doubling or tripling the normal steroid dose 1 hour before the procedure is often recommended. For those patients on low doses for short periods of time (i.e., less than 1 month), no supplementation is generally warranted. Again, in an emergency situation, increasing the steroid dose before the procedure may decrease the chances of acute adrenal crisis. If emergency treatment is not needed, consultation with the physician before treatment is best.

Management of the patient in an acute adrenal insufficiency crisis is as follows:

1. Terminate periodontal treatment.
2. Summon medical assistance.
3. Give oxygen.
4. Monitor vital signs.
5. Place the patient in a supine position.
6. Administer 100 mg of hydrocortisone sodium succinate (Solu-Cortef) intravenously for 30 seconds or intramuscularly.

RENAL DISEASES

The most common causes of renal failure are glomerulonephritis, pyelonephritis, kidney cystic disease, renovascular disease, drug nephropathy, obstructive uropathy, and hypertension.[31,74] Renal failure may result in severe electrolyte imbalances, cardiac arrhythmias, pulmonary congestion, congestive heart failure, and prolonged bleeding.[35] Because the dental management of patients with renal disease may need to be drastically altered, physician consultation is necessary to determine the stage of renal disease, regimen for medical management, and alterations in periodontal therapy. The patient in chronic renal failure has a progressive disease that ultimately may require kidney transplantation or dialysis. It is preferable to treat the patient before, rather than after, transplant or dialysis. The following treatment modifications should be used:

1. Consult the patient's physician.
2. Monitor blood pressure (patients in end-stage renal failure are usually hypertensive).
3. Check laboratory values: partial thromboplastin time, prothrombin time, bleeding time, and platelet count; hematocrit; blood urea nitrogen (do not treat if less than 60 mg/dl); and serum creatinine (do not treat if less than 1.5 mg/dl).
4. Eliminate areas of oral infection to prevent systemic infection.
   - Good oral hygiene should be established.
   - Periodontal treatment should aim at eliminating inflammation or infection and providing easy maintenance. Questionable teeth should be extracted if medical parameters permit.
   - Frequent recall appointments should be scheduled.
5. Drugs that are nephrotoxic or metabolized by the kidney should not be given (e.g., phenacetin, tetracycline, aminoglycoside antibiotics). Acetaminophen may be used for analgesia and diazepam may be used for sedation. Local anesthetics such as lidocaine are generally safe.[35,51]

The patient who is receiving dialysis requires treatment planning modifications.[31] The three modes of dialysis are intermittent peritoneal dialysis (IPD), chronic ambulatory peritoneal dialysis (CAPD), and hemodialysis. Only hemodialysis patients require special precautions. These patients have a high incidence of viral hepatitis, anemia, and prolonged hemorrhage. The risk for hemorrhage is related to anticoagulation during dialysis, platelet trauma from dialysis, and the uremia that develops with renal failure.[35] Hemodialysis patients have either an internal arteriovenous fistula or an external arteriovenous shunt. This shunt is often located in the arm and must be protected from trauma. Thus in addition to guidelines for patients with chronic renal disease, the following recommendation are made for those on hemodialysis:

1. Screen for hepatitis B and hepatitis C antigens and antibody before any treatment.
2. Provide antibiotic prophylaxis to prevent endarteritis of the arteriovenous fistula or shunt. (IPD and CAPD patients do not generally require prophylactic antibiotics).
3. Patients receive heparin anticoagulation on the day of hemodialysis. Therefore provide periodontal treatment on the day *after* dialysis, when the effects of heparinization have subsided. Hemodialysis treatments are generally performed 3 or 4 times a week. (IPD and CAPD patients are not systemically heparinized; therefore they usually do not have the potential bleeding problems associated with hemodialysis.)
4. Be careful to protect the hemodialysis shunt or fistula when the patient is in the dental chair. If the shunt or fistula is placed in the arm, do not cramp the limb; *blood pressure readings should be taken from the other arm.* Do not use the limb for the injection of medication. Patients with leg shunts should avoid sitting with the leg dependent for longer than 1 hour. If appointments last longer, allow the patient to walk about for a few minutes and then resume therapy.
5. Refer the patient to the physician if uremic problems develop, such as uremic stomatitis. Refer to the physician if oral infections do not resolve promptly to prevent systemic dissemination.

The renal transplant patient's greatest foe is infection. Transplant patients take immunosuppressive drugs that greatly reduce resistance to infection.[51] Excessive bleeding may occur during or after periodontal treatment due to drug-induced thrombocytopenia, anticoagulation, or both. A periodontal abscess is a potentially life-threatening situation. For this reason, a dental team approach should be used *before* transplantation to determine which teeth can be easily maintained. Many organ transplant centers now include dental examination in their standard pretransplant protocol. Teeth with severe bone and attachment loss, furcation invasion, periodontal abscesses, or extensive surgical requirements should be extracted, leaving an easily maintainable dentition. In addition to the recommendations for patients with chronic renal failure, the following should be considered for the renal transplant patient:

1. Hepatitis B and C screening.
2. Determination of level of immunocompromise derived from antirejection drug therapy.
3. Prophylactic antibiotics (using American Heart Association recommendations). Not all transplant patients require antibiotic coverage, and physician consultation is warranted before prescribing.

LIVER DISEASES

Liver diseases may range from mild to complete failure. Major causes of liver disease include drug toxicity, cirrhosis, viral infections (e.g., hepatitis B and C), neoplasms, and biliary tract disorders.[73] Because the liver is the site of production for most of the clotting factors, excessive bleeding during or after periodontal treatment may occur in patients with severe liver disease. Many drugs are metabolized in the liver; thus liver disease alters normal drug metabolism. Treatment recommendations for patients with liver disease include the following:

1. Consultation with the physician concerning current stage of disease, risk for bleeding, potential drugs to be prescribed during treatment, and required alterations to periodontal therapy.
2. Screening for hepatitis B and C.
3. Check laboratory values for prothrombin time and partial thromboplastin time.

PULMONARY DISEASES

The periodontal treatment of a patient with pulmonary disease may require alteration depending on the nature and the severity of the respiratory problem. Pulmonary diseases range from obstructive lung diseases (e.g., asthma, emphysema, bronchitis, and acute obstruction) to restrictive ventilatory disorders that are due to muscle weakness, scarring, obesity, or any condition that could interfere with effective lung ventilation.[47,53] Combined restrictive-obstructive lung disease may also develop.

The clinician should be aware of the signs and symptoms of pulmonary disease, such as increased respiratory rate, cyanosis, clubbing of the fingers, chronic cough, chest pain, hemoptysis, dyspnea or orthopnea, and wheezing. Patients with these problems should be referred for medical evaluation and treatment. Most patients with chronic lung disease may undergo routine periodontal therapy if they are receiving adequate medical management. Caution should be practiced in relation to any treatment that may depress respiratory function.

Acute respiratory distress may be caused by slight airway obstruction or depression of respiratory function. Because of their limited vital lung capacity, these patients also have decreased cough effectiveness.[56] They must continually deal with the mental anxiety caused by air hunger and alter their position in attempts to improve their ventilatory efficiency.

The following guidelines should be used during periodontal therapy:

1. Identify and refer patients with signs and symptoms of pulmonary disease to their physicians.
2. In patients with known pulmonary disease, consult with their physicians regarding medications (antibiotics, steroids, chemotherapeutic agents) and the degree and severity of pulmonary disease.
3. Avoid elicitation of respiratory depression or distress:
   - Minimize the stress of a periodontal appointment. The patient with emphysema should be treated in the afternoon, several hours after sleep, to allow for airway clearance.
   - Avoid medications that could cause respiratory depression (e.g., narcotics, sedatives, and general anesthetics).
   - Avoid bilateral mandibular block anesthesia, which could cause increased airway obstruction.
   - Position the patient to allow maximal ventilatory efficiency, be careful to prevent physical airway obstruction, keep the patient's throat clear, and avoid excess periodontal packing.
4. In a patient with a history of asthma, make sure the patient's medication (inhaler) is available.
5. Patients with active fungal or bacterial respiratory diseases should not be treated unless the periodontal procedure is an emergency.

IMMUNOSUPPRESSION AND CHEMOTHERAPY

Immunosuppressed patients have impaired host defenses as a result of an underlying immunodeficiency or drug administration (primarily related to organ transplantation or cancer chemotherapy).[38,55] Because chemotherapy is often cytotoxic to bone marrow, destruction of platelets and red and white blood cells results in thrombocytopenia, anemia, and leukopenia. Immunosuppressed individuals are at greatly increased risk for infection, and even minor periodontal infections can become life threatening if immune suppression is severe. Intraorally, bacterial, viral, and fungal infections may manifest. Patients receiving bone marrow transplantation require special attention because these patients receive very high-dose chemotherapy and are particularly susceptible to dissemination of oral infections.

Treatment in these patients should be directed toward the prevention of oral complications that could be life threatening. The greatest potential for infection occurs during periods of extreme immunosuppression; therefore treatment should be conservative and palliative. It is always preferable to evaluate the patient before initiation of chemotherapy.[38,55] Teeth having a poor prognosis should be extracted, with thorough debridement of remaining teeth to minimize the microbial load. The clinician must teach and emphasize the importance of good oral hygiene. Antimicrobial rinses such as chlorhexidine are recommended, especially for patients with chemotherapy-induced mucositis, to prevent secondary infection.

Chemotherapy is usually performed in cycles, with each cycle lasting several days followed by intervening periods of myelosuppression and recovery. If periodontal therapy is needed during chemotherapy, it is best done the day *before* chemotherapy is given, when white cell counts are relatively high. Coordination with the oncologist is critical. Dental treatment should be done when white cell counts are above 2000/mm^3, with an absolute granulocyte count of 1000 to 1500/mm^3.[35]

RADIATION THERAPY

The use of radiotherapy, alone or in conjunction with surgical resection, is common in the treatment of head and neck tumors. The side effects of ionizing radiation include dramatic perioral changes of significant concern to dental health personnel.[39,54] The extent and severity of mucositis, dermatitis, xerostomia, dysphagia, gustatory alteration, radiation caries, vascular changes, trismus, temporomandibular joint degeneration, and periodontal change depend on a myriad of radiation factors: the type of radiation used, fields of irradiation, number of ports, types of tissues in the fields, and dosage.[59]

Patients scheduled to receive head and neck radiation therapy require dental consultation *at the earliest possible time* to reduce the morbidity of the known perioral side effects. Preirradiation treatment depends on the patient's prognosis, compliance, and residual dentition in addition to the fields, ports, dose, and immediacy of radiotherapy. The initial visit should include panoramic and intraoral radiographs, a clinical dental examination, a periodontal evaluation, and a physician consultation. The physician should be asked about the amount of radiation to be administered, extent and location of the lesion, nature of any surgical procedures already performed or to be performed, number of radiation ports, exact fields to be irradiated, mode of radiation therapy, and patient's prognosis (i.e., the likelihood of metastasis). Preirradiation treatment should commence immediately after the physician consultation. The first decision that should be made relates to possible extractions because radiation can cause side effects that interfere with healing.

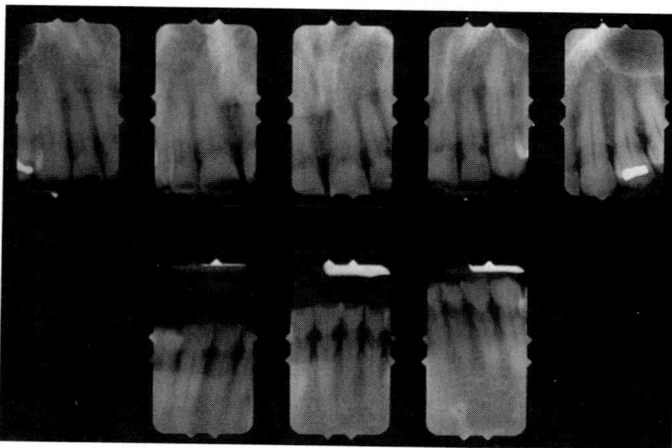

Fig. 38-2 Radiographs of the anterior teeth of a 52-year-old man with postirradiation caries. Patient received 6000-cGy radiation to the posterior mandible and base of tongue for squamous cell carcinoma. Radiation caries developed within 1 year of radiation treatment, affecting the cervical areas and incisal edges of the anterior teeth.

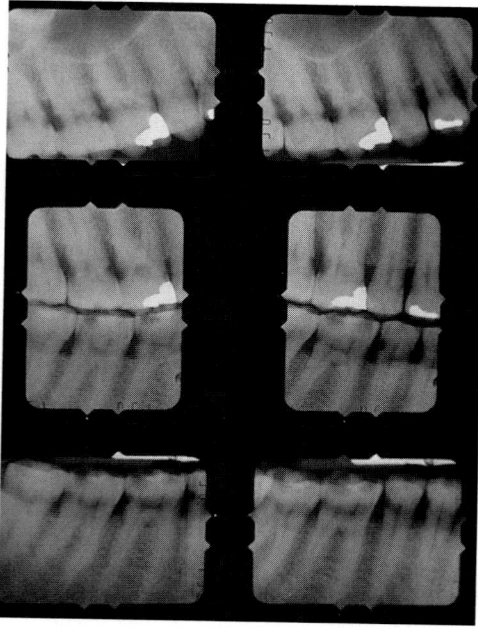

Fig. 38-3 Radiographs of the posterior sextants of the same patient as in Fig. 38-2. Caries affects the cervical areas and cusp tips of the posterior teeth.

For head and neck squamous cell carcinomas, the radiation dose is usually 5000 to 7000 cGy (centigrays; 1 cGy = 1 rad) delivered in a fractionated method (150 to 200 cGy/day over a 6- to 7-week course).[6,39] This is considered full-course radiation treatment, and the degree of perioral side effects depends on which tissues are irradiated; that is, the radiation fields. If this dose is administered to the salivary gland tissues, xerostomia will ensue. The parotid is the most radiosensitive of the salivary glands; saliva may become extremely viscous or nonexistent, depending on the dose delivered to the particular gland. Xerostomia causes a decrease in the normal salivary cleansing mechanisms, buffering capacity of saliva, and pH of oral fluids.[39] Oral bacterial populations shift to preponderantly cariogenic forms (e.g., *Streptococcus mutans, Actinomyces* spp., and *Lactobacillus* spp.). Radiation-induced caries may progress very rapidly and affects primarily smooth tooth surfaces (Figs. 38-2 and 38-3).

High-dose radiation therapy results in hypovascularity of irradiated tissues with a reduction in wound healing capacity.[54] Most severe among the resulting oral complications is osteoradionecrosis (ORN). Decreased vascularity renders the bone less capable of resolving trauma or infection. Such events may cause severe destruction of bone. The risk of ORN continues for the remainder of the patient's life and does not decrease with time.[33]

Periodontal disease can be a precipitating factor in ORN.[8,21] Tooth extraction after radiation treatment involves a high risk of developing ORN, and surgical flap procedures are generally discouraged after radiation. For these reasons, it is important that the clinician address the patient's periodontal disease *before* radiation begins, whenever possible. Teeth that are nonrestorable or severely periodontally diseased should be extracted, ideally at least 2 weeks before radiation.[39] Extractions should be performed in a manner that allows primary closure. Mucoperiosteal flaps should be gently elevated; teeth should be extracted in segments; alveolectomy should be performed, allowing no rough bony spicules to remain; and primary closure should be provided without tension. It is unnecessary to extract teeth that can be retained with conservative restorative, endodontic, or periodontal therapy. However, prudence dictates extraction of questionable teeth because periodontal treatment after irradiation may be limited to nonsurgical forms of therapy. Flap surgery or extraction of teeth after radiation may lead to ORN. Management of ORN is often difficult and costly, involving progressively more aggressive treatment if bone does not respond to conservative therapy. Costly hyperbaric oxygen therapy is frequently required for complete resolution.

During radiation therapy, patients should receive weekly prophylaxis, oral hygiene instruction, and professionally applied fluoride treatments unless mucositis prevents such treatment. Patients should be instructed to brush daily with a 0.4% stannous or 1.0% sodium fluoride gel. Custom gel trays allow optimum fluoride application.[39] All remaining teeth should receive thorough debridement (scaling and root planing).

Postirradiation follow-up consists of palliative treatment given as indicated. Viscous lidocaine may be prescribed for painful mucositis, and salivary substitutes may be given for xerostomia. Daily topical fluoride application and oral hygiene are the best means of preventing radiation caries in the long-term aspect. A long-term, 3-month recall interval is ideal.

PROSTHETIC JOINT REPLACEMENT

The main treatment consideration for patients with prosthetic joint replacements relates to the potential need for antibiotic prophylaxis before periodontal therapy. Currently, there is no scientific evidence that prophylactic antibiotics prevent late prosthetic joint infections, which might occur from transient bacteremia induced by dental treatment.[16,35] Furthermore, although dental-induced bacteremia could theoretically cause prosthetic joint infection, very few reports demonstrate dental treatment as a source of joint infection, and none of these actually document a cause-and-effect relationship.[13,67] Thus the American Dental Association, American Academy of Orthopaedic Surgeons, American Academy of Oral Medicine, and British Society for Antimicrobial Chemotherapy all agree that routine antibiotic prophylaxis before dental treatment is not indicated for most patients with prosthetic joint replacements.[1,13,19,67] However, prophylaxis is indicated for almost all patients within the first 2 years after joint replacement and for so-called "high-risk" patients including those with previous prosthetic joint infections, immunosuppression, rheumatoid arthritis, systemic lupus erythematosis, type 1 diabetes, hemophilia, and malnourishment.[1] Importantly, patients with severe periodontal disease or other potential dental infections are considered by many authors to be high-risk, and antibiotic prophylaxis may be indicated for these patients before dental treatment.[41,67]

Although the evidence demonstrates no need for antibiotic prophylaxis in most patients, many orthopedic surgeons still prefer such treatment.[60] This is most likely due to the high morbidity and potential mortality rates associated with prosthetic joint infections. Consultation with the patient's orthopedic surgeon before periodontal treatment is in the patient's best interest and may help assess the risk for joint infection relative to current dental status and type of periodontal treatment planned. Because individuals with significant periodontal disease are considered "high risk," antibiotic prophylaxis before treatment is common in the periodontal practice. Suggested antibiotic regimens are found in Table 38-7.[1]

TABLE 38-7

Antibiotic Regimens for Prevention of Prosthetic Joint Infections

Patient Characteristics	Drug Regimen
Patients *not* allergic to penicillins	Cephalexin, cephradine, or amoxicillin: 2 g orally 1 hour before dental procedure
Patients allergic to penicillins	Clindamycin: 600 mg orally 1 hour before dental procedure
Patients *not* allergic to penicillins but unable to take oral medication	Cefazolin 1 g or Ampicillin 2 g intramuscularly or intravenously 1 hour before dental procedure
Patients allergic to penicillins and unable to take oral medications	Clindamycin 600 mg intravenously 1 hour before dental procedure (must be diluted and injected slowly)

See reference 2.

PREGNANCY

The aim of periodontal therapy for the pregnant patient is to minimize the potential exaggerated inflammatory response related to pregnancy-associated hormonal alterations. Meticulous plaque control, scaling, root planing, and polishing should be the only nonemergency periodontal procedures performed.

The second trimester is the safest time to perform treatment. However, long, stressful appointments and periodontal surgical procedures should be delayed until the postpartum period. As the uterus increases in size during the second and third trimesters, obstruction of the vena cava and aorta may occur if the patient is placed in a supine position. The reduction in return cardiac blood supply may cause supine hypotensive syndrome, with decreased placental perfusion.[65] Decreasing blood pressure, syncope, and loss of consciousness may occur. This can be prevented by placing the patient on her left side or simply by elevating the right hip 5 to 6 inches during treatment. Appointments should be short, and the patient should be allowed to change positions frequently. A fully reclined position should be avoided if possible.

Other precautions during pregnancy relate to the potential toxic or teratogenic effects of therapy on the fetus. Ideally, no medications should be prescribed. However, analgesics, antibiotics, local anesthetics, and other drugs may be required during pregnancy, depending on the patient's needs. All drugs should be reviewed for potential adverse effects on the fetus prior to prescribing.[35,65]

Use of dental radiographs during pregnancy should be

TABLE 38-8

Laboratory Tests for Bleeding Disorders

	HEMOSTATIC			
	Vascular	**Platelet**	**Coagulation**	**Lytic**
Tests	1. Tourniquet test N: 10 petechiae Abn: >10 petechiae	1. Platelet count N: 150,000–300,000/mm^3 Abn: Thrombocytopenia = <100,000/mm^3 Clinical bleeding occurs at <80,000/mm^3 Spontaneous bleeding occurs at <20,000/mm^3	1. Prothrombin time (measures extrinsic and common pathways: Factors I, II, V, VII, and X) N: 11–14 s (depending on laboratory) Measured against a control Prothrombin time is reported as *INR* (International Normalized Ratio); Normal INR = 1.0 Abn: INR > 1.5	1. Euglobulin clot lysis time N: <90 min Abn: >90 min
	2. Bleeding time N: 1–6 min Abn: >6 min	2. Bleeding time 3. Clot retraction 4. Complete blood cell count	2. Partial thromboplastin time (measures intrinsic and common pathways: Factors III, IX, XI, and low levels of Factors I, II, V, X, and XII) N: 25–40 s (depending on laboratory) Measured against a control Abn: >1.5 times normal 3. Clotting (coagulation) time N: 30–40 min Abn: >1 hr	
Clinical disease association	*Vascular (capillary) wall defect* Rule out: • Thrombocytopenia • Purpuras • Telangiectasia • Aspirin or NSAID therapy • Leukemia • Renal dialysis	*Thrombocytopenia* Rule out: • Vascular wall defect • Acute/chronic leukemia • Aplastic anemia • Liver disease • Renal dialysis	*All three tests:* • Liver disease • Warfarin therapy • Aspirin or NSAID therapy • Malabsorption syndrome or long-term antibiotic therapy (lack of vitamin K utilization) *Prothrombin time:* • Factor VII deficiency *Partial thromboplastic time:* • Hemophilia • Renal dialysis	Increase in fibrinolytic activity

Abn, Abnormal; *N,* normal.

kept to a minimum, as they should for all patients. The small amount of radiation exposure during diagnostic dental radiography poses little, if any, risk to the fetus as long as the mother is properly shielded.[2,65] The American Dental Association has stated that "normal radiographic guidelines do not need to be altered because of pregnancy."[2] Use of a properly positioned lead apron is an absolute requirement (see also Chapter 37).

HEMORRHAGIC DISORDERS

Patients with a history of bleeding problems caused by disease or drugs should be managed so as to minimize risks of hemorrhage. Identification of these patients via the health history, clinical examination, and clinical laboratory tests is paramount. Health questioning should cover (1) history of bleeding after previous surgery or trauma, (2) past and present drug history, (3) history of bleeding problems among relatives, and (4) illnesses associated with potential bleeding problems.

Clinical examinations should detect the existence of jaundice, ecchymosis, spider telangiectasia, hemarthrosis, petechiae, hemorrhagic vesicles, spontaneous gingival bleeding, or gingival hyperplasia. Laboratory tests should include methods to measure the hemostatic, coagulation, or lytic phases of the clotting mechanism, depending on clues regarding which phase is involved (Table 38-8). These tests include bleeding time, tourniquet test, complete blood cell count, prothrombin time, partial thromboplastin time, and coagulation time. Bleeding disorders may be classified as coagulation disorders, thrombocytopenic purpuras, or nonthrombocytopenic purpuras.

Coagulation Disorders

The main inherited coagulation disorders include hemophilias A and B and von Willebrand's disease (Table 38-9). Hemophilia A results in a deficiency of coagulation factor VIII, and the clinical severity of the disorder depends on the level of factor VIII remaining.[45] Severe hemophiliacs with less than 1% of normal factor VIII levels may have severe bleeding on the slightest provocation, whereas more moderate hemophiliacs (1% to 5% factor VIII) have less frequent spontaneous hemorrhage but still bleed with minimal trauma.[35] Mild hemophiliacs (6% to 30% factor VIII) rarely bleed spontaneously but may still have hemorrhage after severe trauma or during surgical procedures. The clinician should consult the patient's physician before dental treatment to determine the risk for bleeding and treatment modifications required. To prevent surgical hemorrhage, factor VIII levels of at least 30% are needed.[35,45] Parenteral 1-deamino-8-D-arginine vasopressin (DDAVP) can be used to raise factor VIII levels 2- to 3-fold in patients with mild or moderate hemophilia. DDAVP has the significant advantage of avoiding the risk of viral disease transmission from factor VIII infusion and is considered the drug of choice in responsive patients. Most moderate and severe hemophiliacs require infusion of factor VIII concentrate before surgical procedures. Before 1985 the risk of viral disease transmission from these infusions was high. In recent years, virally safe, highly purified monoclonal antibody or recombinant DNA factor VIII products have come into widespread use.

Hemophilia B, or Christmas disease, results in a deficiency of factor IX. The severity of the disorder depends on the relative amount of existing factor IX. Surgical therapy requires a factor IX level of 30% to 50% and is usually achieved by administration of purified prothrombin complex concentrates or factor IX concentrates.[45]

von Willebrand's disease results from a deficiency of von Willebrand factor, which mediates adhesion of platelets to the injured vessel wall and is required for primary hemostasis. von Willebrand factor also carries the coagulant portion of factor VIII in the plasma. The disorder

TABLE 38-9

Inherited Coagulation Disorders

Hemophilia Type	Prolonged	Normal	Treatment
A	Partial thromboplastin time	Prothrombin time Bleeding time	DDAVP Factor VIII concentrate or cryoprecipitate Fresh frozen plasma Fresh whole blood Epsilon-aminocaproic acid (EACA) Tranexamic acid
B	Partial thromboplastin time	Prothrombin time Bleeding time	Purified prothrombin complex concentrates Factor IX concentrates Fresh frozen plasma
von Willebrand's disease	Bleeding time Partial thromboplastin time Variable Factor VIII deficiency	Prothrombin time Platelet count	DDAVP Factor VIII concentrate or cryoprecipitate

has three major subtypes with a wide range of clinical severity. In fact, many cases of von Willebrand's disease go undiagnosed, and bleeding during dental treatment may be the first sign of the underlying disease. More severe forms require preoperative factor VIII concentrate or cryoprecipitate infusion. Milder forms respond favorably to administration of DDAVP before periodontal surgery or tooth extraction.[45,46] Periodontal treatment may be performed in patients with these coagulation disorders, provided that sufficient precautions are taken. Probing, scaling, and prophylaxis can usually be done without medical modification. More invasive treatment such as block local anesthesia, root planing, or surgery dictate prior physician consultation.

During treatment, local measures to ensure clot formation and stability are of major importance. Complete wound closure and application of pressure will reduce hemorrhage. Antihemostatic agents such as oxidized cellulose or purified bovine collagen may be placed over surgical sites or into extraction sockets. The antifibrinolytic agent epsilon-aminocaproic acid (EACA), given orally or intravenously, is a potent inhibitor of initial clot dissolution.[28] Tranexamic acid is a more potent antifibrinolytic agent than EACA and has been shown to prevent excessive oral hemorrhage after periodontal surgery and tooth extraction.[49] It is available in a mouthrinse form that may be used either alone or in combination with systemic tranexamic acid for several days after surgery.[61]

Not all coagulation disorders are hereditary. Liver disease may affect all phases of blood clotting because most coagulation factors are synthesized and removed by the liver. Long-term alcohol abusers or chronic hepatitis patients often demonstrate inadequate coagulation. Coagulation may be impaired by vitamin K deficiency, often caused by malabsorption syndromes, or by prolonged antibiotic administration, which alters the intestinal microflora that produces vitamin K. Dental treatment planning for patients with liver disease should include the following:

1. Physician consultation.
2. Laboratory evaluations: prothrombin time, bleeding time, platelet count, and partial thromboplastin time (in patients in later stages of liver disease).
3. Conservative, nonsurgical periodontal therapy, whenever possible.
4. If surgery is required (may require hospitalization):
   - INR (prothrombin time) should generally be <2.0. For simple surgical procedures, INR < 2.5 is generally safe.[27]
   - Platelet count should be >80,000/mm^3.

Perhaps the most common cause of abnormal coagulation is drug therapy. Patients with prosthetic heart valves or histories of myocardial infarction, stroke, or thromboembolism are frequently placed on anticoagulant therapy using coumarin derivatives such as dicumarol and warfarin.[27,32] These drugs are vitamin K antagonists that decrease production of vitamin K-dependent coagulation factors II, VII, IX, and X. The effectiveness of anticoagulation therapy is monitored via the prothrombin time. The recommended level of anticoagulation for most patients is an INR of 2.0 to 3.0, with prosthetic heart valve patients generally in the 2.5 to 3.5 range.[27] Periodontal treatment should be altered as follows:

1. Consult the patient's physician to determine the nature of the underlying medical problem and the degree of required anticoagulation.
2. The procedure to be done determines the acceptable INR. Infiltration anesthesia, scaling, and root planing may be done safely in patients with an INR <3.0. Block anesthesia, minor periodontal surgery, and simple extractions usually require an INR <2.0. Complex surgery or multiple extractions may require an INR <1.5.
3. The physician should be consulted about discontinuing or reducing anticoagulant dosage until the desired INR is achieved. Frequently, the anticoagulant is discontinued for 2 to 3 days before periodontal treatment (the clearance half-life of warfarin is 36 to 42 hours) and the INR is checked on the day of therapy. If the INR is within the acceptable target range, the procedure is done and the anticoagulant is resumed immediately after treatment.
4. Careful technique and complete wound closure are paramount. For all procedures, application of pressure can minimize hemorrhage. Use of oxidized cellulose, microfibrillar collagen, topical thrombin, and tranexamic acid should be considered for persistent bleeding.

Aspirin interferes with normal platelet aggregation and can result in prolonged bleeding. Because it binds irreversibly to platelets, the effects of aspirin last at least 4 to 7 days. It is generally used in small doses of 325 mg or less per day, which usually does not alter bleeding time. However, higher doses may increase bleeding time and predispose the patient to postoperative bleeding.[35] For patients taking more than 325 mg of aspirin per day, the aspirin should be discontinued at least 7 to 10 days before periodontal therapy in consultation with the physician. Nonsteroidal antiinflammatory drugs (NSAIDs) such as ibuprofen also inhibit platelet function. Because they bind reversibly, the effect is transitory, lasting only a short time after the last drug dose. The bleeding time is used when questions about the potential effect of aspirin or NSAIDs exist. Aspirin should not be prescribed for patients who are receiving anticoagulation therapy or have illnesses related to bleeding tendencies.

Heparin is generally used for short-term anticoagulation and is given intravenously (usually in a hospital environment). It is a powerful anticoagulant with a duration of action of 4 to 8 hours. Periodontal treatment is rarely required while a patient is taking heparin.

Thrombocytopenic Purpuras

Thrombocytopenia is defined as a platelet count <100,000/mm^3. Bleeding due to thrombocytopenia may be seen with idiopathic thrombocytopenic purpuras, radiation therapy, myelosuppressive drug therapy (e.g., chemotherapy), leukemia, or infections. Pupuras are hemorrhagic diseases characterized by extravasation of blood into the tissues under the skin or mucosa, producing spontaneous petechiae (small red patches) or ecchymoses (bruises).

Periodontal therapy for patients with thrombocytopenia should be directed toward reducing inflammation by removing local irritants to avoid the need for more aggressive therapy.[35,45] Oral hygiene instructions and frequent maintenance visits are paramount. Physician referral is indicated for a definitive diagnosis and to determine any alterations in planned therapy. Scaling and root planing is generally safe unless platelet counts are <60,000/mm^3. No surgical procedures should be performed unless the platelet count is >80,000/mm^3. Platelet transfusion may be required before surgery. Surgical technique should be as atraumatic as possible, and local hemostatic measures should be applied.

Nonthrombocytopenic Purpuras

Nonthrombocytopenic purpuras occur as a result of either vascular wall fragility or thrombasthenia (impaired platelet aggregation). The former may result from a multitude of causes: hypersensitivity reactions, scurvy, infections, chemicals (phenacetin and aspirin), dysproteinemia, and several others. Thrombasthenia occurs in uremia, Glanzmann's disease, aspirin ingestion, and von Willebrand's disease.[45] Both kinds of nonthrombocytopenic purpuras may result in immediate bleeding after gingival injury. Treatment consists primarily of direct pressure applied for at least 15 minutes. This initial pressure should control the bleeding unless coagulation times are abnormal or reinjury occurs. Surgical therapy should be avoided unless the qualitative and quantitative platelet problems are resolved.

BLOOD DYSCRASIAS

Numerous disorders of red and white blood cells may affect the course of periodontal therapy. Alterations in wound healing, bleeding, tissue appearance, and susceptibility to infection may occur. Clinicians should be aware of the clinical signs and symptoms of blood dyscrasias, availability of screening laboratory tests, and need for physician referral.

Leukemia

Altered periodontal treatment for patients with leukemia is based on such patients' enhanced susceptibility to infections, bleeding tendency, and the effects of chemotherapy.[35] The treatment plan for these patients is as follows:

1. Refer the patient for medical evaluation and treatment. Close cooperation with the physician is required.
2. Before chemotherapy, a complete periodontal treatment plan should be developed with a physician (see the section on treatment for patients receiving chemotherapy).
   - Monitor hematologic laboratory values daily: bleeding time, coagulation time, prothrombin time, and platelet count.
   - Administer antibiotic coverage before any periodontal treatment because infection is a major concern.
   - Extract all hopeless, nonmaintainable, or potentially infectious teeth at least 10 days before the initiation of chemotherapy, if systemic conditions allow.
   - Periodontal debridement (scaling and root planing) should be performed and thorough oral hygiene instructions given if the patient's condition allows. Twice-daily rinsing with 0.12% chlorhexidine gluconate is recommended after oral hygiene procedures. Recognize the potential for bleeding due to thrombocytopenia. Use pressure and topical hemostatic agents as indicated.
3. During the acute phases of leukemia, patients should receive only emergency periodontal care. Any source of potential infection must be eliminated to prevent systemic dissemination. Antibiotic therapy is frequently the treatment of choice, combined with nonsurgical or surgical debridement as indicated.
4. Oral ulcerations or mucositis are treated palliatively with agents such as viscous lidocaine. Systemic antibiotics may be indicated to prevent secondary infection.
5. Oral candidiasis is common in the leukemic patient and can be treated with nystatin suspensions (100,000 U/ml 4 times daily) or clotrimazole vaginal suppositories (10 mg 4 to 5 times daily).[39]
6. For patients with chronic leukemia and those in remission, scaling and root planing can be performed without complication but periodontal surgery should be avoided if possible.
   - Platelet count and bleeding time should be measured on the day of the procedure. If either is low, postpone the appointment and refer the patient to a physician.

Agranulocytosis

Patients with agranulocytosis (cyclic neutropenia and granulocytopenia) have an increased susceptibility to infection. The total white blood cell count is reduced, and granular leukocytes (neutrophils, eosinophils, and/or basophils) are reduced or disappear. These disorders are often marked by early, severe periodontal destruction.[70] When possible, periodontal treatment should be done during periods of disease remission. At such times, treatment should be as conservative as possible while reducing potential sources of systemic infection. After physician consultation, severely affected teeth should be extracted. Oral hygiene instruction should include use of chlorhexidine mouthrinses twice daily. Scaling and root planing should be performed carefully under antibiotic protection.

INFECTIOUS DISEASES

Because many infectious diseases are occult in nature, and because medical histories are often inaccurate or incomplete, all periodontal patients should be treated as though they have an infectious disease. Protection of patients, clinicians, and office staff requires use of universal (standard) precautions for each and every patient, maximizing prevention of infection and cross-contamination. This section provides a brief discussion of hepatitis, human immunodeficiency virus (HIV) and acquired immunodeficiency syndrome (AIDS), and tuberculosis in relation to the precautions required in periodontal therapy.

Hepatitis

To date, six distinct viruses causing viral hepatitis have been identified: hepatitis A, B, C, D, E, and G viruses.[12,23] These forms of viral hepatitis differ in their virology, epidemiology, and prophylaxis (Table 38-10). Because the majority of hepatitis infections are undiagnosed, the clinician must be aware of high-risk groups such as renal dialysis patients, health care workers, immunosuppressed patients, patients who have received multiple blood transfusions, homosexuals, drug users, and institutionalized patients.

Hepatitis A and E are both self-limiting infections with no associated chronic liver disease. These viruses are primarily transmitted via the fecal-oral route. HAV transmission in the U.S. usually occurs due to close personal household, sexual or daycare center contact. Conversely, HEV is transmitted mainly through fecally contaminated drinking water and is thus relatively uncommon in the U.S. Currently a vaccination is available to protect against HAV infection but not HEV infection.

Hepatitis B infection may result in chronic liver disease and a chronic carrier state. Chronic HBV infection develops in about 5% to 10% of infected individuals, with much higher rates among infants and children. Because it is transmitted primarily through a hematogenous route, HBV is a major concern for health care workers. Among health care workers, the highest rates of HBV infection are found among dentists and oral surgeons.[23] Percutaneous or permucosal injury with contaminated instruments or needles is the most common route of infection in the dental office. The hepatitis B vaccine is recommended for all health care workers.

Hepatitis D virus is a defective virus that requires the presence of HBV for its survival, replication, and infectivity. The HDV genetic material is packaged within the HBV surface antigen coating. Thus prevention of HDV infection is similar to prevention for HBV and relies strongly on HBV vaccination. Once antibody titers to HBV are elevated to a protective level, the patient is also protected against HDV infection.

Hepatitis C is probably the most serious of all viral hepatitis infections due to its high chronic infection rate. Only 15% of patients infected with HCV recover completely; 85% develop chronic HCV infection, which dramatically increases the risk for cirrhosis, hepatocellular carcinoma, and liver failure. In fact, HCV infection is the leading cause of liver transplantation in the U.S. Unfortunately, no vaccine is available for HCV. Because HCV is transmitted primarily via a percutaneous or permucosal route, health care workers are at risk from injury with contaminated instruments.

Hepatitis G is a newly discovered virus, and its epidemiology and virology are not clearly understood at this time. HGV rarely occurs as a solitary infection, usually appearing as a coinfection with hepatitis A, B, or C. HGV is known to be transmitted via the blood.

The following guidelines are offered for treating hepatitis patients:

1. If the disease, regardless of type, is active, do not provide periodontal therapy unless the situation is an emergency. In an emergency case, follow the protocol for HB_sAg (HBV surface antigen)-positive patients.
2. For patients with a past history of hepatitis, consult the physician to determine the type of hepatitis, course and length of the disease, mode of transmission, and any chronic liver disease or viral carrier state.
3. For recovered hepatitis A or E patients, perform routine periodontal care.
4. For recovered hepatitis B and D patients, consult with the physician and order HB_sAg and anti-HB_s (antibody to HBV surface antigen) laboratory tests.
   - If HB_sAg and anti-HB_s tests are negative but hepatitis B virus is suspected, order another HB_s determination.
   - Patients who are HB_sAg positive are probably infective (chronic carriers); the degree of infectivity is measured via an HB_sAg determination.
   - Patients who are anti-HB_s positive may be treated routinely (they have antibody to the HB_s antigen).
   - Patients who are HB_sAg negative may be treated routinely.
5. For hepatitis C patients, consult with the physician to determine the patient's risk for transmissibility and current status of chronic liver disease.
6. If a patient with active hepatitis, positive HB_sAg (HBV carrier) status or positive HCV carrier status requires emergency treatment, use the following precautions:
   - Consult the patient's physician regarding status.
   - If bleeding is likely during or after treatment, measure prothrombin time and bleeding time. Hepatitis may alter coagulation; alter treatment accordingly.
   - All personnel in clinical contact with the patient should use full barrier technique, including masks, gloves, glasses or eye shields, and disposable gowns.
   - Use as many disposable covers as possible, covering light handles, drawer handles, and bracket trays. Headrest covers should also be used.
   - All disposable items (gauze, floss, saliva ejectors, masks, gowns, gloves, etc.) should be placed in one lined wastebasket. After treatment, these items and all disposable covers should be bagged, labeled, and disposed of, following proper guidelines for biohazardous waste.
   - Aseptic technique should be followed at all times. Minimize aerosol production by not using ultrasonic instrumentation, air syringe, or high-speed handpieces; remember that saliva contains a distillate of the virus. Prerinsing with chlorhexidine gluconate for 30 seconds is highly recommended.
   - When the procedure is completed, all equipment should be scrubbed and sterilized. If an item cannot be sterilized or disposed of, it should not be used.

If a percutaneous or permucosal injury occurs during dental treatment of a HBV carrier, current Centers for

TABLE 38-10

Comparison of Hepatitis Viruses

	A	B	C	D	E	G
Source	Feces	Blood and body fluids	Blood and body fluids	Blood and body fluids	Feces	Blood
Primary Modes of Transmission	Fecal-oral	Percutaneous/ permucosal; sexual	Percutaneous/ permucosal	Percutaneous/ permucosal (occurs only after previous infection with HBV or as a coinfection with HBV)	Fecal-oral	Percutaneous (usually occurs as coinfection with other hepatitis viruses)
Incubation Period	15–50 days	50–160 days	15–150 days	15–150 days	15–60 days	Unknown
Risk of Chronic Infection	No chronic infection	Varies with age: Adults 5% to 10%; children 25% to 50%; infants >85%	Very high (>85%)	5% when acquired as a coinfection with HBV; >70% when acquired as a second infection in a chronic HBV carrier	No chronic infection	Unknown whether chronic infection occurs
Protective Immunity after Infection?	Yes: anti-HAV antibody	Usually: antibody to core antigen, e-antigen and surface antigen are produced; anti-HB surface antigen antibody is most protective; chronic carrier state exists	No: anti-HCV antibody is produced but is usually not protective	Because HDV infection requires previous infection or coinfection with HBV, protective immmunity is similar to Hepatitis B	Unknown	Unknown
Vaccine Available?	Yes	Yes	No	Yes (HBV vaccine protects against HDV)	No	No

Disease Control and Prevention (CDCP) guidelines recommend administration of hepatitis B immune globulin (HBIG).[10] The HBV vaccine should also be administered if the injured individual has not previously received it. Unfortunately, postexposure prophylaxis with immune globulin or antiviral agents is generally ineffective if a percutaneous injury occurs during treatment of a hepatitis C carrier.[9,12]

HIV and AIDS

Since the beginning of the AIDS epidemic, a wide range of oral lesions have been associated with HIV infection. These lesions are discussed in Chapters 29 and 51.

As with hepatitis, not all HIV-infected patients know that they are infected when they report for dental treatment. Furthermore, individuals with known HIV infection may not admit their status on the medical history. Therefore every patient receiving dental treatment should be managed as a potentially infected person, using universal precautions for all therapy.

Extensive periodontal treatment plans must be considered in light of their relationship to the patient's systemic health, prognosis, and survival time.[35] There are large variations in progression of HIV disease among individuals, and selection of an appropriate treatment plan depends on the state of the patient's overall health. Although there appear to be few contraindications to routine dental treatment for many HIV-infected patients, the periodontal treatment plan is influenced by the patient's overall systemic health and coincident oral infections or diseases. An awareness of oral disorders associated with HIV infection may allow the clinician to recognize previously undiagnosed disease or modify treatment protocols appropriately.

Tuberculosis

The patient with tuberculosis should receive emergency care only, following the guidelines listed in the section on hepatitis. If the patient has completed chemotherapy, his or her physician should be consulted regarding infectivity and the results of sputum cultures for *Mycobacterium tuberculosis*. When medical clearance has been given and the sputum culture results are negative, these patients may be treated normally. Any patient who gives a history of poor medical follow-up (e.g., lack of yearly chest radiographs) or shows signs or symptoms indicative of tuberculosis should be referred for evaluation. Adequate treatment of tuberculosis requires a minimum of 18 months, and thorough posttreatment follow-up should include chest radiographs, sputum cultures, and a review of the patient's symptoms by the physician at least every 12 months.

REFERENCES

1. American Dental Association, American Academy of Orthopaedic Surgeons: Advisory Statement: Antibiotic prophylaxis for dental patients with total joint replacements. J Am Dent Assoc 1997; 128:1004.
2. American Dental Association Council on Dental Materials, Instruments, and Equipment: Recommendations in radiographic practices: An update, 1988. J Am Dent Assoc 1989; 118:115.
3. American Diabetes Association: Report of the Expert Committee on the Diagnosis and Classification of Diabetes Mellitus. Diabetes Care 1997; 20:1183.
4. Barco CT: Prevention of infective endocarditis: A review of the medical and dental literature. J Periodontol 1991; 62:510.
5. Black HR: The coronary artery disease paradox. Am J Hypertens 1996; 9(4 Pt 3):s2.
6. Blaha PJ, Reeve CM: Periodontal treatment for patients with cancer. Curr Opin Periodontol 1994; 64.
7. Burt VL, Whelton P, Roccella EJ, et al: Prevalence of hypertension in the U.S. adult population: Results from the third National Health and Nutrition Examination Survey, 1988–1991. Hypertension 1995; 25:303.
8. Carl W: Local radiation and systemic chemotherapy: Preventing and managing the oral complications. J Am Dent Assoc 1993; 124:119.
9. Centers for Disease Control and Prevention: Recommendations for follow-up of health-care workers after occupational exposure to hepatitis C virus. MMWR 1997; 46:603.
10. Centers for Disease Control and Prevention: Immunization of health-care workers: Recommendation of the advisory committee on immunization practices (ACIP) and the hospital infection control practices advisory committee (HICPAC). MMWR 1997; 46(RR-18):1.
11. Christgau M, Palitzsch KD, Schmalz G, et al: Healing response to non-surgical periodontal therapy in patients with diabetes mellitus: clinical, microbiological, and immunological results. J Clin Periodontol 1998; 25:112.
12. Cleveland JL, Gooch BF, Shearer BG, et al: Risk and prevention of hepatitis C virus infection. Implications for dentistry. J Am Dent Assoc 1999; 130:641.
13. Council on Dental Therapeutics: Management of dental patients with prosthetic joints. J Am Dent Assoc 1990; 121:537.
14. Dajani AS, Taubert KA, Wilson W, et al: Prevention of bacterial endocarditis. Recommendations by the American Heart Association. JAMA 1997; 277:1794.
15. Dajani AS, Taubert KA, Wilson W, et al: Prevention of bacterial endocarditis. Recommendations by the American Heart Association. J Am Dent Assoc 1997;128:1142.
16. Deacon JM, Pagliaro AJ, Zelicof SB, et al: Current concepts review—Prophylactic use of antibiotics for procedures after total joint replacement. J Bone Joint Surg 1996; 78-A:1755.
17. Diabetes Control and Complications Trial Research Group: The effect of intensive treatment of diabetes on the development and progression of long-term complications in insulin-dependent diabetes mellitus. N Engl J Med 1993; 329:977.
18. Diabetes Control and Complications Trial Research Group: Hypoglycemia in the diabetes control and complications trial. Diabetes 1997; 46:271.
19. Eskinazi D, Rathbun W: Is systemic antimicrobial prophylaxis justified in dental patients with prosthetic joints? Oral Surg Oral Med Oral Pathol 1988; 66:430.
20. Findler M, Garfunkel AA, Galili D: Review of very high-risk patients in the dental setting. Compendium Contin Educ Dent 1994; 15:58.
21. Galler C, Epstein JB, Guze KA, et al: The development of osteoradionecrosis from sites of periodontal disease activity: report of 3 cases. J Periodontol 1992; 63:310.
22. Genco RJ, Offenbacher S, Beck J, et al: Cardiovascular diseases and oral infections. In: Rose LF, Genco RJ, Mealey BL,

et al (eds): Periodontal Medicine. Toronto, BC Decker Inc., 1999.
23. Gillchrist JA. Hepatitis viruses A, B, C, D, E and G: Implications for dental personnel. J Am Dent Assoc 1999; 130:509.
24. Glick M: Glucocorticosteroid replacement therapy: A literature review and suggested replacement therapy. Oral Surg Oral Med Oral Pathol 1989; 67:614.
25. Glick M: New guidelines for prevention, detection, evaluation and treatment of high blood pressure. J Am Dent Assoc 1998; 129:1588.
26. Herman WW, Konzelman JL: Angina: An update for dentistry. J Am Dent Assoc 1996; 127:98.
27. Herman WW, Konzelman JL, Sutley SH: Current perspectives on dental patients receiving coumarin anticoagulant therapy. J Am Dent Assoc 1997; 128:327.
28. Johnson WT, Leary JM: Management of dental patients with bleeding disorders: Review and update. Oral Surg Oral Med Oral Pathol 1988; 66:297.
29. Joint National Committee on Prevention, Detection, Evaluation, and Treatment of High Blood Pressure: The fifth report of the Joint National Committee on Prevention, Detection, Evaluation, and Treatment of High Blood Pressure (JNC V). Arch Intern Med 1993; 153:154.
30. Joint National Committee on Prevention, Detection, Evaluation, and Treatment of High Blood Pressure: The sixth report of the Joint National Committee on Prevention, Detection, Evaluation, and Treatment of High Blood Pressure (JNC VI). Bethesda, Md, National Institutes of Health/National Heart Lung, and Blood Institute, 1997. NIH publication 98-4080.
31. Levy HM: Dental considerations for the patient receiving dialysis for renal failure. Spec Care Dent 1988; 8:34.
32. Martinowitz U, Mazar AL, Taicher S, et al: Dental extraction for patients on oral anticoagulant therapy. Oral Surg Oral Med Oral Pathol 1990; 70:274.
33. Marx RE, Johnson RP: Studies in the radiobiology of osteoradionecrosis and their clinical significance. Oral Surg Oral Med Oral Pathol 1987; 64:379.
34. Matsuura H: The systemic management of cardiovascular risk patients in dentistry. Anes Pain Control Dent 1993; 2:49.
35. Mealey BL: Periodontal implications: Medically compromised patients. Ann Periodontol 1996; 1:256.
36. Mealey BL: Impact of advances in diabetes care on dental treatment of the diabetic patient. Compendium Contin Educ Dent 1998; 19:41.
37. Mealey BL: Diabetes mellitus. In: Rose LF, Genco RJ, Mealey BL, et al (eds): Periodontal Medicine. Toronto, BC Decker Inc., 1999.
38. Mealey BL, Semba SE, Hallmon WW: Dentistry and the cancer patient: Part 1. Oral manifestations and complications of chemotherapy. Compendium Contin Educ Dent 1994; 15:1252.
39. Mealey BL, Semba SE, Hallmon WW: The head and neck radiotherapy patient: Part 2. Management of oral complications. Compendium Contin Educ Dent 1994; 15:442.
40. Muzyka BC, Glick M: The hypertensive dental patient. J Am Dent Assoc 1997; 128:1109.
41. Norden CW: Antibiotic prophylaxis in orthopedic surgery. Rev Infect Dis 1991; 13(Suppl. 10):s842.
42. Ostuni E: Stroke and the dental patient. J Am Dent Assoc 1994; 125:721.
43. Packer M: Therapeutic options in the management of chronic heart failure: Is there a drug of first choice? Circulation 1989; 79:198.
44. Pallasch TJ, Slots J: Antibiotic prophylaxis and the medically compromised patient. Periodontol 2000 1996; 10:107.
45. Patton LL, Ship JA: Treatment of patients with bleeding disorders. Dent Clin North Am 1994; 38:465.
46. Petrover MG, Cohen CI: The use of desmopressin in the management of two patients with von Willebrand's disease undergoing periodontal surgery. 2 case reports. J Periodontol 1990; 61:239.
47. Phillips YY, Hnatiuk OW: Diagnosing and monitoring the clinical source of chronic obstructive pulmonary disease. Respir Care Clin N Am 1998; 4:371.
48. Raab FJ, Schaffer EM, Guillaume-Cornelissen G, et al: Interpreting vital sign profiles for maximizing patient safety during dental visits. J Am Dent Assoc 1998; 129:461.
49. Ramstrom G, Sindet-Pedersen S, Hall G, et al: Prevention of postsurgical bleeding in oral surgery using tranexamic acid without dose modification of oral anticoagulants. J Oral Maxillofac Surg 1993; 51:1211.
50. Replogle K, Reader A, Nist R, et al: Cardiovascular effects of intraosseous injections of 2 percent lidocaine with 1:100,000 epinephrine and 3 percent mepivacaine. J Am Dent Assoc 1999; 130:649.
51. Rhodus NL, Little JW: Dental management of the renal transplant patient. Compendium Contin Educ Dent 1993; 14:518.
52. Rose LF: Medical evaluation. In: Rose LF, Genco RJ, Mealey BL, et al (eds): Periodontal Medicine. Toronto, BC Decker, Inc., 1999.
53. Scannapieco FA: Respiratory diseases. In: Rose LF, Genco RJ, Mealey BL, et al (eds): Periodontal Medicine. Toronto, BC Decker, Inc., 1999.
54. Semba SE, Mealey BL, Hallmon WW: The head and neck radiotherapy patient: Part 1. Oral manifestations of radiation therapy. Compendium Contin Educ Dent 1994; 15:250.
55. Semba SE, Mealey BL, Hallmon WW: Dentistry and the cancer patient: Part 2. Oral health management of the chemotherapy patient. Compendium Contin Educ Dent 1994; 15:1378.
56. Shapiro BA: Clinical Application of Respiratory Care, ed 4. Chicago, Year Book Medical, 1991.
57. Shapiro R, Carroll PB, Tzakis A, et al: Adrenal reserve in renal transplant recipients with cyclosporine/azathioprine/prednisone immunosuppression. Transplantation 1990; 49:1011.
58. Sherman RG, Lasseter DH: Pharmacologic management of patients with diseases of the endocrine system. Dent Clin North Am 1996; 40:727.
59. Shrout MK: Managing patients undergoing radiation. J Am Dent Assoc 1991; 122:69.
60. Shrout MK, Scarbrough F, Powell BJ: Dental care and the prosthetic joint patient: A survey of orthopedic surgeons and general dentists. J Am Dent Assoc 1994; 125:429.
61. Sindet-Pedersen S, Stenbjerg S, Ingerslev J: Control of gingival hemorrhage in hemophilic patients by inhibition of fibrinolysis with tranexamic acid. J Periodont Res 1988; 23:72.
62. Slots J, Rosling BG, Genco RJ: Suppression of penicillin resistant oral *Actinobacillus actinomycetemcomitans* with tetracycline. Considerations in endocarditis prophylaxis. J Periodontol 1983; 54:193.
63. Smith GN, Pashley DH: Periodontal ligament injection: Evaluation of systemic effects. Oral Surg Oral Med Oral Pathol 1983; 56:571.
64. Smolensky MH: Chronobiology and chronotherapeutics: Applications to cardiovascular medicine. Am J Hypertens 1996; 9(4 Pt 3):s11.
65. Tarsitano BF, Rollings RE: The pregnant patient: Evaluation and management. Gen Dent 1993; 41:226.
66. Tervonen T, Karjalainen K: Periodontal disease related to diabetic status. A pilot study of the response to periodontal therapy in type 1 diabetes. J Clin Periodontol 1997; 24:505.

67. Thyne GM, Ferguson JW: Antibiotic prophylaxis during dental treatment in patients with prosthetic joints. J Bone Joint Surg (Br) 1991; 73B:191.
68. U.K. Prospective Diabetes Study (UKPDS) Group: Intensive blood glucose control with sulphonylureas or insulin compared with conventional treatment and risk of complications in patients with type 2 diabetes (UKPDS 33). Lancet 1998; 352:837.
69. Umino M, Nagao M: Systemic diseases in elderly dental patients. Int Dent J 1993; 43:213.
70. Watanabe K: Prepubertal periodontitis: A review of diagnostic criteria, pathogenesis, and differential diagnosis. J Periodont Res 1990; 25:31.
71. Westfelt E, Rylander H, Blohme G, et al: The effect of periodontal therapy in diabetics. Results after 5 years. J Clin Periodontol 1996; 23:92
72. Yagiela JA: Adverse drug interactions in dental practice: Interactions associated with vasoconstrictors. J Am Dent Assoc 1999; 130:701.
73. Ziccardi VB, Abubaker AO, Sotereanos GC, et al: Maxillofacial considerations in orthotopic liver transplantation. Oral Surg Oral Med Oral Pathol 1991; 71:21.
74. Ziccardi VB, Saini J, Demas PN, et al: Management of the oral and maxillofacial surgery patient with end-stage renal disease. J Oral Maxillofac Surg 1992; 50:1207.

Periodontal Treatment for Older Adults

Denise J. Fedele and Linda C. Niessen

CHAPTER

CHAPTER OUTLINE

During the late 20th century, the proportion of older adults experienced significant growth with greater increases expected in the 21st century. Currently, almost 70% of older adults have natural teeth.[14] The future trend will be more people with more teeth at risk for periodontal disease. Aging does not cause disease; however, age is associated with more disease. This association was addressed by Jim Beck at the 1996 World Workshop on Periodontics: "It may be that risk factors do change as people or at least the relative importance of risk factors change."

The focus of this chapter is to provide the reader with information on the interrelationship between aging and oral health, with emphasis on periodontal health.

DEMOGRAPHICS

Population Distributions

In 1990, 4% of the U.S. population, or 3.1 million people, were age 65 or older. By 1994, these numbers grew to 13%, or 33.2 million people. From 2001 to 2010, persons aged 65+ years will grow by 13%, aged 85+ years by 29%, and aged 100+ years by 65%. In the first half of the 21st century, the U.S. population is expected to increase by 42%. Fig. 39-1 shows that during the same time period, people aged 65+ years are expected to increase 126%, aged 85+ years by 316%, and centenarians (100+) 956%.[20]

The growth in the older population is the result of the dramatic increase in life expectancy during the past century. Average life expectancy was 47 years in 1900 and 75 years by 1990. In 2000, life expectancy (at birth) was projected to be 77 years. People who reached the age of 65 in 1990 had an average of 17 remaining years of life expectancy.[18,20]

Health Status

Despite the advances in modern medicine that have increased life expectancy, the number of older adults with acute and chronic diseases continues to increase.[20] Visual

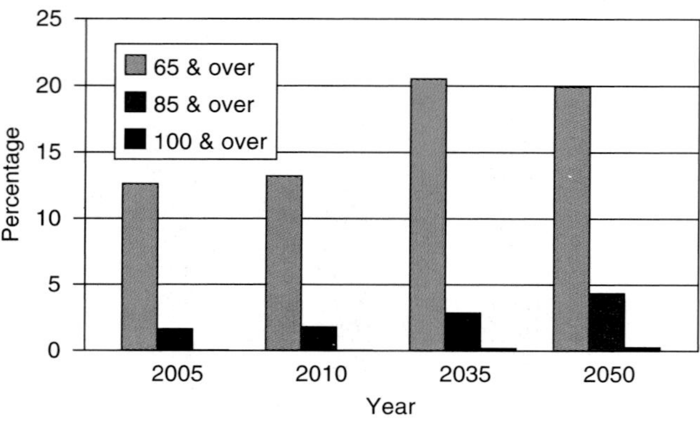

Fig. 39-1 Projected U.S. population trends for older adults. (From US Department of Commerce, Bureau of the Census: Report, Jan 20, 1998. Available at *www.census.gov*.)

TABLE 39-1

Percentage Dentate by Age and Gender, U.S., 1988–91

Age Group	All Persons	Gender	
		Male	Female
50–54	88	90	86
55–59	82	82	83
60–64	76	77	76
65–69	74	73	75
70–74	69	71	67
75+	56	53	58

See reference 14.

impairments, cataracts, glaucoma, and hearing impairments increase in frequency with advancing age.[21] Nearly half of people aged 65+ years have arthritis.[21] Most older adults have at least one chronic condition and many have several chronic conditions.[2] In 1994 the number of chronic conditions that occurred most often per 100 older persons were as follows: arthritis (50), hypertension (36), heart disease (32), hearing impairments (29), cataracts (17), orthopedic impairments (16), sinusitis (15), and diabetes (10).[2] Heart disease remains the leading cause of death among older adults. Approximately 7 in 10 deaths among older adults were caused by heart disease, cancer, or stroke.[20]

The prevalence of sensory impairments and arthritis can have dramatic influences on the oral health of older adults. It is more difficult for older adults with hearing, visual, and dexterity limitations to effectively communicate oral health care needs and concerns and perform good oral hygiene.

Social and Psychologic Issues Affecting Dental Treatment

The education level of older adults is increasing. In 1995, only 64% of noninstitutional older adults completed at least high school and 13% possessed a bachelor's degree. By the year 2015, it is estimated that 76% of older adults will have completed at least high school, with 20% obtaining a bachelor's degree. Those with higher education tend to be better off financially than those with low education. Poverty is less prevalent today among older adults for all race, gender, and ethnic groups.[19,20] In general, older adults have the highest disposable income of all age groups and they spend more money on luxury items such as vacations and automobiles.[23] Higher educational achievement with lower poverty levels suggests an increase in demand for oral health care among older adults.[10]

Dentate Status

Over the past several decades, the prevalence of tooth loss and edentulism has been declining in the U.S. Table 39-1 shows the most current estimates of tooth loss and retention in the U.S. These data indicate that 75% of adults aged 65 to 69 years are dentate and just over half of adults aged 75+ years are dentate.[14]

Periodontal Status

Recent data suggest that older adults who retain teeth are likely to be less susceptible to periodontitis.[6] Advanced periodontal disease among older adults is not as common as once thought.[6] Moderate levels of attachment loss are seen in a high proportion of older adults; however, severe loss is detected in only a small proportion of older adults.[12] The amount of periodontal disease that is associated with age does not appear to be clinically significant, and it is unclear whether the higher prevalence of periodontal disease is a function of age or time.[12] Figs. 39-2 to 39-4 illustrate periodontal disease data from Phase I of the Third National Health and Nutrition Examination Survey (NHANES III) conducted in the U.S. from 1988 to 1991.[5] Fig. 39-2 shows that gingival recession increases with advancing age, with one third (35%) of persons aged 55 to 84 years and less than half (46%) of persons aged 85+ years having 3 mm or more of gingival recession. Fig. 39-3 shows that pocket depth of 6 mm or greater was detected in 7% of persons aged 45 to 54 years, 8% of persons aged 55 to 64 years, and 7% of persons aged 65+ years. Attachment loss, which is displayed in Fig. 39-4, increases with age. Less than half of persons aged 65+ years had loss of attachment measuring 5 mm or greater.

The prevalence of periodontal disease increases with age and appears to be age associated.[4] Age increases the risk for periodontal destruction but is probably consistent with successful aging, not pathology.[12] Periodontal disease in older adults is probably not due to greater susceptibility but instead is the result of cumulative disease progression over time.[6]

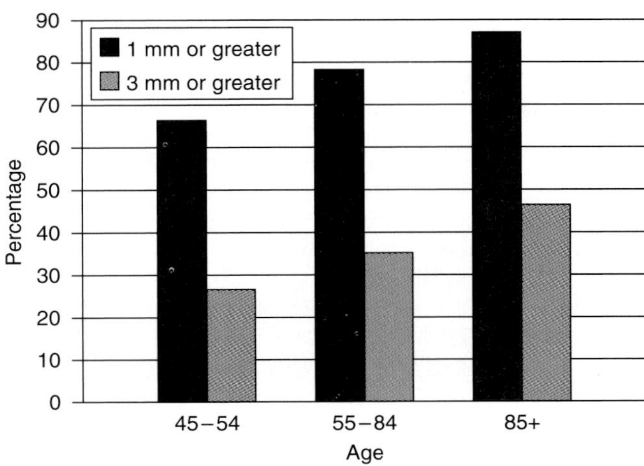

Fig. 39-2 Percentage of persons with gingival recession, 1988–91. (From Brown LJ, Brunelle JA, Kingman A: Periodontal status in the United States, 1988–1991: Prevalence, extent, and demographic variation. J Dent Res 1996; 75(Spec Iss):672.)

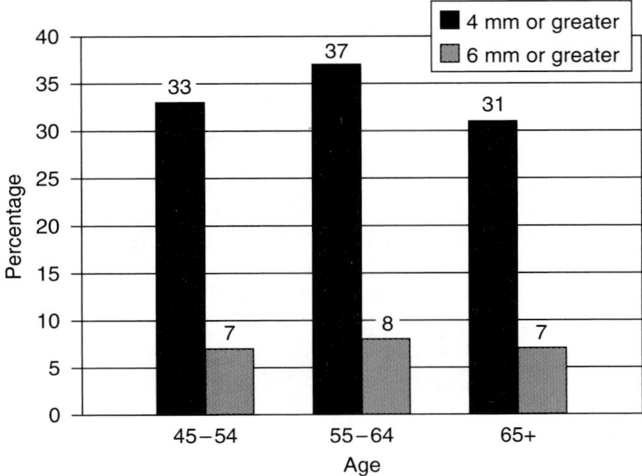

Fig. 39-3 Percentage of persons with pocket depths by age, 1988–91. (From Brown LJ, Brunelle JA, Kingman A: Periodontal status in the United States, 1988–1991: Prevalence, extent, and demographic variation. J Dent Res 1996; 75(Spec Iss):672.)

Caries Status

Root caries is a disease that is particular to older adults. Exposed root surfaces in combination with compromised health status and use of multiple medications make older adults at high risk for root caries. Caries examinations from the Phase I of NHANES III indicate that root caries prevalence increased greatly with age. Decayed or filled root surfaces were detected in 47% of persons aged 65 to 74 years and in 55.9% of persons 75+ years.[27]

Dental Visits

Dental visits by older adults are correlated with having teeth, not age.[23] Data from the 1995 Behavioral Risk Factor Surveillance System (BRFSS), which is a continuous state-based, random-digit-dialed telephone survey of the U.S. noninstitutional population aged 18+ years, indicate that older adults are frequent users of dental services. Of all persons responding to the oral health section, 69% reported having a dental visit in the past year. Among adults aged 65+ years, 62% reported having a dental visit during the previous year. However, 75% of adults aged 65+ years with natural teeth reported a dental visit in the past year.[7] Dental expenditure data indicate that older adults have a higher cost per visit than younger persons and are willing to make a significant investment in dental care.[23]

Xerostomia

Saliva plays an essential role in maintaining oral health. Many older adults take medications for chronic medical conditions and disorders. More than 500 prescription and over-the-counter medications are associated with decreased saliva, dry mouth, and xerostomia. The medications most often associated with xerostomia and decreased saliva are the tricyclic antidepressants, antihistamines, antihypertensives, and diuretics. Medication use is frequently associated with dry mouth; however, certain medical diseases, disorders, or conditions such as radiation treatment for oral, head, neck, and thyroid cancers; Sjögren's syndrome; poorly controlled diabetes; bone marrow transplantation; thyroid disorders; and depression are also associated with dry mouth.[9]

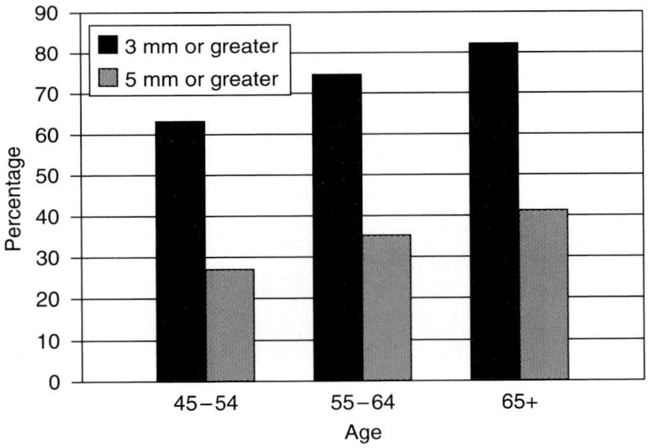

Fig. 39-4 Percentage with loss of attachment by age, 1988–91. (From Brown LJ, Brunelle JA, Kingman A: Periodontal status in the United States, 1988–1991: Prevalence, extent, and demographic variation. J Dent Res 1996; 75(Spec Iss):672.)

Medications that induce xerostomia may also be associated with compromised chewing, speaking, tasting, or swallowing and increased risk for caries, periodontal disease, and candidiasis.

Candidiasis

The overproliferation of *Candida albicans* and its infiltration into the oral mucosal layers results in a pathogenic infection. The causes can be both local and systemic, and the infection is collectively termed *candidiasis*.[11]

Any condition compromising a patient's immune system can be considered a risk factor for candidiasis. Oral candidiasis can occur with long-term use of medications such as antibiotics, steroid therapies, or chemotherapy. Diabetes mellitus, head and neck radiation therapy, and human immunodeficiency virus (HIV) are risk factors for acute pseudomembranous candida. Pseudomembranous candida presents as white lesions that can be wiped away with gauze, leaving an erythematous area.[11]

Chronic atrophic candidiasis presents most commonly as an erythematous area under a maxillary denture and is associated with poor oral hygiene. In patients without a prosthesis, chronic atrophic candidiasis may present as a generalized redness or even generalized burning of the mouth.[11]

Chronic atrophic candidiasis, or angular cheilitis, can also manifest itself in the creases or commissures of the lips. This occurs when a patient has a tendency to pool saliva around the corners of the mouth or constantly lick the lips in some cases.[11]

TABLE 39-2

Top 20 Drugs Prescribed in the U.S., 1998

Product	Drug Class
1. Premarin Tabs	Estrogen hormone
2. Synthroid	Thyroid hormone
3. Trimox	Antibiotic
4. Hydrocodone w/APAP	Combination narcotic analgesic
5. Prozac	Antidepressant/SSRI
6. Prilosec	Antisecretory compound/GI acid
7. Zithromax	Antibiotic
8. Lipitor	HMG-CoA reductase inhibitor
9. Norvasc	Calcium channel blocker
10. Claritin	H1-receptor antagonist/antihistamine
11. Lanoxin	Cardiac glycoside
12. Zoloft	Antidepressant/SSRI
13. Albuterol Aerosol	β2-agonist bronchodilator
14. Paxil	Antidepressant/SSRI
15. Amoxicillin	Antibiotic
16. Prempro	Estrogen and progestin combination
17. Zestril	ACE inhibitor
18. Vasotec	ACE inhibitor
19. Augmentin	Antibiotic
20. Cephalexin	Antibiotic

From Zoeller J: The top 200 drugs. Am Druggist 1999; 216:2.

DENTAL AND MEDICAL ASSESSMENTS

Review of Dental History

At the very least, the review should include past restorative, periodontal, and other dental treatment; head and neck cancer and its treatment; allergies, oral hygiene care techniques; tobacco and alcohol use; and any difficulties or problems associated with dental treatment. In addition, the dental history should review past injuries, the individual's perception of past and future dental treatment outcomes, the fluoride status of the drinking water (bottled, well, community), and the type of toothpaste used (fluoride versus nonfluoride).

Review of Medical History

The medical history should be detailed and include a careful review of past and current medical and mental conditions including allergies and invasive procedures. The review should focus on a careful evaluation of systemic diseases and disorders, particularly those that influence dental treatment such as bleeding disorders and use of anticoagulants, diabetes, heart valve problems, certain cardiovascular conditions, stroke, artificial joints, and use of corticosteroids. A consultation with the individual's physician is advisable, especially for individuals with medical problems or if complicated or invasive procedures are planned. Although obtaining a complete medical history may take longer with older adults, the dialogue between the dentist and the patient often yields valuable medical, psychologic, and dental treatment information.

Review of Medication Use

Older adults are high users of prescription and over-the-counter medications. Table 39-2 lists the top 20 drugs prescribed in the U.S. in 1998. Many medications used by older adults can have a negative impact on oral health. To obtain a complete list of prescription and over-the-counter medications, ask patients to bring each medication bottle or package to the dental office. This helps not only obtain a complete medication list but also provides additional information such as medication dose and number of physicians prescribing medications.

Assessment of Risk

The American Society of Anesthesiologists established a useful tool to predict risk of surgical mortality.[3,16] The tool (Box 39-1) stratifies patients into five categories, adjusts for age by not allowing an older adult to be assigned into Class I, and has been validated for patients aged 80+ years. This classification system was originally designed to assess surgical risk under general anesthesia; however, it is also currently used to assess risk before diagnostic testing and outpatient surgery. Dentists can use this tool for patient assessment before invasive periodontal procedures.[16]

In addition to assessing medical risk, the dentist should evaluate the risk factors that influence the progression of periodontal disease. The prognostic risk factors that influence periodontal therapy are smoking, genetic susceptibility, compliance, and diabetes.[25]

Intraoral and Extraoral Examination

In addition to assessing past dental treatment, tooth loss, restorations, past dental interventions, dental caries, and periodontal status, the comprehensive dental examination should include a complete head and neck examination of soft tissues. Oral and pharyngeal cancer is an age-related oral disease with serious consequences.

Skin of the face and neck should be inspected and palpated for lesions, enlarged lymph nodes, or both. Intraorally, the lips, cheeks, tongue, gingiva, floor of mouth, palate, retromolar trigon, and oropharynx should be inspected and palpated to detect soft tissue abnormalities, particularly red or white patches, ulcerations, or swellings.

The risk for oral and pharyngeal cancer increases with age, tobacco use, frequent use of alcohol, and exposure to sunlight (lip). Oral cancer is treatable if discovered and treated early. Oral and pharyngeal cancer detected at later stages can cause disfigurement, loss of function, decreased quality of life, and death. Surveillance, Epidemiology, and End Results (SEER) data indicate that more than 50% of tongue and floor of mouth cancers had metastasized to a distant site at time of diagnosis.[17] In addition, over the last 25 years, the 5-year survival rate of oral cancer has not improved.[17] Oral and pharyngeal cancer lesions may not be painful. Oral cancer may appear as an ulceration, a swelling, or a red or white sore that does not heal within 1 to 2 weeks. Other signs of oral cancer may be swollen lymph nodes and difficulty swallowing and speaking.[8]

PERIODONTAL DISEASES IN OLDER ADULTS

Etiology

The relationship between age and periodontal disease is age associated and not a consequence of aging.[4] Periodontal disease in older adults is commonly referred to as *chronic periodontitis*.[11,16] Because periodontitis is a chronic disease, much of the ravages of the disease detected in older adults results from an accumulation of the disease over time. Research has shown that the advanced stages of periodontitis are less prevalent than the moderate stages in the older-adult population.[5,11,16] One theory is that many sites of advanced periodontal disease have resulted in tooth loss earlier in life, suggesting that older age is not a risk factor for periodontal disease.[11,16]

Little evidence is available as to whether the risk factors for periodontal disease differ with age.[4] General health status, immune status, diabetes, nutrition, smoking, genetics, medications, mental health status, salivary flow, functional deficits, or finances may possibly modify the relationship between periodontal disease and age.[4,25]

Some medications that are frequently prescribed to older adults can alter the gingival tissues. Steroid-induced gingivitis has been associated with postmenopausal women on steroid therapy. Gingival overgrowth can be induced by certain medications such as cyclosporines, calcium channel blockers, and anticonvulsants (e.g., nifedipine or phenytoin) in the presence of poor oral hygiene. This gingival overgrowth further decreases a person's ability to maintain good oral hygiene.[11]

Relationship to Systemic Disease

A recent review of the literature conducted by Loesche indicates poor oral health has been associated with medical conditions such as aspiration pneumonia and cardiovascular disease. In particular, periodontal disease can be associated with coronary heart disease and cerebrovascular accidents.[13] In addition, the Surgeon General's Report on Oral Health emphasizes that animal and population-based studies demonstrate an association between periodontal disease and diabetes, cardiovascular disease, and stroke.[22]

PERIODONTAL TREATMENT PLANNING

Generally, periodontal disease in older adults is not a rapidly progressive disease but often presents as long-standing chronic disease. Because periodontal disease

BOX 39-1

American Society of Anesthesiologists (ASA) Classification of Physical Status

1. A normal healthy patient.
2. A patient with mild systemic disease.
3. A patient with severe systemic disease that limits activity but is not incapacitating.
4. A patient with an incapacitating systemic disease that is a constant threat to life.
5. A moribund patient not expected to survive 24 hours with or without operation.

E. Precede an emergency operation with an E.

See reference 3.

has periods of exacerbation and remission, understanding and documenting periods of active disease versus quiescent periods is essential to the formulation of the treatment plan and prognosis.[16]

Periodontal disease must be diagnosed regardless of age. The goal of periodontal treatment for both young and old patients is to preserve function and eliminate or prevent the progression of inflammatory disease.[24] Several factors must be considered during treatment planning for older individuals.[16] Periodontal healing and recurrence of disease are not influenced by age.[4] Factors to consider are medical and mental health status, medications, functional status, and lifestyle behaviors that influence periodontal treatment, outcome, or progression of disease.[24] Periodontal disease severity, medical and mental status, medications, function, ability to perform oral hygiene procedures, and the individual's ability to tolerate treatment should be evaluated and considered during treatment planning.[16] The risks and benefits of both surgical and nonsurgical therapy should be considered.[16] Also important is the amount of remaining periodontal support or past periodontal destruction, tooth type, number of occlusal contacts, and individual patient preferences.[24] Dental implants are a reliable replacement for missing teeth in older adults.[26] Age alone is not a contraindication for implant placement.

For older adults, a nonsurgical approach is often the first treatment choice.[24] Depending on the nature and extent of periodontal disease, surgical therapy may be indicated.[16,24] Surgical technique should minimize the amount of additional root exposure.[24] Individuals responding best to surgical therapy are those who are able to maintain the surgical result.[16] Age alone is not a contraindication to surgery.[16] For individuals who are not able to comply with treatment, have poor oral hygiene, or are medically or mentally compromised or functionally impaired, palliative supportive periodontal care instead of surgical periodontal treatment is often the optimal treatment approach.[24]

A common goal for all older adults is to decrease bacteria through oral hygiene and mechanical debridement. Clinical trials involving older adults show that the development or progression of periodontal disease can be prevented or arrested by the control of plaque. For certain patients, topical antibiotic therapy may complement repeated subgingival instrumentation during supportive care. Oral hygiene maintenance should also focus on root surfaces susceptible to caries.[24]

PREVENTION OF PERIODONTAL DISEASE AND MAINTENANCE OF PERIODONTAL HEALTH IN OLDER ADULTS

For both younger and older persons, the most important factor determining a successful outcome of periodontal treatment is plaque control and frequency of professional care.[24] Advanced age does not decrease plaque control; however, older adults may have difficulty performing adequate oral hygiene because of compromised health, mental status, medications, and altered mobility and dexterity.[24] Older adults may change toothbrush habits due to disabilities such as hemiplegia secondary to CVA, visual difficulties, dementia, and arthritis. The newer, lightweight, electric-powered toothbrushes may be more beneficial than a manual toothbrush for older adults with physical and sensory limitations. The proportion of people who report flossing decreases with age >40 years.[23] This may be partly due to impairment of fine motor skills secondary to disease or injury. Interproximal brushes, shaped wooden toothpicks, or mechanical flossing devices often can be used in place of traditional flossing with satisfactory outcomes.

Chemotherapeutic Agents

Antiplaque Agents

Patients who are unable to adequately remove plaque secondary to disease or disability may benefit from antiplaque agents such as chlorhexidine and Listerine or its generic counterparts.[16,23]

Chlorhexidine is a cationic bisbiguanide that has been used as a broad-spectrum antiseptic in medicine since the 1950s. In Europe, a 0.2% concentration of chlorhexidine has been used for years as a preventive and therapeutic agent.[16,23] Chlorhexidine binding to oral structures results in substantivity. It is either bacteriostatic or bactericidal depending on the dose. Some adverse effects of chlorhexidine include an increase in calculus formation, staining of teeth, dysgeusia (altered taste), and permanent staining of teeth.[1] Chlorhexidine is a prescription rinse for short-term use (<6 months); long-term use (>6 months) has not been extensively studied.[23] The American Dental Association (ADA) Council on Dental Therapeutics has approved chlorhexidine to help prevent and reduce supragingival plaque and gingivitis.[1,23] Although chlorhexidine has not been studied in older adults, outcomes in younger persons, including those with disabilities, suggest that it is also effective in older adults. Chlorhexidine may be particularly useful for older adults who have difficulty with plaque removal and those who take phenytoin, calcium channel blockers, and cyclosporins and are at risk for gingival hyperplasia.[16,23]

Listerine antiseptic and its generic counterparts are approved by the ADA Council on Dental Therapeutics to help prevent and reduce supragingival plaque and gingivitis.[16,23] The active ingredients in Listerine are methyl salicylate and three essential oils (eucalyptol, thymol, and menthol).[1,23] Listerine has been shown to be effective in reducing plaque and gingivitis when compared with placebo rinses in young healthy adults. Listerine, which is high in alcohol (ranging from 21.6% to 26.9%), may exacerbate xerostomia and is generally contraindicated in patients under treatment for alcoholism who take Antabuse (disulfiram). Listerine may benefit patients who do not tolerate the taste or staining of chlorhexidine, is sold over the counter, and is less expensive and easier to obtain than chlorhexidine.[16,23]

Fluoride. Fluoride, nature's cavity fighter, is the most effective caries preventive agent currently available. Fluoride's effects are to (1) reduce enamel solubility; (2) promote remineralization of early carious lesions; (3) bactericidally affect metabolic process of bacterial plaque.[16,23]

Topical fluorides are recommended for the prevention and treatment of dental caries. Over-the-counter fluorides include fluoride dentifrices, rinses, and gels that contain concentrations of 230 to 1500 PPM fluoride ions. Prescription 1.1% neutral sodium fluoride gels are available with a fluoride concentration of 5000 PPM fluoride ion. Professionally applied fluoride gel, foam, or varnish products are between 9050 and 22,600 PPM fluoride ion.[1]

Saliva Substitutes. Saliva substitutes, which are intended to match the chemical and physical traits of saliva, are available to relieve the symptoms of dry mouth. Their composition is varied; however, they usually contain salt ions, a flavoring agent, paraben (preservative), cellulose derivative or animal mucins, and fluoride. The ADA's seal of approval has been granted for some artificial saliva products such as Saliva Substitute and Salivart.[1] Most saliva substitutes can be used ad libitum by patients and are dispensed in spray bottle, rinse/swish bottle, or oral swabstick.[1,23] In addition, products such as dry mouth toothpastes and moisturizing gels are also available.

Patients with dry mouth may also benefit by stimulating saliva flow with sugarless candies and sugarless gum. Xylitol chewing gum has been shown to have anticariogenic properties in children. Although no studies have confirmed the effectiveness of xylitol gum in preventing caries in adults, patients with high root caries prevalence and xerostomia may benefit from chewing xylitol gum.[15]

CONCLUSION

Future oral health care trends will see increased numbers of older adults seeking periodontal therapy. Dental practitioners of the 21st century should be comfortable providing comprehensive periodontal care for this segment of the population. Aging dental patients have particular oral and general health conditions that dentists should be familiar with detecting, consulting, and treating. Medical diseases and conditions that occur more often with age may require modification to periodontal preventive tools as well as the planning and treatment phases of periodontal care.

REFERENCES

1. ADA Guide to Dental Therapeutics, ed 2. American Dental Association. Chicago, ADA Publishing, 2000.
2. Administration on Aging: A profile of older Americans, 1998. Available at *http://www.aoa.dhhs.gov.*
3. American Society of Anesthesiologists: New classification of physical status. Anesthesiology 1963; 24:111.
4. Beck JD: Periodontal implications: Older adults. Ann Periodontol 1996; 1:322.
5. Brown LJ, Brunelle JA, Kingman A: Periodontal status in the United States, 1988–1991: Prevalence, extent, and demographic variation. J Dent Res 1996; 75(Spec Iss):672.
6. Burt BA, Eklund SA: Dentistry, Dental Practice, and the Community. Philadelphia, Saunders, 1999.
7. Centers for Disease Control and Prevention: Dental service use and dental insurance coverage—United States, behavioral risk factor surveillance system, 1995. MMWR 1997; 46(50):1199.
8. Fedele DJ, Jones JA, Niessen LC: Oral cancer screening in the elderly. J Am Geriatr Soc 1991; 39(9):920.
9. Fox PC: Management of dry mouth. Dent Clin North Am 1997; 41(4):863.
10. Jones JA, Fedele DJ, Bolden AJ, et al: Gains in dental care use not shared by minority elders, 1994. J Public Health Dent 1994; 54:39.
11. Gibson G, Niessen LC: Aging and the oral cavity. In: Cassel CK, Cohen HJ, Larson EB, et al (eds): Geriatric Medicine. New York, Springer-Verlag, 1997.
12. Locker D, Slade GD, Murray H: Epidemiology of periodontal disease among older adults: A review. Periodontology 2000 1998; 16:16.
13. Loesche WJ, Lopatin DE: Interaction between periodontal disease, medical disease and immunity in the older individual. Periodontology 2000 1998; 16:80.
14. Marcus SE, Drury TF, Brown LJ, et al: Tooth retention and tooth loss in the permanent dentition of adults: United States, 1988–1991. J Dent Res 1996; 75(Spec Iss):684.
15. Niessen LC, Gibson G: Oral health for a lifetime: Preventive strategies for the older adult. Quintessence Int 1997; 28(9):626.
16. Suzuki JB, Niessen LC, Fedele DJ: Periodontal diseases in the older adult. In: Papas AS, Niessen LC, Chauncey HH (eds): Geriatric Dentistry: Aging and Oral Health. St Louis, Mosby, 1991.
17. Shiboski CH, Shiboski SC, Silverman S, Jr: Trends in oral cancer rates in the United States, 1973–1996. Comm Dent Oral Epidemiol 2000; 28:249.
18. US Bureau of the Census: Statistical Abstract of the United States: 1996, 116th ed. Washington, DC, The Bureau, 1996.
19. US Department of Commerce, Economics and Statistics Administration, Bureau of the Census: Aging in the United States—Past, Present, and Future. Washington, DC, National Institute on Aging, July 1997.
20. US Department of Commerce, Bureau of the Census: Report, Jan 20, 1998. Available at *http://www.census.gov.*
21. US Department of Health and Human Services, Public Health Service: Current estimates from the National Health Interview Survey, 1991. Series 10, No. 184, DHHS Pub No. (PHS) 93-1512, Hyattsville, MD, December 1992.
22. US Department of Health and Human Services: Oral Health in America: A Report of the Surgeon General. Rockville, MD, US Department of Health and Human Services, National Institute of Dental and Craniofacial Research, National Institutes of Health, 2000 (NIH Publication No. 00-4713).
23. Wells LM, Kolavic S, Niessen LC, et al: Caring for older adults: Maintaining oral health for a lifetime. In: Hardin JF: Clark's Clinical Dentistry, vol 1. Philadelphia, JB Lippincott, 1996.
24. Wennstrom JL: Treatment of periodontal disease in older adults. Periodontology 2000 1998; 16:106.
25. Wilson TG: Using risk assessment to customized periodontal treatment. CDA Journal 1999; 27(8):627.
26. Wilson TG, Higginbottom FL: Periodontal disease and dental implants in older adults. J Esthetic Dent 1998; 10:265.
27. Winn DM, Brunelle JA, Selwitz RH, et al: Coronal and root caries in the dentition of adults in the United States, 1988–1991. J Dent Res 1996; 75(Spec Iss):642.

Treatment of Refractory Periodontitis, Aggressive Periodontitis, Necrotizing Ulcerative Periodontitis, and Periodontitis Associated with Systemic Diseases

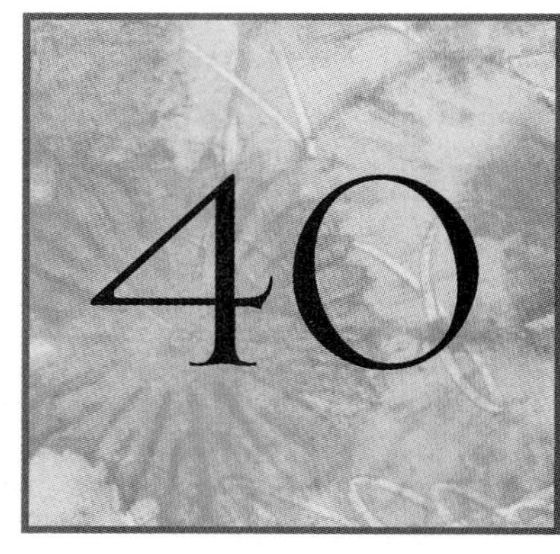

CHAPTER

Richard J. Nagy and Michael G. Newman

CHAPTER OUTLINE

The majority of patients with the commonly encountered forms of chronic periodontitis usually respond well to conventional therapies. Typically, these include nonsurgical débridement and possibly surgery in some patients, followed by adequate long-term maintenance. However, some patients (as many as 17%) with atypical and less frequently encountered types of periodontitis do not respond to these conventional treatment approaches. The major classifications of these atypical forms of periodontitis are refractory, aggressive, necrotizing ulcerative, and periodontitis associated with systemic diseases.[13,23]

The treatment of all of these types of periodontitis is complex and often requires the use of the most intensive and comprehensive therapeutic modalities. Because these patients do not respond "normally" to conventional methods, the logical question is whether there are problems associated with their host response systems. Although there have been many attempts to clarify the immunologic profile of these patients, there have been no major or definitive breakthroughs important for improving the outcomes of therapy. The best treatment for these patients appears to be the combination of a thorough root débridement with or without surgical access, antimicrobial therapy and a closely monitored supportive periodontal therapy maintenance program. Bacterial identification appears to be of value for treatment in these patients, because the information can be used to determine the antibiotic susceptibility of suspected pathogens. Similarly, other bacterial tests have been used to monitor the microflora that recolonize after treatment.

DIAGNOSIS OF REFRACTORY PERIODONTITIS

Although refractory periodontitis is not a currently accepted diagnosis (see Chapter 4), many patients fail to respond to conventional therapy, and their management will be discussed. A diagnosis of refractory periodontitis requires the gathering of baseline data and a subsequent evaluation. This is the major way in which the clinician can determine the normality of the patient's response to treatment (see Chapter 27). A few individuals may appear for the first time with unusually severe forms of periodontal destruction for their age. In these cases the initial diagnosis is not refractory periodontitis, but one of the other aggressive diseases discussed later in this chapter.

A patient with refractory periodontitis often does not have any distinguishing clinical characteristics on initial examination compared with other types of periodontitis. Therefore the initial treatment would follow conventional therapeutic modalities for chronic periodontitis.

After treatment, the differential diagnosis of refractory periodontitis should exclude the following:

1. *Improperly treated periodontitis.* Most forms of periodontitis can be treated effectively with currently available modalities if such modalities are performed properly. If, during a posttreatment examination, it is determined that the patient has not adequately responded to treatment, it must be determined whether the therapy was correctly implemented. The only way to rule out inadequately treated periodontitis is to perform the most thorough treatment available. Treatment to eradicate or control all etiologic factors and use of the most advanced techniques is essential.
2. *Periodontitis associated with poor plaque control by the patient.* Because plaque control is a prerequisite for the success of periodontal treatments,[27,34,35] special attention should be paid to the careful evaluation of plaque control before deciding on classifying a case as refractory periodontitis. Truly refractory periodontitis presupposes a type of periodontal disease that is far more nonresponsive or tenacious than the usual cases. A patient who does not comply with adequate oral hygiene procedures may also be viewed by many clinicians as a failure of the dental professional to adequately motivate, educate, and control the patient. If considered from this perspective, these cases should be included in the "improperly treated periodontitis" category.
3. *Endodontic lesions.* The presence of endodontic involvement should be suspected and ruled out before a diagnosis of refractory periodontitis is made. The clinician should suspect an endodontic etiology especially in those patients with localized recurrent disease.

A true case of refractory periodontitis can be diagnosed if loss of attachment has occurred after well-executed treatment and plaque removal has been performed by both the clinician and the patient and all etiologic agents have been controlled.

TREATMENT MODALITIES

Refractory Periodontitis

Estimates of prognosis and treatment predictability must be based on the evidence available from the literature and the clinician's own experience.[25] The first step in the treatment of refractory periodontitis with antimicrobial therapy must be microbial diagnostic and susceptibility tests. These microbiologic tests include culture analysis, microscopic assessment, nucleic acid probe analysis, restriction endonuclease analysis, detection of bacterial antigens and enzymes, and analysis using polymerase chain reaction. The results of these tests provide information about the presence and relative percentages of suspected periodontal pathogens and, more importantly, determine the organism's sensitivity to specific antimicrobials. This information enables the clinician to make the most informed and appropriate decision about antibiotic selection.

A combination of thorough root débridement and systemic antibiotic treatment can reduce bleeding on probing, suppuration, pocket depth, and incidence of active lesions and can suppress or eliminate periodontal pathogens in patients who present with refractory periodontitis. Mechanical débridement with scaling and root planing can reduce total supra- and subgingival bacterial masses, but major pathogens such as *Actinobacillus actinomycetemcomitans* may escape the effect of treatment due to their ability to invade periodontal tissues or to reside in furcations or other tooth structures outside the reach of hand instruments or due to poor host defense mechanisms. Surgical treatment may also eliminate the marginal tissues that might be invaded by bacteria.[36] In addition, the morphology of the gingival tissues should be modified to facilitate daily plaque removal by the patient.

Systemic antibiotic therapy aims to reinforce mechanical periodontal treatment and support the host defense system in overcoming the infection by killing subgingival pathogens that remain after conventional mechanical periodontal therapy. Antibiotic therapy in the treatment of refractory periodontitis is based on the results obtained from microbial diagnostic tests. Many antibiotics have been used according to the target microflora (Table 40-1) with various degrees of success.[12] For refractory periodontitis patients who fail to respond to initial antibiotic therapy, subsequent treatment should include antimicrobial susceptibility testing of the remaining flora, which is accomplished through culturing only.

Patients diagnosed as having refractory periodontitis often present with a history of tetracycline therapy and microflora that is relatively resistant to this drug, owing

TABLE 40-1

Antibiotic Therapy in the Treatment of Refractory or Rapidly Progressive Periodontitis

Associated Microflora	Antibiotic of Choice
Gram-positive organisms	Amoxicillin-clavulanate potassium (Augmentin)[6,44]
Gram-negative organisms	Clindamycin[11,12,43,44]
Nonoral gram-negative facultative rods	Ciprofloxacin[22]
Pseudomonads, staphylococci	
Black-pigmented bacteria and spirochetes	Metronidazole[11,39]
Prevotella intermedia, Porphyromonas gingivalis	Tetracycline[30]
A. actinomycetemcomitans	Metronidazole/amoxicillin[11,39]
	Metronidazole/Ciprofloxacin
	Tetracycline[20,28]
P. gingivalis	Azithromycin[29]

to the frequent use of this antibiotic.[16,24,42,44] Tetracycline-resistant bacteria containing the Tet m gene for resistance have been isolated from patients with refractory periodontitis.[28] However, some patients with refractory periodontitis may still benefit from the use of tetracycline or one of its derivatives.

Cases of refractory periodontitis in which the associated microflora consists primarily of gram-positive microorganisms have been successfully treated with amoxicillin-clavulanate potassium. Many efforts have been made to establish the most appropriate regimen of antibiotic therapy for these patients. Similar antimicrobials, consisting of 250 mg amoxicillin and 125 mg potassium clavulanate, have been administered three times daily for 14 days along with scaling and root planing and produced a reduction in attachment loss for at least 12 months. A regimen of one capsule containing the same amount of drug every 6 hours for 2 weeks, with intrasulcular full-mouth lavage with a 10% povidone-iodine solution and chlorhexidine mouthwash rinses twice daily, showed a reduction in attachment loss that persisted at approximately 34 months.[6] A regimen of 500 mg metronidazole three times daily for 7 days was shown to be effective in treating refractory periodontitis in patients who were culture positive for *Bacteroides forsythus* in the absence of *A. actinomycetemcomitans*.[45]

Clindamycin is a potent antibiotic that penetrates well into gingival fluid, although it is not usually effective against *A. actinomycetemcomitans* and *Eikenella corrodens*.[41] However, it has been demonstrated to be effective in controlling the extent and rate of disease progression in refractory cases in patients who have a microflora susceptible to this antibiotic.[11,22,43] A regimen of clindamycin hydrochloride 150 mg four times daily for 7 days combined with scaling and root planing produced a decrease in the incidence of disease activity from an annual rate of 8% to 0.5% of sites per patient.[11] Clindamycin should be prescribed with caution due to the potential for pseudomembranous colitis from superinfections with *Clostridium difficile*. Azithromycin may be effective in refractory periodontitis in patients infected with *Porphyromonas gingivalis*.[29]

Combinations of antibiotic therapy may offer greater promise as adjunctive treatment for the management of refractory periodontitis.[1,7,24] The rationale is based on the diversity of putative pathogens[10,39] and the fact that no single antibiotic is bactericidal for all known pathogens. Combination antibiotic therapy may help broaden the antimicrobial range of the therapeutic regimen beyond that attained by any single antibiotic. Other advantages include lowering the dose of individual antibiotics by exploiting possible synergy between two drugs against targeted organisms. In addition, combination therapy may prevent or forestall the emergence of bacterial resistance.

Many combinations of antibiotics (e.g., metronidazole [Augmentin][7,17] or metronidazole/amoxicillin for the treatment of *A. actinomycetemcomitans*–associated periodontitis; metronidazole/doxycycline for the prevention of recurrent periodontitis; metronidazole/ciprofloxacin[32] for the treatment of recurrent cases containing a microflora associated with enteric rods and pseudomonads; and amoxicillin/doxycycline[24] in the treatment of *A. actinomycetemcomitans*– and/or *Porphyromonas gingivalis*–associated periodontitis) have demonstrated significant improvement in the clinical aspects of the disease.[24]

Some cases of refractory periodontitis may not respond to a given antibiotic regimen. When this occurs, the clinician should consider a different antimicrobial therapy based on microbial susceptibility analysis. At this point in the therapy, strong consideration should be given to consulting with the patient's physician for an evaluation of a possible host immune system deficiency or a metabolic problem such as diabetes.

Although there have been no studies of the treatment of refractory periodontitis with local delivery systems, it is possible that this method could be used in localized forms of this disease, particularly localized aggressive periodontal diseases. The advantage of local therapy is that smaller dosages of topical chemotherapy can be delivered inside the pocket, avoiding the side effects of systemic antibacterial agents. These local therapies are in the forms of gels, fibers, or chips.[8,9,15]

Another approach for treating refractory periodontitis and other forms of periodontal disease is through modulation of the host response by subantimicrobial or nonsteroidal antiinflammatory drugs (NSAIDs) in conjunction with conventional therapy. The use of low-dose doxycycline may aid in preventing the destruction of the periodontal attachment through controlling the activation of matrix metalloproteinases, primarily collagenase and gelatinase, from both infiltrating and resident cells of the periodontium, primarily the neutrophils.[38] Other agents such as flurbiprofen, indomethacin, and naproxen may reduce inflammatory mediator production during chronic periodontal disease.[14] Further research needs to be done to substantiate the effects of these agents.

The approach to restorative treatment for these patients should be made based on one single premise: *Plan for future tooth loss.* The teeth with the best prognosis should be identified and considered when planning the restorative work. However, the predictive value of the traditional prognosis categorization can be as low as 43% in patients with refractory periodontitis.[13] The lower cuspids and first premolars are generally more resistant to loss. As a rule, an extensive fixed prosthesis should be avoided, and removable partial dentures should be planned in such a way as to allow for the addition of teeth. The use of dental implants should be considered with great caution, especially in partially edentulous patients.

Although a cause-and-effect relationship has not yet been established between periodontitis and periimplantitis, a relationship between the microflora associated with periodontal and peri-implant pockets, has been described.[20,31,33] The combination of implants and periodontally diseased teeth may be possible, but the risks involved should be clearly explained to the patient and avoided until the patient's disease is stabilized.

Aggressive Periodontitis

The prognosis for patients with aggressive periodontitis (formerly early onset periodontitis) depends on whether the disease is generalized or localized and on the degree of destruction present at the time of examination. The generalized forms, which are usually associated with some systemic disease (see Chapter 28), have a worse prognosis than the localized forms. Aggressive periodontitis rarely undergoes spontaneous remission. It is important to obtain earlier radiographs to assess the stage of the disease.

The following treatments for localized aggressive periodontitis have been attempted in the past, with various degrees of success:

1. *Extraction.* After the involved teeth, usually the first molars, have been extracted, uneventful healing ensues. The enlargement of the maxillary sinus has been mentioned as an unfavorable sequela that would make future treatment of neighboring teeth difficult.[2] Transplantation of developing third molars to the sockets of previously extracted first molars has also been attempted.
2. *Standard periodontal therapy.* Such therapy has included scaling and root planing, curettage, flap surgery with and without bone grafts, root amputations, hemisections, occlusal adjustment, and strict plaque control.[3,37] However, response has been unpredictable. Frequent maintenance visits appear to be most important.[19,40]
3. *Antibiotic therapy.* In the late 1970s and early 1980s, the identification of *A. actinomycetemcomitans* as a major culprit and the discovery that this organism penetrates the tissues clarified the pathogenesis and provided a more solid basis for therapy.[5] Several authors have reported success using antibiotics as adjuncts to standard therapy. Genco and colleagues[10] reported the treatment of localized aggressive periodontitis with scaling and root planing plus tetracycline (250 mg four times daily for 14 days every 8 weeks). Measurements of vertical defects were made at intervals of up to 18 months after the initiation of therapy. Bone loss had stopped, and one third of the defects demonstrated an increase in bone level, whereas in the control group, bone loss continued.

Liljenberg and Lindhe[18] treated patients with localized aggressive periodontitis with tetracycline (250 mg four times daily for 2 weeks), modified Widman flaps, and periodic recall visits (one visit every month for 6 months, then one visit every 3 months). The lesions healed more rapidly and more completely than similar lesions in patients with chronic periodontitis. These investigators reevaluated their results after 5 years and found that the treatment had resulted in resolution of gingival inflammation, gain of clinical attachment, and refill of bone in angular defects.[19]

Several investigators have noted excellent bone fill in cases of localized aggressive periodontitis treated with tetracycline plus flap surgery and placement of grafts.[21,46] Figs. 40-1 and 40-2 show pretreatment destruction and bone repair in a patient treated by Barnett and Baker.[4]

The lack of response of juvenile periodontitis to local therapy alone has been interpreted as the result of the presence of *A. actinomycetemcomitans* in the tissues,[5,36] where it remains after therapy to reinfect the pocket. The systemic use of antibiotics is needed to eliminate bacteria from the tissues.[22]

Current Approach to Therapy. Patients who are diagnosed as having an early form of aggressive periodontitis may respond to standard periodontal therapy. In general, the earlier the disease is diagnosed (as determined by less destruction), the more conservative the therapy may be and the more predictable the outcome.

In almost all cases, systemic tetracycline (250 mg of tetracycline hydrochloride four times daily for at least 1 week) should be given in conjunction with local mechanical therapy. If surgery is indicated, systemic tetracycline should be prescribed, with the patient instructed to begin taking the antibiotic approximately 1 hour before surgery. Doxycycline 100 mg/day may also be used. Chlorhexidine rinses should also be prescribed and continued for several weeks to aid healing and augment plaque control.

In refractory localized aggressive periodontitis cases, tetracycline-resistant *Actinobacillus* species have been suspected. After performing antibiotic susceptibility tests, the clinician may consider a combination of amoxicillin and metronidazole, similar to the regimen suggested for refractory periodontitis patients.[7,30,39]

Generalized Aggressive Periodontitis

In general the treatment of patients with generalized forms of aggressive periodontitis should be very similar to that of patients with refractory forms of the disease. To date, there are no available data that suggest any alterations in the approach used for refractory forms of the disease.

The rate of disease progression may be faster in these younger individuals, and therefore the clinician should monitor such patients more often. Close collaboration between members of the treatment team, which includes the periodontist, the general dentist, the dental hygienist, and the patient's physician, is required.

It is important to monitor and observe the patient's overall physical status, as weight loss, mental depression, and malaise have been reported in patients with generalized aggressive periodontitis. Similarly, flare-ups of proliferative gingival inflammation can be observed early when the patient is on a frequent monitoring cycle. Currently, monitoring every 3 weeks or less is suggested while the disease is in an active phase.

Necrotizing Ulcerative Periodontitis

Patients with necrotizing ulcerative periodontitis (NUP) are unusual and should be treated in consultation with the physician. As indicated in Chapter 27, these patients often have an underlying predisposing systemic factor that renders the patient susceptible to necrosis of the periodontal structures. It is mandatory that these patients be treated aggressively. This includes a medical evaluation and local, topical, and systemic antimicrobials based on the results of laboratory tests.

These patients often harbor bacteria, fungi, viruses, and other non-oral microorganisms, making the selection

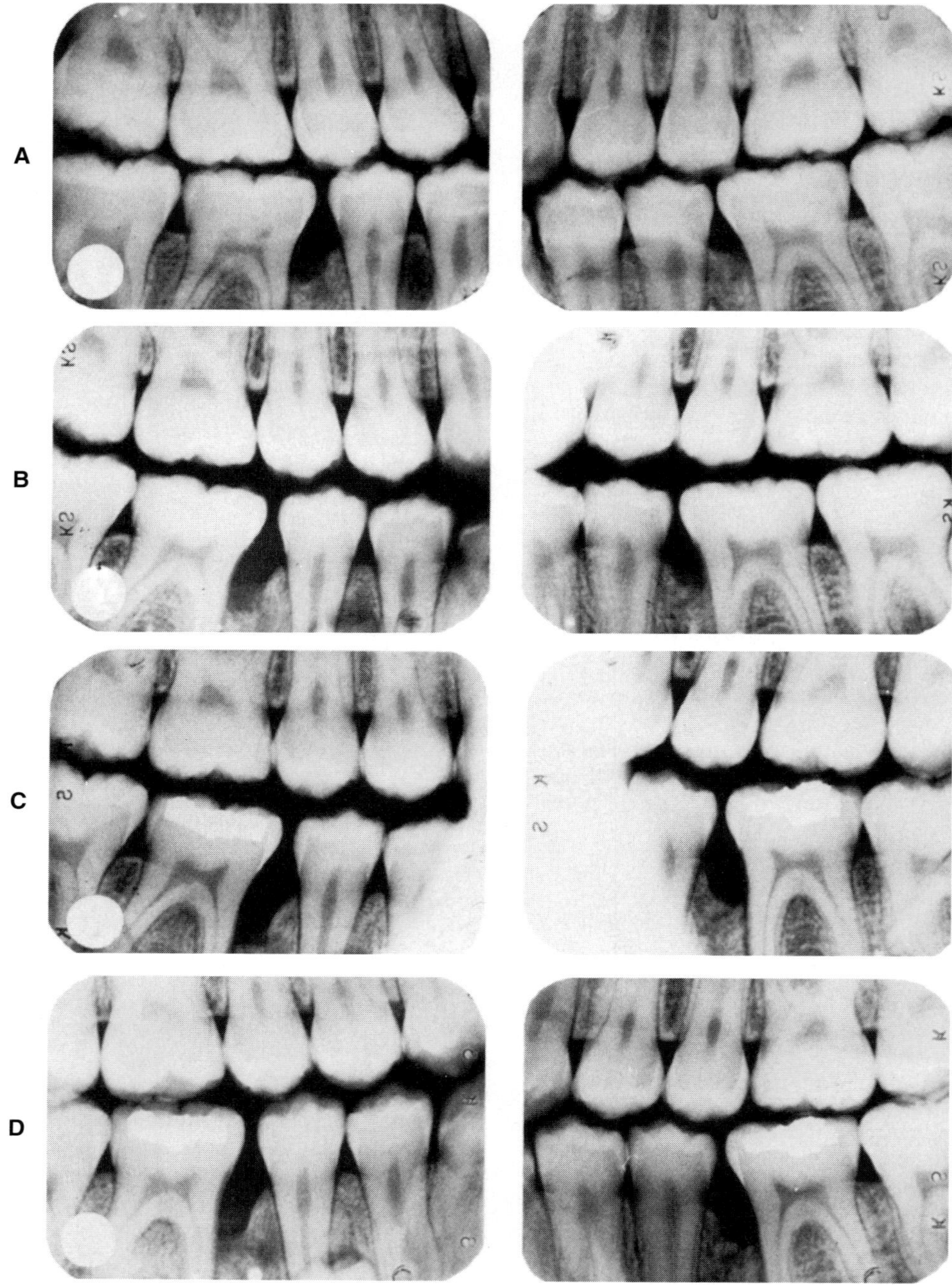

Fig. 40-1 Radiographs depicting progression of the osseous lesion in a case of localized aggressive periodontitis (formerly localized juvenile periodontitis). **A,** January 29, 1979; **B,** August 16, 1979; **C,** February 22, 1980; **D,** May 15, 1981. Note the progressive deterioration of the osseous level. (From Barnett ML, Baker RL: The formation and healing of osseous lesions in a patient with localized juvenile periodontitis. Case report. J Periodontol 1983; 54:148.)

of treatment complicated. Oral hygiene for these patients is complicated by the sometimes painful tissues. In such cases, irrigation with diluted cleansing and antibacterial agents can be of some benefit. The treatment of acquired immunodeficiency syndrome (AIDS)–associated NUP is presented in Chapter 51.

Periodontitis Associated with Systemic Disease

Several systemic diseases appear to predispose the individuals who have them to periodontitis which may be of the aggressive type (see Chapter 28), but which may differ considerably from the aggressive forms described previously. Treatment considerations, however, are similar.

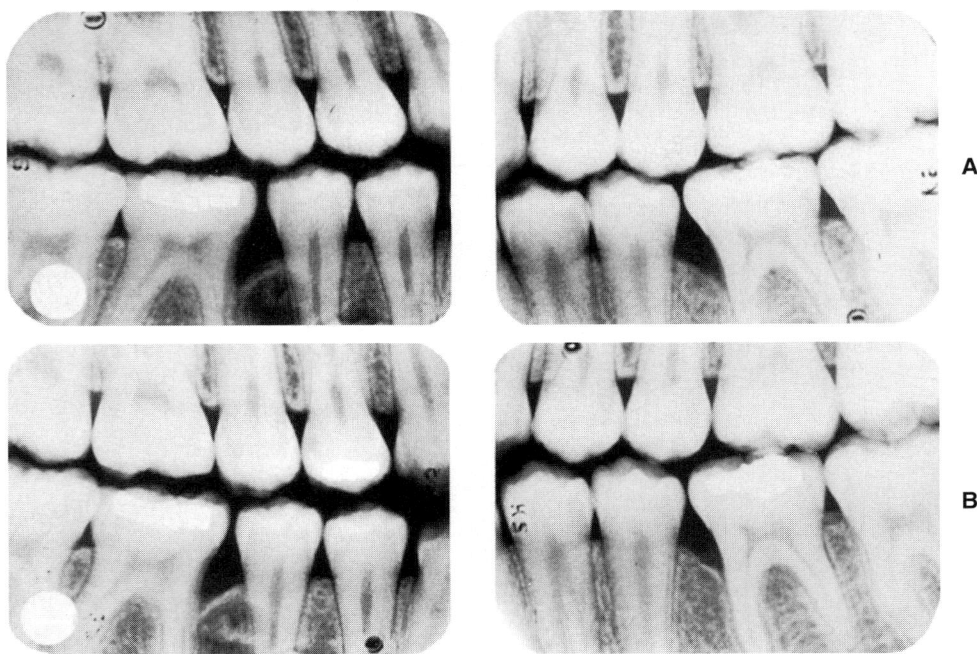

Fig. 40-2 Postoperative radiographs of the patient shown in Fig. 40-1. **A,** November 6, 1981; **B,** March 3, 1982. Treatment consisted of oral hygiene instruction; scaling and root planing concurrently with 1 g of tetracycline per day for 2 weeks; and, finally, modified Widman flaps. (From Barnett ML, Baker RL: The formation and healing of osseous lesions in a patient with localized juvenile periodontitis. Case report. J Periodontol 1983; 54:148.)

This includes a medical evaluation and local, topical, and systemic antimicrobials based on the results of laboratory tests. It is mandatory that these patients be treated aggressively.

TREATMENT ALGORITHM

Individualizing treatment based on information about the patient's bacteria can be difficult because (1) patients with the same clinical presentation can have great differences in their periodontal microflora and (2) patients with the same microflora can have great variations in their clinical presentations.[25]

Fig. 40-3 shows a decision pathway, or algorithm, for a patient with refractory periodontitis. This algorithm can also be used as a general guide for many types of patients with aggressive forms of disease considered in this chapter.[26] It begins with the identification of the patient's disease (A) or nondisease (B) status. The presence of periodontal disease (A) guides the clinician to perform a series of treatments (C) that usually begins with scaling and root planing and often continues to periodontal surgery.[6]

After treatment, reevaluation of the patient (D) is done to determine whether the patient is stable (E) or not stable (F). At this stage, the patient presents with a combination of clinical signs that are a result of an etiologic agent interacting with a predisposing factor to produce the patient's observed clinical status. As an example, we will use the presence of periodontal pathogens as the target etiologic factor. There are four possible conditions that describe the patient's status (Boxes 1, 2, 3, and 4 in Fig. 40-4).

Fig. 40-4, Box 1 represents a situation in which both clinical signs of disease and periodontal pathogens are present. Clinical therapy is strongly recommended, because the tooth is clearly at risk for progression of disease.

Fig. 40-4, Box 2 indicates a situation in which clinical signs of disease are present in the absence of periodontal pathogens as detected by the particular test used for the patient. In this case, treatment should be performed. The rationale for this decision is based on the presence of disease and the fact the particular test used in this case may have "missed" some pathologic organisms because it was not designed to detect them. Similarly, in this group of patients, unusual microorganisms may be encountered, and initial testing may not be sufficient. Thus the clinical status dictates the course of treatment.

Fig. 40-4, Box 3 represents the inverse of Box 2. In this case, periodontal pathogens are present in the absence of clinical signs. The presence of pathogens puts the site, and therefore the tooth, at risk and suggests a worse prognosis. Treatment may vary considerably among patients but is aimed at the elimination of pathogens. This situation may be encountered after initial treatment is rendered and follow-up monitoring is used to determine the status of the previously diseased site.

At periodic reevaluation (see Fig. 40-3), patients can also be "completely" stable (E), a situation in which no

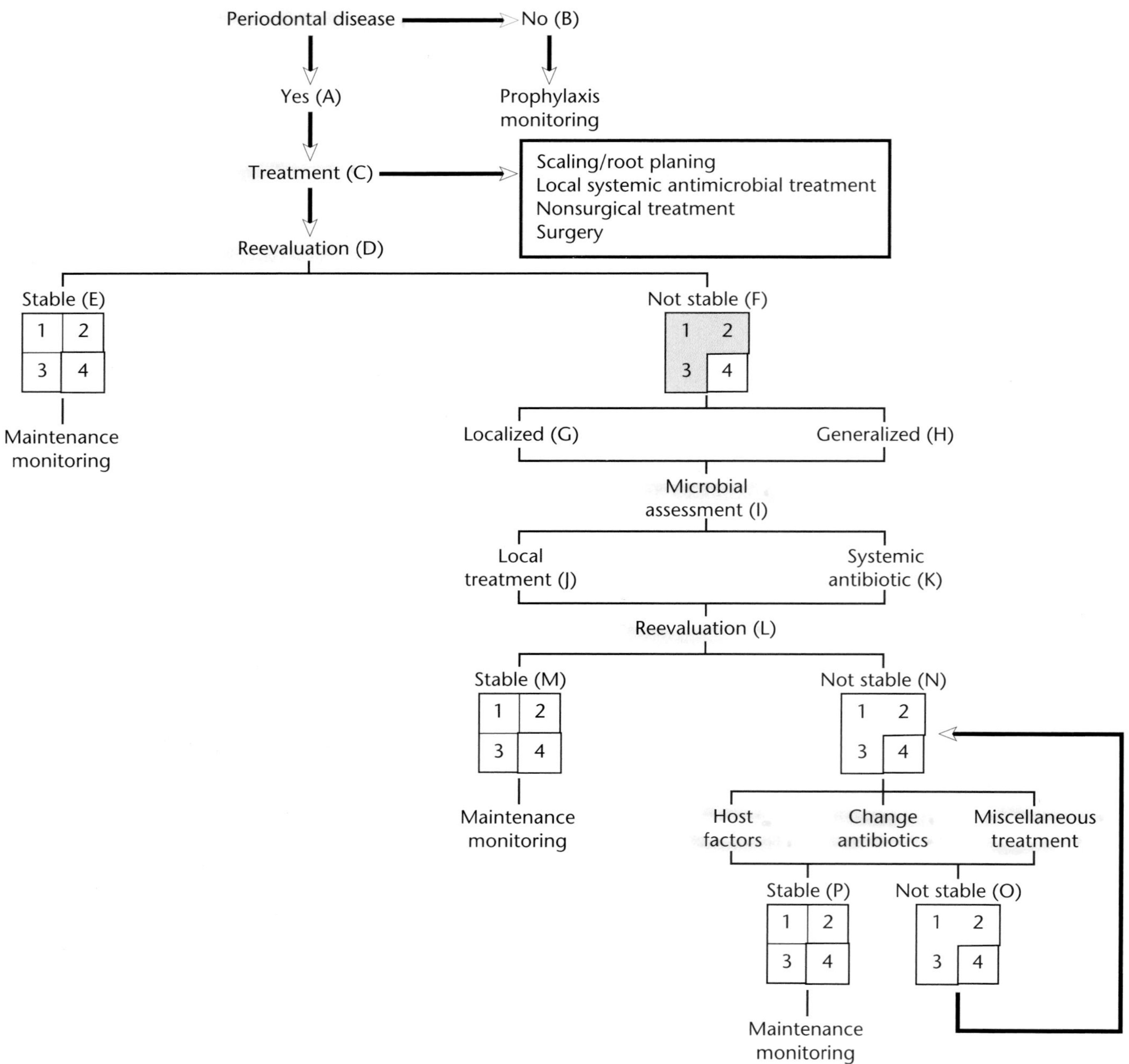

Fig. 40-3 Decision pathway.

pathogens or clinical signs of disease (i.e., bleeding on probing, loss of attachment, or loss of bone) are found (see Fig. 40-4, *Box 4*). Therefore normal maintenance and monitoring are indicated.

In the three unstable situations (see Fig. 40-4, *Boxes 1, 2, and 3*), it is important to assess whether the manifestations of the disease are localized (G) or generalized (H). As stated previously, microbial assessment (I) is recommended.

Local treatment (J) can consist of a variety of procedures, including topical chlorhexidine and local drug delivery. In cases of generalized manifestations, a systemic antibiotic (K) can be suggested based on the results of microbial testing. Topical chlorhexidine should also be prescribed during systemic antibiotic therapy.

Once again, the clinician should reevaluate (L) to judge whether the patient is stable (M), and therefore ready for maintenance (supportive periodontal treatment [SPT]), or whether disease is still present (N). The clinician should evaluate a possible deficiency of the host immune system by consulting the patient's physician, and a different antibiotic regimen may be considered. If disease persists (O), the clinician must try to block the triggers of the disease process by employing

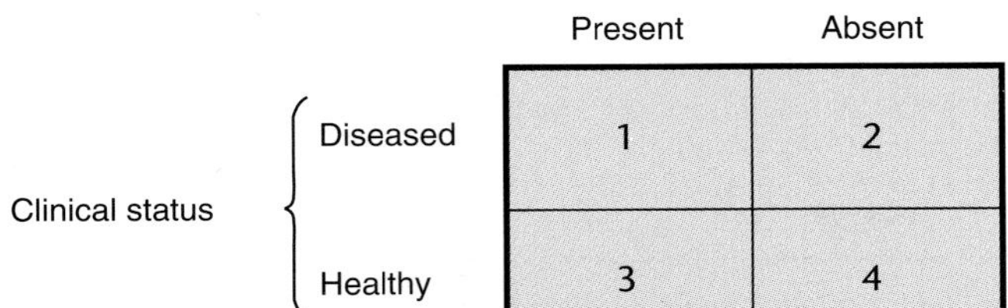

Fig. 40-4 Four possible combinations of the patient's microbial and clinical status. *1,* Clinical signs of disease present/pathogens present. *2,* Clinical signs of disease present/pathogens absent. *3,* Clinical signs of disease absent (healthy)/pathogens present. *4,* Clinical signs of disease absent (healthy)/pathogens absent. (Adapted from Newman MG, Kornman KS, Holtzman S: Association of clinical risk factors with treatment outcomes. J Periodontol 1994; 65:489.)

trial-and-error approaches to treatment, which can be frustrating and often unsuccessful. When such treatment is unsuccessful, the disease is labeled refractory or treatment resistant.

If the patient responds to treatment (P), maintenance and monitoring are preferred on a regular basis.

MAINTENANCE

A supportive periodontal therapy program aimed at early detection and treatment of sites that begin to lose attachment should be established. The duration between these recall visits is usually short during the first period after the patient's evaluation, generally no longer than 3 months.

Patients with refractory periodontitis, when transferred to maintenance care, must have a stable periodontal status, similar to the situation presented in Fig. 40-4, *Box 4*. The maintenance visit should consist of examination and evaluation of the patient's current oral health; thorough root débridement, followed by prophylaxis; and a review of oral hygiene instructions. When signs of disease recur, monitoring with bacterial testing is recommended.

REFERENCES

1. Atiken S, Birek P, Kulkarni GV, et al: Serial doxycycline and metronidazole in prevention of recurrent periodontitis in high-risk patients. J Periodontol 1993; 63:87.
2. Baer PN, Everett FG: The maxillary sinus as a problem in the therapy of periodontosis. J Periodontol 1970; 41:476.
3. Baer PN, Socransky SS: Periodontosis: Case report with long-term follow-up. Periodont Case Rep 1979; 1:1.
4. Barnett ML, Baker RL: The formation and healing of osseous lesions in a patient with localized juvenile periodontitis. Case report. J Periodontol 1983; 4(suppl):148.
5. Carranza FA Jr, Saglie FR, Newman MG, et al: Scanning and transmission electron microscopic study of tissue-invading microorganisms in localized juvenile periodontitis. J Periodontol 1983; 54:598.
6. Collins JG, Offenbacher S, Arnold RR: Effects of a combination of therapy to eliminate Porphyromonas gingivalis in refractory periodontitis. J Periodontol 1993; 64:98.
7. Flemmig TF, Milian E, Karch H, et al: Differential clinical treatment outcome after systemic metronidazole and amoxicillin in patients harboring Actinobacillus actinomycetemcomitans and/or Porphyromonas gingivalis. J Clin Periodontol 1998; 25:380.
8. Fourmousis I, Tonetti MS, Mombelli A, et al: Evaluation of tetracycline fiber therapy with digital image analysis. J Clin Periodontol 1998; 25:737–745.
9. Garrett S, Johnson L, Drisko CH, et al: Two multi-center studies evaluating locally delivered doxycycline hyclate, placebo control, oral hygiene, and scaling and root planing in the treatment of periodontitis. J Periodontol 1999; 70:490.
10. Genco RJ, Ciancio SC, Rosling B: Treatment of localized juvenile periodontitis. Abstract. J Dent Res 1981; 60:527.
11. Gordon J, Walker C, Hovliaras C, et al: Efficacy of clindamycin hydrochloride in refractory periodontitis: 24-month results. J Periodontol 1990; 61:689.
12. Gordon JM, Walker CB: Current status of systemic antibiotic usage in destructive periodontal disease. J Periodontol 1993;64(8 suppl):760.
13. Hirschfeld L, Wasserman B: A long-term survey of tooth loss in 600 treated periodontal patients. J Periodontol 1978; 49:225.
14. Howell T, Williams R: Pharmacologic blocking of host response as an adjunct in the management of periodontal disease: A research update (position paper). Chicago, American Academy of Periodontology, 1992.
15. Killoy WJ: The use of locally delivered chlorhexidine in the treatment of periodontitis. Clinical results. J Clin Periodontol 1998; 25:953–958.
16. Kornman KS, Karl EH: The effect of long-term, low-dose tetracycline therapy on the subgingival microflora in refractory adult periodontitis. J Periodontol 1982; 53:604.
17. Kornman KS, Newman MG, Flemmig T, et al: Treatment of refractory periodontitis with metronidazole plus amoxicillin or Augmentin. Abstract 403. J Dent Res 1989; 68(special issue): 917.
18. Liljenberg B, Lindhe J: Juvenile periodontitis. Some microbiological, histopathological and clinical characteristics. J Clin Periodontol 1980; 7:48.
19. Lindhe J, Liljenberg B: Treatment of localized juvenile periodontitis. Results after 5 years. J Clin Periodontol 1984; 11:399.
20. Listgarten MA, Lai CH, Young V: Microbial composition and pattern of antibiotic resistance in subgingival microbial samples from patients with refractory periodontitis. J Periodontol 1993; 64:155.
21. Mabry T, Yukna R, Sepe W: Freeze-dried bone allografts with tetracycline in the treatment of juvenile periodontitis. J Periodontol 1985; 56:74.
22. Magnusson I, Low SB, McArthur WP, Marks RG, et al: Treatment of subjects with refractory periodontal disease. J Clin Periodontol 1994; 21:628.
23. McFall WT: Tooth loss in 100 treated patients with periodontal disease in a long-term study. J Clin Periodontol 1982; 53:539.
24. Matisko MW, Bissada NF: Short-term sequential administration of amoxicillin/clavulanate potassium and doxycycline in the treatment of recurrent/progressive periodontitis. J Periodontol 1993; 64:553.
25. Newman MG, Kornman K, Holtzman S: Association of clinical risk factors with treatment outcomes. J Periodontol 1994; 65:489.
26. Newman MG, Marinho VC: Assessing bacterial risk factors for periodontitis and peri-implantitis: Using evidence to enhance outcomes. Compend Contin Educ Dent 1994; 15(8):958.

27. Nyman S, Lindhe J, Rosling B: Periodontal surgery in plaque-infected dentitions. J Clin Periodontol 1977; 4:240.
28. Olsvik B, Teniver FC: Tetracycline resistance in periodontal pathogens. Clin Infect Dis 1993; 16(suppl 4):8310.
29. Pajukanta R: In vitro antimicrobial susceptibility of Porphyromonas gingival is to azythromycin, a novel macrolide. Oral Microbiol Immunol 1993; 8:325.
30. Pavicic MJ, van Winkelhoff AJ, Pavivic-Temming YA, et al: Metronidazole susceptibility factors in Actinobacillus actinomycetemcomitans. J Antimicrob Chemother 1995; 35:263.
31. Quiryen M, Listgarten MA: The distribution of bacterial morphotypes around natural teeth and titanium implants ad modum BrAnemark. Clin Oral Impl Res 1990; 1:8.
32. Rams TE, Feik D, Slots J: Ciprofloxacin/metronidazole treatment of recurrent adult periodontitis. Abstract 1708. J Dent Res 1992; 71(special issue):319.
33. Rams TE, Link CC Jr: Microbiology of failing dental implants in humans: Electron microscopy observations. J Oral Implantol 1993; 11:93.
34. Rosling B, Nyman SF, Lindhe J: The effect of systemic plaque control on bone regeneration in infrabony pockets. J Clin Periodontol 1976; 3:38.
35. Rosling B, Nyman SF, Lindhe J, et al: The healing potential of the periodontal tissues following different techniques of periodontal surgery in plaque-free dentitions: A 2-year study. J Clin Periodontol 1976; 3:233.
36. Saglie FR, Carranza FA Jr, Newman MG, et al: Identification of tissue invading bacteria in human periodontal disease. J Periodont Res 1982; 17:452.
37. Tanner ACR, Socransky SS, Goodson M: Microbiota of periodontal pockets losing crestal alveolar bone. J Periodontol Res 1984; 19:279.
38. Thomas JG; Metheny RJ; Karakiozis JM: Long-term sub-antimicrobial doxycycline (Periostat) as adjunctive management in adult periodontitis: effects on subgingival bacterial population dynamics. Adv Dent Res 1998; 12:32.
39. van Winklehoff AJ, Tijhof CJ, de Graaff: Microbial and clinical results of metronidazole plus amoxicillin therapy in *Actinobacillus actinomycetemcomitans*–associated periodontitis. J Periodontol 1992; 63:52.
40. Waerhaug J: Subgingival plaque and loss of attachment in periodontosis as evaluated on extracted teeth. J Periodontol 1977; 48:125.
41. Walker CB, Gordon JM, Socransky SS: Antibiotic susceptibility testing on subgingival plaque samples. J Clin Periodontol 1983; 10:422.
42. Walker CB, Pappas JD, Tyler KZ, Cohen JM: Antibiotic susceptibilities to eight antimicrobial agents. J Periodontol 1985; 56(suppl):67.
43. Walker C, Gordon J: The effect of clindamycin on the microbiota associated with refractory periodontitis. J Periodontol 1990; 61:692.
44. Walker CB, Gordon JM, Magnusson I, et al: A role for antibiotics in the treatment of refractory periodontitis. J Periodontol 1993; 64:772.
45. Winkel EG, Van Winkelhoff AJ, Timmerman MF, et al: Effects of metronidazole in patients with "refractory" periodontitis associated with *Bacteroides forsythus*. J Clin Periodontol 1997; 24:573.
46. Yukna R, Sepe W: Clinical evaluation of localized periodontosis defects with freeze-dried bone allografts combined with local and systemic tetracyclines. Internat J Periodont Restor Dent 1982; 5:9.

SECTION II

Periodontal Instrumentation

Henry H. Takei

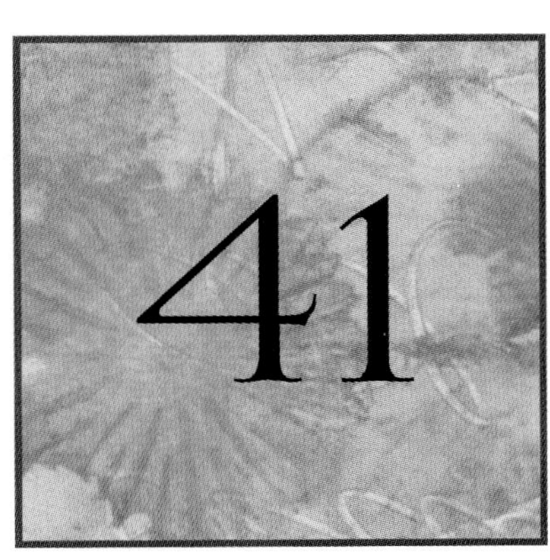

CHAPTER

The Periodontal Instrumentarium

Anna M. Pattison, Gordon L. Pattison, and Henry H. Takei*

CHAPTER OUTLINE

Periodontal instruments are designed for specific purposes, such as removing calculus, planing root surfaces, curetting the gingiva, or removing diseased tissue. On first investigation, the variety of instruments available for similar purposes appears confusing. With experience, however, clinicians select a relatively small set that fulfills all requirements.

CLASSIFICATION OF PERIODONTAL INSTRUMENTS

Periodontal instruments are classified according to the purposes they serve as follows:

1. *Periodontal probes* are used to locate, measure, and mark pockets, as well as determine their course on individual tooth surfaces.
2. *Explorers* are used to locate calculus deposits and caries.
3. *Scaling, root planing, and curettage instruments* are used for removal of plaque and calcified deposits from the crown and root of a tooth, removal of altered cementum from the subgingival root surface, and débridement of the soft tissue lining the pocket. Scaling and curettage instruments are classified as follows:
   - *Sickle scalers* are heavy instruments used to remove supragingival calculus.
   - *Curettes* are fine instruments used for subgingival scaling, root planing, and removal of the soft tissue lining the pocket.
   - *Hoe, chisel, and file scalers* are used to remove tenacious subgingival calculus and altered cementum. Their use is limited compared with that of curettes.

* Material in this chapter was drawn freely from Pattison A, Pattison G: Periodontal Instrumentation, ed 2. Reprinted by permission of Pearson Education, Inc., Upper Saddle River, NJ.

- *Ultrasonic and sonic instruments* are used for scaling and cleansing tooth surfaces and curetting the soft tissue wall of the periodontal pocket.[7,8,15]

4. The *periodontal endoscope* is used to visualize deep subgingivally in pockets and furcations enabling the detection of deposits.
5. *Cleansing and polishing instruments* such as rubber cups, brushes, and dental tape are used to clean and polish tooth surfaces. Also available are air-powder abrasive systems for tooth polishing.

The wearing and cutting qualities of some types of steel used in periodontal instruments have been tested,[17,18,33] but specifications vary among manufacturers.[33] Stainless steel is used most commonly in instrument manufacture. High-carbon steel instruments are also available and are considered by some clinicians to be superior.

Each group of instruments has characteristic features; individual therapists often develop variations with which they operate most effectively. Small instruments are recommended to fit into pockets without injuring the soft tissues.[22,35]

The parts of each instrument, referred to as the working end, shank, and handle, are shown in Fig. 41-1.

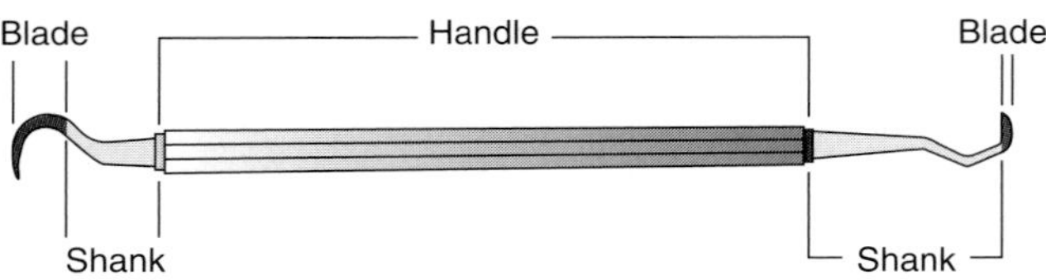

Fig. 41-1 Parts of a typical periodontal instrument.

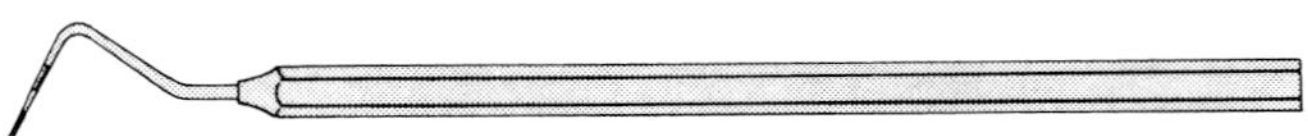

Fig. 41-2 The periodontal probe is composed of the handle, shank, and calibrated working end.

Periodontal Probes

Periodontal probes are used to measure the depth of pockets and to determine their configuration. The typical probe is a tapered, rodlike instrument calibrated in millimeters, with a blunt, rounded tip (Fig. 41-2). There are several other designs with various millimeter calibrations. The World Health Organization (WHO) probe has millimeter markings and a small round ball at the tip (Fig. 41-3). Ideally, these probes are thin, and the shank is angled to allow easy insertion into the pocket. Furcation areas can best be evaluated with the curved, blunt Nabers probe (Fig. 41-4).

When measuring a pocket, the probe is inserted with a firm, gentle pressure to the bottom of the pocket. The shank should be aligned with the long axis of the tooth surface to be probed. Several measurements are made to determine the level of attachment along the surface of the tooth.

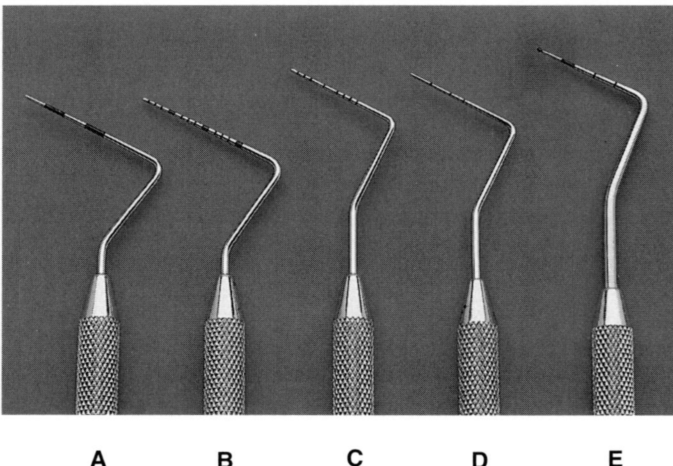

A B C D E

Fig. 41-3 Types of periodontal probes. **A,** The Marquis color-coded probe. Calibrations are in 3-mm sections. **B,** The UNC-15 probe, a 15-mm-long probe with millimeter markings at each millimeter and color coding at the 5th, 10th, and 15th mm. **C,** The University of Michigan "O" probe, with Williams markings (at 1, 2, 3, 5, 7, 8, 9, and 10 mm). **D,** The Michigan "O" probe with markings at 3, 6, and 8 mm. **E,** The WHO (World Health Organization) probe, which has a 0.5 mm ball at the tip and millimeter markings at 3.5, 8.5, and 11.5 millimeters and color coding from 3.5 to 5.5 mm.

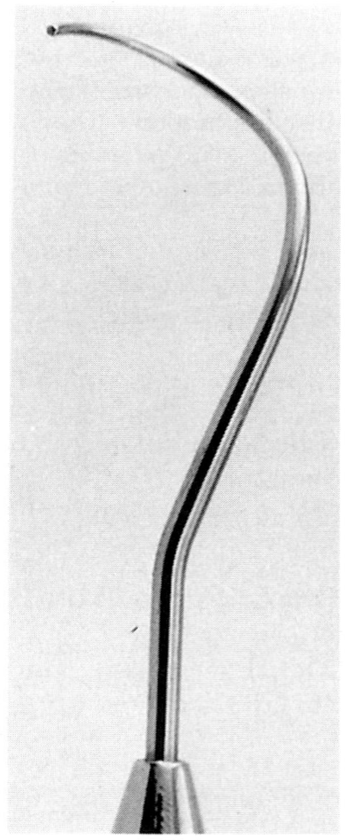

Fig. 41-4 The curved Nabers probe for detection of furcation areas.

Explorers

Explorers are used to locate subgingival deposits and carious areas and to check the smoothness of the root surfaces after root planing. Explorers are designed with different shapes and angles for a variety of uses. Some of the most commonly used explorers are shown in Fig. 41-5, and their uses and limitations are shown in Fig. 41-6. The periodontal probe can also be useful in the detection of subgingival deposits (see Fig. 41-6).

Scaling and Curettage Instruments

Scaling and curettage instruments are illustrated in Fig. 41-7.

Sickle Scalers (Supragingival Scalers). Sickle scalers have a flat surface and two cutting edges that converge in a sharply pointed tip. The shape of the instrument makes the tip strong so that it will not break off during use (Fig. 41-8). The sickle is used primarily to remove supragingival calculus (Fig. 41-9). Because of the design of this instrument, it is difficult to insert a large sickle blade under the gingiva without damaging the surrounding gingival tissues (Fig. 41-10). Small, curved sickle scaler blades such as the 204SD can be inserted under ledges of calculus a few mm below the gingiva. Sickle scalers are used with a pull stroke.

It is important to note that sickle scalers with the same basic design can be obtained with different blade sizes and shank types to adapt to specific uses. The U15/30 (Fig. 41-11), Ball, and Indiana University sickles are large. The Jaquette sickles #1, 2, and 3 have medium-size blades. The curved 204 sickles are available with large, medium, or small blades. The Nevi 2 posterior

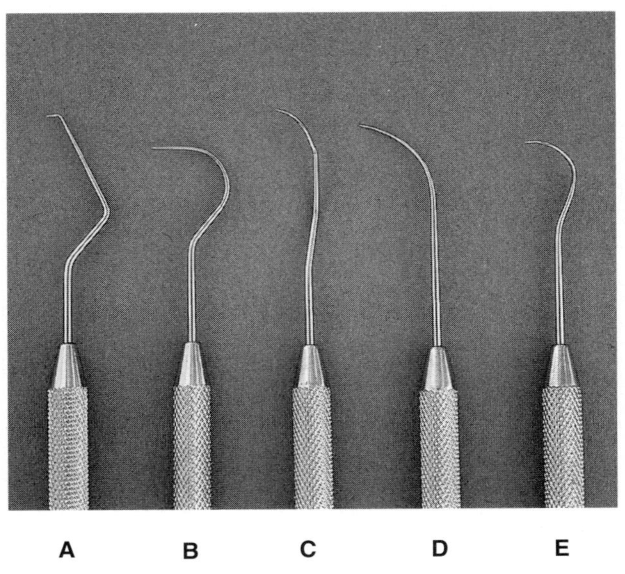

Fig. 41-5 Five typical explorers. **A,** #17; **B,** #23; **C,** EXD 11–12; **D,** #3; **E,** #3CH Pigtail.

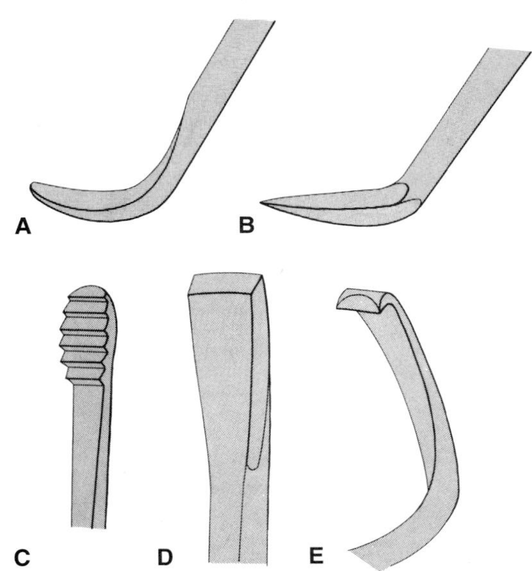

Fig. 41-7 The five basic scaling instruments. **A,** Curette; **B,** sickle; **C,** file; **D,** chisel; **E,** hoe.

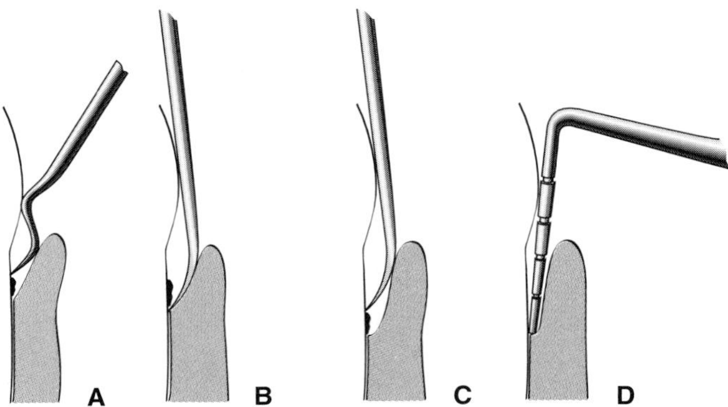

Fig. 41-6 Insertion of two types of explorers and a probe in a pocket for calculus detection. **A,** The limitations of the pigtail explorer in a deep pocket. **B,** Insertion of the #3 explorer. **C,** Limitations of the #3 explorer. **D,** Insertion of the probe.

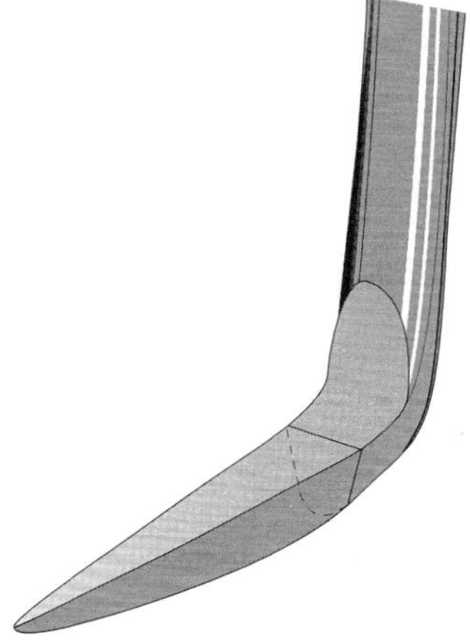

Fig. 41-8 Basic characteristics of a sickle scaler: triangular shape, double-cutting edge, and pointed tip.

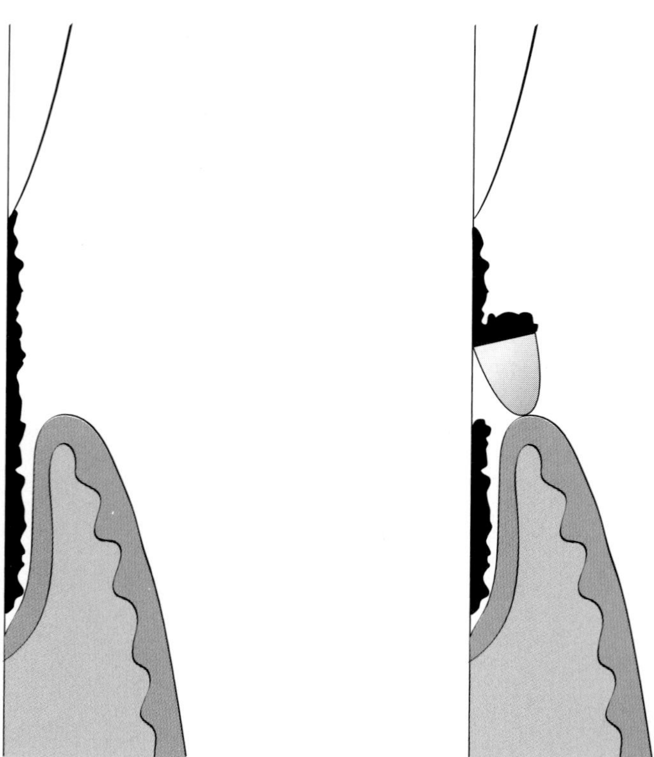

Fig. 41-9 Use of a sickle scaler for removal of supragingival calculus.

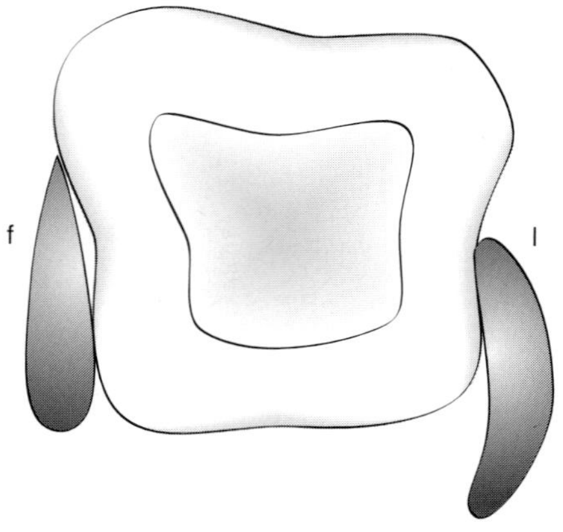

Fig. 41-10 Subgingival adaptation around the root is better with the curette than with the sickle. *f*, facial; *l*, lingual.

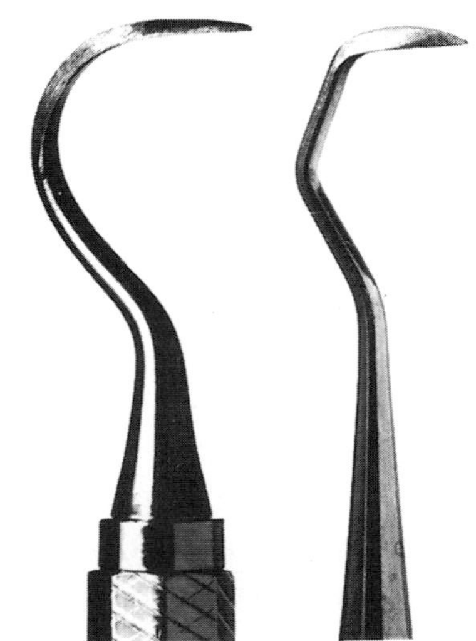

Fig. 41-11 Both ends of a U15/30 scaler.

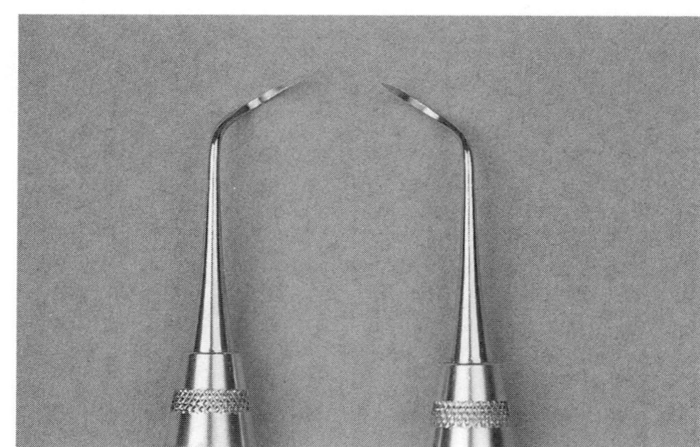

Fig. 41-12 Both ends of a NEVI 2 posterior sickle scaler.

sickle scaler is a new design that is thin enough to be inserted several mm subgingivally for removal of moderate ledges of calculus (Fig. 41-12). The selection of these instruments should be based on the area to be scaled. Sickles with straight shanks are designed for use on anterior teeth and premolars. Sickle scalers with contra-angled shanks adapt to posterior teeth.

Curettes. The curette is the instrument of choice for removing deep subgingival calculus, root planing altered cementum, and removing the soft tissue lining the periodontal pocket (Fig. 41-13). Each working end has a cutting edge on both sides of the blade and a rounded toe. The curette is finer than the sickle scalers and does not have any sharp points or corners other than the cutting edges of the blade (Fig. 41-14). Therefore curettes can be adapted and provide good access to deep pockets, with minimal soft tissue trauma (see Fig. 41-10). In cross section, the blade appears semicircular with a convex base. The lateral border of the convex base forms a cutting edge with the face of the semicircular blade. There are cutting edges on both sides of the blade. Both single- and double-end curettes may be obtained, depending on the preference of the operator.

As shown in Fig. 41-10, the curved blade and rounded toe of the curette allow the blade to adapt better to the root surface, unlike the straight design and pointed end of a sickle scaler, which can cause tissue laceration and trauma. There are two basic types of curettes: universal and area-specific.

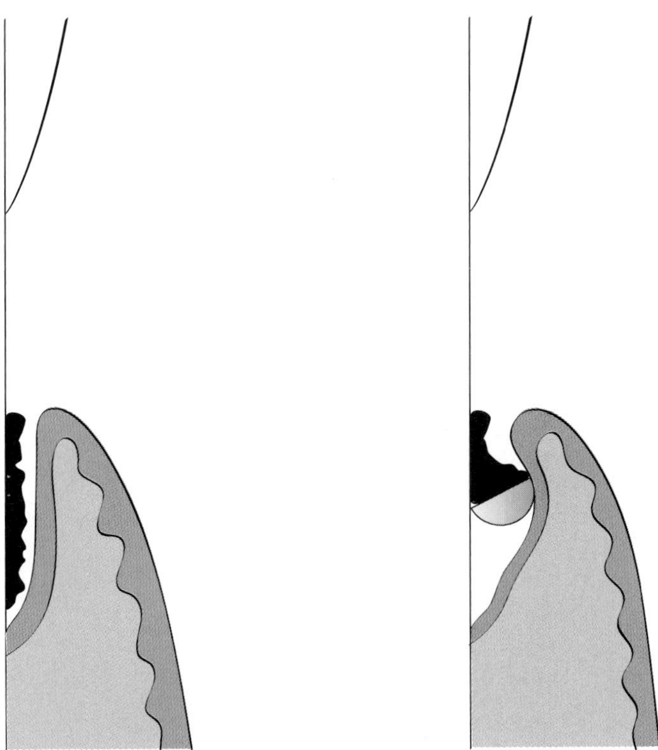

Fig. 41-13 The curette is the instrument of choice for subgingival scaling and root planing.

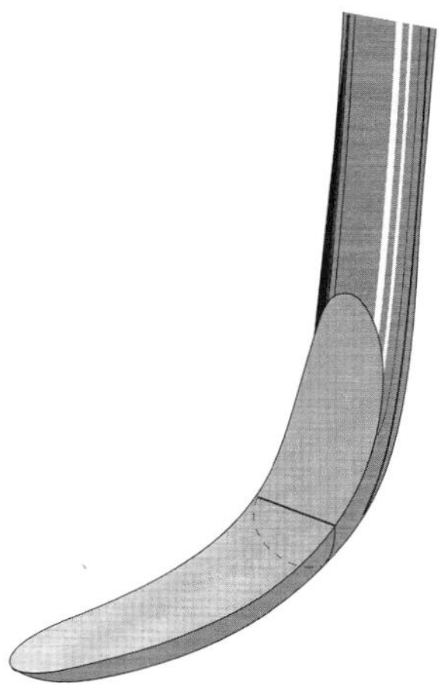

Fig. 41-14 Basic characteristics of a curette: spoon-shaped blade and rounded tip.

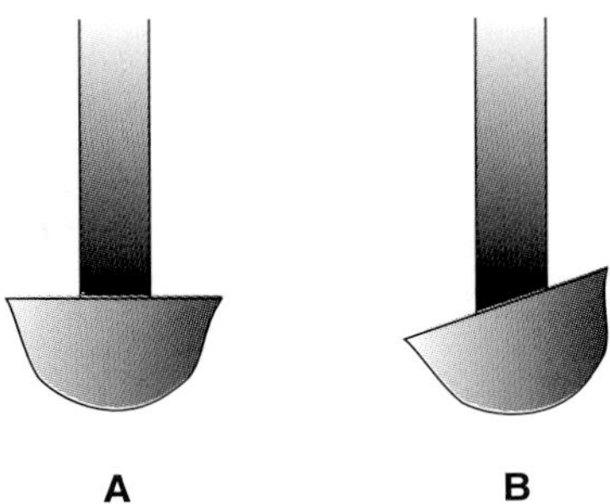

Fig. 41-15 Principal types of curettes as seen from the toe of the instrument. **A,** Universal curette. **B,** Gracey curette. Note the offset blade angulation of the Gracey curette.

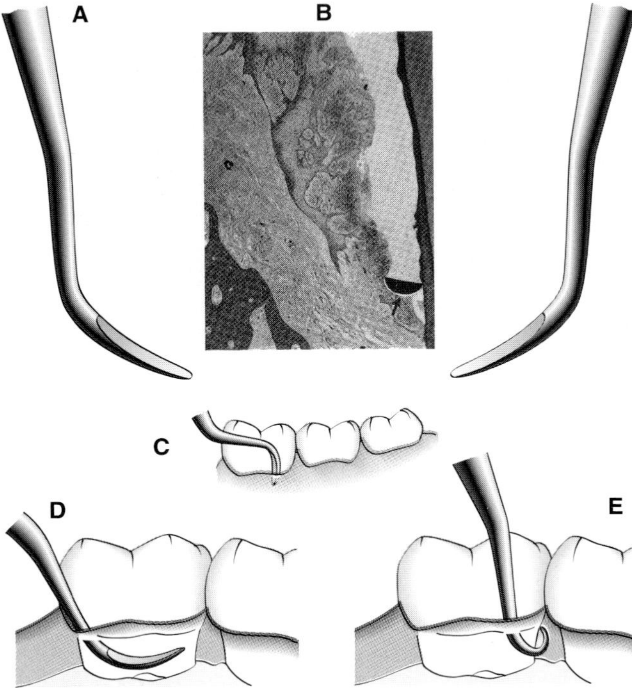

Fig. 41-16 A, Double-ended curette for the removal of subgingival calculus. **B,** Cross section of the curette blade (*arrow*) against the cemental wall of a deep periodontal pocket. **C,** Curette in position at the base of a periodontal pocket on the facial surface of a mandibular molar. **D,** Curette inserted in a pocket with the tip directed apically. **E,** Curette in position at the base of a pocket on the distal surface of the mandibular molar.

Universal Curettes. Universal curettes have cutting edges that may be inserted in most areas of the dentition by altering and adapting the finger rest, fulcrum, and hand position of the operator. The blade size and the angle and length of the shank may vary, but the face of the blade of every universal curette is at a 90-degree angle (perpendicular) to the lower shank when seen in cross section from the tip (Fig. 41-15, *A*). The blade of the universal curette is curved in one direction from the head of the blade to the toe. The Barnhart curettes #1-2 and 5-6 and the Columbia curettes #13-14, 2R-2L, and 4R-4L (Figs. 41-16 and 41-17) are examples of universal curettes.

Area-Specific Curettes

GRACEY CURETTES. Gracey curettes are representative of the area-specific curettes, a set of several instruments designed and angled to adapt to specific anatomic areas of the dentition (Fig. 41-18).

> These curettes and their modifications are probably the best instruments for subgingival scaling and root planing because they provide the best adaptation to complex root anatomy.

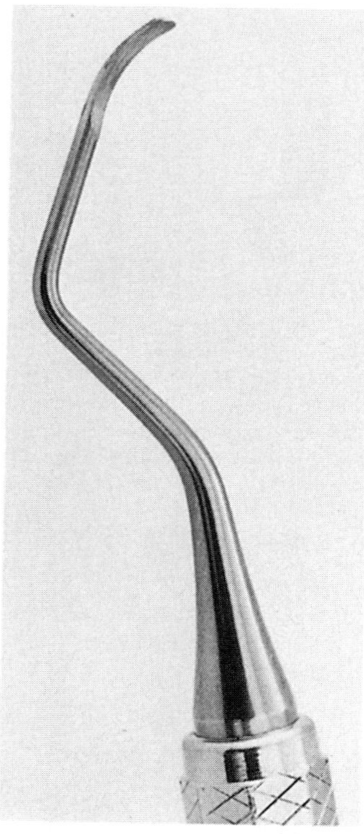

Fig. 41-17 Columbia #4R-4L universal curette.

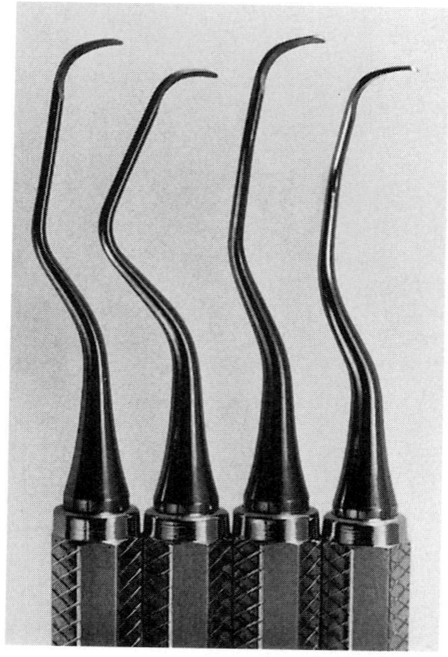

Fig. 41-18 Reduced set of Gracey curettes. From left, #5-6, #7-8, #11-12, and #13-14.

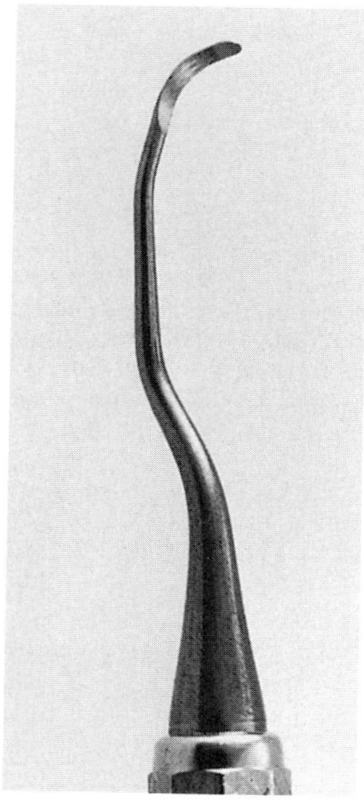

Fig. 41-19 Gracey #11-12 curette. Note the double turn of the shank.

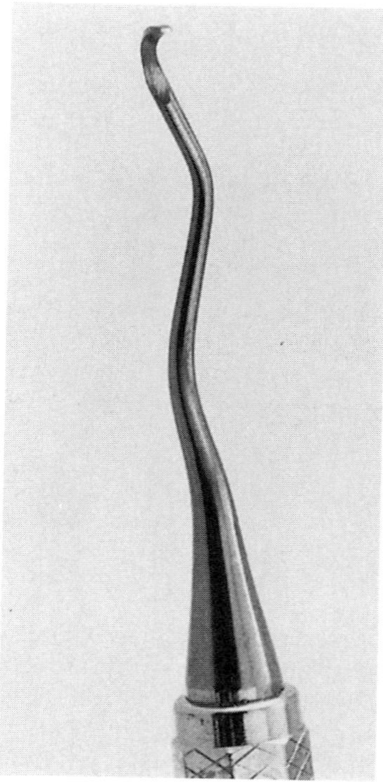

Fig. 41-20 Gracey #13-14 curette. Note the acute turn of the blade.

Double-ended Gracey curettes are paired in the following manner:

Gracey #1-2 and 3-4: Anterior teeth
Gracey #5-6: Anterior teeth and premolars
Gracey #7-8 and 9-10: Posterior teeth: facial and lingual
Gracey #11-12: Posterior teeth: mesial (Fig. 41-19)
Gracey #13-14: Posterior teeth: distal (Fig. 41-20)

Single-ended Gracey curettes can also be obtained; for these curettes a set comprises 14 instruments. Although these curettes are designed to be used in specific areas described above, an experienced operator can adapt each instrument for use in several different areas by altering the position of his or her hand and the position of the patient.

The Gracey curettes also differ from the universal curettes in that the blade is not at a 90-degree angle to the lower shank. The term *offset blade* is used to describe Gracey curettes, because they are angled approximately 60 to 70 degrees from the lower shank (see Fig. 41-15, *B*). This unique angulation allows the blade to be inserted in the precise position necessary for subgingival scaling and root planing, provided that the lower shank is parallel with the long axis of the tooth surface being scaled.

Area-specific curettes also have a curved blade. Whereas the blade of the universal curette is curved in one direction, the Gracey blade is curved from head to toe and also along the side of the cutting edge (Fig. 41-21). Thus only a pull stroke can be used. Some of the major differences between Gracey (area-specific) curettes and universal curettes are listed in Table 41-1.

Gracey curettes are available with either a "rigid" or a "finishing" type of shank. The rigid Gracey has a larger, stronger, and less flexible shank and blade than the standard finishing Gracey. The rigid shank makes it possible to remove moderate-to-heavy calculus without having to employ a separate set of heavy scalers such as sickles and hoes. Although some clinicians prefer the enhanced tactile sensitivity that the flexible shank of the finishing Gracey provides, both types of Graceys are suitable for root planing.

Recent additions to the Gracey curette set have been the Gracey #15-16 (Fig. 41-22) and 17-18. The Gracey #15-16 is a modification of the standard 11-12 and is designed for the mesial surfaces of posterior teeth. It consists of a Gracey #11-12 blade combined with the more acutely angled #13-14 shank. When the clinician is using an intraoral finger rest, it is often difficult to position the lower shank of the Gracey #11-12 so that it is parallel with the mesial surfaces of the posterior teeth, especially on the mandibular molars. The new shank angulation of the Gracey #15-16 allows better adaptation to posterior mesial surfaces from a front position with intraoral rests. If alternative fulcrums such as extraoral or opposite-arch rests are used, the Gracey #11-12 works well, and the new #15-16 is not essential. The Gracey #17-18 is a modification of the #13-14. It has a terminal shank elongated by 3 mm and a more accentuated angulation of the shank to provide complete occlusal clearance and better

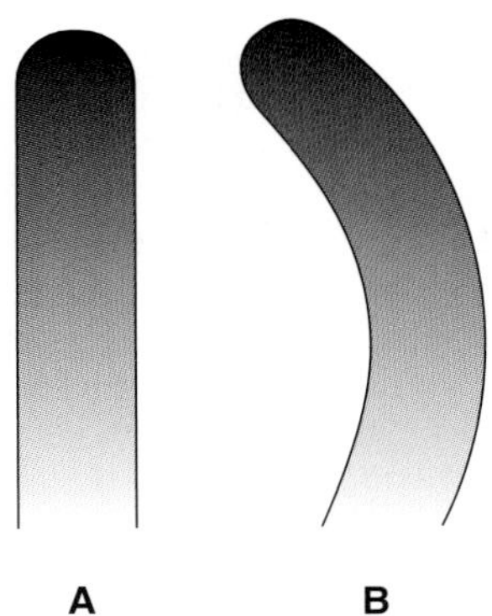

Fig. 41-21 **A,** Universal curette as seen from the blade. Note that the blade is straight. **B,** Gracey curette as seen from the blade. The blade is curved; only the convex cutting edge is used.

TABLE 41-1

Comparison of Specific (Gracey) and Universal Curettes

	Gracey Curette	Universal Curette
Area of use	Set of many curettes designed for specific areas and surfaces	One curette designed for all areas and surfaces
Cutting Edge		
Use	*One cutting edge used;* work with outer edge only	Both cutting edges used; work with either outer or inner edge
Curvature	*Curved in two planes:* blade curves up and to the side	Curved in one plane: blade curves up, not to side
Blade angle	*Offset blade*: face of blade beveled at 60 degrees to shank	Not offset: face of blade beveled at 90 degrees to shank

Modified from Pattison G, Pattison A: Periodontal Instrumentation, ed 2. Norwalk, CT, Appleton & Lange, 1992.

access to all posterior distal surfaces. The horizontal handle position minimizes interference from opposing arches and allows a more relaxed hand position when scaling distal surfaces. In addition, the blade is 1 mm shorter to allow better adaptation of the blade to distal tooth surfaces.

EXTENDED SHANK CURETTES. Extended shank curettes such as the Hu-Friedy After Five curettes are modifications of the standard Gracey curette design. The terminal shank is 3 mm longer, allowing extension into deeper periodontal pockets of 5 mm or more (Figs. 41-23 and 41-24). Other features include a thinned blade for smoother subgingival insertion and reduced tissue distention and a large-diameter, tapered shank. All standard Gracey numbers except for the #9-10 (i.e., #1-2, 3-4, 5-6, 7-8, 11-12, 13-14) are available in the After Five series. The After Five curettes are available in finishing or rigid designs. For heavy or tenacious calculus removal, rigid After Fives should be used. For light scaling or deplaquing in a periodontal maintenance patient, the thinner, finishing After Fives will insert subgingivally more easily.

MINI-BLADED CURETTES. Mini-bladed curettes such as the Hu-Friedy Mini Five curettes are modifications of the After Five curettes. They feature blades that are half the length of the After Five or standard Gracey curettes (Fig. 41-25). The shorter blade allows easier insertion and adaptation in deep, narrow pockets; furcations; developmental grooves; line angles; and deep, tight, facial, lingual, or palatal pockets. In any area where root morphology or tight tissue prevents full insertion of the standard Gracey or After Five blade, the Mini Five curettes can be used with vertical strokes, with reduced tissue distention, and without tissue trauma (Fig. 41-26). In the past, the only solution in most of these areas of difficult access was to use the Gracey curettes with a toe-down horizontal stroke. The Mini Five curettes, along with other short-bladed instruments relatively recently introduced, open a new chapter in the history of root instrumentation by allowing access to areas that previously were extremely difficult or impossible to reach with standard instruments. The Mini Five curettes are available in both the finishing and rigid designs. Rigid Mini Fives are recommended for calculus removal. The more flexible shanked, finishing Mini Fives are appropriate for light scaling and deplaquing in periodontal maintenance patients with tight pockets. As with the After Fives, the Mini Fives are available in all standard Gracey numbers except for the #9-10.

The Gracey Curvettes. The Gracey curvettes are another set of four mini-bladed curettes; the Sub-0 and the #1-2 are used for anteriors and premolars, the #11-12 is used for posterior mesial surfaces, and the #13-14 is used for posterior distal surfaces. The blade length of these instruments is 50% shorter than that of the conventional Gracey curette, and the blade has been curved slightly upward (Fig. 41-27). This curvature allows the Gracey curvettes to adapt more closely to the tooth surface than any other curettes, especially on the anterior teeth and online angles (Fig. 41-28). However, this curvature also carries the potential for gouging or grooving into the root surfaces on the proximal surfaces of the posterior teeth when the Gracey curvette #11-12 or 13-14 is used. Additional features that represent improvements on the standard Gracey curettes are a precision-balanced blade tip in direct alignment with the handle, a blade tip perpendicular to the handle, and a shank closer to parallel with the handle.

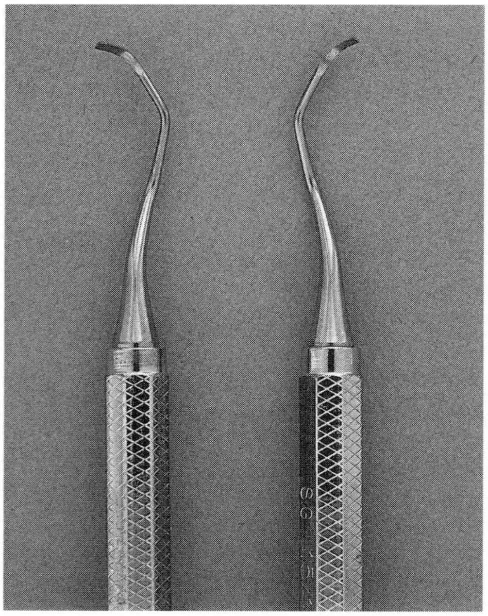

Fig. 41-22 Gracey #15-16. New Gracey curette, designed for mesioposterior surfaces, combines a Gracey #11-12 blade with a Gracey #13-14 shank.

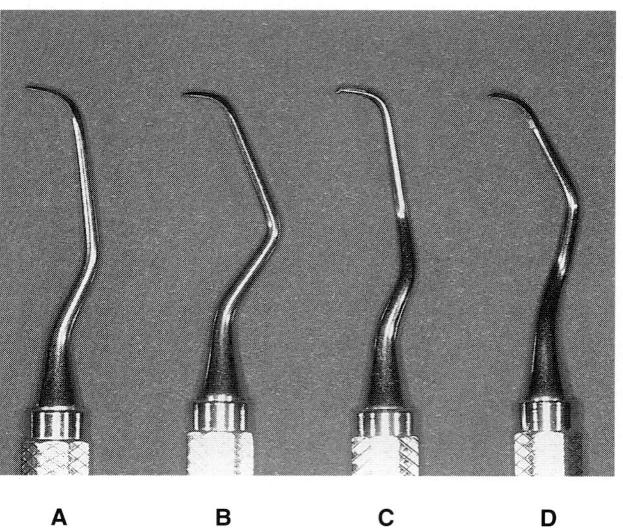

Fig. 41-23 After Five curette. Note the extra 3 mm in the terminal shank of the After Five curette compared with the standard Gracey curette. **A,** #5-6; **B,** #7-8; **C,** #11-12; **D,** #13-14.

For many years, the Morse scaler, a miniature sickle, was the only mini-bladed instrument available. However, the mini-bladed curettes have largely replaced this instrument (Fig. 41-29).

Langer and Mini-Langer Curettes. This set of three curettes combines the shank design of the standard Gracey #5-6, 11-12 and 13-14 curettes with a universal blade honed at 90 degrees rather than the offset blade of the Gracey curette. This marriage of the Gracey and universal curette designs allows the advantages of the area-specific shank to be combined with the versatility of

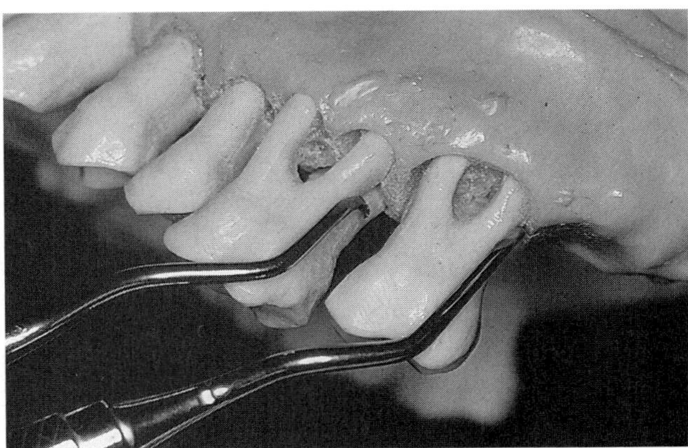

Fig. 41-24 Comparison of the After Five curette with standard Gracey curette. Rigid Gracey #13-14 adapted to the distal surface of the first molar and rigid After Five #13-14 adapted to the distal surface of the second molar. Notice the extra long shank of the After Five, which allows deeper insertion and better access.

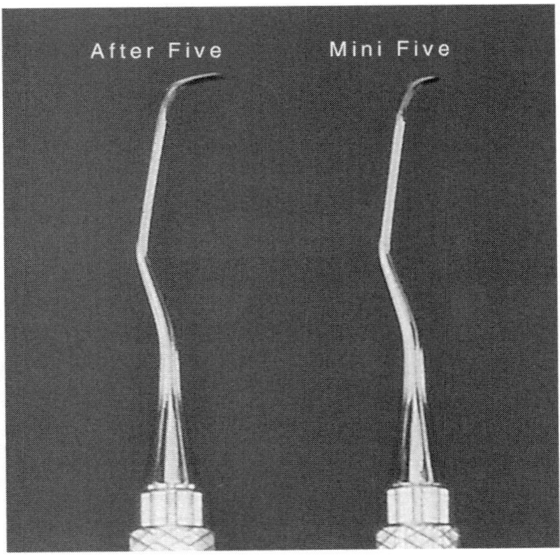

Fig. 41-25 Comparison of the After Five curette and the Mini Five curette. The shorter Mini Five blade (half the length) allows increased access and reduced tissue trauma.

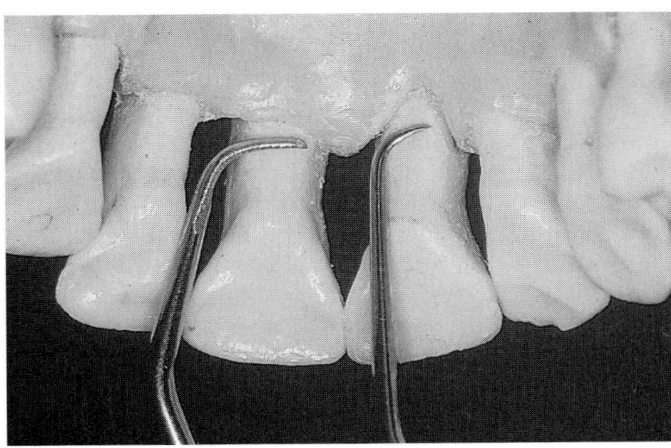

Fig. 41-26 Comparison of a standard rigid Gracey #5-6 with a rigid Mini Five #5-6 on the palatal surfaces of the maxillary central incisors. The Mini Five can be inserted to the base of these tight anterior pockets and used with a straight vertical stroke. A standard Gracey or After Five usually cannot be inserted vertically in this area because the blade is too long.

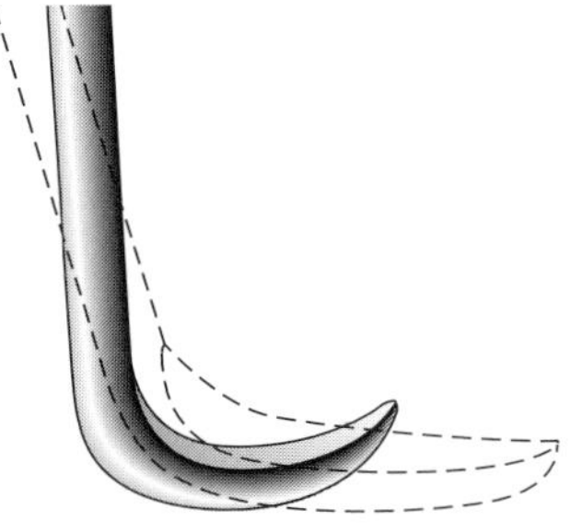

Fig. 41-27 Gracey Curvette blade. This diagram shows the 50% shorter blade of the Gracey Curvette superimposed on the standard Gracey curette blade (*dotted lines*). Notice the upward curvature of the Curvette blade and blade tip. (Redrawn from Pattison G, Pattison A: Periodontal Instrumentation, ed 2. Norwalk, CT, Appleton & Lange, 1992.)

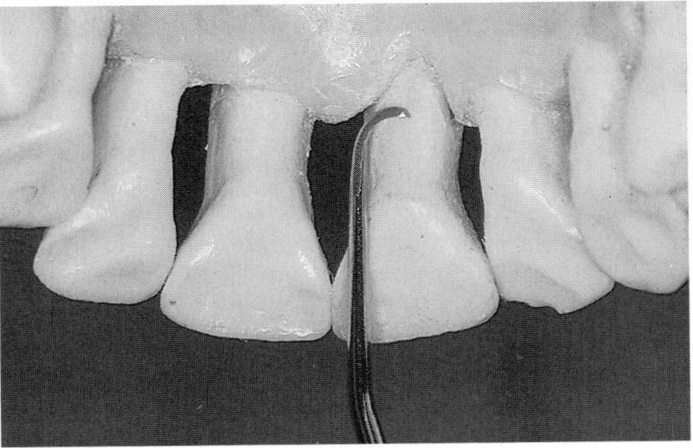

Fig. 41-28 Gracey Curvette Sub-0. Curvette Sub-0 on the palatal surface of a maxillary central. The long shank and short, curved, and blunted tip make this a superior instrument for deep anterior pockets. This curette provides excellent blade adaptation to the narrow root curvatures of the maxillary and mandibular anterior teeth.

the universal curette blade. The Langer #5-6 curette adapts to the mesials and distals of anterior teeth; the Langer #1-2 curette (Gracey #11-12 shank) adapts to the mesial and distal surfaces of mandibular posterior teeth; and the Langer #3-4 curette (Gracey #13-14 shank) adapts to the mesial and distal surfaces of maxillary posterior teeth (Fig. 41-30). These instruments can be adapted to both the mesial and distal tooth surfaces without changing instruments. The standard Langer curette shanks are heavier than a finishing Gracey but less rigid than the rigid Gracey. They are also available with either rigid or finishing shanks and can be obtained in the extended shank (After Five) and mini-bladed (Mini Five) versions.

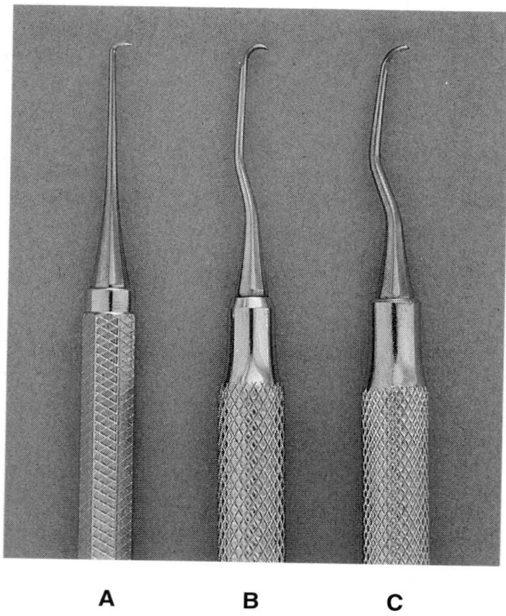

A B C

Fig. 41-29 Comparison of mini-bladed instruments. Four different mini-bladed instruments designed for use on the maxillary and mandibular anteriors. **A,** Morse sickle scaler; **B,** Gracey Curvette Sub-0; **C,** Mini Five #5-6.

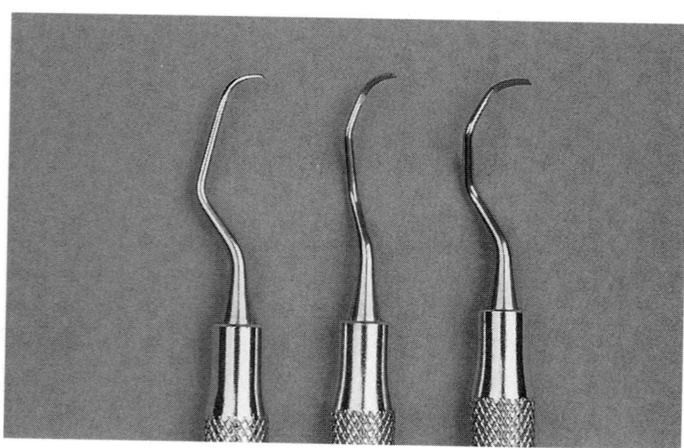

Fig. 41-30 Langer curettes combine Gracey-type shanks with universal curette blades; from left to right: #5-6, #1-2, #3-4.

Schwartz Periotrievers. The Schwartz Periotrievers are a set of two double-ended, highly magnetized instruments designed for the retrieval of broken instrument tips from the periodontal pocket (Figs. 41-31 and 41-32). They are indispensable when the clinician has broken a curette tip in a furcation or deep pocket.[29]

Plastic Instruments for Implants. Several different companies are manufacturing plastic instruments for use on titanium and other implant abutment materials. It is imperative that plastic rather than metal instruments be used to avoid scarring and permanent damage to the implants (Figs. 41-33 and 41-34).[5,6,8,10,13,20,28]

Hoe Scalers. Hoe scalers are used for scaling of ledges or rings of calculus (Fig. 41-35). The blade is bent at a 99-degree angle; the cutting edge is formed by the junction of the flattened terminal surface with the inner aspect of the blade. The cutting edge is beveled at 45 degrees. The blade is slightly bowed so that it can maintain contact at two points on a convex surface. The back of the blade is rounded, and the blade has been reduced

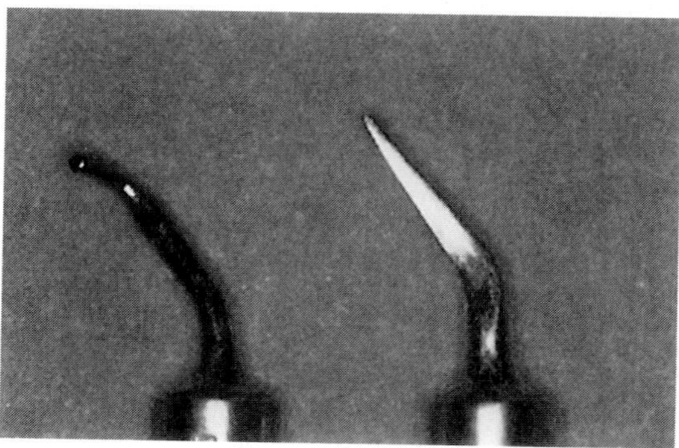

Fig. 41-31 Schwartz Periotriever tip designs. The long blade is for general use in pockets, and the contra-angled tip is for use in furcations. (From Pattison G, Pattison A: Periodontal Instrumentation, ed 2. Norwalk, CT, Appleton & Lange, 1992.)

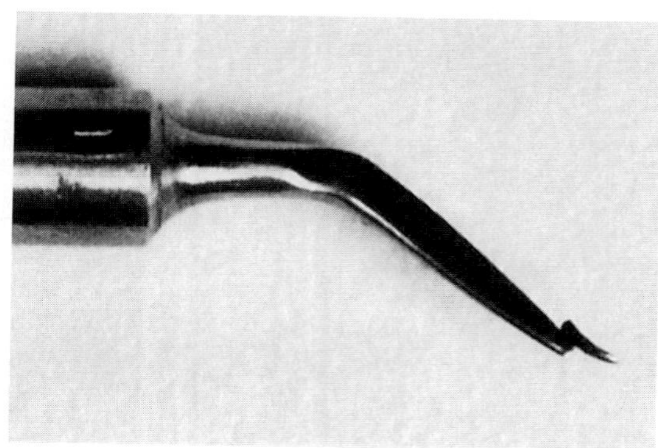

Fig. 41-32 Broken instrument tip attached to the magnetic tip of the Schwartz Periotriever. (From Pattison G, Pattison A: Periodontal Instrumentation, ed 2. Norwalk, CT, Appleton & Lange, 1992.)

to minimal thickness to permit access to the roots without interference from the adjacent tissues.

Hoe scalers are used in the following manner:

1. The blade is inserted to the base of the periodontal pocket so that it makes two-point contact with the tooth (see Fig. 41-35). This stabilizes the instrument and prevents nicking of the root.
2. The instrument is activated with a firm pull stroke toward the crown, with every effort being made to preserve the two-point contact with the tooth.

McCall's hoe scalers #3, 4, 5, 6, 7, and 8 are a set of six hoe scalers designed to provide access to all tooth surfaces. Each instrument has a different angle between the shank and handle.

Files. Files have a series of blades on a base (Fig. 41-36). Their primary function is to fracture or crush tenacious calculus. Files can easily gouge and roughen root surfaces when used improperly. Therefore they are not suitable for fine scaling and root planing. Mini-bladed curettes are currently preferred for areas where files were once commonly used. Files are sometimes used for removing overhanging margins of dental restorations.

Chisel Scalers. The chisel scaler, designed for the proximal surfaces of teeth too closely spaced to permit the use of other scalers, is usually used in the anterior part of the mouth. It is a double-ended instrument with a curved shank at one end and a straight shank at the other (see Fig. 41-36); the blades are slightly curved and have a straight cutting edge beveled at 45 degrees.

The chisel is inserted from the facial surface. The slight curve of the blade makes it possible to stabilize it against the proximal surface, whereas the cutting edge engages the calculus without nicking the tooth. The instrument is activated with a push motion while the side of the blade is held firmly against the root.

Ultrasonic and Sonic Instruments. Ultrasonic instruments may be used for removing plaque, scaling, curetting, and removing stain.[7,8,15,36] The two types of ultrasonic units are magnetostrictive and piezoelectric. In both types, alternating electrical current generates oscillations in materials in the handpiece that cause the scaler tip to vibrate. Depending on the manufacturer, these ultrasonic vibrations at the tip of the instruments of both types range from 20,000 to 45,000 cycles/second (also referred to as *Hertz* [Hz]). In magnetostrictive units (Fig. 41-37), the pattern of vibration of the tip is elliptical, which means that all sides of the tip are active and will work when adapted to the tooth. In piezoelectric units (Fig. 41-38), the pattern of vibration of the tip is linear, or back and forth, meaning that the two sides of the tip are the most active (see Chapter 43).

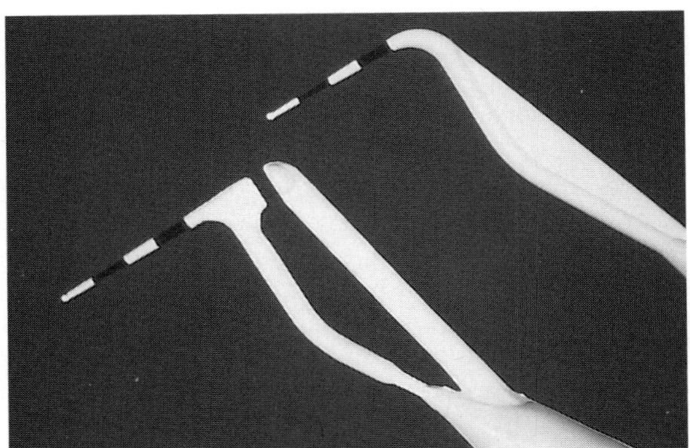

Fig. 41-33 Plastic probes. (Courtesy Professional Dental Technologies, Inc., Batesville, AR.)

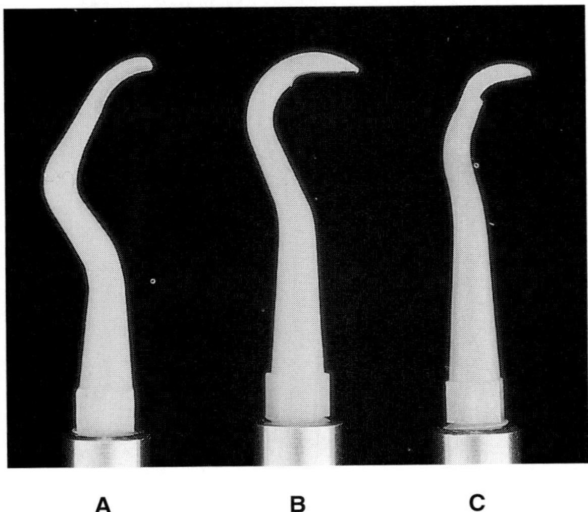

Fig. 41-34 Implacare implant instruments. These implant instruments from the Hu-Friedy Company have autoclavable stainless steel handles and three different cone-socket plastic tip designs. **A,** The Columbia 4R-4L curette tip; **B,** The H6-H7 sickle scaler tip; **C,** The 204S sickle scaler tip.

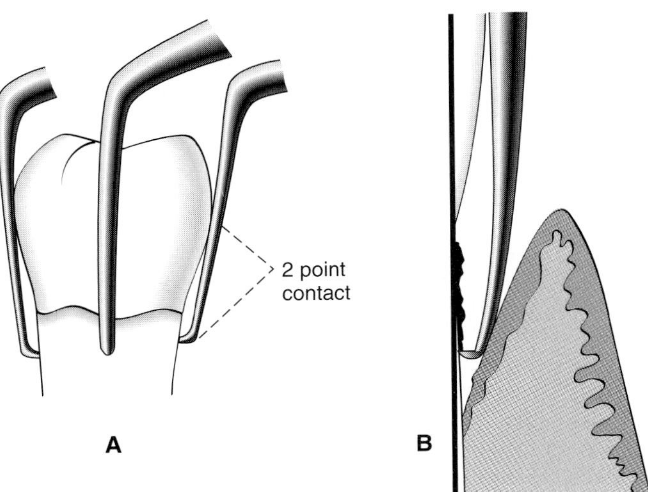

Fig. 41-35 Hoe scalers. **A,** Hoe scalers designed for different tooth surfaces, showing "two-point" contact. **B,** Hoe scaler in a periodontal pocket. The back of the blade is rounded for easier access. The instrument contacts the tooth at two points for stability.

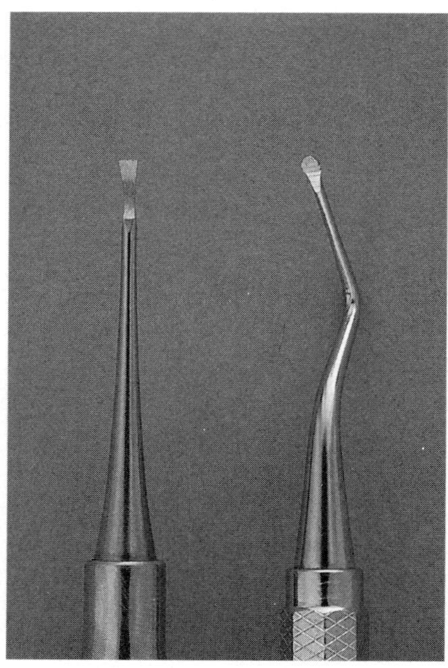

Fig. 41-36 Chisel scaler and file scaler.

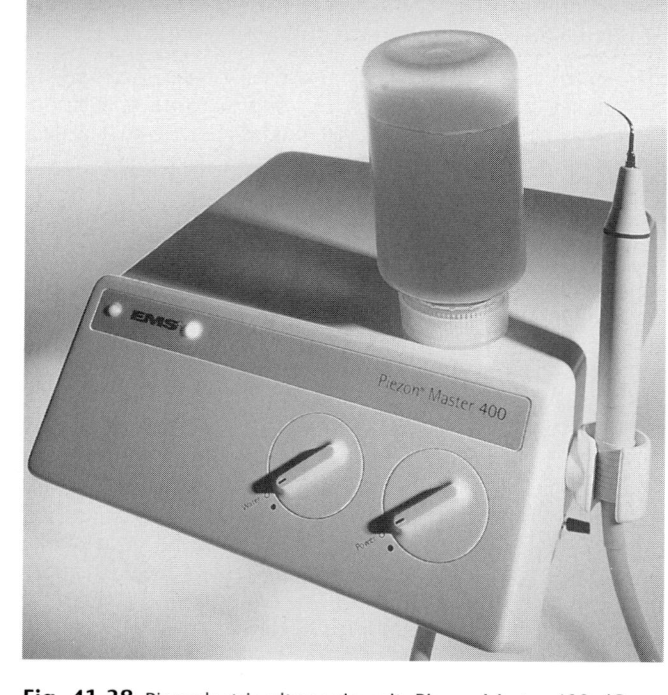

Fig. 41-38 Piezoelectric ultrasonic unit. Piezon Master 400. (Courtesy EMS—Electromedical Systems, Dallas, TX.)

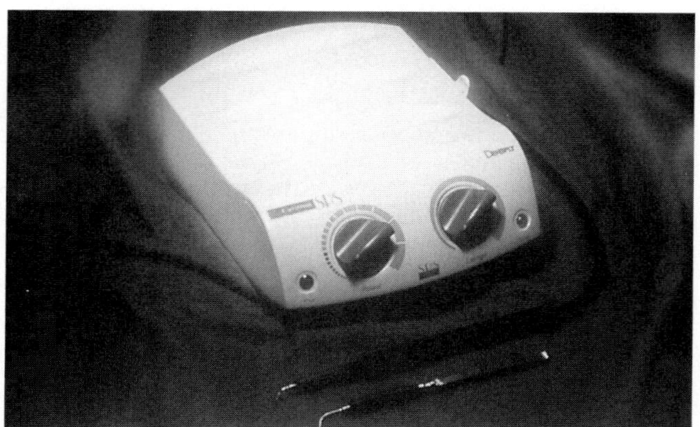

Fig. 41-37 Magnetostrictive ultrasonic unit. The Cavitron SPS ultrasonic scaler. (Courtesy Dentsply International Inc., York, PA.)

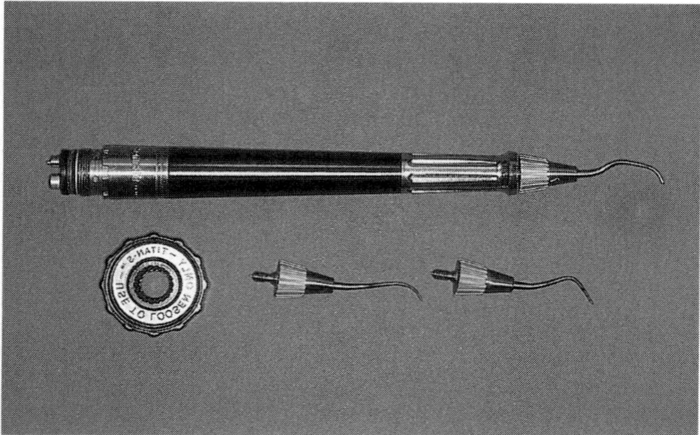

Fig. 41-39 Sonic scaler. The Titan-S sonic scaler from Star Dental Products, Valley Forge, PA.

Sonic units consist of a handpiece that attaches to a compressed air line and uses a variety of specially designed tips (Fig. 41-39). Vibrations at the sonic tip range from 2000 to 6500 cycles per second, which provides less power for calculus removal than ultrasonic units.

A comparison of the three types of power-driven scalers is shown in Table 41-2.

Ultrasonic and sonic tips with different shapes are available for scaling, curetting, root planing, and débriding during periodontal surgery (Fig. 41-40). For many years, only large, bulky tips designed for supragingival removal of heavy calculus were available. In recent years, however, thinner, more delicate tips designed for subgingival debridement have become available[15] (Fig. 41-41). All tips are designed to operate in a wet field and have attached water outlets. The spray is directed at the end of the tip to dissipate the heat generated by the ultrasonic vibrations. Within the water droplets of this spray mist are tiny vacuum bubbles that quickly collapse, releasing energy in a process known as *cavitation*. The cavitating water spray also serves to flush calculus, plaque, and debris dislodged by the vibrating tip from the pocket. Sonic units do not release heat the way ultrasonic units do, but they still have water for cooling and flushing away debris.

TABLE 41-2

Comparison of Sonic and Ultrasonic Scaling Units

		ULTRASONIC	
	Sonic	**Magnetostrictive**	**Piezoelectric**
Advantages			
Calculus removal	good	excellent	excellent
Treatment time	low	low	low
Tip action	orbital	elliptical	linear
Tip adaptability	fair	fair	fair
Patient comfort	good	good	good
Asepsis	good	good	good
Operator control	good	good	good
Space requirement	low	high	high
Disadvantages			
Enamel abrasion	medium	medium	medium
Tissue abrasion	low	low	low
Cemental roughening	medium	medium	medium
Restoration damage	medium	medium	medium
Heat production	low	high	high
Cost	medium	high	high
Maintenance	medium	high	high
Noise level	high	medium	medium

NOTE: This table is meant merely as a guide to choosing power-operated instruments. The clinician is advised to investigate the various types and models of sonic and ultrasonic scaling devices, because technical improvements and changes have affected and will continue to affect the way powered instruments are used in dentistry.

From Perry DA, Beemsterboer P, Carranza FA: Techniques and Theory of Periodontal Instrumentation. Philadelphia, WB Saunders, 1990.

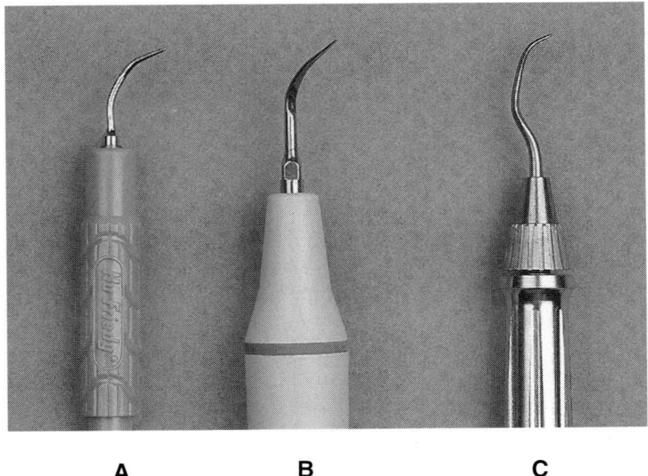

A B C

Fig. 41-40. Ultrasonic and sonic tips. **A,** Triple bend 1000 insert from Dentsply Cavitron, York, PA. **B,** Ultrasonic insert for the EMS scaler. **C,** Sonic insert for the Titan-S.

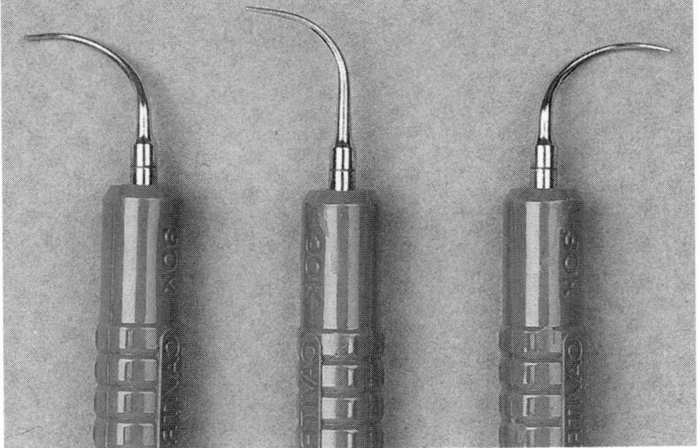

Fig. 41-41 Cavitron FSI® Slim Line ultrasonic tips. Thin inserts from Dentsply Cavitron allow better insertion into deep periodontal pockets and furcations.

The Dental Endoscope. A dental endoscope has been introduced recently for use subgingivally in the diagnosis and treatment of periodontal disease (Fig 41-42). Produced by DentalView, Inc. and called the *Perioscopy System®*, it consists of a 0.99 mm-diameter reusable fiberoptic endoscope over which is fitted a disposable, sterile sheath. The fiberoptic endoscope fits onto periodontal probes and ultrasonic instruments that have been designed to accept it (Fig 41-43). The sheath delivers water irrigation that flushes the pocket while the

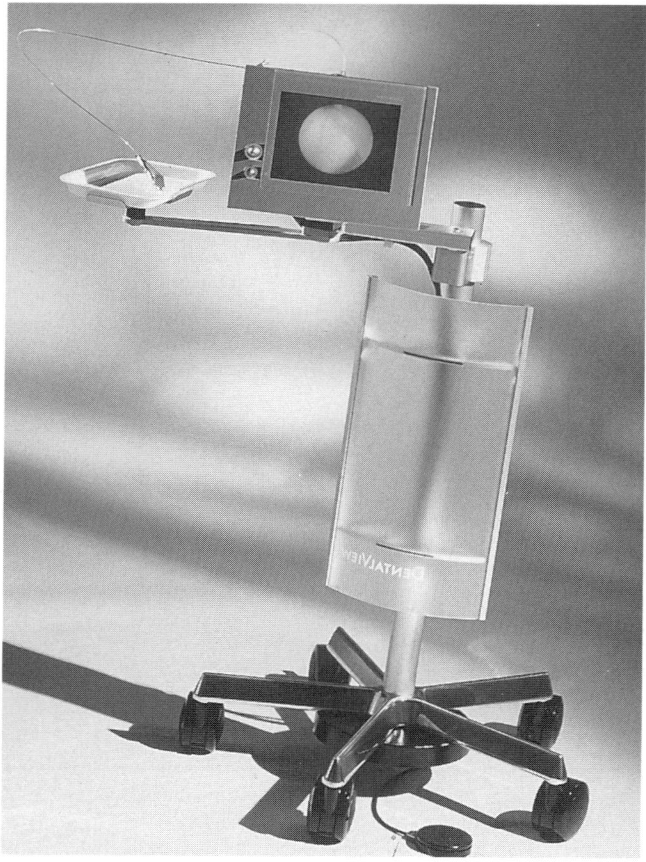

Fig. 41-42 The Perioscopy® System, dental endoscope. (Courtesy DentalView, Inc., Irvine, CA.)

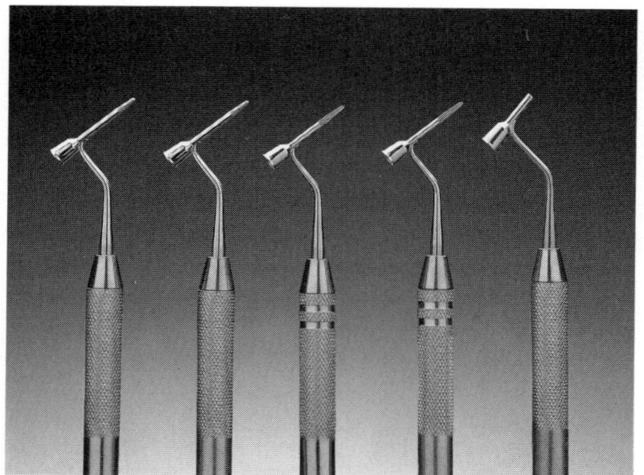

Fig. 41-43 Viewing periodontal explorers (left/right/full viewing) for the Perioscopy® system. (Courtesy DentalView, Inc., Irvine, CA.)

endoscope is in use and keeps the field clear. The fiberoptic endoscope attaches to a medical grade charged coupled device (CCD) video camera and light source that produces an image on a flat panel video monitor for viewing during subgingival exploration and instrumentation. This

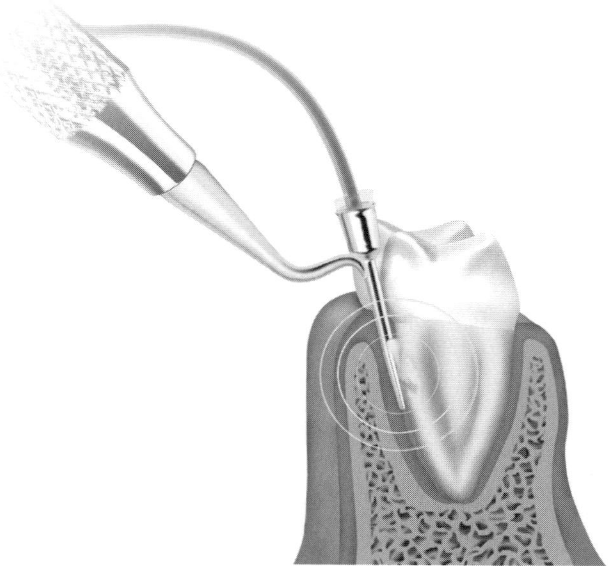

Fig. 41-44 Perioscope® instrumentation permits deep subgingival visualization in pockets and furcations. (Courtesy DentalView, Inc., Irvine, CA.)

device allows clear visualization deep subgingivally in pockets and in furcations (Fig. 41-44). It enables the operator to detect the presence and location of subgingival deposits and guides the operator in their thorough removal. Magnification ranges from 24× to 46×, enabling visualization of even minute deposits of plaque and calculus. Using this device, it is possible to achieve levels of root debridement and cleanliness that are much more difficult or impossible to produce without it. The Perioscopy System® can also be used to evaluate subgingivally for caries, defective restorations, root fractures, and resorption.

The EVA System. Probably the most efficient and least traumatic instruments for correcting overhanging or overcontoured proximal alloy and resin restorations are the motor-driven diamond files of the EVA prophylaxis instrument. These files, which come in symmetric pairs, are made of aluminum in the shape of a wedge protruding from a shaft; one side of the wedge is diamond coated; the other side is smooth. The files can be mounted on a special dental handpiece attachment that generates reciprocating strokes of variable frequency. When the unit is activated interproximally with the diamond-coated side of the file touching the restoration and the smooth side adjacent to the papilla, the oscillating file swiftly planes the contour of the restoration and reduces it to the desired shape.

Cleansing and Polishing Instruments

Rubber Cups. Rubber cups consist of a rubber shell with or without webbed configurations in the hollow interior (Fig. 41-45). They are used in the handpiece with a special prophylaxis angle. The handpiece, prophylaxis angle, and rubber cup must be sterilized after each

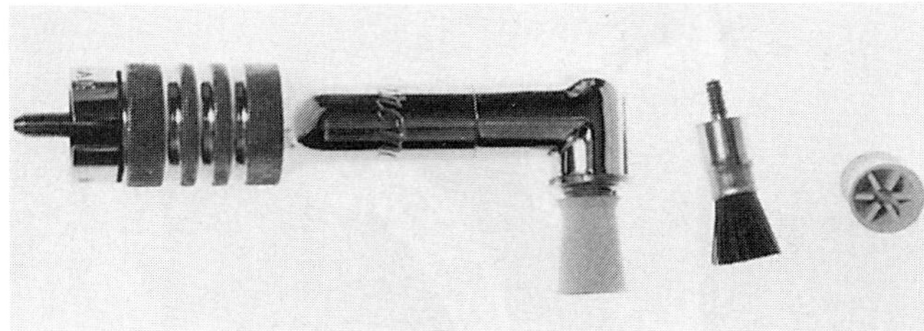

Fig. 41-45 Prophylaxis handpiece with rubber cup and brush.

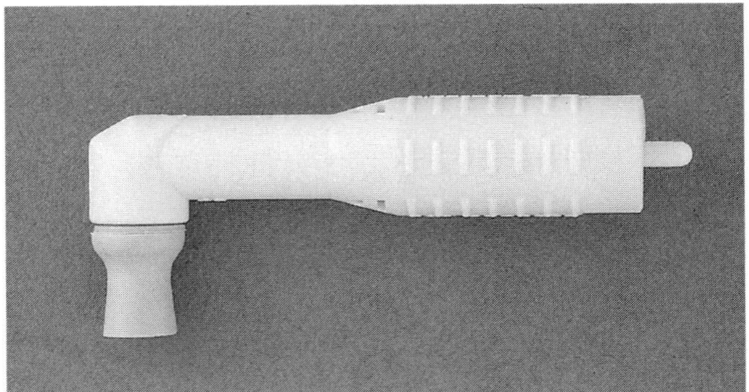

Fig. 41-46 Disposable plastic prophylaxis angle with rubber cup.

patient use, or a disposable plastic prophylaxis angle and rubber cup (Fig. 41-46) may be used and then discarded. A good cleansing and polishing paste that contains fluoride should be used and kept moist to minimize frictional heat as the cup revolves. Polishing pastes are available in fine, medium, or coarse grits and are packaged in small, convenient, single-use containers. Aggressive use of the rubber cup with any abrasive may remove the layer of cementum, which is thin in the cervical area.

Bristle Brushes. Bristle brushes are available in wheel and cup shapes (see Fig. 41-45). The brush is used in the handpiece with a polishing paste. Because the bristles are stiff, use of the brush should be confined to the crown to avoid injuring the cementum and the gingiva.

Dental Tape. Dental tape with polishing paste is used for polishing proximal surfaces that are inaccessible to other polishing instruments. The tape is passed interproximally while being kept at a right angle to the long axis of the tooth and is activated with a firm labiolingual motion. Particular care is taken to avoid injury to the gingiva. The area should be cleansed with warm water to remove all remnants of paste.

Air-Powder Polishing. In the early 1980s, a specially designed handpiece was introduced that delivers an air-powered slurry of warm water and sodium bicarbonate; this instrument is called the *Prophy-Jet* (Fig. 41-47). This system is effective for the removal of extrinsic stains and soft deposits. The slurry removes stains rapidly and efficiently by mechanical abrasion and provides warm water for rinsing and lavage. The flow rate of abrasive cleansing power can be adjusted to increase the amount of powder for heavier stain removal.

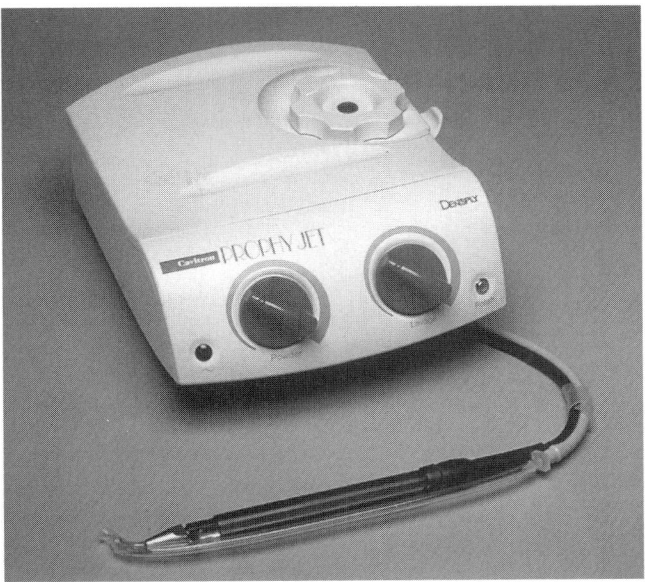

Fig. 41-47 Prophy-Jet air-powder polishing device. (Courtesy Dentsply International, Inc., York, PA.)

The results of studies on the abrasive effect of the air-powder polishing device on cementum and dentin show that tooth substance can be lost.[4,23] Damage to gingival tissue is transient and insignificant clinically, but amalgam restorations, composite resins, cements, and other nonmetallic materials can be roughened.[2,9,19,23] Air-powder polishing can be used safely on titanium implant surfaces.[16,26]

Patients with medical histories of respiratory illnesses, hypertension, hemodialysis, sodium-restricted diets and those on medications affecting the electrolyte balance are not candidates for the use of the air-powder polishing device.[25,32,34] Patients with infectious diseases should not be treated with this device because of the large quantity of aerosol created. A preprocedural rinse with 0.12% chlorhexidine gluconate should be used to minimize the microbial content of the aerosol.[3] High speed evacuation should also be used to eliminate as much of the aerosol as possible.[14]

SURGICAL INSTRUMENTS

Periodontal surgery is accomplished with numerous instruments; Fig. 41-48 shows a typical surgical cassette. Periodontal surgical instruments are classified as follows:

1. Excisional and incisional instruments
2. Surgical curettes and sickles
3. Periosteal elevators
4. Surgical chisels
5. Surgical files
6. Scissors
7. Hemostats and tissue forceps

A

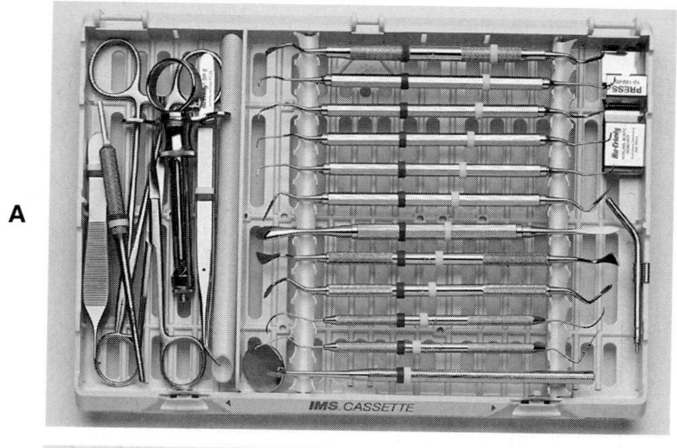

B

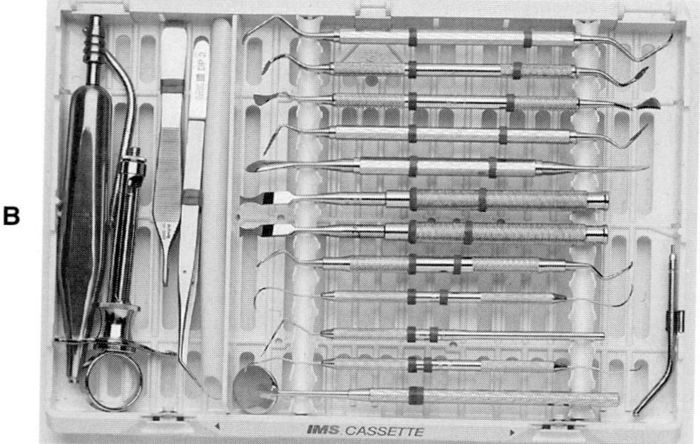

C

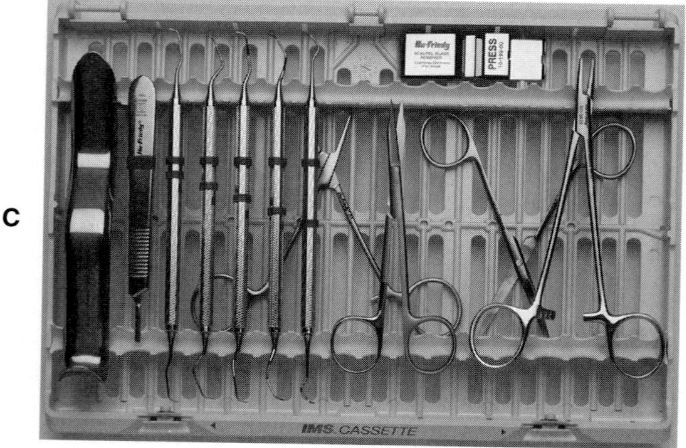

Fig. 41-48 Instrument cassettes for periodontal surgery. Cassettes shown in **A** and **B** are to be used together for involved cases, while the cassette shown in **C** is a reduced set for simple cases. Additional instruments may be used according to individual preferences and case requirements. **A,** Mirror, explorer, probe, furcation probe, chisels, periosteal elevator, file, knives, surgical curette, dressing pliers, tissue pliers, aspirator tip. **B,** Retractor, scalpel handle, root planing curettes, universal curette, hemostat, scissors, needleholders, suture scissors, scalpel blade remover. **C,** Simplified set: mirror, explorer-probe, furcation probe, knives, periosteal elevator, file, root planing curettes, universal curette, chisel, scalpel handle, dressing pliers, tissue pliers, needleholder, scissors, scalpel blade remover. (Courtesy Hu-Friedy Instrument Company, Chicago.)

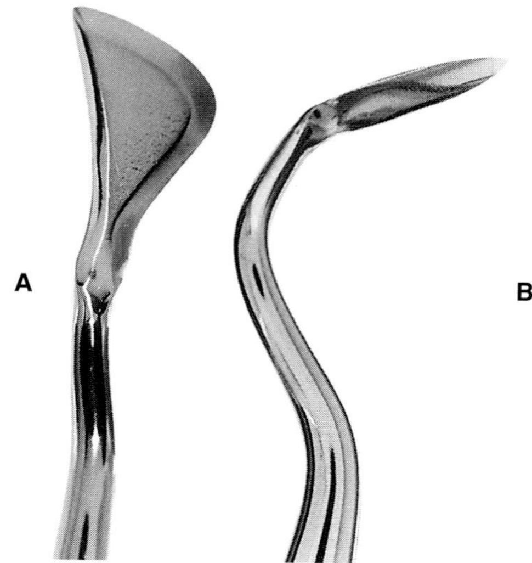

Fig. 41-49 Gingivectomy knives. **A,** Kirkland knife. **B,** Orban interdental knife.

Excisional and Incisional Instruments

Periodontal Knives (Gingivectomy Knives). The Kirkland knife is representative of knives commonly used for gingivectomy. These knives can be obtained as either double-ended or single-ended instruments. The entire periphery of these kidney-shaped knives is the cutting edge (Fig. 41-49, *A*).

Interdental Knives. The Orban knife #1-2 (Fig. 41-49, *B*) and the Merrifield knife #1, 2, 3, and 4 are examples of knives used for interdental areas. These spear-shaped knives have cutting edges on both sides of the blade and are designed with either double-ended or single-ended blades.

Surgical Blades. Scalpel blades of different shapes and sizes are used in periodontal surgery. The most commonly used blades are #12D, 15, and 15C (Fig. 41-50). The #12D blade is a beak-shaped blade with cutting edges on both sides, allowing the operator to engage narrow, restricted areas with both pushing and pulling cutting motions. The #15 blade is used for thinning flaps and for all-around use. The #15C blade, a narrower version of the #15 blade, is useful for making the initial, scalloping type incision. The slim design of this blade allows for incising into the narrow interdental portion of the flap. All of these blades are discarded after one use.

Electrosurgery (Radiosurgery) Techniques and Instrumentation. The term *electrosurgery* or *radiosurgery*[30] is currently used to identify surgical techniques performed on soft tissue using controlled high-frequency electrical (radio) currents in the range of 1.5 to 7.5 million cycles per second or megahertz (Fig. 41-51). There are three classes of active electrodes: single-wire electrodes for incising or excising; loop electrodes for planing tissue; and heavy, bulkier electrodes for coagulation procedures.[11,21]

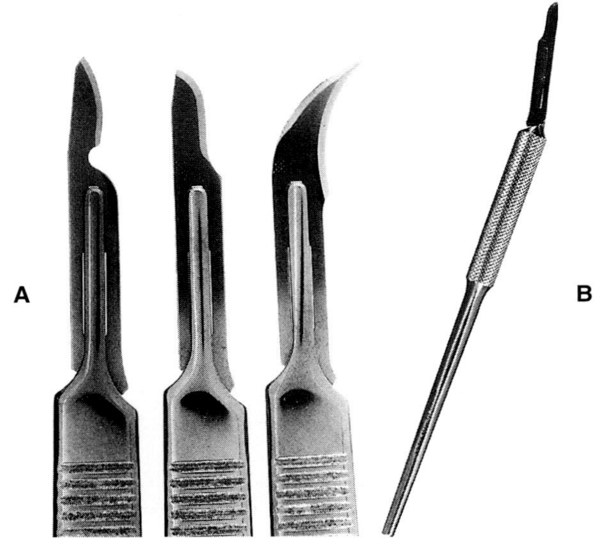

Fig. 41-50 Surgical blades. **A,** #15*C,* 15, and 12*D.* **B,** Contra-angled scalpel handle.

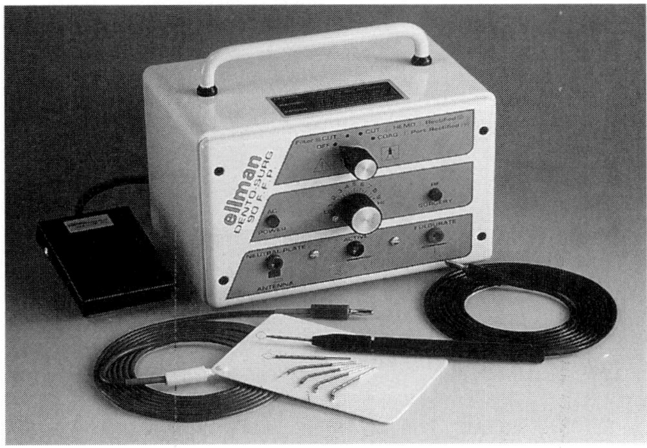

Fig. 41-51 Radiosurgical (electrosurgical) unit. Dento-Surg 90 FFP (Courtesy Ellman International Inc., Hewlett, NY.)

The four basic types of electrosurgical techniques are electrosection, electrocoagulation, electrofulguration, and electrodesiccation.

Electrosection, also referred to as *electrotomy* or *acusection,* is used for incisions, excisions, and tissue planing. Incisions and excisions are performed with single-wire active electrodes that can be bent or adapted to accomplish any type of cutting procedure.

Electrocoagulation provides a wide range of coagulation or hemorrhage control obtained by using the electrocoagulation current. Electrocoagulation can prevent bleeding or hemorrhage at the initial entry into soft tissue, but it cannot stop bleeding after blood is present. All forms of hemorrhage must be stopped first by some form of direct pressure (e.g., air, compress, or hemostat). After bleeding has momentarily stopped, final sealing of the capillaries or large vessels can be accomplished by a short application of the electrocoagulation current. The active electrodes used for coagulation are much bulkier than the fine tungsten wire used for electrosection.

Electrosection and electrocoagulation are the procedures most commonly used in all areas of dentistry. The two monoterminal techniques, electrofulguration and electrodesiccation, are not in general use in dentistry.

The most important basic rule of electrosurgery is: *always keep the tip moving.* Prolonged or repeated application of current to tissue induces heat accumulation and undesired tissue destruction, whereas interrupted application at intervals adequate for tissue cooling (5 to 10 seconds) reduces or eliminates heat buildup. Electrosurgery is not intended to destroy tissue; it is a controllable means of sculpturing or modifying oral soft tissue with little discomfort and hemorrhage for the patient.

The indications for electrosurgery in periodontal therapy and a description of wound healing after electrosurgery are presented in Chapter 58. Electrosurgery is contraindicated for patients who have noncompatible or poorly shielded cardiac pacemakers.

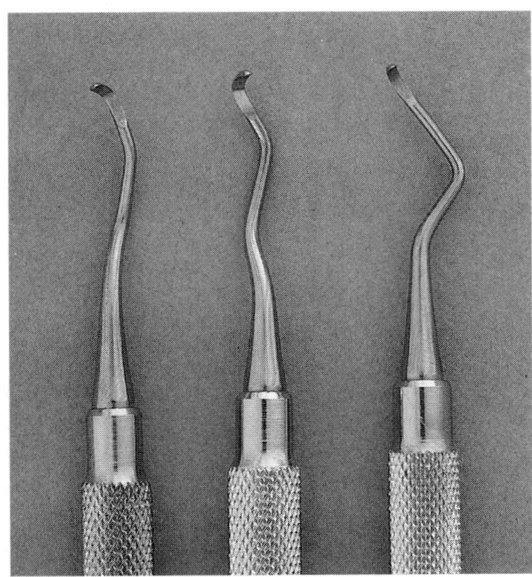

Fig. 41-52 Kramer heavy surgical curettes #1, 2, and 3.

Surgical Curettes and Sickles

Larger and heavier curettes and sickles are often needed during surgery for the removal of granulation tissue, fibrous interdental tissues, and tenacious subgingival deposits. The Kramer curettes #1, 2, and 3 (Fig. 41-52) and the Kirkland surgical instruments are heavy curettes, whereas the Ball scaler #B2-B3 is a popular heavy sickle. The wider, heavier blades of these instruments make them suitable for surgical procedures.

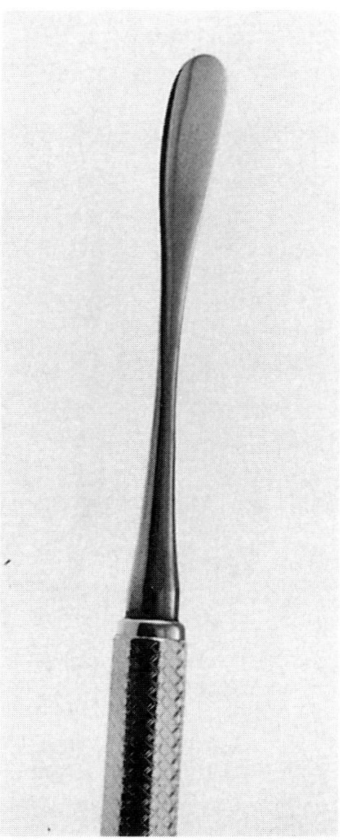

Fig. 41-53 Glickman periosteal elevator #24G.

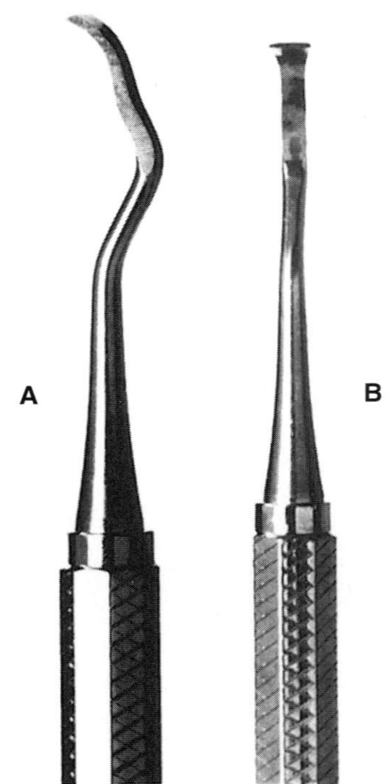

Fig. 41-54 Lateral **(A)** and frontal **(B)** views of a surgical hoe.

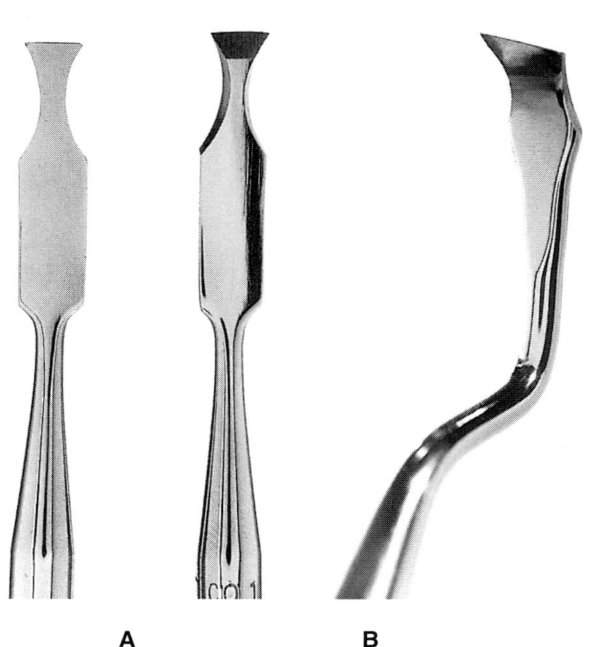

Fig. 41-55 Surgical chisels. **A,** Ochsenbein chisels. **B,** Rhodes chisel.

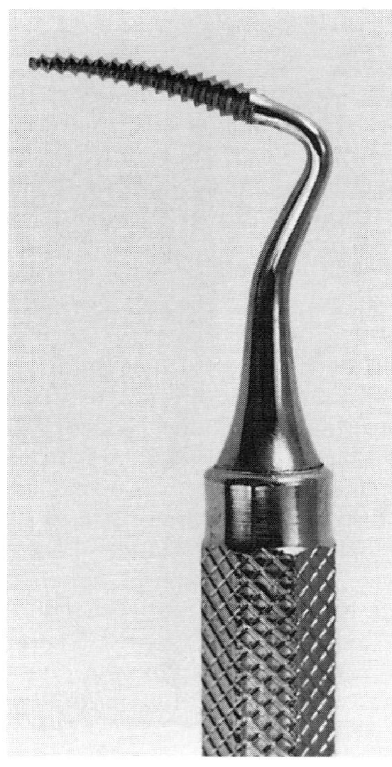

Fig. 41-56 Schluger #9-10 surgical file.

Periosteal Elevators

These instruments are necessary to reflect and move the flap after the incision has been made for flap surgery. The #24G (Fig. 41-53) and the Goldman-Fox #14 are well-designed periosteal elevators.

Surgical Chisels and Hoes

Chisels and hoes are used during periodontal surgery for removing and reshaping bone. The hoe shown in Fig. 41-54 has a curved shank and blade, whereas the Wiedelstadt and Todd-Gilmore chisels are straight shanked. The surgical hoe has a flattened, fishtail-shaped blade with a pronounced convexity in its terminal portion. The cutting edge is beveled with rounded edges and projects beyond the long axis of the handle to preserve the effectiveness of the instrument when the blade is reduced by sharpening. The surgical hoe is generally used for detaching pocket walls after the gingivectomy incision, but it is also useful for smoothing root and bone surfaces made accessible by any surgical procedure. The Ochsenbein #1-2 (Fig. 41-55, *A*) is a useful chisel with a semicircular indentation on both sides of the shank that allows the instrument to engage around the tooth and into the interdental area. Surgical hoes are usually used with a pull stroke, whereas chisels are engaged with a push stroke. The Rhodes chisel is shown in Fig. 41-55, *B*.

Surgical Files

Periodontal surgical files are used primarily to smooth rough bony ledges and to remove all areas of bone. The Schluger (Fig. 41-56) and Sugarman files are similar in design and can be used with a push-and-pull stroke, primarily in the interdental areas.

Scissors and Nippers

Scissors and nippers are used in periodontal surgery for such purposes as removing tabs of tissue during gingivectomy, trimming the margins of flaps, enlarging incisions in periodontal abscesses, and removing muscle attachments in mucogingival surgery. There are many types, and the choice is a matter of individual preference. Fig. 41-57 shows the Goldman-Fox #16 scissors with a curved beveled blade with serrations and the nippers.

Needleholders

Needleholders are used to suture the flap at the desired position after the surgical procedure has been completed. The regular type of needleholder is illustrated in Figure 41-58, *A,* whereas Fig. 41-58, *B* shows the Castroviejo needleholder, which is used for delicate, precise techniques requiring quick and easy release and grasp of the suture.

SHARPENING OF PERIODONTAL INSTRUMENTS

It is impossible to carry out periodontal procedures efficiently with dull instruments. A sharp instrument cuts more precisely and quickly than a dull instrument. To do its job at all, a dull instrument must be held more firmly and pressed harder than a sharp instrument. This reduces tactile sensitivity and increases the possibility that the instrument will inadvertently slip. *Therefore to avoid*

A

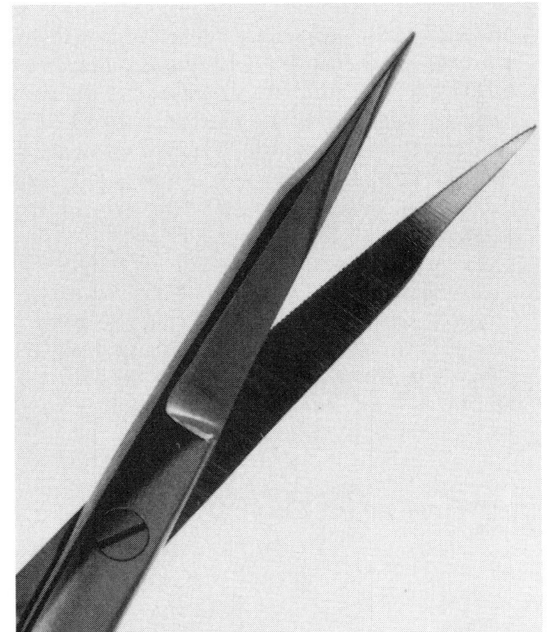

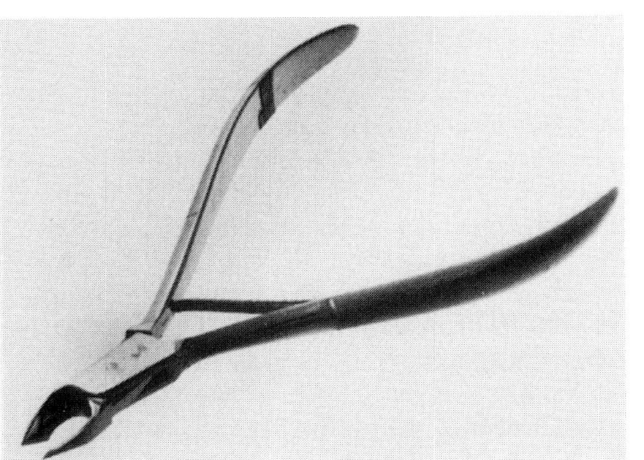

B

Fig. 41-57 A, Goldman-Fox #16 scissors. **B,** Nippers.

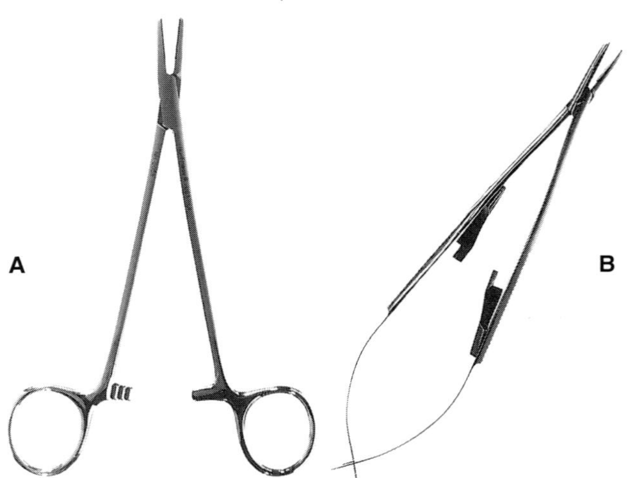

Fig. 41-58 **A,** Conventional needleholder. **B,** Castroviejo needleholder.

wasting time and operating haphazardly, clinicians must be thoroughly familiar with the principles of sharpening and able to apply them to produce a keen cutting edge on the instruments they are using. Development of this skill requires patience and practice, but clinical excellence cannot be attained without it.

SHARPNESS AND HOW TO EVALUATE IT

The cutting edge of an instrument is formed by the angular junction of two surfaces of its blade. The cutting edges of a curette, for example, are formed where the face of the blade meets the lateral surfaces (Fig. 41-59).

When the instrument is sharp, this junction is a fine line running the length of the cutting edge. As the instrument is used, metal is worn away at the cutting edge, and the junction of the face and lateral surface becomes rounded or dulled[1,18] (Fig. 41-60). Thus the cutting edge becomes a rounded surface rather than an acute angle. This is why a dull instrument cuts less efficiently and requires more pressure to do its job.[12]

Sharpness can be evaluated by sight and touch in one of the following ways:

1. When a dull instrument is held under a light, the rounded surface of its cutting edge reflects light back to the observer. It appears as a bright line running the length of the cutting edge (Fig. 41-61). The acutely angled cutting edge of a sharp instrument, on the other hand, has no surface area to reflect light. When a sharp instrument is held under a light, no bright line can be observed (see Fig. 41-59).
2. Tactile evaluation of sharpness is performed by drawing the instrument lightly across an acrylic rod known as a *sharpening "test stick."* A dull instrument will slide smoothly, without "biting" into the surface and raising a light shaving as a sharp instrument would.[36]

The Objective of Sharpening

The objective of sharpening is to restore the fine, thin, linear cutting edge of the instrument. This is done by grinding the surfaces of the blade until their junction is once again sharply angular rather than rounded. For any given instrument, several sharpening techniques may produce this result. A technique is acceptable if it produces a sharp cutting edge without unduly wearing the instrument or altering its original design. To maintain the original design, the operator must understand the location and course of the cutting edges and the angles between the surfaces that form them. It is important to restore the cutting edge without distorting the original angles of the instrument. When these angles have been altered, the instrument does not function as it was designed to function, which limits its effectiveness.

Sharpening Stones

Sharpening stones may be quarried from natural mineral deposits or produced artificially. In either case, the surface of the stone is made up of abrasive crystals that are harder than the metal of the instrument to be sharpened. Coarse stones have larger particles and cut more rapidly; they are used on instruments that are dull. Finer stones with smaller crystals cut more slowly and are reserved for final sharpening to produce a finer edge and for sharpening instruments that are only slightly dull.[27,31] India and Arkansas oilstones are examples of natural abrasive stones. Carborundum, ruby, and ceramic stones are synthetically produced (Fig. 41-62).

Sharpening stones can also be categorized by their method of use.

Mounted Rotary Stones. These stones are mounted on a metal mandrel and used in a motor-driven handpiece. They may be cylindric, conical, or disc shaped. These stones are generally not recommended for routine use, because (1) they are difficult to control precisely and can ruin the shape of the instrument, (2) they tend to wear down the instrument quickly, and (3) they can generate quite a bit of frictional heat, which may affect the temper of the instrument.

Unmounted Stones. These come in a variety of sizes and shapes. Some are rectangular with flat or grooved surfaces, whereas others are cylindric or cone shaped. Unmounted stones may be used in two ways: the instrument may be stabilized and held stationary while the stone is drawn across it, or the stone may be stabilized and held stationary while the instrument is drawn across it.

Principles of Sharpening

1. Choose a stone suitable for the instrument to be sharpened—one that is of an appropriate shape and abrasiveness.
2. Use a sterilized sharpening stone if the instrument to be sharpened will not be resterilized before it is used on a patient.

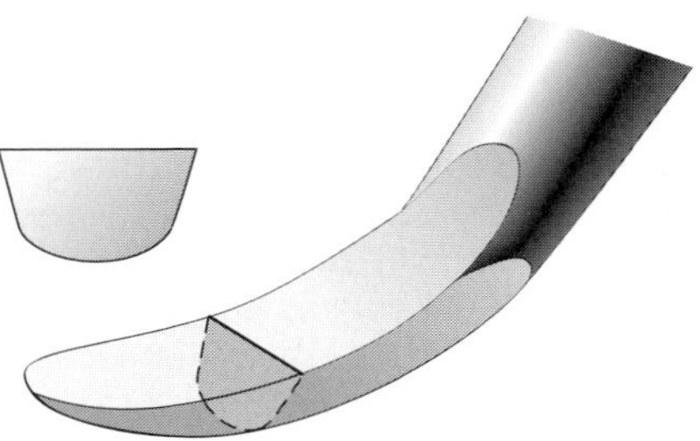

Fig. 41-59 The cutting edge of a curette is formed by the angular junction of the face and the lateral surfaces of the instrument. When the instrument is sharp, the cutting edge is a fine line.

Fig. 41-60 The cutting edge of a dull curette is rounded.

3. Establish the proper angle between the sharpening stone and the surface of the instrument on the basis of an understanding of its design.
4. Maintain a stable, firm grasp of both the instrument and the sharpening stone. This ensures that the proper angulation is maintained throughout the controlled sharpening stroke. In this manner, the entire surface of the instrument can be reduced evenly, and the cutting edge is not improperly beveled.
5. Avoid excessive pressure. Heavy pressure causes the stone to grind the surface of the instrument more quickly and may shorten the instrument's life unnecessarily.
6. Avoid the formation of a "wire edge," characterized by minute filamentous projections of metal extending as a roughened ledge from the sharpened cutting edge.[1,12,24,36] When the instrument is used on root surfaces, these projections produce a grooved surface rather than a smooth surface. A wire edge is produced when the direction of the sharpening stroke is away from, rather than into or toward, the cutting edge.[1,24] When back-and-forth or up-and-down sharpening strokes are used, formation of a wire edge can be avoided by finishing with a down stroke toward the cutting edge.[18]
7. Lubricate the stone during sharpening. This minimizes clogging of the abrasive surface of the sharpening stone with metal particles removed from the instrument.[12,24,36] It also reduces heat produced by friction. Oil should be used for natural stones and water for synthetic stones.
8. Sharpen instruments at the first sign of dullness. A grossly dull instrument is inefficient and requires more pressure when used, which hinders control. Furthermore, sharpening such an instrument requires the removal of a great deal of metal to produce a sharp cutting edge. This shortens the effective life of the instrument.

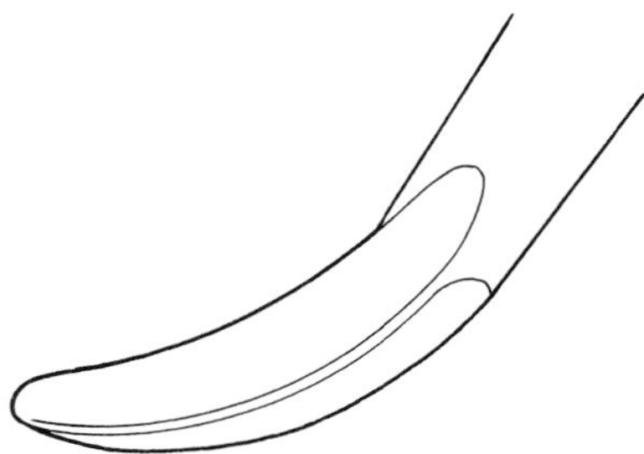

Fig. 41-61 Light reflected from the rounded cutting edge of a dull instrument appears as a bright line.

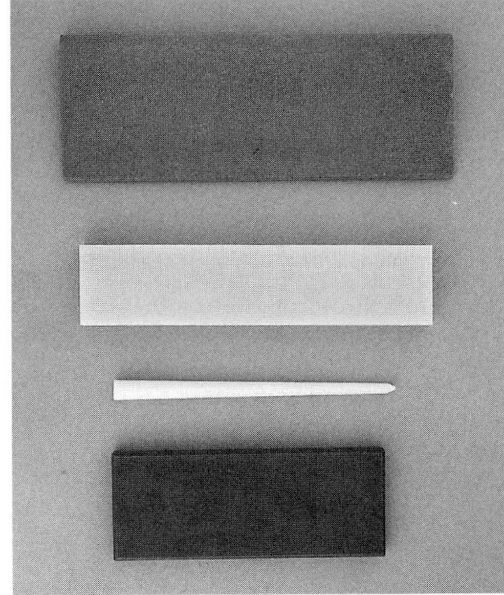

Fig. 41-62 Sharpening stones. *Top to bottom,* A flat India stone, a flat Arkansas stone, a cone-shaped Arkansas stone, and a ceramic stone.

Sharpening Individual Instruments

Universal Curettes. Several techniques will produce a properly sharpened curette. Regardless of the technique used, the clinician must keep in mind that the angle between the face of the blade and the lateral surface of any curette is 70 to 80 degrees (Fig. 41-63). This is the most effective design for removing calculus and root planing. Changing this angle distorts the design of the instrument and makes it less effective. A cutting edge of less than 70 degrees is quite sharp but also thin (Fig. 41-64). It wears down quickly and becomes dull. A cutting edge of 90 degrees or more requires heavy lateral pressure to remove deposits. Calculus removal with such an instrument is often incomplete, and root planing cannot be done effectively (see Fig. 41-64).

The following technique is recommended because it enables the clinician to visualize the critical 70- to

80-degree angle easily and thereby consistently restores an effective cutting edge:

Sharpening the Lateral Surface. When a flat, hand-held stone is correctly applied to the lateral surface of a curette to maintain the 70- to 80-degree angle, the angle between the face of the blade and the surface of the stone will be 100 to 110 degrees (see Fig. 41-63). This can best be visualized by holding the curette so that the face of the blade is parallel with the floor. A palm grasp should be used and the upper arm braced against the body for support.

1. Apply the sharpening stone to the lateral surface of the curette so that the angle between the face of the blade and the stone is 100 to 110 degrees (Fig. 41-65; see Fig. 41-63).
2. Beginning at the shank end of the cutting edge and working toward the toe, activate the stone with short up-and-down strokes. Use consistent, light pressure and keep the stone continuously in contact with the blade. Make sure that the 100- to 110-degree angle is constantly maintained (see Fig. 41-65).
3. Check for sharpness as previously described, and continue sharpening as necessary. To prevent the toe of the curette from becoming pointed, sharpen the entire blade from shank end to toe. When approaching the toe, be sure to sharpen around it to preserve its rounded form (Fig. 41-66).
4. As the stone is moved along the cutting edge, finish each section with a down stroke into or toward the cutting edge. This will minimize the formation of a wire edge. Check the cutting edge under a light.
5. Sharpening the curette in this manner tends to flatten the lateral surface. This can be corrected by lightly grinding the lateral surface and the back of the instrument, away from the cutting edge, each time the instrument is sharpened.
6. When one edge has been properly sharpened, the opposite cutting edge can be sharpened in the same manner.

Sharpening the Face of the Blade. This may be done by moving a hand-held cylindric or cone-shaped stone back and forth across the face of the blade. A similar stone mounted in a hand-piece may also be used by applying it to the face of the blade with the stone rotating toward the toe. These methods are not recommended for routine use for the following reasons:

1. The angulation between the instrument and the stone is difficult to maintain, and therefore the blade may be improperly beveled (Fig. 41-67).[1]

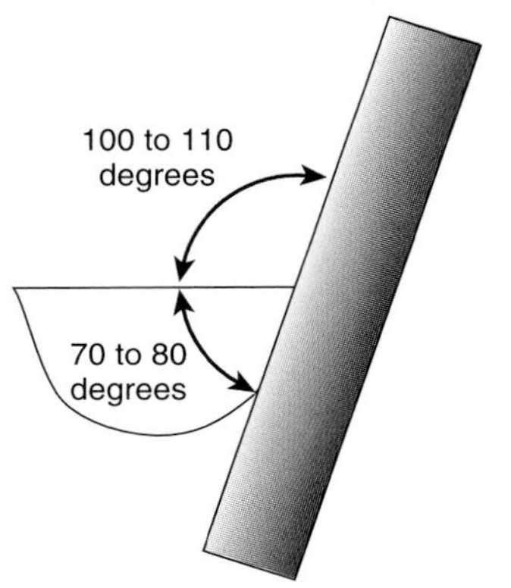

Fig. 41-63 When the sharpening stone forms a 100- to 110-degree angle with the face of the blade, the 70- to 80-degree angle between the face and the lateral surface is automatically preserved.

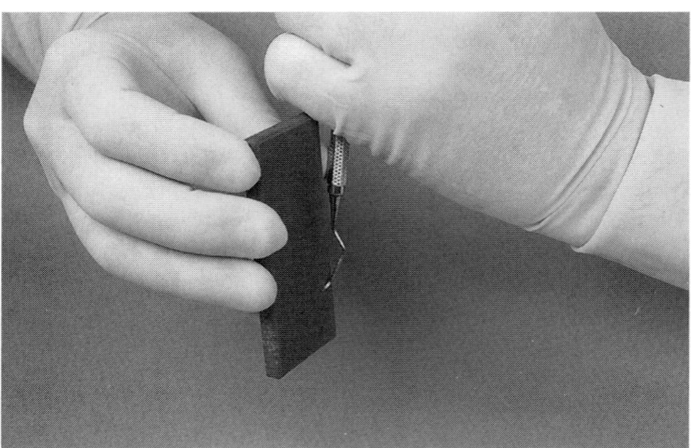

Fig. 41-65 Using a palm grasp, one holds the universal curette so that the face of the blade is parallel to the floor. The stone makes a 100- to 110-degree angle with the face of the blade.

Fig. 41-64 At the left is a properly sharpened curette that maintains a 70- to 80-degree angle between its face and lateral surface. The curette in the center has been sharpened so that one of its cutting edges is less than 70 degrees. This fine edge is quite sharp but dulls easily. One of the cutting edges of the curette on the right has been sharpened to 90 degrees. Heavy lateral pressure must be applied to the tooth to remove deposits with such an instrument.

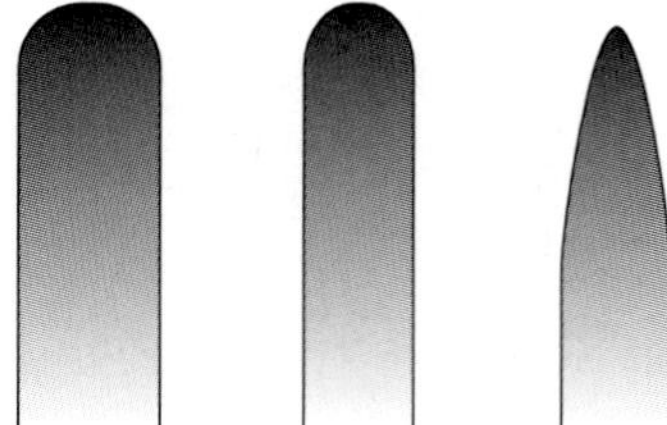

Fig. 41-66 At the left is a new, unsharpened curette viewed from directly above the face of the blade. The curette in the center has been correctly sharpened to maintain the rounded toe. The curette at the right has been incorrectly sharpened, producing a pointed toe.

2. Sharpening the face of the blade narrows the working end from face to back. This weakens the blade and makes it likely to bend or break while in use[1,18,24,29] (see Fig. 41-67).
3. Sharpening the face of the blade with a handheld stone using a back-and-forth motion produces a wire edge that interferes with the sharpness of the blade.[1]

Area-Specific (Gracey) Curettes. Like a universal curette, a Gracey curette has an angle of 70 to 80 degrees between the face and lateral surface of its blade. Therefore the technique described for sharpening a universal curette can be used to sharpen a Gracey curette. However, several unique design features that distinguish a Gracey from a universal curette must be understood to avoid distorting the design of the instrument while sharpening (see Gracey Curettes, pp. 571–574).

Gracey curettes have what is known as an *offset blade* (i.e., the face of the blade is not perpendicular to the shank of the instrument, as it is on a universal curette, but is offset at a 70-degree angle [Fig. 41-68]). A Gracey curette is further distinguished by the curvature of its cutting edges. When viewed from directly above the face of the blade, the cutting edges of a universal curette extend in straight lines from shank to toe; both cutting edges can be used for scaling and root planing. The cutting edges of a Gracey curette, on the other hand, curve gently from shank to toe, and only the larger, outer cutting edge is used for scaling and root planing (Fig. 41-69).

With these points in mind, a Gracey curette is sharpened in the following manner:

1. Hold the curette so that the face of the blade is parallel with the floor. Because the blade is offset, the shank of the instrument will not be perpendicular to the floor, as it is with universal curettes (Fig. 41-70).
2. Identify the edge to be sharpened. Remember that only one cutting edge is used, so only that edge must be sharpened. Apply the stone to the lateral surface so that the angle between the face of the blade and the stone is 100 to 110 degrees.
3. Activate short up-and-down strokes, working from the shank end of the blade to the curved toe. Finish with a down stroke.
4. Remember that the cutting edge is curved. Preserve the curve by turning the stone while sharpening from shank to toe. If the stone is kept in one place for too many strokes, the blade will be flattened (Fig. 41-71).
5. Evaluate sharpness as previously described. Continue sharpening as necessary.

Extended Shank and Mini-Bladed Gracey Curettes. Extended shank Gracey curettes such as the After Fives are sharpened in exactly the same manner as the standard Gracey curettes. Although the terminal shank is 3 mm longer, the blade size and shape are

Fig. 41-67 Angulation is difficult to control when sharpening the face of the blade and often results in unwanted beveling, as shown at the left. Sharpening the face also weakens the blade by narrowing it from face to back, as shown at the right.

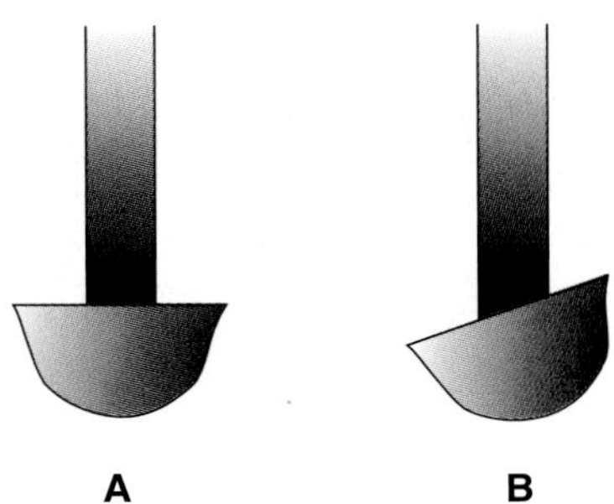

Fig. 41-68 A, The face of a universal curette is at 90 degrees to its shank. **B,** The face of a Gracey curette is offset, forming a 70-degree angle with its shank.

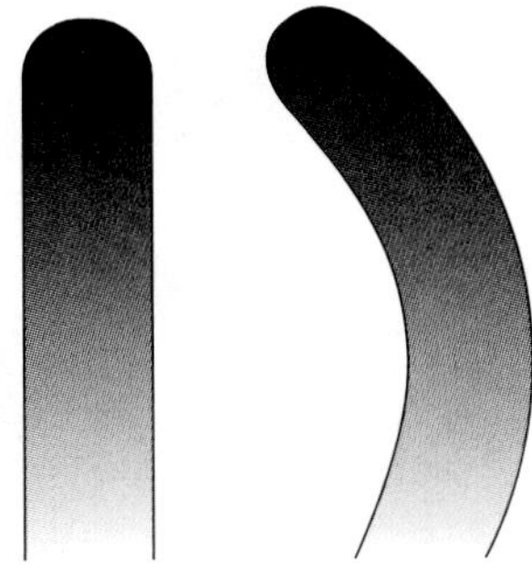

Fig. 41-69 The cutting edges of a universal curette extend straight from shank to toe. The cutting edges of a Gracey curette gently curve from shank to toe. Only the larger, outer cutting edge at the right is used for scaling and needs to be sharpened.

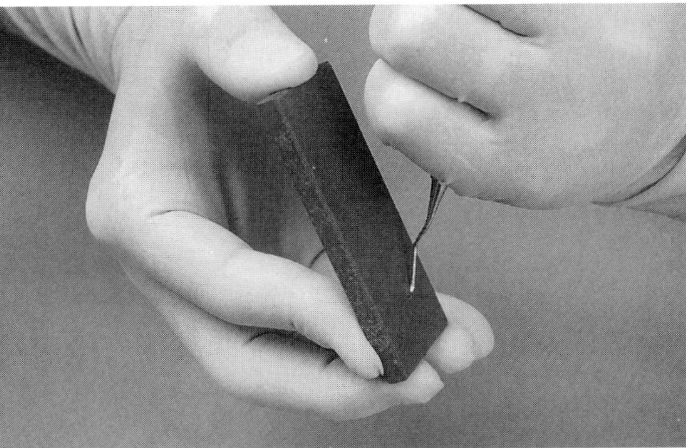

Fig. 41-70 Note that when a Gracey curette is held in proper sharpening position, its shank is not perpendicular to the floor, owing to its offset blade angle. The stone meets the blade at an angle of 100 to 110 degrees. Compare this position with the sharpening position of a universal curette, as shown in Fig. 41-65.

very similar, and therefore, there is no difference in the sharpening technique.

Mini-bladed Gracey curettes such as the Mini Fives or Gracey Curvettes are also sharpened with the same technique. These blades are only half the length of a standard Gracey blade, but the angle between the face and the lateral surface of the blade is still 70 to 80 degrees. However, sharpening too heavily or too often around the toe of a mini-bladed curette should be avoided to prevent excessive shortening of the blade.

Sickle Scalers. The two types of sickle scalers are the straight sickle and curved sickle. On a straight sickle, the face of the blade is flat from shank to tip, whereas on a curved sickle, the face of the blade forms a gentle curve (Fig. 41-72). The straight and curved sickles have similar cross-sectional designs, however. As in the curette, the angle between the face of the blade and the lateral surface of a sickle is 70 to 80 degrees (Fig. 41-73). When a sharpening stone is correctly applied to the lateral surface to preserve this angle, the angle between the face of the blade and the surface of the stone is 100 to 110 degrees. With this in mind, the sickle scaler can be sharpened in a manner much like that described for the curette except that the sickle has a sharp, pointed toe that must not be rounded.

A large, flat stone may also be used to sharpen sickles (Fig. 41-74). The stone is stabilized on a table or cabinet with the left hand. The sickle is held in the right hand with a modified pen grasp and applied to the stone so that the angle between the face of the blade and the stone is 100 to 110 degrees. The fourth finger is placed on the right-hand edge of the stone to stabilize and guide the sharpening movement. The right hand then pushes and pulls the sickle across the surface of the stone. To avoid a wire edge, finish with a pull stroke, being sure that the proper angulation is always maintained.

Chisels and Hoes. Chisels have a single, straight cutting edge that is perpendicular to the shank. The face of the blade is continuous with the shank of the instrument, which may be directly in line with the handle or slightly curved. The end of the blade is beveled at 45 degrees to form the cutting edge.

To sharpen a chisel, stabilize a flat sharpening stone on a flat surface. Grasp the instrument with a modified

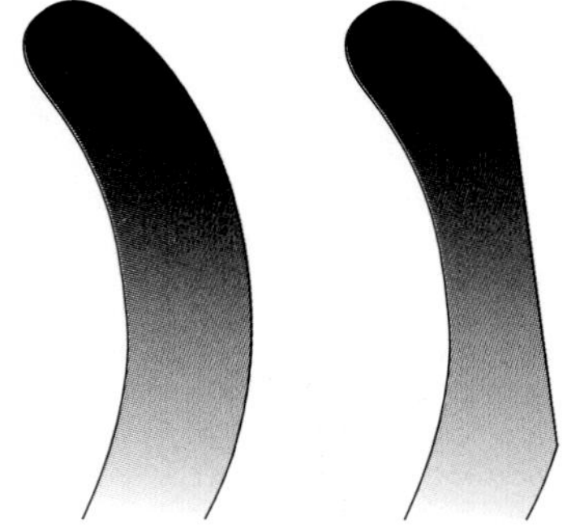

Fig. 41-71 The Gracey curette on the left has been properly sharpened to maintain a symmetric curve on its outer cutting edge. For the curette on the right, the sharpening stone was activated too long in one place, thereby flattening the blade.

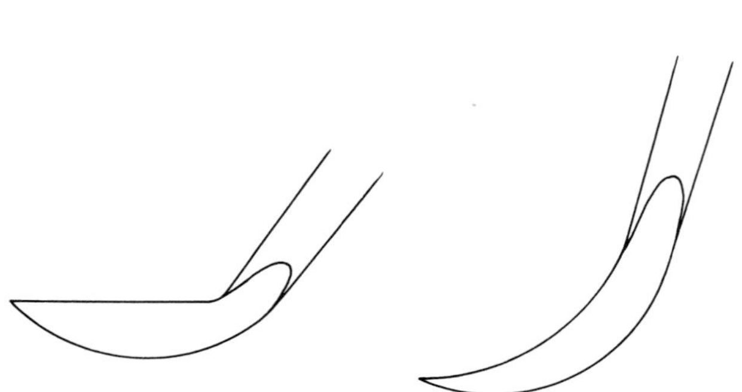

Fig. 41-72 The face of the blade on a straight sickle is flat from shank to tip, whereas on the curved sickle the blade face forms a gentle arc.

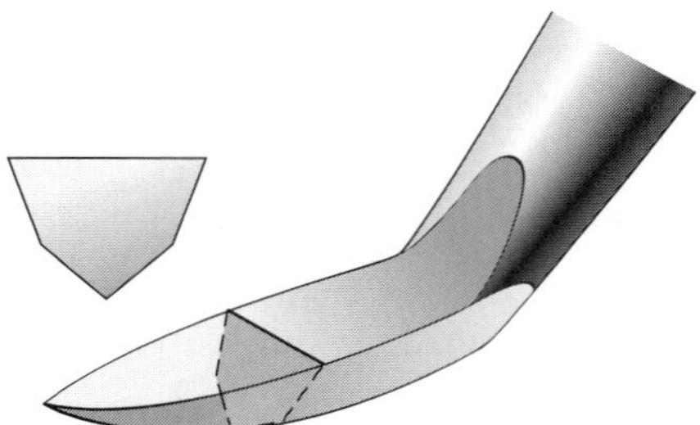

Fig. 41-73 Like the curette, the sickle has an angle of 70 to 80 degrees between the face of the blade and the lateral surface.

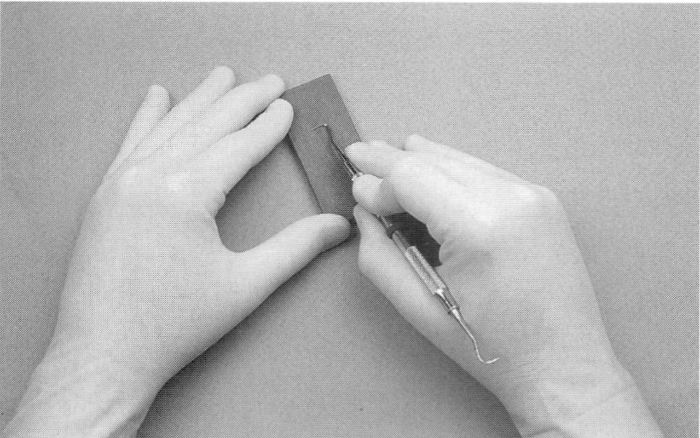

Fig. 41-74 A large, flat stone may also be used to sharpen the sickle. The stone is stabilized on a flat surface. The fourth finger of the right hand guides the sharpening stroke as the instrument is pulled across the face of the stone toward the operator.

pen grasp. Establish a finger rest with the pads of the third and fourth fingers against the straight edge of the sharpening stone. Apply the flat beveled surface of the chisel to the surface of the stone. If the entire surface of the bevel is contacting the stone, then the 45-degree angle between the beveled surface and the face of the blade will be maintained and the design of the instrument will not be altered (Figs. 41-75 and 41-76).

Using moderate, steady pressure, with the hand and arm acting as a unit and the finger resting on the edge of the stone as a guide, push the instrument across the surface of the sharpening stone. Release pressure slightly and draw the instrument back to its starting point. Repeat the sharpening stroke until a sharp edge has been obtained. Remember to finish with a push stroke to prevent the formation of a wire edge. Check for sharpness as previously described. Examine the instrument carefully to be sure that its design has not been inadvertently altered.

Back-action surgical chisels and hoe scalers are sharpened with exactly the same technique described for chisels except that a pull stroke is used rather than a push stroke (Fig. 41-77).

Periodontal Knives. There are two general types of periodontal knives. The first type includes the disposable scalpel blades that come prepackaged. They are presharpened and sterilized by the manufacturer. These are not resharpened when they become dull but are discarded and replaced.

The second type of periodontal knives is reusable and must be sharpened when they become dull. The most commonly used knives in this group are the flat-bladed gingivectomy knives (e.g., the Kirkland knives #15K and 16K) and the narrow, pointed interproximal knives.

FLAT-BLADED GINGIVECTOMY KNIVES. These knives have broad, flat blades that are nearly perpendicular to the lower shank of the instrument. The curved cutting edge extends around the entire outer edge of the blade and is formed by bevels on both the front and back surfaces of the blade (Fig. 41-78).

When sharpening these instruments, only the bevel on the back surface of the instrument needs be ground. This can be done by drawing the blade across a stationary flat sharpening stone or by holding the instrument stationary and drawing the stone across its blade.

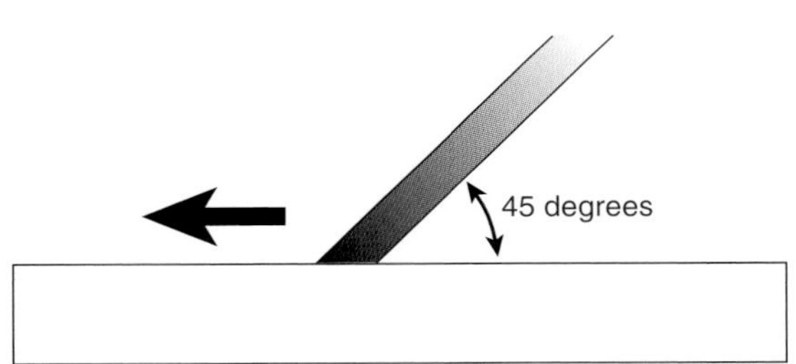

Fig. 41-75 When the entire bevel on a chisel contacts the sharpening stone, the angle between the instrument and the stone is 45 degrees. The cutting edge will be properly sharpened if this angle is maintained as the instrument is pushed across the stone.

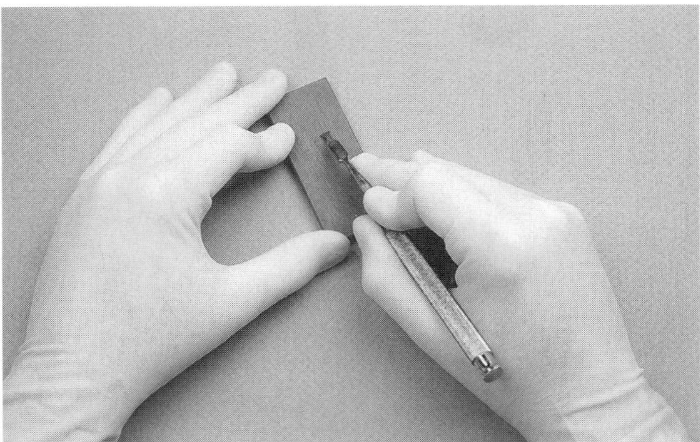

Fig. 41-76 The chisel is also sharpened on a stationary flat sharpening stone.

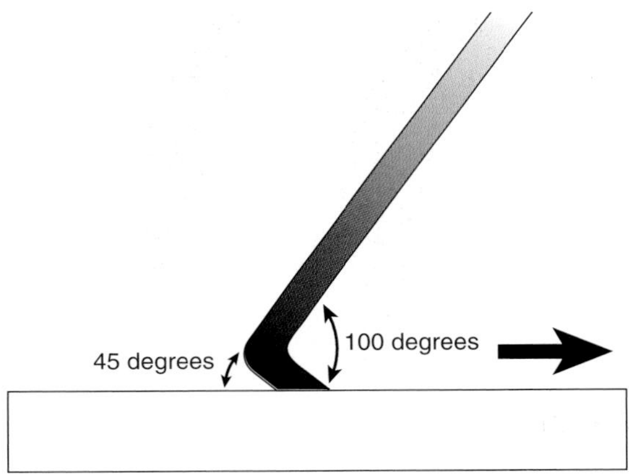

Fig. 41-77 Back-action chisels and hoes are sharpened with a pull stroke.

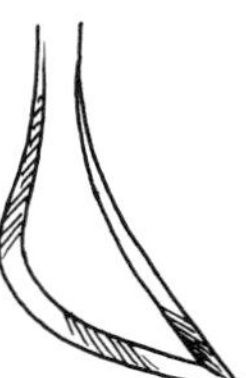

Fig. 41-78 Flat-bladed gingivectomy knives such as this Kirkland knife have a cutting edge that extends around the entire blade. The entire cutting edge must be sharpened.

INTERPROXIMAL KNIVES. The blades of interproximal knives have two long, straight cutting edges that come together at the sharply pointed tip of the instrument. The cutting edges are formed by bevels on the front and back surfaces of the blade. The entire blade is roughly perpendicular to the lower shank of the instrument (Fig. 41-79).

As with the flat-bladed gingivectomy knives, only the bevels on the back surface of the interproximal knives need to be sharpened. Again, this can be accomplished by drawing the instrument across a stationary stone or by holding the instrument stationary and moving the stone across it.

Stationary Stone Technique. Stabilize a flat sharpening stone on a flat surface. Grasp the handle of the instrument with a modified pen grasp, and apply the bevel on the back surface of the blade to the flat surface of the sharpening stone. With moderate pressure, pull the instrument toward you (Fig. 41-80 and Fig. 41-81). Release pressure slightly and return to the starting point. Begin at one end of the cutting edge and continue around the blade by rolling the handle of the instrument slightly between the thumb and the first and second fingers. Finish each section of the blade with a pull stroke to prevent formation of a wire edge. Check for sharpness as described previously.

Stationary Instrument Technique. Grasp the instrument with the palm. Apply the flat surface of a hand-held sharpening stone to the bevel on the back surface of the blade (Fig. 41-82). Begin at one end of the cutting edge and, with moderate pressure, draw the stone back and forth across the instrument. To prevent the formation of a wire edge, finish each section with a stroke into or toward the cutting edge. Proceed around the entire length of the cutting edge by gradually rotating the instrument and the stone in relation to one another.

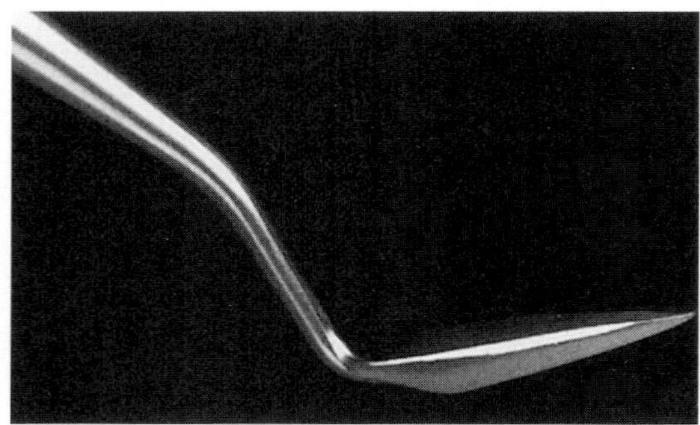

Fig. 41-79 The two cutting edges of an interproximal knife are formed by bevels on the front and back surfaces of the blade.

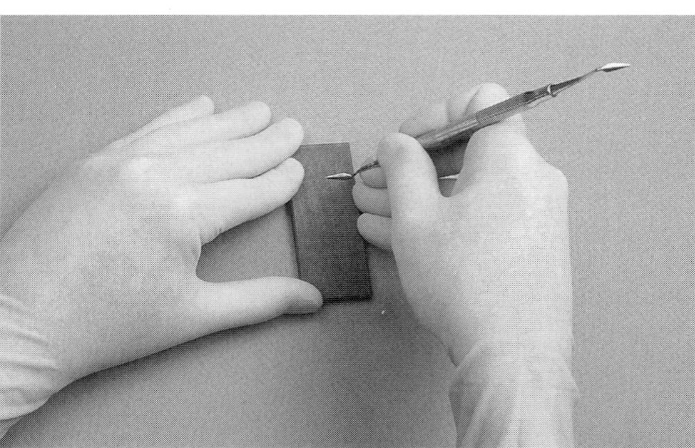

Fig. 41-81 The interproximal knife may be sharpened on a flat stationary stone. The blade is drawn toward the operator.

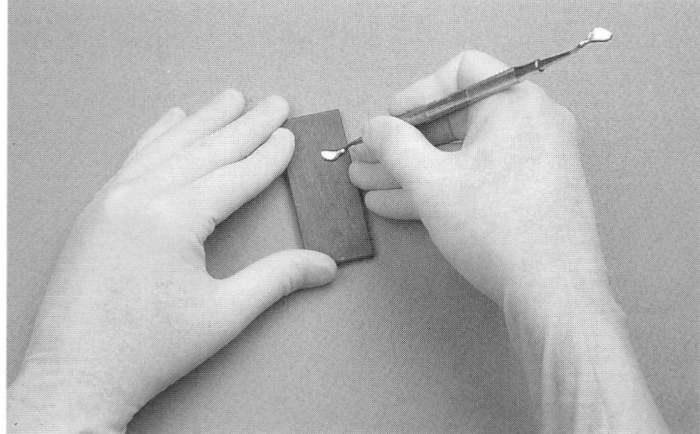

Fig. 41-80 The gingivectomy knife may be sharpened on a stationary flat stone. The instrument is held with a modified pen grasp. The fourth finger guides the sharpening stroke as the instrument is rolled between the fingers so that all sections of the blade are sharpened.

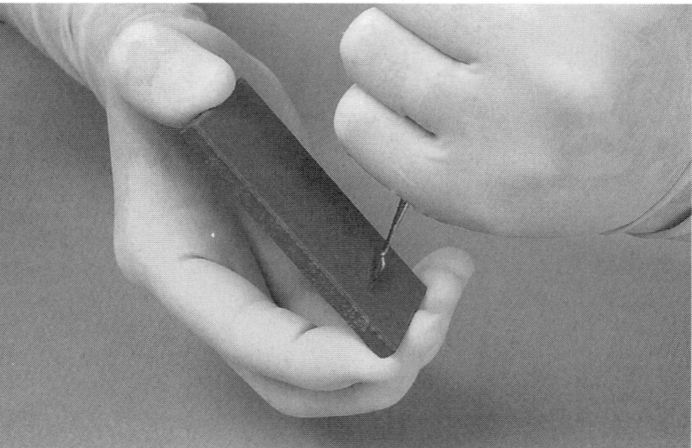

Fig. 41-82 The interproximal knife may also be sharpened with a hand-held stone. The instrument is held with a palm grasp, and the stone is applied to the entire cutting edge.

REFERENCES

1. Antonini CJ, Brady JM, Levin MP, et al: Scanning electron microscope study of scalers. J Periodontol 1977; 48:45.
2. Barnes C, Hayes E, Leinfelder K: Effects of an air abrasive polishing system on restored surfaces. Gen Dent 1987; 35:186.
3. Bay N, Overman P, Krust-Bray K, Cobb C, et al: Effectiveness of antimicrobial mouthrinses on aerosols produced by an air polisher. J Dent Hyg 1993; 67:312.
4. Berkstein S, Reiff RL, McKinney JF, et al: Supragingival root surface removal during maintenance procedures utilizing an air-powder abrasive system or hand scaling. An in vitro study. J Periodontol 1987; 58:327.
5. Brookshire FV, Nagy WW, Dhuru VB, et al: The qualitative effects of various types of hygiene instrumentation on commercially pure titanium and titanium alloy implant abutments: an in vitro and scanning electron microscope study. J Prosthet Dent 1997; 78(3):286.
6. Cross-Poline GN, Shaklee RL, Stach DJ: Effect of implant curets on titanium implant surfaces. Am J Dent 1997; 10(1):41.
7. Drisko CL: Scaling and root planing without overinstrumentation: hand versus power-driven scalers. Curr Opin Periodontol 1993; 78.
8. Drisko CL, Cochran DL, Blieden T, et al: Position paper: sonic and ultrasonic scalers in periodontics. Research, Science and Therapy Committee of the American Academy of Periodontology. J Periodontol 2000; 71(11):1792.
9. Eliades GC, Tzoutzas JG, Vougiouklakis GJ: Surface alterations on dental restorative materials subjected to an air-powder abrasive instrument. J Prosthet Dent 1991; 65(1):27.
10. Fox SC, Moriarty JD, Kusy RP: The effects of scaling a titanium implant surface with metal and plastic instruments: an in vitro study. J Periodontol 1990; (8):485.
11. Gnanasekhar JD, al-Duwairi YS: Electrosurgery in dentistry. Quintessence Int 1998; 29(10):649.
12. Green E, Seyer PC: Sharpening Curets and Sickle Scalers, ed 2. Berkeley, CA, Praxis, 1972.
13. Hallmon WW, Waldrop TC, Meffert RM, et al: A comparative study of the effects of metallic, nonmetallic, and sonic instrumentation on titanium abutment surfaces. Int J Oral Maxillofac Implants. 1996; 11(1):96.
14. Harrel SK, Barnes JB, Rivera-Hidalgo F: Aerosol reduction during air polishing. Quintessence Int 1999; 30(9):623.
15. Holbrook T, Low S: Power-driven scaling and polishing instruments. In Hardin JF (ed): Clarke's Clinical Dentistry. Philadelphia, JB Lippincott, 1991.
16. Koka S, Han J, Razzoog ME, et al: The effects of two air-powder abrasive prophylaxis systems on the surface of machined titanium: a pilot study. Implant Dent 1992; 1(4):259.
17. Lindhe J: Evaluation of periodontal scalers. II. Wear following standardized or diagonal cutting tests. Odontol Revy 1966; 17:121.
18. Lindhe J, Jacobson L: Evaluation of periodontal scalers. I. Wear following clinical use. Odontol Revy 1966; 17:1.
19. Lubow RM, Cooley RL: Effect of air-powder abrasive instrument on restorative materials. J Prosthet Dent 1986; 55:462.
20. Mengel R, Buns CE, Mengel C, et al: An in vitro study of the treatment of implant surfaces with different instruments. Int J Oral Maxillofac Implants. 1998; 13(1):91.
21. Moore DA: Electrosurgery in dentistry: Past and present. Gen Dent. 1995; 43(5):460.
22. Orban B, Manella VB: A macroscopic and microscopic study of instruments designed for root planing. J Periodontol 1956; 27:120.
23. Orton GS: Clinical use of an air-powder abrasive system. Dent Hyg 1987; 75:513.
24. Paquette OE, Levin MP: The sharpening of scaling instruments. I. An examination of principles. J Periodontol 1977; 48:163.
25. Rawson RD, Nelson BN, Jewell BD, et al: Alkalosis as a potential complication of air polishing systems. A pilot study. Dent Hyg 1985; 59:500.
26. Razzoog ME, Koka S: In vitro analysis of the effects of two air-abrasive prophylaxis systems and inlet air pressure on the surface of titanium abutment cylinders. J Prosthodont 1994; 3(2):103.
27. Rossi R, Smukler H: A scanning electron microscope study comparing the effectiveness of different types of sharpening stones and curets. J Peridontol 1995; 66(11):956.
28. Ruhling A, Kocher T, Kreusch J, et al: Treatment of subgingival implant surfaces with Teflon-coated sonic and ultrasonic scaler tips and various implant curettes. An in vitro study. Clin Oral Implants Res 1994; 5(1):19.
29. Schwartz M: The prevention and management of the broken curet. Compend Contin Educ Dent 1998; 19(4):418–420, 422, 424.
30. Sherman JA: Oral Radiosurgery: An Illustrated Clinical Guide, ed 2. London, Martin Dunitz, 1997.
31. Smith BA, Setter MS, Caffesse RG, et al: The effect of sharpening stones upon curette surface roughness. Quintessence Int 1987; 18:603.
32. Snyder JA, McVay JT, Brown FH, et al: The effect of air abrasive polishing on blood pH and electrolyte concentrations in healthy mongrel dogs. J Periodontol 1990; 64:81.
33. Stach DJ, Cross-Poline GN, Newmand SM, et al: Effect of repeated sterilization and ultrasonic cleaning on curet blades. J Dent Hyg. 1995; 69(1):31.
34. Suzuki JB, Delisle AL: Pulmonary actinomycosis of periodontal origin. J Periodontol 1984; 55:581.
35. Waerhaug J, Arno A, Lovdal A: The dimension of instruments for removal of subgingival calculus. J Periodontol 1954; 25:281.
36. Wilkins EM: Clinical Practice of the Dental Hygienist, ed 7. Baltimore, Williams & Wilkins, 1994.

Manual Instrumentation

*Gordon L. Pattison and Anna M. Pattison**

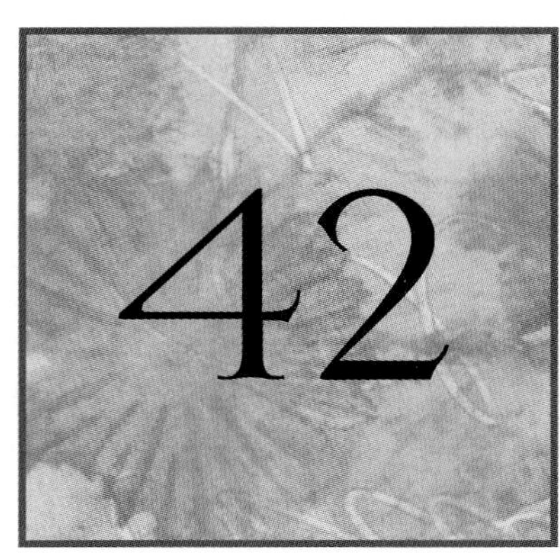

CHAPTER

CHAPTER OUTLINE

GENERAL PRINCIPLES OF INSTRUMENTATION

Effective instrumentation is governed by a number of general principles that are common to all periodontal instruments. Proper position of the patient and the operator, illumination and retraction for optimal visibility, and sharp instruments are fundamental prerequisites. A constant awareness of tooth and root morphologic features and of the condition of the periodontal tissues is also essential. Knowledge of instrument design enables the clinician to efficiently select the proper instrument for the procedure and the area in which it will be performed. In addition to these principles, the basic concepts of grasp, finger rest, adaptation, angulation, and stroke must be understood before clinical instrument-handling skills can be mastered.

Accessibility (Positioning of Patient and Operator)

Accessibility facilitates thoroughness of instrumentation. The position of the patient and operator should provide maximal accessibility to the area of operation. Inadequate accessibility impedes thorough instrumentation, prematurely tires the operator, and diminishes his or her effectiveness.

The clinician should be seated on a comfortable operating stool that has been positioned so that his or her feet are flat on the floor with the thighs parallel to the floor. The clinician should be able to observe the field of operation while keeping the back straight and the head erect.

The patient should be in a supine position and placed so that the mouth is close to the resting elbow of the clinician. For instrumentation of the maxillary arch, the patient should be asked to raise his or her chin slightly to provide optimal visibility and accessibility. For instrumentation on the mandibular arch, it may be necessary to raise the back of the chair slightly and request that the patient lower his or her chin until the mandible is parallel to the floor. This will especially facilitate work on the lingual surfaces of the mandibular anterior teeth.

Visibility, Illumination, and Retraction

Whenever possible, direct vision with direct illumination from the dental light is most desirable (Fig. 42-1). If this is not possible, indirect vision may be obtained by using the mouth mirror (Fig. 42-2), and indirect illumination may be obtained by using the mirror to reflect light to where it is needed (Fig. 42-3). Indirect vision and indirect illumination are often used simultaneously (Fig. 42-4).

Retraction provides visibility, accessibility, and illumination. Depending on the location of the area of operation, the fingers and/or the mirror are used for retraction. The mirror may be used for retraction of the cheeks

* Material in this chapter was drawn freely from Pattison A, Pattison G: Periodontal Instrumentation, ed 2. Reprinted by permission of Pearson Education, Inc., Upper Saddle River, NJ.

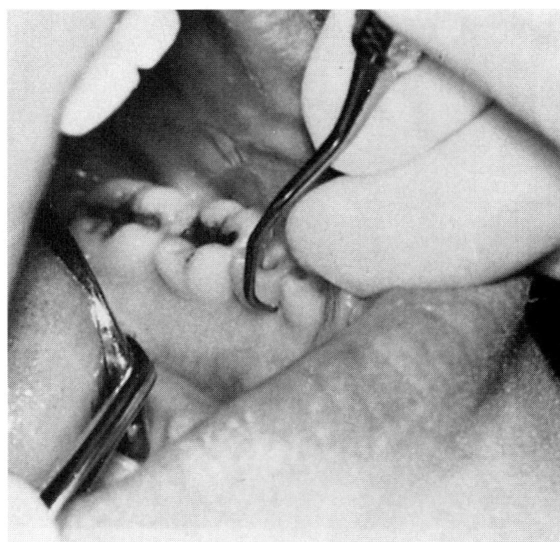

Fig. 42-1 Direct vision and direct illumination in the mandibular left premolar area.

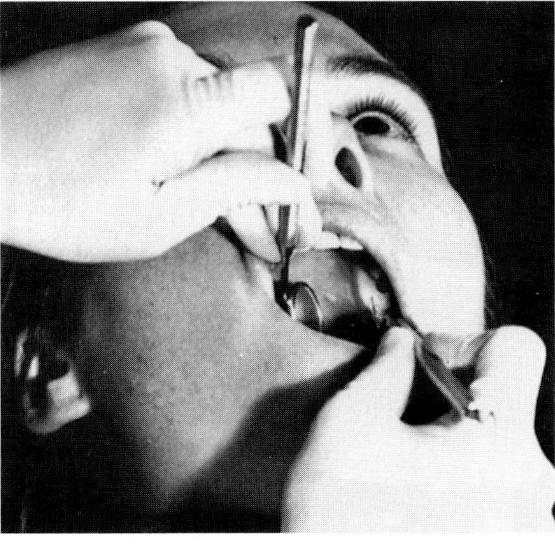

Fig. 42-3 Indirect illumination using the mirror to reflect light onto the maxillary left posterior lingual region.

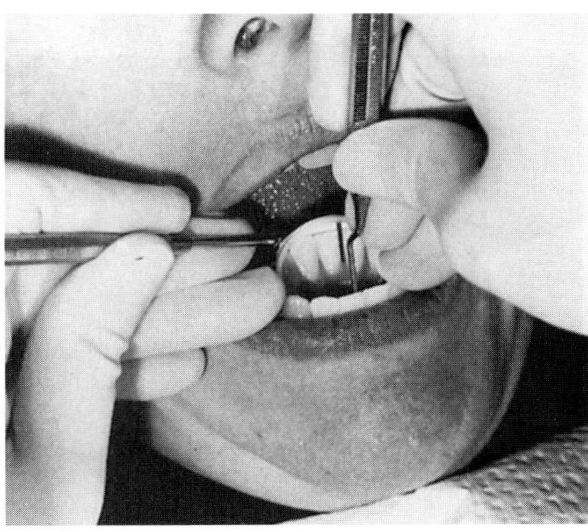

Fig. 42-2 Indirect vision using the mirror for the lingual surfaces of the mandibular anterior teeth.

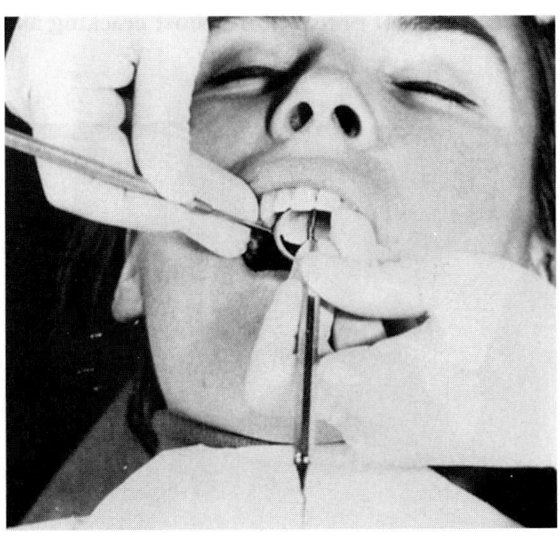

Fig. 42-4 Combination of indirect illumination and indirect vision for the lingual surfaces of the maxillary anterior teeth.

or the tongue; the index finger is used for retraction of the lips or cheeks. The following methods are effective for retraction:

1. Use of the mirror to deflect the cheek while the fingers of the nonoperating hand retract the lips and protect the angle of the mouth from irritation by the mirror handle
2. Use of the mirror alone to retract the lips and cheek (Fig. 42-5)
3. Use of the fingers of the nonoperating hand to retract the lips (Fig. 42-6)
4. Use of the mirror to retract the tongue (Fig. 42-7)
5. Combinations of the preceding methods

When retracting, care should be taken to avoid irritation to the angles of the mouth. If the lips and skin are dry, softening the lips with petroleum jelly before instrumentation is begun is a helpful precaution against cracking and bleeding. Careful retraction is especially important for patients with a history of recurrent *herpes labialis,* because these patients may easily develop herpetic lesions after instrumentation.

Condition of Instruments (Sharpness)

Before any instrumentation, all instruments should be inspected to make sure that they are clean, sterile, and in good condition. The working ends of pointed or bladed

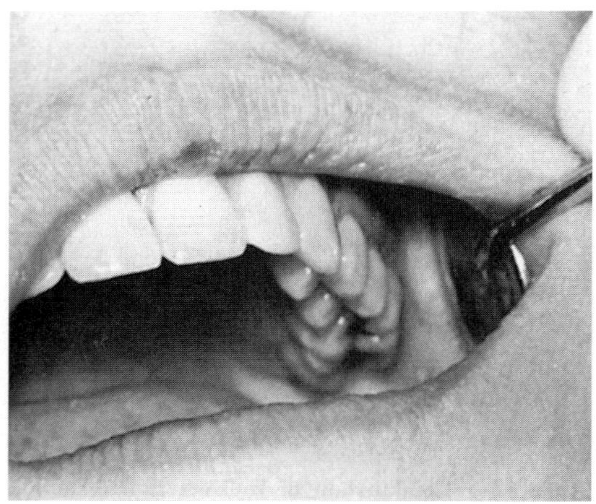

Fig. 42-5 Retracting the cheek with the mirror.

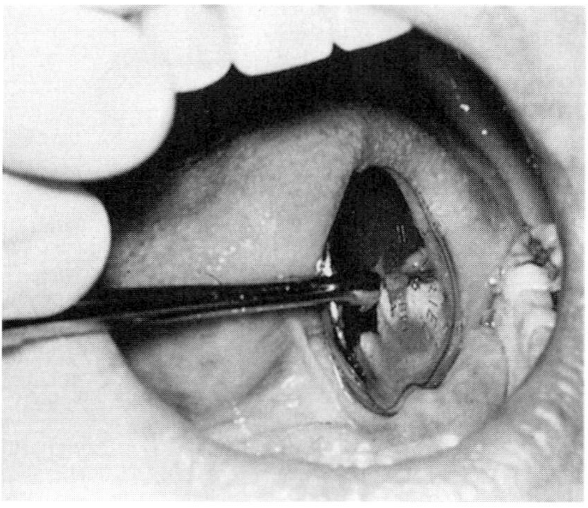

Fig. 42-7 Retracting the tongue with the mirror.

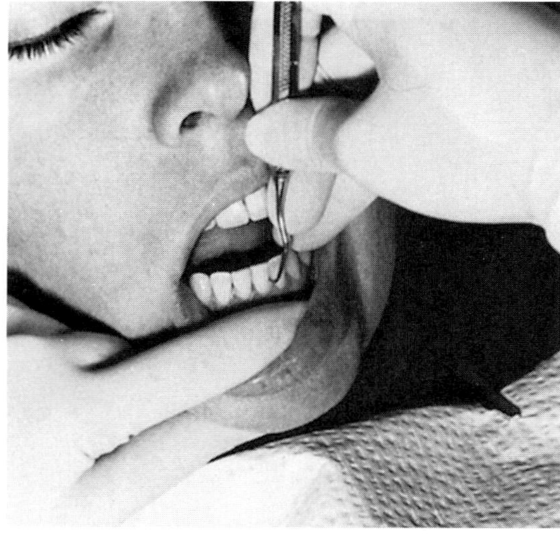

Fig. 42-6 Retracting the lip with the index finger of the nonoperating hand.

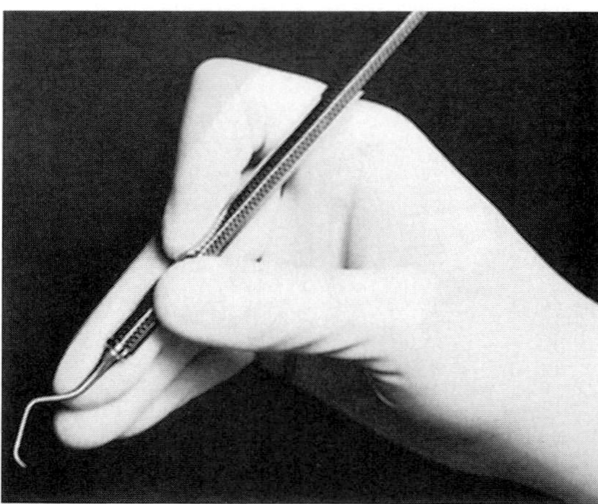

Fig. 42-8 Modified pen grasp. The pad of the middle finger rests on the shank.

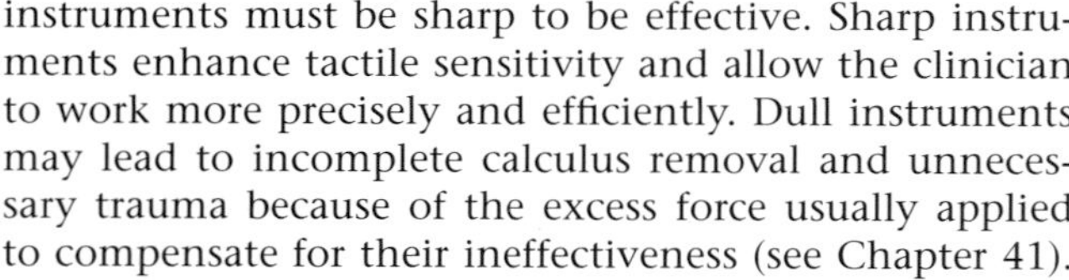

instruments must be sharp to be effective. Sharp instruments enhance tactile sensitivity and allow the clinician to work more precisely and efficiently. Dull instruments may lead to incomplete calculus removal and unnecessary trauma because of the excess force usually applied to compensate for their ineffectiveness (see Chapter 41).

Maintaining a Clean Field

Despite good visibility, illumination, and retraction, instrumentation can be hampered if the operative field is obscured by saliva, blood, and debris. The pooling of saliva interferes with visibility during instrumentation and impedes control because a firm finger rest cannot be established on wet, slippery tooth surfaces. Adequate suction is essential and can be achieved with a saliva ejector or, if working with an assistant, an aspirator.

Gingival bleeding is an unavoidable consequence of subgingival instrumentation. In areas of inflammation this is not necessarily an indication of trauma from incorrect technique; instead, it indicates ulceration of the pocket epithelium. Blood and debris can be removed from the operative field with suction and by wiping or blotting with gauze squares. The operative field should also be flushed occasionally with water.

Compressed air and gauze squares can be used to facilitate visual inspection of tooth surfaces just below the gingival margin during instrumentation. A jet of air directed into the pocket deflects a retractable gingival margin. Retractable tissue can also be deflected away from the tooth by gently packing the edge of a gauze square into the pocket with the back of a curette. Immediately after the gauze is removed, the subgingival area should be clean, dry, and clearly visible for a brief interval.

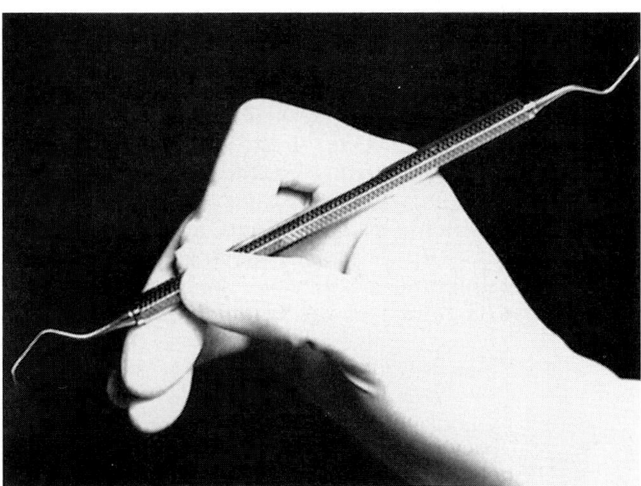

Fig. 42-9 Standard pen grasp. The side of the middle finger rests on the shank.

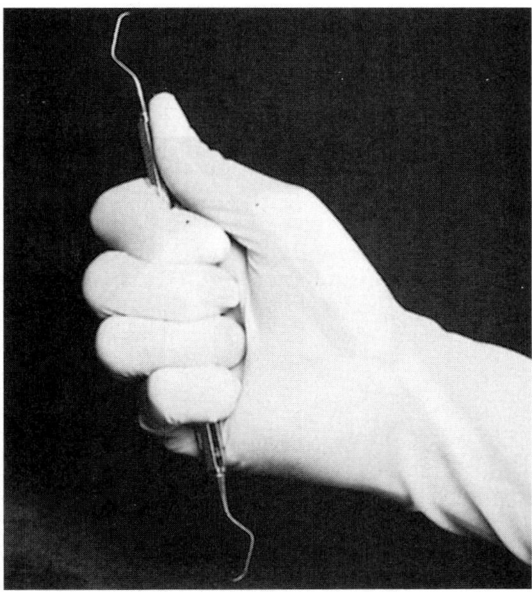

Fig. 42-10 Palm and thumb grasp, used for stabilizing instruments during sharpening.

Instrument Stabilization

Stability of the instrument and the hand is the primary requisite for controlled instrumentation. Stability and control are essential for effective instrumentation and avoidance of injury to the patient or clinician. The two factors of major importance in providing stability are the instrument grasp and the finger rest.

Instrument Grasp. A proper grasp is essential for precise control of movements made during periodontal instrumentation. The most effective and stable grasp for all periodontal instruments is the *modified pen grasp* (Fig. 42-8). Although other grasps are possible, this modification of the standard pen grasp (Fig. 42-9) ensures the greatest control in performing intraoral procedures.

> The thumb, index finger, and middle finger are used to hold the instrument as a pen is held, but the middle finger is positioned so that the side of the pad next to the fingernail is resting on the instrument shank. The index finger is bent at the second joint from the finger tip and is positioned well above the middle finger on the same side of the handle.

The pad of the thumb is placed midway between the middle and index fingers on the opposite side of the handle. This creates a triangle of forces, or tripod effect, that enhances control because it counteracts the tendency of the instrument to turn uncontrollably between the fingers when scaling force is applied to the tooth. This stable modified pen grasp enhances control because it enables the clinician to roll the instrument in precise degrees with the thumb against the index and middle fingers to adapt the blade to the slightest changes in tooth contour. The modified pen grasp also enhances tactile sensitivity, because slight irregularities on the tooth surface are best perceived when the tactile-sensitive pad of the middle finger is placed on the shank of the instrument.

The *palm and thumb grasp* (Fig. 42-10) is useful for stabilizing instruments during sharpening and for manipulating air and water syringes, but it is not recommended for periodontal instrumentation. Maneuverability and tactile sensitivity are so inhibited by this grasp that it is unsuitable for the precise, controlled movements necessary during periodontal procedures.

Finger Rest. The finger rest serves to stabilize the hand and the instrument by providing a firm fulcrum as movements are made to activate the instrument. A good finger rest prevents injury and laceration of the gingiva and surrounding tissues by poorly controlled instruments. The fourth (ring) finger is preferred by most clinicians for the finger rest. Although it is possible to use the third (middle) finger for the finger rest, this is not recommended, because it restricts the arc of movement during the activation of strokes and severely curtails the use of the middle finger for both control and tactile sensitivity. Maximal control is achieved when the middle finger is kept between the instrument shank and the fourth finger. This "built-up" fulcrum is an integral part of the wrist-forearm action that activates the powerful working stroke for calculus removal. Whenever possible, these two fingers should be kept together to work as a one-unit fulcrum during scaling and root planing. Separation of the middle and fourth fingers during scaling strokes results in a loss of power and control because it forces the clinician to rely solely on finger flexing for activation of the instrument.

Finger rests may be generally classified as intraoral finger rests or extraoral fulcrums. Intraoral finger rests on tooth surfaces ideally are established close to the working area. Variations of intraoral finger rests and extraoral fulcrums are used whenever good angulation and a sufficient arc of movement cannot be achieved by a finger rest close to the working area. The following examples illustrate the different variations of the intraoral finger rest:

1. *Conventional:* The finger rest is established on tooth surfaces immediately adjacent to the working area (Fig. 42-11).
2. *Cross-arch:* The finger rest is established on tooth surfaces on the other side of the same arch (Fig. 42-12).
3. *Opposite-arch:* The finger rest is established on tooth surfaces on the opposite arch (e.g., mandibular arch finger rest for instrumentation on the maxillary arch) (Fig. 42-13).

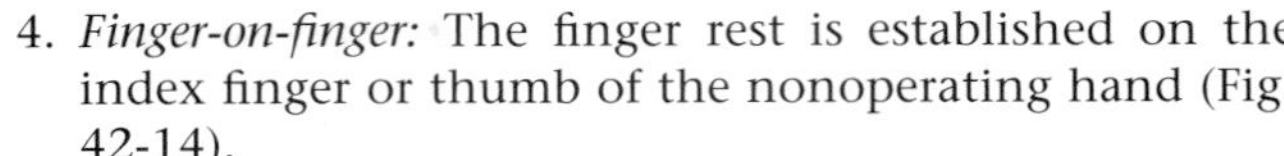

4. *Finger-on-finger:* The finger rest is established on the index finger or thumb of the nonoperating hand (Fig. 42-14).

Extraoral fulcrums are essential for effective instrumentation of some aspects of the maxillary posterior teeth. When properly established, they allow optimal access and angulation while providing adequate stabilization. Extraoral fulcrums are not finger rests in the literal sense, because the tips or pads of the fingers are not used for extraoral fulcrums as they are for intraoral finger rests. Instead, as much of the front or back surface of

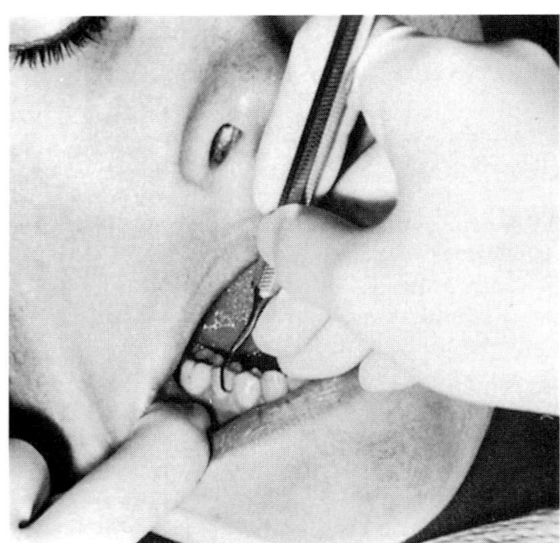

Fig. 42-11 Intraoral conventional finger rest. The fourth finger rests on the occlusal surfaces of adjacent teeth.

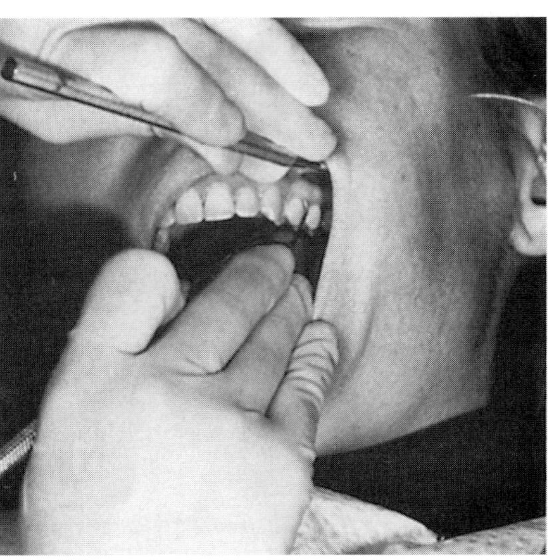

Fig. 42-13 Intraoral opposite-arch finger rest. The fourth finger rests on the mandibular teeth while the maxillary posterior teeth are instrumented.

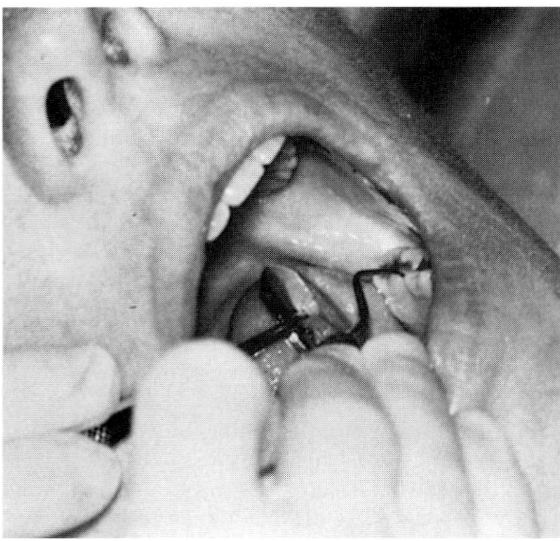

Fig. 42-12 Intraoral cross-arch finger rest. The fourth finger rests on the incisal surfaces of teeth on the opposite side of the same arch.

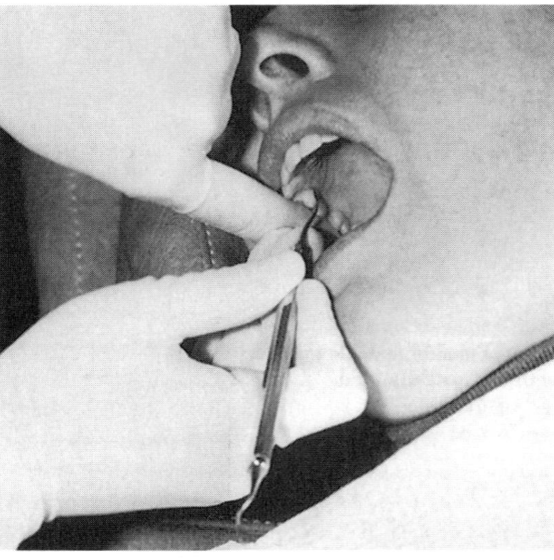

Fig. 42-14 Intraoral finger-on-finger rest. The fourth finger rests on the index finger of the nonoperating hand.

the fingers as possible is placed on the patient's face to provide the greatest degree of stability. The two most commonly used extraoral fulcrums are as follows:

1. *Palm-up:* The palm-up fulcrum is established by resting the backs of the middle and fourth fingers on the skin overlying the lateral aspect of the mandible on the right side of the face (Fig. 42-15).
2. *Palm-down*: The palm-down fulcrum is established by resting the front surfaces of the middle and fourth fingers on the skin overlying the lateral aspect of the mandible on the left side of the face (Fig. 42-16).

Both intraoral finger rests and extraoral fulcrums may be reinforced by applying the index finger or thumb of the nonoperating hand to the handle or shank of the instrument for added control and pressure against the tooth. The reinforcing finger is usually employed for opposite-arch or extraoral fulcrums when precise control and pressure are compromised by the longer distance between the fulcrum and the working end of the instrument. Fig. 42-17 shows the index finger-reinforced rest, and Fig. 42-18 shows the thumb-reinforced rest.

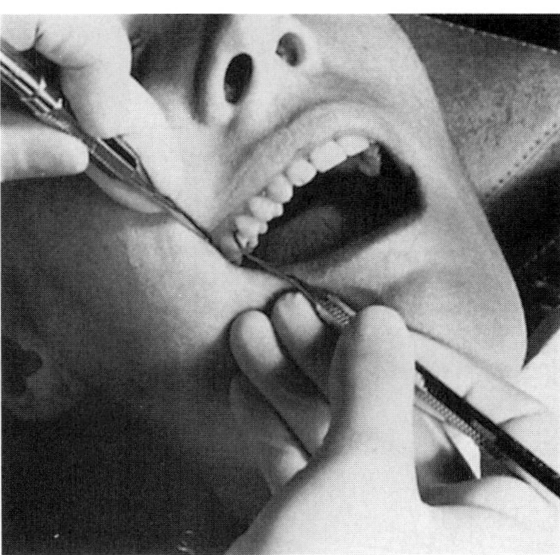

Fig. 42-15 Extraoral palm-up fulcrum. The backs of the fingers rest on the right lateral aspect of the mandible while the maxillary right posterior teeth are instrumented.

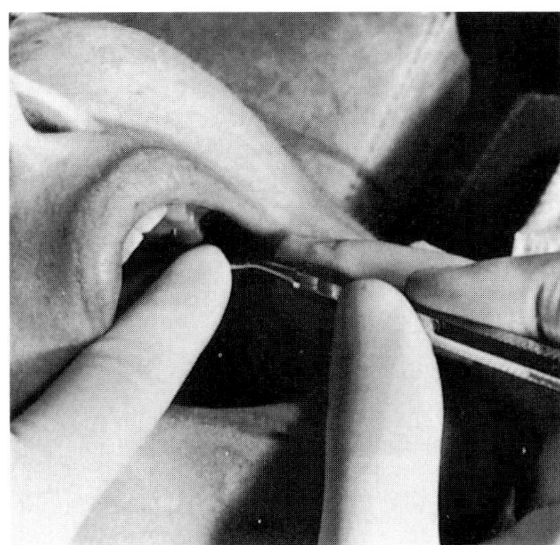

Fig. 42-17 Index finger-reinforced rest. The index finger is placed on the shank for pressure and control in the maxillary left posterior lingual region.

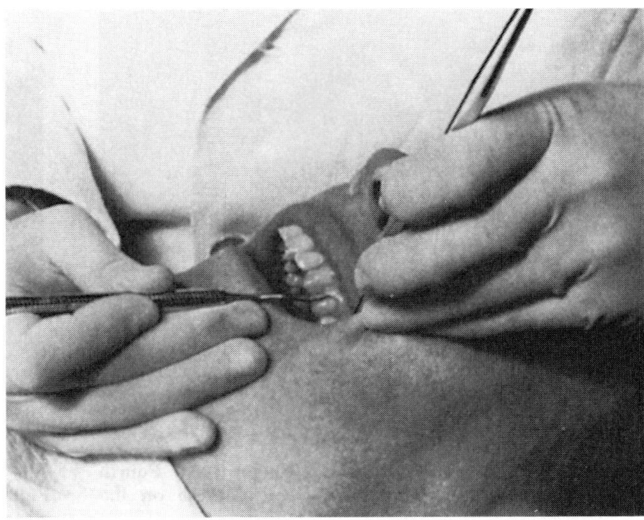

Fig. 42-16 Extraoral palm-down fulcrum. The front surfaces of the fingers rest on the left lateral aspect of the mandible while the maxillary left posterior teeth are instrumented.

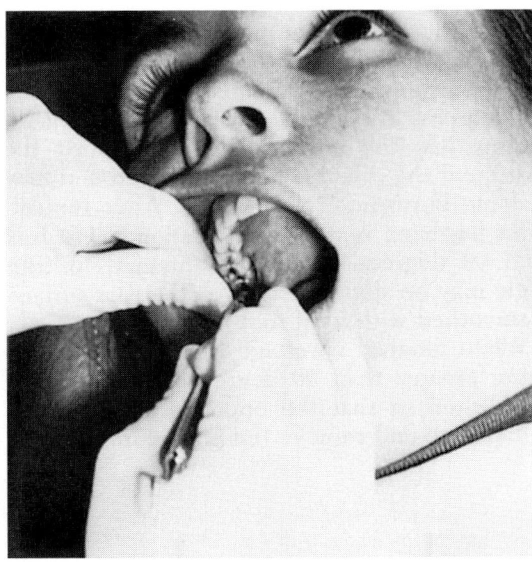

Fig. 42-18 Thumb-reinforced rest. The thumb is placed on the handle for control in the maxillary right posterior lingual region.

Instrument Activation

Adaptation. Adaptation refers to the manner in which the working end of a periodontal instrument is placed against the surface of a tooth. The objective of adaptation is to make the working end of the instrument conform to the contour of the tooth surface. Precise adaptation must be maintained with all instruments to avoid trauma to the soft tissues and root surfaces and to ensure maximum effectiveness of instrumentation.

Correct adaptation of the probe is quite simple. The tip and side of the probe should be flush against the tooth surface as vertical strokes are activated within the crevice. Bladed instruments such as curettes and sharp-pointed instruments such as explorers are more difficult to adapt. The ends of these instruments are sharp and can lacerate tissue, so adaptation in subgingival areas becomes especially important. The lower third of the working end, which is the last few millimeters adjacent to the toe or tip, must be kept in constant contact with the tooth while it is moving over varying tooth contours (Fig. 42-19). Precise adaptation is maintained by carefully rolling the handle of the instrument against the index and middle fingers with the thumb. This rotates the instrument in slight degrees so that the toe or tip leads into concavities and around convexities. On convex surfaces such as line angles, it is not possible to adapt more than 1 or 2 mm of the working end against the tooth. Even on what appear to be broader, flatter surfaces, no more than 1 or 2 mm of the working end can be adapted, because the tooth surface, although it may seem flat, is actually slightly curved.

If only the middle third of the working end is adapted on a convex surface so that the blade contacts the tooth at a tangent, the toe or sharp tip will jut out into soft tissue, causing trauma and discomfort (Fig. 42-20). If the instrument is adapted so that only the toe or tip is in contact, the soft tissue can be distended or compressed by the back of the working end, also causing trauma and discomfort. A curette that is improperly adapted in this manner can be particularly damaging, because the toe can gouge or groove the root surface.

Angulation. *Angulation* refers to the angle between the face of a bladed instrument and the tooth surface. It may also be called the tooth-blade relationship.

Correct angulation is essential for effective calculus removal. For subgingival insertion of a bladed instrument such as a curette, angulation should be as close to 0 degree as possible (Fig. 42-21). The end of the instrument can be inserted to the base of the pocket more easily with the face of the blade flush against the tooth. During scaling and root planing, optimal angulation is between 45 and 90 degrees (see Fig. 42-21). The exact blade angulation depends on the amount and nature of the calculus, the procedure being performed, and the condition of the tissue. Blade angulation is diminished or closed by tilting the lower shank of the instrument toward the tooth. It is increased or opened by tilting the lower shank away from the tooth. During scaling strokes on heavy, tenacious calculus, angulation should be just less than 90 degrees so that the cutting edge "bites" into the calculus. With angulation of less than 45 degrees, the cutting edge will not bite into or engage the calculus properly (see Fig. 42-21). Instead, it will slide over the calculus, smoothing or "burnishing" it. If angulation is more than 90 degrees, the lateral surface of the blade, rather than the cutting edge, will be against the tooth, and the calculus will not be removed and may become burnished (see Fig. 42-21). After the calculus has been removed, angulation of just less than 90 degrees may be maintained, or the angle may be slightly closed as the root surface is smoothed with light root planing strokes.

When gingival curettage is indicated, angulation greater than 90 degrees is deliberately established so that the cutting edge will engage and remove the pocket lining (see Fig. 42-21).

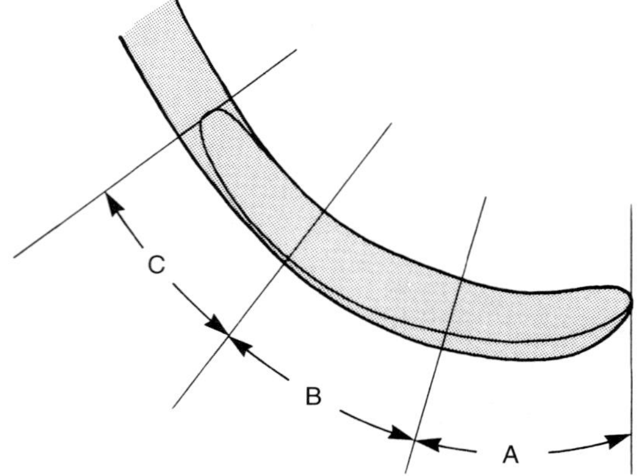

Fig. 42-19 Gracey curette blade divided into three segments: the lower one third of the blade, consisting of the terminal few millimeters adjacent to the toe **(A)**; the middle one third **(B)**; and the upper one third, which is adjacent to the shank **(C)**.

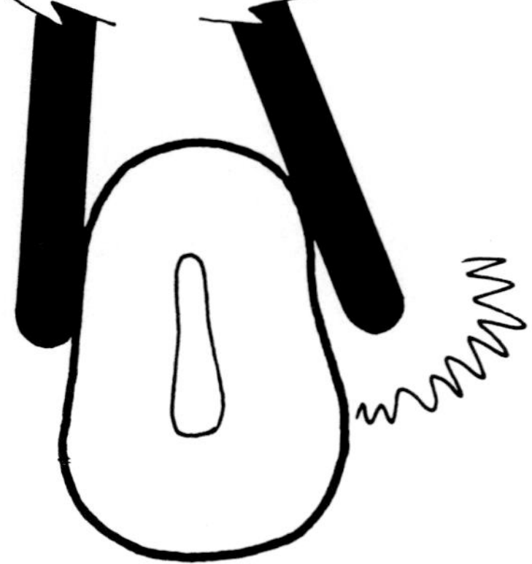

Fig. 42-20 Blade adaptation. The curette on the left is properly adapted to the root surface. The curette on the right is incorrectly adapted; the toe juts out, lacerating the soft tissues.

Lateral Pressure. *Lateral pressure* refers to the pressure created when force is applied against the surface of a tooth with the cutting edge of a bladed instrument. The exact amount of pressure applied must be varied according to the nature of the calculus and according to whether the stroke is intended for initial scaling to remove calculus or for root planing to smooth the root surface.

Lateral pressure may be firm, moderate, or light. When removing calculus, lateral pressure is applied firmly or moderately initially and is progressively diminished until light lateral pressure is applied for the final root planing strokes. When insufficient lateral pressure is applied for the removal of heavy calculus, rough ledges or lumps may be shaved to thin, smooth sheets of burnished calculus that are difficult to detect and remove. This burnishing effect often occurs in areas of developmental depressions and along the cementoenamel junction (CEJ).

Although firm lateral pressure is necessary for the thorough removal of calculus, indiscriminate, unwarranted, or uncontrolled application of heavy forces during instrumentation should be avoided. Repeated application of excessively heavy strokes often nicks or gouges the root surface.

The careful application of varied and controlled amounts of lateral pressure during instrumentation is an integral part of effective scaling and root planing techniques and is absolutely critical to the success of both of these procedures.

Strokes. Three basic types of strokes are used during instrumentation: the exploratory stroke, the scaling stroke, and the root planing stroke. Any of these basic strokes may be activated by a pull or a push motion in a vertical, oblique, or horizontal direction (Fig. 42-22). Vertical and oblique strokes are used most frequently. Horizontal strokes are used selectively on line angles or deep pockets that cannot be negotiated with vertical or oblique strokes. The direction, length, pressure, and number of strokes necessary for either scaling or root planing are determined by four major factors: gingival position and tone, pocket depth and shape, tooth contour, and the amount and nature of the calculus or roughness.

The **exploratory stroke** is a light, "feeling" stroke that is used with probes and explorers to evaluate the dimensions of the pocket and to detect calculus and irregularities of the tooth surface. With bladed instruments such as the curette, the exploratory stroke is alternated with scaling and root planing strokes for these same purposes of evaluation and detection. The instrument is grasped lightly and adapted with light pressure against the tooth to achieve maximal tactile sensitivity.

The **scaling stroke** is a short, powerful pull stroke that is used with bladed instruments for the removal of both supragingival and subgingival calculus. The muscles of the fingers and hands are tensed to establish a secure grasp, and lateral pressure is firmly applied against the tooth surface. The cutting edge engages the apical border of the calculus and dislodges it with a firm movement in a coronal direction. The scaling motion should be initiated in the forearm and transmitted from the wrist to the hand with a slight flexing of the fingers. Rotation of the wrist is synchronized with movement of the forearm. The scaling stroke is not initiated in the wrist or fingers, nor is it carried out independently without the use of the forearm.

It is possible to initiate the scaling motion by rotating the wrist and forearm or by flexing the fingers. The use of wrist and forearm action versus finger motion has long been debated among clinicians. Perhaps the strong opinions on both sides should be the most valid indication that there is a time and a place for each. Neither method can be advocated exclusively, because a careful analysis of effective scaling and root planing technique

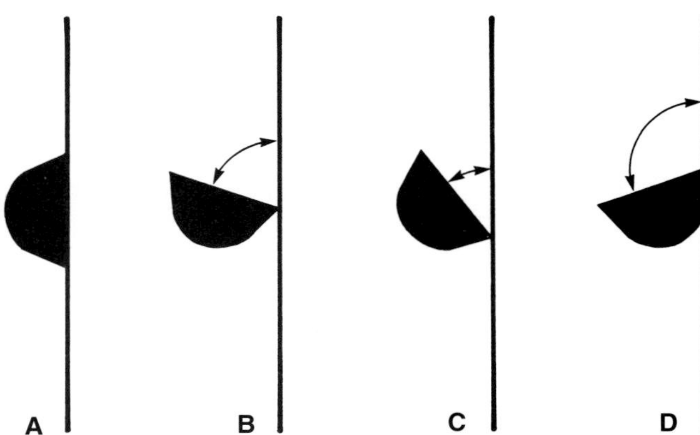

Fig. 42-21 Blade angulation. **A,** 0 degrees: correct angulation for blade insertion. **B,** 45 to 90 degrees: correct angulation for scaling and root planing. **C,** Less than 45 degrees: incorrect angulation for scaling and root planing. **D,** More than 90 degrees: incorrect angulation for scaling and root planing, correct angulation for gingival curettage.

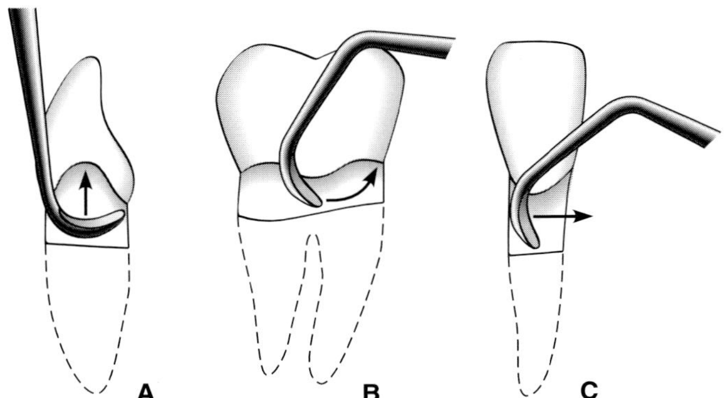

Fig. 42-22 Three basic stroke directions. **A,** Vertical; **B,** oblique; **C,** horizontal.

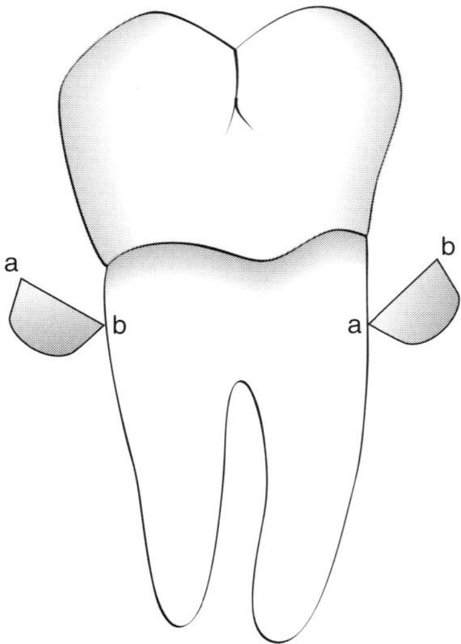

Fig. 42-23 Adaptation of the universal curette on a posterior tooth. Cross-sectional representations of the same universal curette blade as its cutting edges *(a and b)* are adapted to the mesial and distal surfaces of a posterior tooth.

reveals that, indeed, both types of stroke activation are necessary for complete instrumentation. The wrist and forearm motion, pivoting in an arc on the finger rest, produces a more powerful stroke and is therefore preferred for scaling. Finger flexing is indicated for precise control over stroke length in areas such as line angles and when horizontal strokes are used on the lingual or facial aspects of narrow-rooted teeth.

The push scaling motion has been advocated by some clinicians. In the push stroke, the instrument engages the lateral or coronal border of the calculus, and the fingers provide a thrust motion that dislodges the deposit. Because the push stroke may force calculus into the supporting tissues, its use, especially in an apical direction, is not recommended.

The **root planing stroke** is a moderate to light pull stroke that is used for final smoothing and planing of the root surface. Although hoes, files, and ultrasonic instruments have been used for root planing, curettes are widely acknowledged to be the most effective and versatile instruments for this procedure.[1-6,8,12-15] The design of the curette, which allows it to be more easily adapted to subgingival tooth contours, makes curettes particularly suitable for root planing in periodontal patients. With a moderately firm grasp, the curette is kept adapted to the tooth with even, lateral pressure. A continuous series of long, overlapping shaving strokes is activated. As the surface becomes smoother and resistance diminishes, lateral pressure is progressively reduced.

Instruments for Scaling and Root Planing

Universal Curettes. The working ends of the universal curette are designed in pairs so that all surfaces of the teeth can be treated with one double-ended instrument or a matched pair of single-ended instruments (see Fig. 42-16).

In any given quadrant, when approaching the tooth from the facial aspect, one end of the universal curette adapts to the mesial surfaces and the other end adapts to the distal surfaces. When approaching from the lingual aspect in the same quadrant, the double-ended universal curette must be turned end for end, because the blades are mirror images. This means that the end that adapts to the mesial surfaces on the facial aspect also adapts to the distal surfaces on the lingual aspect, and vice versa. Both ends of the universal curette are used to instrument the anterior teeth. On posterior teeth, however, owing to the limited access to distal surfaces, a single working end can be used to treat both mesial and distal surfaces by using both of its cutting edges. To do this, the instrument is first adapted to the mesial surface with the handle nearly parallel to the mesial surface. Because the face of the universal curette blade is honed at 90 degrees to the lower shank, if the lower shank is positioned so that it is absolutely parallel to the surface being instrumented, the tooth-blade angulation is 90 degrees. To close this angle and thus obtain proper working angulation, the lower shank must be tilted slightly toward the tooth. The distal surface of the same posterior tooth can be instrumented with the opposite cutting edge of the same blade. This cutting edge can be adapted at proper working angulation by positioning the handle so that it is *perpendicular* to the distal surface (Fig. 42-23).

When adapting the universal curette blade, as much of the cutting edge as possible should be in contact with the tooth surface, except on narrow convex surfaces such as line angles. Although the entire cutting edge should contact the tooth, pressure should be concentrated on the lower third of the blade during scaling strokes. During root planing strokes, however, lateral pressure should be distributed evenly along the cutting edge.

The primary advantage of these curettes is that they are designed to be used universally on all tooth surfaces, in all regions of the mouth. However, universal curettes have limited adaptability for the treatment of deep pockets in which apical migration of the attachment has exposed furcations, root convexities, and developmental depressions. For this reason, the Gracey curettes and the new modifications of Gracey curettes, which are area specific and specially designed for subgingival scaling and root planing in periodontal patients, are preferred by many clinicians.

Gracey Curettes. Gracey curettes (see Fig. 42-18) are a set of area-specific instruments that were designed by Dr. Clayton H. Gracey of Michigan in the mid-1930s. Four design features make the Gracey curettes unique: (1) they are area specific, (2) only one cutting edge on each blade is used, (3) the blade is curved in two planes, and (4) the blade is "offset." (These features have been summarized in Table 41-1.) Each of these features directly influences the manner in which the Gracey curettes are used and should be discussed individually.

AREA SPECIFICITY. There are seven pairs of curettes in the set. The Gracey curettes #1-2 and 3-4 are used on anterior teeth. The Gracey #5-6 may be used on both anterior and premolar teeth. The facial and lingual surfaces of posterior teeth are instrumented with Gracey curettes #7-8 and 9-10. The Gracey #11-12 is designed for mesial surfaces of posterior teeth, and the #13-14 adapts to the distal surfaces of posterior teeth. Although these guidelines for areas of use were originally established by Dr. Clayton H. Gracey, it is possible to use a Gracey curette in an area of the mouth other than the one for which it was specifically designed if the general principles regarding these curettes are understood and applied. Gracey curettes need not be reserved exclusively for periodontal patients. In fact, many clinicians prefer Gracey curettes for general scaling because of their excellent adaptability.

SINGLE CUTTING EDGE USED. Like a universal curette, the Gracey curette has a blade with two cutting edges. Unlike the universal curette, however, the Gracey instrument is designed so that only one cutting edge is used. To determine which of the two is the correct cutting edge to adapt to the tooth, the blade should be held face up and parallel to the floor. When viewed from this angle, the blade can be seen to curve to the side. One cutting edge forms a larger outer curve and the other forms a shorter, small inner curve. The larger outer curve, which has also been described as the inferior cutting edge or as the cutting edge farther away from the handle, is the correct cutting edge (Fig. 42-24).

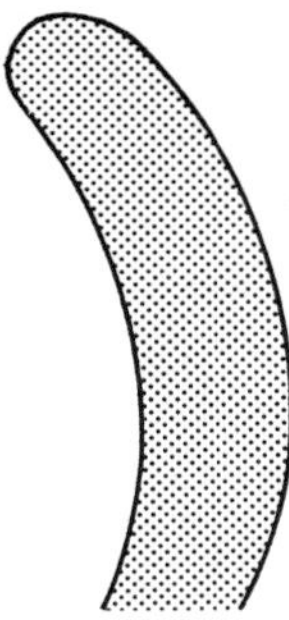

Fig. 42-24 Determining the correct cutting edge of a Gracey curette. When viewed from directly above the face of the blade, the correct cutting edge is the one forming the larger, outer curve on the right.

BLADE CURVES IN TWO PLANES. Like the toe of the universal curette, the toe of the Gracey curette curves upward. However, the toe of the Gracey curette also curves to the side, as mentioned in the preceding discussion. This unique curvature enhances the blade's adaptation to convexities and concavities as the working end is advanced around the tooth. Only the lower third or half of the Gracey blade is in contact with the tooth during instrumentation. The cutting edge of a universal curette blade, on the other hand, is straight and does not curve to the side. This makes it less adaptable to root concavities.

OFFSET BLADE. Gracey curette blades are honed at an offset angle, which means that the face of the blade is not perpendicular to the lower shank as it is on a universal curette. Instead, Gracey curettes are designed so that the tooth-blade working angulation is 60 to 70 degrees when the lower shank is held parallel to the tooth surface. Gracey curettes were originally designed to be used with push strokes and were beveled to provide a tooth-blade angulation of 40 degrees when the lower shank was parallel to the tooth surface; for many years, Gracey curettes were available only in this form. Currently Gracey curettes are available not only in the original push design, but also in a modified version to be used with pull strokes. It is important to understand this when purchasing Gracey curettes to avoid obtaining instruments that are not properly designed for pull strokes. If Gracey curettes that are designed to be used with push strokes are used with pull strokes instead, they are likely to burnish calculus rather than completely remove it. The design of the Gracey curette was modified in response to requests from clinicians who liked the shank design and adaptability of the original Gracey instruments but were opposed to the use of push strokes for scaling and root planing. The push stroke is not recommended, especially for the novice clinician, because it is likely to cause undue trauma to the junctional epithelium and to embed fragments of dislodged calculus in the soft tissues.

PRINCIPLES OF USE. The following general principles of use of the Gracey curettes are essentially the same as those for the universal curette; italicized principles apply only to Gracey curettes:

1. *Determine the correct cutting edge.* The correct cutting edge should be determined by visually inspecting the blade and confirmed by lightly adapting the chosen cutting edge to the tooth with the lower shank parallel to the surface of the tooth. With the toe pointed in the direction to be scaled (e.g., mesially with a #7-8 curette), only the back of the blade can be seen if the correct cutting edge has been selected (Fig. 42-25). If the wrong cutting edge has been adopted, the flat, shiny face of the blade will be seen instead (Fig. 42-26).
2. *Make sure the lower shank is parallel to the surface to be instrumented.* The lower shank of a Gracey curette is that portion of the shank between the blade and the first bend in the shank. Parallelism of the handle or upper shank is not an acceptable guide with Gracey curettes, because the angulations of the shanks vary. On anterior teeth, the lower shank of the Gracey #1-2, 3-4, or 5-6 should be parallel to the mesial, distal, facial, or lingual surfaces of the teeth (Fig. 42-27). On posterior teeth the lower shank of the #7-8 or 9-10 should be parallel to the facial or lingual surfaces of the teeth (Fig. 42-28); the lower shank of the #11-12 should be parallel to the mesial surfaces of the teeth (Fig. 42-29); and the lower shank of the #13-14 should be parallel to the distal surfaces of the teeth (Fig. 42-30).
3. When using intraoral finger rests, keep the fourth and middle fingers together in a built-up fulcrum for maximum control and wrist-arm action.
4. Use extraoral fulcrums or mandibular finger rests for optimal angulation when working on the maxillary posterior teeth.
5. Concentrate on using the lower third of the cutting edge for calculus removal, especially on line angles or when attempting to remove a calculus ledge by breaking it away in sections, beginning at the lateral edge.
6. Allow the wrist and forearm to carry the burden of the stroke, rather than flexing the fingers.

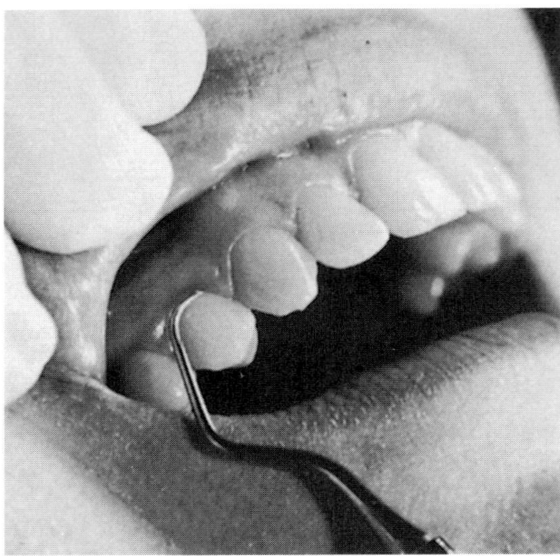

Fig. 42-25 Correct cutting edge of a Gracey curette adapted to the tooth.

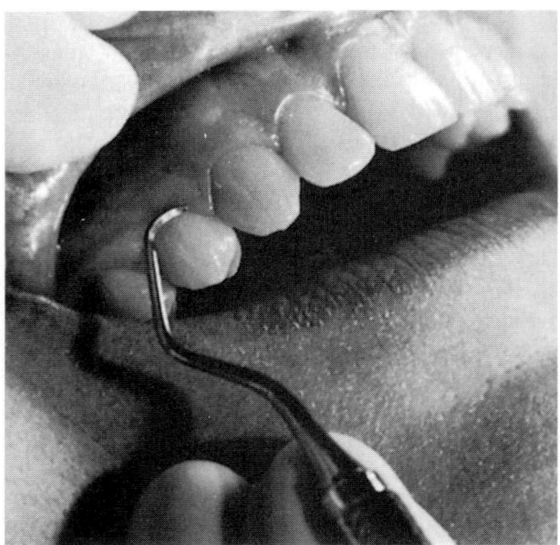

Fig. 42-26 Incorrect cutting edge of a Gracey curette adapted to the tooth.

7. Roll the handle slightly between the thumb and fingers to keep the blade adapted as the working end is advanced around line angles and into concavities.
8. Modulate lateral pressure from firm to moderate to light depending on the nature of the calculus, and reduce pressure as the transition is made from scaling to root planing strokes.

EXTENDED SHANK GRACEY CURETTES. Extended shank Gracey curettes such as the After Five curettes are 3 mm longer in the terminal shank than the standard Gracey curettes but are used with the same technique (see Fig. 41-23). They are most useful for deep pockets on maxillary and mandibular posterior teeth, where the longer terminal shank allows better access, especially to deep mesial and distal pockets (see Fig. 41-24). Although the longer lower shank makes access easier while using a conventional intraoral finger rest, the use of an extraoral fulcrum allows better access and adaptation to all of the maxillary posterior teeth. After Five curettes with rigid shanks should be used for scaling of heavy calculus; those with regular, finishing shanks should be used for periodontal maintenance patients with deep residual pockets.

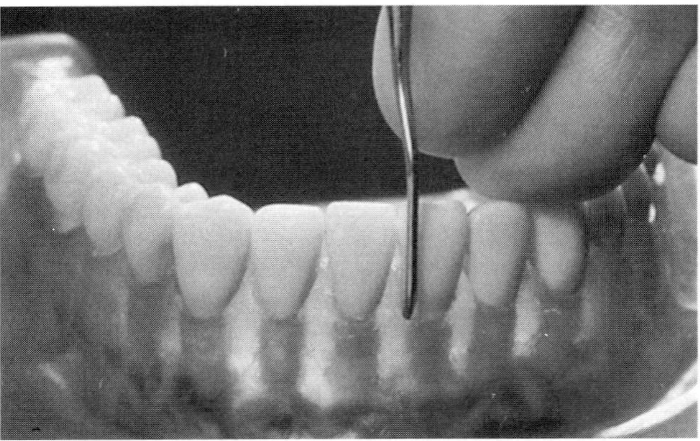

Fig. 42-27 Gracey #5-6 curette adapted to an anterior tooth.

MINI-BLADED GRACEY CURETTES. Mini-bladed Gracey curettes such as the Mini Five curettes and the Gracey Curvette curettes have a terminal shank that is 3 mm longer than the standard Gracey curettes and a blade that is 50% shorter (see Fig. 42-26 and Fig. 42-27). These mini-bladed instruments are generally used in the same manner as the Gracey curettes except for the following specific differences:

1. Mini-bladed curettes should not be used routinely in place of standard Gracey or After Five curettes. Instead, they should be used to supplement conventional curettes and ultrasonic instruments in areas of difficult access such as furcations; line angles; and deep, tight, or narrow pockets.
2. Large #4 handles are recommended for any mini-bladed instruments, because the larger diameter of the handles allows better control of the small blades.
3. Mini-bladed curettes can be used to scale with the toe directed either mesially or distally. In fact, the Mini Five curettes often adapt more effectively to the root curvatures of many posterior teeth when the blade is inserted with the toe pointed distally and strokes are activated from the mesial toward the distal line angle (Fig. 42-31).
4. Use rigid shank mini-bladed curettes for calculus removal. Use the thinner, standard shank mini-bladed curettes for deplaquing during maintenance.
5. When using mini-bladed curettes for calculus removal, use intraoral finger rests close to the working area. When performing light root planing or deplaquing, either intraoral or extraoral rests may be used. Extraoral rests are usually necessary to gain access to deep pockets on maxillary second and third molars.

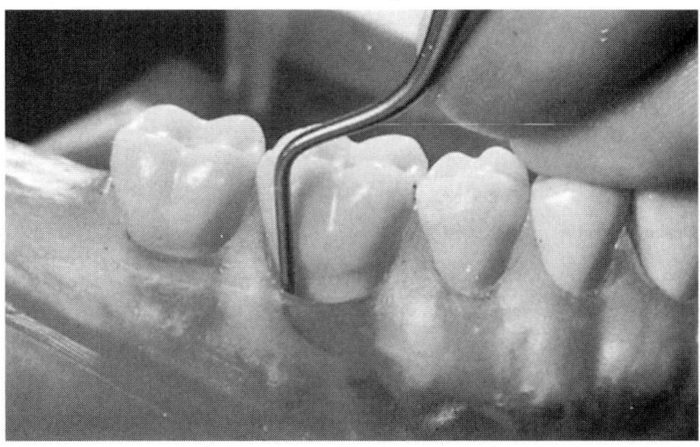

Fig. 42-28 Gracey #7-8 curette adapted to the facial surface of a posterior tooth.

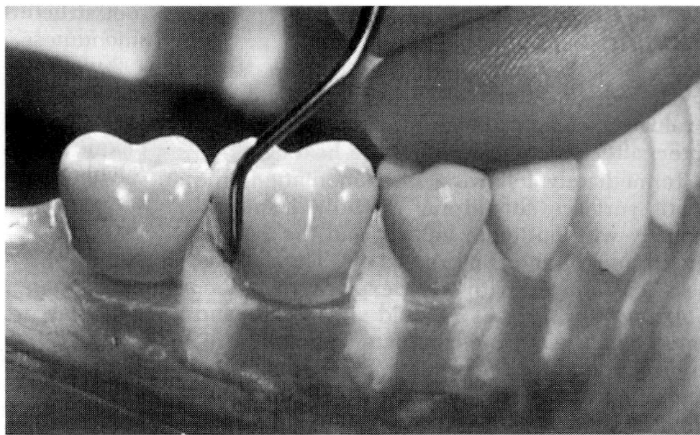

Fig. 42-30 Gracey #13-14 curette adapted to the distal surface of a posterior tooth.

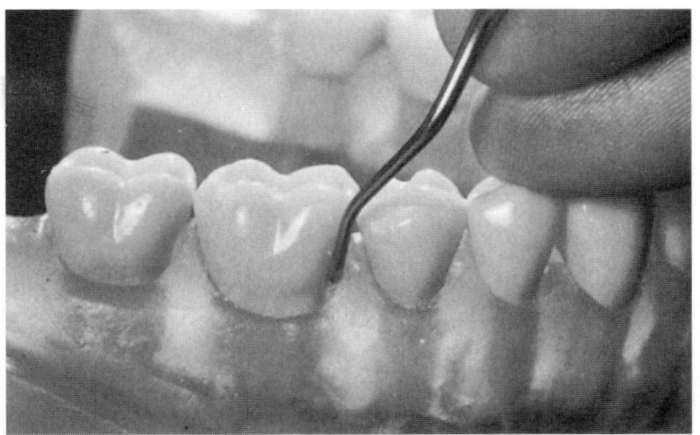

Fig. 42-29 Gracey #11-12 curette adapted to the mesial surface of a posterior tooth.

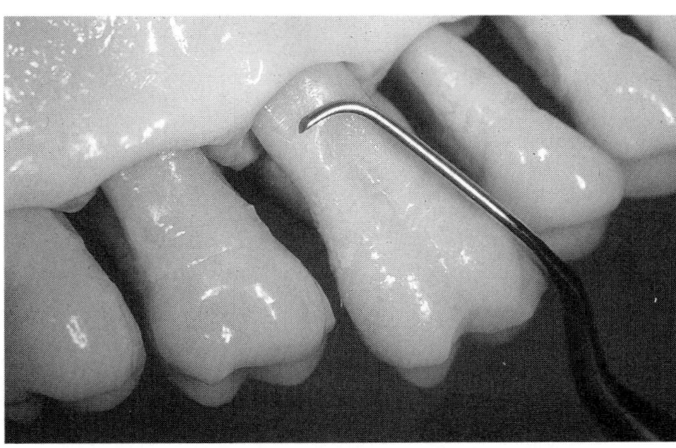

Fig. 42-31 Mini Five 13/14 curette adapted to the palatal surface of a maxillary molar with the toe directed distally.

6. Mini Fives are generally used with straight vertical strokes. They may also be used with oblique or horizontal strokes but due to the shortness of the blade, these strokes might not extend far enough subgingivally unless the tissue is very retractable. Horizontal strokes with the Mini Fives are most effective when used in the CEJ or in developmental depressions just below it.

When properly used, mini-bladed Gracey curettes allow unprecedented access and effectiveness for both nonsurgical and surgical root débridement. One study has shown that Gracey Curvette curettes performed better than standard Gracey curettes in deep anterior pockets.[7] In areas such as line angles; furcations; and narrow, curved, facial, or palatal root surfaces, these miniature curettes provide excellent adaptation with better tactile sensitivity than modified slim ultrasonic tips. Studies have shown that Gracey Curvette curettes performed better than ultrasonic slim tips on deep mandibular anterior pockets, furcations and furcation entrances.[9,10] No comparison of hand instruments and modified slim ultrasonic tips can be made unless mini-bladed curettes have been fully employed. To date, some research has been done to compare the effectiveness of mini-bladed instruments with the modified slim ultrasonic tips. There is a need for more of these studies to be performed *in vivo* to guide clinicians in the optimal utilization of these new types of instruments.[11]

REFERENCES

1. Barnes JE, Schaffer EM: Subgingival root planing: A comparison using files, hoes, and curets. J Periodontol 1960; 31:300.
2. Garnick JJ, Dent J: A scanning electron micrographical study of root surfaces and subgingival bacteria after hand scaling and ultrasonic instrumentation. J Periodontol 1989; 60:441.
3. Garrett JS: Effects of non-surgical periodontal therapy on periodontitis in humans. A review. J Clin Periodontol 1983; 10:515.
4. Green E, Ramfjord SR: Tooth roughness after subgingival root planing. J Periodontol 1966; 37:396.

5. Greenstein G: Nonsurgical periodontal therapy in 2000: A literature review. J Am Dent Assoc 2000; 131(111):1580.
6. Kerry GJ: Roughness of root surfaces after use of ultrasonic instruments and hand curets. J Periodontol 1967; 38:340.
7. Landry C, Long B, Singer D, et al: Comparison between a short and a conventional blade periodontal curet: an in vitro study. J Clin Periodontol 1999; 26(8):548.
8. Orban B, Manella V: Macroscopic and microscopic study of instruments designed for root planing. J Periodontol 1956; 27:120.
9. Otero-Cagide FJ, Long BA: Comparative in vitro effectiveness of closed root débridement with fine instruments on specific areas of mandibular first molar furcations. I. Root trunk and furcation entrance. J Periodontol 1997; 68(11):1093.
10. Otero-Cagide FJ, Long BA: Comparative in vitro effectiveness of closed root débridement with fine instruments on specific areas of mandibular first molar furcations. I. Furcation area. J Periodontol 1997; 68(11):1098.
11. Pattison AM: The use of hand instruments in supportive periodontal treatment. Periodontol 2000 1996; 12:71.
12. Schlageter L, Rateitschak-Pluss EM, Schwarz JP: Root surface smoothness or roughness following open débridement. An *in vivo* study. J Clin Periodontol 1996; 23(5):460.
13. Schaffer EM: Histologic results of root curettage on human teeth. J Periodontol 1956; 27:269.
14. Van Volkinburg J, Green E, Armitage G: The nature of root surfaces after curette, cavitron, and alpha-sonic instrumentation. J Periodont Res 1976; 11:374.
15. Wilkinson RF, Maybury J: Scanning electron microscopy of the root surface following instrumentation. J Periodontol 1973; 44:559.

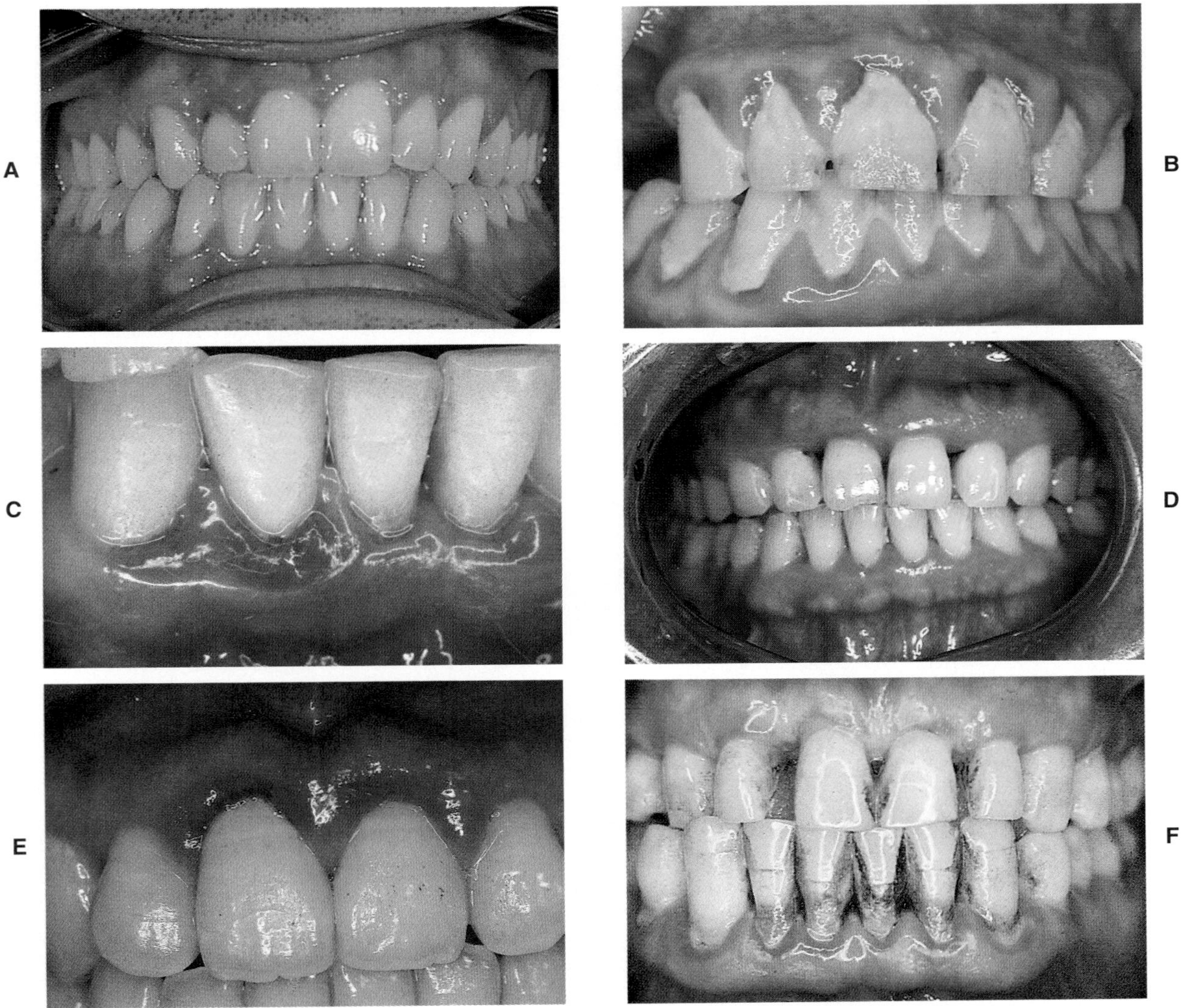

Color Fig. 30-1 **A,** Incipient marginal gingivitis. Note the slight puffiness and bleeding *(arrow)* around the upper right lateral incisor. **B,** Edematous type of gingival inflammation. Note the loss of stippling, increase in size, abundant plaque and materia alba, and change in color. **C,** Close-up view of edematous type of gingival inflammation. Note the red, shiny, smooth gingiva. **D,** Fibrocytic type gingival inflammation. Pockets of moderate depth are present, but the gingiva retains its stippling in some areas. **E,** Severe generalized gingival inflammation and inflammatory gingival enlargement. **F,** Fibrotic gingival inflammation. Note the abundant calculus and the gingival recession. The patient has pockets of moderate-to-severe depth in the mandibular anterior teeth and more shallow pockets in the maxillary teeth.

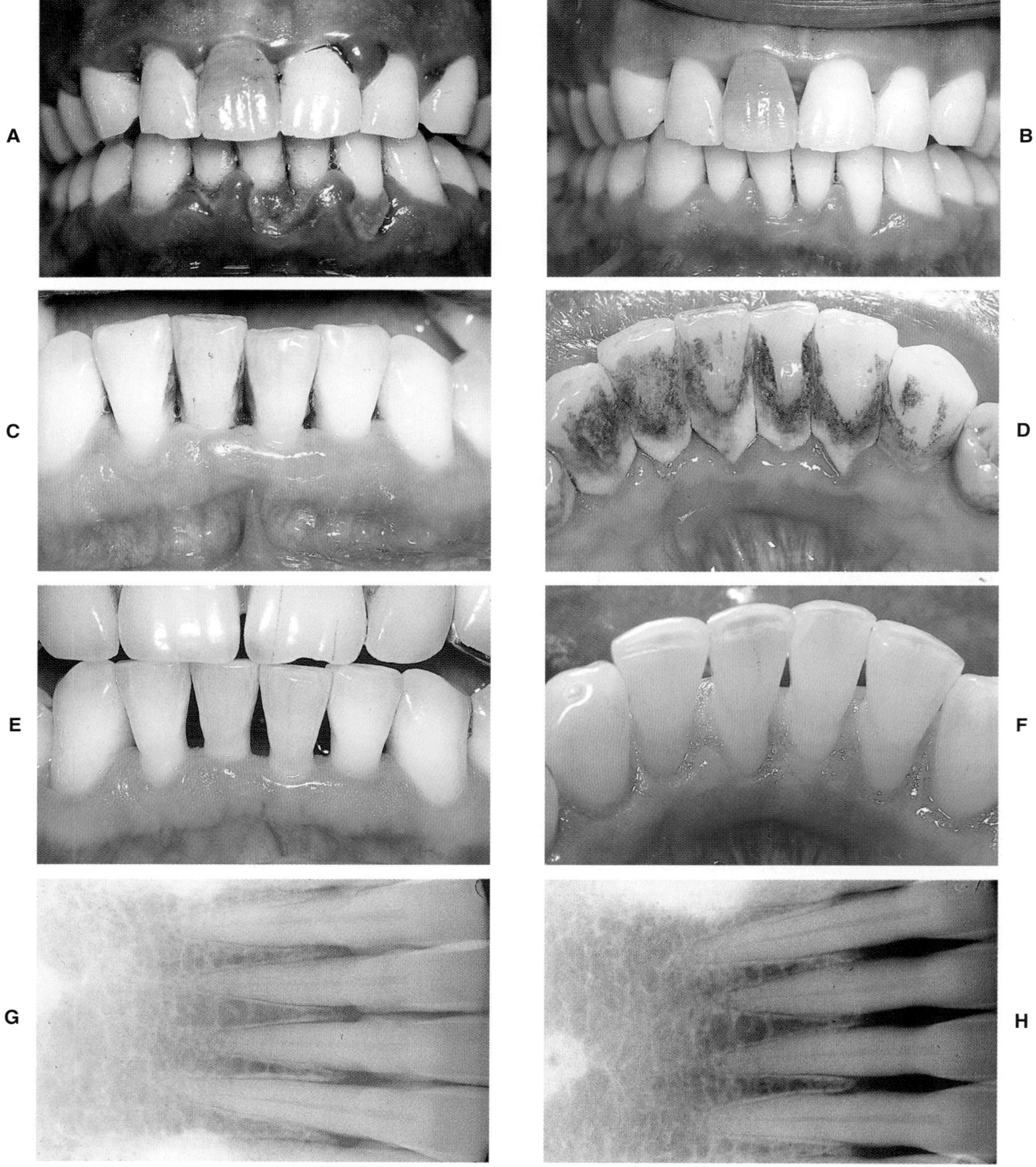

Color Fig. 48-1 Results of Phase I therapy. **A and B,** Severe chronic periodontitis. **A,** Severe chronic periodontitis characterized by deep pockets, attachment loss, and severe swelling and redness of the gingiva. **B,** Healing results, 3 weeks after elimination of irritants. Tissue has returned to a more normal contour with redness and swelling dramatically reduced. **C to H,** Moderate chronic periodontitis. **C,** Patient presenting with moderate attachment loss and probe depths in the 4- to 6-mm range. Note the gingiva appears pink because it is fibrotic and the inflammation is deep in the periodontal pockets. **D,** Lingual view pretreatment with more visible inflammation and heavy deposits of calculus. **E and F,** The same areas with significant improvement in gingival health 18 months after scaling, root planing, and plaque control therapy were provided; the patient returned for regular maintenance visits. **G,** Presenting radiograph of the lower anterior teeth. **H,** Radiograph taken 18 months after Phase I therapy and maintenance. The follow-up radiograph shows no increase in bone loss during the 18 months.

Sonic and Ultrasonic Instrumentation

Gregor J. Petersilka and Thomas F. Flemmig

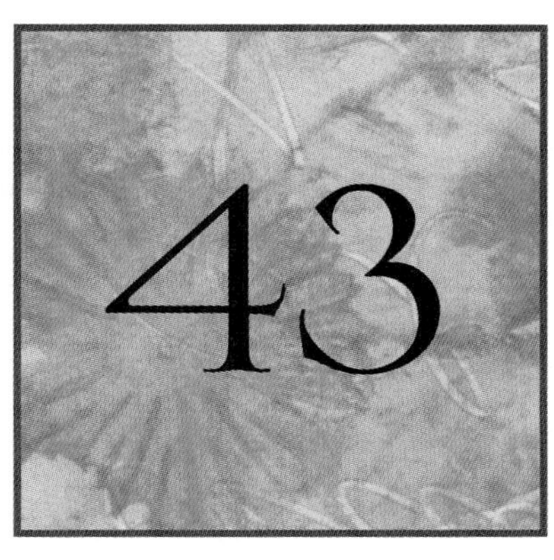

CHAPTER

CHAPTER OUTLINE

One of the central components of periodontal therapy is the removal of the subgingival bacterial biofilm and calculus that act as reservoirs for periodontopathogenic microrganisms. Traditionally, root surface debridement has been carried out with hand instruments such as curettes. Hand instrumentation is technically demanding, time consuming, tiring, and uncomfortable for both the operator and the patient, and as a result, numerous power-driven scalers have been developed during the last decades. Until recently, their use was mostly limited to supragingival debridement due to bulky working tips. Technologic advances and new designs of ultrasonic and sonic scalers have transformed the role of power-driven oscillating instruments in periodontal therapy. The probelike, slender instrument tips allow efficient instrumentation of deep periodontal pockets with increased patient comfort and less operator fatigue[10,12,25,54] (Fig. 43-1). Consequently, power-driven instrumentation has now become an accepted treatment modality in periodontal therapy.

SONIC SCALERS AND MAGNETOSTRICTIVE AND PIEZOELECTRIC ULTRASONIC SCALERS

Oscillating scaler systems can be divided into sonic scalers and magnetostrictive and piezoelectric ultrasonic scalers. Sonic scaler hand-pieces were invented during the 1960s (e.g., Densonic scaler, Titan S, KaVo Sonicflex)[62] and operate by compressed air from the dental unit. A rotating cam within the instrument hand-piece generates vibrations with frequencies in the range of 6000 Hz to 9000 Hz (Fig. 43-2). The vibrations are conducted to the scaler tip, which then oscillates, depending on the air pressure input, with an amplitude of up to 1000 μm in an almost circular motion[20,29,34,59] (Fig. 43-3). Due to this oscillation pattern, irrespective of the adaptation of the tip to the root surface (i.e., mesial, distal, or buccal), plaque and calculus are removed by a tapping motion, which is one of the major advantages of the sonic scalers over the ultrasonic scalers (Fig. 43-4).

Magnetostrictive ultrasonic scalers (e.g., Dentsply Cavitron, Odontosson) were introduced in the 1950s[62] and are either driven by a metal stack consisting of nickel-iron alloy strips or a Ferrite Insert inserted into a hand-piece (Figs. 43-5 and 43-6). Inside the hand-piece a live coil generates an alternating electromagnetic field that leads to expansion or contraction of the ferromagnetic material. The resulting vibrations are conducted to the scaler tip, causing oscillations with amplitudes of 13 to 72 μm and an elliptical motion pattern at frequencies of 20,000 Hz to 45,000 Hz.[34] Thus depending on the angulation of the scaler tip in relation to the root surface, a

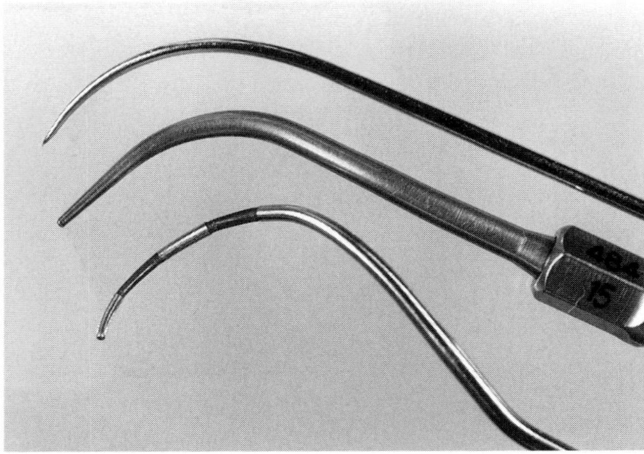

Fig. 43-1 Slender ultrasonic and sonic scaler tips allowing subgingival debridement with oscillating scalers. *Top to bottom,* Explorer EXS 3A, Sonic Scaler tip, Nabers furcation Probe.

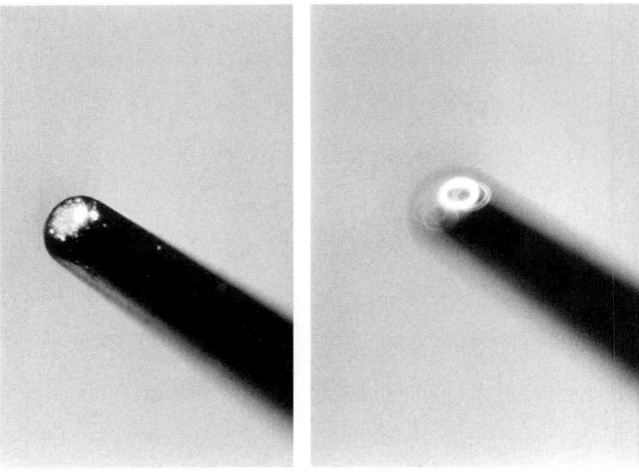

Fig. 43-3 Photomicrograph of a sonic scaler tip seen perpendicular to the very end of the tip. *Left,* Tip at rest, showing distinct reflections of a light beam. *Right,* Oscillating tip; reflections describe a circular motion pattern of the oscillation. (Courtesy Dr. B. Ehmke, University of Münster, Germany.)

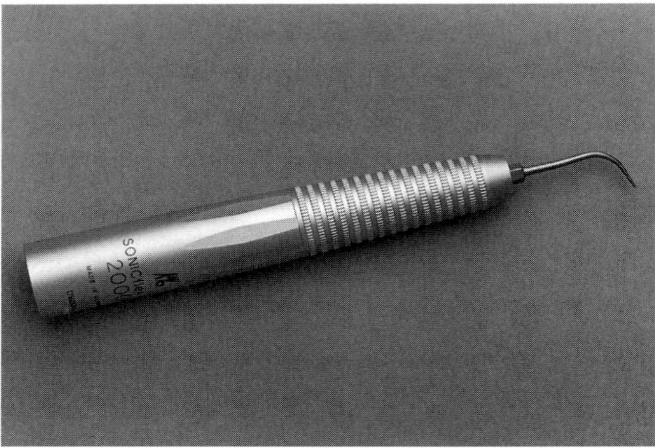

Fig. 43-2 Sonic scaler hand-piece fitted with slim scaler tip (Type KaVo Sonicflex Lux 2000).

more or less pronounced hammering or scraping motion pattern will result (Fig. 43-4).

Piezoelectric scalers (e.g., Amdent, EMS Piezon Master, Satellec Suprasson) also oscillate with frequencies of 20,000 to 45,000 Hz (Fig. 43-7). The vibration is generated by changes in the dimension of a quartz crystal caused by the application of an alternating current. The resulting oscillation mode of the piezoelectric scaler tip is strictly linear with amplitudes up to 72 μm.[34] The mode of action of the tip is either of a tapping or a scraping nature, depending on the direction of the scaler tip toward the root surface (see Fig. 43-4). Instrument power setting of magnetostrictive and piezoelectric ultrasonic scalers can be adjusted by the operator. A higher power setting increases the amplitude of tip oscillation, however, with a constant and stable tip oscillation frequency and motion pattern.

Safety and Efficacy of Oscillating Scalers

It is imperative to adjust the amount of substance removal and, consequently, the use of sonic and ultrasonic scaler tips, according to the appropriate phase of periodontal therapy. In initial periodontal therapy an instrument needs to efficiently and rapidly remove tenacious calculus, whereas in maintenance therapy the instruments should efficiently remove bacterial biofilms while minimizing root substance removal.[9,35,52] In particular, during repeated maintenance visits, even minimal substance loss may accumulate over time and may lead to severe root damage. Factors influencing the amount of root substance removed during hand instrumentation have been well evaluated.[11,61] Assuming a correct angulation of the curette, the number of scaling strokes and the lateral force applied represent the two main parameters influencing the efficacy of hand instruments. However, using power-driven oscillating scalers, the instruments' efficacy and safety also depends on instrumentation time, lateral force, scaler tip angulation, and instrument power setting. In addition, the interactions of the working parameters create a highly complex pattern of substance removal. More detailed information regarding the influence of certain working parameters root substance loss for different oscillating scaler systems was gained by *in vitro* studies.[17-19] For sonic scalers (KaVo Sonicflex Lux 2000, KaVo, Biberach, Germany), lateral force showed the same impact on substance loss as scaler tip angulation. Assuming that a defect depth of 0.5 mm, resulting from repeated subgingival scaling over 10 years of maintenance, is clinically acceptable and the same surfaces are always scaled, the average defect depth per year should not exceed 50 μm. With respect to instrument safety, a resulting defect depth of 50 μm after 40-second instrumentation time (average time spent for debridement of a root surface during maintenance within 1

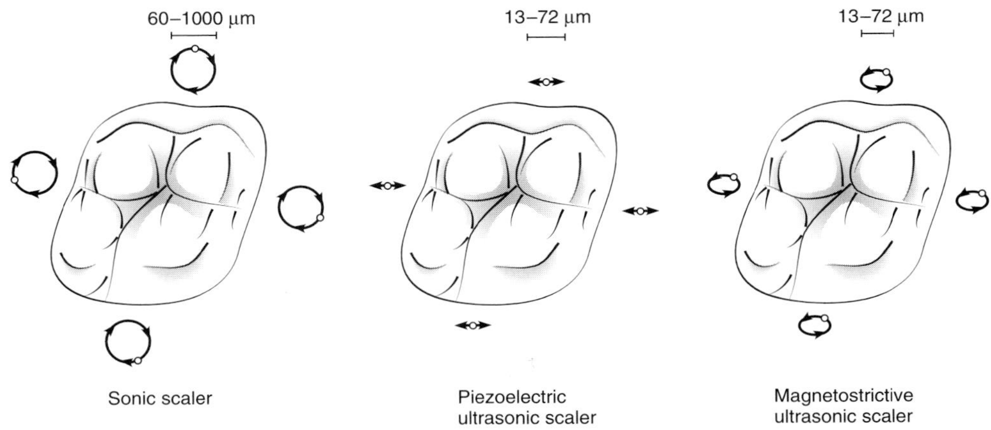

Fig. 43-4 Schematic drawing showing the differences between the different oscillation patterns of oscillating scaler systems. *Left,* Sonic scaler; *center,* Piezoelectric ultrasonic scaler; *right,* Magnetostrictive ultrasonic scaler. (Modified from Petersilka GJ, Flemmig TF: Subgingival root surface treatment using sonic and ultrasonic scalers. Parodontologie 1999; 3:233.)

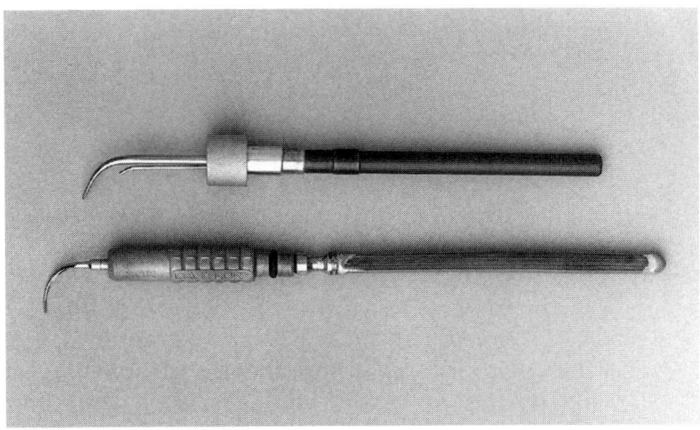

Fig. 43-5 Insert used for magnetostrictive ultrasonic scalers. *Top,* Ferrite Insert (Odontosson) and metal alloy stack insert (Dentsply).

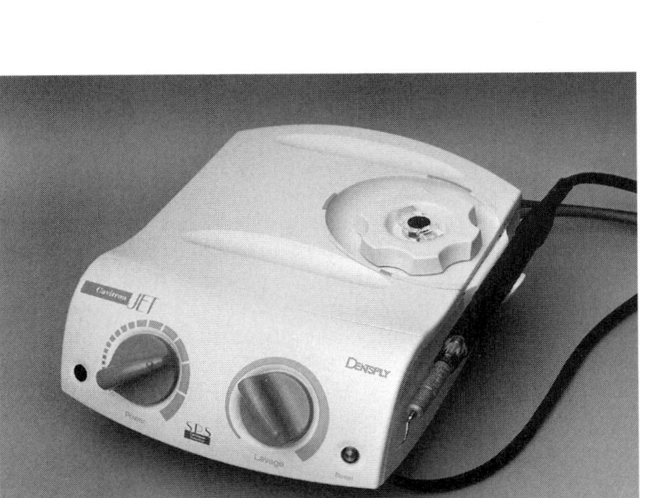

Fig. 43-6 Magnetostrictive ultrasonic scaling unit (Type Dentsply Cavijet SLS. (Courtesy Dentsply International, Inc., York, PA).

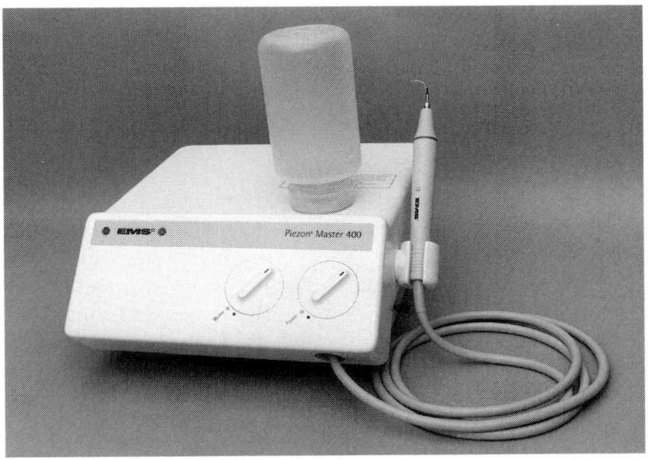

Fig. 43-7 Piezoelectric ultrasonic scaler unit (EMS Piezon master 400. (Courtesy Electromedical Systems, Dallas, TX.)

year)[2] may be acceptable. Thus these instruments can be used safely if the scaler tip is angulated parallel to the root surface and the forces applied do not exceed 2N (Fig. 43-8). However, all other parameter combinations can lead to severe root damage.

In magnetostrictive ultrasonic scalers, tip angulation and lateral force also have an almost identical influence on substance removal. For all instrument power settings, assessed higher angulations and lateral forces resulted in greater defect depths. By contrast, an increasing instrument power setting does not lead to a pronounced increase in defect depth. The critical defect depth of 50 μm can only be maintained if the scaler tip is angulated absolutely parallel to the root surface and the forces used do not exceed 1N (see Fig. 43-8).

As piezoelectric ultrasonic scalers show a linear oscillation pattern, root substance removal from these

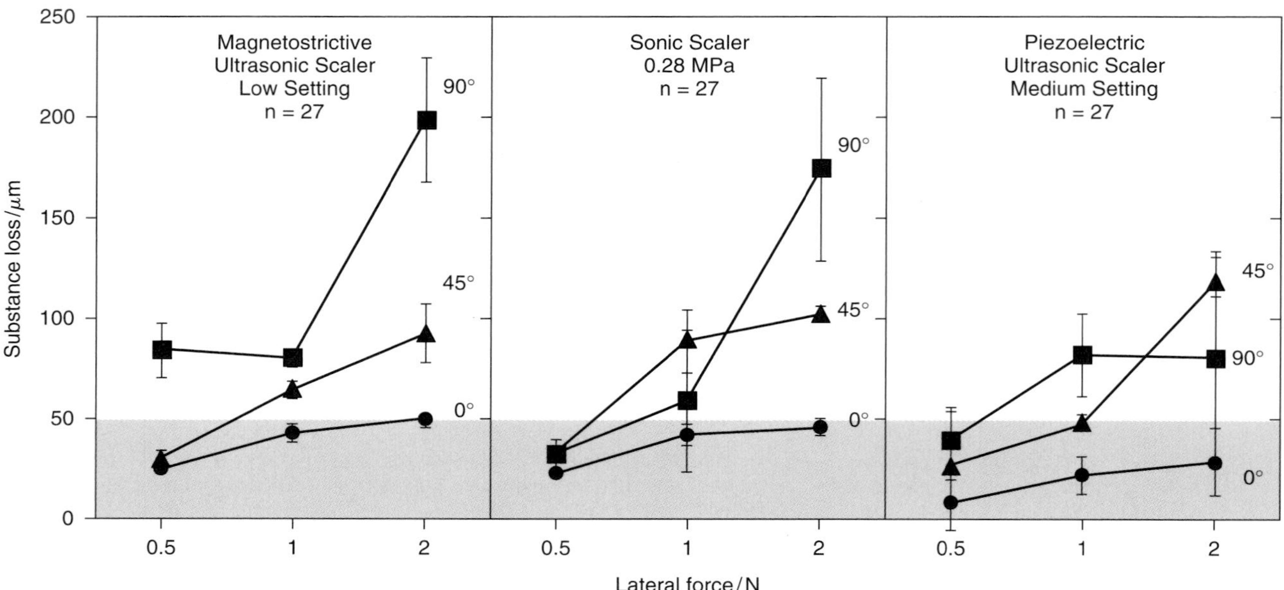

Fig. 43-8 Defect depth after 40-s instrumentation time with a piezoelectric scaler *(right),* sonic scaler *(center)* and magnetostrictive ultrasonic scaler *(left).* The critical defect depth of 50 μm is marked by the shaded area. (From Flemmig T, Petersilka G, Mehl A, et al: Working parameters of a sonic scaler influencing root substance removal in vitro. Clin Oral Invest 1997; 1:55.)

instruments is mostly influenced by scaler tip angulation. The greatest increment in defect depth was found with increasing tip angulation from 45 degrees to 90 degrees. In contrast, lateral force and the instrument power setting do not substantially influence substance loss. However, if the tip is angulated parallel to the root surface, the critical defect depth can be maintained below 50 μm, even if higher application forces up to 2N are used (Fig. 43-9).

Comparing the efficacy of oscillating scalers revealed that magnetostrictive ultrasonic scalers remove a larger amount of root substance at all power settings than the piezoelectric ultrasonic scaler. The efficacy of the sonic scaler is comparable to the efficacy of a magnetostrictive scaler at low power setting or to the efficacy of the piezoelectric scaler at medium power settings.[44]

Principles of Sonic and Ultrasonic Instrumentation

Indications. Indications and contraindications for sonic and ultrasonic scaling do not substantially differ from those given for the use of hand instruments in initial and supportive periodontal therapy. Clinical studies have shown that achievable attachment gain and pocket probing depth reduction after the use of hand instruments and sonic or different types of ultrasonic scalers are identical.[2,31,33] Numerous attempts have been made to investigate the quality—that is, the degree of roughness or root substance after different scaling modalities.[1,14,23,24,26,32,36,41,48,55] However, results are equivocal and difficult to compare as study designs and results vary greatly.

In addition, the quality of root surfaces after debridement is of reduced importance, as are the clinical results of root surface instrumentation. Subgingival root surface roughness does not seem to interfere with healing after scaling and root planing.[39,56] Thus it does not appear useful to reinstrument root surfaces with hand instruments after a clinically detectable smooth surface has been created with sonic or ultrasonic scalers. Complete instrumentation of molar furcational aspects is difficult to achieve either with hand or power-driven scalers.[16,28,42,43,56] This may be due to the fact that the average width of molar furcational entrances is smaller than the working end of conventional curets.[5] Additionally, even if access with small hand instruments is possible, it is difficult to implement proper working strokes within a furcation in the limited space available. Slim sonic or ultrasonic scaler tips allow access to the furcation and have been shown to be superior to hand instruments in cleaning furcation areas *in vitro.*[31,40]

Sonic and ultrasonic scalers should not be used when treating patients with transmissible diseases, since aerosol and splatter caused by sonic and ultrasonic scalers[21] are a potential health hazard to the operating dental staff.[4,22] Although the amount of microbial content in an aerosol generated during supragingival ultrasonic scaling may be reduced by using a preprocedural antiseptics rinse,[15,21] subgingival scaling procedures always result in the dispersion of blood. Thus splatter and aerosol still might be contaminated with pathogenic microorganisms. A careful operative technique and the use of high volume evacuators aid in minimizing the aerosol dispersion[47] and therefore are of high importance for infection control. Since magnetostrictive ultrasonic scalers

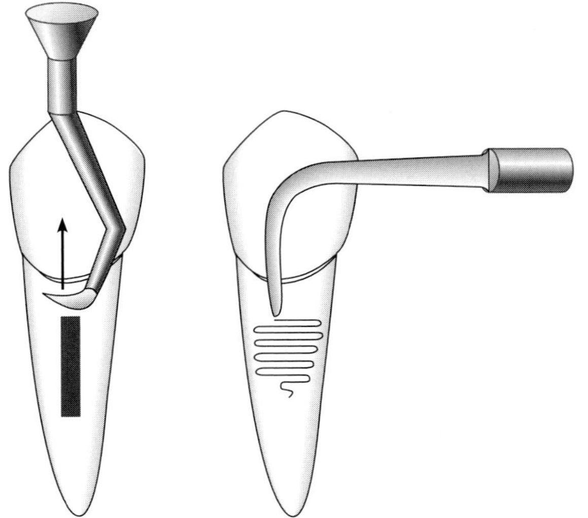

Fig. 43-9 Schematic drawing of the different patterns of the cleaning action of hand instruments versus power-driven oscillating scalers. *Left,* Using a hand curette allows a sectionwide cleaning of contaminated root surfaces. *Right,* Complete root surface debridement with oscillating scalers is achieved by carrying out serpentine-like, overlapping horizontal strokes in corono-apical direction. (Modified from Petersilka GJ, Flemmig TF: Subgingival root surface treatment using sonic and ultrasonic scalers. Parodontologie, 1999; 3:233.)

may interfere with some cardiac pacemakers, their use is also not recommended in affected patients due to health concerns.

Patient and Operator Positioning

Patient and operator positioning for sonic and ultrasonic instrumentation follow the same principles as for hand instrumentation. For instrumentation of the upper arch, the patient is seated in a supine position with the chin slightly lifted up. The backrest of the dental chair should be in approximately 45-degree angulation to the floor if treatment is carried out in the mandible. A slight lowering of the patient's chin allows good visibility to the lingual aspects of the lower front teeth. Good patient positioning should allow the operator to be seated upright; whenever necessary, indirect view or illumination by the use of dental mirrors should be used.

Site Evaluation

Before each scaling procedure, the clinician should carry out a thorough evaluation of the sites to be treated. This includes evaluation of pocket probing depth, root surface anatomy, and morphology (i.e., detection of surface irregularities such as calculus, furcations, or invaginations), as well as an adequate interpretation of radiographic findings. In combination with detailed anatomic knowledge, the operator should be able to develop a three dimensional picture of the periodontal pocket topography.

The Role of Coolant in Subgingival Sonic and Ultrasonic Scaling

The high frequency oscillation of sonic and ultrasonic scaler tips generates heat which necessitates the application of a cooling irrigation fluid to keep the tissues surrounding the scaler tip within a physiologic temperature range.[37] A flow rate of at least 14 ml/min to 23 ml/min cooling agent[22] appears to be sufficient to prevent thermal damages in periodontal pockets as the penetration of the coolant used correlates well with the depth of the pocket treated.[38] However, positioning of high volume evacuators close to the tip reduces the amount of coolant reaching the site being scaled and may lead to excessive heat generation.

Since only little lateral dispersion of the irrigation fluid from the scaler tip occurs, bacterial biofilm removal *in vivo* is most likely caused by mechanical disruption due to the oscillating tip. Possible cleaning mechanisms due to microstreaming effects or cavitation caused by collapsing microbubbles formed within the coolant surrounding the oscillating ultrasonic scalers tip have been detected *in vitro*.[27,57–60] In addition, cell disruption due to ultrasonic scaling has been shown in filamentous and rod-shaped bacteria.[3] However, these effects have not been proven to occur subgingivally, and cavitation is not likely to have an *in vitro* antimicrobial effect on periodontopathogenic bacteria such as *Actinobacillus actinomycetemcomitans* or *Porphyromonas gingivalis*.[50]

Several studies have evaluated the possible advantageous effects of the use of antimicrobials as a coolant. Although povidone-iodine solutions used as adjunctive irrigation liquid during ultrasonic scaling have been reported to have favorable clinical and microbiologic effects, there is a lack of clinically relevant attachment gain.[49] In addition, delivery of low concentration (0.1% to 0.2 %) chlorhexidine digluconate solutions as an irrigant during ultrasonic or sonic scaling does not appear to have relevant long-term benefits.[7,46,51,53] Therefore the use of antimicrobials cannot be considered as scientifically warranted at this time.

Instrument Power Setting

The power setting of sonic and ultrasonic scalers influences the amplitude of tip oscillation. Therefore a high instrument setting may generate pronounced aerosol and splatter formation and might reduce the volume of cooling agent that is delivered into the periodontal pocket. As treatment outcome is not significantly altered by instrument power setting[8] and high instrument power setting might facilitate unnecessary root substance removal,[17–19] power setting should be reduced to a low or medium level whenever possible.

Instrument Grasp and Finger Rest

To allow maximum instrument stabilization the instrument hand-piece should be held using a modified pen

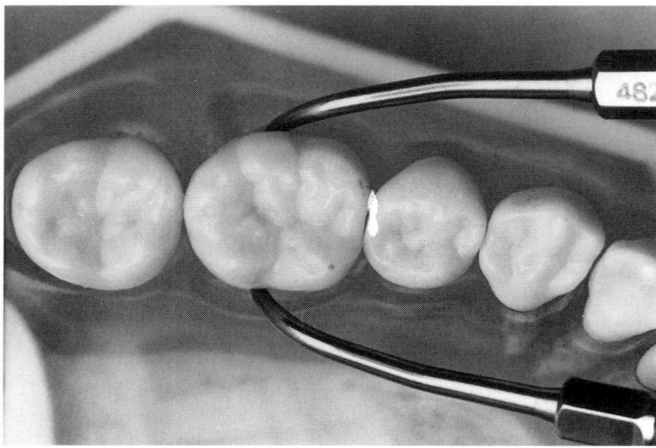

Fig. 43-10 Sample of scaler tip systems showing a left and right offset angulation. Note the correct application of the scaler tips to the root surface as the convex part is applied to the root surface only.

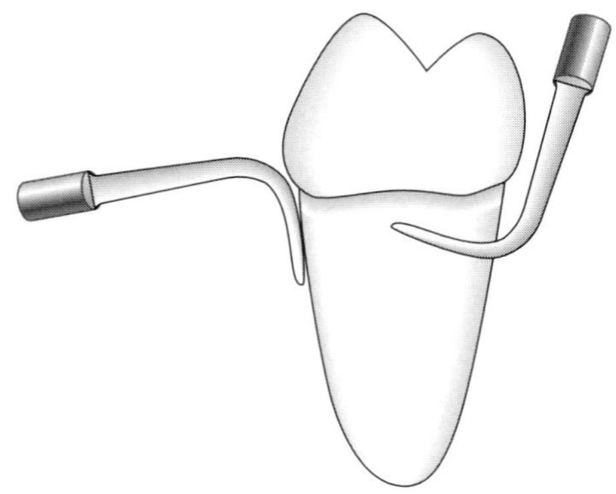

Fig. 43-11 Systematic approach of cleaning a root surface with slim scaler tips. The tip is applied parallel to the long axis of the tooth. Additionally, an oblique insertion of the tip for cleaning the contralateral interdental surface is recommended. Irrespective of the orientation to the long axis of the tooth, the tip needs to be applied parallel to the root surface treated to avoid root surface damage. (Modified from Petersilka GJ, Flemmig TF: Subgingival root surface treatment using sonic and ultrasonic scalers. Parodontologie 1999; 3:233.)

grasp. With hand instrumentation an intraoral finger rest is recommended for instrumentation of teeth in the lower arch and in the upper front segment. An extraoral palm rest should be chosen while instrumenting maxillary posterior teeth, with the back of the hand in the right maxillary area or with the palm of the hand in the left area respectively.

Systematic Approach

Studies to date have failed to confirm that power-driven root instrumentation is much more rapid than hand instrumentation.[2,30,55] Experienced operators have been shown to instrument root surfaces more thoroughly,[6,13,16,28] so a systematic approach in learning the use of power-driven instruments is necessary to achieve the best clinical results. The application and implementation of sonic and ultrasonic instruments is different from that required for hand instrumentation. Plaque and calculus removal with hand instruments is achieved by carrying out a series of overlapping vertical strokes around the circumference of the tooth. Because the contact surface between a rounded power-driven scaler tip and the spherical root surface is rather small, thorough mechanical debridement can only be attained by a series of overlapping horizontal serpentine-like strokes in a coronal-apical direction (Fig 43-10). Using the appropriate working parameters and instrument settings, roots should be instrumented with the scaler tip in constant motion until the surface feels smooth and clean. The use of an explorer helps detect residual calculus and prevents inadvertent root overinstrumentation. To allow sufficient access to all tooth surfaces within the whole dentition, most sonic and ultrasonic scaler systems operate with two different working tips showing a left and right offset angulation (Fig. 43-10). For the use of these slim instruments it is of utmost importance that they be inserted into the pocket in a manner in which the convex working surface of the tip is in contact to the root (Fig. 43-11).[45] Using the concave side as a working surface bears the risk that the instrument tip will be applied perpendicular to the root surface leading to unnecessary gauging and root surface damage. The left bent tip is used for the instrumentation of the maxillary right posterior facial aspect, the maxillary front teeth palatal aspect and the maxillary left palatal aspect (Fig. 43-12). In addition, the contralateral approximal tooth surfaces may be cleaned with the same left offset tip inserted in an almost oblique/horizontal position (see Fig. 43-11). The right offset tip is used to instrument the remaining areas to be treated (see Fig. 43-12). For instrumentation in the mandible the left offset tip should be used for the right lingual molar area, the lower buccal frontal segment, and the lower left buccal posterior area. As in the maxilla, the right bent tip is used for the instrumentation of the corresponding sites remaining to be treated (see Fig. 43-11).

By using this systematic approach, a complete and efficient instrumentation of the entire dentition is attainable and both patient and operator will benefit from the use of sonic and ultrasonic scalers.

REFERENCES

1. Allen E, Rhoads R: Effects of high-speed periodontal instruments on tooth surfaces. J Periodontol 1963; 34:352.
2. Badersten A, Nilvéus R, Egelberg J: Effect of nonsurgical periodontal therapy. I. J Clin Periodontol 1981; 8:57.
3. Baehni P, Thilo B, Chapuis B, et al: Effects of ultrasonic and sonic scalers on dental plaque microflora *in vitro* and *in vivo*. J Clin Periodontol 1992; 19:455.
4. Barnes JB, Harrel SK, Rivera-Hidalgo F: Blood contamination of the aerosols produced by in vivo use of ultrasonic scalers. J Periodontol 1998; 69:434.
5. Bower RC: Furcation morphology relative to periodontal treatment. Furcation entrance architecture. J Periodontol 1979; 50:23.

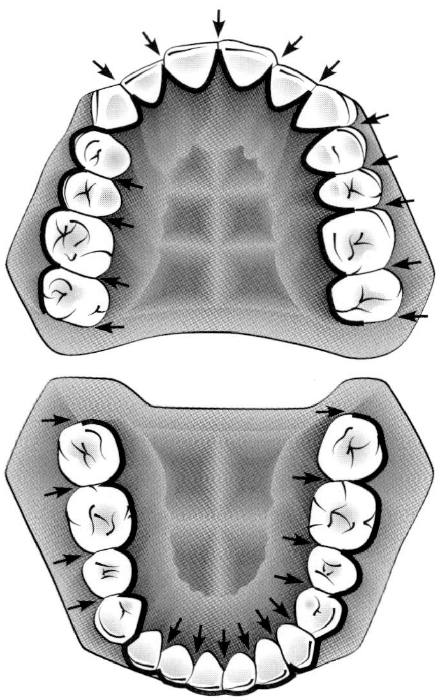
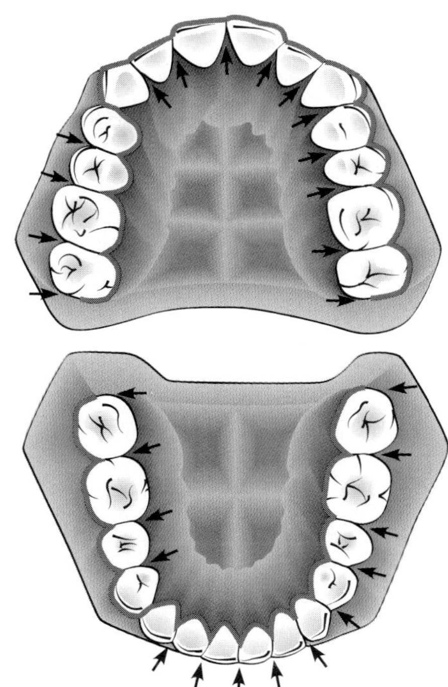

Fig. 43-12 Areas of the dentition to be débrided with area indicated by red line *(left)* or the area indicated by green line *(right)* offset angulated tips. The approximal areas indicated by arrows might be treated with the scaler tip inserted horizontally, but parallel to the root surface. (Modified from Petersilka GJ, Flemmig TF: Subgingival root surface treatment using sonic and ultrasonic scalers. Parodontologie 1999; 3:233.)

6. Brayer WK, Mellonig JT, Duinlap RM, et al: Scaling and root planing effectiveness: The effect of root surface access and operator experience. J Periodontol 1989; 60:67.
7. Chapple ILC, Walmsley AD, Saxby MS, et al: Effect of subgingival irrigation with chlorhexidine during ultrasonic scaling. J Periodontol 1992; 63:812.
8. Chapple ILC, Walmsley AD, Saxby MS, et al: Effect of instrument power setting during ultrasonic scaling upon treatment outcome. J Periodontol 1995; 66:56.
9. Cheetham WA, Wilson M, Kieser JB: Root surface debridement: An *in vitro* assessment. J Clin Periodontol 1988; 15:288.
10. Clifford LR, Needleman IG, Chan YK: Comparison of periodontal pocket penetration by conventional and microultrasonic inserts. J Clin Periodontol 1996; 26:124.
11. Coldiron NB, Yukna RA, Weir J, et al: A quantitative study of cementum removal with hand curettes. J Periodontol 1990; 61:293–299.
12. Dragoo M: A clinical evaluation of hand and ultrasonic instruments on subgingival debridement. I. With unmodified and modified ultrasonic inserts. Int J Perio Res Dent 1992; 12:311.
13. Eaton KA, Kieser JB, Davies RM: The removal of root substance deposits. J Clin Periodontol 1985; 12:141.
14. Ewen S, Scopp I, Witkin R, et al: A comparative study of ultrasonic generators and hand instruments. J Periodontol 1976; 47:82.
15. Fine DH, Mendieta C, Barnett ML, et al: Efficacy of preprocedural rinsing with an antiseptic in reducing viable bacteria in dental aerosols. J Periodontol 1992; 63:821.
16. Fleischer HC, Mellonig JT, Brayer WK, et al: Scaling and root planing efficacy in multirooted teeth. J Periodontol 1989; 60:402.
17. Flemmig T, Petersilka G, Mehl A, et al: Working parameters of a sonic scaler influencing root substance removal *in vitro*. Clin Oral Invest 1997; 1:55.
18. Flemmig T, Petersilka G, Mehl A, et al: The effect of working parameters on root substance removal using a piezoelectric ultrasonic scaler *in vitro*. J Clin Periodontol 1998; 25:158.
19. Flemmig T, Petersilka G, Mehl A, et al: Working parameters of a magnetostrictive ultrasonic scaler influencing root substance removal in vitro. J Periodontol 1998; 69:547.
20. Gankerseer EJ, Walmsley AD: Preliminary investigation into the performance of a sonic scaler. J Periodontol 1987; 8:780.
21. Gross KB, Overman PR, Cobb C, et al: Aerosol generation by two ultrasonic scalers and one sonic scaler. A comparative study. J Dent Hyg 1992; 66:314.
22. Harrel SK, Barnes JB, Rivera-Hidalgo F: Reduction of aerosols produced by ultrasonic scalers. J Periodontol 1996; 67:28.
23. Jones S, Lozdan J, Boyde A: Tooth surfaces treated *in situ* with periodontal instruments. Scanning electron microscopic studies. Br Dent J 1972; 132:57.
24. Jotikashtira N, Lie T, Leknes K: Comparative *in vitro* studies of sonic, ultrasonic and reciprocating scaling instruments. J Clin Periodontol 1992; 19:560.
25. Kawanami M, Sugaya T, Kato S, et al: Efficacy of an ultrasonic scaler with a periodontal probe-type tip in deep periodontal pockets. Adv Dent Res 1988; 2:405.
26. Kerry G: Roughness of root surfaces after use of ultrasonic instruments and hand curettes. J Periodontol 1967; 38:340.
27. Khambay BS, Walmsley AD: Acoustic microstreaming: Detection and measurement around ultrasonic scalers. J Periodontol 1999; 70:626.
28. Kocher T, Rühling A, Momsen H, et al: Effectiveness of subgingival instrumentation with power-driven instruments in the hands of experienced an inexperienced operators. A study on manikins. J Clin Periodontol 1997; 24:498.

29. Kocher T, Plagmann HC: The diamond-coated sonic scaler tip. I. Oscillation pattern of different sonic scalers. Int J Periodont Rest Dent 1997; 17:393.
30. Laurell L, Petterson B: Periodontal healing after treatment with the Titan-S sonic scaler or hand instruments. Swed Dent J 1988; 12:187.
31. Leon LE, Vogel RI: A comparison of the effectiveness of hand scaling and ultrasonic debridement in furcations as evaluated by differential dark-field microscopy. J Periodontol 1987; 58:86.
32. Lie T, Meyer K: Calculus removal and loss of tooth substance in response to different periodontal instruments: A scanning electron microscope study. J Clin Periodontol 1977; 4:340.
33. Loos B, Kiger R, Egelberg J: An evaluation of basic periodontal therapy using sonic and ultrasonic scalers. J Clin Periodontol 1987; 14:25.
34. Menne A, Griesinger H, Jepsen S, et al: Vibration characteristics of oscillating scalers. J Dent Res 1994; 73:434.
35. Moore J, Wilson M, Kieser JB: The distribution of bacterial lipopolysaccharide (endotoxin) in relation to periodontally involved root surfaces. J Clin Periodontol 1986; 13:748.
36. Moskow B, Bressmann E: Cemental response to ultrasonic and hand instrumentation. J Am Dent Ass 1964; 68:698.
37. Nicoll BK, Peters RJ: Heat generation during ultrasonic instrumentation of dentin as affected by different irrigation methods. J Periodontol 1998; 69:884.
38. Nosal G, Scheidt M, O'Neal R, et al: The penetration of lavage solution into the periodontal pocket during ultrasonic instrumentation. J Periodontol 1991; 62:554.
39. Oberholzer R, Rateitschak K: Root cleaning or root smoothing. An *in vivo* study. J Clin Periodontol 1996; 23:326.
40. Oda S, Ishikawa I: *In vitro* effectiveness of a newly designed ultrasonic scaler tip for furcation areas. J Periodontol 1989; 60:634.
41. Pameijer C, Stallard R, Hiep N: Surface characteristics of teeth following periodontal instrumentation: A scanning electron microscope study. J Periodontol 1972; 43:628.
42. Parashis AO, Anagnou-Vareltzides A, Demetriou N: Calculus removal from multirooted teeth with and without surgical access. I. Efficacy on external and furcation surfaces in relation to probing depth. J Clin Periodontol 1993; 20:294.
43. Parashis AO, Anagnou-Vareltzides A, Demetriou N: Calculus removal from multirooted teeth with and without surgical access. II. Comparison between external and furcation surfaces and effect of furcation entrance width. J Clin Periodontol 1993; 20:294.
44. Petersilka GJ, Flemmig TF, Mehl A, et al: Comparison of root substance removal by magnetostrictive and piezoelectric ultrasonic and sonic scalers *in vitro*. J Clin Periodontol 1997; 24(abstr 70):864.
45. Petersilka GJ, Flemmig TF: Subgingival root surface treatment using sonic- and ultrasonic scalers. Parodontologie 1999; 3:233.
46. Reynolds MA, Lavigne CK, Minah GE, et al: Clinical effects of simultaneous ultrasonic scaling and subgingival irrigation with chlorhexidine. Mediating influence of periodontal probing depth. J Clin Periodontol 1992; 19:595.
47. Rivera-Hidalgo F, Barnes JB, Harrel SK: Aerosol and splatter production by focused spray and standard ultrasonic inserts. J Periodontol 1999; 70:473.
48. Rosenberg R, Ash M: The effect of root roughness on plaque accumulation and gingival inflammation. J Periodontol 1974; 45:146.
49. Rosling BG, Slots J, Christersson LA, et al: Topical antimicrobial therapy and diagnosis of subgingival bacteria in the management of periodontal disease. J Clin Periodontol 1986, 13:975.
50. Schenk G, Flemmig TF, Lob S, et al: Lack of antimicrobial effect on periodontopathogenic bacteria by ultrasonic and sonic scalers *in vitro*. J Clin Periodontol 1999; 27(2):116.
51. Shiloah J, Patters MR: DNA probe analysis of selected periodontal pathogens following scaling, root planing, and intrapocket irrigation. J Periodontol 1994; 65:568.
52. Smart GJ, Wilson M, Davies EH, et al: The assessment of ultrasonic root surface debridement by determination of residual endotoxin levels. J Clin Periodontol 1990; 17:174.
53. Taggart JA, Palmer RM, Wilson RF: A clinical and microbiological comparison of the effects of water and 0.02% chlorhexidine as coolants during ultrasonic scaling and root planing. J Clin Periodontol 1999; 17:32.
54. Torfason T, Kiger R, Selvig A, et al: Clinical improvement of gingival conditions following ultrasonic versus hand instrumentation of periodontal pockets. J Clin Periodontol 1979; 6:165.
55. Van Volkinburg J, Green E, Armitage G: The nature of root surfaces after curette, Cavitron and alpha-sonic instrumentation. J Periodont Res 1976; 11:374.
56. Waerhaugh J: Effect of rough surfaces upon gingival tissues. Int Dent J 1956; 45:322.
57. Waerhaugh J: The furcation problem. Etiology, pathogenesis, diagnosis, therapy and prognosis. J Clin Periodontol 1980; 7:73.
58. Walmsley AD, Laird WRE, Williams AR: A model system to demonstrate the role of cavitational activity in ultrasonic scaling. J Dent Res 1984; 63:1162.
59. Walmsley AD, Laird WRE, Williams AR: Dental plaque removal by cavitational activity during ultrasonic scaling. J Clin Periodontol 1988; 15:539.
60. Walmsley AD, Walsh TF, Laird WRE, et al: Effects of cavitational activity on the root surface of the teeth during ultrasonic scaling. J Clin Periodontol 1990; 17:306–312.
61. Zappa U, Smith B, Simona C, et al: Root substance removal by scaling and root planing. J Periodontol 1991; 62:750–754.
62. Zinner DD: Recent ultrasonic dental studies, including periodontia, without the use of an abrasive. JADA 1955; 59:636–639.

Supragingival and Subgingival Irrigation

Thomas F. Flemmig

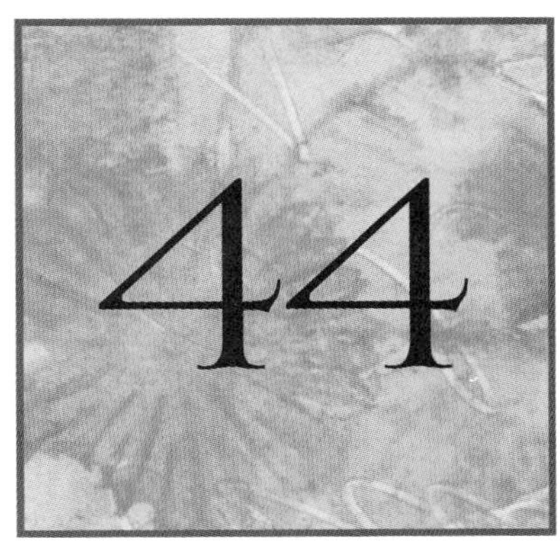

CHAPTER

Chapter Outline

In the treatment of periodontal diseases, irrigation is used as a lavage to flush away the bacteria that are in contact with the periodontal tissues. Irrigation is a nonspecific reduction of plaque bacteria. The two types of irrigation are supragingival and subgingival irrigation. They vary by the depth to which the irrigant is projected into the gingival or periodontal pocket. In supragingival irrigation, the irrigant penetrates 29% to 71% of shallow pockets, and 44% to 68% of moderately deep and deep pockets[9,21] compared with 75% to 93% of the periodontal pocket that is penetrated by subgingival irrigation.[9,12,30] Mouth rinses penetrate only 4% of the pocket depth and are therefore largely restricted to the supragingival area[55] (Fig. 44-1).

IRRIGATOR DEVICES

A number of irrigators offered today vary by irrigation pressure, water stream characteristics, and jet type design. A syringe can also be used for delivering a solution to irrigate the pocket (Fig. 44-2). Monojet or multistreamed jet tips are available for supragingival irrigation, as well as blunted cannulae with end or side parts for subgingival irrigation. In most units the irrigation pressure is produced by an electrical pump and is delivered in a continuous or pulsating stream. The alternating compression and decompression phases in pulsating irrigators may facilitate the displacement of plaque bacteria.[7] A continuous flow of water during irrigation causes constant tissue compression and may impair removal of bacteria. The majority of information available on the therapeutic effects of supragingival irrigation are based on studies using pulsating monojet irrigators, and multistreamed irrigators have been insufficiently examined to date. For this reason, pulsating monojet irrigators are preferred for supragingival irrigation.

SUPRAGINGIVAL IRRIGATION

Supragingival irrigation is usually performed once or twice daily by the patient as an adjunct to toothbrushing and flossing. The irrigator's nozzle should be positioned at some distance from the gingival margin and the jet stream lined perpendicular to the long axis of the teeth to achieve optimal subgingival penetration of an irrigant[21] (Fig. 44-3). Irrigation pressures of 540 kPa to 620 kPa (80 psi to 90 psi) can be tolerated without adverse effects.[8,9] No histologic alteration of the gingiva has been observed after supragingival irrigation at a pressure of 410 kPa (60 psi).[6]

Supragingival Irrigation as a Monotherapy

Supragingival irrigation with water alone does not sufficiently prevent plaque accumulation nor gingivitis. In this respect, supragingival irrigation is clearly inferior to mechanical plaque control such as using conventional oral hygiene measures.[33] Thus supragingival irrigation

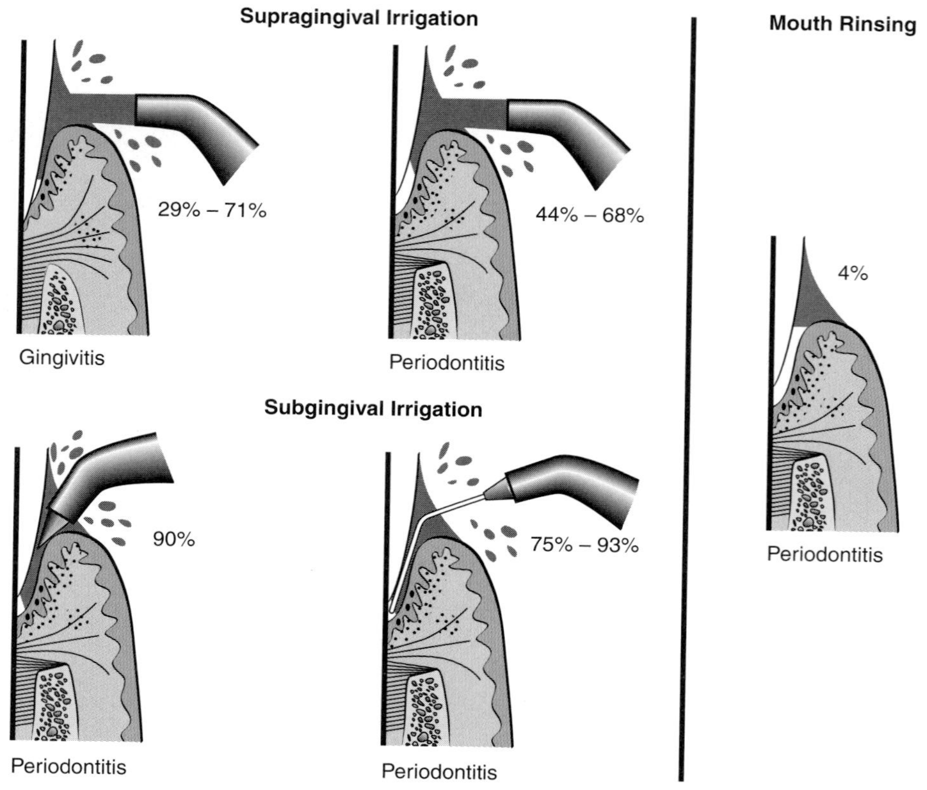

Fig. 44-1 Subgingival penetration of solutions delivered by supragingival or subgingival irrigation and rinsing in percent of pocket depth.

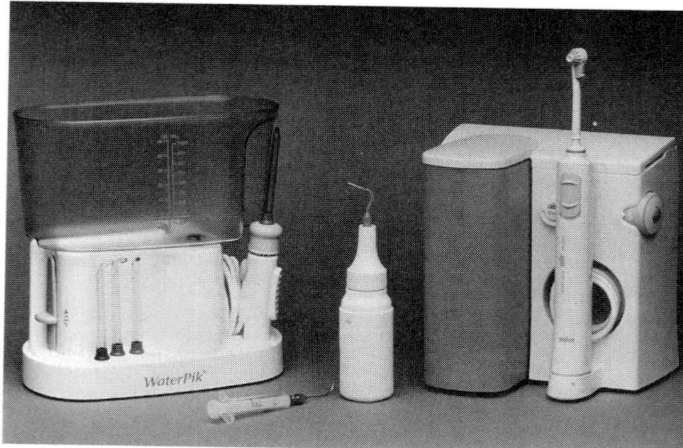

Fig. 44-2 Devices for supra- and subgingival irrigation.

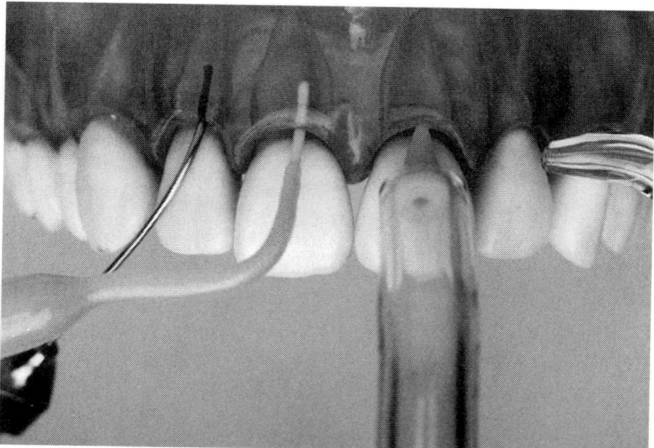

Fig. 44-3 Positioning of various irrigator tips for supragingival *(extreme right)* and subgingival irrigation *(others)*.

cannot replace toothbrushing and should only be used as an adjunct to toothbrushing and interdental cleaning.

Supragingival Water Irrigation and Toothbrushing

Although earlier studies concerning supragingival water irrigation as an adjunct to toothbrushing yielded controversial results,[18,22,32,33] recent studies have clearly demonstrated that this method in conjunction with toothbrushing can improve the periodontal health in patients with gingivitis and/or periodontitis, particularly for patients with clinical signs of gingival inflammation and/or poor oral hygiene[13,25,26,34,49] (Fig. 44-4). However, patients with low plaque scores (i.e., good oral hygiene) have no additional benefit from supragingival irrigation[26,33] (Fig. 44-5).

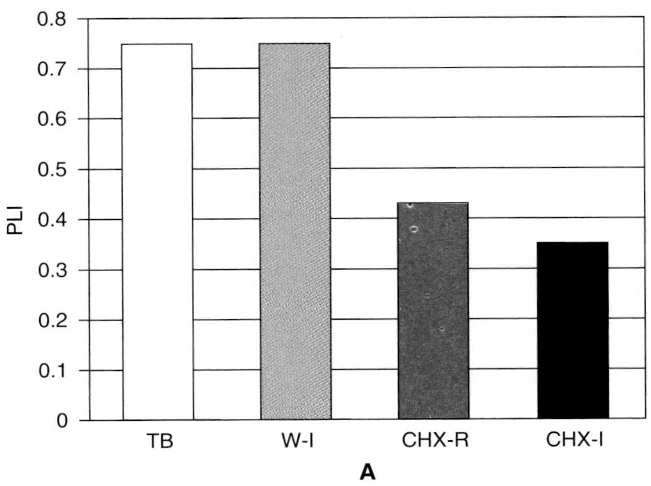

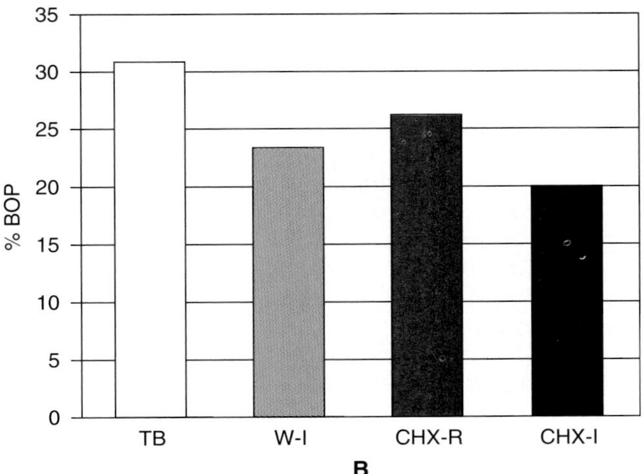

Fig. 44-4 Covariance adjusted mean plaque index scores (PLI) and percent of sites with bleeding on probing (BOP) in patients with naturally occurring gingivitis after 6 months of adjunctive irrigation. Supragingival irrigation was performed with 500 ml water (W-I) or 300 ml of water immediately followed by irrigation of 200 ml 0.06% chlorhexidine digluconate (CHX-I). Adjunctive rinsing with 15 ml of 0.12% chlorhexidine digluconate for 30 seconds twice daily (CHX-R) and toothbrushing alone (TB) were used as positive and negative controls, respectively. All groups performed regular tooth brushing.[25]

The therapeutic effects of supragingival irrigation with water on gingival inflammation is considerable and has been shown to be equivalent to twice daily mouth rinsing with 0.12% chlorhexidine digluconate solution in patients with gingivitis[25] (see Fig. 44-4). Daily supragingival irrigation with water after initial therapy may also improve gingival health among patients with periodontitis.[3] In patients receiving regular supportive periodontal therapy, daily supragingival irrigation with water can significantly reduce gingival inflammation and bleeding on probing.[26,49] Interestingly, supragingival irrigation with water has only limited effects on plaque scores—that is, supragingival plaque mass or the composition of the subgingival microflora.[17,20,25,26,48]

Earlier reports of direct bactericidal effects from irrigation resulting in the reduction of bacterial cell contents[11] have not been confirmed. Thus it may be possible that supragingival irrigation reduces gingival inflammation without altering the supra- and subgingival plaque. Although the responsible mechanism for the antiinflammatory effect is not clearly known, it can be assumed that through supragingival irrigation, there is a dilution or a removal of bacterial toxins, an interference with plaque maturation, or a possibility that the unattached plaque may be washed away. One may also speculate that the additional bacteremia caused by supragingival irrigation[23,57] may stimulate the production of specific antibodies directed against periodontal pathogens.[62] Such antibodies have been shown to be protective and reduce periodontal disease progression.[5,29]

Antimicrobial Agents and Toothbrushing

Enhanced penetration of antimicrobials into the periodontal pocket delivered by supragingival irrigation has been speculated to better control the subgingival microflora compared to mouth rinsing.[9,21,55] The minimal effective dosage for once daily supragingival irrigation with chlorhexidine digluconate has been established to be 400 ml of a 0.02% solution.[39]

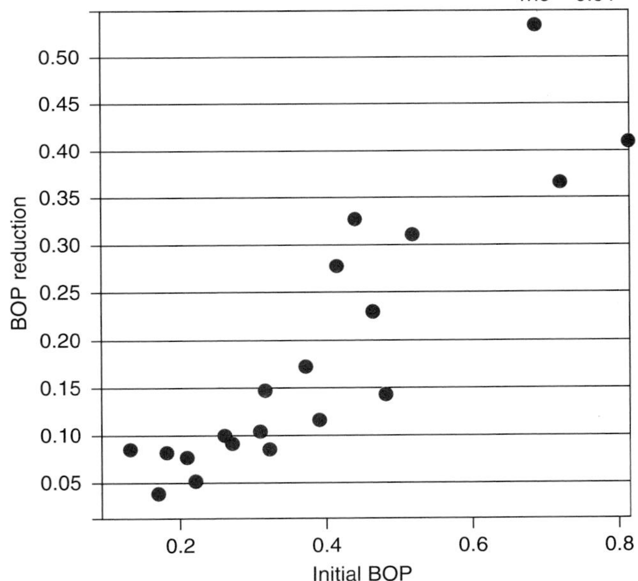

Fig. 44-5 Correlation between the reduction of bleeding on probing by adjunctive supragingival irrigation with water and initial bleeding on probing score.

In patients with gingivitis using antimicrobials with supragingival irrigation (e.g., 200 ml of 0.06% chlorhexidine digluconate), there is a greater reduction of gingival inflammation compared to irrigation with only water[13,25] or mouth rinsing with antimicrobials.[25,38,54] The superior antiinflammatory effects of supragingival irrigation with 0.06% chlorhexidine digluconate is also accompanied by a reduction of supragingival plaque and black-pigmented bacteria, as well as other gram negative anaerobic rods in the subgingival plaque.[48] However, not all antimicrobial agents are beneficial as an irrigant. The use of 0.00225% sanguinaria solution or a solution of thymol, menthol, eucalyptus, and methylsalicilate as an irrigant did not improve the therapeutic effects of the supragingival irrigation when compared with water or a placebo irrigant.[16,54]

Gingival health was significantly improved in patients with periodontitis after scaling and supragingival irrigation with 0.2% chlorhexidine digluconate or 0.02% stannous fluoride compared to only supragingival irrigation with water.[8,70] Lower concentrations of chlorhexidine digluconate (0.02%) or metronidazole (0.05%) solution used over 4 weeks after initial therapy in patients with periodontitis demonstrated no differences in reducing gingival inflammation compared with supragingival irrigation with water.[3]

The relatively high daily dosage of chlorhexidine digluconate needed for supragingival irrigation is also financially more costly compared with mouth rinsing.[2,28,44] Thus the incremental benefit of using an antimicrobial agent versus water for supragingival irrigation and delivering an antimicrobial agent by supragingival irrigation compared with application by mouth rinsing should be weighed against the long-term costs.

It is noteworthy that there is a significant elevation of calculus formation, tooth and tongue staining, and taste impairment that occurs from the long-term use of chlorhexidine digluconate[25,40] (Fig. 44-6). In addition, few patients tolerate the esthetically compromising brown teeth stains that may appear over time with prolonged use. Although chlorhexidine digluconate may be safely applied long term,[44] its side effects have usually limited its use to short periods.

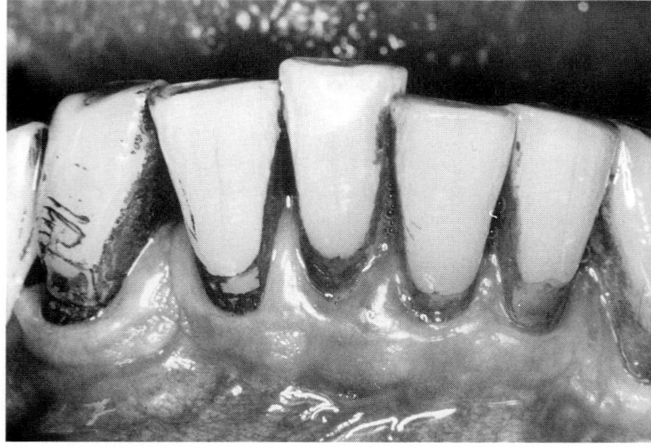

Fig. 44-6 Extrinsic tooth staining after long-term application of chlorhexidine digluconate.

SUBGINGIVAL IRRIGATION

Numerous studies have assessed the potential benefit of subgingival irrigation using various irrigants in the treatment of periodontitis; however, its benefit remains questionable due to controversial results.[27,59] To penetrate the periodontal pocket near its base by 75% to 93%,[9,12,30] rubber tip nozzles are positioned at the gingival margin[12] or blunted cannulas with an end or side port are inserted into the periodontal pocket[30] (see Fig. 44-3). Ejection site pressures at the opening of various tip designs have been demonstrated to range from 0.7 kPa to 35 kPa (0.1 psi to 5 psi) and were lowest in side port systems.[9,41] Care should be taken not to block the opening of the canula to prevent excessive pressure buildup. Irrigating devices similar to those employed for supragingival irrigation or syringes have been used for the delivery of solutions. Similar subgingival penetration can be achieved using the side or end port cannulas.[41]

Several factors limit the irrigant from reaching the base of the pocket. The lateral dispersion of the subgingivally irrigated solution [51] and the presence of calculus deposits impair the subgingival penetration into deep pockets of 7 to 10 mm.[41] To bring the irrigant into contact with all root surfaces, scaling and root planing should precede subgingival irrigation, and irrigation should be performed circumferentially. Practical considerations, as well as patient dexterity and compliance, dictate that the use of cannulas be limited to professionals, whereas rubber tip irrigators can be applied by the patient. However, it has been reported that some instructed patients may be able to successfully use a blunted canula for subgingival irrigation.[1,74] Patient-applied subgingival irrigation can be performed on a daily basis, whereas professionally performed irrigation requires the patient to visit the dentist and is therefore limited to several applications per year.

Subgingival Irrigation as a Monotherapy for Periodontitis

Several studies have demonstrated that subgingival irrigation with antimicrobial agents (e.g., 0.2% chlorhexidine digluconate solution, 1% chlorhexidine digluconate gel, 0.4% or 1.6% stannous fluoride, 0.5% tetracycline HCl, 7% tetrapotassium peroxydiphosphate, 3% hydrogen peroxide, or 0.5% metronidazole) resulted in a transient reduction of spirochetes, motile bacteria, and/or black-pigmented anaerobic rods in subgingival plaque. However, a rebound to pretreatment levels occurred within 1 to 8 weeks.[31,37,42,43,47,58,60,72,73] Clinically, supragingival plaque scores were reduced and periodontal health was somewhat improved after subgingival irrigation.[10,24,31,37,42,43,47,58,60,63,71,73] However, no difference was found between an antimicrobial agent or saline as the subgingival irrigant.[31,35,37,43,71,73] When compared with scaling and root planing, subgingival irrigation as a monotherapy had only limited effects on the subgingival microflora with low clinical benefits.[42,43,58,71,73] Therefore applying subgingival irrigation with water or antimicrobial agents as the sole therapeutic method is insufficient to treat periodontitis and should not be performed in lieu of scaling and root planing.

Antimicrobial Agents and Scaling and Root Planing

It is well documented that mechanical debridement of deep pockets is often incomplete with residual subgingival plaque and/or calculus remaining in the pocket.[14,56,66] The rationale for subgingival irrigation with an antimicrobial agent after scaling and root planing is based on the assumption that bacteria left behind during mechanical debridement could be killed by the so-applied antimicrobial solution. However, several factors impede the efficacy of antimicrobial agents delivered into the periodontal pocket.

Due to the outwardly directed gingival crevicular fluid flow, antimicrobial agents irrigated subgingivally may not be in contact with the subgingival microflora long enough to be effective. The half-life time of subgingivally injected agents has been shown to be approximately 13 minutes.[53] After subgingival irrigation for 5 minutes with 0.12% chlorhexidine, no chlorhexidine at antimicrobially effective levels remained in the periodontal pocket.[64]

Chlorhexidine digluconate inhibits the majority of subgingival bacteria in vitro at concentrations attainable in vivo[4,68] and may be inactivated when in contact with blood components in the periodontal pocket.[52] A 0.5% chlorhexidine digluconate solution required a longer contact time to eliminate periodontal pathogens in the presence of serum.[52] Considering the biofilm structure of subgingival plaque[61] and its effect on the activity of antimicrobial agents, it becomes rather unlikely that subgingivally irrigated solutions have a profound effect on the subgingival microflora. For example, when *Streptococcus sanguis* was exposed to 0.2% chlorhexidine digluconate or 0.05% cetylpyridinium chloride, no viable bacteria were detected after 5 minutes of exposure of planktonic cells. However, the same bacterium was shown to survive in biofilms even after exposure to chlorhexidine digluconate or cetylpyridinium chloride for 4 hours.[75] Also, 50 to 5000 times higher concentrations of antimicrobials are needed to kill bacteria that are embeded in a biofilm compared with planktonic bacteria.[36,50] These considerations may explain why subgingival irrigation with 0.12% chlorhexidine digluconate is of limited benefit as an adjunct to scaling and root planing.[10,46,65,71,72]

Only subgingival irrigation with 50 mg/ml to 100 mg/ml tetracycline HCl for 5 minutes per tooth after scaling and root planing results in an effective release of tetracycline HCl from root surfaces at antimicrobial concentrations over 4 to 7 days due to the binding of tetracycline to the root surface.[15,64] Some improvements in clinical attachment gain over scaling and root planing alone have also been reported.

The preponderance of information available to date, however, gives little evidence that suggests that adjunctive subgingival irrigation has a substantial long-term benefit beyond its use in scaling and root planing.

SAFETY OF IRRIGATION

Supragingival irrigation appears to be a safe method of treatment. Daily supragingival irrigation with water has shown no clinically significant adverse effects over longer observation periods.[25,26,49] In addition, no micromorphologic changes of periodontal tissues after supragingival irrigation have been found.[6] There has only been one recent report on extensive tissue necrosis and permanent loss of alveolar bone after subgingival irrigation with 2% stannous fluoride.[62]

It is important to know that the use of irrigators like toothbrushing and subgingival scaling[23,57] can cause transient bacteremia. Although the incidence of transient bacteremia after toothbrushing or subgingival scaling is not significantly increased by supragingival irrigation[67,69] or subgingival irrigation,[45] it may be prudent not to recommend irrigation for patients requiring premedication for bacterial endocarditis.[19]

REFERENCES

1. Asari AM, Newman HN, Wilson M, et al: 0.1%/0.2% commercial chlorhexidine solution as subgingival irrigants in chronic periodontitis. J Clin Periodontol 1996; 23:320.
2. Axelsson P, Lindhe J: Efficacy of mouthrinses in inhibiting dental plaque and gingivitis. J Clin Periodontol 1987; 14:205.
3. Aziz-Gandour IA, Newman HN: The effects of a simplified oral hygiene regime plus supragingival irrigation with chlorhexidine or metronidazole on chronic inflammatory periodontal disease. J Clin Periodontol 1986; 13:228.
4. Baker PJ, Coburn RA, Genco RJ, et al: Structural determinants of activity of chlorhexidine and alkyl bisbiguanides against the human oral flora. J Dent Res 1987; 66:1099.
5. Beikler T, Karch H, Ehmke B, et al: Protective effect of serum antibodies against a 110-kilodalton protein of Actinobacillus actinomycetemcomitans following periodontal therapy. Oral Microbiol Immunol 1999; 14:281.
6. Bhaskar SN, Cutright DE, Frisch J: Effect of high pressure water jet on oral mucosa of varied density. J Periodontol 1969; 40:593.
7. Bhaskar SN, Cutright DE, Gross A, et al: Water jet devices in dental practice. J Periodontol 1971; 42:658.
8. Boyd RL, Leggott P, Quinn R, et al: Effect of self-administered daily irrigation with 0.02% SnF_2 on periodontal disease activity. J Clin Periodontol 1985; 12:420.
9. Boyd RL, Hollander BN, Eakle WS: Comparison of a subgingivally placed cannula oral irrigator tip with a supragingivally placed standard irrigator tip. J Clin Periodontol 1992; 19:340.
10. Braatz L, Garrett S, Claffey N, et al: Antimicrobial irrigation of deep pockets to supplement non-surgical periodontal therapy. II. Daily irrigation. J Clin Periodontol 1985; 12:630.
11. Brady JM, Gray WA, Bhaskar SN: Electron microscopic study of the effect of water jet lavage devices on dental plaque. J Dent Res 1973; 52:1310.
12. Braun RE, Ciancio SG: Subgingival delivery by an oral irrigation device. J Periodontol 1992; 63:469.
13. Brownstein CN, Briggs SD, Schweitzer KL, et al: Irrigation with chlorhexidine to resolve naturally occurring gingivitis. A methodologic study. J Clin Periodontol 1990; 17:588.
14. Caffessee RG, Sweeny PL, Smith BA: Scaling and root planing with and without periodontal flap surgery. J Clin Periodontol 1986; 13:205.
15. Christersson LA, Norderyd OM, Puchalsky CS: Topical application of tetracycline-HCl in human periodontitis. J Clin Periodontol 1993; 20:88.
16. Ciancio SG, Mather ML, Zambon JJ, et al: Effect of chemotherapeutic agent delivered by an oral irrigation device on plaque, gingivitis, and subgingival microflora. J Periodontol 1989; 60:310.

17. Cobb CM, Rodgers RL, Killoy WJ: Ultrastructural examination of human periodontal pockets following the use of an oral irrigation device in vivo. J Periodontol 1988; 59:155.
18. Covin NR, Lainson PA, Belding JH, et al: The effects of stimulating the gingiva by a pulsating water device. J Periodontol 1973; 44:286.
19. Dajani AS, Taubert KA, Wilson W: Prevention of bacterial endocarditis. Recommendations by the American Heart Association. JAMA 1997; 277:1794.
20. Drisko GL, White CL, Killoy WJ, et al: Comparison of darkfield microscopy and a flagella stain for monitoring the effect of a Water Pik on bacterial motility. J Periodontol 1987; 58:381.
21. Eakle WS, Ford C, Boyd RL: Depth of penetration in periodontal pockets with oral irrigation. J Clin Periodontol 1986; 13:39.
22. Emslie RD: The value of oral hygiene. Br Dent J 1964; 117:373.
23. Felix J, Rosen S, App G: Detection of bacteremia after use of an oral irrigation device in subjects with periodontitis. J Periodontol 1971; 42:785.
24. Fine JB, Harper DS, Gordon JM, et al: Short-term microbiological and clinical effects of subgingival irrigation with an antimicrobial mouthrinse. J Periodontol 1994; 65:30.
25. Flemmig TF, Newman MG, Doherty FM, et al: Supragingival irrigation with 0.06% chlorhexidine in naturally occurring gingivitis. I. 6-month clinical observations. J Periodontol 1990; 61:112.
26. Flemmig TF, Epp B, Funkenhauser Z, et al: Adjunctive supragingival irrigation with acetylsalicylic acid in periodontal supportive therapy. J Clin Periodontol 1995; 22:427.
27. Greenstein G: Subgingival irrigations ability to enhance periodontal status. J Periodontol 1987; 58:827.
28. Grossman E, Meckel AH, Isaacs R, et al: A clinical comparison of antibacterial mouthrinses: Effects of chlorhexidine, phenotics, and sanguinarine on dental plaque and gingivitis. J Periodontol 1989; 60:435.
29. Gunsolley JC, Burmeister JA, Tew JG, et al: Relationship of serum antibody to attachment level patterns in young adults with juvenile periodontitis or generalized severe periodontitis. J Periodontol 1987; 58:314.
30. Hardy JH, Newman HN, Strhan JD: Direct irrigation and subgingival plaque. J Clin Periodontol 1982; 9:57.
31. Haskel F, Faquenasi J, Yussim I: Effects of subgingival chlorhexidine irrigation in chronic moderate periodontitis. J Periodontol 1986; 57:305.
32. Hoover DR, Robinson HB: The comparative effectiveness of a pulsating oral irrigator as an adjunct in maintaining oral health. J Periodontol 1971; 42:37.
33. Hugoson A: The effect of the Water Pik device on the development of plaque and gingivitis. J Clin Periodontol 1978; 5:95.
34. Jolkovsky DL, Waki MY, Newman MG, et al: Clinical and microbiological effects of subgingival and gingival marginal irrigation with chlorhexidine gluconate. J Periodontol 1990; 61:663.
35. Kalaitzakis CJ, Tynelius-Bratthall G, Attstrom R: Clinical and microbiological effects of subgingival application of a chlorhexidine gel in chronic periodontitis. A pilot study. Swed Dent J 1993; 17:129.
36. Khoury AE, Lam K, Ellis B, et al: Prevention and control of bacterial infections associated with medical devices. Am Soc Artif Intern Organs 1992; 38:M174.
37. Lander PE, Newcomb GM, Seymour GJ, et al: The antimicrobial and clinical effects of a single subgingival irrigation of chlorhexidine in advanced periodontal lesions. J Clin Periodontol 1986; 13:74.
38. Lang NP, Raber K: Use of oral irrigators as vehicles for the application of antimicrobial agents in chemical plaque control. J Clin Periodontol 1981; 8:177.
39. Lang NP, Ramseier-Grossman K: Optimal dosage of chlorhexidine digluconate in chemical plaque control when applied by the oral irrigator. J Clin Periodontol 1981; 8:189.
40. Lang NP, Catalanotto FA, Knöpfli RU, et al: Quality-specific taste impairment following the application of chlorhexidine gluconate mouthrinse. J Clin Periodontol 1988; 15:43.
41. Larner JR, Greenstein G: Effect of calculus and irrigator tip design on depth of subgingival irrigation. Int J Periodontics Restorative Dent 1993; 13:288.
42. Lazzaro AJ, Bissada NF: Clinical and microbiologic changes following the irrigation of periodontal pockets with metronidazole or stannous fluoride. Periodont Case Rep 1989; 11:12.
43. Listgarten MA, Grossberg D, Schwimer C, et al: Effect of subgingival irrigation with tetrapotassium peroxydiphosphate on scaled and untreated periodontal pockets. J Periodontol 1989; 60:4.
44. Löe H, Schiött CR, Glavind L, et al: Two years oral use of chlorhexidine in man. I. General design and clinical effects. J Periodont Res 1976; 17:135.
45. Lofthus JE, Waki MY, Jolkovsky DL, et al: Bacteremia following subgingival irrigation and scaling and root planing. J Periodontol 1991; 62:602.
46. MacAlpine R, Magnusson I, Kiger R, et al: Antimicrobial irrigation of deep pockets to supplement oral hygiene instruction and root débridement. J Clin Periodontol 1985; 12:568.
47. Mazza JE, Newman MG, Sims TN: Clinical and antimicrobial effect of stannous fluoride on periodontitis. J Clin Periodontol 1981; 8:203.
48. Newman MG, Flemmig TF, Nachnani S, et al: Irrigation with 0.06% chlorhexidine in naturally occurring gingivitis. II. 6-month microbiological observations. J Periodontol 1990; 61:427.
49. Newman MG, Cattabriga M, Etienne D, et al: Effectiveness of adjunctive irrigation in early periodontitis: Multi-center evaluation. J Periodontol 1994; 65:224.
50. Nickel JC, Ruseka I, Wright JB, et al: Tobramycin resistance of *Pseudomonas aeruginosa* cells growing in a biofilm on urinary catheter material. Antimicrob Agents Chemother 1985; 27:619.
51. Nosal G, Scheidt MJ, O'Neal R, et al: The penetration of lavage solution into the periodontal pocket during ultrasonic instrumentation. J Periodontol 1991; 62:554.
52. Oosterwaal PJ, Mikx FH, van den Brink ME, et al: Bactericidal concentrations of chlorhexidine-digluconate, amine fluoride gel and stannous fluoride gel for subgingival bacteria tested in serum at short contact times. J Periodont Res 1989; 24:155.
53. Oosterwaal PJ, Mikx FH, Renggli HH: Clearance of a topically applied fluorescein gel from periodontal pockets. J Clin Periodontol 1990; 17:613.
54. Parsons LG, Thomas LG, Southard GL, et al: Effect of sanguinaria extract on established plaque and gingivitis when supragingivally delivered as a manual rinse or under pressure in an oral irrigator. J Clin Periodontol 1987; 14:381.
55. Pitcher GR, Newman HN, Strahen JD: Access to subgingival plaque by disclosing agents using mouthrinsing and direct irrigation. J Clin Periodontol 1980; 7:300.
56. Rabbani GM, Ash MM, Caffesse RG: The effectiveness of subgingival scaling and root planing in calculus removal. J Periodontol 1981; 52:119.
57. Rahn R, Shah PM, Schäfer V, et al: Endokarditis-risiko bei anwendung von mundduschen [Endocarditits risk following use of irrigators]. ZWR 1990; 99:266.

58. Schmid E, Kornman KS, Tinanoff N: Changes of subgingival total colony-forming units and black-pigmented *Bacteroides* after a single irrigation of periodontal pockets with 1.64% SnF2. J Periodontol 1985; 56:330.
59. Shiloah J, Hovious LA: The role of subgingival irrigations in the treatment of periodontitis. J Periodontol 1993; 64:835.
60. Silverstein L, Bissada N, Manouchehr-puor M, et al: Clinical and microbiological effects of local tetracycline irrigation of periodontitis. J Periodontol 1988; 59:301.
61. Singleton S, Treloar R, Warren P: Methods for microscopic characterization of oral biofilms: analysis of colonization, microstructure, and molecular transport phenomena. Adv Dent Res 1997; 11:133.
62. Sjostrom S, Kalfas S: Tissue necrosis after subgingival irrigation with fluoride solution. J Clin Periodontol 1999; 26:257.
63. Southard S, Drisko CL, Killoy WF: The effects of 2% chlorhexidine digluconate irrigation on the levels of Bacteroides gingivalis in periodontal pockets. J Periodontol 1989; 60:302.
64. Stabholz A, Kettering J, Aprecio R, et al: Retention of antimicrobial activity by human root surfaces after in situ subgingival irrigation with tetracycline HCl or chlorhexidine. J Periodontol 1993; 64:137.
65. Stabholz A, Nicholas AA, Zimmerman GJ, et al: Clinical and antimicrobial effects of a single episode of subgingival irrigation with tetracycline HCl or chlorhexidine in deep periodontal pockets. J Clin Periodontol 1998; 25:794.
66. Stambough RV, Dragoo M, Smith DM: The limits of subgingival scaling, Int J Perio & Rest Dent 1981; 1:31.
67. Tamimi H, Thomassen P, Moser Jr E: Bacteremia study using a water irrigation device. J Periodontol 1969; 40:424.
68. Wade WG, Addy W: In vitro activity of a chlorhexidine-containing mouthwash against subgingival bacteria. J Periodontol 1989; 60:521.
69. Waki MY, Jolkovsky DL, Lofthus JE, et al: Effects of subgingival irrigation on the incidence of bacteremia following scaling and root planing. J Periodontol 1990; 61:405.
70. Walsh TF, Glenwright HD, Hull PS: Clinical effects of pulsed oral irrigation with 0.2% chlorhexidine digluconate in patients with adult periodontitis. J Clin Periodontol 1992; 19:245.
71. Wennstrom JL, Heijl L, Dahlen G, et al: Periodic subgingival antimicrobial irrigation of periodontal pockets. I. Clinical observations. J Clin Periodontol 1987; 14:541.
72. Wennstrom JL, Dahlen G, Grondahl K, et al: Periodic subgingival antimicrobial irrigation of periodontal pockets. II. Microbiological and radiographical observations. J Clin Periodontol 1987; 14:573.
73. Westling M, Tynelius-Bratthall G: Microbiological and clinical short-term effects of repeated intracrevicular chlorhexidine rinsings. J Periodontal Res 1984: 19(2):202.
74. Wiedes SG, Newman HN, Strahan JD: Stannous fluoride and subgingival chlorhexidine irrigation in the control of plaque and chronic periodontitis. J Clin Periodontol 1983; 10:172.
75. Wilson M, Patel H, Fletcher J: Susceptibility of biofilms of Streptococcus sanguis to chlorhexidine gluconate and cetylpyridinium chloride. Oral Microbiol Immunol 1996; 11:188.

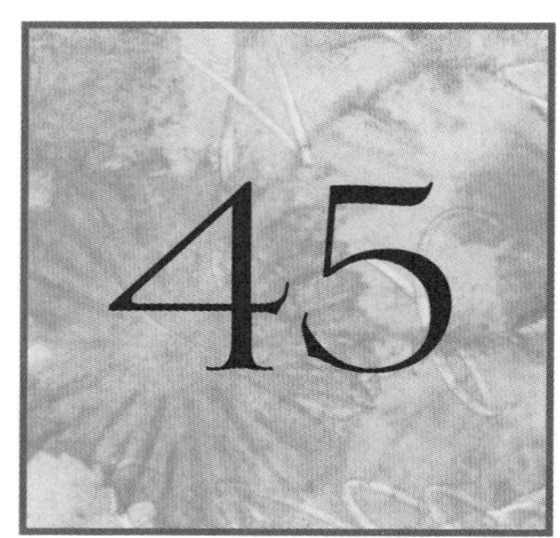

CHAPTER

Treatment of Acute Gingival Disease

Perry R. Klokkevold

Chapter Outline

The treatment of acute gingival disease entails the alleviation of the acute symptoms and elimination of all other periodontal disease, chronic and acute, throughout the oral cavity. Treatment is not complete as long as periodontal pathologic changes or factors capable of causing them are present.

TREATMENT OF ACUTE NECROTIZING ULCERATIVE GINGIVITIS

Necrotizing ulcerative gingivitis (NUG) can occur in a mouth essentially free of any other gingival involvement or be superimposed on underlying chronic gingival disease. Treatment should include the alleviation of the acute symptoms and the correction of the underlying chronic gingival disease. The former is the simplest part of the treatment, whereas the latter requires more comprehensive procedures.

The treatment of NUG consists of (1) alleviation of the acute inflammation plus treatment of chronic disease either underlying the acute involvement or elsewhere in the oral cavity, (2) alleviation of generalized toxic symptoms such as fever and malaise, and (3) correction of systemic conditions that contribute to the initiation or progress of the gingival changes. Chapter 51 provides further information on the management and treatment of NUG in patients with acquired immunodeficiency syndrome (AIDS).

Treatment

Treatment of NUG should follow an orderly sequence, as described in the following paragraphs.

First Visit. At the first visit, the clinician should obtain a general impression of the patient's background, including information regarding recent illness, living conditions, dietary background, type of employment, hours of rest, and mental stress. The patient's general appearance should be observed, as well as apparent nutritional status and responsiveness or lassitude, and his or her temperature should be taken. The submaxillary and submental areas should be palpated to detect enlarged lymph glands.

The oral cavity is examined for the characteristic lesion of NUG (see Chapters 19 and 27), its distribution, and the possible involvement of the oropharyngeal region. Oral hygiene is evaluated; the presence of pericoronal flaps, periodontal pockets, and local irritants is determined. A bacterial smear may be made from the material in the involved areas, but this is merely corroboratory and is not to be relied on for diagnosis.

The patient is questioned regarding the history of the acute disease and its onset and duration. Is it recurrent? Are the recurrences associated with specific factors such as menstruation, particular foods, exhaustion, or mental stress? Has there been any previous treatment? When and for how long? One should also inquire as to the type of treatment received and the patient's impression regarding its effect.

Treatment during this initial visit is confined to the acutely involved areas, which are isolated with cotton rolls and dried. A topical anesthesia is applied, and after 2 or 3 minutes the areas are gently swabbed with a cotton pellet to remove the pseudomembrane and nonattached surface debris. Each cotton pellet is used in a small area and is then discarded; sweeping motions over large areas with a single pellet are not recommended. After the area is cleansed with warm water, the superficial calculus is removed. Ultrasonic scalers are very useful for this purpose, since they do not elicit pain, and the water jet aids in the lavage of the area.

Subgingival scaling and curettage are contraindicated at this time because of the possibility of extending the infection to deeper tissues, and also of causing a bacteremia. *Unless an emergency exists, procedures such as extractions or periodontal surgery are postponed until the patient has been symptom free for a period of 4 weeks, to minimize the likelihood of exacerbating the acute symptoms.*

The patient is also told to rinse the mouth every 2 hours with a glassful of an equal mixture of warm water and 3% hydrogen peroxide. Twice-daily rinses with 0.12% chlorhexidine are also very effective.

Patients with moderate or severe NUG and local lymphadenopathy or other systemic symptoms are placed on an antibiotic regimen of penicillin, 500 mg orally every 6 hours. For penicillin-sensitive patients, other antibiotics, such as erythromycin (500 mg every 6 hours) are prescribed. Metronidazole (500 mg twice times daily for 7 days), is also effective. Antibiotics are continued until the systemic complications or the local lymphadenopathy have subsided.

Patients are told to report back to the clinician in 1 to 2 days. The patient should be advised of the extent of total treatment the condition requires and warned that treatment is not complete when pain stops. He or she should be informed of the presence of chronic gingival or periodontal disease, which must be eliminated to prevent recurrence of the acute symptoms.

INSTRUCTIONS TO THE PATIENT. The patient is discharged with the following instructions:

1. Avoid tobacco, alcohol, and condiments.
2. Rinse with a glassful of an equal mixture of 3% hydrogen peroxide and warm water every 2 hours and/or twice daily with 0.12 % chlorhexidine solution.
3. Pursue usual activities, but avoid excessive physical exertion or prolonged exposure to the sun as required in golf, tennis, swimming, or sunbathing.
4. Confine toothbrushing to the removal of surface debris with a bland dentifrice; overzealous brushing and the use of dental floss or interdental cleaners will be painful. Chlorhexidine mouth rinses are also very helpful in controlling plaque throughout the mouth.

Second Visit. At the second visit, 1 to 2 days later, the patient's condition is usually improved; the pain is diminished or no longer present. The gingival margins of the involved areas are erythematous, but without a superficial pseudomembrane.

Scaling is performed if sensitivity permits. Shrinkage of the gingiva may expose previously covered calculus, which is gently removed. The instructions to the patient are the same as those given previously.

Third Visit. At the next visit, 1 to 2 days after the second, the patient should be essentially symptom free. There may still be some erythema in the involved areas, and the gingiva may be slightly painful on tactile stimulation (Fig. 45-1). Scaling and root planing are repeated. The patient is instructed in plaque control procedures (see Chapter 49), which are essential for the success of the treatment and the maintenance of periodontal health. The hydrogen peroxide rinses are discontinued, but chlorhexidine rinses can be maintained for two or three weeks.

Subsequent Visits. In subsequent visits, the tooth surfaces in the involved areas are scaled and smoothed, and plaque control by the patient is checked and corrected if necessary.

Unfortunately, treatment is often stopped at this time because the acute condition has subsided, but this is when comprehensive treatment of the patient's chronic periodontal problem should start. Appointments are scheduled for the treatment of chronic gingivitis, periodontal pockets, and pericoronal flaps, as well as for the elimination of all forms of local irritation.

Patients without gingival disease other than the treated acute involvement are dismissed for 1 week. If the condition is satisfactory at that time, the patient is dismissed for 1 month, at which time the schedule for subsequent recall visits is determined according to the patient's needs.

Gingival Changes with Healing

The characteristic lesion of NUG undergoes the following changes in the course of healing in response to treatment:

1. Removal of the surface pseudomembrane exposes the underlying red, hemorrhagic, craterlike depressions in the gingiva.

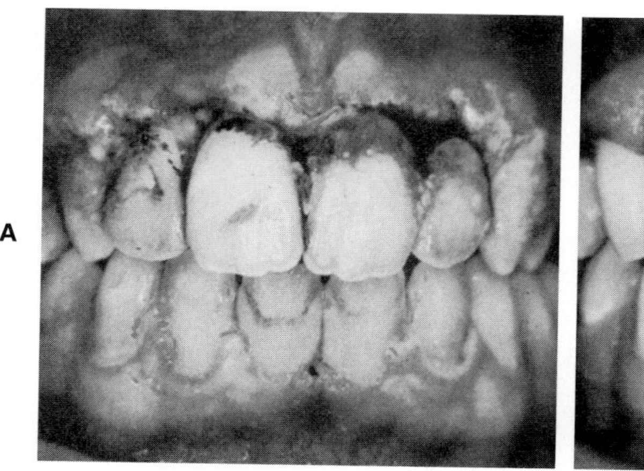

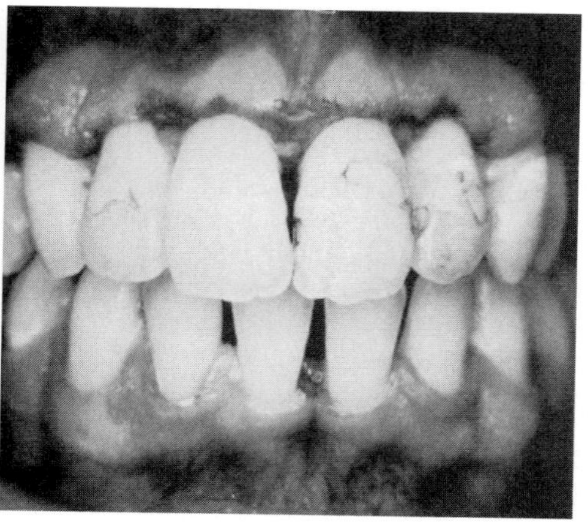

Fig. 45-1 Initial response to treatment of acute necrotizing ulcerative gingivitis (NUG). **A,** Severe acute necrotizing ulcerative gingivitis. **B,** Third day after treatment. There is still some erythema, but the condition is markedly improved.

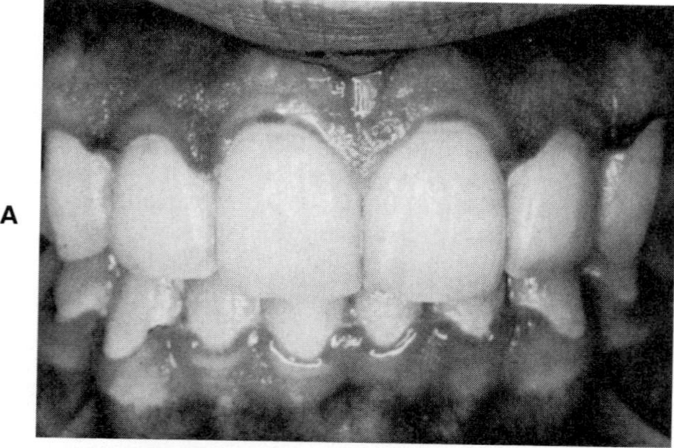

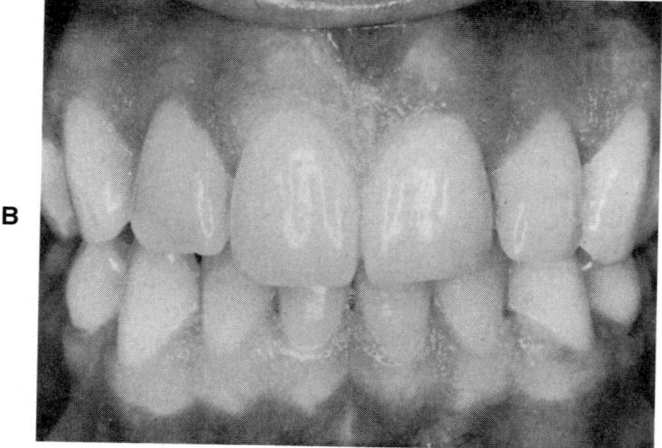

Fig. 45-2 Treatment of acute NUG. **A,** Before treatment. Note the characteristic interdental lesions. **B,** After treatment, showing restoration of healthy gingival contour.

2. In the next stage the bulk and redness of the crater margins are reduced, but the surface remains shiny (see Fig. 45-1).
3. This is followed by the early signs of restoration of normal gingival contour and color.
4. In the final stage the normal gingival color, consistency, surface texture, and contour are restored. Portions of the root exposed by the acute disease are covered by healthy gingiva (Figs. 45-2 and 45-3). When the menstrual period occurs in the course of treatment, there is a tendency toward exacerbation of the acute signs and symptoms, giving the appearance of a relapse. Patients should be informed of this possibility and spared unnecessary anxiety regarding their oral condition.

Additional Treatment Considerations

Contouring of the Gingiva as an Adjunctive Procedure. Even in cases of severe gingival necrosis, healing ordinarily leads to restoration of the normal gingival contour (Fig. 45-4). However, if the teeth are irregularly aligned, healing sometimes results in the formation of a shelflike gingival margin, which favors the retention of plaque and the recurrence of gingival inflammation. This can be corrected by reshaping the gingiva surgically or with electrosurgery (Fig. 45-5). Effective plaque control by the patient is particularly important to establish and maintain the normal gingival contour in areas of tooth irregularity.

Surgical Procedures. Tooth extraction or periodontal surgery should be postponed until 4 weeks after the acute signs and symptoms of NUG have subsided. If emergency surgery is required in the presence of acute symptoms, prophylactic chemotherapy with systemic penicillin or other antibiotics is indicated to prevent worsening or spreading of the acute disease.

Role of Drugs. A large variety of drugs have been used topically in the treatment of NUG.[2] Topical drug therapy is only an adjunctive measure; *no drug, when used alone, can be considered complete therapy.*

Escharotic drugs such as phenol, silver nitrate, and chromic acid should not be used. They are necrotizing agents that alleviate the painful symptoms by destroying the nerve endings in the gingiva. They also destroy the young cells necessary for repair and delay healing. Their repeated use results in the loss of gingival tissue, which is not restored when the disease subsides.[3]

SYSTEMIC ANTIBIOTICS. *Antibiotics are administered systemically only in patients with toxic systemic complications or local adenopathy.* They are not recommended in NUG patients who do not have these complications.

When used, systemic antibiotics also reduce the oral bacterial flora and alleviate the oral symptoms,[10,11] but they are only an adjunct to the complete local treatment the disease requires. Patients treated by systemic antibiotics alone should be cautioned that the acute painful symptoms may recur after the drug is discontinued.

SUPPORTIVE SYSTEMIC TREATMENT. In addition to systemic antibiotics, supportive treatment consists of copious fluid consumption and administration of analgesics for relief of pain. Bed rest is necessary for patients with toxic systemic complications such as high fever, malaise, anorexia, and general debility.

NUTRITIONAL SUPPLEMENTS. The rationale for nutritional supplements in the treatment of NUG is based on the following:

1. Lesions resembling those of NUG have been produced experimentally in animals with certain nutritional deficiencies (see Chapter 12).
2. It is possible that difficulty in chewing raw fruits and vegetables in a painful condition such as NUG could lead to the selection of a diet inadequate in vitamins B and C.
3. Isolated clinical studies[4,6] report fewer recurrences when local treatment of NUG is supplemented with vitamin B or vitamin C.

When the intake of water-soluble vitamins B and C has been severely curtailed because of pain in NUG, nutritional supplements may be indicated along with local treatment to ward off deficiencies of the aforementioned vitamins. Under such circumstances the patient may be given a standard multivitamin preparation combined with a therapeutic dose of vitamins B and C.

The patient should be placed on a natural diet with the required detergent action and nutritional content as soon as the oral condition permits. Nutritional supplements may be discontinued after 2 months.

Local procedures are the keystone of the treatment of necrotizing ulcerative gingivitis. Inflammation is a local conditioning factor that impairs the nutrition of the gingiva regardless of the systemic nutritional status. Local irritants should be eliminated to foster normal metabolic and reparative processes in the gingiva. Persistent or recurrent NUG is more likely to be caused by the failure to remove local irritants and by inadequate plaque control than by nutritional deficiency.

Sequelae of Inadequate Treatment

Persistent or "Unresponsive" Cases. If the clinician finds it necessary to change from drug to drug in

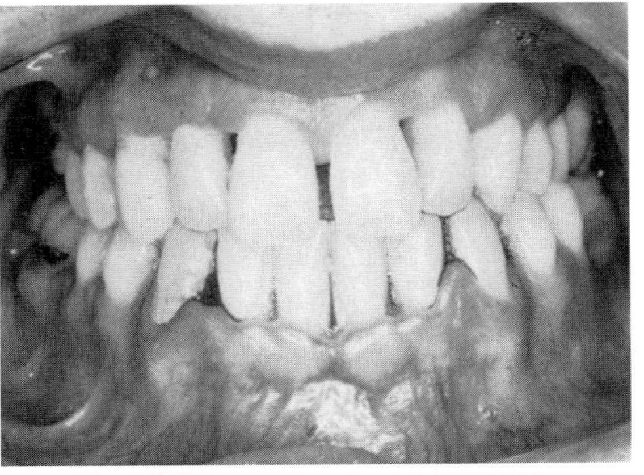
A

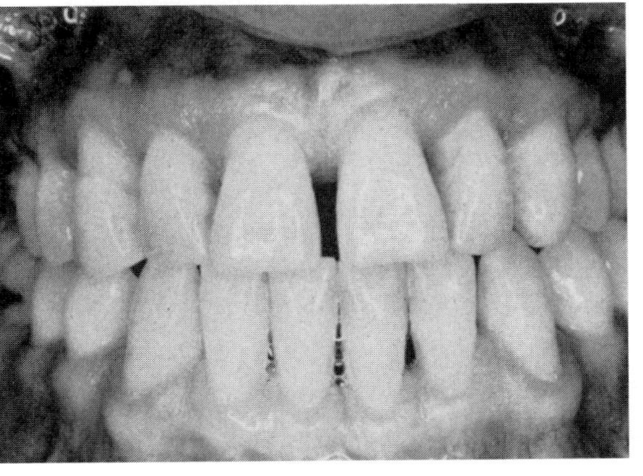
B

Fig. 45-3 Physiologic contour and new attachment of gingiva after treatment of acute NUG. **A,** Acute NUG showing the characteristic punched-out eroded gingival margin with surface pseudomembrane. **B,** After treatment. Note the restoration of physiologic gingival contour and reattachment of the gingiva to the surfaces of the mandibular teeth, which had been exposed by the disease.

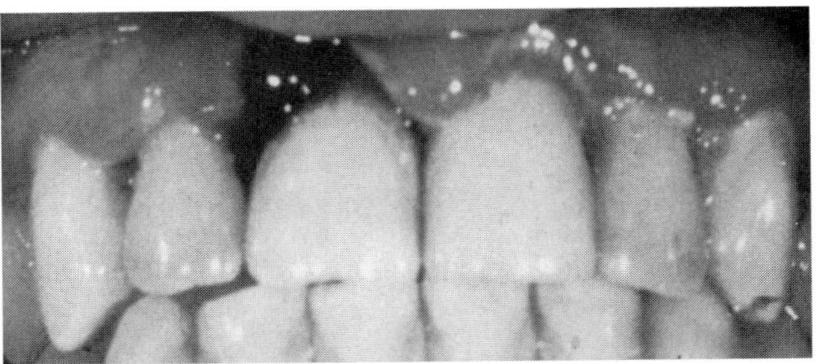
A

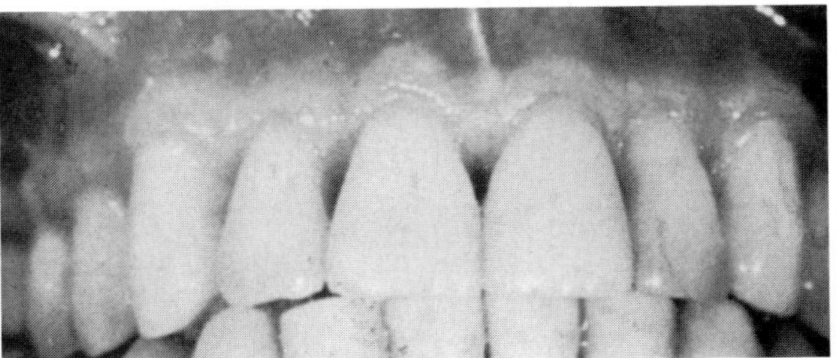
B

Fig. 45-4 Gingival healing after treatment. **A,** Before treatment. Severe acute necrotizing ulcerative gingivitis with crater formation. **B,** After treatment. Note the restored gingival contour.

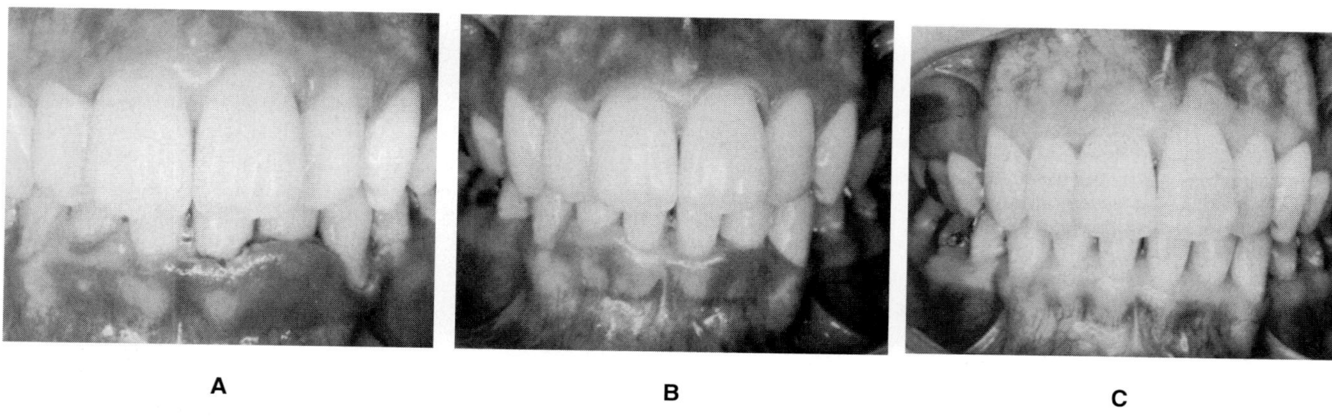

Fig. 45-5 Reshaping the gingiva in the treatment of acute NUG. **A,** Before treatment, showing bulbous gingiva and interdental necrosis in the mandibular anterior area. **B,** After treatment. Gingival contours still undesirable. **C,** Final result. Physiologic contours obtained by reshaping the gingiva.

an effort to relieve a "stubborn" case of NUG, something is wrong with the overall treatment regimen that is not likely to be corrected by changing drugs. When confronted with such a problem, the following should be completed:

1. All local drug therapy should be discontinued so that the condition may be studied in an uncomplicated state.
2. Careful differential diagnosis is undertaken to rule out diseases that resemble NUG (see Chapter 12).
3. A search is made for contributing local and systemic etiologic factors that may have been overlooked.
4. Special attention is given to instructing the patient in plaque control before undertaking comprehensive local treatment.

Recurrent Necrotizing Ulcerative Gingivitis. The following factors should be explored in patients with recurrent NUG:

1. *Inadequate local therapy.* Too often, treatment is discontinued when the symptoms have subsided, without eliminating the chronic gingival disease and periodontal pockets that remain after the superficial acute condition is relieved. Persistent chronic inflammation causes degenerative changes that predispose the gingiva to recurrence of acute involvement.
2. *Pericoronal flap.* Recurrent acute involvement in the mandibular anterior area is often associated with persistent pericoronal inflammation arising from difficult eruption of third molars.[7] The anterior involvement is less likely to recur after the third molar situation is corrected.
3. *Anterior overbite.* Marked overbite is often a contributing factor in the recurrence of disease in the anterior region. When the incisal edges of the maxillary teeth impinge on the labial gingival margin or the mandibular teeth strike the palatal gingiva, the resultant tissue injury predisposes the gingiva to recurrent acute disease. Less severe overbite produces food impaction and gingival trauma. Correction of the overbite is necessary for the complete treatment of NUG.

Inadequate plaque control and *heavy use of tobacco* are also common causes of recurrent disease.

TREATMENT OF ACUTE PERICORONITIS

The treatment of pericoronitis depends on the severity of the inflammation, the systemic complications, and the advisability of retaining the involved tooth. All pericoronal flaps should be viewed with suspicion. Persistent symptom-free pericoronal flaps should be removed as a preventive measure against subsequent acute involvement.

The treatment of acute pericoronitis consists of (1) gently flushing the area with warm water to remove debris and exudate and (2) swabbing with antiseptic after elevating the flap gently from the tooth with a scaler. The underlying debris is removed, and the area is flushed with warm water (Fig. 45-6). Antibiotics can be prescribed in severe cases. If the gingival flap is swollen and fluctuant, an anteroposterior incision to establish drainage is made with a #15 blade.

After the acute symptoms have subsided, a determination is made as to whether the tooth is to be retained or extracted. The decision is governed by the likelihood of further eruption into a good functional position. Bone loss on the distal surface of the second molars is a hazard following the extraction of partially or completely impacted third molars,[1] and the problem is significantly greater if the third molars are extracted after the roots are formed or in patients older than their early twenties. To reduce the risk of bone loss around second molars, partially or completely impacted third molars should be extracted as early as possible in their development.

If it is decided to retain the tooth, the pericoronal flap is removed using periodontal knives or electrosurgery (Fig. 44-6). It is necessary to remove the tissue distal to the tooth, as well as the flap on the occlusal surface. Incising only the occlusal portion of the flap leaves a deep distal pocket, which invites recurrence of acute pericoronal involvement.

After the tissue is removed, a periodontal pack is applied. The pack may be retained by bringing it forward along the facial and lingual surfaces into the interproximal space between the second and third molars. The pack is removed after 1 week.

Pericoronitis and Necrotizing Ulcerative Gingivitis

Pericoronitis and NUG pericoronal flaps that are chronically inflamed may become the sites of NUG. The disease is treated in the same manner as elsewhere in the mouth; after the acute symptoms have subsided, the flap is removed. Pericoronal flaps are often referred to as *primary incubation zones* in NUG; their elimination is one of many measures required to minimize the likelihood of recurrent disease.

TREATMENT OF ACUTE HERPETIC GINGIVOSTOMATITIS

Primary infection with herpes simplex virus in the oral cavity results in a condition known as acute herpetic gingivostomatitis, which is an oral infection often, accompanied by systemic symptoms (see Chapter 19). This infection typically occurs in children, but it can and does occur in adults as well. It runs a 7- to 10-day course and heals without scars. A recurrent herpetic episode may be precipitated in individuals with a history of herpes virus infections and by respiratory infections, sunlight exposure, fever, trauma, exposure to chemicals, and emotional stress.

Various medications have been used to treat herpes gingivostomatitis with little success; these have included local applications of escharotics, vitamins, radiation and antibiotics. Limited success was initially reported with the use of herpesvirus-specific drugs, such as acyclovir ointment.[8] However, a recent clinical report has suggested good results using systemic acyclovir to prevent (or lessen the severity of) recurrent herpes virus infection associated with dental treatment.[12] The patient, who was known to have recurrent infections after dental treatment, did not experience any recurrence when treated with acyclovir. Most strains of herpes virus are susceptible to acyclovir, and it has been suggested that topical application of acyclovir is useful in decreasing the spread and severity of the infection.

Treatment consists of palliative measures to make the patient comfortable until the disease runs its course. Plaque, food debris and superficial calculus are removed to reduce gingival inflammation, which complicates the acute herpetic involvement. Extensive periodontal therapy should be postponed until the acute symptoms subside to avoid the possibility of exacerbation (Fig. 45-7). For symptomatic relief, especially before meals, topical local anesthetic, such as lidocaine hydrochloride viscous solution can be applied to the affected areas. Before each meal the patient should rinse with 1 tablespoon of this solution. If the patient is experiencing pain of longer duration, aspirin or a nonsteroidal antiinflammatory agent can be given systemically.

Local or systemic application of antibiotics is sometimes advised to prevent opportunistic infection of ulcerations. This is especially true in the immune compromised individual. If the condition does not resolve within a 2-week period, the patient should be referred to a physician for medical consultation.[5]

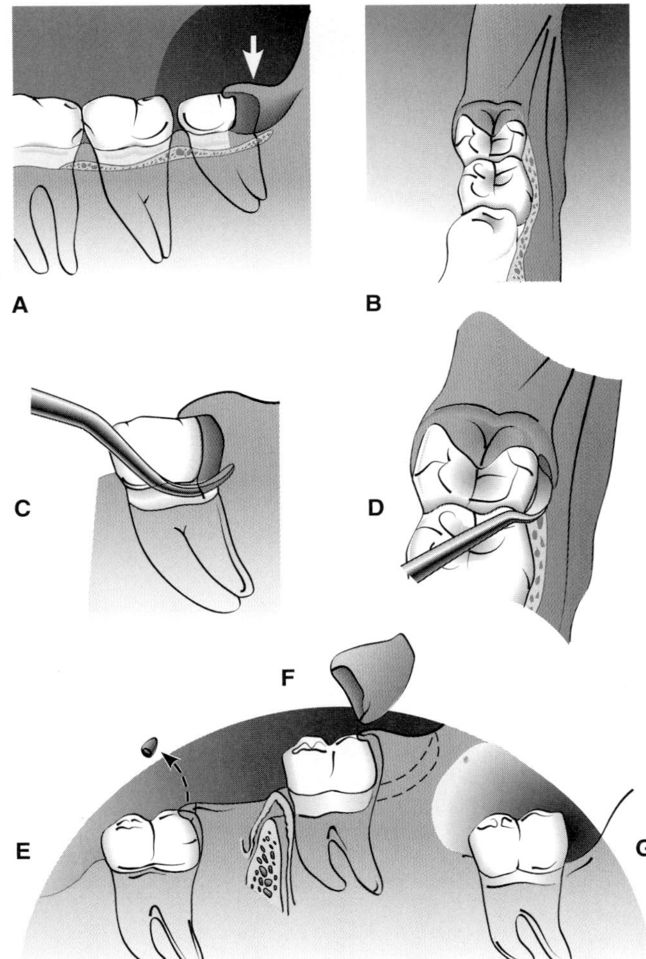

Fig. 45-6 Treatment of acute pericoronitis. **A,** Inflamed pericoronal flap *(arrow)* in relation to the mandibular third molar. **B,** Anterior view of third molar and flap. **C,** Lateral view with scaler in position to gently remove debris under flap. **D,** Anterior view of scaler in position. **E,** Removal of section of the gingiva distal to the third molar, after the acute symptoms subside. The line of incision is indicated by the broken line. **F,** Appearance of the healed area. **G,** Incorrect removal of the tip of the flap, permitting the deep pocket to remain distal to the molar.

The patient should be informed that the disease is contagious at certain stages such as when vesicles are present (highest viral titer). All individuals exposed to an infected patient should take precautions. Herpetic infection of a clinician's finger, referred to as *herpetic whitlow,* can occur if a seronegative clinician becomes infected with a patient's herpetic lesions.[8,9]

Supportive Treatment

Supportive measures include copious fluid intake and systemic antibiotic therapy for the management of toxic systemic complications. For the relief of pain, aspirin is usually sufficient. A dosage of 325 mg to 650 mg every 4 hours may be prescribed for adults, with smaller doses used for children.

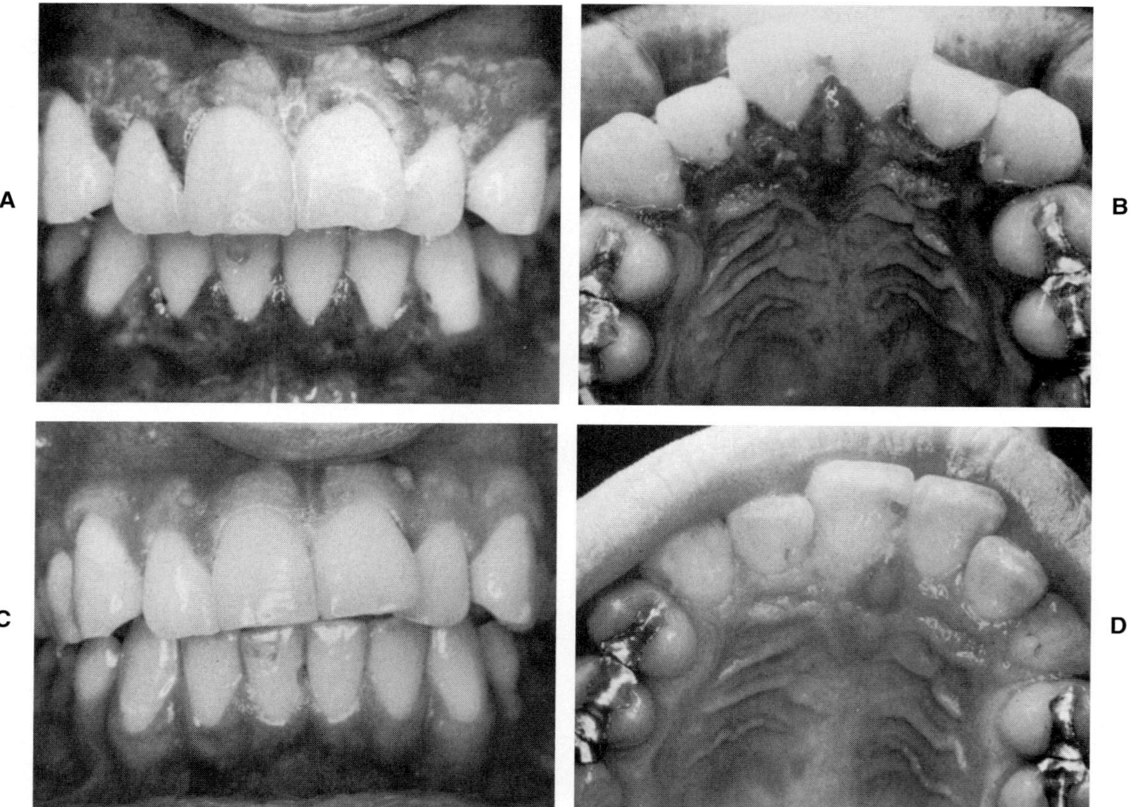

Fig. 45-7 Treatment of acute herpetic gingivostomatitis. **A,** Before treatment. Note diffuse erythema and surface vesicles. **B,** Before treatment, lingual view, showing gingival edema and ruptured vesicle on palate. **C,** One month after treatment, showing restoration of normal gingival contour and stippling. **D,** One month after treatment, lingual view.

REFERENCES

1. Ash Jr MM, Costich ER, Hayward JR: A study of periodontal hazards of third molars. J Periodontol 1962; 33:209.
2. Burket LW: Oral Medicine, ed 3. Philadelphia, JB Lippincott, 1946.
3. Glickman I, Johannessen LB: The effect of a six per cent solution of chromic acid on the gingiva of the albino rat—a correlated gross, biomicroscopic, and histologic study. J Am Dent Assoc 1950; 41:674.
4. King JD: Nutritional and other factors in "trench mouth" with special reference to the nicotinic acid component of the vitamin B2 complex. Br Dent J 1943; 74:113.
5. Langlais RP, Miller CS: Color Atlas of Common Oral Diseases, ed 2. New York, Williams & Wilkins, 1998.
6. Linghorne WJ, McIntosh WG, Tice JW, et al: The relation of ascorbic acid intake to gingivitis. J Can Dent Assoc 1946; 12:49.
7. Mitchell DF, Baker BR: Topical antibiotic control of necrotizing gingivitis. J Periodontol 1968; 39:81.
8. Regezi JA, Sciubba JJ: Oral Pathology: Clinical-Pathologic Correlations. WB Saunders, Philadelphia, 1989.
9. Snyder ML, Church DH, Rickles NH: Primary herpes infection of right second finger. Oral Surg 1969; 27:598.
10. Wade AB, Blake GC, Manson JD, et al: Treatment of the acute phase of ulcerative gingivitis (Vincent's type). Br Dent J 1963; 115:372.
11. Wade AB, Blake G, Mirza K: Effectiveness of metronidazole in treating the acute phase of ulcerative gingivitis. Dent Pract 1966; 16:440.
12. Williamson RT: Diagnosis and management of recurrent herpes simplex induced by fixed prosthodontic tissue management: a clinical report. J Prosthet Dent 1999; 82:1.

Treatment of the Periodontal Abscess

Henry H. Takei

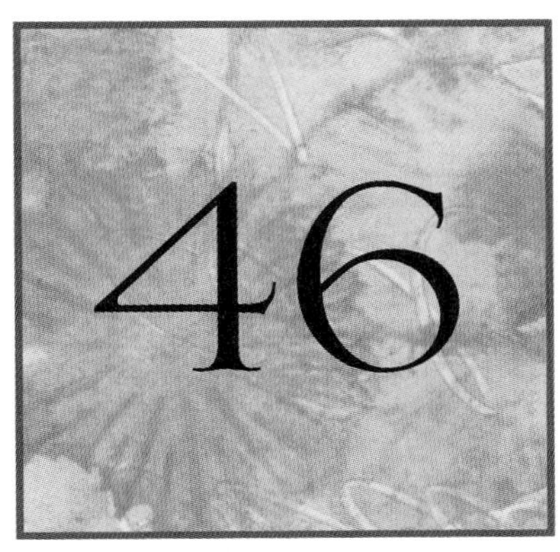

CHAPTER

CHAPTER OUTLINE

Periodontal abscesses are commonly encountered in patients with deep pockets. They are an acute exacerbation of a preexisting pocket resulting from exudates and purulent material being entrapped in the pocket with no pathway for drainage. Abscesses may be acute or chronic. *Acute abscesses* are painful, edematous, red, shiny ovoid elevations of the gingival margin, the attached gingiva, or both. After their purulent content is partially exuded, they become chronic. *Chronic abscesses* may produce a dull pain and may at times become acute (see Chapter 30).

THE ACUTE PERIODONTAL ABSCESS

To undertake the proper course of therapy, it is essential to establish the differential diagnosis between a periodontal and a pulpal abscess. Box 46-1 compares the symptoms associated with the two lesions.

Treatment

The purpose of treatment of an acute abscess is to alleviate the pain, control the spread of infection, and establish drainage.[1] The patient's general systemic response should be evaluated. Rise in temperature, feverish appearance, and a feeling of malaise should be noted and a proper antibiotic regimen started if necessary.

Drainage can be established through the pocket or by means of an incision from the outer surface. The former is preferable.

Drainage through the Pocket. The area is anesthetized topically and, if necessary, local anesthesia is injected around the periphery of the abscess. Care is taken not to inject into the swelling itself. A flat instrument or a probe is carefully introduced into the pocket in an attempt to distend the pocket wall for drainage. A curette can then be gently inserted into the pocket to further drain and gently curette the mass of tissue internally.

Drainage through an External Incision. The abscess is isolated and dried with gauze sponges. After the application of topical anesthesia, local anesthesia is injected around the periphery of the abscess.

A #15 blade is used to make a vertical incision through the most fluctuant part of the swelling, extending to an area just apical to the abscess (Fig. 46-1). A curette or periosteal elevator is used to gently elevate the tissue to create drainage and curette the granulomatous tissue in the internal aspect of the abscess. The external aspect of the abscess is gently pushed to drain the remaining purulent material and approximate the wound edges. Sutures are usually not required.

After the drainage stops, the area is dried and painted with an antiseptic. Patients without systemic complications are instructed to rinse often with a solution of 1 tsp salt in a glass of warm water and to return for follow-up evaluation the next day. In addition to the rinses, penicillin or other antibiotics are prescribed for patients with elevated temperatures. The patient is also instructed to avoid exertion and is placed on a copious fluid diet.

BOX 46-1

Differences between Periodontal and Pulpal Abscesses

Periodontal Abscess	*Pulpal Abscess*
The abscess is associated with a preexisting periodontal pocket, caries, or both.	The abscess is associated with deep restoration.
A pulp test may be vital.	A pulp test may be nonvital.
Swelling is generalized and located around the involved tooth and gingival margin, seldom with a fistulous tract.	Swelling is localized, often with a fistulous opening in the apical area. This may be located away from the offending tooth.
Pain is usually dull, constant, and less severe than in a periapical abscess. The pain is localized and the patient usually can locate the offending tooth.	Pain is usually severe, throbbing, and may last for days. The patient may not be able to locate the offending tooth.
Pain associated with the movement or percussion is not as severe as with a pulpal abscess.	Pain associated with tooth movement or percussion can be severe.

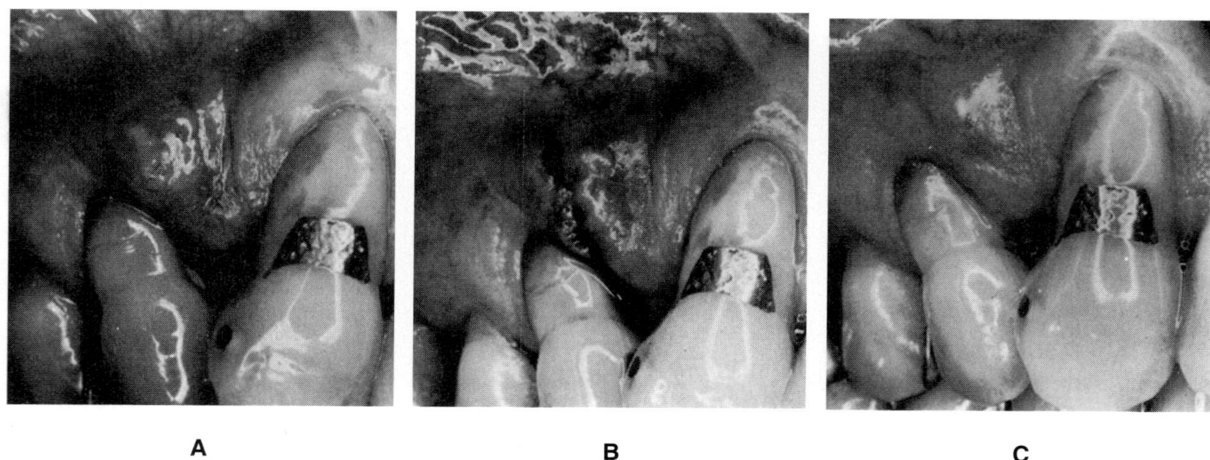

Fig. 46-1 Incision of an acute periodontal abscess. **A,** Fluctuant acute periodontal abscess. **B,** Abscess incised. **C,** After acute signs subside.

If necessary, bed rest is recommended. Analgesics are prescribed for pain.

The next day, the swelling is generally markedly reduced or absent and the symptoms should have subsided. If acute symptoms persist, the patient is instructed to continue the regimen prescribed the previous day and to return in 24 hours. The symptoms invariably disappear by this time, and the lesion is ready for the usual treatment of a chronic periodontal abscess.

THE GINGIVAL ABSCESS

In contrast to the periodontal abscess, which involves the supporting tissues, the gingival abscess is a lesion of the marginal or interdental gingiva, usually produced by an impacted foreign object. It is treated as follows:

Under topical and local infiltrative anesthesia, the fluctuant area of the lesion is incised with a #15 blade, and the incision is gently widened to permit drainage. The area is cleansed with warm water and covered with a gauze pad. After bleeding stops, the patient is dismissed for 24 hours and instructed to rinse every 2 hours with a glassful of warm water.

When the patient returns, the lesion is generally reduced in size and free of symptoms. A topical anesthetic is applied, and the area is scaled. If the residual size of the lesion is too great, it is removed surgically.

THE CHRONIC PERIODONTAL ABSCESS

After adequate drainage, antibiotic treatment, or both, the acute abscess becomes chronic. Some cases have drained spontaneously and the patient is then diagnosed as having a chronic abscess. Further treatment is similar to that of a periodontal pocket.

REFERENCE

1. Manson JD: Periodontics, ed 3. Philadelphia, Lea & Febiger, 1975.

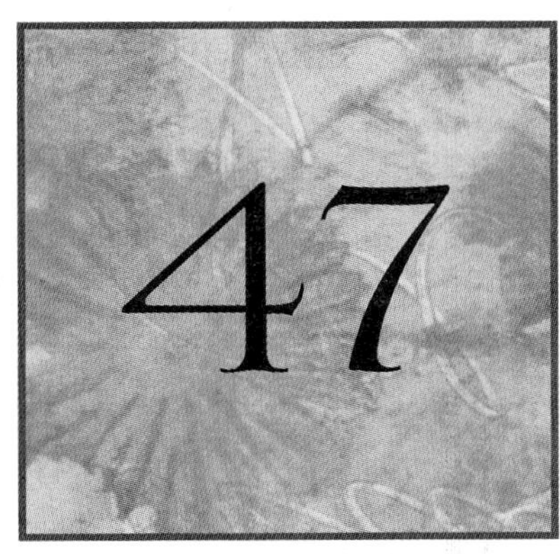

CHAPTER

Scaling and Root Planing

Gordon L. Pattison and Anna M. Pattison*

CHAPTER OUTLINE

PRINCIPLES OF SCALING AND ROOT PLANING

Definitions and Rationale

Scaling is the process by which plaque and calculus are removed from both supragingival and subgingival tooth surfaces. No deliberate attempt is made to remove tooth substance along with the calculus. *Root planing* is the process by which residual embedded calculus and portions of cementum are removed from the roots to produce a smooth, hard, clean surface.

The primary objective of scaling and root planing is to restore gingival health by completely removing elements that provoke gingival inflammation (i.e., plaque, calculus, and endotoxin) from the tooth surface (see Color Fig. 48-1). Instrumentation has been shown to dramatically reduce the numbers of subgingival microorganisms and produce a shift in the composition of subgingival plaque from one with high numbers of gram-negative anaerobes to one dominated by gram-positive facultative bacteria that are compatible with health.[66,68,77,97,100,108,110] After thorough scaling and root planing, a profound reduction of spirochetes, motile rods, and putative pathogens such as *Actinobacillus actinomycetemcomitans, Porphyromonas gingivalis,* and *Prevotella intermedia* and an increase in coccoid cells occur.[68,97,103,108,120,127] These changes in the microbiota are accompanied by a reduction or elimination of inflammation clinically.[9,35,37,49,52,67,92,93] This positive microbial change must be sustained by the periodic scaling and root planing performed during supportive periodontal therapy.[6,14,64,67,90,108,124]

Scaling and root planing are not separate procedures. All the principles of scaling apply equally to root planing. The difference between scaling and root planing is only a matter of degree. The nature of the tooth surface determines the degree to which the surface must be scaled or planed.

Plaque and calculus on enamel surfaces provoke gingival inflammation. Unless they are grooved or pitted, enamel surfaces are relatively smooth and uniform. When plaque and calculus form on enamel, the deposits are usually superficially attached to the surface and are not locked into irregularities. Scaling alone is sufficient to completely remove plaque and calculus from enamel, leaving a smooth, clean surface.

Root surfaces exposed to plaque and calculus pose a

* Material in this chapter was drawn freely from Pattison AM, Pattison GL: Periodontal Instrumentation, ed 2. Upper Saddle River, NJ. Prentice Hall, 1992.

different problem. *Deposits of calculus on root surfaces are frequently embedded in cemental irregularities.*[1,17,76,105,128] *When dentin is exposed, plaque bacteria may invade dentinal tubules.*[1] *Therefore scaling alone is insufficient to remove them, and a portion of the root surface must be removed to eliminate these deposits.* Furthermore, when the root surface is exposed to plaque and the pocket environment, its surface is contaminated by toxic substances, notably endotoxins.[2,3,44] Recent evidence suggests that these toxic substances are only superficially attached to the root and do not permeate it deeply.[18,19,47,48,75,79,80,111] Removal of extensive amounts of dentin and cementum is not necessary to render the roots free of toxins and should be avoided.[35,67,90] However, where cementum is thin, instrumentation may expose dentin. Although this is not the aim of treatment, it may be unavoidable.[104,119]

Scaling and root planing should not be thought of as separate procedures unrelated to the rest of the treatment plan. They belong in the initial phase of an orderly sequence of treatment. After careful analysis of a case, the number of appointments needed to complete this phase of treatment is estimated. Patients with small amounts of calculus and relatively healthy tissues can be treated in one appointment. Most other patients require several treatment sessions. The dentist should estimate the number of appointments needed on the basis of the number of teeth in the mouth, severity of inflammation, amount and location of calculus, depth and activity of pockets, presence of furcation invasions, patient's comprehension of and compliance with oral hygiene instructions, and need for local anesthesia. Recent research indicates that completing initial scaling and root planing in one or two long appointments rather than four shorter quadrant scaling appointments may be advantageous.[74,94,95] This removes pathogens from the entire mouth as quickly as possible so that they are not present to reinfect previously instrumented areas.

When the rationale for scaling and root planing is thoroughly understood, it becomes apparent that mastery of these skills is essential to the ultimate success of any course of periodontal therapy. Of all clinical dental procedures, subgingival scaling and root planing in deep pockets are the most difficult and exacting skills to master. It has been argued that such proficiency in instrumentation cannot be attained; therefore periodontal surgery is necessary to gain access to root surfaces. Others have argued that although proficiency is possible, it need not be developed because access to the roots can be gained more easily with surgery. However, without mastering subgingival scaling and root planing skills, the clinician will be severely hampered and unable to treat adequately those patients for whom surgery is contraindicated.

Detection Skills

Good visual and tactile detection skills are required for the accurate initial assessment of the extent and nature of deposits and root irregularities before scaling and root planing. Valid evaluation of results of instrumentation depends on these detection skills.

Visual examination of supragingival and subgingival calculus just below the gingival margin is not difficult with good lighting and a clean field. Light deposits of supragingival calculus are often difficult to see when they are wet with saliva. Compressed air may be used to dry supragingival calculus until it is chalky white and readily visible. Air also may be directed into the pocket in a steady stream to deflect the marginal gingiva away from the tooth so that subgingival deposits near the surface can be seen.

Tactile exploration of the tooth surfaces in subgingival areas of pocket depth, furcations, and developmental depressions is much more difficult than visual examination of supragingival areas and requires the skilled use of a fine-pointed explorer or probe. The explorer or probe is held with a light but stable modified pen grasp. This provides maximal tactile sensitivity for detection of subgingival calculus and other irregularities. The pads of the thumb and fingers, especially the middle finger, should perceive the slight vibrations conducted through the instrument shank and handle as irregularities in the tooth surface are encountered.

After a stable finger rest is established, the tip of the instrument is carefully inserted subgingivally to the base of the pocket. Light exploratory strokes are activated vertically on the root surface. When calculus is encountered, the tip of the instrument should be advanced apically over the deposit until the termination of the calculus on the root is felt. The distance between the apical edge of the calculus and the bottom of the pocket usually ranges from 0.2 to 1.0 mm. The tip is adapted closely to the tooth to ensure the greatest degree of tactile sensitivity and avoid tissue trauma. When a proximal surface is being explored, strokes must be extended at least halfway across that surface past the contact area to ensure complete detection of interproximal deposits. When an explorer is used at line angles, convexities, and concavities, the handle of the instrument must be rolled slightly between the thumb and fingers to keep the tip constantly adapted to the changes in tooth contour.

Although exploration technique and good tactile sensitivity are important, interpreting various degrees of roughness and making clinical judgments based on these interpretations also require much expertise. The beginning student usually has difficulty detecting fine calculus and altered cementum. Such detection must begin with the recognition of ledges, lumps, or spurs of calculus, then smaller spicules, then slight roughness, and finally a slight graininess that feels like a sticky coating or film covering the tooth surface. Overhanging or deficient margins of dental restorations, caries, decalcification, and root roughness caused by previous instrumentation are all commonly found during exploration. These and other irregularities must be recognized and differentiated from subgingival calculus. Because this requires a great deal of experience and a high degree of tactile sensitivity, many clinicians agree that the development of detection skills is as important as the mastery of scaling and root planing technique.

Supragingival Scaling Technique

Supragingival calculus is generally less tenacious and less calcified than subgingival calculus. Because instrumentation is performed coronal to the gingival margin, scaling strokes are not confined by the surrounding tissues. This makes adaptation and angulation easier. It also allows direct visibility as well as a freedom of movement not possible during subgingival scaling.

Sickles, curettes, and ultrasonic and sonic instruments are most commonly used for the removal of supragingival calculus. Hoes and chisels are less frequently used. To perform supragingival scaling, the sickle or curette is held with a modified pen grasp, and a firm finger rest is established on the teeth adjacent to the working area. The blade is adapted with an angulation of slightly less than 90 degrees to the surface being scaled. The cutting edge should engage the apical margin of the supragingival calculus while short, powerful, overlapping scaling strokes are activated coronally in a vertical or an oblique direction. The sharply pointed tip of the sickle can easily lacerate marginal tissue or gouge exposed root surfaces, so careful adaptation is especially important when this instrument is being used. The tooth surface is instrumented until it is visually and tactilely free of all supragingival deposits. If the tissue is retractable enough to allow easy insertion of the bulky blade, the sickle may be used slightly below the free gingival margin. If the sickle is used in this manner, final scaling and root planing with the curette should always follow.

Subgingival Scaling and Root Planing Technique

Subgingival scaling and root planing are far more complex and difficult to perform than supragingival scaling. Subgingival calculus is usually harder than supragingival calculus and is often locked into root irregularities, making it more tenacious and therefore more difficult to remove.[17,76,105,128] The overlying tissue creates significant problems in subgingival instrumentation. Vision is obscured by the bleeding that inevitably occurs during instrumentation and by the tissue itself. The clinician must rely heavily on tactile sensitivity to detect calculus and irregularities, guide the instrument blade during scaling and root planing, and evaluate the results of instrumentation.

In addition, the adjacent pocket wall limits the direction and length of the strokes. The confines of the soft tissue make careful adaptation to tooth contours imperative to avoid trauma. Such precise adaptation cannot be accomplished without a thorough knowledge of tooth morphologic features. The clinician must form a mental image of the tooth surface to anticipate variations in contour, continually confirming or modifying the image in response to tactile sensations and visual cues such as the position of the instrument handle and shank. The clinician then must instantaneously adjust the adaptation and angulation of the working end to the tooth. It is this complex and precise coordination of visual, mental, and manual skills that makes subgingival instrumentation one of the most difficult of all dental skills. *The curette is preferred by most clinicians for subgingival scaling and root planing because of the advantages afforded by its design.* Its curved blade, rounded toe, and curved back allow the curette to be inserted to the base of the pocket and adapted to variations in tooth contour with minimal tissue displacement and trauma.

Sickles, hoes, files, and ultrasonic instruments also are used for subgingival scaling of heavy calculus. Some small files such as the Hirschfeld file may be inserted to the base of the pocket to crush or initially fracture tenacious deposits. Larger files, hoes, sickles, and standard ultrasonic tips for supragingival use are too bulky and cannot easily be inserted into deep pockets or areas where tissue is firm and fibrotic. Hoes and files are not able to produce as smooth a surface as curettes.[12,104] Hoes, files, and standard large ultrasonic tips are all more hazardous than the curette in terms of trauma to the root surface and surrounding tissues.[12,85,104] Although thin ultrasonic tips designed for scaling of deep pockets and furcations can be inserted more easily subgingivally, they must be used on low power.[31,32,45] When low-power scaling is performed on heavy calculus or tenacious sheets of calculus, thin ultrasonic tips are likely to burnish the calculus rather than thoroughly remove it. Therefore ultrasonic scaling should be followed by careful assessment with an explorer and further instrumentation with curettes when necessary.

Subgingival scaling and root planing are accomplished with either universal or area-specific (Gracey) curettes using the following basic procedure: The curette is held with a modified pen grasp, and a stable finger rest is established. The correct cutting edge is slightly adapted to the tooth, with the lower shank kept parallel to the tooth surface. The lower shank is moved toward the tooth so that the face of the blade is nearly flush with the tooth surface. The blade is then inserted under the gingiva and advanced to the base of the pocket by a light exploratory stroke. When the cutting edge reaches the base of the pocket, a working angulation of between 45 and 90 degrees is established, and pressure is applied laterally against the tooth surface. Calculus is removed by a series of controlled, overlapping, short, powerful strokes primarily using wrist-arm motion (Fig. 47-1). As calculus is removed, resistance to the passage of the cutting edge diminishes until only a slight roughness remains. Longer, lighter root planing strokes are then activated with less lateral pressure until the root surface is completely smooth and hard. The instrument handle must be rolled carefully between the thumb and fingers to keep the blade adapted closely to the tooth surface as line angles, developmental depressions, and other changes in tooth contour are followed. Scaling and root planing strokes should be confined to the portion of the tooth where calculus or altered cementum is found. This zone is known as the *instrumentation zone*. Sweeping the instrument over the crown where it is not needed wastes operating time, dulls the instrument, and causes loss of control.

The amount of lateral pressure applied to the tooth surface depends on the nature of the calculus and whether the strokes are for initial calculus removal or final root planing. If heavy lateral pressure is continued after the bulk of calculus has been removed and the blade is repeatedly readapted with short, choppy strokes, the result will be a root surface roughened by numerous nicks and gouges, resembling the rippled surface of a washboard.[89] If heavy lateral pressure is continued with long, even strokes, the result will be excessive removal of root structure, producing a smooth but "ditched" or "riffled" root surface. To avoid these hazards of overinstrumentation,

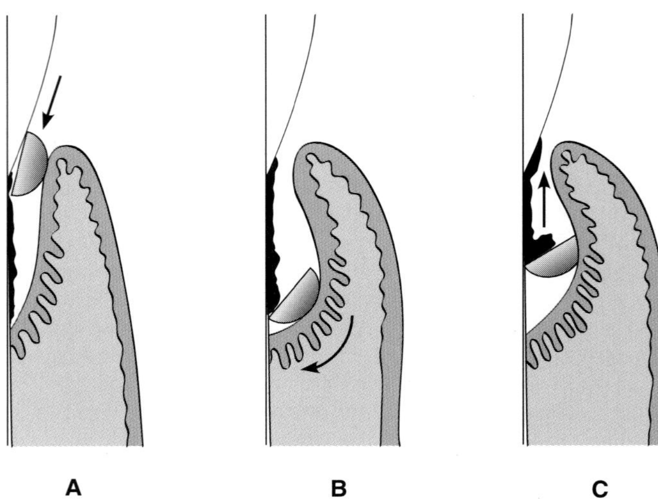

Fig. 47-1 Subgingival scaling procedure. **A,** Curette inserted with the face of the blade flush against the tooth. **B,** Working angulation (45 to 90 degrees) is established at the base of the pocket. **C,** Lateral pressure is applied, and the scaling stroke is activated in the coronal direction.

a deliberate transition from short, powerful scaling strokes to longer, lighter root planing strokes must be made as soon as the calculus and initial roughness have been eliminated.

When scaling strokes are used to remove calculus, force can be maximized by concentrating lateral pressure onto the lower third of the blade (see Fig. 42-19). This small section, the terminal few millimeters of the blade, is positioned slightly apical to the lateral edge of the deposit, and a short vertical or oblique stroke is used to split the calculus from the tooth surface. Without withdrawing the instrument from the pocket, the lower third of the blade is advanced laterally and repositioned to engage the next portion of the remaining deposit. Another vertical or oblique stroke is made, slightly overlapping the previous stroke. This process is repeated in a series of powerful scaling strokes until the entire deposit has been removed. The overlapping of these pathways or "channels" of instrumentation[89] ensures that the entire instrumentation zone is covered (Fig. 47-2).

Engaging a large, tenacious ledge or piece of calculus with the entire length of the cutting edge is not recommended because the force is distributed through a longer section of the cutting edge rather than concentrated. Far more lateral pressure is required to dislodge the entire deposit in one stroke. Although some clinicians may possess the strength to remove calculus completely in this manner, the heavier forces required diminish tactile sensitivity and contribute to a loss of control that results in tissue trauma. A single heavy stroke usually is not sufficient to remove calculus entirely. Instead, the blade skips over or skims the surface of the deposit. Subsequent strokes made with the entire cutting edge tend to shave the deposit down layer by layer. When a series of these repeated whittling strokes is applied, the calculus may be reduced to a thin, smooth, burnished sheet that is difficult to distinguish from the surrounding root surface.

A common error in instrumenting proximal surfaces is failing to reach the midproximal region apical to the contact. This area is relatively inaccessible, and the technique requires more skill than instrumentation of buccal or lingual surfaces. It is extremely important to extend strokes at least halfway across the proximal surface so that no calculus or roughness remains in the interproximal area. With properly designed curettes, this can be accomplished by keeping the lower shank of the curette parallel with the long axis of the tooth (Fig. 47-3). With the lower shank parallel to the long axis, the blade of the curette will reach the base of the pocket and the toe will extend beyond the midline as strokes are advanced across the proximal surface. This extension of strokes beyond the midline ensures thorough exploration and instrumentation of these surfaces. If the lower shank is angled or tilted away from the tooth, the toe will move toward the contact area. Because this prevents the blade from reaching the base of the pocket, calculus apical to the contact will not be detected or removed. Strokes will be hampered because the toe tends to become lodged in the contact. If the instrument is angled or tilted too far toward the tooth, the lower shank will hit the tooth or the contact area, preventing extension of strokes to the mid-proximal region (see Fig. 47-3).

The relationship between the location of the finger rest and the working area is important for two reasons. First, the finger rest or fulcrum must be positioned to allow the lower shank of the instrument to be parallel or nearly parallel to the tooth surface being treated. This parallelism is a fundamental requirement for optimal working angulation. Second, the finger rest must be positioned to enable the operator to use wrist-arm motion to activate strokes. On some aspects of the maxillary posterior teeth, these requirements can be met only with the use of extraoral or opposite-arch fulcrums. When intraoral finger rests are used in other regions of the mouth, the finger rest must be close enough to the working area to fulfill these two requirements. A finger rest that is established too far from the working area forces the clinician to separate the middle finger from the fourth finger in an effort to obtain parallelism and proper angulation. Effective wrist-arm motion is possible only when these two fingers are kept together in a built-up fulcrum. Separation of the fingers commits the clinician to the exclusive use of finger flexing for the activation of strokes.

As instrumentation proceeds from one tooth to the next, the body position of the operator and the location of the finger rest must be frequently adjusted or changed to allow parallelism and wrist-arm motion. Various approaches to instrumentation in different areas of the mouth are illustrated here. The examples shown provide maximal efficiency for the clinician and comfort for the patient. For most areas, more than one approach is presented. Other approaches are possible and are acceptable if they provide equal efficiency and comfort. The following approaches may be used:

Maxillary right posterior sextant: facial aspect (Fig. 47-4).
Operator position: Side position.
Illumination: Direct.
Visibility: Direct (indirect for distal surfaces of molars).

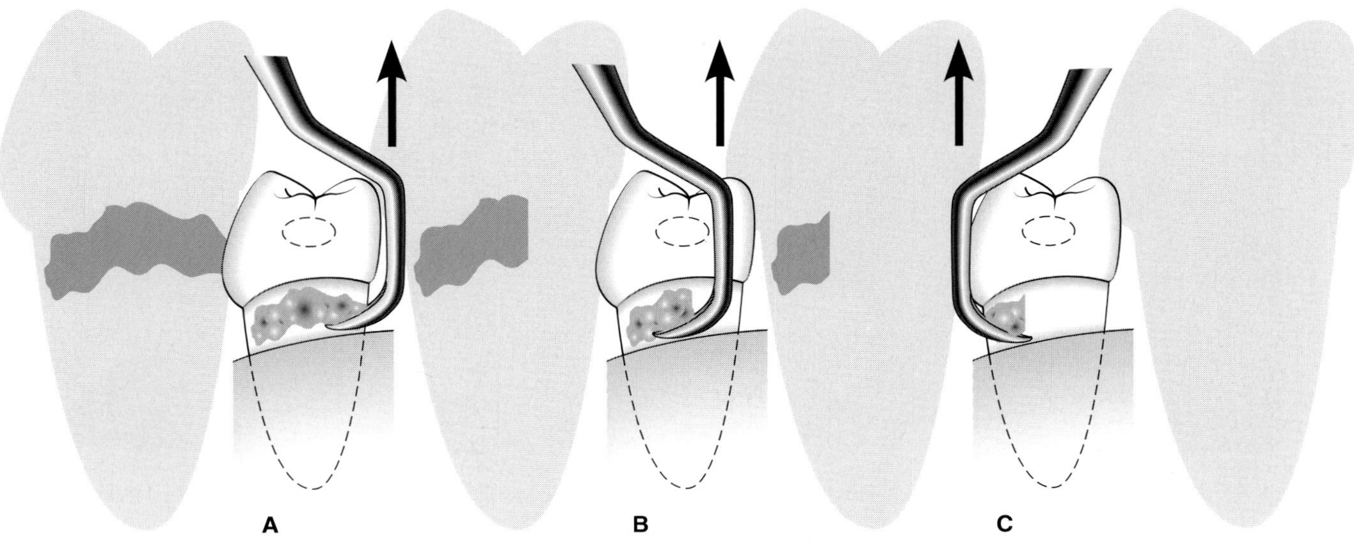

Fig. 47-2 Instrumentation for calculus removal. **A,** Calculus is removed by engaging the apical or lateral edge of the deposit with the cutting edge of a scaler; vertical movement of the instrument will remove the fragment of calculus engaged by the instrument, as seen in the shaded drawing. **B,** The instrument is moved laterally and again engages the edge of the calculus, overlapping the previous stroke to some extent; the shaded drawing shows further removal. **C,** The final portion of the deposit is engaged and removed. Note how in an interdental space the operation is performed by entering facially and lingually.

Retraction: Mirror or index finger of the nonoperating hand.
Finger rest: Extraoral, palm up. Backs of the middle and fourth fingers on the lateral aspect of the mandible on the right side of the face.

Maxillary right posterior sextant, premolar region only: facial aspect (Fig. 47-5).
Operator position: Side or back position.
Illumination: Direct.
Visibility: Direct.
Retraction: Mirror or index finger of the nonoperating hand.
Finger rest: Intraoral, palm up. Fourth finger on the occlusal surfaces of the adjacent maxillary posterior teeth.

Maxillary right posterior sextant: lingual aspect (Fig. 47-6).
Operator position: Side or front position.
Illumination: Direct and indirect.
Visibility: Direct or indirect.
Retraction: None.
Finger rest: Extraoral, palm up. Backs of the middle and fourth fingers on the lateral aspect of the mandible on the right side of the face.

Maxillary right posterior sextant: lingual aspect (Fig. 47-7).
Operator position: Front position.
Illumination: Direct.
Visibility: Direct.
Retraction: None.
Finger rest: Intraoral, palm up, finger-on-finger. Index finger of the nonoperating hand on the occlusal surfaces of the maxillary right posterior teeth; fourth finger of the operating hand or the index finger of nonoperating hand.

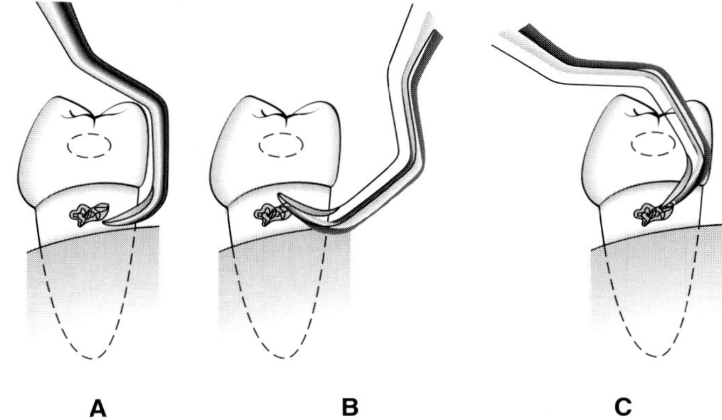

Fig. 47-3 Shank position for scaling proximal surfaces. **A,** Correct shank position, parallel with the long axis of the tooth. **B,** Incorrect shank position, tilted away from the tooth. **C,** Incorrect shank position, tilted too far toward the tooth. Sextant: lingual aspect.

Maxillary anterior sextant: facial aspect, surfaces away from the operator (Fig. 47-8).
Operator position: Back position.
Illumination: Direct.
Visibility: Direct.
Retraction: Index finger of the nonoperating hand.
Finger rest: Intraoral, palm up. Fourth finger on the incisal edges or occlusal surfaces of adjacent maxillary teeth.

Maxillary anterior sextant: facial aspect, surfaces toward the operator (Fig. 47-9).
Operator position: Front position.

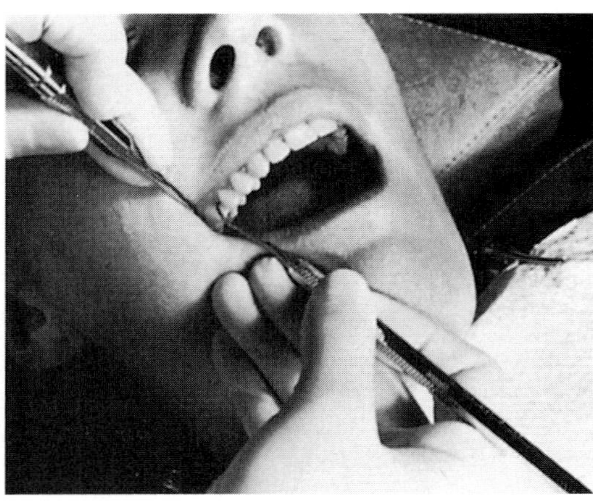

Fig. 47-4 Maxillary right posterior sextant: facial aspect.

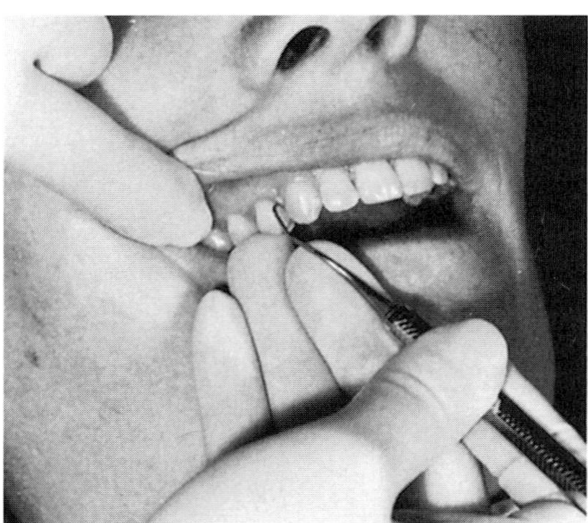

Fig. 47-5 Maxillary right posterior sextant, premolar region only: facial aspect.

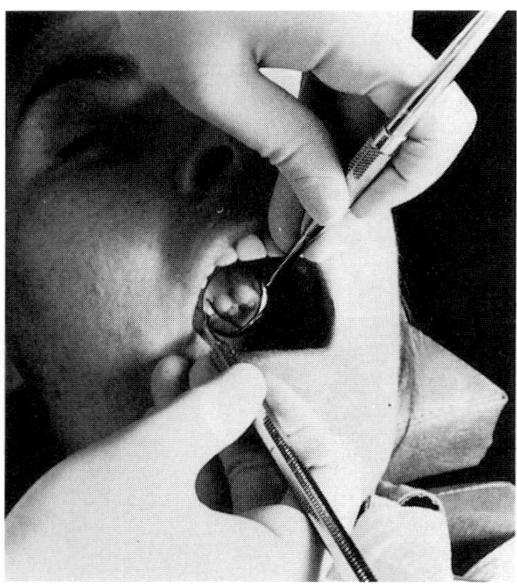

Fig. 47-6 Maxillary right posterior sextant: lingual aspect.

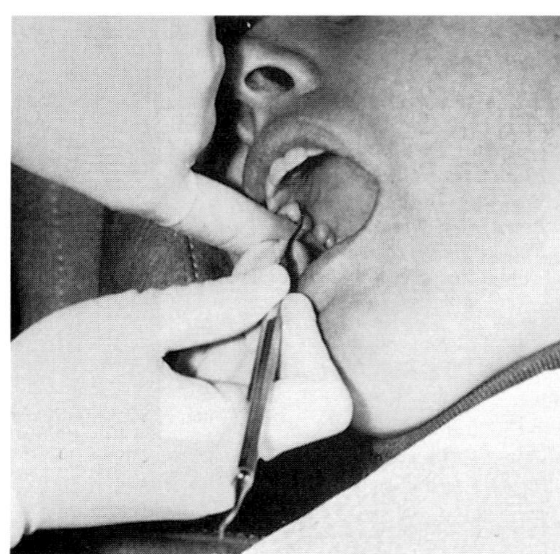

Fig. 47-7 Maxillary right posterior sextant: lingual aspect.

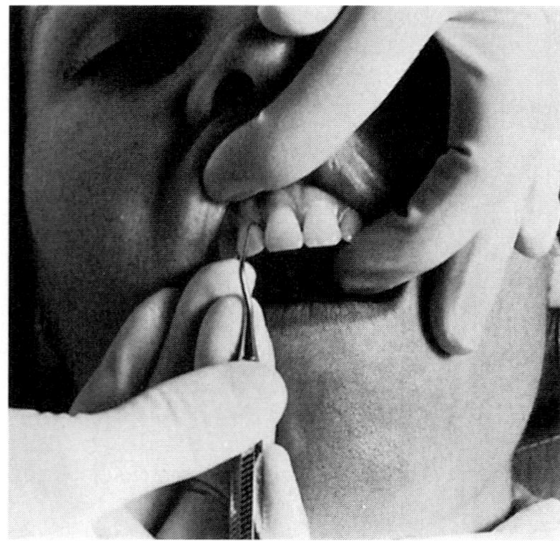

Fig. 47-8 Maxillary anterior sextant: facial aspect, surfaces away from the operator.

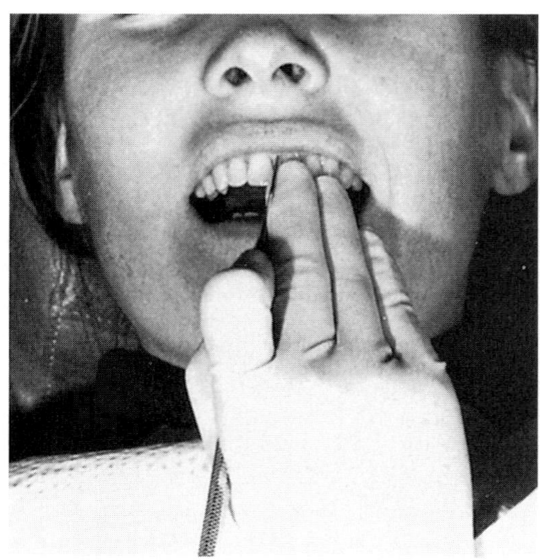

Fig. 47-9 Maxillary anterior sextant: facial aspect, surfaces toward the operator.

Illumination: Direct.
Visibility: Direct.
Retraction: Index finger of the nonoperating hand.
Finger rest: Intraoral, palm down. Fourth finger on the incisal edges or the occlusal or facial surfaces of adjacent maxillary teeth.

Maxillary anterior sextant: lingual aspect, surfaces away from the operator (surfaces toward the operator are scaled from a front position) (Fig. 47-10).
Operator position: Back position.
Illumination: Indirect.
Visibility: Indirect.
Retraction: None.
Finger rest: Intraoral, palm up. Fourth finger on the incisal edges or occlusal surfaces of adjacent maxillary teeth.

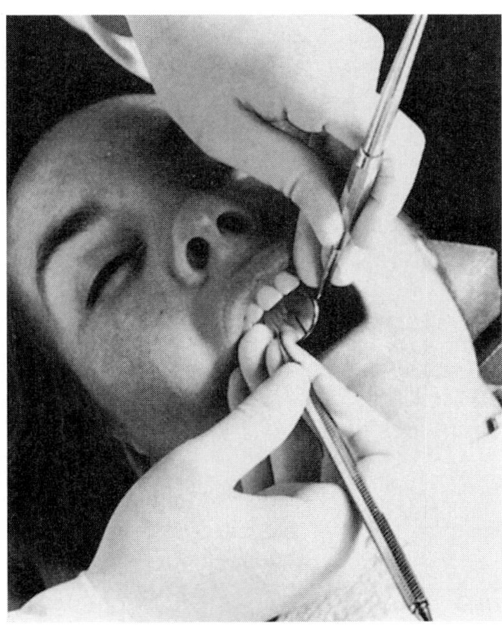

Fig. 47-10 Maxillary anterior sextant: lingual aspect, surfaces away from the operator (surfaces toward the operator are scaled from a front postion).

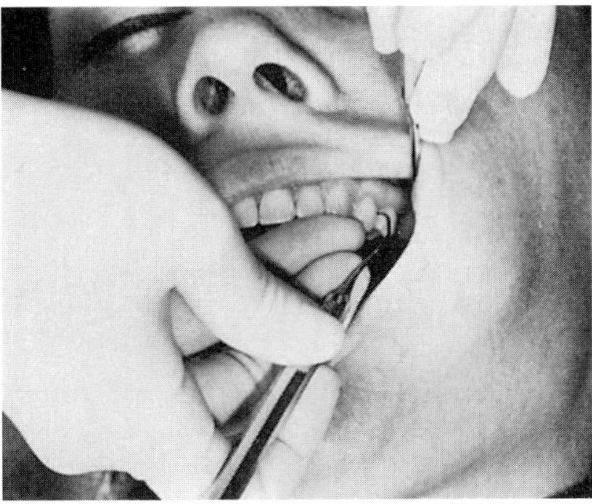

Fig. 47-12 Maxillary left posterior sextant: facial aspect.

Maxillary left posterior sextant: facial aspect (Fig. 47-11).
Operator position: Side or back position.
Illumination: Direct or indirect.
Visibility: Direct or indirect.
Retraction: Mirror.
Finger rest: Extraoral, palm down. Front surfaces of the middle and fourth fingers on the lateral aspect of the mandible on the left side of the face.

Maxillary left posterior sextant: facial aspect (Fig. 47-12).
Operator position: Back or side position.
Illumination: Direct or indirect.
Visibility: Direct or indirect.
Retraction: Mirror.
Finger rest: Intraoral, palm up. Fourth finger on the incisal edges or occlusal surfaces of adjacent maxillary teeth.

Maxillary left posterior sextant: lingual aspect (Fig. 47-13).
Operator position: Front position.
Illumination: Direct.

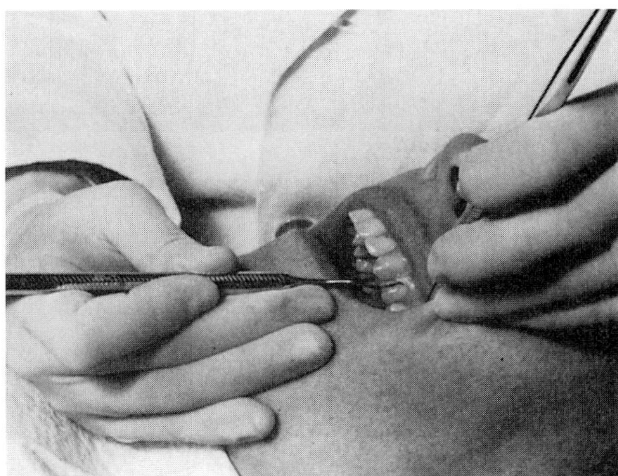

Fig. 47-11 Maxillary left posterior sextant: facial aspect.

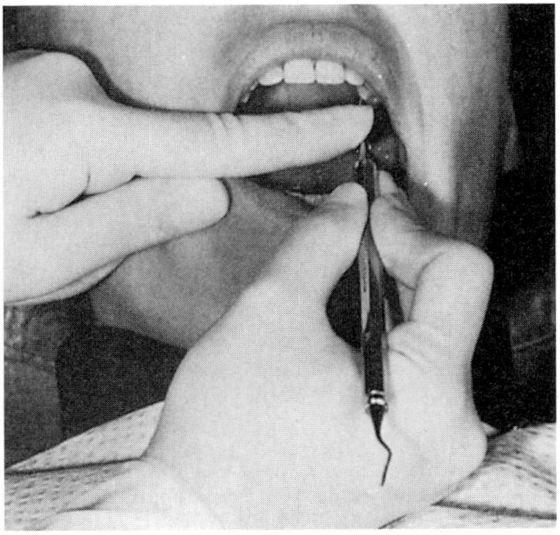

Fig. 47-13 Maxillary left posterior sextant: lingual aspect.

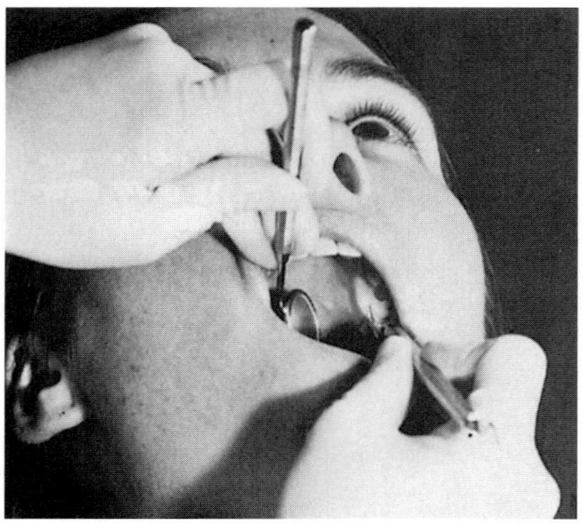

Fig. 47-14 Maxillary left posterior sextant: lingual aspect.

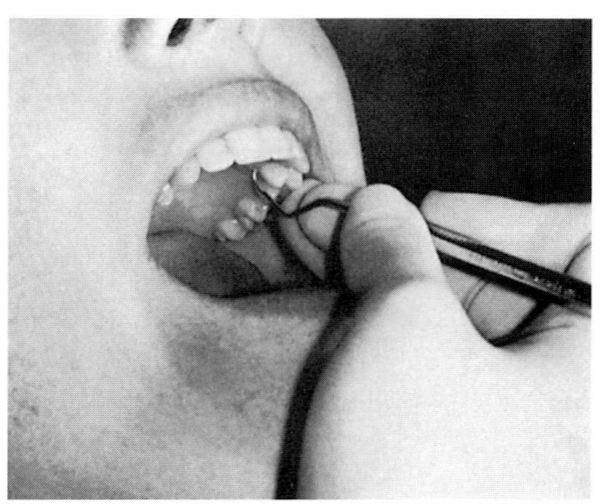

Fig. 47-15 Maxillary left posterior sextant: lingual aspect.

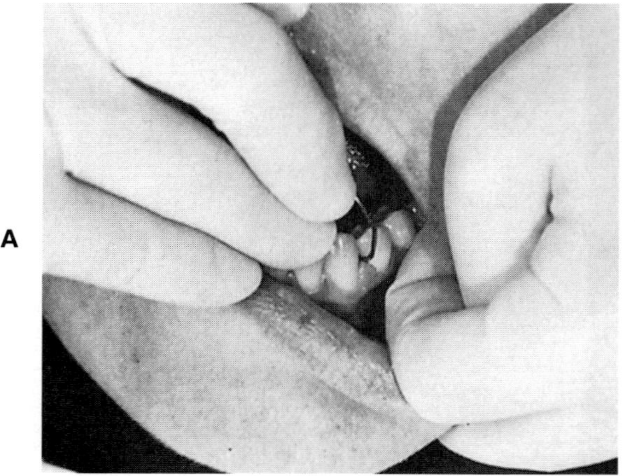

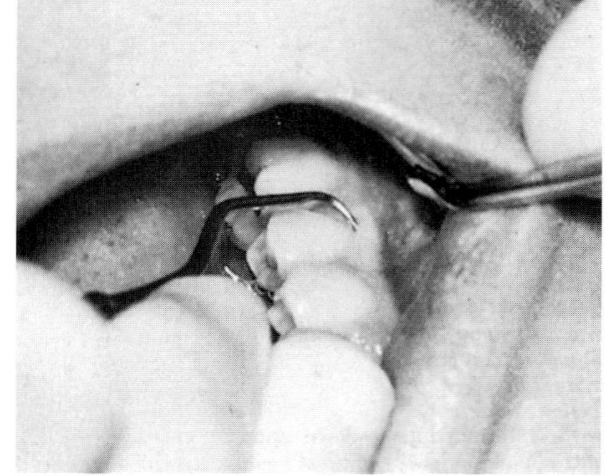

Fig. 47-16 Mandibular left posterior sextant: facial aspect.

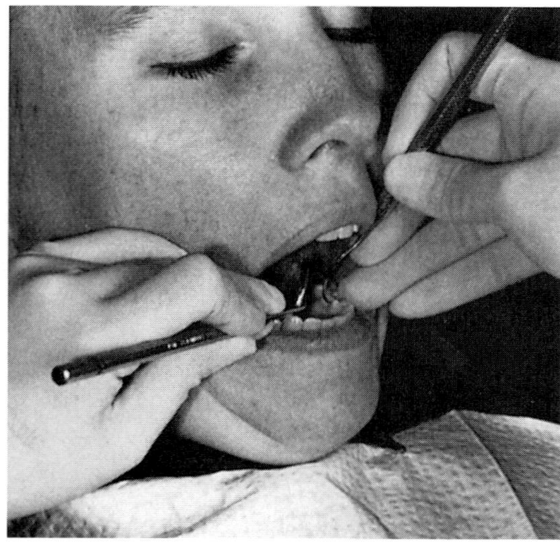

Fig. 47-17 Mandibular left posterior sextant: lingual aspect.

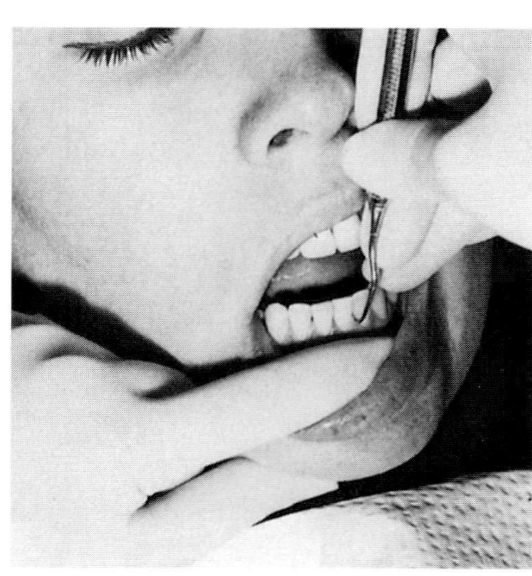

Fig. 47-18 Mandibular anterior sextant: facial aspect, surfaces toward the operator.

Visibility: Direct.
Retraction: None.
Finger rest: Intraoral, palm down, opposite arch, reinforced. Fourth finger on the incisal edges of the mandibular anterior teeth or the facial surfaces of the mandibular premolars, reinforced with the index finger of the nonoperating hand.

Maxillary left posterior sextant: lingual aspect (Fig. 47-14).
Operator position: Front position.
Illumination: Direct and indirect.
Visibility: Direct and indirect.
Retraction: None.
Finger rest: Extraoral, palm down. Front surfaces of the middle and fourth fingers on the lateral aspect of the mandible on the left side of the face. The nonoperating hand holds the mirror for indirect illumination.

Maxillary left posterior sextant: lingual aspect (Fig. 47-15).
Operator position: Side or front position.
Illumination: Direct.
Visibility: Direct.
Retraction: None.
Finger rest: Intraoral, palm up. Fourth finger on the occlusal surfaces of adjacent maxillary teeth.

Mandibular left posterior sextant: facial aspect (Fig. 47-16).
Operator position: Side or back position.
Illumination: Direct.
Visibility: Direct or indirect.
Retraction: Index finger or mirror of the nonoperating hand.
Finger rest: Intraoral, palm down. Fourth finger on the incisal edges or the occlusal or facial surfaces of adjacent mandibular teeth.

Mandibular left posterior sextant: lingual aspect (Fig. 47-17).
Operator position: Front or side position.
Illumination: Direct and indirect.
Visibility: Direct.
Retraction: Mirror retracts tongue.
Finger rest: Intraoral, palm down. Fourth finger on the incisal edges or the occlusal surfaces of adjacent mandibular teeth.

Mandibular anterior sextant: facial aspect, surfaces toward the operator (Fig. 47-18).
Operator position: Front position.
Illumination: Direct.
Visibility: Direct.
Retraction: Index finger of the nonoperating hand.
Finger rest: Intraoral, palm down. Fourth finger on the incisal edges or the occlusal surfaces of adjacent mandibular teeth.

Mandibular anterior sextant: facial aspect, surfaces away from the operator (Fig. 47-19).
Operator position: Back position.
Illumination: Direct.
Visibility: Direct.
Retraction: Index finger or thumb of the nonoperating hand.
Finger rest: Intraoral, palm down. Fourth finger on the incisal edges or the occlusal surfaces of adjacent mandibular teeth.

Mandibular anterior sextant: lingual aspect, surfaces away from the operator (Fig. 47-20).
Operator position: Back position.
Illumination: Direct and indirect.
Visibility: Direct and indirect.
Retraction: Mirror retracts tongue.
Finger rest: Intraoral, palm down. Fourth finger on the incisal edges or the occlusal surfaces of adjacent mandibular teeth.

Mandibular anterior sextant: lingual aspect, surfaces toward the operator (Fig. 47-21).
Operator position: Front position.
Illumination: Direct and indirect.
Visibility: Direct and indirect.
Retraction: Mirror retracts tongue.
Finger rest: Intraoral, palm down. Fourth finger on the incisal edges or the occlusal surfaces of adjacent mandibular teeth.

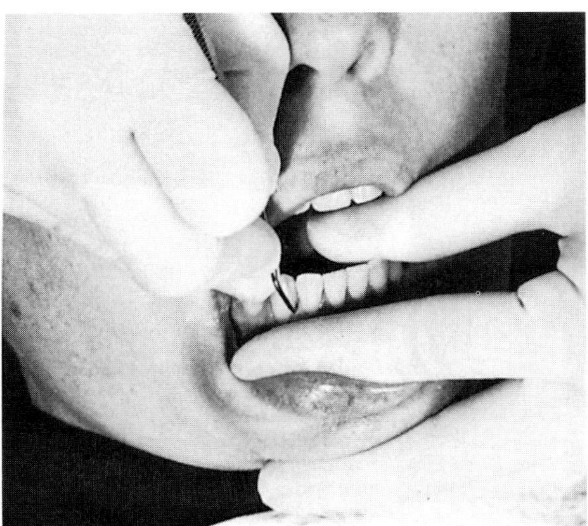

Fig. 47-19 Mandibular anterior sextant: facial aspect, surfaces away from the operator.

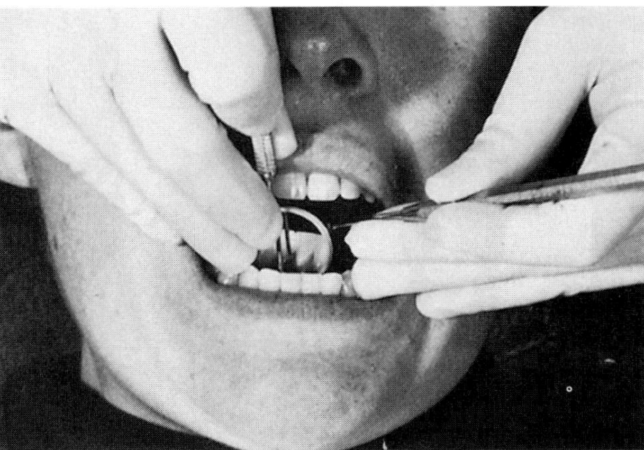

Fig. 47-20 Mandibular anterior sextant: lingual aspect, surfaces away from the operator.

Mandibular right posterior sextant: facial aspect (Fig. 47-22).
Operator position: Side or front position.
Illumination: Direct.
Visibility: Direct.
Retraction: Mirror or index finger of the nonoperating hand.
Finger rest: Intraoral, palm down. Fourth finger on the incisal edges or the occlusal surfaces of adjacent mandibular teeth.

Mandibular right posterior sextant: lingual aspect (Fig. 47-23).
Operator position: Front position.
Illumination: Direct and indirect.
Visibility: Direct and indirect.
Retraction: Mirror retracts tongue.
Finger rest: Intraoral, palm down. Fourth finger on the incisal edges or the occlusal surfaces of adjacent mandibular teeth.

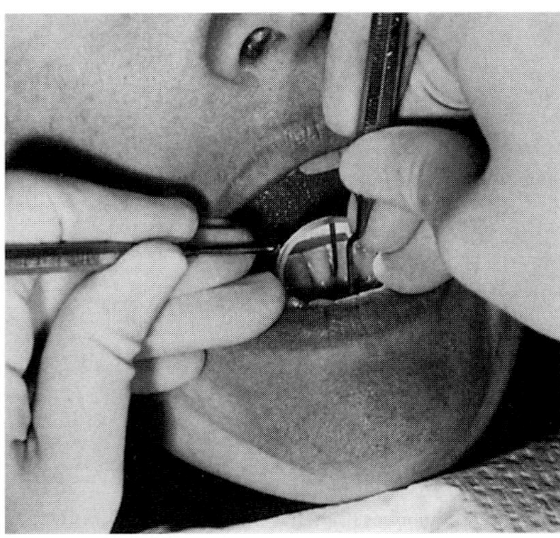

Fig. 47-21 Mandibular anterior sextant: lingual aspect, surfaces toward the operator.

Ultrasonic Scaling

Ultrasonic Scaling Instruments. Ultrasonic instruments have been used as a valuable adjunct to conventional hand instrumentation for many years. Until relatively recently, all ultrasonic tips were large and bulky, making them generally suitable only for supragingival scaling or subgingival scaling where tissue was inflamed and retractable. However, newly designed, thin ultrasonic tips have allowed better access to subgingival areas previously accessible only with hand instruments.[20] It is important to understand this historical perspective when attempting to interpret the literature comparing the effects of hand and ultrasonic instruments on root surfaces. Earlier studies using older tip designs generally showed that ultrasonic instruments left a rougher, more damaged surface than curettes.[4,22,35,36,51,53,114,119,126] More recent studies, especially those using the newer, thinner tips, show that ultrasonic instruments can produce root surfaces as smooth or smoother than can be produced by curettes.[30,31,34,98] Whether these relative degrees of smoothness are important has not been clearly established.[35,45,54,61,81,107] It is evident, however, that both methods of instrumentation are able to provide satisfactory clinical results as measured by removal of plaque and calculus, reduction of bacteria, reduction of inflammation and pocket depth, and gain in clinical attachment.[6–10,28,37,65,83,92,114,117] Ultrasonic instruments have been shown to be more effective than hand instruments at reducing spirochetes and motile rods in class II and III furcations.[62] Recently, two in vitro studies found that ultrasonic and sonic scalers do not kill periodontopathic bacteria by vibrational energy but rather suggest an antimicrobial effect from an increase in temperature.[82,106] Other in vitro studies found that Gracey Curvette curets were more effective than slim ultrasonic inserts in de-

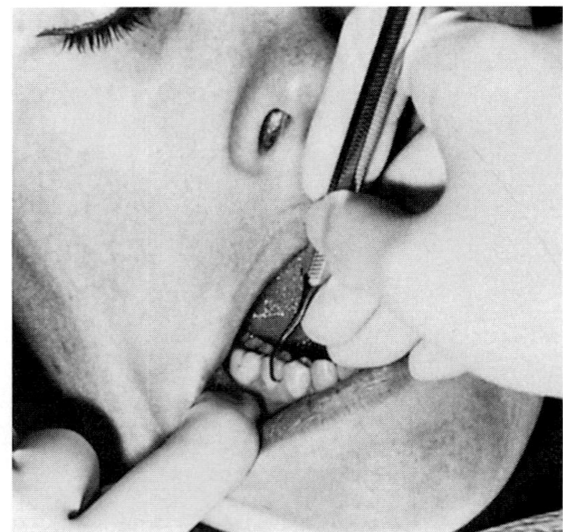

Fig. 47-22 Mandibular right posterior sextant: facial aspect.

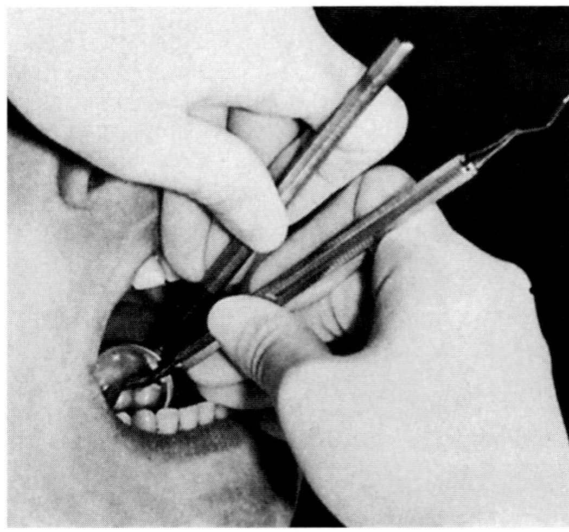

Fig. 47-23 Mandibular right posterior sextant: lingual aspect.

briding root trunks, furcation entrances, and furcation areas of mandibular first molars.[86,87]

The selection of either ultrasonic or hand instrumentation should be determined by the clinician's preference and experience and the needs of each patient. The success of either treatment method is determined by the time devoted to the procedure and the thoroughness of root debridement. In practice, clinicians commonly use a combination of both ultrasonic and hand instrumentation to achieve thorough debridement.

The vibrational energy produced by the ultrasonic instrument makes it useful for removing heavy, tenacious deposits of calculus and stain. Such deposits can be removed more quickly and with less effort ultrasonically than manually. When ultrasonic instruments are properly manipulated, less tissue trauma and therefore less postoperative discomfort occur. This makes ultrasonic instrumentation useful for initial debridement in patients with acute painful conditions such as necrotizing ulcerative gingivitis. This same quality can be used to advantage with the new, thin ultrasonic tips for subgingival root debridement and deplaquing in maintenance patients with residual pocket depth. Ultrasonic scaling devices also have been used for gingival curettage and to remove overhangs and excess cement after cementing orthodontic appliances. Opinions differ regarding the effectiveness of ultrasonic instruments for removing stain compared with conventional polishing methods.[5,16]

Some definite contraindications to the use of ultrasonic and sonic scaling devices exist. No one with a cardiac pacemaker should be exposed to ultrasonic instruments.[70] Patients with known communicable diseases that can be transmitted by aerosols should not be treated with ultrasonic or sonic scaling devices. The water spray creates a contaminated aerosol that fills the operating area, exposing personnel and surfaces.[58,78] Even when treating patients without known communicable diseases, it is especially important that proper infection control measures be observed (i.e., use of protective clothing, eyewear, masks, and gloves) and proper surface decontamination be performed afterward. Prerinsing for 1 minute with an antimicrobial mouthwash such as 0.12% chlorhexidine significantly reduces the number of bacteria in the aerosol for approximately 1 hour.[121] Patients at risk for respiratory disease should not be treated with ultrasonic or sonic devices; these include patients who are immunosuppressed or suffer from chronic pulmonary disorders.[109,115] Finally, metal ultrasonic and sonic inserts are contraindicated for titanium implants, which can be etched or gouged, and for porcelain or bonded restorations, which can be fractured or removed.[15,29,59,96,122] Plastic-tipped ultrasonic and sonic inserts that do not cause damage to titanium implants are available.[57] Also, Teflon-coated sonic scaler tips have been developed for titanium implants and for deplaqueing and subgingival polishing of root surfaces.[55,56,102]

Ultrasonic Scaling Technique. Ultrasonic instrumentation is accomplished with a light touch and light pressure, keeping the tip parallel to the tooth surface and constantly in motion.[31,45,91] Leaving the tip in one place for too long or using the point of the tip against the tooth can produce gouging and roughening of the root surface or overheating of the tooth.[30] Using a lower-power setting and applying only slight pressure reduces the volume and depth of tooth structure removal.[22,91] The working end of the ultrasonic instrument must come in contact with the calculus deposit to fracture and remove it. As with hand instruments, instrument adaptation to the tooth is critical to success. The working tip must contact all aspects of the root surface to thoroughly remove plaque and toxins. Although as much as 10 mm or more of the length of the ultrasonic tip vibrates, only a small portion of it can be adapted to contact the curved root surface at any one time or point. As with hand instruments, a series of rapid, overlapping strokes must be activated to ensure complete root coverage.[45] However, these rapid, light strokes with a blunt, vibrating working end impair tactile sensitivity, and the constant water spray necessary for the operation of the instrument hampers visibility. For these reasons, during ultrasonic instrumentation, the tooth surface should be frequently examined with an explorer to evaluate the completeness of debridement.

The aerosol produced by sonic and ultrasonic instrumentation may contain potentially infectious bloodborne and airborne pathogens.[5,38–40,46,58,72,73,99,118] Pneumococci, staphylococci, alpha hemolytic streptococci, and *Mycobacterium tuberculosis* are among the bacteria that have been found in dental aerosols.[50,63] Aerosols also subject dental personnel and patients to many viruses including herpes simplex virus, hepatitis virus, influenza virus, common cold viruses, Epstein-Barr virus, and cytomegalovirus.[20–26,69,116] Of additional concern are pathogens that do not originate from patients but are from the contaminated waterlines of the dental unit or the ultrasonic device.[27,33,88] Putative pathogens such as *Pseudomonas* sp. and *Legionella pneumophilia* have been isolated from dental unit water and can become aerosolized by an ultrasonic scaler.[27,33,38,84] Aerosol from ultrasonic instrumentation always contains blood[11,71] and lingers in the air for 30 minutes or longer in the entire operatory and in areas of the dental office outside the operatory.[58,60,72,73] Unprotected patients may be more susceptible to infection from the aerosol than dental personnel who are wearing protective barriers such as masks, gloves, eyewear and clinical clothing.[13,20,109] High-speed evacuation, preprocedural rinsing with chlorhexidine, flushing of the handpiece and waterlines or a self-contained sterile water source, thorough disinfection of environmental surfaces, and adequate ventilation and air filtration units with HEPA (High Efficiency Particulate Air) filters (Honeywell Environmental Air Control Inc., Hagerstown, MD) are all important precautions to minimize the potential hazards of ultrasonic aerosols.[41–43,101]

With these points in mind, the ultrasonic device is used in the following manner:

1. Thoroughly wipe the ultrasonic unit with a disinfectant. Use a sterile, autoclavable ultrasonic handpiece or wipe the handpiece with disinfectant. Cover the ultrasonic unit or control knobs and the handpiece with plastic or latex barriers. Flush the waterlines and handpiece for 2 minutes to decrease the number of microorganisms in the lines.[125] Use waterline filters or sterile water whenever possible.

2. Direct the patient to rinse for 1 minute with an antimicrobial mouthrinse such as 0.12% chlorhexidine to reduce the contaminated aerosol.[121,125]
3. The clinician and the assistant should wear protective eyewear and masks and use high-speed evacuation to minimize inhalation of the contaminated aerosol produced during instrumentation.[41–43]
4. Turn on the unit, select an insert, place it into the handpiece, and then adjust the water control knob to produce a light mist of water at the working tip. Adequate aspiration is necessary to remove this water as it accumulates in the mouth. The power setting should begin on low and be adjusted no higher than necessary to remove calculus. Medium- to high-power settings have been shown to cause damage to roots when the tip is not parallel to the root surface.
5. The instrument is grasped with a light pen or modified pen grasp, and a finger rest or extraoral fulcrum should be established to allow a very light, featherlike touch. Extraoral hand rests should be used for the maxillary teeth. For the mandibular teeth, either intraoral or extraoral fulcrums may be used.
6. Use short, light, vertical, horizontal, or oblique overlapping strokes. Keep the working tip adapted to the tooth surface as it is passed over the deposit. Heavy lateral pressure is unnecessary because the vibrational energy of the instrument dislodges the calculus. However, the working end must touch the deposit for this to occur.
7. The working end should be kept in constant motion, and the tip should be kept parallel to the tooth surface or at no more than a 15-degree angle to avoid etching or grooving the tooth surface.[125]
8. The instrument should be switched off periodically to allow for aspiration of water, and the tooth surface should be examined frequently with an explorer.
9. Any remaining irregularities of the root surface may be removed with sharp standard or mini-bladed curettes if necessary.

Evaluation

The adequacy of scaling and root planing is evaluated when the procedure is performed and again later, after a period of soft tissue healing.

Immediately after instrumentation, the tooth surfaces should be carefully inspected visually with optimal lighting and the aid of a mouth mirror and compressed air; they also should be examined with a fine explorer or probe. Subgingival surfaces should be hard and smooth. Although complete removal of calculus is definitely necessary for the health of the adjacent soft tissue,[123] little documented evidence that root smoothness is necessary is available.[35,37,117] Nevertheless, relative smoothness is still the best immediate clinical indication that calculus has been completely removed.[35]

Although smoothness is the criterion by which scaling and root planing are immediately evaluated, the ultimate evaluation is based on tissue response.[123] Clinical evaluation of the soft tissue response to scaling and root planing, including probing, should not be conducted earlier than 2 weeks postoperatively. Reepithelialization of the wounds created during instrumentation takes 1 to 2 weeks.[112,113] Until then, gingival bleeding on probing can be expected even when calculus has been completely removed because the soft tissue wound is not epithelialized. Any gingival bleeding on probing noted after this interval is more likely to be due to persistent inflammation produced by residual deposits that were not removed during the initial procedure or inadequate plaque control. Positive clinical changes after instrumentation often continue for weeks or months. For this reason, a longer period of evaluation may be indicated before deciding whether to intervene with further instrumentation or surgery.[21]

Occasionally the clinician may find that some slight root roughness remains after scaling and root planing.[53,114,126] If sound principles of instrumentation have been followed, the roughness may not be calculus. Because calculus removal, not root smoothness per se, has been shown to be necessary for tissue health, it might be more prudent in such a case to stop short of perfect smoothness and reevaluate the patient's tissue response after 2 to 4 weeks or longer. This avoids overinstrumentation and removal of excessive root structure in the pursuit of smoothness for its own sake. If the tissue is healthy after an interval of 2 to 4 weeks or longer, no further root planing is necessary. If the tissue is inflamed, the clinician must determine to what extent this is due to plaque accumulation or the presence of residual calculus and to what degree further root planing is necessary.

REFERENCES

1. Adriaens P, Edwards C, DeBoever J, et al: Ultrastructural observations on bacterial invasion in cementum and radicular dentin of periodontally diseased human teeth. J Periodontol 1988; 59:493.
2. Aleo J, DeRenzis F, Farber P: In vitro attachment of human gingival fibroblasts to root surfaces. J Periodontol 1975; 46:639.
3. Aleo J, DeRenzis F, Farber P, et al: The presence and biological activity of cementum-bound endotoxin. J Periodontol 1974; 45:672.
4. Allen EF, Rhoads RH: Effects of high-speed periodontal instruments on tooth surfaces. J Periodontol 1963; 34:352.
5. Ashimoto A, Chen C, Bakker I, et al: Polymerase chain reaction detection of 8 putative periodontal pathogens in subgingival plaque of gingivitis and advanced periodontitis lesions. Oral Microbiol Immunol 1996; 11(4):266.
6. Axelsson P, Lindhe J: Effect of controlled oral hygiene procedures on caries and periodontal disease in adults. Results after 6 years. J Clin Periodontol 1981; 8:239.
7. Baderstein A, Nilveus R, Egelberg J: Effect of nonsurgical periodontal therapy. I. Moderately advanced periodontitis. J Clin Periodontol 1981; 8:57.
8. Baderstein A, Nilveus R, Egelberg J: 4-year observations of basic periodontal therapy. J Clin Periodontol 1987; 14:438.
9. Baderstein A, Nilveus R, Egelberg J: Scores of plaque, bleeding, suppuration, and probing depth to predict probing attachment loss. 5 years of observation following nonsurgical periodontal therapy. J Clin Periodontol 1990; 17:102.
10. Baehni P, Thilo P, Chapuis B, et al: Effects of ultrasonic and sonic scalers on dental plaque microflora in vitro and in vivo. J Clin Periodontol 1992; 19:455.
11. Barnes JB, Harrel SK, Rivera-Hidalgo F: Blood contamination of the aerosols produced by in vivo use of ultrasonic scalers. J Periodontol 1998; 69:434.

12. Barnes JE, Schaffer EM: Subgingival root planing: A comparison using files, hoes, and curets. J Periodontol 1960; 31:300.
13. Basu MK, Browne RM, Potts AJ, et al: A survey of aerosol-related symptoms in dental hygienists. J Soc Occup Med 1988; 38(1–2):23.
14. Becker W, Berg LE, Becker BE: Long-term evaluation of periodontal treatment and maintenance in 95 patients. Int J Periodontics Restorative Dent 1984; 4:54.
15. Bjornson EJ, Collins DE, Engler WO: Surface alteration of composite resins after curette, ultrasonic and sonic instrumentation: An in vitro study. Quintessence Int 1990; 21:381.
16. Burman LR, Alderman NE, Ewen SJ: Clinical application of ultrasonic vibrations for supragingival calculus and stain removal. J Dent Med 1968; 13:156.
17. Canis MF, Kramer GM, Pameijer CM: Calculus attachment. Review of the literature and findings. J Periodontol 1979; 50:406.
18. Checchi L, Pelliccioni GA: Hand versus ultrasonic instrumentation in the removal of endotoxin from root surface in vitro. J Periodontol 1998; 59:398.
19. Cheetham WA, Wilson M, Kieser JB: Root surface debridement—An in vitro assessment. J Clin Periodontol 1988; 15:228.
20. Chen SK, Vesley D, Brosseau LM, et al: Evaluation of single-use masks and respirators for protection of health care workers against mycobacterial aerosols. Am J Infect Control 1994; 22(2):65.
21. Claffey N: Decision making in periodontal therapy: The reevaluation. J Clin Periodontol 1991; 18:364.
22. Clark S, Group H, Mabler D: The effect of ultrasonic instrumentation on root surfaces. J Periodontol 1968; 39:125.
23. Contreras A, Slots J: Active cytomegalovirus infection in human periodontitis. Oral Microbiol Immunol 1998; 13(4):225.
24. Contreras A, Slots J: Herpesviruses in human periodontal disease. J Periodontal Res 2000; 35(1):3.
25. Contreras A, Slots J: Mammalian viruses in human periodontitis. Oral Microbiol Immunol 1996; 11(6):381.
26. Contreras A, Umeda M, Chen C, et al: Relationship between herpesviruses and adult periodontitis and periodontopathic bacteria. J Periodontol 1999; 70(5):478.
27. Council on Dental Materials, Instruments and Equipment, American Dental Association: Dental units and water retraction. J Am Dent Assoc 1988; 16:417.
28. Copulos TA, Low SB, Walker CB, et al: Comparative analysis between a modified ultrasonic tip and hand instruments on clinical parameters of periodontal disease. J Periodontol 1993; 64:694.
29. Cutler BJ, Goldstein GR, Simonelli G: The effect of dental prophylaxis instruments on the surface roughness of metals used for metal ceramic crowns. J Prosthet Dent 1995; 73:219.
30. Dragoo MR: A clinical evaluation of hand and ultrasonic instruments on subgingival debridement. Part I. With unmodified and modified ultrasonic inserts. Int J Periodontol 1992; 12:311.
31. Drisko CL: Scaling and root planing without overinstrumentation: Hand versus power-driven scalers. Curr Opin Periodontol 1993; 3:78.
32. Drisko CL, Cochran DL, Blieden T, et al: Position paper: sonic and ultrasonic scalers in periodontics. Research, Science and Therapy Committee of the American Academy of Periodontology. J Periodontol 2000; 71(11):1792.
33. Fitzgibbon EJ, Bartzokas CA, Martin MV, et al: The source, frequency and extent of bacterial contamination of dental unit water systems. Br Dent J 1984; 157:98.
34. Garnick JJ, Dent J: A scanning electron micrographical study of root surfaces and subgingival bacteria after hand scaling and ultrasonic instrumentation. J Periodontol 1989; 60:441.
35. Garrett JS: Effects of nonsurgical periodontal therapy on periodontitis in humans. A review. J Clin Periodontol 1983; 10:515.
36. Green E, Ramfjord SR: Tooth roughness after subgingival root planing. J Periodontol 1966; 37:396.
37. Greenstein G: Nonsurgical periodontal therapy in 2000: A literature review. J Am Dent Assoc 2000; 131(111):1580.
38. Gross A, Devine MJ, Cutright DE: Microbial contamination of dental units and ultrasonic scalers. J Periodontol 1976; 47:670.
39. Gross KB, Overman PR, Cobb C, et al: Aerosol generation by two ultrasonic scalers and one sonic scaler. A comparative study. J Dent Hyg 1992; 66:314.
40. Haffajee AD, Socransky SS: Microbial etiological agents of destructive periodontal diseases. Periodontol 2000 1994; 5:78.
41. Hannan MM, Azadian BS, Gazzard BG, et al: Hospital infection control in an era of HIV infection and multi-drug resistant tuberculosis. J Hosp Infect 2000; 44(1):5.
42. Harrel SK, Barnes JB, Rivera-Hidalgo F: Reduction of aerosols produced by ultrasonic scalers. J Periodontol 1996; 67:28.
43. Harrel SK, Barnes JB, Rivera-Hidalgo F: Aerosol and splatter contamination from the operative site during ultrasonic scaling. J Am Dent Assoc 1998; 129(9):1241.
44. Hatfield CG, Baumhammers A: Cytotoxic effects of periodontally involved surfaces of human teeth. Arch Oral Biol 1971; 16:465.
45. Holbrook T, Low S: Power-driven scaling and polishing instruments. Clin Dent 1989; 3:1.
46. Holbrook WP, Muir KF, MacPhee IT, et al: Bacteriological investigation of the aerosol from ultrasonic scalers. Br Dent J 1978; 144:245.
47. Hughes FJ, Auger DW, Smales FC: Investigation of the distribution of cementum-associated lipopolysaccharides in periodontal disease with scanning electron microscope immunohistochemistry. J Periodont Res 1988; 23:100.
48. Hughes FJ, Smales FC: Immunohistochemical investigation of the presence and distribution of cementum-associated lipopolysaccharides in periodontal disease. J Periodont Res 1986; 21:660.
49. Hughes TP, Caffesse RG: Gingival changes following scaling root planing and oral hygiene. A biometric evaluation. J Periodontol 1978: 49:245.
50. Jokit W (ed): Zinsser's Microbiology, ed 20. Norwalk, CT, Appleton & Lange, 1992.
51. Johnson WN, Wilson JR: The application of the ultrasonic dental units to scaling procedures. J Periodontol 1957; 28:264.
52. Kaldahl WB, Kalkwarf KL, Patil KD, et al: Long-term evaluation of periodontal therapy: I. Response to 4 therapeutic modalities. J Periodontol 1996; 67:93.
53. Kerry GJ: Roughness of root surfaces after use of ultrasonic instruments and hand curets. J Periodontol 1967; 38:340.
54. Khatiblou FA, Ghodssi A: Root surface smoothness or roughness in periodontal treatment. A clinical study. J Peridontol 1983; 54(6):365.
55. Kocher T, Konig J, Hansen P, et al: Subgingival polishing compared to scaling with steel curettes: a clinical pilot study. J Clin Periodontol 2001; 28(2):194.
56. Kocher T, Langenbeck M, Ruhling A, et al: Subgingival polishing with a Teflon-coated sonic scaler insert in comparison to conventional instruments as assessed on extracted teeth. (I) Residual deposits. J Clin Periodontol 2000; 27(4):243.

57. Kwan J, Zablotsky MH, Meffert RM: Implant maintenance using a modified ultrasonic instrument. J Dent Hyg 1990; 64:422.
58. Larato DC, Ruskin PF, Martin A: Effect of an ultrasonic scaler on bacterial counts in air. J Periodontol 1967; 38:550.
59. Lee S-Y, Lai Y-L, Morgano SM: Effects of ultrasonic scaling and periodontal curettage on surface roughness of porcelain. J Prothet Dent 1995; 73:227.
60. Legnani P, Checchi L, Pelliccioni GA, et al: Atmospheric contamination during dental procedures. Quintessence Int 1994; 25(6):435.
61. Leknes KN, Lie T, Wikesjo UM, et al: Influence of tooth instrumentation roughness on subgingival microbial colonization. J Periodontol 1994; 65(4):303.
62. Leon LE, Vogel RI: A comparison of the effectiveness of hand scaling and ultrasonic debridement in furcations as evaluated by differential dark-field microscopy. J Periodontol 1987; 58:86.
63. Lever MS, Williams A, Bennett AM: Survival of mycobacterial species in aerosols generated from artificial saliva. Lett Appl Microbiol 2000; 31(3):238.
64. Lindhe J, Nyman S: Long-term maintenance of patients treated for advanced periodontal disease. J Clin Periodontol 1984; 11:504.
65. Lindhe J, Nyman S, Karring T: Scaling and root planing in shallow pockets. J Clin Periodontol 1982; 9:415.
66. Listgarten MA, Lindhe J, Hellden L: Effect of tetracycline and/or scaling on human periodontal disease. Clinical microbiological and histological observations. J Clin Periodontol 1978; 5:246.
67. Lowenguth RA, Greenstein G: Clinical and microbiological response to nonsurgical mechanical periodontal therapy. Periodontol 2000 1995; 9:14.
68. Magnusson I, Lindhe J, Yoneyama T, et al: Recolonization of a subgingival microbiota following scaling in deep pockets. J Clin Periodontol 1984; 11:193.
69. Michalowicz BS, Ronderos M, Camara-Silva R, et al: Human herpesviruses and *Porphyromonas gingivalis* are associated with juvenile periodontitis. J Periodontol 2000; 71(6):981.
70. Miller CS, Leonelli FM, Latham E: Selective interference with pacemaker activity by electrical dental devices. Oral Surg Oral Med Oral Pathol Oral Radiol Endod 1998; 85:33.
71. Miller RL: Characteristics of blood-containing aerosols generated by common powered dental instruments. Am Ind Hyg Assoc J 1995; 56(7):670.
72. Miller RL, Micik RE: Air pollution and its control in the dental office. Dent Clin North Am 1978; 22:453.
73. Miller RL, Micik RE, Abel C, et al: Studies on dental aerobiology: II. Microbial splatter discharged from the oral cavity of dental patients. J Dent Res 1971; 50:621.
74. Mongardini C, Van Steenberghe D, Dekeyser C, et al: One stage full- versus partial-mouth disinfection in the treatment of chronic adult or generalized early-onset periodontitis. I. Long-term clinical observations. J Periodontol 1999; 70(6):632.
75. Moore J, Wilson M, Kieser JB: The distribution of bacterial lipopolysaccharide (endotoxin) in relation to periodontally involved root surfaces, J Clin Periodontol 1986; 13:748.
76. Moskow BS: Calculus attachment in cemental separations. J Periodontol 1969; 40:125.
77. Mousques T, Listgarten MA, Phillips RW: Effect of scaling and root planing on the composition of human subgingival microbial flora. J Periodont Res 1980; 7:199.
78. Muir KF, Ross PW, MacPhee IT, et al: Reduction of microbial contamination from ultrasonic scalers. Br Dent J 1978; 145:760.
79. Nakib NM, Bissada NF, Simmelink JW, et al: Endotoxin penetration into root cementum of periodontally healthy and diseased human teeth. J Periodontol 1982; 53:368.
80. Nyman S, Westfelt E, Sarhed G, et al: Role of "diseased" root cementum in healing following treatment of periodontal disease: A clinical study. J Clin Periodontol 1988; 15:464.
81. Oberholzer R, Rateitschak KH: Root cleaning or root smoothing. An in vivo study. J Clin Periodontol 1996; 23(4):326.
82. O'Leary R, Sved AM, Davies EH, et al: The bactericidal effects of dental ultrasound on *Actinobacillus actinomycetemcomitans* and *Porphyromonas gingivalis*. An in vitro investigation. J Clin Periodontol 1997; 24(6):432.
83. Oosterwall PJ, Matee MI, Mikx FHM, et al: The effect of subgingival debridement with hand and ultrasonic instruments on subgingival microflora. J Clin Periodontol 1987; 14:528.
84. Oppenheim BA, Sefton AM, Gill ON, et al: Widespread *Legionella pneumophila* contamination of dental stations in a dental school without apparent human infection. Epidemiol Infect 1987; 99(1):159.
85. Orban B, Manella V: Macroscopic and microscopic study of instruments designed for root planing. J Periodontol 1956; 27:120.
86. Otero-Cagide FJ, Long BA: Comparative in vitro effectiveness of closed root debridement with fine instruments on specific areas of mandibular first molar furcations. I. Root trunk and furcation entrance. J Periodontol 1997; 68(11):1093.
87. Otero-Cagide FJ, Long BA: Comparative in vitro effectiveness of closed root debridement with fine instruments on specific areas of mandibular first molar furcations. I. Furcation area. J Periodontol 1997; 68(11):1098.
88. Pankhurst CL, Johnson NW, Woods RG: Microbial contamination of dental unit waterlines: The scientific argument. Int Dent J 1998; 48(4):359.
89. Parr R, Green E, Madsen L, et al: Subgingival Scaling and Root Planing. Berkeley, CA, Praxis Publishing, 1976.
90. Pattison AM: The use of hand instruments in supportive periodontal treatment. Periodontol 2000 1996; 12:71.
91. Petersilka GJ, Flemmig TF, Mehl A, et al: Comparison of root substance removal by magnetostrictive and piezoelectric ultrasonic and sonic scalers in vitro. J Clin Periodontol 1997; 24:864.
92. Pihlstrom BL, McHugh RB, Oliphant TH, et al: Comparison of surgical and nonsurgical treatment of periodontal disease. A review of current studies and additional results after $6\frac{1}{2}$ years. J Clin Periodontol 1983; 10:524.
93. Proye M, Caton J, Polson A: Initial healing of periodontal pockets after a single episode of root planing monitored by controlled probing force. J Periodontol 1982; 53:296.
94. Quirynen M, Mongardini C, de Soete M, et al: The role of chlorhexidine in the one-stage full-mouth disinfection treatment of patients with advanced adult periodontitis. Long-term clinical and microbiological observations. J Clin Periodontol 2000; 27(8):578.
95. Quirynen M, Mongardini C, Pauwels M, et al: One stage full- versus partial-mouth disinfection in the treatment of chronic adult or generalized early-onset periodontitis. II. Long-term impact on microbial load. J Periodontol 1999; 70(6):646.
96. Rajstein J, Tal M: The effects of ultrasonic scaling on the surface of Class V amalgam restorations—A scanning electron microscope study. J Oral Rehabil 1984; 11:299.
97. Renvert S, Wikström M, Dahlén G, et al: Effect of root debridement on the elimination of *Actinobacillus actinomycetemcomitans* and *Bacteroides gingivalis* from periodontal pockets. J Clin Periodontol 1990; 17:345.
98. Ritz L, Hefti AF, Rateitschak KH: An in vitro investigation on the loss of root substance in scaling with various instruments. J Clin Peridontol 1991; 18:643.

99. Rivera-Hidalgo F, Barnes JB, Harrel SK: Aerosol and splatter production by focused spray and standard ultrasonic inserts. J Periodontol 1999; 70:473.
100. Rosenberg ES, Evian CI, Listgarten M: The composition of the subgingival microbiota after periodontal therapy. J Periodontol 1981; 52:435.
101. Rutala WA, Jones SM, Worthington JM, et al: Efficacy of portable filtration units in reducing aerosolized particles in the size range of *Mycobacterium tuberculosis*. Infect Control Hosp Epidemiol 1995; 16(7):391.
102. Ruhling, A, Kocher T, Kreusch J, et al: Treatment of subgingival implant surfaces with Teflon-coated sonic and ultrasonic scaler tips and various implant curettes. An in vitro study. Clin Oral Implants Res 1994; 5(1):19.
103. Sbordone L, Ramaglia L, Guletta E, et al: Recolonization of the subgingival microflora after scaling and root planing in human periodontitis. J Periodontol 1990; 61:579.
104. Schaffer EM: Histologic results of root curettage on human teeth. J Periodontol 1956; 27:269.
105. Selvig KA: Attachment of plaque and calculus to tooth surfaces. J Periodont Res 1970; 5:8.
106. Schenk G, Flemmig TF, Lob S, et al: Lack of antimicrobial effect on periodontopathic bacteria by ultrasonic and sonic scalers in vitro. J Clin Periodontol 2000; 27(2):116.
107. Schlageter L, Rateitschak-Pluss EM, Schwarz JP: Root surface smoothness or roughness following open debridement. An in vivo study. J Clin Periodontol 1996; 23(5):460.
108. Shiloah J, Patters M: Repopulation of periodontal pockets by microbial pathogens in the absence of supportive therapy. J Peridontol 1996; 67:130.
109. Shreve WB, Hoerman KC, Trautwein CA: Illness in patients following exposure to dental aerosols. J Public Health Dent 1972; 32(1):34.
110. Slots J, Mashimo P, Levine MJ, et al: Periodontal therapy in humans. I. Microbiological and clinical effects of a single course of periodontal scaling and root planing, and of adjunctive tetracycline therapy. J Periodontol 1979; 50:495.
111. Smart GJ, Wilson M, Davis EH, et al: The assessment of ultrasonic root surface debridement by determination of residual endotoxin levels. J Clin Periodontol 1990; 17:174.
112. Stahl SS, Slavkin HC, Yamada L, et al: Speculations about gingival repair. J Periodontol 1972; 43:395.
113. Stahl SS, Weiner JM, Benjamin S, et al: Soft tissue healing following curettage and root planing. J Periodontol 1971; 42:678.
114. Stende GW, Schaffer EM: A comparison of ultrasonic and hand scaling. J Periodontol 1961; 32:312.
115. Suzuki JB, Delisle AL: Pulmonary *Actinomycosis* of periodontal origin. J Periodontol 1984; 55:581.
116. Ting M, Contreras A, Slots J: Herpesvirus in localized juvenile periodontitis. J Periodontal Res 2000; 35(1):17.
117. Torfason T, Kiger R, Selvig KA, et al: Clinical improvement of gingival conditions following ultrasonic versus hand instrumentation of periodontal pockets. J Clin Periodontol 1979; 6:165.
118. Umeda M, Contreras A, Chen C, et al: The utility of whole saliva to detect the oral presence of periodontopathic bacteria. J Periodontol 1998; 69(7):828.
119. Van Volkinburg J, Green E, Armitage G: The nature of root surfaces after curette, cavitron, and alpha-sonic instrumentation. J Periodont Res 1976; 11:374.
120. van Winkelhoff AJ, van der Velden U, de Graaff J: Microbial succession in recolonizing deep periodontal pockets after a single course of supra- and subgingival debridement. J Clin Periodontol 1988; 15:116.
121. Veksler AE, Kayrouz GA, Newman MG: Reduction of salivary bacteria by pre-procedural rinses with chlorhexidine 0.12%. J Periodontol 1991; 62:649.
122. Vermilyea SG, Prasanna MK, Agar JR: Effect of ultrasonic cleaning and air polishing on porcelain labial margin restorations. J Prosthet Dent 1994; 71:447.
123. Waerhaug J: Healing of the dentoepithelial junction following subgingival plaque control. J Periodontol 1978; 49:1.
124. Westfelt E, Nyman S, Socransky SS, et al: Significance of frequency of professional tooth cleaning following periodontal surgery. J Clin Periodontol 1983; 10:148.
125. Wilkins EM: Clinical Practice of the Dental Hygienist, ed 7. Philadelphia, Williams & Wilkins, 1994.
126. Wilkinson RF, Maybury J: Scanning electron microscopy of the root surface following instrumentation. J Periodontol 1973; 44:559.
127. Ximenez-Fyvie LA, Haffajee AD, Socransky SS: Comparison of the microbiota of supra- and subgingival plaque in health and periodontitis. J Clin Periodontol 2000; 27(9):648.
128. Zander HA: The attachment of calculus to root surfaces. J Periodontol 1953; 24:16.

Phase I Periodontal Therapy

Dorothy A. Perry and Max O. Schmid

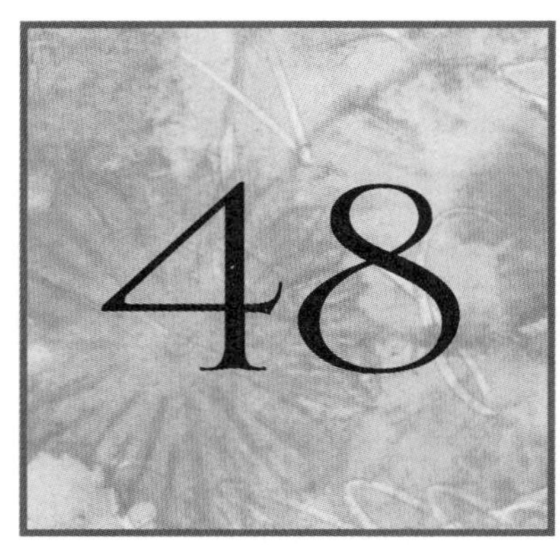

CHAPTER

CHAPTER OUTLINE

Phase I therapy is the first step in the chronologic sequence of procedures that constitute periodontal treatment. The objective of Phase I therapy is to alter or eliminate the microbial etiology and contributing factors for gingival and periodontal diseases. The result is the arresting of the progression of disease and preservation of the dentition in a state of health, comfort, and function with appropriate esthetics.[1] Phase I therapy is referred to by a number of names, including *initial therapy*,[1] *nonsurgical periodontal therapy*,[12] *cause-related therapy*,[8] and the *etiotropic phase of therapy*.[16] All terms refer to the procedures performed to treat gingival and periodontal infections, up to and including tissue reevaluation.

RATIONALE

The reduction and elimination of etiologic and contributing factors in periodontal treatment is achieved by complete removal of calculus, correction of defective restorations, treatment of carious lesions, and institution of a comprehensive daily plaque control regimen.[3,5,7,9,14] The initial phase of therapy is provided to all patients with periodontal pockets who later will be evaluated for surgical intervention and those with gingivitis or mild chronic periodontitis who are unlikely to need surgical treatment. The procedures included in Phase I therapy may be the only procedures required to solve the patient's periodontal problems, or they may constitute the preparatory phase for surgical therapy. Color Fig. 48-1 shows the results of Phase I therapy for two different periodontal patients.

Phase I therapy is a critical aspect of periodontal treatment. Data from clinical research indicate that the long-term success of periodontal treatment depends predominantly on maintaining the results achieved with Phase I therapy and much less on any specific surgical procedures. In addition, Phase I therapy provides an opportunity for the dentist to evaluate tissue response and the patient's attitude toward periodontal care, both of which are crucial to the overall success of treatment.

Phase I therapy has many specific goals that go well beyond the control of inflammation and pocket reduction by mechanical means. The American Academy of Periodontology has included the following aspects in the Parameters of Care for Phase I Therapy[1]:

1. Evaluation and alteration of patient systemic risk factors. These include, among others, systemic diseases and conditions, smoking, substance abuse, and use of medications. Consultation with the patient's physician may be a necessary part of Phase I therapy.
2. Plaque control performed by the patient (see Chapter 49).
3. Removal of microbial plaque and calculus from the surfaces of the teeth (see Chapters 42 and 43).
4. Appropriate use of antimicrobial agents and devices including necessary plaque sampling and antibiotic sensitivity testing (see Chapters 44 and 50).

5. Control or elimination of contributing local factors including the following:
   A. Treatment of poorly fitting restorations
   B. Correction of poorly fitting prosthetic devices
   C. Restoration of carious lesions
   D. Odontoplasty
   E. Tooth movement
   F. Treatment of food impaction areas
   G. Treatment of occlusal trauma
   H. Extraction of hopeless teeth

Based on the knowledge that microbial plaque harbors the primary pathogens of gingival inflammation, the specific aim of Phase I therapy for every patient is effective plaque control. This is accomplished by establishing an effective daily plaque control regimen for the patient, removing calculus, and eliminating rough and irregular tooth surfaces, including treating carious lesions. Effective plaque control is the key objective of every therapeutic periodontal procedure, but it is best accomplished if tooth surfaces are free of rough deposits and irregular contours so that they are readily accessible to oral hygiene aids.

Caries control and treatment of active carious lesions is an often-overlooked aspect of Phase I therapy. Caries is now recognized as an infection.[2] As such, carious must be temporized, with removal of the infectious process and improved tooth contours established to maximize the healing achieved during the scaling and root planing treatment. Frank carious lesions, particularly Class V lesions in the cervical areas of teeth and those on root surfaces, provide a reservoir for bacteria and can contribute to the repopulation of the periodontal plaque. The cavities themselves are receptacles where plaque is sheltered from even the most energetic mechanical plaque removal. For these reasons it is imperative that caries control and at least temporization of carious lesions be completed during Phase I therapy.

After careful analysis of the case and diagnosis of the specific periodontal condition presented, the dentist determines the treatment plan for the scaling and root planing portion of Phase I therapy. This is an estimate of the procedures and number of appointments needed to complete the initial phase of therapy after carious lesions are controlled. Patients with small amounts of calculus and relatively healthy tissues can be treated in one appointment. Most patients require several treatment sessions to complete debridement of tooth surfaces. The dentist should estimate the number of appointments needed on the basis of the conditions presented by each individual patient. In addition to the number of times the patient must be seen, some consideration should be given to control of infectious organisms during the period of active Phase I treatment. One option for scheduling appointments is one or two longer appointments on consecutive days, while the patient is on an aggressive prescribed regimen of antimicrobial agents, then follow-up appointments during healing. This treatment sequence has been referred to as anti-infective or disinfection treatment.[10,13] Data from these studies indicated that improvements in probing depths and reduction of periodontal pathogens were somewhat greater for the group using antimicrobial adjuncts. As our understanding of the best use of antimicrobial agents increases, treatment plans undoubtedly will evolve to maximize therapeutic results.

A number of specific conditions need to be considered in formulating the treatment plan for each patient. The individual patient considerations relating to the development of the Phase I therapy treatment plan and sequence include the following[15]:

- General health and tolerance of treatment
- Number of teeth present
- Amount of supragingival calculus
- Amount of subgingival calculus
- Probing pocket depths (amount of attachment loss is less significant than depth of pockets for determining the treatment plan)
- Furcation involvement
- Alignment of teeth
- Margins of restorations
- Developmental anomalies
- Physical barriers to access (i.e., limited opening or tendency to gag)
- Patient cooperation
- Patient sensitivity (requiring use of anesthesia or analgesia)

RESULTS

Phase I therapy is a complex and individualized treatment. It requires detailed analysis of each patient's disease and contributing factors and customized therapy. The treatments common to all Phase I therapy are patient plaque control, caries control, and scaling and root planing to remove supragingival calculus, subgingival calculus, and plaque deposits. Plaque control performed by the patient at home is complex and requires changing lifelong habits. It is difficult to achieve and varies among individual patients, but strategies for success exist. Plaque control education and motivation are presented in Chapter 49.

Scaling and root planing therapy has been studied extensively to evaluate its effects on periodontal disease. A review of studies evaluating the effects of scaling and root planing indicate that the treatment is both effective and reliable.[6] Studies ranging from 1 month to 2 years in length demonstrate up to 80% reductions in bleeding on probing and mean probing depth reductions in the range of 2 to 3 mm. Others have demonstrated that the number of pockets 4 mm in depth or greater was reduced by 52% to 80%. Several of these studies also compared the relative healing result using hand instrumentation and ultrasonic or sonic instruments for scaling and root planing. No difference in healing was identified based on the type of instruments used to provide the treatment.[6] Additional individual treatment such as caries control and correction of ill-fitting restorations only augment the positive results of healing gained through good plaque control and scaling and root planing. Fig. 48-1 shows the effects of an overhanging amalgam restoration on the gingiva. Maximal healing from scaling and root planing is not possible with local

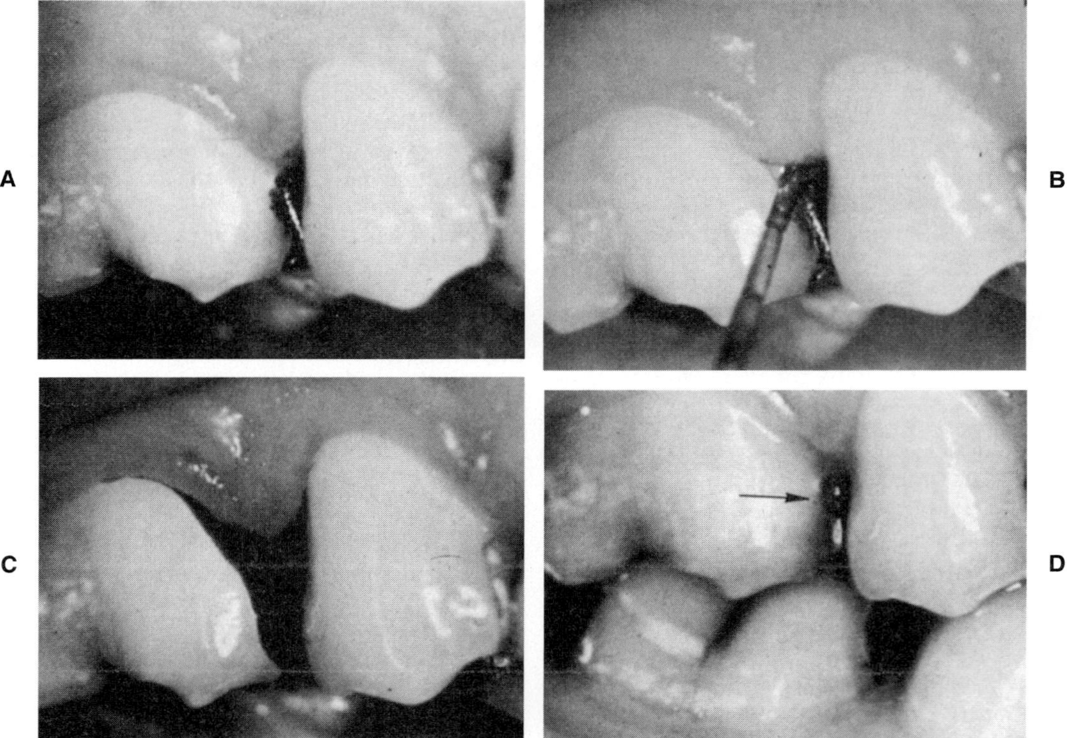

Fig. 48-1 Effect of an overhanging amalgam margin on the interproximal gingiva of a maxillary first molar. **A,** Clinical appearance of rough, irregular, and overcontoured amalgam. **B,** Gentle probing of the interproximal pocket. **C,** Extreme amount of bleeding elicited by gentle probing in the area is indicative of severe inflammation in the area. **D,** Clinical appearance of recontoured restoration *(arrow)*.

conditions that retain plaque and provide reservoirs for repopulation of periodontal pathogens.

REEVALUATION

Reevaluation of the periodontal case should occur about 4 weeks after the completion of the scaling and root planing procedures. This permits time for both epithelial and connective tissue healing, correction of conditions such as overhanging margins, and sufficient practice with oral hygiene skills so that the dentist can accurately assess the periodontal condition at the end of Phase I therapy.

Gingival inflammation is usually substantially reduced or eliminated within 3 to 4 weeks after removal of calculus and local irritants. Healing consists of the formation of a long junctional epithelium rather than new connective tissue attachment to the root surfaces. The attachment epithelium reappears within 1 to 2 weeks. Gradual reductions in inflammatory cell population, crevicular fluid flow, and repair of connective tissue result in reduction of the clinical signs of inflammation, with less redness and swelling.[6]

Transient root hypersensitivity and recession of the gingival margins frequently accompany the healing process. Patients should be warned at the outset of treatment that these results may happen, otherwise it may come as an unpleasant surprise. These unexpected and uncomfortable consequences may result in distrust and loss of motivation to continue therapy, so it is important that patients be educated about the consequences at the outset of treatment.

The periodontal tissues must be carefully reexamined to determine the need for further therapy. Pockets must be reprobed to decide whether surgical intervention in indicated. However, additional improvement through surgery can be expected only if Phase I therapy has been successful. Therefore surgical treatment of periodontal pockets should be attempted only if the patient is exercising effective plaque control and the gingiva is free of overt inflammation.

DECISION TO REFER FOR SPECIALIST TREATMENT

The goal of this textbook is to prepare general dentists to manage most periodontal care required in their practices. The preface to the 8th edition of this textbook states:

> *The periodontal care of the public is primarily the concern of the general dentist, and that the general dentist cannot disregard his or her responsibility to provide periodontal care for all patients. The extremely high incidence of periodontal problems in the population makes it impossible for the small number of specialists*

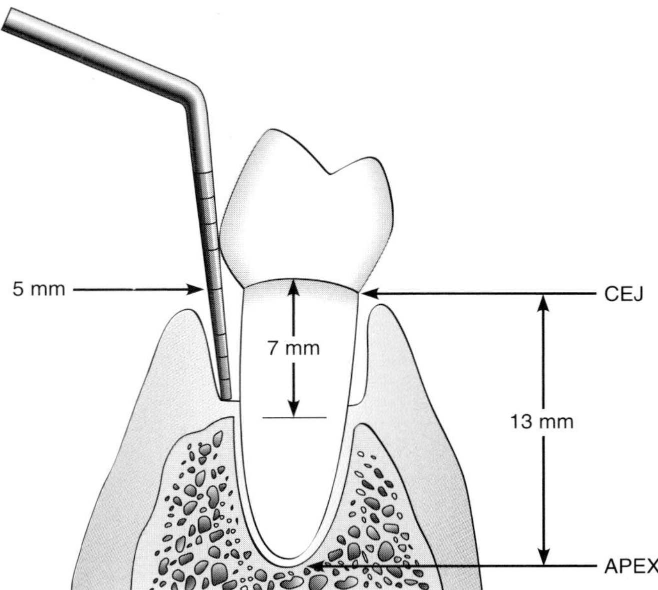

Fig. 48-2 The 5-mm standard for referral to a periodontist is based on root length, probing depth, and attachment loss. The standard serves as a reasonable guideline to trigger further analysis of the case and possible need for specialist care. (Redrawn from Armitage G (ed): Periodontal Maintenance Therapy. Berkeley, CA, Praxis, 1974.)

in periodontics to cope with them; in addition, the close relationship between periodontal and restorative dental therapies makes it very important for the general dentist to have a thorough knowledge of periodontics. A well-trained group of periodontists who specialized in the diagnosis and treatment of severe or unusual problems should serve only to supplement the general dental care available to our population.[4]

The question remains when to refer a patient for specialist periodontal care. With a few patients the disease is so severe or unusual in presentation that referral to a periodontist is obvious. Many cases are treatable in the general dentist's office and likely to heal sufficiently after Phase I therapy so that no further treatment intervention is required beyond routine maintenance. Any patient who does not clearly fall into either category has been called a *candidate for referral*.[11] The 5-mm standard has been proposed as a guideline for referral. If the patient at reevaluation has apical migration of the epithelial attachment, probing depths of greater than 5 mm, or both, then referral should be considered. The 5-mm standard has been suggested because the typical root length is about 13 mm (Fig. 48-2). The probe, when inserted into the 5-mm pocket, rests near the epithelial attachment, which is normally about 1 mm thick. The crest of the bone supporting the tooth would then be 7 mm apical to the cementoenamel junction (CEJ), demonstrating loss of approximately half the bone support for the tooth. Specialist care could help preserve the tooth in this situation by eliminating deep pockets and regenerating support for the tooth.

In addition to the 5-mm standard, other factors must be considered in the decision to refer. These include the following:

1. Extent of disease: The deeper the pockets, the stronger the indication for referral.
2. Root length: Short roots are more seriously jeopardized by 5 mm of clinical attachment loss than long roots.
3. Hypermobility, which suggests a more guarded prognosis.
4. Difficulty of scaling and root planing: The presence of deep pockets and furcations make local treatment much more difficult.
5. Restorative work: Long-term prognosis of the tooth is an important consideration in planning extensive restorative work.
6. Age of the patient: The younger the patient with extensive attachment loss, the more aggressive the disease process is likely to be.
7. Resolution by shrinkage: Some tissue such as thick, fibrotic gingiva do not resolve as well as thinner, edematous gingiva when edema subsides, leaving deeper probing depths.

The success in treating advanced periodontal disease generally occurs in patients with 6- to 8-mm probing depths and/or attachment loss. Specialists have limited success when depths are 9 mm or greater, so early referral of advanced cases is likely to provide the best results. Each patient is unique, and the decision process for each patient is complex. The considerations presented in this section should give the reader some guidance in making referral decisions.

REFERENCES

1. Ad Hoc Committee on the Parameters of Care: Phase I Therapy. American Academy of Peridontology. J Periodontol 2000; 71(suppl):856.
2. Anderson MH, Bales DJ, Omnell K-A: Modern management of dental caires: The cutting edge is not the dental bur. J Amer Dent Assoc 1993; 124:37.
3. Axelsson P, Lindhe J: The effect of a preventive programme on dental plaque, gingivitis and caries in school children. Results after one and two years. J Clin Periodontol 1974; 1:126.
4. Carranza FA, Jr, Newman MG: Preface. In: Carranza FA, Jr, Newman MG (eds): Clinical Periodontology, ed 8. Philadelphia, Saunders, 1996.
5. Chawla TN, Nanda RS, Kapoor KK: Dental prophylaxis procedures in control of periodontal disease in Lucknow (rural). Indian J Periodontol 1975; 46:498.
6. Cobb CM: Non-surgical pocket therapy: Mechanical. Ann Periodontol 1996: 1:443.
7. Lightner LM, O'Leary TJ, Drake RB, et al: Preventive periodontics treatment procedures: Results over 46 months. J Periodontol 1971; 42:555.
8. Lindhe J: Textbook of Clinical Periodontology. Philadelphia, Saunders, 1983.
9. Lindhe J, Kock G: The effect of supervised oral hygiene on the gingiva of children. Progression and inhibition of gingivitis. J Periodont Res 1966; 1:260.

10. Mongardini C, van Steenberghe D, Dekeyser C, et al: One stage full- versus partial-mouth disinfection in the treatment of chronic adult or generalized early-onset periodontitis. I. Long-term clinical observations. J Periodontol 1999; 70:632.
11. Parr RW, Pipe P, Watts T: Shall I refer? In: Armitage G (ed): Periodontal Maintenance Therapy, ed 2. Berkeley, CA, Praxis, 1982.
12. Perry DA, Beemsterboer PB, Taggart EJ: Periodontology for the Dental Hygienist. Philadelphia, Saunders, 2001.
13. Quirynen M, Mongardini C, Pauwels M, et al: One stage full- versus partial-mouth disinfection in the treatment of chronic adult or generalized early-onset periodontitis. II. Long-term impact on microbial load. J Periodontol 1999; 70:646.
14. Suomi JD, Greene JC, Vermillion JR, et al: The effect of controlled oral hygiene procedures on the progression of periodontal disease in adults: Results after third and final year. J Peridontol 1971; 42:152.
15. Treatment planning for the periodontal patient. In: Perry DA, Beemsterboer PB, Taggart EJ: Periodontology for the Dental Hygienist. Philadelphia, Saunders, 2001.
16. Wilkins EM: Clinical Practice of the Dental Hygienist. Philadelphia, Lea & Febiger, 1989.

Plaque Control for the Periodontal Patient

Dorothy A. Perry

CHAPTER

CHAPTER OUTLINE

Plaque control is the removal of dental plaque on a regular basis and the prevention of its accumulation on the teeth and adjacent gingival surfaces. It is a critical component of dental practice, permitting long-term success of periodontal and dental care. This widely held view is reflected in the following policy statement adopted in 1998 European Workshop on Mechanical Plaque Control: "Forty years of experimental research, clinical trials, and demonstration projects in different geographical and social settings have confirmed that effective removal of dental plaque is essential to dental and periodontal health throughout life."[122]

In 1965, Löe and co-workers conducted the classic study demonstrating the relationship between plaque accumulation and the development of experimental gingivitis in humans. Dental plaque was allowed to accumulate in the absence of any plaque control procedures, resulting in the development of gingivitis in all subjects within 7 to 21 days. The composition of bacteria also shifted so that gram-negative organisms predominated in dental plaque associated with gingival inflammation. In addition, it was shown that the gingivitis was reversible. Daily removal of dental plaque led to resolution of the gingival inflammation in just a few days.[103] Good supragingival plaque control has also been shown to retard calculus formation and affect the growth and composition of subgingival plaque.[126] Carefully performed daily home plaque control, combined with frequent professionally delivered plaque removal, has been demonstrated to reduce supragingival plaque, decrease the total number of microorganisms in moderately deep pockets, including furcation areas, and greatly reduce the number of subgingival sites with *Porphyromonas gingivalis*, a significant periodontal pathogen.[74] Thus plaque control is an effective way of treating and preventing gingivitis and is a critical part of all the procedures involved in the treatment and prevention of periodontal diseases.[23]

Although all patients need to adopt good plaque control practices, periodontal patients are considered more "at risk" than the general dental patient population. Their plaque control is critical because they have active infections or have had previously treated disease. In either case, periodontal patients have demonstrated susceptibility to periodontal infections. The tissue destruction they experience creates sites and defects susceptible to further breakdown.[88] The role of other risk factors for periodontal infections, such as smoking, genetic predisposition, or systemic disease, also are very important but not easily quantified. In reality, the control of these other risk factors is often beyond the control of the clinician, requiring the focus on this one well-established etiologic factor, dental plaque. Plaque control and preventive procedures can be relied upon to improve periodontal infections; however, the resolution of disease also depends on the type of periodontal infection and the presence of additional risk factors.[55]

The dental profession relies on mechanical plaque control (i.e., daily cleaning with a toothbrush and other oral hygiene aids) as the most dependable way of achieving oral health benefits for all dental patients including periodontal patients. Plaque growth occurs within hours and must be completely removed at the very least every 48 hours in periodontally healthy subjects to prevent inflammation.[140] Toothbrushing is a completely accepted part of daily life and good oral hygiene practice. However, plaque control by toothbrushing alone is not sufficient to control gingival and periodontal diseases because periodontal lesions are predominantly interdental.[88] It has been demonstrated in healthy subjects that plaque formation begins on the interproximal surfaces where the toothbrush does not reach. Masses of plaque first develop in the molar and premolar areas, followed by the proximal surfaces of the anterior teeth and the facial surfaces of the molars and premolars. Lingual surfaces accumulate the least amount of plaque. In terms of removing plaque, subjects consistently leave more plaque on the posterior teeth than the anterior teeth, and interproximal surfaces retain the highest amounts of plaque.[140] The plaque control efforts of periodontal patients are further complicated by defects in gingival architecture and long, exposed root surfaces.

The optimal frequency for plaque removal by periodontal patients has not been determined, but it is reasonable to expect periodontal patients to completely remove plaque from the teeth at least once every 24 hours due to patient susceptibility to disease and complexity of the task.[4] Taken together, these findings suggest plaque control efforts must focus on more than simply improved toothbrushing. Periodontal patients must concentrate on cleaning interproximal areas and be encouraged to adopt significantly more difficult and time-consuming oral hygiene habits that must be performed daily.

Chemical inhibitors of plaque and calculus incorporated in mouthwashes or dentifrices also play an important role in plaque control. Fluorides are essential for caries control. These products have been highly marketed and are commonly used as adjunctive agents to mechanical techniques. These medicaments, as with any drug, should be recommended and prescribed according to the needs of individual patients. Chemical plaque control is a rapidly growing field and will become even more significant for periodontal patients and practices in the future as increasingly effective products become available.

Plaque control is one of the key elements of the practice of dentistry. It permits each patient to assume responsibility for his or her own oral health on a daily basis. Without it, optimal oral health through periodontal treatment cannot be attained or preserved. Every patient in every dental practice should be educated about plaque control and encouraged to perform a personalized program on a daily basis. Good plaque control facilitates the return to health for patients with gingival and periodontal diseases, prevents tooth decay, and preserves oral health for a lifetime.

THE TOOTHBRUSH

The bristle toothbrush appeared about the year 1600 in China, was first patented in America in 1857, and has since undergone little change. Generally, toothbrushes vary in size and design as well as in length, hardness, and arrangement of the bristles (Fig. 49-1).[134] The American Dental Association has described the range of dimensions of acceptable brushes: a brushing surface 1 to 1.25 inches (25.4 to 31.8 mm) long and $\frac{5}{16}$ to $\frac{3}{8}$ inch (7.9 to 9.5 mm) wide, 2 to 4 rows of bristles, and 5 to 12 tufts per row.[2] A toothbrush should be able to reach and efficiently clean most areas of the teeth.

Some toothbrush manufacturers claim superiority of design for such things as minor modifications of bristle placement, length, or stiffness. These claims are primarily based on demonstrations of plaque removal that are shown to be statistically significantly superior to comparable toothbrushes in one or more clinical studies. However, the research does not show significant differences in gingivitis scores or bleeding indices, the more important measures of improved gingival health. It is questionable whether slight differences in measurements of plaque removal are in fact clinically significant because no toothbrush and few toothbrushers remove all plaque. A recent study of four different commercially available toothbrush designs compared plaque removal at a single brushing. All four toothbrushes removed plaque equally and the authors concluded that no one design was superior to others.[33]

In terms of recommending a particular toothbrush, superiority of clinical significance has not been demonstrated for any one type of toothbrush. Ease of manipulation by the patient is an important factor in brush selection, as is the patient's perception that the brush works well. The effectiveness of and potential injury from different types of brushes depend to a great degree on how the brushes are used.[26] Data from in vitro studies of abrasion by different manual toothbrushes suggest that differences in the brush design permitting the bristles to carry more toothpaste while brushing contribute to abrasion more than brush bristles themselves.[41] The

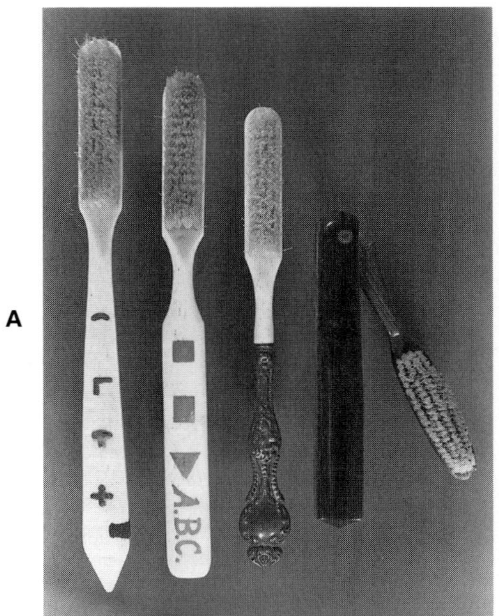

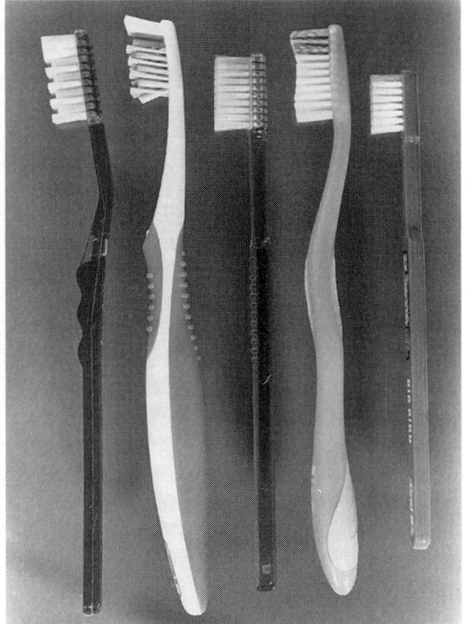

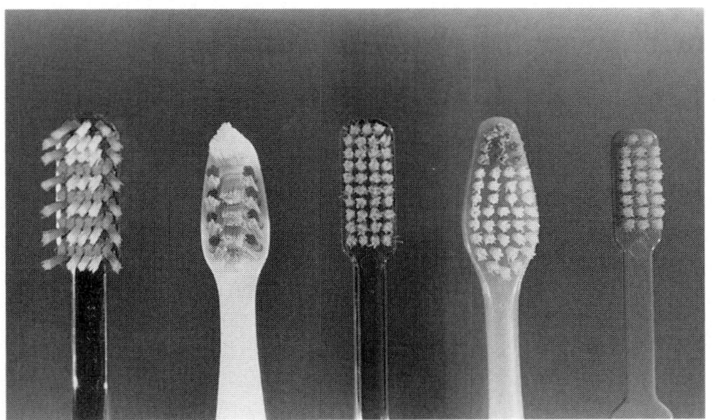

Fig. 49-1 Manual toothbrushes. **A,** Toothbrushes from the 19th and 20th centuries, two with ivory handles from about 1890 *(left),* one with a sterling silver handle *(center),* and an early travel brush with a plastic handle from about 1930 *(right).* The ivory-handled brushes belonged to dental students who used the handles to practice cutting preparations and using filling materials. The designs are "filled" with either gold foil or amalgam. **B,** A variety of toothbrushes are available; note the variation in brush head and handle design. **C,** Close-up view of brush heads showing various bristle configurations. (Antique brushes from the UCSF School of Dentistry Historical Collection, courtesy Dean Charles N. Bertolami, San Francisco, Calif.)

type of brush is largely a matter of individual preference. However, there is common agreement that use of a hard toothbrush, vigorous horizontal brushing, and possibly use of very abrasive dentifrice may lead to cervical abrasions of teeth and recession of gingiva.[81]

Recently, some novel designs intended to make brushing easier and hard-to-reach areas more accessible have been described. One has curved bristles on both sides of the brush head and shorter bristles running down the center. It is designed to brush buccal, lingual, and occlusal/incisal surfaces of the teeth at one time. One study demonstrating its plaque removal ability showed statistically significant differences between the curved bristles and a conventional brush, but absolute differences were slight.[30] Another design featured a U-shaped head with bristles that would also reach buccal, lingual, and occlusal/incisal surfaces at one time. This study also showed slight differences in plaque removal favoring the new design over a conventional brush and a powered toothbrush. It did not evaluate changes in gingival condition.[155] The notion of brushing all reachable surfaces of the teeth at one time is attractive, and these inventive brush designs may be useful for some patients to achieve better plaque control. There is no reason to discourage use of any particular device, especially if the patient likes it and uses it more or better than a conventional brush. There may well be a truly better design in the hands of any individual patient that results in better plaque removal and improved gingival health.

Two kinds of bristle material are used in toothbrushes: natural bristles from hogs and artificial filaments made predominantly of nylon. Both types remove plaque, and nylon bristles vastly predominates in the market.[21] However, in terms of homogeneity of the material, uniformity of bristle size, elasticity, resistance to fracture, and repulsion of water and debris, nylon filaments are clearly superior. Because of their tubular form, natural bristles are significantly more susceptible to fraying, breaking, contamination with diluted microbial debris, softening, and loss of elasticity. Patients accustomed to the softness of an older natural bristle brush can traumatize the gingiva when using a new brush with comparable vigor. It is helpful to point this out when a patient changes from natural to nylon bristles.

Toothbrush bristles are grouped in tufts that are usually arranged in three or four rows. Multitufted toothbrushes contain more bristles and may clean more efficiently than skimpier brushes. Rounded bristle ends cause fewer scratches on the gingiva than flat cut bristles with sharp ends.[37,134] The question of the most desirable bristle hardness is not settled. Bristle hardness is proportional to the square of the diameter and inversely proportional to the square of bristle length.[70] Diameters of commonly used bristles range from 0.007 inch (0.2 mm) for soft brushes to 0.012 inch (0.3 mm) for medium brushes and 0.014 inch (0.4 mm) for hard brushes.[76] Soft bristle brushes of the type described by Bass[18] have gained wide acceptance. Bass recommended a straight handle and nylon bristles 0.007 inch (0.2 mm) in diameter and 0.406 inch (10.3 mm) long, with rounded ends, arranged in three rows of tufts, six evenly spaced tufts per row, with 80 to 86 bristles per tuft. For children, the brush is smaller, with thinner (0.005 inch or 0.1 mm) and shorter (0.344 inch or 8.7 mm) bristles.[18]

Opinions regarding the merits of hard and soft bristles are based on studies carried out under differing conditions; these studies are often inconclusive and contradict one another.[77] Soft bristles are more flexible, clean beneath the gingival margin when used with a sulcus brushing technique,[17] and reach further onto the proximal tooth surfaces.[57] Use of hard-bristled toothbrushes is associated with more gingival recession, and frequent brushers who use hard bristles have more recession than those who use soft bristles.[86] However, the manner in which a brush is used and the abrasiveness of the dentifrice affect the action and abrasion to a greater degree than the bristle hardness itself.[1,109] Bristle hardness does not significantly affect wear on enamel surfaces.[128]

Overzealous brushing can lead to gingival recession; bacteremia, especially in patients with pronounced gingivitis; wedge-shaped defects in the cervical area of root surfaces[56,127]; and painful ulceration of the gingiva.[120] This type of brushing should be identified and discouraged.

To maintain cleaning effectiveness, toothbrushes must be replaced periodically. Wear patterns differ widely among individuals, but with conscientious, regular use, most brushes show signs of wear within a few months. If all the bristles are flattened after 1 week, brushing is probably quite vigorous; if the bristles are still straight after 6 months, either the brushing is done very gently or the brush has not been used every day. The amount of force used to brush does not appear to be critical in plaque removal.[144] Nor does the amount of visible bristle wear appear to affect plaque removal function for up to 9 weeks.[36] Unfortunately, people tend to use toothbrushes as long as possible, often long after the bristles are quite worn. Toothbrushes with wear reminders (e.g., a blue dye on some of the bristles) are currently available. The dye fades with use and can be helpful in reminding patients to replace their toothbrushes periodically.

The preference of handle characteristics is a matter of individual taste. The handle should fit comfortably in the palm of the hand; it may be straight or angled, thick or thin (see Fig. 49-1). Brushes with modest angulation between the head and the handle are available, and some clinical evidence supports the idea that these brush handles improve access for plaque removal under supervised brushing conditions.[81] In fact, a recent study described a toothbrush with a double angulation of the neck of the handle and demonstrated significantly more plaque reduction, especially on the buccal and lingual surfaces.[87] The clinical significance of these findings has not been determined, but it is reasonable to surmise that modifications improving access may help some patients to brush more effectively.

For most patients, short-headed brushes with straight-cut, round-ended, soft to medium nylon bristles arranged in three or four rows of tufts are recommended. However, if a patient perceives any benefit from a particular brush design characteristic, use of that brush should be encouraged.

POWERED TOOTHBRUSHES

Electrically powered toothbrushes were invented in 1939 and intended to make plaque control easier for patients to master. The first powered toothbrushes were designed to mimic hand toothbrushing techniques using back-and-forth motions. Some were subsequently designed with circular or elliptic motions, and some with combinations of motions. Today, many types of powered toothbrushes designed for home use are available, some with reciprocating bristle tufts (Fig. 49-2) and brushes that use low-frequency acoustic energy to enhance cleaning ability. Powered toothbrushes that have shaped tips designed for interproximal cleaning are also available (Fig. 49-3).

All powered toothbrushes rely on mechanical contact between the bristles and the tooth to remove plaque. The addition of low-frequency acoustic energy generates dynamic fluid movement and provides cleaning slightly away from the bristle tips. The vibrations have also been shown to interfere with bacterial adherence to oral surfaces. Neither the sonic vibrations nor the mechanical motion of powered toothbrushes has been shown to affect bacterial cell viability.[106]

One review suggested that acoustic microstreaming, hydrodynamic shear forces that may disrupt plaque, are the likely mechanism of action for these powered brushes. The authors noted that most comparison studies between powered toothbrushes, manual toothbrushes, or other powered devices demonstrate, at best, slightly improved plaque removal for the device of interest in short-term clinical trials. Although this permits advertising claims of superiority, improved oral health for all patients or all periodontal patients has not been

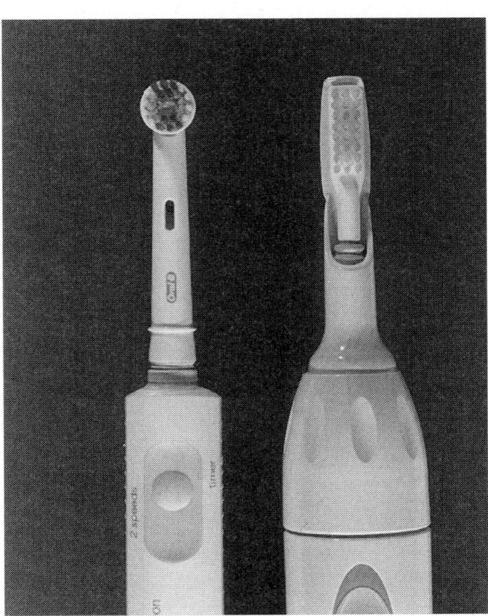

Fig. 49-2 Powered toothbrush designs offer options in head shape and size.

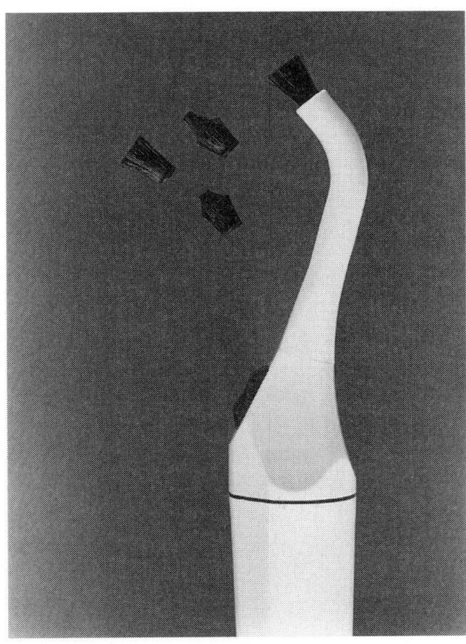

Fig. 49-3 Powered toothbrush with shaped tips can be used for interproximal cleaning and other difficult areas around the teeth.

demonstrated. Patient acceptance of powered toothbrushes is good. A recent study reported that 88.9% of patients introduced to a powered toothbrush would continue to use it.[148] Patients quit using powered toothbrushes after about 5 or 6 months, presumably when the novelty has worn off.[73] However, modern powered toothbrushes with additional features such as sonic technology to reach further onto proximal surfaces and timers to remind patients to brush longer are considered by some to be superior to manual brushes.[145]

Regardless of the type of device, the best plaque removal results are obtained when the patient is instructed in its proper use. This assures that the moving bristles have to be placed correctly around the mouth.[11,145] In fact, instructional videos have been shown to be an effective way of educating patients on the proper use of powered toothbrushes.[123]

Patients who can develop the ability to use a toothbrush properly usually do equally well with a manual or a powered toothbrush. Less diligent brushers do better with powered toothbrushes, which generate stroke motions automatically and require less operator effort.[60] Powered toothbrushes have been shown to improve oral health for: (1) children and adolescents, (2) children with physical or mental disabilities, (3) hospitalized patients, including older adults who need to have their teeth cleaned by caregivers, and (4) patients with fixed orthodontic appliances. They have not been shown to routinely provide benefits for patients with rheumatoid arthritis, children who are well-motivated brushers, and patients with chronic periodontitis.[73]

Powered toothbrushes are not generally superior to manual ones. Although some researchers have reported that powered toothbrushes remove more plaque than manual toothbrushes, reduce calculus accumulation, and improve gingival health,[101,108] other authors have reported that the same brushes failed to perform better than comparisons.[14,15,54,60,112,145] Identified improvements tend to be slight and localized in terms of improved gingival health,[5] but more plaque is typically removed from proximal surfaces using the newer devices.[143] One interesting study demonstrated reductions in gingival fluid flow for patients with moderate periodontal disease when the sonic toothbrush was used over an 8-week period. The authors suggested the sonic toothbrush might have some effect on inflammation beyond that achieved by manual toothbrushing.[116] Generally, powered toothbrushes are at least as good for plaque removal as manual brushes. If a powered toothbrush can be helpful to a particular patient, it should be recommended and encouraged.

No specific toothbrush can be singled out as clearly superior for the routine removal of dental plaque from the teeth when measured by improvement in gingival health. Requirements for a good toothbrush differ greatly among individuals, and any toothbrush, including powered toothbrushes, should be recommended after considering factors such as patient interest, morphology of the dentition, periodontal health, and manual dexterity. Because of the wide acceptance of oral hygiene principles first reported by Bass,[17,18] the one brush probably most commonly recommended by dentists appears to be the four-row, multitufted, soft, nylon, handheld toothbrush. This style of brush is certainly adequate but does not fit the needs or provide the best choice for every patient in every practice.

Powered toothbrushes can be valuable replacements for manual brushes if used regularly and properly. They are particularly useful for cleaning proximal surfaces and for people with limited dexterity, children who like them, and caregivers of ill patients. Some patients simply prefer powered toothbrushes and are more compliant with oral hygiene procedures when using them.

DENTIFRICES

Dentifrices aid in cleaning and polishing tooth surfaces. They are used mostly in the form of pastes, although tooth powders and gels are also available. Dentifrices are made up of abrasives such as silicon oxides, aluminum oxides, and granular polyvinyl chlorides; water; humectants; soap or detergent; flavoring and sweetening agents; therapeutic agents such as fluorides and pyrophosphates; and coloring agents and preservatives.[71]

Dentifrices should be sufficiently abrasive for satisfactory cleansing and polishing but should provide a margin of safety to protect the aggressive toothbrusher from wearing away root structure and soft restorative materials.[130] Abrasives, commonly in the form of insoluble inorganic salts, make up 20% to 40% of a dentifrice. The proper use of a dentifrice can enhance the abrasive action of a toothbrush as much as 40 times.[109] Tooth powders contain about 95% abrasives and are five times more abrasive than pastes. The abrasive quality of dentifrices affects enamel, but abrasion is more of a concern for patients with exposed roots because dentin is abraded 25 times faster and cementum 35 times faster than enamel. This can lead to root surface abrasion and root sensitivity.[139] Existing literature suggests that hard tissue damage from oral hygiene procedures is mainly due to abrasive dentifrices, whereas gingival lesions can be produced by the toothbrush alone[120,128] (Fig. 49-4).

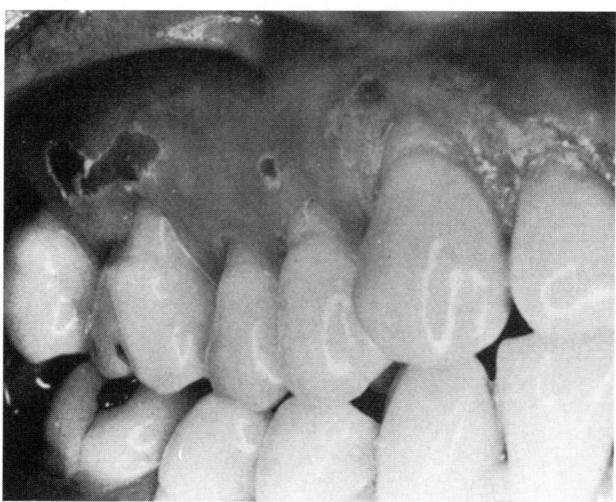

Fig. 49-4 Vigorous tooth brushing with an abrasive dentifrice can result in trauma and wearing away of the tooth surfaces, especially root surfaces, and contribute to gingival recession.

Abrasions are more prevalent on maxillary than on mandibular teeth and are found more frequently on the left than on the right half of the dental arch.[46] This suggests that access and right- or left-handedness may also contribute to the abrasion. Dentifrices that provide the effectiveness required for plaque control with a minimum of abrasion are preferable.

There is considerable interest in improving dentifrices by using them as vehicles for chemotherapeutic agents to inhibit plaque, calculus, caries, or root hypersensitivity. The pronounced caries-preventive effect of fluorides incorporated in dentifrices has been proved beyond question.[138] To achieve this effect, free fluoride ions must be available in the paste, not bound to the ingredients in the abrasive system. The American Dental Association (ADA) Council on Scientific Affairs[3] (formerly the Council on Dental Therapeutics) has voluntarily evaluated fluoride dentifrices. Several toothpastes have been found to have fluoride available in the correct amount (1000 to 1100 ppm), along with clinical studies documenting their caries reduction effects. Toothpaste products that have been tested by the ADA and have been determined to have fluoride ion available in the appropriate amount carry the ADA seal of approval for caries control and can be relied on to provide caries protection.

Substances such as chlorhexidine,[45] penicillin, dibasic ammonium phosphate, vaccines, vitamins, chlorophyll, and formaldehyde have proved to be of little therapeutic value in toothpastes. Tartar control toothpastes with the active ingredient pyrophosphate are currently available. This ingredient interferes with crystal formation in calculus and does not affect the fluoride ion in the paste or increase tooth sensitivity. This type of dentifrice has reduced the formation of new supragingival calculus by 30% or more.[83,107,154] These pastes are beneficial only for supragingival calculus. They do not affect subgingival calculus formation or gingival inflammation. To achieve the greatest effect from anti-calculus toothpaste, the patient's teeth must be cleaned and completely free of supragingival calculus when starting to use the product daily. The inhibitory effect will only work against the deposition of new calculus.

TOOTHBRUSHING METHODS

Many methods for brushing the teeth have been described and promoted as being efficient and effective. These methods can be categorized primarily according to the pattern of motion when brushing[81]:

Roll: The roll method[6] or modified Stillman[78] technique
Vibratory: The Stillman,[137] Charters,[29] or Bass[17] techniques
Circular: The Fones[53] technique
Vertical: The Leonard technique[96]
Horizontal: The scrub technique[150]

Controlled studies evaluating the effectiveness of the most common brushing techniques have not demonstrated any clear superiority for any one method. The scrub technique is probably the simplest and most common method of brushing. Patients with periodontal disease are most frequently taught a sulcular brushing technique using a vibratory motion to improve access in the gingival areas. The roll technique seems to be the least effective method, perhaps because it generates only intermittent pressure against the teeth compared with the sustained force applied with the sulcular and scrub techniques.[22]

Three common methods of brushing the teeth are presented here; any of them, if properly performed, can provide excellent plaque control. The goal of brushing is

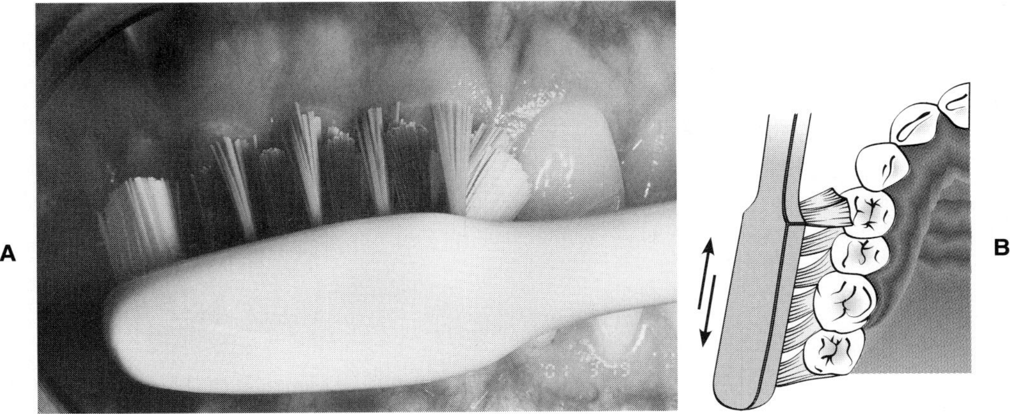

Fig. 49-5 Bass method. **A,** Place the toothbrush so that the bristles are angled approximately 45 degrees from the tooth surfaces. **B,** Start at the most distal tooth in the arch and use a vibrating, back-and-forth motion to brush.

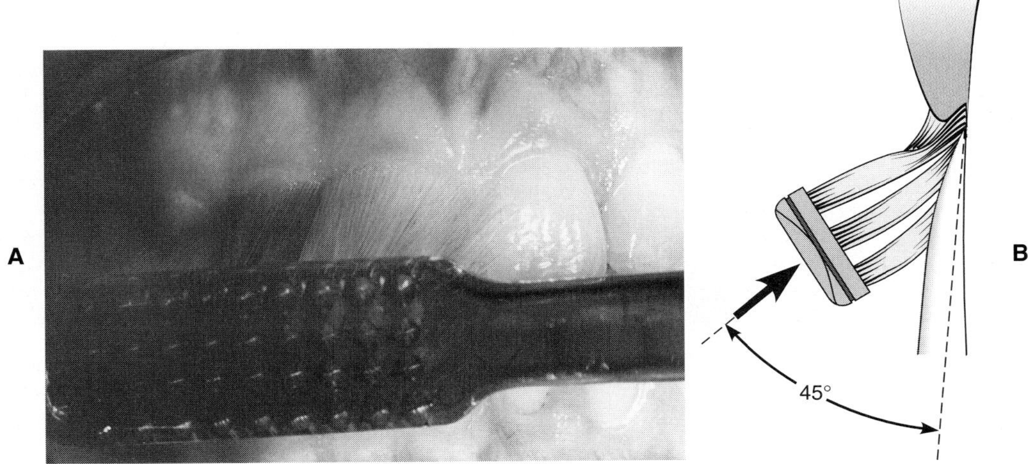

Fig. 49-6 Bass method. **A,** Proper position of the brush in the mouth aims the bristle tips toward the gingival margin. **B,** Diagrams shows the ideal placement, which could permit slight subgingival penetration of the bristle tips.

to remove as much plaque from the accessible tooth surfaces as possible. The best brushing method for each patient is determined when forming an individualized and complete plaque control program. It also should be remembered that brushing with a powered toothbrush is an equally good alternative.

The Bass Method

Technique. Place the head of a soft brush parallel with the occlusal plane, with the brush head covering three to four teeth, beginning at the most distal tooth in the arch.[17] Place the bristles at the gingival margin, establishing an angle of 45 degrees to the long axis of the teeth. Exert gentle vibratory pressure, using short back-and-forth motions without dislodging the tips of the bristles. This motion forces the bristle ends into the gingival sulcus area (Fig. 49-5) as well as partially into the interproximal embrasures. The pressure should produce perceptible blanching of the gingiva (Fig. 49-6). Complete approximately 20 strokes in the same position. This repeated motion cleans the tooth surfaces, concentrating on the apical third of the clinical crowns, the gingival sulci, and as far onto the proximal surfaces as the bristles can reach. Lift the brush, move it to the adjacent teeth, and repeat the process for the next three or four teeth.

Continue around the arch, brushing about three teeth at a time, then use the same method to brush the lingual surfaces (Figs. 49-7 and 49-8). After completing the maxillary arch, move the brush to the mandibular arch and brush in the same manner until the entire dentition is completed. To help reach the lingual surfaces of the anterior teeth if the brush seems too large, insert the brush vertically (Figs. 49-9 and 49-10). Press the end of the

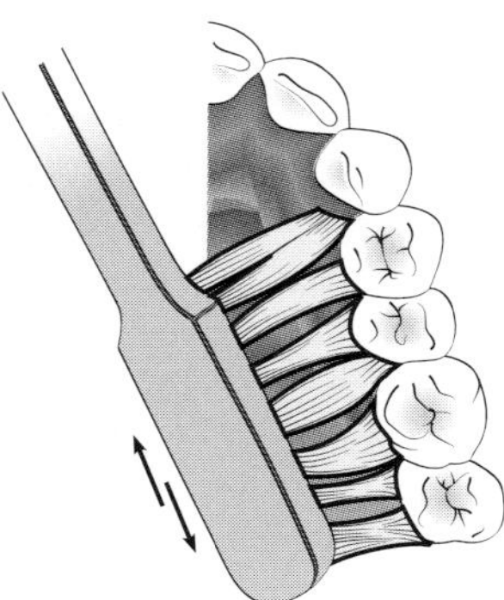

Fig. 49-7 Bass method. The correct palatal position on molars and premolars is with the bristle tips at the gingival margin as shown in the diagram, not on the occlusal surfaces.

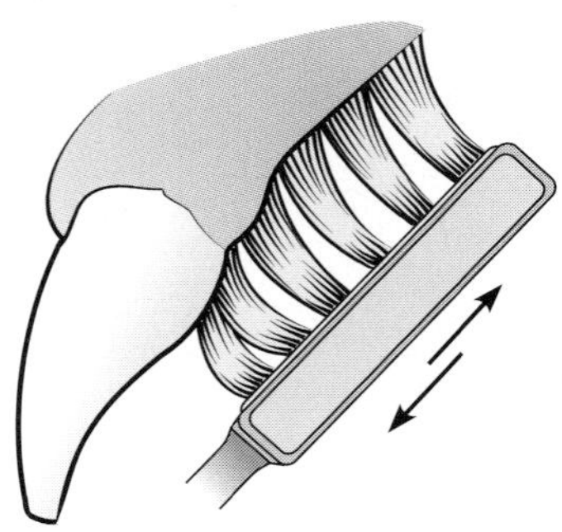

Fig. 49-9 Bass method. Adjusting the palatal position of the toothbrush on incisors, as shown in the diagram, may provide better access for plaque removal.

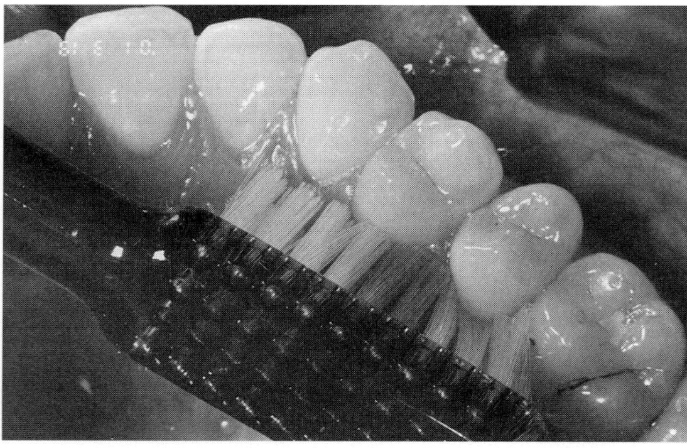

Fig. 49-8 Bass method. Palatal position of the soft toothbrush on the molars and premolars permits bristle tip penetration into the interproximal areas and possibly slightly subgingivally.

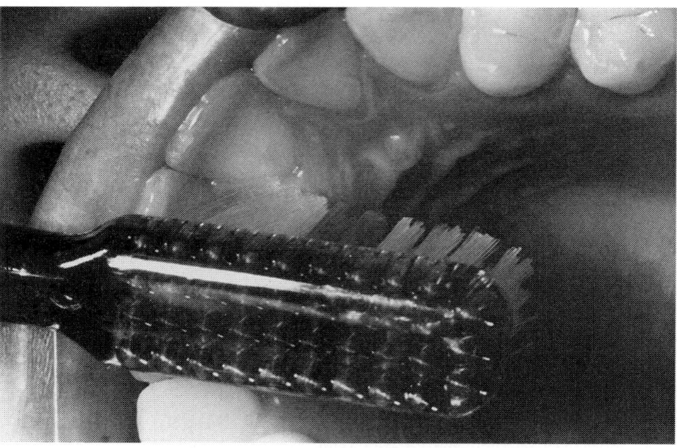

Fig. 49-10 Bass method. Placement of the bristles on the palatal surfaces of the incisor teeth can be difficult and often requires this modified approach.

brush into the gingival sulcus area and proximal surfaces at a 45-degree angle to the long axis of the teeth and brush with multiple short vibratory strokes.

Press the bristles firmly into the pits and fissures of the occlusal surfaces (Fig. 49-11) and brush with about 20 short back-and-forth strokes. Use this technique and brush a few teeth at a time until all posterior teeth in all four quadrants are cleaned.

The Bass technique requires patience and placement of the toothbrush in many different positions to cover the full dentition. Patients need to be instructed to brush in a controlled and systematic sequence to optimize plaque removal.

The Bass method has certain advantages over other techniques, as follows:

1. The short back-and-forth motion is easy to master because it is a simple movement familiar to most patients who brush using a scrub technique.
2. It concentrates the cleaning action on the cervical and interproximal portions of the teeth, where microbial plaque is most likely to have accumulated.

The Bass technique is efficient and can be recommended for any patient with or without periodontal involvement.

The Modified Stillman Method

The modified Stillman method[78,137] requires that the brush be placed with the bristle ends resting partly on the cervical portion of the teeth and partly on the adjacent gingiva, pointing in an apical direction and at an oblique angle to the long axis of the teeth (Fig. 49-12). Apply pressure against the gingival margin to produce a perceptible blanching. Then move the brush about 20 short back-and-forth strokes while simultaneously moving it coronally along the attached gingiva, the gingival margin, and the tooth surface. A soft or medium multitufted brush should be used with this technique to minimize trauma to the gingiva.

This process must be repeated on all tooth surfaces, proceeding systematically around the mouth. To reach the lingual surfaces of the maxillary and mandibular incisors, the handle of the brush can be held in a vertical position,

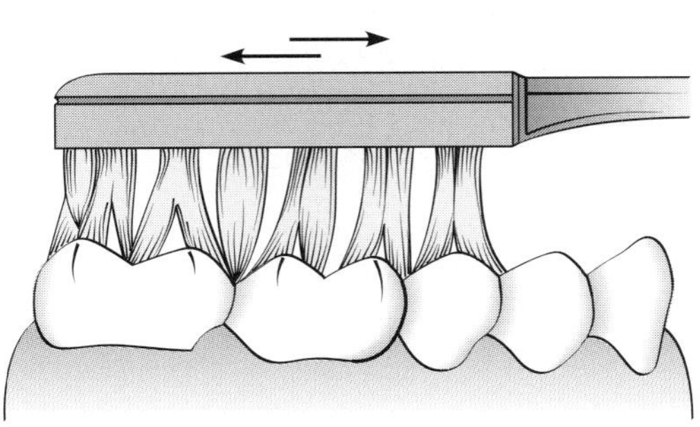

Fig. 49-11 This brush position on occlusal surfaces of the teeth is used with any technique, including the Bass, Stillman, or Charters method.

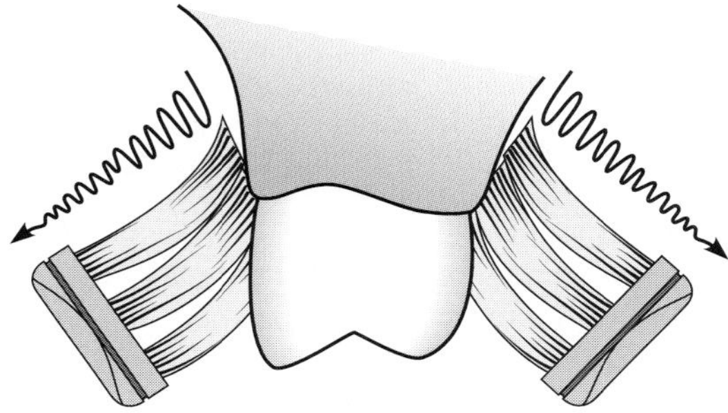

Fig. 49-12 Modified Stillman method. This method requires placement of the sides of the bristles against the teeth and gingiva while moving the brush with short, back-and-forth strokes in a coronal direction.

engaging the end of the brush. With this technique, the sides rather than the ends of the bristles do the work. The bristles tend not to penetrate into the gingival sulcus.

The occlusal surfaces of molars and premolars are cleaned with the bristles placed perpendicular to the occlusal plane and penetrating into the grooves and interproximal embrasures (see Fig. 49-11).

The modified Stillman method may be recommended for cleaning in areas with progressing gingival recession and root exposure to minimize abrasive tissue destruction.

The Charters Method

The Charters method[29] requires placement of a soft or medium multitufted brush on the teeth with the bristles pointed toward the crown at a 45-degree angle to the long axis of the teeth (Fig. 49-13). The sides of the bristles should be flexed against the gingiva, and a back-and-forth vibratory motion used to brush. The technique was designed to gently massage the gingiva, so the bristle tips should not drag across the gingiva. The bristle tips should be placed in the pits and fissures, and short back-and-forth strokes should be used to clean the occlusal surfaces (see Fig. 49-11). The procedures are repeated systematically until all surfaces are cleaned.

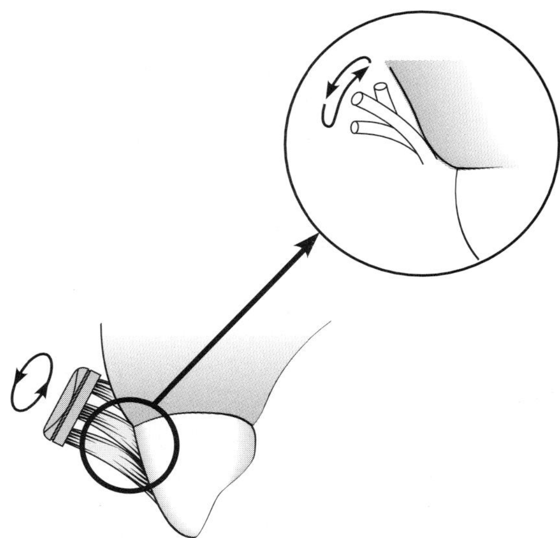

Fig. 49-13 Charters method. The Charters method requires that the bristles be pressed against the sides of the teeth and gingiva. The brush is moved with short circular or back-and-forth strokes.

The Charters method provides gentle plaque removal. This technique can be recommended for cleaning in areas of healing wounds after periodontal surgery.

Methods of Cleaning with Powered Toothbrushes

The various mechanical motions built into powered toothbrushes do not require special techniques of application. The patient need only concentrate on placing the brush head next to the teeth at the gingival margin and proceeding systematically around the dentition.[144] Additional placement adjustments can be made to clean difficult areas, such as the distal surfaces of the third molars, furcations, or gingival clefts. The methods described for manual brushing are also suitable for application with powered toothbrushes (Fig. 49-14).

INTERDENTAL CLEANING AIDS

Any toothbrush, regardless of the brushing method used, does not completely remove interdental plaque. This is true both in individuals with healthy periodontal conditions and those with periodontal destruction resulting in open embrasures.[58,63,131] Interdental plaque removal is crucial to augment the effects of tooth brushing because, as previously noted, the majority of dental and periodontal disease originates in interproximal areas. Other conditions found in periodontal and gingival diseases also demand an emphasis on interproximal cleaning. The gingival tissues are swollen in the presence of gingival inflammation, rendering the self-cleansing mechanisms of the mouth less effective than in a healthy periodontium. Also, tissue destruction associated with periodontal disease may leave large open spaces between teeth and long-exposed root surfaces with anatomical concavities and furcations. These are difficult areas to

A

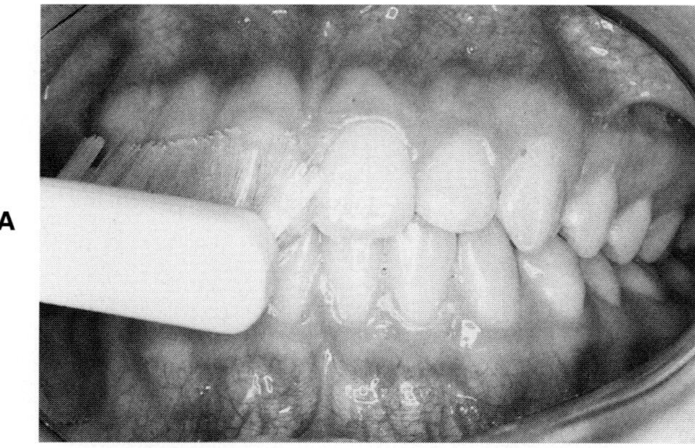

B

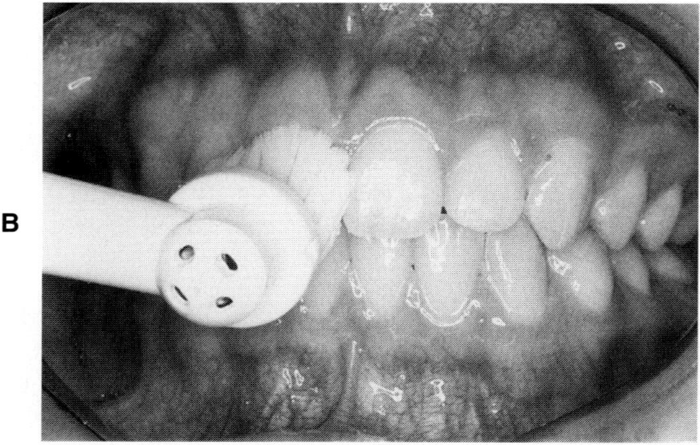

Fig. 49-14 Positioning of the powered toothbrush head and bristle tips so that they reach the gingival margin is critical to achieving the most effective cleaning results. **A,** Straight head placement. **B,** Round head placement.

clean and only poorly accessible to the toothbrush.[88] Interdental cleaning should occur every day for the same rationale as brushing daily.[4]

The purpose of interdental cleaning is to remove plaque, not to dislodge fibrous threads of food wedged between teeth. Although interdental cleaning does dislodge food fragments, correcting proximal tooth contacts and plunger cusps is required to stop chronic food impaction.

The specific aids required for interproximal cleaning depend on various criteria such as the size of the interdental spaces, the presence of furcations, tooth alignment, and the presence of orthodontic appliances or fixed prostheses.

Among the numerous aids available, dental floss and interdental cleaners such as wooden or plastic tips and interdental brushes are commonly recommended.

Dental Floss

Dental floss is the most widely recommended tool for removing plaque from proximal tooth surfaces.[59] Floss is available as a multifilament nylon yarn that is twisted or nontwisted, bonded or nonbonded, waxed or unwaxed, and thick or thin. Monofilament flosses made of a Teflon-type material are preferred by some individuals because they are slick and do not fray. A variety of individual factors determine the choice of dental floss, such as the tightness of tooth contacts, roughness of proximal surfaces, and patient's manual dexterity, not the superiority of any one product. Clinical research so far has not been able to show any significant differences in the ability of the various types of floss to remove dental plaque; they all work equally well.[51,75,84,85,128] In the past, waxed dental floss was thought to leave a waxy film on proximal surfaces, thus contributing to plaque accumulation and gingivitis. It has been shown, however, that wax is not deposited on tooth surfaces[121] and that improvement in gingival health is unrelated to the type of floss used.[51] Therefore recommendations about type of floss should be based on ease of use and personal preference.

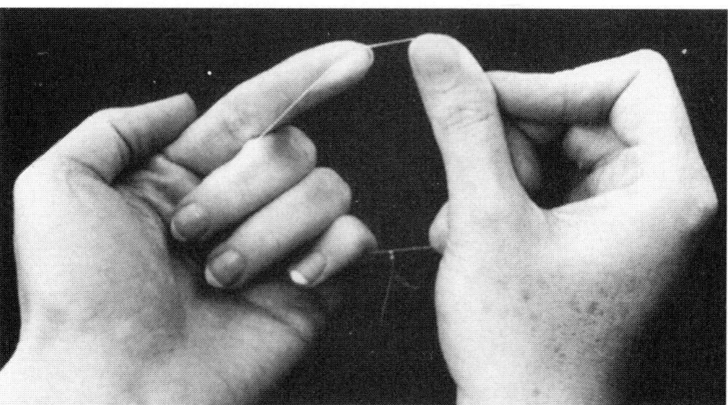

Fig. 49-15 Dental floss may be held securely in the fingers or tied in a loop.

Technique. The floss must contact the proximal surface from line angle to line angle to clean effectively. It must also clean the entire proximal surface, not just be slipped apical to the contact area. The following description is a primer in floss technique:

- Start with a piece of floss long enough to grasp securely; 12 to 18 inches is usually sufficient. It may be wrapped around the fingers, or the ends may be tied together in a loop.
- Stretch the floss tightly between the thumb and forefinger (Fig. 49-15), or between both forefingers, and pass it gently through each contact area with a firm back-and-forth motion. Do not snap the floss past the contact area, because this may injure the interdental gingiva. In fact, zealous snapping of floss through contact areas creates proximal grooves in the gingiva.
- Once the floss is apical to the contact area between the teeth, wrap the floss around the proximal surface of one tooth, and slip it under the marginal gingiva. Move the floss firmly along the tooth up to the contact area and gently down into the sulcus again, repeating this up-and-down stroke several times (Fig. 49-16). Then move the floss across the interdental gingiva and repeat the procedure on the proximal surface of the adjacent tooth.

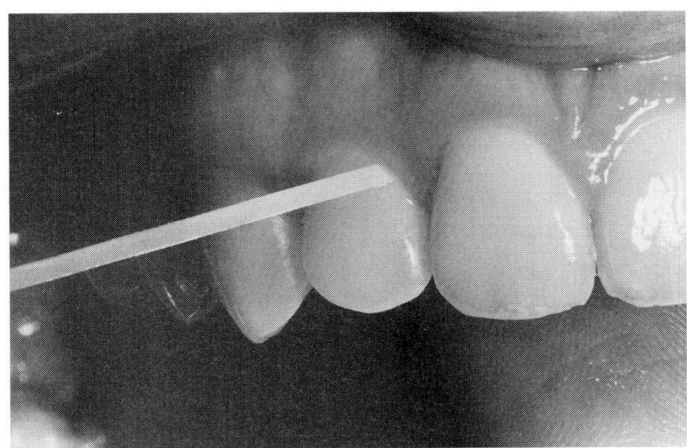

Fig. 49-16 Dental floss technique. The floss is slipped between the contact area of the teeth (in this case teeth #7 and #8), wrapped around proximal surface, and removes plaque by using several up-and-down strokes. The process must be repeated for the distal surface of tooth #8.

- Continue through the whole dentition, including the distal surface of the last tooth in each quadrant. When the working portion of the floss becomes soiled or begins to shred, move to a fresh portion of floss.

Flossing can be made easier by using a floss holder (Fig. 49-17, *A*). Although use of such devices can be more time consuming than finger flossing, they are helpful for patients lacking manual dexterity and for nursing personnel assisting handicapped and hospitalized patients in cleaning their teeth. A floss holder should possess these features: (1) one or two forks that are rigid enough to keep the floss taut when penetrating into tight contact areas, and (2) an effective and simple mounting mechanism to hold the floss firmly in place. The disadvantage of floss tools is that they must be rethreaded whenever the floss becomes soiled or begins to shred.

Disposable, single-use floss holders with prethreaded floss are available and may be useful for some patients. Short-term clinical evidence suggests that plaque reduction and improvement in gingivitis scores are similar for individuals instructed in the use of disposable floss devices when compared with scores for those instructed in finger flossing (see Fig. 49-17, *B*).[27,135]

Powered flossing devices are also available (Fig. 49-18). These devices have a single bristle that moves in a circular motion. The devices have been shown to be safe and effective but no better at plaque removal than finger flossing.[34,64]

The establishment of a lifelong habit of flossing the teeth is difficult to achieve for both patients and dentists, regardless of whether one uses a tool or flosses with the fingers. In fact, the daily use of floss is universally low. It was recently reported that only about 8% of 12- to 16-year olds in Great Britain floss daily,[105] a number similar to other countries.[88] An analysis of the British adolescents showed that daily flossing was correlated to frequent hand washing and bathing and having recently visited the dentist.[105] No information is available about the establishment of long-term flossing habits comparing the various tools to finger flossing. However, the tools may be useful to help some individuals begin flossing or make flossing possible if they have limited dexterity. The benefits of interproximal cleaning using dental floss are undisputed. Proper manipulation of floss requires good dexterity and repeated reinforcement.

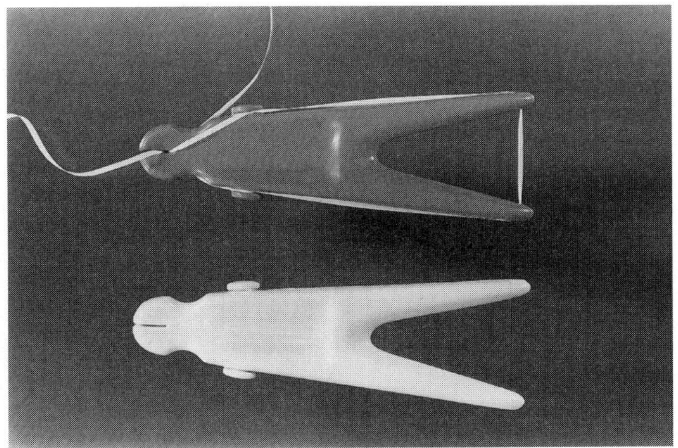

A

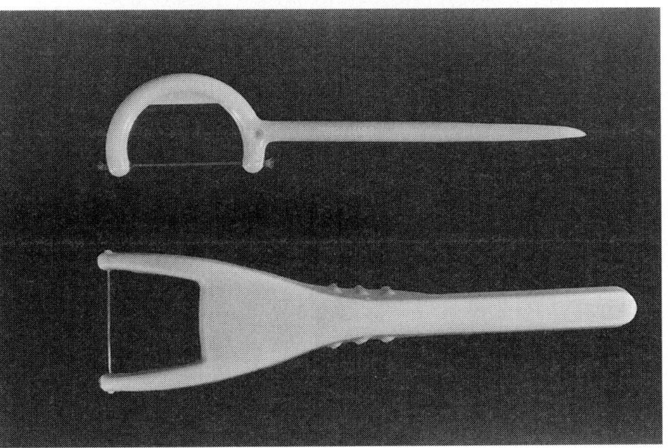

B

Fig. 49-17 Floss holders can simplify the manipulation of dental floss. **A,** Reusable floss tools require stringing the floss around a series of knobs and grooves to secure it. **B,** Disposable floss tools have prestrung floss and are easy to use, but the floss may shred and break, requiring several tools to complete flossing the teeth.

Interdental Cleaning Devices

Dental floss is probably the most effective dental hygiene aid for cleaning in narrow gingival embrasures that are occupied by intact papillae and bordered by tight contact zones. Concave root surfaces and furcations that are often present in periodontal patients who have experienced significant attachment loss and recession are not as thoroughly cleaned with dental floss alone. A comparison study of dental floss and interdental brushes used by patients with moderate to severe periodontal disease showed that the interproximal brushes removed slightly more interproximal plaque. However, no difference was

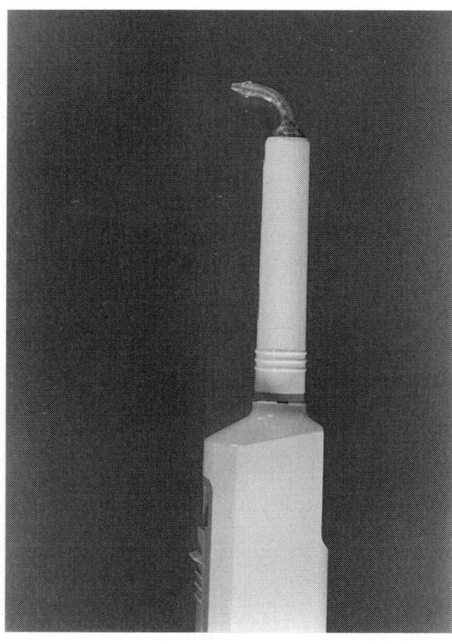

Fig. 49-18 A powered flossing device can be easier to use than hand-held floss. The tip is inserted into the proximal space, and a bristle or wand comes out of the tip and moves in a circular motion when the device is turned on. The bristle mechanically removes the plaque.

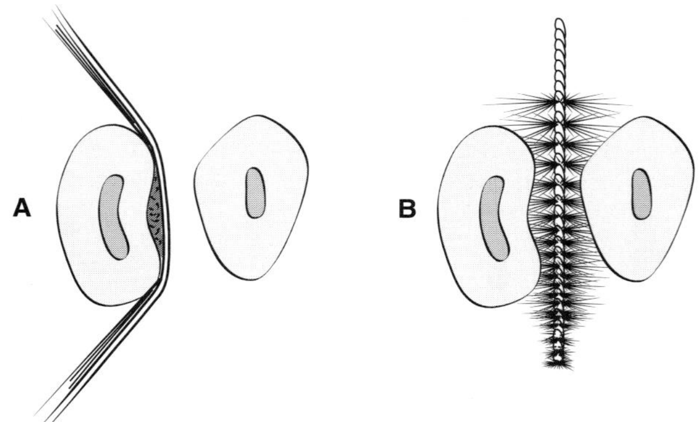

Fig. 49-19 Cleaning of concave or irregular proximal tooth surfaces. Dental floss **(A)** may be less effective than an interdental brush **(B)** on long root surfaces with concavities.

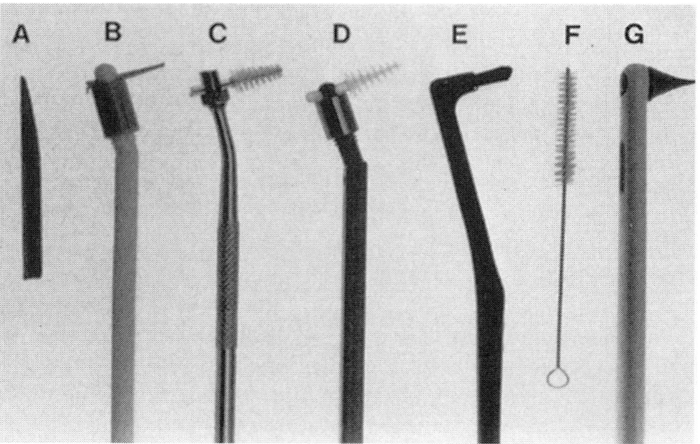

Fig. 49-20 A large variety of interproximal cleaning devices are available: wooden tips **(A and B)**, interproximal brushes **(C–F)**, and rubber tip stimulators **(G)**.

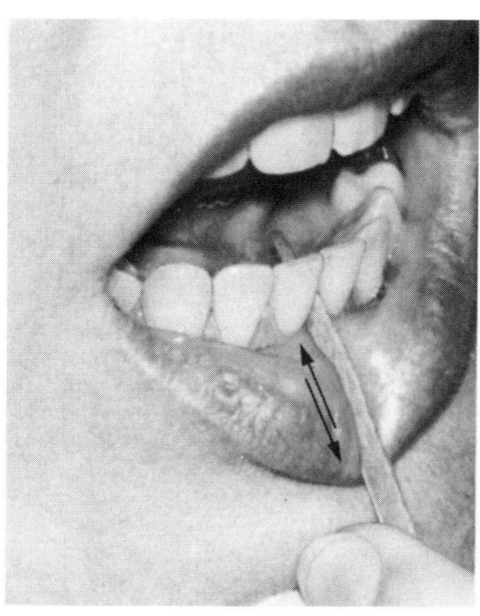

Fig. 49-21 Triangular wooden tip. The tip is inserted between the teeth, with the triangular portion resting on the gingival papilla, and is moved in and out. This device is popular but is very difficult to use on posterior teeth and from the lingual aspect of all teeth.

seen in probe depth reductions or bleeding indices. In addition, the interdental brushes were considered by the subjects to be easier to use than dental floss.[31] Therefore other cleaning aids that are easy to handle and adaptable to irregular and long, exposed root surfaces (Fig. 49-19) can be recommended for proximal cleaning of teeth when interdental spaces permit access.[88] This type of gingival architecture and root exposure is commonly found in periodontal patients.

A wide variety of interdental cleaning devices are available for removing soft debris from tooth surfaces that are not accessible to a full-size toothbrush and dental floss (Fig. 49-20). The most common types are small conical or cylindric brushes, tapered wooden toothpicks that are round or triangular in cross-section, and single-tufted brushes. Many interdental devices can be attached to a handle for convenient manipulation around the teeth and in posterior areas. Clinical research has shown that the devices are effective on lingual and facial tooth surfaces as well as on proximal surfaces.[88,131,146]

Interdental Brushes. Interdental brushes are cone-shaped or cylindric brushes made of bristles mounted on a handle (see Fig. 49-20, *C* and *D*), single-tufted brushes

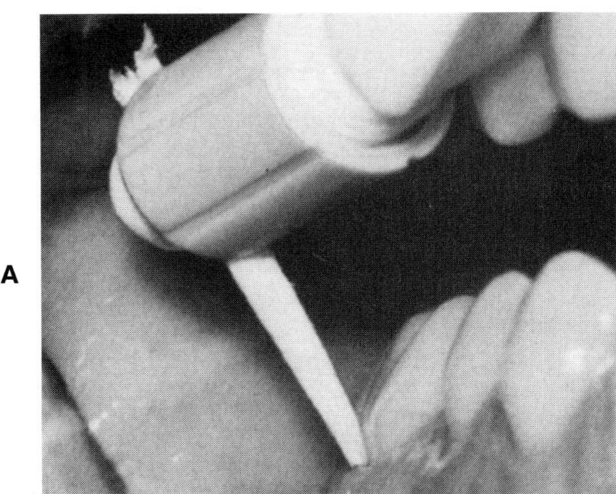
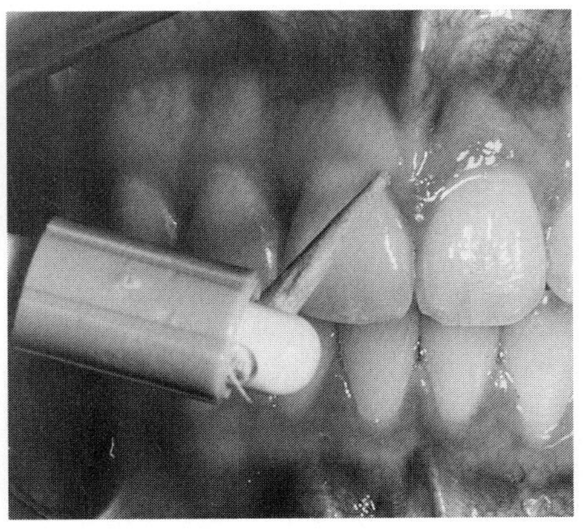

Fig. 49-22 Wooden toothpick. **A,** The tip is a common wooden toothpick held in a handle and broken off. It is used to clean subgingivally and reach into periodontal pockets. **B,** The tip can also be used to clean along the gingival margins of the teeth and reach under the gingiva.

(see Fig. 49-20, *E*), or small cylindric brushes (see Fig. 49-20, *F*). Interdental brushes are particularly suitable for cleaning large, irregular, or concave tooth surfaces adjacent to wide interdental spaces.

Technique. Interdental brushes of any style are inserted through interproximal spaces and moved back and forth between the teeth with short strokes. For most efficient cleaning, it is probably best to select the diameter of brush that is slightly larger than the gingival embrasures to be cleaned. This size permits bristles to exert pressure on both proximal tooth surfaces, working their way into concavities on the roots. Single-tufted brushes are highly effective on the lingual surface of mandibular molars and premolars, where the tongue often impedes a regular toothbrush, and may provide access to furcation areas and isolated areas of deep recession.

Wooden or Rubber Tips. Wooden tips are used either with or without a handle (Fig. 49-20, *A* and *B*). Access is easier from the buccal surfaces for those tips without handles, primarily in the anterior and bicuspid areas. Rubber tips come mounted on handles or the ends of toothbrushes and can easily be adapted to all proximal surfaces in the mouth. Various plastic tips are also available and can be used in a manner similar to wooden tips. Both rubber and plastic tips can be rinsed and reused and easily carried in a pocket or purse, features that are attractive to some patients.

Technique. Soft, triangular wooden picks or plastic alternatives are placed in the interdental space in such a way that the base of the triangle rests on the gingiva and the sides are in contact with the proximal tooth surfaces (Fig. 49-21). The pick is then repeatedly moved in and out of the embrasure, removing soft deposits from the teeth and mechanically stimulating the papillary gingiva. The disadvantage of the triangular toothpick is that it is very hard to access any surfaces other than the facial surfaces in the more anterior region of the mouth.

Rubber tips should be placed into the embrasure space and used in a circular motion. They can be applied to interproximal spaces and other defects throughout the mouth and are easily adaptable to lingual surfaces.

Conventional toothpicks can also be used for interproximal cleaning. They have the advantage of being a common device and readily available in most homes. Toothpicks can be attached to commercially available handles for better access to posterior and lingual areas or used as bought (Fig. 49-20, *B*). Once mounted on the handle, the toothpick is broken off so that it is only 6 or 7 mm long. The tip of the toothpick is used to trace along the gingival margin and into the proximal areas from both the facial and lingual surfaces throughout the mouth. Plaque can also be removed by using the sides in a manner similar to a wooden pick (Fig. 49-22, *A*) or the tip of the toothpick (Fig. 49-22, *B*). This device is particularly efficient for cleaning along the gingival margin[59] and into periodontal pockets and furcations.

Conclusions. A large and changing variety of interdental cleaning aids are available for patients. Experience and patient preference will help you determine which are best for any particular situation. It is important to remember that brushing alone is not sufficient for plaque removal and that some interproximal device needs to be used routinely by the patient in the daily plaque control regimen. In general, the largest brush or device that fits into a space will clean most efficiently, and obviously, the devices the patient likes will be most used.

Embrasure spaces vary greatly in size and shape. A representation of three types of embrasures and the kind of interdental cleaner often recommended for each is shown in Fig. 49-23. As a general rule, the larger the space, the larger the device that should be used. However, some devices are more difficult to assemble and use than others, so a favorite tool of one individual may be impossible for another to use. It is useful to have a variety of aids available so that you and the patient can decide what fits best and is easiest to use. Often the patient requires three components to the plaque control routine; a brushing method, dental floss to clean subgingivally and tight embrasure spaces, and an interdental aid for larger interdental spaces and furcations. Typically, the routine of complete plaque removal with the brush and required interproximal aids takes the periodontal patient up to 30 minutes every day.

GINGIVAL MASSAGE

Massaging the gingiva with a toothbrush or an interdental cleaning devices produces epithelial thickening, increased keratinization, and increased mitotic activity in the epithelium and connective tissue.[26,28,61,136] The increased keratinization occurs on the oral gingiva and not on the areas more vulnerable to microbial attack, the sulcular epithelium and the interdental areas where the gingival col is present. It has never been demonstrated that epithelial thickening, increased keratinization, and blood circulation provide protection against microorganisms and other local irritants and thus are beneficial or necessary for gingival health.[62] The improved gingival health associated with interdental stimulation is far more likely the result of plaque removal rather than gingival massage. In addition, studies of chemotherapeutic mouthrinses containing chlorhexidine have shown that gingival health can be maintained for periods of time in the absence of any mechanical oral hygiene procedure.[102] These data underscore the importance of emphasizing altering or removing plaque rather than stimulating or thickening the keratinized surface in the plaque control program.

Toothbrushing methods designed to massage the gingiva and devices such as the rubber tip stimulator (see Fig. 49-21, *G*) result in plaque removal in addition to massage. The plaque removal effect is likely far more important to periodontal health.

ORAL IRRIGATION DEVICES

Supragingival Irrigation

Oral irrigators for daily home use by patients work by directing a high-pressure, steady or pulsating stream of water through a nozzle to the tooth surfaces (see also Chapter 44). Most commonly, a device with a built-in pump generates the pressure (Fig. 49-24, *A*), but other devices attach to the water faucet. Oral irrigators clean nonadherent bacteria and debris from the oral cavity more effectively than toothbrushes and mouthrinses. They are particularly helpful for removing debris from inaccessible areas around orthodontic appliances and fixed prostheses. When used as adjuncts to toothbrushing, these devices can have a beneficial effect on periodontal health by retarding the accumulation of plaque and calculus[80,100,125] and by reducing inflammation and pocket depth.[25,125]

Oral irrigation has been shown to disrupt and detoxify subgingival plaque and can be useful in delivering antimicrobial agents into periodontal pockets.[114] Irrigation can be supragingival or subgingival. Daily supragingival irrigation with a dilute antiseptic, chlorhexidine, for 6 months resulted in significant reductions in bleeding and gingivitis compared with water irrigation and chlorhexidine rinse controls. Irrigation with water alone also reduced gingivitis significantly but not as much as the dilute chlorhexidine.[52]

Technique. The common home-use irrigator tip is a plastic nozzle with a 90-degree bend at the tip (Fig. 49-24, *B*), attached to a pump providing pulsating beads of water at speeds regulated by a dial. Patients should be instructed to aim the pulsating jet across the proximal papilla, hold it there for 10 to 15 seconds, then trace along the gingival margin to the next proximal space and repeat the procedure. By the time the patient has

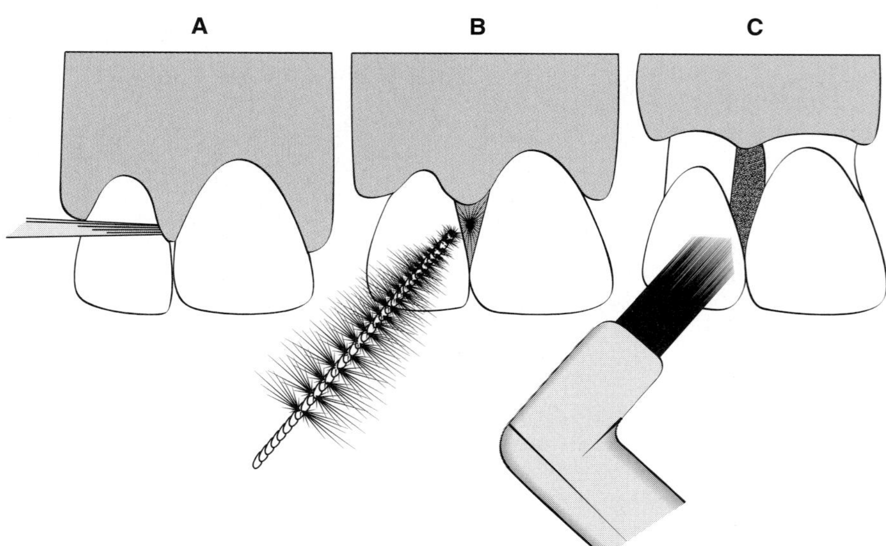

Fig. 49-23 Interproximal embrasure spaces vary greatly in patients with periodontal disease. In general, embrasures with no gingival recession are adequately cleaned using dental floss **(A)**; larger spaces with exposed root surfaces require the use of an interproximal brush **(B)**; and single-tufted brushes clean efficiently in interproximal spaces with no papillae **(C)**.

irrigated all the proximal spaces in the full dentition, the irrigator reservoir will be empty. The irrigator should be used from both the buccal surface and lingual surface. This cleaning must be done while leaning across the bathroom sink because water will drip down the patient's arm. Patients with gingival inflammation usually start at lower pressure and then can increase the pressure comfortably to about medium as tissue health improves. Some individuals like to use the device on the highest pressure setting, with no reported harm. Patient comfort should be the guide for pressure setting.

Subgingival Irrigation

Subgingival irrigation performed both in the dental office or by the patient at home, particularly employing antimicrobial agents, has been shown to provide some site-specific therapy. It is performed by aiming or placing the irrigation tip into the periodontal pocket, attempting to insert the tip at least 3 mm. This is achieved by using a soft rubber tip at home or a canula in the dental office (Fig. 49-24, *C* and *D*).[40] Irrigation performed in the dental office, also called *lavage* or *flushing of the periodontal pocket,* as a one-time treatment after scaling and root planing has not been shown to improve clinical healing. It was reported that the flushing of untreated periodontal pockets with stannous fluoride resulted in slowed regrowth of subgingival bacteria.[111] However, other studies have not confirmed this effect. Data from clinical studies of flushing immediately after scaling and root planing do not show improved gingival healing and do not support its use as providing consistent therapeutic results.[67,132]

Subgingival irrigation performed with an oral irrigator using chlorhexidine diluted to one-third strength, performed regularly at home after scaling, root planing, and in-office irrigation therapy, has produced significant gingival improvement compared with controls.[82] These documented improvements in gingival health, along with other positive clinical results,[67,132] suggest that patients can and should use subgingival irrigation at least once daily in difficult sites such as furcations and residual pockets. Currently available subgingival irrigation tips have been shown to disrupt plaque about half the depth of pockets, up to 7 mm, much further apically than a toothbrush or floss can reach.[42]

Currently, two types of irrigator tips are useful for subgingival irrigation (see Fig. 49-24, *C* and *D*). One is

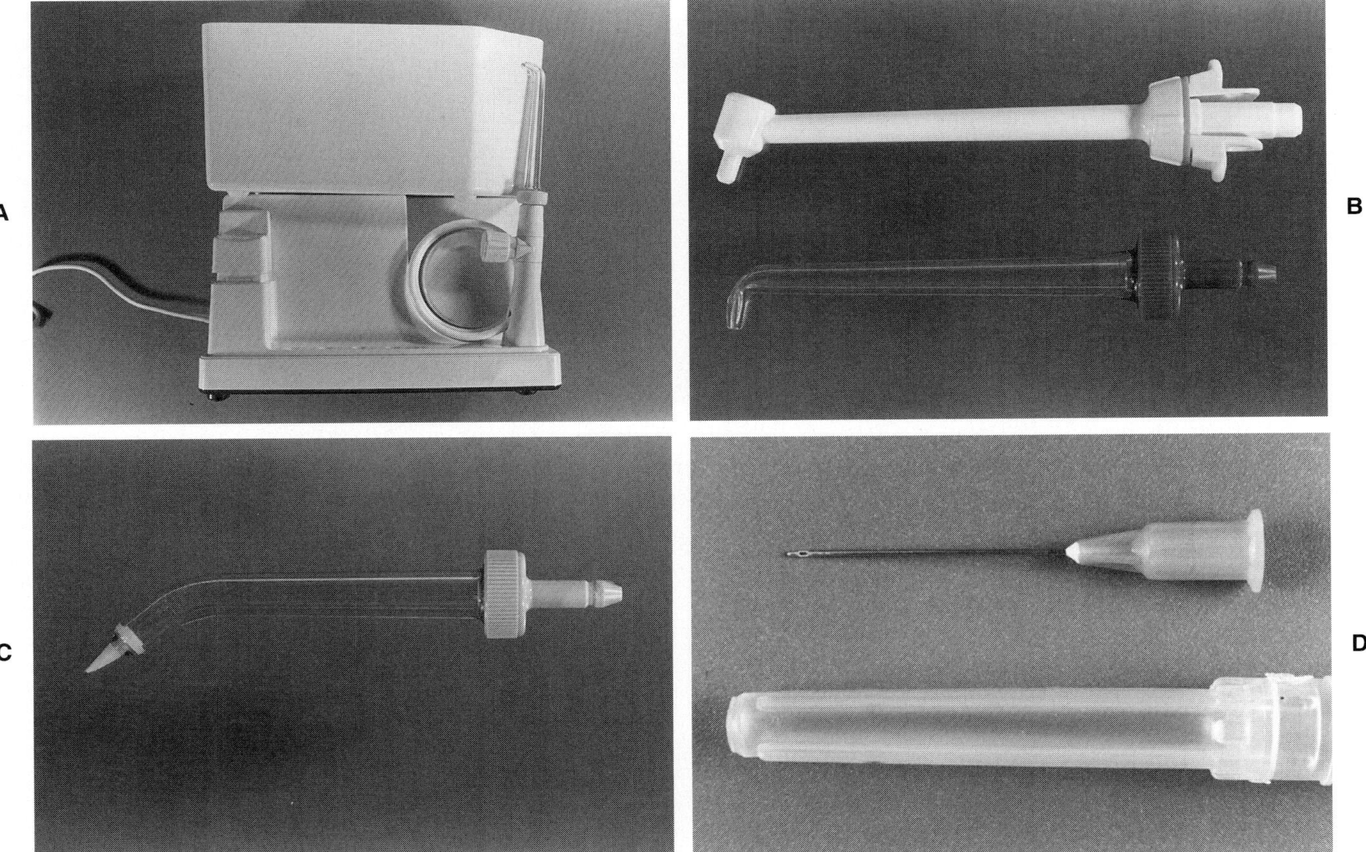

Fig. 49-24 Oral irrigation. **A,** The most common devices have a built-in pump and reservoir. **B,** Conventional plastic tips are used for daily supragingival irrigation at home by the patient. **C,** A soft rubber tip is used for daily subgingival irrigation by the patient at home. **D,** A canula tip is used for subgingival irrigation by the dentist or dental hygienist in the office.

the cannula type tip recommended for office use, and the other is a soft rubber tip for patient use at home. Both reduce the pressure and flow of the pulsating jet of water. Effective penetration of irrigant of up to 70% in laboratory simulation has been shown when using the cannula tip for deeper pockets.[79] Similar results have been reported for the soft rubber tip.[24] The soft rubber tip, designed to irrigate at low pressure and reduced flow, is recommended for patient use at home.[32]

One cautionary note must be considered. Transient bacteremia has been reported after water irrigation in patients with periodontitis[50] and patients on periodontal maintenance.[147] However, bacteremia has also been found after toothbrushing[118] and is known to occur in some significant number of patients after scaling alone.[147] According to the Council on Dental Therapeutics of the ADA, bacteremia also can occur in the absence of dental procedures.[35] Therefore dentists should make every attempt to reduce gingival inflammation in susceptible patients by the use of toothbrushes, floss, and antiseptic mouthrinses. Subgingival irrigation at home is not the oral hygiene procedure of choice for patients requiring antibiotic prophylaxis before dental treatment, particularly if extensive inflammation is present.[40] Supragingival irrigation used in combination with toothbrushing and other interdental cleaning aids is acceptable and can result in improved clinical health.

CARIES CONTROL FOR THE PERIODONTAL PATIENT

Dental caries, particularly root caries, can be a problem for periodontal patients because of attachment loss associated with the disease process and periodontal therapeutic procedures. Root caries develops through a process similar to coronal caries, involving the alternating cycle of demineralization and remineralization of the surfaces.[149] The process requires the fermentation of carbohydrates in the plaque by oral bacteria, resulting in loss of mineral from the root surface. *Lactobacilli* and *Streptococci* species are involved in the root caries process, similar to coronal caries.[47] The major difference is the amount of organic material in the root surfaces is greater than in enamel, so once the demineralization has occurred, the organic matrix—mostly collagen—is exposed. Organic material is then further broken down by bacterial enzymes, resulting in destruction of the root surface.[47]

Fluoride works primarily by topical effects to prevent and reverse the caries process, whether in enamel, cementum, or dentin. Low concentrations of topical fluoride inhibit demineralization, enhance remineralization, and inhibit the enzyme activity in bacteria by acidifying the cells.[48,49]

Topical application of fluorides has been demonstrated to prevent and reverse root surface carious lesions in vitro.[149] Adult patients benefit from the prevention and reversal of root caries provided by low-concentration topical fluoride delivered by toothpastes or other topical applications.[48] It also has been demonstrated that the use of fluoride dentifrice containing 5000 ppm fluoride was more effective in reversing active root caries lesions than the fluoride level of 1100 ppm found in conventional toothpastes.[19]

Periodontal patients require appropriate use of topical fluorides in the daily plaque control regimen to protect and remineralize both exposed root surfaces and coronal surfaces of teeth.

CHEMICAL PLAQUE CONTROL

Mechanical plaque removal remains the primary method used to prevent dental diseases and maintain oral health. However, an improved understanding of the infectious nature of dental diseases has dramatically revitalized interest in chemical methods of plaque control.

The ADA Council on Scientific Affairs has adopted a program for acceptance of plaque control agents. The agents must be evaluated in placebo-controlled clinical trials of 6 months or longer that demonstrate significantly improved gingival health compared with controls. To date, the ADA has accepted two agents for treatment of gingivitis: prescription solutions of chlorhexidine digluconate mouthrinse and nonprescription essential oil mouthrinse.

Chlorhexidine

The agent that has shown the most positive results to date is chlorhexidine, a diguanidohexane with pronounced antiseptic properties. The initial finding that two daily rinses with 10 ml of a 0.2% aqueous solution of chlorhexidine digluconate almost completely inhibited the development of dental plaque, calculus, and gingivitis in the human model for experimental gingivitis[63] has been confirmed by several other clinical investigations. Clinical studies of several months' duration have reported plaque reductions of 45% to 61% and, more importantly, gingivitis reductions of 27% to 67%.[68,92] The 0.12% chlorhexidine digluconate preparation is an equally effective agent currently available in the U.S. for reducing plaque and gingivitis.[7,90]

Local, reversible side effects to chlorhexidine use may occur, primarily brown staining of the teeth, tongue, and silicate and resin restorations[92] and transient impairment of taste perception.[104] Chlorhexidine has very low systemic toxic activity in humans, has not produced any appreciable resistance of oral microorganisms, and has not been associated with any teratogenic alterations.[90] The preparation contains 12% alcohol, which is of concern to clinicians and patients who know that regular use of alcohol increases the risk of oropharyngeal cancer. However, an extensive review of the available epidemiologic evidence associating alcohol-containing mouthrinse preparations with cancer concluded that existing data do not support this association.[44] Regardless, many patients continue to express this concern or simply do not wish to consume alcohol in any form.

Essential Oil Mouthrinse

Essential oil mouthrinses contain thymol, eucalyptol, menthol, and mythyl salicylate.[7] They have been evaluated in three long-term clinical studies and demonstrate plaque reductions of 20% to 35% and gingivitis reductions of 25% to 35%.[39,65,89] This type of mouthrinse has a long history of daily use and safety dating back to the 19th century, and many patients have used the products for decades. These products also contain alcohol (up to 24% depending on the preparation), so some patients and clinicians are reluctant to use them.

Other Products

One preparation containing triclosan has shown some effectiveness in reducing plaque and gingivitis. It is available in toothpaste form, and the active ingredient is more effective in combination with zinc citrate or a copolymer of methoxyethylene.[69]

Several other mouthrinse products on the market have shown some evidence of plaque reduction, although long-term improvement in gingival health has not been substantiated. These include stannous fluoride,[98,152] cetylpyridinium chloride (quaternary ammonia compounds),[12,13] and sanguinarine.[110,119] Evidence suggests that these and other available mouthrinse products do not possess the antimicrobial potential of either chlorhexidine products or essential oil preparations. Also available are mouthrinse preparations with no alcohol content, which may be preferable for some patients. However, any of these mouthrinse products can be useful for patients who perceive benefits from the preparations.

One type of agent has been marketed as a prebrushing mouthrinse to improve the effectiveness of toothbrushing. The active ingredient is sodium benzoate. Research to support its effectiveness is contradictory, but the preponderance of evidence suggests that using a prebrushing rinse is no more effective than brushing alone.[20,21]

Chemical plaque control has been shown to be effective for both plaque reduction and improved wound healing after periodontal surgery.[129] Both chlorhexidine[9] and essential oil[153] mouthrinses have significant positive effects when prescribed for use after periodontal surgery for periods of 1 to 4 weeks.

Recommendations

Mechanical plaque control is necessary and not replaceable by chemical plaque control. Fluoride toothpastes are an essential part of any long-term plaque control program. Appropriate topical preparations of fluoride such as mouthrinses and higher concentration gels should be used as needed for caries control. The addition of antimicrobial mouthrinses will likely reduce gingivitis in periodontal patients.[7] Chlorhexidine rinses are very effective agents[69] and can be used to augment plaque control during Phase I therapy, for patients with recurrent problems, for ineffective plaque control for any reason, for some uncommon oral mucous membrane diseases, and for use after periodontal or oral surgery. Essential oil mouthrinses are also effective but to a lesser degree.[69] They may be advantageous because they have fewer side effects and are available without a prescription. Oral irrigators used with dilute solutions of effective antimicrobial agents can improve daily plaque control by patients.[43] The use of other agents such as cosmetic mouthrinses and prebrushing rinses should not be discouraged if patients perceive benefits from them, but they should not be used to replace proven mechanical and chemical means of plaque removal. Active recommendation of the use of all adjunctive agents should be based on evidence of efficacy and confirmed by clinical research on patients.

DISCLOSING AGENTS

Disclosing agents are solutions or wafers capable of staining bacterial deposits on the surfaces of teeth, tongue, and gingiva. They are excellent oral hygiene aids because they can provide the patient with an educational and motivational tool to improve the efficiency of plaque control procedures[10] (Fig. 49-25).

Solutions and wafers are available commercially. Solutions are applied to the teeth as concentrates on cotton swabs or diluted as rinses. They usually produce heavy staining of bacterial plaque, gingiva, tongue, lips, and fingers, as well as the sink. Wafers are crushed between the teeth and swished around the mouth for a few seconds and then spit out. Either should be used in the office for plaque control instruction and dispensed as needed for home use to aid periodontal patients in evaluating the effectiveness of their oral hygiene routines.

FREQUENCY OF PLAQUE REMOVAL

In the controlled and supervised environment of clinical research, where well-trained individuals remove all visible plaque, gingival health can be maintained by one thorough cleaning exercise with brush, floss, and toothpicks every 24 to 48 hours.[81,88,91] Most patients, however, fall far short of this goal. The average cleaning lasts less than 2 minutes every day and removes only 40% of plaque.[38] Several studies report improved plaque removal and therefore improved periodontal health associated with increasing the frequency of brushing up to twice per day.[81,113] Cleaning three or more times per day does not appear to further improve periodontal conditions. Cleaning once a day with all necessary tools is sufficient if it is performed meticulously. If plaque control is not adequate, a second brushing will help.

Recommendation

Emphasis must be placed on the efficiency of complete plaque removal at least once per day, rather than the frequency of brushing alone. However, poor performance of plaque removal can be improved by brushing twice per day.

PLAQUE CONTROL INSTRUCTION

In periodontal therapy, plaque control has two important purposes: to minimize gingival inflammation and to prevent the recurrence or progression of periodontal disease. Daily mechanical removal of plaque by the patient, including the use of appropriate antimicrobial agents, appears to be the only practical means for improving oral hygiene on a long-term basis. The process requires motivation on the part of the patient, education, and

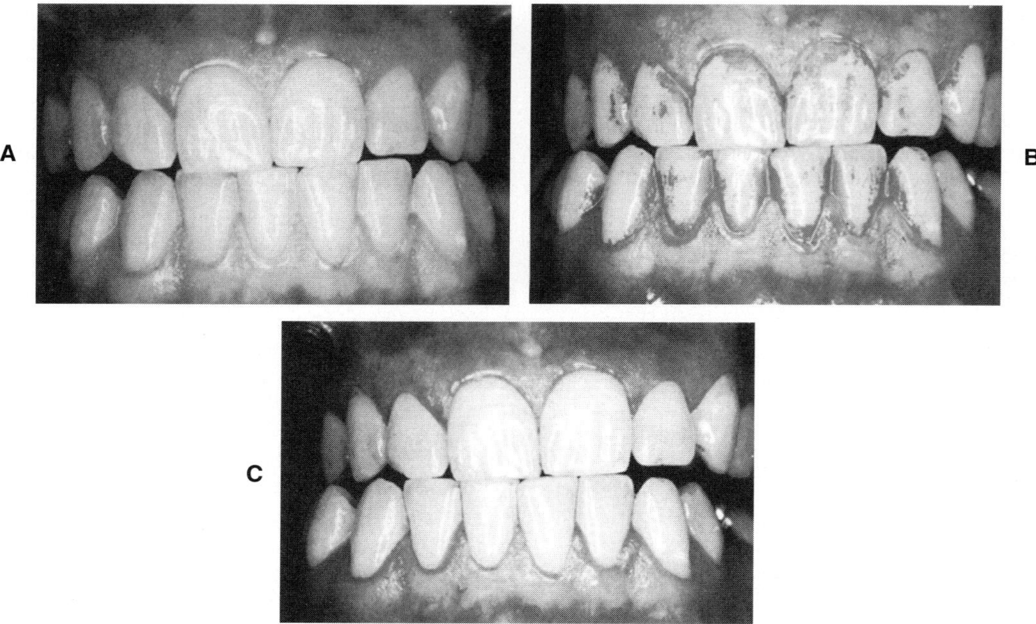

Fig. 49-25 Effect of a disclosing agent. **A,** Unstained. **B,** Plaque shows as dark-red particulate matter when stained with a disclosing dye. **C,** The absence of plaque is dramatically demonstrated by restaining the teeth after mechanical plaque control procedures.

instruction, followed by encouragement and reinforcement. An example of a plaque control record that permits repeated measures and comparison over time is presented in Fig. 49-26.

Motivation for Effective Plaque Control

Undoubtedly, mechanical oral hygiene practices, whether or not they are supplemented with chemical plaque control, are key in the restoration of health and prevention of disease in dentistry. This is true for the two major oral health diseases, dental caries and periodontal disease.[94] Although this chapter has focused on plaque control for patients with periodontal disease, appropriate use of fluoride products to promote remineralization of tooth surfaces and deter demineralization are also essential elements in all individual plaque control programs. These must be used along with appropriate mechanical implements and disinfecting solutions.

Once the patient and clinician have determined the appropriate regimen, changing and augmenting patient behavior remains a significant challenge. Motivating patients to perform effective plaque control is one of the most critical and difficult elements of long-term success in periodontal therapy. It requires both the patient's commitment to adopting new habits of daily plaque control and regular return visits for maintenance and reinforcement.

Patient noncompliance with both prescribed oral hygiene regimens and regular return visits is a common occurrence in dental practice. To give a sense of the magnitude of the problem with plaque control devices, it has been shown that patients stop using interproximal cleaning aids in a very short period of time. Heasman and co-workers followed 100 patients who had been treated for moderate to severe periodontal disease.[72] All had been taught to use one or more interdental cleaning aids, but only 20% used the aids after 6 months. Of those who had started using three devices, one third had stopped all interdental cleaning at 6 months; the others used one or two of the aids. The situation is no better when looking at patient willingness to return for office visits. One study of private patients in a dental clinic showed very disappointing compliance with recall maintenance, the long-term reinforcement and prevention of recurrence aspects of periodontal care. Of 1280 patients, most of whom had periodontal surgery in multiple sites after intensive scaling, root planing, and plaque control instruction, 25% never returned for a follow-up visit. Only 40% returned regularly.[115] Wilson reported that 67% of periodontal patients were noncompliant with return visits in a 20-year retrospective of a private periodontal practice.[151]

Yet motivating patients to adopt new habits and return for office visits is not an impossible task. To be successful, the patient must be:

1. Receptive: Required to understand the concepts of the pathogenesis, treatment, and prevention of periodontal disease.
2. Willing to change the habits of a lifetime: Necessary to adopt a successful, self-administered daily plaque control regimen.
3. Able to make behavioral changes: Required to adjust the hierarchy of a person's beliefs, practices, and values to accommodate the required new oral hygiene habits and return for regular periodontal maintenance visits.

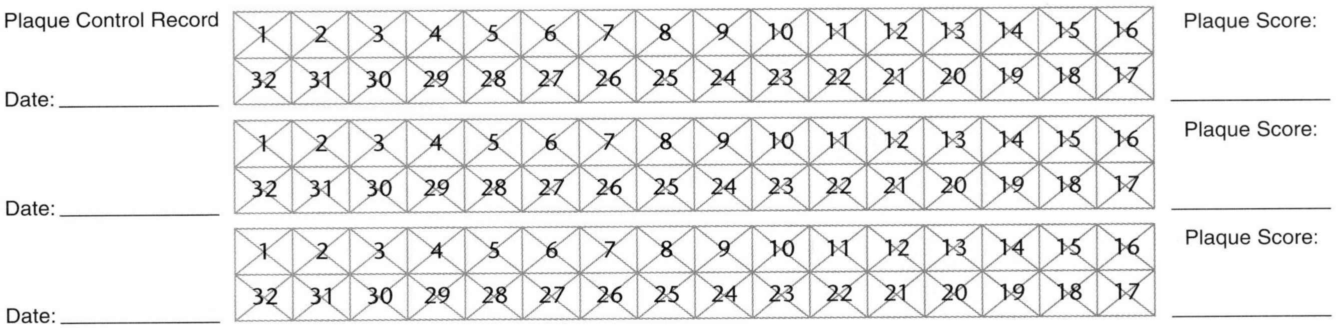

Plaque Control Record	1	2	3	4	5	6	7	8	9	10	11	12	13	14	15	16	Plaque Score:
Date: ______________	32	31	30	29	28	27	26	25	24	23	22	21	20	19	18	17	______________
	1	2	3	4	5	6	7	8	9	10	11	12	13	14	15	16	Plaque Score:
Date: ______________	32	31	30	29	28	27	26	25	24	23	22	21	20	19	18	17	______________
	1	2	3	4	5	6	7	8	9	10	11	12	13	14	15	16	Plaque Score:
Date: ______________	32	31	30	29	28	27	26	25	24	23	22	21	20	19	18	17	______________

Fig. 49-26 The plaque control record can be an effective motivator for patients. This form permits easy comparison of scores over time. (Courtesy Dean Charles N. Bertolami, UCSF School of Dentistry, San Francisco, Calif.)

The patient must understand what periodontal disease is, what its effects are, that he or she is susceptible to it, and what his or her responsibility is in achieving and maintaining oral health. Manual skills must be developed and used to establish an effective plaque control regimen. In addition, the benefits of a clean mouth must be understood. The patient must both learn and adopt the required plaque control measures and return for periodic recall treatment to achieve long-term health benefits.[124] If not, long-term success of treatment is far less likely and can lead to frustration for both the dentist and the patient. Changes in the habits of individuals' entire lives are difficult to achieve but essential. This process begins with educating the patient, developing an acceptable plaque control strategy, and reinforcing positive changes in behavior.

Education

Many patients believe that visits to the dental office for periodontal care will eliminate the disease process. It is incumbent on the dentist to educate and inform the patient to reinforce patient responsibility for long-term success of therapy and cure. Patient-administered plaque control currently is the most important preventive and therapeutic procedure in periodontal therapy. Our health-conscious society is an advantage with regard to patient education. Most patients know what gingivitis is because they have heard about it on television or read about it in magazines. They are willing to spend time and money to try new products such as toothbrushes and mouthrinses. Each patient education experience must be individualized according to need and level of understanding.

Patients must be informed that periodic assessment and debridement of the teeth in the dental office are required to prevent recurrence of periodontal diseases and identify problems that may arise. These procedures work best if combined with individualized oral hygiene procedures practiced daily at home. Therefore time spent in the dental office teaching the patient how to perform plaque control procedures is as central to ongoing care as scaling the teeth. The purpose of the recall visit is **not** to remove plaque because plaque forms every day. Patients sometimes have the concept that "cleanings" by the dentist or dental hygienist once every few months are sufficient for plaque removal and disease control. It must be explained that dental visits two or three times a year are only part of the maintenance needed; effective daily home plaque control is the rest. This information gives each patient responsibility for health care and control over the disease process. Only the combination of regular office visits with conscientious home care significantly reduces gingivitis and loss of supporting periodontal tissues over the long term.[99,141]

The periodontal patient should be shown that periodontal disease has manifested itself in his or her own mouth. Stained dental plaque, the bleeding of inflamed gingiva, and demonstrations of the periodontal probe inserted into pockets are impressive and convincing demonstrations of the presence of pathogens and symptoms of disease. It also is of educational value to a patient to have his or her oral cleanliness and periodontal condition recorded periodically.[16] The patient and the dentist can use this as feedback information about the level of performance and positive reinforcement for improvement. The Plaque Control Record and the Bleeding Points Index are simple indices and are commonly used for patient reinforcement.

Plaque Control Record (the O'Leary Index).[117]

Disclosing solution is applied to all supragingival tooth surfaces. After the patient has rinsed to remove excess dye, each tooth surface (except occlusal surfaces) is examined for the presence or absence of stained deposits at the dentogingival junction, four surfaces for each tooth. Plaque, if present, is indicated on the appropriate box in a diagram. After all teeth have been scored, the index is calculated by dividing the number of surfaces with plaque by the total number of surfaces scored and then multiplied by 100 to get a percentage of surfaces with plaque present. A reasonable goal for patients is 10% or fewer surfaces with plaque, unless plaque is always present in the same areas. If so, special instructions should be directed toward improving performance in those areas. It is extremely difficult to achieve a perfect score of 0, so patients should be rewarded for approaching it.

Some commonly used plaque indices do not require staining the teeth, such as the Plaque Index of Silness and Löe.[133] These may seem more convenient to use and possibly more acceptable to patients, but they have some disadvantages for patient education. Identification of plaque is not as quick and easy for the clinician's record making, and because plaque is not stained, it is not highlighted for the patient to see and remove.

Bleeding Points Index.[95] The Bleeding Points Index provides an evaluation of bleeding gingiva around each tooth in the patient's mouth. Retract the cheek, and place the periodontal probe 1 mm into the sulcus or pocket at the distal aspect of the most posterior tooth in the quadrant. Carry the probe lightly across the length of the sulcus to the mesial interproximal area on the facial aspect. Continue along all the teeth in the quadrant from the facial aspect. Wait 30 seconds, and record the presence of bleeding on the distal, facial, and mesial surfaces on the chart. Repeat on the lingual-palatal aspect, recording bleeding only for the direct lingual surface, not for the mesial or distal surfaces. This results in four separate scores for each tooth and does not score the mesial and distal surfaces twice. Repeat the steps for each quadrant.

The percentage of the number of bleeding surfaces is then calculated to provide the patient's score. Divide the number of surfaces that bled by the total number of tooth surfaces (4 per tooth) and convert the number to a percentage by multiplying by 100.

This index is designed to demonstrate bleeding gingiva rather than the presence of plaque. Again, a goal of 10% or fewer bleeding points is good, but 0 is ideal. If a few bleeding points repeatedly occur in the same areas, plaque control for those areas should be reinforced or modified.

Significance of Plaque Scores and Bleeding Scores. Plaque scores are helpful as indicators of patient compliance and success with daily plaque control procedures. They once were used as an educational tool to demonstrate improvement in patient technique and give positive reinforcement. However, plaque levels themselves do not necessarily reflect gingival health or risk of disease progression, even though plaque is highly correlated with the presence of gingivitis.[103] In terms of predicting success in controlling inflammation and reducing the chance of disease progression, bleeding is by far the better indicator. Bleeding on probing is not the most specific and sensitive of measures of health; however, it has a strong negative correlation to disease progression. If bleeding is absent at any given site in the mouth, reflecting good plaque control and disease management, the chance that periodontal disease will progress is unlikely.[93]

Instruction and Demonstration

Patients can reduce the incidence of plaque and gingivitis with repeated instruction and encouragement far more effectively than with self-acquired oral hygiene habits.[66,141] However, instruction in how to clean teeth must be more than a cursory chairside demonstration of the use of a toothbrush. It is a painstaking procedure that requires patient participation, careful supervision with correction of mistakes, and reinforcement during return visits until the patient demonstrates that he or she has developed the necessary proficiency.[8,97]

One useful strategy for introducing plaque control to the periodontal patient includes several elements. At the first instruction visit, the patient should be given a new toothbrush, an interdental cleaner, and a disclosing agent. The patient's plaque should be disclosed. Small amounts of dental plaque are difficult for the patient to see if not disclosed (see Fig. 49-25, *A*); heavier accumulations of plaque and debris may be visible as gray, yellow, or white material on the teeth, along the gingival margin, and in faciolingual embrasures. Then a disclosing solution or wafer is used to stain the invisible plaque. After a brief water rinse to remove excess dye and stained saliva, which would obscure the view of the teeth, the stained plaque and pellicle can be clearly demonstrated to the patient (see Fig. 49-25, *B*). Polished dental restorations do not take up the stain, but the oral mucosa and the lips may retain it for up to several hours. Covering the lips lightly with petroleum jelly before using the dye is helpful.

Toothbrushing should be demonstrated in the patient's mouth while he or she observes with a hand mirror. The patient then takes over and repeats the procedures on his or her own teeth with the instructor giving assistance, correction, and positive reinforcement.

Repeat the demonstration and instruction process with dental floss and interdental cleaning aids according to the patient's needs. The teeth can be restained to evaluate the efficiency of plaque removal, but even after vigorous cleaning, some stain usually remains on proximal surfaces (see Fig. 49-25, *C*). Teaching videos and pamphlets can be used to augment personalized instruction, but they are not a substitute; reminder pamphlets may be useful for the patient to take home.

The patient should be given the hygiene aids necessary to get started. He or she must be encouraged to clean the teeth at least once a day, with thorough attention to all areas. Home care procedures on a full dentition take 5 to 10 minutes; in complex periodontal maintenance cases, such procedures may require up to 30 minutes. The patient should set aside a convenient time and place in his or her daily schedule to perform the procedures reliably every day.

Subsequent instruction visits should be used to reinforce or modify previous instructions, periodically recording the state of gingival health and amount of plaque.

In general, some strategies will help improve patient compliance. These include the following:

- Providing clinician encouragement
- Demonstrating how devices should work
- Providing samples
- Showing improvements
- Generally using positive reinforcement[142]

In addition, some strategies are sure not to work. These include the following:

- Showing insensitivity to patient needs and situation
- Instructing at the end of the appointment, when the

plaque has either been removed by the clinician or the patient is exhausted or sore

- Failing to provide reinforcement at subsequent appointments
- Handing the patient too many tools
- Relying only on a pamphlet to provide education

Reinforcement and encouragement should be given often to help patients modify long-standing habits, adopt new ones, and understand that their plaque control is also important to the clinician.

Sensitivity to patient needs, patience on the clinician's part, and positive reinforcement are the secrets of success in plaque control instruction.

SUMMARY

1. All patients require the regular use of a toothbrush, either manual or electric, at least once per day. The brushing method should include access to the gingival margin of all accessible surfaces and extension as far onto the proximal surfaces as possible.
2. Dental floss should be used in all interdental spaces that are filled with gingiva. The technique requires wrapping the floss around the proximal surfaces and inserting the floss as far subgingivally as possible. Flossing may be accomplished either with a tool or by using the fingers.
3. Interdental aids such as interproximal brushes, wooden tips, rubber tips, or toothpicks should be used in all areas where the toothbrush and floss techniques cannot adequately remove the plaque. This includes large embrasure spaces and furcation areas.
4. All periodontal patients should use some form of low-concentration topical fluoride on a daily basis, a fluoride containing dentifrice at the very least. Topical rinses and gels may be required if the patient demonstrates a risk of caries or history of root caries.
5. Daily home-delivered subgingival irrigation may be a good choice for reduction of inflammation and maintenance for patients with residual deep pockets and those who struggle with mechanical interproximal cleaning devices. The effectiveness of irrigation is enhanced by the addition of chlorhexidine or essential oil mouthrinse to the irrigation water.
6. Chemical antimicrobial agents such as chlorhexidine or essential oil mouthwashes can be prescribed to disinfect the patient's mouth and control the infection. They may be continued indefinitely, as no specific duration of time for use of these products has been recommended. In fact, many patients have used essential oil mouthrinses for years. The staining of teeth and taste alteration side effects may limit patient use of these products.
7. Reinforcement of daily plaque control practices and routine visits to the dental office for maintenance care are essential to successful plaque control and long term success of therapy.

REFERENCES

1. Abrasivity of current dentifrices: Report of the Council of Dental Therapeutics. J Am Dent Assoc 1970; 81:1177.
2. Accepted Dental Therapeutics, ed 3. Chicago, American Dental Association, 1969–1970.
3. ADA Council on Scientific Affairs. 2001; www.ada.org.
4. Addy M, Adriaens P: Consensus report of group A epidemiology and etiology of periodontal diseases and the role of plaque control in dental caries. In: Lang NP, Ättstrom R, Löe H (eds): Proceedings of the European Workshop on Mechanical Plaque Control. Chicago, Quintessence, 1998.
5. Ainamo J, Xie Q, Ainamo A, et al: Assessment of the effect of an oscillating/rotating electric toothbrush on oral health: A 12-month longitudinal study. J Clin Periodontol 1997; 24:28.
6. American Academy of Periodontology, Committee Report: The tooth brush and methods of cleaning the teeth. Dent Items Int 1920; 42:193.
7. American Academy of Periodontology: Treatment of gingivitis and periodontitis position paper. J Periodontol 1997; 68:1246.
8. Anderson JL: Integration of plaque control into the practice of dentistry. Dent Clin North Am 1972; 16:621.
9. Anderson L, Sanz M, Newman MG, et al: Clinical effects of a 0.12% chlorhexidine mouthrinse on periodontal surgical wounds without periodontal dressing. J Dent Res 1988; 67:329(abst 1728).
10. Arnim SS: The use of disclosing agents for measuring tooth cleanliness. J Periodontol 1963; 34:227.
11. Ash MM: A review of the problems and results of studies on manual and power toothbrushes. J Periodontol 1964; 35:202.
12. Ashley FP, Skinner A, Jackson P, et al: The effect of a 0.1% cetylpyridinium chloride mouthrinse on plaque and gingivitis in adult subjects. Br Dent J 1984; 157:191.
13. Ashley FP, Skinner A, Jackson PY, et al: Effect of a 0.1% cetylpyridinium chloride mouthrinse on the accumulation and biochemical composition of dental plaque in young adults. Caries Res 1984; 18:465.
14. Axelsson P, Lindhe J: The effect of a preventive programme on dental plaque, gingivitis and caries in school children: Results after one and two years. J Clin Periodontol 1974; 1:126.
15. Barnes CM, Russell CM, Weatherford III TW: A comparison of the efficacy of 2 powered toothbrushes in affecting plaque accumulation, gingivitis, and gingival bleeding. J Periodontol 1999; 70:840.
16. Barrikman R, Penhall O: Graphing indexes reduce plaque. J Am Dent Assoc 1973; 87:1404.
17. Bass CC: An effective method of personal oral hygiene. Part II. J La State Med Soc 1954; 106:100.
18. Bass CC: The optimum characteristics of toothbrushes for personal oral hygiene. Dent Items Int 1948; 70:697.
19. Baysan A, Lynch E, Ellwood R, et al: Reversal of primary root caries using dentifrices containing 5000 and 1100 ppm fluoride. Caries Res 2001; 35:41.
20. Beiswander BB, Mallott MC, Mau MS, et al: The relative plaque removal effect of a prebrushing mouthrinse. J Am Dent Assoc 1990; 120:190.
21. Binney A, Addy M, Newcombe RG: The plaque removal effects of single rinsings and brushings. J Periodontol 1993; 64:181.
22. Bjorn H, Lindhe J: On the mechanics of toothbrushing. Odont Revy 1966; 17:9.
23. Brandtzaeg P: The significance of oral hygiene in the prevention of dental diseases. Odont T 1964; 72:460.
24. Braun RE, Ciancio SG: Subgingival delivery by an oral irrigation device. J Periodontol 1992; 63:469.
25. Cantor MT, Stahl SS: Interdental col tissue responses to the use of a water pressure device. J Periodontol 1969; 40:292.

26. Cantor MT, Stahl SS: The effects of various interdental stimulators upon the keratinization of the interdental col. Periodontics 1965; 3:243.
27. Carter-Hanson C, Gadbury-Amyot C, Killoy WJ: Comparison of the plaque removal efficacy of a new flossing aid (Quik-Floss) to finger flossing. J Clin Periodontol 1996; 23:873.
28. Castenfelt T: Toothbrushing and Massage in Periodontal Disease. An Experimental Clinical Histologic Study. Stockholm, Nordisk Rotegravyr, 1952.
29. Charters WJ: Eliminating mouth infections with the toothbrush and other stimulating instruments. Dent Digest 1932; 38:130.
30. Chava VK: An evaluation of the efficacy of a curved bristle and conventional toothbrush. A comparative clinical study. J Periodontol 2000; 71:785.
31. Christou V, Timmerman MF, Van der Velden U, et al: Comparison of different approaches of interdental oral hygiene: Interdental brushes versus dental floss. J Periodontol 1998; 69:759.
32. Ciancio SC: Clinical benefits of powered subgingival irrigation. Biol Ther Dentist 1992; 8:13.
33. Claydon N, Addy M: Comparative single-use plaque removal by toothbrushes of different designs. J Clin Periodontol 1996; 23:1112.
34. Cronin M, Dembling W, et al: An investigation of the efficacy and safety of a new electric interdental plaque remover for the reduction of interproximal plaque and gingivitis. J Clin Dent 1996; 7:74.
35. Dajani AS, Taubert KA, Wilson W, et al: Prevention of bacterial endocarditis: Recommentations by the American Heart Association. J Am Dent Assoc 1997; 128:1142.
36. Daly CG, Chapple CC, Cameron AC: Effect of toothbrush wear on plaque control. J Clin Periodontol 1996; 23:45.
37. Danser MM, Timmerman MF, Ijzerman Y, et al: Evaluation of the incidence of gingival abrasion as a result of toothbrushing. J Clin Periodontol 1998; 25:701.
38. de la Rosa MR, Guerra JZ, Johnston DA, et al: Plaque growth and removal with daily toothbrushing. J Periodontol 1979; 50:661.
39. de Paola LG, Overholser CD, Meiller TF, et al: Chemotherapeutic reduction of plaque and gingivitis development, a 6 month investigation. J Dent Res 1986; 65:274(abst 941).
40. Drisko CH: Nonsurgical periodontal therapy: Pharmacotherapeutics. Ann Periodontol 1996; 1:491.
41. Dyer D, Addy M, Newcombe RG: Studies in vitro of abrasion by different manual toothbrush heads and a standard toothpaste. J Clin Periodontol 2000; 27:99.
42. Eakle WS, Ford C, Boyd RL: Depth of penetration in periodontal pockets with oral irrigation. J Clin Periodontol 1986; 13:39.
43. Echeverria JJ: Managing the use of oral hygiene aids to prevent damage: Effects and sequelae of the incorrect use of mechanical plaque removal devices. In: Lang NP, Attstrom R, Löe H (eds): Proceedings of the European Workshop on Mechanical Plaque Control. Chicago, Quintessence, 1998.
44. Elmore JG, Horwitz JI: Oral cancer and mouthwash use: Evaluation of the epidemiologic evidence. Otolaryngol Head Neck Surg 1995; 113:253.
45. Eriksen HM, Gjermo P, Johansen JR: Results from two years' use of chlorhexidine (CH)-containing dentifrices. Helv Odontol Acta 1973; 17:52.
46. Ervin JC, Bucher ET: Prevalence of tooth root exposure and abrasion among dental patients. Dent Items Int 1944; 66:7601.
47. Featherstone JDB: Fluoride, remineralization and root caries. Am J Dent 1994; 7:271.
48. Featherstone JDB: Prevention and reversal of dental caries: Role of low level fluoride. Comm Dent Oral Epidemiol 1999; 27:31.
49. Featherstone JDB: The science and practice of caries prevention. J Amer Dent Assoc 2000; 131:887.
50. Felix JA, Rosen S, App GR: Detection of bacteremia after the use of an oral irrigation device in subjects with periodontitis. J Periodontol 1971; 42:785.
51. Finkelstein P, Grossman E: The effectiveness of dental floss in reducing gingival inflammation. J Dent Res 1979; 58:1034.
52. Flemmig TF, Newman MG, Doherty FM, et al: Supragingival irrigation with 0.06% chlorhexidine in naturally occurring gingivitis. I. Six month clinical observations. J Periodontol 1990; 61:112.
53. Fones AC: Mouth Hygiene, ed 4. Philadelphia, Lea & Febiger, 1934.
54. Forgas-Brockmann LB, Carter-Hanson C, Killoy WJ: The effects of an ultrasonic toothbrush on plaque accumulation and gingival inflammation. J Clin Periodontol 1998; 25:375.
55. Garmyn P, van Steenberghe D, Quirynen M: In: Lang NP, Ättstrom R, Löe H (eds): Proceedings of the European Workshop on Mechanical Plaque Control. Chicago, Quintessence, 1998.
56. Gillette WB, Van House RL: Ill effects of improper oral hygiene procedures. J Am Dent Assoc 1980; 101:476.
57. Gilson CM, Charbeneau GT, Hill HC: A comparison of physical properties of several soft toothbrushes. J Mich Dent Assoc 1969; 51:347.
58. Gjermo P, Flotra L: The effect of different methods of interdental cleaning. J Periodont Res 1970; 5:230.
59. Gjermo P, Flotra L: The plaque removing effect of dental floss and toothpicks: A group comparison study. J Periodont Res 1969; 4:170(abst).
60. Glass RL: A clinical study of hand and electric toothbrushing. J Periodontol 1965; 36:322.
61. Glickman I, Petralis R, Marks R: The effect of powered toothbrushing and interdental stimulation upon microscopic inflammation and surface keratinization of the interdental gingiva. J Periodontol 1965; 36:108.
62. Glickman I, Petralis R, Marks R: The effect of powered toothbrushing plus interdental stimulation upon the severity of gingivitis. J Periodontol 1964; 35:519.
63. Goldman HM: The effect of single and multiple toothbrushing in the normal and periodontally involved dentition. Oral Surg 1956; 9:203.
64. Gordon JM, et al: A clinical study of the safety and efficacy of a novel electric interdental cleaning device. J Clin Dent 1996; 7:70.
65. Gordon JM, Lamster IV, Seiger MC: Efficacy of Listerine antiseptic in inhibiting the development of plaque and gingivitis. J Clin Periodontol 1985; 12:697.
66. Gravelle HR, Shackelford NF, Lovett JT: The oral hygiene of high school students as affected by three different educational programs. J Public Health Dent 1967; 27:91.
67. Greenstein G: Effects of subgingival irrigation on periodontal status. J Periodontol 1987; 58:827.
68. Grossman E, Reiter G, Sturzenberger OP, et al: Six-month study of the effects of a chlorhexidine mouthrinse on gingivitis in adults. J Periodont Res 1986; 21(Suppl):33.
69. Hancock EP: Prevention. Ann Periodontol 1996; 1:223.
70. Harrington JH, Terry IA: Automatic and hand toothbrushing abrasion studies. J Am Dent Assoc 1964; 68:343.
71. Harris NO: Dentifrices, mouth rinses, and oral irrigators. In: Harris NO, Christen AG (eds): Primary Preventive Dentistry, ed 3. East Norwalk, CT, Appleton & Lange, 1991.

72. Heasman PA, Jacobs DJ, Chapple IL: An evaluation of the effectiveness and patient compliance with plaque control methods in the prevention of periodontal disease. J Clin Prev Dent 1989; 11:24.
73. Heasman PA, McCracken GI: Powered toothbrushes: A review of clinical trials. J Clin Periodontol 1999; 26:407.
74. Hellstrom M-K, Ramberg P, Krok L, et al: The effects of supragingival plaque control on subgingival microflora in human periodontitis. J Clin Periodontol 1996; 23:934.
75. Hill HC, Levi PA, Glickman I: The effects of waxed and unwaxed dental floss on interdental plaque accumulation and interdental gingival health. J Periodontol 1973; 44:411.
76. Hine MK: Toothbrush. Int Dent J 1956; 6:15.
77. Hiniker JJ, Forscher BK: The effect of toothbrush type on gingival health. J Periodontol 1954; 25:40.
78. Hirschfeld I: The toothbrush, its use and abuse. Dent Items Int 1931; 3:833.
79. Hollander BN, Boyd RL, Eakle WS: Comparison of subgingivally placed cannula oral irrigator tip with a supragingivally placed standard irrigator tip. J Clin Periodontol 1992; 19:340.
80. Hoover DR, Robinson HBG, Billingsley A: The comparative effectiveness of the Water-Pik in a noninstructed population. J Periodontol 1968; 39:43(abst).
81. Jepson S: The role of manual toothbrushes in effective plaque control; advantages and limitations. In: Lang NP, Ättstrom R, Löe H (eds): Proceedings of the European Workshop on Mechanical Plaque Control. Chicago, Quintessence, 1998.
82. Jolkovsky DL, Waki MY, Newman MN, et al: Clinical and microbiological effects of subgingival and gingival marginal irrigation with chlorhexidine gluconate. J Periodontol 1990; 61:663.
83. Kazmierczak M, Mather M, Ciancio S, et al: A clinical evaluation of anticalculus dentifrices. J Clin Preventive Dent 1990; 12:13–17.
84. Keller SE, Manson-Hing LR: Clearance studies of proximal tooth surfaces. Part II. In vivo removal of interproximal plaque. Ala J Med Sci 1969; 6:266.
85. Keller SE, Manson-Hing LR: Clearance studies of proximal tooth surfaces. Parts III and IV. In vivo removal of interproximal plaque. Ala J Med Sci 1969; 6:399.
86. Khocht A, Simon G, Person P, et al: Gingival recession in relation to history of hard toothbrush use. J Periodontol 1993; 64:900–905.
87. Kieser J: Groeneveld H: A clinical evaluation of a novel toothbrush design. J Clin Periodontol 1997; 24:419.
88. Kinane DF: The role of interdental cleaning in effective plaque control: need for interdental cleaning in primary and secondary prevention. In: Proceedings of the European Workshop on Mechanical Plaque Control. Chicago, Quintessence, 1998.
89. Lamster IB, Alfano MC, Seiger MC, et al: The effect of Listerine antiseptic on reduction of existing plaque and gingivitis. J Clin Prev Dent 1983; 5:12.
90. Lang NP, Brecx MC: Chlorhexidine digluconate—an agent for chemical plaque control and prevention of gingival inflammation. J Periodont Res 1986; 21(Suppl):74.
91. Lang NP, Cumming BR, Löe H: Toothbrushing frequency as it relates to plaque development and gingival health. J Periodontol 1973; 44:396.
92. Lang NP, Hotz P, Graf H, et al: Effects of supervised chlorhexidine mouthrinses in children. A longitudinal clinical trial. J Periodont Res 1982; 17:101.
93. Lang NP, Joss A, Orsanic T, et al: Bleeding on probing: a predictor for the progression of periodontal diseases? J Clin Periodontol 1986; 13:590.
94. Lang NP: Preface. In: Lang NP, Ättstrom R, Löe H (eds): Proceedings of the European Workshop on Mechanical Plaque Control. Chicago, Quintessence, 1998.
95. Lenox JA, Kopczyk RA: A clinical system for scoring a patient's oral hygiene performance. J Am Dent Assoc 1973; 86:849.
96. Leonard JF: Conservative treatment of periodontoclasia. J Am Dent Assoc 1939; 26:1308.
97. Less W: Mechanics of teaching plaque control. Dent Clin North Am 1972; 16:647.
98. Leverett DH, McHugh WD, Jensen DE: Effect of daily rinsing with stannous fluoride on plaque and gingivitis: Final report. J Dent Res 1984; 63:1083.
99. Lindhe J, Nyman S: The effect of plaque control and surgical pocket elimination on the establishment and maintenance of periodontal health. A longitudinal study of periodontal therapy in cases of advanced disease. J Clin Periodontol 1975; 2:67.
100. Lobene RR: The effect of a pulsed water pressure cleaning device on oral health. J Periodontol 1969; 40:667.
101. Lobene RR: The effect of an automatic toothbrush on gingival health. J Periodontol 1964; 35:137.
102. Löe H, Schiott CR: The effect of mouthrinses and topical application of chlorhexidine on the development of dental plaque and gingivitis in man. J Periodont Res 1970; 5:79.
103. Löe H, Theilade E, Jensen SB: Experimental gingivitis in man. J Periodontol 1965; 36:177.
104. Löe H: Does chlorhexidine have a place in the prophylaxis of dental disease? J Periodont Res 1973; 8(suppl 12):93.
105. Macgregor IDM, Balding JW, Regis D: Flossing behaviour in English adolescents. J Clin Periodontol 1998; 25:291.
106. MacNeill S, Walter DM, Day A, et al: Sonic and mechanical toothbrushes an in vitro study showing altered microbial surface structures but lack of effect on viability. J Clin Periodontol 1998; 25:988.
107. Mallatt ME, Beiswanger BB, Stookey GK, et al: Influence of soluble pyrophosphates on calculus formation in adults. J Dent Res 1985; 64:1159.
108. Manhold JH: Gingival tissue health with hand and power brushing: A retrospective with corroborative studies. J Periodontol 1967; 38:23.
109. Manly RS, Brudevold F: Relative abrasiveness of natural and synthetic toothbrush bristles on cementum and dentin. J Am Dent Assoc 1957; 55:779.
110. Mauriello SM, Bader JD: Six-month effects of a sanguinarine dentifrice on plaque and gingivitis. J Periodontol 1988; 59:238.
111. Mazza JE, Newman MG, Simms TN: Clinical and microbial effect of stannous fluoride on periodontitis. J Clin Periodontol 1981; 8:203.
112. McKendrick AJW, Barbenel LMH, McHugh WD: A two-year comparison of hand and electric toothbrushes. J Periodont Res 1968; 3:224.
113. McKendrick AJW, Barbenel LMH, McHugh WD: The influence of time of examination, eating, smoking, and frequency of brushing on the oral debris index. J Periodont Res 1970; 5:205.
114. Mueller-Joseph LM, Davis C, Jones B: Oral irrigation and antimicrobial plaque control. In: Woodall IR (ed): Comprehensive Dental Hygiene Care, ed 4. St Louis, Mosby, 1993.
115. Novaes AB, Novaes AB Jr, Moraes N, et al: Compliance with supportive periodontal therapy. J Periodontol 1996; 67:213.
116. O'Beirne G, Johnson RH, Persson GR, et al: Efficacy of a sonic toothbrush on inflammation and probing depth in adult periodontitis. J Periodontol 1996; 67:900.
117. O'Leary TJ, Drake RB, Naylor JE: The plaque control record. J Periodontol 1972; 43:38.

118. O'Leary TJ, Shafer WG, Swenson HM, et al: Possible penetration of crevicular tissue from oral hygiene procedures. II. Use of the toothbrush. J Periodontol 1970; 41:158.
119. Parsons LG, Thomas LG, Southard GL, et al: Effect of sanguinaria extract on established plaque and gingivitis when supragingivally delivered as a manual rinse or under pressure in an oral irrigator. J Clin Periodontol 1987; 14:381.
120. Pattison GA: Self-inflicted gingival injuries: Literature review and case report. J Periodontol 1983; 54:299.
121. Perry DA, Pattison G: The investigation of wax residue on tooth surfaces after the use of waxed dental floss. Dent Hygiene 1986; 60:16.
122. Proceedings of the European Workshop on Mechanical Plaque Control (Lang NP, Ättstrom R, Löe H, eds.) Chicago, Quintessence, 1998.
123. Renton-Harper P, Addy M, Warren P, et al: Comparison of video and written instructions for plaque removal by an oscillating/rotating/reciprocating electric toothbrush. J Clin Periodontol 1999; 26:752.
124. Renvert S, Glavind L: Individualized instruction and compliance in oral hygiene practices: recommendations and means of delivery. In: Lang NP, Ättstrom R, Löe H, (eds): Proceedings of the European Workshop on Mechanical Plaque Control. Chicago, Quintessence, 1998.
125. Robinson HBG, Hoover PR: The comparative effectiveness of a pulsating oral irrigator as an adjunct in maintaining oral health. J Periodontol 1971; 42:37.
126. Sanders WE, Robinson HBG: The effect of toothbrushing on deposition of calculus. J Periodontol 1962; 33:386.
127. Sangnes G, Gjermo P: Prevalence of oral soft and hard tissue lesions related to mechanical tooth cleaning procedures. Commun Dent Oral Epidemiol 1976; 4:77.
128. Sangnes G: Traumatization of teeth and gingiva related to habitual tooth cleaning procedures. J Clin Periodontol 1976; 3:94.
129. Sanz M, Herrera D: Role of oral hygiene during the healing phase of periodontal therapy. In: Lang NP, Ättstrom R, Löe H (eds): Proceedings of the European Workshop on Mechanical Plaque Control. Chicago, Quintessence, 1998.
130. Saxton CA: The effects of dentifrices on the appearance of the tooth surface observed with the scanning electron microscope. J Periodont Res 1976; 11:74.
131. Schmid MO, Balmelli O, Saxer UP: The plaque removing effect of a toothbrush, dental floss and a toothpick. J Clin Periodontol 1976; 3:157.
132. Shiloah J, Hovious LA: The role of subgingival irrigations in the treatment of periodontitis. J Periodontol 1993; 64:835.
133. Silness J, Löe H: Periodontal disease in pregnancy: II. Correlation between oral hygiene and periodontal condition. Acta Odontol Scand 1964; 22:121.
134. Silverstone LM, Featherstone MJ: A scanning electron microscope study of the end rounding of bristles in eight toothbrush types. Quint Int 1988;19:87.
135. Spolsky VA, Perry DA, Meng Z, et al: Evaluating the efficacy of a new flossing aid. J Clin Periodontol 1993; 20:490.
136. Stahl SS, Wachtel N, DeCastro C, et al: The effect of toothbrushing on the keratinization of the gingiva. J Periodontol 1953; 24:20.
137. Stillman PR: A philosophy of the treatment of periodontal disease. Dent Digest 1932; 38:314.
138. Stookey G: Are all fluoride dentifrices the same? In: Wei SHY (ed): Clinical Uses of Fluorides. Philadelphia, Lea & Febiger, 1985.
139. Stookey GK, Muhler JC: Laboratory studies concerning the enamel and dentin abrasion properties of common dentifrice polishing agents. J Dent Res 1968; 47:524.
140. Straub AM, Salvi GE, Lang NP: Supragingival plaque formation in the human dentition. In: Lang NP, Ättstrom R, Löe H (eds): Proceedings of the European Workshop on Mechanical Plaque Control. Chicago, Quintessence, 1998.
141. Suomi JD, Green JC, Vermillion JR, et al: The effect of controlled oral hygiene procedures on the progression of periodontal disease in adults: Results after two years. J Periodontol 1969; 40:416.
142. Tedesco LA, Keffler MA, Davis EL, et al: Effect of a social cognitive intervention no oral health status, behavior reports, and cognition. J Periodontol 1992; 63:567.
143. Tritten CB, Armitage GA: Comparison of a sonic and a manual toothbrush for efficacy in supragingival plaque removal and reduction of gingivitis. J Clin Periodontol 1996; 23:641.
144. van der Weijden GA, Timmerman MF, Danser MM, et al: Relationship between the plaque removal efficacy of a natural toothbrush and brushing force. J Clin Periodontol 1998; 25:413.
145. van der Weijden GA, Timmerman MF, Danser MM, et al: The role of electric toothbrushes: advantages and limitations. In: Lang NP, Ättstrom R, Löe H (eds): Proceedings of the European Workshop on Mechanical Plaque Control. Chicago, Quintessence, 1998.
146. Waerhaug J. The interdental brush and its place in operative and crown and bridge dentistry. J Oral Rehabil 1976; 3:107.
147. Waki MY, Jolkovsky DL, Otomo-Corgel J, et al: Effects of subgingival irrigation on bacteremia following scaling and root planing. J Periodontol 1990; 61:405.
148. Warren PR, Ray TS, Cugini M, et al: A practice-based study of a power toothbrush: assessment of effectiveness and acceptance. J Am Dent Assoc 2000; 131:389.
149. Wefel JS: Root caries histopathology and chemistry. Am J Dent 1994; 7:261.
150. Wilkins EM: Oral disease control: toothbrushes and toothbrushing. In: Clinical Practice of the Dental Hygienist, ed 6. Philadelphia, Lea & Febiger, 1992.
151. Wilson TG Jr, Glover ME, Schoen J, et al: Compliance with maintenance therapy in a private dental practice. J Periodontol 1984; 55:468.
152. Yankell SL: Toothbrushing and toothbrushing techniques. In: Harris NO, Christen AG (eds): Primary Preventive Dentistry, ed 3. East Norwalk, CT, Appleton & Lange, 1991.
153. Yukna RA, Broxson AW, Mayer ET, et al: Comparison of Listerine mouthwash and periodontal dressing following periodontal flap surgery. Clin Prev Dent 1986; 4:14.
154. Zacheri WA, Pheiffer HJ, Swancar JR: The effect of soluble pyrophosphates on dental calculus in adults. J Am Dent Assoc 1985; 110:737.
155. Zimmer S, Didner B, Roulet J-F: Clinical study on the plaque-removing ability of a new triple-headed toothbrush. J Clin Periodontol 1999; 26:281.

Chemotherapeutic Agents in the Treatment of Periodontal Diseases

David L. Jolkovsky and Sebastian G. Ciancio

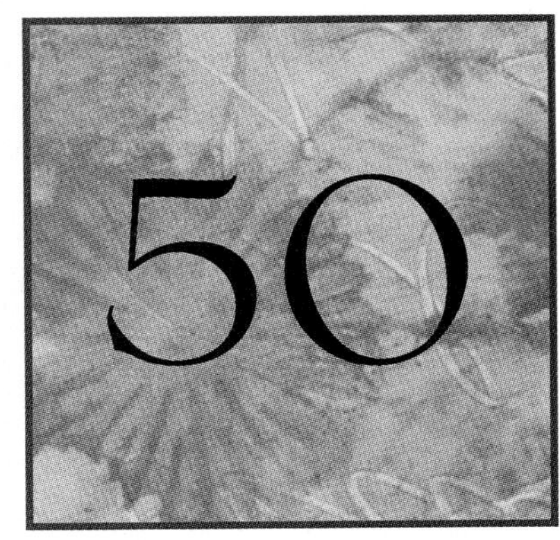

CHAPTER

CHAPTER OUTLINE

The various periodontal diseases result from susceptible hosts having their periodontal tissues colonized by specific oral pathogens in numbers sufficient to overwhelm their tissue defenses. Clinical success in the treatment of these diseases thus requires reduction of the bacterial load or enhancement of the host tissues' ability to defend or repair itself. Traditionally, the foundations of clinical success include education of patients in daily oral hygiene; surgical and nonsurgical mechanical root debridement to remove subgingival bacteria and their accretions from root surfaces; and supportive periodontal therapy generally at 3- to 6-month intervals. In certain types of periodontal disease including chronic advanced periodontitis, refractory periodontitis, aggressive periodontitis, and periodontitis as a manifestations of systemic diseases, adjunctive chemotherapeutic agents may be necessary to control the disease process.[3] This chapter reviews the indications and use of chemotherapeutic agents in the treatment of periodontal disease.

Chemotherapeutic agent is a general term for a chemical substance that provides a clinical therapeutic benefit. This term does not specify in what way the agent aids in attaining a clinical benefit. Clinical benefits can be derived through antimicrobial actions or an increase in the host's resistance. An **antimicrobial agent** is a chemotherapeutic agent that works by reducing the number of bacteria present. **Antibiotics** are a naturally occurring, semisynthetic or synthetic type of antimicrobial agent that destroys or inhibits the growth of selective microorganisms, generally at low concentrations. **Antiseptics** are chemical antimicrobial agents that are applied topically or subgingivally to mucous membranes, wounds, or intact dermal surfaces to destroy microorganisms and inhibit their reproduction or metabolism.[18] In dentistry, antiseptics are widely used as the active ingredient in antiplaque and antigingivitis mouthrinses and dentifrices. **Disinfectants,** a subcategory of antiseptics, are antimicrobial agents that are generally applied to inanimate surfaces to destroy microorganisms.[18]

Chemotherapeutic agents can be administered *locally, orally, or parenterally.* In either case, their purpose is to reduce the number of bacteria present in the diseased periodontal pocket. *Systemic* antibiotics may be a necessary adjunct in controlling bacterial infection because bacteria can invade periodontal tissues, making mechanical therapy alone sometimes ineffective.[11,15,60] *Local administration* of antimicrobial agents, generally directly in the pocket, has the potential to provide greater concentrations directly to the infected area and reduce possible systemic side effects.

A single chemotherapeutic agent can have a dual mechanism of action. For instance, tetracycline is a chemotherapeutic agent that can reduce collagen and bone destruction through its ability to inhibit the enzyme collagenase. As an antibiotic agent, it also can reduce periodontal pathogens in periodontal tissues.[17,18] Additionally, tetracyclines have been shown to be effective when administered systemically and applied locally.

SYSTEMIC ADMINISTRATION OF ANTIBIOTICS

The treatment of periodontal diseases is based on the infectious nature of these diseases (Table 50-1). Ideally, the causative microorganism(s) should be identified and the most effective agent selected using antibiotic sensitivity tests. Although this appears simple, the difficulty lies primarily in identifying specific etiologic microorganism(s) rather than microorganisms simply associated with various periodontal disorders.[16,17]

The possible clinical benefits of administering antibiotics to help control periodontal disease must be weighed against possible adverse reactions. Some adverse reactions include allergic/anaphylactic reactions, superinfections of opportunistic bacteria, development of resistant bacteria, interactions with other medications, upset stomach nausea, and vomiting.[38] Common and indiscriminate use of antibiotics worldwide has contributed to increasing numbers of resistant bacterial strains over the last 15 to 20 years, and this trend is likely to continue given the widespread use of antibiotics.[77] The overuse, misuse, and widespread prophylactic application of antimicrobial drugs are some of the factors that have led to the emergence of resistant microorganisms. Increasing levels of resistance of subgingival microflora to antibiotics has been correlated with the increased use of antibiotics in individual countries.[73]

An ideal antibiotic for use in prevention and treatment of periodontal diseases should be specific for periodontal pathogens, allogenic and nontoxic, substantive,

TABLE 50-1

Antibiotics Used to Treat Periodontal Diseases: Their Major Features and Indications

Category/Family	Agent(s) Used to Treat Periodontal Diseases	Major Features	Indications
Penicillin	Amoxicillin	Extended spectrum of antimicrobial activity, excellent oral adsorption; used systemically.	LAP, GAP, MRP, RP.
	Augmentin	Effective against penicillinase producing microorganisms; used systemically.	
Tetracycline	Minocycline	Effective against broad spectrum of microorganisms; used systemically and applied locally (subgingivally).	
	Doxycycline	Effective against broad spectrum of microorganisms; used systemically and applied locally (subgingivally); chemotherapeutically used in subantimicrobial dose for host modulation (Periostat).	
	Tetracycline	Effective against broad spectrum of microorganisms; applied locally (subgingivally) in fiber (Actisite).	
Quinolone	Ciprofloxacin	Effective against gram-negative rods, promotes health-associated microflora.	
Macrolide	Azithromycin	Concentrates at sites of inflammation; used systemically.	
Lincomycin derivative	Clindamycin	Used in penicillin-allergic patients; effective against anaerobic bacteria; used systemically.	
Nitroimidazole	Metronidazole	Effective against anaerobic bacteria; used systemically and applied locally (subgingivally) as a gel.	LAP, GAP, MRP, RP, AP, NUG.

CP, Chronic periodontitis; *LAP,* localized aggressive periodontitis; *GAP,* generalized aggressive periodontitis; *MRP,* medically related periodontitis; *NUG,* necrotizing ulcerative periodontitis; *RP,* refractory periodontitis.

not in general use for treatment of other diseases, and inexpensive.[26] Currently, an ideal antibiotic for the treatment of periodontal diseases does not exist.[38] Although oral bacteria are susceptible to many antibiotics, no single antibiotic at concentrations achieved in body fluids inhibits all putative periodontal pathogens.[81] Indeed, a combination of antibiotics may be necessary to eliminate all putative pathogens from some periodontal pockets[57] (Table 50-2).

Guidelines for use of antibiotics in periodontal therapy include the following:

1. The *clinical diagnosis* and situation dictate the need for possible antibiotic therapy as an adjunct in controlling active periodontal disease (Fig. 50-1). The patient's diagnosis can change over time. For instance, a patient that presents with generalized slight chronic periodontitis can return to a diagnosis of periodontal health after initial therapy. However, if this patient has been treated appropriately and continues to have active disease, the diagnosis can change to refractory periodontitis.
2. Continuing disease activity, as measured by continuing attachment loss, purulent exudate, and/or continuing periodontal pockets of ≥5 mm[43,44] that bleed on probing, is an indication for microbial analysis and further periodontal therapy.
3. When used to treat periodontal disease, antibiotics are selected based on the microbial composition of the plaque, the patient's medical status and the current medications.[38]
4. Microbiologic sampling is performed according to the instructions of the reference microbiologic laboratory. Commonly, the samples are taken at the beginning of an appointment before instrumentation of the pocket. Supragingival plaque is removed and an endodontic paper point is inserted subgingivally into the deepest pocket(s) present to absorb bacteria in the loosely associated plaque. This endodontic point is placed in reduced transfer fluid and sent overnight to the laboratory. The laboratory will then send the referring dentist a report that includes the pathogens present and any appropriate antibiotic regimen.
5. Plaque sampling can be performed at the initial examination, root planing, reevaluation, or supportive periodontal therapy appointment. As noted previously, clinical indications for microbial testing include aggressive forms of periodontal disease, diseases refractory to standard mechanical therapy, and periodontitis associated with systemic conditions (see Fig. 50-1).
6. Antibiotics have been shown to have value in reducing the need for periodontal surgery in patients with chronic periodontitis.[47]
7. Antibiotic therapy should **not** be used as a monotherapy (Figs. 50-1 and 50-2). That is, it must be part of the comprehensive periodontal treatment plan. This therapy should have debridement of root surfaces, optimal oral hygiene, and frequent supportive periodontal therapy at the center of therapy. Other chemotherapeutic adjuncts include locally placed subgingival antimicrobial agents, subgingival ultrasonic irrigation with iodophors during root debridement, chlorhexidine rinse after debridement for 2 weeks, and home intraoral irrigation with or without chemotherapeutic agents.[38] Chlorhexidine gluconate is effective as an antiplaque rinse, but its antimicrobial activity is greatly reduced in the presence of organic matter in the subgingival periodontal pocket. However, povidone-iodine (Betadine) is an effective antibacterial agent when used directly into the periodontal pocket, even at low concentrations.[38,59] Povidone-iodine must be used with caution in patients sensitive to iodine, although the sensitization rate is low.[52] It also should be used with caution in patients who are pregnant or lactating.[14]
8. Slots and co-workers have described a series of steps using antimicrobial agents for enhancing regenerative healing. They recommend starting antibiotics 1 to 2 days before surgery and continuing for a total of at least 8 days.[38,54,62]

TABLE 50-2

Common Antibiotic Regimens Used in Treating Periodontal Diseases[38]

	Regimen	Duration
Single Agent		
Metronidazole	250–500 mg 3 times daily	8 days
Ciprofloxacin	500 mg 2 times daily	8 days
Clindamycin	300 mg 2 times daily	8 days
Combination Therapy		
Metronidazole/amoxicillin	250 mg of each 3 times daily	8 days
Metronidazole/ciprofloxacin	500 mg of each 2 times daily	8 days

These regimens are prescribed with a review of the patient's medical history, periodontal diagnosis, and antimicrobial testing. Consult *Mosby's GenRx*[61] or manufacturer's guidelines for contraindications and precautions.

Tetracyclines

Tetracyclines have been widely used in the treatment of periodontal diseases. They have been frequently used in treating refractory periodontitis, including localized aggressive periodontitis (see Table 50-1). Tetracyclines have the ability to concentrate in the periodontal tissues and inhibit the growth of *Actinobacillus actinomycetemcomitans*. In addition, they exert an anticollagenase effect that can inhibit tissue destruction and may aid bone regeneration (see Host Modulation).

Pharmacology. The tetracyclines are a group of antibiotics produced naturally from certain species of *Streptomyces* or derived semisynthetically. These antibiotics are bacteriostatic and are effective against rapidly multiplying bacteria. They generally are more effective against gram-positive bacteria than gram-negative bacteria.[83]

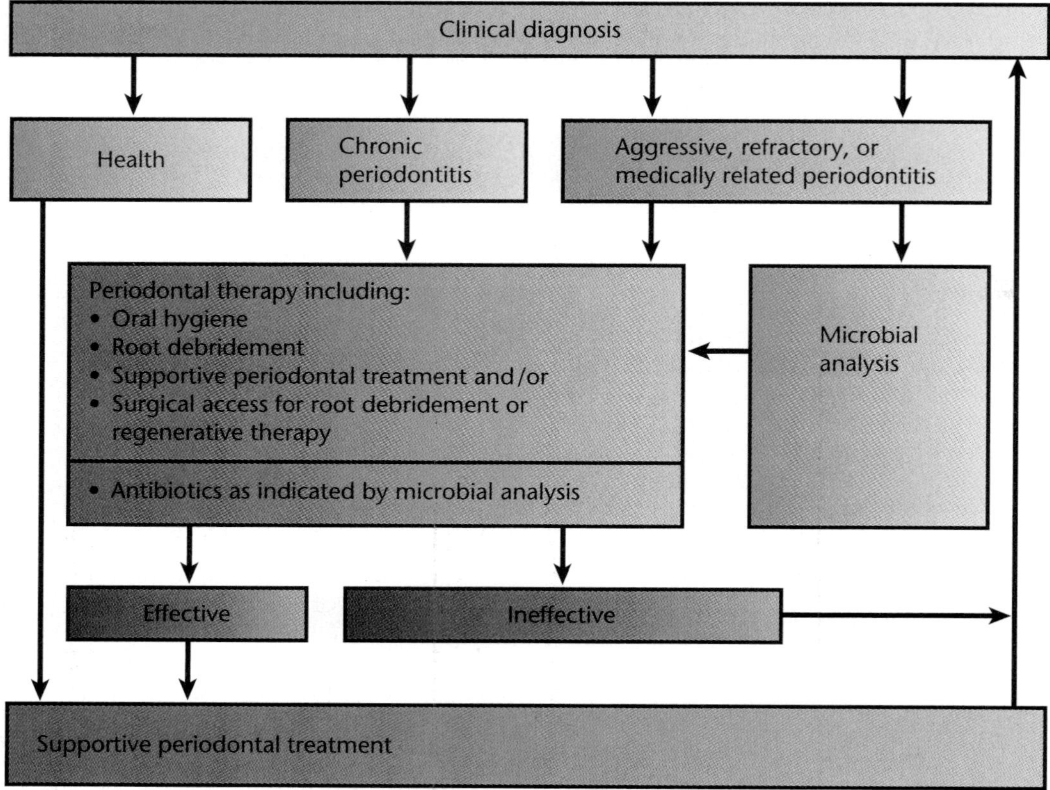

Fig. 50-1 Guidelines for use of antimicrobial therapy.

Tetracyclines are effective in treating periodontal diseases in part because their concentration in the gingival crevice is 2 to 10 times that in serum.[2,5,31] This allows a high drug concentration to be delivered into periodontal pockets. In addition, several studies have demonstrated that tetracyclines at a low gingival crevicular fluid concentration (2 to 4 μg/ml) are very effective against many periodontal pathogens.[6,7,81]

Clinical Use. Tetracyclines have been investigated as adjuncts in the treatment of localized aggressive periodontitis (LAP). *A. actinomycetemcomitans* is a frequent causative microorganism in LAP and is tissue invasive. Therefore mechanical removal of calculus and plaque from root surfaces may not eliminate this bacterium from the periodontal tissues. Systemic tetracycline can eliminate tissue bacteria and has been shown to arrest bone loss and suppress *A. actinomycetemcomitans* levels in conjunction with scaling and root planing.[63,64] This combined form of therapy allows mechanical removal of root surface deposits and elimination of pathogenic bacteria from within the tissues. Increased posttreatment bone levels have been noted using this method.[25,63]

Long-term use of low doses of tetracyclines has been advocated in the past. One long-term study of patients taking low doses of tetracycline (250 mg per day for 2 to 7 years) showed persistence of deep pockets that did not bleed on probing. These sites contained high proportions of tetracycline-resistant, gram-negative rods (i.e., *Fusobacterium nucleatum*). After the antibiotic was discontinued, the flora was characteristic of sites with disease.[42] Therefore it is not advisable to engage in long-term regimens of tetracyclines because of the possible development of resistant bacterial strains. Although commonly used in the past as antimicrobial agents, especially for localized aggressive periodontitis and other types of aggressive periodontitis, tetracyclines now tend to be replaced by more effective combination antibiotics.[38,73]

Specific Agents. Tetracycline, minocycline, and doxycycline—all semisynthetic members of the tetracycline group—have been used in periodontal therapy.

TETRACYCLINE. Tetracycline requires administration of 250 mg qid. It is inexpensive, but compliance may be reduced by having to take four capsules per day.

MINOCYCLINE. Minocycline is effective against a broad spectrum of microorganisms. In patients with adult periodontitis, it suppresses spirochetes and motile rods as effectively as scaling and root planing, with suppression remaining evident for up to 3 months after therapy. Minocycline can be given twice a day, thus facilitating compliance when compared with tetracycline. Although it is associated with less photo- and renal toxicity than tetracycline, it may cause reversible vertigo. Minocycline administered in a dosage of 200 mg per day for 1 week results in a reduction in total bacterial counts,

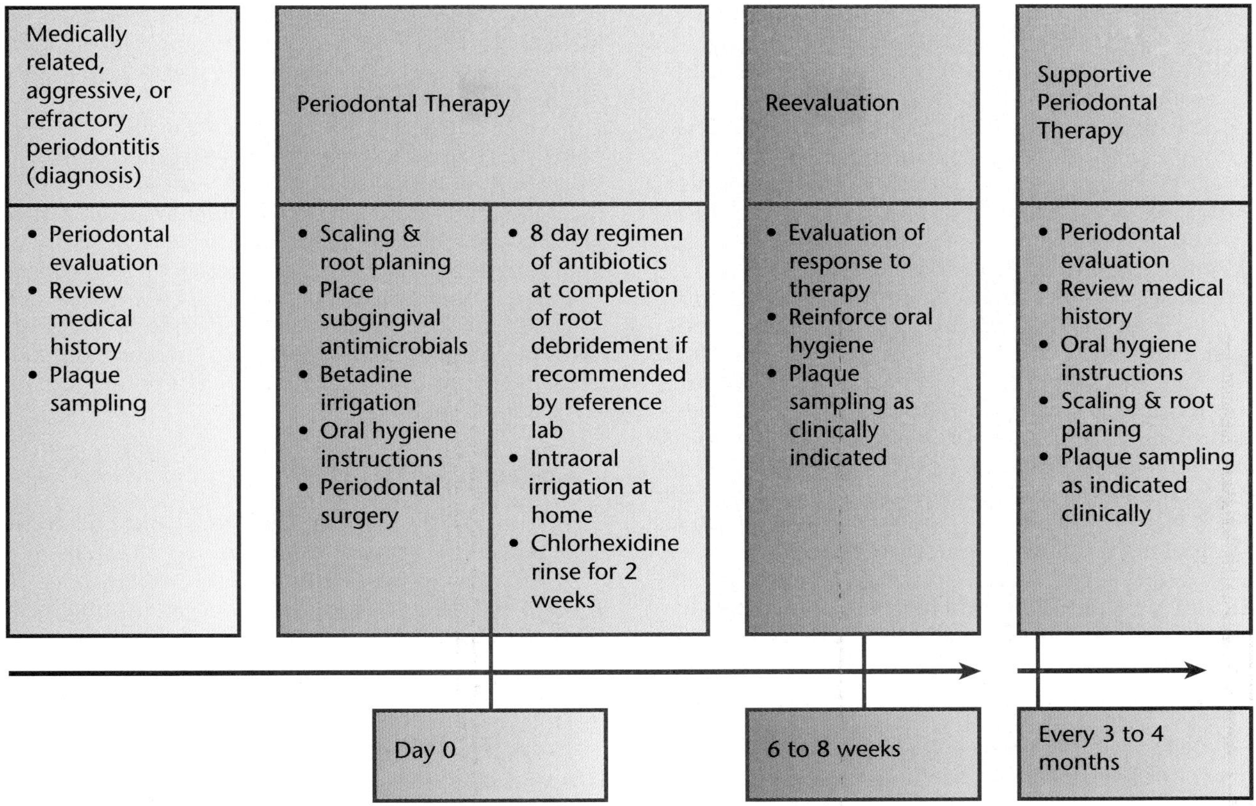

Fig. 50-2 Sequencing of antimicrobial agents. (Adapted from Jorgensen MG, Slots J: Practical antimicrobial periodontal therapy. Compend Contin Educ Dent 2000; 21:111.)

complete elimination of spirochetes for periods of up to 2 months, and improvement in all clinical parameters.[20]

DOXYCYCLINE. Doxycycline has the same spectrum of activity as minocycline and may be equally as effective.[17] Because it can be given only once daily, patients may be more compliant. Compliance is also favored because its absorption from the gastrointestinal tract is not altered by calcium, metal ions, or antacids, as is absorption of other tetracyclines. The recommended dosage when used as an antimicrobial agent is 100 mg twice daily the first day, then 100 mg once daily. To reduce gastrointestinal upset, 50 mg can be taken twice daily. When used in a subantimicrobial dose to inhibit collagenase, it is recommended in a 20-mg dose twice daily[13] (see Host Modulation).

Metronidazole

Pharmacology. Metronidazole is a nitroimidazole compound developed in France to treat protozoal infections. It is bactericidal to anaerobic organisms and is believed to disrupt bacterial DNA synthesis in conditions in which a low reduction potential is present. Metronidazole is not the drug of choice for treating *A. actinomycetemcomitans* infections, but it may be effective at therapeutic levels owing to its hydroxy metabolite. However, it is effective against *A. actinomycetemcomitans* when used in combination with other antibiotics.[56,57] Metronidazole is also effective against anaerobes such as *Porphyromonas gingivalis* and *Prevotella intermedia*.[34]

Clinical Usage. Metronidazole has been used clinically to treat gingivitis, acute necrotizing ulcerative gingivitis, chronic periodontitis, and aggressive periodontitis. It has been used as monotherapy and also in combination with both root planing and surgery or with other antibiotics. Metronidazole has been used successfully for treating necrotizing ulcerative gingivitis.[48]

Studies in humans[46,47] have demonstrated the efficacy of metronidazole in the treatment of gingivitis and periodontitis. A single dose of metronidazole (250 mg orally) appears in both serum and gingival fluid in sufficient quantities to inhibit a wide range of suspected periodontal pathogens. Administered systemically (750 to 1000 mg/day for 2 weeks), this drug reduces the growth of anaerobic flora, including spirochetes, and decreases the clinical and histopathologic signs of periodontitis.[46] The most commonly prescribed regimen is 250 mg tid for 7 days.[48] Loesche and co-workers found that 250 mg of metronidazole given three times daily for 1 week was of benefit to patients with a diagnosed anaerobic periodontal infection. In this study, an infection was considered anaerobic when spirochetes composed 20% or more of the total microbial count. Metronidazole used as a supplement to rigorous scaling and root planing resulted in a significantly reduced need for surgery when compared with root planing alone. The bacteriologic data of this study showed that only the spirochete count was significantly reduced.[47] Currently, the critical level of spirochetes needed to diagnose an anaerobic infection, the appropriate time to give metronidazole, and the ideal dosage or duration of therapy are unknown.[34]

As monotherapy (no concurrent root planing), metronidazole is inferior and at best only equivalent to root planing. Therefore if metronidazole is used, it should not be administered as monotherapy.

Metronidazole offers some benefit in the treatment of refractory periodontitis, particularly when used in combination with amoxicillin. The existence of refractory periodontitis as a diagnostic category indicates that some patients do not respond to conventional therapy, including root planing, surgery, or both. Soder and co-workers showed that metronidazole was more effective than placebo in the management of sites unresponsive to root planing.[65] Nevertheless, many patients still had sites that bled on probing despite metronidazole therapy.

Studies have suggested that when combined with amoxicillin or amoxicillin-clavulanate potassium (Augmentin), metronidazole may be of value in the management of patients with localized aggressive or refractory periodontitis (see later discussion).

Side Effects. Metronidazole has an antabuse effect when alcohol is ingested. The response is generally proportional to the amount ingested and can result in severe cramps, nausea, and vomiting. Products containing alcohol should be avoided during therapy and for at least 1 day after therapy is discontinued. Metronidazole also inhibits warfarin metabolism. Patients undergoing anticoagulant therapy should avoid metronidazole because it prolongs prothrombin time.[34] It also should be avoided in patients who are taking lithium.

Penicillins

Pharmacology. Penicillins are the drugs of choice for the treatment of many serious infections in humans and are the most widely used antibiotics. Penicillins are natural and semisynthetic derivatives of broth cultures of the *Penicillium* mold. They inhibit bacterial cell wall production and therefore are bactericidal.

Clinical Usage. Penicillins other than amoxicillin and amoxicillin-clavulanate potassium (Augmentin) have not been evaluated, and their use in periodontal therapy does not appear to be justified.[82]

Side Effects. Penicillins may induce allergic reactions and bacterial resistance; up to 10% of patients may be allergic to penicillin.

Amoxicillin. Amoxicillin is a semisynthetic penicillin with an extended antimicrobial spectrum that includes gram-positive and gram-negative bacteria. It demonstrates excellent absorption after oral administration. Amoxicillin is susceptible to penicillinase, a β-lactamase produced by certain bacteria that breaks the penicillin ring structure and thereby renders penicillins ineffective.[82]

Amoxicillin may be useful in the management of patients with aggressive periodontitis, both in the localized and generalized forms. Recommended dosage is 500 mg tid for 8 days.[38,39]

Amoxicillin–Clavulanate (Augmentin). The combination of amoxicillin with clavulanate potassium makes Augmentin resistant to penicillinase enzymes produced by some bacteria. Augmentin may be useful in the management of patients with refractory or localized aggressive periodontitis.[57] Bueno and co-workers reported that Augmentin arrested alveolar bone loss in patients with periodontal disease that was refractory to treatment with other antibiotics including tetracycline, metronidazole, and clindamycin.[10]

Cephalosporins

Pharmacology. The family of β-lactams known as *cephalosporins* is similar in action and structure to penicillins. They are frequently used in medicine and are resistant to a number of β-lactamases normally active against penicillin.

Clinical Usage. Cephalosporins are generally not used to treat dental-related infections. The penicillins are superior to cephalosporins in their range of action against periodontopathic bacteria.

Side Effects. Patients allergic to penicillins must be considered allergic to all β-lactam products. Rashes, urticaria, fever, and gastrointestinal upset have been associated with cephalosporins.[78]

Clindamycin

Pharmacology. Clindamycin is effective against anaerobic bacteria.[71] It is effective in situations in which the patient is allergic to penicillin.

Clinical Usage. Clindamycin has shown efficacy in patients with periodontitis refractory to tetracycline therapy. Walker and co-workers[80] have shown aid in stabilizing refractory patients. Dosage used in their studies was 150 mg qid for 10 days. Jorgensen and Slots have recommended a regimen of 300 mg twice daily for 8 days.[39]

Side Effects. Clindamycin has been associated with pseudomembranous colitis more often than other antibiotics, thereby limiting its use. When needed, however, it can be used with caution. Diarrhea or cramping that develops during the use of clindamycin may be indicative of cholitis, and clindamycin should be discontinued. If symptoms persist, the patient should be referred to an internist.

Ciprofloxacin

Pharmacology. Ciprofloxacin is a quinolone active against gram-negative rods, including all facultative and some anaerobic putative periodontal pathogens.

Clinical Usage. Because it demonstrates minimal effect on *Streptococcus* species, which are associated with periodontal health,[56] ciprofloxacin therapy may facilitate the establishment of a microflora associated with periodontal health. At present, ciprofloxacin is the only antibiotic in periodontal therapy to which all strains of *A. actinomycetemcomitans* are susceptible. It also has been used in combination with metronidazole.[56]

Side Effects. Nausea, headache, and abdominal discomfort have been associated with ciprofloxacin. Quinolones inhibit the metabolism of theophylline, and caffeine and concurrent administration can produce toxicity. Quinolones have also been reported to enhance the effect of warfarin and other anticoagulants.[78]

Macrolides

Pharmacology. Macrolide antibiotics contain a many-membered lactone ring to which one or more deoxy sugars are attached. They inhibit protein synthesis by binding to the 50 S ribosomal subunits of sensitive microorganisms. They can be bacteriostatic or bactericidal, depending on the concentration of the drug and the nature of the microorganism.

Clinical Usage. **Erythromycin** does not concentrate in gingival crevicular fluid, and it is not effective against most putative periodontal pathogens. For these reasons, it is not recommended as an adjunct to periodontal therapy. **Spiramycin** is active against gram-positive organisms; it is excreted in high concentrations in saliva. It is used as an adjunct to periodontal treatment in Canada and Europe but is not available in the U.S. Several studies have shown benefits, as measured by the Gingival Index, the Plaque Index, pocket depth, and crevicular fluid flow[50,68] when spiramycin was prescribed in advanced periodontal disease. In addition, it is a safe, nontoxic drug with few and infrequent side effects and is not in general use for medical problems.[28] **Azithromycin (Zithromax)** is a member of the azalide class of macrolides. It is effective against anaerobes and gram-negative bacilli. After an oral dosage of 500 mg once daily for three consecutive days, significant levels of azithromycin can be detected in most tissues for 7 to 10 days.[8] The concentration of azithromycin in tissue specimens from periodontal lesions is significantly higher than that of normal gingiva.[49] It has been proposed that azithromycin penetrates fibroblasts and phagocytes in concentrations 100 to 200 times greater than that of the extracellular compartment. The azithromycin is actively transported to sites of inflammation by phagocytes and then released directly into the sites of inflammation as the phagocytes rupture during phagocytosis.[27,36] Therapeutic use requires a single dose of 250 mg per day for 5 days after an initial loading dose of 500.[78]

SERIAL AND COMBINATION ANTIBIOTIC THERAPY

Rationale

Because periodontal infections may contain a wide diversity of bacteria, no single antibiotic is effective against all putative pathogens. Indeed, differences exist in the microbial flora associated with the various periodontal disease syndromes.[80] These "mixed" infections can include a variety of aerobic, microaerophilic, and anaerobic bacteria, both gram negative and gram positive. In these instances, it may be necessary to use more than one antibiotic, either serially or in combination.[57] However, before combinations of antibiotics are used, the periodontal pathogen(s) being treated must be identified and antibiotic susceptibility testing performed.

Clinical Use

Antibiotics that are *bacteriostatic* (e.g., tetracycline) generally require rapidly dividing microorganisms to be effective. They do not function well if a *bactericidal* antibiotic (e.g., amoxicillin) is given concurrently. *When both types of drugs are required, they are best given serially, not in combination.*

Rams and Slots reviewed combination therapy using systemic metronidazole along with amoxicillin, Augmentin, or ciprofloxacin.[57] The metronidazole–amoxicillin and metronidazole–Augmentin combinations provided excellent elimination of many organisms in adult and localized aggressive periodontitis that had been treated unsuccessfully with tetracyclines and mechanical debridement. These drugs have an additive effect regarding suppression of *A. actinomycetemcomitans.* Tinoco and coworkers[69] found metronidazole and amoxicillin to be clinically effective in treating localized aggressive periodontitis, although 50% of patients harbored *A. actinomycetemcomitans* one year later. Metronidazole–ciprofloxacin combination is effective against *A. actinomycetemcomitans.* Metronidazole targets obligate anaerobes, and ciprofloxacin targets facultative anaerobes. This is a powerful combination against mixed infections. Studies of this drug combination in the treatment of refractory periodontitis have documented marked clinical improvement. This combination may provide a *therapeutic benefit* by reducing or eliminating pathogenic organisms and a *prophylactic benefit* by giving rise to a predominantly streptococcal microflora.[56]

Systemic antibiotic therapy combined with mechanical therapy appears valuable in the treatment of recalcitrant periodontal infections and localized aggressive periodontitis infections involving *A. actinomycetemcomitans.* Antibiotic treatment should be reserved for specific subsets of periodontal patients who do not respond to conventional therapy. Selection of specific agents should be guided by the results of cultures and sensitivity tests for subgingival plaque microorganisms.

HOST MODULATION

Doxycycline Hyclate

The U.S. Food and Drug Administration recently granted marketing approval for doxycycline hyclate (Periostat) for the adjunctive treatment of periodontitis. Periostat, available as a 20-mg capsule of doxycycline hyclate, is prescribed for use by patients twice daily. The mechanism of action is by suppression of the activity of collagenase, particularly that produced by polymorphonuclear leukocytes. A schematic diagram of the role of matrix metalloproteinases in the progression of periodontal

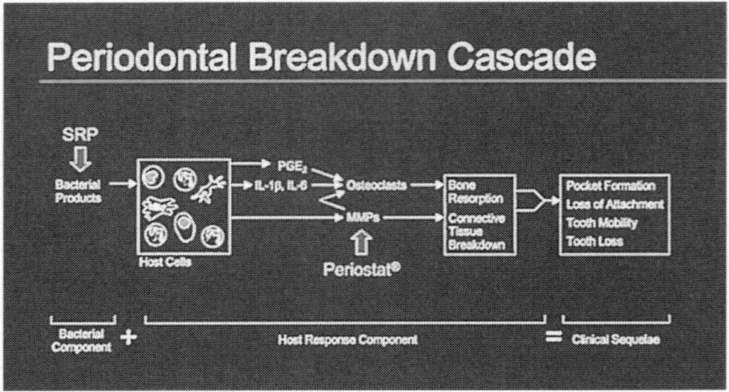

Fig. 50-3 Matrix metalloproteinases in the progression of periodontal disease.

disease is seen in Fig. 50-3. Although this drug is in the antibiotic family, it does not produce antibacterial effects because the dose of 20 mg twice daily is too low to affect bacteria. As a result, resistance to this medication has not been seen.

Four double-blind, clinical, multicenter studies of more than 650 patients have demonstrated that doxycycline hyclate improves the effectiveness of professional periodontal care and slows the progression of the disease process. The results of the first three studies showed that doxycycline hyclate resulted in approximately a 50% improvement in clinical attachment levels in pockets with probing depths (PD) of 4 to 6 mm and a 34% improvement in pockets with probing depths ≥7 mm. It was also noted that attachment loss was prevented in sites with normal probing depths (0 to 3 mm), whereas the placebo groups lost 0.13 mm at 12 months ($p = 0.05$).[12,19]

A recent study by Caton and co-workers has shown statistically significant reductions in probing depths and increases in clinical attachment levels with adjunctive Periostat in conjunction with root planing at 3-, 6-, and 9-month evaluations compared with placebo groups undergoing root planing alone.[13] Although statistically significant, the net changes were considered limited alterations in patients with moderate to severe chronic periodontitis.[4]

Results of safety studies showed the use of 20-mg Periostat BID either with or without mechanical therapy (SRP) did not exert an antimicrobial effect on the periodontal microflora and did not result in a detrimental shift in the normal flora. The colonization or overgrowth of the periodontal pocket by bacteria resistant to doxycycline, tetracycline, minocycline, amoxicillin, erythromycin, or clindamycin has not been observed. In addition, no evidence of any tendency toward the acquisition of multiantibiotic resistance was found.[21,76]

Nonsteroidal Antiinflammatory Drugs

It is only relatively recently that the role of the host's inflammatory system in periodontal disease has begun to be understood. Following activation of inflammatory cells in the periodontium by bacteria, phospholipids in the plasma membranes of cells are acted on by phospholipase. This leads to the liberation of free arachidonic acid,[58] which then can be metabolized into prostaglandins, thromboxanes, and prostacycline by the enzyme cyclooxygenase. The lipoxygenase pathway can produce leukotrienes and hydroxyeicosatetraenoic acids from arachidonic acid. Strong evidence suggests that cyclooxygenase pathway products (e.g., prostaglandins) may be important mediators of some pathologic events occurring in periodontal disease.[58] Therefore modulation of the host's inflammatory response to bacteria may alter the incidence and severity of periodontal disease. Nonsteroidal antiinflammatory drugs (NSAIDs) may be of therapeutic value in treating periodontal disease because of their ability to interfere with arachidonic acid metabolism and thereby inhibit the inflammatory process. This expectation has been validated in studies in both animals and humans.[23,55,75,86,88] Some NSAIDs have been shown to affect the response of polymorphonuclear neutrophils (PMNs) to inflammation not related to prostaglandin inhibition.[22,40] Beneficial effects of NSAIDs have also been found after topical application.[35,74,85] Drugs such as flurbiprofen, ibuprofen, mefenamic acid, and naproxen have been studied.

Flurbiprofen appears to be an NSAID worthy of further investigation. It inhibits PMN migration, reduces vascular permeability, and inhibits platelet aggregation by inhibiting cyclooxygenase.[35] In a 3-year study, Williams and co-workers reported that flurbiprofen significantly inhibited radiographic alveolar bone loss when compared with placebo. Unfortunately, by 24 months, the difference in the rate of bone loss had disappeared.[84] This group also reported a return to baseline in the rate of bone loss after treatment with flurbiprofen was discontinued.[87]

LOCAL DELIVERY OF ANTIBIOTICS

The limitations of mouthrinsing and irrigation have prompted research for the development of alternative delivery systems. Recently, advances in delivery technology have resulted in the controlled release of drugs (Table 50-3). The requirements for treating periodontal disease include a means for targeting an antimicrobial to infection sites and sustaining its localized concentration at effective levels for a sufficient time while concurrently evoking minimal or no side effects.

Tetracycline-Containing Fibers (Actisite)

The first local delivery product available in the U.S., one which has been extensively studied, is an ethylene/vinyl acetate copolymer fiber, diameter 0.5 mm, containing tetracycline, 12.7 mg/9 inches (Actisite tetracycline fiber; manufactured by Alza Corporation, Palo Alto, CA; distributed by Procter & Gamble Co., Cincinnati, OH) (Fig. 50-4). When packed into a periodontal pocket, it is well tolerated by oral tissues, and for 10 days it sustains tetracycline concentrations exceeding 1300 μg/ml, well beyond the 32 to 64 μg/ml required to inhibit the growth of pathogens isolated from periodontal pockets.[70,79] In contrast, crevicular fluid concentrations of only 4 to 8 μg/ml are reported after systemic tetracycline administration, 250 mg four times daily for 10 days (total oral dose, 10 g).[32]

Studies demonstrate that tetracycline fibers applied with or without scaling and root planing reduce probing

TABLE 50-3

Currently Available or Investigational, Locally Delivered Antimicrobials for Periodontal Therapy

Product	Antimicrobial Agent	FDA Clearance	Dosage Form	Manufacturer
Actisite	Tetracycline	Yes	Nonresorbable fiber	Alza Corp., Palo Alto, CA
Arestin	Minocycline	No	Biodegradable powder in syringe	Orapharma Corp., Warminster, PA
Atridox	Doxycycline	Yes	Biodegradable mixture in syringe	Atrix Labs, Ft. Collins, CO
Dentamycin, Perio Cline	Minocycline	No	Biodegradable mixture in syringe	Sunstar Corp., Tokyo, Japan
Elyzol	Metronidazole	No	Biodegradable mixture in syringe	Dumex Corp., Copenhagen, Denmark
PerioChip	Chlorhexidine	Yes	Biodegradable device	Dexcel Pharma, Inc., Jerusalem, Israel

depth, bleeding on probing, and periodontal pathogens and provide gains in clinical attachment level. Such effects are significantly better than those attained with scaling and root planing alone or with placebo fibers. In a 2-month study, compared with scaling and root planing, the fibers used alone have provided more than a 60% greater improvement in probing depth and clinical attachment level than scaling alone.[29]

No change in antibiotic resistance to tetracycline has been found following tetracycline fiber therapy among the tested putative periodontal pathogens.[30] Disadvantages of the fiber include the length of time required for placement (10 minutes or more per tooth), the considerable learning curve required to gain proficiency at placement, and the need for a second patient appointment 10 days after placement for removal of the fiber. Also, placement of fibers around 12 or more teeth has resulted in oral candidiasis in a few cases.

Another study suggested that rinsing with 0.12% chlorhexidine (Peridex; Zila Pharmaceuticals, Inc., Phoenix, AZ) after fiber placement had a synergistic effect, enhancing the reduction of bacterial pathogens.[53]

Evaluation of the effect of tetracycline fibers on root surfaces, using fluorescent light and scanning electron microscopy,[51] showed superficial penetration of tetracycline, with minor penetration into dental tubules, and a few areas of demineralized root surface. Scanning electron microscopic observations made in this study also revealed reductions in the subgingival microbial flora on the root surfaces of teeth treated with the fibers versus the control specimens.

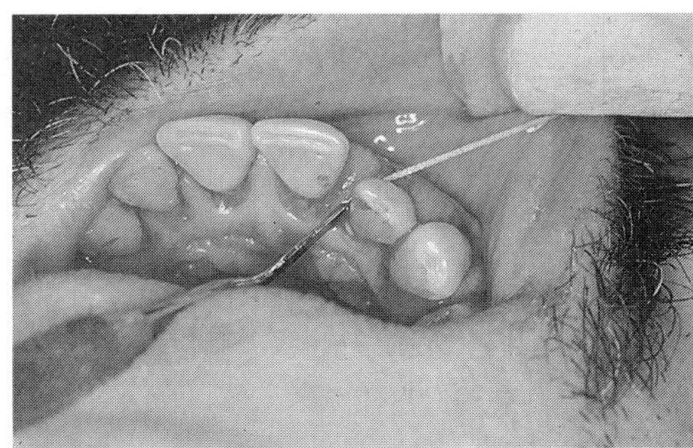

Fig. 50-4 Placement of Actisite fiber.

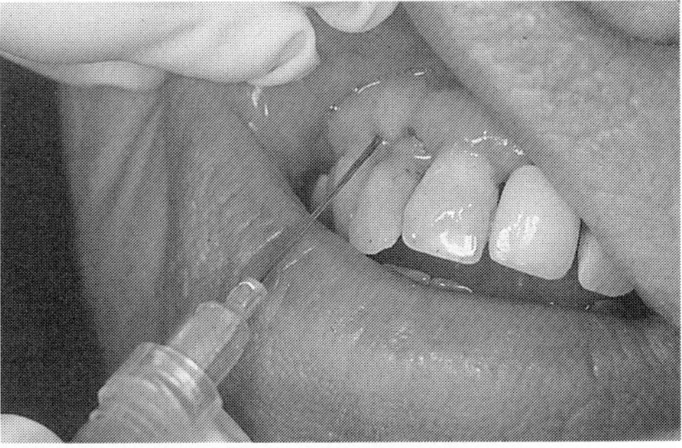

Fig. 50-5 Placement of Atridox gel.

Subgingival Delivery of Doxycycline (Atridox)

Atridox® (manufactured by Atrix Laboratories, Fort Collins, CO; licensed for marketing by Block Drug, Inc., Jersey City, NJ) is a gel system that incorporates the antibiotic doxycycline (10%) in a syringeable gel system (Fig. 50-5). Atridox is cleared by the FDA for sale in the U.S.

In a 9-month multicenter study of 180 patients, treatment with Atridox alone was more effective than the other treatments at all time periods, with the exception of the 3-month clinical attachment level value. For the Atridox group, the reduction in clinical attachment level at 9 months showed a gain of 0.4 mm compared with vehicle control, the reduction in probing depth was 0.6 mm greater than vehicle control, and the reduction of bleeding on probing was 0.2 units greater than vehicle control. The differences were clinically small but statistically significant. Although resistance was not evaluated in this study, the local application of doxycycline has

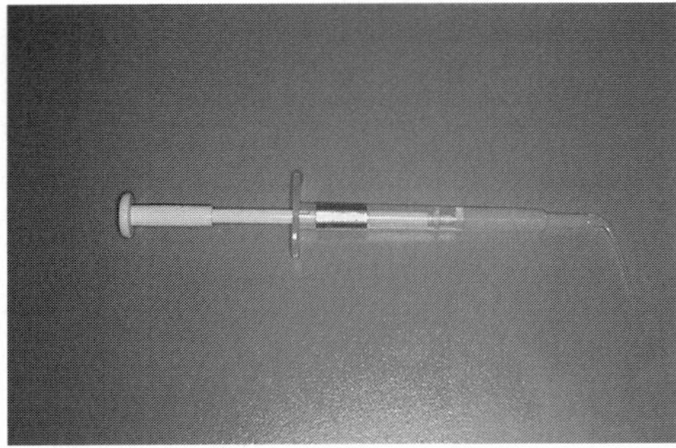

Fig. 50-6 Minocycline syringable gel.

previously been reported to show transient increases in resistance in oral microbes and no overgrowth of foreign pathogens.[45]

Data also has been reported from two multicenter clinical trials, each studying 411 patients with moderate to severe periodontitis.[24] At baseline, patients were randomized to one of four treatment groups: Atridox, vehicle control, oral hygiene only, and scaling and root planing. Sites with probing depth ≥5 mm that bled on probing were treated at baseline and then again with the same treatment at 4 months. Clinical assessments were made for 9 months, measuring clinical attachment level, probing depth, and bleeding on probing. All treatment groups in both studies showed clinical improvements from baseline over the 9-month period. The results for all parameters measured were significantly better in the Atridox group compared with vehicle control and oral hygiene only. Compared with scaling and root planing, the effects of Atridox as a monotherapy on clinical attachment level gain and probing depth reduction were equivalent.

Subgingival Delivery System for Minocycline (Dentamycin and PerioCline)

A subgingival delivery system of 2% (w/w) minocycline hydrochloride (Dentamycin, Cyanamid International, Lederle Division, Wayne, NJ; PerioCline, SunStar, Osaka, Japan) is available in many countries for use as an adjunct to subgingival debridement. This system is a syringeable gel suspension delivery formulation (Fig. 50-6).

In a four-center, double-blind, randomized trial, patients with periodontal pockets at least 5 mm deep were selected, and either 2% minocycline gel or vehicle were applied once every 2 weeks for four applications following initial scaling and root planing.[72] A total of 343 teeth (976 sites) were included in the minocycline group, with 299 teeth (810 sites) in the control group.

Reductions in *P. gingivalis* and *P. intermedia* at weeks 2, 4, 6, and 12 and at weeks 6 and 12 for *A. actinomycetemcomitans* were statistically significant. These results demonstrated the advantages of supplementing standard subgingival debridement with minocycline gel application.

The three primary clinical efficacy variables in this study were probing depth, clinical attachment level, and bleeding index. There was a trend toward clinical improvement in both the treatment groups for all three measures, and the reduction in probing depth was significantly greater with minocycline gel.

When sites with probing depth of at least 7 mm and significant bleeding at baseline were considered, the improvements were greater than with 5-mm pockets. The improvements with minocycline were statistically significantly better than the vehicle-control group.

Applications of 2% minocycline were also evaluated in a 3-month study in 30 patients.[33] Active or placebo gel was placed subgingivally at planed sites in each subject according to a double-blind protocol, immediately after scaling and root planing and 2 and 4 weeks later. Differences between groups in mean probing depth did not reach statistical significance at any visit, but mean clinical attachment levels were different in favor of the minocycline group ($p < 0.05$) at both reassessments. A difference was found in the number of sites that bled after deep probing at 12 weeks, favoring the minocycline group ($p < 0.05$). This product (2% minocycline) is not available in the U.S.

Subgingival Delivery of Metronidazole

A topical medication (Elyzol; Dumex, Copenhagen, Denmark) containing an oil-based metronidazole 25% dental gel (glyceryl mono-oleate and sesame oil) has been tested in a number of studies.[1] It is applied in viscous consistency to the pocket, where it is liquidized by the body heat and then hardens again forming crystals in contact with water. As a precursor, the preparation contains metronidazole-benzoate, which is converted into the active substance by esterases in the crevicular fluid. Two 25% gel applications at a 1-week interval have been used in clinical studies.[41]

Studies of the metronidazole gel have shown it to be equivalent to scaling and root planing but have not shown adjunctive benefits in conjunction with scaling and root planing. For example, a recent 6-month study of 30 patients showed the following[67]: The treatment consisted of two applications of the dental gel in two randomly selected quadrants at 1-week intervals as well as simultaneous subgingival scaling of the remaining quadrants. Oral hygiene instructions were given on day 21. Statistical analyses showed that both treatments were effective in reducing probing depth and bleeding on probing over the 6-month period. At the end of the follow-up period, the mean reduction in probing depth was 1.3 mm after gel treatment and 1.5 mm after subgingival scaling. Bleeding on probing was reduced by 35% and 42%, respectively. No significant differences between the two treatments were detected. Dark-field microscopy showed a shift towards a seemingly more healthy microflora for both treatment modalities; this effect persisted throughout the 6-month period.

A large, multicenter study of 206 subjects investigated two applications of this gel in two randomly selected quadrants versus two quadrants of scaling.[1] Probing depths were reduced by 1.2 mm in the gel and 1.5 mm in the scaling group. At 6 months, the differences between treatments were statistically but not clinically significant. Also, bleeding on probing was reduced by 88% for both treatment groups.

LOCAL DELIVERY OF AN ANTISEPTIC AGENT

A resorbable delivery system (Periochip) has been tested for the subgingival placement of chlorhexidine gluconate with positive clinical results. It is a small chip (4.0 × 5.0 × 0.35 mm) composed of a biodegradable hydrolyzed gelatin matrix, cross-linked with glutaraldehyde and also containing glycerin and water, into which 2.5 mg chlorhexidine gluconate has been incorporated per chip. This delivery system releases chlorhexidine and maintains drug concentrations in the gingival crevicular fluid greater than 100 μg/ml for at least 7 days,[66] concentrations well above the tolerance of most oral bacteria.[9] Because the chip biodegrades in 7 to 10 days, a second appointment for removal is not needed.

Two multicenter, randomized, double-blind, parallel group, controlled clinical trials of this chip were conducted in the U.S. with a total of 447 patients in 10 centers.[37] In these studies, patients received a supragingival prophylaxis for up to 1 hour, followed by scaling and root planing for 1 hour. Chips were placed in target sites with probing depth of 5 to 8 mm at baseline that bled on probing and again at 3 and 6 months if probing depth remained ≥5 mm. Sites in control-group subjects received either a placebo chip (inactive) with scaling and root planing or scaling and root planing alone. Sites in test-group subjects received either a chlorhexidine chip (active) with scaling and root planing or scaling and root planing alone (to maintain the study blind). Examinations were performed at baseline and again at 3, 6, and 9 months. At 9 months, significant decreases in probing depth from baseline favoring the active chip compared with controls were observed: chlorhexidine chip with scaling and root planing, −0.95 ± 0.05 mm; placebo chip with scaling and root planing, −0.69 ± 0.05 mm ($p = 0.001$); scaling and root planing alone, −0.65 ± 0.05 mm ($p = 0.00001$). Although statistically significant, the net clinical changes were limited. The proportion of pocket sites with a probing depth reduction of 2 mm or more was increased in the chlorhexidine chip group (30%) compared with scaling and root planing alone (16%), a difference which was statistically significant on a per patient basis ($p < 0.0001$).

No signs of staining were noted in any of the above three studies as a result of the "chlorhexidine chip" treatment, as measured by a stain index. Adverse effects were minimal, with a few patients who complained of slight pain and swelling in the first 24 hours after chip placement.

REFERENCES

1. Ainamo J, Lie T, Ellingsen BH, et al: Clinical responses to subgingival application of a metronidazole 25% gel compared to the effect of subgingival scaling in adult periodontitis. J Clin Periodontol 1992; 19(Part II):723.
2. Alger FA, Solt CW, Vuddhankanok S, et al: The histologic evaluation of new attachment in periodontally diseased human roots treated with tetracycline-hydrochloride and fibronectin. J Periodontol 1990; 61:447.
3. American Academy of Periodontology: Parameters of care. J Periodontol 2000; 71(suppl):847.
4. American Academy of Periodontology Statement (Committee on Research, Science, and Therapy). October 1998.
5. Bader HI, Goldhaber P: The passage of intravenously administered tetracycline into the gingival sulcus of dogs. J Oral Ther Pharmacol 1968; 2:324.
6. Baker PJ, Evans RT, Slots J, et al: Antibiotic susceptibility of anaerobic bacteria from the oral cavity. J Dent Res 1985; 65:1233.
7. Baker PJ, Evans RT, Slots J, et al: Susceptibility of human oral anaerobic bacteria to antibiotics suitable for topical use. J Clin Periodontol 1985; 12:201.
8. Blandizzi C, Tecla M, Lupetti A, et al: Periodontal tissue disposition of azithromycin in patients affected by chronic inflammatory periodontal diseases. J Periodontol 1999; 70:960.
9. Briner WW, Kayrouz GA, Chanak MX: Comparative antimicrobial effectiveness of a substantive (0.12% chlorhexidine) and a nonsubstantive (phenolic) mouthrinse in vivo and in vitro. Compend Contin Educ Dent 1994; 15:1158.
10. Bueno L, Walker C, Van Ness W, et al: Effect of augmentin on microbiota associated with refractory periodontitis. Abstract 1064. J Dent Res 1988; 67:246.
11. Carranza FA Jr, Saglie R, Newman MG, et al: Scanning and transmission electron microscopic study of tissue-invading microorganisms in localized juvenile periodontitis. J Periodontol 1983; 54:598.
12. Caton J, Bleiden T, Adams D, et al: Subantimicrobial doxycycline therapy for periodontits (Abstract). J Dent Res 1997; 76:1307.
13. Caton JG, Ciancio SG, Blieden TM, et al: Treatment with subantimicrobial dose doxycycline improves the efficacy of scaling and root planing in patients with adult periodontitis. J Periodontol 2000; 71:521.
14. Chanoine, J, Boulvain M, Bourdoux, D, et al: Increased recall rate at screening for congenital hypothyroidism in breast fed infants born to iodine overloaded mothers. Arch Dis Child 1988; 63:1207.
15. Christersson LA, Slots J, Rosling BG, et al: Microbiological and clinical effects of surgical treatment of localized juvenile periodontitis. J Clin Periodontol 1985; 12:465.
16. Ciancio SG: Use of antibiotics in periodontal therapy. In: Newman MG, Goodman A (eds): Antibiotics in Dentistry. Chicago, Quintessence, 1983.
17. Ciancio SG: Antibiotics in periodontal therapy. In: Newman MG, Kornman K (eds): Antibiotic/Antimicrobial Use in Dental Practice. Chicago, Quintessence, 1990.
18. Ciancio SG: Antiseptics and antibiotics as chemotherapeutic agents for periodontitis management. Compend Contin Educ Dent 2000; 21:59.
19. Ciancio SG, Adams D, Blieden T, et al: Subantimicrobial dose doxycycline: A new adjunctive therapy for adult periodontitis. Presented at the annual meeting of the American Academy of Periodontology, Boston, MA, September 1998.
20. Ciancio SG, Slots J, Reynolds HS, et al: The effect of shortterm administration of minocycline HCl administration on gingival inflammation and subgingival microflora. J Periodontol 1982; 53:557.
21. Crout R, Adams D, Blieden T, et al: Safety of doxycycline hyclate 20 mg bid in patients with adult periodontitis. Presented at the annual meeting of the American Academy of Periodontology, Boston, MA, September, 1998.
22. Edelson H, Kaplan H, Korchak H: Differing effects of nonsteroidal anti-inflammatory agents on neutrophil functions. Clin Res 1982; 30:469A.
23. Feldman R, Szeto B, Chauncey H, et al: Nonsteroidal antiinflammatory drugs in the reduction of human alveolar bone loss. J Clin Periodontol 1983; 10:131.
24. Garrett S, Adams D, Bandt C, et al: Two multicenter clinical trials of subgingival doxycycline in the treatment of periodontitis. J Dent Res 1997; 76:153(Abstr #1113).

25. Genco RJ, Cianciola JJ, Rosling H: Treatment of localized juvenile periodontitis. Abstract 872. J Dent Res 1981; 60:527.
26. Gibson W: Antibiotics and periodontal disease: A selective review of the literature. J Am Dent Assoc 1982; 104:213.
27. Gladue RP, Snyder ME: Intracellular accumulation of azithromycin by cultured human fibroblasts. Antimicrob Agents Chemother 1990; 34:1056.
28. Gold SI: Combined therapy in the treatment of periodontosis: Case report. Periodont Case Rep 1979; 1:12.
29. Goodson JM, Cugini M, Kent RL, et al: Multicenter evaluation of tetracycline fiber therapy: II. Clinical response. J Periodont Res 1991; 26:371.
30. Goodson JM, Tanner A: Antibiotic resistance of the subgingival microbiota following local tetracycline therapy. Oral Microbiol Immunol 1992; 7:113.
31. Gordon JM, Walker CB, Murphy JC: Concentration of tetracycline in human gingival fluid after single doses. J Clin Periodontol 1981; 8:117.
32. Gordon JM, Walker CB, Murphy CJ, et al: Tetracycline: levels achievable in gingival crevice fluid and in vitro effect on subgingival organisms. Part I. Concentrations in crevicular fluid after repeated doses. J Periodontol 1981; 52:609.
33. Grace MA, Watts TLP, Wilson RF, et al: A randomized controlled trial of a 2% minocycline gel as an adjunct to non-surgical periodontal treatment, using a design with multiple matching criteria. J Clin Periodontol 1997; 24:249.
34. Greenstein G: The role of metronidazole in the treatment of periodontal diseases. J Periodontol 1993; 1:1.
35. Heasam PA, Benn DK, Kelly PJ, et al: The use of topical flurbiprofen as an adjunct to non-surgical management of periodontal disease. J Clin Periodontol 1993; 20:457.
36. Hoepelman IM, Schneider MME: Azithromycin: The first of the tissue-selective azalides. Int J Antimicrob Agents 1995; 5:145.
37. Jeffcoat M, Bray KS, Ciancio SG, et al: Adjunctive use of a subgingival controlled-release chlorhexidine chip reduces probing depth and improves attachment level compared with scaling and root planing alone. J Periodontol 1998; 69:989.
38. Jorgensen MG, Slots J: Practical antimicrobial periodontal therapy. Compend Contin Educ Dent 2000; 21:111.
39. Jorgensen MG, Slots J: Responsible use of antimicrobials in periodontics. J Cal Dent Assoc 2000; 28:185.
40. Kaplan H, Edelson H, Korchak H, et al: Effects of nonsteroidal anti-inflammatory agents on neutrophil functions in vitro and in vivo. Biochem Pharmacol 1984; 33:371.
41. Klinge B, Attström R, Karring T, et al: 3 regimes of topical metronidazole compared with subgingival scaling on periodontal pathology in adults. J Clin Periodontol 1992; 19 (Part II):708.
42. Kornman KS, Karl EH: The effect of long-term low-dose tetracycline therapy on the subgingival microflora in refractory adult periodontitis. J Periodontol 1982; 53:604.
43. Lang NP, Adler R, Joss A, et al: The absence of bleeding on probing. An indicator of periodontal stability. J Clin Periodontol 1990; 17:714.
44. Lang NP, Joss A, Orsanic T, et al: Bleeding on probing. A predictor for the progression of periodontal disease? J Clin Periodontol 1986; 13:590.
45. Larsen T: Occurrence of doxycycline-resistant bacteria in the oral cavity after local administration of doxycycline in patients with periodontal disease. Scand J Infect Dis 1991; 23:89.
46. Lekovic V, Kenney EB, Carranza FA Jr, et al: Effect of metronidazole on human periodontal disease. A clinical and microbiologic study. J Periodontol 1983; 54:476.
47. Loesche WJ, Giordano JR, Hujoel P, et al: Metronidazole in periodontitis: Reduced need for surgery. J Clin Periodontol 1992; 19:103.
48. Lozdan J, Sheiham A, Pearlman BA, et al: The use of nitrimidazine in the treatment of acute ulcerative gingivitis. A double-blind controlled trial. Br Dent J 1971; 130:294.
49. Malizia T, Tejada MR, Ghelardi E, et al: Periodontal tissue disposition of azithromycin. J Periodontol 1997; 68:1206.
50. Mills WH, Thompson GW, Beagrie GS: Clinical evaluation of spiramycin and erythromycin in control of periodontal disease. J Clin Periodontol 1979; 6:308.
51. Morrison SL, Cobb CM, Kazakos GM, et al: Root surface characteristics associated with subgingival placement of monolithic tetracycline-impregnated fibers. J Periodontol 1992; 63:137.
52. Neidner R: Cytotoxicity and sensitization of povidone-iodine and other frequently used anti-infective agents. Dermatology 1997; 195(suppl):89.
53. Niederman R, Holborow D, Tonetti M, et al: Reinfection of periodontal sites following tetracycline fiber therapy. J Dent Res 1990; 69:277(Abstr 1345).
54. Nowzari H, McDonald ES, Flynn J, et al: The dynamics of microbial colonization of barrier membranes for guided tissue regeneration. J Periodontol 1996; 67:694.
55. Offenbacher S, Braswell L, Loos A, et al: Effects of flurbiprophen on the progression of periodontitis in *Macaca mulatta.* J Periodont Res 1987; 22:473.
56. Rams TE, Feik D, Slots J: Ciprofloxacin/metronidazole treatment of recurrent adult periodontitis. Abstract. J Dent Res 1992; 71:319.
57. Rams TE, Slots J: Antibiotics in periodontal therapy: An update. Compend Contin Educ Dent 1992; 13:1130.
58. Research, Science and Therapy Committee: Pharmacologic blocking of host responses as an adjunct in the management of periodontal diseases: A research update. Chicago, American Academy of Periodontology, 1992.
59. Rosling BG, Slots J, Christersson LA, et al: Topical antimicrobial therapy and diagnosis of subgingival bacteria in the management of inflammatory periodontal disease. J Clin Periodontol 1986; 13:975.
60. Saglie FR, Carranza FA Jr, Newman MG, et al: Identification of tissue invading bacteria in human periodontal disease. J Periodont Res 1982; 17:452.
61. Schrefer J (pub): Mosby's GENRx, ed 10. St Louis, Mosby, 2001.
62. Slots J, McDonald ES, Nowzari H: Infectious aspects of periodontal regeneration. Periodontol 2000 1999; 19:164.
63. Slots J, Rams TE: Antibiotics and periodontal therapy: Advantages and disadvantages. J Clin Periodontol 1990; 17:479.
64. Slots J, Rosling BG: Suppression of periodontopathic microflora in localized juvenile periodontitis by systemic tetracycline. J Clin Periodontol 1983; 10:465.
65. Soder P, Frithiof L, Wikner S, et al: The effects of systemic metronidazole after non-surgical treatment in moderate and advanced periodontitis in young adults. J Periodontol 1990; 61:281.
66. Soskolne WA, Heasman PA, Stabholz A, et al: Sustained local delivery of chlorhexidine in the treatment of periodontitis: a multi-center study. J Periodontol 1997; 68:32.
67. Stelzel M, Flores-De-Jacoby L: Topical metronidazole application compared with subgingival scaling. A clinical and microbiological study on recall patients. J Clin Periodontol 1996; 23:24.
68. Sznajder N, Piovano S, Bernat MI, et al: Effect of spiramycin therapy on human periodontal disease. J Clin Periodontol 1987; 22:255.
69. Tinoco EM, Beldi M, Campedelli F, et al: Clinical and microbiologic effects of adjunctive antibiotics in treatment of localized aggressive periodontitis. A controlled clinical study. J Periodontol 1998; 69:1355.
70. Tonetti M, Cugini AM, Goodson JM: Zero order delivery with periodontal placement of tetracycline loaded ethylene vinyl acetate fibers. J Periodontal Res 1990; 25:243.

71. Tyler K, Walker CB, Gordon J, et al: Evaluation of clindamycin in adult refractory periodontitis: Antimicrobial susceptibilities. Abstract 1667. J Dent Res 1985; 64 (special issue):360.
72. Van Steenberghe D, Bercy P, Kohl J: Subgingival minocycline hydrochloride ointment in moderate to severe chronic adult periodontitis: A randomized, double-blind, vehicle-controlled, multicenter study. J Periodontol 1993; 64:637.
73. Van Winkelhoff AJ, Gonzales DH, Winkel EG, et al: Antimicrobial resistance in the subgingival microflora in patients with adult periodontitis. A comparison between the Netherlands and Spain. J Clin Perio 2000; 27:79.
74. Vogel R, Schneider L, Goteinter D: The effects of a topical nonsteroidal anti-inflammatory drug on ligature induced periodontal disease in the squirrel monkey. J Clin Periodontol 1986; 12:139.
75. Waite I, Saxon C, Young A, et al: The periodontal status of subjects receiving nonsteroidal anti-inflammatory drugs. J Periodont Res 1981; 16:100.
76. Walker C, Thomas J: The effect of subantimicrobial doses of doxycycline on the microbial flora and antibiotic resistance in patients with adult periodontitis. Presented at the annual meeting of the American Academy of Periodontology, Boston, MA, September, 1998.
77. Walker CB: The acquisition of resistance of antibiotic resistance in the periodontal microflora. Periodontol 2000 1996; 10:79.
78. Walker CB: Selected antimicrobial agents: Mechanisms of action, side effects and drug interactions. Periodontol 2000 1996; 10:12.
79. Walker CB, Cordon JM, Mcquilkin SJ, et al: Tetracycline: Levels achievable in gingival crevice fluid and in vitro effect on subgingival organisms. Part II. Susceptibilities of periodontal bacteria. J Periodontol 1981; 52:613.
80. Walker CB, Gordon JM, Magnusson I, et al: A role for antibiotics in the treatment of refractory periodontitis. J Periodontol 1993; 64:772.
81. Walker CB, Gordon JM, Socransky SS: Antibiotic susceptibility testing of subgingival plaque samples. J Clin Periodontol 1983; 10:422.
82. Weinstein L: Antimicrobial agents: Penicillins and cephalosporins. In: Goodman LS, Gilman A (eds): The Pharmachological Basis of Therapeutics, ed 5. New York, Macmillan, 1975.
83. Weinstein L: Antimicrobial agents: Tetracyclines and chloramphenicol. In: Goodman LS, Gilman A (eds): The Pharmachological Basis of Therapeutics, ed 5. New York, Macmillan, 1975.
84. Williams RC, Jeffcoat MK, Howell T, et al: Altering the progression of human alveolar bone loss with the non-steroidal anti-inflammatory drug flurbiprofen. J Periodontol 1989; 60:485.
85. Williams RC, Jeffcoat MK, Howell T, et al: Ibuprofen: An inhibitor of alveolar bone resorption in beagles. J Periodont Res 1988; 23:225.
86. Williams RC, Jeffcoat MK, Howell T, et al: Indomethacin or flurbiprofen treatment of periodontitis in beagles: Comparison of effect on bone loss. J Periodont Res 1987; 22:403.
87. Williams RC, Jeffcoat MK, Howell T, et al: Three year trial of flurbiprofen treatment in humans: Post-treatment period. Abstract #1617. J Dent Res 1991; 70:448.
88. Williams RC, Jeffcoat MK, Wechter WJ, et al: Flurbiprofen: A potent inhibitor of alveolar bone resorption in beagles. Science 1985; 227:640.

CHAPTER

Periodontal Management of HIV-Infected Patients

Terry D. Rees

CHAPTER OUTLINE

Acquired immunodeficiency syndrome (AIDS) is a universal epidemic that significantly affects dental practice, regardless of geographic location. The oral cavity is a frequent site for clinical manifestations of the disease. The ability to recognize and manage the oral manifestations of this disease is an important part of dental practice. The dentist should be prepared to assist human immunodeficiency virus (HIV)-infected patients in maintenance of oral health throughout the course of their disease.

The detection and diagnosis of oral lesions in HIV-positive patients was described in Chapter 29. The clinical management of these conditions, with particular emphasis on periodontal conditions, is presented in this chapter.

PERIODONTAL TREATMENT PROTOCOL

To safely and effectively provide periodontal therapy to HIV-infected individuals, several treatment considerations are important.

Health Status

The patient's health status should be determined from the health history, physical evaluation, and consultation with his or her physician. Treatment decisions will vary depending on the patient's state of health. For example, delayed wound healing and increased risk of postoperative infection are possible complicating factors in AIDS patients, but neither concern should significantly alter treatment planning in an otherwise healthy, asymptomatic, HIV-infected patient with a normal or near-normal CD4 count and a low viral bioload.[21,29,36] It is important to obtain information regarding the patient's immune status. What is the $CD4^+$ T4 lymphocyte level? What is the current viral load? How do current $CD4^+$ T4 cell and viral load counts differ from previous evaluations? How often are such tests performed? How long ago was the HIV infection identified? Is it possible to identify the approximate date of original exposure? Is there a history of drug abuse, sexually transmitted diseases, multiple infections, or other factors that might alter immune response? For example, does the patient have a history of chronic hepatitis B, hepatitis C, neutropenia, thrombocytopenia, nutritional deficiency, or adrenocorticoid insufficiency? What medications is the patient taking? Does the patient describe or present with possible adverse side effects from medications being taken?

Infection Control Measures

Clinical management of HIV-infected periodontal patients requires strict adherence to established methods of infection control, based on guidance from the American Dental Association (ADA) and the Centers for Disease Control and Prevention (CDC).[5] Compliance, especially with universal precautions, will eliminate or minimize risks to patients and the dental staff.[28,33] Immunocompromised patients are potentially at risk for acquiring as well as transmitting infections in the dental office or other health care facility.[4,27,31,53]

Goals of Therapy

A thorough oral examination will determine the patient's dental treatment needs. The primary goals of dental therapy should be the restoration and maintenance of oral health, comfort, and function. At the very least, periodontal treatment goals should be directed toward control of HIV-associated mucosal diseases such as chronic candidiasis and recurrent oral ulcerations. Acute periodontal and dental infections should be managed, and the patient should receive detailed instructions in performance of effective oral hygiene procedures.[47] Conservative, nonsurgical periodontal therapy should be a treatment option for virtually all HIV-positive patients, and performance of elective surgical periodontal procedures to include implant placement has been reported.[15,30] Necrotizing ulcerative periodontitis (NUP) or necrotizing ulcerative stomatitis (NUS) can be severely destructive to periodontal structures, but a history of these conditions does not automatically dictate extraction of involved teeth unless the patient is unable to maintain effective oral hygiene in affected areas. Decisions regarding elective periodontal procedures should be made with the informed consent of the patient and after medical consultation, when possible.

Supportive Periodontal Therapy

It is imperative that the patient maintain meticulous personal oral hygiene. In addition, periodontal maintenance recall visits should be conducted at short intervals (2 to 3 months) and any progressive periodontal disease treated vigorously. As mentioned earlier, however, systemic antibiotic therapy should be administered with caution. Blood and other medical laboratory tests may be required to monitor the patient's overall health status, and close consultation and coordination with the patient's physician are necessary.

Psychologic Factors

HIV infection of neuronal cells may affect brain function and lead to outright dementia. This may profoundly influence the responsiveness of affected patients to dental treatment. However, psychologic factors are numerous in virtually all HIV-infected patients, even in the absence of neuronal lesions. Patients may be greatly concerned with maintenance of medical confidentiality, and such confidentiality must be upheld. Coping with a life-threatening disease may elicit depression, anxiety, and anger in such patients, and this anger may be directed toward the dentist and the staff.[1] It is important to display concern and understanding for the patient's situation. Treatment should be provided in a calm, relaxed atmosphere, and stress to the patient must be minimized.[1]

The dentist should be prepared to advise and counsel patients on their oral health status. Dentists often encounter HIV-infected patients who are unaware of their disease status. Early diagnosis and treatment of HIV infection can have a profound effect on the patient's life expectancy and quality of life, and the dentist should be prepared to assist the patient in obtaining testing.[41] Any patient with oral lesions suggestive of HIV infection should be informed of the findings and, if appropriate, questioned regarding any previous exposure to HIV. If HIV testing is requested, it must be accompanied by patient counseling. For this reason, such tests might best be obtained through medical referral. However, if the dentist elects to request testing for HIV antibody, the patient must be informed. In most circumstances, written informed consent is desirable prior to testing.

ORAL CANDIDIASIS

Early oral lesions of HIV-related candidiasis are usually responsive to topical antifungal therapy (Fig. 51-1). More advanced lesions, including hyperplastic candidiasis, may require systemic antifungal drugs; systemic therapy is mandatory for esophageal candidiasis (Fig. 51-2).[42,51]

With any therapy, lesions tend to recur after the drug is discontinued, and resistant strains of candidal organisms have been described, especially with the use of systemic agents.[8,42,48,51] Box 51-1 identifies therapeutic agents commonly prescribed for treatment of candidal infections. Most oral topical antifungal agents contain large quantities of sucrose, which may be cariogenic after long-term use. For this reason, some authorities recommend oral use of vaginal tablets because they do not contain sucrose. However, such tablets are relatively low in active units (100,000) versus usual oral dosages of 200,000 to 600,000 units. Sucrose-free nystatin is also available in a powder form, which may be mixed extemporaneously with water at each use ($\frac{1}{8}$ tsp powder to $\frac{1}{2}$ glass water). Recently, sucrose-free oral suspensions of itraconazole and amphotericin B oral rinse have become available. To date, no comparative studies have been performed regarding the effectiveness of these products. Amphotericin B oral suspension is more effective against *Candida albicans* than other species. Patients should be instructed to rinse with the oral suspension for several minutes, then swallow.[34] Fluconazole oral suspension has been reported to be more effective as an antifungal than liquid nystatin.[35] Chlorhexidine and cetylpyridinium chloride oral rinses may also be of some prophylactic value against oral candidal infection.[10,14]

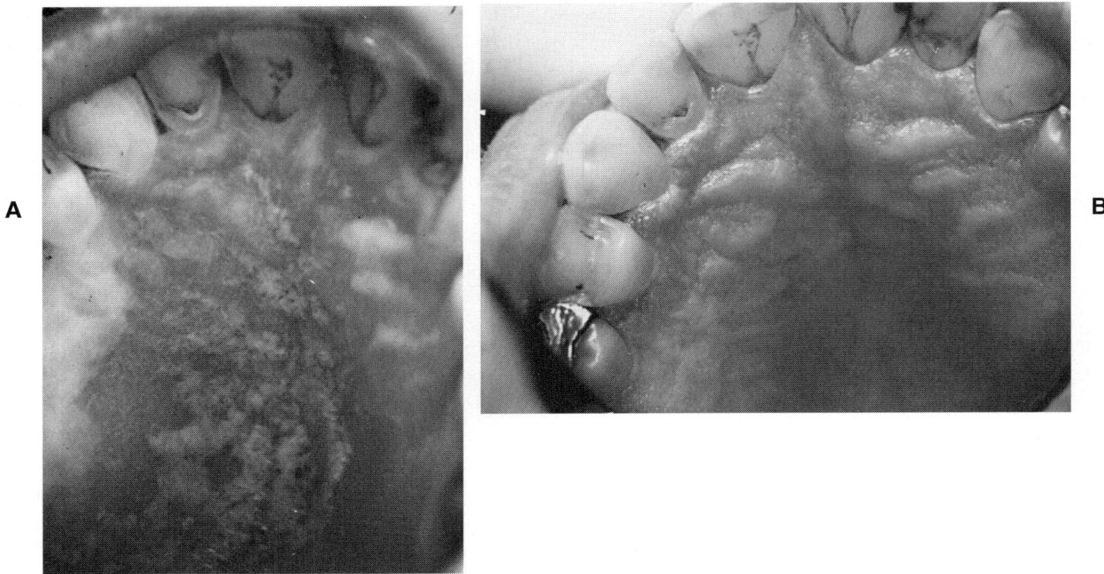

Fig. 51-1 Erythematous and pseudomembranous candidiasis. **A,** Before treatment. **B,** Resolution after 1 week of topical clotrimazole therapy.

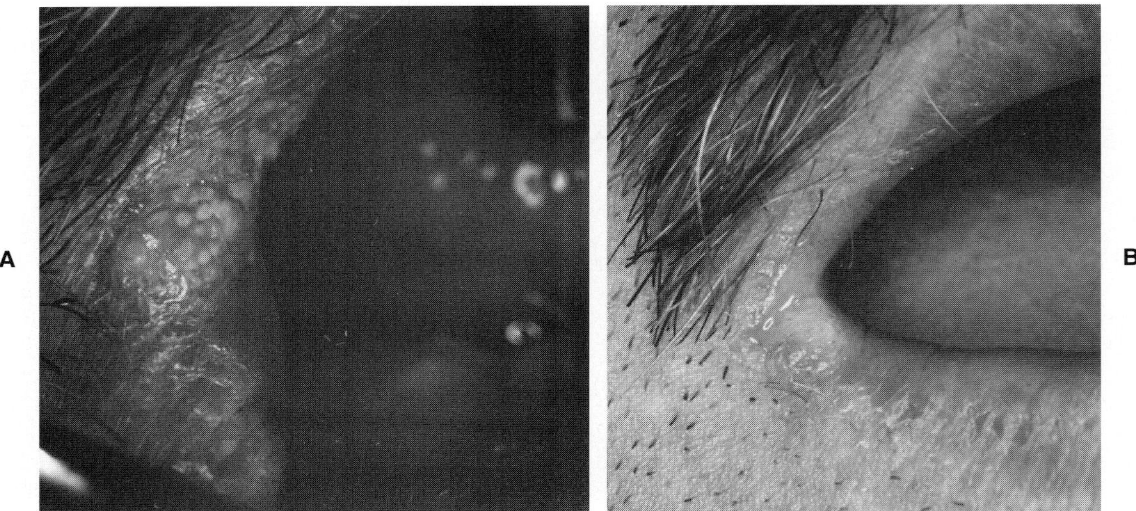

Fig. 51-2 Marked hyperplastic candidiasis in corner of mouth. **A,** Before treatment. **B,** After 2 weeks of systemic fluconazole therapy.

Long-term prophylactic effectiveness of once-weekly systemic fluconazole also has been described.[10,42]

Systemic antifungal agents such as ketoconazole, fluconazole, itraconazole and amphotericin B are effective in treatment of oral candidiasis (see Box 51-1). Ketoconazole may be the agent of choice when systemic therapy is required.[8,46] As mentioned before, however, resistant strains of candidal organisms may develop with prolonged use of any systemic agent, potentially rendering the drugs ineffective against life-threatening candidal infections in the later stages of immune suppression.[3] In addition, significant adverse side effects may occur. As an example, long-term use of ketoconazole may induce liver damage in individuals with preexistent liver disease. The increased risk of chronic hepatitis B or hepatitis C infection in immunosuppressed individuals may put some patients at risk for ketoconazole-induced liver damage. If ketoconazole is prescribed, patients should receive liver function tests at baseline and at least monthly during therapy. The drug is contraindicated if the patient's aspartate transaminase (AST) level is greater than 2.5 times normal.[51] Ketoconazole absorption also may be hampered by the gastropathy experienced by many HIV-infected individuals.[25]

BOX 51-1

Commonly Prescribed Antifungal Therapeutic Agents for Oral Candidiasis

Topical Drugs

1. Clotrimazole (Mycelex), 10-mg tablets: Dissolve in mouth 3–5 tablets daily for 7–14 days.
2. Nystatin (Mycostatin, Nilstat).
   - (a) Oral suspension.
     - 100,000 U/ml: Disp 240 ml.
     - Rinse with 1 tsp (5 ml) qid.
   - (b) Oral suspension (extemporaneous).
     - Disp 2–4 billion U.
     - Mix $\frac{1}{8}$ tsp (500,000 U) in 4 oz water ($\frac{1}{2}$ cup).
     - Rinse 4 times daily.
     - *Note*: Extemporaneous nystatin is sucrose free.
   - (c) Tablets (500,000 U): Dissolve 1 tablet in mouth, 4–5 times daily.
   - (d) Pastilles (200,000 U): Dissolve 1–2 pastilles in mouth, 4–5 times daily.
   - (e) Vaginal tablets (100,000 U): Dissolve 1 tablet in mouth tid.
     - *Note*: Vaginal troches are sucrose free.
   - (f) Ointment (for angular cheilitis), 15-g tube: Apply to affected area 3–4 times daily.
3. Clotrimazole ointment, 15-g tube: Apply to affected area qid.
4. Miconazole 2% ointment, 15-g tube: Apply to affected area qid.
5. Itraconazole oral suspension (Sporanox), 100–200 mg, once daily for 7–28 days.
6. Fluconazole oral suspension (Diflucan), 200 mg of first day followed by 100 mg once daily for at least 2 weeks.
7. Amphotericin B oral suspension (Fungizone), 100 mg, four times daily for 2 weeks.

Systemic Drugs

1. Ketoconazole (Nyzoral), 200-mg tablets: Take 2 tablets immediately, then 1–2 tablets daily with food for 5–14 days.
2. Fluconazole (Diflucan), 100-mg tablets: Take 2 tablets immediately, then 1 tablet daily for 7–14 days.
3. Itraconazole (Sporanox), 100-mg capsules: 200 mg once daily with meals for 4 weeks IDS and neutropenic patients.

A 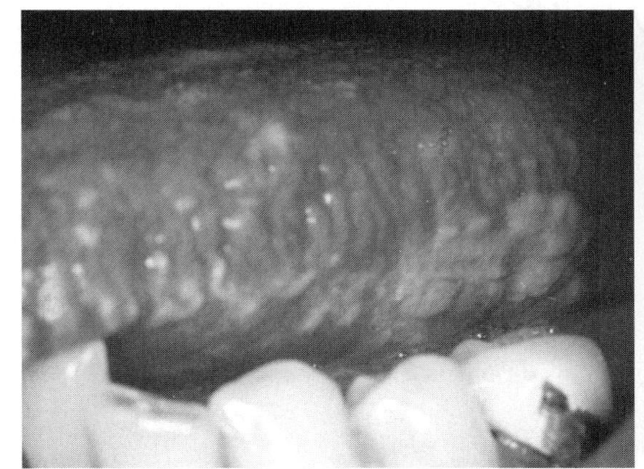

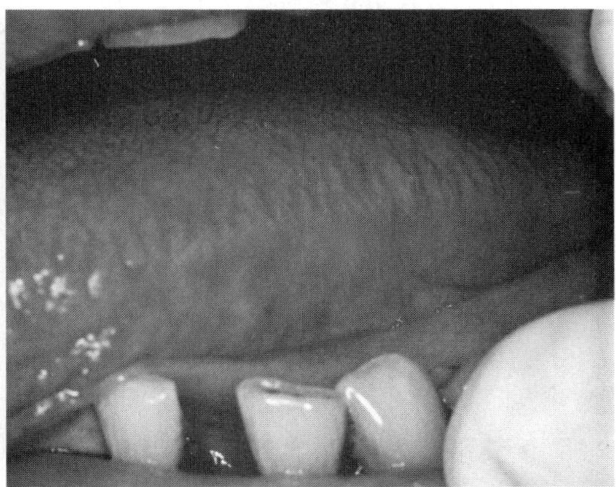 B

Fig. 51-3 Oral hairy leukoplakia of 2 years' duration. **A,** Before treatment. **B,** Unexpected remission after initiation of zidovudine therapy.

ORAL HAIRY LEUKOPLAKIA

At present, there appears to be little advantage in treating oral hairy leukoplakia (OHL) in most patients. Lesions can be successfully removed, however, with laser or conventional surgery. Resolution has been reported after therapy with zidovudine (Fig. 51-3) or topical retinoids, but systemic antiviral agents such as acyclovir may elicit remission more predictably (Fig. 51-4), although lesions reappear when antiviral therapy is discontinued.[2,38,40]

Clinical impressions suggest that the incidence of OHL has been markedly reduced since the advent of multidrug antiviral therapy for HIV infection.

KAPOSI'S SARCOMA

Although Kaposi's sarcoma (KS) has been the most common tumor encountered in HIV-positive individuals, its incidence may be markedly decreasing since the advent of multidrug antiviral therapy.[49] Treatment of oral KS may

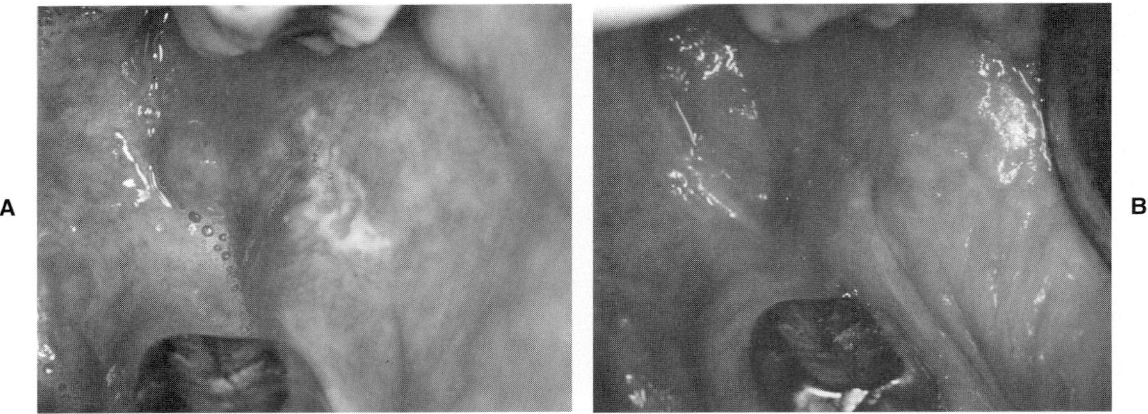

Fig. 51-4 Oral hairy leukoplakia of left buccal mucosa. **A,** Before treatment. **B,** Remission after initiation of systemic acyclovir therapy.

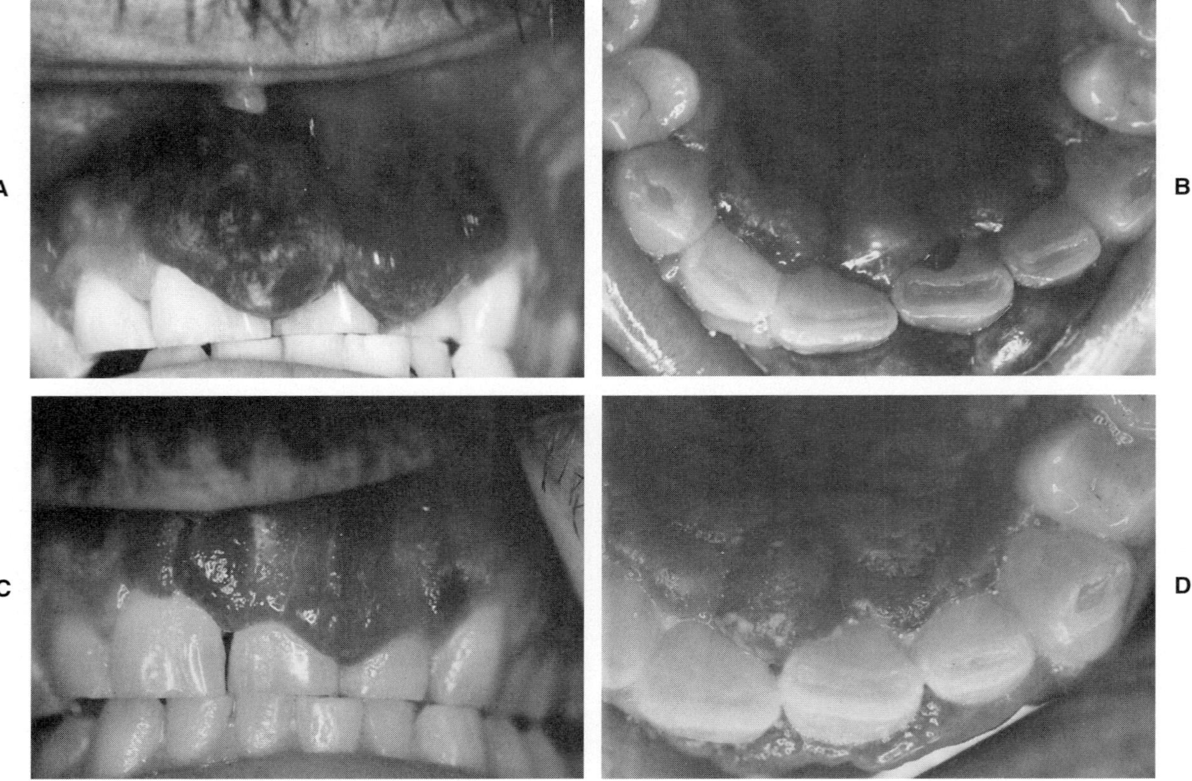

Fig. 51-5 Kaposi's sarcoma of maxillary anterior region. **A,** Anterior facial gingiva before treatment. **B,** Palate before treatment. **C,** Partial resolution of facial gingival lesion after two vinblastine injections. **D,** Partial resolution of palatal lesion. Patient was satisfied with results and declined additional therapy.

include use of antiretroviral agents, laser excision, radiation therapy, or intralesional injection with vinblastine (Fig. 51-5), interferon α, or other chemotherapeutic drugs.[11,12,13,40,43,49] Nichols et al[32] described the successful use of intralesional injections of vinblastine at a dosage of 0.1 mg/cm2 using a 0.2 mg/ml solution of vinblastine sulfate in saline. In responsive patients, treatment was repeated at 2-week intervals until resolution or stabilization of the lesions. Side effects included some posttreatment pain and occasional ulceration of the lesions, but in general the therapy was well tolerated. Total resolution was achieved in 70% of 82 intraoral KS lesions with one to six treatments. Lesions tended to recur, however, thus indicating that treatment probably should be reserved for

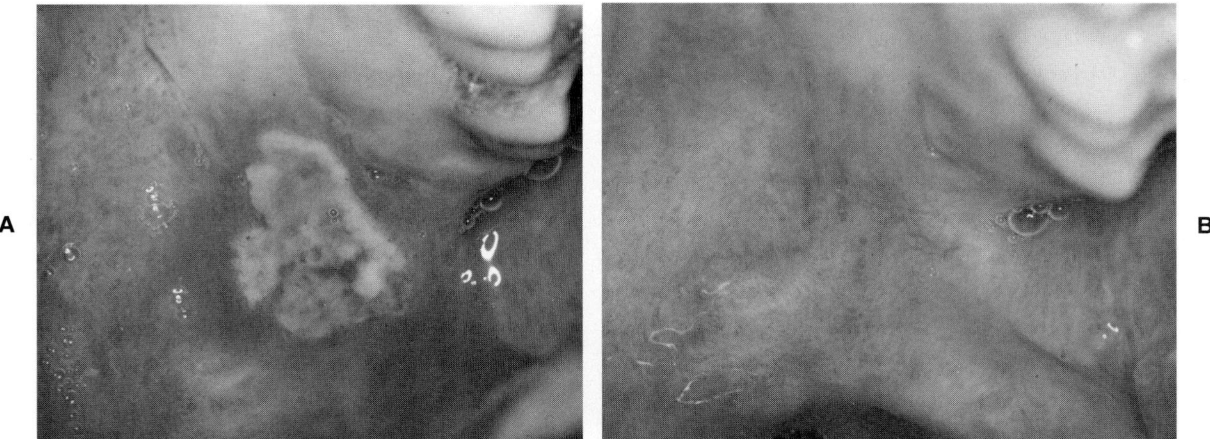

Fig. 51-6 Major aphthae of soft palate in a 28-year-old HIV-positive man. **A,** Before treatment. **B,** Remission of lesion 1 week after prescribing topical corticosteroids.

oral KS lesions that are easily traumatized or interfere with chewing or swallowing. On some occasions, treatment may be indicated when KS lesions create an unsightly appearance on the lips or in the anterior oral cavity.

Destructive periodontitis has also been reported in conjunction with gingival KS. In such instances, scaling and root planing and other periodontal therapy may be indicated in addition to intralesional or systemic chemotherapy.[43,48]

BACILLARY (EPITHELIOID) ANGIOMATOSIS

Treatment of bacillary angiomatosis consists of broad-spectrum antibiotics such as erythromycin or doxycycline in conjunction with conservative periodontal therapy and possibly excision of the lesion.[16,18,30]

NONSPECIFIC ORAL ULCERATIONS AND RECURRENT APHTHAE

Recent evidence indicates that many nonspecific oral ulcerations may be of viral origin with herpes simplex, Epstein-Barr virus, and cytomegalovirus being most common.[37] For this reason, the practitioner should consider viral culturing of such lesions and the use of antiviral agents in treatment where appropriate.

Oral viral infections in immunocompromised individuals are often treated with acyclovir (200 to 800 mg administered five times daily for at least 10 days). Subsequent daily maintenance therapy (200 mg two to five times daily) may be required to prevent recurrence. Resistant viral strains are treated with foscarnet, ganciclovir, or valacyclovir hydrochloride.[48,50]

Topical corticosteroid therapy (fluocinonide gel applied three to six times daily) is safe and efficacious for treatment of recurrent aphthous ulcer or other mucosal lesions in immunocompromised individuals[17,48] (Fig. 51-6). However, topical corticosteroids may predispose immunocompromised individuals to candidiasis. Consequently, prophylactic antifungal medications should be prescribed.

On occasion, large aphthae in HIV-positive individuals may prove resistant to conventional topical therapy. In this event, systemic corticosteroids (prednisone 40 to 60 mg daily) (Fig. 51-7) or alternative therapy (thalidomide, levamisole, pentoxifylline, or others) must be considered.[6,17,19,24,45]

These agents may have significant side effects, however, and the clinician should remain alert for any evidence suggestive of an adverse drug reaction or adverse interaction with currently prescribed medications.[22] It should be noted that virtually all antiviral agents used in treatment of HIV infection have the potential for adverse side effects or drug interactions. For these reasons, the dental clinician should consider topical therapy as long as it is effective.

PERIODONTAL DISEASE IN HIV-POSITIVE INDIVIDUALS

As described in Chapter 29, gingival and periodontal manifestations may be found in HIV-positive individuals. The former include linear gingival erythema and necrotizing ulcerative gingivitis (NUG), both of which may develop into rapidly progressive necrotizing ulcerative stomatitis (NUS) or necrotizing ulcerative periodontitis (NUP).[9] Management of these conditions should be preceded by a thorough medical evaluation, including determination of the CD4 and viral load status, in consultation with the treating physician.

Linear Gingival Erythema

LGE is often refractory to treatment, but lesions may undergo spontaneous remission. Recent evidence suggests that LGE may result from a chronic infection with *C. albicans* or other candidal strains.[52] The recommended management of this condition is as follows:

Step 1: Instruct the patient in performance of meticulous oral hygiene.
Step 2: Scale and polish affected areas, and perform subgingival irrigation with chlorhexidine.

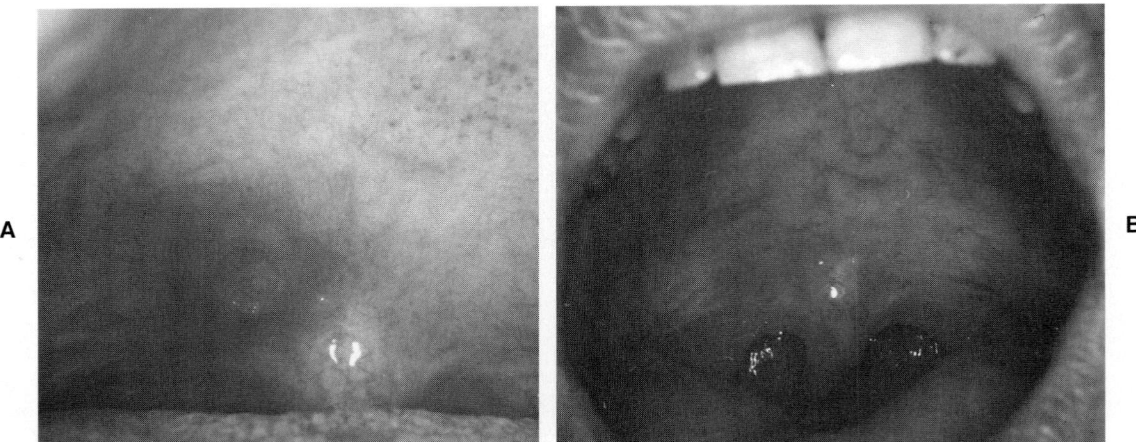

Fig. 51-7 Persistent ulceration of soft palate. **A,** Lesion was refractory to topical corticosteroids. **B,** Healing after 1 week of systemic corticosteroid therapy (40 mg prednisone daily).

Step 3: Prescribe chlorhexidine gluconate mouthrinse.
Step 4: Reevaluate the patient in 2 to 3 weeks. If lesions persist, evaluate for possible candidiasis. Consider empiric administration of a systemic antifungal agent such as fluconazole for 7 to 10 days.
Step 5: Re-treat if necessary.
Step 6: Place the patient on 2- to 3-month recall.

Necrotizing Ulcerative Gingivitis

There is no consensus on whether the incidence of NUG increases in HIV-positive patients.[23] The treatment of this condition in these individuals does not differ from that in HIV-negative individuals (see Chapter 45). Basic treatment may consist of cleaning and debridement of affected areas with a cotton pellet soaked in peroxide after application of a topical anesthetic. Escharotic oral rinses such as hydrogen peroxide should only rarely be used, however, for any patient and are especially contraindicated in immunocompromised individuals. The patient should be seen daily or every other day for the first week; debridement of affected areas is repeated at each visit, and plaque control methods are gradually introduced. A meticulous plaque control program should be taught and started as soon as the sensitivity of the area allows it.

The patient should avoid tobacco, alcohol, and condiments. An antimicrobial mouthrinse such as chlorhexidine gluconate 0.12% is prescribed.

Systemic antibiotics such as metronidazole or amoxicillin may be prescribed for patients with moderate to severe tissue destruction, localized lymphadenopathy or systemic symptoms, or both. The use of prophylactic antifungal medication should be considered if antibiotics are prescribed.

The periodontium should be reevaluated 1 month after resolution of acute symptoms to assess the results of treatment and determine the need for further therapy.

Necrotizing Ulcerative Stomatitis

NUS may be severely destructive and acutely painful. It is characterized by necrosis of significant areas of oral soft tissue and underlying bone. It may occur separately or as an extension of NUP[9,20] and is commonly associated with severe depression of $CD4^+$ immune cells and an increased viral load.

Treatment may include prescription of an antibiotic such as metronidazole and use of an antimicrobial mouthrinse such as chlorhexidine gluconate. If osseous necrosis is present, it is often necessary to remove the affected bone to promote wound healing.[55]

Necrotizing Ulcerative Periodontitis

Therapy for NUP includes local debridement, scaling and root planing, in-office irrigation with an effective antimicrobial agent such as chlorhexidine gluconate or povidone iodine (Betadine), and establishment of meticulous oral hygiene, including home use of antimicrobial rinses or irrigation[20,26,39,54] (Color Fig. 51-1 and Fig. 51-8).

This therapeutic approach is based on reports involving only a small number of patients.[39] In severe NUP, antibiotic therapy may be necessary but should be used with caution in HIV-infected patients to avoid an opportunistic and potentially serious localized candidiasis or even candidal septicemia.[3] If an antibiotic is necessary, metronidazole (250 mg, with two tablets taken immediately and then one tablet qid for 5 to 7 days) is the drug of choice. Prophylactic prescription of a topical or systemic antifungal agent is prudent if an antibiotic is used.

Conventional periodontitis should be managed based on the considerations outlined in "Periodontal Treatment Protocol."

REFERENCES

1. Asher RS, McDowell JD, Winquist H: HIV-related neuropsychiatric changes: Concerns for dental professionals. J Am Dent Assoc 1993; 124:80.

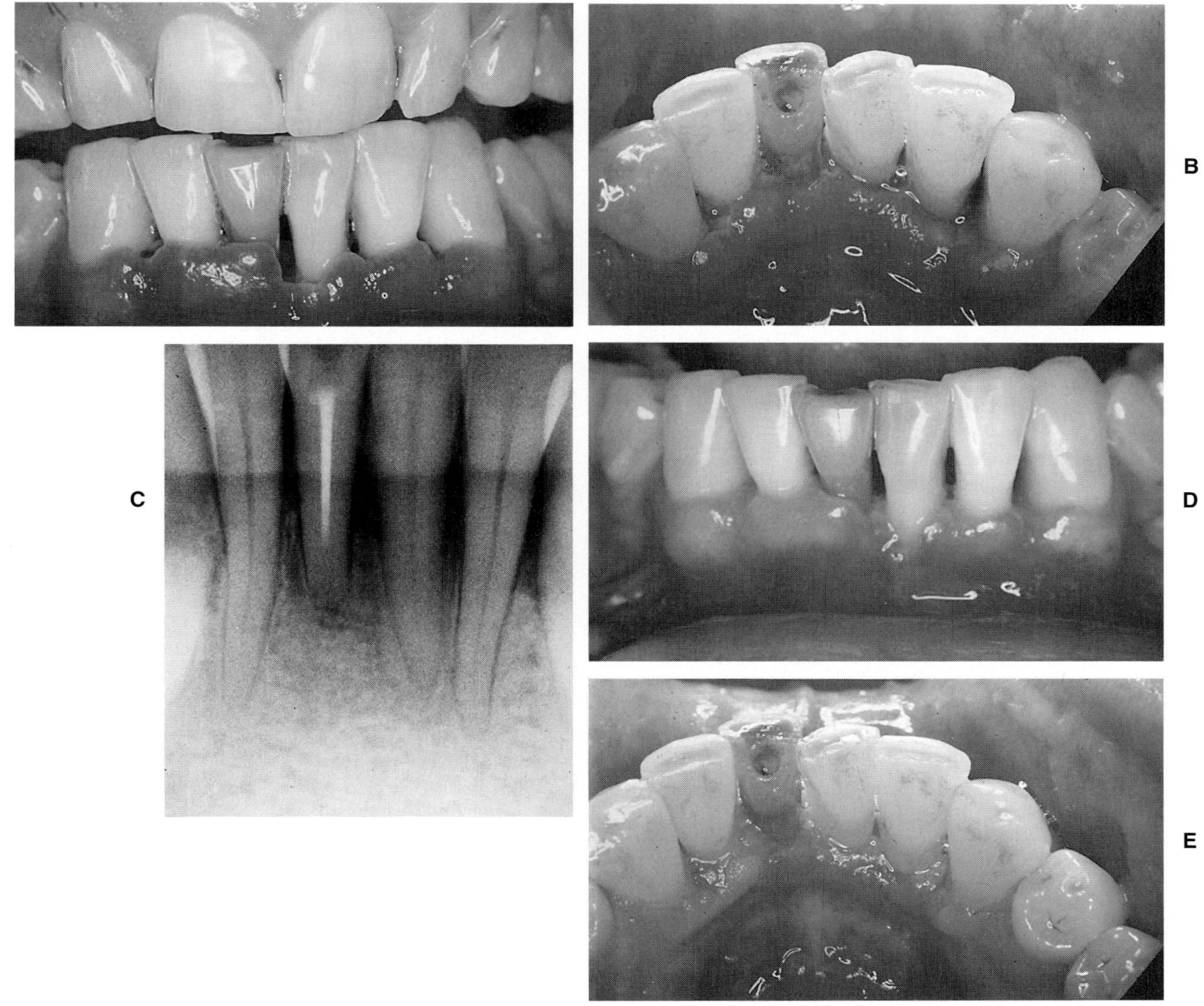

Fig. 51-8 Localized necrotizing ulcerative periodontitis in a 43-year-old HIV-positive man. **A,** Facial view. **B,** Lingual view. **C,** Radiographic view of the mandibular anterior. **D,** Resolution 48 hours after initiation of periodontal therapy. Facial view. **E,** Resolution. Lingual view.

2. Brockmeyer NH, Kreugfelder E, Martins L, et al: Zidovudine therapy of asymptomatic HIV-1-infected patients and combined Zidovudine-acyclovir therapy of HIV-1-infected patients with oral hairy leukoplakia. J Infect Dermatol 1989; 92:647.
3. Casado JL, Quereda C, Oliva J, et al: Candidal meningitis in HIV-infected patients: Analysis of 14 cases. Clin Infect Dis 1997; 25:673.
4. Centers for Disease Control: Case-control study of HIV seroconversion in health-care workers after percutaneous exposure to HIV-infected blood—France, United Kingdom and United States. January 1988–August 1994. MMWR 1995; 44:929.
5. Centers for Disease Control: Recommended infection-control practices for dentistry, 1993. MMWR 1993; 42(RR-8):1.
6. Chandrasekhar J, Liem AA, Cox NH, et al: Oxypentifylline in the management of recurrent aphthous oral ulcers. Oral Surg Oral Med Oral Pathol Oral Radiol Endod 1999; 87:564.
7. Clerici M, Piconi S, Balotta C, et al: Pentoxifylline improves cell-mediated immunity and reduces human immunodeficiency virus (HIV) plasma viremia in asymptomatic HIV-seropositive persons. J Infect Dis 1997; 175:1210.
8. Dis Dios P, Hermida AO, Alvarez CM, et al: Fluconazole-resistant oral candidosis in HIV-infected patients. AIDS 1995; 9:809.
9. European Community Clearinghouse on Oral Problems Related to HIV Infection and WHO Collaborating Centre on Oral Manifestations of the Immunodeficiency Virus: Classification and diagnostic criteria for oral lesions in HIV infection. J Oral Pathol Med 1993; 22:289.
10. Epstein JB: Antifungal therapy in oropharyngeal mycotic infections. Oral Surg Oral Med Oral Pathol 1990; 69:32.
11. Epstein JB, Lozada-Nur F, McLeod A, et al: Oral Kaposi's sarcoma in acquired immunodeficiency syndrome: Review of management and report of the efficacy of intralesional vinblastine. Cancer 1989; 64:2424.

12. Epstein JB, Scully C: HIV infection: Clinical features and treatment of 33 homosexual men with Kaposi's sarcoma. Oral Med Oral Surg Oral Pathol 1991; 71:38.
13. Ficarra G, Berson AM, Silverman S Jr, et al: Kaposi's sarcoma of the oral cavity: A study of 134 patients with a review of the pathogenesis, epidemiology, clinical aspects and treatment. Oral Surg Oral Med Oral Pathol 1988; 66:543.
14. Giuliana G, Pizzo G, Milici ME, et al: In vitro activities of antimicrobial agents against *Candida* species. Oral Surg Oral Med Oral Pathol Oral Radiol Endod 1999; 87:44.
15. Glick M: Clinical protocol for treating patients with HIV disease. Gen Dent 1990; 38:418.
16. Glick M, Cleveland DB: Oral mucosal bacillary epitheloid angiomatosis in a patient with AIDS associated with rapid alveolar bone loss: A case report. J Oral Pathol Med 1993; 22:235.
17. Glick M, Muzyka BC: Alternative therapies for major aphthous ulcers in AIDS patients. J Am Dent Assoc 1992; 123:61.
18. Glick M, Holmstrop P: HIV infection and periodontal diseases. Periodontal Medicine. In: Genco R, Mealey B, Rose L (eds): Hamilton, Canada, 2000, Decker.
19. Gorin I, Vilette B, Gehanno P, et al:. Thalidomide in hyperalgic pharyngeal ulceration of AIDS. Lancet 1990; 335:1343.
20. Grassi M, Williams CA, Winkler JR, et al: Management of HIV-associated periodontal diseases. In: Robertson PB, Greenspan JS (eds): Oral Manifestations of AIDS. Littleton, MA, PSG, 1988.
21. Hammer SM: Advances in antiretroviral therapy and viral load monitoring. AIDS 1996; 10(Suppl 3):S1.
22. Haslett P, Tramontana J, Burroughs M, et al: Adverse reactions to thalidomide in patients infected with human immunodeficiency virus. Clin Infect Dis 1997; 24:1223.
23. Horning GM, Cohen ME: Necrotizing ulcerative gingivitis, periodontitis and stomatitis: Clinical staging and predisposing factors. J Periodontol 1995; 66:990.
24. Jacobson JM, Greenspan JS, Spritzler J, et al: Thalidomide for the treatment of oral aphthous ulcers in patients with human immunodeficiency virus infection. N Engl J Med 1997; 336:1487.
25. Lake-Bakaar G, Tom W, Lake-Bakaar D, et al: Gastropathy and ketoconazole malabsorption in the acquired immunodeficiency syndrome (AIDS). Ann Intern Med 1988; 109:471.
26. Levine RA, Glick M: Rapidly progressive periodontitis as an important clinical marker for HIV disease. Compend Contin Educ Dent 1991; XII(7):478.
27. Lot F, Seguier J-C, Fegueux S, et al: Probably transmission of HIV from an orthopedic surgeon to a patient in France. Ann Intern Med 1999; 130:1.
28. Mandel ID: Occupational risks in dentistry: Comforts and concerns. J Am Dent Assoc 1993; 124:41.
29. Margiotta V, Campisi G, Mancuso S, et al: HIV infection: Oral lesions, CD4+ cell count and viral load in an Italian study population. J Oral Pathol Med 1999; 28:173.
30. Mealey BL: Periodontal implications: Medically compromised patients. Ann Periodontol 1996; 1:256.
31. Molinari JA: HIV, health care workers and patients: How to ensure safety in the dental office. J Am Dent Assoc 1993; 124:51.
32. Nichols CM, Flaitz CM, Hicks MJ: Treating Kaposi's lesions in the HIV-infected patient. J Am Dent Assoc 1993; 124:78.
33. Olsen RJ, Lynch P, Coyle MB, et al: Examination gloves as barriers to hand contamination in clinical practice. JAMA 1993; 270(3):350.
34. Pons V, Greenspan D, Lozada-Nur F, et al: Oropharyngeal candidiasis in patients with AIDS: Randomized comparison of fluconazole versus nystatin oral suspensions. Clin Infect Dis 1997; 24:1204.
35. Physicians Desk Reference: Fungisone oral suspension. Health Care Series 1998; 97:1.
36. Porter SR, Scully C, Luker J: Complications of dental surgery in persons with HIV disease. Oral Surg Oral Med Oral Pathol 1993; 75:165.
37. Regezi JA, Eversole LR, Barker BF, et al: Herpes simplex and cytomegalovirus coinfected oral ulcers in HIV-positive patients. Oral Surg Oral Med Oral Pathol Oral Radiol Endod 1996; 81:55.
38. Reichart PA, Langford A, Gelderblom HR, et al: Oral hairy leukoplakia: Observations in 95 cases and review of the literature. J Oral Pathol Med 1989; 18:410.
39. Robinson P: Periodontal diseases and HIV infection. J Clin Periodontol 1992; 19:609.
40. Saiag P, Pavlovic M, Clerici T, et al: Treatment of early AIDS-related Kaposi's sarcoma with oral all-*trans*-retinoic acid: Results of a sequential non-randomized phase II trial. AIDS 1998; 12:2169.
41. Schulman DJ: The dentist, HIV and the law. CDA J 1993; 21(9):45.
42. Schuman P, Capps L, Peng G, et al: Weekly fluconazole for the prevention of mucosal candidiasis in women with HIV infection. Ann Int Med 1997; 126:689.
43. Shibosky CH, Winkler JR: Gingival Kaposi's sarcoma and periodontitis. Oral Med Oral Surg Oral Pathol 1991; 76:38.
44. Shibosky CH, Winkler JR: Gingival Kaposi's sarcoma and periodontitis. Oral Surg Oral Med Oral Pathol 1993; 76:49.
45. Silverman S: Color Atlas of Oral Manifestations of AIDS. Toronto, Decker, 1989.
46. Silverman S Jr, Gallo JW, McKnight ML, et al: Clinical characteristics and management responses in 85 HIV-infected patients with oral candidiasis. Oral Surg Oral Med Oral Pathol Oral Radiol Endod 1996; 82:402.
47. Stevenson GC: Removable prosthodontics and the HIV-infected patient: Assessment and treatment planning. Dental Alliance AIDS/HIV Care 1996; 3(1):8.
48. Tavitian A, Raufman JP, Rosenthal LE, et al: Ketoconazole-resistant candida esophagitis in patients with acquired immune deficiency syndrome. Gastroenterology 1986; 90:443.
49. Tomlinson DR, Coker RJ, Fisher M: Management and treatment of Kaposi's sarcoma in AIDS. Int J STD AIDS 1996; 7:466.
50. United States Pharmacopeial Convention Inc: Drug information for the health care professional, ed 19. World Color Book Services, Taunton. 1999.
51. Ustianowski AP, Leake H, Evans S: Outpatient therapy of HIV-associated oral and oesophageal candidosis. Int J STD AIDS 1997; 8:592.
52. Velegraki A, Nicolatou O, Theodoridou M, et al: Pediatric AIDS-related linear gingival erythema: A form of erythematous candidiasis? J Oral Pathol Med 1999; 28:178.
53. Verrusio AC: Risk of transmission of the human immunodeficiency virus to health care workers exposed to HIV-infected patients: A review. J Am Dent Assoc 1989; 118:339.
54. Winkler JR, Murray PA, Grassi M, et al: Diagnosis and management of HIV-associated periodontal lesions. J Am Dent Assoc 1989; 120(suppl):S25.
55. Winkler JR, Murray PA, Hammerle C: Gangrenous stomatitis in AIDS. Lancet 1989; 2(8454):108.

Occlusal Evaluation and Therapy in the Management of Periodontal Disease

Carol A. Bibb

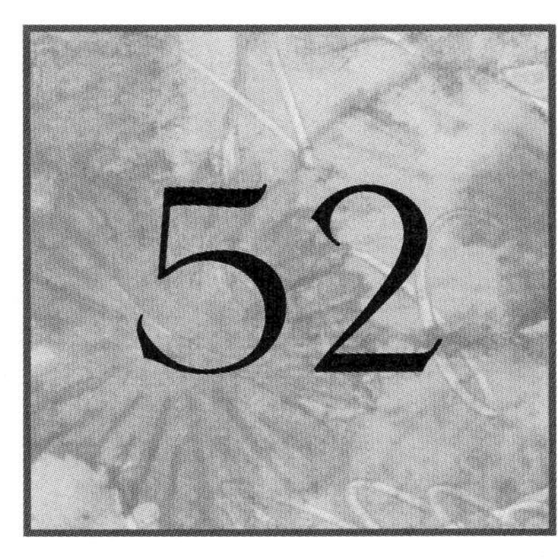

CHAPTER

Chapter Outline

An understanding of the principles of occlusion and the relationship to oral health and disease is necessary for all dental clinicians. Unfortunately, no other discipline in dentistry has been so complicated by confusion and controversy. Historically, occlusal relationships have been considered largely from a morphologic rather than a biologic perspective. This approach has led to an overemphasis on occlusal scheme and jaw position without adequate consideration of the functional status of the patient's entire masticatory system.

The current resurgence of interest in occlusion[18,19,27] coincides with the Institute of Medicine's recommendation that the dental profession make use of scientific evidence, outcomes research, and formal consensus processes when devising practice guidelines.[12] As a result, we now have the opportunity and responsibility to move away from practice based on empiric experience toward practice based on scientific evidence. Application of this approach to the field of occlusion has already begun to have, and is expected to continue to have, a significant impact on clinical practice and an improved standard of patient care, including for those patients undergoing periodontal therapy.[14,19,20]

Contemporary definitions of occlusion reflect the importance of structure-function relationships in biologic systems. For example, McNeill[29] defines *occlusion* as the functional relationship between the components of the masticatory system, including the teeth, supporting tissues, neuromuscular system, temporomandibular joints, and craniofacial skeleton. An important corollary of this definition is that the occlusion is a dynamic relationship and must be defined physiologically as well as morphologically. The clinical application of this definition is that the occlusion cannot be evaluated or treated in isolation. Instead, each component of the masticatory system must be fully understood along with its potential for adaptation and pathophysiology as well as interactions with the other components. This chapter presents a biologic rationale and practical guidelines for evaluating jaw function status and occlusion in the context of the management of periodontal disease.

TERMINOLOGY

The complexity surrounding occlusal concepts has been compounded by an abundance of heterogeneous terminology requiring definition and clarification. The key

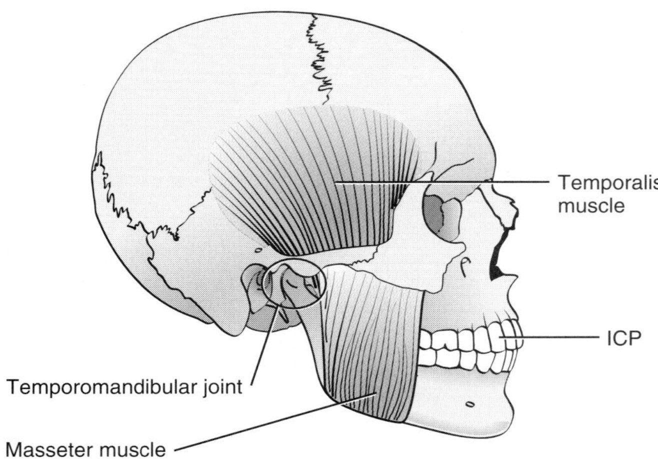

Fig. 52-1 Functional anatomy of the masticatory system shown in sagittal view: the temporomandibular joint *(circled),* the masseter and temporalis muscles, and the dental occlusion in ICP.

terms used in this chapter, along with common synonyms, are defined as follows:

Intercuspal position (ICP): The position of the mandible when there is maximal intercuspation between the maxillary and mandibular teeth. *Synonym:* centric occlusion.

Muscular contact position (MCP): The position of the mandible when lifted into contact from resting position.

Excursive movement: Any movement of the mandible away from ICP.

Laterotrusion: Movement of the mandible laterally to the right or left from ICP. *Synonym:* working movement.

Laterotrusive side: The side of either dental arch corresponding to the side of the mandible moving away from the midline. *Synonym:* working side.

Mediotrusive side: The side of either dental arch corresponding to the side of the mandible moving toward the midline. *Synonym:* balancing side, nonworking side.

Protrusion: Movement of the mandible anteriorly from ICP.

Retrusion: Movement of the mandible posteriorly from ICP.

Retruded position: The most cranial position of the mandible along the retruded path of closure. *Synonym:* centric relation.

Guidance: Pattern of opposing tooth contact during excursive movements of the mandible. The teeth making such contact cause separation of the other teeth. *Synonym:* disclusion.

Interference: Any contact, in ICP or excursions, that prevents the remaining occlusal surfaces from achieving stable contact. *Synonym:* supracontact.

FUNCTIONAL ANATOMY OF THE MASTICATORY SYSTEM

An understanding of the biologic basis of occlusal function requires that the teeth, temporomandibular joints (TMJs), and muscles of mastication be considered as a functional unit (Fig. 52-1). These structures developed together during embryogenesis and postnatal growth, and perturbations to one component in the system would be expected to influence other components to undergo either adaptive or pathologic changes. Therefore the clinician must recognize that it is inappropriate to consider any component in isolation and instead must include all components of the system and their functional interactions as part of any evaluation.

BIOLOGIC BASIS OF OCCLUSAL FUNCTION

The ideal occlusal relationships depicted in textbook diagrams and on typodont models have served as the primary focus of traditional dental education. In reality, such ideal tooth contact relationships are uncommon in natural dentitions,[2,17,22,35,43] and a variety of occlusal schemes, including chronic excursive interferences,[1,32,33,42] are clinically acceptable.

In addition, it is now recognized that the occlusion is a dynamic relationship reflecting an equilibrium between the various components of the masticatory system.[29] Therefore the functional status of an individual's occlusion is more clinically significant than its morphology.

A widely accepted physiologic classification of occlusion is as follows:

A **physiologic occlusion** is present when no signs of dysfunction or disease are present and no treatment is indicated.

A **nonphysiologic (or traumatic) occlusion** is associated with dysfunction or disease due to tissue injury, and treatment may be indicated. In this text, the term *trauma from occlusion* is applied to periodontal tissue injury due to occlusal forces.

A **therapeutic occlusion** is the result of specific interventions designed to treat dysfunction or disease.

Maintenance of a physiologic occlusion requires favorable structure-function relationships and optimal tissue adaptation throughout the masticatory system. The anatomic features that contribute to a physiologic occlusion and should be the goal in a therapeutic occlusion[29] include a stable end-point of mandibular closure, bilateral distribution of occlusal forces across many posterior teeth, and axial loading of these teeth. When occlusal forces are distributed optimally, the occlusion will be stable by objective criteria and is likely to be subjectively comfortable for the patient.

The signs and symptoms of a nonphysiologic occlusion include damaged teeth and restorations, abnormal mobility, fremitus, a widened periodontal ligament, pain, and a subjective sense of bite discomfort. As emphasized in Chapter 24, *the criterion that determines whether an occlusion is traumatic is whether it produces periodontal injury, not how the teeth occlude. Alternatively, many so-called malocclusions do not produce discomfort or injury and therefore are not traumatic occlusions by definition.*

Adverse tooth loading due to increased force or frequency can result from many factors. One cause is missing or shifting teeth, leading to alterations in arch form and alignment. This situation is frequently seen in patients who have lost teeth due to untreated periodontal disease. In general, occlusal changes that occur gradually are more likely to give the tissue time to adapt, whereas acute occlusal changes, including iatrogenic changes introduced by faulty restorative dentistry, are more likely to produce injury.

Parafunctional habits such as bruxism are another potential cause of occlusal trauma. *Bruxism* is defined as diurnal or nocturnal parafunctional activity including clenching, bracing, gnashing, and grinding of the teeth. Although there is no association between bruxism and gingival inflammation[7] or periodontitis,[15,16] bruxism definitely has the potential to cause tooth wear, fracture, and periodontal and muscle pain and is a major cause of mobility.[34] There is no significant evidence that malocclusions or interferences are causal factors in bruxism,[9] and occlusal adjustment has not proven to be an effective means of treatment.[3,21] Instead, the maxillary stabilization appliance is generally considered the most effective means of managing bruxism.[6]

Chapter 24 provides a detailed description of the response of the periodontium to occlusal forces and discusses the relationship of trauma from occlusion to the etiology and progression of periodontal disease. The literature on this topic includes numerous experimental animal model studies[10,11,23–25,30,38,39,43] in which the challenge is to make clinically relevant extrapolations to human periodontal disease. The current consensus is that trauma from occlusion has the potential to alter disease severity and prognosis. However, the therapeutic priority is to control inflammation, and this must be successful for healing of the periodontal tissues to occur.[14,30,31,36,37,43] Therefore it is recommended that occlusal interventions be deferred until inflammation is controlled and reevaluation determines that any residual mobility is the result of adverse tooth loading rather than decreased support.[13,19,20]

CLINICAL EVALUATION PROCEDURES

The current standard of care requires that a screening evaluation for temporomandibular disorders (TMD) be included in all routine dental examinations.[26] This screening should occur early in the physical evaluation of the patient to ensure that subsequent examination and treatment procedures will not have an adverse impact on preexisting TMDs. In addition, a valid examination of the occlusion requires that the patient's jaw function status be within normal limits.

TMD Screening Examination

The recommended screening examination includes health history questions focused on jaw function status, a brief history, and a cursory examination expected to take approximately 5 minutes. The generally accepted components of this examination[26] are shown in Box 52-1.

BOX 52-1

TMD Screening Evaluation

1. Maximal interincisal opening
2. Opening-closing pathway
3. Auscultation for TMJ sounds
4. Palpation for TMJ tenderness
5. Palpation for muscle tenderness

Interincisal opening: The patient is instructed to "open as wide as possible" while a millimeter ruler is placed on the lower incisors. The interincisal distance is recorded in millimeters (mm).

Opening pathway: The opening/closing pathway is observed, and any deviations from a midline path are diagrammed.

TMJ sounds: Light finger pressure is applied bilaterally over the TMJs while the patient is asked to open and close. Joint sounds are classified as discrete clicks or diffuse grating sounds, termed *crepitus.* The location of the sound in the opening/closing cycle and any associated pain or mechanical disruption should be documented.

TMJ tenderness: Light bilateral palpation over the lateral aspect of the condyles is used to elicit TMJ tenderness if present. It should be recorded as mild, moderate, or severe. The patient should be asked to compare right and left sides for calibration purposes.

Muscle tenderness: The masseter (origin and insertion) and temporalis (anterior and middle) muscles are examined bilaterally using moderate finger pressure. Sites of muscle pain should be localized and described as mild, moderate, and severe on an appropriate anatomic diagram. The most common error is to apply insufficient pressure, so the patient should be advised to expect some discomfort and instructed to differentiate pressure from pain. It is also helpful to ask the patient to compare right and left sides for calibration purposes.

Intraoral Evaluation of Occlusion

In addition to collecting standard data on static occlusal relationships, a functional evaluation of the occlusion (Box 52-2) should be carried out. This includes an assessment of ICP stability, the quality of mandibular movements, and tooth mobility and wear.

Intercuspal position: The patient should be able to close into ICP consistently from MCP without searching for a stable or comfortable bite. The most efficient way to locate zones of ICP contact is to place mylar strips between the teeth and ask the patient to "close and

BOX 52-2

Intraoral Occlusal Evaluation

1. Identification of ICP zones of contact
2. Guidance in excursive movements
3. Tooth mobility
4. Attrition

hold." The presence or absence of contacts should be documented for the molars, premolars, canines, and incisors. More detailed information on the specific sites of ICP contacts can be obtained by using occlusal indicator wax or marking ribbon.

Excursive movements: The quality of tooth contact patterns during mandibular movements out of ICP are observed by asking the patient to move into protrusion and right and left laterotrusion. Mylar strips are useful for verifying tooth contact patterns during excursions.

Tooth mobility: Mobility is recorded as part of the initial occlusal evaluation and to monitor any changes over time. (See Chapter 30 for additional details.)

Attrition: Attrition is defined as wear due to tooth-to-tooth contact. A certain amount of physiologic attrition is normal. However, accelerated attrition should be noted, including the location of significant wear facets.

Role of Articulated Casts

Articulated dental casts are not necessary for a functional evaluation of the occlusion. In specific cases, they may be required for pretreatment documentation of occlusal relationships, localization of wear facets, trial occlusal adjustments, and monitoring of the progression of occlusal changes.

INTERPRETATION AND TREATMENT PLANNING

TMD Screening

The goal of the TMD screening examination is to determine whether jaw function status is sufficiently within the normal range to permit examination procedures and treatment to proceed without provoking or exacerbating symptoms. Therefore the clinical significance of the findings will be considered in this context.

A suggested practical approach is to use the screening examination findings to place the patient in one of the following three categories:

1. The jaw function status is determined to be within normal limits; there are no contraindications to proceeding with further examination and treatment procedures. A patient in this category will have no complaints or significant history of jaw pain or dysfunction, an interincisal opening of at least 40 mm, no significant joint or muscle tenderness, and minimal joint sounds.
2. Certain findings should alert the clinician to the potential for aggravating benign problems, especially with wide opening during long appointments. Examples include a history of jaw problems after long appointments, several sites of mild to moderate muscle tenderness, or a previously benign TMJ click. In these cases the patients should be advised of the need to notify the clinician if symptoms develop or progress. Use of a bite block, shortened appointments, and longer intervals between appointments may also be indicated.
3. Significant findings indicate the need for a more comprehensive evaluation or referral prior to any nonemergency treatment. Examples include a restricted interincisal opening, significant pain on jaw use, severe joint or muscle pain, and progressive locking episodes, such as after wide opening. It should be obvious that continuing with nonemergency treatment would be difficult and likely to exacerbate these problems. Furthermore, evaluation of the occlusion will not be valid unless the patient's jaw function status is determined to be within normal limits.

BOX 52-3

Requirements for Occlusal Stability

1. Intercuspal position
   - Light or absent anterior contacts
   - Well-distributed posterior contacts
   - Coupled contacts between opposing teeth
   - Cross tooth stabilization
   - Forces directed along long axis of each tooth
2. Smooth excursive movements without interferences
3. No trauma from occlusion
4. Favorable subjective response to occlusal form and function

It is important to emphasize that the prevalence of TMD signs and symptoms in adult subjects ranges from 28% to 86% in various studies,[40] but it has been estimated that only 5% to 7% are in need of TMD treatment.[41] In triaging patients as described previously, significant pain or dysfunction and progression of symptoms are the key determinants. Furthermore, clinicians treating older adults should be aware that a high prevalence of crepitus and jaw opening of less than 40 mm has been reported in older individuals compared with young adults.[4] These signs were not associated with pain or disability and do not contraindicate treatment.[4] However, they may have an impact on providing dental care to this age group.

Occlusal Evaluation

The findings from the occlusal examination should be reviewed in the context of the definitions of physiologic

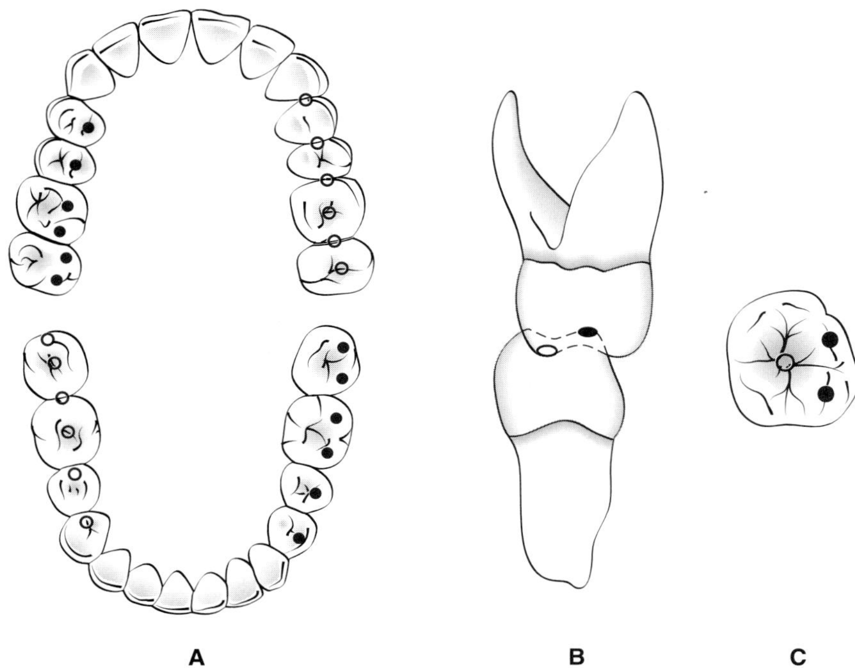

Fig. 52-2 **A,** Sites of ICP contact on supporting cusps *(solid circles)* and corresponding vertical stops *(open circles)*. Cross tooth stabilization is shown on proximal **(B)** and occlusal views **(C)**. Note the direction of occlusal forces along the long axis of the teeth shown in **B**.

and nonphysiologic occlusions. The most significant concern is whether the occlusion meets the requirements for occlusal stability (Box 52-3). Specific requirements for stability of posterior teeth in ICP are illustrated in Fig. 52-2.

OCCLUSAL THERAPY

The purpose of occlusal therapy is to establish stable functional relationships favorable to the oral health of the patient, including the periodontium. A variety of procedures could contribute to this objective: interocclusal appliance therapy, occlusal adjustment, restorative procedures, orthodontic tooth movement, and orthognathic surgery.

Some overall guidelines apply to occlusal therapy in general. First, there should be a sound biologic rationale for the intervention. Second, occlusal interventions should be considered an adjunct to periodontal therapy. Third, significant irreversible occlusal changes should be considered in the context of the restorative care planned for the patient. Finally, it is imperative that a thorough, informed consent be provided to the patient. With respect to periodontal management, it is critical that the patient understand that the goal of the occlusal intervention is to increase stability and comfort, *not* to treat the periodontal disease.

The contributions of restorative dentistry and orthodontic tooth movement to the management of the periodontal patient are covered elsewhere in this book. Therefore the role of occlusal adjustment and interocclusal appliance therapy is the primary focus of this discussion.

Occlusal Adjustment

Occlusal adjustment, or coronoplasty, is the selective reshaping of occlusal surfaces with the goal of establishing a stable, nontraumatic occlusion. The resulting occlusion should meet the requirements for occlusal stability described previously and would be termed a *therapeutic occlusion*. Many categories of occlusal adjustment exist, ranging from the altering of contours of a single tooth to major full mouth equilibration to the retruded position.

Occlusal adjustment procedures have been used extensively in the past for treating a variety of problems including occlusal trauma, TMD symptoms, bruxism, and headache. However, occlusal adjustment is an invasive, irreversible intervention. Therefore in the current climate of evidence-based practice, the prudent clinician is encouraged to question the scientific evidence in support of such therapy. Specifically, does the evidence support a causal relationship between occlusal factors and the condition being treated? What is the evidence that occlusal adjustment is therapeutically beneficial for the condition being treated?

In the case of TMD, the evidence leads to the conclusion that occlusal adjustment as an irreversible treatment modality should rarely be considered as a primary component of TMD treatment and never as a preventive measure.[26] Similarly, there is no evidence that occlusal adjustment is useful in the management of bruxism.[3,21]

The role of occlusal adjustment in the management of periodontal disease is more complex because both periodontitis and trauma from occlusion can lead to tooth mobility. In one randomized clinical trial with a two-year follow-up,[5] it was concluded that occlusal adjustment resulted in a more favorable attachment level but no differences in reduction of mobility or pocket depth. Clearly, additional well-designed outcome studies designed to evaluate the effects of occlusal adjustment on healing after periodontal therapy are needed. These studies should include variables such as timing of the occlusal intervention in the therapeutic sequence, the response of individual teeth rather than dentitions, and long term follow-up.

Until these issues are resolved, it is recommended that occlusal adjustment generally be deferred until inflammation is controlled, time is allowed for tissue healing, and reevaluation determines that any residual mobility is the result of adverse tooth loading rather than decreased support.[13,19,20] Exceptions to this recommendation include the need to address pain or dysfunction clearly determined to be the result of occlusal trauma.

A major consideration prior to occlusal adjustment is the restorative needs of the patient. For example, the benefits of placing provisional restorations with optimal contours and well-adjusted occlusal surfaces should not be overlooked. This approach offers the opportunity to restore occlusal stability by distributing forces as well as to evaluate the response of the periodontium to the anticipated restoration of the patient's dentition.

For cases in which occlusal adjustment has been determined the best approach, the procedure must be preceded by good informed consent,[8] and trial adjustment on accurately mounted diagnostic casts is recommended. Clark[8] and McNeill[28] have provided detailed practical protocols for occlusal adjustment procedures.

Interocclusal Appliance Therapy

Interocclusal appliances, generally fabricated of hard acrylic resin, have the advantage of providing a reversible means of redistributing occlusal forces and minimizing excessive force on individual teeth. A full-coverage, maxillary stabilization appliance is particularly useful in managing bruxism as part of an overall comprehensive treatment plan for the patient. Providing such an appliance to the periodontal patient is likely to contribute to an overall sense of bite comfort in addition to minimizing the destructive consequences of bruxism. Clark[6] has provided an excellent description of design, delivery, adjustment, and postinsertion instructions for such an appliance.

SUMMARY

Evaluation and management of the periodontal patient must include a thorough examination of the masticatory system, including a TMD screening exam and functional evaluation of the occlusion. Occlusal interventions should be considered an adjunct to periodontal therapy, reversible when possible, and planned in the context of the restorative needs of the patient.

REFERENCES

1. Agerberg G, Sandstrom R: Frequency of occlusal interferences: A clinical study in teenagers and young adults. J Prosthet Dent 1988; 59:212.
2. Anderson JR, Myers GE: Natural contacts in centric occlusion in 32 adults. J Dent Res 1971; 50:7.
3. Bailey JO Jr, Rugh JD: Effect of occlusal adjustment on bruxism as monitored by nocturnal EMG recordings. Abstract 199. J Dent Res 1980; 59:317.
4. Bibb CA, Atchison KA, Pullinger AG, et al: Jaw function status in an elderly community sample. Community Dent Oral Epidemiol 1995; 23:303.
5. Burgett FG, Ramfjord SP, Nissle RR, et al: A randomized trial of occlusal adjustment in the treatment of periodontitis patients. J Clin Periodontol 1992; 19:381.
6. Clark GT: Interocclusal appliance therapy. In: Mohl ND, Zarb GA, Carlsson GE, et al (eds): A Textbook of Occlusion. Chicago, Quintessence, 1988.
7. Clark GT, Love R: The effect of gingival inflammation on nocturnal masseter muscle activity. J Am Dent Assoc 1981; 102:319.
8. Clark GT, Mohl ND, Riggs RR: Occlusal adjustment therapy. In: Mohl ND, Zarb GA, Carlsson GE, et al (eds): A Textbook of Occlusion. Chicago, Quintessence, 1988.
9. Clark GT, Tsukiyama Y, Baba K, et al: Sixty-eight years of experimental interference studies: what have we learned? J Prosthet Dent 1999; 82:704.
10. Ericsson I, Giargia M, Linde J, et al: Progression of periodontal tissue destruction at splinted/non-splinted teeth: An experimental study in the dog. J Clin Periodontol 1993; 10:693.
11. Ericsson I, Lindhe J: Lack of effect of trauma from occlusion on the recurrence of experimental periodontitis. J Clin Periodontol 1977; 4:115.
12. Field MJ (ed): Dental Education at the Crossroads. Washington, DC, National Academy Press, 1995.
13. Fleszar TJ, Knowles JW, Morrison EC, et al: Tooth mobility and periodontal therapy. J Clin Periodontol 1980; 7:495.
14. Gher ME: Changing concepts. The effect of occlusion on periodontitis. Dent Clin North Am 1998; 2:285.
15. Hanamura H, Houston F, Rylander H, et al: Periodontal status and bruxism. A comparative study of patients with periodontal disease and occlusal parafunctions. J Periodontol 1987; 58:173.
16. Hellsing G: Functional adaptation to changes in vertical dimension. J Prosthet Dent 1984; 52:867.
17. Hochman N, Ehrlich J: Tooth contact location in intercuspal position. Quintess Int 1987; 18:193.
18. J Calif Dent Assoc 2000; vol 28 (entire issue).
19. Kao RT: The role of occlusion in periodontal disease. In: McNeill C (ed): Science and Practice of Occlusion. Chicago, Quintessence, 1997.
20. Kao RT, Chu R, Curtis D: Occlusal considerations in determining treatment prognosis. J Calif Dent Assoc 2000; 28:760.
21. Kardachi BJR, Bailey JO Jr, Ash MM Jr: A comparison of biofeedback and occlusal adjustment on bruxism. J Periodontol 1978; 49:367.
22. Korioth TWP: Number and location of occlusal contacts in intercuspal position. J Prosthet Dent 1990; 64:206.
23. Lindhe J, Ericsson I: Effect of longstanding jiggling on experimental marginal periodontitis in the beagle dog. J Clin Periodontol 1982; 9:497.
24. Lindhe J, Ericsson I: The effect of elimination of jiggling forces on periodontically exposed teeth in the dog. J Periodontol 1982; 53:562.
25. Lindhe J, Svanberg G: Influence of trauma from occlusion on progression of experimental periodontitis in the beagle dog. J Clin Periodontol 1974; 1:3.
26. McNeill C (ed): Temporomandibular Disorders: Guidelines for Classification, Assessment, and Management. Chicago, Quintessence, 1993.

27. McNeill C (ed): Science and Practice of Occlusion. Chicago, Quintessence, 1997.
28. McNeill C: Selective tooth grinding and equilibration. In: McNeill C (ed): Science and Practice of Occlusion. Chicago, Quintessence, 1997.
29. McNeill C: Occlusion: What it is and what it is not. J Calif Dent Assoc 2000; 28:748.
30. Meitner S: Co-destructive factors of marginal periodontitis and repetitive mechanical injury. J Dent Res 1975; 54:78.
31. Miyata T, Kobayashi Y, Araki H, et al: The influence of controlled occlusal overload on peri-implant tissue. Int J Oral Maxillofac Implants 1998; 13:677.
32. Nilner M: Prevalence of functional disturbances and diseases of the stomatognathic system in 15–18 year-olds. Swed Dent J 1981; 5:189.
33. Nilner M, Lassing S-A: Prevalence of functional disturbances and diseases of the stomatognathic system in 7–14 year-olds. Swed Dent J 1981; 5:173.
34. Pavone BW: Bruxism and its effect on the natural teeth. J Pros Dent 1985; 53:692.
35. Plasmans PJJM, Knipers L, Vollenbrock HR, et al: The occlusal status of molars. J Prosthet Dent 1988; 60:500.
36. Polson AM: The relative importance of plaque and occlusion in periodontal disease. J Clin Periodontol 1986; 13:923.
37. Polson AM, Adams RA, Zander HA: Osseous repair in the presence of active tooth hypermobility. J Clin Periodontol 1983; 10:370.
38. Polson AM, Meitner SW, Zander HA: Trauma and progression of marginal periodontitis in squirrel monkeys. III. Adaptation of interproximal alveolar bone to repetitive injury. J Periodont Res 1976; 11:279.
39. Polson AM, Meitner SW, Zander HA: Trauma and progression of marginal periodontitis in squirrel monkeys. IV. Reversibility of bone loss due to trauma alone and trauma superimposed upon periodontitis. J Periodont Res 1976; 11:290.
40. Rugh JD, Solberg WK: Oral health status in the United States: Temporomandibular disorders. J Dent Educ 1985; 49:398.
41. Solberg WK: Epidemiology, Incidence, and Prevalence of Temporomandibular Disorders: A Review. In: The President's Conference on the Examination, Diagnosis, and Management of Temporomandibular Disorders. Chicago, American Dental Association, 1983.
42. Tipton RT, Rinchuse DJ: The relationship between static occlusion and functional occlusion in a dental school population. Angle Orthodont 1991; 61:57.
43. Zander HA, Polson AM: Present status of occlusion and occlusal therapy in periodontics. J Periodontol 1977; 48:540.

The Role of Orthodontics as an Adjunct to Periodontal Therapy

Vincent G. Kokich

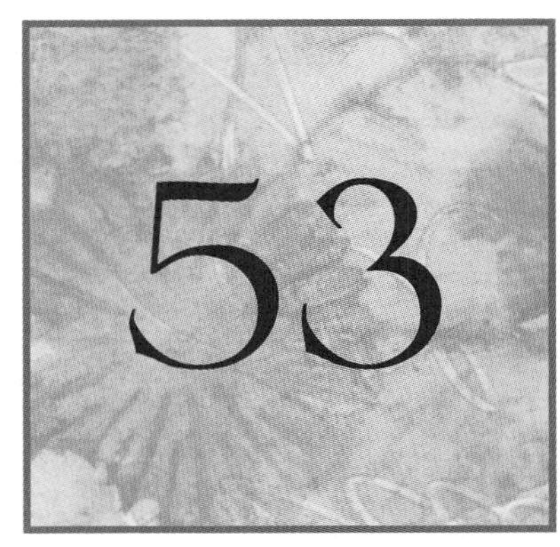

CHAPTER

Chapter Outline

Orthodontic tooth movement may be a substantial benefit to the adult periorestorative patient. Many adults who seek routine restorative dentistry have problems with tooth malposition that compromise their ability to adequately clean and maintain their dentitions. If these individuals also are susceptible to periodontal disease, tooth malposition could be an exacerbating factor that could cause premature loss of specific teeth. Orthodontic appliances have become smaller, less noticeable, and easier to maintain during orthodontic therapy. Many adults are taking advantage of the opportunity to have their teeth aligned to improve the esthetics of their smiles. If these individuals also have underlying gingival or osseous periodontal defects, these defects often can be improved during orthodontic therapy if the orthodontist is aware of the situation and designs the appropriate tooth movement. In addition, implants have become a major part of the treatment plan for many adults with missing teeth. If adjacent teeth have drifted into edentulous spaces, orthodontics is often helpful to provide the ideal amount of space for implants and subsequent restorations. This chapter shows the ways in which adjunctive orthodontic therapy can enhance the periodontal health and restorability of teeth.

BENEFITS OF ORTHODONTICS FOR A PERIODONTAL PATIENT

Orthodontic therapy can provide several benefits to the adult periodontal patient. The following six factors should be considered:

1. Aligning crowded or malposed maxillary or mandibular anterior teeth permits the adult patient better access to adequately clean all surfaces of their teeth. This could be a tremendous advantage for patients who are susceptible to periodontal bone loss or do not have the dexterity to adequately maintain their oral hygiene.
2. Vertical orthodontic tooth repositioning can improve certain types of osseous defects in periodontal patients. Often, the tooth movement eliminates the need for resective osseous surgery.

3. Orthodontic treatment can improve the esthetic relationship of the maxillary gingival margin levels before restorative dentistry. Aligning the gingival margins orthodontically avoids gingival recontouring, which potentially could require bone removal and exposure of the roots of the teeth.
4. The *fourth* benefit of orthodontics is for the patient who has suffered a severe fracture of a maxillary anterior tooth, which requires forced eruption to permit adequate restoration of the root. In this situation, erupting the root allows the crown preparation to have sufficient resistance form and retention for the final restoration.
5. Orthodontic treatment allows open gingival embrasures to be corrected to regain lost papilla. If these open gingival embrasures are located in the maxillary anterior region, they can be unaesthetic. In most patients, these areas can be corrected with a combination of orthodontic root movement, tooth reshaping, and/or restoration.
6. Orthodontic treatment could improve adjacent tooth position before implant placement or tooth replacement. This is especially true for the patient who has been missing teeth for several years and has drifting and tipping of the adjacent dentition.

PREORTHODONTIC OSSEOUS SURGERY

The extent of the osseous surgery depends on the type of defect (i.e., crater, hemiseptal defect, three-wall defect, and/or furcation lesion). The prudent clinician knows which defects can be improved with orthodontic treatment and which defects require preorthodontic, periodontal, surgical intervention.

Osseous Craters

An osseous crater is an interproximal, two-wall defect that does not improve with orthodontic treatment. Some shallow craters (i.e., 4- to 5-mm pocket) may be maintainable nonsurgically during orthodontic treatment. However, if surgical correction is necessary, this type of osseous lesion can easily be eliminated by reshaping the defect[12,15] and reducing the pocket depth (Fig. 53-1) (see Chapter 62). This in turn enhances the ability to maintain these interproximal areas during orthodontic treatment. The need for surgery is based on the patient's response to initial root planing, the patient's periodontal resistance, the location of the defect, and the predictability of maintaining defects nonsurgically while the patient is wearing orthodontic appliances.

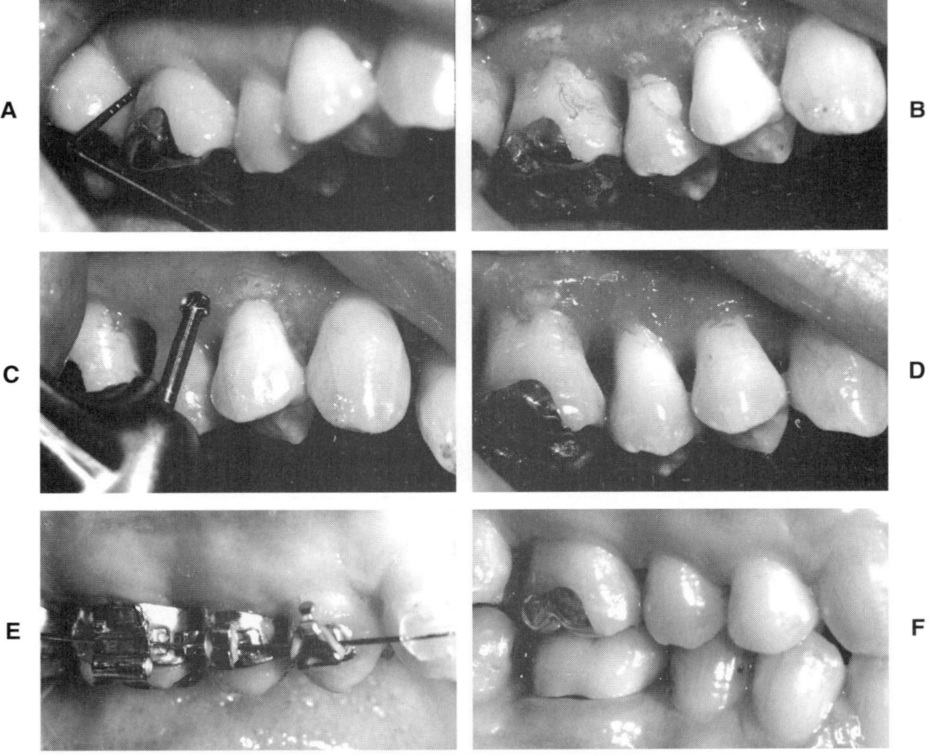

Fig. 53-1 This patient had a 6-mm probing defect distal to the maxillary right first molar **(A)**. When this area was flapped **(B)**, a cratering defect was apparent. Osseous surgery was used to alter the bony architecture on the buccal and lingual to eliminate the defect **(C and D)**. After 6 weeks, the probing pocket defect had been reduced to 3 mm, and orthodontic appliances were placed on the teeth **(E)**. By eliminating the crater before orthodontics, the patient could maintain the area during and after orthodontics **(F)**.

Three-Wall Intrabony Defects

Three-wall defects are amenable to pocket reduction with regenerative periodontal therapy.[1] Bone grafts using either autogenous bone from the surgical site or allografts along with the use of resorbable membranes have been successful in filling three-wall defects.[14] If the result of periodontal therapy is stable (Fig. 53-2) 3 to 6 months after periodontal surgery, orthodontic treatment may be initiated.

ORTHODONTIC TREATMENT OF OSSEOUS DEFECTS

Hemiseptal Defects

Hemiseptal defects are one- or two-wall osseous defects that often are found around mesially tipped teeth (Fig. 53-3) or teeth that have supererupted (Fig. 53-4). Usually, these defects can be eliminated with the appropriate orthodontic treatment. In the case of the tipped tooth, uprighting[2,5] and eruption of the tooth levels the bony defect. If the tooth is supererupted, intrusion and leveling of the adjacent cementoenamel junctions can help level the osseous defect.

It is imperative that periodontal inflammation be controlled before orthodontic treatment. This usually can be achieved with initial debridement and rarely requires any preorthodontic surgery. After the completion of orthodontic treatment, these teeth should be stabilized for at least 6 months and reassessed periodontally. Often, the pocket has been reduced or eliminated and no further periodontal treatment is needed. It would be injudicious to perform preorthodontic osseous corrective surgery in such lesions if orthodontics is part of the overall treatment plan.

In the periodontally healthy patient, orthodontic brackets are positioned on the posterior teeth relative to the marginal ridges and cusps. However, some adult patients may have marginal ridge discrepancies caused by uneven tooth eruption. When marginal ridge discrepancies are encountered, the decision as to where to place the bracket or band is not determined by the anatomy of the tooth. In these situations, it is important to assess these teeth radiographically to determine the interproximal bone level.

If the bone level is oriented in the same direction as the marginal ridge discrepancy, then leveling the marginal ridges will level the bone. However, if the bone level is flat between adjacent teeth (see Fig. 53-4) and the marginal ridges are at significantly different levels, correction of the marginal ridge discrepancy orthodontically produces a hemiseptal defect in the bone. This could cause a periodontal pocket between the two teeth.

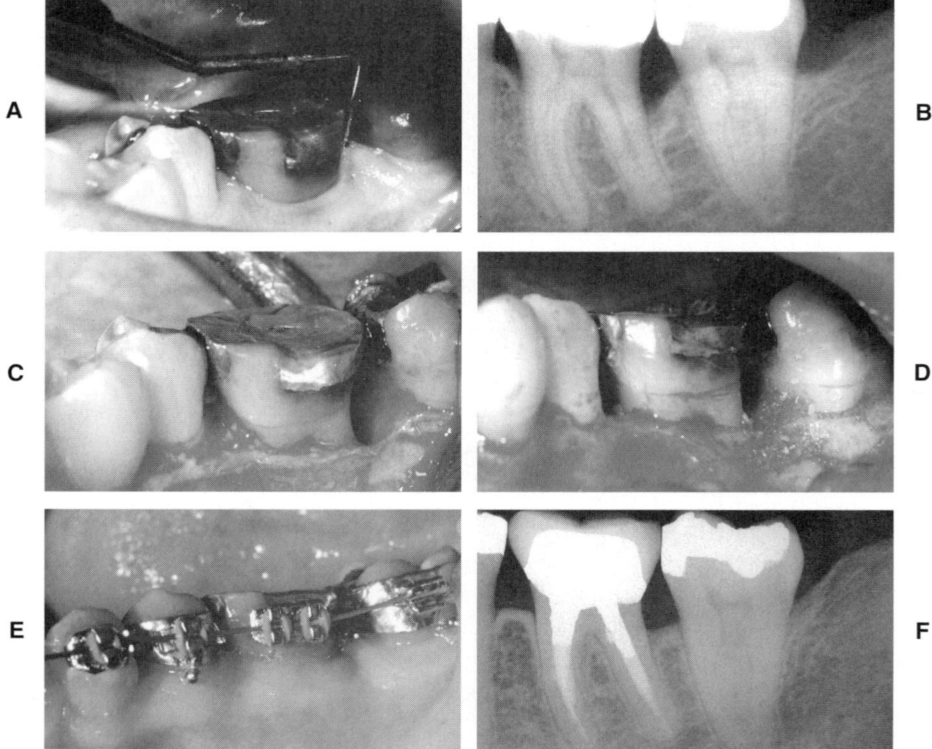

Fig. 53-2 This patient had a significant periodontal pocket **(A)** distal to the mandibular right first molar. A periapical radiograph **(B)** confirmed the osseous defect. A flap was elevated **(C)**, revealing a deep, three-wall osseous defect. Freeze-dried bone **(D)** was placed in the defect 6 months after the bone graft. Orthodontic treatment was initiated **(E)**. The final periapical radiograph shows that the preorthodontic bone graft helped regenerate bone and eliminate the defect distal to the molar **(F)**.

If the bone is flat and a marginal ridge discrepancy is present, the orthodontist should not level the marginal ridges orthodontically. In these situations, it may be necessary to equilibrate the crown of the tooth (see Fig. 53-4). For some patients, the latter technique may require endodontic therapy and restoration of the tooth because of the required amount of reduction of the length of the crown. This approach is acceptable if the treatment results in a more favorable bone contour between the teeth.

In some patients, a discrepancy may exist between both the marginal ridges and the bony levels between two teeth. However, these discrepancies may not be of equal magnitude. In these patients, orthodontic leveling of the bone may still leave a discrepancy in the marginal ridges (Fig. 53-5). In these situations, the crowns of the teeth should not be used as a guide for completing orthodontic therapy. The bone should be leveled orthodontically and any remaining discrepancies between the marginal ridges should be equilibrated. This method produces the best occlusal result and improves the periodontal health.

During orthodontic treatment, when teeth are being extruded to level hemiseptal defects, the patient should be monitored regularly. Initially, the hemiseptal defect has a greater sulcular depth and is more difficult for the patient to clean. As the defect is ameliorated through tooth extrusion, interproximal cleaning becomes easier. The patient should be recalled every 2 to 3 months during the leveling process to control inflammation in the interproximal region.

Advanced Horizontal Bone Loss

After orthodontic treatment has been planned, one of the most important factors that determine the outcome of orthodontic therapy is the location of the bands and brackets on the teeth. In a periodontally healthy individual, the position of the brackets is usually determined by the anatomy of the crowns of the teeth. Anterior brackets should be positioned relative to the incisal edges. Posterior bands or brackets are positioned relative to the marginal ridges. If the incisal edges and marginal ridges are at the correct level, the cementoenamel junction (CEJ) will also be at the same level. This relationship creates a flat, bony contour between the teeth. However, if a patient has underlying periodontal problems and significant alveolar bone loss around certain teeth, using the anatomy of the crown to determine bracket placement is not appropriate (Fig. 53-6).

In a patient with advanced horizontal bone loss, the bone level may have receded several millimeters from

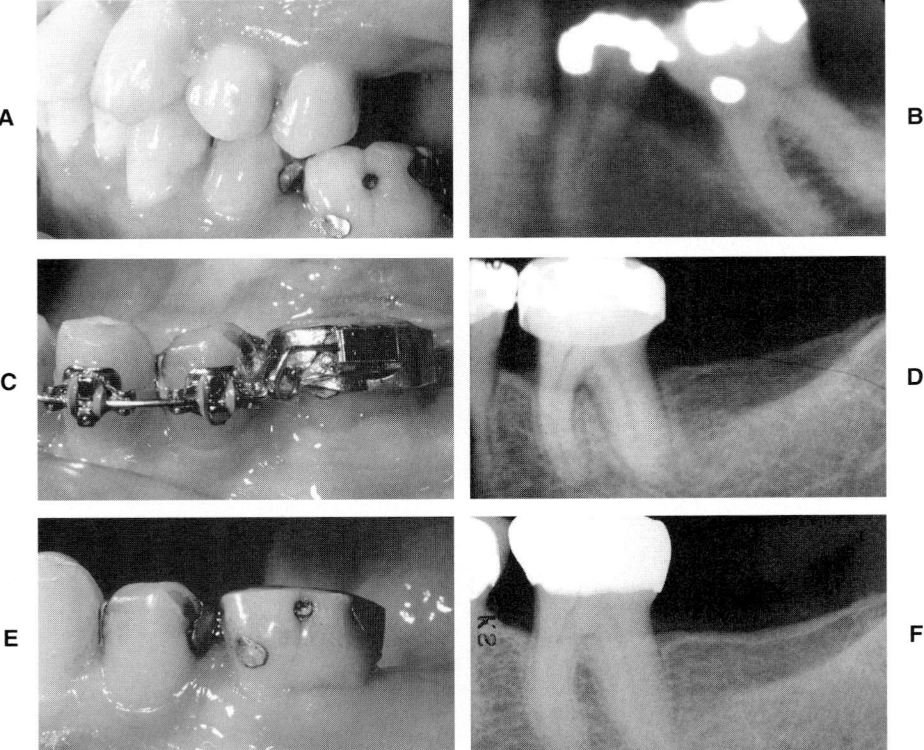

Fig. 53-3 This patient was missing the mandibular left second premolar, and the first molar had tipped mesially **(A)**. A pretreatment periapical radiograph **(B)** revealed a significant hemiseptal osseous defect on the mesial of the molar. To eliminate the defect, the molar was erupted and the occlusal surface was equilibrated **(C)**. The eruption was stopped when the bone defect was leveled **(D)**. The posttreatment intraoral photograph **(E)** and periapical radiograph **(F)** show that the periodontal health had been improved by correcting the hemiseptal defect orthodontically.

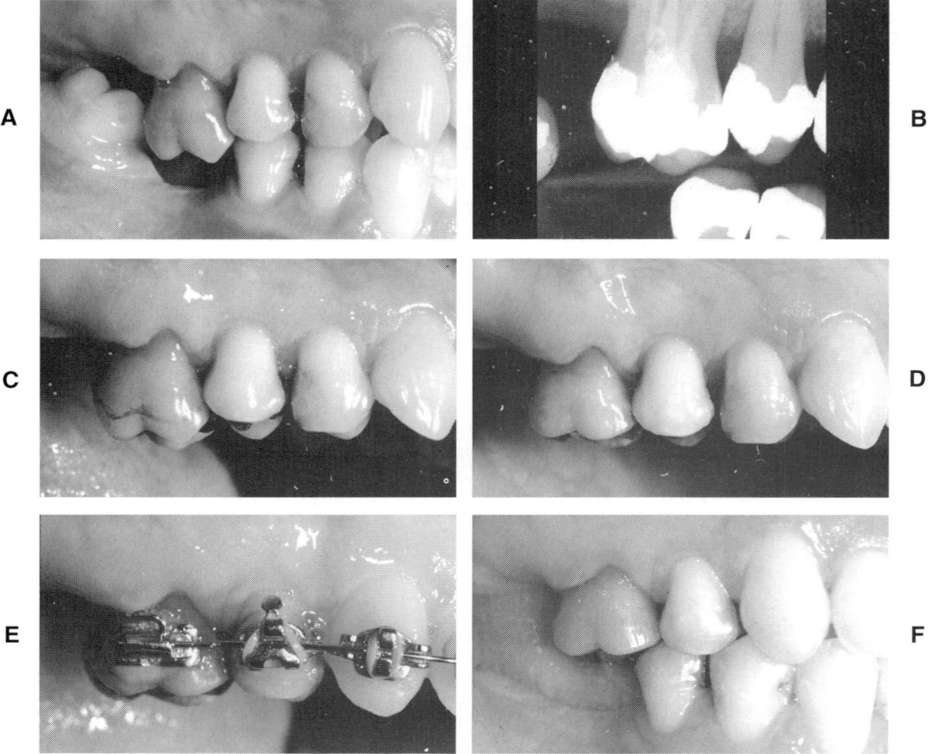

Fig. 53-4 This patient showed overeruption of the maxillary right first molar and a marginal ridge defect between the second premolar and first molar **(A)**. A pretreatment periapical radiograph **(B)** showed that the interproximal bone was flat. To avoid creating a hemiseptal defect, the occlusal surface of the first molar was equilibrated **(C and D)** and the malocclusion was corrected orthodontically **(E and F)**.

the CEJ. As this occurs, the crown-to-root ratio becomes less favorable. By aligning the crowns of the teeth, the clinician may perpetuate tooth mobility by maintaining an unfavorable crown-to-root ratio. In addition, by aligning the crowns of the teeth and disregarding the bone level, significant bone discrepancies occur between healthy and periodontally diseased roots. This could require periodontal surgery to ameliorate the discrepancies.

Many of these problems can be corrected by using the bone level as a guide to position the brackets on the teeth (see Fig. 53-6). In these situations, the crowns of the teeth may require considerable equilibration. If the tooth is vital, the equilibration should be performed gradually to allow the pulp to form secondary dentin and insulate the tooth during the equilibration process. The goal of equilibration and creative bracket placement is to provide a more favorable bony architecture as well as a more favorable crown-to-root ratio. In some of these patients, the periodontal defects that were apparent initially may not require periodontal surgery after orthodontic treatment.

Furcation Defects

Furcation defects can be classified as incipient (Class I), moderate (Class II), or advanced (Class III). These lesions require special attention in the patient undergoing orthodontic treatment. Often, the molars require bands with tubes and other attachments that impede the patient's access to the buccal furcation for home care and instrumentation at the time of recall.

Furcation lesions require special consideration because they are the most difficult lesions to maintain and can worsen during orthodontic therapy. These patients need to be maintained on a 2- to 3-month recall schedule. Detailed instrumentation of these furcations helps minimize further periodontal breakdown.

If a patient with a Class III furcation defect will be undergoing orthodontic treatment, a possible method for treating the furcation is to eliminate it by hemisecting the crown and root of the tooth (Fig. 53-7). However, this procedure requires endodontic, periodontal, and restorative treatment. If the patient will be undergoing orthodontic treatment, it is advisable to perform the orthodontic treatment first. This is especially true if the roots of the teeth will not be moved apart. In these patients, the molar to be hemisected remains intact during orthodontics (see Fig. 53-7). This patient would require 2- or 3-month recall visits to ensure that the furcation defect does not lose bone during orthodontic treatment. Keeping the tooth intact during the orthodontics simplifies the concentration of tooth movement for the orthodontist. After orthodontics, endodontic therapy is

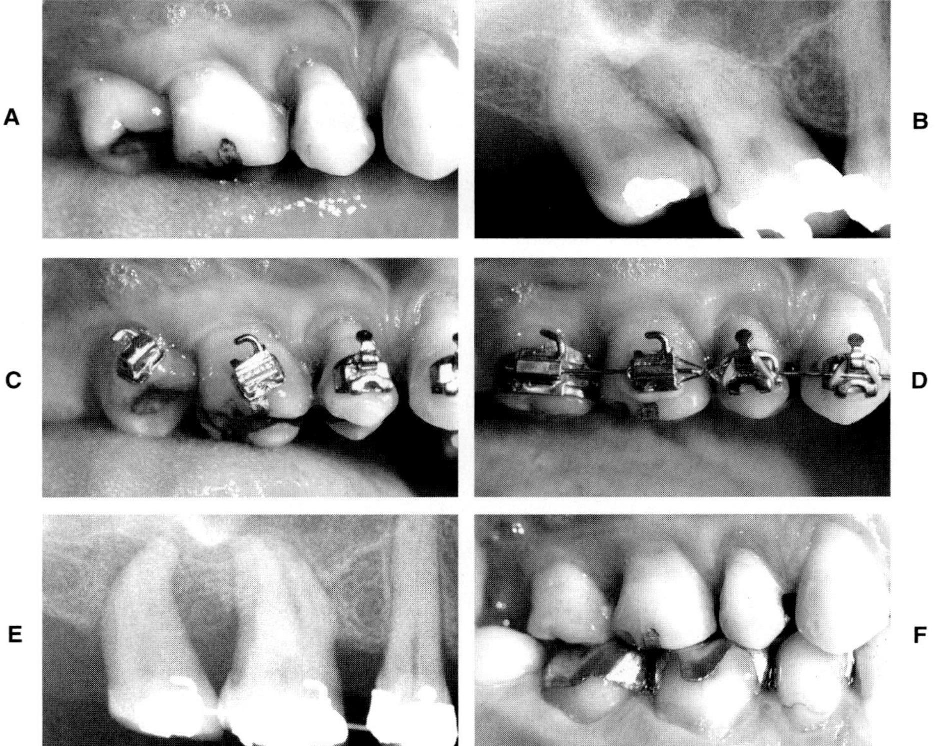

Fig. 53-5 Before orthodontic treatment, this patient had significant mesial tipping of the maxillary right first and second molars, causing marginal ridge discrepancies **(A)**. The tipping produced root proximity between the molars **(B)**. To eliminate the root proximity, the brackets were placed perpendicular to the long axis of the teeth **(C)**. This method of bracket placement facilitated root alignment and elimination of the root proximity as well as leveling of the marginal ridge discrepancies **(D, E, and F)**.

required (followed by periodontal surgery) to divide the tooth.

In some patients requiring hemisection of a mandibular molar with a Class III furcation, pushing the roots apart during orthodontic treatment may be advantageous (Fig. 53-8). If the hemisected molar will be used as an abutment for a bridge after orthodontics, moving the roots apart orthodontically permits a favorable restoration and splinting across the adjacent edentulous spaces.

In the latter situation, hemisection, endodontic therapy, and periodontal surgery must be completed before the start of orthodontic treatment. After these procedures have been completed, bands or brackets can be placed on the root fragments and coil springs used to separate the roots. The amount of separation is determined by the size of the adjacent edentulous spaces and the occlusion in the opposing arch. About 7 or 8 mm may be created between the roots of the hemisected molar. This process eliminates the original furcation problem and allows the patient to clean the area with greater efficiency.

In some molars with Class III furcation defects, the tooth may have short roots, advanced bone loss, fused roots, or other problems that prevent hemisection and crowning of the remaining roots. In these patients (Fig. 53-9), extracting the root with a furcation defect and placing an implant may be more advisable.[11] If this type of plan has been adopted, the timing of the extraction and placement of the implant can occur at any time relative to the orthodontic treatment. In some situations, the implant could be used as an anchor to facilitate prerestorative orthodontic treatment (see Fig. 53-9).

The implant must remain embedded in bone for 4 to 6 months after placement before it can be loaded as an orthodontic anchor. It must be placed precisely so that it not only provides an anchor for tooth movement but also may be used an eventual abutment for a crown or fixed bridge. If the implant will not be used as an anchor for orthodontic movement, it may be placed after the orthodontic treatment has been completed. Considerations regarding timing are determined by the restorative treatment plan.

Root Proximity

When roots of posterior teeth are in close proximity, the ability to maintain periodontal health and accessibility for restoration of adjacent teeth may be compromised.[4] However, if the patient were undergoing orthodontic therapy, the roots can be moved apart and bone will be formed between the adjacent roots (see Fig. 53-5). This opens the embrasure beneath the tooth contact, provides additional bone support, and enhances the patient's access to the interproximal region for hygiene.

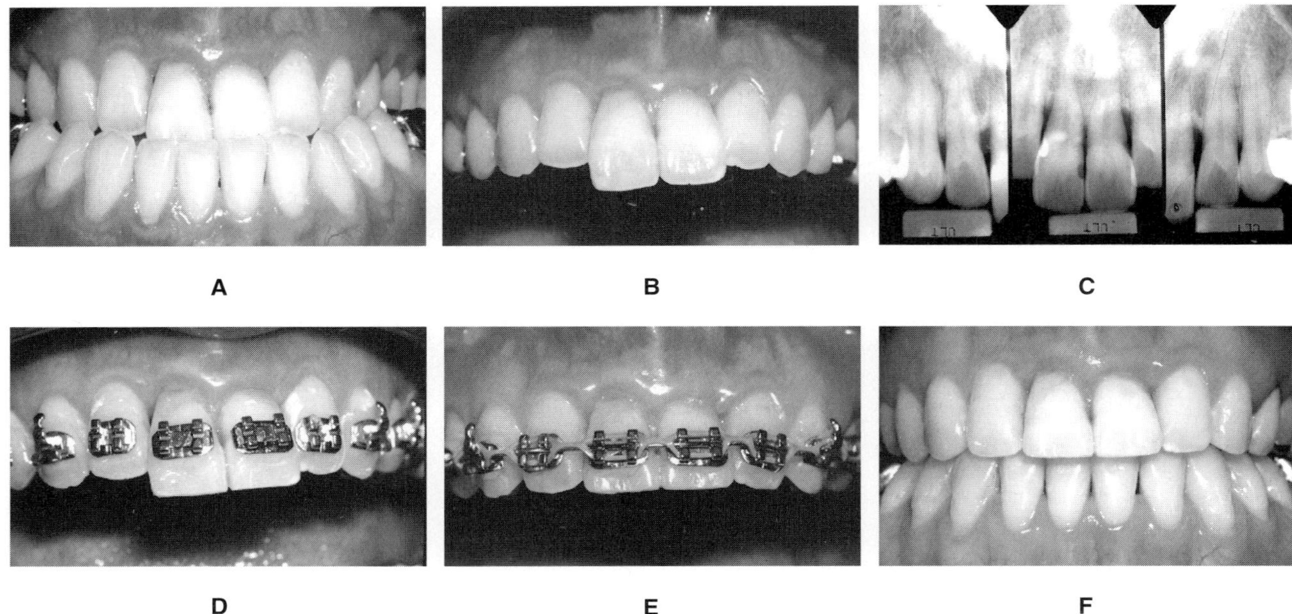

Fig. 53-6 Before orthodontic treatment, this patient had a significant Class III malocclusion **(A)**. The maxillary central incisors had overerupted **(B)** relative to the occlusal plane. A pretreatment periapical radiograph **(C)** showed that significant horizontal bone loss had occurred. To avoid creating a vertical periodontal defect by intruding the central incisors, the brackets were placed to maintain the bone height **(D)**. The incisal edges of the centrals were equilibrated **(E)**, and the orthodontic treatment was completed without intruding the incisors **(F)**.

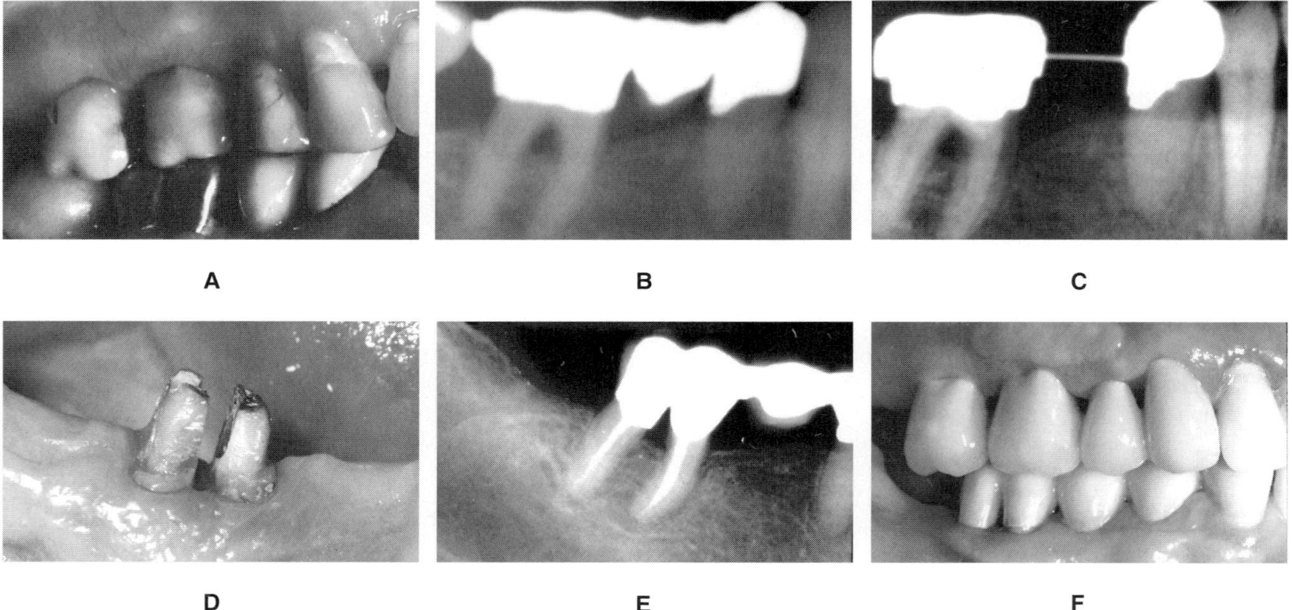

Fig. 53-7 This patient had a Class III furcation defect before orthodontic treatment **(A and B)**. Orthodontic treatment was performed **(C)**, and the furcation defect was maintained by the periodontist on 2-month recalls until after orthodontic treatment. After appliance removal, the tooth was hemisected **(D)**, and the roots were restored, and splinted together **(E)**. The final periapical radiograph **(F)** shows that the furcation defect has been eliminated by hemisecting and restoring the two root fragments.

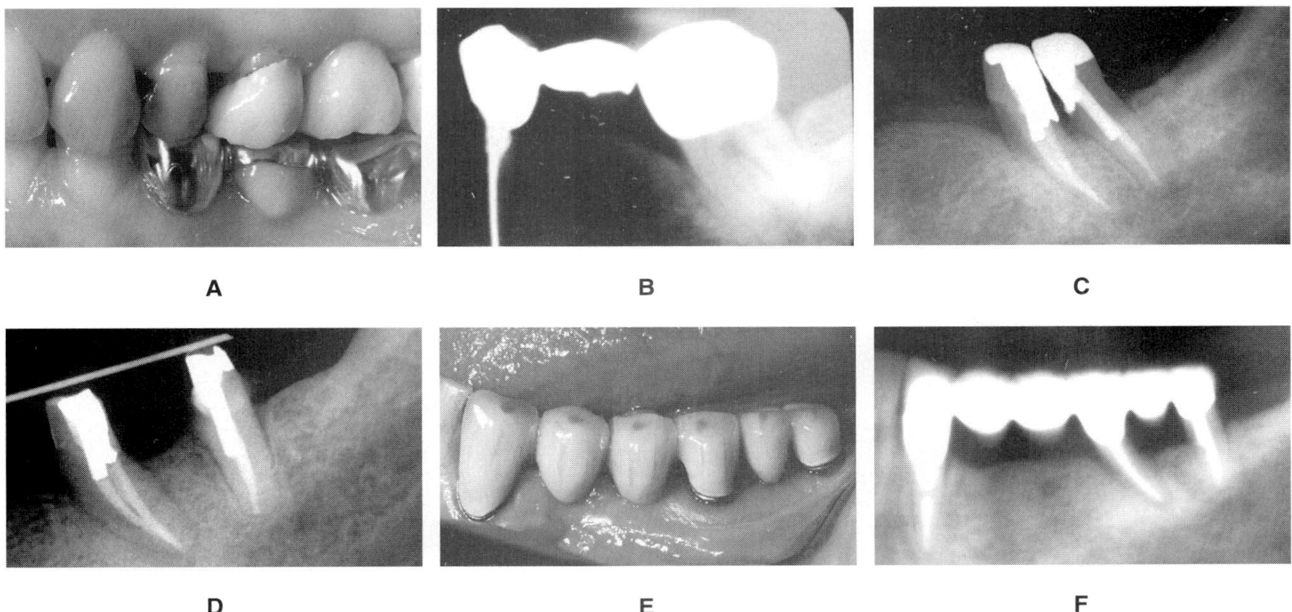

Fig. 53-8 Before orthodontic treatment, this patient had a Class III furcation defect in the mandibular left second molar **(A and B)**. Because the patient had an edentulous space mesial to the molar, the tooth was hemisected **(C),** and the root fragments were separated orthodontically **(D)**. After orthodontic treatment, the root fragments were used as abutments to stabilize a multiunit posterior bridge **(E and F)**.

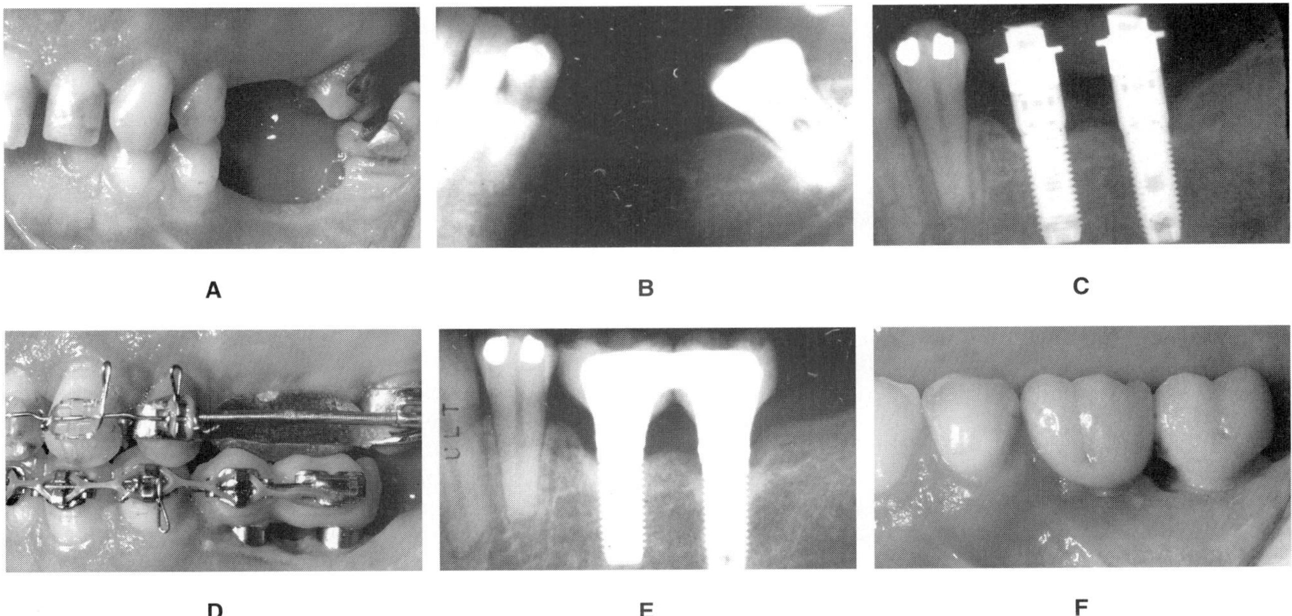

Fig. 53-9 This patient was missing several teeth in the mandibular left posterior quadrant **(A)**. The mandibular left third molar had a Class III furcation defect and short roots **(B)**. The third molar was extracted and two implants were placed in the mandibular left posterior quadrant **(C)**. The implants were used as anchors to facilitate orthodontic treatment **(D)** and help reestablish the left posterior occlusion **(E and F)**.

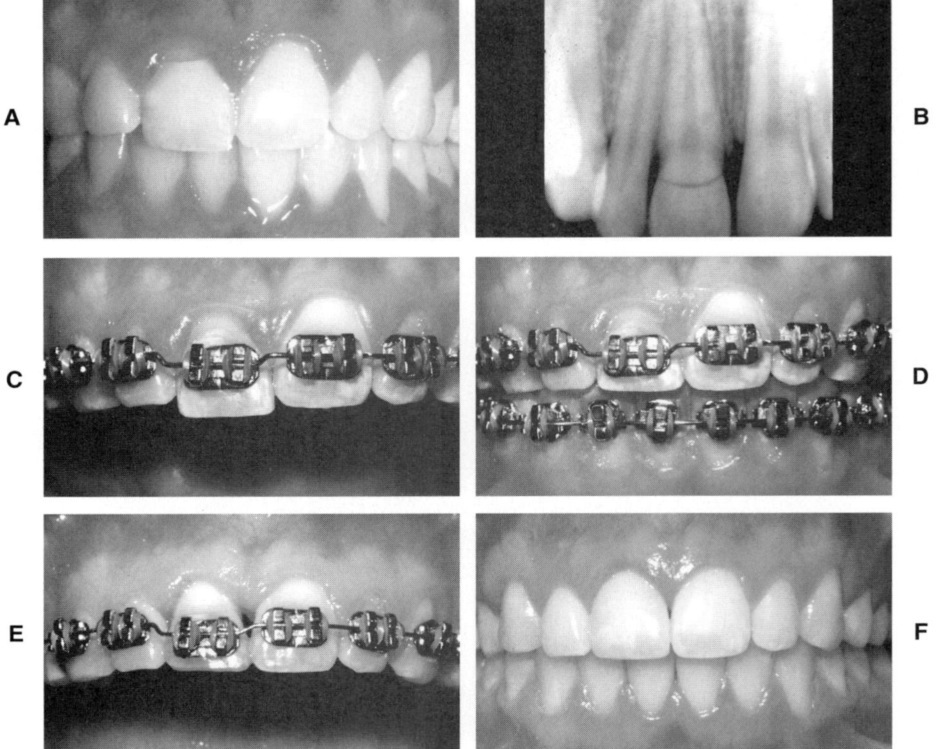

Fig. 53-10 This patient had a severe fracture of the maxillary right central incisor **(A)** that extended apical to the level of the alveolar crest on the lingual **(B)**. To restore the tooth adequately and avoid impinging on the periodontium, the fractured root was extruded 4 mm **(C)**. As the tooth erupted, the gingival margin followed the tooth **(D)**. Gingival surgery was required to lengthen the crown of the central incisor **(E)** so that the final restoration had sufficient ferrule for resistance and retention and the appropriate gingival margin relationship with the adjacent central incisor **(F)**.

This generally improves the periodontal health of this area.

If orthodontic treatment will be used to move roots apart, this plan must be known before bracket placement. It is advantageous to place the brackets so that the orthodontic movement to separate the roots will begin with the initial archwires (see Fig. 53-5). Therefore brackets must be placed obliquely to facilitate this process. To determine the progress of orthodontic root separation, radiographs are needed to monitor the status. Generally, 2 to 3 mm of root separation provides adequate bone and embrasure space to improve periodontal health. During this time, the patient should be maintained to ensure that a favorable bone response occurs as the roots are moved apart. In addition, these patients need occasional occlusal adjustment to recontour the crown because the roots are moving apart. As this occurs, the crowns may develop an unusual occlusal contact with the opposing arch. This should be equilibrated to improve the occlusion.

Fractured Teeth/Forced Eruption

Occasionally, children and adolescents may fall and accidentally injure their anterior teeth. If the injuries are minor and result in small fractures of enamel, these can be restored with light-cured composite or porcelain veneers. However, in some situations, the fracture may extend beneath the level of the gingival margin and terminate at the level of the alveolar ridge (Fig. 53-10). In these situations, restoration of the fractured crown is impossible because the tooth preparation would extend to the level of the bone. This overextension of the crown margin could result in an invasion of the biologic width of the tooth and cause persistent inflammation of the marginal gingiva. It may be beneficial in such cases to erupt the fractured root out of the bone and move the fracture margin coronally so that it can be properly restored.[7] However, if the fracture extends too far apically, it may be better to extract the tooth and replace it with an implant or bridge. Six criteria determine whether the tooth should be forcibly erupted or extracted.

1. *Root length:* Is the root long enough so that a one-to-one crown-root ratio will be preserved after the root has been erupted? To determine the answer to this question, the clinician must know how far to erupt the root. If a tooth fracture extends to the level of the bone, it must be erupted 4 mm. The first 2.5 mm moves the fracture margin far enough away from the bone to prevent a biologic width problem. The other 1.5 mm provides the proper amount of ferrule for

adequate resistance form of the crown preparation. Therefore if the root is fractured to the bone level and must be erupted 4 mm, the periapical radiograph must be evaluated (see Fig. 53-10) and 4 mm subtracted from the end of the fractured tooth root. The length of the residual root should be compared with the length of the eventual crown on this tooth. The root-to-crown ratio should be about 1:1. If the root-to-crown ratio is less than this amount, there may be too little root remaining in the bone for stability. In the latter situation, it may be prudent to extract the root and place a bridge or implant.

2. *Root form:* The shape of the root should be broad and nontapering, rather than thin and tapered. A thin, tapered root provides a narrower cervical region after the tooth has been erupted 4 mm. This could compromise the esthetic appearance of the final restoration. The internal root form is also important. If the root canal is wide, the distance between the external root surface and root canal filling will be narrow. In these situations, the walls of the crown preparation are thin, which could result in early fracture of the restored root. The root canal should not be more than one third of the overall width of the root. In this way, the root could still provide adequate strength for the final restoration.
3. *Level of the fracture:* If the entire crown is fractured 2 to 3 mm apical to the level of the alveolar bone, it is difficult, if not impossible, to attach to the root to erupt it.
4. *Relative importance of the tooth:* If the patient were 70 years of age and both adjacent teeth had prosthetic crowns, then it could be more prudent to construct a fixed bridge. However, if the patient is 15 years of age and the adjacent teeth were unrestored, then forced eruption would be much more conservative and appropriate.
5. *Esthetics:* If the patient has a high lip line and displays 2 to 3 mm of gingiva when smiling, then any type of restoration in this area will be more obvious. In this situation, keeping the patient's own tooth would be much more esthetic than any type of implant or prosthetic replacement.
6. *Endo/perio prognosis:* If the tooth has a significant periodontal defect, it may not be possible to retain the root. In addition, if the tooth root has a vertical fracture, the prognosis would be poor and extraction of the tooth would be the proper course of therapy.

If all these factors are favorable, then forced eruption of the fractured root is indicated. The orthodontic mechanics necessary to erupt the tooth can vary from elastic traction to orthodontic banding and bracketing. If a large portion of the tooth is still present, then orthodontic bracketing is necessary. If the entire crown has fractured, leaving only the root, then elastic traction from a bonded bar may be possible. The root may be erupted rapidly or slowly. If the movement is performed rapidly, the alveolar bone will be left behind temporarily and a circumferential fiberotomy may be performed to prevent bone from following the erupted root. However, if the root is erupted slowly, the bone follows the tooth. In this situation, the erupted root requires crown lengthening to expose the correct amount of tooth to create the proper ferrule, resistance form, and retention for the final restoration.

After the tooth root has been erupted, it must be stabilized to prevent it from intruding back into the alveolus. The reason for reintrusion is the orientation of the principal fibers of the periodontium. During forced eruption, the periodontal fibers become oriented obliquely and stretched as the root moves coronally. These fibers eventually reorient themselves after about 6 months. Before this occurs, the root can reintrude significantly. Therefore if this type of treatment is performed, an adequate period of stabilization is necessary to avoid significant relapse and reintrusion of the root.

As the root erupts, the gingiva move coronally with the tooth. As a result, the clinical crown length becomes shorter after extrusion (see Fig. 53-10). In addition, the gingival margin may be positioned more incisally than the adjacent teeth. In these situations, gingival surgery is necessary to create ideal gingival margin heights. The type of surgery varies depending on whether bone removal is necessary. If bone has followed the root during eruption, a flap is elevated and the appropriate amount of bone is removed to match the bone height of the adjacent teeth. If the bone level is flat between adjacent teeth, a simple excisional gingivectomy corrects the gingival margin discrepancy.

After gingival surgery, an open gingival embrasure may exist between the erupted root and adjacent teeth (see Fig. 53-10). The space occurs because the narrower root portion of the erupted tooth has been moved into the oral cavity. This space may be closed in two different ways. One method involves overcontouring of the replacement restoration. The other method involves reshaping of the crown of the tooth and movement of the root to close the space. This latter method often helps improve the overall shape of the final crown on the restored tooth.

Hopeless Teeth Maintained for Orthodontic Anchorage

Patients with advanced periodontal disease may have specific teeth diagnosed as hopeless, which would be extracted before orthodontics (Fig. 53-11). However, these teeth can be useful for orthodontic anchorage if the periodontal inflammation can be controlled. In moderate to advanced cases, some periodontal surgery may be indicated around a hopeless tooth. Flaps are reflected for debridement of the roots to control inflammation around the hopeless tooth during the orthodontic process. The important factor is to maintain the health of the bone around the adjacent teeth. Periodontal recall is imperative during the process.

After orthodontic treatment, there is a six-month period of stabilization before reevaluating the periodontal status. Occasionally, the hopeless tooth may be so improved after orthodontic treatment that it is retained. However, in most cases, the hopeless tooth requires extraction, especially if other restorations are planned in the segment. Again, these decisions require reevaluation by the clinician.

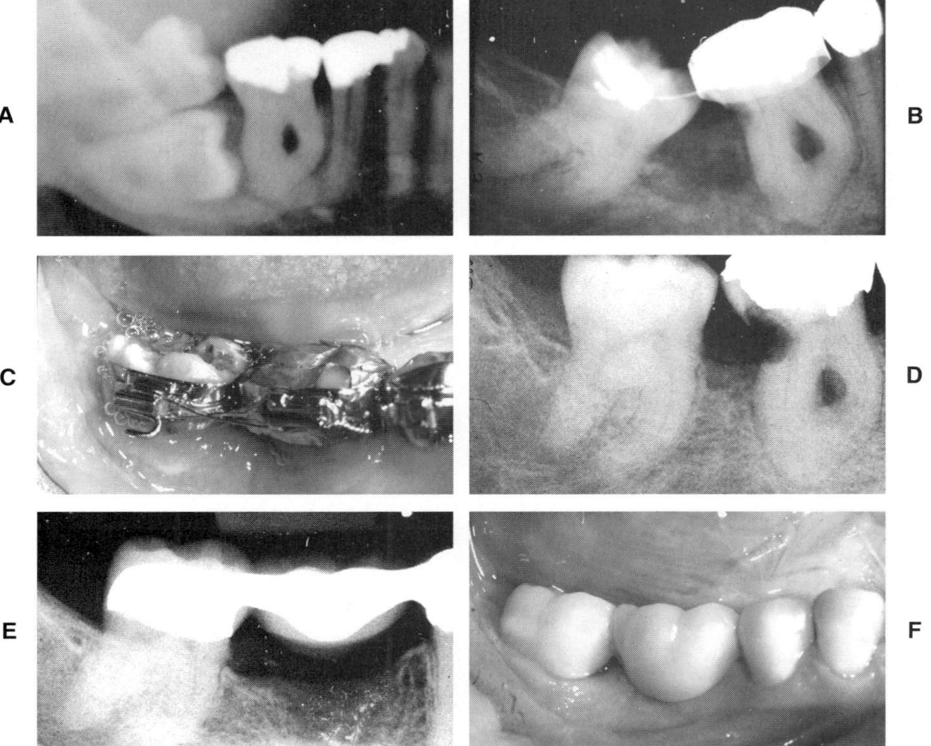

Fig. 53-11 This patient had an impacted mandibular right second molar **(A)**. The mandibular right first molar was periodontally hopeless because of an advanced Class III furcation defect. The impacted second molar was extracted, but the first molar was maintained as an anchor to help upright the third molar orthodontically **(B, C, and D)**. After orthodontic uprighting of the third molar, the first molar was extracted and a bridge was placed to restore the edentulous space **(E and F)**.

ORTHODONTIC TREATMENT OF GINGIVAL DISCREPANCIES

Uneven Gingival Margins

The relationship of the gingival margins of the six maxillary anterior teeth plays an important role in the esthetic appearance of the crowns. Four factors contribute to ideal gingival form.

1. The gingival margins of the two central incisors should be at the same level.
2. The gingival margins of the central incisors should be positioned more apically than the lateral incisors and at the same level as the canines.[13]
3. The contour of the labial gingival margins should mimic the CEJs of the teeth.
4. A papilla should exist between each tooth, and the height of the tip of the papilla is usually halfway between the incisal edge and the labial gingival height of contour over the center of each anterior tooth. Therefore the gingival papilla occupies half of the interproximal contact, and the adjacent teeth form the other half of the contact.

However, some patients may have gingival margin discrepancies between adjacent teeth (Fig. 53-12). These discrepancies could be caused by abrasion of the incisal edges or delayed migration of the gingival margins. When gingival margin discrepancies are present, the proper solution for the problem must be determined: orthodontic movement to reposition the gingival margins or surgical correction of gingival margin discrepancies.

To make the correct decision, it is necessary to evaluate four criteria. First, the relationship between the gingival margin of the maxillary central incisors and the patient's lip line should be assessed when the patient smiles. If a gingival margin discrepancy is present but the discrepancy is not exposed, it does not require correction.

If a gingival margin discrepancy is apparent, the second step is to evaluate the labial sulcular depth over the two central incisors. If the shorter tooth has a deeper sulcus, excisional gingivectomy may be appropriate to move the gingival margin of the shorter tooth apically. However, if the sulcular depths of the short and long incisors are equivalent, gingival surgery does not correct the problem.

The third step is to evaluate the relationship between the shortest central incisor and the adjacent lateral incisors. If the shortest central is still longer than the lateral incisors, the other possibility is to extrude the longer central incisor and equilibrate the incisal edge. This moves the gingival margin coronally and eliminates the gingival margin discrepancy. However, if the shortest central is shorter than the laterals, this technique would

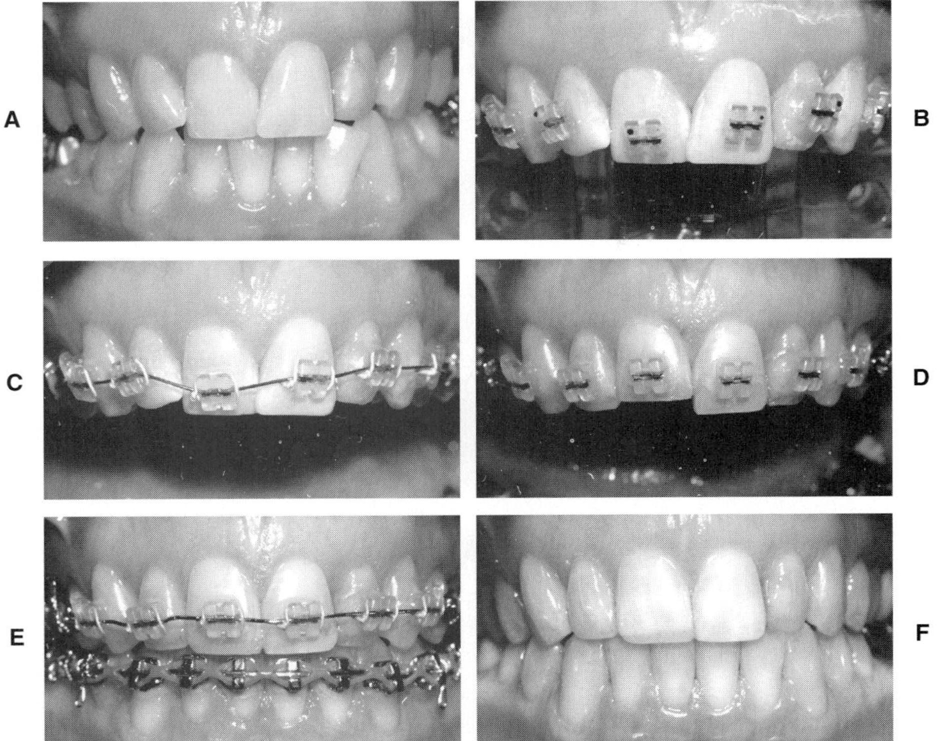

Fig. 53-12 This patient had a protrusive bruxing habit that had resulted in abrasion and overeruption of the maxillary right central incisor **(A)**. The objective was to level the gingival margins during orthodontic therapy. Although gingival surgery was a possibility, the labial sulcular depth of the maxillary right central incisor was only 1 mm, and the CEJ was located at the bottom of the sulcus. Therefore the best solution involved positioning the orthodontic brackets to facilitate intrusion of the right central incisor **(B, C, and D)**. This permitted the restorative dentist to restore the portion of the tooth that the patient had abraded **(E)**, resulting in the correct gingival margin levels and crown lengths at the end of treatment **(F)**.

produce an unaesthetic relationship between the gingival margins of the central and lateral incisors.

The fourth step is to determine whether the incisal edges have been abraded. This is best accomplished by evaluating the teeth from an incisal perspective. If one incisal edge is thicker labiolingually than the adjacent tooth, this may indicate that it has been abraded and the tooth has overerupted. In such cases, the best method of correcting the gingival margin discrepancy is to intrude the short central incisor (see Fig. 53-12). This method moves the gingival margin apically and permits restoration of the incisal edges.[3,6,8–10] The intrusion should be accomplished at least 6 months before appliance removal. This allows reorientation of the principal fibers of the periodontium and avoids reextrusion of the central incisor(s) after appliance removal.

Significant Abrasion and Overeruption

Occasionally, patients have destructive dental habits such as a protrusive bruxing habit that could result in significant wear of the maxillary and mandibular incisors and compensatory overeruption of these teeth (Fig. 53-13). The restoration of these abraded teeth is often impossible because of the lack of crown length to achieve adequate retention and resistance form for the crown preparations. Two options are available. One option is extensive crown lengthening by elevating a flap, removing sufficient bone, and apically positioning the flap to expose adequate tooth length for crown preparation. However, this type of procedure is contraindicated in the patient with short tapered roots because it could adversely affect the final root to crown ratio and potentially open gingival embrasures between the anterior teeth.

The other option for improving the restorability of these short abraded teeth is to orthodontically intrude the teeth and move the gingival margins apically (see Fig. 53-13). It is possible to intrude up to four maxillary incisors by using the posterior teeth as anchorage during the intrusion process. This process is accomplished by placing the orthodontic brackets as close to the incisal edges of the maxillary incisors as possible. The brackets are placed in their normal position on the canines and remaining posterior teeth. The patient's posterior occlusion resists the eruption of the posterior teeth, and the incisors gradually intrude and move the gingival margins and the crowns apically. This creates the restorative space necessary to temporarily restore the incisal edges of these teeth and then eventually place the final crowns.

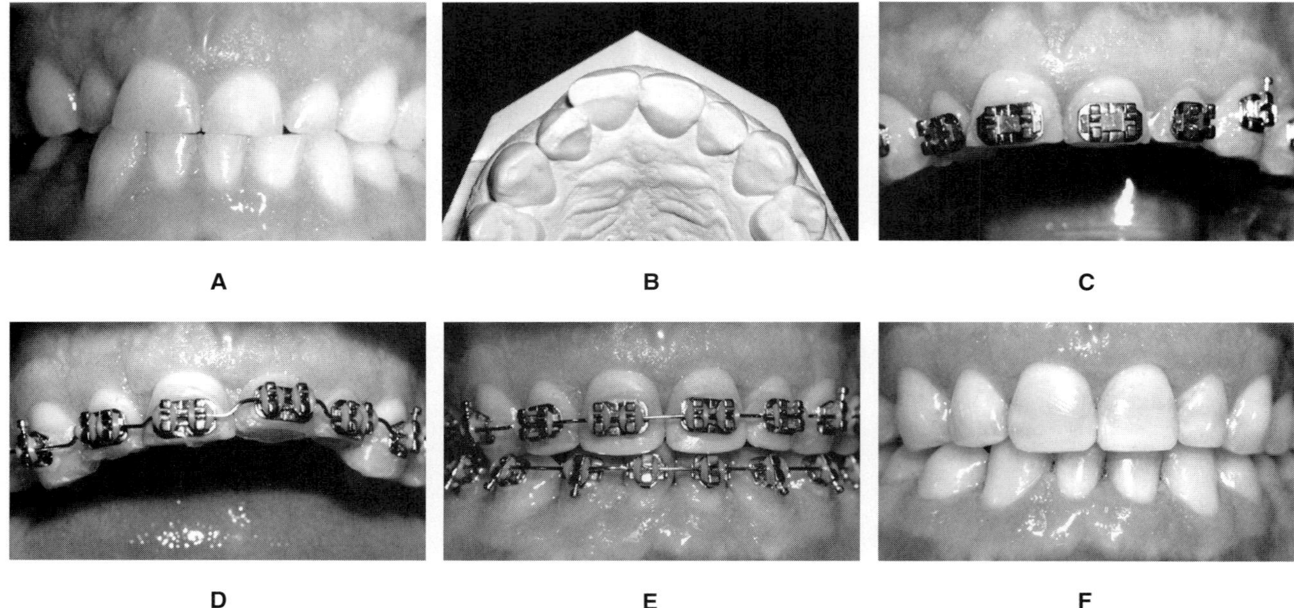

Fig. 53-13 This patient had a protrusive bruxing habit that had caused severe abrasion of the maxillary anterior teeth, resulting in the loss of over half of the crown length of the incisors **(A and B)**. Two possible options existed for gaining crown length to restore the incisors. One possibility was an apically positioned flap with osseous recontouring, which would expose the roots of the teeth. The less destructive option was to intrude the four incisors orthodontically, level the gingival margins **(C and D)**, and allow the dentist to restore the abraded incisal edges **(E and F)**. The orthodontic option was clearly successful and desirable in this patient.

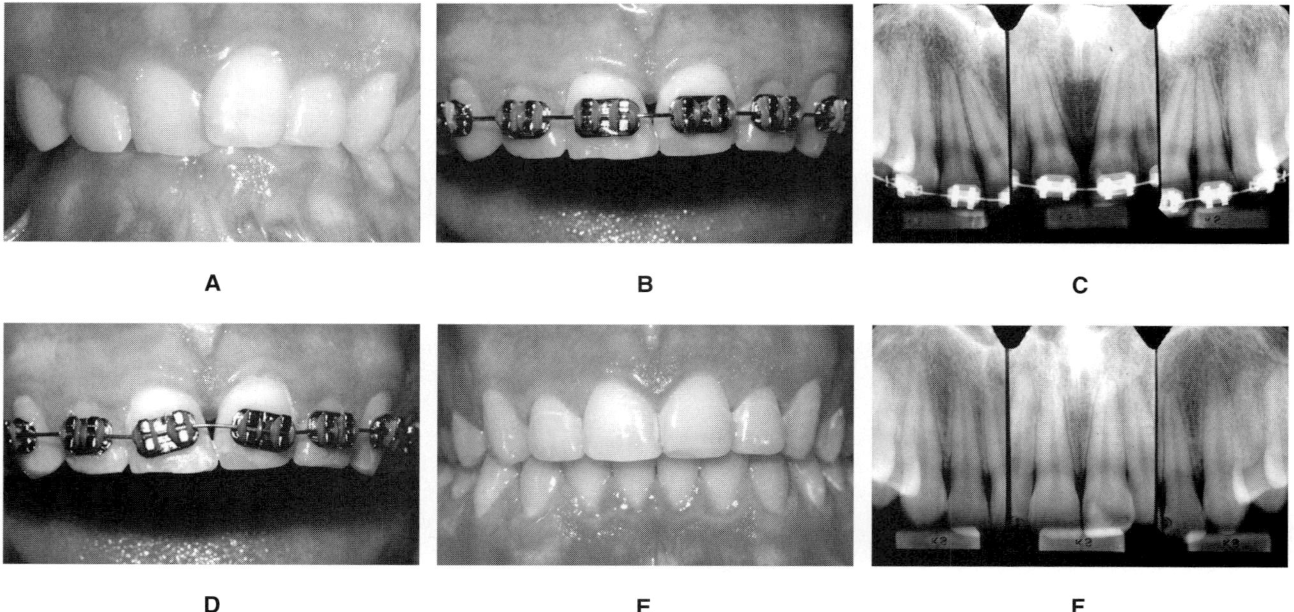

Fig. 53-14 This patient initially had overlapped maxillary central incisors **(A)**, and after initial orthodontic alignment of the teeth, an open gingival embrasure appeared between the centrals **(B)**. A radiograph showed that the open embrasure was caused by divergence of the central incisor roots **(C)**. To correct the problem, the central incisor brackets were repositioned **(D)**, and the roots were moved together. This required restoration of the incisal edges after orthodontics **(E)** because these teeth had worn unevenly before orthodontic therapy. As the roots were paralleled **(F)**, the tooth contact moved gingivally and the papilla moved incisally, resulting in the elimination of the open gingival embrasure.

When abraded teeth are significantly intruded, it is necessary to hold these teeth for at least 6 months in the intruded position with either the orthodontic brackets, archwires, or both, or some type of bonded retainer. The principal fibers of the periodontium must accommodate to the new intruded position, a process that could take a minimum of 6 months in most adult patients. Orthodontic intrusion of severely abraded and overerupted teeth is usually a distinct advantage over periodontal crown lengthening unless the patient has extremely long and broad roots or has had extensive horizontal periodontal bone loss.

Open Gingival Embrasures

The presence of a papilla between the maxillary central incisors is a key esthetic factor in any individual. Occasionally, adults have open gingival embrasures or lack gingival papillae between their central incisors. These unaesthetic areas are often difficult to resolve with periodontal therapy. However, orthodontic treatment can correct many of these open gingival embrasures. This open space is usually due to one of three causes: tooth shape, root angulation, or periodontal bone loss.[9]

The interproximal contact between the maxillary central incisors consists of two parts. One portion is the tooth contact, and the other is the papilla. The ratio of papilla to contact is 1:1. Half of the space is occupied by papilla, and half is formed by the tooth contact. If the patient has an open embrasure, the first aspect that must be evaluated is whether the problem is due to the papilla or the tooth contact. If the papilla is the problem, then the cause is usually a lack of bone support due to an underlying periodontal problem.

In some situations, a deficient papilla can be improved with orthodontic treatment. By closing open contacts, the interproximal gingiva can be squeezed and moved incisally. This type of movement may help create a more esthetic papilla between two teeth despite alveolar bone loss. Another possibility is to erupt adjacent teeth when the interproximal bone level is positioned apically.

Most open embrasures between the central incisors are due to problems with tooth contact. The first step in the diagnosis of this problem is to evaluate a periapical radiograph of the central incisors. If the root angulation is divergent, then the brackets should be repositioned so the root position can be corrected (Fig. 53-14). In these situations, the incisal edges may be uneven and require restoration with either composite or porcelain restorations. If the periapical radiograph shows that the roots are in their correct relationship, then the open gingival embrasure is due to a triangular tooth shape (Fig. 53-15).

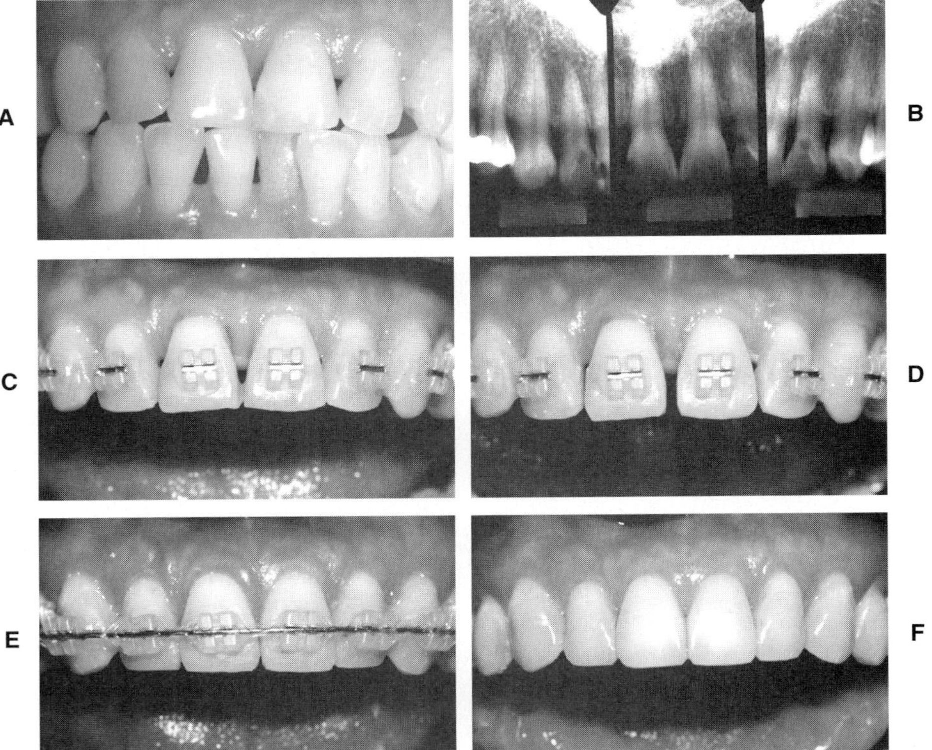

Fig. 53-15 This patient initially had triangular-shaped central incisors **(A and B)**, which produced an open gingival embrasure after orthodontic alignment **(C)**. Because the roots of the central incisors were parallel with one another, the appropriate solution for the open gingival embrasure was to recontour the mesial surfaces of the central incisors **(D)**. As the diastema was closed **(E)**, the tooth contact moved gingivally and the papilla moved incisally, resulting in the elimination of the open gingival embrasure **(F)**.

If the shape of the tooth is the problem, two solutions are possible. One possibility is to restore the open gingival embrasure. The other option is to reshape the tooth by flattening the incisal contact and closing the space (see Fig. 53-15). This results in lengthening of the contact until it meets the papilla. In addition, if the embrasure space is large, closing the space squeezes the papilla between the central incisors. This helps create a 1:1 ratio between the contact and papilla and restores uniformity to the heights between the midline and adjacent papillae.

SUMMARY

This chapter has discussed and illustrated the benefits of integrating orthodontics and periodontics in the management of adult patients with underlying periodontal defects. The key to treating these types of patients is communication and proper diagnosis before orthodontic therapy as well as continued dialogue during orthodontic treatment. Not all periodontal problems are treated in the same way. This chapter has provided a framework for the integration of orthodontics to solve periodontal problems.

REFERENCES

1. Becker W, Becker BE: Treatment of mandibular 3-wall intrabony defects by flap debridement and expanded polytetrafluoroethylene barrier membranes. Long-term evaluation of 32 treated patients. J Periodontol 1993; 64:1138.
2. Brown IA: The effect of orthodontic therapy on certain types of periodontal defects. I. Clinical findings. J Periodontol 1973; 44:742.
3. Chiche G, Kokich V, Caudill R: Diagnosis and treatment planning of esthetic problems. In: Pinault A, Chiche G (eds): Esthetics in Fixed Prosthodontics. Chicago, Quintessence, 1994.
4. Gould MSE, Picton DCA: The relation between irregularities of the teeth and periodontal disease. Br Dent J 1966; 121:21.
5. Ingber J: Forced eruption: Part I. A method of treating isolated one and two wall infrabony osseous defects; rationale and case report. J Periodontal 1974; 45:199.
6. Kokich V: Enhancing restorative, esthetic and periodontal results with orthodontic therapy, In: Schluger S, Youdelis R, Page R, et al (eds): Periodontal Therapy. Philadelphia, Lea & Febiger, 1990.
7. Kokich V, Nappen D, Shapiro P: Gingival contour and clinical crown length: Their effects on the esthetic appearance of maxillary anterior teeth. Am J Orthod 1984; 86:89.
8. Kokich V: Anterior dental esthetics: An orthodontic perspective. I. Crown length. J Esthet Dent 1993; 5:19.
9. Kokich V: Esthetics and vertical tooth position: The orthodontic possibilities. Compendium Cont Ed Dent 1997; 18:1225.
10. Kokich V: Esthetics: The orthodontic-periodontic-restorative connection. Semin Orthod 1996; 2:21.
11. Kramer GM: Surgical alternatives in regenerative therapy of the periodontium. Int J Periodont Rest Dent 1992; 12:11.
12. Ochsenbein C, Ross S: A re-evaluation of osseous surgery. Dent Clin North Am 1969; 13:87.
13. Rufenacht C: Structural esthetic rules. In: Rufenacht C (ed): Fundamental of Esthetics. Chicago, Quintessence, 1990.
14. Schallhorn R, McClain P: Combined osseous composite grafting, root conditioning and guided tissue regeneration. Int J Periodont Rest Dent 1988; 8:9.
15. Schluger S: Osseous resection: A basic principle in periodontal surgery. Oral Surg 1949; 2:316.

SECTION V

Periodontal Surgical Phase

Henry H. Takei

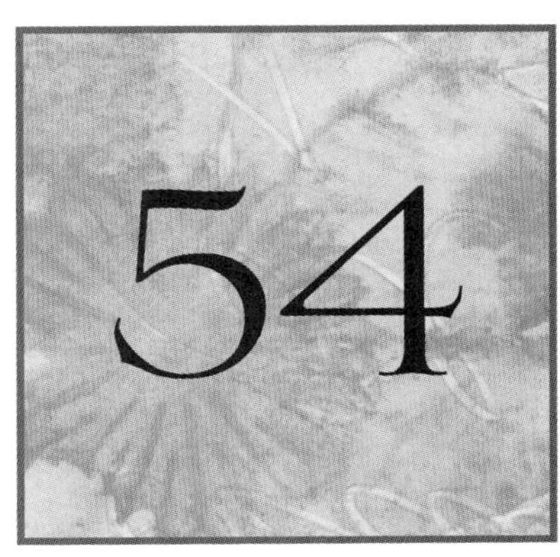

CHAPTER

The Surgical Phase of Therapy

Henry H. Takei and Fermin A. Carranza

CHAPTER OUTLINE

Although in a strict sense, all instrumental therapy can be considered surgical, this chapter refers only to those techniques that include the intentional severing or incising of gingival tissue* with the following purposes:

- Controlling or eliminating periodontal disease.
- Correcting anatomic conditions that may favor periodontal disease, impair esthetics, or impede the placement of correct prosthetics.
- Placing implants to replace lost teeth and improving the environment for their placement and function.

* Scaling and root planing are not included because these procedures do not *intentionally* act on the gingival tissue.

OBJECTIVES OF THE SURGICAL PHASE

The surgical phase of periodontal therapy seeks the following:

1. Improvement of the prognosis of teeth and their replacements.
2. Improvement of esthetics.

The surgical phase consists of techniques performed for pocket therapy and for the correction of related morphologic problems, namely mucogingival defects. In many cases, procedures are combined so that one surgical intervention fulfills both objectives.

The purpose of surgical pocket therapy is to eliminate the pathologic changes in the pocket walls; to create a stable, easily maintainable state; and, if possible, to promote periodontal regeneration. To fulfill these objectives, surgical techniques 1) increase accessibility to the

BOX 54-1

Periodontal Surgery

Pocket Reduction Surgery

Resective (gingivectomy, apically displaced flap and undisplaced flap with or without osseous resection)

Regenerative (flaps with grafts, membranes, etc.)

Correction of Anatomic/Morphologic Defects

Plastic surgery techniques to widen attached gingiva (free gingival grafts, and other techniques, etc.)

Esthetic surgery (root coverage, re-creation of gingival papillae)

Preprosthetic techniques (crown lengthening, ridge augmentation, vestibular deepening)

Placement of dental implants, including techniques for site development for implants (guided bone regeneration, sinus grafts)

root surface, making it possible to remove all irritants; 2) reduce or eliminate pocket depth, making it possible for the patient to maintain the root surfaces free of plaque; and 3) reshape soft and hard tissues to attain a harmonious topography. Pocket reduction surgery seeks to reduce pocket depth by either resective or regenerative means or often by a combination of both methods. Chapters 60 to 64 describe the different techniques used for these purposes.

The second objective of the surgical phase of periodontal therapy is the correction of anatomic morphologic defects that may favor plaque accumulation and pocket recurrence or impair esthetics. It is important to understand that these procedures are not directed to treat disease but aim to alter the gingival and mucosal tissues to correct defects that may predispose to disease. They are performed on noninflamed tissues and in the absence of periodontal pockets.

Three types of techniques fall into this category: the *plastic surgery techniques* used to create or widen the attached gingiva by placing grafts of various types, the *esthetic surgery techniques* used to cover denuded roots and to recreate lost papillae, and the *preprosthetic techniques,* the purpose of which is the adaptation of the periodontal and neighboring tissues to receive prosthetic replacements and which include crown lengthening, ridge augmentation, and vestibular deepening. The plastic and esthetic surgery techniques are presented in Chapter 66 and the preprosthetic techniques in Chapter 74.

In addition, periodontal surgical techniques for the placement of dental implants are available. These involve not only the implant placement techniques but also a variety of surgical procedures to adapt the neighboring tissues, such as the sinus floor or the mandibular nerve canal, for subsequent placement of the implant (Box 54-1). These methods are discusssed in Chapters 70 and 71.

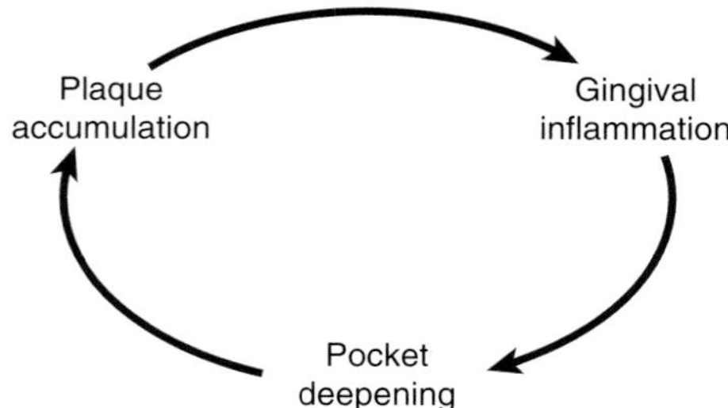

Fig. 54-1 Accumulation of plaque leads to gingival inflammation and pocket deepening, which in turn increases the area of plaque accumulation.

Surgical Pocket Therapy

Surgical pocket therapy can be directed toward 1) access surgery to ensure the removal of irritants from the tooth surface or 2) elimination, or reduction of the depth of, the periodontal pocket.

The effectiveness of periodontal therapy is predicated on success in completely eliminating calculus, plaque, and diseased cementum from the tooth surface. Numerous investigations have shown that the difficulty of this task increases as the pocket becomes deeper.[2,5] The presence of irregularities on the root surface also increase the difficulty of the procedure. As the pocket gets deeper, the surface to be scaled increases, more irregularities appear on the root surface, and accessibility is impaired[11,15]; the presence of furcation involvements sometimes creates insurmountable problems (see Chapter 64).

All these problems can be reduced by resecting or displacing the soft tissue wall of the pocket, thereby increasing the visibility and accessibility of the root surface.[3] The flap approach and the gingivectomy technique attain this result.

The need to eliminate or reduce the depth of the pocket is another important consideration. Pocket elimination consists of reducing the depth of periodontal pockets to that of a physiologic sulcus to enable cleansing by the patient. By proper case selection, both resective techniques and regenerative techniques can be used to accomplish this goal. The presence of a pocket produces areas that are impossible for the patient to keep clean, and therefore the vicious circle depicted in Fig. 54-1 is established.

Results of Pocket Therapy

A periodontal pocket can be in an active state or a period of inactivity or quiescence. An active pocket is one under which bone is being lost (Fig. 54-2, *top left*). It often can be diagnosed clinically by bleeding, either spontaneously or on probing. After Phase I therapy, the inflammatory changes in the pocket wall subside, rendering the pocket inactive and reducing its depth (see Fig. 54-2, *top center*). The extent of this reduction depends on the depth before treatment and the degree to which the depth is the result of the edematous and inflammatory component of the pocket wall.

Whether the pocket remains inactive depends on its depth and the individual characteristics of the plaque components and the host response. Recurrence of the initial activity is likely.

Inactive pockets can sometimes heal with a long junctional epithelium (see Fig. 54-2, *top right*). However, this condition also may be unstable, and the chance of recurrence and reformation of the original pocket is always present because the epithelial union to the tooth is weak. However, one study in monkeys has shown that the long junctional epithelial union may be as resistant to plaque infection as a normal connective tissue attachment.[9]

Studies have shown that inactive pockets can be maintained for long periods with little loss of attachment by means of frequent scaling and root planing procedures.[6,10,12] A more reliable and stable result is obtained, however, by transforming the pocket into a healthy sulcus. The bottom of the healthy sulcus can be located either where the bottom of the pocket was localized or coronal to it. In the first case, there is no gain of attachment (see Fig. 54-2, *bottom left*) and the area of the root that was previously the tooth wall of the pocket becomes exposed. This does not mean that the periodontal treatment has caused recession, but rather that it has uncovered the recession previously induced by the disease.

The healthy sulcus can also be located coronal to the bottom of the preexistent pocket (Fig. 54-2, *bottom center* and *right*). This is conducive to a restored marginal periodontium; the result is a sulcus of normal depth with gain of attachment. The creation of a healthy sulcus and a restored periodontium is termed *regeneration* and entails a total restoration of the status that existed before periodontal disease began. This is, of course, the ideal result of treatment.

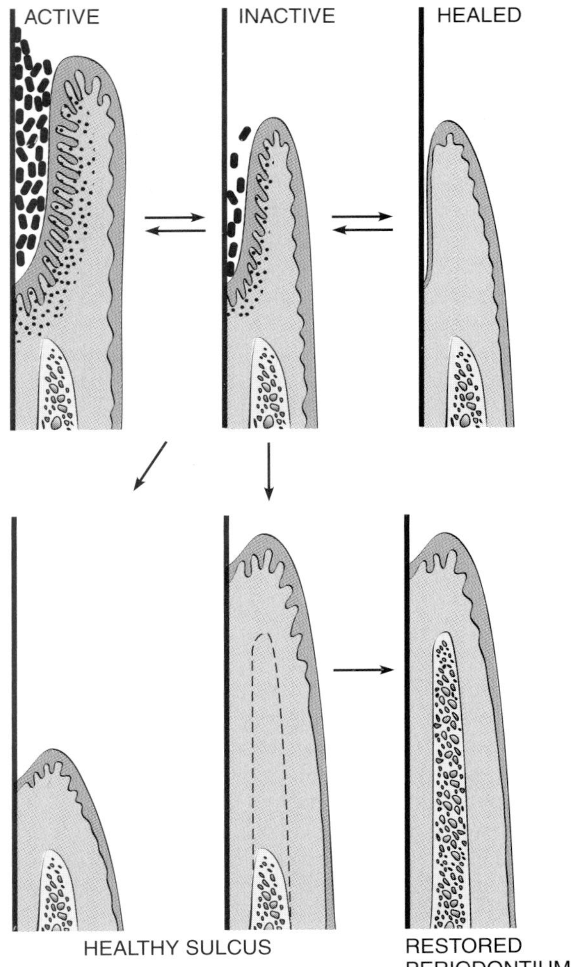

Fig. 54-2 Possible results of pocket therapy. An active pocket can become inactive and heal by means of a long junctional epithelium. Surgical pocket therapy can result in a healthy sulcus, with or without gain of attachment. Improved gingival attachment promotes restoration of bone height, with reformation of periodontal ligament fibers and layers of cementum.

POCKET ELIMINATION VERSUS POCKET MAINTENANCE

Pocket elimination (depth reduction to gingival sulcus levels) has traditionally been considered one of the main goals of periodontal therapy. It was considered vital because of the need to improve accessibility to root surfaces for the therapist during treatment and for the patient after healing. It is now the prevalent opinion that while in general the presence of deep pockets after therapy represents a greater risk of disease progression than shallow sites, individual probing depths per se are not good predictors of future clinical attachment loss.[5] The absence of deep pockets in treated patients is, on the other hand, an excellent predictor of a stable periodontium.[5]

Longitudinal studies of different therapeutic modalities, carried out in the last quarter century, have given somewhat conflicting results,[7,16] probably because of inherent problems created by the "split-mouth" design. In general, however, after surgical therapy, pockets that rebound to a shallow or moderate depth can be maintained in a healthy state and without radiographic evidence of advancing bone loss by maintenance visits consisting of scaling and root planing, with oral hygiene reinforcement performed at regular intervals of not more than 3 months. In these cases the residual pocket can be examined with a thin periodontal probe, but no pain, exudate, or bleeding results; this appears to indicate that no plaque has formed on the subgingival root surfaces.

These findings do not alter the indications for periodontal surgery because the results obtained are based on surgical exposure of the root surfaces for a thorough and complete elimination of irritants. They do, however, emphasize the importance of the maintenance phase and the close monitoring of both level of attachment and pocket depth, together with the other clinical variables (bleeding, exudation, and tooth mobility). *The transformation of the initial deep, active pocket into a shallower, inactive, maintainable one requires some form of definitive pocket therapy and constant supervision thereafter.*

Pocket depth is an extremely useful and widely employed clinical determination, but it must be evaluated together with level of attachment and the presence of bleeding, exudation, and pain. The most important variable for evaluating whether a pocket (or deep sulcus) is progressive is the level of attachment, which is measured in millimeters from the cementoenamel junction; it is the apical displacement of the level of attachment that places the tooth in jeopardy, not the increase in pocket depth, which may be due to coronal displacement of the gingival margin.

Pocket depth remains an important clinical variable on which decisions about treatment selection can be based in part. Lindhe and colleagues compared the effect of root planing alone and in conjunction with a modified Widman flap on the resultant level of attachment and in relation to initial pocket depth.[8] They reported that scaling and root planing procedures induce loss of attachment if performed in pockets shallower than 2.9 mm, whereas gain of attachment occurs in deeper pockets. The modified Widman flap induces loss of attachment if done in pockets shallower than 4.2 mm but results in a greater gain of attachment than root planing in pockets deeper than 4.2 mm. The loss is a true loss of connective tissue attachment, whereas the gain can be considered a false gain owing to reduced penetrability of connective tissues apical to the bottom of the pocket after treatment.[9,17]

Furthermore, probing depths established following active therapy and healing (approximately 6 months after treatment) can be maintained unchanged or reduced even further during a maintenance care period involving careful prophylaxis once every 3 months.[8]

Ramfjord and associates[12] and Rosling and colleagues[13] showed that, regardless of the surgical technique used for pocket therapy, a certain pocket depth recurs. *Therefore maintenance of this depth without any further loss of attachment becomes the goal.*

REEVALUATION AFTER PHASE I THERAPY

The longitudinal studies mentioned previously[5] have noted that all patients should be treated initially with scaling and root planing and that a final decision on the need for periodontal surgery should be made only after a thorough evaluation of the effects of Phase I therapy. The assessment is generally made no less than 1 to 3 months and sometimes as much as 9 months after the completion of Phase I therapy.[1] This reevaluation of the periodontal condition should include reprobing the entire mouth, with rechecking for the presence of calculus, root caries, defective restorations, and all signs of persistent inflammation.

CRITICAL ZONES IN POCKET SURGERY

Criteria for the selection of one of the different surgical techniques for pocket therapy are based on clinical findings in the soft tissue pocket wall, tooth surface, underlying bone, and attached gingiva.

Zone 1: The Soft Tissue Wall

The morphologic features, thickness, and topography of the soft tissue pocket wall and persistence of inflammatory changes in it should be determined.

Zone 2: The Tooth Surface

The presence of deposits and alterations on the cementum surface and the accessibility of the root surface to instrumentation should be identified. Phase I therapy should have solved many, if not all, of the problems on the tooth surface. Evaluation of the results of Phase I therapy should determine the need for further therapy and the method to be used.

Zone 3: The Bone

The shape and height of the alveolar bone next to the pocket wall should be established by careful probing and clinicoradiographic examination. Bony craters, horizontal or angular bone losses, and other bone deformities are important criteria for the selection of the treatment technique.

Zone 4: The Attached Gingiva

The presence or absence of an adequate band of attached gingiva is a factor to be considered when selecting the pocket treatment method. Diagnostic techniques for mucogingival problems are described in Chapter 66. An inadequate attached gingiva may be due to a high frenum attachment, marked gingival recession, or a deep pocket that reaches the level of the mucogingival junction. All of these possible conditions should be explored and their influence on pocket therapy determined.

INDICATIONS FOR PERIODONTAL SURGERY

The following findings may indicate the need for a surgical phase of therapy:

1. Areas with irregular bony contours, deep craters, and other defects usually require a surgical approach.
2. Pockets on teeth in which a complete removal of root irritants is not considered clinically possible may call for surgery. This occurs frequently in molar and premolar areas.
3. In cases of furcation involvement of Grade II or III, a surgical approach ensures the removal of irritants; any necessary root resection or hemisection also requires surgical intervention.
4. Intrabony pockets on distal areas of last molars, frequently complicated by mucogingival problems, are usually unresponsive to nonsurgical methods.
5. Persistent inflammation in areas with moderate to deep pockets may require a surgical approach. In areas with shallow pockets or normal sulci, persistent inflammation may point to the presence of a mucogingival problem that needs a surgical solution.

METHODS OF POCKET THERAPY

The methods for pocket therapy can be classified under three main headings:

1. **New attachment techniques** offer the ideal result because they eliminate pocket depth by reuniting the gingiva to the tooth at a position coronal to the bottom of the preexisting pocket. New attachment is

usually associated with filling in of bone and regeneration of periodontal ligament and cementum.
2. **Removal of the pocket wall** is the most common method. The wall of the pocket consists of soft tissue and may also include bone in the case of intrabony pockets. It can be removed by the following:
   - **Retraction or shrinkage,** in which scaling and root planing procedures resolve the inflammatory process and the gingiva therefore shrinks, reducing the pocket depth.
   - **Surgical removal** performed by the gingivectomy technique or by means of an undisplaced flap.
   - **Apical displacement** with an apically displaced flap.
3. **Removal of the tooth side of the pocket,** which is accomplished by tooth extraction or by partial tooth extraction (hemisection or root resection).

The techniques, what they accomplish, and the factors governing their selection are presented in Chapters 58 to 64.

Criteria for Method Selection

Scientific criteria to establish the indications for each technique are difficult to determine. Longitudinal studies following a significant number of cases over a number of years, standardizing multiple factors and many variables, would be needed. Clinical experience, however, has suggested the criteria for selecting the method to be used to treat the pocket in individual cases. The selection of a technique for treatment of a particular periodontal lesion is based on a number of considerations.

1. Characteristics of the pocket: depth, relation to bone, and configuration.
2. Accessibility to instrumentation, including presence of furcation involvements.
3. Existence of mucogingival problems.
4. Response to Phase I therapy.
5. Patient cooperation, including ability to perform effective oral hygiene and, for smokers, willingness to stop their habit at least temporarily (i.e., a few weeks).
6. Age and general health of the patient.
7. Overall diagnosis of the case: various types of gingival enlargement and types of periodontitis (chronic marginal periodontitis, localized aggressive periodontitis, generalized aggressive periodontitis, and so forth).
8. Esthetic considerations.
9. Previous periodontal treatments.

Each of these variables is analyzed in relation to the pocket therapy techniques available, and a specific technique is selected. Of the many techniques, the one that would most successfully solve the problems with the fewest undesirable effects should be chosen. **Clinicians who adhere to one technique to solve all problems do not use to the advantage of the patient the wide repertoire of techniques at their disposal.**

Therapy for Gingival Pockets. Two factors are taken into consideration: 1) the character of the pocket wall and 2) the pocket accessibility. The pocket wall can be either edematous or fibrotic. Edematous tissue shrinks after the elimination of local factors, thereby reducing or totally eliminating pocket depth. Therefore scaling and root planing is the technique of choice in these cases.

Pockets with a fibrotic wall are not appreciably reduced in depth after scaling and root planing. They therefore are eliminated surgically. Until recently, gingivectomy was the only technique available; it solves the problem successfully, but in cases of marked gingival enlargement (e.g., severe phenytoin enlargement), it may leave a large wound that goes through a painful and prolonged healing process. In these cases, a modified flap technique can adequately solve the problem with fewer postoperative problems (see Chapter 59).

Therapy for Slight Periodontitis. In slight or incipient periodontitis, bone loss has occurred to a small degree and pockets are shallow to moderate. In these cases, a conservative approach and adequate oral hygiene generally suffice to control the disease. Incipient periodontitis occurring as recurrence in previously treated sites may require a thorough analysis of the causes for the recurrence and, on occasions, a surgical approach to correct them.

Therapy for Moderate to Severe Periodontitis in the Anterior Sector. The anterior teeth are important esthetically; therefore the techniques that induce the least amount of visual root exposure should be considered first. However, the importance of esthetics may be different for different patients, and nonelimination of the pocket may place the tooth in jeopardy. The final decision may have to be a compromise between health and esthetics, not attaining ideal results in either respect.

Anterior teeth offer some advantages to a conservative approach. First, they are all single rooted and easily accessible; second, patient's compliance and thoroughness in plaque control are easier to attain. **Therefore scaling and root planing is the technique of choice for the anterior teeth.**

Sometimes, however, a surgical technique may be necessary owing to the need for improved accessibility for root planing or regenerative surgery of osseous defects. The **papilla preservation flap** can be used for both purposes and also offers a better postoperative result with less recession and reduced soft tissue crater formation interproximally.[14] **It is the first choice when a surgical approach is needed.**

When the teeth are too close interproximally, the papilla preservation technique may not be feasible, and a technique that splits the papilla will have to be used. The **sulcular incision flap** offers good esthetic results and is the next choice.

When esthetics are not the primary consideration, the so-called **modified Widman flap** can be chosen. This technique uses an internal bevel incision about 1 to 2 mm from the gingival margin without thinning the flap and may result in some small recession.

In some infrequent cases, bone contouring may be needed despite the resultant root exposure. The technique of choice is the **apically displaced flap with bone contouring.**

Therapy for Moderate to Severe Periodontitis in the Posterior Area. Treatment for premolars and molars usually poses no esthetic problem but frequently involves difficult accessibility. Bone defects are more frequent than in the anterior sector, and root morphologic features, particularly in relation to furcations, may offer unsurmountable problems for instrumentation in a close field. Therefore surgery is frequently indicated in this region.

The purpose of surgery in the posterior area is either enhanced accessibility or the need for definitive pocket reduction requiring osseous surgery. Accessibility can be obtained by either the undisplaced or apically displaced flap.

Most cases of moderate to severe periodontitis have developed osseous defects that require some degree of osseous remodeling or regenerative procedures. When osseous defects amenable to regeneration are present, the **papilla preservation flap is the technique of choice** because it better protects the interproximal areas where defects are frequently present. **Second and third choices are the sulcular flap and the modified Widman flap, maintaining as much of the papilla as possible.**

When osseous defects with no possibility of reconstruction, such as interdental craters, are present, the technique of choice is the **flap with osseous contouring.**

Surgical Techniques for Correction of Morphologic Defects. The objectives and rationale for the techniques performed to correct morphologic defects (mucogingival, esthetic and preprosthetic) are given in Chapter 66.

Surgical Techniques for Implant Placement and Related Problems. The objectives and rationale for these techniques are described in Chapter 70.

REFERENCES

1. Badersten A, Nilveus R, Egelberg J: Effect of nonsurgical periodontal therapy. II. Severely advanced periodontitis. J Clin Periodontol 1984; 11:63.
2. Bower RC: Furcation morphology relative to periodontal treatment. Furcation root surface anatomy. J Periodontol 1979; 50:366.
3. Caffesse RG, Sweeney PL, Smith BA: Scaling and root planing with and without periodontal flap surgery. J Clin Periodontol 1986; 11:205.
4. Gher ME, Vernino AR: Root morphology—Clinical significance in pathogenesis and treatment of periodontal disease. J Am Dent Assoc 1980; l0l:627.
5. Greensteifl G: Contemporary interpretation of probing depth assessment: Diagnostic and therapeutic implications. A literature review. J Periodontol 1997; 68:1194.
6. Hill RW, Ramfjord SP, Morrison GC, et al: Four types of periodontal treatment compared over two years. J Periodontol 1981; 52:655.
7. Kaldahl WB, Kalkwarf KL, Patil KD: A review of longitudinal studies that compared periodontal therapies. J Periodontol 1993; 64:243.
8. Lindhe J, Socransky SS, Nyman S, et al: Critical probing depths in periodontal therapy. J Clin Periodontol 1982; 9:323.
9. Magnusson I, Runstad L, Nyman S, et al: A long junctional epithelium—A locus minoris resistentiae in plaque infection. J Clin Periodontol 1983; 10:333.
10. Pihlstrom BL, Ortiz Campos C, McHugh RB: A randomized four-year study of periodontal therapy. J Periodontol 1981; 52:227.
11. Rabbani GM, Ash MM, Caffesse RG: The effectiveness of subgingival scaling and root planing in calculus removal. J Periodontol 1981; 52:119.
12. Ramfjord SP, Knowles JW, Nissle RR, et al: Results following three modalities of periodontal therapy. J Periodontol 1975; 12:522.
13. Rosling B, Nyman S, Lindhe J, et al: The healing potential of the periodontal tissues following different techniques of periodontal surgery in plaque-free dentitions. A 2-year clinical study. J Clin Periodontol 1976; 3:233.
14. Takei HH, Han T J, Carranza FA Jr, et al: Flap technique for periodontal bone implants—The papilla preservation technique. J Periodontol 1985; 56:204.
15. Waerhaug J: Healing of the dentoepithelial junction following subgingival plaque control. II. As observed on extracted teeth. J Periodontol 1978; 40:119.
16. Weeks PR: Pros and cons of periodontal pocket elimination procedures. J Western Soc Periodontol 1980; 28:4.
17. Westfelt E, Bragd L, Socransky SS, et al: Improved periodontal conditions following therapy. J Clin Periodontol 1985; 12:283.

General Principles of Periodontal Surgery

Perry R. Klokkevold, Fermin A. Carranza, and Henry H. Takei

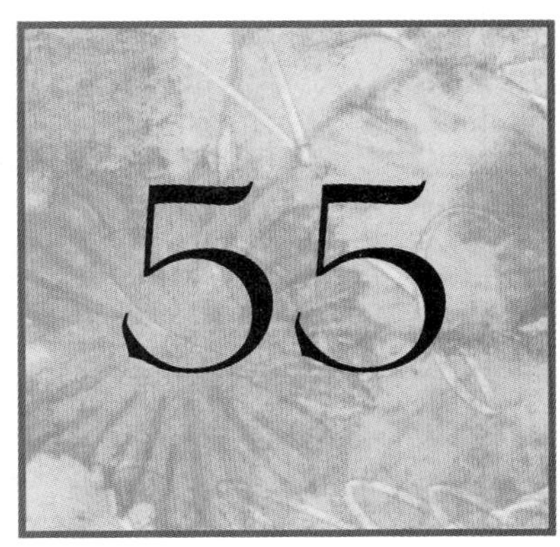

CHAPTER

CHAPTER OUTLINE

All surgical procedures should be very carefully planned. The patient should be adequately prepared medically, psychologically, and practically for all aspects of the intervention. This chapter covers the preparation of the patient and the general considerations common to all periodontal surgical techniques. Complications that may occur during or after surgery are also discussed.

Surgical periodontal procedures are usually performed in the dental office. Hospital periodontal surgery is discussed at the end of this chapter.

OUTPATIENT SURGERY

Preparation of the Patient

Reevaluation after Phase I Therapy. Almost every patient undergoes the so-called initial or preparatory phase of therapy, which basically consists of thorough scaling and root planing and removing all irritants responsible for the periodontal inflammation. These procedures 1) eliminate some lesions entirely; 2) render the tissues more firm and consistent, thus permitting a more accurate and delicate surgery; and 3) acquaint the patient with the office and the operator and assistants, thereby reducing the patient's apprehension and fear.

The reevaluation phase consists of reprobing and reexamining all the pertinent findings that previously indicated the need for the surgical procedure. Persistence of these findings confirms the indication for surgery. The number of surgical procedures, expected outcome, and postoperative care necessary are all decided beforehand. These are discussed with the patient and a final decision is made, incorporating any necessary adjustments to the original plan.

Premedication.* For patients who are not medically compromised, the value of administering antibiotics routinely for periodontal surgery has not been

* Precautions to be taken with medically compromised patients can be found in Chapter 38.

clearly demonstrated,[27] although some studies have reported reduced postoperative complications including reduced pain and swelling when antibiotics are given before periodontal surgery and continuing for 4 to 7 days after surgery.[4,12,20,30]

The prophylactic use of antibiotics in patients who are otherwise healthy has been advocated for bone-grafting procedures and has been claimed to enhance the chances of new attachment. Although the rationale for such use appears logical, no research evidence is available to support it. In any case, the risks inherent in the administration of antibiotics should be evaluated together with the potential benefits.

Other presurgical medications include administration of a nonsteroidal, antiinflammatory drug such as ibuprofen (Motrin) 1 hour before the procedure and one oral rinse with 0.12% chlorhexidine gluconate (Peridex or PerioGard).[36]

Smoking. The deleterious effect of smoking on healing of periodontal wounds has been amply documented[19,31,40] (see also Chapter 14). Patients should be clearly informed of this fact and requested to quit or stop smoking for a minimum of 3 to 4 weeks after the procedure. For patients who are unwilling to follow this advice, an alternate treatment plan not including highly sophisticated techniques such as regenerative procedures and mucogingival and esthetic techniques should be considered.

Informed Consent. The patient should be informed at the time of the initial visit about the diagnosis, prognosis, the different possible treatments with their expected results, and all pros and cons of each approach. At the time of surgery, the patient should again be informed, verbally and in writing, of the procedure to be performed, and he or she should indicate agreement by signing the consent form.

Emergency Equipment

The operator, all assistants, and office personnel should be trained to handle all the possible emergencies that may arise. Drugs and equipment for emergency use should be readily available at all times.

The most common emergency is *syncope* or a transient loss of consciousness due to a reduction in cerebral blood flow. The most common cause is fear and anxiety. Syncope is usually preceded by a feeling of weakness, and then the patient develops pallor, sweating, coldness of the extremities, dizziness, and slowing of the pulse. The patient should be placed in a supine position with the legs elevated; tight clothes should be loosened, and a wide-open airway ensured. Administration of oxygen is also useful. Unconsciousness persists for a few minutes. A history of previous syncopal attacks during dental appointments should be explored before treatment is begun, and, if these are reported, extra efforts to relieve the patient's fear and anxiety should be made. The reader is referred to other texts[3] for a complete analysis of this important topic.

Measures to Prevent Transmission of Infection

In recent years, the danger of transmitting infections to the dental team or other patients has become apparent, particularly with the threat of acquired immune deficiency syndrome (AIDS) and hepatitis B. Universal precautions, including protective attire, and barrier techniques are strongly recommended and often required by law. They include the use of disposable sterile gloves, surgical masks, and protective eyewear. All surfaces possibly contaminated with blood or saliva that cannot be sterilized (such as light handles and unit syringes) must be covered with aluminum foil or plastic wrap. Aerosol-producing devices, such as the Cavitron, should not be used on patients with suspected infections, and their use should be kept to a minimum in all other patients. Special care should be taken when using and disposing of sharp items such as needles and scalpel blades.

Sedation and Anesthesia

Periodontal surgery should be performed painlessly. The patient should be assured of this at the outset and throughout the procedure. The most reliable means of providing painless surgery is the effective administration of local anesthesia. The area to be treated should be thoroughly anesthetized by means of regional block and local infiltration injections. Injections directly into the interdental papillae may also be helpful.

Apprehensive and neurotic patients require special management with antianxiety or sedative hypnotic agents. Modalities for the administration of these agents include inhalation, oral, intramuscular, and intravenous routes. The specific agents and modality of administration selected is based on the desired level of sedation, anticipated length of the procedure, and overall condition of the patient. Specifically, the medical history and physical and emotional status of the patient should be taken into consideration when selecting agents and techniques to be employed.

Perhaps the simplest, least invasive method to alleviate anxiety in the dental office is nitrous oxide and oxygen inhalation sedation. For many individuals, this is quite effective. Advantages include a quick onset of action, the ability to adjust the level of sedation throughout the procedure, a rapid recovery, and little or no concern for postoperative impairment of sensory or motor function. Disadvantages are few. A small percentage of patients will not achieve the desired effect. This is especially true for the mentally impaired individual because nitrous oxide and oxygen sedation requires some level of patient cooperation. Overall, inhalation sedation with nitrous oxide and oxygen is a safe, effective and reliable means of reducing mild anxiety.

For individuals with mild to moderate anxiety, oral administration of a benzodiazepine can be effective in decreasing anxiety and producing a level of relaxation. Oral administration of a sedative agent can be more effective than inhalation anesthesia because the level of sedation achieved may be more profound. Disadvantages of oral sedative administration include incomplete recovery, an inability to control the level of sedation, and a prolonged period of impaired sensory and motor skills. A variety of benzodiazepine agents are available for oral administration. See Table 55-1 for a brief description of commonly used benzodiazepine agents, including dosage, onset of action, and duration of effect (half-life).

Intravenous (IV) administration of a benzodiazepine, alone or in combination with other agents, can be used to achieve a greater level of sedation in individuals with moderate to severe levels of anxiety. Furthermore, the onset of action of intravenous sedation is almost immediate and the level of sedation can be titrated, on an individual basis, to the desired effect. The recovery period depends on the half-life of the agent used and the amount given. The operator should receive formal training in the techniques of sedation; this often is required by law. A thorough understanding of the indications, contraindications, and risks of these agents is required.[3] The reader is referred to other texts for a more detailed discussion of conscious sedation techniques.[25]

Tissue Management

1. *Operate gently and carefully.* In addition to being most considerate to the patient, this is also the most effective way to operate. Tissue manipulation should be precise, deliberate, and gentle. Thoroughness is essential, but roughness must be avoided because it produces excessive tissue injury, causes postoperative discomfort, and delays healing.
2. *Observe the patient at all times.* It is essential to pay careful attention to the patient's reactions. Facial expressions, pallor, and perspiration are some distinct signs that may indicate the patient is experiencing pain, anxiety, or fear. The doctor's responsiveness to these signs can be the difference between success and failure.
3. *Be certain the instruments are sharp.* Instruments must be sharp to be effective; successful treatment is not possible without sharp instruments. Dull instruments inflict unnecessary trauma due to poor cutting and excessive force applied to compensate for their ineffectiveness. A sterile sharpening stone should be available on the operating table at all times.

Scaling and Root Planing

Although scaling and root planing has been performed previously as part of Phase I therapy, all exposed root surfaces should be carefully explored and planed as needed as part of the surgical procedure. In particular, areas of difficult access such as furcations or deep pockets often have rough areas or even calculus that was undetected during the preparatory sessions. The assistant who is retracting the tissues and using the aspirator should also check for the presence of calculus and the smoothness of each surface from a different angle.

Hemostasis

Hemostasis is an important aspect of periodontal surgery because good intraoperative control of bleeding permits an accurate visualization of the extent of disease, pattern of bone destruction, and anatomy and condition of the root surfaces. It provides the operator with a clear view of the surgical site, which is essential for wound debridement and scaling and root planing. In addition, good hemostasis also prevents excessive loss of blood into the mouth, oropharynx, and stomach.

Periodontal surgery can produce profuse bleeding, especially during the initial incisions and flap reflection. After flap reflection and removal of granulation tissue, bleeding disappears or is considerably reduced. Typically, control of intraoperative bleeding can be managed with aspiration. Continuous suctioning of the surgical site with an aspirator is indispensable for performing periodontal surgery. Application of pressure to the surgical wound with moist gauze can be a helpful adjunct to control site specific bleeding. Intraoperative bleeding that is not controlled with these simple methods may indicate a more serious problem and require additional control measures.

Excessive hemorrhaging following initial incisions and flap reflection may be due to laceration of venules, arterioles, or larger vessels. Fortunately, the laceration of medium or large vessels is rare because incisions near highly vascular anatomic areas such as the posterior mandible (lingual and inferior alveolar arteries), and the posterior, mid-palatal regions (greater palatine arteries) are avoided in incision and flap design. Proper design of the flaps, taking into consideration these areas, avoids accidents (see Chapter 56). However, even when all anatomic precautions are taken, it is possible to cause bleeding from medium or large vessels because anatomic variations do occur and may result in inadvertent laceration. If a medium or large vessel is lacerated, a suture around the bleeding end may be necessary to control

TABLE 55-1

Oral Benzodiazepine Agents Commonly Used for Perioperative Antianxiety and Sedation

Generic	Proprietary	Adult Dose (mg)	Onset (Hours)	Half-Life (Hours)
Alprazolam	Xanax	0.25–0.5	1–2	12–15
Diazepam	Valium	2–10	0.5–2	30–70
Lorazepam	Ativan	1–4	1–6	10–18
Triazolam	Halcion	0.125–0.5	1–2	1.5–5.5

hemorrhage. Pressure should be applied through the tissue to determine the location that will stop blood flow in the severed vessel. Then a suture can be passed through the tissue and tied to restrict blood flow.

It is also possible to have excessive bleeding from a surgical wound due to incisions across a capillary plexus. Minor areas of persistent bleeding from capillaries can be stopped by applying cold pressure to the site with moist gauze (soaked in sterile ice water) for several minutes. The use of a local anesthetic with a vasoconstrictor may also be useful in controlling minor bleeding from the periodontal flap. Both of these methods act via vasoconstriction, thus reducing the flow of blood through incised small vessels and capillaries. This action is relatively short lived and should not be relied on for long-term hemostasis. It is important to avoid the use of vasoconstrictors to control bleeding prior to sending a patient home. If a more serious bleeding problem exists or a firm blood clot is not established, bleeding is likely to reoccur when the vasoconstrictor has metabolized and the patient is no longer in the office.

For slow, constant blood flow and oozing, hemostasis may be achieved with hemostatic agents. Table 55-2 describes available, absorbable hemostatic agents useful in the control of bleeding.

Absorbable gelatin sponge (Gelfoam), oxydized cellulose (Oxycel), oxidized regenerated cellulose (Surgicel Absorbable Hemostat), and microfibrillar collagen hemostat (Collacote, Collatape, Collaplug) are useful hemostatic agents for the control of capillaries, small blood vessels, and deep wound bleeding.

Absorbable gelatin sponge is a porous matrix prepared from pork skin that helps stabilize a normal blood clot. The sponge can be cut to the desired dimensions and either sutured in place or positioned within the wound (e.g., extraction socket). It is absorbed in 4 to 6 weeks.

Oxydized cellulose is a chemically modified form of surgical gauze that forms an artificial clot. The material is friable and can be difficult to keep in place. It absorbs in 1 to 6 weeks.

Oxydized regenerated cellulose is prepared from cellulose by reaction with alkali to form a chemically pure, more uniform structure than oxidized cellulose. The material is prepared in a cloth or thin gauze form that can be cut to the desired size and sutured or layered on the bleeding surface. It can be used as a surface dressing because it

TABLE 55-2

Absorbable Hemostatic Agents

Generic Name	Brand Name	Directions	Adverse Effects	Precautions
Absorbable gelatin sponge	Gelfoam	May be cut into various sizes and applied to bleeding surfaces.	May form nidus for infection or abscess.	Should not be overpacked into extraction site or wound—may interfere with healing.
Oxidized cellulose	Oxycel	Most effective when applied to wound dry as opposed to moistened.	May cause foreign body reaction.	Extremely friable and difficult to place; should not be used adjacent to bone—impairs bone regeneration; should not be used as a surface dressing—inhibits epithelialization.
Oxidized regenerated cellulose	Surgicel Absorbable Hemostat	May be cut to various shapes and positioned over bleeding sites; thick or excessive amounts should not be used.	Encapsulation, cyst formation, and foreign body reaction possible.	Should not be placed in deep wounds—may physically interfere with wound healing and bone formation.
Microfibrillar collagen hemostat	Collacote, Collatape, Collaplug	May be cut to shape and applied to bleeding surface.	May potentiate abscess formation, hematoma, and wound dehiscence; possible allergic reaction or foreign body reaction.	May interfere with wound healing; placement in extraction sockets has been associated with increased pain.
Thrombin	Thrombostat	May be applied topically to bleeding surface.	Allergic reaction can occur in patients with known sensitivity to bovine materials.	Must not be injected into tissues or vasculature because it can cause severe (possibly fatal) clotting.

does not impair epithelialization, and it is bactericidal against many gram-negative and gram-positive microorganisms, both aerobic and anaerobic. Caution should be used when wounds are infected or have an increased potential to becoming infected (e.g., immunocompromised patients) because the absorbable hemostatic agents can serve as a nidus for infection.

Thrombin is a drug capable of hastening the process of blood clotting. It is intended for topical use only because is applied as a liquid or powder. Thrombin should never be injected into tissues because it can cause serious, even fatal intravascular coagulation. Also, because thrombin is a bovine-derived material, caution should be used for any patient with known allergic reaction to bovine products.

Finally, it is imperative to recognize that excessive bleeding may be due to systemic disorders, including but not limited to platelet deficiencies, coagulation defects, medications, and hypertension. As a precaution, all surgical patients should be asked about current medications that may contribute to bleeding, any family history of bleeding disorders, and hypertension. *All* patients, regardless of health history, should have their blood pressure evaluated prior to surgery, and anyone diagnosed with hypertension must be advised to see a physician before surgery. Patients with known or suspected bleeding deficiencies or disorders must be carefully evaluated before any surgical procedure. A consultation with the patient's physician is recommended and laboratory tests should be done to assess the risk of bleeding. It may be necessary to refer the patient to a hematologist for a comprehensive work-up.

Periodontal Dressings (Periodontal Packs)

In most cases, after the surgical periodontal procedures are completed, the area is covered with a surgical pack. In general, dressings have no curative properties; they assist healing by protecting the tissue rather than providing "healing factors." The pack minimizes the likelihood of postoperative infection and hemorrhage, facilitates healing by preventing surface trauma during mastication, and protects against pain induced by contact of the wound with food or the tongue during mastication. For a complete literature review on this subject, the reader is referred to the work by Sachs et al.[35]

Zinc Oxide–Eugenol Packs. Packs based on the reaction of zinc oxide and eugenol include the Wondr-Pak developed by Ward[43] in 1923 and several others that modified Ward's original formula. The addition of accelerators such as zinc acetate gives the dressing a better working time.

Zinc oxide–eugenol dressings are supplied as a liquid and a powder that are mixed prior to use. Eugenol in this type of pack may induce an allergic reaction that produces reddening of the area and burning pain in some patients.

Noneugenol Packs. The reaction between a metallic oxide and fatty acids is the basis for Coe-Pak, which is the most widely used dressing in the U.S. This is supplied in two tubes, the contents of which are mixed immediately before use until a uniform color is obtained. One tube contains zinc oxide, an oil (for plasticity), a gum (for cohesiveness), and lorothidol (a fungicide); the other tube contains liquid coconut fatty acids thickened with colophony resin (or rosin) and chlorothymol (a bacteriostatic agent).[35,37] This dressing does not contain asbestos or eugenol, thereby avoiding the problems associated with these substances.

Other noneugenol packs include cyanoacrylates[6,18,23] and tissue conditioners (methacrylate gels).[2] However, these are not commonly used.

Retention of Packs. Periodontal dressings are usually kept in place mechanically by interlocking in interdental spaces and joining the lingual and facial portions of the pack.

In isolated teeth or when several teeth in an arch are missing, retention of the pack may be difficult. Numerous reinforcements and splints and stents for this purpose have been described.[16,17,44] Placement of dental floss tied loosely around the teeth enhances retention of the pack.

Antibacterial Properties of Packs. Improved healing and patient comfort with less odor and taste[6] have been obtained by incorporating antibiotics in the pack. Bacitracin,[5] oxytetracycline (Terramycin),[13] neomycin, and nitrofurazone have been tried, but all may produce hypersensitivity reactions. The emergence of resistant organisms and opportunistic infection have been reported.[33]

Incorporation of tetracycline powder in Coe-Pak is generally recommended, particularly when long and traumatic surgeries are performed.

Allergy. Contact allergy to eugenol and rosin has been reported.[32]

Preparation and Application of the Periodontal Dressing. Zinc oxide packs are mixed with eugenol or noneugenol liquids on a wax paper pad with a wooden tongue depressor. The powder is gradually incorporated with the liquid until a thick paste is formed.

Coe-Pak is prepared by mixing equal lengths of paste from tubes containing the accelerator and the base until the resulting paste is a uniform color. A capsule of tetracycline powder can be added at this time. The pack is then placed in a cup of water at room temperature. In 2 to 3 minutes, the paste loses its tackiness (Fig. 55-1) and can be handled and molded; it remains workable for 15 to 20 minutes. Working time can be shortened by adding a small amount of zinc oxide to the accelerator (pink paste) before spatulating.

The pack is then rolled into two strips approximately the length of the treated area. The end of one strip is bent into a hook shape and fitted around the distal surface of the last tooth, approaching it from the distal surface (Fig. 55-2, *A*). The remainder of the strip is brought forward along the facial surface to the midline and gently pressed into place along the gingival margin and interproximally. The second strip is applied from the lingual surface. It is joined to the pack at the distal surface

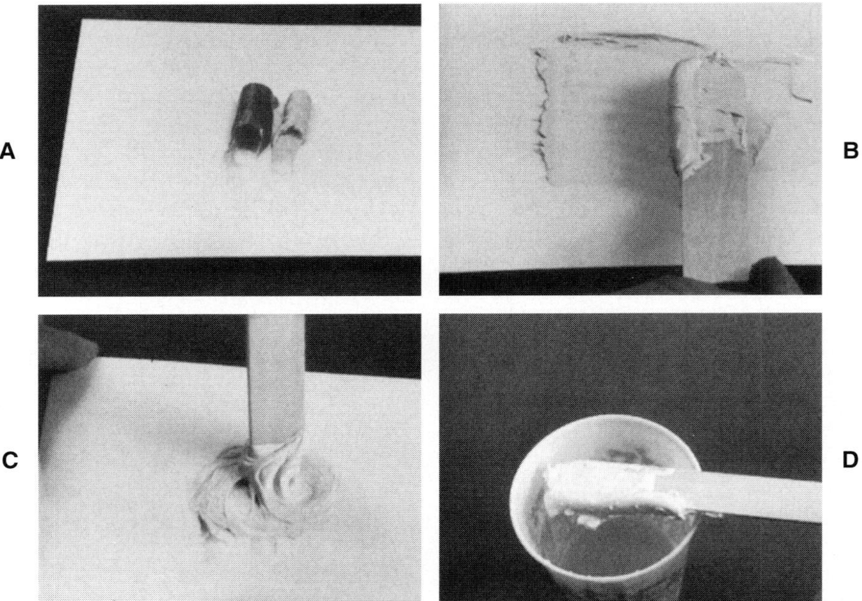

Fig. 55-1 Preparing the surgical pack (Coe-Pak). **A,** Equal lengths of the two pastes are placed on a paper pad. **B,** Pastes are mixed with a wooden tongue depressor for 2 or 3 minutes until the paste loses its tackiness **(C)**. **D,** Paste is placed in a paper cup of water at room temperature. With lubricated fingers, it is then rolled into cylinders and placed on the surgical wound.

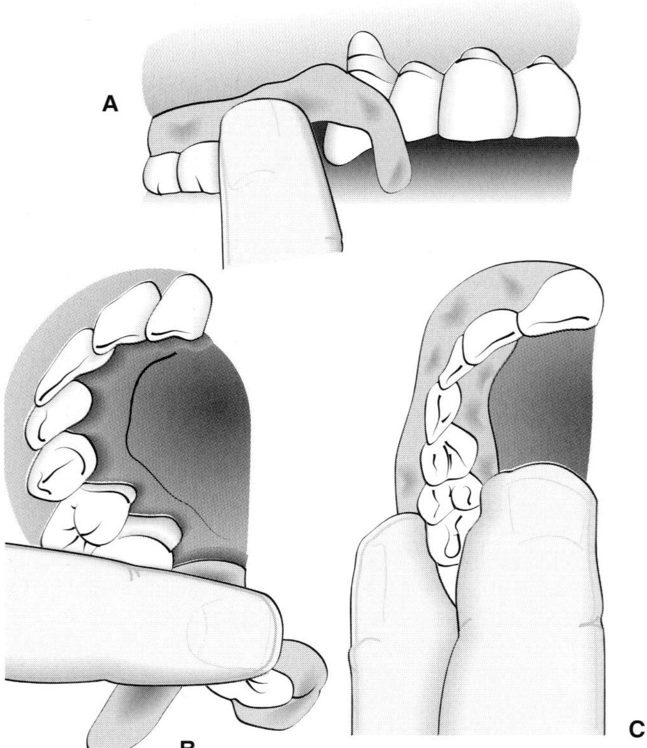

Fig. 55-2 Inserting the periodontal pack. **A,** A strip of pack is hooked around the last molar and pressed into place anteriorly. **B,** The lingual pack is joined to the facial strip at the distal surface of the last molar and fitted into place anteriorly. **C,** Gentle pressure on the facial and lingual surfaces joins the pack interproximally.

of the last tooth, then brought forward along the gingival margin to the midline (Fig. 55-2, *B*). The strips are joined interproximally by applying gentle pressure on the facial and lingual surfaces of the pack (Fig. 55-2, *C*). For isolated teeth separated by edentulous spaces, the pack should be made continuous from tooth to tooth, covering the edentulous areas (Fig. 55-3).

When split flaps have been performed, the area should be covered with tin foil to protect the sutures before placing the pack (see Chapter 60).

The pack should cover the gingiva, but overextensions onto uninvolved mucosa should be avoided. *Excess pack irritates the mucobuccal fold and floor of the mouth and interferes with the tongue.* Overextension also jeopardizes the remainder of the pack because the excess tends to break off, taking pack from the operated area with it. *Pack that interferes with the occlusion should be trimmed away before the patient is dismissed* (Fig. 55-4). Failure to do this causes discomfort and jeopardizes retention of the pack.

The operator should ask the patient to move the tongue forcibly out and to each side, and the cheek and lips should be displaced in all directions to mold the pack while it is still soft. After the pack has set, it should be trimmed to eliminate all excess.

As a general rule, the pack is kept on for 1 week after surgery. This guideline is based on the usual timetable of healing and clinical experience. It is not a rigid requirement; the period may be extended, or the area may be repacked for an additional week.

Fragments of the surface of the pack may come off during the week, but this presents no problem. If a portion of the pack is lost from the operated area and the

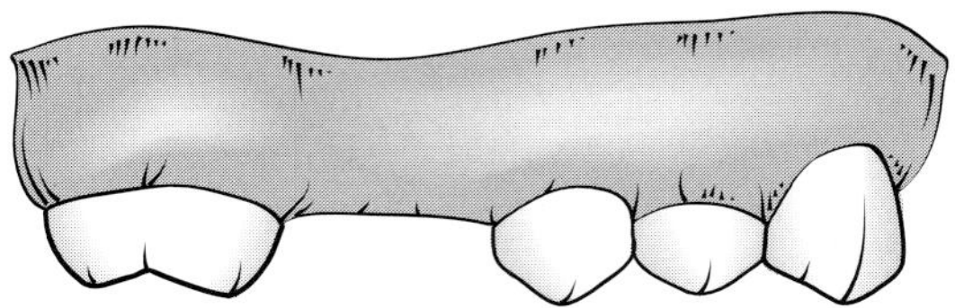

Fig. 55-3 Continuous pack covers the edentulous space.

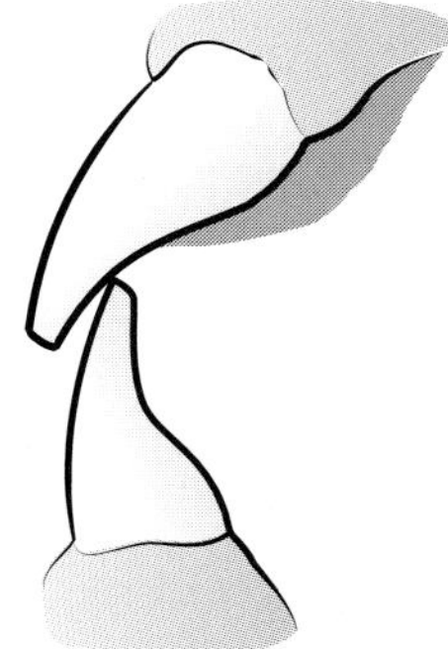

Fig. 55-4 The pack should not interfere with the occlusion.

patient is uncomfortable, it is usually best to repack the area. The clinician should remove the remaining pack, wash the area with warm water, and apply a topical anesthetic before replacing the pack, which is then retained for 1 week. Again, patients may develop pain from an overextended margin that irritates the vestibule, floor of the mouth, or tongue. The excess pack should be trimmed away, making sure that the new margin is not rough, before the patient is dismissed.

Instructions for the Patient after Surgery

After the pack is placed, printed instructions are given to the patient to be read before he or she leaves the chair (Box 55-1).

The First Postoperative Week

Properly performed, periodontal surgery presents no serious postoperative problems. Patients should be told to rinse with 0.12% chlorhexidine gluconate (Peridex, PerioGard) immediately after the surgical procedure and twice daily thereafter until normal plaque control technique can be resumed.[28,36,42] The following complications may arise in the first postoperative week, although they are the exception rather than the rule:

1. *Persistent bleeding after surgery.* The pack is removed, the bleeding points are located, and the bleeding is stopped with pressure, electrosurgery, or electrocautery. After the bleeding is stopped, the area is repacked.
2. *Sensitivity to percussion.* Sensitivity to percussion may be caused by the extension of inflammation into the periodontal ligament. The patient should be questioned regarding the progress of the symptoms. Gradually diminishing severity is a favorable sign. The pack should be removed and the gingiva checked for localized areas of infection or irritation, which should be cleaned or incised to provide drainage. Particles of calculus that may have been overlooked should be removed. Relieving the occlusion is usually helpful. Sensitivity to percussion may also be caused by excess pack, which interferes with the occlusion. Removal of the excess usually corrects the condition.
3. *Swelling.* Sometimes within the first 2 postoperative days, patients report a soft, painless swelling of the cheek in the area of operation. Lymph node enlargement may occur, and the temperature may be slightly elevated. The area of operation itself is usually symptom free. This type of involvement results from a localized inflammatory reaction to the operative procedure. It generally subsides by the fourth postoperative day, without necessitating removal of the pack. If swelling persists, becomes worse, or is associated with increased pain, then amoxyicillin, 500 mg should be taken every 8 hours for 1 week, and the patient should also be instructed to apply moist heat intermittently over the area. The antibiotic should also be used as a prophylactic measure after the next operation, starting before the surgical appointment.
4. *Feeling of weakness.* Occasionally, patients report having experienced a "washed-out," weakened feeling for about 24 hours after the operation. This represents a systemic reaction to a transient bacteremia induced by the operative procedure. It is prevented by premedication with amoxycillin, 500 mg every 8 hours, beginning 24 hours before the next operation and continuing for a 5-day postoperative period.

Removal of the Periodontal Pack and Return Visit Care

When the patient returns after 1 week, the pack is taken off by inserting a surgical hoe along the margin and exerting gentle lateral pressure. Pieces of pack retained interproximally and particles adhering to the tooth surfaces are removed with scalers. Particles may be enmeshed in the cut surface and should be carefully picked off with fine cotton pliers. The entire area is rinsed with peroxide to remove superficial debris.

Findings at Pack Removal. The following are usual when the pack is removed:

If a *gingivectomy* has been performed, the cut surface is covered with a friable meshwork of new epithelium, which should not be disturbed. If calculus has not been completely removed, red, beadlike protuberances of granulation tissue will persist. The granulation tissue must be removed with a curette, exposing the calculus so that it can be removed and the root can be planed. Removal of the granulation tissue without removal of calculus is followed by recurrence.

After a *flap operation,* the areas corresponding to the incisions are epithelialized but may bleed readily when touched; they should not be disturbed. Pockets should not be probed.

BOX 55-1

Patient Instructions after Surgery

Instructions for ___________ (Patient's Name)

The following information on your gum operation has been prepared to answer questions you may have about how to take care of your mouth. Please read the instructions carefully; our patients have found them very helpful.

Although there will be little or no discomfort when the anesthesia wears off, you should take two acetaminophen (Tylenol) tablets every 6 hours for the first 24 hours. After that, take the same medication if you have some discomfort. Do not take aspirin, as this may increase bleeding.

We have placed a periodontal pack over your gums to protect them from irritation. The pack prevents pain, aids healing, and enables you to carry on most of your usual activities in comfort. The pack will harden in a few hours, after which it can withstand most of the forces of chewing without breaking off. It may take a little while to become accustomed to it.

The pack should remain in place until it is removed in the office at the next appointment. If particles of the pack chip off during the week, do not be concerned as long as you do not have pain. If a piece of the pack breaks off and you are in pain, or if a rough edge irritates your tongue or cheek, please call the office. The problem can be easily remedied by replacing the pack.

For the first 3 hours after the operation, avoid hot foods to permit the pack to harden. It is also convenient to avoid hot liquids during the first 24 hours. You can eat anything you can manage, but try to chew on the nonoperated side of your mouth. Semisolid or finely minced foods are suggested. Avoid citrus fruits or fruit juices, highly spiced foods, and alcoholic beverages; these will cause pain. Food supplements, or vitamins are generally not necessary.

Do not smoke. The heat and smoke will irritate your gums, and the immunologic effects of nicotine will delay healing and prevent a completely successful outcome of the procedure performed. If at all possible, use this opportunity to give up smoking. In addition to all other well-known health risks, smokers have more gum disease than nonsmokers.

Do not brush over the pack. Brush and floss the areas of the mouth not covered by the pack, as normal. Use chlorhexidine (Peridex, PerioGard) mouthrinses after brushing (the prescription for this mouthrinse has been given to you).

During the first day, apply ice intermittently on the face over the operated area. It is also beneficial to suck on ice chips intermittently during the first 24 hours. These methods will keep tissues cool and reduce inflammation and swelling.

You may experience a slight feeling of weakness or chills during the first 24 hours. This should not be cause for alarm but should be reported at the next visit. *Follow your regular daily activities, but avoid excessive exertion of any type.* Golf, tennis, skiing, bowling, swimming, or sunbathing should be postponed for a few days after the operation.

Swelling is not unusual, particularly in areas that required extensive surgical procedures. The swelling generally begins 1 to 2 days after the operation and subsides gradually in 3 or 4 days. If this occurs, apply moist heat over the operated area. If the swelling is painful or appears to become worse, please call the office.

Occasional blood stains in the saliva may occur for the first 4 or 5 hours after the operation. This is not unusual and will correct itself. If there is considerable bleeding beyond this, take a piece of gauze, form it into the shape of a U, hold it in the thumb and index finger, apply it to both sides of the pack, and hold it there under pressure for 20 minutes. Do not remove it during this period to examine it. If the bleeding does not stop at the end of 20 minutes, please contact the office. *Do not try to stop bleeding by rinsing.*

After the pack is removed, the gums most likely will bleed more than they did before the operation. This is perfectly normal in the early stage of healing and will gradually subside. Do not stop cleaning because of it.

If any other problems arise, please call the office.

The facial and lingual mucosa may be covered with a grayish-yellow or white granular layer of food debris that has seeped under the pack. This is easily removed with a moist cotton pellet. The root surfaces may be sensitive to a probe or to thermal changes, and the teeth may be stained.

Fragments of calculus delay healing. Each root surface should be rechecked visually to be certain that no calculus is present. Sometimes the color of the calculus is similar to that of the root. The grooves on proximal root surfaces and the furcations are areas in which calculus is likely to be overlooked.

Repacking. After the pack is removed, it is usually not necessary to replace it. However, it is advisable to repack for an additional week for patients with 1) a low pain threshold who are particularly uncomfortable when the pack is removed, 2) unusually extensive periodontal involvement, or 3) slow healing. Clinical judgement helps in deciding whether to repack the area or leave the initial pack on longer than 1 week.

Tooth Mobility. Tooth mobility is increased immediately after surgery,[8] but it diminishes below the pretreatment level by the fourth week.[24]

Care of the Mouth between Periodontal Surgery Procedures

Care of the mouth by the patient between the treatment of the first and the final areas, as well as after surgery is completed, is extremely important.[45] These measures should begin after the pack is removed from the first operation. The patient has been through a presurgical period of instructed plaque control and should be reinstructed at this time.

Vigorous brushing is not feasible during the first week after the pack is removed. However, the patient is informed that plaque and food accumulation retard healing and is advised to try to keep the area as clean as possible by the gentle use of soft toothbrushes and light water irrigation. Rinsing with a chlorhexidine mouthwash or its topical application with cotton-tipped applicators (Q-tips) is indicated for the first few postoperative weeks, particularly in advanced cases. Brushing is introduced when healing of the tissues permits it; the vigor of the overall hygiene regimen is increased as healing progresses. Patients should be told that there be more gingival bleeding will most likely occur than before the operation, that it is perfectly normal and will subside as healing progresses, and that it should not deter them from following their oral hygiene regimen.

Management of Postoperative Pain

Periodontal surgery performed following the basic principles outlined here should produce only minor pain and discomfort.[38] One study of 304 consecutive periodontal surgical interventions revealed that 51.3% of the patients reported minimal or no postoperative pain, and only 4.6% reported severe pain. Of these, only 20.1% took five or more doses of analgesic.[11] The same study showed that mucogingival procedures result in six times more discomfort and osseous surgery in 3.5 times more discomfort than plastic gingival surgery. In the few cases in which severe pain may be present, its control then becomes an important part of patient management.[27]

A common source of postoperative pain is overextension of the periodontal pack onto the soft tissue beyond the mucogingival junction or onto the frena. Overextended packs cause localized areas of edema, usually noticed 1 to 2 days after surgery. Removal of excess pack is followed by resolution in about 24 hours. Extensive and excessively prolonged exposure and dryness of bone also induce severe pain.

For most healthy patients, a preoperative dose of ibuprofen (600 to 800 mg) followed by one tablet every 8 hours for 24 to 48 hours is very effective in reducing discomfort after periodontal therapy. Patients are advised to continue taking ibuprofen or change to acetaminophen if needed thereafter. If pain persists, acetaminophen plus codeine (Tylenol #3) can be prescribed.

Caution should be used in prescribing or dispensing ibuprofen to patients with hypertension controlled by medications because it can interfere with the effectiveness of the medication.

When severe postoperative pain is present, the patient should be seen at the office on an emergency basis. The area is anesthetized by infiltration or topically, the pack is removed, and the wound is examined. Postoperative pain related to infection is accompanied by localized lymphadenopathy and a slight elevation in temperature. It should be treated with systemic antibiotics and analgesics.

Treatment of Sensitive Roots. Root hypersensitivity is a relatively common problem in periodontal practice. It may occur spontaneously when the root becomes exposed as a result of gingival recession or pocket formation, or it may appear after scaling and root planing and surgical procedures.* It is manifested as pain induced by cold or hot temperature, more commonly cold; by citrus fruits or sweets; or by contact with a toothbrush or a dental instrument.

Root sensitivity occurs more frequently in the cervical area of the root, where the cementum is extremely thin. Scaling and root planing procedures remove this thin cementum, inducing the hypersensitivity.

Transmission of stimuli from the surface of the dentin to the nerve endings located in the dental pulp or in the pulpal region of the dentin could occur through the odontoblastic process or owing to a hydrodynamic mechanism (displacement of dentinal fluid). The latter process seems more likely and would explain the importance of burnishing desensitizing agents to obturate the dentinal tubule.

An important factor for reducing or eliminating hypersensitivity is adequate plaque control. However, hypersensitivity may prevent plaque control, and therefore a vicious circle of escalating hypersensitivity and plaque accumulation may be created.

---

* For a complete review of the literature, see Curro FA: Tooth hypersensitivity. Dent Clin North Am 1990; 34(3):403.[10]

DESENSITIZING AGENTS. A number of agents have been proposed to control root hypersensitivity. Clinical evaluation of the many agents proposed is difficult because 1) measuring and comparing pain between different persons is difficult, 2) hypersensitivity disappears by itself after a time, and 3) desensitizing agents usually take a few weeks to act.

The patient should be informed about the possibility of root hypersensitivity before treatment is undertaken. The following information on how to cope with the problem should also be given to the patient:

1. Hypersensitivity appears as a result of the exposure of dentin, which is inevitable if calculus and plaque and their products, buried in the root, are to be removed.
2. Hypersensitivity slowly disappears over a few weeks.
3. Plaque control is important for the reduction of hypersensitivity.
4. Desensitizing agents do not produce immediate relief. They have to be used for several days or even weeks to produce results.

Desensitizing agents can be applied by the patient at home or by the dentist or hygienist in the dental office. The most likely mechanism of action is the reduction in the diameter of the dentinal tubules so as to limit the displacement of fluid in them. According to Trowbridge and Silver,[40] this can be attained by 1) formation of a smear layer produced by burnishing the exposed surface, 2) topical application of agents that form insoluble precipitates within the tubules, 3) impregnation of tubules with plastic resins, or 4) sealing of the tubules with plastic resins.

Agents used by the Patient. The most common agents used by the patient for oral hygiene are dentifrices. Although many dentifrice products contain fluoride, additional active ingredients for desensitization are strontium chloride, potassium nitrate and sodium citrate. The following dentifrices have been approved by the American Dental Association for desensitizing purposes: Sensodyne, and Thermodent, which contain strontium chloride[7,9,34]; Crest Sensitivity Protection, Denquel, and Promise, which contain potassium nitrate[1,9]; and Protect, which contains sodium citrate. Fluoride rinsing solutions and gels can also be used after the usual plaque control procedures.[39]

Patients should be aware that several factors must be considered in the treatment of tooth hypersensitivity, including the history and severity of the problem as well as the physical findings of the tooth or teeth involved. A proper diagnosis is required before any treatment can be initiated so that pathologic causes of pain (e.g., caries, cracked tooth, pulpitis) can be ruled out before attempting to treat hypersensitivity. Desensitizing agents act via the precipitation of crystalline salts on the dentin surface, which block dentinal tubules. Patients must be aware that their use will not prove to be effective unless used continuously for a period of at least 2 weeks.

Agents used in the Dental Office. Box 55-2 lists various office treatments for the desensitization of hypersensitive dentin. These products and treatments aim to decrease hypersensitivity via blocking dentinal tubules with either a crystalline salt precipitation or an applied coating (varnish or bonding agent) on the root surface. The reader is again referred to the Towbridge and Silver[41] for a more detailed consideration of these methods.

Several agents have been used to precipitate crystalline salts on the dentin surface in an attempt to occlude the dentinal tubules. Fluoride solutions and pastes historically have been the agents of choice. In addition to their antisensitivity properties, they have the advantage of anticaries activity, which is particularly important for patients with a tendency to develop root caries. However, certain agents such as chlorhexidine, decrease the ability of fluoride to bind with calcium on the root surfaces.[1] Thus it is important to advise patients not to rinse or eat for 1 hour after a desensitizing treatment. Currently, potassium and ferric oxalate solutions are the preferred agents. They form insoluble calcium oxalate crystals that occlude the dentinal tubules.[26,28] Potassium oxalate is available under the name *Protect* and ferric oxalate under the name *Sensodyne Sealant.* Special applicators have been developed for their use.

A newer method of treatment for hypersensitive dentin is the use of varnishes or dentin bonding agents to occlude dentinal tubules. Newer restorative materials, such as glass-ionomer cements and dentine bonding agents, are still under investigation, but when the tooth needs recontouring or difficult cases do not respond to other treatments, the dentist may choose to use a restorative material. Resin primers alone could be promising, but the effects are not permanent and investigations are ongoing.[14]

Despite some successes in decreasing dentin hypersensitivity, it is important to note that these "dental office" treatments have not been a predictable means of solving hypersensitivity and the success achieved is often short lived. The crystalline salts and/or varnishes and

BOX 55-2

Office Treatments for Dentinal Hypersensitivity

- Cavity varnishes
- Antiinflammatory agents
- Treatments that partially obturate dentinal tubules
  - Burnishing of dentin
  - Silver nitrate
  - Zinc chloride–potassium ferrocyanide
  - Formalin
  - Calcium compounds
    - Calcium hydroxide
    - Dibasic calcium phosphate
  - Fluoride compounds
    - Sodium fluoride
    - Stannous fluoride
  - Iontophoresis
  - Strontium chloride
  - Potassium oxalate
- Restorative resins
- Dentin bonding agents

From Trowbridge HO, Silver DR: A review of current approaches to in-office management of tooth hypersensitivity. Dent Clin North Am 1990; 34(3):566.

sealants can be washed away over time, and hypersensitivity may return. When this occurs, patients can have sensitive root surfaces treated again.

Recently, attempts have been made to improve the success and longevity of these treatments using lasers. Low-level laser "melting" of the dentin surface appears to seal dentinal tubules without damage to the pulp.[15,21] Finally, in a combined treatment modality, the Nd:YAG laser has been used to congeal fluoride varnish on root surfaces. This in vitro study demonstrated that the laser treated fluoride varnish resisted removal by electric toothbrushing, with 90% of tubules remaining blocked while in the controls (no laser treatment) the fluoride varnish was almost completely brushed away.[22] Despite these convincing preliminary results, more research is needed before laser treatment can be considered an effective and predictable means of desensitization. Furthermore, laser treatment is expensive and has the potential to cause pulp damage.

HOSPITAL PERIODONTAL SURGERY

Ordinarily, periodontal surgery is an office procedure performed in quadrants or sextants, usually at biweekly or longer intervals. Under certain circumstances, however, it is in the best interest of the patient to treat the mouth in one operation with the patient treated in a hospital operating room under general anesthesia. Indications for hospital periodontal surgery include optimal control and management of apprehension, convenience for individuals who cannot endure multiple visits to complete surgical treatment, and patient protection.

Indications

The Apprehensive Patient. Gentleness, understanding, and preoperative sedation usually suffice to calm the fears of most patients. For some patients, however, the prospect of a series of surgical procedures is sufficiently stressful to trigger disturbances that jeopardize the well-being of the patient and hamper treatment. Explaining that the treatment at the hospital will be performed painlessly and that it will be accomplished by a level of anesthesia that is neither practical nor safe for patients in a dental office is an important step in allaying their fears. The thought of completing the necessary surgical procedures in one session rather than in repeated visits is an added comfort to the patient because it eliminates the prospect of repeated anxiety in anticipation of each treatment.

Patient Convenience. With complete mouth surgery, there is less stress for the patient and less time involved in postoperative care. For patients whose occupation entails considerable contact with the public, surgery performed at biweekly intervals sometimes presents a special problem. It means that for a period of several weeks, some area of the mouth will be covered by a periodontal pack. With the complete mouth technique, the pack is ordinarily retained for only 1 week. Patients find this an acceptable alternative to several weeks of discomfort in different areas of the mouth and multiple dressing applications. For a variety of other reasons, patients may desire to attend to their surgical needs in one session under optimal conditions.

Patient Protection. Some patients have systemic conditions that are not severe enough to contraindicate elective surgery but may require special precautions best provided in a hospital setting. This includes some patients with cardiovascular disease, abnormal bleeding tendencies, or hyperthyroidism; those undergoing prolonged steroid therapy; and those with a history of rheumatic fever.

The purpose of hospitalization is to protect patients by anticipating their special needs, not to perform periodontal surgery when it is contraindicated by the patient's general condition. For some patients, elective surgery is contraindicated regardless of whether it is performed in the dental office or hospital. When consultation with the patient's physician leads to this decision, palliative periodontal therapy, in the form of scaling and root planing if permissible, is the necessary compromise.

Premedication. Patients should be given a sedative the night before surgery. Benzodiazepines work well for most patients, allowing the patient to sleep well the night before surgery. If the patient is extremely nervous about the procedure, it is also helpful to advise them to take a benzodiazepine on the morning of surgery. This ensures that they will be rested and as relaxed as possible before surgery.

Patients with systemic problems (history of rheumatic fever, cardiovascular problems, etc.) are premedicated as needed (see Chapter 38).

Anesthesia. Local or general anesthesia[25] may be used. Local anesthesia is the method of choice, except for especially apprehensive patients. It permits unhampered movement of the head, which is necessary for optimal visibility and accessibility to the various root surfaces. Local anesthesia is used in the same manner as for routine periodontal surgery.

When general anesthesia is indicated, it is administered by an anesthesiologist. It is important that the patient also receive local anesthesia, administered as for routine periodontal surgery, to ensure comfort for the patient and reduced bleeding during the procedure. The judicious use of local anesthetics to block regional nerves allows the level of sedation or general anesthesia to be lighter. Hence the entire operation is performed with a wider margin of safety.

The Operation

Surgery in the operating room is performed on the operating table with the patient lying down and the table either positioned flat or with the head inclined up to 30 degrees. Some operating rooms are equipped with dental chairs that can be used either flat or up to 30 degrees. When general anesthesia is used, it is advisable to delay placing the periodontal dressing until the patient has recovered sufficiently to have a demonstrable cough reflex. Periodontal dressings placed before the end of general anesthesia can be displaced during the recovery period and pose serious risks of blocking the airway.

Postoperative Instructions

After a full recovery from general anesthesia, most patients can be discharged home with a responsible adult. The effects of general anesthesia and sedative agents make the patient drowsy for hours, recommending adult supervision at home for up to 24 hours after surgery. The typical postoperative instructions should be given to the responsible adult and the patient should be scheduled for a postoperative visit in 1 week.

REFERENCES

1. ADA Guide to Dental Therapeutics, ed 1. Chicago, ADA, 1998.
2. Addy M, Douglas WH: A chlorhexidine-containing methacrylic gel as a periodontal dressing. J Periodontol 1975; 46:465.
3. Allen GD: Dental Anesthesia and Analgesia (Local and General), ed 3. Baltimore, Williams & Wilkins, 1984.
4. Ariaudo AA: The efficacy of antibiotics in periodontal surgery. J Periodontol 1969; 40:150.
5. Baer PN, Goldman HM, Scigliano J: Studies on a bacitracin periodontal dressing. Oral Surg 1958; 11:712.
6. Baer PN, Summer CF III, Miller G: Periodontal dressings. Dent Clin North Am 1969; 13:181.
7. Blitzer B: A consideration of the possible causes of dental hypersensitivity: Treatment by a strontium ion dentifrice. Periodontics 1967; 5:318.
8. Burch J, Conroy CW, Ferris RT: Tooth mobility following gingivectomy. A study of gingival support of the teeth. Periodontics 1960; 6:90.
9. Collins JF, Gingold J, Stanley H, et al: Reducing dentinal hypersensitivity with strontium chloride and potassium nitrate. Gen Dent 1984; 32:40.
10. Curro FA: Tooth hypersensitivity. Dent Clin North Am 1990; 34(3):403.
11. Curtis JW Jr, McLain JB, Hutchinson RA: The incidence and severity of complications and pain following periodontal surgery. J Periodontol 1985; 56:597.
12. Dal Pra DJ, Strahan JD: A clinical evaluation of the benefits of a course of oral penicillin following periodontal surgery. Aust Dent J 1972; 17:219.
13. Fraleigh CM: An evaluation of topical Terramycin in post-gingivectomy pack. J Periodontol 1956; 27:201.
14. Gangarosa LP Sr: Current strategies for dentist-applied treatment in the management of hypersensitive dentine. Arch Oral Biol 1994; 39(Suppl):101S.
15. Gerschman JA, Ruben J, Gebart-Eaglemont J: Low-level laser therapy for dentinal tooth hypersensitivity. Aust Dent J 1994; 39:353.
16. Hirschfeld AS, Wassermen BH: Retention of periodontal packs. J Periodontol 1958; 29:199.
17. Holmes CH: Periodontal pack on single tooth retained by acrylic splint. J Am Dent Assoc 1962; 64:831.
18. Javelet J, Torabinejad M, Danforth A: Isobutyl cyanoacrylate: A clinical and histological comparison with sutures in closing mucosal incisions in monkeys. Oral Surg 1985; 59:91.
19. Jones JK, Triplett RG: The relationship of cigarette smoking to impaired intraoral wound healing: A review of evidence and implications for patient care. J Oral Maxillofac Surg 1992; 50:237.
20. Kidd EA, Wade AB: Penicillin control of swelling and pain after periodontal osseous surgery. J Clin Periodontol 1974; 1:52.
21. Lan WH, Liu HC: Treatment of dentin hypersensitivity by Nd:YAG laser. J Clin Laser Med Surg 1996; 14:89.
22. Lan WH, Liu HC, Lin CP: The combined occluding effect of sodium fluoride varnish and Nd:YAG laser irradiation on human dentinal tubules. J Endod. 1999; 25:424.
23. Levin MP, Cutright DE, Bhaskar SN: Cyanoacrylate as a periodontal dressing. J Oral Med 1975; 30:40.
24. Majewski I, Sponholz H: Ergebnisse nach parodonal therapeutischen Massnahmen unter besonderer Berucksichtigung der Zahnbeweglichkeitssung mit dem Makroperiodontometer nach Muhlemann. Zahnaerztl Rundsch 1966; 75:57.
25. Malamed SF: Sedation. A Guide to Patient Management, ed 7. St Louis, Mosby, in press.
26. Miller JT, Shannon KL, Kilyore WG, et al: Use of water-free stannous fluoride–containing gel in the control of dental hypersensitivity. J Periodontol 1969; 40:490.
27. Murphy NC, DeMarco TJ: Controlling pain in periodontal patients. Dent Survey 1979; 55:46.
28. Newman MG, Sanz M, Nachnani S, et al: Effect of 0.12% chlorhexidine on bacterial recolonization after periodontal surgery. J Periodontol 1989; 60:577.
29. Pack PO, Haber J: The incidence of clinical infection after periodontal surgery. A retrospective study. J Periodontol 1983; 54:441.
30. Pendrill K, Reddy J: The use of prophylactic penicillin in periodontal surgery. J Periodontol 1980; 51:44.
31. Preber H, Bergstrom J: Effect of cigarette smoking on periodontal healing following surgical therapy. J Clin Periodontol 1990; 17:324.
32. Romanow I: Allergic reactions to periodontal pack. J Periodontol 1957; 28:151.
33. Romanow I: Relationship of moniliasis to the presence of antibiotics in periodontal packs. Periodontics 1964; 2:298.
34. Ross MR: Hypersensitive teeth: Effect of strontium chloride in a compatible dentifrice. J Periodontol 1961; 32:49.
35. Sachs HA, Fanroush A, Checchi L, et al: Current status of periodontal dressings. J Periodontol 1984; 55:689.
36. Sanz M, Newman MG, Anderson L, et al: Clinical enhancement of post-periodontal surgical therapy by 0.12 per cent chlorhexidine gluconate mouthrinse. J Periodontol 1989; 60:570.
37. Smith DC: A materialistic look at periodontal packs. Dent Pract Dent Rec 1970; 20:273.
38. Strahan JD, Glenwright HD: Pain experience in periodontal surgery. J Periodont Res 1967; 1:163.
39. Tarbet WJ, Silverman G, Stolman JW, et al: A clinical evaluation of a new treatment for dentinal hypersensitivity. J Periodontol 1980; 51:535.
40. Tonetti MS, Pini Prato G, Cortellini P: Effect of cigarette smoking on periodontal healing following GTR in infrabony pockets. A preliminary retrospective study. J Clin Periodontol 1995; 22:229.
41. Trowbridge HO, Silver DR: A review of current approaches to in-office management of tooth hypersensitivity. Dent Clin North Am 1990; 34:583.
42. Vaughan ME, Garnick JJ: The effect of 0.125 per cent chlorhexidine rinse on inflammation after periodontal surgery. J Periodontol 1989; 60:704.
43. Ward AW: Inharmonious cusp relation as a factor in periodontoclasia. J Am Dent Assoc 1923; 10:471.
44. Watts TAP, Combe EC: Adhesion of periodontal dressings to enamel in vitro. J Clin Periodontol 1980; 7:62.
45. Westfelt E, Nyman S, Socransky SS: Significance of frequency of professional cleaning for healing following periodontal surgery. J Clin Periodontol 1983; 10:148.

Surgical Anatomy of the Periodontium and Related Structures

Fermin A. Carranza

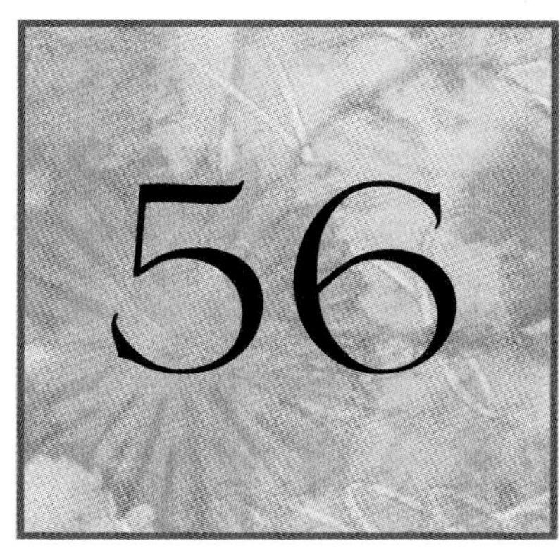

CHAPTER

CHAPTER OUTLINE

A sound knowledge of the anatomy of the periodontium and the hard and soft structures that surround it is essential to determine the scope and possibilities of surgical periodontal procedures and minimize their risks. Bones, muscles, blood vessels, and nerves, as well as the anatomic spaces located in the vicinity of the periodontal surgical field, are particularly important. Only those features of periodontal relevance are mentioned in this chapter; the reader is referred to books on oral anatomy[3,4] for a more comprehensive description of these structures.

MANDIBLE

The mandible is a horseshoe-shaped bone connected to the skull by the temporomandibular joints. It presents several landmarks of great surgical importance.

The *mandibular canal,* occupied by the inferior alveolar nerve and vessels, begins at the mandibular foramen on the medial surface of the mandibular ramus and curves downward and forward, becoming horizontal below the apices of the molars (Fig. 56-1). The distance from the canal to the apices of the molars is shorter in the third molar area and increases as it goes forward. In the premolar area, the canal divides in two: the incisive canal, which continues horizontally to the midline, and the mental canal, which turns upward and opens in the mental foramen.

The author is grateful to Dr. Andrew D. Dixon for his constructive analysis of this chapter.

The *mental foramen,* from which the mental nerve and vessels emerge, is located on the buccal surface of the mandible below the apices of the premolars, sometimes closer to the second premolar and usually halfway between the lower border of the mandible and the alveolar margin (Fig. 56-2). The opening of the mental foramen faces upward and distally, with its posterosuperior border slanting gradually to the bone surface. As it emerges, the mental nerve divides into three branches. One branch of the nerve turns forward and downward to supply the skin of the chin. The other two branches course anteriorly and upward to supply the skin and mucous membrane of the lower lip and the mucosa of the labial alveolar surface.

Surgical trauma to the mental nerve can produce paresthesia of the lip, which recovers slowly. Familiarity with the location and appearance of the mental nerve reduces the likelihood of injury (Fig. 56-3).

In partially or totally edentulous jaws, the disappearance of the alveolar portion of the mandible brings the mandibular canal closer to the superior border. When these patients are evaluated for placement of implants, the distance between the canal and the superior surface of the bone must be carefully determined to avoid surgical injury to the nerve.

The *lingual nerve,* along with the inferior alveolar nerve, is a branch of the posterior division of the mandibular nerve and descends along the mandibular ramus medial to and in front of the inferior alveolar nerve. It lies close to the surface of the oral mucosa in the third molar area and goes deeper as it goes forward

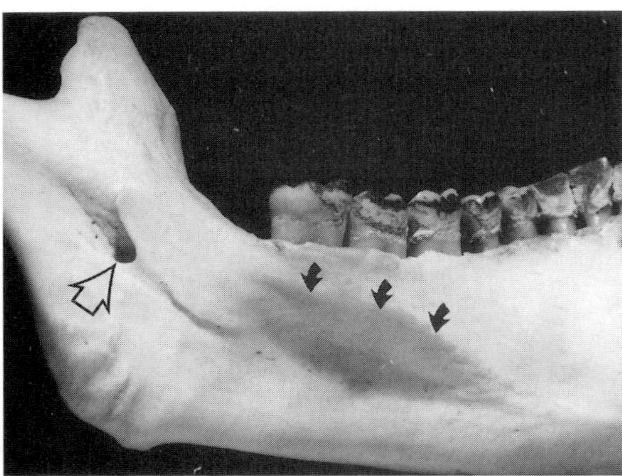

Fig. 56-1 Mandible, lingual surface view. Note the lingual or mandibular foramen *(open arrow)* where the inferior alveolar nerve enters the mandibular canal and the mylohyoid ridge *(solid arrows).*

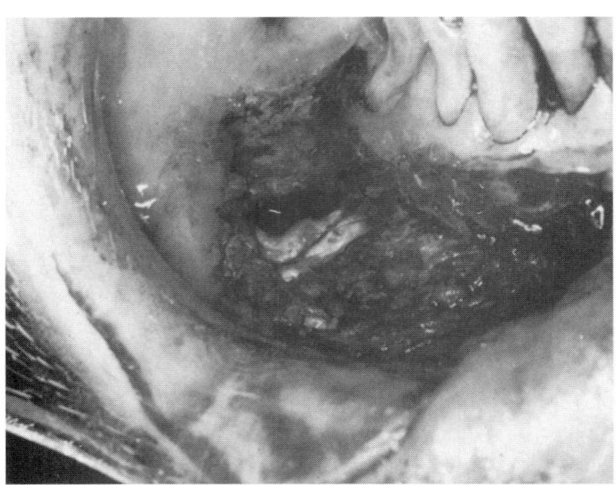

Fig. 56-3 Mental nerve emerging from the foramen in the premolar area.

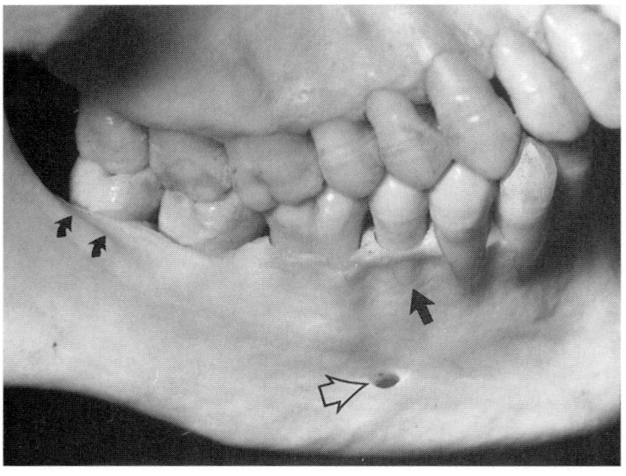

Fig. 56-2 Mandible, facial surface view. Note the location of the mental foramen *(open arrow),* slightly distal and apical to the apex of the second premolar, and the shelflike area in the region of the molars *(curved solid arrows),* created by the external oblique ridge. Note also the fenestration present in the second premolar *(straight solid arrow).*

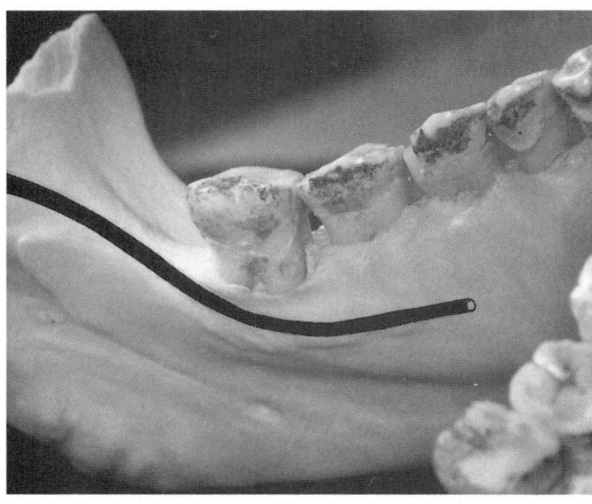

Fig. 56-4 Lingual view of the mandible showing the pathway of the lingual nerve, which goes near the gingiva in the third molar area and then continues forward, going deeper and medially.

(Fig. 56-4; see also Fig. 56-18). It can be damaged during anesthetic injections and during oral surgery procedures such as third molar extractions.[7] Less commonly, it may be injured when a periodontal partial thickness flap is raised in the third molar region or releasing incisions are made.

The *alveolar process,* which provides the supporting bone to the teeth, has a narrower distal curvature than the body of the mandible (Fig. 56-5), creating a flat surface in the posterior area between the teeth and the anterior border of the ramus. This results in the formation of the *external oblique ridge,* which runs downward and forward to the region of the second or first molar (Fig. 56-6), creating a shelflike bony area. Resective osseous therapy may be difficult or impossible in this area owing to the amount of bone that would have to be removed.

Distal to the third molar, the external oblique ridge circumscribes the *retromolar triangle* (see Fig. 56-6). This region is occupied by glandular and adipose tissue covered by unattached nonkeratinized mucosa. If sufficient space exists distal to the last molar, a band of attached gingiva may be present; only in such a case can a distal wedge operation be performed.

The inner side of the body of the mandible is traversed obliquely by the *mylohyoid ridge,* which starts close to the alveolar margin in the third molar area and continues anteriorly, increasing its distance from the osseous margin as it goes forward (Fig. 56-7). The mylohy-

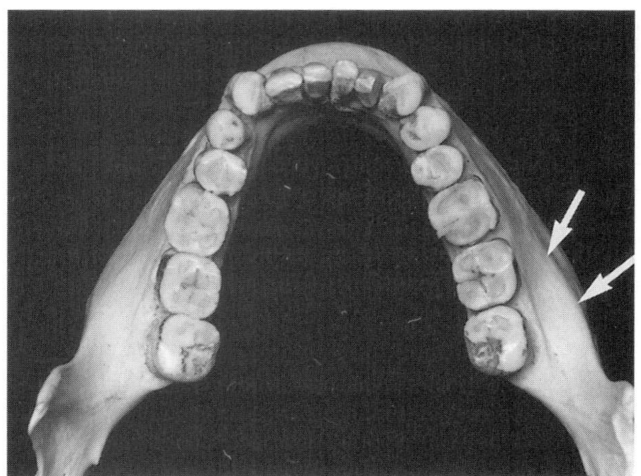

Fig. 56-5 Occlusal view of mandible. Note the shelf created in the facial molar areas by the external oblique ridge. Arrows on the right show the attachment of the buccinator muscle.

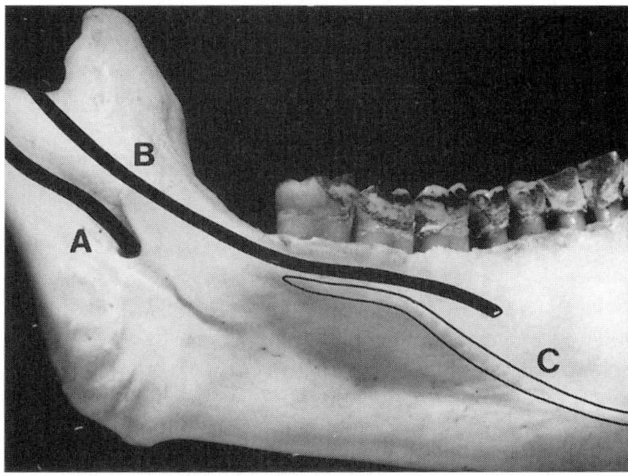

Fig. 56-7 Mandible: lingual view showing the inferior alveolar nerve entering the mandibular canal *(A)*, the lingual nerve traversing near the lingual surface of the third molar *(B)*, and inferiorly, the attachment of the mylohyoid muscle *(C)*.

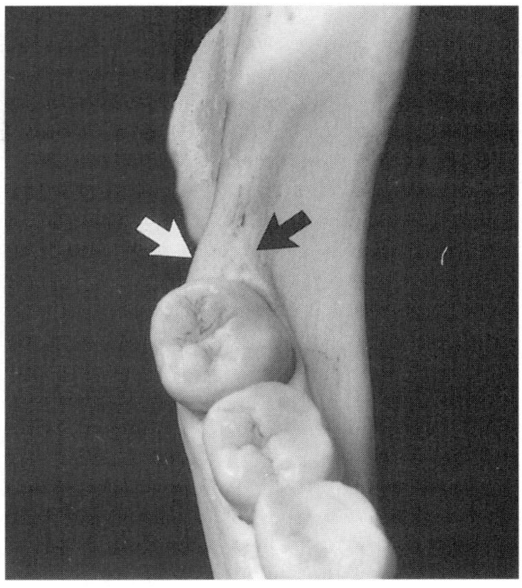

Fig. 56-6 Mandible: occlusal view of ramus and molars. Note the retromolar triangle area distal to the third molar *(arrows)*.

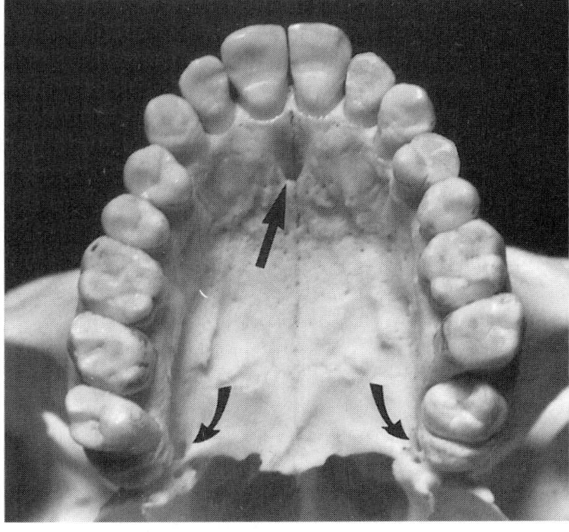

Fig. 56-8 Occlusal view of maxilla and palatine bone. Note the opening of the incisive canal or anterior palatine foramen *(straight arrow)* and the greater palatine foramen *(curved arrows)*.

oid muscle, inserted at this ridge, separates the sublingual space, located more anteriorly and superiorly, from the submandibular space, located more posteriorly and inferiorly (see Fig. 56-18).

MAXILLA

The maxilla is a paired bone that is hollowed out by the maxillary sinus and has four processes: the *alveolar process*, which contains the sockets for the upper teeth; the *palatine process*, which extends horizontally to meet its counterpart from the other maxilla at the midline intermaxillary suture, and posteriorly with the horizontal plate of the palatine bone to form the hard palate; the *zygomatic process*, which extends laterally from the area of the first molar and determines the depth of the vestibular fornix; and the *frontal process*, which extends in an ascending direction and articulates with the frontal bone at the frontomaxillary suture.

The terminal branches of the nasopalatine nerve and vessels pass through the *incisive canal*, which opens in the midline anterior area of the palate (Fig. 56-8). The mucosa overlying the incisive canal presents a slight protuberance called the *incisive papilla*. Vessels emerging through the incisive canal are of small caliber, and their surgical interference is of little consequence.

The *greater palatine foramen* opens 3 to 4 mm anterior to the posterior border of the hard palate (Fig. 56-9). The

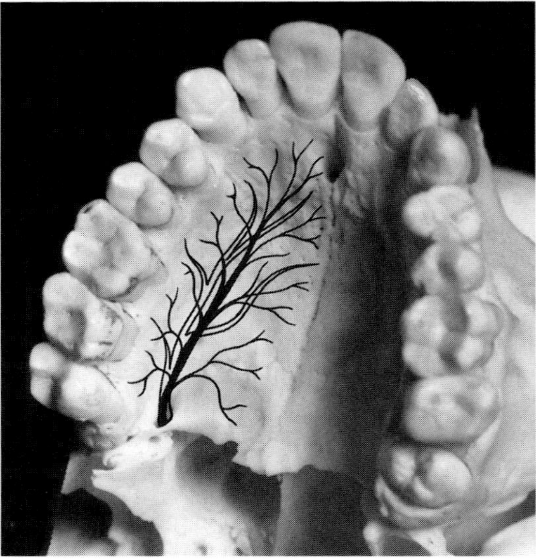

Fig. 56-9 Occlusolateral view of palate showing nerves and vessels emerging from the greater palatine foramen and continuing anteriorly on the palate.

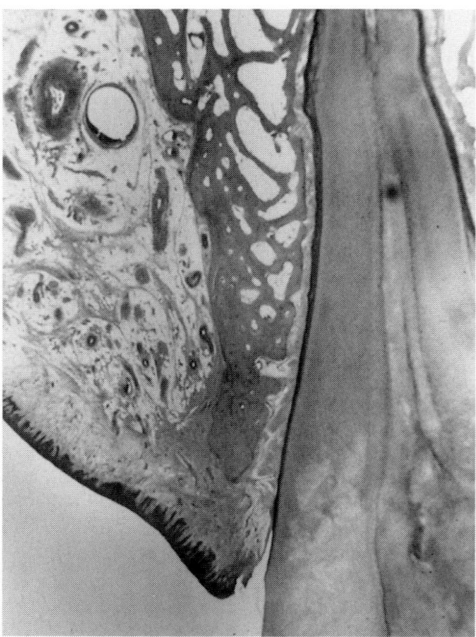

Fig. 56-10 Histologic frontal section of human palate at the level of the first molar, showing the location of vessels and nerve, surrounded by adipose and glandular tissue.

greater palatine nerve and vessels emerge through this foramen and run anteriorly in the submucosa of the palate, between the palatal and alveolar processes (Fig. 56-10). Palatal flaps and donor sites for gingival grafts should be carefully performed and selected to avoid invading these areas, as profuse hemorrhages may ensue, particularly if vessels are damaged at the palatine foramen.

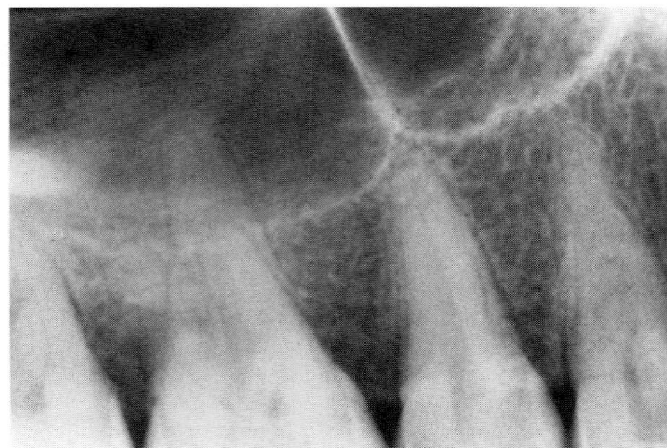

Fig. 56-11 Radiograph of upper molars and premolars, with the maxillary sinus apparently near the apices.

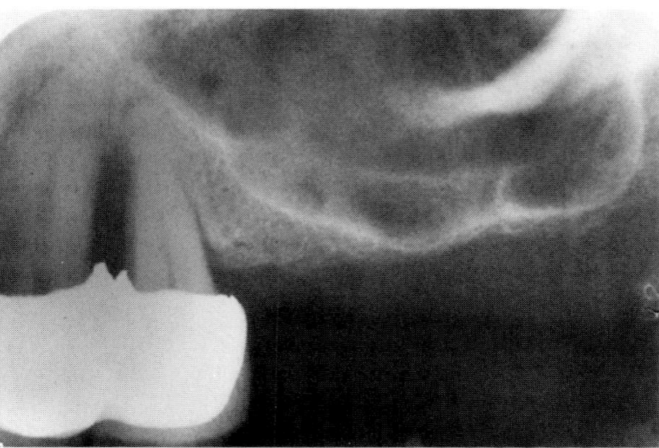

Fig. 56-12 Radiograph of edentulous molar maxillary area, with the sinus very close to the surface.

The mucous membrane covering the hard palate is firmly attached to the underlying bone. The submucous layer of the palate posterior to the first molars contains the *palatal glands,* which are more compact in the soft palate and extend anteriorly, filling the gap between the mucosal connective tissue and the periosteum and protecting the underlying vessels and nerve (see Fig. 56-17).

The area distal to the last molar is called the *maxillary tuberosity* and consists of the posteroinferior angle of the infratemporal surface of the maxilla; medially it articulates with the pyramidal process of the palatine bone. It is covered by fibrous connective tissue and contains the terminal branches of the middle and posterior palatine nerves. Excision of the area for distal wedge surgery may reach medially to the tensor palati muscle, which comes from the greater wing of the sphenoid bone and ends in a tendon that forms the palatine aponeurosis, which expands, fanlike, to attach to the posterior border of the hard palate.

The body of the maxilla is occupied by the *maxillary sinus* or *antrum,* which is a hollow pyramidal area with its base toward the nose and lined by respiratory epithelium. The inferior wall of the maxillary sinus is

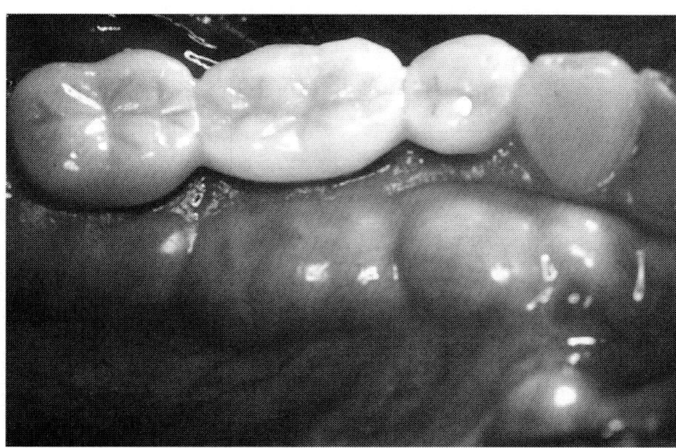

Fig. 56-13 Clinical photograph of mandibular torus.

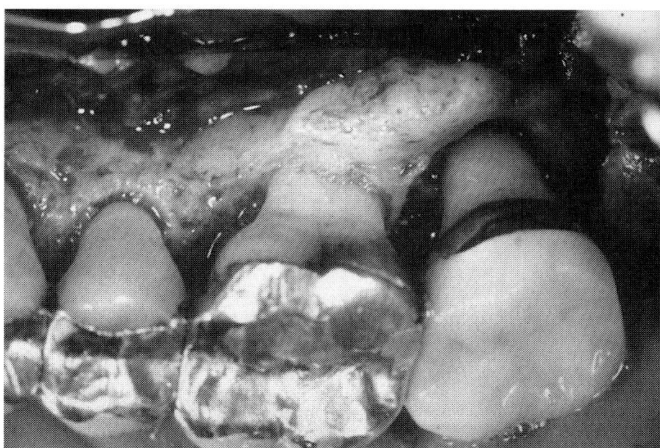

Fig. 56-15 Clinical photograph after flap elevation, showing a palatal torus located near the osseous margin. Note also the circumferential bone loss around the second molar.

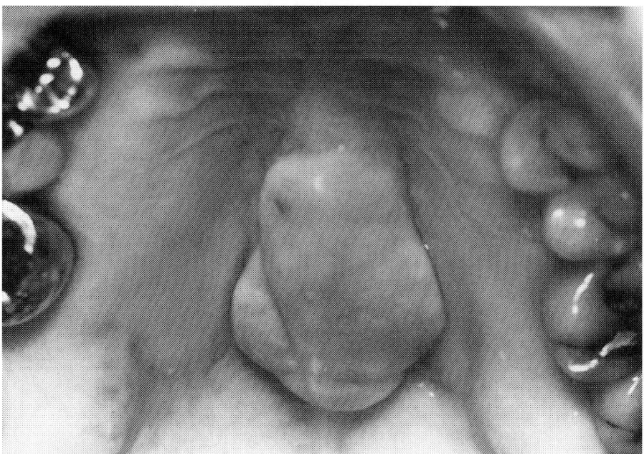

Fig. 56-14 Clinical photograph of palatal torus, located in the midline of the palate.

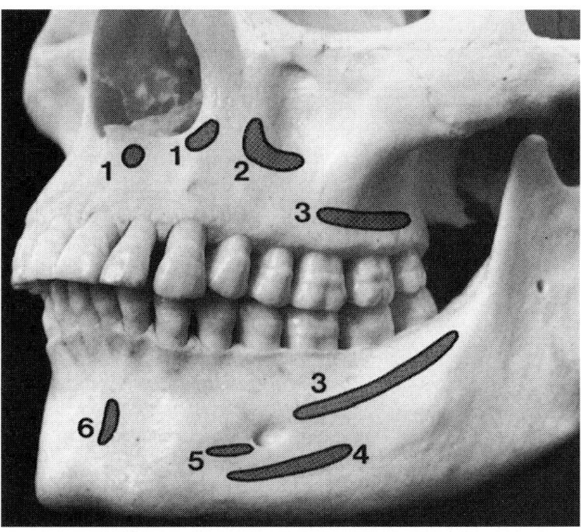

Fig. 56-16 Muscle attachments that may be encountered in mucogingival surgery. *1,* Nasalis; *2,* levator anguli oris; *3,* buccinator; *4,* depressor anguli oris; *5,* depressor labii inferioris; *6,* mentalis.

frequently separated from the apices and roots of the maxillary posterior teeth by a thin, bony plate (Fig. 56-11). In edentulous posterior areas the maxillary sinus bony wall may be only a thin plate in intimate contact with the alveolar mucosa (Fig. 56-12). Adequate determination of the extension of the maxillary sinus into the surgical site is important to avoid creating an oroantral communication, particularly in relation to the placement of implants. In edentulous jaws, determining the amount of available bone in the anterior area, below the floor of the nasal cavity, is also critical.

Both the maxilla and the mandible may have exostoses or tori, which are considered to be within the normal range of anatomic variation. Sometimes they may hinder the removal of plaque by the patient and may have to be removed to improve the prognosis of neighboring teeth. The most common location of a *mandibular torus* is in the lingual area of canine and premolars, above the mylohyoid muscle (Fig. 56-13). *Maxillary tori* are usually located in the midline of the hard palate (Fig. 56-14); smaller tori may be seen over the palatal roots of the molars (Fig. 56-15).

MUSCLES

Several muscles may be encountered when performing periodontal flaps, particularly in mucogingival surgery. These are the *mentalis, incisivus labii inferioris, depressor labii inferioris, depressor anguli oris (triangularis), incisivus labii superioris,* and *buccinator.* Their bony attachment is shown in Fig. 56-16, and they provide mobility to the lips and cheeks.

ANATOMIC SPACES

Several anatomic spaces or compartments are found close to the operative field of periodontal surgery. These spaces contain loose connective tissue but can be easily distended by inflammatory fluid and infection.

Surgical invasion of these areas may result in dangerous infections and should be carefully avoided. Some of

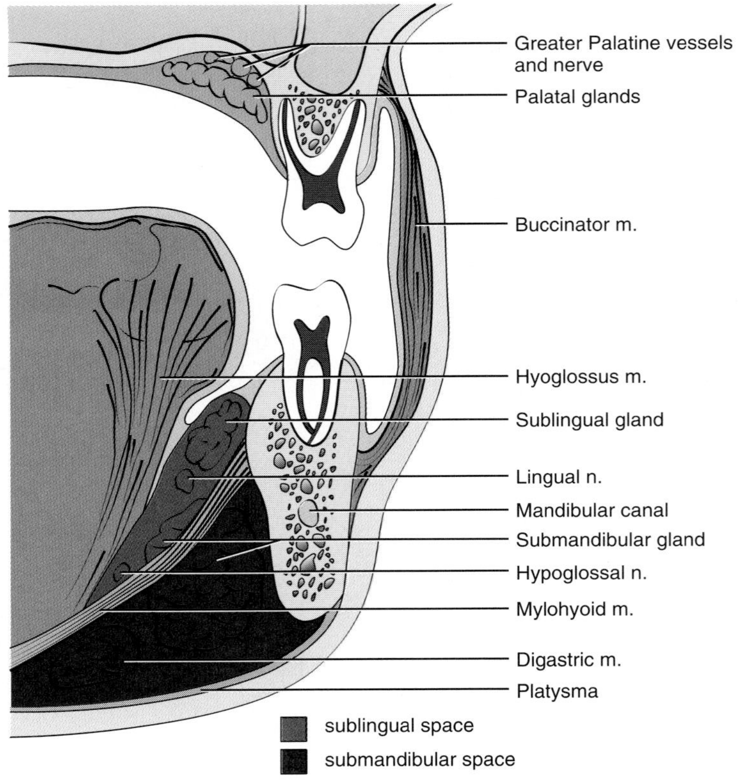

Fig. 56-17 Diagram of a frontal section of the human head at the level of the first molars, depicting the most important structures in relation to periodontal surgery. Note the location of the sublingual space, submandibular space, and greater palatine nerve and vessels.

these spaces are briefly described here. For further information, the reader is referred to other sources.[2,5,6,9,10]

The *canine fossa* contains varying amounts of connective tissue and fat and is bounded superiorly by the quadratus labii superioris muscle, anteriorly by the orbicularis oris, and posteriorly by the buccinator. Infection of this area results in swelling of the upper lip, obliterating the nasolabial fold, and of the upper and lower eyelids, closing the eye.

The *buccal space* is located between the buccinator and the masseter muscles. Infection of this area results in swelling of the cheek but may extend to the temporal space or the submandibular space, with which the buccal space communicates.

The *mental* or *mentalis space* is located in the region of the mental symphysis, where the mental muscle, depressor muscle of the lower lip, and depressor muscle of the corner of the mouth are attached. Infection of this area results in large swelling of the chin, extending downward.

The *masticator space* contains the masseter muscle, pterygoid muscles, tendon of insertion of the temporalis muscle, and mandibular ramus and posterior part of the body of the mandible. Infection of this area results in swelling of the face and severe trismus and pain. If the abscess occupies the deepest part of this compartment, facial swelling may not be obvious but the patient may complain of pain and trismus. Patients may also have difficulty and discomfort when moving the tongue and swallowing.

The *sublingual space* is located below the oral mucosa in the anterior part of the floor of the mouth and contains the sublingual gland and its excretory duct, the submandibular or Wharton's duct, and is traversed by the lingual nerve and vessels and hypoglossal nerve (Fig. 56-17). Its boundaries are the geniohyoid and genioglossus muscles medially and the lingual surface of the mandible and below the mylohyoid muscle laterally and anteriorly (Fig. 56-18). Infection of this area raises the floor of the mouth and displaces the tongue, resulting in pain and difficulty in swallowing but little facial swelling.

The *submental space* is found between the mylohyoid muscle superiorly and the platysma inferiorly. It is bounded laterally by the mandible and posteriorly by the hyoid bone, and it is traversed by the anterior belly of the digastric muscle. Infections of this area arise from the region of the mandibular anterior teeth and result in swelling of the submental region; they become more dangerous as they proceed posteriorly.

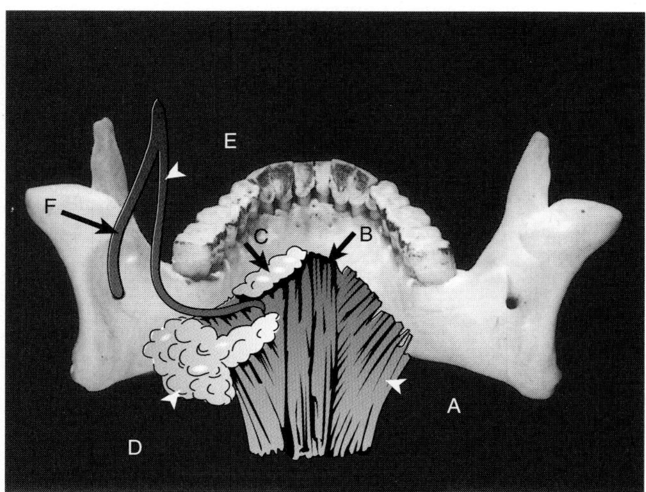

Fig. 56-18 Posterior view of mandible, showing the attachment of the mylohyoid muscles *(A)*; geniohyoid muscles *(B)*; sublingual gland *(C)*; submandibular gland *(D)*, which extends below and also to some extent above the mylohyoid muscle; and sublingual *(E)* and inferior alveolar *(F)* nerves.

The *submandibular space* is found external to the sublingual space, below the mylohyoid and hyoglossus muscles (see Figs. 50-17 and 50-18). This space contains the submandibular gland, which extends partially above the mylohyoid muscle, thus communicating with the sublingual space, and numerous lymph nodes. Infections of this area originate in the molar or premolar area and result in swelling that obliterates the submandibular line and pain when swallowing. Ludwig's angina is a severe form of infection of this space that may extend to the sublingual and submental spaces; it results in hardening of the floor of the mouth and may lead to asphyxiation from edema of the neck and glottis. Although the bacteriology of these infections has not been completely determined, they are presumed to be mixed infections with an important anaerobic component.[1,8]

REFERENCES

1. Bartlett JG, Gorbach SL: Anaerobic infections of the head and neck. Otolaryngol Clin North Am 1976; 9:655.
2. Clarke MA, Bueltmann KW: Anatomical considerations in periodontal surgery. J Periodontol 1971; 42:610.
3. Dixon AD: Anatomy for Students of Dentistry, ed 5. New York, Churchill Livingstone, 1986.
4. DuBrul EL: Sicher and DuBrul's Oral Anatomy, ed 8. St Louis, Ishiyaku EuroAmerica, 1988.
5. Gregg JM: Surgical anatomy. In: Laskin DM: Oral and Maxillofacial Surgery. Vol 1. St Louis, Mosby, 1980.
6. Hollinshead WH: Anatomy for Surgeons. Vol 1: The Head and Neck. New York, Hoeber-Harper, 1954.
7. Kiesselbach JE, Chamberlain JG: Clinical and anatomic observations on the relationship of the lingual nerve to the mandibular third molar region. J Oral Maxillofac Surg 1984; 42:565.
8. Mulligan ME: Ear, nose, throat, and head and neck infections. In: Finegold SM, George WL (eds): Anaerobic Infections in Humans. San Diego, Academic Press, 1989.
9. Spilka CJ: Pathways of dental infections. J Oral Surg 1966; 24:111.
10. Topazian RG, Goldberg MH: Oral and Maxillofacial Infections, ed 3. Philadelphia, Saunders, 1994.

Gingival Curettage

Fermin A. Carranza and Henry H. Takei

CHAPTER

CHAPTER OUTLINE

The word *curettage* is used in periodontics to mean the scraping of the gingival wall of a periodontal pocket to separate diseased soft tissue. *Scaling* refers to the removal of deposits from the root surface, whereas *planing* means smoothing the root to remove infected and necrotic tooth substance. Scaling and root planing may inadvertently include various degrees of curettage. However, they are different procedures, with different rationales and indications, and should be considered separate parts of periodontal treatment.

A differentiation has been made between gingival and subgingival curettage (Fig. 57-1). *Gingival curettage* consists of the removal of the inflamed soft tissue lateral to the pocket wall, whereas *subgingival curettage* refers to the procedure that is performed apical to the epithelial attachment, severing the connective tissue attachment down to the osseous crest.

It should also be understood that some degree of curettage is done unintentionally when scaling and root planing is performed. This is called *inadvertent curettage*. This chapter refers to the purposeful curettage performed during the same visit as scaling and root planing or as a separate operation; its aim is to reduce pocket depth by enhancing gingival shrinkage, new connective tissue attachment, or both.

RATIONALE

Curettage accomplishes the removal of the chronically inflamed granulation tissue that forms in the lateral wall of the periodontal pocket. This tissue, in addition to the usual components of granulation tissues (fibroblastic and angioblastic proliferation), contains areas of chronic inflammation and may also have pieces of dislodged calculus and bacterial colonies. The latter may perpetuate the pathologic features of the tissue and hinder healing.

This inflamed granulation tissue is lined by epithelium, and deep strands of epithelium penetrate into the tissue. The presence of this epithelium is construed as a barrier to the attachment of new fibers in the area.

When the root is thoroughly planed, the major source of bacteria disappears and the pocket pathologic changes resolve with no need to eliminate the inflamed granulation tissue by curettage. The existing granulation tissue is slowly resorbed; the bacteria present, in the absence of replenishment of their numbers by the pocket plaque,

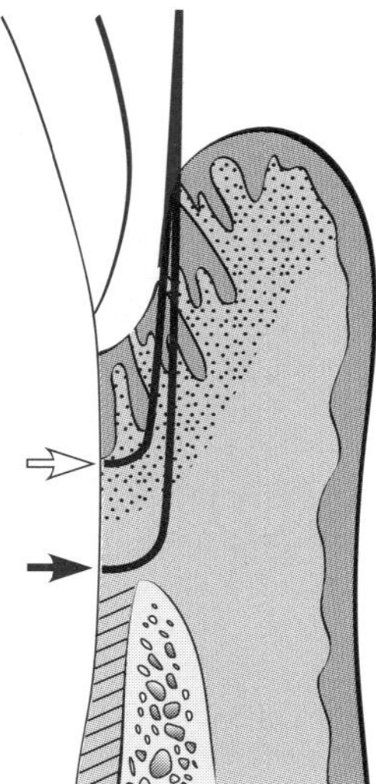

Fig. 57-1 Extent of gingival curettage *(white arrow)* and subgingival curettage *(black arrow).*

are destroyed by the defense mechanisms of the host. *Therefore the need for curettage just to eliminate the inflamed granulation tissue appears questionable.** It has been shown that scaling and root planing with additional curettage does not improve the condition of the periodontal tissues beyond the improvement caused by scaling and root planing alone.

Curettage may also eliminate all or most of the epithelium that lines the pocket wall and the underlying junctional epithelium. This purpose of curettage is still valid, particularly when an attempt is made at new attachment, as occurs in intrabony pockets. However, opinions differ regarding whether scaling and curettage consistently remove the pocket lining and the junctional epithelium. Some investigators report that scaling and root planing tear the epithelial lining of the pocket without removing either it or the junctional epithelium,[15] but both epithelial structures,[3,4,14] sometimes including underlying inflamed connective tissue,[16] are removed by curettage. Other investigators report that the removal of the pocket lining and junctional epithelium by curettage is not complete.[23,25,26]

Curettage and Esthetics

The awareness of esthetics in periodontal therapy has become an integral part of care in the modern practice of periodontics. In the past, pocket elimination was the primary goal of therapy, and little regard was given to the esthetic result. Maximal, rapid shrinkage of gingival tissue was the aim to eliminate the pocket. Currently, esthetics is a major consideration of therapy, particularly in the anterior maxilla (teeth #6 to 11), and *requires preservation of the interdental papilla.*

When regenerative therapy is not possible, every effort should be made to minimize shrinkage or loss of the interdental papilla. A compromise therapy that is feasible in the anterior maxilla, where access is not difficult, consists of thorough subgingival root planing, attempting not to detach the connective tissue beneath the pocket and *avoiding gingival curettage.* The granulation tissue in the lateral wall of the pocket, in an environment free of plaque and calculus, becomes connective tissue, thereby minimizing shrinkage. Thus although complete pocket elimination is not accomplished, the inflammatory changes are reduced or eliminated while the interdental papilla and the esthetic appearance of the area are preserved.

Surgical techniques specially designed to preserve the interdental papilla, such as the papilla preservation technique (see Chapter 60), result in better esthetic appearance of the anterior maxilla than do aggressive scaling and curettage of the area.

Another important precaution refers to root planing apical to the base of the pocket. The removal of the junctional epithelium and disruption of the connective tissue attachment exposes the nondiseased portion of the cementum. Root planing in this area of nondiseased cementum may result in excessive shrinkage of the gingiva, increasing recession or requiring "new attachment" where no disease previously existed.

INDICATIONS

Indications for curettage are very limited. It can be used after scaling and root planing for the following purposes:

1. Curettage can be performed as part of new attachment attempts in moderately deep intrabony pockets located in accessible areas where a type of "closed" surgery is deemed advisable. However, technical difficulties and inadequate accessibility frequently contraindicate such surgery.
2. Curettage can be done as a nondefinitive procedure to reduce inflammation prior to pocket elimination using other methods or in patients in whom more aggressive surgical techniques (e.g., flaps) are contraindicated owing to age, systemic problems, psychologic problems, and so forth. It should be understood that in these patients, the goal of pocket elimination is compromised and prognosis is impaired. The clinician should resort to this approach only when the indicated surgical techniques cannot be performed, and both the clinician and the patient must have a clear understanding of its limitations.
3. Curettage is also frequently performed on recall visits[20] as a method of maintenance treatment for areas of recurrent inflammation and pocket depth, particularly where pocket reduction surgery has previously been performed. Careful probing should establish the

* This should not be confused with elimination of granulation tissue during flap surgery. The reason for the latter is to remove the bleeding tissue that obstructs the view and does not allow the necessary examination of the root surface and the bone morphology. Thus removal of granulation tissue during surgery is done for technical rather than biologic reasons.

extent of the required root planing and curettage to avoid unnecessary shrinkage, pocket formation, or both.

PROCEDURE

Basic Technique

Curettage does not eliminate the causes of inflammation (i.e., bacterial plaque and deposits). *Therefore it should always be preceded by scaling and root planing, which is the basic periodontal therapy procedure.*

Scaling and root planing is described in detail in Chapters 42 and 47. The use of local infiltrative anesthesia for this procedure is optional. However, gingival curettage always requires some type of local anesthesia.

The curette is selected so that the cutting edge will be against the tissue (e.g., the Gracey No. 13-14 is used for mesial surfaces and the Gracey No. 11-12 for distal surfaces). Curettage can also be performed with a 4R-4L Columbia Universal curette. The instrument is inserted so as to engage the inner lining of the pocket wall and is carried along the soft tissue, usually in a horizontal stroke (Fig. 57-2). The pocket wall may be supported by gentle finger pressure on the external surface. The curette is then placed under the cut edge of the junctional epithelium to undermine it.

In subgingival curettage, the tissues attached between the bottom of the pocket and the alveolar crest are removed with a scooping motion of the curette to the tooth surface (Fig. 57-3). The area is flushed to remove debris, and the tissue is partly adapted to the tooth by gentle finger pressure. Sometimes suturing of separated papillae and application of a periodontal pack may be indicated.

Other Techniques

Other techniques for gingival curettage include the excisional new attachment procedure, ultrasonic curettage, and the use of caustic drugs:

Excisional New Attachment Procedure (ENAP). ENAP has been developed and used by the U.S. Naval Dental Corps.[19,29,30] It is a definitive subgingival curettage procedure performed with a knife. The technique is as follows:

1. After adequate anesthesia, an internal bevel incision is made from the margin of the free gingiva apically to a point below the bottom of the pocket (Fig. 57-4). The incision is carried interproximally on both the facial and the lingual sides, attempting to retain as much interproximal tissue as possible. The intention is to cut the inner portion of the soft tissue wall of the pocket, all around the tooth.
2. Remove the excised tissue with a curette, and carefully root plane all exposed cementum to a smooth, hard consistency. Preserve all connective tissue fibers that remain attached to the root surface.
3. Approximate the wound edges; if they do not meet passively, recontour the bone until good adaptation of the wound edges is achieved. Place sutures and a periodontal dressing.

Ultrasonic Curettage. The use of ultrasonic devices has been recommended for gingival curettage.[17] When applied to the gingiva of experimental animals, ultrasonic vibrations disrupt tissue continuity, lift off epithelium, dismember collagen bundles, and alter the morphologic features of fibroblast nuclei.[10] Ultrasound is effective for debriding the epithelial lining of periodontal pockets[10]; it results in a narrow band of necrotic tissue (microcauterization), which strips off the inner lining of the pocket.

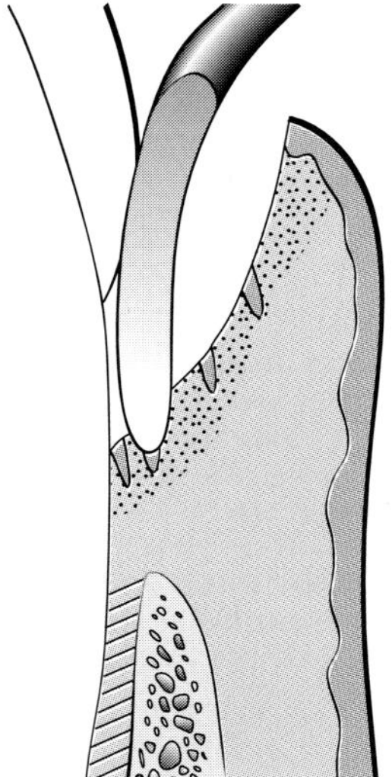

Fig. 57-2 Gingival curettage performed with a horizontal stroke of the curette.

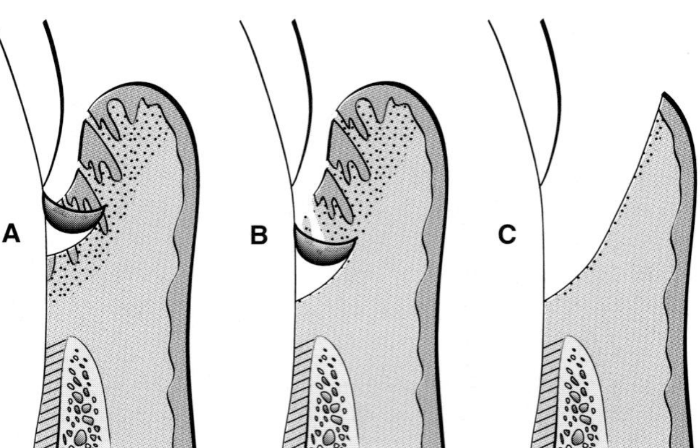

Fig. 57-3 Subgingival curettage. **A,** Elimination of pocket lining. **B,** Elimination of junctional epithelium and granulation tissue. **C,** Procedure completed.

The Morse scaler-shaped and rod-shaped ultrasonic instruments are used for this purpose. Some investigators found ultrasonic instruments to be as effective as manual instruments for curettage[17,22,31] but resulted in less inflammation and less removal of underlying connective tissue. The gingiva can be made more rigid for ultrasonic curettage by injecting anesthetic solution directly into it.[7]

Caustic Drugs. Since early in the development of periodontal procedures,[24,28] the use of caustic drugs has been recommended to induce a chemical curettage of the lateral wall of the pocket or even the selective elimination of the epithelium. Drugs such as sodium sulfide, alkaline sodium hypochlorite solution (Antiformin),[5,11,12] and phenol[1,6] have been proposed and then discarded after studies showed their ineffectiveness.[2,9,12] The extent of tissue destruction with these drugs cannot be controlled, and they may increase rather than reduce the amount of tissue to be removed by enzymes and phagocytes.

HEALING AFTER SCALING AND CURETTAGE

Immediately after curettage, a blood clot fills the pocket area, which is totally or partially devoid of epithelial lining. Hemorrhage is also present in the tissues with dilated capillaries, and abundant polymorphonuclear leukocytes appear shortly thereafter on the wound surface. This is followed by a rapid proliferation of granulation tissue, with a decrease in the number of small blood vessels as the tissue matures.

Restoration and epithelialization of the sulcus generally require from 2 to 7 days,[13,16,18,26] and restoration of the junctional epithelium occurs in animals as early as 5 days after treatment. Immature collagen fibers appear within 21 days. Healthy gingival fibers inadvertently severed from the tooth and tears in the epithelium[15,21] are repaired in the healing process. Several investigators have reported that in monkeys[8,29] and humans[27] treated by scaling procedures and curettage, healing results in the formation of a long, thin junctional epithelium with no new connective tissue attachment. Sometimes this long epithelium is interrupted by "windows" of connective tissue attachment.[8]

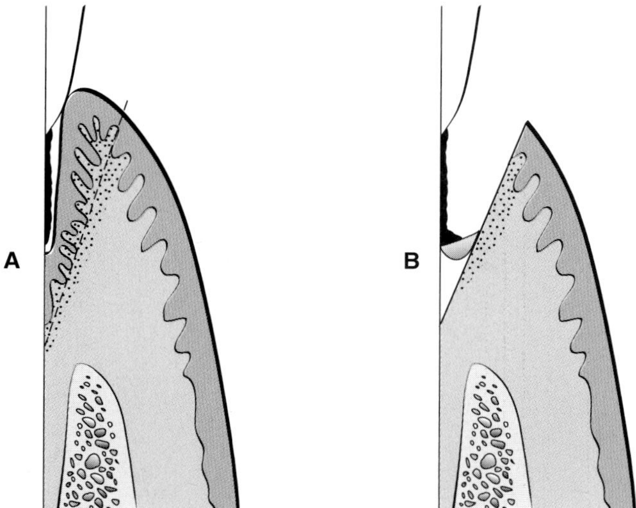

Fig. 57-4 Excisional new attachment procedure. **A,** Internal bevel incision to point below bottom of pocket. **B,** After excision of tissue, scaling and root planing are performed.

CLINICAL APPEARANCE AFTER SCALING AND CURETTAGE

Immediately after scaling and curettage, the gingiva appears hemorrhagic and bright red.

After 1 week, the gingiva appears reduced in height owing to an apical shift in the position of the gingival margin. The gingiva is also slightly redder than normal, but much less so than on previous days.

After 2 weeks and with proper oral hygiene by the patient, the normal color, consistency, surface texture, and contour of the gingiva are attained, and the gingival margin is well adapted to the tooth.

REFERENCES

1. Barkann A: A conservative technique for the eradication of a pyorrhea product. J Am Dent Assoc 1939; 26:61.
2. Beube FE: An experimental study of the use of sodium sulphide solution in treatment of periodontal pockets. J Periodontol 1939; 10:49.
3. Beube FE: Treatment methods for marginal gingivitis and periodontitis. Texas Dent J 1953; 71:427.
4. Blass JL, Lite T: Gingival healing following surgical curettage: A histopathologic study. NY Dent J 1959; 25:127.
5. Box KF: Periodontal disease and treatment. J Ontario Dent Assoc 1952; 29:194.
6. Bunting RW: The control and treatment of pyorrhea by subgingival surgery. J Am Dent Assoc 1928; 15:119.
7. Burman LR, Alderman LE, Ewen SJ: Clinical application of ultrasonic vibrations for supragingival calculus and stain removal. J Dent Med 1958; 13:156.
8. Caton JC, Zander HA: The attachment between tooth and gingival tissues after periodic root planing and soft tissue curettage. J Periodontol 1979; 50:462.
9. Glickman J, Patur B: Histologic study of the effect of Antiformin on the soft tissue wall of periodontal pockets in humans. J Am Dent Assoc 1955; 51:420.
10. Goldman HM: Histologic assay of healing following ultrasonic curettage versus hand instrument curettage. Oral Med Oral Pathol 1961; 14:925.
11. Hunter HA: A study of tissues treated with Antiformin citric acid. J Can Dent Assoc 1955; 21:344.
12. Johnson RW, Waerhaug J: Effect of Antiformin on gingival tissue. J Periodontol 1956; 27:24.
13. Kon S, Novaes AB, Ruben MP, et al: Visualization of microvascularization of the healing periodontal wound. II. Curettage. J Periodontol 1969; 40:96.
14. Morris ML: The removal of the pocket and attachment epithelium in humans: A histological study. J Periodontol 1954; 25:7.
15. Moskow BS: The response of the gingival sulcus to instrumentation: A histologic investigation. I. The scaling procedure. J Periodontol 1962; 33:282.
16. Moskow BS: The response of the gingival sulcus to instru-

mentation: A histologic investigation. II. Gingival curettage. J Periodontol 1964; 35:112.
17. Nadler H: Removal of crevicular epithelium by ultrasonic curettes. J Periodontol 1962; 33:220.
18. O'Bannon JY: The gingival tissues before and after scaling the teeth. J Periodontol 1964; 35:69.
19. Periodontics Syllabus: NAVED P5110. US Naval Dental Corps, 1975, pp 113–115.
20. Ramfjord SP, Ash MM Jr: Periodontology and Periodontics. Philadelphia, Saunders, 1979.
21. Ramfjord SP, Kiester G: The gingival sulcus and the periodontal pocket immediately following scaling of the teeth. J Periodontol 1954; 25:167.
22. Sanderson AD: Gingival curettage by hand and ultrasonic instruments—A histologic comparison. J Periodontol 1966; 37:279.
23. Sato M: Histopathological study of the healing process after surgical treatment for alveolar pyorrhea. Bull Tokyo Dent College 1960; 1:71.
24. Stewart H: Partial removal of cementum and decalcification of tooth in the treatment of pyorrhea alveolaris. Dent Cosmos 1899; 41:617.
25. Stone S, Ramfjord SP, Waldron J: Scaling and gingival curettage—A radioautographic study. J Periodontol 1966; 37:415.
26. Waerhaug J: Microscopic demonstration of tissue reaction incident to removal of subgingival calculus. J Periodontol 1955; 26:26.
27. Waerhaug J: Healing of the dentoepithelial junction following subgingival plaque control. I. As observed in human biopsy material. J Periodontol 1978; 49:1.
28. Younger WJ: Some of the latest phases in implantations and other procedures. Dent Cosmos 1893; 35:102.
29. Yukna RA: A clinical and histological study of healing following the excisional new attachment procedure in rhesus monkeys. J Periodontol 1976; 47:701.
30. Yukna RA, Bowers GM, Lawrence JJ, et al: A clinical study of healing in humans following the excisional new attachment procedure. J Periodontol 1976; 47:696.
31. Zach L, Cohen G: The histologic response to ultrasonic curettage. J Dent Res 1961; 40:751.

The Gingivectomy Technique

Fermin A. Carranza

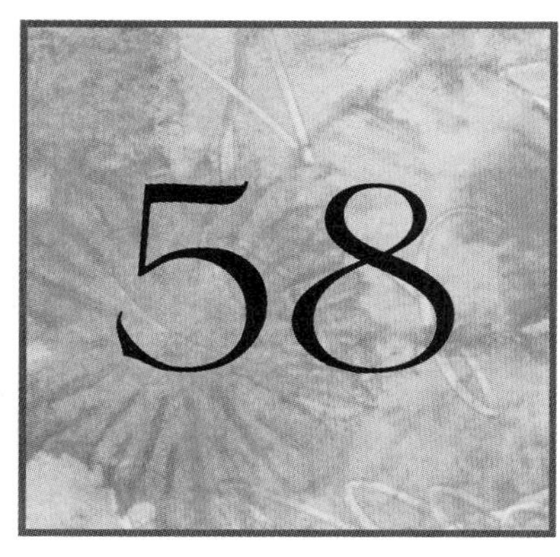

CHAPTER

CHAPTER OUTLINE

Gingivectomy means excision of the gingiva. By removing the pocket wall, gingivectomy provides visibility and accessibility for complete calculus removal and thorough smoothing of the roots (Fig. 58-1), creating a favorable environment for gingival healing and restoration of a physiologic gingival contour.

The gingivectomy technique was widely performed in the past. Improved understanding of healing mechanisms and the development of more sophisticated flap methods have relegated the gingivectomy to a lesser role in the current repertoire of available techniques. However, it remains an effective form of treatment when indicated (Fig. 58-2).

INDICATIONS AND CONTRAINDICATIONS

The gingivectomy technique may be performed for:

1. Elimination of suprabony pockets, regardless of their depth, if the pocket wall is fibrous and firm
2. Elimination of gingival enlargements
3. Elimination of suprabony periodontal abscesses[8]

Contraindications include the following:

1. The need for bone surgery or examination of the bone shape and morphology
2. Situations in which the bottom of the pocket is apical to the mucogingival junction
3. Esthetic considerations, particularly in the anterior maxilla

The gingivectomy technique may be performed by means of scalpels, electrodes, laser beams, or chemicals. All these techniques will be reviewed, although the surgical method is the only one recommended.

SURGICAL GINGIVECTOMY

Step 1: The pockets on each surface are explored with a periodontal probe and marked with a pocket marker (Figs. 58-3 and 58-4). Each pocket is marked in several areas to outline its course on each surface.

Step 2: Periodontal knives (e.g., Kirkland knives) are used for incisions on the facial and lingual surfaces and those distal to the terminal tooth in the arch. Orban periodontal knives are used for supplemental interdental incisions, if necessary, and Bard-Parker knives #11 and 12 and scissors are used as auxiliary instruments.

The incision is started apical to the points marking the course of the pockets[27,31] and is directed coronally to a point between the base of the pocket and the crest of the bone. It should be as close as possible to the bone without exposing it to remove the soft tissue coronal to the bone. Exposure of bone is undesirable. If it occurs, healing usually presents no problem if the area is adequately covered by the periodontal pack.

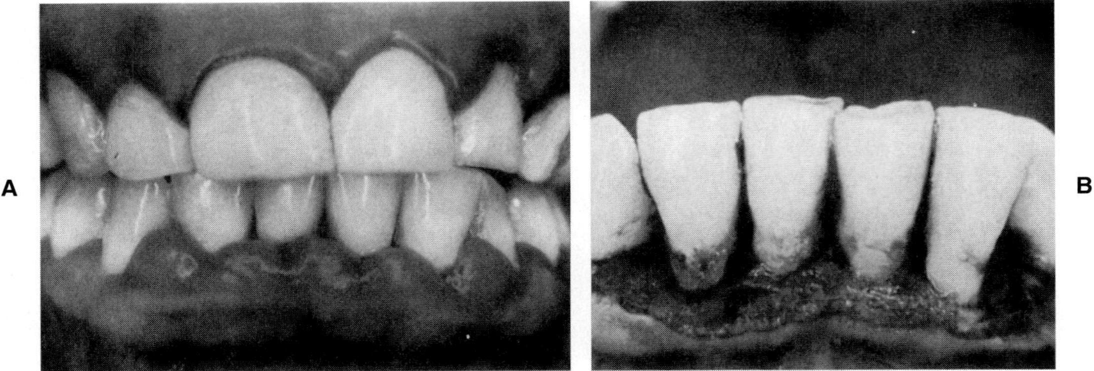

Fig. 58-1 Visibility and accessibility of calculus. **A,** Gingival enlargement. **B,** Removal of diseased gingiva exposes calculus. (Phase I therapy is sometimes omitted when the indication for a gingivectomy is obvious. It can never be omitted when a flap appears to be indicated.)

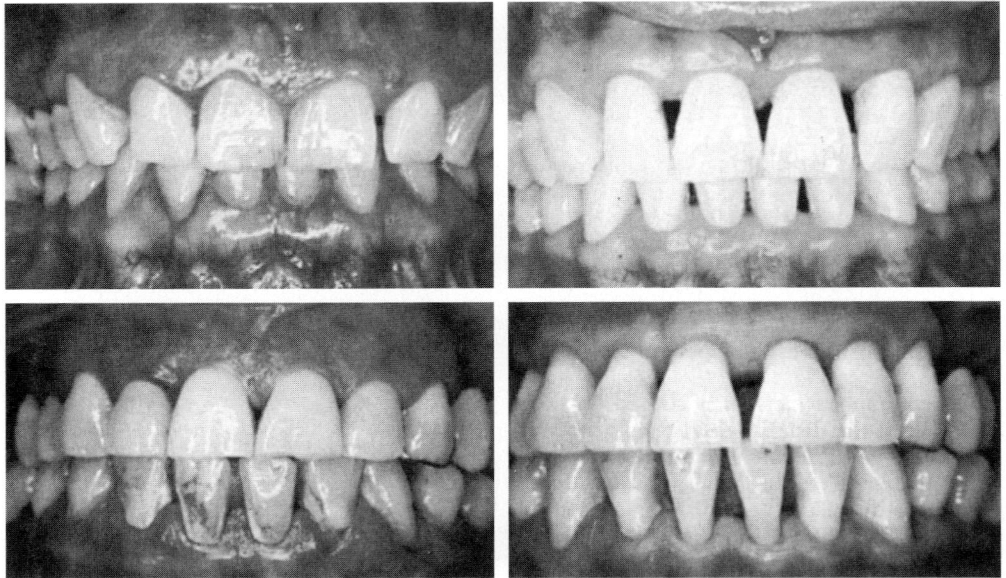

Fig. 58-2 Results obtained by treating suprabony pockets of different depths with gingivectomy. *Left,* Before treatment. *Right,* After treatment.

Discontinuous or continuous incisions may be used. Fig. 58-5 shows the design of each of these two incisions. *The incision should be beveled at approximately 45 degrees to the tooth surface and should recreate, as far as possible, the normal festooned pattern of the gingiva.* Failure to bevel leaves a broad, fibrous plateau that takes more time than is ordinarily required to develop a physiologic contour. In the interim, plaque and food accumulation may lead to recurrence of pockets.

Step 3: Remove the excised pocket wall, clean the area, and closely examine the root surface. The most apical zone consists of a bandlike light zone where the tissues were attached, and coronally to it some calculus remnants, root caries, or root resorption may be found. Granulation tissue may be seen on the excised soft tissue (Fig. 58-6).

Step 4: Carefully curette out the granulation tissue and remove any remaining calculus and necrotic cementum so as to leave a smooth and clean surface.

Step 5: Cover the area with a surgical pack (see Chapter 55).

Gingivoplasty

Gingivoplasty is similar to gingivectomy, but its purpose is different. Gingivectomy is performed to eliminate periodontal pockets and includes reshaping as part of the technique. Gingivoplasty is a reshaping of the gingiva to create physiologic gingival contours, with the sole purpose of recontouring the gingiva in the absence of pockets.

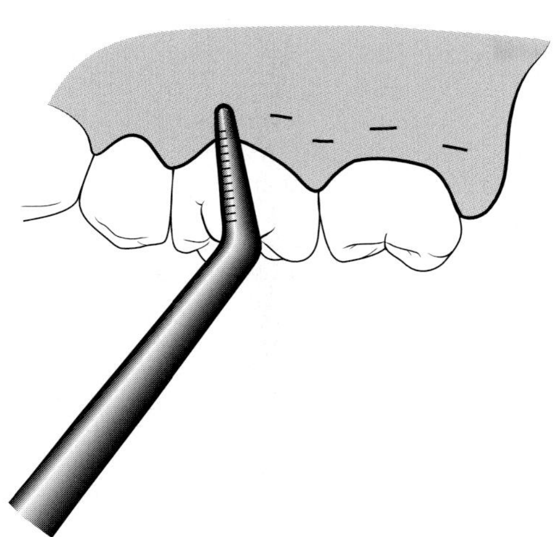

Fig. 58-3 Pocket marker makes pinpoint perforations that indicate pocket depth.

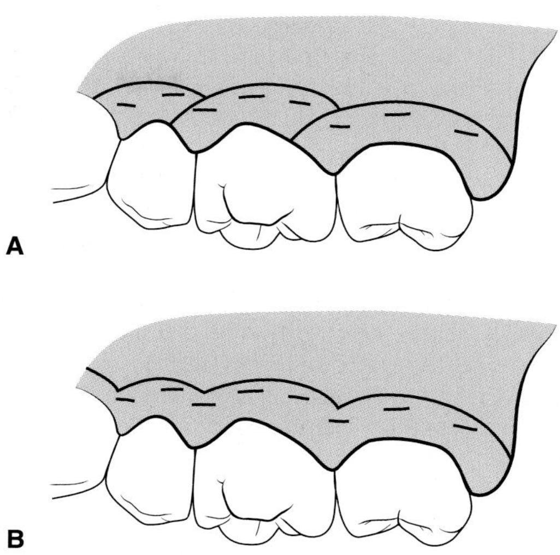

Fig. 58-5 A, Discontinuous incision apical to bottom of the pocket indicated by pinpoint markings. **B,** Continuous incision begins on the molar and extends anteriorly without interruption.

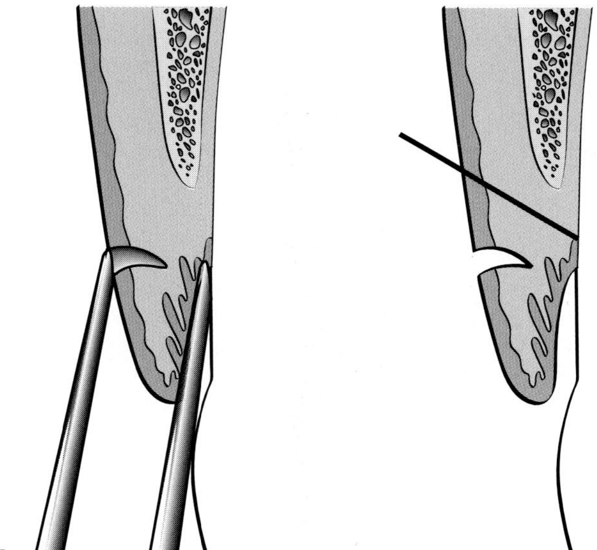

Fig. 58-4 Marking the depth of suprabony pocket. **A,** Pocket marker in position. **B,** Beveled incision extends apical to the perforation made by the pocket marker.

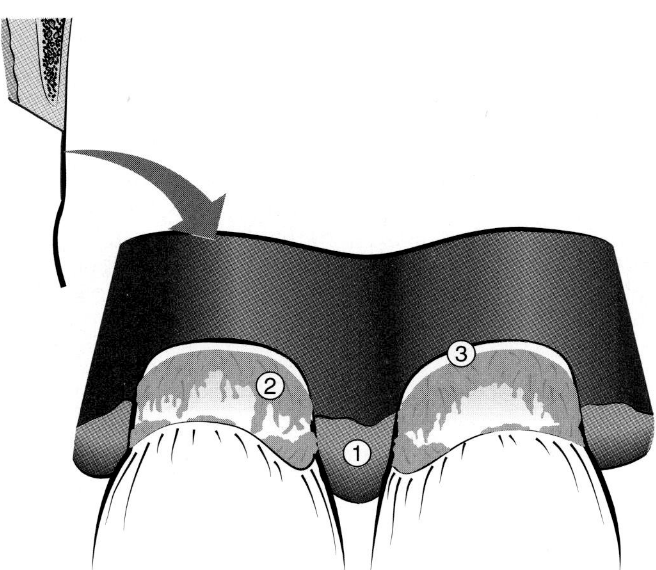

Fig. 58-6 Field of operation immediately after removing pocket wall. *1,* Granulation tissue; *2,* calculus and other root deposits; *3,* clear space where bottom of the pocket was attached.

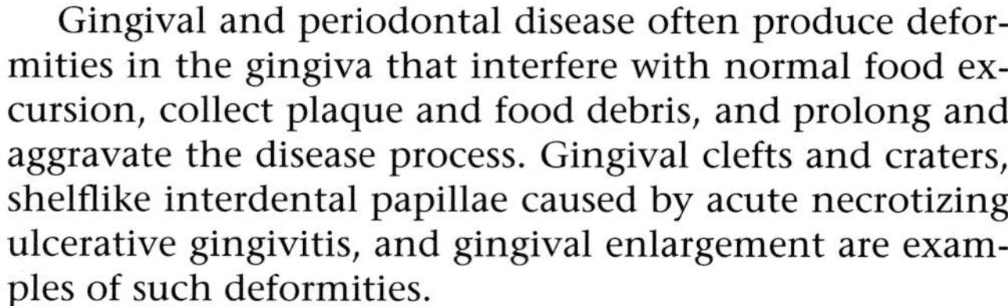

Gingival and periodontal disease often produce deformities in the gingiva that interfere with normal food excursion, collect plaque and food debris, and prolong and aggravate the disease process. Gingival clefts and craters, shelflike interdental papillae caused by acute necrotizing ulcerative gingivitis, and gingival enlargement are examples of such deformities.

Gingivoplasty may be done with a periodontal knife, a scalpel, rotary coarse diamond stones,[6] or electrodes.[5] It consists of procedures that resemble those performed in festooning artificial dentures; namely, tapering the gingival margin, creating a scalloped marginal outline, thinning the attached gingiva, and creating vertical interdental grooves and shaping the interdental papillae to provide sluiceways for the passage of food.

Healing after Surgical Gingivectomy

The initial response is the formation of a protective surface clot; the underlying tissue becomes acutely inflamed, with some necrosis. The clot is then replaced by granulation tissue. By 24 hours, there is an increase in new connective tissue cells, mainly angioblasts, just beneath the surface layer of inflammation and necrosis; by the third day, numerous young fibroblasts are located in the area.[26] The highly vascular granulation tissue grows coronally, creating a new free gingival margin and sulcus.[22] Capillaries derived from blood vessels of the periodontal ligament migrate into the granulation tissue, and within 2 weeks they connect with gingival vessels.[32]

After 12 to 24 hours, epithelial cells at the margins of the wound start to migrate over the granulation tissue, separating it from the contaminated surface layer of the clot. Epithelial activity at the margins reaches a peak in 24 to 36 hours[5]; the new epithelial cells arise from the basal and deeper spinous layers of the wound edge epithelium and migrate over the wound over a fibrin layer that is later resorbed and replaced by a connective tissue bed.[14] The epithelial cells advance by a tumbling action, with the cells becoming fixed to the substrate by hemidesmosomes and a new basement lamina.[15]

Surface epithelization is generally complete after 5 to 14 days. During the first 4 weeks after gingivectomy, keratinization is less than it was prior to surgery. Complete epithelial repair takes about 1 month.[29] Vasodilation and vascularity begin to decrease after the fourth day of healing and appear to be almost normal by the 16th day.[19] Complete repair of the connective tissue takes about 7 weeks.[29]

The flow of gingival fluid in humans is initially increased after gingivectomy and diminishes as healing progresses.[1,28] Maximal flow is reached after 1 week, coinciding with the time of maximal inflammation.

Although the tissue changes that occur in postgingivectomy healing are the same in all individuals, the time required for complete healing varies considerably, depending on the area of the cut surface and interference from local irritation and infection. In patients with physiologic gingival melanosis, the pigmentation is diminished in the healed gingiva.

GINGIVECTOMY BY ELECTROSURGERY

Advantages

Electrosurgery permits an adequate contouring of the tissue and controls hemorrhage.[9,21]

Disadvantages

Electrosurgery cannot be used in patients who have noncompatible or poorly shielded cardiac pacemakers. The treatment causes an unpleasant odor. If the electrosurgery point touches the bone, irreparable damage can be done[2,9,12,25]; furthermore, the heat generated by injudicious use can cause tissue damage and loss of periodontal support when the electrode is used close to bone. When the electrode touches the root, areas of cementum burn are produced.[33] *Therefore the use of electrosurgery should be limited to superficial procedures such as removal of gingival enlargements, gingivoplasty, relocation of frenum and muscle attachments, and incision of periodontal abscesses and pericoronal flaps; extreme care should be exercised to avoid contacting the tooth surface. It should not be used for procedures that involve proximity to the bone, such as flap operations, or mucogingival surgery.*

Technique

The removal of gingival enlargements and gingivoplasty[21] is performed with the needle electrode, supplemented by the small ovoid loop or the diamond-shaped electrodes for festooning. A blended cutting and coagulating (fully rectified) current is used. In all reshaping procedures, the electrode is activated and moved in a concise "shaving" motion.

In the treatment of acute periodontal abscesses, the incision to establish drainage can be made with the needle electrode without exerting painful pressure. The incision remains open because the edges are sealed by the current. After the acute symptoms subside, the regular procedure for the treatment of the periodontal abscess is followed (see Chapter 46).

For hemostasis, the ball electrode is used. Hemorrhage must be controlled by direct pressure (via air, compress, or hemostat) first; then the surface is lightly touched with a coagulating current. Electrosurgery is helpful for the control of isolated bleeding points. Bleeding areas located interproximally are reached with a thin, bar-shaped electrode.

Frenum and muscle attachments can be relocated to facilitate pocket elimination using a loop electrode. For this purpose, the frenum or muscle is stretched and sectioned with the loop electrode and a coagulating current. For cases of acute pericoronitis, drainage may be obtained by incising the flap with a bent needle electrode. A loop electrode is used to remove the flap after the acute symptoms subside.

Healing after Electrosurgery

Some investigators report no significant differences in gingival healing after resection by electrosurgery and resection with periodontal knives[6,18]; other researchers find delayed healing, greater reduction in gingival height, and more bone injury after electrosurgery.[25] There appears to be little difference in the results obtained after shallow gingival resection with electrosurgery and that with periodontal knives. *However, when used for deep resections close to bone, electrosurgery can produce gingival recession, bone necrosis and sequestration, loss of bone height, furcation exposure, and tooth mobility, which do not occur with the use of periodontal knives.*[2,9]

LASER GINGIVECTOMY

The lasers most commonly used in dentistry are the carbon dioxide (CO_2) and the neodymium:yttrium-aluminum-garnet (Nd:YAG), which have wavelengths of 10,600 nm and 1064 nm, respectively, both in the infrared range; they must be combined with other types of visible lasers for the beam to be seen and aimed.

The CO_2 laser beam has been used for the excision of gingival growths,[3,23] although healing is delayed when compared with healing after conventional scalpel gingivectomy.[11,17,24] The use of laser beam for oral surgery requires precautionary measures to avoid reflecting the beam on instrument surfaces, which could result in injury to neighboring tissues and the eyes of the operator.

At present, the use of lasers for periodontal surgery is not supported by research and is therefore discouraged. The use of lasers for other periodontal purposes, such as subgingival curettage is equally unsubstantiated and is also not recommended.

GINGIVECTOMY BY CHEMOSURGERY

Techniques to remove the gingiva using chemicals, such as 5% paraformaldehyde[20] or potassium hydroxide,[16] have been described in the past but are not currently used. They are presented here to provide a historical perspective.

The chemical gingivectomy has the following disadvantages:

1. The depth of action cannot be controlled, and therefore healthy attached tissue underlying the pocket may be injured.
2. Gingival remodeling cannot be accomplished effectively.
3. Epithelialization and reformation of the junctional epithelium and reestablishment of the alveolar crest fiber system are slower in chemically treated gingival wounds than in those produced by a scalpel.[30]

The use of chemical methods therefore is not recommended.

REFERENCES

1. Arnold R, Lunstad G, Bissada N, et al: Alterations in crevicular fluid flow during healing following gingival surgery. J Periodont Res 1966; 1:303.
2. Azzi R, Kenney EB, Tsao TF, et al: The effect of electrosurgery upon alveolar bone. J Periodontol 1983; 54:96.
3. Barak S, Kaplan H: The CO_2 laser in the surgical excision of gingival hyperplasia caused by nifedipine. J Clin Periodontol 1988; 15:633.
4. Eisenmann D, Malone WF, and Kusek J: Electron microscopic evaluation of electrosurgery. Oral Surg 1970; 29:660.
5. Engler WO, Ramfjord S, Hiniker JJ: Healing following simple gingivectomy. A tritiated thymidine radioautographic study. I. Epithelialization. J Periodontol 1966; 37:289.
6. Fisher SE, Frame JW, Browne RM, et al: A comparative histological study of wound healing following CO_2 laser and conventional surgical excision of the buccal mucosa. Arch Oral Biol 1983; 28:287.
7. Flocken JE: Electrosurgical management of soft tissues and restoration dentistry. Dent Clin North Am 1980; 24:247.
8. Glickman I: The results obtained with the unembellished gingivectomy technique in a clinical study in humans. J Periodontol 1956; 27:247.
9. Glickman I, Imber LR: Comparison of gingival resection with electrosurgery and periodontal knives: a biometric and histologic study. J Periodontol 1970; 41:142.
10. Goldman HM: The development of physiologic gingival contours by gingivoplasty. Oral Surg 1950; 3:879.
11. Gottsegen R, Ammons WF Jr: Research in Lasers in Periodontics. Position Paper. Chicago, American Academy of Periodontology, May 1992.
12. Henning F: Healing of gingivectomy wounds in the rat: Reestablishment of the epithelial seal. J Periodontol 1968; 39:265.
13. Henning F: Epithelial mitotic activity after gingivectomy. Relationship to reattachment. J Periodont Res 1969; 4:319.
14. Innes PB: An electron microscopic study of the regeneration of gingival epithelium following gingivectomy in the dog. J Periodont Res 1970; 5:196.
15. Krawczyk WS: A pattern of epithelial cell migration during wound healing. J Cell Biol 1971; 49:247.
16. Löe H: Chemical gingivectomy. Effect of potassium hydroxide on periodontal tissues. Acta Odontol Scand 1961; 19:517.
17. Loumanen M: A comparative study of healing of laser and scalpel incision wounds in rat oral mucosa. Scand J Dent Res 1987; 95:65.
18. Malone WF, Eisenmann D, Kusck J: Interceptive periodontics with electrosurgery. J Prosthet Dent 1969; 22:555.
19. Novaes AB, Kon S, Ruben MP, et al: Visualization of the microvascularization of the healing periodontal wound. III. Gingivectomy. J Periodontol 1969; 40:359.
20. Orban B: New methods in periodontal treatment. Bur 1942; 42:116.
21. Oringer MJ: Electrosurgery for definitive conservative modern periodontal therapy. Dent Clin North Am 1969; 13:53.
22. Persson PA: The healing process in the marginal periodontium after gingivectomy with special regard to the regeneration of epithelium (an experimental study on dogs). Odontol T 1959; 67:593.
23. Pick RM, Pecaro BC, Silberman CJ: The laser gingivectomy: The use of CO_2 laser for the removal of phenytoin hyperplasia. J Periodontol 1985; 56:492.
24. Pogrel MA, Yen CK, Hanser LS: A comparison of carbon dioxide laser, liquid nitrogen cryosurgery and scalpel wound in healing. Oral Surg Med Pathol 1990; 69:269.
25. Pope JW, Gargiulo AW, Staffileno H, et al: Effects of electrosurgery on wound healing in dogs. Periodontics 1968; 6:30.
26. Ramfjord SP, Engler WD, Hiniker JJ: A radiographic study of healing following simple gingivectomy. II. The connective tissue. J Periodontol 1966; 37:179.
27. Ritchey B, Orban B: The periodontal pocket. J Periodontol 1952; 23:199.
28. Sandalli P, Wade AB: Alterations in crevicular fluid flow during healing following gingivectomy and flap procedures. J Periodont Res 1969; 4:314.
29. Stanton G, Levy M, Stahl SS: Collagen restoration in healing human gingiva. J Dent Res 1969; 48:27.
30. Tonna E, Stahl SS: A polarized light microscopic study of rat periodontal ligament following surgical and chemical gingival trauma. Helv Odontol Acta 1967; 11:90.
31. Waerhaug J: Depth of incision in gingivectomy. Oral Surg 1955; 8:707.
32. Watanabe Y, Suzuki S: An experimental study in capillary vascularization in the periodontal tissue following gingivectomy or flap operation. J Dent Res 1963; 42:758.
33. Wilhelmsen NR, Ramfjord SP, Blankenship JR: Effects of electrosurgery on the gingival attachment in Rhesus monkeys. J Periodontol 1976; 47:160.

Treatment of Gingival Enlargement

Paulo M. Camargo and Fermin A. Carranza

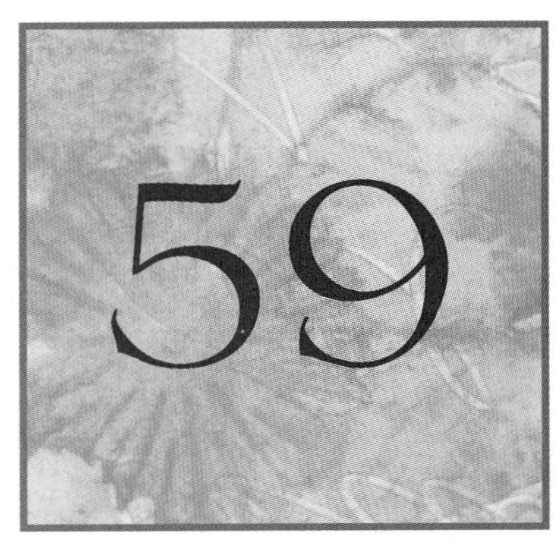

CHAPTER

CHAPTER OUTLINE

Treatment of gingival enlargement is based on an understanding of the cause and underlying pathologic changes (see Chapter 18). Gingival enlargements are of special concern to the patient and the dentist because they pose problems in plaque control, function (including mastication, tooth eruption and speech), and esthetics. Because gingival enlargements differ in cause, treatment of each type is best considered individually.

TREATMENT OF CHRONIC INFLAMMATORY ENLARGEMENT

Chronic inflammatory enlargements, which are soft and discolored and are caused principally by edema and cellular infiltration, are treated by *scaling and root planing,* provided the size of the enlargement does not interfere with complete removal of deposits from the involved tooth surfaces.

When chronic inflammatory gingival enlargements include a significant fibrotic component that does not undergo shrinkage after scaling and root planing or are of such size that they obscure deposits on the tooth surfaces and interfere with access to them, *surgical removal* is the treatment of choice. Two techniques are available for this purpose: gingivectomy and flap operation.

Selection of the appropriate technique depends on the size of the enlargement and character of the tissue. When the enlarged gingiva remains soft and friable even after scaling and root planing, a gingivectomy is used to remove it because a flap requires a firmer tissue to adequately perform the incisions and other steps in the technique (Fig. 59-1). However, if the gingivectomy incision removes all the attached gingiva, creating a mucogingival problem, then a flap operation is indicated.

Tumorlike inflammatory enlargements are treated by gingivectomy as follows: Under local anesthesia, the tooth surfaces beneath the mass are scaled to remove calculus and other debris. The lesion is separated from the mucosa at its base with a #12 Bard-Parker blade. If the lesion extends interproximally, the interdental gingiva is included in the incision to ensure exposure of irritating root deposits. After the lesion is removed, the involved root surfaces are scaled and planed and the area is cleansed with warm water. A periodontal pack is applied and removed after a week, at which time the patient is instructed in plaque control (Fig. 59-2, *A* and *B*).

The Flap Operation

See Chapters 60 and 61 and the following discussion of the flap technique for drug-induced enlargements.

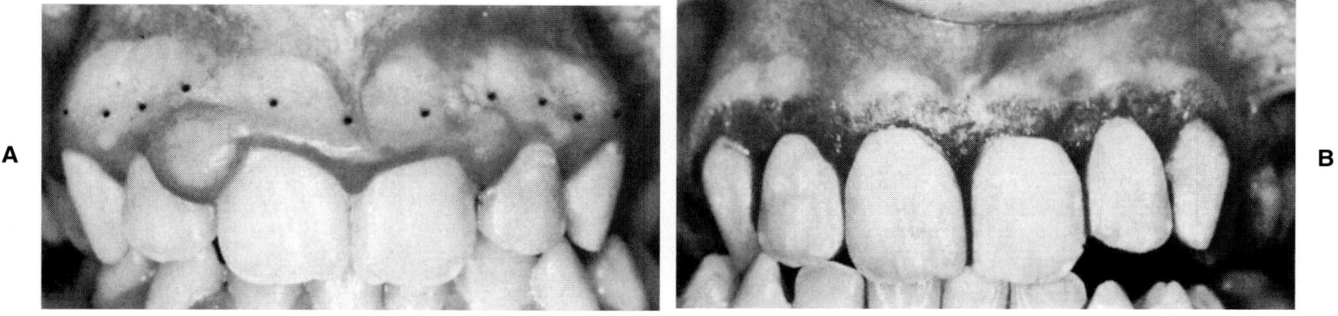

Fig. 59-1 Gingivectomy incision for gingival enlargement. **A,** Chronic inflammatory gingival enlargement with tumorlike area. Pinpoint markings outline the extent of the enlargement. Note the amount of attached gingiva remaining. **B,** Enlarged gingiva removed. Note the beveled incision.

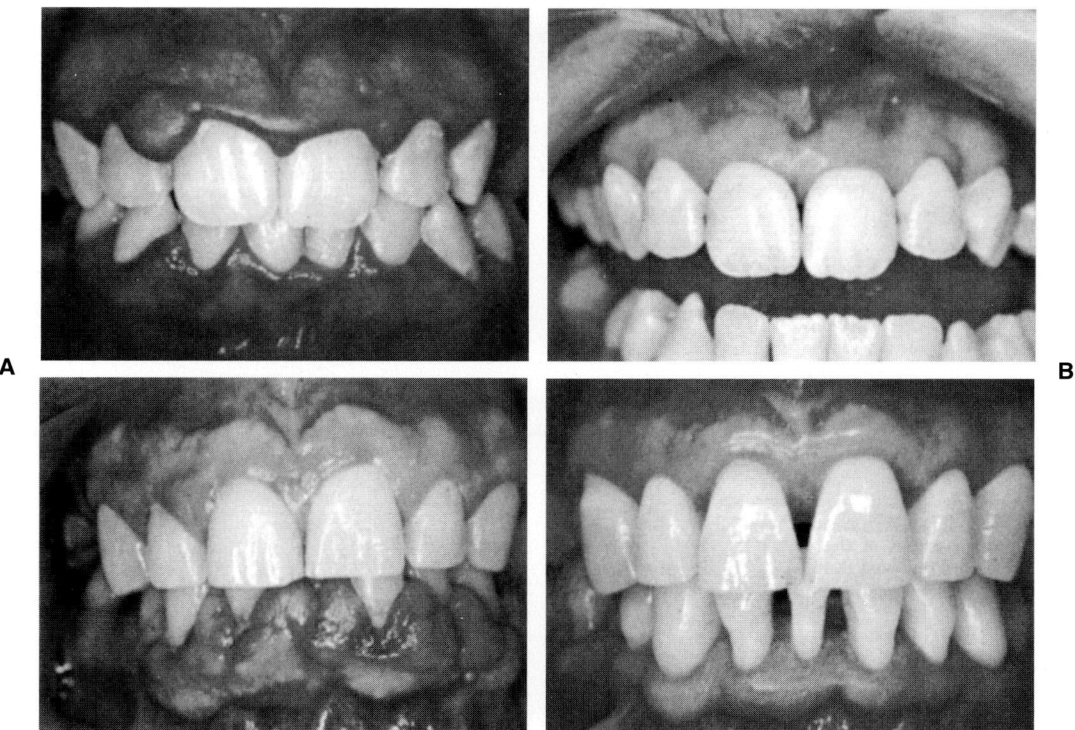

Fig. 59-2 **A,** Chronic inflammatory gingival enlargement associated with mouth breathing. **B,** Appearance after treatment.

TREATMENT OF PERIODONTAL AND GINGIVAL ABSCESSES

The reader is referred to Chapter 46, "Treatment of the Periodontal Abscess," for a more complete discussion of this topic.

TREATMENT OF DRUG-ASSOCIATED GINGIVAL ENLARGEMENT

Gingival enlargement has been associated with the administration of three different types of drugs: anticonvulsants, calcium channel blockers, and the immunosupressant cyclosporine. A comprehensive review of the clinical and microscopic features, and pathogenesis of gingival enlargement induced by the above-mentioned drugs is provided in Chapter 18.

Examination of cases of drug-induced gingival enlargement reveals the overgrown tissues to have two components: a *fibrotic* one, which is caused by the drug, and an *inflammatory* one that is induced by bacterial plaque. Although the two components (fibrotic and inflammatory) present in the enlarged gingiva are the result of distinct pathologic processes, they almost always are observed in combination. The role of bacterial plaque in the overall pathogenesis of drug-induced gingival enlargement is not clear. Some studies indicate that plaque is a prerequisite for gingival enlargement,[8] whereas others suggest that the presence of plaque is a consequence of its accumulation due to the enlarged gingiva.

Treatment Options

Treatment of drug-induced gingival enlargement should be based on the medication being used and the clinical features of the case.

First, consideration should be given to the possibility of discontinuing the drug[6,9] or changing medication. These possibilities should be examined with the patient's physician. Simple discontinuation of the offending drug is usually not a practical option, but its substitution for another medication might be. If any drug substitution is attempted, it is important to allow for a 6- to 12-month period of time to elapse between discontinuation of the offending drug and the possible resolution of gingival enlargement before a decision to implement surgical treatment is made.

Alternative medications to phenytoin include carbamazepine[5] and valproic acid, both of which have been reported to have a lesser impact in inducing gingival enlargement.

For patients on nifedipine, which has a reported prevalence of gingival enlargement of up to 44%, other calcium channel blockers such as diltiazem or verapamil

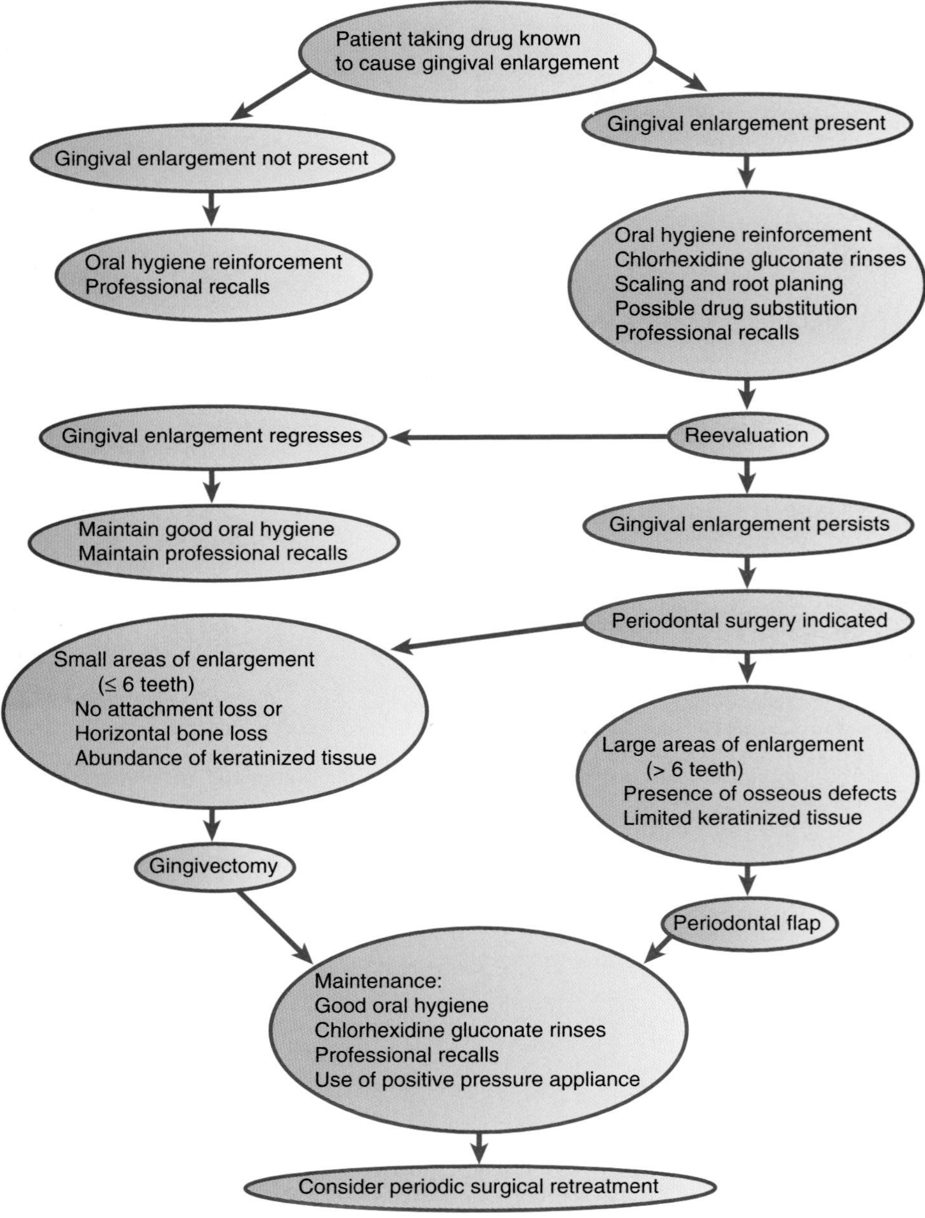

Fig. 59-3 Decision tree for treatment of drug-induced gingival enlargements.

may be viable alternatives, and their reported prevalence of gingival enlargement is 20% and 4%, respectively.[3,7,11] Also, consideration may be given to the use of another class of antihypertensive medications rather than calcium channel blockers, none of which are known to induce gingival enlargement.

Drug substitutions for cyclosporine are more limited. Recently, it has been shown that cyclosporine-induced gingival enlargement can spontaneously resolve if the drug is substituted by tracolimus.[10] There is also preliminary evidence that the antibiotic azithromycin may aid in decreasing the severity of cyclosporine-induced gingival enlargement.[17]

Second, the clinician should emphasize plaque control as the first step in the treatment of drug-induced gingival enlargement. Despite the fact that the exact role played by bacterial plaque is not well understood, there is evidence that good oral hygiene and frequent professional removal of plaque decreases the degree of gingival enlargement present and improves overall gingival health.[6,8,16] The presence of drug-induced enlargement is associated with pseudo-pocket formation, frequently with abundant plaque accumulation, which raises the possibility of periodontitis to develop; meticulous plaque control therefore helps maintain attachment levels. Also, adequate plaque control may aid in preventing or retarding the recurrence of gingival enlargement in surgically treated cases.

Third, in some cases, gingival enlargement persists after careful consideration of the above-mentioned approaches. These cases need to be treated by surgery, either gingivectomy or the periodontal flap. A decision tree outlining the sequence of events and options in the treatment of gingival enlargement is presented in Fig. 59-3.

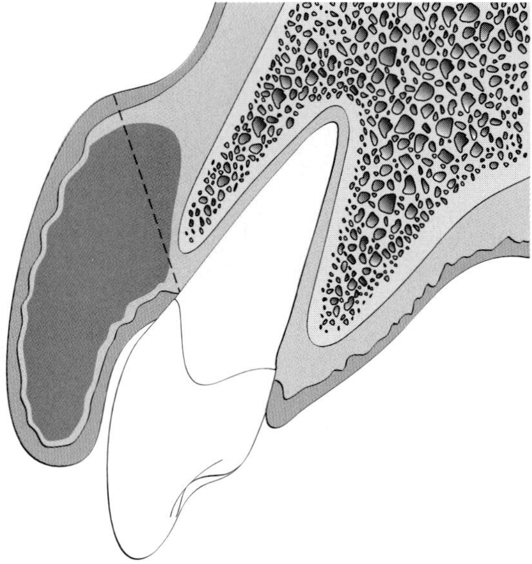

Fig. 59-4 The gingivectomy technique as used in treating drug-induced gingival enlargement cases. The dotted line represents the external bevel incision, and the shaded area corresponds to the tissue to be excised. Gingivectomy incision may not remove the entire hyperplastic tissue *(shaded area)* and may leave a wide wound of exposed connective tissue.

Gingivectomy has the advantage of simplicity and quickness but presents the disadvantages of more postoperative discomfort and increased chance of postoperative bleeding. It also sacrifices keratinized tissue and does not allow for osseous recontouring. The clinician's decision between the two surgical techniques available must consider the extension of the area to be operated, the presence of periodontitis and osseous defects, and the location of the base of the pockets in relation to the mucogingival junction.

In general, small areas (up to 6 teeth) of drug-induced gingival enlargement with no evidence of attachment loss (and therefore no anticipated need for osseous surgery) can be effectively treated with the gingivectomy technique. An important consideration is the amount of keratinized tissue present, remembering that at least 3 mm in the apicocoronal direction should remain after the surgery is completed.

The gingivectomy technique is described in detail in Chapter 58. Fig. 59-4 depicts diagrammatically the procedure, and Fig. 59-5 illustrates a case of cyclosporine-induced gingival enlargement treated with the gingivectomy technique.

Gingivectomy/gingivoplasty can also be performed via electrosurgery or a laser device. The advantages and disadvantages of these techniques are presented in Chapter 58.

The Flap Technique. Larger areas of gingival enlargement (more than 6 teeth) or areas where attachment loss and osseous defects are present should be treated by the flap technique, as should any situation in which the gingivectomy technique may create a mucogingival problem.

The periodontal flap technique used for the treatment of gingival enlargements is a simple variation of the one used to treat periodontitis, described in Chapters 60 and 61. Fig. 59-6 shows the basic steps in the technique, described as follows:

1. After anesthetizing the area, sounding of the underlying alveolar bone is performed with a periodontal probe to determine the presence and extent of osseous defects.
2. With a #15 Bard-Parker blade, the initial scalloped internal bevel incision is made at least 3 mm coronal to the mucogingival junction, including the creation of new interdental papillae.
3. The same blade is used to thin the gingival tissues in a buccolingual direction to the mucogingival junction. At this point the blade establishes contact with the alveolar bone, and a full-thickness or a split-thickness flap is elevated.
4. Using an Orban knife, the base of each papilla connecting the facial and the lingual incisions is incised.
5. The excised marginal and interdental tissue are removed with curettes.
6. Tissue tabs are removed, the roots are thoroughly scaled and planed, and the bone is recontoured as needed.
7. The flap is replaced and, if necessary, trimmed to exactly reach the bone-tooth junction. The flap is then

sutured with an interrupted or a continuous mattress technique, and the area is covered with periodontal dressing.

Sutures and pack are removed after 1 week, and the patient is instructed to start plaque control methods. Usually it is convenient to have the patient use chlorhexidine mouthrinses once or twice daily for 2 to 4 weeks. Fig. 59-7 illustrates a case treated with the flap technique.

Recurrence of drug-induced gingival enlargements is a reality in surgically treated cases.[14] As stated previously, meticulous home care,[4,12] chlorhexidine gluconate rinses,[15] and professional cleanings can decrease the speed and the degree to which recurrence occurs. A hard, natural rubber, fitted bite guard worn at night sometimes assists in the control of recurrence.[1,2]

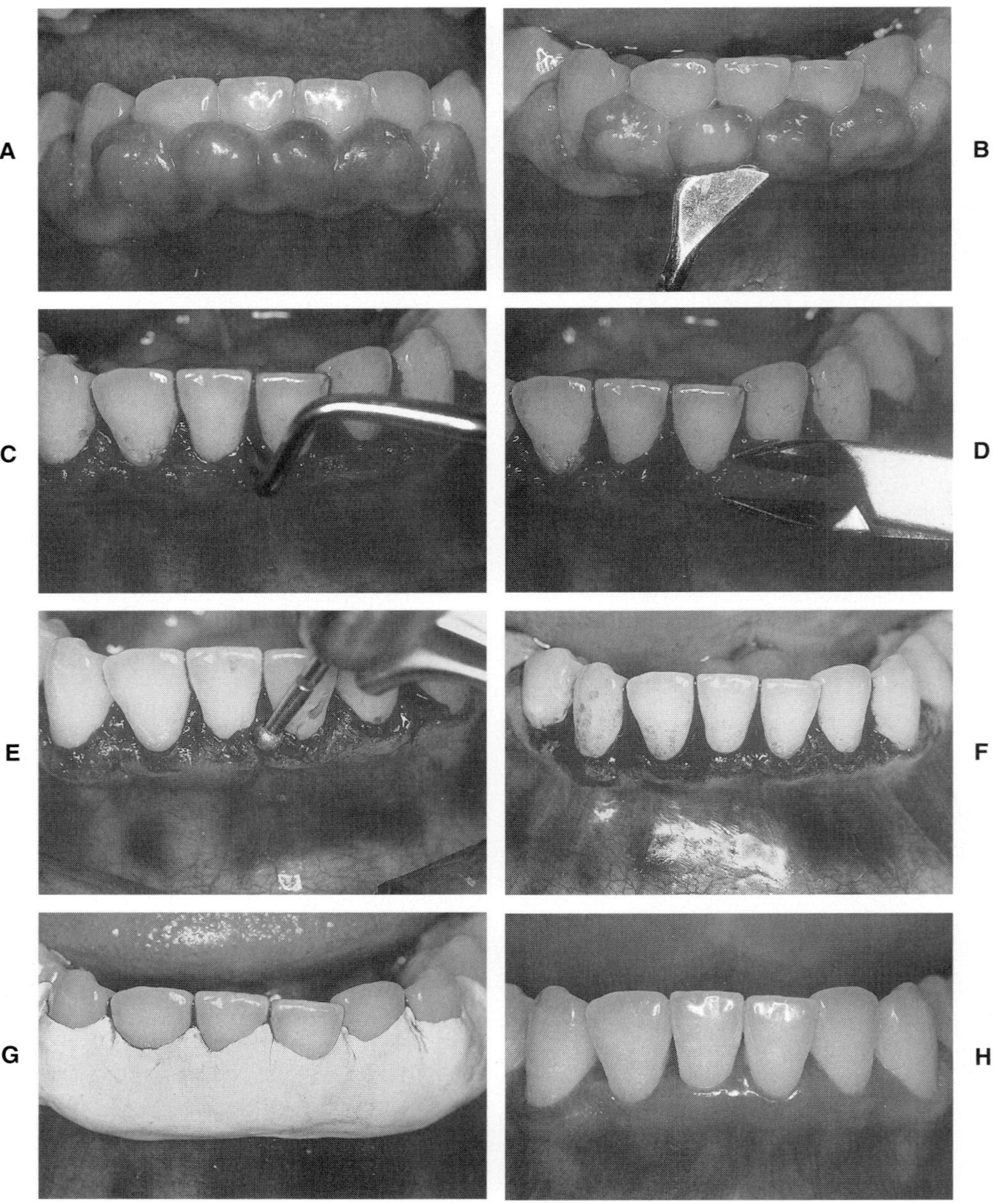

Fig. 59-5 Surgical treatment of cyclosporin-induced gingival enlargement using the gingivectomy technique on a 16-year-old girl who had received a kidney allograft 2 years previously. **A,** Presence of enlarged gingival tissues and pseudo-pocket formation; no attachment loss or evidence of vertical bone loss existed. **B,** Initial external bevel incision performed with a Kirkland knife. **C,** Interproximal tissue release achieved with an Orban knife. **D and E,** Gingivoplasty performed with tissue nippers and a round diamond at high speed with abundant refrigeration. **F,** Aspect of the surgical wound at the conclusion of the surgical procedure. **G,** Placement of noneugenol periodontal dressing. **H,** Surgical area 3 months postoperatively. Note the successful elimination of enlarged gingival tissue, restoration of a physiologic gingival contour, and maintenance of an adequate band of keratinized tissue.

Recurrence may occur as early as 3 to 6 months after the surgical treatment, but in general, surgical results are maintained for at least 12 months. One study[13] examined the recurrence of cyclosporine-induced gingival enlargement after treatment with the periodontal flap or gingivectomy and determined that increased pocket depth return is slower with the flap as revealed by 6-month postsurgical examination. Recurrence of periodontal tissue increased thickness, however, has not been objectively evaluated.

TREATMENT OF LEUKEMIC GINGIVAL ENLARGEMENT

Leukemic enlargement occurs in acute or subacute leukemia and is uncommon in the chronic leukemic state. The medical care of leukemic patients is often complicated by gingival enlargement with superimposed painful acute necrotizing ulcerative gingivitis, which interferes with eating and creates toxic systemic reactions. Bleeding and clotting times and platelet count of the patient should be checked and the hematologist consulted before periodontal treatment is instituted (see Chapter 38).

Treatment of acute gingival involvement is described in Chapter 45. After acute symptoms subside, attention is directed to correction of the gingival enlargement. The rationale is to remove the local irritating factors to control the inflammatory component of the enlargement.

The enlargement is treated by scaling and root planing carried out in stages under topical anesthesia. The initial treatment consists of gently removing all loose accumulations with cotton pellets, performing superficial scaling, and instructing the patient in oral hygiene for plaque control, which should include, at least initially, daily use of chlorhexidine mouthwashes. Oral hygiene procedures are extremely important in these cases and should be performed by the nurse if necessary.

Progressively deeper scalings are carried out at subsequent visits. Treatments are confined to a small area of the mouth to facilitate control of bleeding. Antibiotics are administered systemically the evening before and for 48 hours after each treatment to reduce the risk of infection.

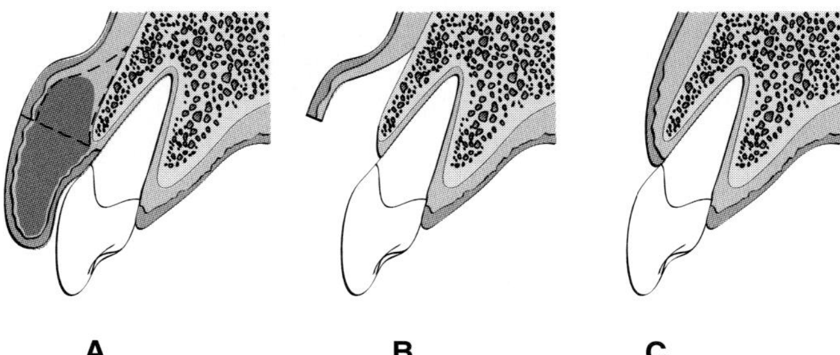

Fig. 59-6 Diagram representative of the periodontal flap for the treatment of drug-induced gingival enlargement. **A,** Initial reverse bevel incision followed by thinning of the enlarged gingival tissue; dotted lines represent incisions and the shaded area represents the tissue portion to be excised. **B,** After flap elevation, the enlarged portion of the gingival tissue is removed. **C,** The flap is placed on top of the alveolar bone and sutured.

TREATMENT OF GINGIVAL ENLARGEMENT IN PREGNANCY

Treatment requires elimination of all local irritants responsible for precipitating the gingival changes in pregnancy. Elimination of local irritants early in pregnancy is a preventive measure against gingival disease, which is preferable to treatment of gingival enlargement after it occurs. Marginal and interdental gingival inflammation and enlargement are treated by scaling and curettage (see Chapters 42 and 47). Treatment of tumorlike gingival enlargements consists of surgical excision and scaling and planing of the tooth surface. The enlargement recurs unless all irritants are removed. Food impaction is frequently an inciting factor.

When to Treat

Gingival lesions in pregnancy should be treated as soon as they are detected, although not necessarily by surgical means. Scaling and root planing procedures and adequate oral hygiene measures may reduce the size of the enlargement. Gingival enlargements do shrink after pregnancy, but they usually do not disappear. After pregnancy, the entire mouth should be reevaluated, a full set of radiographs taken, and the necessary treatment undertaken.

Lesions should be removed surgically during pregnancy only if they interfere with mastication or produce an esthetic disfigurement that the patient wishes removed.

In pregnancy, the emphasis should be on 1) preventing gingival disease before it occurs and 2) treating existing gingival disease before it worsens. All patients should be seen as early as possible in pregnancy. Those without gingival disease should be checked for potential sources of local irritation and should be instructed in plaque control procedures. Those with gingival disease should be treated promptly, before the conditioning effect of pregnancy on the gingiva becomes manifest. Precautions necessary for periodontal treatment of pregnant women are presented in Chapter 37.

Every pregnant patient should be scheduled for periodic dental visits, the importance of which in the prevention of serious periodontal disturbances should be stressed.

TREATMENT OF GINGIVAL ENLARGEMENT IN PUBERTY

Gingival enlargement in puberty is treated by performing scaling and curettage, removing all sources of irritation, and controlling plaque. Surgical removal may be required in severe cases. The problem in these patients is recurrence due to poor oral hygiene.

RECURRENCE OF GINGIVAL ENLARGEMENT

Recurrence after treatment is the most common problem in the management of gingival enlargement. Residual local irritation and systemic or hereditary conditions causing noninflammatory gingival hyperplasia are the responsible factors.

Recurrence of chronic inflammatory enlargement immediately after treatment indicates that all irritants have

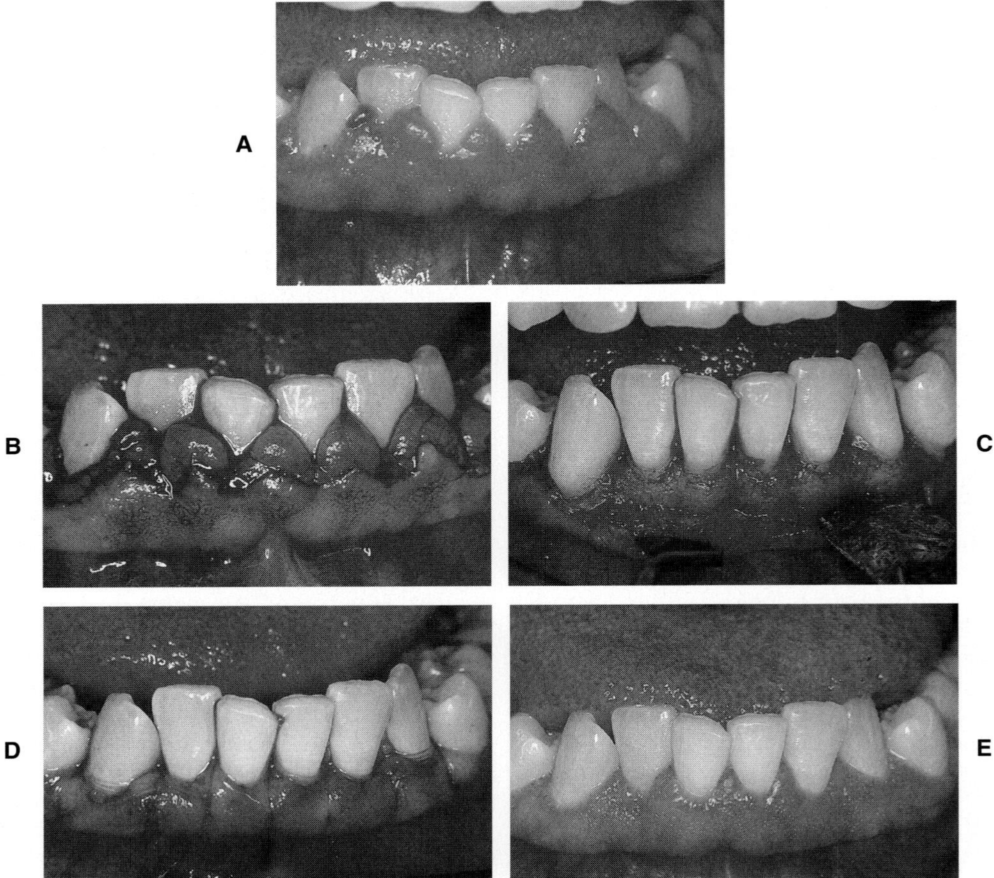

Fig. 59-7 Treatment of a case of a combined cyclosporin- and nifedipine-induced gingival enlargement with a periodontal flap on a 35-year-old female who had received a kidney allograft $3\frac{1}{2}$ years previously. **A,** Presurgical clinical aspect of the lower anterior teeth, showing severe gingival enlargement. **B,** Initial scalloped reverse bevel incision, including maintenance of keratinized tissue and creation of surgical papillae. **C,** Elevation of a full thickness flap and removal of the inner portion of the previously thinned gingival tissue; after scaling and root planing, osseous recontouring can be performed if necessary. **D,** The flap is positioned on top of the alveolar crest. **E,** Postsurgical aspect of the treated area at 12 months; note the reduction of enlarged tissue volume and acceptable gingival health.

not been removed. Contributory local conditions, such as food impaction and overhanging margins of restorations, are commonly overlooked. If the enlargement recurs after healing is complete and normal contour is attained, inadequate plaque control by the patient is the most common cause.

Recurrence during the healing period is manifested as red, beadlike, granulomatous masses that bleed on slight provocation. This is a proliferative vascular inflammatory response to local irritation, usually a fragment of calculus on the root. The condition is corrected by removing the granulation tissue and scaling and planing the root surface.

Familial, hereditary, or idiopathic gingival enlargement recurs after surgical removal, even if all local irritants have been removed. The enlargement can be maintained at minimal size by preventing secondary inflammatory involvement.

The use of escharotic drugs has been recommended in the past for the removal of gingival enlargements, but its use is currently *not* recommended. The destructive action of the drugs is difficult to control; injury to healthy tissue and root surfaces, delayed healing, and excessive postoperative pain are complications that can be avoided when the gingiva is removed with periodontal knives and scalpels or by electrosurgery.

REFERENCES

1. Aiman R: The use of positive pressure mouthpiece as a new therapy for Dilantin gingival hyperplasia. Chron Omaha Dent Soc 1968; 131:244.
2. Babcock JR: The successful use of a new therapy for Dilantin gingival hyperplasia. Periodontics 1965; 3:196.
3. Barclay S, Thomason JM, Idle JR, et al: The incidence and severity of nifedipine-induced gingival overgrowth. J Clin Periodontol 1992; 19:311.
4. Ciancio SG, Yaffe SJ, Catz CC: Gingival hyperplasia and diphenylhydantoin. J Periodontol 1972; 43:411.
5. Dahilof G, Preber H, Eliasson S, et al: Periodontal condition of epileptic adults treated with phenytoin or carbamazepine. Epilepsia 1993; 34:960.

6. Dongari A, O'Donnell HT, Langlais RP: Drug-induced gingival overgrowth. Oral Surg Oral Med Oral Path 1993; 76:543.
7. Fattore L, Stablein M, Bredfelt G, et al: Gingival hyperplasia: A side effect of nifedipine and diltiazem. Spec Care Dent 1991; 11:107.
8. Hall WB: Dilantin hyperplasia: A preventable lesion. J Periodont Res 1969; 4:36.
9. Harel-Raviv M, Eckler M, Lalani K, et al: Nifedipine-induced gingival hyperplasia. A comprehensive review and analysis. Oral Surg Oral Med Oral Path Oral Radiol Endod 1995; 79:115.
10. Hernandez G, Arriba L, Lucas M, et al: Reduction of severe gingival overgrowth in a kidney transplant patient by replacing cyclosporin A with tracolimus. J Periodontol 2000; 71:1630.
11. Nery EB, Edson RG, Lee KK, et al: Prevalence of nifedipine-induced gingival hyperplasia. J Periodontol 1995; 66:572.
12. Nishikawa S, Tada H, Hamasaki A, et al: Nifedipine-induced gingival hyperplasia: A clinical and in vitro study. J Periodontol 1991; 62:30.
13. Pilloni A, Camargo PM, Carere M, et al: Surgical treatment of cyclosporine A- and nifedipine-induced gingival enlargement. J Periodontol 1998; 69:791.
14. Rees TD, Levine RA: Systemic drugs as a risk factor for periodontal disease initiation and progression. Compend Cont Educ Dent 1995; 16:20.
15. Saravia ME, Svirsky JA, Friedman R: Chlorhexidine as an oral hygiene adjunct for cyclosporine-induced gingival hyperplasia. J Dent Child 1990; 57:366.
16. Seymour RA, Jacobs DJ: Cyclosporin and the gingival tissues. J Clin Periodontol 1992; 19:1.
17. Wahlstrom E, Zamora JU, Teichman S: Improvement in cyclosporin-associated gingival hyperplasia with azithromycin therapy. N Eng J Med 1995; 332:753.

The Periodontal Flap

Henry H. Takei and Fermin A. Carranza

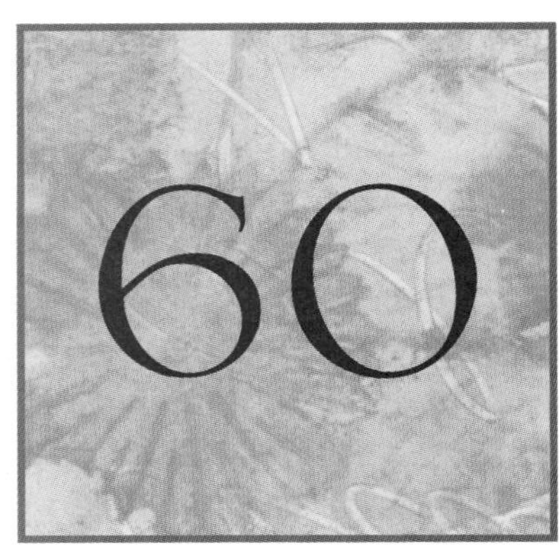

CHAPTER

CHAPTER OUTLINE

A periodontal flap is a section of gingiva and/or mucosa surgically separated from the underlying tissues to provide visibility of and access to the bone and root surface. The flap also allows the gingiva to be displaced to a different location in patients with mucogingival involvement (Color Fig. 60-1).

CLASSIFICATION OF FLAPS

Periodontal flaps can be classified based on the following:

- Bone exposure after flap reflection
- Placement of the flap after surgery
- Management of the papilla

Based on bone exposure after reflection, the flaps are classified as either full thickness (mucoperiosteal) or partial thickness (mucosal) flaps (Fig. 60-1).

In full thickness flaps, all the soft tissue, including the periosteum, is reflected to expose the underlying bone. This complete exposure of, and access to, the underlying bone is indicated when resective osseous surgery is contemplated.

The partial thickness flap includes only the epithelium and a layer of the underlying connective tissue. The bone remains covered by a layer of connective tissue, including the periosteum. This type of flap is also called the *split thickness flap*. The partial thickness flap is indicated when the flap is to be positioned apically or when the operator does not desire to expose bone.

There are conflicting data regarding the advisability of uncovering the bone when this is not actually needed. When bone is stripped of its periosteum, a loss of marginal bone occurs, and this loss is prevented when the periosteum is left on the bone.[4] The differences, however, are usually not clinically significant,[7] although sometimes they may be (Fig. 60-2). The partial thickness flap may be necessary in cases in which the crestal bone margin is thin and is exposed when the flap is placed apically, or when dehiscences or fenestrations are present. The periosteum left on the bone may also be used for suturing the flap when it is displaced apically.

Based on flap placement after surgery, flaps are classified as 1) *nondisplaced flaps,* when the flap is returned and sutured in its original position; or 2) *displaced flaps* that are placed apically, coronally, or laterally to their original position. Both full thickness and partial thickness flaps can be displaced, but to do so, the attached gingiva has to be totally separated from the underlying bone, thereby enabling the unattached portion of the gingiva to be moveable. However, palatal flaps cannot be displaced owing to the absence of unattached gingiva.

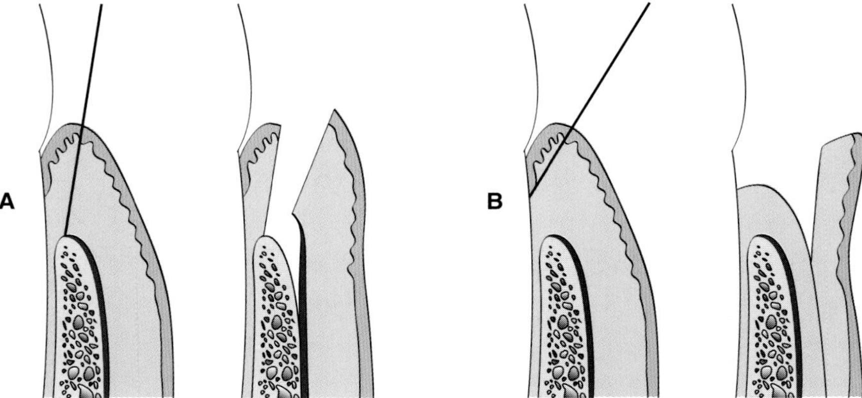

Fig. 60-1 **A,** Diagram of the internal bevel incision (first incision) to reflect a full thickness (mucoperiosteal) flap. Note that the incision ends on the bone to allow for the reflection of the entire flap. **B,** Diagram of the internal bevel incision to reflect a partial thickness flap. Note that the incision ends on the root surface to preserve the periosteum on the bone.

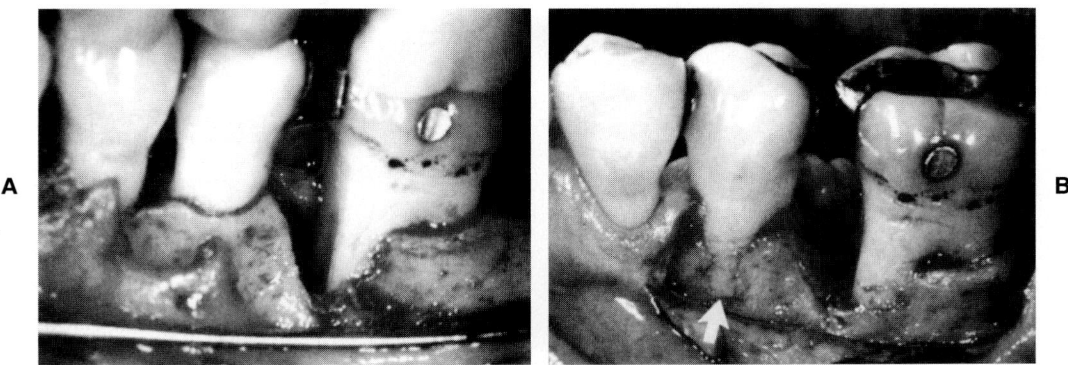

Fig. 60-2 Loss of marginal bone as a result of uncovering the osseous crest. **A,** Mucoperiosteal flap elevated as part of a clinical study. **B,** Reentry performed 6 months later reveals loss of marginal bone facial to second premolar *(arrow).* (Courtesy Dr. Silvia Oreamuno; San Jose, Costa Rica.)

Apically displaced flaps have the important advantage of preserving the outer portion of the pocket wall and transforming it into attached gingiva. Therefore they accomplish the double objective of eliminating the pocket and increasing the width of the attached gingiva.

Based on management of the papilla, flaps can be conventional or papilla preservation flaps. In the conventional flap the interdental papilla is split beneath the contact point of the two approximating teeth to allow reflection of buccal and lingual flaps. The incision is usually scalloped to maintain gingival morphology with as much papilla as possible. The conventional flap is used when 1) the interdental spaces are too narrow, thereby precluding the possibility of preserving the papilla, and 2) when the flap is to be displaced.

Conventional flaps include the modified Widman flap, the undisplaced flap, the apically displaced flap, and the flap for regenerative procedures. These techniques are described in detail in Chapter 61.

The papilla preservation flap incorporates the entire papilla in one of the flaps by means of crevicular interdental incisions to sever the connective tissue attachment and a horizontal incision at the base of the papilla, leaving it connected to one of the flaps.

DESIGN OF THE FLAP

The design of the flap is dictated by the surgical judgement of the operator and may depend on the objectives of the operation. The degree of access to the underlying bone and root surfaces necessary and the final position of the flap must be considered in designing the flap. Preservation of good blood supply to the flap is an important consideration.

Two basic flap designs are used. Depending on how the interdental papilla is dealt with, flaps can either split the papilla (conventional flap) or preserve it (papilla preservation flap).

In the conventional flap operation, the incisions for the facial and the lingual or palatal flap reach the tip of

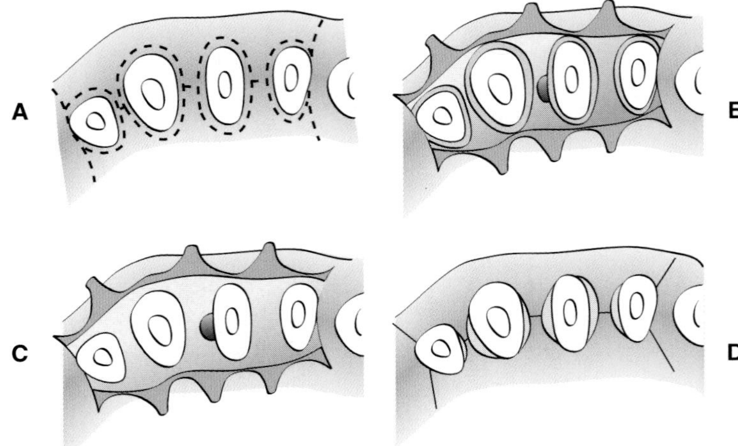

Fig. 60-3 Flap design for the conventional or traditional flap technique. **A,** Design of the incisions: the internal bevel incision, splitting the papilla, and the vertical incisions are drawn in interrupted lines. **B,** The flap has been elevated, and the wedge of tissue next to the tooth is still in place. **C,** All marginal tissue has been removed, exposing the underlying bone (see defect in one space). **D,** Tissue returned to its original positron. Proximal areas are not totally covered.

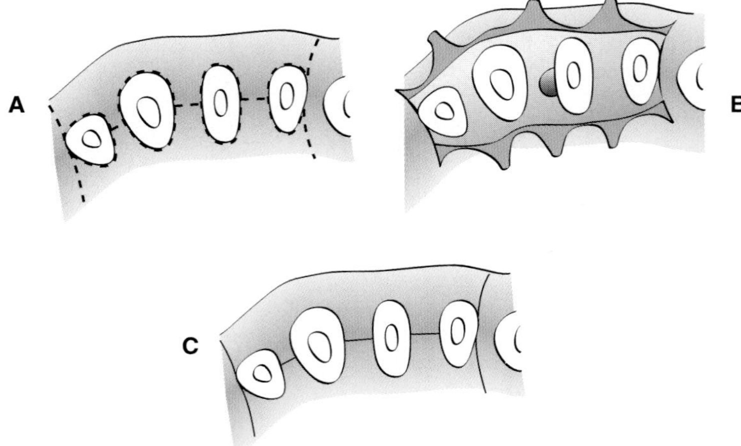

Fig. 60-4 Flap design for a sulcular incision flap. **A,** Design of the incisions: the sulcular incisions and the vertical incisions are depicted by interrupted lines. **B,** The flap has been elevated, exposing the underlying bone (see defect in one space). **C,** Tissue returned to its original position covers the entire interdental spaces.

the interdental papilla or its vicinity, thereby splitting the papilla into a facial half and a lingual or palatal half (Figs. 60-3 and 60-4).

The entire surgical procedure should be planned in every detail before the intervention is begun. This should include the type of flap, exact location and type of incisions, management of the underlying bone, and final closure of the flap and sutures. Although some details may be modified during the actual performance of the procedure, detailed planning allows for a better clinical result.

INCISIONS

Horizontal Incisions

Periodontal flaps use horizontal and vertical incisions. Horizontal incisions are directed along the margin of the gingiva in a mesial or a distal direction (Fig. 60-5). Two types of horizontal incisions have been recommended: the internal bevel incision,[6] which starts at a distance from the gingival margin and is aimed at the bone crest, and the crevicular incision, which starts at the bottom of the pocket and is directed to the bone margin. In

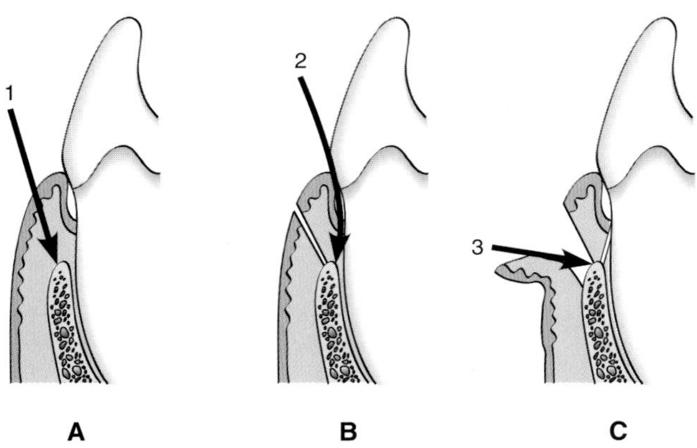

Fig. 60-5 A to C, The first (internal bevel), second (crevicular), and third (interdental) incisions are the three incisions necessary for flap surgery.

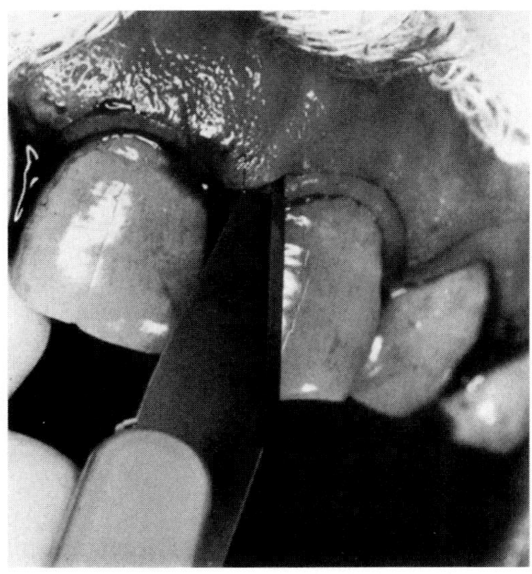

Fig. 60-6 Position of knife in performing internal bevel incision.

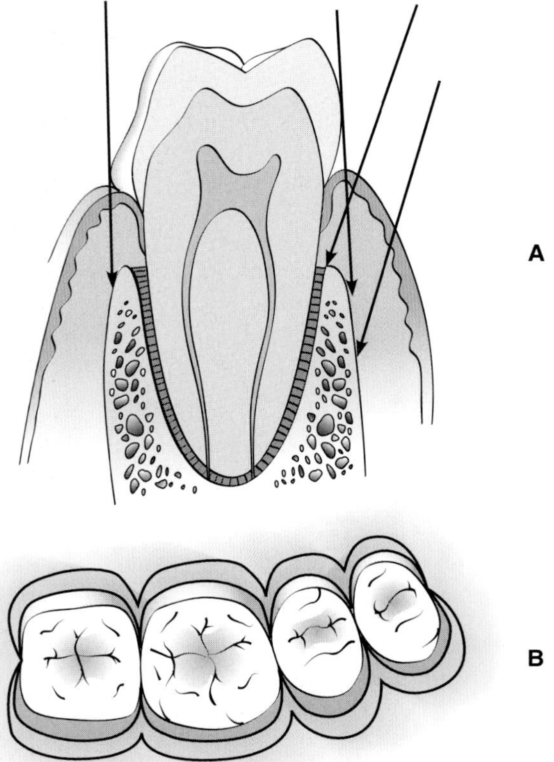

Fig. 60-7 A, The internal bevel (first) incision can be made at varying locations and angles according to the different anatomic and pocket situations. **B,** An occlusal view of the different locations where the internal bevel incision can be made. Note the scalloped shape of the incisions.

addition, the interdental incision is performed after the flap is elevated.

The *internal bevel incision* is basic to most periodontal flap procedures. It is the incision from which the flap is reflected to expose the underlying bone and root. The internal bevel incision accomplishes three important objectives: 1) it removes the pocket lining; 2) it conserves the relatively uninvolved outer surface of the gingiva, which, if apically positioned, becomes attached gingiva; and 3) it produces a sharp, thin flap margin for adaptation to the bone-tooth junction. This incision has also been termed the first incision because it is the initial incision in the reflection of a periodontal flap, and the reverse bevel incision, because its bevel is in reverse direction from that of the gingivectomy incision. The #11 or #15 surgical scalpel is used most commonly. That portion of the gingiva left around the tooth contains the epithelium of the pocket lining and the adjacent granulomatous tissue. It is discarded after the crevicular (second) and interdental (third) incisions are performed (see Fig. 60-5).

The internal bevel incision starts from a designated area on the gingiva and is directed to an area at or near the crest of the bone (Fig. 60-6). The starting point on the gingiva is determined by whether the flap is apically displaced or not displaced (Fig. 60-7).

The *crevicular incision,* also termed the second incision, is made from the base of the pocket to the crest of the bone (Fig. 60-8). This incision, together with the initial reverse bevel incision, forms a V-shaped wedge ending at or near the crest of bone; this wedge of tissue contains most of the inflamed and granulomatous areas that constitute the lateral wall of the pocket, as well as the junctional epithelium and the connective tissue fibers that still persist between the bottom of the pocket and the crest of the bone. The incision is carried around the entire tooth. The beak-shaped #12D blade is usually used for this incision.

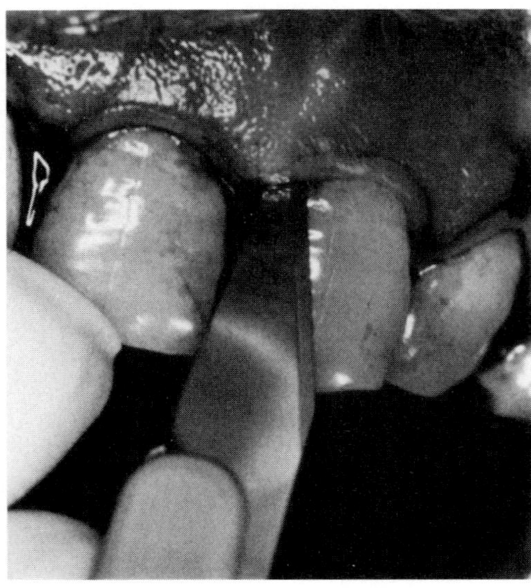

Fig. 60-8 Position of knife in performing crevicular incision.

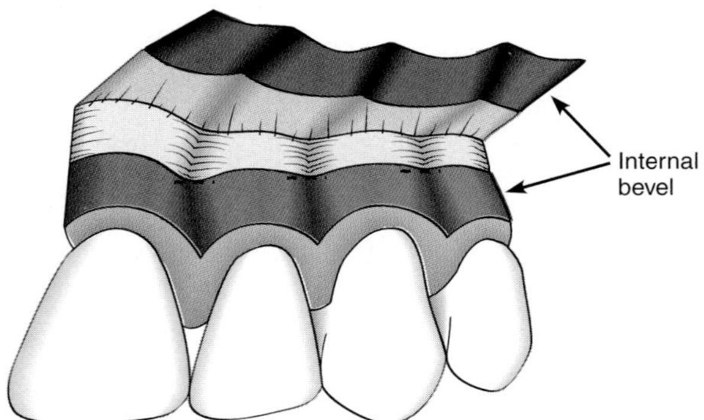

Fig. 60-9 After the flap has been elevated, a wedge of tissue remains on the teeth, attached by the base of the papillae. An interdental incision along the horizontal lines seen in the interdental spaces will sever these connections.

A periosteal elevator is inserted into the initial internal bevel incision, and the flap is separated from the bone. The most apical end of the internal bevel incision is more exposed and visible. With this access, the surgeon is able to make the third or *interdental incision* to separate the collar of gingiva that is left around the tooth. The Orban knife is usually used for this incision. The incision is made not only around the facial and lingual radicular area but also interdentally, connecting the facial and lingual segments, to completely free the gingiva around the tooth (Fig. 60-9; see Fig. 60-5).

These three incisions allow the removal of the gingiva around the tooth (i.e., the pocket epithelium and the adjacent granulomatous tissue). A curette or a large scaler (U15/30) can be used for this purpose. After removal of the large pieces of tissue, the remaining connective tissue in the osseous lesion should be carefully curetted out so that the entire root and the bone surface adjacent to the teeth can be observed.

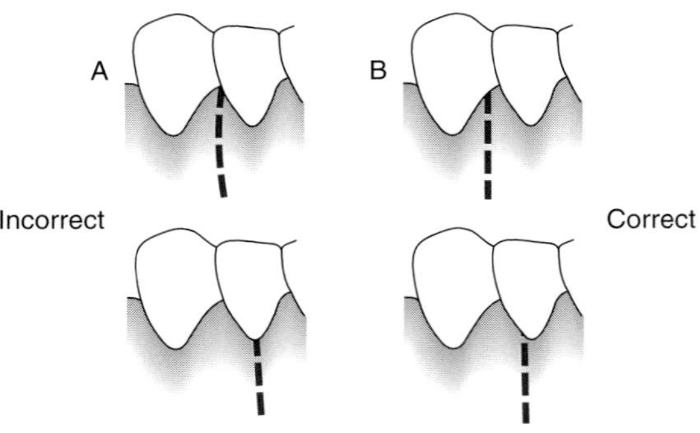

Fig. 60-10 Incorrect **(A)** and correct **(B)** locations of a vertical incision. This incision should be made at the line angles to prevent splitting of a papilla or incising directly over a radicular surface.

Flaps can be reflected using only the horizontal incision if sufficient access can be obtained by this means and if apical, lateral, or coronal displacement of the flap is not anticipated. If no vertical incisions are made, the flap is called an *envelope flap*.

Vertical Incisions

Vertical or oblique releasing incisions can be used on one or both ends of the horizontal incision, depending on the design and purpose of the flap. Vertical incisions at both ends are necessary if the flap is to be apically displaced. Vertical incisions must extend beyond the mucogingival line, reaching the alveolar mucosa, to allow for the release of the flap to be displaced (see Chapter 61).

In general, vertical incisions in the lingual and palatal areas are avoided. Facial vertical incisions should not be made in the center of an interdental papilla or over the radicular surface of a tooth. Incisions should be made at the line angles of a tooth either to include the papilla in the flap or to avoid it completely (Fig. 60-10). The vertical incision should also be designed so as to avoid short flaps (mesiodistal) with long, apically directed horizontal incisions because these could jeopardize the blood supply to the flap.

Several investigators[1,2,11,12] proposed the so-called interdental denudation procedure, which consists of horizontal, internal bevel, nonscalloped incisions to remove the gingival papillae and denude the interdental space. This technique completely eliminates the inflamed interdental areas, which heal by secondary intention, and results in excellent gingival contour. It is contraindicated when bone grafts are used.

ELEVATION OF THE FLAP

When a full thickness flap is desired, the reflection is accomplished by blunt dissection. A periosteal elevator is used to separate the mucoperiosteum from the bone by moving it mesially, distally, and apically until the desired reflection is accomplished (Fig. 60-11).

Sharp dissection is necessary to reflect a partial thickness flap. A surgical scalpel (#11 or #15) is used (Fig. 60-12).

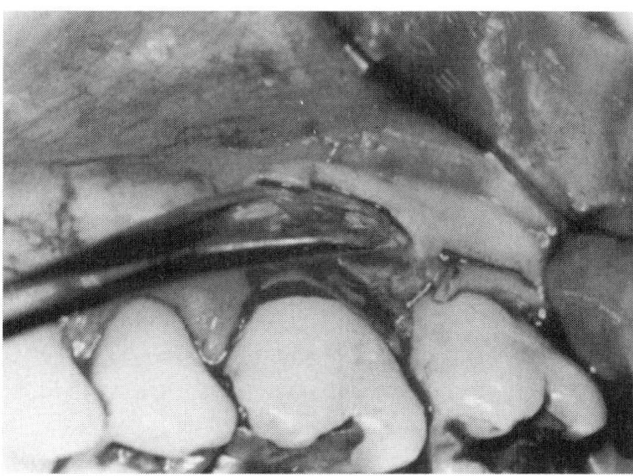

Fig. 60-11 Elevation of the flap with a periosteal elevator to obtain a full thickness flap.

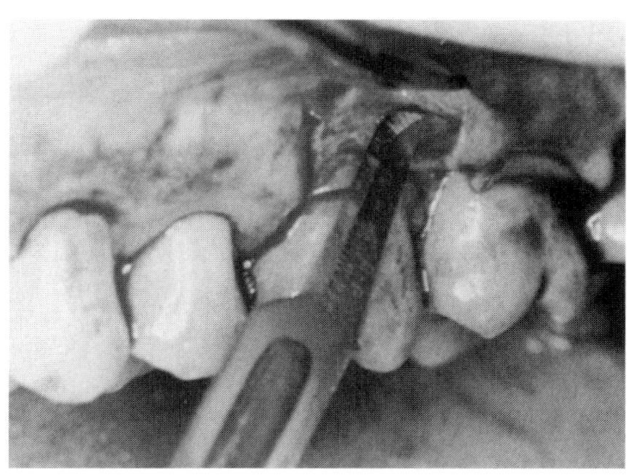

Fig. 60-12 Elevation of the flap with a Bard-Parker knife to obtain a split thickness flap.

A combination of full and partial thickness flaps can often be indicated to obtain the advantages of both. The flap is started as a full thickness procedure, and then a partial thickness flap is made at the apical portion. In this way the coronal portion of the bone, which may be subject to osseous remodeling, is exposed while the remaining bone remains protected by its periosteum.

SUTURING TECHNIQUES

After all the necessary procedures are completed, the area is reexamined and cleansed, and the flap is placed in the desired position, where it should remain without tension. It is convenient to keep it in place with light pressure with a piece of gauze so that a blood clot can form. The purpose of suturing is to maintain the flap in the desired position until healing has progressed to the point where sutures are no longer needed.

There are many types of sutures, suture needles, and materials.[5,10] Suture materials may be either nonresorbable or resorbable, and they may be further categorized as braided or monofilaments. The resorbable sutures have gained popularity since they enhance patient comfort and eliminate suture removal appointments. The monofilament type of suture alleviates the "wicking effect" of braided sutures that may allow bacteria from the oral cavity to be drawn through the suture to the deeper areas of the wound. Box 60-1 is a classification of the sutures available today:

The nonresorbable, braided silk suture was the most commonly used in the past due to its ease of use and low cost. The expanded polytetrafluoroethylene synthetic monofilament is an excellent nonresorbable suture widely used today.

The most commonly used resorbable sutures are the natural, plain gut and the chromic gut. Both are monofilaments and are processed from purified collagen of either sheep or cattle intestines. The chromic suture is a plain gut suture processed with chromic salts to make it resistant to enzymatic resorption, thereby increasing the resorption time. The synthetic resorbable sutures are also often used.

BOX 60-1

Sutures for Periodontal Flaps

Nonabsorbable
Silk: braided
Nylon: monofilament (Ethilon)
EPTfe: monofilament (Gore-tex)
Polyester: braided (Ethibond)

Absorbable
Surgical: gut
Plain gut; monofilament (30 days)
Chromic gut; monofilament (45–60 days)

Synthetic
Polyglycolic: braided (16–20 days)
(Vicryl; Ethicon)
(Dexon; Davis & Geck)
Polyglecaprone: monofilament (90–120 days)
(Monocryl; Ethicon)
Polyglyconate: monofilament (Maxon)

Technique

The needle is held with the needle holder and should enter the tissues at right angles and no less than 2 to 3 mm from the incision. The needle is then carried through the tissue, following the needle's curvature. The knot should not be placed over the incision.

The periodontal flap is closed either with independent sutures or with continuous, independent sling sutures. The latter method eliminates the pulling of the buccal and lingual or palatal flaps together and instead, uses the teeth as an anchor for the flaps. There is less tendency for the flaps to buckle, and the forces on the flaps are better distributed.

Sutures of any kind placed in the interdental papillae should enter and exit the tissue at a point located below

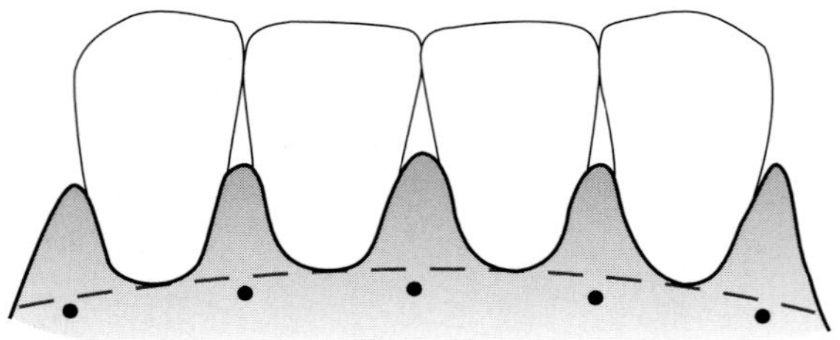

Fig. 60-13 Placement of suture in the interdental space below the base of an imaginary triangle in the papilla.

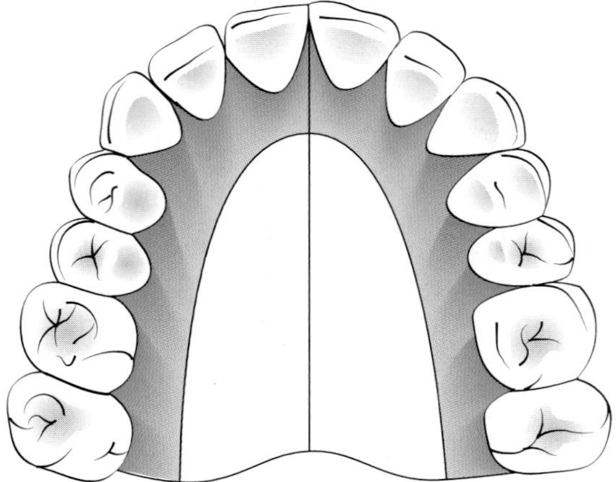

Fig. 60-14 Placement of sutures for closing a palatal flap. For slightly or moderately elevated flaps, the sutures are placed in shaded areas; for more substantial elevation of the flap, they are placed in the central (unshaded) area of their palate.

the imaginary line that forms the base of the triangle of the interdental papilla (Fig. 60-13). The location of sutures for closure of a palatal flap depend on the extent of flap elevation that has been performed. The flap is divided in four quadrants as depicted in Fig. 60-14. If the elevation of the flap is slight or moderate, the sutures can be placed in the quadrant closest to the teeth. If the flap elevation is substantial, the sutures should be placed in the central quadrants of the palate.

One may or may not use periodontal dressings. When the flaps are not apically displaced, it is not necessary to use dressings other than for patient comfort.

Ligation

Interdental Ligation. Two types of interdental ligation can be used: the director loop suture (Fig. 60-15) and the figure-eight suture (Fig. 60-16). In the figure-eight suture, there is thread between the two flaps. This suture is therefore used when the flaps are not in close apposition because of apical flap position or nonscalloped incisions. It is simpler to perform than the direct ligation. The direct suture permits a better closure of the interdental papilla and should be performed when bone grafts are used or when close apposition of the scalloped incision is required.

Sling Ligation. The sling ligation can be used for a flap on one surface of a tooth that involves two interdental spaces (Fig. 60-17).

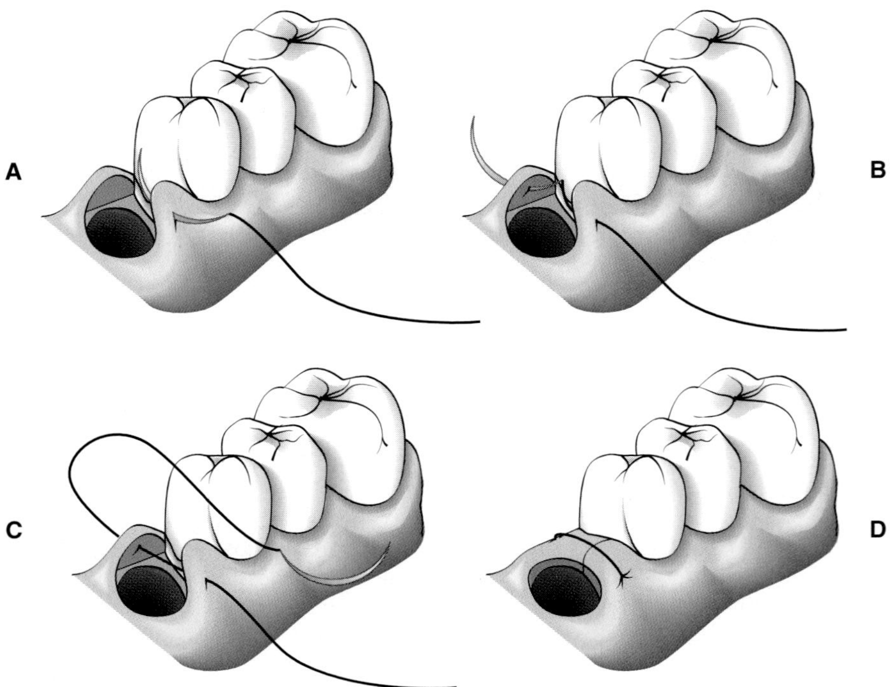

Fig. 60-15 A simple loop suture is used to approximate the buccal and lingual flaps. **A,** The needle penetrates the outer surface of the first flap. **B,** The undersurface of the opposite flap is engaged, and the suture is brought back to the initial side **(C),** where the knot is tied **(D).**

Types of Sutures

Horizontal Mattress Suture. This suture is often used for the interproximal areas of diastemata or for wide interdental spaces to properly adapt the interproximal papilla against the bone. Two sutures are often necessary. The horizontal mattress suture can be incorporated with continuous, independent sling sutures, as shown in Fig. 60-18.

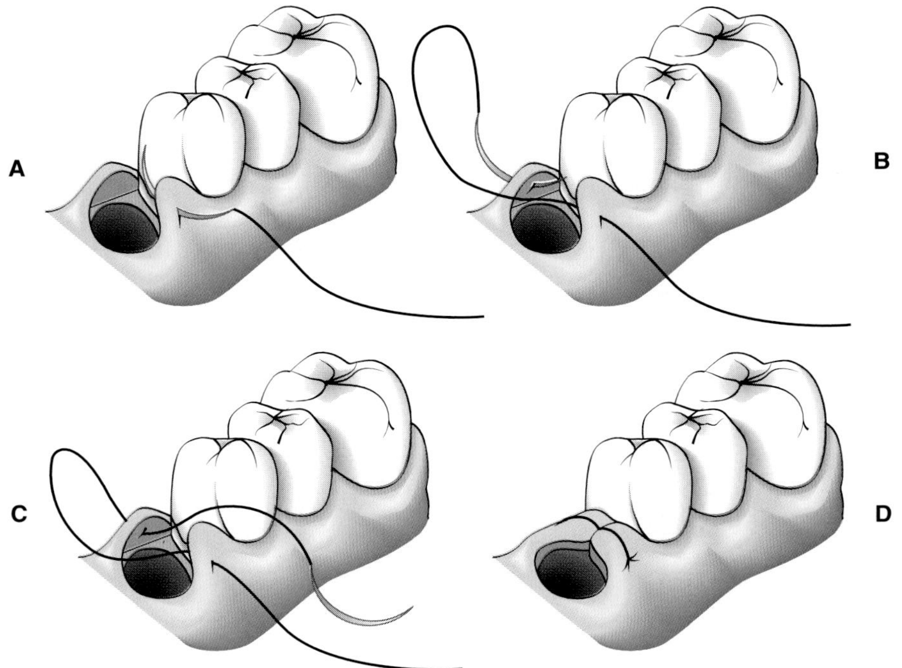

Fig. 60-16 An interrupted figure-eight suture is used to approximate the buccal and lingual flaps. The needle penetrates the outer surface of the first flap **(A)** and the outer surface of the opposite flap **(B).** The suture is brought back to the first flap **(C),** and the knot is tied **(D).**

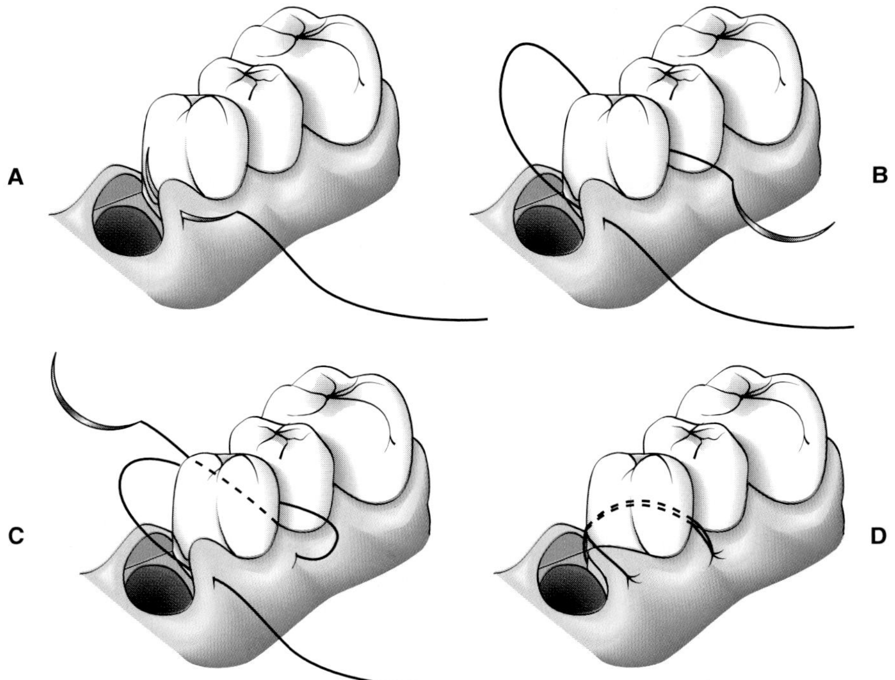

Fig. 60-17 A single, interrupted sling suture is used to adapt the flap around the tooth. **A,** The needle engages the outer surface of the flap and encircles the tooth **(B). C,** The outer surface of the same flap of the adjacent interdental area is engaged. **D,** the suture is returned to the initial site and the knot tied.

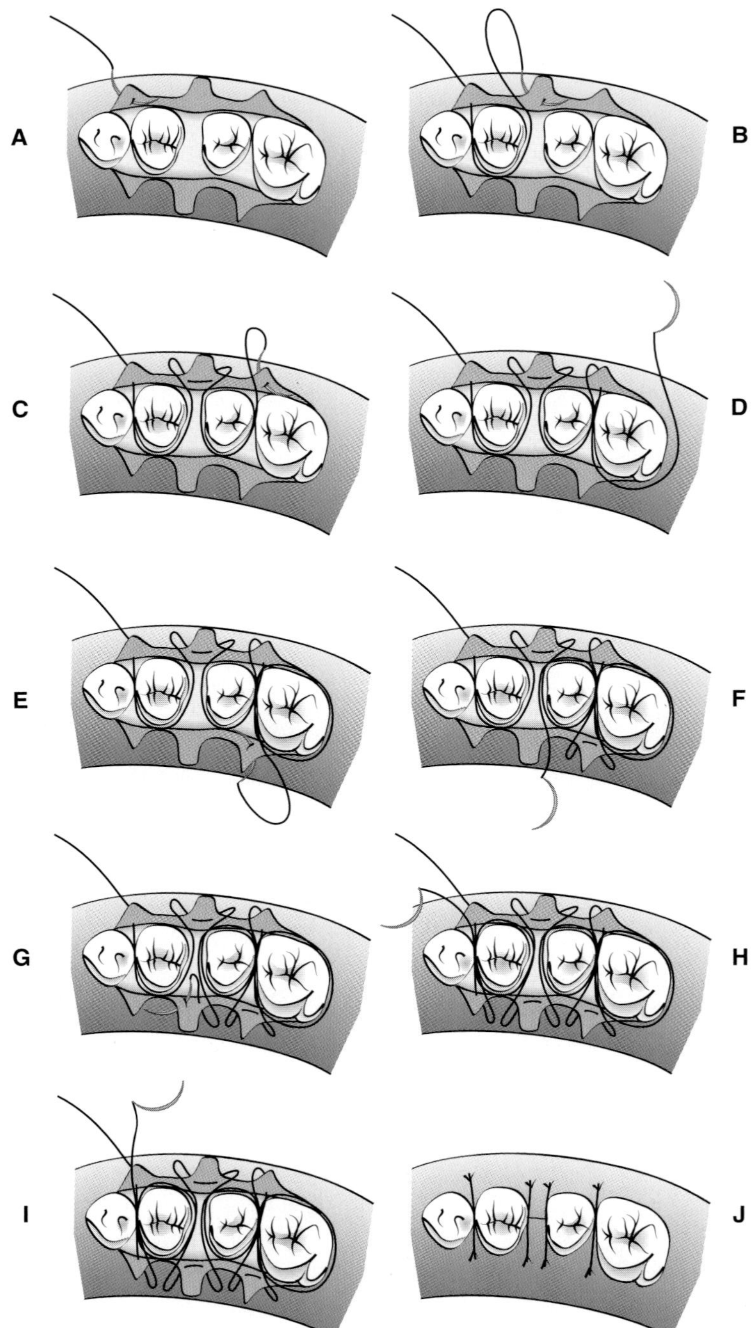

Fig. 60-18 **A,** Continuous, independent sling suture using a horizontal mattress suture around diastemata or wide interdental areas **(B and C)**. This mattress suture is utilized on both the buccal **(D)** and the lingual **(E and F)** surfaces. Continuation of suture on lingual surfaces **(G to I)** and completed suture **(J)**.

The penetration of the needle is performed in such a way that the mesial and distal edges of the papilla lie snugly against the bone. The needle enters the outer surface of the gingiva and crosses the undersurface of the gingiva horizontally. The mattress sutures should not be close together at the midpoint of the base of the papilla. The needle reappears on the outer surface at the other base of the papilla and continues around the tooth with the sling sutures.

Continuous Independent Sling Suture. This is used when there is both a facial and a lingual flap involving many teeth. The suture is initiated on the facial papilla closest to the midline, because this is the easiest place to position the final knot (Fig. 60-19). A continuous sling suture is laced for each papilla on the facial surface. When the last tooth is reached, the suture is anchored around it to prevent any pulling of the facial sutures when the lingual flap is sutured around the teeth

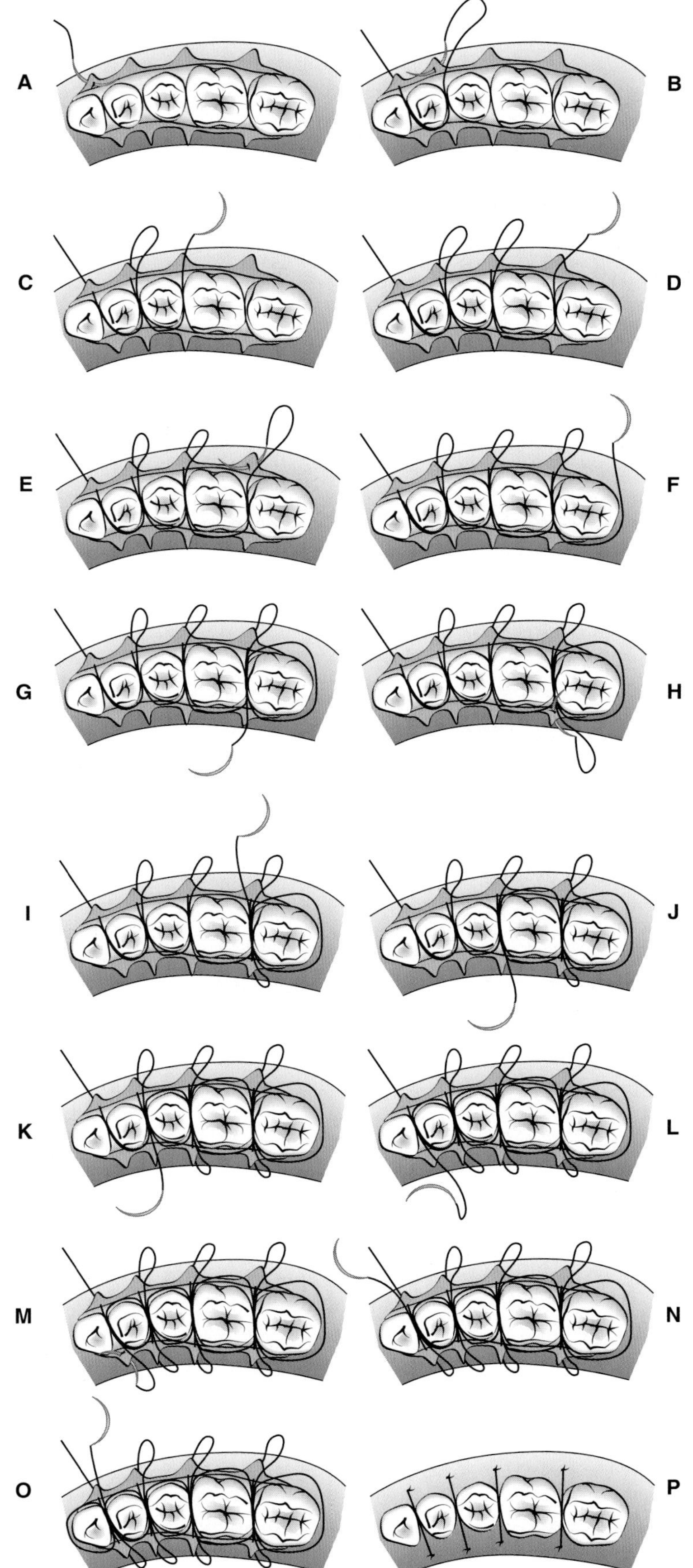

Fig. 60-19 The continuous, independent sling suture is used to adapt the buccal and lingual flaps without tying the buccal flap to the lingual flap. The teeth are used to suspend each flap against the bone. It is important to anchor the suture on the two teeth at the beginning and end of the flap so that the suture will not pull the buccal flap to the lingual flap.

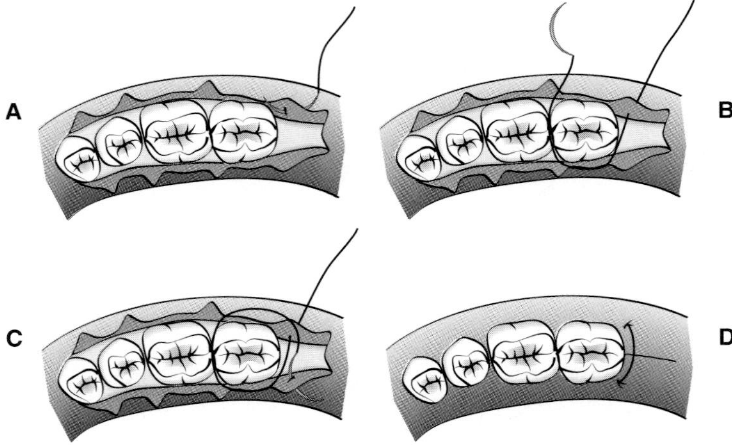

Fig. 60-20 A to D, Distal wedge suture. This suture is also used to close flaps that are mesial or distal to a lone-standing tooth.

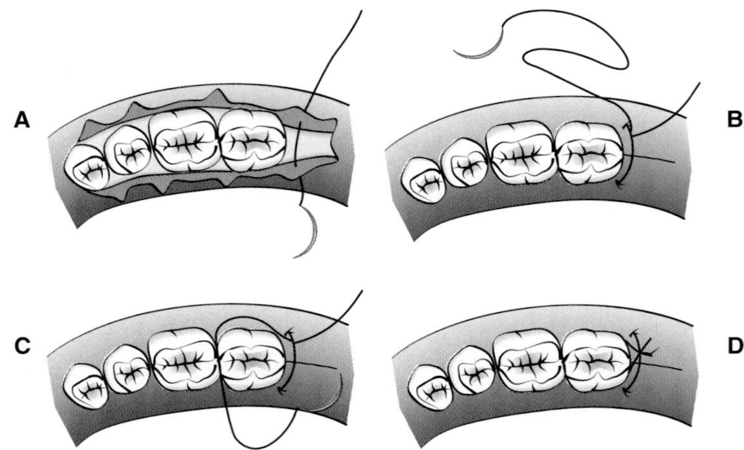

Fig. 60-21 The closed anchor suture, another technique to suture distal wedges.

in a similar fashion. The suture is again anchored around the last tooth before tying the final knot.

This type of suture does not produce a pull on the lingual flap when the latter is sutured. The two flaps are completely independent of each other owing to the anchoring around both the initial and the final tooth. The flaps are tied to the teeth and not to each other because of the sling sutures.

This type of suturing is especially appropriate for the maxillary arch because the palatal gingiva is attached and fibrous, whereas the facial tissue is thinner and mobile.

Anchor Suture. The closing of a flap mesial or distal to a tooth, as in the mesial or distal wedge procedures, is best accomplished by the anchor suture. This suture closes the facial and lingual flaps and adapts them tightly against the tooth. The needle is placed at the line angle area of the facial or lingual flap adjacent to the tooth, anchored around the tooth, passed beneath the opposite flap, and tied. The anchor suture can be repeated for each area that requires it (Fig. 60-20).

Closed Anchor Suture. Another technique to close a flap located in an edentulous area mesial or distal to a tooth consists of tying a direct suture that closes the proximal flap, carrying one of the threads around the tooth to anchor the tissue against the tooth, and then tying the two threads (Fig. 60-21).

Periosteal Suture. This type of suture is used to hold in place apically displaced partial thickness flaps. There are two types of periosteal sutures: the holding suture and the closing suture. The holding suture is a horizontal mattress suture placed at the base of the displaced flap to secure it into the new position. Closing sutures are used to secure the flap edges to the periosteum. Both types of periosteal sutures are shown in Fig. 60-22.

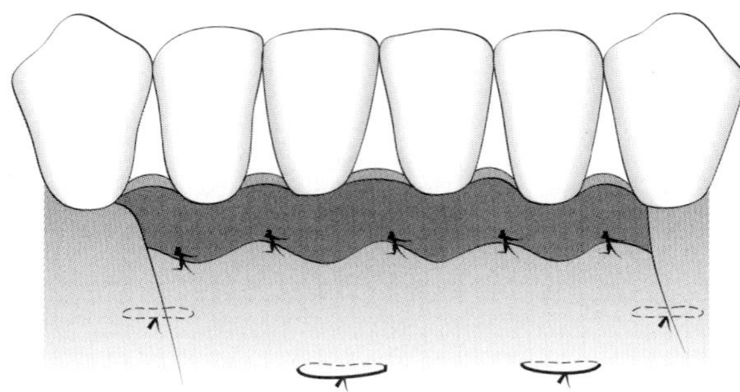

Fig. 60-22 Periosteal sutures for an apically displaced flap. Holding sutures, shown at the bottom, are done first, followed by the closing sutures, shown at the coronal edge of the flap.

HEALING AFTER FLAP SURGERY

Immediately after suturing (0 to 24 hours), a connection between the flap and the tooth or bone surface is established by a blood clot, which consists of a fibrin reticulum with many polymorphonuclear leukocytes, erythrocytes, debris of injured cells, and capillaries at the edge of the wound.[3] A bacteria and an exudate or transudate also result from tissue injury.

One to 3 days after flap surgery, the space between the flap and the tooth or bone is thinner, and epithelial cells migrate over the border of the flap, usually contacting the tooth at this time. When the flap is closely adapted to the alveolar process, there is only a minimal inflammatory response.[3]

One week after surgery, an epithelial attachment to the root has been established by means of hemidesmosomes and a basal lamina. The blood clot is replaced by granulation tissue derived from the gingival connective tissue, the bone marrow, and the periodontal ligament.

Two weeks after surgery, collagen fibers begin to appear parallel to the tooth surface.[3] Union of the flap to the tooth is still weak, owing to the presence of immature collagen fibers, although the clinical aspect may be almost normal.

One month after surgery, a fully epithelialized gingival crevice with a well-defined epithelial attachment is present. There is a beginning functional arrangement of the supracrestal fibers.

Full-thickness flaps, which denude the bone, result in a superficial bone necrosis at 1 to 3 days; osteoclastic resorption follows and reaches a peak at 4 to 6 days, declining thereafter.[13] This results in a loss of bone of about 1 mm[3,16]; the bone loss is greater if the bone is thin.[14,15]

Osteoplasty (thinning of the buccal bone) using diamond burs, included as part of the surgical technique, results in areas of bone necrosis with reduction in bone height, which is later remodeled by new bone formation. Therefore the final shape of the crest is determined more by osseous remodeling than by surgical reshaping.[8] This may not be the case when osseous remodeling does not include excessive thinning of the radicular bone.[9] Bone repair reaches its peak at 3 to 4 weeks.[15]

Loss of bone occurs in the initial healing stages both in radicular bone and in interdental bone areas. However, in interdental areas, which have cancellous bone, the subsequent repair stage results in total restitution without any loss of bone; whereas in radicular bone, particularly if thin and unsupported by cancellous bone, bone repair results in loss of marginal bone.[15]

REFERENCES

1. Barkann L: A conservative surgical technique for the eradication of pyorrhea pockets. J Am Dent Assoc 1939; 26:61.
2. Beube FE: Interdental tissue resection: An experimental study of a surgical technique which aids in repair of the periodontal tissues to their original contour and function. Oral Surg 1947; 33:497.
3. Caffesse RG, Ramfjord SP, Nasjleti CE: Reverse bevel periodontal flaps in monkeys. J Periodontol 1968; 39:219.
4. Carranza Jr FA, Carraro JJ: Effect of removal of periosteum on postoperative result of mucogingival surgery. J Periodontol 1963; 34:223.
5. Dahlberg WH: Incisions and suturing: Some basic considerations about each in periodontal flap surgery. Dent Clin North Am 1969; 113:149.
6. Friedman N: Mucogingival surgery: The apically repositioned flap. J Periodontol 1962; 33:328.
7. Hoag PM, Wood DL, Donnenfeld OW, et al: Alveolar crest reduction following full and partial thickness flaps. J Periodontol 1972; 43:141.
8. Lobene RR, Glickman I: The response of alveolar bone to grinding with rotary stones. J Periodontol 1963; 34:105.
9. Matherson DG: An evaluation of healing following periodontal osseous surgery in monkeys. Int J Periodont Restor Dent 1988; 8:9.
10. Morris ML: Suturing techniques in periodontal surgery. Periodontics 1965; 3:84.
11. Prichard JF: Present state of the interdental denudation procedure. J Periodontol 1977; 48:566.
12. Ratcliff PA, Raust GT: Interproximal denudation: A conservative approach to osseous surgery. Dent Clin North Am 1964; 8:121.
13. Staffileno H, Wentz FE, Orban BJ: Histologic study of healing of split thickness flap surgery in dogs. J Periodontol 1962; 33:56.
14. Wilderman MN: Exposure of bone in periodontal surgery. Dent Clin North Am 1964; 8:23.
15. Wilderman MN, Pennel BM, King K, et al: Histogenesis of repair following osseous surgery. J Periodontol 1970; 41:551.

The Flap Technique for Pocket Therapy

Fermin A. Carranza and Henry H. Takei

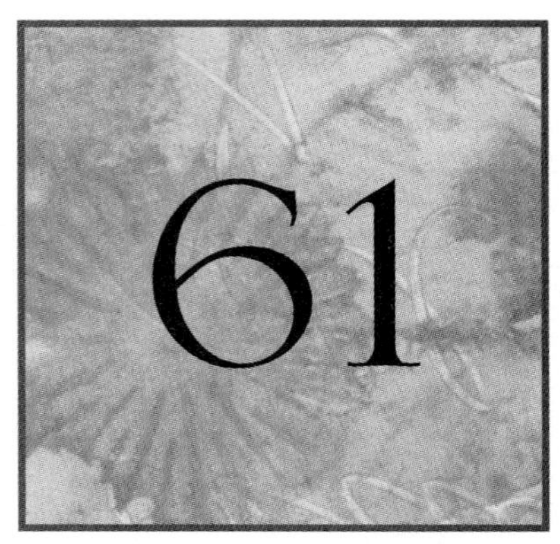

CHAPTER

CHAPTER OUTLINE

Several techniques can be used for the treatment of periodontal pockets. The periodontal flap is one of the most commonly employed procedures, particularly for moderate and deep pockets in posterior areas (see Chapter 54).

Flaps are used for pocket therapy to accomplish the following:

1. Increase accessibility to root deposits
2. Eliminate or reduce pocket depth by resection of the pocket wall
3. Expose the area to perform regenerative methods

To fulfill these purposes several flap techniques are available and in current use.

The modified Widman flap facilitates instrumentation but does not attempt to reduce pocket depth. Two flap techniques have as their main purpose the reduction or elimination of pocket depth: the now-displaced flap and the apically displaced flap. The decision of whether to perform one or the other depends on two important anatomical landmarks: pocket depth and the location of the mucogingival junction. These landmarks establish the presence and width of the attached gingiva, which is the basis for the decision.

The *modified Widman flap* has been described for exposing the root surfaces for meticulous instrumentation and for removal of the pocket lining[6]; it is not intended to eliminate or reduce pocket depth, except for the reduction that occurs in healing by tissue shrinkage.

The *undisplaced (unrepositioned) flap,* in addition to improving accessibility for instrumentation, removes the pocket wall, thereby reducing or eliminating the pocket. This is essentially an excisional procedure of the gingiva.

The *apically displaced flap* also improves accessibility and eliminates the pocket, but does the latter by apically positioning the soft tissue wall of the pocket.[2] Therefore it preserves and/or increases the width of the attached gingiva by transforming the previously unattached keratinized pocket wall into attached tissue. This increase in width of the band of attached gingiva is supposedly based on an apical shift of the mucogingival junction, which includes apical displacement of the muscle attachments. A study made before and 18 years after apically displaced flaps failed to show a permanent relocation of the mucogingival junction.[1] All three techniques use the basic incisions described in Chapter 60: the internal bevel incision, the crevicular incision, and the interdental incision. However, there are important variations in the way in which these incisions are performed for the different types of flaps.

The modified Widman flap does not intend to remove the pocket wall, but it does eliminate the pocket lining. Therefore the internal bevel incision starts close (no more than 1 to 2 mm apically) to the gingival margin and follows the normal scalloping of the gingival margin (Figs. 61-1 and 61-2).

For the apically displaced flap, the pocket wall also must be preserved to be positioned apically while its lining is removed. The purpose of this surgical technique is to preserve the maximum amount of keratinized gingiva of the pocket wall to displace it apically and transform it into attached gingiva. For this reason, the internal bevel incision should be made as close to the tooth as possible (0.5 to 1.0 mm) (see Fig. 61-1).

There is no need to determine where the bottom of the pocket is in relation to the incision, as one would for the undisplaced flap; the flap is placed approximately at the tooth-bone junction by apically displacing the flap. Its final position is not determined by the placement of this first incision.

For an undisplaced flap, however, the internal bevel incision is initiated at or near a point just coronal to the projection of the bottom of the pocket on the outer surface of the gingiva (see Fig. 61-1). This incision can be accomplished only if there is sufficient attached gingiva remaining apical to the incision. Therefore the two anatomic landmarks, pocket depth and location of the mucogingival junction, must be considered to evaluate the amount of attached gingiva that remains.

Because the pocket wall is not displaced apically, the initial incision should also eliminate the pocket wall. If the incision is made too close to the tooth, it will not eliminate the pocket wall and may result in the recreation of a soft tissue pocket. If the tissue is thick it should also be thinned by the initial incision to cover the bone properly during flap closure. Proper placement of the flap during closure is essential to prevent either recurrence of pockets or bone exposure; placement is determined by where this first incision is placed. The internal bevel incision should be scalloped to preserve, as much as possible, the interdental papilla (see Fig. 61-2). This allows better coverage of the bone at both the radicular and the interdental areas.

If the surgeon contemplates osseous surgery, the first incision should be placed in such a way as to compensate for the removal of bone tissue so that the flap ends at the tooth-bone junction.

The *techniques used for regenerative purposes* are the papilla preservation flap and the flap using only crevicular or pocket incisions, to retain the maximum amount of gingival tissue, including the papilla, for graft or membrane coverage.

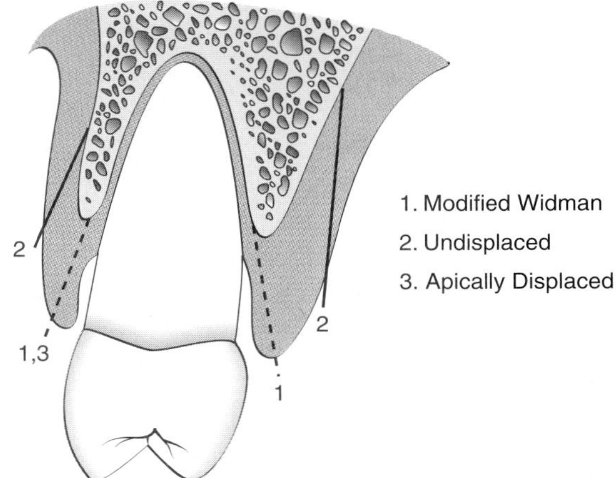

Fig. 61-1 Locations of the internal bevel incisions for the different types of flaps.

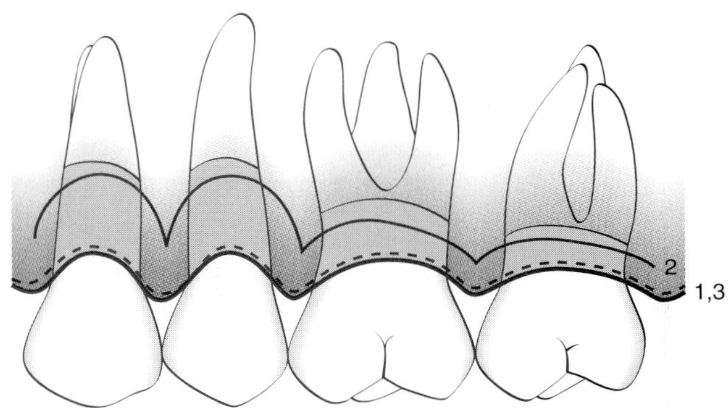

Fig. 61-2 Scallopings required for the different types of flaps.

THE MODIFIED WIDMAN FLAP

In 1965, Morris revived a technique described early in this century in the periodontal literature; he called it the *unrepositioned mucoperiosteal flap*.[4] Essentially the same procedure was presented in 1974 by Ramfjord and Nissle who called it the *modified Widman flap* (Fig. 61-3).[6] This technique offers the possibility of establishing an intimate postoperative adaptation of healthy collagenous connective tissue to tooth surfaces[5,6] and provides access for adequate instrumentation of the root surfaces and immediate closure of the area. The following is an outline of this technique:

Step 1: The initial incision is an internal bevel incision to the alveolar crest starting 0.5 to 1 mm away from the gingival margin (see Fig. 61-3, *C*). Scalloping

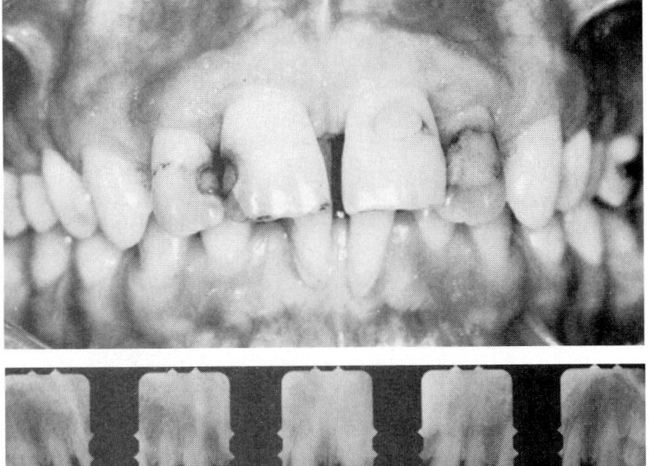

Fig. 61-3 The modified Widman flap technique. **A,** Facial view before surgery. Probing of pockets revealed interproximal depths ranging from 4 to 8 mm and facial and palatal depths of 2 to 5 mm. **B,** Radiographic survey of area. Note generalized horizontal bone loss.

Continued

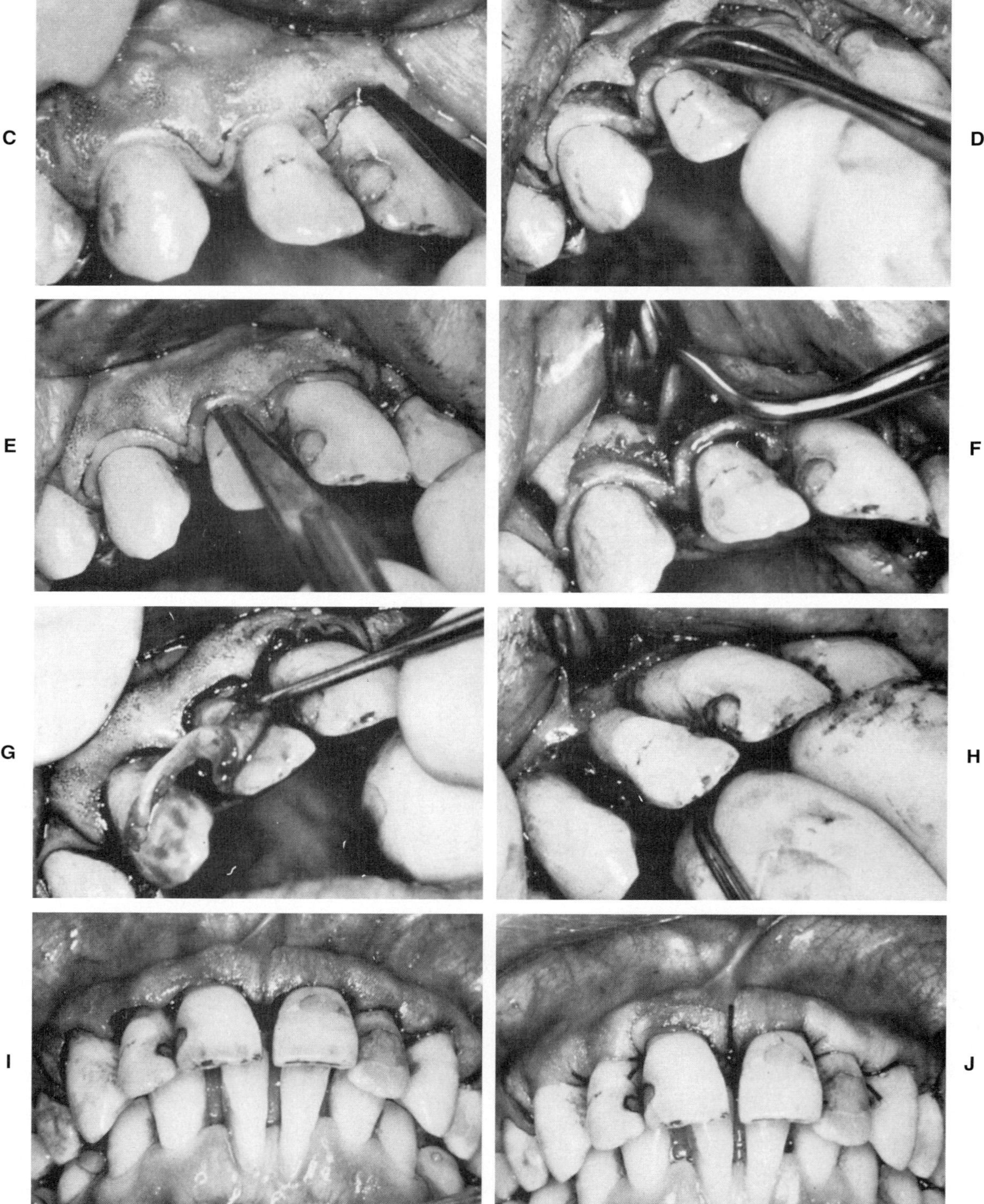

Fig. 61-3, cont'd The modified Widman flap technique. **C,** Internal bevel incision. **D,** Elevation of the flap, leaving a wedge of tissue still attached by its base. **E,** Crevicular incision. **F,** Interdental incision sectioning the base of the papilla. **G,** Removal of tissue. **H,** Exposure of root surfaces and marginal bone; root planing and removal of remaining calculus. **I,** Replacement of flap in its original position. **J,** Interdental sutures in place. (Courtesy Dr. Raul G. Caffesse, Houston, TX.)

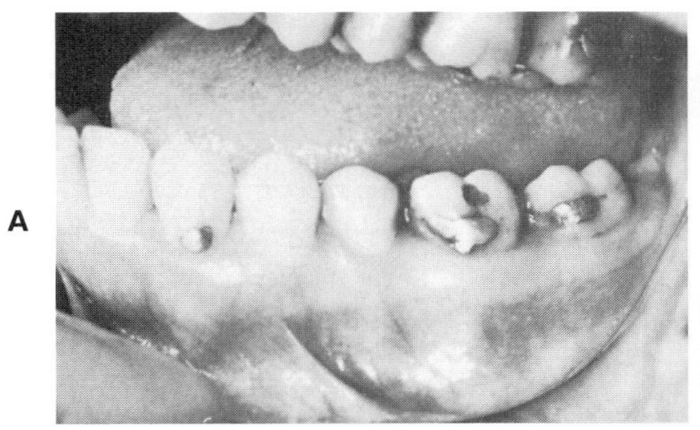

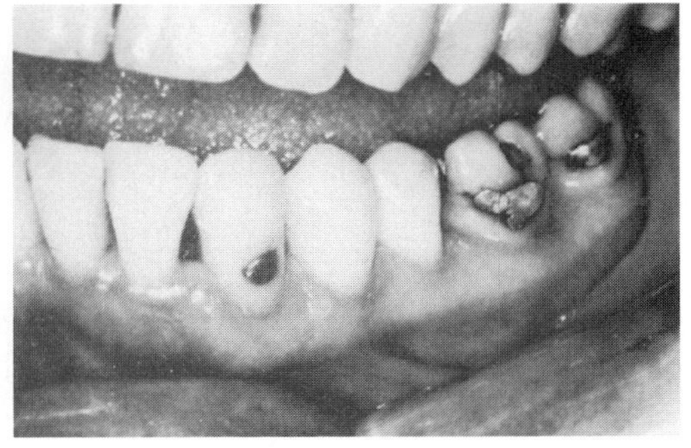

Fig. 61-4 A patient before **(A)** and after **(B)** treatment by means of Widman flaps. Note the reduction in gingival height and concomitant pocket depth. (Courtesy Dr. Raul G. Caffesse, Houston, TX.)

follows the gingival margin. Care should be taken to insert the blade in such a way that the papilla is left with a thickness similar to that of the remaining facial flap. Vertical relaxing incisions are usually not needed.

Step 2: The gingiva is reflected with a periosteal elevator (Fig. 61-3, *D*).

Step 3: A crevicular incision is made from the bottom of the pocket to the bone, circumscribing the triangular wedge of tissue containing the pocket lining (Fig. 61-3, *E*).

Step 4: After the flap is reflected, a third incision is made in the interdental spaces coronal to the bone with a curette or an interproximal knife, and the gingival collar is removed (Fig. 61-3, *F* and *G*).

Step 5: Tissue tags and granulation tissue are removed with a curette. The root surfaces are checked, and then scaled and planed if needed (Fig. 61-3, *H*). Residual periodontal fibers attached to the tooth surface should not be disturbed.

Step 6: Bone architecture is not corrected except if it prevents good tissue adaptation to the necks of the teeth. Every effort is made to adapt the facial and lingual interproximal tissue adjacent to each other in such a way that no interproximal bone remains exposed at the time of suturing (Fig. 61-3, *I*). The flaps may be thinned to allow for close adaptation of the gingiva around the entire circumference of the tooth and to each other interproximally.

Step 7: Interrupted direct sutures are placed in each interdental space (Fig. 61-3, *J*) and covered with tetracycline (Achromycin) ointment and with a periodontal surgical pack.

Ramfjord and colleagues performed an extensive longitudinal study comparing the Widman procedure, as modified by them, with the curettage technique and the pocket elimination methods that include bone contouring when needed.[6] The patients were assigned randomly to one of the techniques, and results were analyzed yearly up to 7 years posttherapy. They reported approximately similar results with the three methods tested. Pocket depth was initially similar for all methods but was maintained at shallower levels with the Widman flap (Fig. 61-4); the attachment level remained higher with the Widman flap.

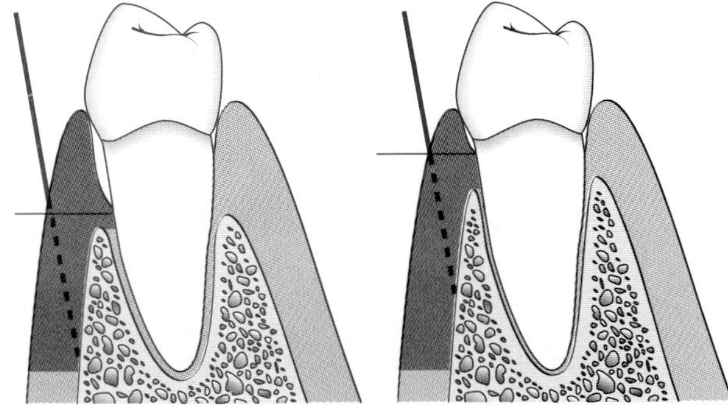

Fig. 61-5 Diagram showing the location of different areas where the internal bevel incision is made in an undisplaced flap. The incision is made at the level of the pocket to discard the tissue coronal to it if there is sufficient remaining attached gingiva.

THE UNDISPLACED FLAP

Currently, the undisplaced flap is perhaps the most commonly performed type of periodontal surgery. It differs from the modified Widman flap in that the soft tissue pocket wall is removed with the initial incision; thus it may be considered an internal bevel gingivectomy. The undisplaced flap and the gingivectomy are the two techniques that surgically remove the pocket wall. To perform this technique without creating a mucogingival problem it should be determined that enough attached gingiva will remain after removal of the pocket wall. The following is an outline of this technique:

Step 1: The pockets are measured with the periodontal probe, and a bleeding point is produced on the outer surface of the gingiva to mark the pocket bottom.

Step 2: The initial, internal bevel incision is made (Fig. 61-5) after the scalloping of the bleeding marks on the gingiva (Fig. 61-6). The incision is usually carried to a point apical to the alveolar crest, depending on the thickness of the tissue. The thicker the tissue, the more apical is the ending point of the incision (see Fig. 61-5). In addition, thinning of the flap should be done with the initial incision because at this time, it is easier to accomplish than later with a loose

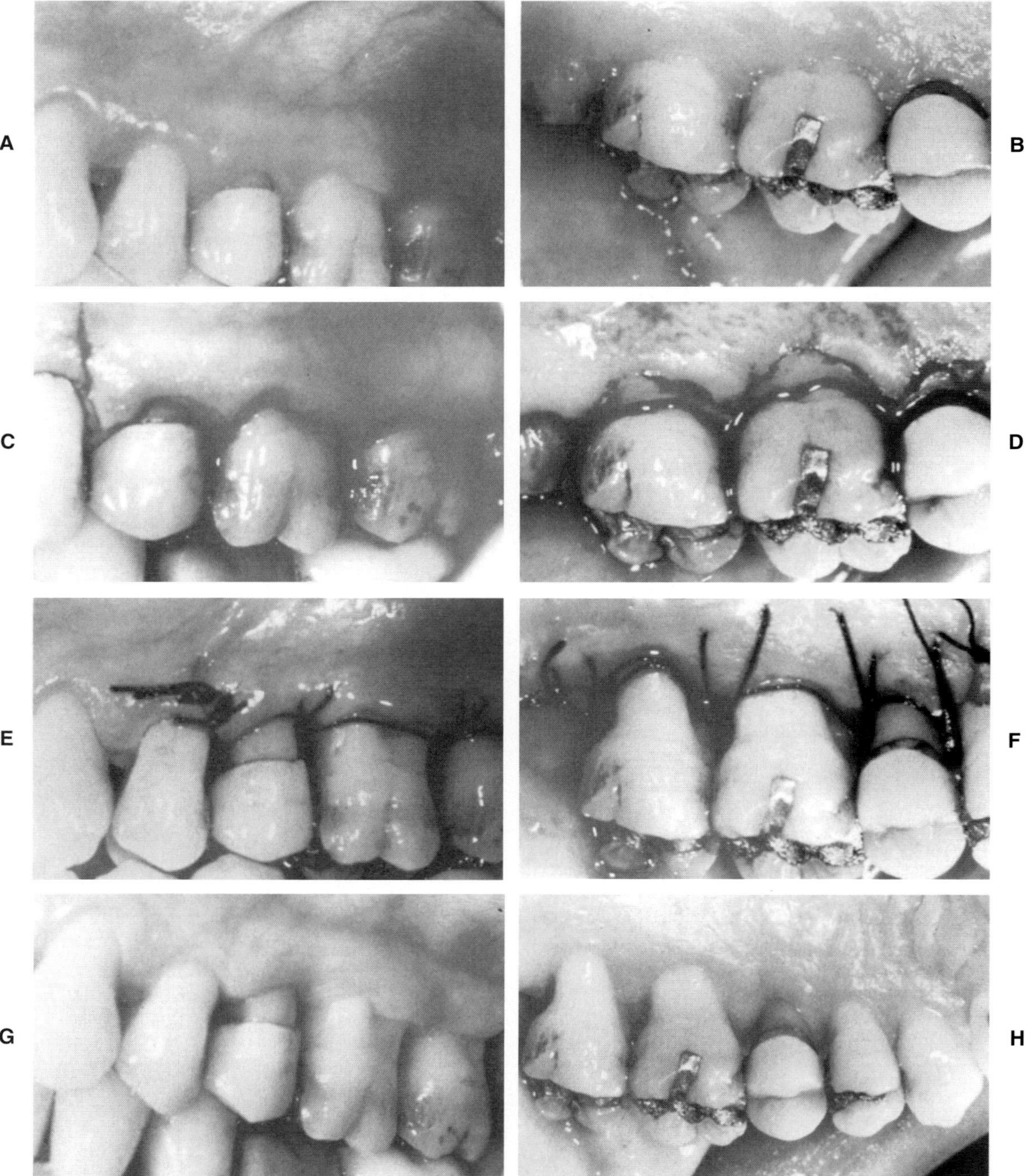

Fig. 61-6 The undisplaced. **A** and **B,** Preoperative facial and palatal views. **C** and **D,** Internal bevel incisions in the facial and palatal aspects. Note the deeper scalloping palatally for the replaced flap. **E** and **F,** After the necessary osseous surgery, the flaps have been sutured. The facial flap is apically displaced, whereas the palatal flap is replaced. **G** and **H,** Ten-week postoperative results. (Courtesy Dr. Silvia Oreamuno, San Jose, Costa Rica.)

reflected flap that is difficult to manage. (Use of this technique in palatal areas is considered in the following discussion.)

Step 3: The second or crevicular incision is made from the bottom of the pocket to the bone to detach the connective tissue from the bone.

Step 4: The flap is reflected with a periosteal elevator (blunt dissection) from the internal bevel incision. Usually there is no need for vertical incisions because the flap is not displaced apically.

Step 5: The interdental incision is made with an interdental knife, separating the connective tissue from the bone.

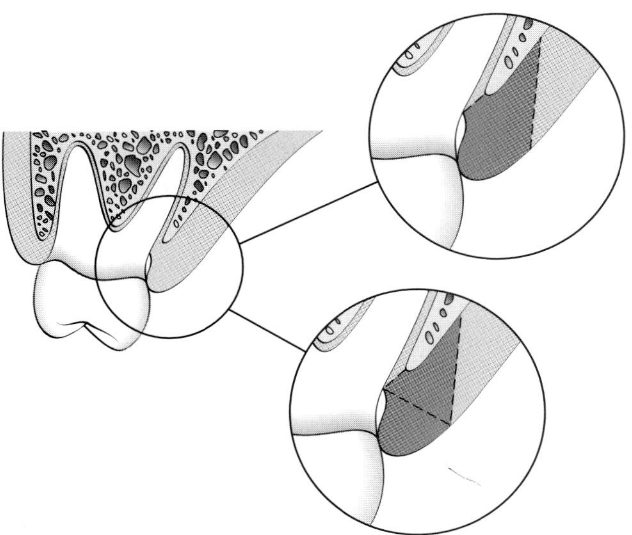

Fig. 61-7 Examples of two methods for eliminating a palatal pocket. One incision is an internal bevel incision made at the area of the apical extent of the pocket. The other procedure uses a gingivectomy incision, which is followed by an internal bevel incision.

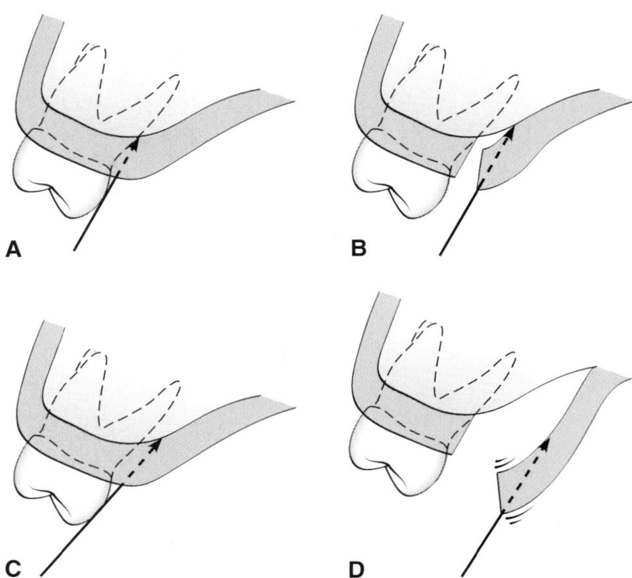

Fig. 61-8 Diagrams illustrating the angle of the internal bevel incision in the palate and the different ways to thin the flap. **A,** The usual angle and direction of the incision. **B,** The thinning of the flap after it has been slightly reflected with a second internal incision. **C,** The beveling and thinning of the flap with the initial incision if the position and contour of the tooth allow. **D,** The problem encountered in thinning the flap once it has been reflected. The flap is too loose and free for proper positioning and incision.

Step 6: The triangular wedge of tissue created by the three incisions is removed with a curette.

Step 7: The area is débrided, removing all tissue tags and granulation tissue using sharp curettes.

Step 8: After the necessary scaling and root planing, the flap edge should rest on the root-bone junction. If this is not the case, due to improper location of the initial incision or to the unexpected need for osseous surgery, the edge of the flap is rescalloped and trimmed to allow the flap edge to end at the root-bone junction.

Step 9: A continuous sling suture is used to secure the facial and the lingual or palatal flaps. This type of suture, using the tooth as an anchor, is advantageous to position and hold the flap edges at the root-bone junction. The area is covered with a periodontal pack.

The Palatal Flap

The surgical approach to the palatal area differs from that for other areas because of the character of the palatal tissue and the anatomy of the area. The palatal tissue is all attached, keratinized tissue and has none of the elastic properties associated with other gingival tissues. Therefore the palatal tissue cannot be apically displaced, nor can a partial (split) thickness flap be accomplished.

The initial incision for the palatal flap should be such that when the flap is sutured, it is precisely adapted at the root-bone junction. It cannot be moved apically or coronally to adapt to the root-bone junction, as can be done with the flaps in other areas. Therefore the location of the initial incision is important for the final placement of the flap.

The palatal tissue may be thin or thick, it may or may not have osseous defects, and the palatal vault may be high or low. These anatomic variations may require changes in the location, angle, and design of the incision.

The initial incision for a flap varies with the anatomic situation. As shown in Fig. 61-7, the initial incision may be the usual internal bevel incision, followed by crevicular and interdental incisions. If the tissue is thick, a horizontal gingivectomy incision may be made, followed by an internal bevel incision that starts at the edge of this incision and ends on the lateral surface of the underlying bone. The placement of the internal bevel incision must be done in such a way that the flap fits around the tooth without exposing the bone.

Before the flap is reflected to the final position for scaling and management of the osseous lesions, its thickness must be checked. Flaps should be thin to adapt to the underlying osseous tissue and provide a thin, knifelike gingival margin. Often flaps, particularly palatal flaps, are too thick; they may have a propensity to separate from the tooth and may delay and complicate healing. It is best to thin the flaps before their complete reflection, because a free, mobile flap is difficult to hold for thinning (Fig. 61-8). A sharp, thin papilla positioned properly around the interdental areas at the tooth-bone junction is essential to prevent recurrence of soft tissue pockets.

The purpose of the palatal flap should be considered before the incision is made. If the intent of the surgery is débridement, the internal bevel incision is planned so that the flap adapts at the root-bone junction when sutured. If osseous resection is necessary, the incision

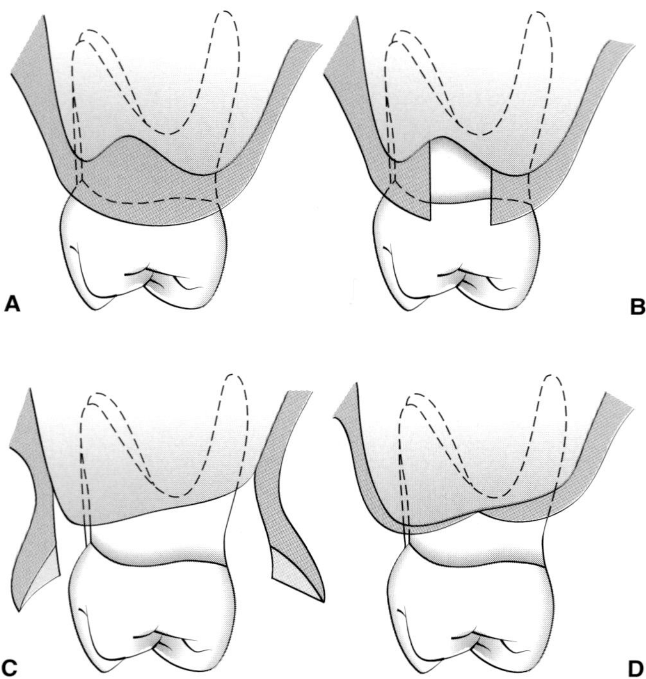

Fig. 61-9 **A,** A distal view of incisions made to eliminate a pocket distal to the maxillary second molar. **B,** Two parallel incisions and the removal of the intervening tissue. **C,** Thinning of the flap and contouring of the bone. **D,** Approximation of the buccal and palatal flaps.

should be planned to compensate for the lowered level of the bone when the flap is closed. Probing and sounding of the osseous level and the depth of the intrabony pocket should be used to determine the position of the incision.

The apical portion of the scalloping should be narrower than the line angle area because the palatal root tapers apically. A rounded scallop results in a palatal flap that does not fit snugly around the root. This procedure should be done before the complete reflection of the palatal flap, as a loose flap is difficult to grasp and stabilize for dissection.

It is sometimes necessary to thin the palatal flap after it has been reflected. This can be accomplished by holding the inner portion of the flap with a mosquito hemostat or Adson forceps as the inner connective tissue is carefully dissected away with a sharp #15 scalpel blade. Care must be taken not to perforate or overthin the flap. The edge of the flap should be thinner than the base; therefore the blade should be angled toward the lateral surface of the palatal bone. The dissected inner connective tissue is removed with a hemostat. As with any flap, the triangular papilla portion (Fig. 61-9) should be thin enough to fit snugly against the bone and into the interdental area.

The principles for the use of vertical releasing incisions are similar to those for using other incisions. Care must be exercised so that the length of the incision is minimal to avoid the numerous vessels located in the palate.

THE APICALLY DISPLACED FLAP

This technique with some variants can be used for one or both of the following purposes: pocket eradication or widening the zone of attached gingiva. Depending on the purpose, it can be a full thickness (mucoperiosteal) or a split thickness (mucosal) flap. The split thickness flap requires more precision and time, and a gingival tissue thick enough to split, but it can be more accurately positioned and sutured in an apical position using a periosteal suturing technique, as follows:

Step 1: An internal bevel incision is made (Fig. 61-10). To preserve as much of the keratinized and attached gingiva as possible, it should be no more than about 1 mm from the crest of the gingiva and directed to the crest of the bone (see Fig. 61-1). The incision is made after the existing scalloping, and there is no need to mark the bottom of the pocket in the external gingival surface because the incision is unrelated to pocket depth. It is also not necessary to accentuate the scallop interdentally, as the flap is displaced apically and not placed interdentally.

Step 2: Crevicular incisions are made, followed by initial elevation of the flap, and then interdental incisions are performed and the wedge of tissue that contains the pocket wall is removed.

Step 3: Vertical incisions are made extending *beyond the mucogingival junction,* if the objective is a full thickness flap it is elevated by blunt dissection with a periosteal elevator. If a split thickness flap is required, it is elevated using sharp dissection with a Bard-Parker knife to split it, leaving a layer of connective tissue, including the periosteum, on the bone.

Step 4: After removal of all granulation tissue, scaling and root planing, and osseous surgery if needed, the flap is displaced apically. It is important that the vertical incisions, and consequently, the flap elevation, reach past the mucogingival junction to provide adequate mobility to the flap for its apical displacement.

Step 5: If a full thickness flap was performed, a sling suture around the tooth prevents the flap from sliding to a position more apical than that desired, and the periodontal dressing can avoid its movement in a coronal direction. A partial thickness flap is sutured to the periosteum using a direct loop suture or a combination of loop and anchor suture. A dry foil is placed over the flap before covering it with the dressing to prevent the introduction of pack under the flap.

After 1 week, dressings and sutures are removed. The area is usually repacked for another week, after which the patient is instructed to use chlorhexidine mouth rinse or to apply chlorhexidine topically with cotton-tipped applicators for another 2 or 3 weeks.

FLAPS FOR REGENERATIVE SURGERY

In current regenerative therapy, either bone grafts, membranes, or a combination of these with or without other agents, are used for a successful outcome (see Chapter 63). The flap design should therefore be set up so that the maximum amount of gingival tissue and

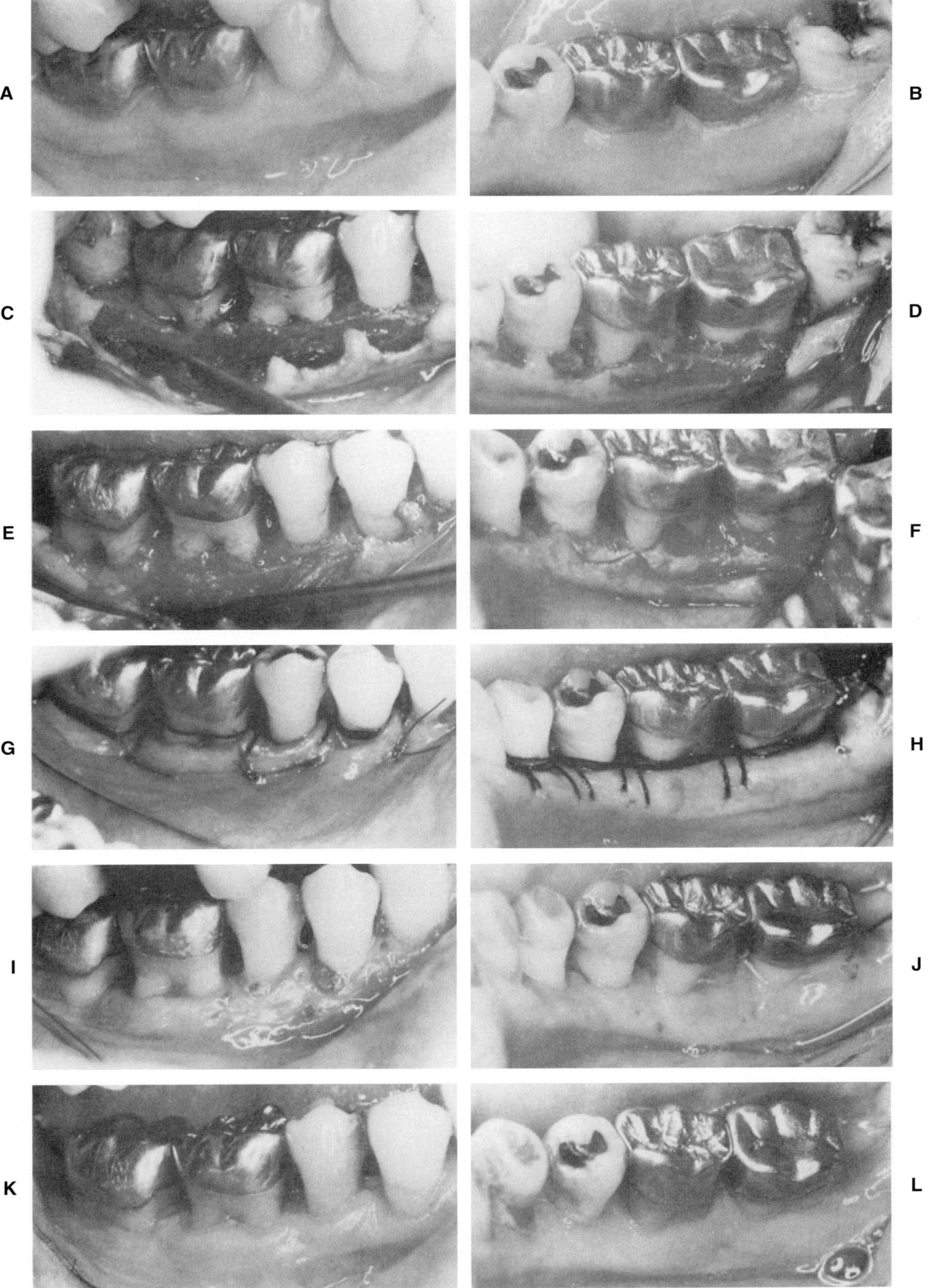

Fig. 61-10 Apically displaced flap. **A** and **B,** Facial and lingual preoperative views. **C** and **D,** Facial and lingual flaps elevated. **E** and **F,** After debridement of the areas. **G** and **H,** Sutures in place. **I** and **J,** Healing after 1 week. **K** and **L,** Healing after 2 months. Note the preservation of attached gingiva displaced to a more apical position.

papilla are retained to cover the material(s) placed in the pocket.

Two flap designs are available for regenerative surgery: the papilla preservation flap and the conventional flap with only crevicular incisions. The flap design of choice is the papilla preservation flap, which retains the entire papilla covering the lesion. However, to use this flap, there must be adequate interdental space to allow the intact papilla to be reflected with the facial or lingual/palatal flap. When the interdental space is very narrow, making it impossible to perform a papilla preservation flap, a conventional flap with only crevicular incisions is made.

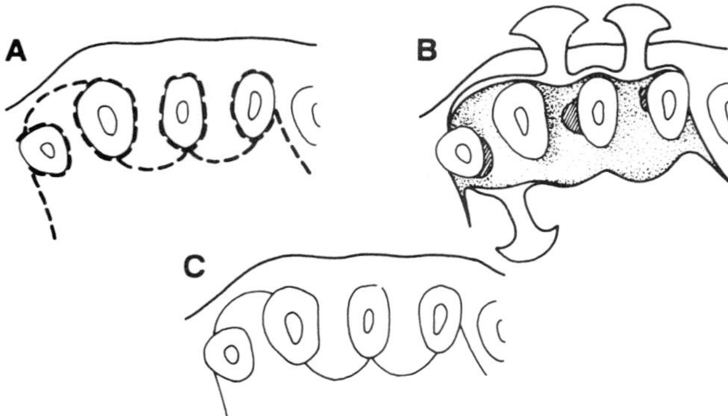

Fig. 61-11 Flap design for a papilla preservation flap. **A,** Incisions for this type of flap are depicted by interrupted lines. The preserved papilla can be incorporated into the facial or the lingual-palatal flap. **B,** The reflected flap exposes the underlying bone. Several osseous defects are seen. **C,** The flap returned to its original position covering the entire interdental spaces.

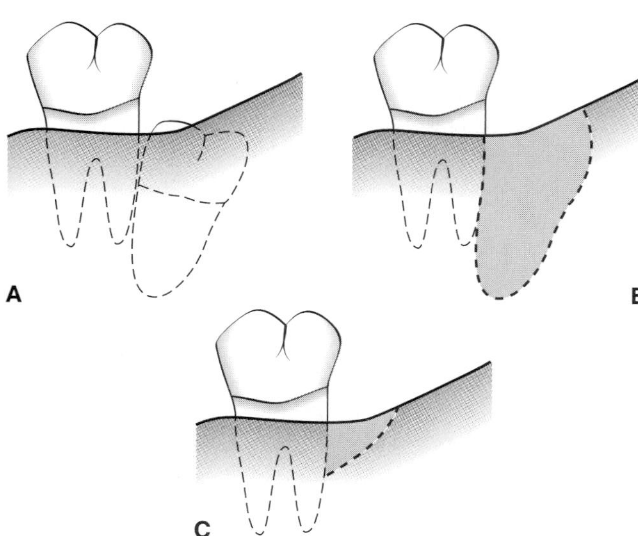

Fig. 61-12 A, The impaction of a third molar distal to a second molar with little or no interdental bone between the two teeth. **B,** Removal of the third molar creates a pocket with little or no bone distal to the second molar. This often leads to a vertical osseous defect distal to the second molar **(C)**.

The Papilla Preservation Flap

The technique for employing a papilla preservation flap is as follows:

Step 1: A crevicular incision is made around each tooth with no incisions across the interdental papilla.

Step 2: The preserved papilla can be incorporated into the facial or lingual/palatal flap, although it is most commonly integrated into the facial flap. In these cases the lingual or palatal incision consists of a semilunar incision across the interdental papilla in its palatal or lingual aspect; this incision dips apically from the line angles of the tooth so that the papillary incision is at least 5 mm from the crest of the papilla.

Step 3: An Orban knife is then introduced into this incision to sever one-half to two-thirds of the base of the interdental papilla. The papilla is then dissected from the lingual or palatal aspect and elevated intact with the facial flap.

Step 4: The flap is reflected without thinning the tissue. These incisions are illustrated in Fig. 61-11 and Color Fig. 60-1.

Conventional Flap for Regenerative Surgery

The technique for employing a conventional flap for regenerative surgery is as follows:

Step 1: Using a #12 blade, incise the tissue at the bottom of the pocket and to the crest of the bone, splitting the papilla below the contact point. Every effort should be made to retain as much tissue as possible to subsequently protect the area.

Step 2: Reflect the flap maintaining it as thick as possible, not attempting to thin it as is done for resective surgery. The maintenance of a thick flap is necessary to prevent exposure of the graft or the membrane due to necrosis of the flap margins.

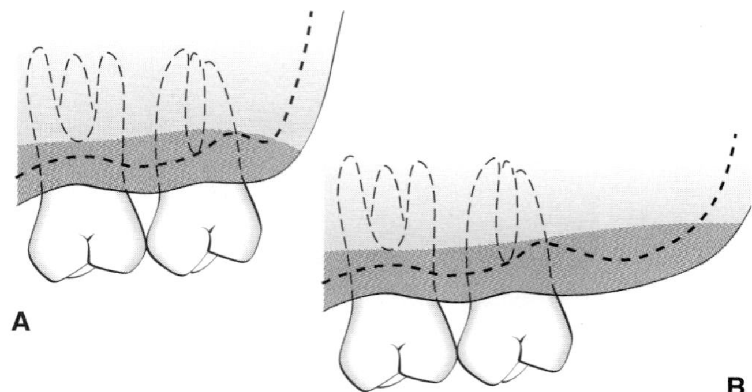

Fig. 61-13 A, Removal of a pocket distal to the maxillary second molar may be difficult if there is minimal attached gingiva. If the bone ascends acutely apically, the removal of this bone may make the procedure easier. **B,** A long distal tuberosity with abundant attached gingiva is an ideal anatomic situation for distal pocket eradication.

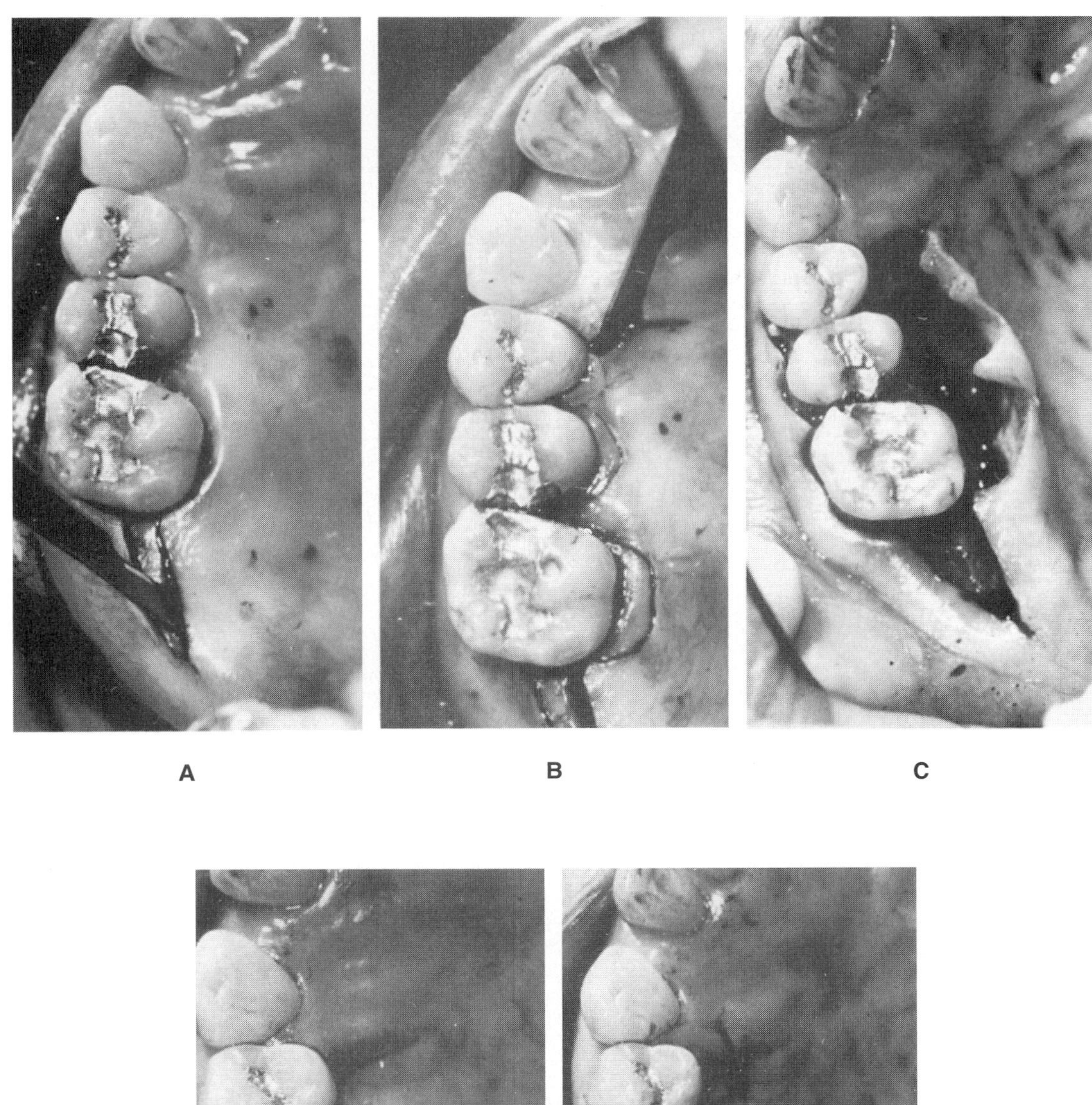

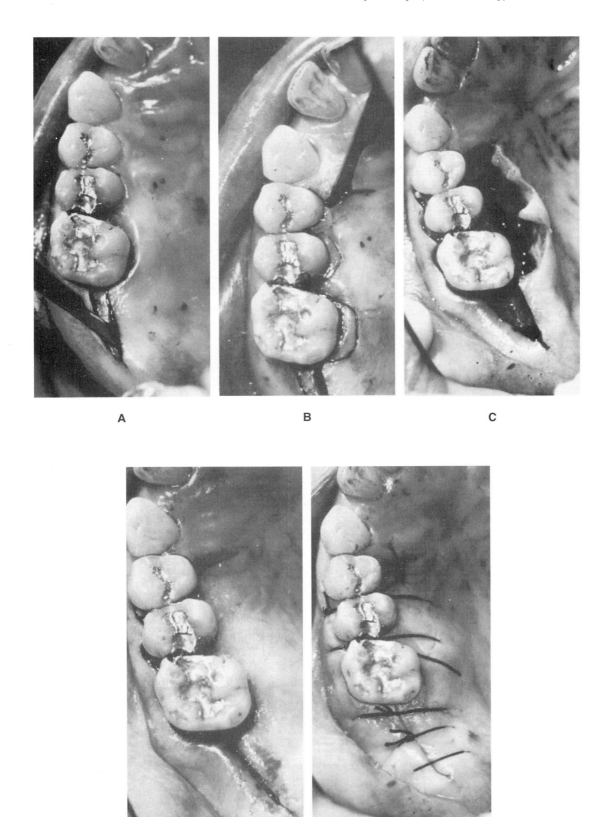

Fig. 61-14 **A,** A distal pocket eradication procedure with the incision distal to the molar. **B,** The scalloped incision around the remaining teeth. **C,** The flap reflected and thinned around the distal incision. **D,** The flap in position prior to suturing. It should be closely approximated. **E,** The flap sutured both distally and over the remaining surgical area.

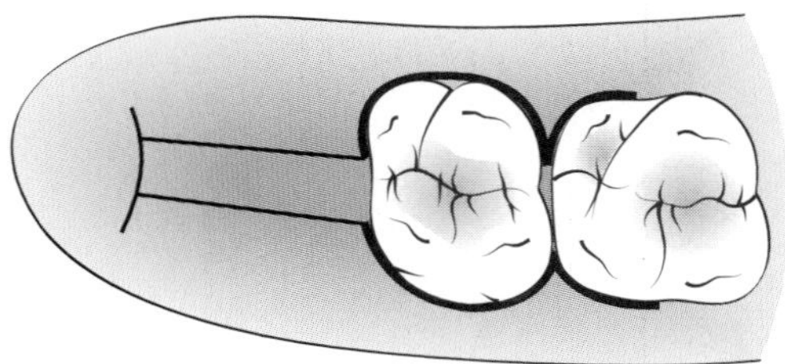

Fig. 61-15 A typical incision design for a surgical procedure distal to the maxillary second molar.

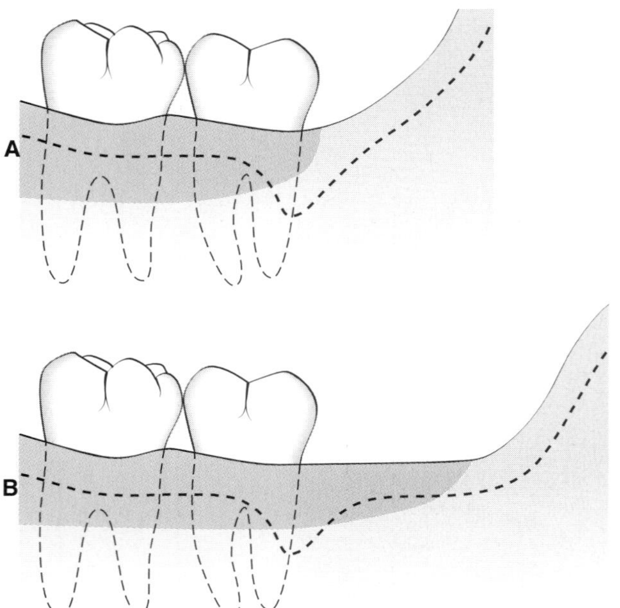

Fig. 61-16 A, Pocket eradication distal to a mandibular second molar with minimal attached gingiva and a close ascending ramus is anatomically difficult. **B,** For surgical procedures distal to a mandibular second molar, abundant attached gingiva and distal space are ideal.

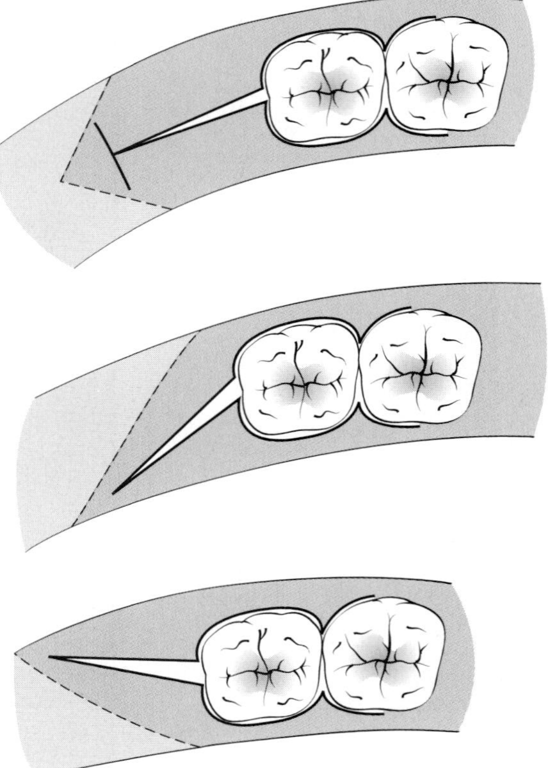

Fig. 61-17 Incision designs for surgical procedures distal to the mandibular second molar. The incision should follow the areas of greatest attached gingiva and underlying bone.

DISTAL MOLAR SURGERY

Treatment of periodontal pockets on the distal surface of terminal molars is often complicated by the presence of bulbous fibrous tissue over the maxillary tuberosity or prominent retromolar pads in the mandible. Deep vertical defects are also commonly present in conjunction with the redundant fibrous tissue. Some of these osseous lesions may result from incomplete repair after the extraction of impacted third molars (Fig. 61-12).

The gingivectomy incision is the most direct approach in treating distal pockets that have adequate attached gingiva and no osseous lesions. However, the flap approach is less traumatic postsurgically, because it produces a primary closure wound rather than the open secondary wound left by a gingivectomy incision. In addition, it results in attached gingiva and provides access for examination and, if needed, correction of the osseous defect. Operations for this purpose were described by Robinson[7] and Braden[2] and modified by several other investigators. Some representative procedures are discussed here.

Maxillary Molars. The treatment of distal pockets on the maxillary arch is usually more simple than the treatment of a similar lesion on the mandibular arch because the tuberosity presents a greater amount of fibrous attached gingiva than does the area of the retromolar pad. In addition, the anatomy of the tuberosity extending distally is more adaptable to pocket elimination than is that of the mandibular molar arch, where the tissue extends coronally. However, the lack of a broad area of attached gingiva and the abruptly ascending tuberosity sometimes complicates therapy (Fig. 61-13).

The following considerations determine the location of the incision for distal molar surgery: accessibility, amount of attached gingiva, pocket depth, and available distance from the distal aspect of the tooth to the end of the tuberosity or retromolar pad.

Technique. Two parallel incisions, beginning at the distal portion of the tooth and extending to the mucogingival junction distal to the tuberosity or retromolar pad, are made (Fig. 61-14). The faciolingual distance between these two incisions depends on the depth of the pocket and the amount of fibrous tissue involved. The deeper the pocket, the greater the distance between the two parallel incisions. It should be noted that when the tissue between the two incisions is removed and the flaps are thinned, the two flap edges must approximate each other at a new apical position without overlapping.

When the depth of the pocket cannot be easily estimated, it is better to err on the conservative side, leaving overlapping flaps rather than too short flaps that result in exposure of bone. When the two flaps overlap after the surgery is completed, they should be placed one over the other and the overlapping portion of one of them is grabbed with a hemostat. Then a sharp knife or scissors is used to cut the excess.

A transversal incision is made at the distal end of the two parallel incisions so that a long, rectangular piece of tissue can be removed. These incisions are usually interconnected with the incisions for the remainder of the surgery in the quadrant involved. The parallel distal incisions should be confined to the attached gingiva because bleeding and flap management become problems when the incision is extended into the alveolar mucosa. If access is difficult, especially if the distance from the distal aspect of the tooth to the mucogingival junction is short, a vertical incision can be made at the end of the parallel incisions.

In treating the tuberosity area, the two distal incisions are usually made at the midline of the tuberosity (Fig. 61-15). In most cases, no attempt is made to undermine the underlying tissue at this time. These incisions are made straight down into the underlying bone where access is difficult. A #12B blade is generally used. It is easier to dissect out the underlying redundant tissue when the flap is partially reflected. When the distal flaps are placed back on the bone, the two flap margins should closely approximate each other.

Mandibular Molars. Incisions for the mandibular arch differ from those used for the tuberosity, owing to differences in the anatomy and histologic features of the areas. The retromolar pad area does not usually present as much fibrous attached gingiva. The keratinized gingiva, if present, may not be found directly distal to the molar. The greatest amount may be distolingual or distofacial and may not be over the bony crest. The ascending ramus of the mandible may also create a short horizontal area distal to the terminal molar (Fig. 61-16). The shorter this area, the more difficult it is to treat any deep distal lesion around the terminal molar.

The two incisions distal to the molar should follow the area with the greatest amount of attached gingiva (Fig. 61-17). Therefore the incisions could be directed distolingually or distofacially, depending on which area has more attached gingiva. Before the flap is completely reflected, it is thinned with a #15 blade. It is easier to thin the flap before it is completely free and mobile. After the reflection of the flap and the removal of the redundant fibrous tissue, any necessary osseous surgery is performed. The flaps are approximated similarly to those in the maxillary tuberosity area.

REFERENCES

1. Ainamo A, Bergenholtz A, Hugoson A, et al: Location of the mucogingival junction 18 years after apically repositioned flap surgery. J Clin Periodontol 1992; 19:49.
2. Braden BE: Deep distal pockets adjacent to terminal teeth. Dent Clin North Am 1969; 13:161.
3. Matelski DE, Hurt WC: The corrective phase: The modified Widman flap. In: Hurt WC (ed): Periodontics in General Practice. Springfield, IL, Charles C Thomas, 1976.
4. Morris ML: The unrepositioned mucoperiosteal flap. Periodontics 1965; 3:147.
5. Ramfjord SP: Present status of the modified Widman flap procedure. J Periodontol 1977; 48:558.
6. Ramfjord SP, Nissle RR: The modified Widman flap. J Periodontol 1974; 45:601.
7. Robinson RE: The distal wedge operation. Periodontics 1966; 4:256.

Resective Osseous Surgery

Thomas N. Sims and Williams Ammons, Jr.

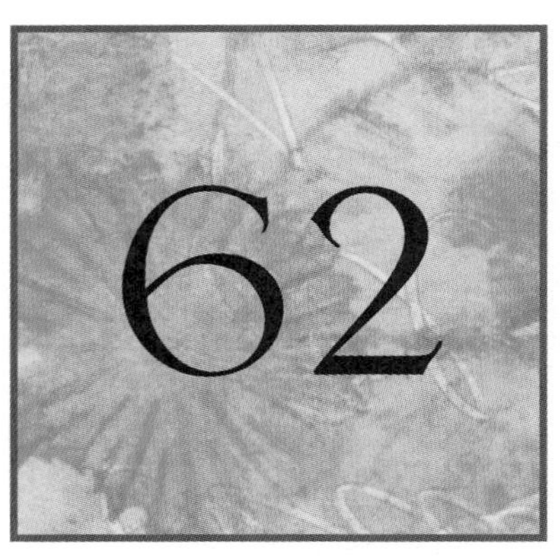

CHAPTER

CHAPTER OUTLINE

The damage resulting from periodontal disease reveals itself in variable destruction of the tooth-supporting bone. Generally, bony deformities are not uniform. They are not indicative of the alveolar housing of the tooth before the disease process, nor do they reflect the overlying gingival architecture. Bone loss has been classified as either horizontal or vertical, but in fact, bone loss is most often a combination of horizontal and vertical loss. Horizontal bone loss generally results in a relative thickening of the marginal alveolar bone, since bone tapers as it approaches its most coronal margin.

The effects of this thickening and the development of vertical defects leave the alveolar bone with countless combinations of bony shapes. If these various topographic changes are to be altered to provide a more physiologic bone pattern, a method for osseous recontouring must be followed.

> Osseous surgery may be defined as the procedure by which changes in the alveolar bone can be accomplished to rid it of deformities induced by the periodontal disease process or other related factors, such as exostosis and tooth supraeruption.

Osseous surgery can be either additive or subtractive in nature. **Additive osseous surgery** includes procedures directed at restoring the alveolar bone to its original level, whereas **subtractive osseous surgery** is designed to restore the form of preexisting alveolar bone to the level existing at the time of surgery or slightly more apical to this level (Fig. 62-1).

Additive osseous surgery brings about the ideal result of periodontal therapy; it implies regeneration of lost bone and reestablishment of the periodontal ligament,

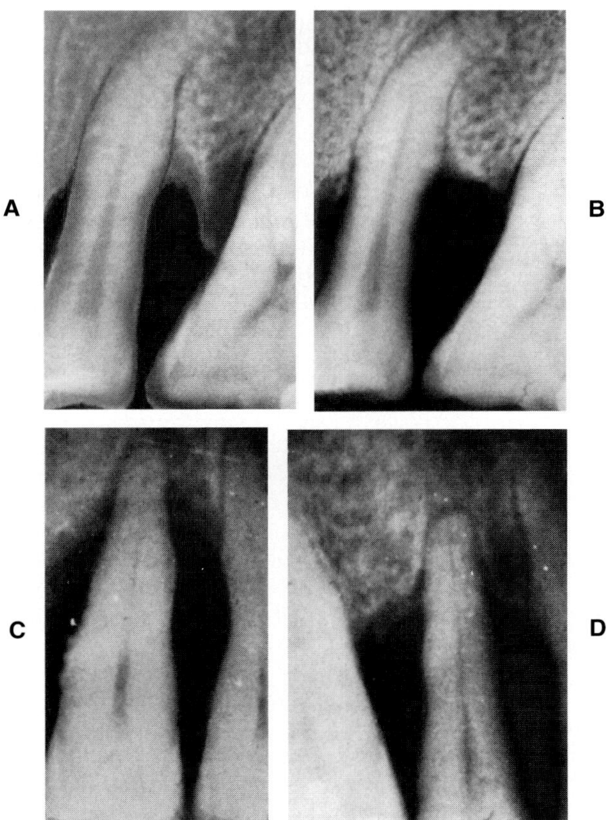

Fig. 62-1 Additive and subtractive osseous surgery. **A,** Before and **B,** immediately after subtractive osseous surgery; the osseous wall of the two adjoining infrabony pockets has been removed. **C,** Before and **D,** 1 year after additive osseous surgery; the area has been flapped and thoroughly instrumented, resulting in regeneration of the interdental and periapical bone. (Courtesy Drs. E. A. Albano and B. O. Barletta; Argentina.)

gingival fibers, and junctional epithelium at a more coronal level. This type of osseous surgery is discussed in Chapter 63.

Subtractive osseous surgery procedures provide an alternative to additive methods and should be resorted to when the latter are not feasible. They are discussed in this chapter.

SELECTION OF TREATMENT TECHNIQUE

The morphology of the osseous defect largely determines the treatment technique to be used. One-wall angular defects usually have to be recontoured surgically. Three-wall defects, particularly if they are narrow and deep, can be successfully treated with techniques that aim at new attachment and bone regeneration. Two-wall angular defects can be treated with either method, depending on their depth, width, and general configuration. Therefore except for one-wall defects, wide and shallow two-wall defects, along with interdental craters, osseous defects are treated with the objective of obtaining optimal repair by natural healing processes.

RATIONALE

Osseous resective surgery necessitates following a series of strict guidelines for proper contouring of alveolar bone and subsequent management of the overlying gingival soft tissues. The specifics of these techniques are discussed later in this chapter. They are quite technique sensitive. The techniques discussed here for osseous resective surgery have limited applicability in very deep intrabony or hemiseptal defects, which could be treated with a different surgical approach, are discussed in Chapter 63. Osseous surgery provides the purest and surest method for reducing pockets with bony discrepancies that are not overly vertical and also remains one of the principal periodontal modalities because of its long-term success and predictability.

Osseous resective surgery is the most predictable pocket reduction technique.[10,12,13] However, more than any other surgical technique, osseous resective surgery is performed at the expense of bony tissue and attachment level.[1,2,8] Thus its value as a surgical approach is limited by the presence, quantity, and shape of the bony tissues and by the amount of attachment loss that is acceptable.

The major rationale for osseous resective surgery is centered on the tenet that discrepancies in level and shapes of the bone and gingiva predispose patients to the recurrence of pocket depth postsurgically.[6] Although this concept is not universally accepted[3,5] and despite the fact that the procedure induces loss of radicular bone in the healing phase, there are cases in which recontouring of bone is the only logical treatment choice. The goal of osseous resective therapy is to reshape the marginal bone to resemble that of the alveolar process undamaged by periodontal disease. The technique is performed in combination with apically positioned flaps, and the procedure eliminates periodontal pocket depth and improves tissue contour to provide a more easily maintainable environment. The relative merits of pocket reduction procedures are discussed in Chapters 33 and 54; this chapter discusses the osseous resective technique and how and where it may be accomplished.

It is proposed that the conversion of the periodontal pocket to a shallow gingival sulcus enhances the patient's ability to remove plaque and oral debris from the dentition. Likewise, the ability of dental professionals to maintain the periodontium in a state free of gingivitis and periodontitis is more predictable in the presence of shallow sulci. The more effective the periodontal maintenance therapy, the greater is the longitudinal stability of the surgical result. The efficacy of osseous surgery therefore is dependent on its ability to affect pocket depth and to promote periodontal maintenance.[11,23,24] The merits of resection vs. other treatment procedures are discussed in Chapter 54 of this text.

NORMAL ALVEOLAR BONE MORPHOLOGY

Knowledge of the morphology of the bony periodontium in a state of health is required to correctly perform resective osseous surgery (Fig. 62-2). The characteristics of a normal bony form are as follows:

1. The interproximal bone is more coronal in position than the labial or lingual/palatal bone and pyramidal in form.
2. The form of the interdental bone is a function of the tooth form and the embrasure width. The more tapered the tooth, the more pyramidal is the bony form. The wider the embrasure, the more flattened is the interdental bone mesiodistally and buccolingually.
3. The position of the bony margin mimics the contours of the cementoenamel junction. The distance from the facial bony margin of the tooth to the interproximal bony crest is more flat in the posterior areas than the anterior. This "scalloping" of the bone on the facials and linguals/palatals is related to tooth and root form, as well as tooth position, within the alveolus. Teeth with prominent roots or that are displaced to the facial or lingual may also have fenestrations or dehiscences (Fig. 62-3). The molar teeth have less scalloping and a more flat profile than bicuspids and incisors. Although these general observations apply to all patients, the bony architecture may vary from patient to patient in the extent of contour, configuration, and thickness. These variations may be both normal and healthy.

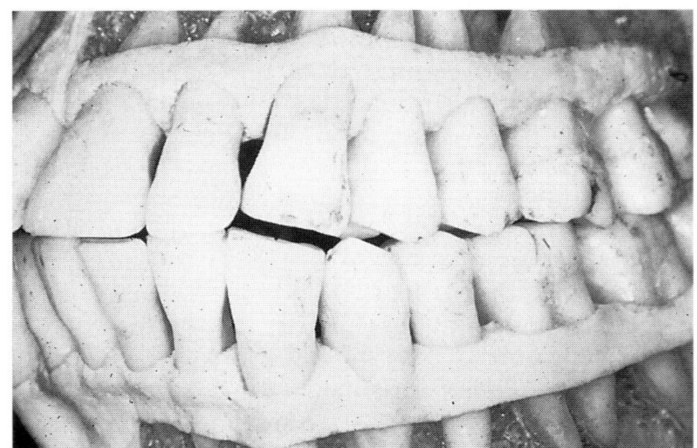

Fig. 62-2 Photograph of a healthy bony periodontium in a skull. Although a slight amount of attachment may have been lost, this skull demonstrates the characteristics of normal form.

TERMINOLOGY

Numerous terms have been developed to describe the topography of the alveolar housing, the procedure for its removal, and the resulting correction. These terms should be clearly defined.

Procedures used to correct osseous defects have been classified in two groups: osteoplasty and ostectomy.[7] **Osteoplasty** refers to reshaping the bone without removing tooth-supporting bone. **Ostectomy** (or *osteoectomy*) includes the removal of tooth-supporting bone. One or both of these procedures may be necessary to produce the desired result.

Terms that describe the bone form after reshaping can refer to morphologic features or to the thoroughness of the reshaping performed. Examples of morphologically descriptive terms include *negative, positive, flat,* and *ideal.* These terms all relate to a preconceived standard of ideal osseous form.

Positive or **negative architecture** refer to the relative position of interdental bone to radicular bone (Fig. 62-4). The architecture is said to be positive if the radicu-

A

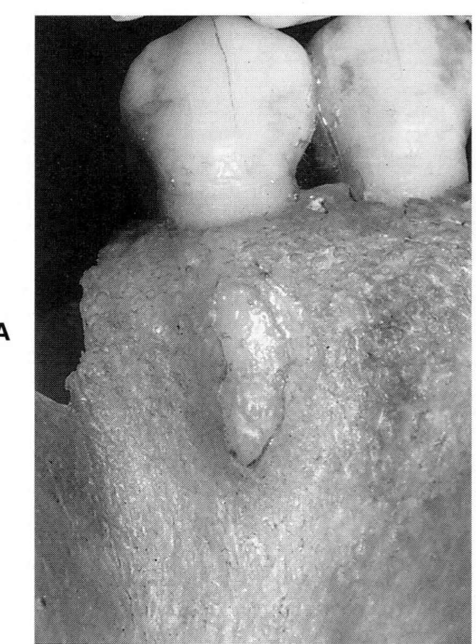

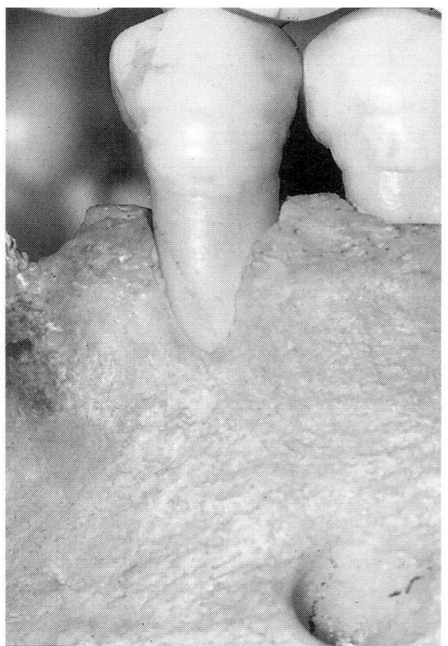

B

Fig. 62-3 The effects of tooth position on facial bony contours. **A,** Bony fenestration; **B,** bony dehiscence. These deformities can and should be detected by palpation, probing and sounding prior to flap surgery.

lar bone is apical to the interdental bone. The bone is said to have negative architecture if the interdental bone is more apical than the radicular bone. **Flat architecture** is the reduction of the interdental bone to the same height as the radicular bone.

Osseous form is considered to be *ideal* when the bone is consistently more coronal on the interproximal surfaces than on the facial and lingual surfaces. The ideal form of the marginal bone has similar interdental height, with gradual, curved slopes between interdental peaks (Fig. 62-5).

Terms that relate to the thoroughness of the osseous reshaping techniques include *definitive* and *compromise.* **Definitive osseous reshaping** implies that further osseous reshaping would not improve the overall result. **Compromise osseous reshaping** indicates a bone pattern that cannot be improved without significant osseous removal that would be detrimental to the overall result. References to compromise and definitive osseous architecture can be useful to the clinician, not as description of morphologic feature, but as terms that express the expected therapeutic result.

FACTORS IN THE SELECTION OF RESECTIVE OSSEOUS SURGERY

The relationship between the depth and configuration of the bony lesion(s) to root morphology and the adjacent teeth determines the extent that bone and attachment is removed during resection. Bony lesions have been classified according to their configuration and number of bony walls.[9] The technique of ostectomy is best applied to patients with early-to-moderate bone loss (2 to 3 mm) with moderate-length root trunks[19] that have bony defects with one or two walls. These shallow-to-moderate bony defects can be effectively managed by osteoplasty and osteoectomy. Patients with advanced attachment loss and deep intrabony defects are not candidates for resection to produce a positive contour. To simulate a normal architectural form, so much bone would have to be removed that the survival of the teeth could be compromised.

Two-walled defects/craters occur at the expense of the interseptal bone. As a result, they have buccal and lingual/palatal walls that extend from one tooth to the adjacent tooth. The interdental loss of bone exposes the proximal aspects of both adjacent teeth. The buccal-lingual interproximal contour that results is opposite to the contour of the cementoenamel junction of the teeth (Fig. 62-6, *A* and *B*). Two-walled defects (craters) are the most common bony defects found in patients with periodontitis.[15,21] If the facial and/or lingual plates of this bone are resected, the resultant interproximal contour would become more flattened or ovate (Fig. 62-6, *C* and *D*). However, confining resection only to ledges and the interproximal lesion results in a facial and lingual bone form in which the interproximal bone is located more apically than is the bone on the facial or lingual aspects of the tooth. This resulting anatomic form is *reversed* or *negative* architecture[18,19,23] (see Fig. 62-6, *C* and *D*).

Although the production of a reversed architecture minimizes the amount of ostectomy that is performed, it is not without consequences.[5] Peaks of bone commonly remain at the facial, lingual/palatal line angles of the teeth (so-called *widow's peaks*). During healing, the soft tissue tends to bridge the embrasure from the most coronal height of the bone on one tooth to the most coronal heights on the adjacent teeth. The result therefore is the tendency to replicate the attachment contour on the

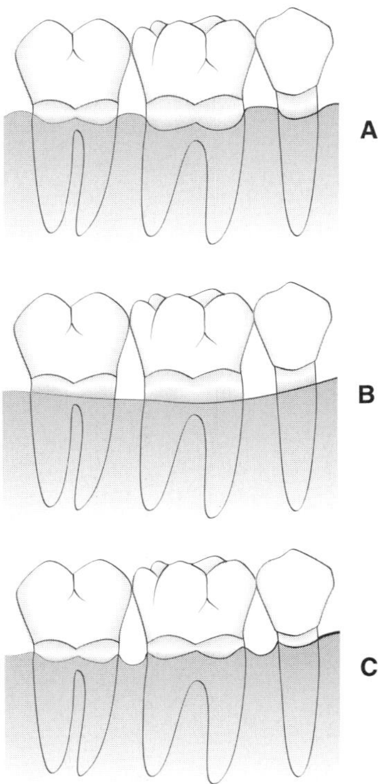

Fig. 62-4 Diagram of types of bony architecture. **A,** a positive bony architecture; **B,** a flat bony architecture; and **C,** a reversed or negative bony form.

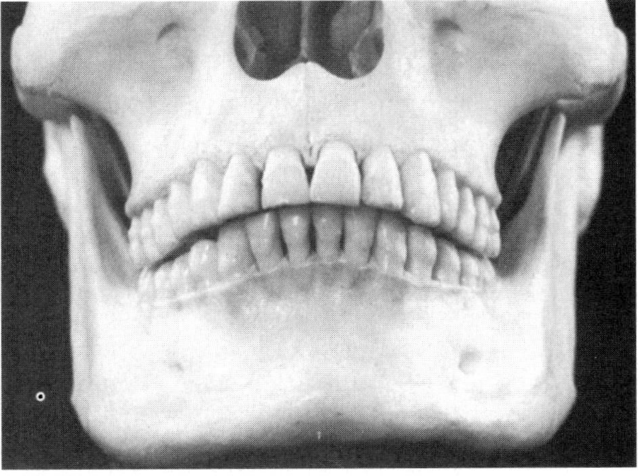

Fig. 62-5 Skull photograph of a healthy periodontium. Note the shape of the alveolar bone housing. This bone is considered to have ideal form. It is more coronal in the interproximal areas, with a gradual slope around and away from the tooth.

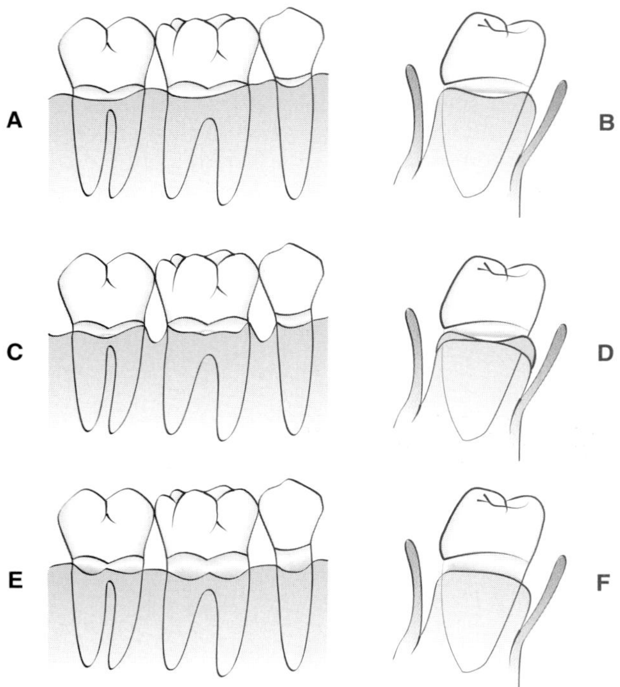

Fig. 62-6 Effect of correction of craters. **A and B,** Diagram of facial and interproximal bony contours after flap reflection. Note the loss of some interproximal bone and cratering. **C and D,** Line angles; this is only osteoplasty and has resulted in a reversed architecture. **E and F,** Ostectomy on the facial and lingual bone and the removal of the residual widow's peaks to produce a positive bony architecture.

tooth. The interproximal soft tissues invest these peaks of bone, which may subsequently resorb with a tendency to rebound without gain in attachment over time. A recurrence of interproximal pocket depth can occur.[23,25]

Ostectomy to a positive architecture requires the removal of the line angle inconsistencies (widow's peaks), as well as some of the facial, lingual and palatal and interproximal bone. The result is a loss of some attachment on the facial and lingual root surfaces but a topography that more closely resembles normal bone form before disease (Fig. 62-6, *E* and *F*). Proponents of osseous resection to create a positive contour believe that this architecture, devoid of sharp angles and spines, is conducive to the formation of a more uniform and reduced soft tissue dimension postoperatively.[18,22] The therapeutic result is less pocket depth and increased ease of periodontal maintenance by the patient, dental hygienist or dentist.

The amount of attachment lost from the use of ostectomy varies with the depth and configuration of the osseous defects that are treated. Osseous resection applied to two-wall intrabony defects (craters), the most common osseous defects, results in attachment loss at the proximal line angles and the facial and lingual aspects of the affected teeth without affecting the base of the pocket. The extent of attachment loss during resection to a positive architecture has been measured. When the technique is properly applied to appropriate patients, the mean reduction in attachment circumferentially around the tooth has been determined to be 0.6 mm at six probing sites.[23] Practically, this means that the technique is best applied to interproximal lesions 1- to 3-mm deep in patients with moderate to long root trunks.[18] Patients with deep, multiwalled defects are not candidates for resective osseous surgery. They are better treated with regenerative therapies or by combining osteoplasty to reduce bony ledges and to facilitate flap closure with new attachment/regeneration procedures.

EXAMINATION AND TREATMENT PLANNING WITH RESECTIVE SURGERY

The potential for the use of resective osseous surgery is usually identified during a comprehensive periodontal examination. Suitable patients display the signs and symptoms of periodontitis (see Chapter 30). The gingiva may be inflamed and deposits of plaque, calculus, and oral debris may be present. An increased flow of crevicular fluid may be detected, and bleeding on probing and exudation are commonly observed.

Periodontal probing and exploration are key aspects of the examination. Careful probing reveals the presence of (1) pocket depth greater than that of a normal gingival sulcus, (2) the location of the base of the pocket relative to the mucogingival junction and attachment level on adjacent teeth, (3) the number of bony walls, and (4) the presence of furcation defects. **Transgingival probing,** or *sounding,* under local anesthesia confirms the extent and configuration of the intrabony component of the pocket or offurcation defects.[6,17]

Routine dental radiographs do not identify the presence of periodontitis, nor do they accurately document the extent of bony defects. The number of bony walls and the presence or extent of bony lesions on the facial/buccal or lingual/palatal walls cannot be accurately determined by radiographs. Well-made radiographs provide useful information about the extent of interproximal bone loss, the presence of angular bone loss, caries, root trunk length, and root morphology. They also facilitate the identification of other dental pathoses that require treatment. In addition, a properly made radiographic survey serves as a means of evaluating the success of therapy and of documenting the longitudinal stability of the patient.[20]

Treatment planning should provide solutions for active periodontal diseases and correction of deformities that result from periodontitis, and it should facilitate the performance of other dental procedures included in a comprehensive dental treatment plan. The extent of periodontal involvement can vary significantly from tooth to tooth in the same patient. The response to therapy from patient to patient may also vary, as may the treatment objectives for the patients. Therefore a treatment plan may encompass a number of steps and/or combinations of procedures in the same surgical area.

After oral hygiene instruction, scaling, and root planing, along with other disease control procedures, the response of the patient to these treatment procedures is evaluated by reexamination and recording the changes that have occurred in the periodontium. Because the extent of periodontal involvement can vary significantly from tooth to tooth in the same patient, the local response to therapy is also variable. The resolution of inflammation and decrease in edema and swelling may have resulted in a return to normal depth and configuration of some pockets and additional therapy beyond periodic maintenance is not required.

The patient with moderate to advanced periodontitis and bony defects, although the overt signs of periodontitis may be reduced, may display a persistence of pocket depth bleeding on probing and suppuration. These signs may indicate the presence of residual plaque and calculus attributable to the difficulty of instrumentation in these deep pockets or an inability or unwillingness of the patient to perform adequate oral hygiene in these sites. Patients with inadequate oral hygiene are not good candidates for periodontal surgery. If the supragingival plaque control is good, and the residual pocket depths are 5 mm or more, such areas may be candidates for periodontal surgery.[14]

Resective osseous surgery is also used to facilitate certain restorative/prosthetic dental procedures. Dental caries can be exposed for restoration, fractured roots of abutment teeth can be exposed for removal, and bony exostoses and ridge deformities can be altered in contour to improve the performance of removable or fixed prostheses (Fig. 62-7, *A* to *D*). Severely decayed teeth or teeth with short anatomic crowns can be lengthened by resection or by a combination of orthodontic tooth extrusion and osseous resection. Such procedures allow the therapist to expose more tooth for restoration, prevent an invasion of the biologic width of attachment, and create a periodontal attachment of normal dimension.[8,16] Resection can also provide a means of producing optimal crown length for cosmetic purposes.

METHODS OF OSSEOUS RESECTIVE SURGERY

The reshaping process is fundamentally an attempt to gradualize the bone sufficiently to allow soft tissue structures to follow the contour of the bone. The soft tissue predictably attaches to the bone within certain specific dimensions. The length and quality of connective tissue and junctional epithelium that reforms in the surgical

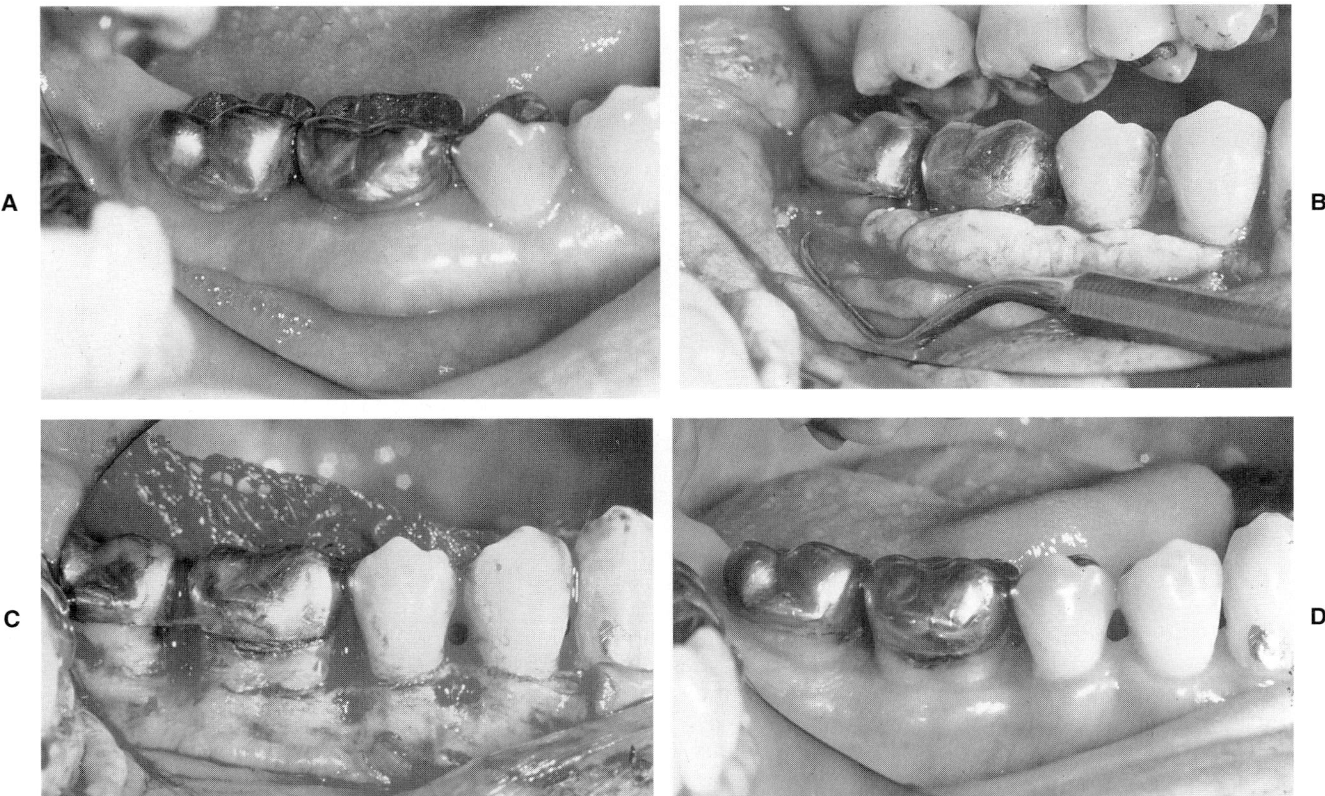

Fig. 62-7 Reduction of bony ledges and exposure of caries by osteoplasty. **A,** Buccal preoperative photograph showing two crowns, exostoses, and caries. **B,** Flap reflected to reveal caries on both molars at the restoration margins, interdental cratering, and a facial exostosis. **C,** Postosseous surgery; the bulk of the bony removal was by osteoplasty with minor ostectomy between the two molars. The caries is now exposed and the crowns lengthened for restoration. **D,** Six weeks postoperative photograph. The plaque control is deficient but the teeth should be readily restorable at this time. (Courtesy Dr. Joseph Schwartz; Portland, Ore.)

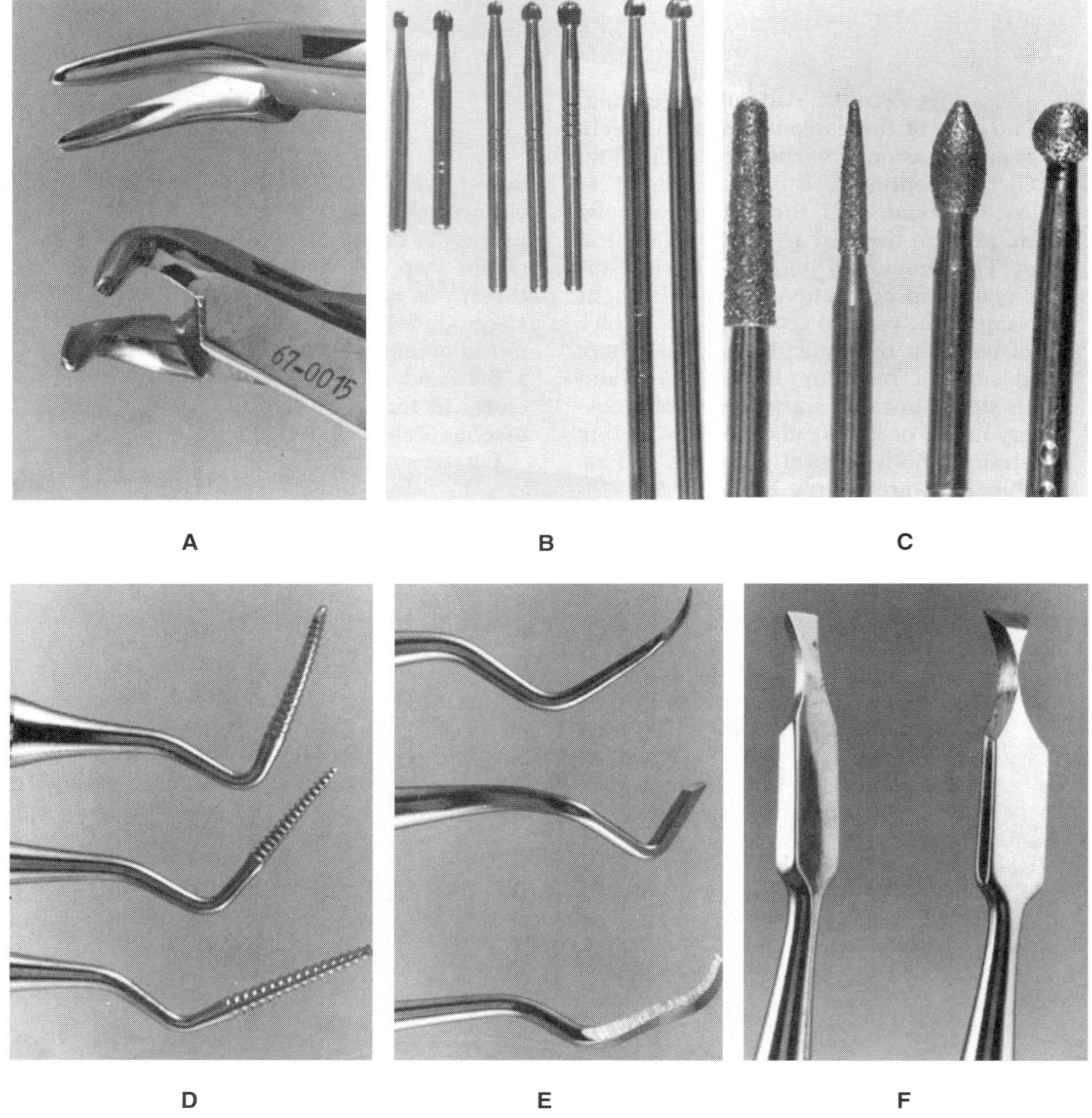

Fig. 62-8 Instruments often used in osseous surgery. **A,** Rongeurs: Friedman (top) and 90-degree Blumenthal (bottom). **B,** Carbide round burrs (left to right): friction grip, surgical-length friction grip, and slow-speed hand-piece. **C,** Diamond burrs. **D,** Interproximal files: Schluger and Sugarman. **E,** Back-action chisels. **F,** Ochsenbein chisels.

site are dependent on numerous factors, including the health of the tissue, the condition of the root surface and the topography, as well as the proximity of the bone surrounding the tooth. Each of these factors must be controlled to the best of the clinician's ability to obtain the optimal result, making osseous resective surgery an extremely precise technique.

It is assumed in this chapter that the gingival tissue has been reflected by the apically positioned flap described in Chapter 60. Reshaping of the bone may necessitate selective changes in gingival height. These changes must be calculated and accounted for in the initial flap design. For this reason, it is important for the clinician to know about the underlying bone tissue before flap reflection. The clinician must gain as much indirect knowledge as possible from soft tissue palpation, radiographic assessment, and transgingival probing, or *sounding.*

Radiographic examination can reveal the existence of angular bone loss in the interdental spaces; these usually coincide with intrabony pockets. The radiograph does not show the number of bony walls of the defect, nor does it determine with any accuracy the presence of angular cone defects on facial or lingual surfaces. Clinical examination and probing determines the presence and depth of periodontal pockets on any surface of any tooth and can also give a general sense of the bony topography, but intrabony pockets can go undetected by probing. Both clinical and radiographic examinations can indicate the presence of intrabony pockets when (1) angular bone

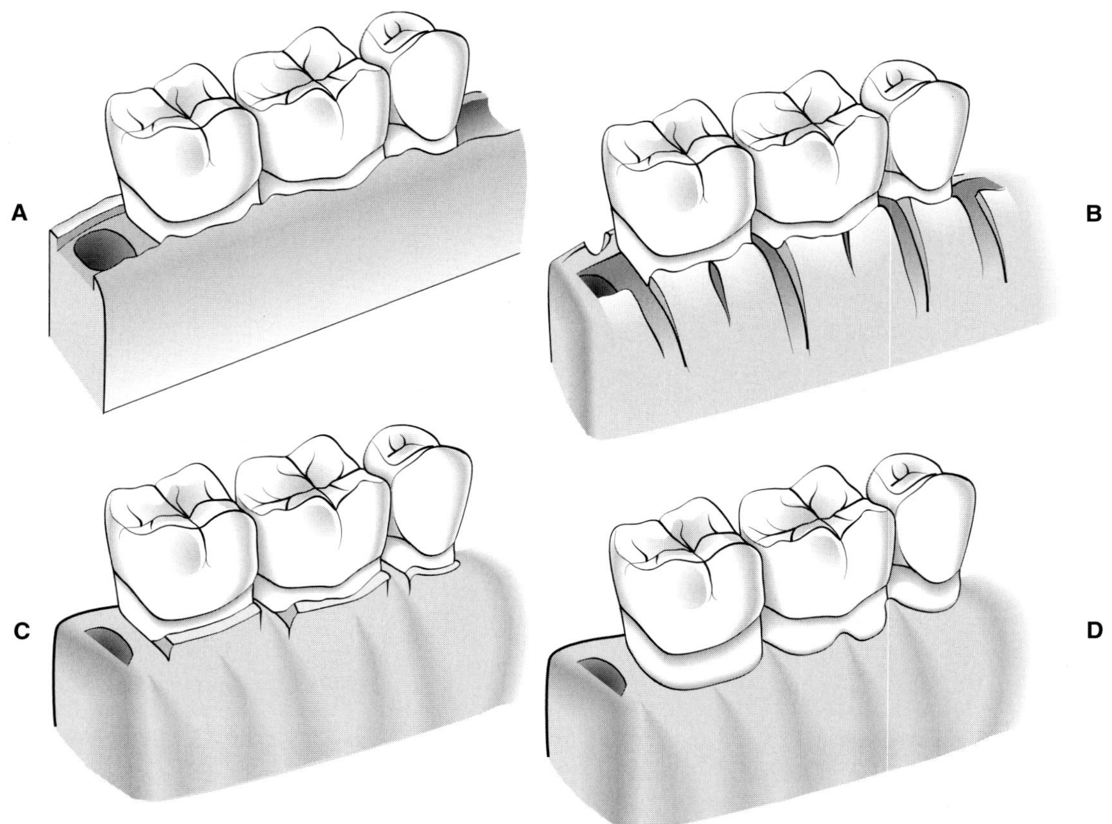

Fig. 62-9 A, Drawing representing the bony topography in moderate periodontitis with interdental craters. **B,** Vertical grooving, the first step in correction by osseous reshaping. **C,** Radicular blending and flattening of interproximal bone. **D,** Gradualizing the marginal bone. Note the area of the furcation on the first molar where the bone is preserved.

loss, (2) irregular bone loss, or (3) pockets of irregular depth in adjacent areas of the same tooth or adjacent teeth are found.

The experienced clinician can use transgingival probing to predict many features of the underlying bony topography. The information thus obtained can change the treatment plan. For example, an area that had been selected for osseous resective surgery may be found to have a narrow defect that was unnoticed in the initial probing and radiographic assessment and is ideal for augmentation procedures. Such findings can and do change the flap design, osseous procedure, and results expected from the surgical intervention. Transgingival probing is extremely useful just before flap reflection. It is necessary to anesthetize the tissue locally before inserting the probe. The probe should be "walked" along the tissue-tooth interface so that the operator can feel the bony topography. The probe may also be passed horizontally through the tissue to provide three-dimensional information regarding bony contours (i.e., thickness, height, and shape of the underlying base). It must be remembered, however, that this information is still "blind," and although it is undoubtedly better than probing alone, it has significant limitations. Nevertheless, this step is recommended immediately before the surgical intervention.

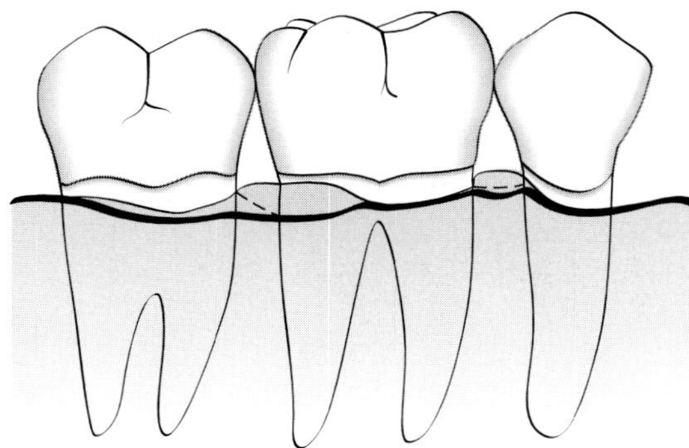

Fig. 62-10 Diagrammatic representation of bone irregularities in periodontal disease. The thick line is the proposed correction of the defect. Note the flattening of the interproximal bone between the molars and the protection of the furcal bone on the first molar. Facial crest height is reduced in both interproximal areas to the depth of the defect.

The situations that can be encountered after periodontal flap reflection vary greatly. When all soft tissue is removed around the teeth, there may be larger exotoses, ledges, troughs, craters, vertical defects, or combinations of any of these. For this reason, each osseous situa-

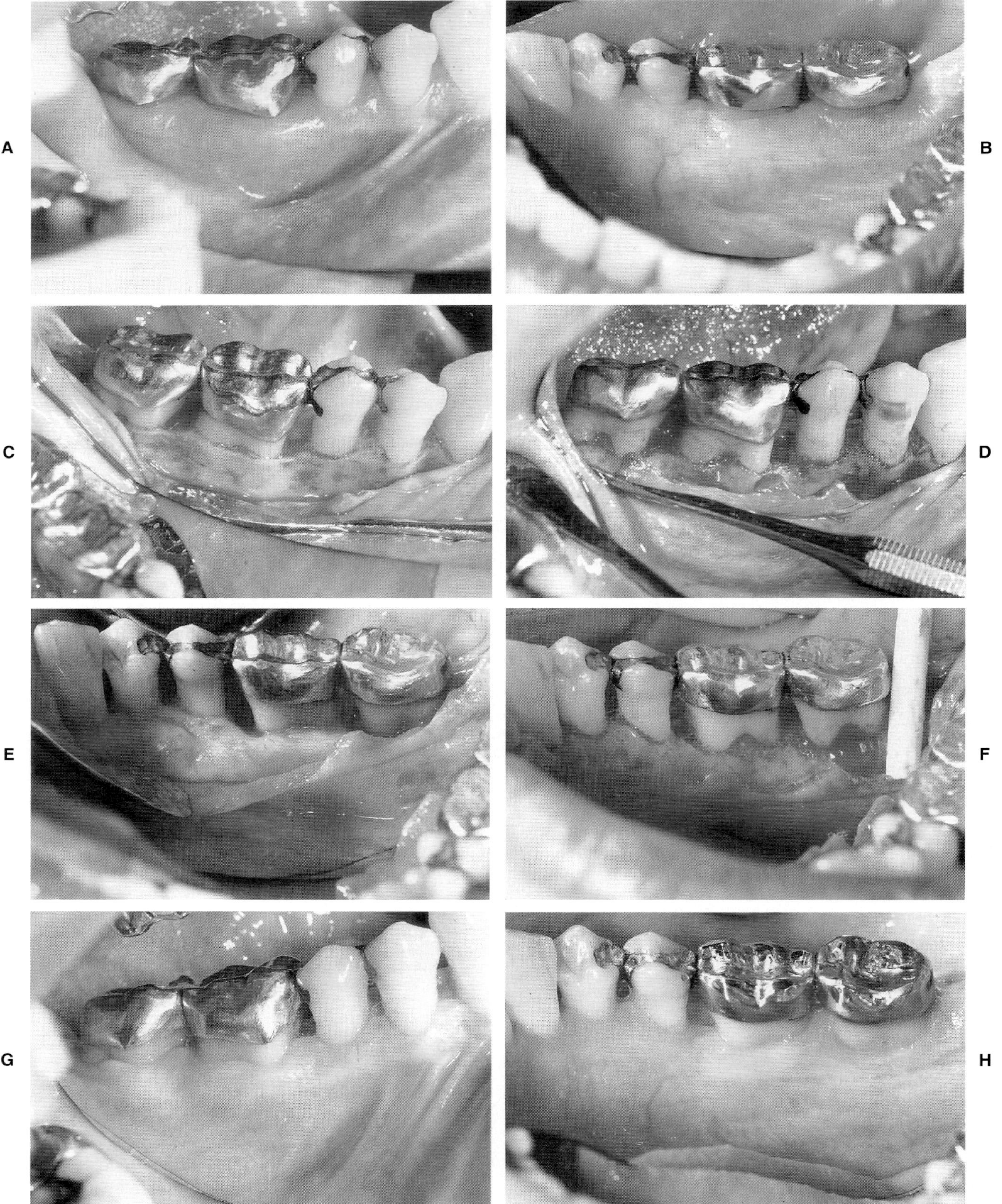

Fig. 62-11 Compromise osseous surgery. **A and B,** Preoperative views of the buccal and lingual surfaces. **C and D,** Pre- and postoperative view of the buccal osseous recontouring class I buccal furcation defects, a moderate crater between the two molars, and a deep 1-2-3 walled defect at the mesial of the first involvements. **D,** The buccal aspects of these lesions were corrected with osteoplasty and a small amount of ostectomy. **E and F,** Pre- and postoperative views of the lingual osseous management. **E,** Notice the combination 1-2-3 wall defect between the second bicuspid and first molar, as well as the irregular pattern of bone loss with ledging. **F,** These defects were corrected by osteoplasty and ostectomy with the exception of the deep defect at the mesial of the molar. This area was resected until the residual defect was of two and three walls only and left to repair. **G and H,** Buccal and lingual 5-year postoperative views of tissue configuration. Note the residual soft tissue defect between the bicuspid and first molar.

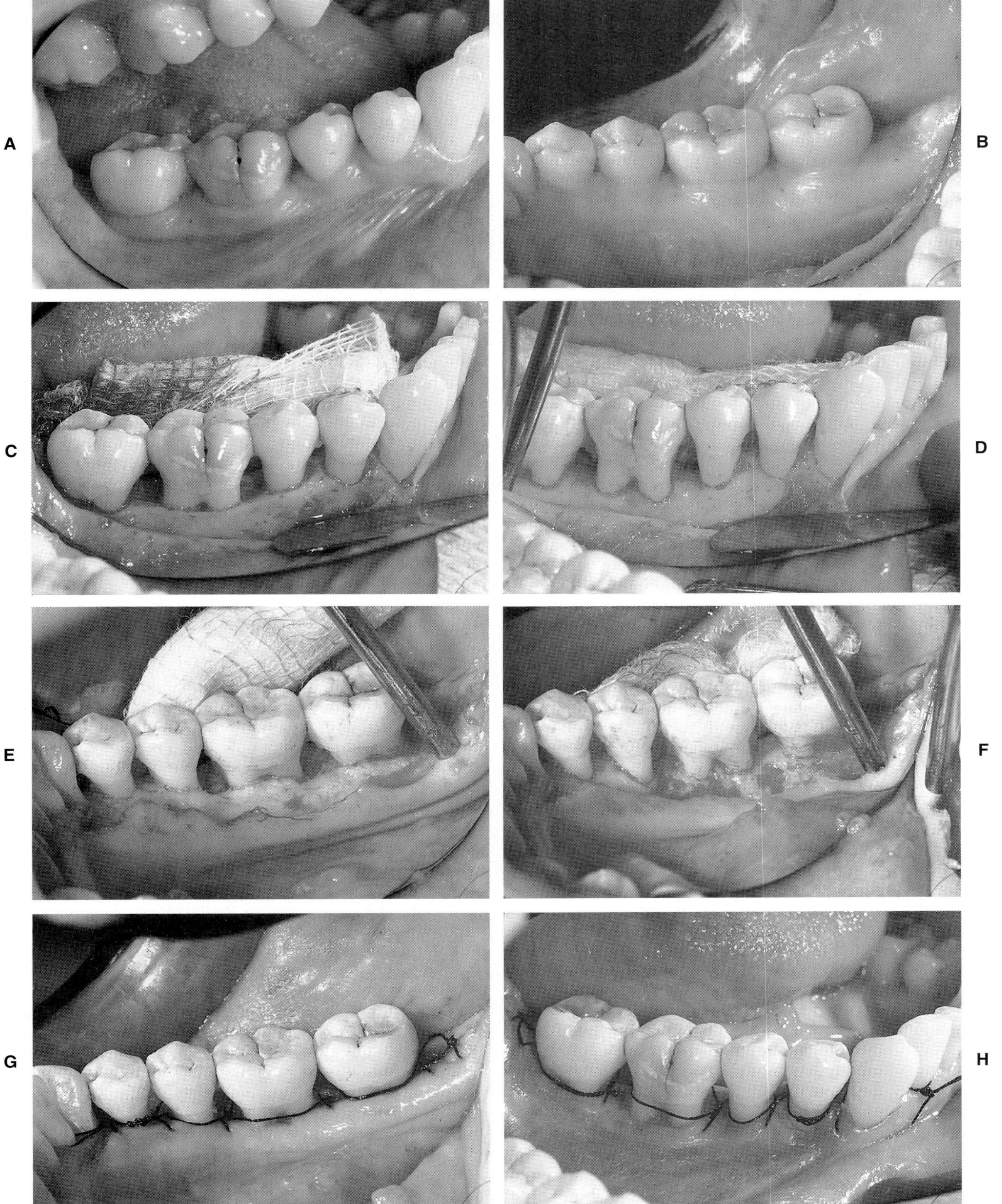

Fig. 62-12 Osteoectomy and osteoplasty to a positive contour with flap placement at the newly created bony crest for minimal pocket depth. **A** and **B,** Buccal and lingual preoperative views. **C and D,** Buccal pre-and postosseous correction. Osteoplasty and osteoectomy used to produce a positive contour. Note the osteoplasty into the buccal furcation of the first molar. This is about the extent of craters that can be corrected to a positive contour in teeth with moderate root trunk length. **E and F,** Lingual pre- and postosseous correction. Osteoplasty and osteoectomy to produce a positive contour. Note the lingual ledge, which was reduced. Such ledges are common in this area. **G and H,** Buccal and lingual flaps sutured with continuous sling sutures to allow placement of the flaps to cover the bony margins.

Continued

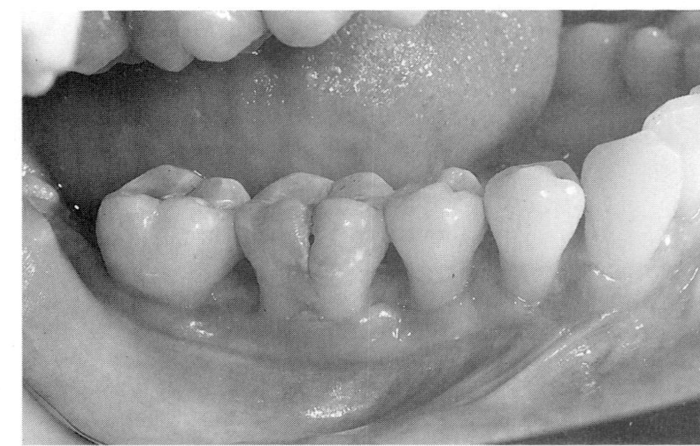

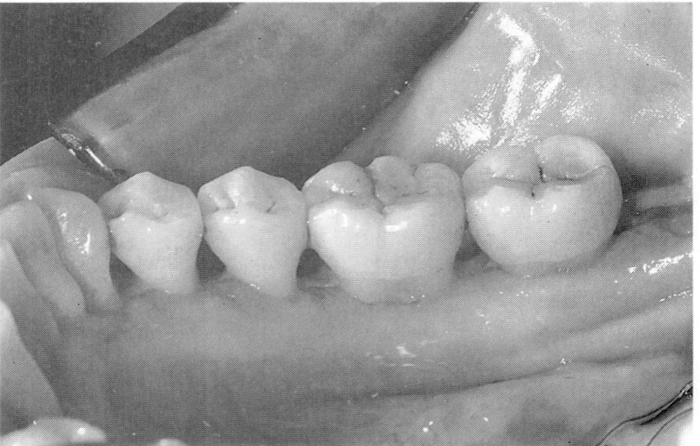

Fig. 62-12, cont'd Osteosectomy and osteoplasty to a positive contour with flap placement at the newly created bony crest for minimal pocket depth. **I and J,** Buccal and lingual 1 week postoperative views. There is a minimal soft tissue thickness, and the interdental areas are granulating in over the positive bony form. Minimal pocket depth results from such management.

tion presents uniquely challenging problems, especially if reshaping to the optimal level is contemplated.

THE OSSEOUS RESECTION TECHNIQUE

Instruments Used

A number of hand and rotary instruments have been used for osseous resective surgery. Some excellent clinicians use only hand instruments and rongeurs, whereas others prefer a combination of hand and rotary instruments. Rotary instruments are useful for the osteoplastic steps outlined previously, whereas hand instruments provide the most precise and safe results with ostectomy procedures. Nevertheless, care and precision are required each step of the way to prevent excessive bone removal or root damage, both of which are irreversible. Fig. 62-8 illustrates some of the instruments commonly used for osseous resective techniques.

Technique

To handle the multitude of clinical situations, the following sequential steps are suggested (Fig. 62-9, *A* to *D*):

1. Vertical grooving
2. Radicular blending
3. Flattening interproximal bone
4. Gradualizing marginal bone

Not all steps are necessary in every case, but the sequencing of the steps in the order given is necessary to expedite the reshaping procedure, as well as to minimize the removal of bone.

Vertical Grooving

Vertical grooving is designed to reduce the thickness of the alveolar housing and to provide relative prominence to the radicular aspects of the teeth (see Fig. 62-9, *B*) and Color Fig. 62-1). It also provides continuity from the interproximal surface onto the radicular surface. It is the first step of the resective process, because it can define the general thickness and subsequent form of the alveolar housing. This step is usually performed with rotary instruments such as round carbide burrs or diamonds. The advantages of vertical grooving are most apparent with thick, bony margins; shallow crater formations; or other areas that require maximal osteoplasty and minimal ostectomy. Vertical grooving is contraindicated in areas with close root proximity or thin alveolar housing.

Radicular Blending

Radicular blending, the second step of the osseous reshaping technique, is an extension of vertical grooving (see Fig. 62-9, *C*). Conceptually, it is an attempt to gradualize the bone over the entire radicular surface to provide the best results from vertical grooving. This provides a smooth, blended surface for good flap adaptation. The indications are the same as for vertical grooving (i.e., thick ledges of bone on the radicular surface, where selective surgical resection is desired). Naturally, this step is not necessary if vertical grooving is very minor or if the radicular bone is thin or fenestrated. Both vertical grooving and radicular blending are purely osteoplastic techniques that do not remove supporting bone. In most situations, they compose the bulk of osseous resective surgery. Classically, shallow crater formations, thick osseous ledges of bone on the radicular surfaces, and class I and early class II furcation involvements are treated almost entirely with these two steps.

Flattening Interproximal Bone

Flattening of the interdental bone requires the removal of very small amounts of supporting bone (Fig. 62-10). It is indicated when interproximal bone levels vary horizontally. By definition, most of the indications for this step are one-walled interproximal defects or so-called hemiseptal defects. The omission of flattening in such cases results in increased pocket depth on the most apical side of the bone loss. This step is typically not

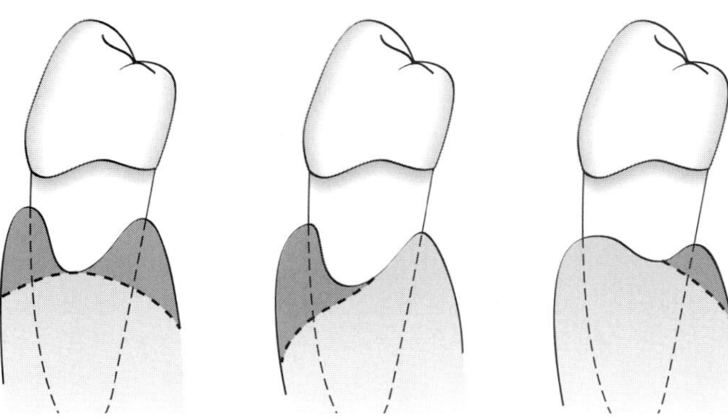

Fig. 62-13 Interproximal craters. The shaded areas illustrate different techniques for the management of such defects. The technique that reduces the least amount of supporting bone is preferable.

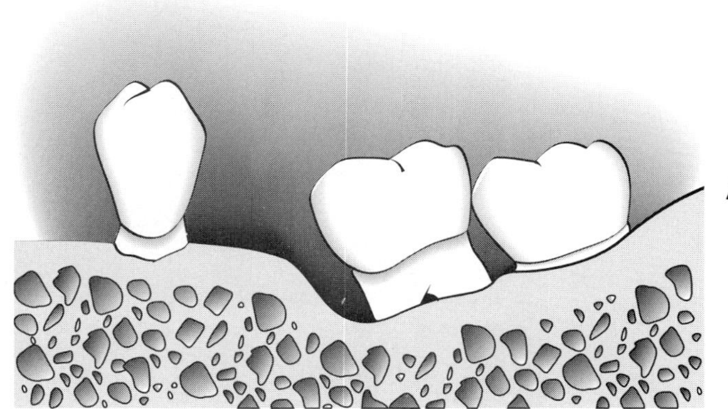

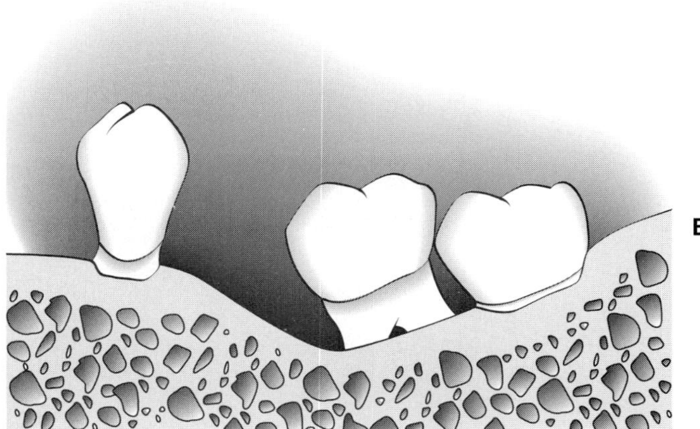

Fig. 62-14 Reduction of a one-wall angular defect. **A,** Angular bone defect mesial to the tilted molar. **B,** Defect reduced by "ramping" angular bone.

necessary in class crater formations or flat interproximal defects. It is best used in defects that have a coronally placed one-walled edge of a predominantly three-walled angular defect, and it can be helpful in obtaining good flap closure and improved healing in the three-walled defect. The limitation of this step, as with osseous resective surgical therapy in general, is in the treatment of advanced lesions. Large hemiseptal defects would require removal of inordinate amounts of bone to provide a flattened architecture, and the operation would be too costly in terms of bony support. Compromised osseous architecture is the only logical solution (Fig. 62-11).

Gradualizing Marginal Bone

The final step in the osseous resective technique is also an ostectomy process. Bone removal is minimal but necessary to provide a sound, regular base for the gingival tissue to follow. Failure to remove small bony discrepancies on the gingival line angles (often called *widow's peaks*) allows the tissue to rise to a higher level than the base of the bone loss in the interdental area (see Fig. 62-9, *C* and *D*). This may make the process of selective recession and subsequent pocket reduction incomplete. This step of the procedure also requires gradualization and blending of the radicular surface (see Fig. 62-10 and Color Fig. 62-1, *C*). The two ostectomy steps should be performed with great care so as not to produce nicks or grooves on the roots. When the radicular bone is thin, it is extremely easy to overdo this step, to the detriment of the entire surgical effort. For this reason, various hand instruments, such as chisels and curettes, are preferable to rotary instruments for gradualizing marginal bone.

FLAP PLACEMENT AND CLOSURE

Following the performance of resection, the flaps are positioned and sutured. Flaps may be replaced to their original position, to cover the new bony margin, or they may be apically positioned. Replacing the flap in areas that previously had deep pockets may result initially in greater postoperative pocket depth, although a selective recession may diminish the depth over time. Positioning the flap apically to expose marginal bone is one method of altering the width of the gingiva (denudation). However, such flap placement results in more postsurgical resorption of bone and patient discomfort than if the newly created bony margin were covered by the flap. Positioning the flap to cover the new margin results in a minimum of postoperative complications and optimal postsurgical pocket depths (Fig. 62-12, *I* and *J*).

Suturing may be accomplished using a variety of different suture materials and suture knots[4] (see Chapter 60). The sutures should be placed with minimal tension to coapt the flaps, prevent their separation, and maintain the position of the flaps. Sutures placed with excessive tension rapidly pull through the tissues.

POSTOPERATIVE MAINTENANCE

Sutures may be removed at varying periods. Nonresorbable sutures such as silk are usually removed after 1 week of healing, although some of the newer synthetic materials may be left for periods of up to 3 weeks or longer without adverse consequences. Resorbable sutures maintain wound approximation for varying periods or 1 to 3 weeks or more, depending on the material of which they are made. At the suture removal appointment

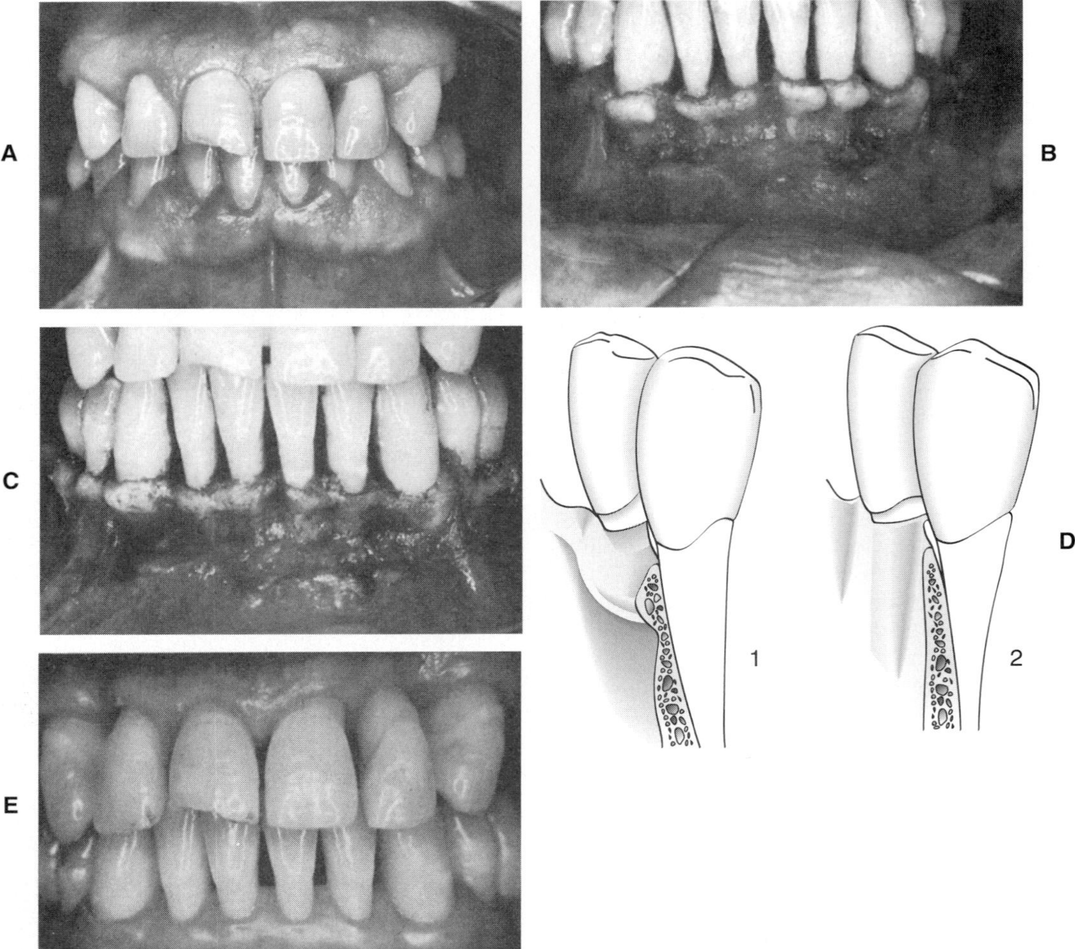

Fig. 62-15 Correction of exotoses by osseous surgery. **A,** Periodontal disease in a patient with bulbous gingival contour in the mandible. **B,** Reflected flap reveals exostoses. **C,** Exostoses reduced, interdental grooves established, and interdental bone tapered inward and toward the crest. **D,** (1) Lateral view, showing exostosis; (2) exostosis reduced and bone recontoured to provide interdental grooves. **E,** After 10 weeks, pockets are eliminated, and physiologic gingival contour is restored. Compare with **A.** (Courtesy of Dr. Charles A. Palioca; Homosassa, Fla.)

the periodontal dressing, if present, is removed, and the surgical site is gently cleansed of debris with a cotton pellet dampened with saline. Nonresorbable sutures are then cut and removed. If sutures of a resorbable material were used, then the area should be inspected carefully to insure that no suture fragments remain. Suture removal should be accomplished without dragging contaminated portions of the suture through the periodontal tissues. This may be accomplished by lightly compressing the soft tissue immediately adjacent to the suture. This exposes (extrudes) a portion of the suture that was previously under the gingival tissues and less likely to be contaminated by plaque. The suture is then cut at the gingival surface. Removal of the pressure from the site results in the cut surface being slightly submerged in the tissue. The sutures are then removed with cotton pliers by pulling the suture from its contaminated end.

After suture removal the surgical site is examined carefully, and any excessive granulation tissue is removed with a sharp curette. The patient is provided with postsurgical maintenance instructions and the instruments needed to maintain the surgical site in a plaque-free state. These instruments should not produce additional trauma to the healing tissues. Many therapists find the use of a plaque-suppressive agent such as chlorhexidine digluconate to be a valuable adjunct to postsurgical maintenance. A second postoperative visit is often performed at the second or third week, and the surgical site is lightly débrided for optimal results. A professional prophylaxis for complete plaque removal should be done every 2 weeks until healing is complete and the patient is maintaining appropriate levels of plaque control.

Healing should proceed uneventfully, with the attachment of the flap to the underlying bone being

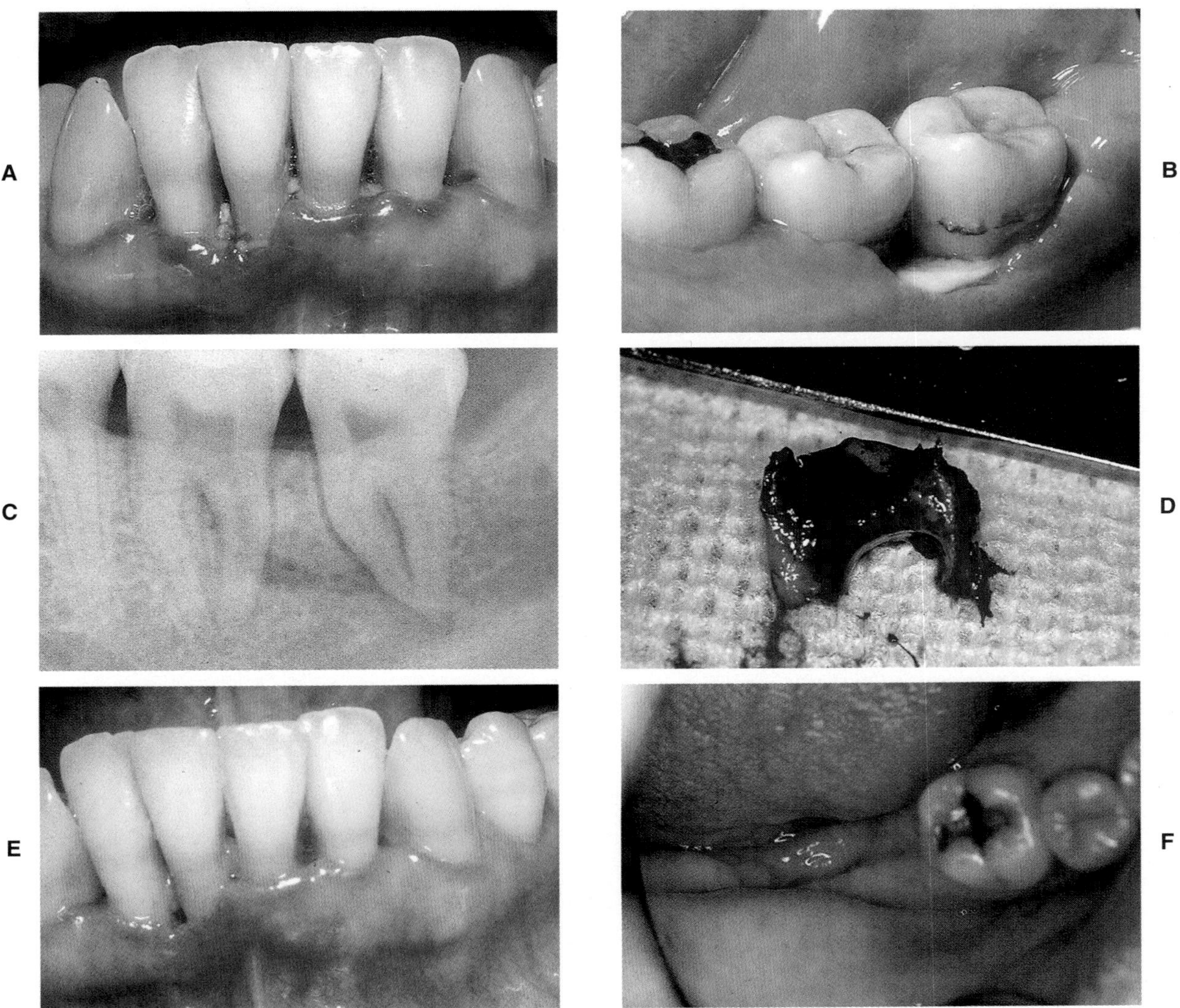

Color Fig. 51-1 Necrotizing ulcerative peridontitis (NUP) in a 28-year-old woman with a CD4 count of 48. **A,** NUP of mandibular anterior region. **B,** Necrotizing stomatitis in mandibular left molar area. **C,** Radiograph of sequestra in mandibular left molar area. **D,** Sequestrae removed in conjunction with extraction of teeth #17 and 18. **E,** Mandibular anterior area 1 week posttreatment. **F,** Mandibular left molar region 2 months postoperatively. Note the uneventful healing.

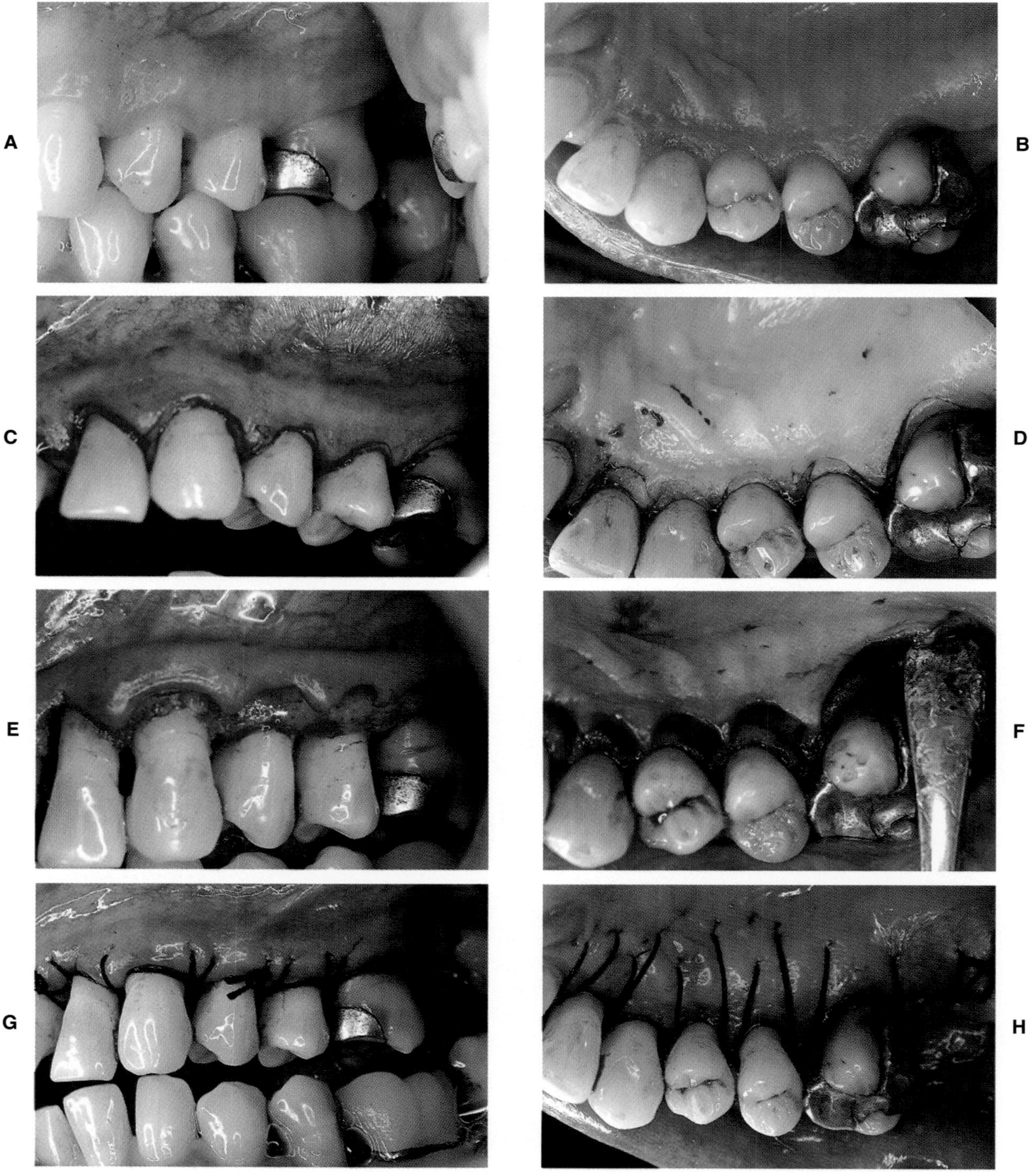

Color Fig. 60-1 The periodontal flap technique. **A,** Facial view and **B,** palatal view of case preoperatively. A thorough scaling and root planing had been performed 6 weeks before. Five- to six-millimeter pockets persisted in palatal areas. **C,** Facial incisions (internal bevel and crevicular) performed. **D,** Palatal incisions performed. Note the scalloping. **E and F,** Facial and palatal flaps elevated. Wedge of marginal tissue not yet removed in the palate. After thorough debridement, the root is examined for any remaining accretions and the bone is examined to determine the need for osseous surgery. **G and H,** Continuous mattress suture in place.

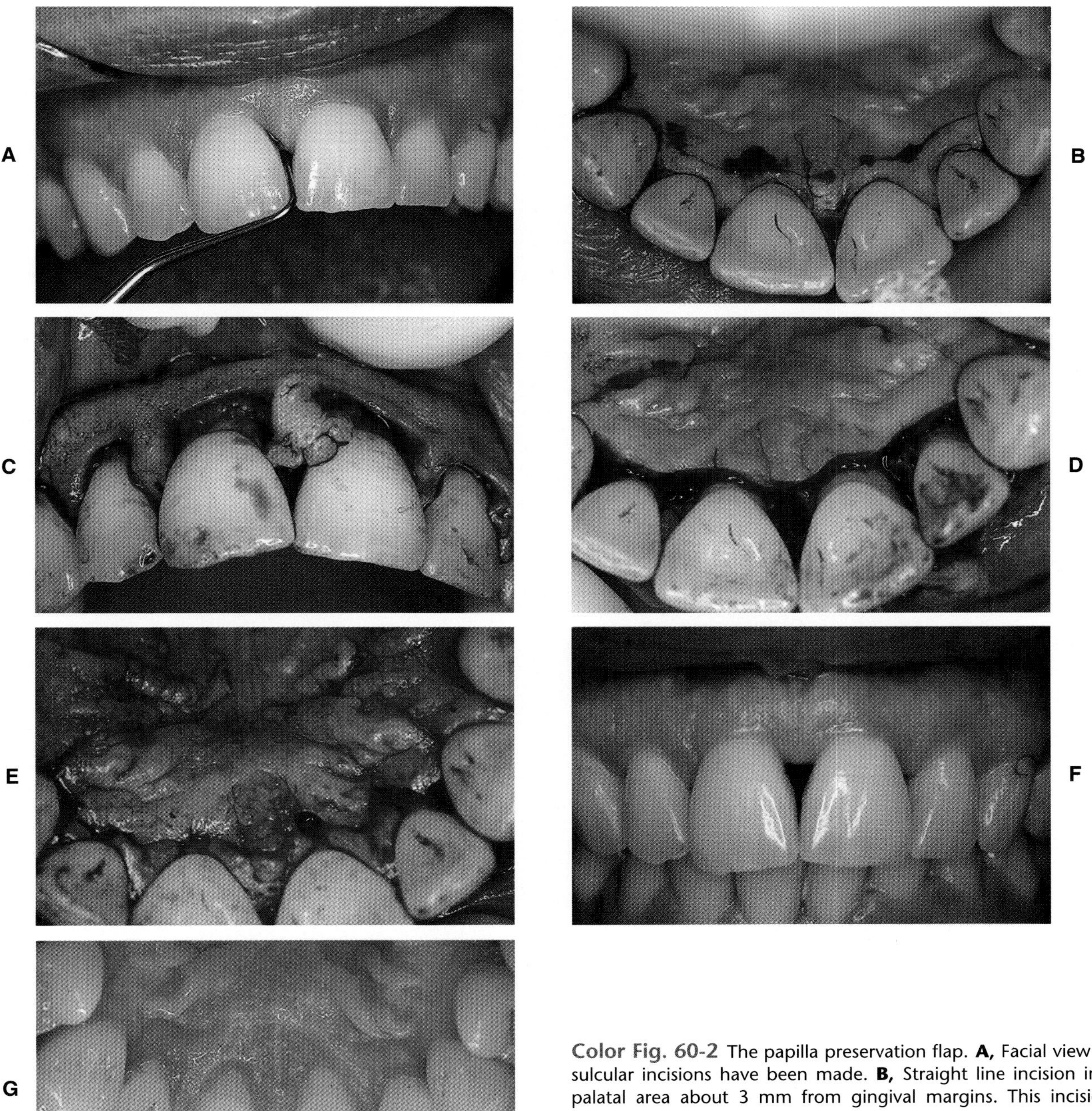

Color Fig. 60-2 The papilla preservation flap. **A,** Facial view after sulcular incisions have been made. **B,** Straight line incision in the palatal area about 3 mm from gingival margins. This incision is then connected to the margins with vertical incisions in the mid-part of each tooth. **C,** The papillae are reflected with the facial flap. **D,** Lingual view after reflection of the flap. **E,** Lingual view after the flap is brought back to its original position. It is then sutured with independent sutures. **F,** Facial view after healing. **G,** Palatal view after healing.

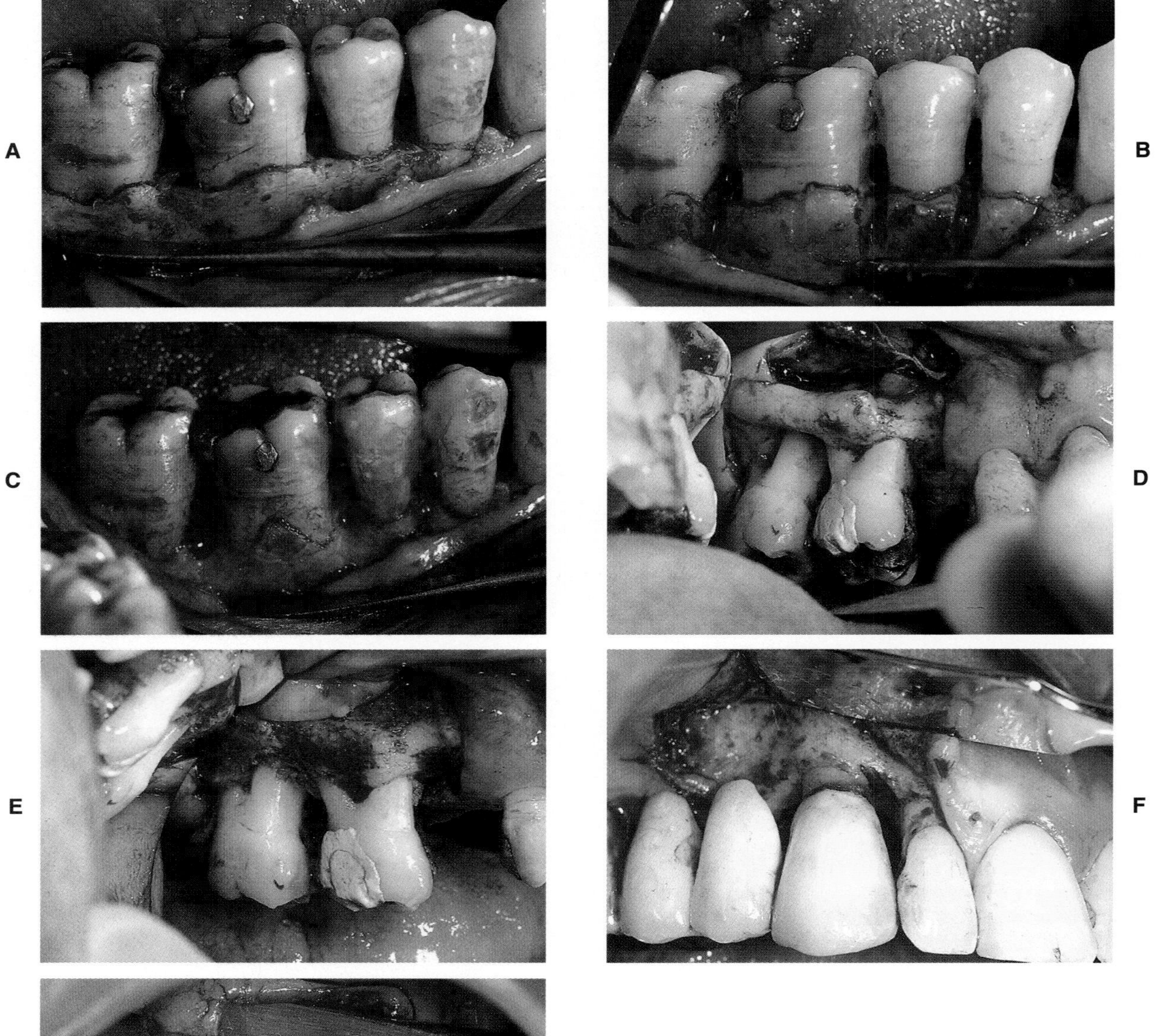

Color Fig. 62-1 Bone contouring in flap surgery. **A–C,** Bone contouring in interdental craters. **D** and **E,** Bone contouring in exotoses. **F** and **G,** Bone contouring in one-wall vertical defect.

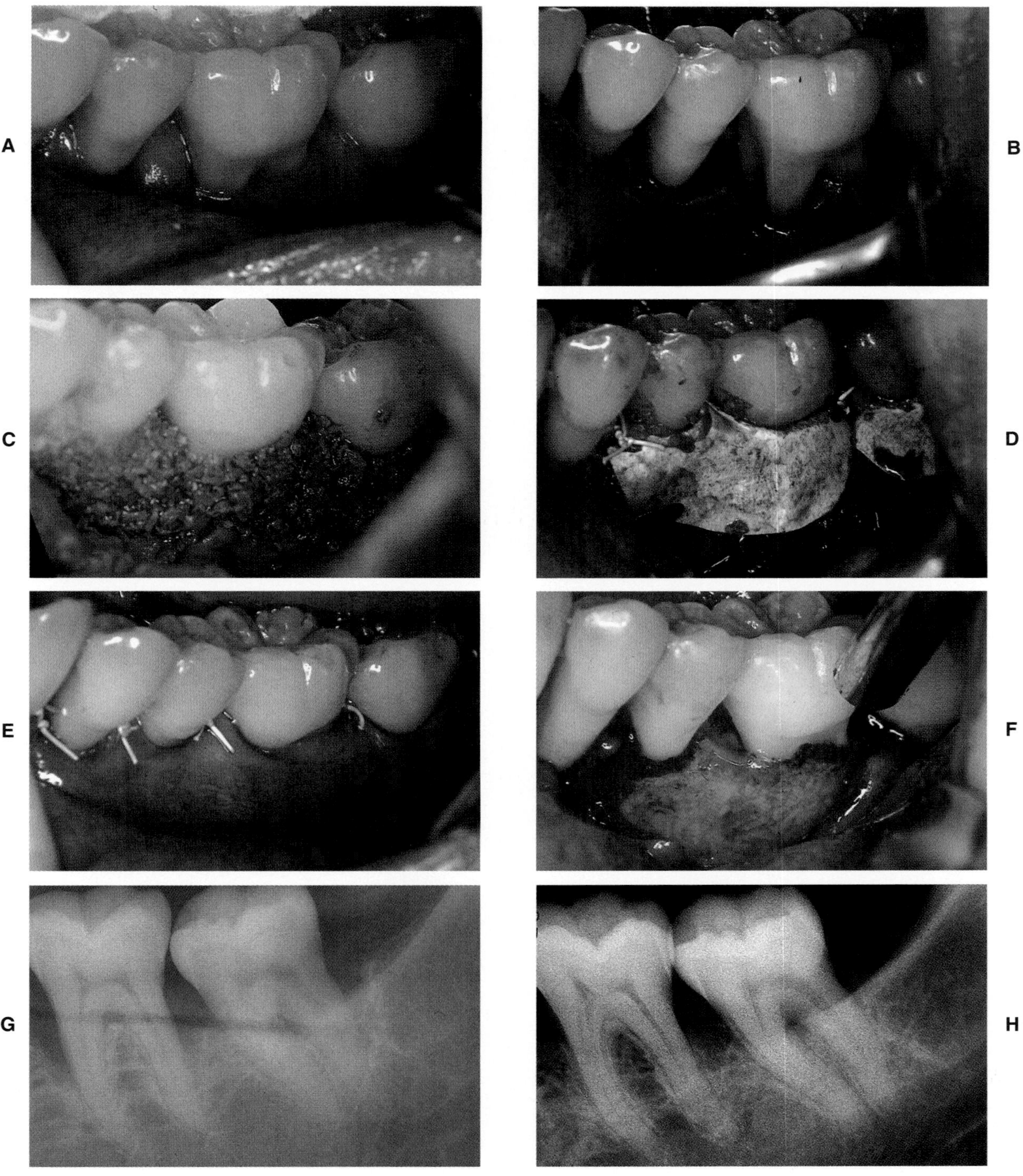

Color Fig. 63-1 **A,** Pretreatment photograph of lower left posterior teeth with marked recession and tissue inflammation. **B,** Underlying extensive crestal bone loss, dehiscence, and intrabony osseous defects. **C,** Bone graft in position approximating the cementoenamel junction of the posterior teeth. **D,** Barrier membranes over the bone grafts. **E,** Flaps coronally positioned and secured over the barrier membranes. **F,** Membrane removal revealing new alveolar bone. **G,** Pretreatment radiograph. **H,** One-year postoperative radiograph depicting new alveolar bone apposition. (From McClain P: Dental Economics 1996; 4:92.)

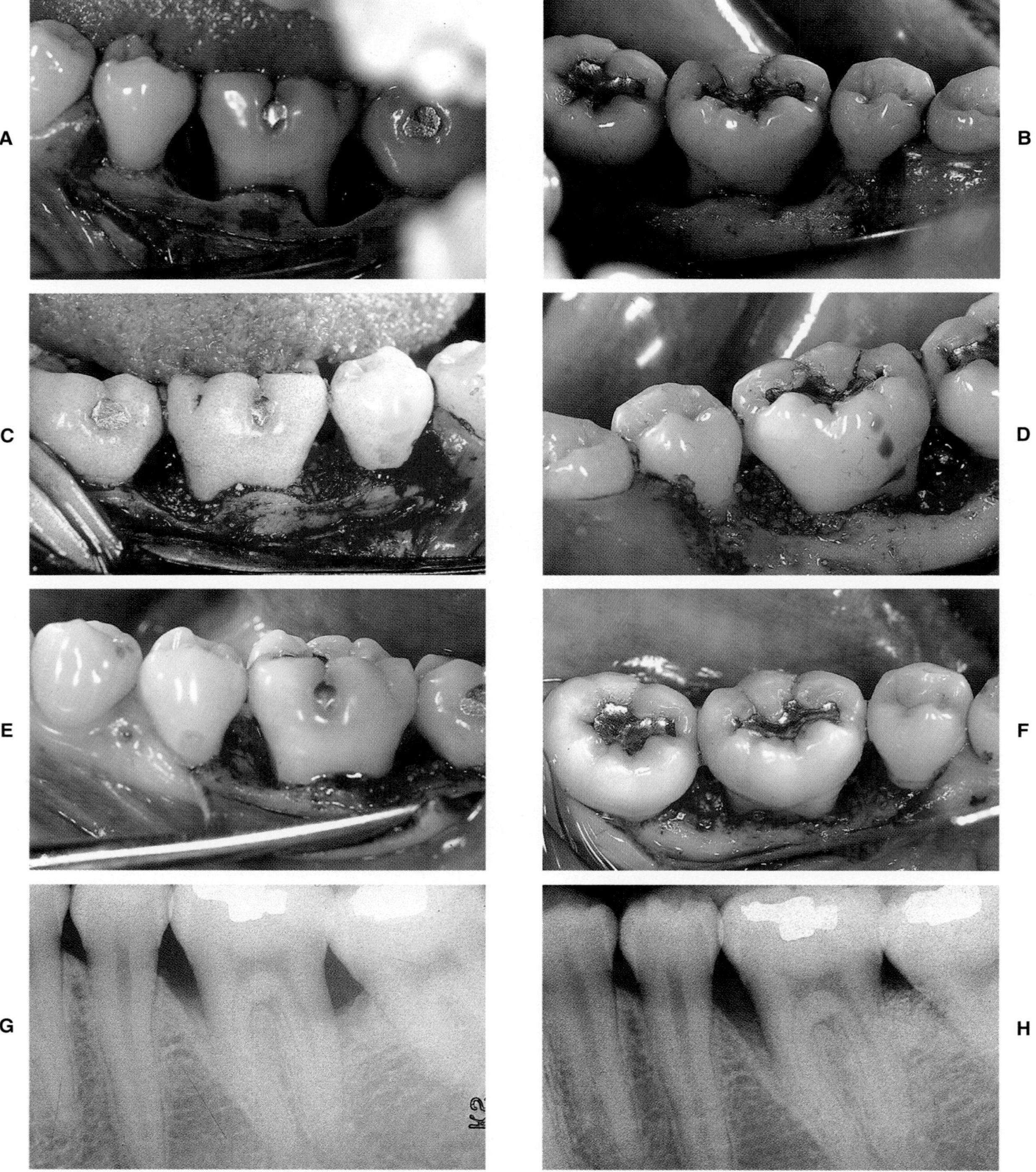

Color Fig. 63-2 Reconstructive periodontics: use of decalcified freeze-dried bone allografts (DFDBA) and porous hydroxyapatite. Facial view **(A)** and lingual view **(B)** of deep vertical lesions mesial and distal to lower first molar, exposed by a flap and debridement. Furcation is not involved. **C and D,** Facial and lingual views, respectively, of lesions filled with DFDBA (mesial defect) and porous hydroxyapatite (distal defect). This case was part of a study comparing both types of bone grafts. **E and F,** Facial and lingual views, respectively, of reentry at 6 months postoperatively, showing total fill of distal defect and partial fill of mesial defect. **G,** Preoperative radiograph. **H,** Radiograph immediately after placement of grafts.

Continued

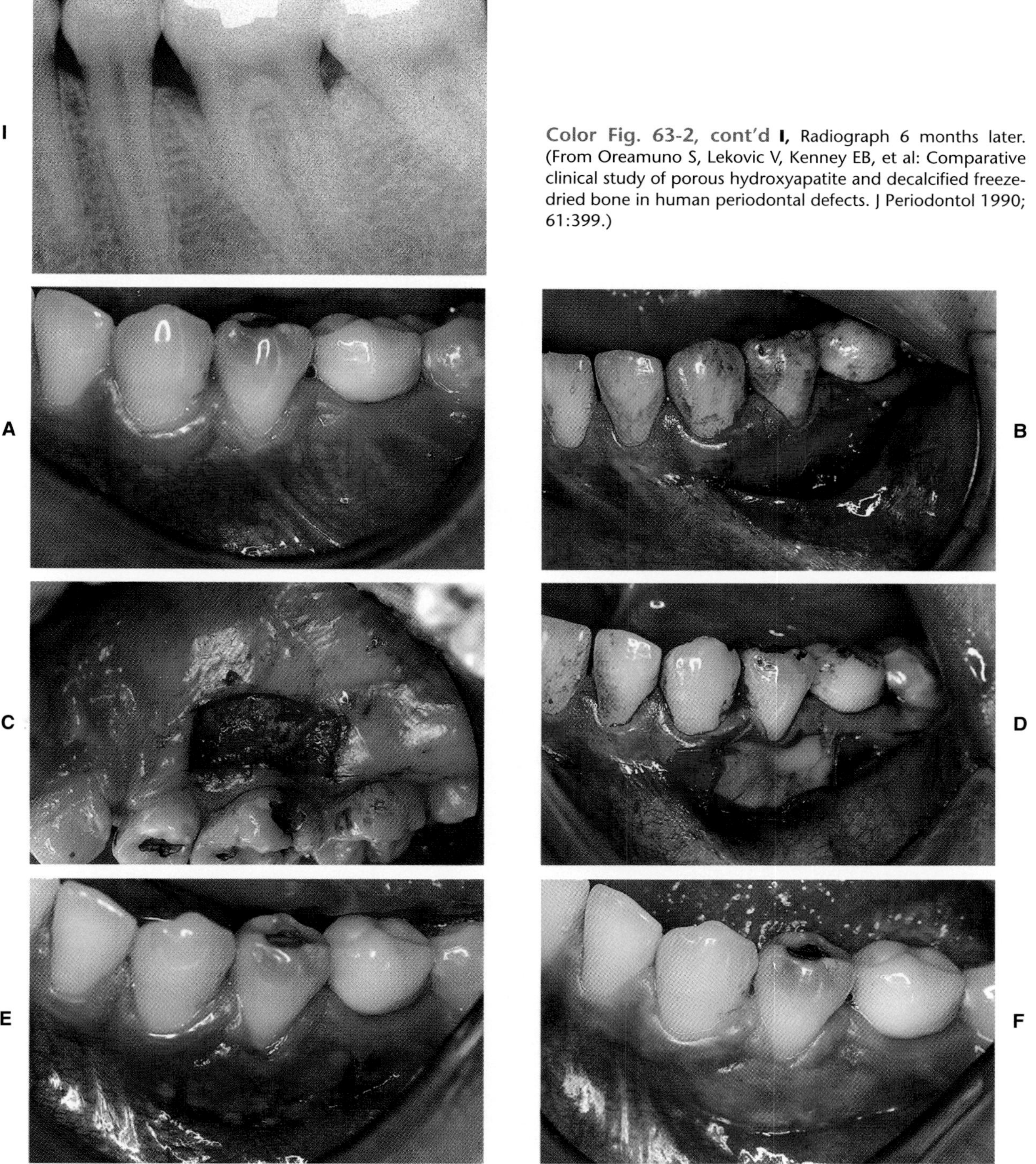

I

A B

C D

E F

Color Fig. 63-2, cont'd I, Radiograph 6 months later. (From Oreamuno S, Lekovic V, Kenney EB, et al: Comparative clinical study of porous hydroxyapatite and decalcified freeze-dried bone in human periodontal defects. J Periodontol 1990; 61:399.)

Color Fig. 66-1 Technique for free gingival grafts. **A,** Lack of attached gingiva and the beginning of recession on the lower second premolar. **B,** Surgical bed prepared and the border of the wound sutured to the periosteum. **C,** Donor site in the palatal area immediately after removal of tissue for grafting. Note the presence of periosteum. **D,** Donor tissue placed on the surgical bed and sutured with catgut. **E,** Recipient site 1 month postoperatively. **F,** Recipient site 3 months postoperatively. Compare with **A.** (Courtesy Dr. Agusti Marfany, St. Julian, Andorra.)

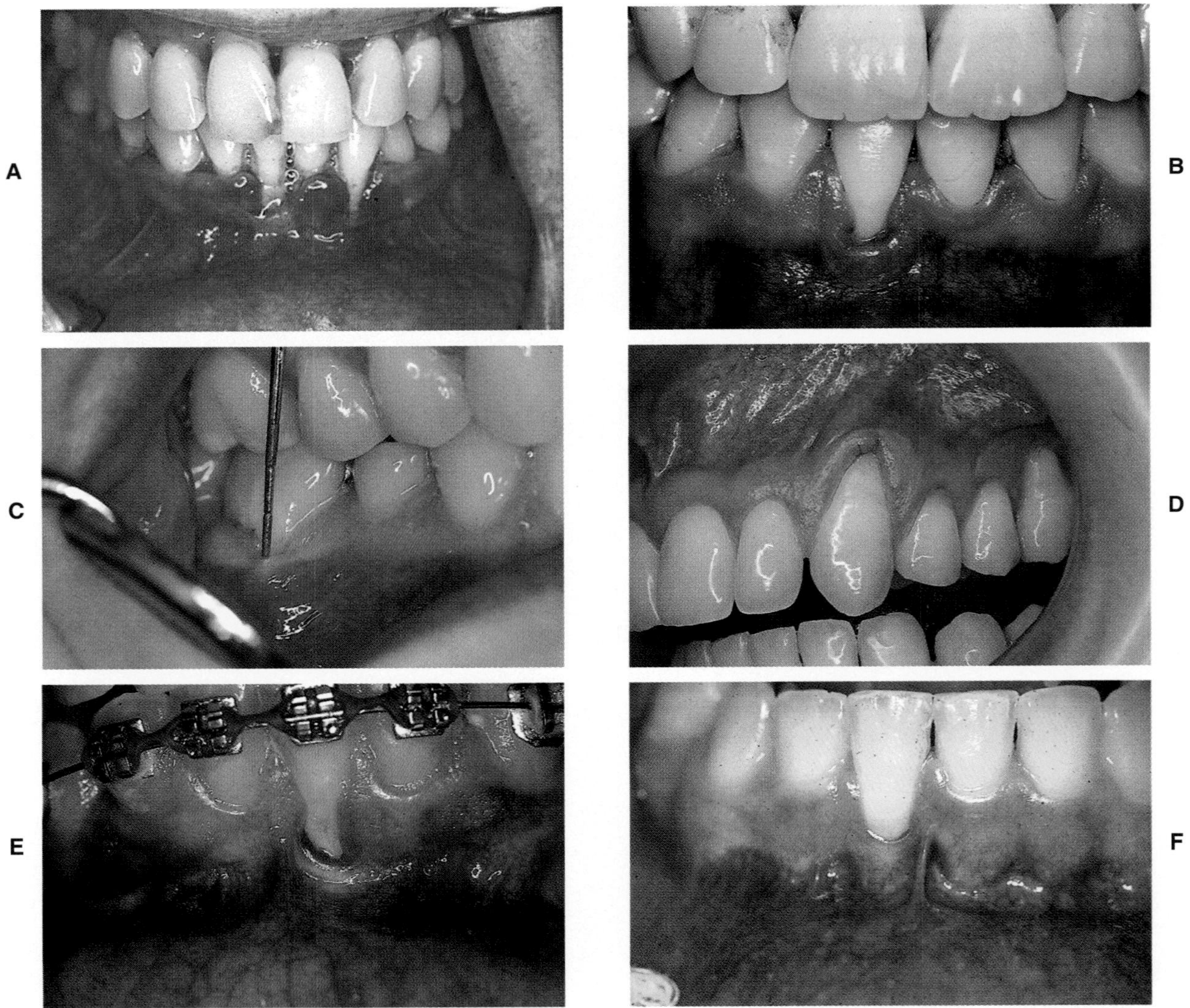

Color Fig. 66-2 Mucogingival defects. **A,** Irregular gingival contours, pocket furcations, and recession with severe gingival inflammation. **B,** Gingival recession and inflammation. Bottom of pocket is beyond mucogingival junction. **C,** Recession on mesiobuccal root of lower first molar. Probe indicates presence of shallow pocket with absence of attached gingiva. **D,** Gingival recession and cleft on upper cuspid. **E,** Advanced gingival recession and inflammation. **F,** After scaling and root planing and adequate plaque control, gingival condition has improved markedly.

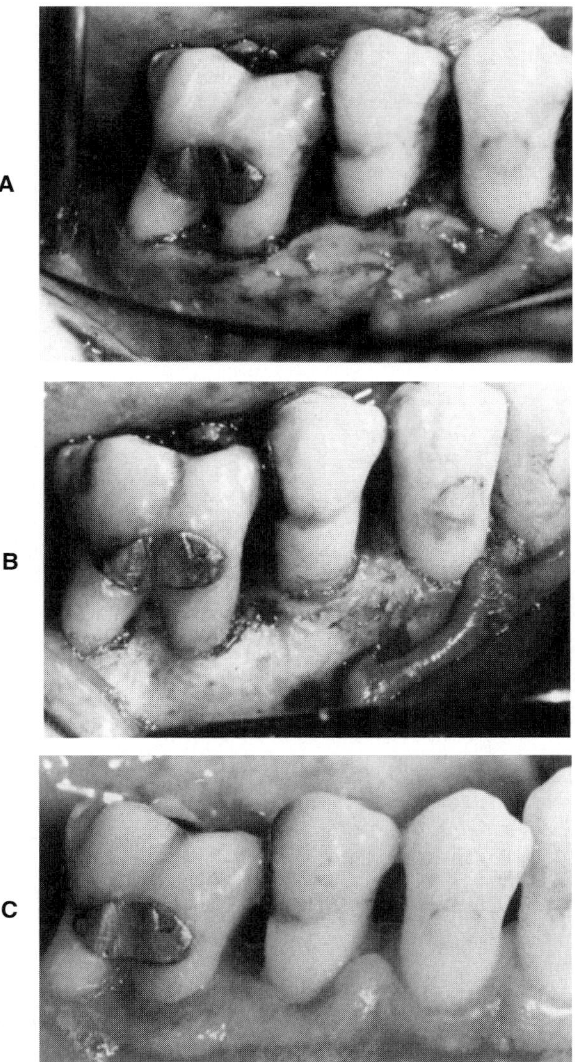

Fig. 62-16 Photographs taken **A,** before osseous surgery and **B,** after osseous management. **C,** Results 3 weeks after surgery.

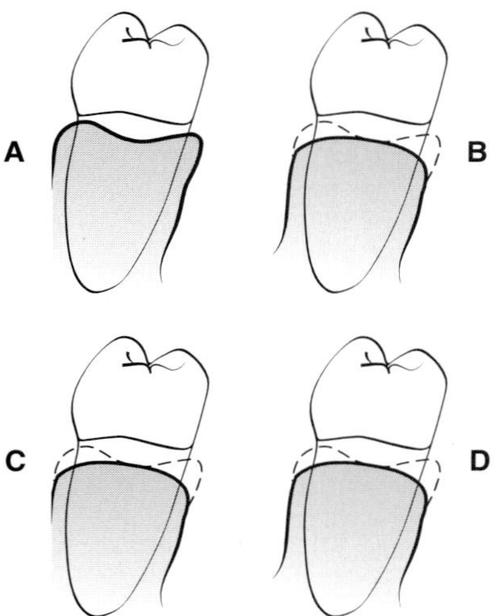

Fig. 62-17 Diagram of crater reduction patterns. **A,** Preoperative bony form after flap reflection. **B,** Reduction of craters to the facial. **C,** Reduction of craters to the lingual. **D,** Reduction of craters to both buccal and lingual.

completed by 14 to 21 days. Maturation and remodeling can continue for up to 6 months. It is usually advisable to wait a minimum period of 6 weeks after the completion of the last surgical area before beginning dental restorations. For those patients with a major cosmetic concern, it is wise to wait as long as possible to achieve a postoperative soft tissue position and sulcus that is stable.

SPECIFIC OSSEOUS RESHAPING SITUATIONS

The osseous corrective procedure that has been described is classically applied to shallow craters with heavy faciolingual ledges (Fig. 62-13). The correction of other osseous defects is also possible; however, careful case selection for definitive osseous surgery is very important.

Correction of one-walled hemiseptal defects requires that the bone be reduced to the level of the most apical portion of the defect. Therefore great care should be taken to select the adequate case. If one-walled defects occur next to an edentulous space, the edentulous ridge is reduced to the level of the osseous defect (Fig. 62-14).

Other situations that complicate osseous correction are exostoses (Fig. 62-15; see Color Fig. 62-1, *D* and *E*), malpositioned teeth, and supraerupted teeth. Each of these situations is best controlled by following the four steps previously outlined. In most situations, the unique feature of the bony profile is well managed by prudently applying the same principles. (Fig. 62-16; see Color Fig. 62-1). However, some situations require deviation from the definitive osseous reshaping technique; examples include dilacerated roots, root proximity, and furcations that would be compromised by osseous surgery.

In the absence of ledges or exostoses, the elimination of the bony lesion begins with reduction of the interdental walls of craters and the one-walled component of angular defects and wells (moats) and grooving into sites of early involvement.[10] The walls of the crater may be reduced at the expense of the buccal, lingual, or both walls (Fig. 62-17). The reduction should be made to remove the least amount of alveolar bone required to produce a satisfactory form, prevent the therapeutic invasion of furcations, and blend the contours with the adjacent teeth. The selective reduction of bony defects by "ramping" the bone to the palatal or lingual to avoid involvement of the furcations has been advocated by Ochsenbein and Bohannan[19] and Tibbetts, Ochsenbein, and Loughlin[24] (Fig. 62-18).

One-walled or hemiseptal defects usually require the removal of some bone from the tooth with the greatest coronal bony height. This removal of bone may result in a significant reduction in attachment on relatively unaffected adjacent teeth to eliminate the defect (see Fig. 62-16, *A* and *B*). However, if a tooth in the surgical field has one-walled defects on both its mesial and distal surfaces and this is recognized during examination, the severely affected tooth may be extruded by orthodontics during disease control treatment to minimize or eliminate the need for resection of bone from the adjacent teeth.

In the presence of heavy ledges of bone, it is usually wise to do osteoplasty first to eliminate any exostoses or reduce the buccal/lingual bulk of the bone (Fig. 62-19). It is common to incorporate a degree of vertical grooving during the reduction of bony ledges, since it facilitates the process of blending the radicular bone into the interproximal areas at the next step.

SUMMARY

Though osseous surgical techniques cannot be applied to every single bony abnormality or topographic modification, clearly it has been demonstrated that properly used osseous surgery can eliminate and modify defects, as well as gradualize excessive bony ledges, irregular alveolar bone, early furcation involvement, excessive bony exostosis, and circumferential defects. When properly performed, osseous resective surgery achieves a physiologic architecture of marginal alveolar bone conducive to gingival flap adaptation with minimal probing depth. The advantages of this surgical modality include a predictable amount of pocket reduction that can enhance oral hygiene and periodic maintenance. It also preserves the width of the attached tissue, while removing granulatous tissue and providing access for débridement of the radicular surfaces. Additionally, recontouring of bony abnormalities, including hemiseptal defects, tori, and ledges, is permitted. Proper assessment for restorative procedures such as crown lengthening and assessment of restorative overhangs and tooth abnormalities such as enamel projections, enamel pearls, perforations, and fractures is also a substantial benefit of osseous resective surgery. All factors lead to the conclusion that osseous resective surgery can be an important technique in the armamentarium necessary to provide a maintainable periodontium for periodontal patients.

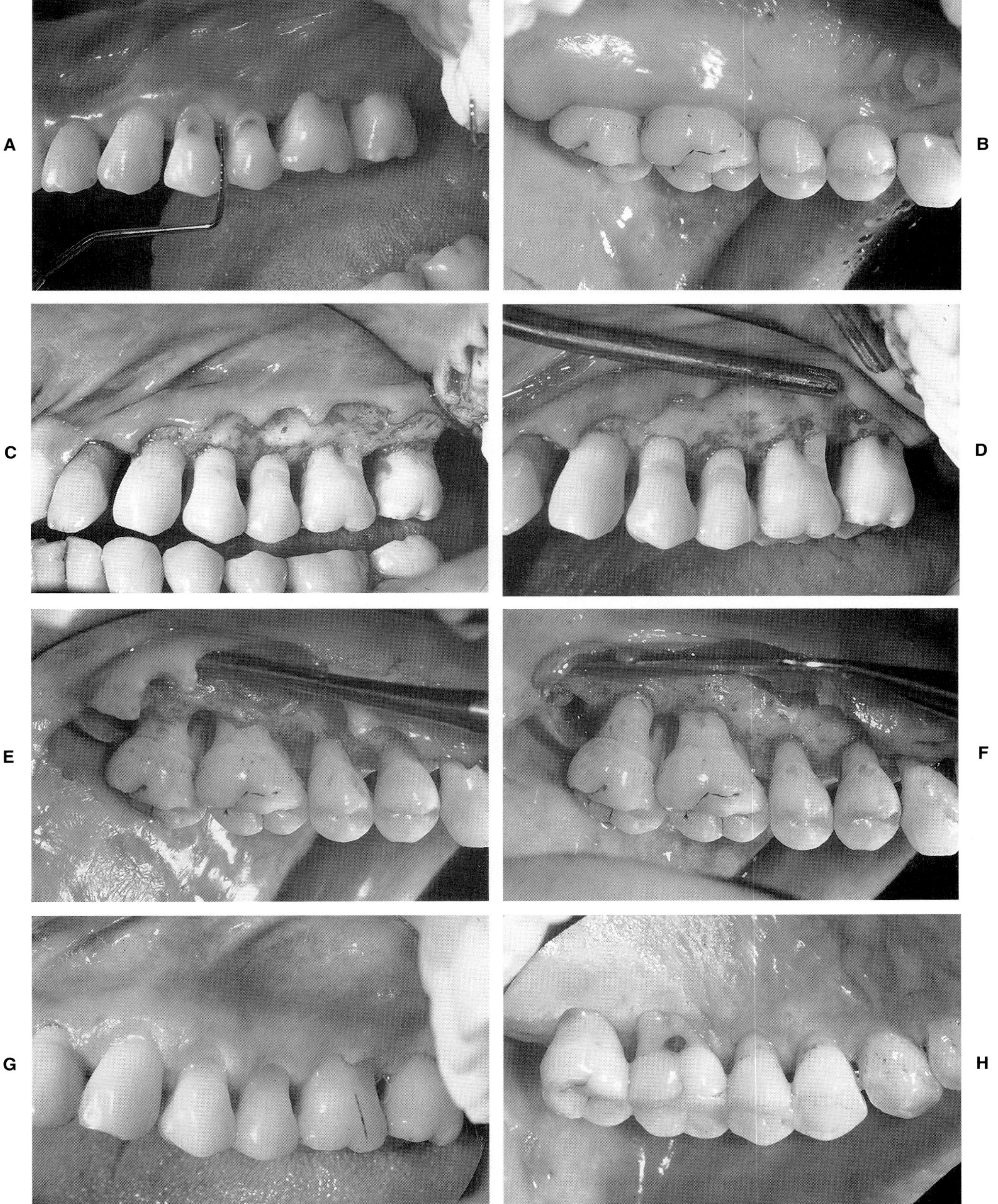

Fig. 62-18 Correction of osseous defects largely to the palatal. **A and B,** Buccal and palatal preoperative views. The patient is 6 weeks post-completion of scaling and root planing. **C and D,** Buccal preosseous and postosseous views. **C,** Note the ledging on the facial of the molars, and one wall defects on both molars. **D,** The postosseous view shows the elimination of these defects by osteoplasty on the ledges and ostectomy of the one wall defects to produce a positive buccal architecture. **E and F,** Palatal preosseous and postosseous views. **E,** Note the pattern of bony loss, which is more severe on the palatal. In addition to the facial one-wall defects, there is an incipient furcation defect at the mesial of the first molar and a class II furcation at the mesial of the second molar. **F,** The configuration of the defects was such that ostectomy was performed on the palatal roots of both molars to produce a compromised architecture. **G and H,** Ten-year postoperative views of the buccal and palatal areas displaying the pattern of soft tissue adaptation to the surgically produced bony form.

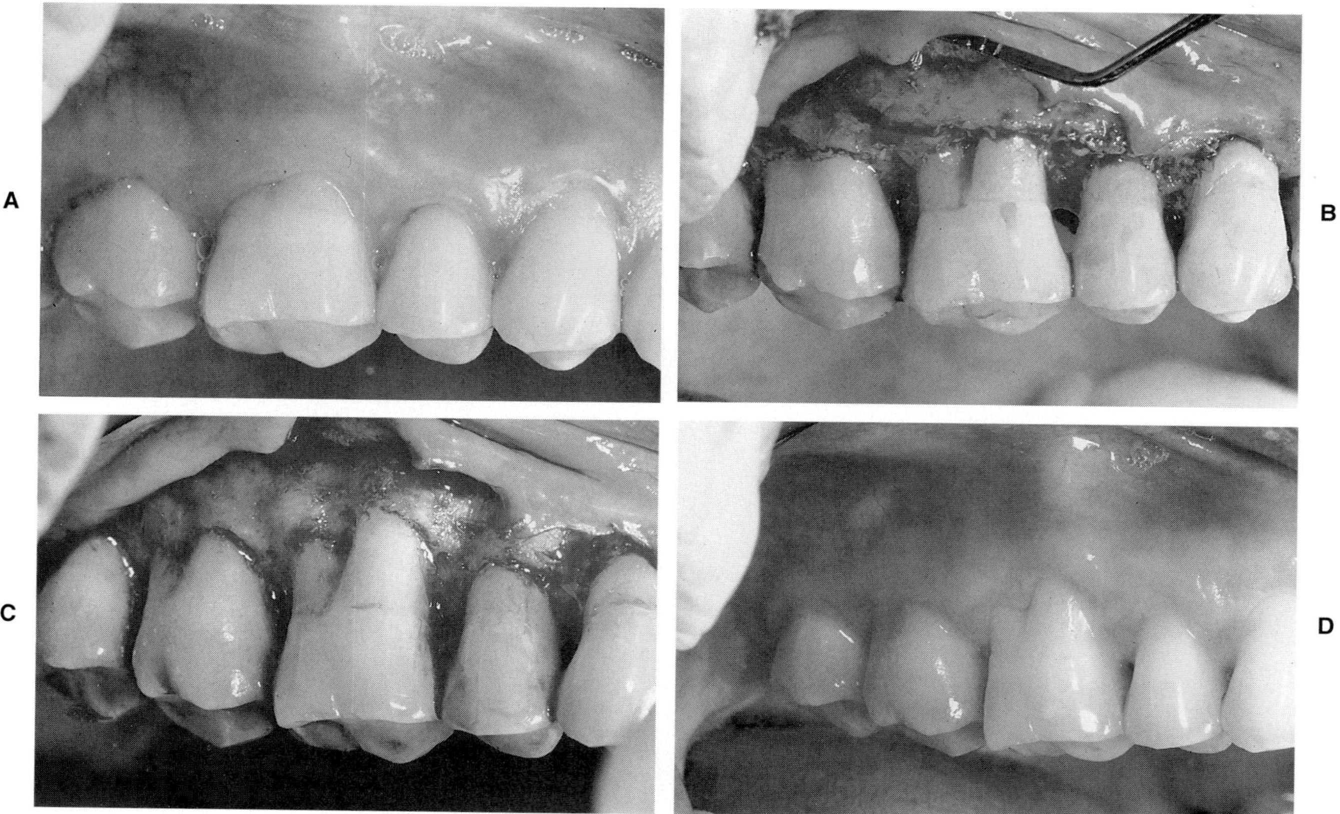

Fig. 62-19 Reduction of bony ledges by osteoplasty before correction of interdental defects. **A,** Buccal preoperative view. **B,** Buccal flap reflection. Note the buccal ledge and the class II buccal furcation. **C,** Buccal correction largely by osteoplasty with minor ostectomy over the root prominence to produce a positive architecture. **D,** Ten-year postoperative view of soft tissue form. Minimal pocket depth is present.

REFERENCES

1. Black GV: Surgical treatment of pockets. In Black AD: Special Dental Pathology, ed 3. Chicago, Medico Dental, 1917.
2. Carranza FA, Carranza FA Jr: The management of the alveolar bone in the treatment of the periodontal pocket. J Periodontol 1956; 27:29.
3. Caton J, Nyman S: Histometric evaluation of periodontal surgery. III. The effect of bone resection on the connective tissue attachment level. J Periodontol 1981; 52:405.
4. Dahlberg WH: Incisions and suturing: Some basic considerations about each in periodontal surgery. Dent Clin N Amer 1969; 13(1):149.
5. Donnenfeld OW, Hoag PM, Weissman DP: A clinical study of the effects of osteoplasty. J Periodontol 1961; 32:131.
6. Easley J: Methods of determining alveolar osseous form. J Periodontol 1967; 38:112.
7. Friedman N: Periodontal osseous surgery: Osteoplasty and osteoectomy periodontol 1955; 26:257.
8. Garguilo AW, Wentz FM, Orban B: Dimensions and relations of the dentogingival junction in humans. J Periodontol 1961; 32:261.
9. Goldman HM, Cohen DW: The infrabony pocket: Classification and treatment. J Periodontol 1958; 29:272.
10. Kaldahl WB, Kalkwarf KL, Patin KD, et al: Evaluation of four modalities of periodontal therapy: Mean probing depth, probing attachment level and recession changes. J Periodontol 1988; 59:783.
11. Kaldahl WB, Kalkwarf KL, Patil KD, et al: Long-term evaluation of periodontal therapy. I. Response to four therapeutic modalities. J Periodontol 1996; 67:93.
12. Kaldahl WB, Kalkwarf KL, Patil KD, et al: Long-term evaluation of periodontal therapy: I. Response to four therapeutic modalities. J Periodontol 1996; 67:103.
13. Knowles J, Burgett F, Nissle R, et al: Results of periodontal treatment related to pocket depth and attachment level. Eight years. J Periodontol 1979; 50:225.
14. Lindhe J, Socransky S, Nyman S, et al: Critical probing depths in peridontal therapy. J Clin Periodontol 1982; 9:323.
15. Manson JD, Nicholson K: The distribution of bone defects in chronic periodontitis. J Periodontol 1974; 45:88.
16. Maynard JG, Wilson RDK: Physiologic dimensions of the periodontium significant to the restorative dentist. J Periodontol 1979; 50:170.
17. Mealey BL, Beybayer MF, Butzin CA, et al: Use of furcal bone sounding to improve the accuracy of furcation diagnosis. J Periodontol 1994; 65:649.

18. Ochsenbein C: A primer for osseous surgery. Int J Perio Rest Dent 1986; 6(1):9.
19. Ochsenbein C, Bohannan HM: The palatal approach to osseous surgery. II. Clinical application. J Periodontol 1964; 35:54.
20. Prichard JF: The roentgenographic depiction of periodontal disease. Periodontics 1973; 3(2).
21. Schluger S: Osseous resection: A basic principle in periodontal surgery. Oral Surg Oral Med Oral Path 1949; 2:316.
22. Schluger S, Yuodelis RA, Page RC, et al: Resective periodontal surgery in pocket elimination. In Periodontal Diseases. Philadelphia, Lea & Febiger, 1990.
23. Selipsky HS: Osseous surgery. How much need we compromise? Dent Clin N Amer 1976; 20(1):79.
24. Tibbetts L, Ochsenbein C, Loughlin D: The lingual approach to osseous surgery. J Periodontol 1976; 20(1):61.
25. Townsend-Olsen C, Ammons WF, Van Belle C: A longitudinal study comparing apically repositioned flaps, with and without osseous surgery. Int J Periodontics Restorative Dent 1985; 5(4):11.

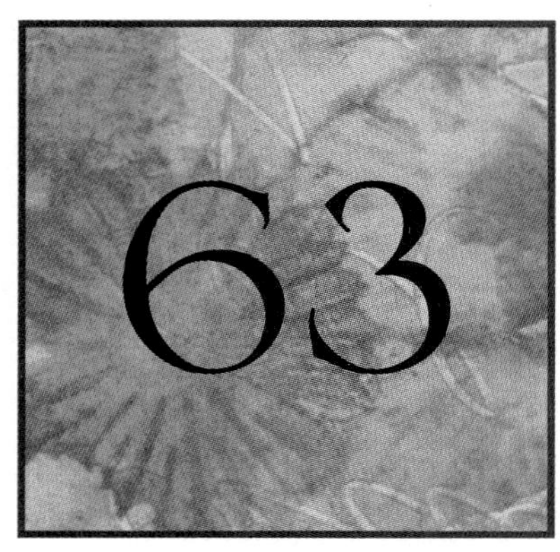

CHAPTER

Regenerative Osseous Surgery

Fermin A. Carranza, Pamela McClain, and Robert Schallhorn

CHAPTER OUTLINE

New attachment with periodontal regeneration is the ideal outcome of therapy because it results in obliteration of the pocket and reconstruction of the marginal periodontium (Color Fig. 63-1; Fig. 63-1). However, the techniques available are not totally dependable, and the following other results of therapy may be seen (Fig. 63-2):

1. Healing with a long junctional epithelium, which can occur even if filling in of bone has occurred.
2. Ankylosis of bone and tooth with resultant root resorption.
3. Recession.
4. Recurrence of the pocket.
5. Any combination of the above.

EVALUATION OF NEW ATTACHMENT AND BONE REGENERATION

It is sometimes difficult in clinical and experimental situations to determine whether new attachment has occurred and the extent to which it has occurred. Evidences of reconstruction of the marginal periodontium can be obtained by clinical, radiographic, surgical reentry, or histologic procedures.[28,99] All these methods have advantages and shortcomings that should be well understood and considered in individual cases and when critically evaluating the literature.

Clinical Methods

Clinical methods consist of comparison of pre- and posttreatment pocket probings and determinations of clinical gingival findings. The probe can be used to determine pocket depth, attachment level, and bone level (see Chapter 30) (Fig. 63-3). Clinical determinations of attachment level are more useful than strict pocket depths because the latter may change as a result of displacement of the gingival margin. Several studies have determined that the depth of penetration of a probe in a periodontal pocket varies according to the degree of inflammatory involvement of the tissues immediately beneath the bottom of the pocket (Fig. 63-4). Therefore even though the forces used may be standardized with pressure-sensitive probes, there is an inherent margin of error in this method that is difficult to overcome. Fowler and colleagues[54] have calculated this error to be 1.2 mm, but it is even greater when furcations are probed.[117]

Bone probing performed under anesthesia is not subject to this error and has been found to be as accurate as bone height measurements made on surgical reentry.[70,144,186]

Measurements of the defect should be made before and after treatment from the same exact point within the defect and with the same angulation of the probe. This reproducibility of probe placement is difficult and

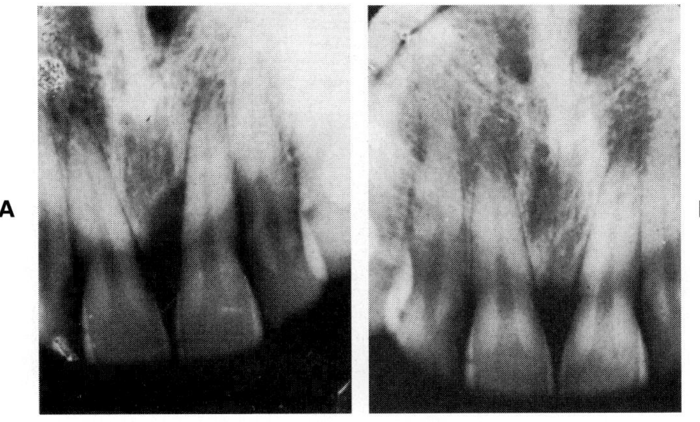

Fig. 63-1 Bone regeneration after closed scaling, root planing, and curettage. Before **(A)** and after **(B)** radiographs are shown. (From Carranza FA Sr: A technique for reattachment. J Periodontol 1954; 25:272.)

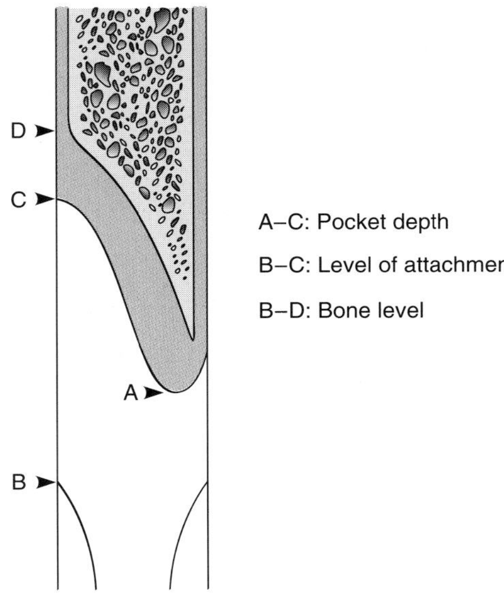

Fig. 63-3 Different types of probings in an interdental space.

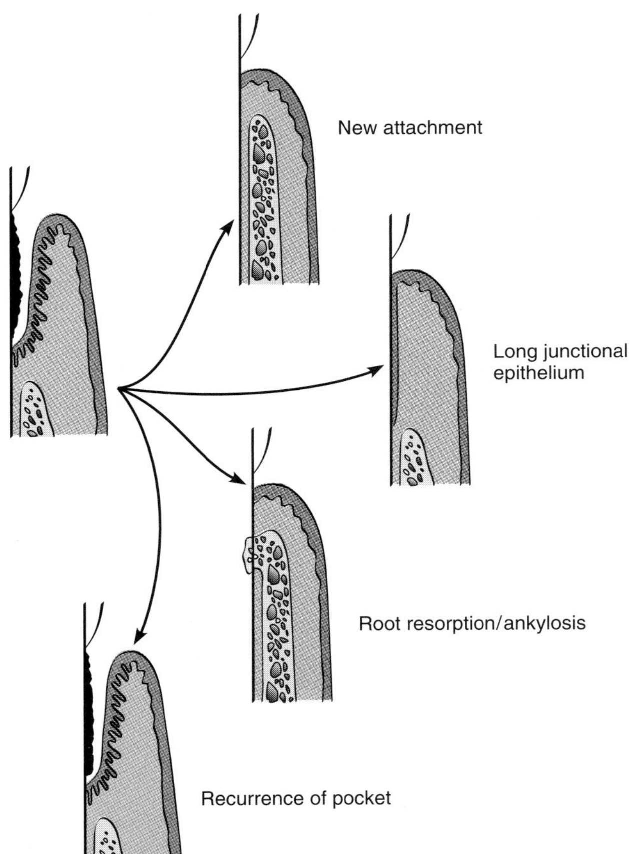

Fig. 63-2 Possible outcomes of therapy.

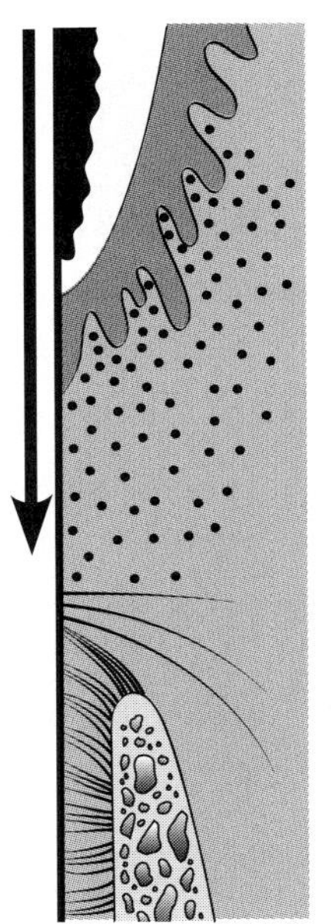

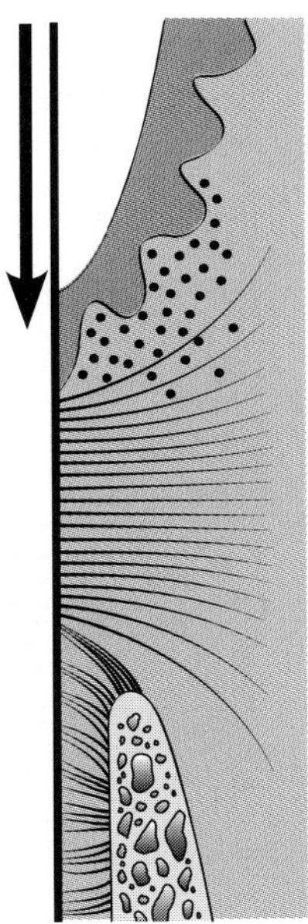

Fig. 63-4 *Left,* Arrow pointing downward depicts penetration of a probe in an untreated periodontal pocket. The probe tip goes past the junctional epithelium and the inflamed tissue and is stopped by the first intact, attached collagen fibers. *Right,* After thorough scaling and root planing, the location of the bottom of the pocket has not changed, but the probe penetrates to only about one third the length of the junctional epithelium (see Chapter 30). *The reduction in probing depth may not reflect a change in attachment level.*

may be facilitated in part by using a grooved stent to guide the introduction of the probe (Fig. 63-5). Preoperative and postoperative comparability of probing measurements that do not use this standardized method may be open to question.

Radiographic Methods

Radiographic evaluation of bone regeneration also requires carefully standardized techniques for reproducible positioning of the film and the tube.[128,148] Even with standardized techniques (see Chapter 34), the radiograph

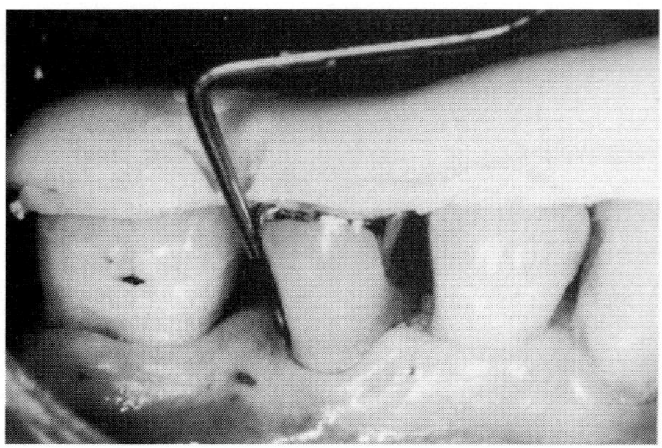

Fig. 63-5 Grooved acrylic stent used in clinical research to standardize the direction of introduction of the probe.

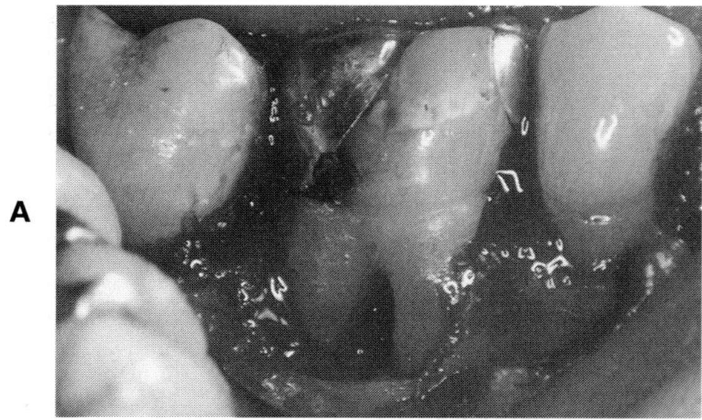

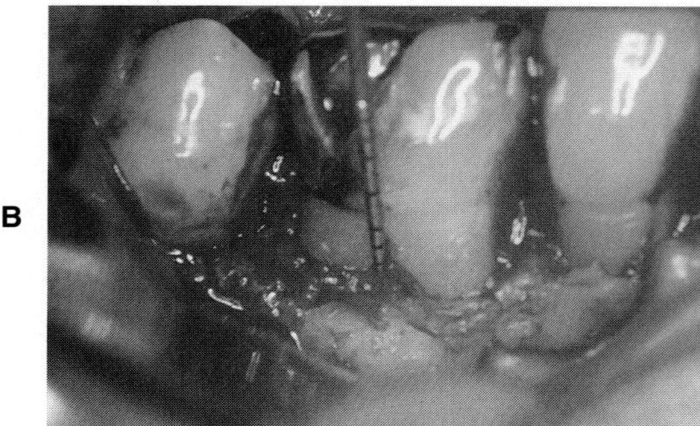

Fig. 63-6 Reentry evidence of bone apposition following regenerative therapy. **A,** Surgical exposure of facial bone dehiscence and furcation defects. **B,** Two-year reentry with tip of probe on new coronal bone height. (From McClain P, Schallhorn RG: The use of combined periodontal regenerative techniques (guest editorial). Int J Periodont Restorative Dent 1993; 13:15.)

does not show the entire topography of the area before or after treatment. Furthermore, thin bone trabeculae may exist before treatment and go undetected radiographically because a certain minimal amount of mineralized tissue must be present to register on the radiograph. Several studies have demonstrated that radiographs, even those taken with standardized methods, are less reliable than clinical probing techniques.[91,178] A comparative study of pretreatment bone levels and posttherapy bone fill with 12-month reentry bone measurements showed that linear

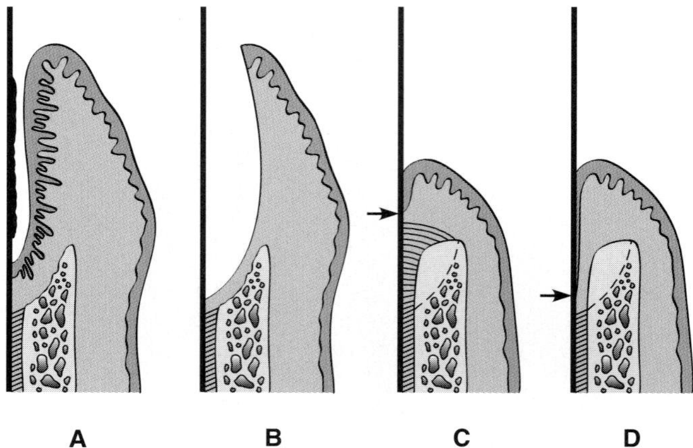

Fig. 63-7 **A,** Periodontal pocket preoperatively. **B,** Periodontal pocket immediately after scaling, root planing, and curettage. **C,** New attachment. The arrow indicates the most apical part of the junctional epithelium. Note regeneration of bone and periodontal ligament. **D,** Healing by long junctional epithelium. Again, the arrow indicates the most apical part of the junctional epithelium. Note that the bone is new but the periodontal ligament is not.

radiographic analysis significantly underestimates pretreatment bone loss and posttreatment bone fill.[181]

Studies with subtraction radiography have enhanced the usefulness of radiographic evaluation.[43,44,190] A comparative study between linear measurement, computer assisted densitometric analysis (CADIA) (see Chapter 34), and a method combining the two reported that the linear-CADIA method offers the highest level of accuracy.[179]

Surgical Reentry

The surgical reentry of a case after a period of healing can give a good view of the state of the bone crest that can be compared with the view taken during the initial surgical intervention and can also be subject to measurements (Fig. 63-6). Models from impressions of the bone taken at the time of the initial surgery and later at reentry can be used to assess the results of therapy. This method is very useful but has two shortcomings: it requires a frequently unnecessary second operation, and it does not show the type of attachment that exists (i.e., new attachment or long junctional epithelium (Fig. 63-7).[31]

Histologic Methods

The type of attachment can be determined only by histologic analysis of tissue blocks obtained from the healed area. Although this method can offer clear evidence of regeneration of the attachment apparatus, it is not without problems. The need to remove a tooth with its periodontium after successful treatment limits this method to volunteers who need the extraction for prosthetic or other reasons and agree to the procedure.

Animal studies can be used to clarify some aspects of the tissue response to different materials. However, species differences should always be remembered when extrapolations to humans are attempted. The compati-

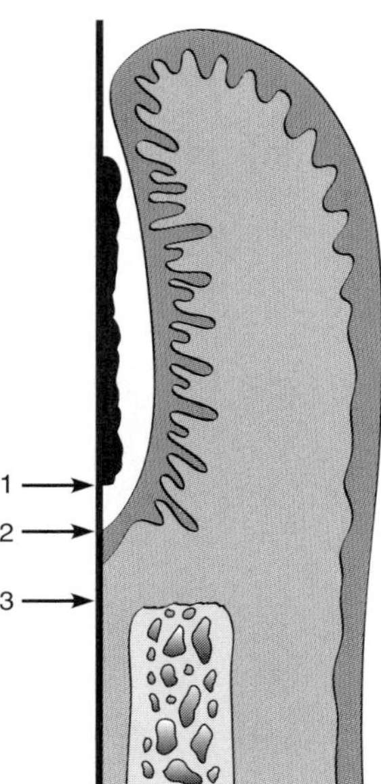

Fig. 63-8 For future histologic reference, notches can be placed clinically at the most apical part of the calculus *(1)* or at the level of the osseous crest *(3)*. However, the real landmark that determines whether new attachment has taken place is the base of the pocket *(2)*.

bility of a material with the tissues can be shown by implanting the substance into the long bones or calvaria of rats or other rodents, but this does not prove the regeneration of periodontal attachment.

Studies of the reconstruction of periodontal structures have been performed in dogs, monkeys, and pigs. Because it is difficult to find naturally occurring periodontal osseous defects that would be adequate for a study, experimentally induced bone defects must be used. Surgically produced bone defects can simulate the shape of osseous periodontal lesions but lack their chronicity and self-sustaining features. They are not exactly similar to naturally occurring disease. They can be allowed to become chronically infected, and then their similarity to chronic natural lesions improves, but they are never identical.[192] However, these studies are useful to establish healing sequences and mechanisms.

In addition, the exact location of the bottom of the pocket must be determined prior to the procedure because the surgical technique opens tissues beyond the bottom of the pocket, and healing below this point does not constitute new attachment. Notches on the root surface must be used to indicate this important point. Because the exact coronal point of the junctional epithelium is lost when surgically opening the area, a decision must be made as to whether to place the notch at the bottom of the calculus or on the crest of the alveolar bone (Figs. 63-8 and 63-9). The former is slightly coronal and the latter slightly apical to the real bottom of the pocket. The bottom of the calculus is a better landmark, but obviously the presence of calculus is required.

Numerous pitfalls are therefore inherent in histologic studies, and their accuracy and reliability should always be very carefully considered.

REGENERATIVE SURGICAL TECHNIQUES

Regenerative periodontics can be subdivided into two major areas: non–graft-associated new attachment and graft-associated new attachment. Many techniques combine both approaches.

All recommended techniques include careful and complete removal of all irritants. Although this can be done in some cases as a closed procedure, in the great majority of cases it should be done after exposure of the area with a flap. Flap design and incisions should follow the description given in Chapter 60 for regenerative flaps. Trauma from occlusion may impair posttreatment healing of the supporting periodontal tissues, reducing the likelihood of new attachment. Occlusal adjustment, if needed, is therefore indicated.

Systemic antibiotics are generally used after regenerative periodontal therapy, although definitive information on the advisabilitty of this measure is still lacking. Case reports have been presented showing extensive regeneration of the periodontal lesions after scaling, root planing, and curettage combined with systemic and local treatment with penicillin or tetracycline in combination with other forms of therapy.[25,120]

Non–Graft-Associated New Attachment

Periodontal reconstruction can be attained without the use of grafts in meticulously treated three-wall defects (intrabony defects) and in periodontal and endodontal abscesses.[25,66,79,122,138] New attachment is more likely to occur when the destructive process has occurred very rapidly (e.g., after treatment of pockets complicated by the formation of acute periodontal abscesses and after treatment of acute necrotizing ulcerative gingivitis).

The following section covers the rationale and technique for the removal of the junctional and pocket epithelium and the prevention of their migration into the healing area after therapy. It also covers the so-called bio-conditioning of the root surface and the use of growth factors and enamel matrix proteins to enhance or direct healing.

Removal of Junctional and Pocket Epithelium.

Since the earliest attempts at periodontal new attachment, the presence of junctional and pocket epithelium has been perceived as a barrier to successful therapy because its presence interferes with the direct apposition of connective tissue and cementum, thus limiting the height to which periodontal fibers can become inserted to the cementum.[76,118,141,193] Several methods have been recommended to remove junctional and pocket epithelia. These include curettage, chemical agents, ultrasonic methods, and surgical techniques.

CURETTAGE. Results of removal of epithelium by means of curettage vary from complete removal to persistence of as much as 50%.[165] It therefore is not a reliable procedure. Ultrasonic methods and rotary abrasive stones have also been used, but their effects cannot be controlled because of the clinician's lack of tactile sense when using these methods

CHEMICAL AGENTS. Chemical agents have also been used to remove pocket epithelium, in most cases in conjunction with curettage. The most commonly used drugs have been sodium sulfide, phenol camphor, antiformin, and sodium hypochlorite. However, the effect of these agents is not limited to the epithelium, and their depth of action cannot be controlled. They are mentioned here for their historical interest.

SURGICAL TECHNIQUES. Surgical techniques have been recommended to eliminate the pocket and junctional epithelia. The *excisional new attachment procedure* consists of an internal bevel incision performed with a surgical knife, followed by removal of the excised tissue.[194] No attempt is made to elevate a flap. After care-

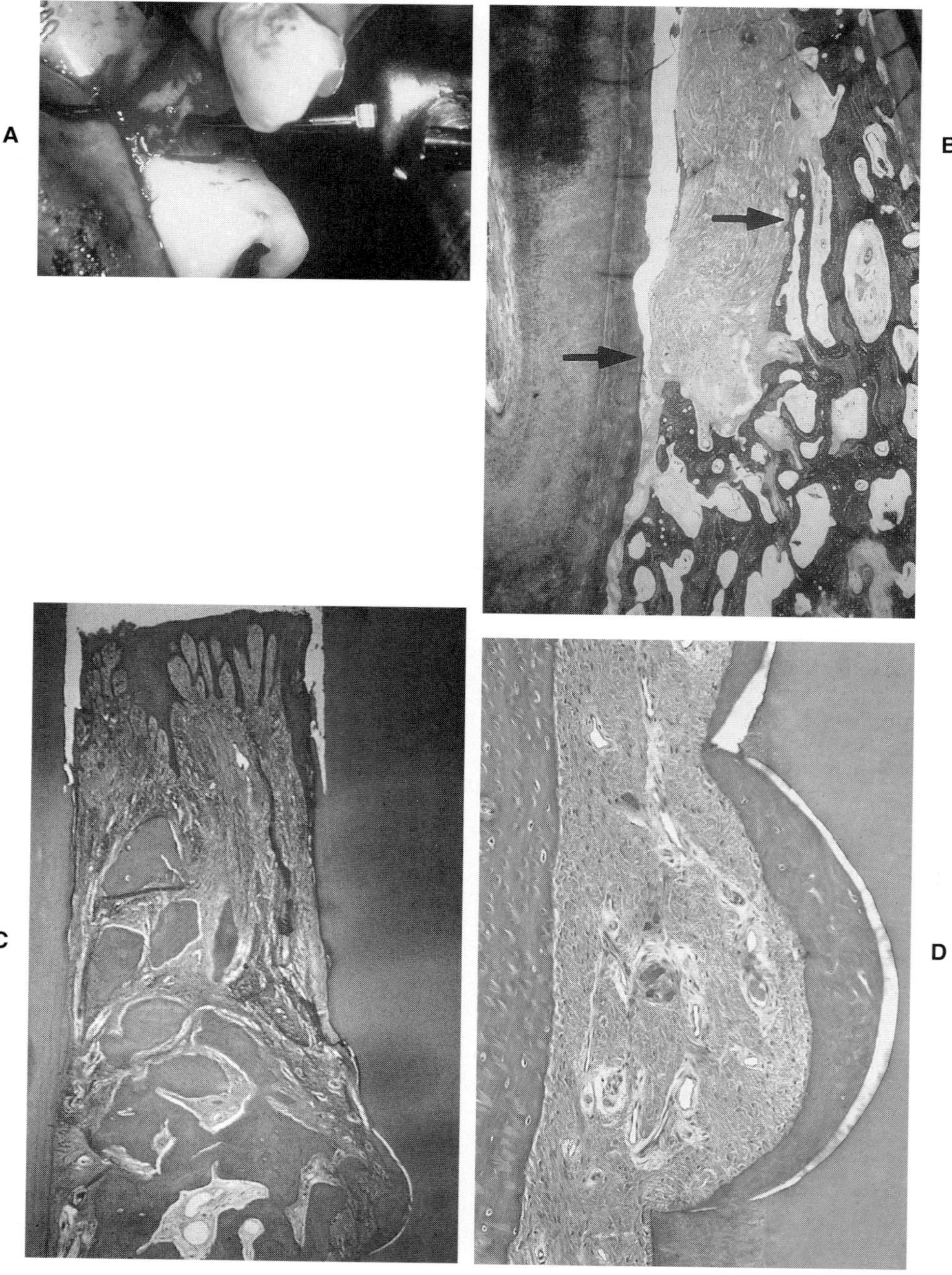

Fig. 63-9 A, Notch being placed through the apical extent of the calculus into the root surface as a histologic marker. **B,** Six-month postoperative histologic block section of control site depicting no regeneration coronal to the reference notch *(arrow)*. **C,** Six-month postoperative histologic block section of experimental site using a demineralized freeze-dried bone allograft depicting regeneration coronal to the crestal bone notch (calculus notch 7 mm apical to crestal notch). **D,** High power of reference notch through calculus at base of defect with new cementum (artifactual split during histologic preparation), bone, and periodontal ligament. (Courtesy Dr. Gerald Bowers, University of Maryland.)

ful scaling and root planing, interproximal sutures are used to close the wound (see Chapter 57).

Glickman and Prichard have advocated performing a *gingivectomy to the crest of the alveolar bone and debriding the defect.*[65,137] Excellent results have been obtained with this technique in uncontrolled human studies.[8,138]

The *modified Widman flap,* as described by Ramfjord and Nissle, is similar to the excisional new attachment procedure but is followed by elevation of a flap for better exposure of the area.[142] It eliminates the pocket epithelium with the internal bevel incision (see Chapter 61).

Another approach to delaying epithelial migration into the healing pocket area has been the use of *coronal displacement of the flap,* which increases the distance between the epithelium and the healing area. This technique is particularly suitable for the treatment of lower molar furcations and has been used mostly in conjunction with citric acid treatment of the roots.[61,102] Periodontal regeneration after the use of this technique has been demonstrated histologically in humans.[171]

Prevention of Epithelial Migration. Elimination of junctional and pocket epithelia may not be sufficient because the epithelium from the excised margin may rapidly proliferate to become interposed between the healing connective tissue and the cementum.

Several investigators have analyzed in animals and humans the effect of excluding the epithelium by amputating the crown of the tooth and covering the root with the flap (*root submergence*).[12,13,17] This experimental technique not only excludes the epithelium but also prevents microbial contamination of the wound during the reparative stages. Successful repair of osseous lesions in the submerged environment was reported, but obviously this method has little or no clinical application.

Another method proposed to prevent or retard the migration of the epithelium consists of total removal of the interdental papilla covering the defect and its replacement with a *free autogenous graft* obtained from the palate.[46] During healing, the epithelium necroses, and its migration is retarded.

GUIDED TISSUE REGENERATION. The method for the prevention of epithelial migration along the cemental wall of the pocket that has gained wide attention is the so-called *guided tissue regeneration (GTR).* This method derives from the classic studies of Nyman, Lindhe, Karring, and Gottlow and is based on the assumption that only the periodontal ligament cells have the potential for regeneration of the attachment apparatus of the tooth.[68,69,125,126] It consists of placing barriers of different types to cover the bone and periodontal ligament, thus temporarily separating them from the gingival epithelium (see Chapter 36). Excluding the epithelium and the gingival connective tissue from the root surface during the postsurgical healing phase not only prevents epithelial migration into the wound but also favors repopulation of the area by cells from the periodontal ligament and the bone.

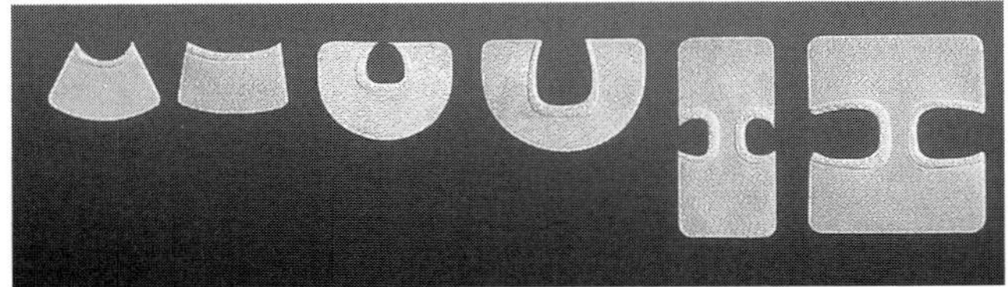

Fig. 63-10 Different shapes and sizes of expanded polytetrafluoroethylene membranes marketed by Gore-Tex (Flagstaff, AZ).

Initial animal experiments using Millipore filters and Teflon membranes resulted in regeneration of cementum and alveolar bone and a functional periodontal ligament.[29,30,33,116] Clinical case reports showed that guided tissue regeneration results in a gain in attachment level, which is not necessarily associated with a buildup of alveolar bone.[9,10] Histologic studies in humans provided evidence of periodontal regeneration in most instances, even in cases of horizontal bone losses.[69,170,174]

The use of polytetrafluoroethylene membranes (Gore-Tex periodontal material, Gore-Tex, Flagstaff, AZ) has been tested in controlled clinical studies in lower molar furcations and has shown statistically significant decreases in pocket depths and improvement in attachment levels after 6 months; bone level measurements have been inconclusive.[94,136] A study on upper molar furcations did not result in significant gain in attachment or bone levels.[115]

The initial membranes developed were nonresorbable and therefore required a second operation, albeit frequently very simple, to remove it. This second operation was done after the initial stages of healing, usually 3 to 6 weeks after the first intervention. This second operation was a significant obstacle in the utilization of the procedure, and therefore resorbable membranes were developed.[189]

The expanded polytetrafluoroethylene membrane (nonresorbable) can be obtained in different shapes and sizes to suit proximal spaces and facial/lingual surfaces of furcations (Fig. 63-10). The technique for its use is as follows (Figs. 63-11):

1. Raise a mucoperiosteal flap with vertical incisions, extending a minimum of two teeth anteriorly and one tooth distally to the tooth being treated.
2. Debride the osseous defect and thoroughly plane the roots.
3. Trim the membrane with sharp scissors to the approximate size of the area being treated. The apical border of the material should extend 3 to 4 mm apical to the margin of the defect and laterally 2 to 3 mm beyond the defect; the occlusal border of the membrane should be placed 2 mm apical to the cementoenamel junction.[10]
4. Suture the membrane tightly around the tooth with a sling suture.
5. Suture the flap back in its original position or slightly coronal to it, using independent sutures interdentally and in the vertical incisions. The flap should cover the membrane completely.
6. The use of periodontal dressings is optional, and the patient is placed on antibiotic therapy for 1 week.

After 4 to 6 weeks, the margin of the membrane becomes exposed. The membrane is removed with a gentle tug 5 weeks after the operation. If it cannot be removed

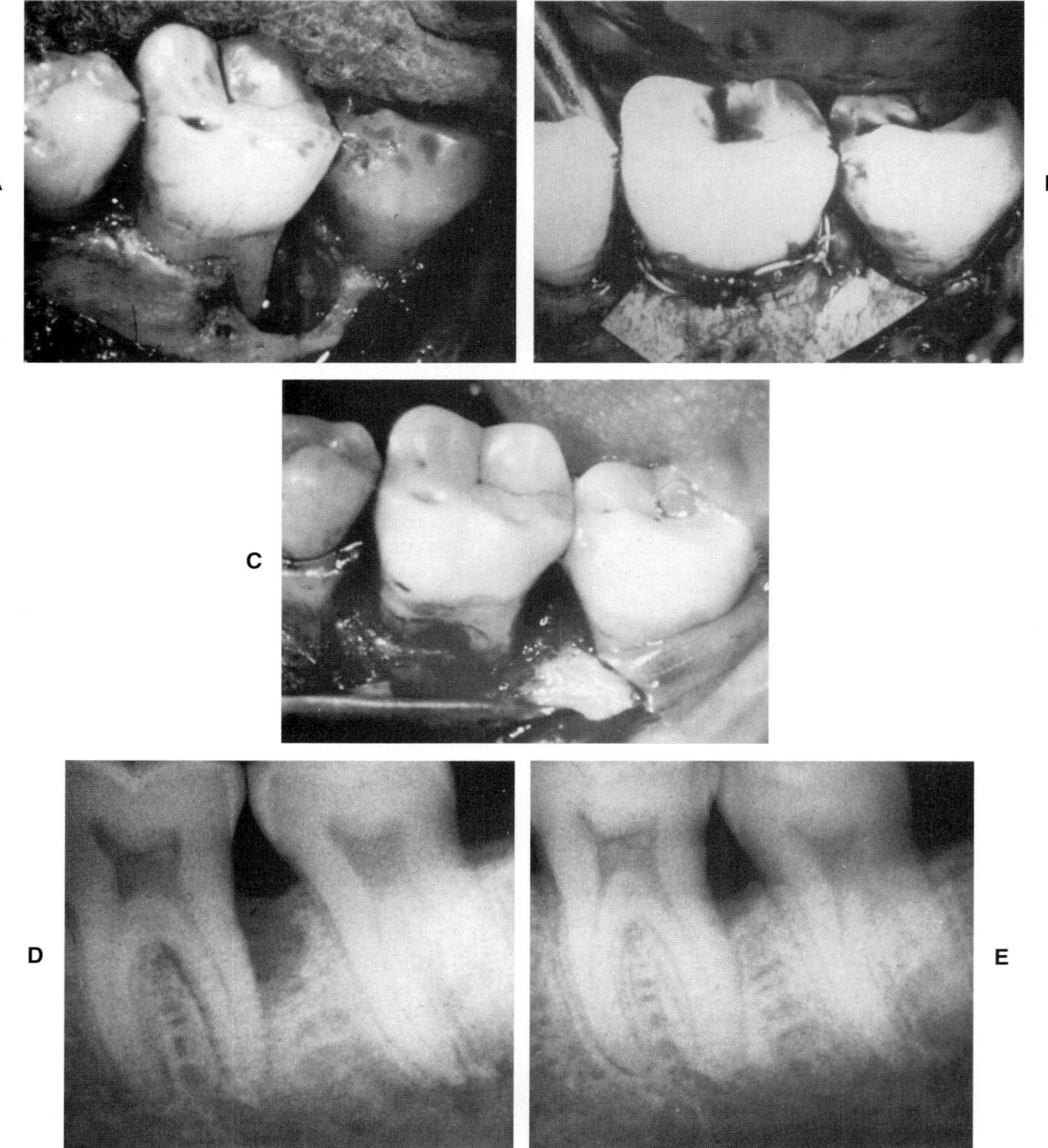

Fig. 63-11 Patient treated according to the principles of guided tissue regeneration. **A,** Deep osseous defect on the distal root of a lower molar. **B,** After thorough instrumentation, the Gore-Tex membrane is placed. **C,** Reentry after 9 months, showing the defect fill. Before **(D)** and after **(E)** radiographs of patient. (Courtesy Drs. Burton Becker and William Becker, Tucson, Ariz.)

easily, the tissues are anesthetized and the material is surgically removed using a miniflap.

The results obtained with the guided tissue regeneration technique are enhanced when the technique is combined with grafts placed in the defects (see Combined Technique).[5,16,92,103]

The Use of Biodegradable Membranes. The search for resorbable membranes included tests with rat collagen, bovine collagen, Cargile membrane derived from the cecum of an ox, polylactic acid, Vycril (polyglactin 910), synthetic skin (Biobrane), and freeze-dried dura mater.[14,15,24,32,52,53,60,100,101,131–133,189,196] Clinical studies with a mixture of copolymers derived from polylactic acid and acetyl tributylcitrate resorbable membranes (Guidor membrane, no longer on the market) and a poly-D,L-lactide-co-glycolide (Resolut membrane, also no longer on the market) have shown significant gains in clinical attachment and bone fill.[34,61,180]

Resorbable membranes marketed in the U.S. as of this writing include: OsseoQuest, Gore Co. (polyglycolic acid, polylactic acid and trimethylene carbonate; resorbs at 6 to 14 months); BioGuide, OsteoHealth Co. (bi-layer porcine-derived collagen); Atrisorb, Block Drug Co.

(polylactic acid gel); and BioMend, Calcitech Co. (bovine Achilles tendon collagen, resorbs in 4 to 18 weeks).

The potential of using autogenous periosteum as a membrane and also to stimulate periodontal regeneration has been explored in two controlled clinical studies, one of grade II furcation involvements in lower molars and another of interdental defects.[90,93] The periosteum was obtained from the patient's palate by means of a window flap. Both studies reported that autogenous periosteal grafts can be used in guided tissue regeneration and result in significant gains in clinical attachment and osseous defect fill.

Clot Stabilization, Wound Protection, and Space Creation. Some investigators have attributed the successful results reported with graft materials, barrier membranes, and coronally displaced flaps to the fact that all protect the wound and create a space for undisturbed and stable maturation of the clot.[62,74,75] This hypothesis suggests that preservation of the root surface–fibrin clot interface prevents apical migration of the gingival epithelium and allows for connective tissue attachment during the early wound healing period.[62,192]

The importance of space creation for bone repair has long been recognized in orthopedic and maxillofacial surgery. Transference of this concept to periodontal therapy has been explored for regeneration techniques and root coverage and treatment of periimplant bone defects. The space is created by using a titanium-reinforced ePTFE membrane to prevent its collapse. For the study of regenerative techniques, these membranes were placed over experimentally created supraalveolar bone defects in dogs and considerable bone regeneration was reported.[164]

Biomodification of the Root Surface. Changes in the tooth surface wall of periodontal pockets (e.g., degeneration of remnants of Sharpey's fibers, accumulation of bacteria and their products, and disintegration of the cementum and dentin) interfere with new attachment. However, these obstacles to new attachment can be eliminated by thorough root planing.

Several substances have been used in attempts to better condition the root surface for attachment of new connective tissue fibers. These include citric acid, fibronectin, and tetracycline.

CITRIC ACID. Studies by Urist showed that the implantation of demineralized dentin matrix into muscle tissue in animals induced mesenchymal cells to differentiate into osteoblasts and started an osteogenic process.[183-185] Following up on this concept, a series of studies applied citric acid to the roots to demineralize the surface, thus inducing cementogenesis and attachment of collagen fibers.

The following actions of citric acid have been reported:

1. Accelerated healing and new cementum formation occur after surgical detachment of the gingival tissues and demineralization of the root surface by means of citric acid.[143]
2. Topically applied citric acid on periodontally diseased root surfaces has no effect on nonplaned roots, but after root planing, the acid produces a 4-mm-deep demineralized zone with exposed collagen fibers.[64]
3. Root-planed, non–acid-treated roots are left with a surface smear layer of microcrystalline debris; citric acid application not only removes the smear layer, exposing the dentinal tubules, but also makes the tubules appear wider and with funnel-shaped orifices.[134]
4. Citric acid has also been shown in vitro to eliminate endotoxins and bacteria from the diseased tooth surface.[39,51]
5. An early fibrin linkage to collagen fibers exposed by the citric acid treatment prevents the epithelium from migrating over treated roots.[135]

This technique has been extensively investigated in animals and humans. Studies in dogs have given encouraging results, especially for the treatment of furcation lesions, but the results in humans have been contradictory.[37,124,143,145,168]

The recommended technique is as follows:

1. Raise a mucoperiosteal flap.
2. Thoroughly instrument the root surface, removing calculus and underlying cementum.
3. Apply cotton pledgets soaked in a saturated solution of citric acid (pH 1), and leave on for 2 to 5 minutes.
4. Remove pledgets, and irrigate root surface profusely with water.
5. Replace the flap and suture.

The use of citric acid has also been recommended in conjunction with coverage of denuded roots using free gingival grafts (see Chapter 66).

FIBRONECTIN. Fibronectin is the glycoprotein that fibroblasts require to attach to root surfaces. The addition of fibronectin to the root surface may promote new attachment.[23,50,176] However, increasing fibronectin above plasma levels produces no obvious advantages. Adding fibronectin and citric acid to lesions treated with GTR in dogs did not improve the results.[22,166]

The effect of a fibrin-fibronectin sealing system on healing of periodontal surgical wounds, particularly in reconstructive procedures, has been investigated.[130] This material is commercially available in Europe as Tissucol. It is a biologic mediator that enhances the tissue response in the early phases of wound healing, prevents separation of the flap, and favors hemostasis and connective tissue regeneration. Clinical trials have been promising, but further research is necessary.[35]

TETRACYCLINE. In vitro treatment of the dentin surfaces with tetracycline increases binding of fibronectin, which in turn stimulates fibroblast attachment and growth while suppressing epithelial cell attachment and migration.[177] It also removes an amorphous surface layer and exposes the dentin tubules.[191] In vivo studies, however, have not shown favorable results.[191] A human study showed a trend for greater connective tissue attachment after tetracycline treatment of roots; tetracycline alone gave better results than when combined with fibronectin.[2]

Polypeptide Growth Factors. Growth factors are polypeptide molecules released by cells in the inflamed area that regulate events in wound healing. They can be considered hormones that are not released into the bloodstream but have only a local action. Growth substances regulate connective tissue cell migration and proliferation and synthesis of proteins and other components of the extracellular matrix.[98]

These factors, primarily secreted by macrophages, endothelial cells, fibroblasts, and platelets, include platelet-derived growth factor (PDGF), insulin-like growth factor (IGF), basic fibroblastic growth factor (bFGF), and transforming growth factor (TGF)-α and -β. Growth factors could be used to control events during periodontal wound healing (e.g., promoting proliferation of fibroblasts from the periodontal ligament and favoring bone formation).[187] Howell and co-workers reported that a single application in human periodontal defects of IGF-I resulted in significant improvement in bone fill above that obtained in controls, while another growth factor tested (PDGF-BB) was not effective.[82]

Enamel Matrix Proteins. Enamel matrix proteins, mainly amelogenin, are secreted by Hertwig's epithelial root sheath during tooth development and induce acellular cementum formation. Based on these observations, they are believed to favor periodontal regeneration.[72]

One enamel matrix protein derivative obtained from developing porcine teeth has been approved by the Food and Drug Administration (FDA) and marketed under the trade name *Emdogain.* The material is a viscous gel obtained by mixing 1 ml of a vehicle solution with a powder and applied with a syringe into the site.

The technique, as described by Mellonig, is as follows[110]:

1. Raise a flap for regenerative purposes (see Chapter 60).
2. Remove all granulation tissue and tissue tags, exposing the underlying bone, and remove all root deposits by hand, ultrasonic scaling, or both.
3. Completely control bleeding within the defect.
4. Demineralize the root surface with citric acid pH 1, or preferably with 24% ethylenediaminetetracetic acid (EDTA Biora) pH 6.7 for 15 seconds. This removes the smear layer and facilitates adherence of the Emdogain.
5. Rinse the wound with saline and apply the gel to fully cover the exposed root surface. Avoid contamination with blood or saliva.
6. Close the wound with sutures. Perfect abutment of the flaps is necessary; if this cannot be obtained, correct the scalloping of the gingival margin or perform a slight osteoplasty. Although placement of the dressing is optional, it may protect the wound.

Systemic antibiotic coverage for 10 to 21 days is recommended (Doxycycline, 100 mg daily).

In a histologic study of 10 defects in 8 patients, Yukna and Mellonig report evidences of regeneration (new cementum, new bone, and new periodontal ligament) in 3 specimens, new attachment (connective tissue attachment/adhesion only) in 3 specimens, and a long junctional epithelium in 4 specimens.[198] No evidence of root resorption or ankylosis was found.

Heijl et al have compared the use of enamel matrix derivatives with a placebo in 33 patients with 34 paired test and control sites, mostly one and two wall defects, followed for 3 years.[78] They found a statistically significant radiographic bone gain of 2.6 mm. Additional studies are needed to assess its potential use in various defects and possible enhancing effect in combined techniques.

Graft Materials and Procedures

Numerous therapeutic grafting modalities for restoring periodontal osseous defects have been investigated. Material to be grafted can be obtained from the same person (autografts), from a different person of the same species (allografts), or from a different species (xenografts).

Bone graft materials are generally evaluated based on their osteogenic, osteoinductive, or osteoconductive potential. *Ostegenesis* refers to the formation or development of new bone by cells contained in the graft; *osteoinduction* is a chemical process by which molecules contained in the graft (bone morphogenetic proteins or BMPs) convert the neighboring cells into osteoblasts, which in turn form bone; and *osteoconduction* is a physical effect by which the matrix of the graft forms a scaffold that favors outside cells to penetrate the graft and form new bone.

Periodontal defects as sites for transplantation differ from osseous cavities surrounded by bony walls. Saliva and bacteria may easily penetrate along the root surface, and epithelial cells may proliferate into the defect, resulting in contamination and possible exfoliation of the grafts. Therefore the principles established to govern transplantation of bone or other materials into closed osseous cavities are not fully applicable to transplantation of bone into periodontal defects.[45]

The considerations that govern the selection of a material have been defined as follows[157]:

Biologic acceptability
Predictability
Clinical feasibility
Minimal operative hazards
Minimal postoperative sequelae
Patient acceptance

It is difficult to find a material with all these characteristics, and to date there is no ideal material or technique.

Graft materials have been developed and tried in many forms. To familiarize the reader with various types of graft material, as defined by either the technique or the material used, a brief discussion of each is provided.

All grafting techniques require presurgical scaling, occlusal adjustment as needed, and exposure of the defect with a full-thickness flap. The flap technique best suited for grafting purposes is the papilla preservation flap because it provides complete coverage of the interdental area after suturing.[175] (See Chapter 60 for a description of the technique.) The use of antibiotics after the procedure is generally recommended.

Autogenous Bone Grafts

BONE FROM INTRAORAL SITES. In 1923, Hegedus attempted to use bone grafts for the reconstruction of bone defects produced by periodontal disease.[77] The method was revived by Nabers and O'Leary in 1965, and numerous efforts have been made since that time to define its indications and technique.[121]

Sources of bone include bone from healing extraction wounds, bone from edentulous ridges, bone trephined from within the jaw without damaging the roots, newly formed bone in wounds especially created for the purpose, and bone removed during osteoplasty and ostectomy.[27,71,78,80,147]

Osseous Coagulum. Robinson described a technique using a mixture of bone dust and blood that he termed *osseous coagulum.*[146] The technique uses small particles ground from cortical bone. The advantage of the particle size is that it provides additional surface area for the interaction of cellular and vascular elements.

Sources of the implant material include the lingual ridge on the mandible, exostoses, edentulous ridges, the bone distal to a terminal tooth, bone removed by osteoplasty or ostectomy, and the lingual surface of the mandible or maxilla at least 5 mm from the roots. Bone is removed with a carbide bur #6 or #8 at speeds between 5000 and 30,000 rpm, placed in a sterile dappen dish or amalgam cloth, and used to fill the defect (Fig. 63-12). The obvious advantage of this technique is the ease of obtaining bone from already exposed surgical sites, and its disadvantages are its relatively low predictability and inability to procure adequate material for large defects.[55] Although notable success has been reported by many individuals, studies documenting the efficacy of the technique are still inconclusive.[36,56,58,146]

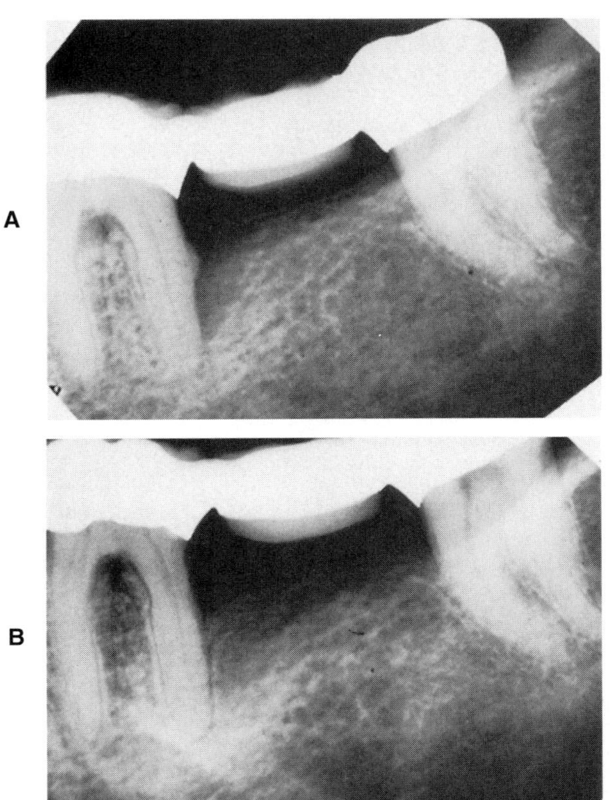

Fig. 63-12 Bone defect on the distal root of a first molar treated with osseous coagulum implants. **A,** Before treatment. **B,** One year after treatment. (Courtesy Dr. R. Earl Robinson.)

Bone Blend. Some disadvantages of osseous coagulum derive from the inability to use aspiration during accumulation of the coagulum; another problem is the unknown quantity and quality of the bone fragments in the collected material. To overcome these problems, the so-called bone blend technique has been proposed.[40]

The bone blend technique uses an autoclaved plastic capsule and pestle. Bone is removed from a predetermined site, triturated in the capsule to a workable, plastic-like mass, and packed into bony defects. Froum and co-workers have found osseous coagulum-bone blend procedures to be at least as effective as iliac autografts and open curettage.[56-58]

Intraoral Cancellous Bone Marrow Transplants. Cancellous bone can be obtained from the maxillary tuberosity, edentulous areas, and healing sockets.[80] The maxillary tuberosity frequently contains a good amount of cancellous bone, particularly if the third molars are not present; also, foci of red marrow are occasionally observed. After a ridge incision is made distally from the last molar, bone is removed with a curved and cutting rongeur. Care should be taken not to extend the incision too far distally to avoid sectioning the tendons of the palatine muscle; also, the location of the maxillary sinus has to be analyzed on the radiograph to avoid cutting into it.

Edentulous ridges can be approached with a flap, and cancellous bone and marrow are removed with curettes. Healing sockets are allowed to heal for 8 to 12 weeks, and the apical portion is used as donor material. The particles are reduced to small pieces (Figs. 61-13 and 61-14).

Bone Swaging. This technique requires the existence of an edentulous area adjacent to the defect from which the bone is pushed into contact with the root surface without fracturing the bone at its base.[48,149] Bone swaging is technically difficult, and its usefulness is limited.

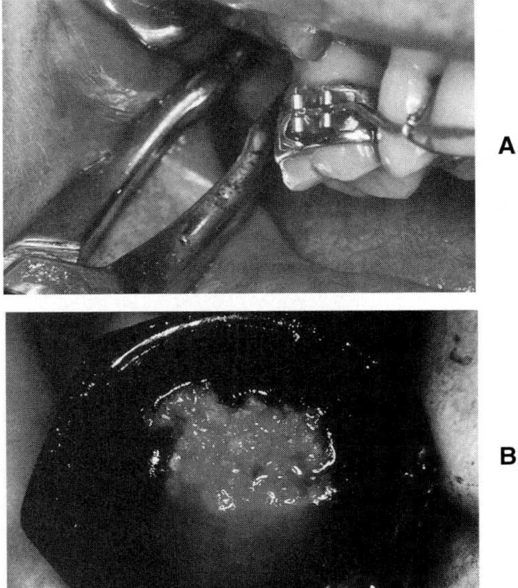

Fig. 63-13 A, Bone being removed from the maxillary tuberosity (creating a "socket") to be used as an intraoral osseous cancellous bone and marrow graft. **B,** Graft materal placed in dappen dish prior to transfer to the graft site.

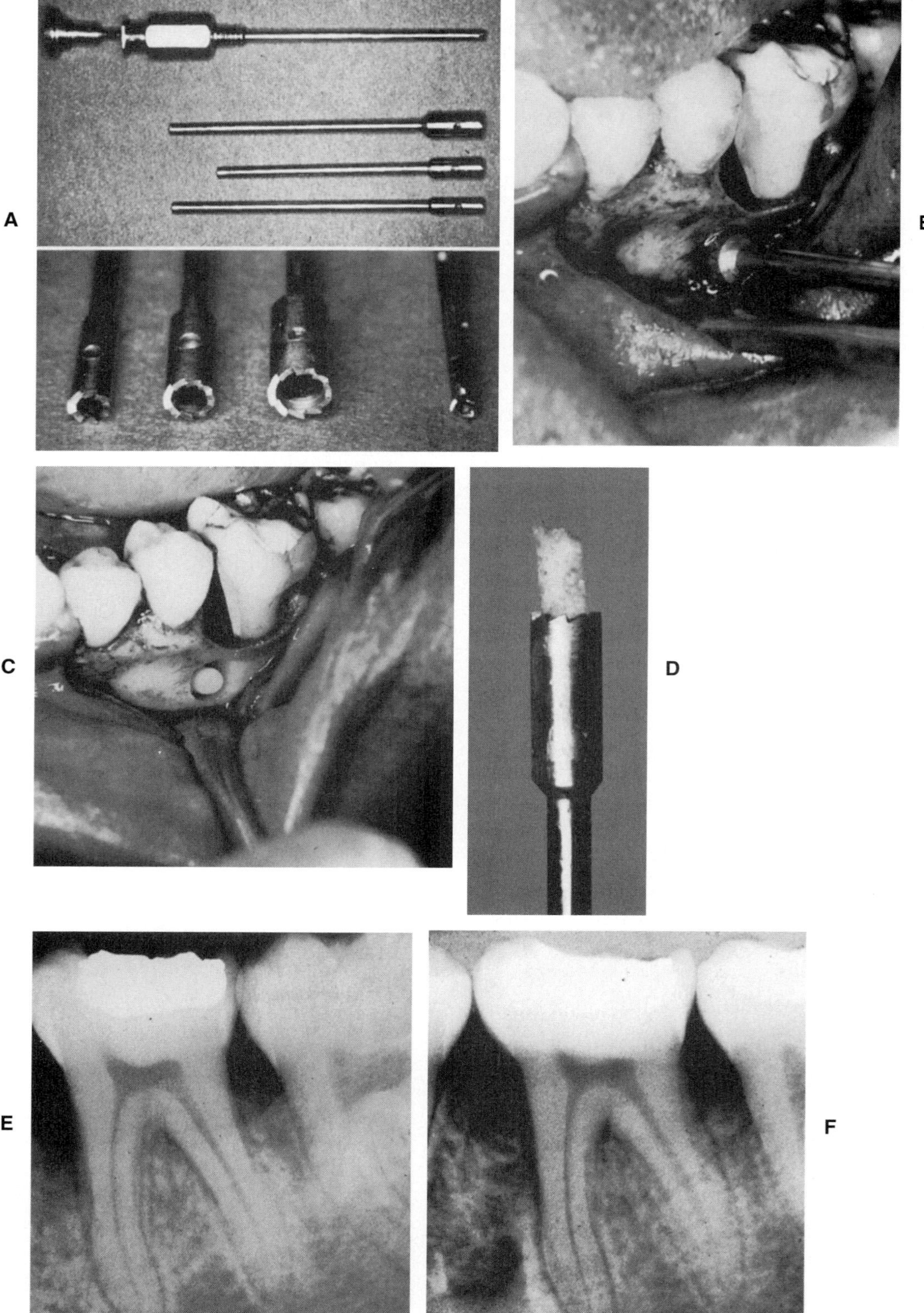

Fig. 63-14 Autogenous bone transplant obtained with trephine. **A,** Trephines: *top,* manual trephine; *center,* different sized power trephines (#2, #4, and #6); *bottom,* orifices of trephines. **B,** Mucoperiosteal flap elevated, showing osseous defect on the mesial surface of the first molar. The trephine is inserted into bone distal to the second molar. **C,** Bone separated by a trephine. **D,** Bone transplant; the cancellous portion is used and the cortical layer is removed. **E,** Radiograph showing an osseous defect on mandibular first molar. **F,** Six months after treatment, showing the osseous defect partially filled with the implant. The radiolucent area in the interdental bone is the donor site of the transplant.

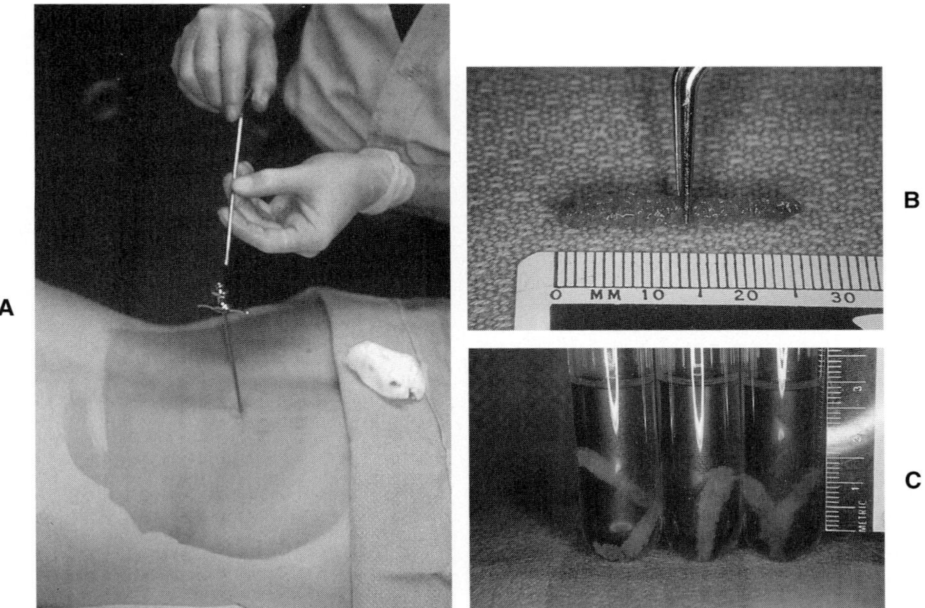

Fig. 63-15 A, Cancellous bone and marrow being procured from the posterior iliac crest with a Westerman-Jensen bone marrow biopsy needle. **B,** One of the cores obtained, approximately 3 × 25 mm in size. **C,** Five cores removed through the same $\frac{1}{4}$-inch incision site through different cortical punctures and placed in a transfer storage media prior to direct placement of frozen storage if periodontal surgery is delayed/staged.

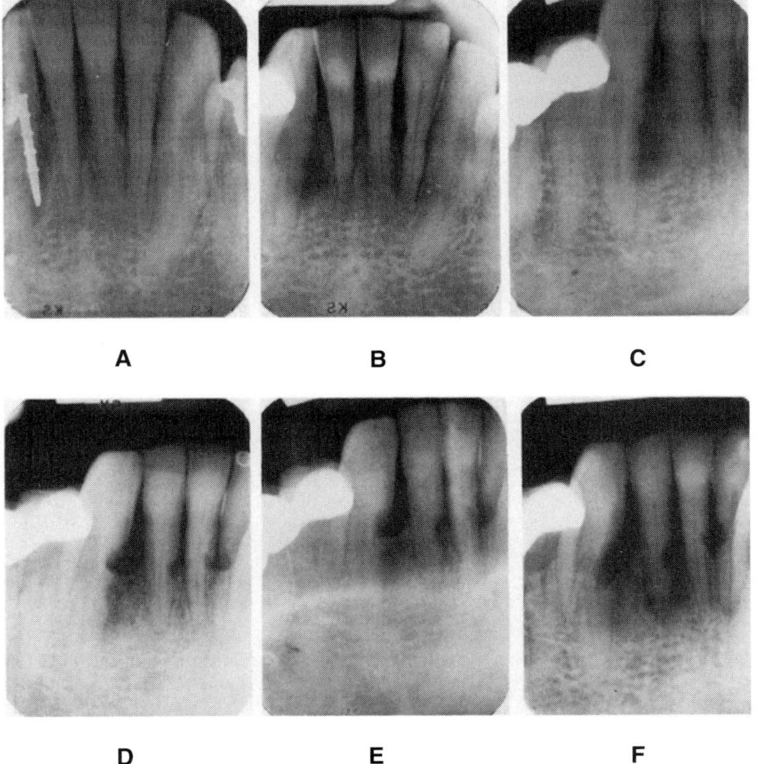

Fig. 63-16 A, November 1973. Radiograph of a patient immediately prior to the placement of a fresh iliac autograft. **B,** Two months later, bone repair is evident. Note the early radiolucent areas on the mesial aspect of the canine. **C,** After 7 months, "bone fill" is occurring, but obvious root resorption is present. **D,** April 1975. Root resorption is apparent on all grafted teeth. Note the obvious degree of fill of the original bone defects. **E,** February 1976. Further involvement. **F,** October 1977. Four years later, root resorption has progressed into the pulp of the lateral incisor, causing a periosteal-endosteal complication.

BONE FROM EXTRAORAL SITES

Iliac Autografts. The use of fresh or preserved iliac cancellous marrow bone has been extensively investigated. This material has been used by orthopedic surgeons for years. Data from human and animal studies support its use, and the technique has proved successful in bony defects with various numbers of walls, in furcations, and even supracrestally to some extent (Fig. 63-15).[11,20,38,41,42,154,155,158] However, owing to problems associated with its use, such as postoperative infection, exfoliation, sequestration; varying rates of healing; root resorption; and rapid recurrence of the defect (Fig. 63-16), in addition to increased patient expense and difficulty in procuring the donor material, the technique is no longer in use.[20,42,156,157]

Allografts. Obtaining donor material for autograft purposes necessitates inflicting surgical trauma on another part of the patient's body. Obviously, it would be to the patient's and therapist's advantage if a suitable substitute could be used for grafting purposes that would offer similar potential for repair and not require the additional surgical removal of donor material from the patient. However, both allografts and xenografts are foreign to the organism and therefore have the potential to provoke an immune response. Attempts have been made to suppress the antigenic potential of allografts and xenografts by radiation, freezing, and chemical treatment.[19]

Bone allografts are commercially available from tissue banks. They are obtained from cortical bone within 12 hours of the death of the donor, defatted, cut in pieces, washed in absolute alcohol, and deep frozen. The material may then be demineralized, and subsequently ground and sieved to a particle size of 250 to 750 mm and freeze dried. Finally, it is vacuum sealed in glass vials.

Numerous steps are also taken to eliminate viral infectivity. These include exclusion of donors from known high-risk groups and various tests on the cadaver tissues to exclude individuals with any type of infection or malignant disease. The material is then treated with chemical agents or strong acids to effectively inactivate the virus, if still present. The risk of human immunodeficiency virus (HIV) infection has been calculated as 1 in 1 million to 8 million and is therefore characterized as highly remote.[114]

UNDECALCIFIED FREEZE-DRIED BONE ALLOGRAFT (FDBA). Several clinical studies by Mellonig, Bowers, and co-workers reported bone fill exceeding 50% in 67% of the defects grafted with FDBA and in 78% of the defects grafted with FDBA plus autogenous bone.[113,150,162] FDBA, however, is considered an osteoconductive material, whereas decalcified FDBA (DFDBA) is considered an

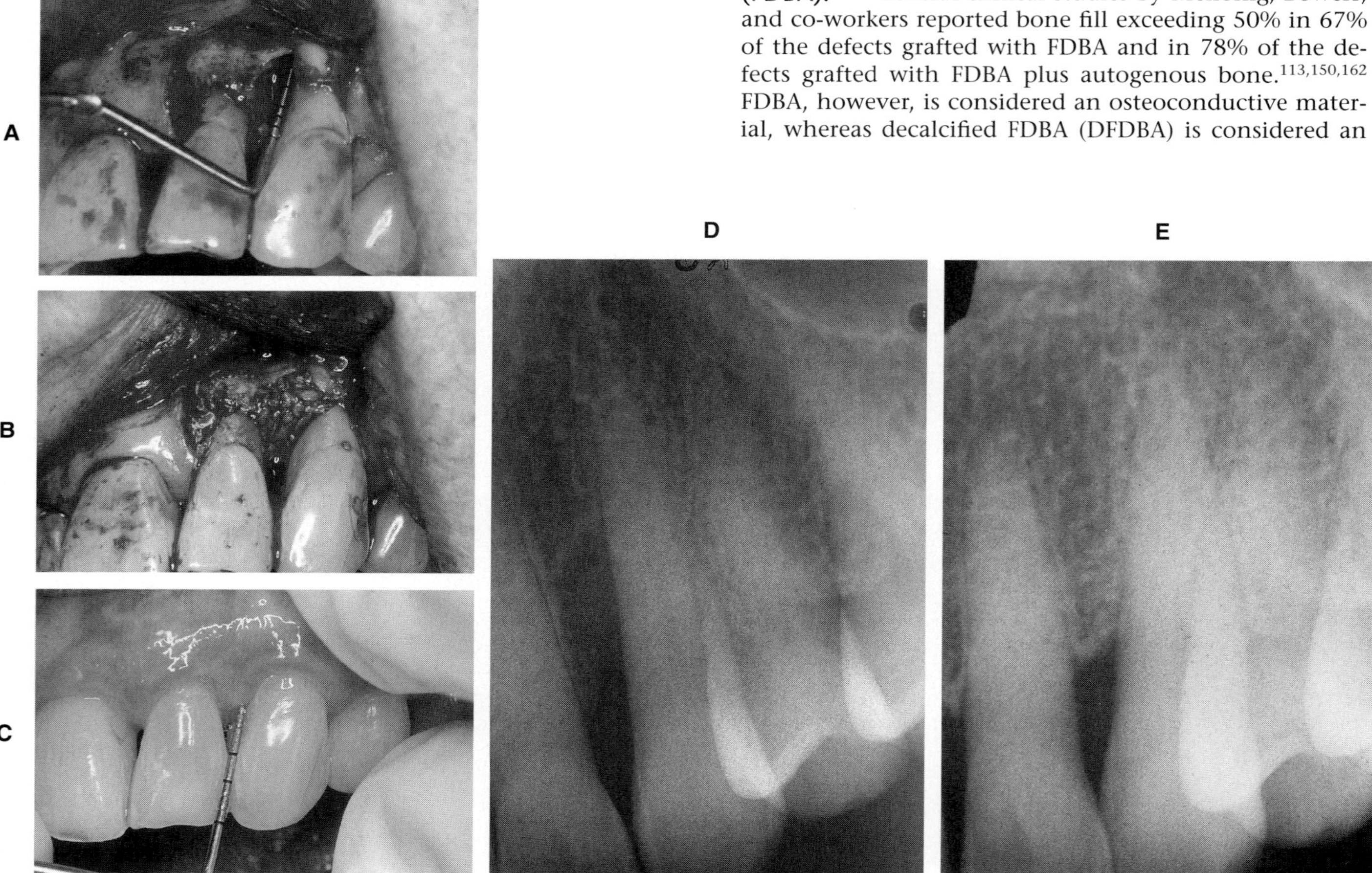

Fig. 63-17 A, Combined mesial two-wall, three-wall intrabony and facial dehiscense osseous defects on tooth #23. **B,** Demineralized freeze-dried bone allograft in place after root and site preparation is completed. **C,** Three-year posttreatment photo of site, depicting slight gingival recession and a 2-mm probing depth. **D,** Preoperative radiograph of site. **E,** Three-year postoperative radiograph suggesting bone fill and stability, which correlates with probing attachment level improvement.

osteoinductive graft. Laboratory studies have found that DFDBA has a higher osteogenic potential than FDBA and is therefore preferred.[109,111,112]

DECALCIFIED FREEZE-DRIED BONE ALLOGRAFTS. Experiments by Urist and co-workers have established the osteogenic potential of DFDBA.[183,184] Demineralization in cold, diluted hydrochloric acid exposes the components of bone matrix, closely associated with collagen fibrils, that have been termed *bone morphogenetic protein* (Figs. 63-17 and 63-18).[185]

In 1975, Libin et al reported three patients with 4 to 10 mm of bone regeneration in periodontal osseous defects.[97] Subsequent clinical studies were made with cancellous DFDBA and cortical DFDBA.[129,139] The latter resulted in more desirable results (2.4 mm versus 1.38 mm of bone fill).

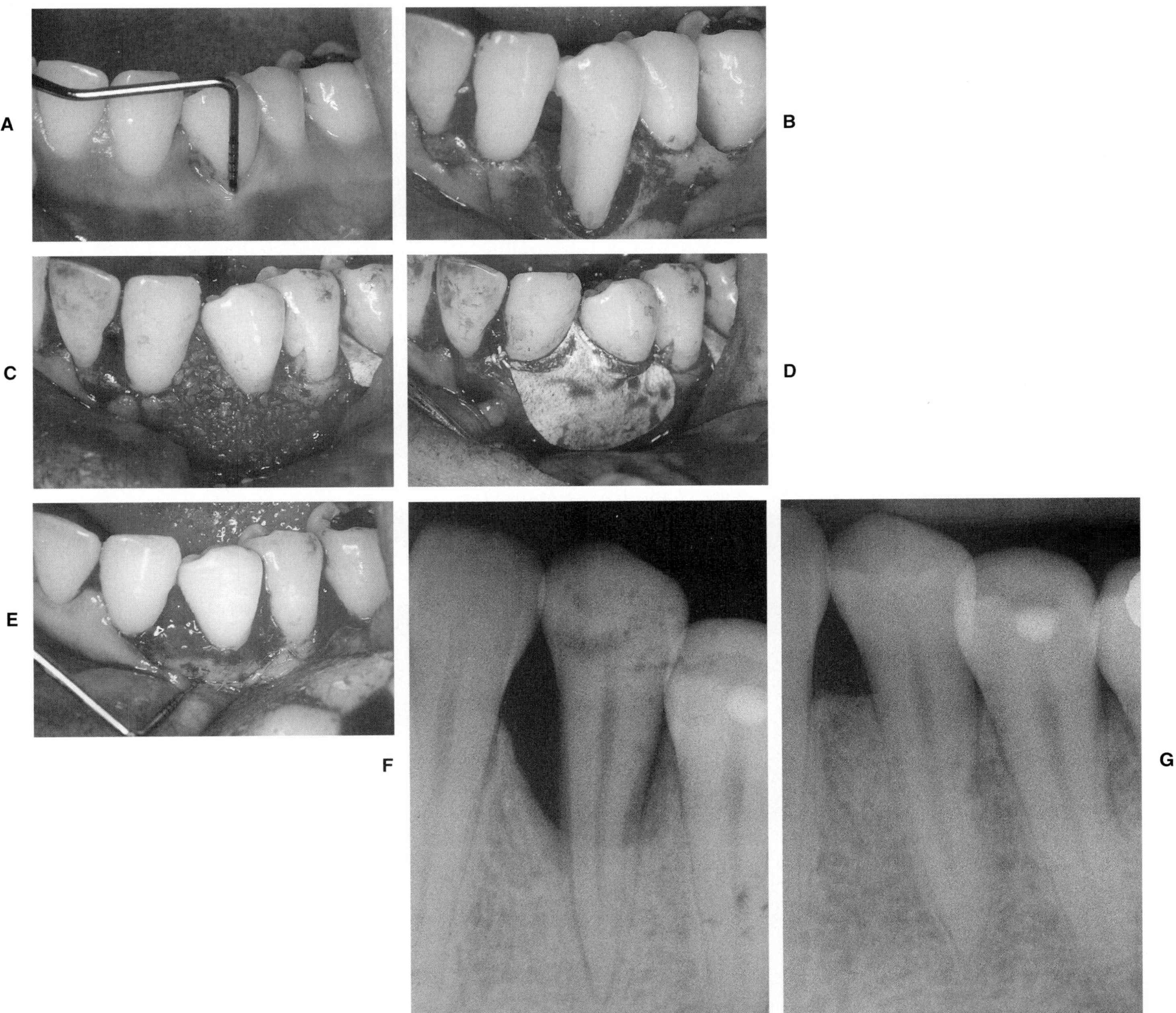

Fig. 63-18 A, Facial aspect of tooth #34 with 9-mm pocket. **B,** Mesial one-wall/hemiseptal intrabony defect and facial dehiscence osseous defect exposed and site debrided. **C,** Bone replacement graft (DFDBA) in position. **D,** Barrier membrane (ePTFE) over bone graft. **E,** Appearance of new tissue at time of membrane removal (6 weeks after surgery) suggestive of new alveolar bone slightly apical to the cementoenamel junction. **F,** Pretreatment radiograph of site. **G,** Two-year postoperative radiograph depicting favorable bone regeneration in the site.

Bowers and associates, in a histologic study in humans, showed new attachment and periodontal regeneration in defects grafted with DFDBA.[17] Mellonig and associates tested DFDBA against autogenous materials in the calvaria of guinea pigs and showed it to have similar osteogenic potential.[111,112]

These studies provided strong evidence that DFDBA in periodontal defects results in significant probing depth reduction, attachment level gain, and osseous regeneration (Color Fig. 63-2); the combination of DFDBA and guided tissue regeneration has also proven very successful.[5,170] However, limitations of the use of DFDBA include the possible, albeit remote, potential of disease transfer from the cadaver.

A bone-inductive protein isolated from the extracellular matrix of human bones, termed *osteogenin,* has been tested in human periodontal defects and seems to enhance osseous regeneration.[18]

Xenografts. *Calf bone* (Boplant), treated by detergent extraction, sterilized, and freeze dried, has been used for the treatment of osseous defects.[7,160,161] *Kiel bone* is calf or ox bone denatured with 20% hydrogen peroxide, dried with acetone, and sterilized with ethylene oxide. *Anorganic bone* is ox bone from which the organic material has been extracted by means of ethylenediamine; it is then sterilized by autoclaving.[106,107] These materials have been tried and discarded for various reasons; they are mentioned here to provide a historical perspective.

Recently, however, Yukna and co-workers have used a natural, anorganic, microporous, bovine-derived hydroxyapatite bone matrix, in combination with a cell-binding polypeptide that is a synthetic clone of the 15 amino acid sequence of type I collagen.[199] The addition of the cell binding polypeptide was shown to enhance the bone regenerative results of the matrix alone in periodontal defects.[199]

Nonbone Graft Materials. In addition to bone graft materials, many nonbone graft materials have been tried for restoration of the periodontium (Fig. 63-19). Among them are sclera, dura, cartilage, cementum, dentin, plaster of Paris, plastic materials, ceramics, and coral-derived materials.[21,47,95,96,123,152] None offers a reliable substitute to bone graft materials; some of these materials are briefly presented here to offer a complete picture of the many attempts that have been made to solve the crucial problem of periodontal regeneration.

SCLERA. Sclera was originally used in periodontal procedures because it is a dense fibrous connective tissue with poor vascularity and minimal cellularity.[87–89] This affords a low incidence of antigenicity and other untoward reactions.[83] In addition, sclera may provide a barrier to apical migration of the junctional epithelium and serve to protect the blood clot during the initial healing period.

Although some studies show that sclera is well accepted by the host and is sometimes invaded by host cells and capillaries and replaced by dense connective tissue, it does not appear to induce osteogenesis or cementogenesis.[49,119,127,182] The available scientific research does not warrant the routine use of sclera in periodontal therapy.

CARTILAGE. Cartilage has been used for repair studies in monkeys and treatment of periodontal defects in humans.[151,153] It can serve as a scaffolding; when so used, new attachment was obtained in 60 of 70 case studies.[153] However, cartilage has received only limited evaluation.

PLASTER OF PARIS. Plaster of Paris (calcium sulfate) is biocompatible and porous, thereby allowing fluid

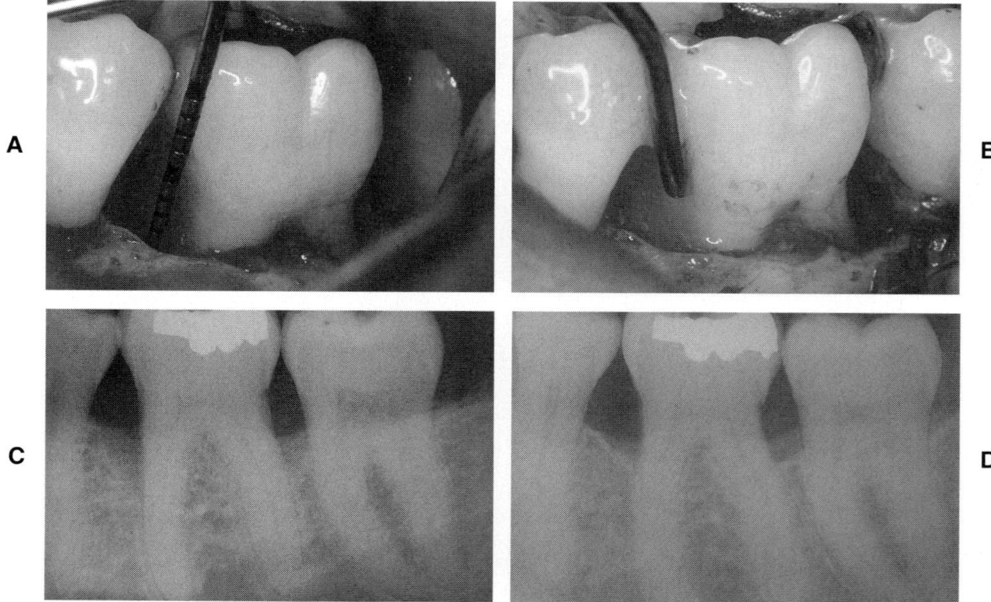

Fig. 63-19 **A,** Surgical exposure of the lower first molar, depicting a deep intrabony defect on the mesial and distal. **B,** Enamel matrix protein placement in site after root preparation. **C,** Preoperative radiograph. **D,** Two-year postoperative radiograph suggesting bone fill.

exchange, which prevents flap necrosis. Plaster of Paris resorbs completely in 1 to 2 weeks. One study in surgically created three-wall defects in dogs showed significant regeneration of bone and cementum.[86] It was found to be useful in one uncontrolled clinical study, but other investigators have reported that it does not induce bone formation.[1,163] One report suggested its use in combination with DFDBA and a Gore-Tex membrane.[167] Its usefulness in human cases, however, has not been proven.

PLASTIC MATERIALS. HTR polymer is a nonresorbable, microporous, biocompatible composite of polymethylmethacrylate and polyhydroxylethylmethacrylate.[195] A clinical 6-month study showed significant defect fill and improved attachment level.[195] Histologically, this material is encapsulated by connective tissue fibers, with no evidence of new attachment.[173]

CALCIUM PHOSPHATE BIOMATERIALS. Several calcium phosphate biomaterials have been tested since the mid-1970s and are currently available for clinical use. Calcium phosphate biomaterials have excellent tissue compatibility and do not elicit any inflammation or foreign body response. These materials are *osteoconductive,* not osteoinductive, meaning that they will induce bone formation when placed next to viable bone but not when surrounded by non–bone-forming tissue such as skin.

Two types of calcium phosphate ceramics have been used:

1. Hydroxyapatite (HA) has a calcium-to-phosphate ratio of 1.67, similar to that found in bone material. HA is generally nonbioresorbable.
2. Tricalcium phosphate (TCP), with a calcium-to-phosphate ratio of 1.5, is mineralogically B-whitlockite. TCP is at least partially bioresorbable.

Case reports and uncontrolled human studies have shown that calcium phosphate bioceramic materials are perfectly tolerated and can result in clinical repair of periodontal lesions. Several controlled studies were conducted on the use of Periograf and Calcitite; clinical results were good, but histologically these materials appeared to be encapsulated by collagen.[59,105,140,197]

BIOACTIVE GLASS. Bioactive glass consists of sodium and calcium salts, phosphates, and silicon dioxide; for its dental applications it is used in the form of irregular particles measuring 90 to 170 μm (PerioGlas, Block Drug Co., Jersey City, NJ) or 300 to 355 μm (BioGran, Ortho Vita, Malvern, PA). When this material comes into contact with tissue fluids, the surface of the particles becomes coated with hydroxycarbonateapatite, incorporates organic ground proteins such as chondroitin sulfate and glycosaminoglycans, and attracts osteoblasts that rapidly form bone.[6]

This material may have potential, and clinical studies are needed to establish its real usefulness.

CORAL-DERIVED MATERIALS. Two different coralline materials have been used in clinical periodontics: natural coral and coral-derived porous hydroxyapatite. Both are biocompatible, but whereas natural coral is resorbed slowly (several months), porous hydroxyapatite is not resorbed or takes years to do so.

Clinical studies on these materials showed pocket reduction, attachment gain, and bone level gain.[81,84,85] The materials have also been studied in conjunction with membranes, with good results.[92,172] Both materials have demonstrated microscopic cementum and bone formation, but their slow resorbability or lack thereof has hindered clinical success in practice.[26,169]

Combined Techniques

The combination of barrier techniques with bone grafts and other methods has been suggested and procedures following these ideas proposed by several authors.[5,73,92,104,108,188] The following technique has been described by Schallhorn and McClain[103,159]:

1. Perform a regenerative type flap. If recession has occurred and/or coronal flap positioning is required for membrane coverage, periosteal separation is performed.
2. The defect is debrided of all granulation tissue and the root surface is planed to remove all remnants of plaque, accretions and other root surface alterations (grooves, notches, caries) employing ultrasonic/sonic, hand, and/or rotary instrumentation.
3. Odontoplasty and/or osteoplasty are performed if required for adequate access to the defect including intraradicular or furcation fundus concavities and/or reduction of enamel projections.
4. The bone graft (typically DFDBA) is prepared in a dappen dish, hydrating it with sterile saline or local anesthetic solution, and if there is no contraindication, is combined with tetracycline (125 mg/0.25 g of DFDBA). After mixing, the dappen dish is covered with a sterile, moistened gauze to prevent drying of the graft.
5. The appropriate membrane (usually ePTFE) is selected and trimmed to fit the desired position and placed on a sterile gauze. Care is taken to prevent contamination by contact with soft tissues or saliva.
6. The area is thoroughly cleansed and isolated, and the regenerative site root surface is treated with cotton pellets soaked in citric acid pH 1 for 3 minutes, taking care that the solution does not go beyond the root and bone surface. The pellets are removed and the site inspected for any residual cotton fibers prior to flushing the site with sterile water or saline.
7. If a sclerotic bone surface exists in the graft site, intramarrow penetration is performed with a $\frac{1}{4}$ round bur.
8. The ligament surface is "scraped" with a periodontal probe to remove any eschar and stimulate bleeding.
9. The DFDBA is packed firmly in the defect using an overfill approach, covering the root trunk and combination or confluent vertical dehiscence or horizontal osseous defects.
10. The custom-fitted membrane is placed over the graft and secured as appropriate.
11. The area is rechecked to ensure that adequate graft material remains in the desired area, and the flap is positioned to cover the membrane and secured with nonabsorbable sutures.
12. A periodontal dressing is passively applied over the surgical area, with Surgicel covering the sutures.

Typical peri- and postoperative medication regimens include, if not contraindicated, 7 to 10 days of antibiotic coverage, which is subsequently extended with doxycycline, 100 mg daily for 2 to 7 weeks; steroid therapy such as methylprednisolone dosepak; and analgesic agents.

Sutures are removed if and when they become loose or no longer aid in tissue position or wound closure. The patient is seen for monitoring and local debridement as needed every 1 to 2 weeks. If a nonresorbable membrane has been used, it is removed 6 to 8 weeks after the operation.

Several studies and case reports have shown excellent results with the combined technique.[5,16,18,92,103,108,159,188]

FACTORS INFLUENCING A SUCCESSFUL OUTCOME

Factors adversely affecting outcomes were assessed in the 1996 evidence-based World Workshop in Periodontics.[63,139] These included the following:

- Inadequate plaque control
- Poor compliance with supportive periodontal therapy
- Smoking
- Other factors such as flap design, defect and root morphology, material employed, flap position, and postoperative management

Other factors possibly influencing outcomes but which lack conclusive evidence at this time include: age, systemic conditions, and use of membranes in patients requiring prophylactic medication.

Other reports have also attempted to delineate variables for case/site selection and management.[3,4] These included: therapist considerations (training and experience), patient factors (systemic conditions, stress level, smoking habits, plaque control, patient compliance, tissue response to presurgical therapy, and age), defect factors (bone height, access, tooth/defect anatomy, space maintenance of membranes employed, and tooth stability), surgical considerations (flap design/management, root preparation and possible biomodification, regenerative materials employed, infection control, etc.), postsurgical management, and supportive periodontal therapy after completion of active therapy.

SUMMARY

The subject of new attachment has received a great deal of attention because of its obvious importance in improving the results of therapy. On the basis of available information, reconstruction of human supporting periodontal tissues is possible in selected sites and patients with the use of autogenous bone grafts and/or freeze dried bone allografts and resorbable or nonresorbable barrier membranes.

The clinician should make an effort to differentiate between those techniques that have been studied in depth and with acceptable results and others that, although promising, are still experimental. Research papers must be critically evaluated for adequacy of controls, selection of cases, methods of evaluation, and long-range postoperative results.

REFERENCES

1. Alderman NE: Sterile plaster of Paris as an implant in the infrabony environment: A preliminary study. J Periodontol 1969; 40:11.
2. Alger FA, Solt CW, Vuddahanok S, et al: The histologic evaluation of new attachment in periodontally diseased human roots treated with tetracycline-hydrochloride and fibronectin. J Periodontol 1990; 61:447.
3. American Academy of Periodontology: Glossary of Periodontal Terms, ed 3. Chicago, American Academy of Periodontology, 1992.
4. American Dental Association, Council on Scientific Affairs: Products designed to regenerate periodontal tissues: Acceptance Program Guidelines. The American Dental Association, July 1997, pp. 1–7.
5. Andereeg CR, Martin SJ, Gray JL, et al: Clinical evaluation of the use of decalcified freeze-dried bone allograft with guided tissue regeneration in the treatment of molar furcation invasions. J Periodontol 1991; 62:264.
6. Andereeg CR, Alexander DC, Freidman M: A bioactive glass particulate in the treatment of molar furcations. J Periodontol 1999; 70:384.
7. Arrocha R, Wittwer J, Gargiulo A: Tissue response to heterogenous bone implantation in dogs. J Periodontol 1968; 39:162.
8. Becker W, Becker BE, Berg L, et al: Clinical and volumetric analysis of three-wall intrabony defects following open flap debridement. J Periodontol 1986; 57:277.
9. Becker W, Becker BE, Berg L, et al: New attachment after treatment with root isolation procedures: Report for treated class III and class II furcations and vertical osseous defects. Int J Periodont Restor Dent 1988; 8(3):9.
10. Becker W, Becker BE, Prichard JF, et al: Root isolation for new attachment procedures—A surgical and suturing method: Three case reports. J Periodontol 1987; 58:819.
11. Bierly JA, Sottosanti JS, Costley JM, et al: An evaluation of the osteogenic potential of marrow. J Periodontol 1975; 46:277.
12. Bjorn H: Experimental studies on reattachment. Dent Pract 1961; 11:351.
13. Bjorn H, Hollender L, Lindhe J: Tissue regeneration in patients with periodontal disease. Odont Rev 1965; 16:317.
14. Blumenthal NM: The use of collagen materials in bone grafted defects to enhance guided tissue regeneration. Periodont Case Rep 1987; 9:16.
15. Blumenthal NM: The use of collagen membranes to guide regeneration of new connective tissue attachment in dogs. J Periodontol 1988; 59:830.
16. Blumenthal NM, Steinberg J: The use of collagen membrane barriers in conjunction with combined demineralized bone-collagen gel implants in human infrabony defects. J Periodontol 1990; 61:319.
17. Bowers GM, Chadroff B, Carnevale R, et al: Histologic evaluation of new attachment apparatus formation in humans. Part III. J Periodontol 1989; 60:683.
18. Bowers G, Felton F, Middleton F, et al: Histologic comparison of regeneration in human intrabony pockets when osteogenin is combined with demineralized freeze-dried bone allograft and with purified bovine collagen. J Periodontol 1991; 62:690.
19. Buring K, Urist MR: Effects of ionizing radiation on the bone induction principle in the matrix of bone implants. Clin Orthop 1967; 55:225.
20. Burnette WE: Fate of the iliac crest graft. J Periodontol 1972; 43:88.
21. Busschopp J, De Boever J: Clinical and histological characteristics of lyophilized allogenic dura mater in periodontal bony defects in humans. J Clin Periodontol 1983; 10:399.

22. Caffesse RG, Nasjleti CE, Anderson GB, et al: Periodontal healing following guided tissue regeneration with citric acid and fibronectin application. J Periodontol 1991; 62:21.
23. Caffesse RG, Smith BA, Nasjleti CE, et al: Cell proliferation after flap surgery, root conditioning and fibronectin application. J Periodontol 1987; 58:661.
24. Card SJ, Caffesse RG, Smith BA, et al: New attachment following the use of a resorbable membrane in the treatment of periodontitis in dogs. Int J Periodont Restor Dent 1989; 9:59.
25. Carranza FA Sr: A technic for reattachment. J Periodontol 1954; 25:272.
26. Carranza FA Jr, Kenney EB, Lekovic V, et al: Histologic study of healing of human periodontal defects after placement of porous hydroxyapatite implants. J Periodontol 1987; 58:682.
27. Carraro JJ, Sznajder N, Alonso CA: Intraoral cancellous bone autografts in treatment of infrabony pockets. J Clin Periodontol 1976; 3:104.
28. Caton JC: Overview of clinical trials on periodontal regeneration. Ann Periodontol 1887; 2:215.
29. Caton JG, DeFuria EL, Polson AM, et al: Periodontal regeneration via selective cell repopulation. J Periodontol 1987; 58:546.
30. Caton J, Wagener C, Polson A, et al: Guided tissue regeneration in interproximal defects in monkeys. Int J Periodont Restor Dent 1992; 12:267.
31. Caton J, Zander H: Osseous repair of an infrabony pocket without new attachment of connective tissue. J Clin Periodontol 1976; 3:54.
32. Chung KM, Salkin LM, Stein MD, et al: Clinical evaluation of a biodegradable collagen membrane in guided tissue regeneration. J Periodontol 1990; 61:732.
33. Claffey N, Hahn R, Egelberg J: Effect of placement of occlusive membranes on root resorption and bone regeneration during healing of circumferential periodontal defects in dogs. J Clin Periodontol 1989; 16:371.
34. Cortellini P, Pini Prato G, Tonetti M: Periodontal regeneration of human infrabony defects with bioresorbable membranes: a controlled clinical study. J Periodontol 1996; 67:217.
35. Cortellini P, Tonetti M, Pini Prato GP: Guided tissue regeneration in infrabony defects with and without a fibrin-fibronectin system: One year reentry procedure and x-ray evaluation (Abstract). J Periodontol 1991; 62:800.
36. Coverly L, Toto P, Gargiulo A: Osseous coagulum: A histologic evaluation. J Periodontol 1975; 46:596.
37. Crigger M, Bogle G, Nilveus R, et al: Effect of topical citric acid application in the healing of experimental furcation defects in dogs. J Periodont Res 1978; 13:538.
38. Cushing M: Autogenous red marrow grafts: Potential for induction of osteogenesis. J Periodontol 1969; 40:492.
39. Daly CG: Antibacterial effect of citric acid treatment of periodontally diseased root surface "in vitro." J Clin Periodontol 1982; 9:386.
40. Diem CR, Bowers GM, Moffitt WC: Bone blending: A technique for osseous implants. J Periodontol 1972; 43:295.
41. Dragoo MR, Irwin RK: A method of procuring cancellous iliac bone utilizing a trephine needle. J Periodontol 1972; 43:82.
42. Dragoo MR, Sullivan HC: A clinical and histologic evaluation of autogenous iliac bone grafts in humans. Part II. External root resorption. J Periodontol 1973; 44:614.
43. Eickholz P, Hausmann E: Evidence for healing of class II and III furcations after GTR therapy: Digital subtraction and clinical measurements. J Periodontol 1997; 68:636.
44. Eickholz P, Hausmann E: Evidence for healing of interproximal intrabony defects after conventional and regenerative therapy: Digital radiography and clinical measurements. J Periodont Res 1998; 33:156.
45. Ellegaard B: Bone grafts in periodontal attachment procedures. J Clin Periodontol 1976; 3:5.
46. Ellegaard B, Karring T, Löe H: Retardation of epithelial migration in new attachment attempts in intrabony defects in monkeys. J Clin Periodontol 1976; 3:23.
47. Ellegaard B, Nielsen IM, Karring T: Lyodura grafts in new attachment procedures. J Dent Res 1976; 55(special issue B):B-304.
48. Ewen SJ: Bone swaging. J Periodontol 1965; 36:57.
49. Feingold JP, Chasens AI, Doyle J, et al: Preserved scleral allografts on periodontal defects in man. II. Histologic evaluation. J Periodontol 1977; 48:4.
50. Fernyhough W, Page RC: Attachment, growth and synthesis of human gingival fibroblasts on demineralized or fibronectin-treated normal and diseased tooth roots. J Periodontol 1983; 54:133.
51. Fine DH, Morris ML, Tabak L, et al: Preliminary characterization of material eluted from the roots of periodontally diseased teeth. J Periodont Res 1980; 15:10.
52. Flanary DB, Twohey SM, Gray JL, et al: The use of a synthetic skin substitute as a physical barrier to enhance healing in human periodontal furcation defects; A follow-up report. J Periodontol 1991; 62:684.
53. Fleisher N, Waal H, Bloom A: Regeneration of lost attachment apparatus in the dog using Vicryl absorbable mesh (Polyglactin 910). Int J Periodont Restor Dent 1988; 8(2):45.
54. Fowler C, Garrett S, Crigger M, et al: Histologic probe position in treated and untreated human periodontal tissues. J Clin Periodontol 1982; 9:373.
55. Freeman E, Turnbull RS: The value of osseous coagulum as a graft material. J Periodont Res 1973; 8:299.
56. Froum SJ: Comparison of different autograft material for obtaining bone fill in human periodontal defects. J Periodontol 1974; 45:240.
57. Froum SJ, Thaler R, Scoop IW, et al: Osseous autografts. I. Clinical responses to bone blend or hip marrow grafts. J Periodontol 1975; 46:515.
58. Froum SJ, Thaler R, Scoop IW, et al: Osseous autografts. II. Histologic responses to osseous coagulum-bone blend grafts. J Periodontol 1975; 46:656.
59. Froum SJ, Kushner L, Scoop IW, et al: Human clinical and histologic responses to Durapatite implants in intraosseous lesions. J Periodontol 1982; 53:719.
60. Gager AH, Schultz AJ: Treatment of periodontal defects with an absorbable membrane (polyglactin 910) with and without osseous grafting: Case reports. J Periodontol 1991; 62:276.
61. Gantes BG, Garrett S: Coronally displaced flaps in reconstructive periodontal therapy. Reconstruct Periodontics 1991; 35(3):495.
62. Garrett S: Early wound healing stability and its importance in periodontal regeneration. In: Polson AM (ed): Periodontal Regeneration: Current Status and Directions. Chicago, Quintessence, 1994.
63. Garrett S: Periodontal regeneration around natural teeth. In: Proceedings of the 1996 World Workshop in Periodontology. Ann Periodontol 1996; 7:621.
64. Garrett S, Crigger M, Egelberg J: Effects of citric acid on diseased root surfaces. J Periodont Res 1978; 13:155.
65. Glickman I: Clinical Periodontology, ed 1. Philadelphia, Saunders, 1953.
66. Goldman H: A rationale for the treatment of the intrabony pocket. One method of treatment-subgingival curettage. J Periodontol 1948; 20:83.
67. Gottlow J: Guided tissue regeneration using bioresorbable and non-resorbable devices: Initial healing and long-term results. J Periodontol 1993; 64:1157.
68. Gottlow J, Nyman S, Lindhe J, et al: New attachment formation as a result of controlled tissue regeneration. J Clin Periodontol 1984; 11:494.

69. Gottlow J, Nyman S, Lindhe J, et al: New attachment formation in human periodontium by guided tissue regeneration. J Clin Periodontol 1986; 13:604.
70. Greenberg J, Laster L, Listgarten MA: Transgingival probing as a potential estimation of alveolar bone level. J Periodontol 1976; 47:514.
71. Halliday DG: The grafting of newly formed autogenous bone in the treatment of osseous defects. J Periodontol 1969; 40:511.
72. Hammarstrom L: Enamel matrix, cementum development and regeneration. J Clin Periodontol 1997; 4:658.
73. Hancock EB: Regenerative procedures. In: Proceedings of the World Workshop in Clinical Periodontics. Chicago, American Academy of Periodontology, 1989.
74. Haney JM, Nilvéus RE, McMillan PJ, et al: Periodontal repair in dogs: expanded polytetrafluoroethylene barrier membranes support wound stabilization and enhance bone regeneration. J Periodontol 1993; 64:883.
75. Hardwick R, Hayes BK, Flynn C: Devices for dentoalveolar regeneration: An up-to-date literature review. J Periodontol 1995; 55:495.
76. Hecker F: Pyorrhea Alveolaris. St Louis, Mosby, 1913.
77. Hegedus Z: The rebuilding of the alveolar process by bone transplantation. Dent Cosmos 1923; 65:736.
78. Heijl L, Heden G, Svardstrom G, et al: Enamel matrix derivative in the treatment of intrabony periodontal defects. J Clin Periodontol 1997; 24:705.
79. Hiatt WH: Periodontal pocket elimination by combined endodontic-periodontic therapy. J Periodontol 1963; 1:153.
80. Hiatt WH, Schallhorn RG: Intraoral transplants of cancellous bone and marrow in periodontal lesions. J Periodontol 1973; 44:194.
81. Hippolyte MP, Fabre D, Peyrol S: Corail et regeneration tissulaire guidée. Aspects histologiques. J Parodontologie 1991; 10:279.
82. Howell TH, Fiorellini JP, Paquette DW, et al: A Phase I/II clinical trial to evaluate a combination of recombinant human platelet-derived growth factor-BB and recombinant human insulin-like growth factor-I in patients with periodontal disease. J Periodontol 1997; 68:1186.
83. Johnson W, Parkhill EM, Grindlay JH: Transplantation of homografts of sclera: Experimental study. Am J Ophthalmol 1962; 54:1019.
84. Kenney EB, Lekovic V, Han T, et al: The use of a porous hydroxylapatite implant in periodontal defects. I. Clinical results after six months. J Periodontol 1985; 56:82.
85. Kenney EB, Lekovic V, Elbaz J-J, et al: The use of a porous hydroxylapatite implant in periodontal defects. II. Treatment of class II furcation lesions in lower molars. J Periodontol 1988; 59:67.
86. Kim CK, Kim HY, Chai JK, et al: Effect of a calcium sulfate implant with calcium sulfate barrier on periodontal healing in 3-wall intrabony defects in dogs. J Periodontol 1998; 69:982.
87. Klingsberg J: Preserved sclera in periodontal surgery. J Periodontol 1972; 43:634.
88. Klingsberg J: Scleral allografts in the repair of periodontal osseous defects. NY State Dent J 1972; 38:418.
89. Klingsberg J: Periodontal scleral grafts and combined grafts of sclera and bone: Two year appraisal. J Periodontol 1974; 45:262.
90. Kwan SK, Lekovic V, Camargo PM, et al: The use of autogenous periosteal grafts as barriers for the treatment of intrabony defects in humans. J Periodontol 1998; 69:1203.
91. Lang NP, Hill RW: Radiographs in periodontics. J Clin Periodontol 1976; 4:16.
92. Lekovic V, Kenney EB, Carranza FA Jr, et al: Treatment of class II furcation defects using porous hydroxyapatite in conjunction with a polytetrafluoroethylene membrane. J Periodontol 1990; 61:575.
93. Lekovic V, Kenney EB, Carranza FA Jr, et al: The use of autogenous periosteal grafts as barriers for the treatment of grade II furcation involvements in lower molars. J Periodontol 1991; 62:775.
94. Lekovic V, Kenney EB, Kovacevic K, et al: Evaluation of guided tissue regeneration in class II furcation defects. A clinical study. J Periodontol 1989; 60:694.
95. Levin MP, Getter L, Cutright DE: A comparison of iliac marrow and biodegradable ceramic in periodontal defects. J Biomed Mater Res 1975; 9:183.
96. Levin MP, Getter L, Adrian J, et al: Healing of periodontal defects with ceramic implants. J Clin Periodontol 1974; 1:197.
97. Libin BM, Ward HL, Fishman LL: Decalcified lyophilized bone allografts for use in human periodontal defects. J Periodontol 1975; 46:51.
98. Lynch SE: The role of growth factors in periodontal repair and regeneration. In: Polson AM (ed): Periodontal Repair and Regeneration. Current Status and Directions. Chicago, Quintessence, 1994.
99. Machtei EE: Outcome variables for the study of periodontal regeneration. Ann Periodontol 1997; 2:229.
100. Magnusson I, Batich C, Collins BR: New attachment formation following controlled tissue regeneration using biodegradable membranes. J Periodontol 1988; 59:1.
101. Magnusson I, Stenberg WV, Batich C, et al: Connective tissue repair in circumferential periodontal defects in dogs following use of a biodegradable membrane. J Clin Periodontol 1990; 17:243.
102. Martin M, Gantes B, Garrett S, et al: Treatment of periodontal furcation defects. (I) Review of the literature and description of a regenerative surgical technique. J Clin Periodontol 1988; 15:227.
103. McClain PK, Schallhorn RG: Long-term assessment of combined osseous composite grafting, root conditioning and guided tissue regeneration. Int J Periodont Restor Dent 1993; 13:9.
104. McClain PK, Schallhorn RG: The use of combined periodontal regenerative techniques (Guest Editorial). J Periodontol 1999; 70:102.
105. Meffert RM, Thomas JR, Hamilton KM, et al: Hydroxylapatite as an alloplastic graft in the treatment of human periodontal osseous defects. J Periodontol 1985; 56:63.
106. Melcher AH: The use of heterogenous anorganic bone in periodontal bone grafting: A preliminary report. I. Dent Assoc South Afr 1958; 13:80.
107. Melcher AH: The use of heterogenous anorganic bone as an implant material in oral procedures. Oral Surg 1962; 15:996.
108. Mellado JR, Salkin LM, Freedman AL, et al: A comparative study of ePTFE membranes with and without decalcified freeze-dried bone allografts for the regeneration of interproximal intraosseous defects. J Periodontol 1995; 66:751.
109. Mellonig JT: Freeze-dried bone allografts in periodontal reconstructive surgery. Dent Clin North Am 1991; 35:505.
110. Mellonig JT: Enamel matrix derivative for periodontal reconstructive surgery: Technique and clinical and histologic case report. Int J Periodont Restor Dent 1999; 19:9.
111. Mellonig JT, Bowers GM, Bailey RC: Comparison of bone graft materials. Part I: New bone formation with autografts and allografts determined by strontium-85. J Periodontol 1981; 52:291.
112. Mellonig JT, Bowers GM, Bailey RC: Comparison of bone graft materials. Part II: New bone formation with autografts and allografts: A histological evaluation. J Periodontol 1981; 52:297.

113. Mellonig JT, Bowers GM, Bright RW, et al: Clinical evaluation of freeze-dried bone allografts in periodontal osseous defects. J Periodontol 1976; 47:125.
114. Mellonig JT, Prewett AB, Moyer MP: HIV inactivation in a bone allograft. J Periodontol 1992; 63:979.
115. Metzler DG, Seamoons BC, Mellonig JT, et al: Clinical evaluation of guided tissue regeneration in the treatment of maxillary class II molar furcation invasions. J Periodontol 1991; 62:353.
116. Minabe M: A critical review of the biologic rationale for guided tissue regeneration. J Periodontol 1991; 62:171.
117. Moriarty JD, Hutchens LH, Scheitler LE: Histological evaluation of periodontal probe penetration in untreated facial molar furcations. J Periodontol 1989; 16:21.
118. Morris ML: Reattachment of periodontal tissue. A critical study. Oral Surg 1949; 2:1194.
119. Moskow BS, Gold SI, Gottsegen R: Effects of scleral collagen upon the healing of experimental osseous wounds. J Periodontol 1976; 47:596.
120. Moskow BS, Tannenbaum P: Enhanced repair and regeneration of periodontal lesions in tetracycline-treated patients. Case reports. J Periodontol 1991; 62:341.
121. Nabers CL, O'Leary TJ: Autogenous bone transplants in the treatment of osseous defects. J Periodontol 1965; 36:5.
122. Nabers JM, Meador HL, Nabers CL, et al: Chronology, an important factor in the repair of osseous defects. Periodontics 1964; 2:304.
123. Nery EB, Lynch KL: Preliminary clinical studies of bioceramic in periodontal osseous defects. J Periodontol 1978; 49:523.
124. Nilveus R, Bogle G, Crigger M, et al: Effect of topical citric acid application in the healing of experimental furcation defects in dogs. 2. Healing after repeated surgery. J Periodont Res 1980; 15:544.
125. Nyman S, Gottlow J, Karring T, et al: The regenerative potential of the periodontal ligament. An experimental study in the monkey. J Clin Periodontol 1982; 9:257.
126. Nyman S, Lindhe J, Karring T, et al: New attachment following surgical treatment of human periodontal disease. J Clin Periodontol 1982; 9:290.
127. Passell MS, Bissada NF: Histomorphologic evaluation of scleral grafts in experimental bony defects. J Periodontol 1975; 46:629.
128. Patur B, Glickman I: Clinical and roentgenographic evaluation of the post-treatment healing of infrabony pockets. J Periodontol 1962; 33:164.
129. Pearson GE, Rosen S, Deporter DA: Preliminary observations on the usefulness of a decalcified freeze-dried cancellous bone allograft material in periodontal surgery. J Periodontol 1981; 52:55.
130. Pini Prato G, Clauser C, Cortellini P: Augmentation of periodontal regeneration response using biologic mediators. In: Polson A: Periodontal Regeneration. Current Status and Directions. Chicago, Quintessence, 1994.
131. Pitaru S, Tal H, Soldinger M, et al: Collagen membranes prevent the apical migration of epithelium during periodontal wound healing. J Periodont Res 1987; 22:331.
132. Pitaru S, Tal H, Soldinger M, et al: Partial regeneration of periodontal tissues using collagen barriers. Initial observations in the canine. J Periodontol 1988; 59:380.
133. Pitaru S, Tal H, Soldinger M, et al: Collagen membranes prevent apical migration of epithelium and support new connective tissue attachment during periodontal wound healing in dogs. J Periodont Res 1989; 24:2467.
134. Polson AM, Frederick GT, Ladenhein S, et al: The production of a root surface smear by instrumentation and its removal by citric acid. J Periodontol 1984; 55:443.
135. Polson AM, Proye MP: Fibrin linkage: A precursor for new attachment. J Periodontol 1983; 54:141.
136. Pontoriero R, Lindhe J, Nyman S, et al: Guided tissue regeneration in degree II furcation-involved mandibular molars. A clinical study. J Clin Periodontol 1988; 15:247.
137. Prichard JF: The intrabony technique as a predictable procedure. J Periodontol 1957; 28:202.
138. Proceedings of the 1996 World Workshop in Periodontology, Consensus Report: Periodontal regeneration around natural teeth. Ann Periodontol 1996; 7:667.
139. Quintero G, Mellonig JT, Gambill VM, et al: A six-month clinical evaluation of decalcified freeze-dried bone allografts in periodontal osseous defects. J Periodontol 1982; 53:726.
140. Rabalais ML, Yukna RA, Mayer ET: Evaluation of Durapatite ceramic as an alloplastic implant in periodontal osseous defects. J Periodontol 1981; 52:680.
141. Ramfjord SP: Experimental periodontal reattachment in rhesus monkeys. J Periodontol 1951; 22:67.
142. Ramfjord SP, Nissle RR: The modified Widman flap. J Periodontol 1974; 45:601.
143. Register AA, Burdick FA: Accelerated reattachment with cementogenesis to dentin, demineralized in situ. II. Defect repair. J Periodontol 1976; 47:497.
144. Renvert S, Badersten A, Nilveus R, et al: Healing after treatment of periodontal osseous defects. I. Comparative study of clinical methods. J Clin Periodontol 1981; 8:387.
145. Renvert S, Egelberg J: Healing after treatment of periodontal intraosseous defects. II. Effect of citric acid conditioning of the root surface. J Clin Periodontol 1981; 8:459.
146. Rivault AF, Toto PD, Levy S, et al: Autogenous bone grafts: Osseous coagulum and osseous retrograde procedures in primates. J Periodontol 1971; 42:787.
147. Robinson RE: Osseous coagulum for bone induction. J Periodontol 1969; 40:503.
148. Rosling B, Hollender L, Nyman S, et al: A radiographic method for assessing changes in alveolar bone height following periodontal therapy. J Clin Periodontol 1975; 2:211.
149. Ross SE, Malamed EH, Amsterdam M: The contiguous autogenous transplant—Its rationale, indications and technique. Periodontics 1966; 4:246.
150. Sanders J, Sepe W, Bowers G, et al: Clinical evaluation of freeze-dried bone allografts in periodontal osseous defects. III. Composite freeze-dried bone allograft with and without autogenous bone. J Periodontol 1983; 54:1.
151. Schaffer EM: Cartilage transplants into periodontium of rhesus monkeys. Oral Surg 1956; 11:1233.
152. Schaffer EM: Cementum and dentine implants in a dog and a rhesus monkey. J Periodontol 1957; 28:125.
153. Schaffer EM: Cartilage grafts in human periodontal pockets. J Periodontol 1958; 29:176.
154. Schallhorn RG: The use of autogenous hip marrow biopsy implants for bony crater defects. J Periodontol 1968; 39:145.
155. Schallhorn RG: Postoperative problems associated with iliac transplants. J Periodontol 1972; 43:3.
156. Schallhorn RG: Osseous grafts in the treatment of periodontal osseous defects. In: Stahl SS (ed): Periodontal Surgery. Biologic Basis and Technique. Springfield, IL, Charles C Thomas, 1976.
157. Schallhorn RG: Present status of osseous grafting procedures. J Periodontol 1977; 48:570.
158. Schallhorn RG, Hiatt WH, Boyce W: Iliac transplants in periodontal therapy. J Periodontol 1970; 41:566.
159. Schallhorn RG, McClain PK: Combined osseous composite grafting, root conditioning, and guided tissue regeneration. Int J Periodont Restor Dent 1988; 8:8.
160. Scoop IW, Kassouny DY, Morgan FH: Bovine bone (Boplant). J Periodontol 1966; 37:400.

161. Scoop IW, Morgan FH, Dooner JJ, et al: Bovine bone (Boplant) implants for infrabony oral lesions (clinical trials in humans). Periodontics 1966; 4:169.
162. Sepe W, Bowers G, Lawrence J, et al: Clinical evaluation of freeze-dried bone allograft in periodontal osseous defects. Part II. J Periodontol 1978; 49:9.
163. Shaffer CD, App GR: The use of plaster of Paris in treating infrabony periodontal defects in humans. J Periodontol 1971; 42:685.
164. Sigurdsson TJ, Hardwick R, Bogle GC, et al: Periodontal repair in dogs: space provision by reinforced ePTFE membranes enhances bone and cementum regeneration in large supraalveolar defects. J Periodontol 1994; 65:350.
165. Smith BA, Echeverri M: The removal of pocket epithelium. A review. J West Soc Periodontol 1984; 32:45.
166. Smith BA, Smith JS, Caffesse RG, et al: Effect of citric acid and various concentrations of fibronectin on healing following periodontal flap surgery in dogs. J Periodontol 1987; 58:667.
167. Sottosanti J: Calcium phosphate: An aid to periodontal, implant and restorative therapy. J Calif Dent Assoc 1992; 20:45.
168. Stahl SS, Froum SJ: Human clinical and histologic repair responses following the use of citric acid in periodontal therapy. J Periodontol 1977; 48:261.
169. Stahl SS, Froum SJ: Histological and clinical responses to porous hydroxylapatite implants in human periodontal defects three to twelve months post-implantation. J Periodontol 1987; 58:689.
170. Stahl SS, Froum SJ: Histologic healing responses in human vertical lesions following the use of osseous allografts and barrier membranes. J Clin Periodontol 1991; 18:149.
171. Stahl SS, Froum SJ: Human suprabony healing responses following root demineralization and coronal flap anchorage. J Clin Periodontol 1991; 18:685.
172. Stahl SS, Froum SJ: Human intrabony lesion response to debridement, porous hydroxylapatite implants and Teflon barrier membranes. J Clin Periodontol 1991; 18:605.
173. Stahl SS, Froum SJ, Tarnow D: Human clinical and histologic responses to the placement of HTR polymer particles in 11 intrabony lesions. J Periodontol 1990; 61:269.
174. Stahl SS, Froum SJ, Tarnow D: Human histologic responses to guided tissue regenerative techniques in intrabony lesions. J Clin Periodontol 1990; 17:191.
175. Takei HH, Han TJ, Carranza FA Jr, et al: Flap technique for periodontal bone implants. Papilla preservation technique. J Periodontol 1985; 56:204.
176. Terranova VP, Martin GR: Molecular factors determining gingival tissue interaction with tooth structure. J Periodont Res 1982; 17:530.
177. Terranova VP, Franzetti LC, Hic S, et al: A biochemical approach to periodontal regeneration: Tetracycline treatment of dentin promotes fibroblast adhesion and growth. J Periodont Res 1986; 21:330.
178. Theilade J: An evaluation of the reliability of radiographs in the measurement of bone loss in periodontal disease. J Periodontol 1960; 31:143.
179. Topback GA, Brunsvold MA, Nummikoski PV, et al: The accuracy of radiographic methods in assessing the outcome of periodontal regenerative therapy. J Periodontol 1999; 70:1479.
180. Tonetti MS, Cortellini P, Suvan JE, et al: Generalizability of the added benefits of guided tissue regeneration in the treatment of deep intrabony defects. Evaluation in a multicenter randomized controlled clinical trial. J Periodontol 1998; 69:1183.
181. Tonetti M, Pini Prato GP, Williams R, et al: Periodontal regeneration of human infrabony defects. III. Diagnostic strategies to detect bone gain. J Periodontol 1993; 64:269.
182. Turnbull RS, Freeman E, Melcher AH: Histological evaluation of the osteogenic capacity of sclera. J Dent Res 1976; 55:972.
183. Urist MR: Bone formation by autoinduction. Science 1965; 150:893.
184. Urist MR: Bone histogenesis and morphogenesis in implants of demineralized enamel and dentin. Oral Surg 1971; 29:38.
185. Urist MR, Strates BS: Bone morphogenetic protein. J Dent Res 1971; 50:1392.
186. Ursell MJ: Relationships between alveolar bone levels measured at surgery, estimated by transgingival probing and clinical attachment level measurements. J Clin Periodontol 1989; 16:81.
187. Van Dyke TE, Lester MA, Shapira L: The role of the host response in periodontal disease progression: Implications for future treatment strategies. J Periodontol 1993; 64:792.
188. Wallace SC, Gellin RG, Miller MC, et al: Guided tissue regeneration with and without decalcified freeze-dried bone in mandibular Class II furcation invasions. J Periodontol 1994; 65:244.
189. Wang HL, McNeil RL: Guided tissue regeneration. Absorbable barriers. Dent Clin North Amer 1998; 42:505.
190. Wenzel A, Warrer K, Karring T: Digital subtraction radiography in assessing bone changes in periodontal defects following guided tissue regeneration. J Clin Periodontol 1992; 19:208.
191. Wikesjö UME, Claffey N, Christersson LA, et al: Repair of periodontal furcation defects in beagle dogs following reconstructive surgery including root surface demineralization with tetracycline hydrochloride and topical fibronectin application. J Clin Periodontol 1988; 15:73.
192. Wikesjö UME, Nilveus R: Periodontal repair in dogs: Effects of wound stabilization in healing. J Periodontol 1990; 61:719.
193. Younger WJ: Some of the latest phases in implantations and other operations. Dent Cosmos 1893; 25:102.
194. Yukna RA: A clinical and histological study of healing following the excisional new attachment procedure in rhesus monkeys. J Periodontol 1976; 47:701.
195. Yukna RA: HTR polymer graft in human periodontal osseous defects. I. 6-months clinical results. J Periodontol 1990; 61:633.
196. Yukna RA: Clinical human comparison of expanded polytetrafluoroethylene barrier membrane and freeze-dried dura mater allografts for guided tissue regeneration of lost periodontal support. I. Mandibular molar class II furcations. J Periodontol 1992; 63:431.
197. Yukna RA, Mayer ET, Brite DV: Longitudinal evaluation of Durapatite ceramic as an alloplastic implant in periodontal osseous defects after three years. J Periodontol 1984; 55:633.
198. Yukna RA, Mellonig JT: Histologic evaluation of periodontal healing in humans following regenerative therapy with enamel matrix derivative. A 10-case series. J Periodontol 2000; 71:752.
199. Yukna RA, Krauser JT, Callan DP, et al: Multi-center clinical comparison of combination anorganic bovine-derived hydroxyapatite matrix (ABM)/cell binding peptide (P-15) and ABM in human periodontal osseous defects, 6-month results. J Periodontol 2000; 71:1671.

Furcation: The Problem and Its Management

William F. Ammons, Jr. and Gerald W. Harrington

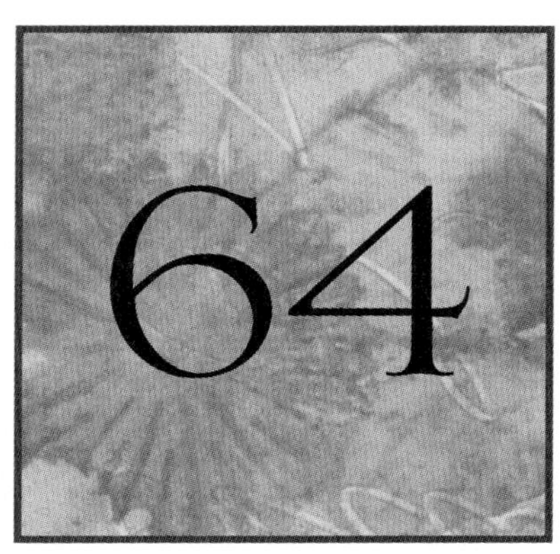

CHAPTER

CHAPTER OUTLINE

The progress of inflammatory periodontal disease, if unabated, ultimately results in attachment loss sufficient enough to affect the bifurcation or trifurcation of multirooted teeth. The furcation is an area of complex anatomic morphology[5,6,10] that may be difficult or impossible to be débrided by routine periodontal instrumentation.[28,33] Routine home care methods may not keep the furcation area free of plaque.[17,22] The presence of furcation involvement is one clinical finding that can lead to a diagnosis of advanced periodontitis and potentially to a less favorable prognosis for the affected tooth or teeth. Furcation involvement therefore presents both diagnostic and therapeutic dilemmas.

ETIOLOGIC FACTORS OF FURCATION PROBLEMS

The primary etiologic factor in the development of furcation defects is bacterial plaque and the inflammatory consequences that result from its long-term presence. The extent of attachment loss required to produce a furcation defect is variable and related to local anatomic factors such as root trunk length, root morphology,[11,27] and local developmental anomalies such as cervical enamel projections.[21,27] Local factors may affect the rate of plaque deposition or complicate the performance of oral hygiene procedures thereby contributing to the development of periodontitis and attachment loss. Studies indicate that prevalence and severity of furcation involvement increase with age.[20,21,33] Dental caries and pulpal death may also affect a tooth with furcation involvement or even the area of the furcation. All of these factors should be considered during the diagnosis, treatment planning and therapy of the patient with furcation defects.

DIAGNOSIS AND CLASSIFICATION OF FURCATION DEFECTS

A thorough clinical examination is the key to diagnosis and treatment planning. Careful probing is required to determine the presence and extent of furcation involvement, the position of the attachment relative to the furca, and the extent and configuration of the furcation defect.[35] Transgingival sounding may further define the anatomy of the furcation defect.[28] The goal of this examination is to identify and classify the extent of furcation involvement and to identify factors that may have contributed to the development of the furcation defect or that could affect treatment outcome. Among these factors are 1) the morphology of the affected tooth, 2) the position of the tooth relative to adjacent teeth, 3) the local anatomy of the alveolar bone, 4) the configuration of any bony defects, and 5) the presence and extent of other dental diseases such as caries and pulpal necrosis.

The dimension of the furcation entrance is variable but usually quite small. Eighty-one percent of furcations have an orifice of 1 mm or less, and 58% are 0.75 mm or less.[5,6] These dimensions, along with the local anatomy[10,11,12] of the furcation area, should be kept in mind in the selections of instruments for probing. A probe of small cross section is required if one is to detect early furcation involvement.

CLASSIFICATION OF FURCATION INVOLVEMENT

The extent and configuration of the furcation defect are factors in both diagnosis and treatment planning. This has led to the development of a number of indices to record furcation involvement. These indices are based on the horizontal measurement of attachment loss in the furcation,[13,17] on a combination of horizontal and vertical measurements,[34] or a combination of these findings with the localized configuration of the bony deformity.[9] Glickman[13] graded furcation involvement into the following four classes (Fig. 64-1, *A–D*):

Grade I: A Grade I furcation involvement is the incipient or early stage of furcation involvement (see Fig. 64-1, *A*). The pocket is suprabony and primarily affects the soft tissues. Early bone loss may have occurred with an increase in probing depth, but radiographic changes are not usually found.

Grade II: Grade II furcation can affect one or more of the furcations of the same tooth. The furcation lesion is

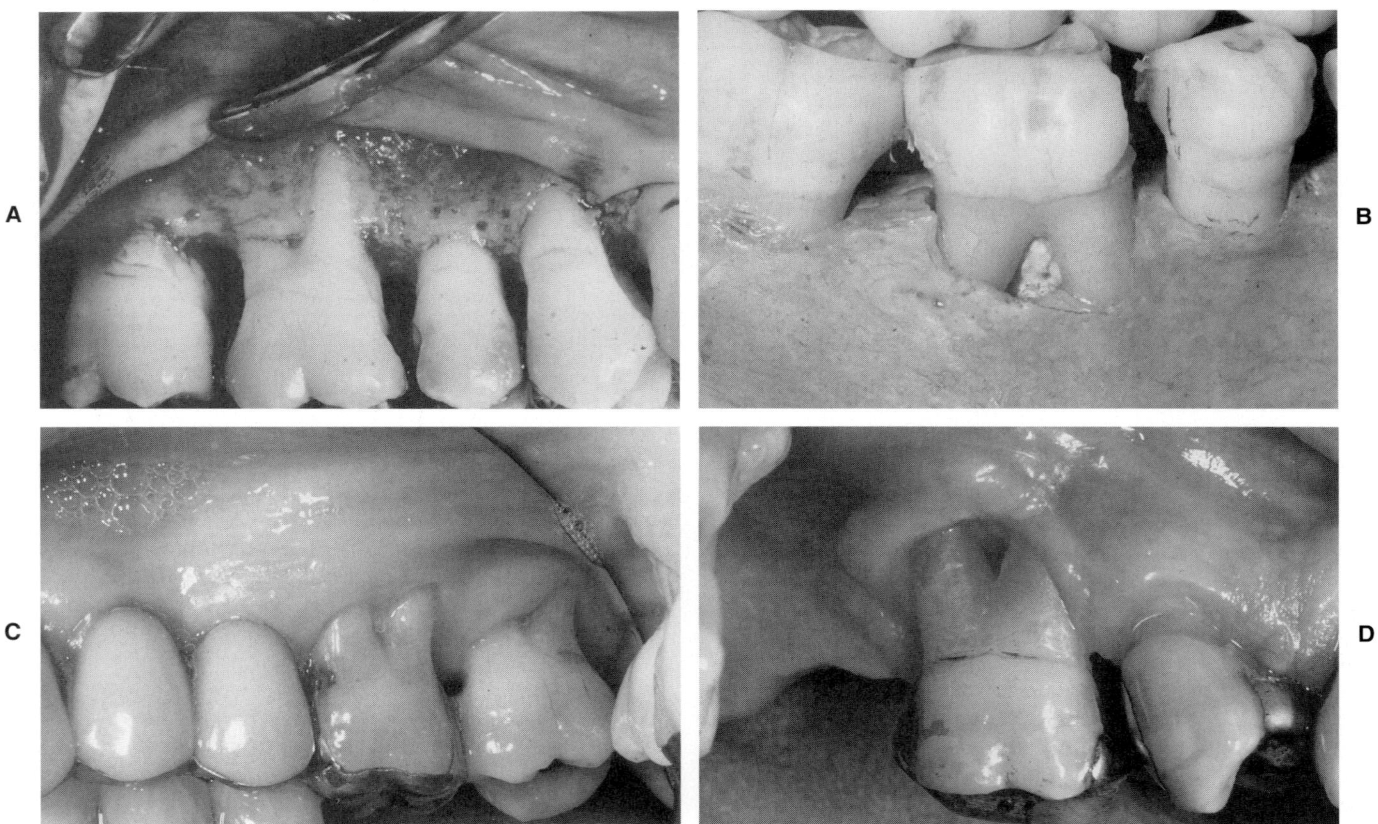

Fig. 64-1 Glickman's classification of furcation involvement. **A,** Grade I furcation involvement. Although the periodontal ligament is visible at the entrance to the furcation, no horizontal component of the furcation is evident on probing. **B,** Grade II furcation in a dried skull. Note both the horizontal and the vertical component of this cul-de-sac. **C,** Grade III furcations on maxillary molars. Probing confirms that the buccal furcation connects with the distal furcation of both of these molars, yet the furcation is filled with soft tissue. **D,** Grade IV furcation. The soft tissues have receded sufficiently to allow direct vision into the furcation of this maxillary molar.

essentially a cul-de-sac (see Fig. 64-1, *B*) with a definite horizontal component. If multiple defects are present, they do not communicate with each other, since a portion of the alveolar bone remains attached to the tooth. The extent of the horizontal probing of the furcation determines whether the defect is early or advanced. Vertical bone loss may be present and represents a therapeutic complication. Radiographs may or may not depict the furcation involvement. This is particularly true of maxillary molars because of the radiographic overlap of the roots. Although in some views the presence of furcation arrows indicate possible furcation involvement (see Chapter 31).

Grade III: In grade III furcations the bone is not attached to the dome of the furcation. In early grade III involvement the opening may be filled with soft tissue and may not be visible. Indeed one may not be able to pass a periodontal probe completely through the furcation because of interference with the bifurcational ridges or facial/lingual bony margins. However, if one adds the buccal and lingual probing dimensions and obtains a cumulative probing measurement that is equal to or greater than the buccal/lingual dimension of the tooth at the furcation orifice, it must be concluded that a grade III furcation exists (see Fig. 64-1, *C*). Properly exposed and angled radiographs of early class III furcations display the defect as a radiolucent area in the crotch of the tooth (see Chapter 32).

Grade IV: In grade IV furcations the interdental bone is destroyed and the soft tissues have receded apically so that the furcation opening is clinically visible. A tunnel therefore exists between the roots of such an affected tooth. The periodontal probe therefore passes readily from one aspect of the tooth to another (see Fig. 64-1, *D*).

Other classification indices: Hamp, Nyman, and Lindhe[17] modified a three-stage classification system by attaching a millimeter measurement to separate the extent of horizontal involvement. Easley and Drennan,[9] and Tarnow and Fletcher[34] have described classification systems that consider both horizontal and vertical attachment loss in classifying the extent of furcation involvement. Consideration of defect configuration and the vertical component of the defect provides additional information that may be useful in planning therapy.

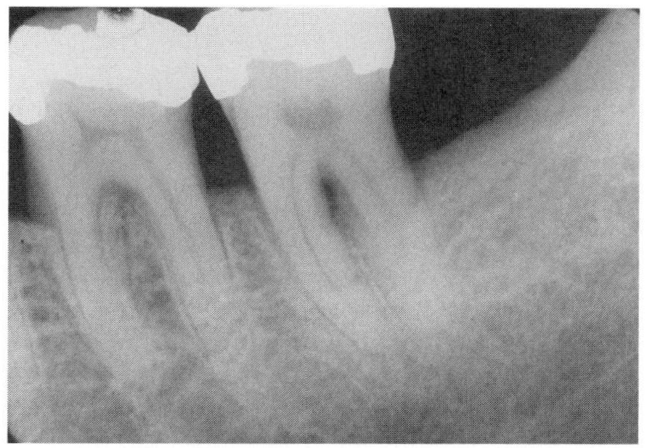

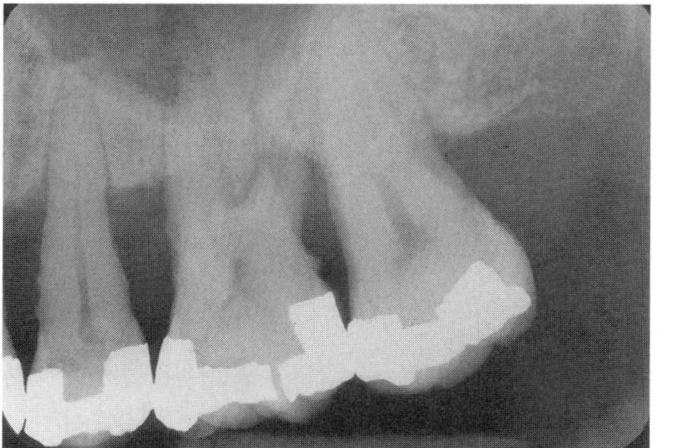

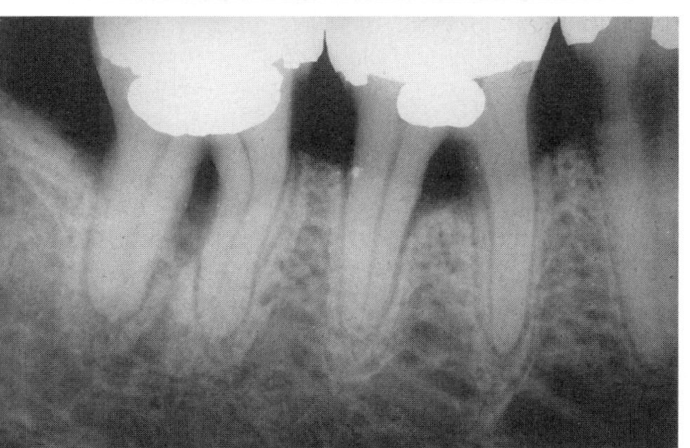

Fig. 64-2 Different degrees of furcation involvement in radiographs. **A,** Grade I furcation on the maxillary first molar and a Grade III furcation on the mandibular second molar. The root approximation on the second molar may be sufficient to impede accurate probing of this defect. **B,** Multiple furcation defects on a maxillary first molar. There is a class I buccal furcation involvement and grade II mesiopalatal and distopalatal furcations. Deep developmental grooves on the maxillary second molar simulate furcation involvement in this molar with fused roots. **C,** Grade III and IV furcations on mandibular molars.

LOCAL ANATOMIC FACTORS IN TREATMENT OF FURCATIONS

Clinical examination of the patient should allow the therapist to identify not only furcation defects but many of the local anatomic factors that may affect the result of therapy (prognosis). Well-made dental radiographs, while not allowing a definitive classification of furcation involvement, provide additional information vital for treatment planning (Fig. 64-2, *A–C*). Important local factors are described in the following section.

The Tooth

During treatment planning, the following anatomic features of the affected teeth should be considered:

Root trunk length: This is a key factor in both the development and treatment of furcation involvement. The distance from the cementoenamel junction to the entrance of the furcation can vary extensively. Teeth may have very short root trunks, moderate length trunks or roots than may be fused to a point near the apex (Fig. 64-3). The combination of root trunk length with the number and configuration of the roots affects both the ease and success of therapy. The shorter the root trunk, the less attachment has to be lost before the furcation is involved. Once the furcation is exposed, teeth with short root trunks may be more accessible to maintenance procedures and the short root trunks may facilitate some surgical procedures. Alternatively teeth with unusually long root trunks or fused roots may not be appropriate candidates for treatment once the furcation has been affected.

Root length: Root length is directly related to the quantity of attachment supporting the tooth. Teeth with long roots trunks and short roots may have lost a majority of their support by the time that the furcation becomes affected.[12,19] Teeth with long roots and short to moderate root trunk length are more readily treated as sufficient attachment remains to meet functional demands.

Root form: The mesial root of most mandibular first and second molars and the mesiofacial root of the maxillary first molar are commonly curved to the distal in the apical third. In addition, the distal aspect of this root is usually heavily fluted. The curvature and fluting may increase the potential for root perforation during endodontics or complicate postplacement during restoration.[1,24] These anatomic features may also result in an increased incidence of vertical root fracture. The size of the mesial radicular pulp may result in removal of the majority of the portion of the tooth during preparation.

Interradicular dimension: The degree of separation of the roots is also an important factor in treatment planning. Closely approximated or fused roots can preclude adequate instrumentation during scaling, root planing, and surgery. Teeth with widely separated roots present more treatment options and are more readily treated.

Anatomy of the furcation: The anatomy of the furcation is complex. The presence of bifurcational ridges, a concavity in the dome,[10] and possible accessory canals[16] complicates not only scaling, root planing, and surgical therapy,[26] but also periodontal maintenance. Odontoplasty to reduce or eliminate these ridges may be required during surgical therapy for an optimum result.

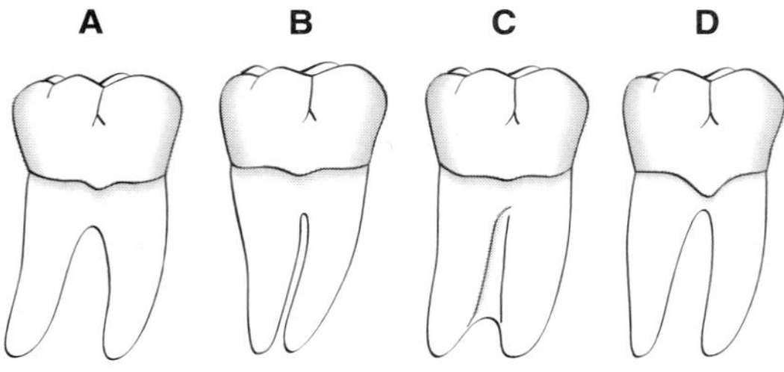

Fig. 64-3 Different anatomic features that may be important in prognosis and treatment of furcation involvement. **A,** Widely separated roots. **B,** Roots are separated but close. **C,** Fused roots separated only in their apical portion. **D,** Presence of enamel projection that may be conducive to early furcation involvement.

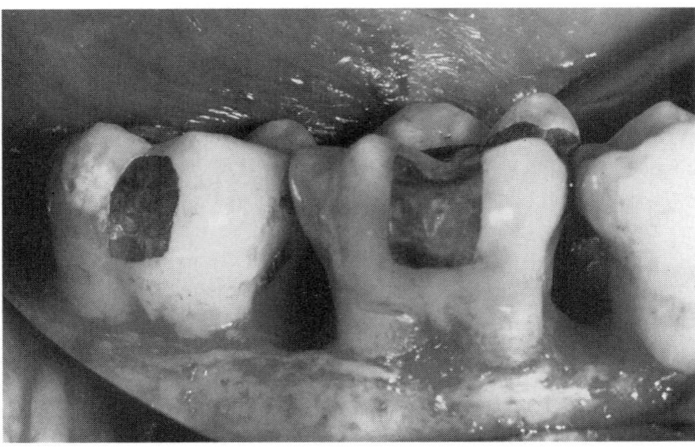

Fig. 64-4 Furcation involvement by grade III cervical enamel projections.

BOX 64-1

Classification of Cervical Enamel Projections

Grade I: The enamel projection extends from the cementoenamel junction of the tooth toward the furcation entrance.
Grade II: The enamel projection approaches the entrance to the furcation. It does not enter the furcation, therefore there is no horizontal component.
Grade III: The enamel project actually extends horizontally into the furcation.

Masters DH, Hoskins SW: Projection of cervical enamel into molar furcations. J Periodontol 1964; 35:49.

Cervical enamel projections: Cervical enamel projections (CEPs) are reported to occur on 8.6% to 28.6% of molars.[25,27,32] The prevalence is highest for mandibular and maxillary second molars. The extent of CEPs was classified by Masters and Hoskins[27] in 1964 (Box 64-1). An example of a grade III CEP is shown in Fig. 64-4. These projections can affect plaque removal, complicate scaling and root planing, and may be a local factor in the development of gingivitis and periodontitis. They should be removed to facilitate maintenance.

THE ANATOMY OF THE BONY LESIONS

Pattern of Attachment Loss

The form of the bony lesions associated with the furcation can vary significantly. Horizontal bone loss can expose the furcation as thin facial/lingual plates of bone that may be totally lost during resorption. Alternatively, areas with thickened bony ledges may persist and predispose to the development of furcations with deep vertical components. The pattern of bone loss on other surfaces of the affected tooth and adjacent teeth must also be considered during treatment planning. The treatment response in deep multiwalled bony defects is different from that in areas of horizontal bone loss. Complex multiwalled defects with deep interradicular vertical components may be candidates for regenerative therapies. Alternatively, molars with advanced attachment loss on only one root may be treated by resective procedures.

OTHER DENTAL FINDINGS

The dental and periodontal condition of the adjacent teeth must be considered during treatment planning for furcation involvement. The combination of furcation involvement and root approximation with an adjacent tooth represents the same problem that exists in furcations without adequate root separation. Such a finding may dictate the removal of the most severely affected tooth or the removal of a root or roots (Fig. 64-5).

The presence of an adequate band of gingiva and a moderate to deep vestibule will facilitate the performance of a surgical procedure should it be indicated.

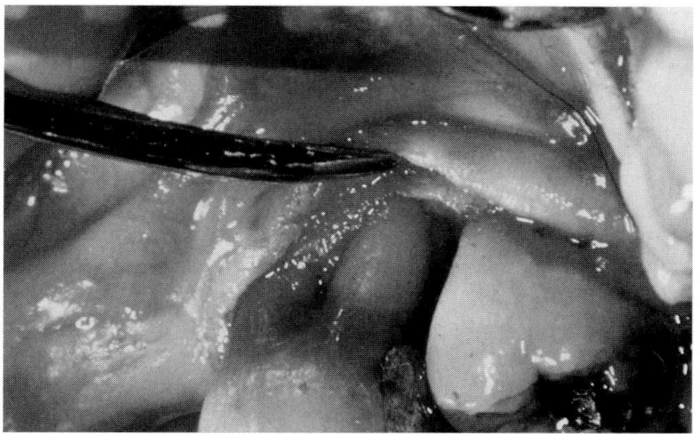

Fig. 64-5 Advanced bone loss, furcation involvement, and root approximation. Note the buccal furcation, which communicates with the distal furcation of a maxillary first molar that also displays advanced attachment loss on the distal root and approximation with the mesial of the maxillary second molar. The patient with such teeth may benefit from root resection of the distobuccal root of the first molar or extraction of the molar.

TREATMENT OF FURCATION DEFECTS

The objectives of furcation therapy are to 1) facilitate maintenance, 2) prevent further attachment loss, and 3) obliterate the furcation defects as a periodontal maintenance problem. The selection of therapeutic mode varies with the class of furcation involvement, the extent and configuration of bone loss, and other anatomic factors.

Therapy for Early Furcation Defects: Class I

Incipient or early furcation defects (class I) are amenable to conservative periodontal therapy. As the pocket is suprabony and has not entered the furcation, oral hygiene, scaling, and root planing are effective.[15] Any thick overhanging margins of restorations, facial grooves, or cervical enamel projections should be eliminated by odontoplasty, recontouring, or replacement. The resolution of inflammation and subsequent repair of the periodontal ligament and bone is usually sufficient to restore periodontal health.

Therapy for Furcation Involvement: Class II

Once a horizontal component to the furcation has developed (class II), therapy becomes more complicated. Shallow horizontal involvement without significant vertical bone loss usually responds favorably to localized flap operation with odontoplasty and osteoplasty. Isolated deep class II furcations may respond to flap procedures with osteoplasty and odontoplasty (Fig. 64-6, *A* and *B*). This

A

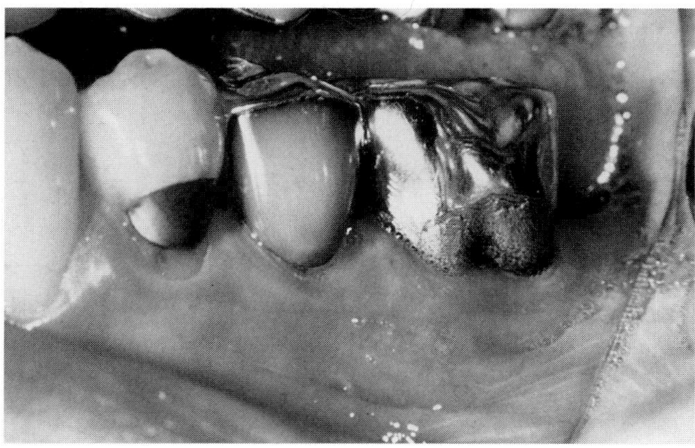

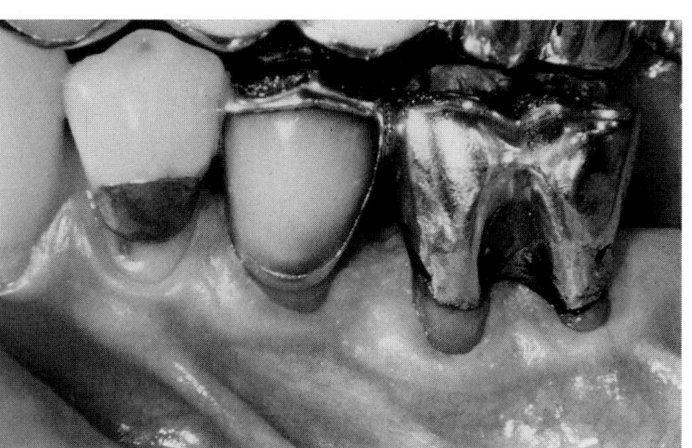

B

Fig. 64-6 Treatment of a grade II furcation by osteoplasty and odontoplasty. **A,** This mandibular first molar has been treated by endodontics and an area of caries in the furcation repaired. A class II furcation is present. **B,** Five year postoperative picture of the results of flap debridement, osteoplasty, and severe odontoplasty. Note the adaptation of the gingiva into the furcation area. (Courtesy Dr. Ronald Rott; Sacramento, Calif.)

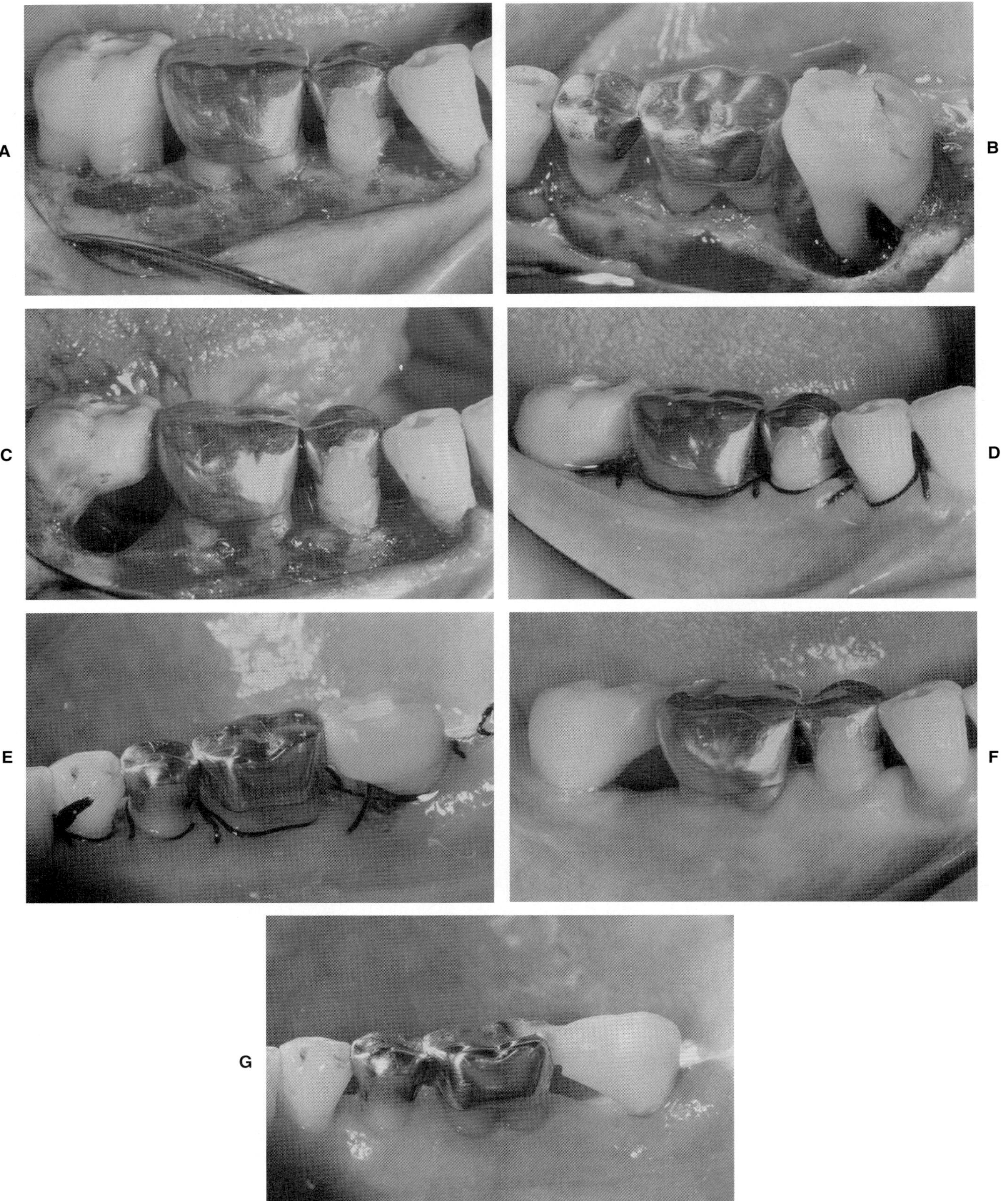
A
B
C
D
E
F
G

Fig. 64-7 Resection of a root with advanced bone loss. **A,** Facial osseous contours. There is an early grade II furcation on the facial of the mandibular first molar and a class III furcation on the mandibular second molar. **B,** Lingual osseous contours. Note the early grade II lingual furcation on the first molar and the deep circumferential bony lesion on the mesial root of the mandibular second molar. **C,** Resection of the mesial root. The mesial portion of the crown was retained to prevent mesial drift of the distal root during healing. The grade II furcations were treated by osteoplasty. **D,** Buccal flaps adapted and sutured. **E,** Lingual flaps adapted and sutured. **F,** Three-month postoperative view of the buccal aspect of this resection. New restorations were subsequently placed. **G,** Three-month postoperative view of the lingual aspect of this resection.

reduces the dome of the furcation and alters gingival contours to facilitate the patient's plaque removal.

Therapy for Advanced Furcation Defects: Class II-IV

The development of a significant horizontal component to one or more furcations of a multirooted tooth (late class II, class III or IV[13]) and/or the development of a deep vertical component to the furca poses additional problems. Nonsurgical treatment is commonly ineffective as the ability to instrument the tooth surfaces adequately is compromised.[30,36] Periodontal surgery, endodontics, and restoration of the tooth may be required to retain the tooth.

SURGICAL THERAPY FOR FURCATION INVOLVEMENT

Root Resection

Root resection may be indicated in multirooted teeth with grade II to IV furcation involvements. Root resection may be performed on vital[18] or endodontically treated teeth. It is preferable, however, to have endodontic therapy completed before resection of a root(s).[14] If this is not possible, then the pulp should be removed, the patency of the canals determined, and the pulp chamber medicated before resection. It is distressing to perform a vital root resection and to subsequently have an untoward event occur such as perforation, fracture of the root, or an inability to instrument the canal.

The indications and contraindications for root resection were well summarized by Bassaraba.[1] In general, teeth planned for root resection should include the following:

1. Teeth that are of critical importance to the overall dental treatment plan.[4] Examples are teeth serving as abutments of fixed or removable restorations for which the loss of the tooth would result in the loss of the prosthesis and entail major prosthetic retreatment.
2. Teeth that have sufficient attachment remaining for function. Molars with advanced bone loss in the interproximal and interradicular zones, unless the lesions have three bony walls, are not candidates for root amputation.
3. Teeth for which there is no more predictable or cost-effective method of therapy. Examples are teeth with furcation defects that have been treated successfully with endodontics but now present with a vertical root fracture, advanced bone loss or caries on bone root.
4. Teeth in patients with good oral hygiene and low activity for caries are suitable candidates. Patients unable or unwilling to perform good oral hygiene and preventive measures are not suitable candidates for root resection or hemisection. Root-resected teeth require endodontic treatment[14] and commonly require cast restorations.

These therapies can represent a sizeable financial investment on the part of the patient in an effort to save the tooth. Alternative therapies and their impact on the overall treatment plan should always be considered and presented to the patient.

Root Resection: Which Root to Remove and Why? A tooth with an isolated furcation defect in an otherwise intact dental segment may present few diagnostic problems. However, the existence of multiple furcation defects of varying severity when combined with generalized advanced periodontitis can be a treatment planning challenge. Careful diagnosis usually allows the therapist to determine the feasibility of root resection and the identification of which root to remove before surgery (Fig. 64-7, *A–G*).

The following is a guide to determining which root should be removed in these cases:

1. Remove the root(s) that will elliminate the furcation and allow the production of a maintainable architecture on the remaining roots.
2. Remove the root with the greatest amount of bone and attachment loss. It is obvious that sufficient periodontal attachment must remain after surgery for the tooth to withstand the functional demands placed on it. Teeth with uniform advanced horizontal bone loss are not candidates for root resection.
3. Remove the root that best contributes to the elimination of periodontal problems on adjacent teeth. For example, a maxillary first molar, with a class III buccal-to-distal furcation is adjacent to a maxillary second molar with a two-walled intrabony defect between the molars and an early class II furcation on the mesial furcation of the second molar. There may or may not be local anatomic factors affecting the teeth. The removal of the distobuccal root of the first molar allows the elimination of the furcation and management of the two-walled intrabony lesion and also facilitates access for instrumentation and maintenance of the second molar (Fig. 64-8).
4. Remove the root with the greatest number of anatomic problems such as severe curvature, developmental grooves, root flutings, or accessory and multiple root canals.
5. Remove the root that least complicates future periodontal maintenance.

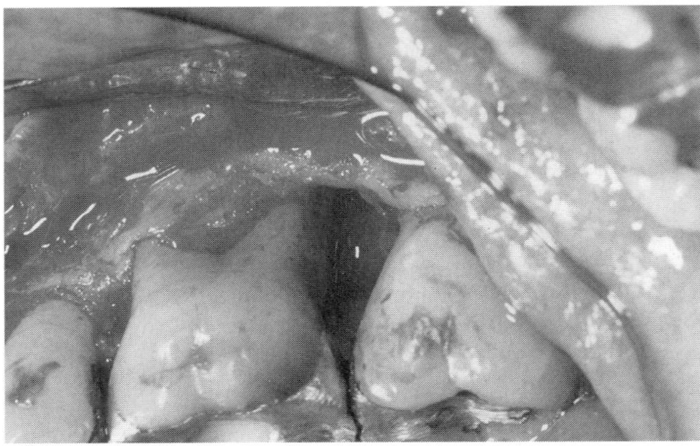

Fig. 64-8 Advanced bone loss on one root with furcation involvement. The majority of the attachment has been lost on the distal surface of this maxillary first molar. A buccal grade I and a deep grade II distal furcation defect is present. A shallow two-walled defect, correctable by osteoplasty and osteoectomy, is present at the mesial of the second molar. Treatment options are root amputation or extraction.

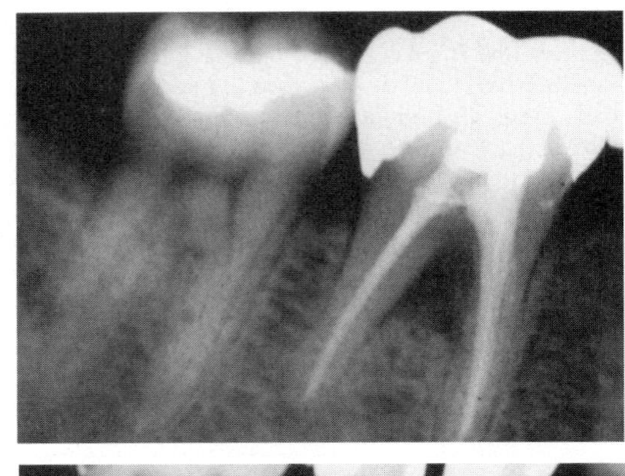

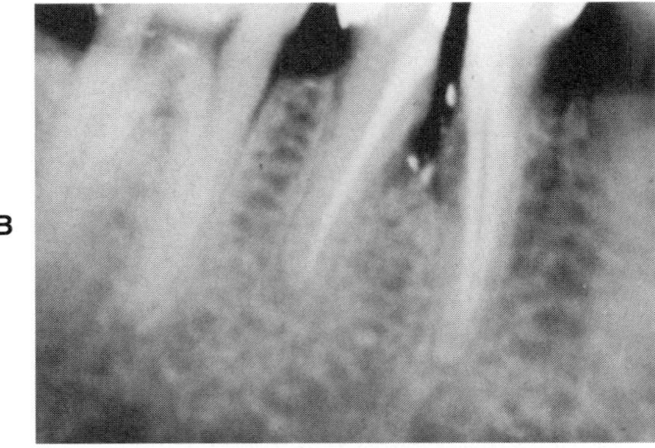

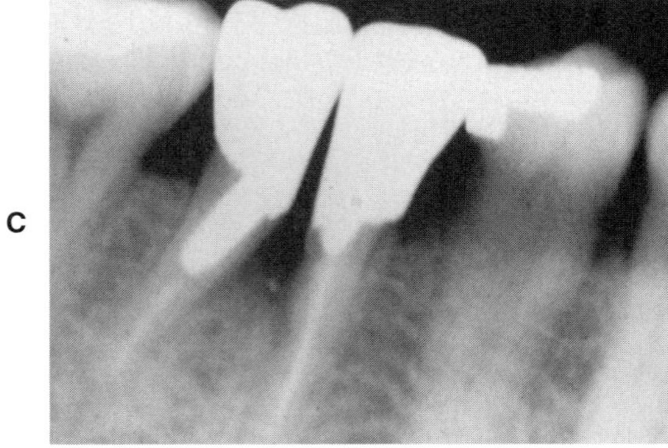

Fig. 64-9 Hemisection.

HEMISECTION

Hemisection is the splitting of a two-rooted tooth into two separate portions. This process has been called *bicuspidization* or *separation* as it changes the molar into two separate roots. It is most likely to be performed on mandibular molars with buccal and lingual class II or III furcation involvements. As with root resection, molars with advanced bone loss in the interproximal and interradicular zones are not good candidates for hemisection. After sectioning of the teeth, one or both roots can be retained. This decision is based on the extent and pattern of bony loss, root trunk and root length, ability to eliminate the osseous defect, and endodontic and restorative considerations. The anatomy of the mesial roots of mandibular molars often leads to their extraction and the retention of the distal root to facilitate both endodontics and restorative dentistry.

The interradicular dimension between the two roots of a tooth to be hemisected is also important. Narrow interradicular zones can complicate the surgical procedure. The retention of both molar roots can complicate the restoration of the tooth, since it may be virtually impossible to finish margins or to provide an adequate embrasure between the two roots for effective oral hygiene and maintenance (Fig. 64-9). Therefore orthodontic separation of the roots is commonly required to allow restoration with adequate embrasure form (Fig. 64-10, *A–D*). The result can be the need for multiple procedures and extensive interdisciplinary therapy. In such patients the availability of other treatment alternatives such as guided tissue/guided bone regeneration or replacement by osseointegrated dental implants should be considered.

THE ROOT RESECTION/ HEMISECTION PROCEDURE

The most commonly performed root resection is the distobuccal root of the maxillary first molar.[2,25] This resection is diagramed in Fig. 64-11, *A–F*. After appropriate local anesthesia, a full-thickness mucoperiosteal flap is elevated. Root resection or hemisection of teeth with advanced attachment loss usually requires opening both facial and lingual/palatal flaps. Chapter 60 of this text describes the process of flap elevation. It is uncommon to be able to resect a root without elevation of a flap. The flap should provide adequate access for visualization and instrumentation and to minimize trauma during the operation.

After débridement the resection of the root begins with the exposure of the furcation on the root to be removed (see Fig. 64-11, *A*). The removal of a small amount of facial or palatal bone may be required to provide access for elevation and facilitate root removal (see Fig. 64-11, *B*). A cut is then directed from just apical to the contact point of the tooth, through the tooth, to the facial

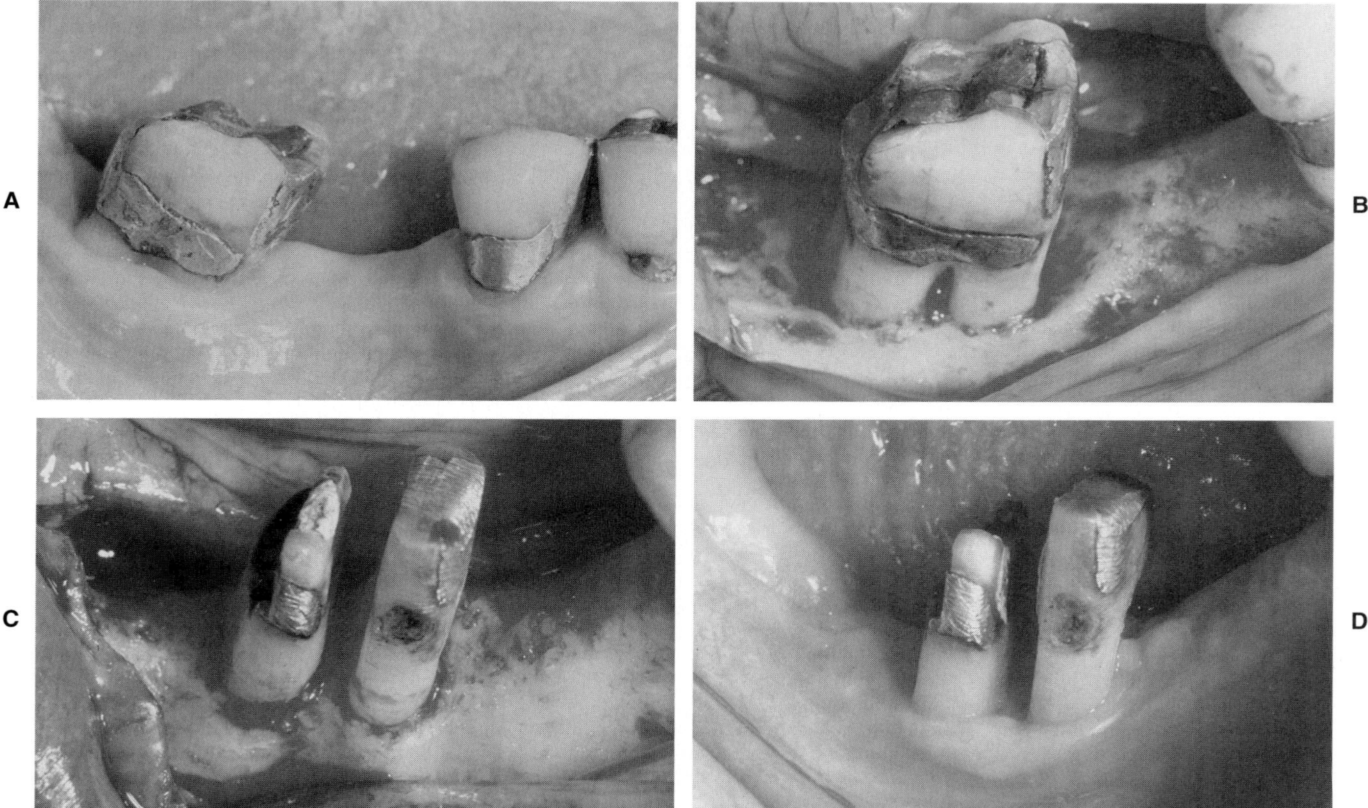

Fig. 64-10 Hemisection and interradicular dimension. **A,** Buccal preoperative view of a mandibular right second molar with a deep grade II buccal furcation and root approximation. **B,** Buccal view of bony lesions with flaps. Note the mesial and distal one-wall bony defects. The lingual furcation was similarly affected. **C,** The molar has been hemisected and partially prepared for temporary crowns. Observe the minimal dimension between the two roots. **D,** Buccal view 3 weeks postoperative. As the embrasure space is minimal, these roots will be separated with orthodontics to facilitate restoration. (Courtesy Dr. Louis Cuccia; Roseville, Calif.)

and distal orifices of the furcation, (see Fig. 64-11, *C*). This cut is made with a high-speed surgical length fissure or cross-cut fissure carbine bur. The placement of a curved periodontal probe into or through the furcation aids in orienting the angle of the resection. For hemisection a vertically oriented cut is made faciolingually through the buccal and lingual developmental grooves of the tooth, through the pulp chamber, and through the furcation. If the sectioning cut passes through a metallic restoration, the metallic portion of the cut should be made before flap elevation. This prevents the contamination of the surgical field with metallic particles.

If a vital root resection is to be performed a more horizontal cut through the root is advisable (see Fig. 64-11, *D*). An oblique cut exposes a large surface area of the radicular pulp and/or dental pulp chamber. This can lead to postoperative pain and can complicate the performance of endodontics. A horizontal cut, although it may complicate root removal, has less postoperative complications. This root stump can be removed by odontoplasty after the completion of endodontic therapy or at the time of tooth preparation.

After sectioning, the root is elevated from its socket (see Fig. 64-11, *E*). Care should be taken not to traumatize bone on the remaining roots or to damage an adjacent tooth. Removal of the root provides visibility to the furcation aspects of the remaining roots and simplifies the débridement of the furcation with hand, rotary, or ultrasonic instruments. If necessary, odontoplasty is performed to remove portions of the developmental ridges and prepare a furcation that is free of any deformity that would enhance plaque retention or adversely affect plaque removal (see Fig. 64-11, *F*).

Patients with advanced periodontitis commonly have root resection performed in conjunction with other surgical procedures. An example of combining root resection and periodontal osseous surgery is shown in Fig. 64-12, *A–I*. The bony lesions that may be present on adjacent teeth are then treated using resective or regenerative therapies. After resection the flap(s) are then approximated to cover any grafted tissues or to slightly cover the bony margins around the tooth. Sutures are then placed to maintain the position of the flaps. The area may or may not be covered with a surgical dressing.

The removal of a root alters the distribution of occlusal forces on the remaining roots. Therefore it is wise

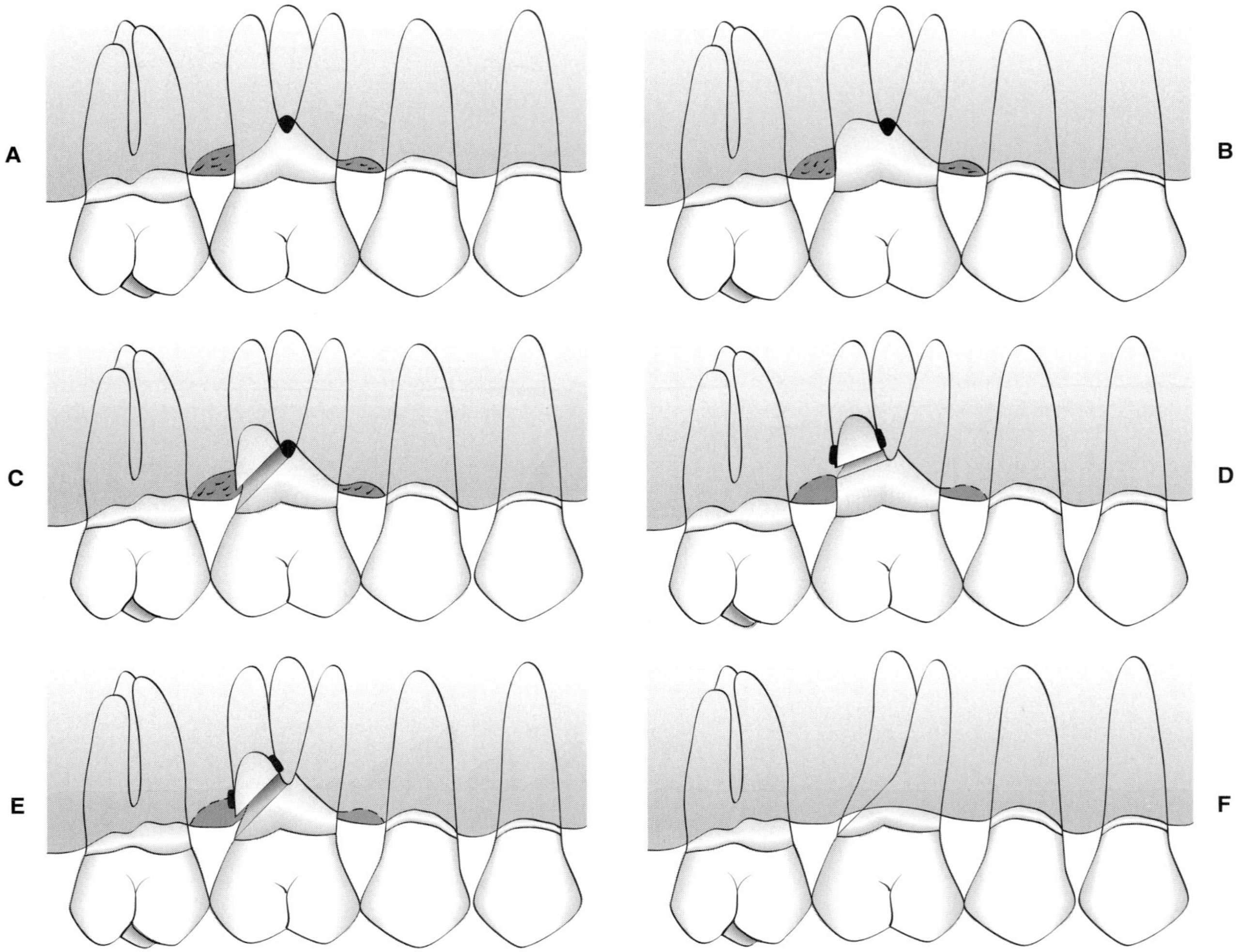

Fig. 64-11 Diagram of a distobuccal root resection of a maxillary first molar. **A,** Pre-operative bony contours with grade II buccal furcation and a crater between the first and second molar. **B,** Removal of bone from the facial of the distobuccal root and exposure of the furcation for instrumentation. **C,** Oblique section that separates the distal root from the mesial and palatal roots of the molar. **D,** More horizontal section that may be used on a vital root amputation as it exposes less of the pulp of the tooth. **E,** Areas of application of instruments to elevate the sectioned root. **F,** Final contours of the resection.

to evaluate the occlusion of teeth from which roots have been resected and if necessary to adjust the occlusion. Centric holds should be maintained, but eccentric forces should be eliminated from the area over the root that was removed. Patients with advanced attachment loss may benefit from temporary stabilization of the resected tooth to prevent movement (Fig. 64-13, *A–I*).

REGENERATION

The periodontal literature has well-documented therapeutic efforts designed to induce new attachment and/or regeneration on molars with furcation defects. Many surgical procedures using a variety of grafting materials have been tested on teeth with different classes of furcation involvement. Some investigators have reported clinical success with these techniques,[23] whereas others have suggested that the use of these materials in class II, III, or IV furcations offers little advantage compared with surgical controls.[3,8,29]

Furcation defects with deep two-walled or significant three-walled components may however be candidates for regeneration procedures. These vertical bony deformities respond favorably to a variety of other surgical procedures such as débridement with or without membranes and bone grafts. Therapies designed to induce new attachment or reattachment are addressed in Chapter 63.

EXTRACTION

The extraction of teeth with through and through furcation defects (class III and IV) and advanced attachment

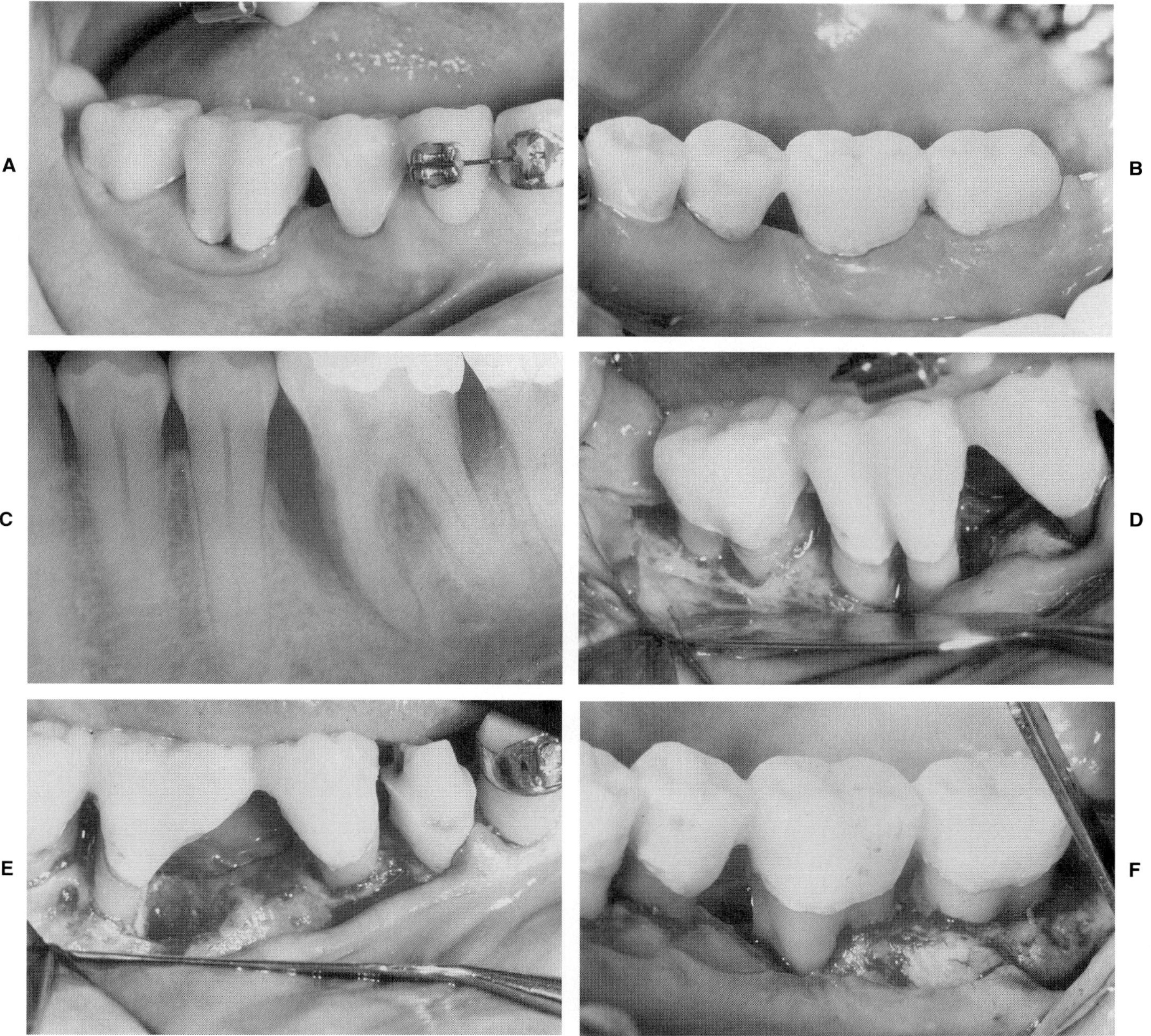

Fig. 64-12 Hemisection combined with osseous surgery to treat furcation defects. **A,** Buccal preoperative view with provisional bridge. **B,** Lingual view with provisional bridge in place. **C,** Radiograph of bony defects. Note the deep mesial bony defect that is largely of one wall and the radiolucent area in the furcation of the first molar indicating a grade II furcation. **D,** Buccal preosseous surgery view. In addition to the furcation involvement there is a root separation problem between the two roots of the first molar. Class II furcations are present on the second molar. **E,** Buccal view postosseous surgery. Mesial root hemisected and removed. The other defects were treated by osteoplasty and osteosectomy. **F,** Lingual pre-osseous view. Note the heavy bony ledging at the lingual of these first and second molars.

(Continued)

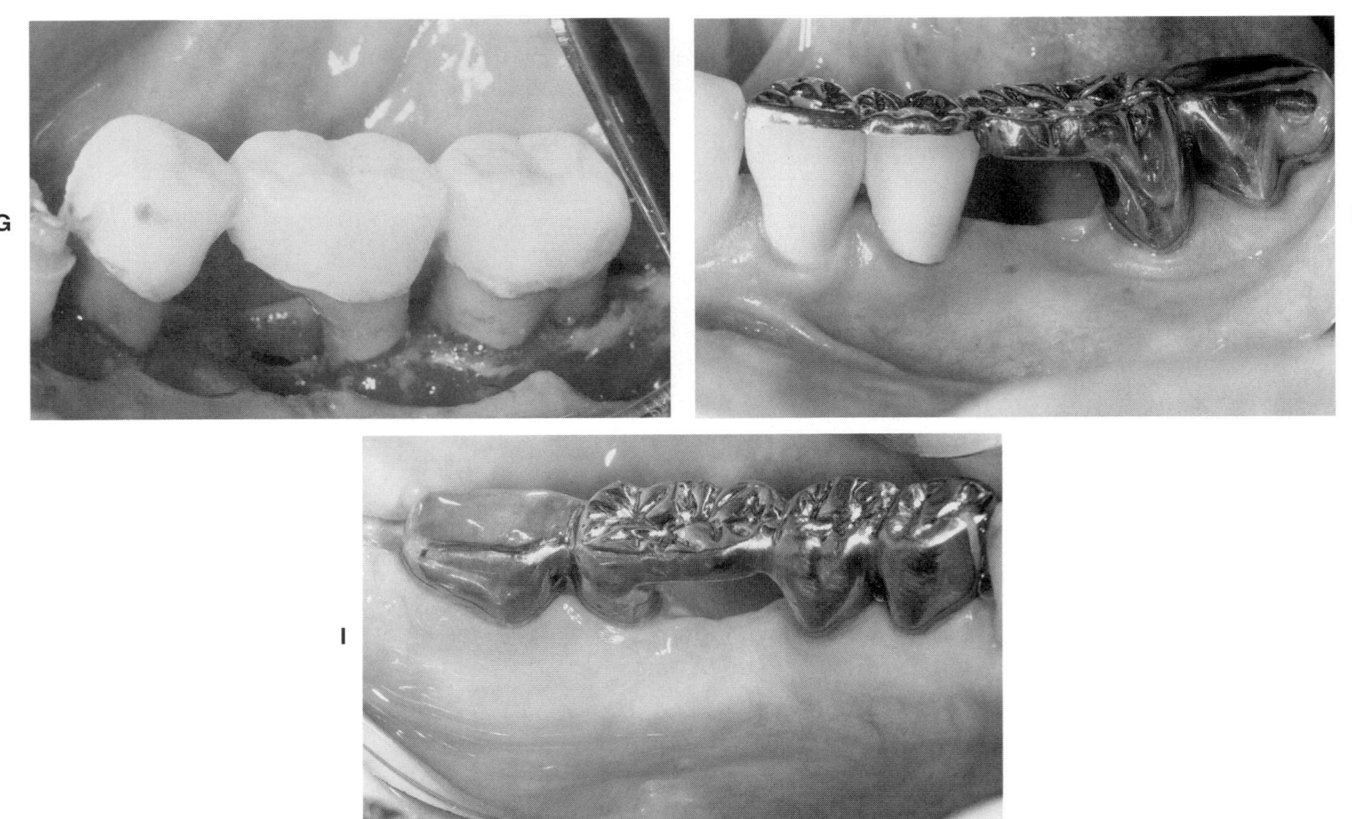

Fig. 64-12 *(Cont'ed)* **G,** Lingual view postosseous surgery. The mesial root has been resected, the bony ledging recontoured, and the grade II furcations treated by osteoplasty. **H,** Buccal view, 10 years posttreatment. **I,** Lingual view, 10 years posttreatment. (Courtesy Dr. Louis Cuccia; Roseville, Calif.)

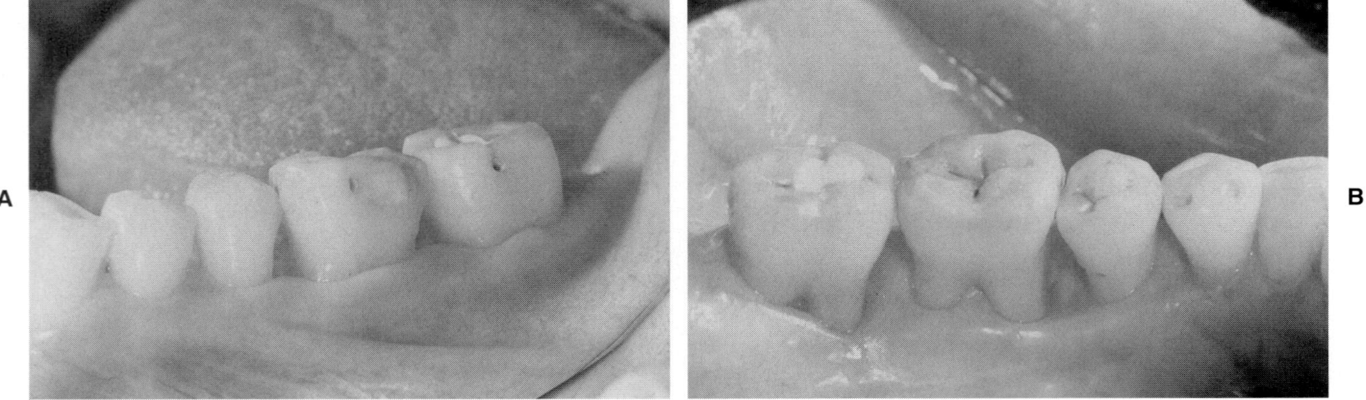

Fig. 64-13 Mesial root resection in the presence of advanced bone loss. **A and B,** Buccal and lingual preoperative views. Note the soft tissue contours that are predictive of the bony defects.

(Continued)

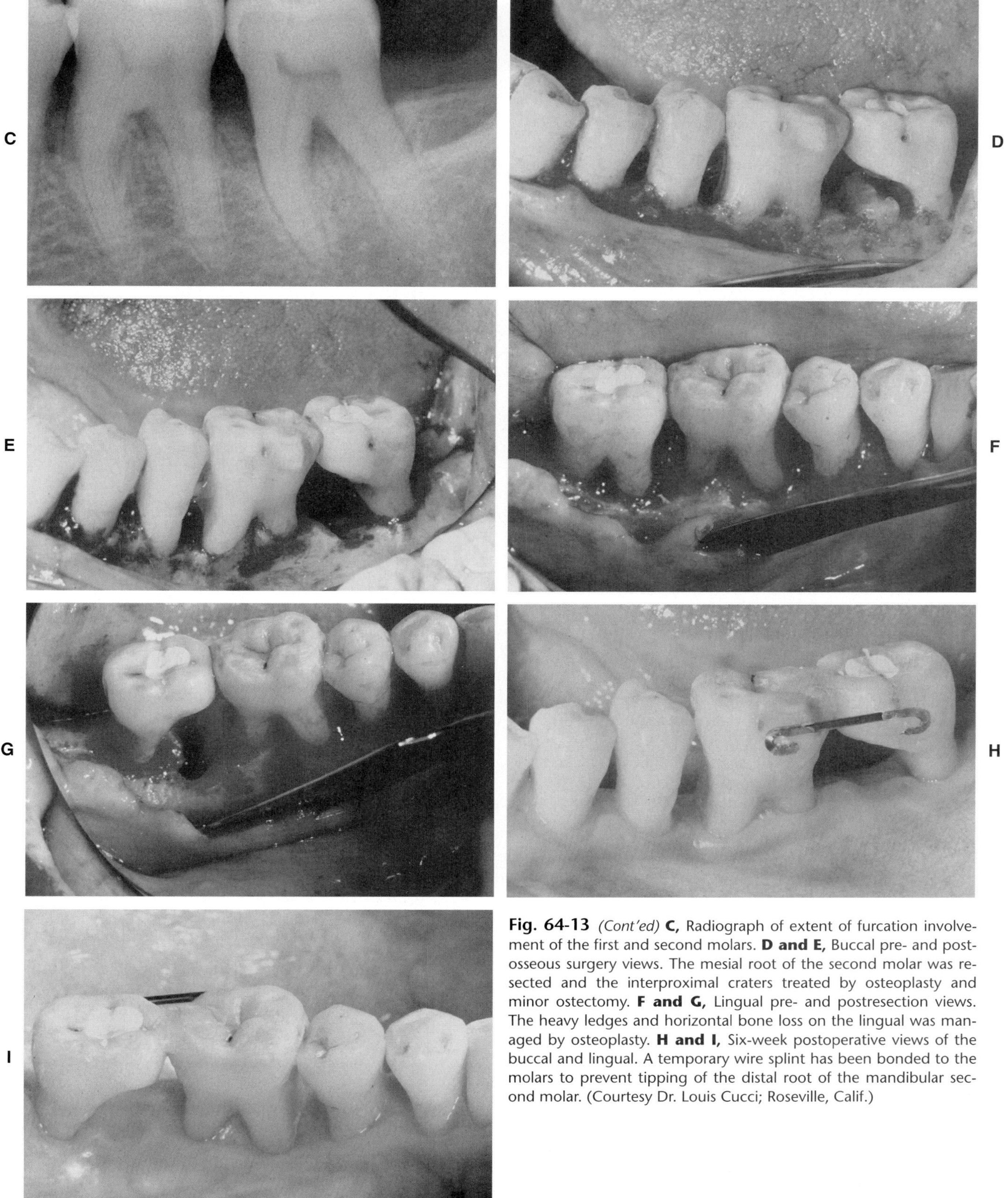

Fig. 64-13 *(Cont'ed)* **C,** Radiograph of extent of furcation involvement of the first and second molars. **D and E,** Buccal pre- and post-osseous surgery views. The mesial root of the second molar was resected and the interproximal craters treated by osteoplasty and minor ostectomy. **F and G,** Lingual pre- and postresection views. The heavy ledges and horizontal bone loss on the lingual was managed by osteoplasty. **H and I,** Six-week postoperative views of the buccal and lingual. A temporary wire splint has been bonded to the molars to prevent tipping of the distal root of the mandibular second molar. (Courtesy Dr. Louis Cucci; Roseville, Calif.)

loss may be the most appropriate therapy for some patients. This is particularly true for individuals who cannot or will not perform adequate plaque control, have a high level of caries activity, will not commit to a suitable maintenance program, or have socioeconomic factors that may preclude more complex therapies. Some patients are reluctant to accept periodontal surgery or even allow the removal of a tooth with advanced furcation involvement even though the long-term prognosis is poor. The patient may elect to forego therapy, opt to treat the area with scaling and root planing or site-specific antibacterial therapies, and delay removal of the tooth until the tooth becomes symptomatic. Although additional attachment loss may occur, it is not uncommon for such teeth to last a significant number of years.[20,31]

The advent of osseointegrated dental implants as an alternative abutment source has had a major impact on the retention of teeth with advanced furcation problems. The high level of predictability of osseointegration may motivate the therapist and patient to consider removal of teeth with a guarded or poor prognosis and to seek an implant-supported prosthetic treatment plan.

PROGNOSIS FOR ROOT RESECTION/HEMISECTION

For many years the presence of significant furcation involvement was deemed to give a tooth a hopeless long-term prognosis. Clinical research, however, has indicated that furcation problems are not as severe a complication as originally suspected if one can prevent the development of caries in the furcation. Relatively simple periodontal therapy is sufficient to maintain these teeth in function for long periods.[20,31] Other investigators have defined the reasons for clinical failure of root-resected or hemisected teeth.[2,24] Their data indicate that recurrent periodontal disease is not a major cause of the failure of these teeth. Investigations of root-resected or hemisected teeth have provided evidence that such teeth can function successfully for long periods.[2,7,24] The keys to long-term success appear to be thorough diagnosis, selection of patients with good oral hygiene, and careful surgical and restorative management.

REFERENCES

1. Bassaraba N: Root amputation and tooth hemisection. Dent Clin N Amer 1969; 13(1):121.
2. Basten CHJ, Ammons WF, Persson R: Long-term evaluation of root resected molars. A retrospective study. Int J Periodontics Restorative Dent 1996; 16(3):207.
3. Becker W, Becker BE, Berg L, et al: New attachment after treatment with root isolation procedures. Report for treated class III and class II furcations and vertical osseous defects. Int J Periodont Restorative Dent 1988; 8(3):9.
4. Black GV: The American System of Dentistry. (Ed: W Litch.) Philadelphia, Lea Brothers, 1886.
5. Bower RC: Furcation morphology relative to periodontal treatment. Furcation root surface anatomy. J Periodontol 1979; 50:366.
6. Bower RC: Furcation morphology relative to periodontal treatment: Furcation entrance architecture. J Periodontol 1979; 50:23.
7. Carnevale G, DiFebo G, Toyelli MP, et al: A retrospective analysis of the periodontal-prosthodontic treatment of molars with interradicular lesions. Int J Periodontics Restorative Dent 1991; 11:188.
8. Demolon IA, Person GR, Ammons WF, et al: Effects of antibiotic treatment on clinical conditions with guided tissue regeneration: one-year results. J Periodontol 1994; 65:713.
9. Easley JR, Drennan GA: Morphological classification of the furca. J Canada Dent Assn 1969; 35(2):104.
10. Everett F, Jump E, Holder T, et al: The intermediate bifurcational ridge: a study of the morphology of the bifurcation of the lower molar. J Dent Res 1958; 37:162.
11. Gher ME, Vernino AR: Root morphology: clinical significance in pathogenesis and treatment of periodontal disease. J Amer Dent Assn 1980; 101:627.
12. Gher ME Jr, Dunlap RW: Linear variation of the root surface area of the maxillary first molar. J Periodontol 1985; 56:39.
13. Glickman I: Clinical Periodontology, ed 1. Philadelphia, Saunders, 1953.
14. Harrington GW: The perio-endo question: differential diagnosis. Dent Clin N Amer 1979; 23(4):673.
15. Goldman HM: Therapy of the incipient bifurcation involvement. J Periodontol 1958; 29:112.
16. Gutmann JL: Prevalence, location and patency of accessory canals in the furcation region of permanent molars. J Periodontol 1978; 49:21.
17. Hamp S-E, Nyman S, Lindhe J: Periodontal treatment of multirooted teeth. Results after 5 years. J Clin Periodontol 1975; 2:126
18. Haskell EW, Stanley HR: A review of vital root resection. Int J Periodont Restorative Dent 1982; 2(6):29.
19. Hermann DW, Gher ME Jr, Dumlap RM, et al: The potential attachment area of the maxillary first molar. J Periodontol 1983; 54:431.
20. Hirschfeld L, Wasserman B: A long-term survey of tooth loss in 600 treated periodontal patients. J Periodontol 1978; 49:225.
21. Hou GL, Tasai CC: Relationship between periodontal furcation involvement and molar cervical enamel projection. J Periodontol 1978; 58:715.
22. Kalkwarf K, Kaldahl W, Patil K, et al: Evaluation of furcation region response to periodontal therapy. J Periodontol 1988; 59:794.
23. Kenney EB, Lekovic V, Elbaz JJ, et al: The use of porous hydroxylapatite implants in periodontal defects. II. Treatment of class II furcation lesions in lower molars. J Periodontol 1988; 59:67.
24. Langer B, Stein SD, Wagenberg B: An evaluation of root resections. A ten-year study. J Periodontol 1981; 52:719.
25. Larato DC: Some anatomical factors related to furcation involvement. J Periodontol 1975; 46:608.
26. Matia JB, Bissada NF, Maybury JE, et al: Efficiency of scaling of the molar furcation area with and without surgical access. Int J Periodont Restorative Dent 1986; 6(6):25.
27. Masters DH, Hoskins SW: Projection of cervical enamel into molar furcations. J Periodontol 1964; 35:49.
28. Mealy BL, Beybayer MF, Butzin CA, et al: Use of furcal bone sounding to improve accuracy of furcation diagnosis. J Periodontol 1994; 65:649.
29. Metzler DG, Seamons BC, Mellonig JT, et al: Clinical evaluation of guided tissue regeneration in the treatment of maxillary class II molar furcation. J Periodontol 1991; 62:353.
30. Parashis AO, Anognou-Vareltzides A, Demetrious N: Calculus removal from multirooted teeth with and without surgical access. I. Efficacy on external and furcation surfaces in relation to probing depth. J Clin Periodontol 1993; 20:63.

31. Ross I, Thompson RH: A long-term study of root retention of maxillary molars with furcation involvement. J Periodontol 1978; 49:238.
32. Tal H: Furcal bony defects in dry mandibles. I. Biometric study. J Periodontol 1982; 53:360.
33. Tal H, Lemmer J: Furcal defects in dry mandibles. II. Severity of furcal defects. J Periodontol 1982; 53:364.
34. Tarnow D, Fletcher P: Classification of the vertical component of furcation involvement. J Periodontol 1984; 55:283.
35. Tibbetts LF: Use of diagnostic probes for detection of periodontal disease. J Amer Dent Assn 1969; 78:549.
36. Wylam JM, Mealey B, Mills MP, et al: The clinical effectiveness of open versus closed scaling and root planing on multi-rooted teeth. J Periodontol 1993; 64:1023.

The Periodontic-Endodontic Continuum

William F. Ammons, Jr. and Gerald W. Harrington

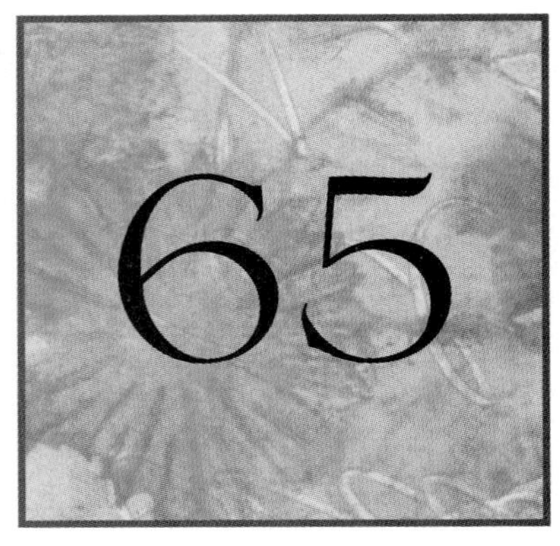

CHAPTER

CHAPTER OUTLINE

The simultaneous existence of pulpal problems and inflammatory periodontal disease can complicate diagnosis and treatment planning and affect the sequence of care to be performed. This is particularly true for the patient with advanced periodontitis, tooth loss and pulpal disease.

ETIOLOGIC FACTORS OF PULPAL DISEASE

The major causes of pulpal inflammation are 1) instrumentation during periodontal, restorative or prosthetic dentistry; 2) the progression of dental caries; and 3) direct, local trauma such as tooth fracture. The extent of inflammation of the pulp and the signs and symptoms that result vary with the severity of the insult and the ability of the host to ameliorate the inflammation that results.

Of these, dental caries is the most common cause of pulpal disease. Bacteria are present in carious enamel and dentin. Although the numbers of bacteria may diminish in the deepest layers of the dentin, the ability of microorganisms and their by-products to penetrate through the dentinal tubules and to provoke pulpal inflammation is well documented.[6,7] Direct exposure of the pulp by caries[21] or sealing infected pulps may alter the process of infection if the pulp is unable to eliminate the bacteria.[6,20] The dynamics of the pulpal reaction is dictated by the virulence of the bacteria, the host response, the effectiveness of pulpal circulation, and the degree of vascular and lymphatic drainage.[42]

Pulpal infection is a polymicrobial process. Although a correlation between causation and any species of bacteria is not currently possible,[2] studies based on culturing suggest that a mean of five bacterial strains may be cultured from infected root canals.[3] The organisms cultured are predominately gram-negative anaerobes.[2,3,10,13,38] As the infective process proceeds the proportion of strict anaerobic-to-facultative organisms and the total number of bacteria increases. The most common organisms associated with pulpitis are listed in Table 65-1.

TABLE 65-1

Bacteria Associated with Pulpitis

Bacteria	Number of Strains	Gram Stain
Eubacterium ssp.	59	Gram-positive, nonmotile
Peptostreptococcus ssp.	54	Gram-positive, nonmotile
Fusobacterium ssp.	50	Gram-negative, nonmotile
Prophyromonas ssp.	32	Gram-negative, nonmotile
Prevotella spp.	45	Gram-negative, nonmotile
Streptococcus spp.	28	Gram-positive, nonmotile
Lactobacillus spp.	24	Gram-positive, nonmotile
Wolinella spp.	18	Gram-negative, motile
Actinomyces spp.	14	Gram-positive rod, nonmotile

Modified from Sundqvist G, Johansson E, Sjogren U: Prevalence of black-pigmented bacteroides species in root canal infections. J Endodon 1989; 15(1):13; and Baumgartner JC, Falkler WA: Bacteria in the apical 5 mm of infected root canals. J Endodon 1991; 17(8):380.

CLASSIFICATION OF PULPAL DISEASE

The correlation between the histology of pulpal disease and the patient's symptoms is poor. Therefore pulpal disease is generally classified based on clinical signs and symptoms rather than on histologic changes.[20,41] Such a classification is illustrated in Box 65-1.

Minor injury such as periodontal root planing or the conservative preparation of a tooth for a restoration may lead to pulpal symptoms. A transient hypersensitivity to thermal stimuli is the most common symptom noted. The application of a thermal stimulus results in a brief, painful response that varies in intensity from mild to severe. The response rapidly disappears after removal of the stimulus. Although permanent pulpal damage may not occur, a transient inflammatory response can lead to the deposition of reparative dentin if odontoblasts are destroyed. The reversibility of inflammation and symptoms, without permanent pulpal damage, has led to a classification of this condition as **reversible pulpitis.**

If the pulp is so affected that the inflammatory lesion cannot be resolved, even though the source of the trauma is eliminated, a progressive degeneration of the pulp results. This progression has been described as being an *irreversible pulpitis.* Irreversible pulpitis may be void of symptoms or it may be associated with intermittent or continuous episodes of spontaneous pain. The application of heat to a tooth with irreversible pulpitis can lead to an immediate painful response that can persist for a prolonged period. Cold may also provoke such a response, although occasionally, the application of cold may provide relief from the pain. A reduced responsiveness of teeth with irreversible pulpitis to thermal stimuli has been claimed, but Mumford found similar pain thresholds in both inflamed and noninflamed pulps.[26]

Irreversible pulpitis ultimately leads to loss of pulpal vitality (necrosis). Necrosis usually results from the same factors that induced the irreversible pulpitis and may lead to an alteration in the patient's symptoms. Not all nonvital teeth display signs and symptoms of pulpal disease and necrotic pulps are commonly asymptomatic. When symptoms do occur, they may be manifested as episodes of spontaneous pain. Testing the pulp with heat may be inconclusive, and a response to cold stimuli is rare.

BOX 65-1

Classification of Pulpal Disease

Reversible pulpitis
Irreversible pulpitis
Hyperplastic pulpitis
Pulpal necrosis

EFFECTS OF PULPAL DISEASE ON THE PERIODONTIUM

Pulpal tissue may be significantly inflamed and yet exert little or no effect on the periodontium. As long as the pulp remains vital it is unlikely that significant changes will occur in the periodontium. Necrosis of the pulp, however, can result in bone resorption and the production of radiolucency at the apex of the tooth, in the furcation or at points along the root[25,34,41,43] (Fig. 65-1). Dental radiographs usually document the presence of apical or lateral lesions.

The lesion that results may be an acute apical lesion or abscess, a more chronic periradicular lesion (cyst or granuloma); or a lesion associated with a lateral or accessory canal. The lesion may remain small, or it can expand sufficiently to destroy a substantial amount of the attachment of the tooth and/or to communicate with a lesion of periodontitis. A classification of periradicular lesions is found in Box 65-2.

The histopathologic structure of the periapical inflammatory lesion is usually a highly vascularized granulation tissue infiltrated to varying degrees by inflammatory cells. Neutrophils may be present near the apical foramen, whereas plasma cells, macrophages, lymphocytes and fibroblasts are increased in the periphery of the lesion.[5,28,39,44] This cellular infiltrate may vary with the nature and intensity of the irritants to the tissues.

Similar lesions may develop adjacent to accessory or lateral canals. These canals form when the epithelial root sheath breaks down before root formation or anasto-

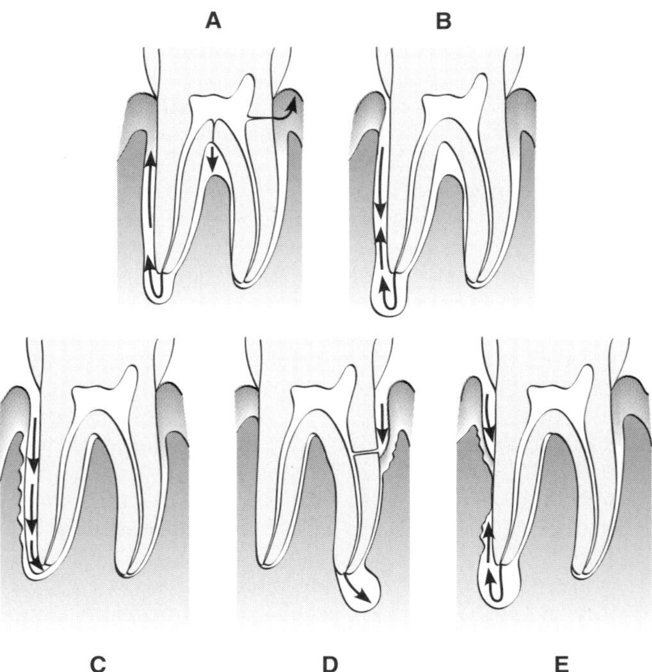

Fig. 65-1 Diagrammatic representation of different types of endoperiodontal problems. **A,** An originally endodontic problem with fistulization from the apex and along the root to the gingiva. Pulpal infection can also spread through accessory canals to the gingiva or to the furcation. **B,** A long-standing periapical lesion draining through the periodontal ligament can become secondarily complicated, leading to a *retrograde periodontitis.* **C,** A periodontal pocket can deepen to the apex and secondarily involve the pulp. **D,** A periodontal pocket can infect the pulp through a lateral canal, and this, in turn, can result in a periapical lesion. **E,** Two independent lesions, periapical and marginal, can coexist and eventually fuse with each other. (Redrawn and modified from Simon JHS, Glick DH, Frank AL: The relationship of endodontic-periodontic lesions. J Periodontol 1972; 43:202.)

BOX 65-2

Classification of Periradicular Lesions

Acute apical periodontitis
Chronic apical periodontitis
Condensing osteitis
Acute apical abscess
Chronic apical abscess

moses between the dental papilla and the dental sac persist. Although many of the anastomoses are blocked or reduced by the formation of dentin or the depositing of cementum, some of the communications between the pulp and periodontium may remain patent in the adult dentition. Lateral canals are usually not visible on x-rays and are most commonly identified only when the root and lateral canal has been filled with a radiopaque material during endodontic therapy

The incidence of accessory and/or lateral canals has been quoted as ranging from 2% to 27%, but the true incidence is unknown.[9,12,43] The majority of these canals occur in the apical portion of the root, with decreased numbers in the furcation area. They are more common in posterior teeth and in the apical portion of the root.[9,22,33] The prevalence of lateral canals in the middle and cervical areas of the root and the prevalence of endodontic-derived lesions in the marginal periodontium via lateral or accessory canals are low. The clinical significance of accessory or lateral canals in spreading infection from the necrotic pulp to the periodontium is therefore unclear. Necrotic pulps apparently exert no effect through the dentinal tubules on the cementum.[1]

EFFECT OF PERIODONTITIS ON THE DENTAL PULP

Although the effects of pulpal disease on the periodontium are well documented, a clear-cut relationship between periodontitis and pulpal involvement is less evident. One may postulate that bacterial and the inflammatory products of periodontitis could gain access to the pulp via accessory canals, apical foramina, or dentinal tubules. This process, the reverse of the effects of a necrotic pulp on the periodontal ligament, has been referred to as *retrograde pulpitis*.[31,35]

However, although inflammatory changes have been reported adjacent to accessory canals exposed by periodontitis, periodontitis rarely produces significant changes in the dental pulp. Neither irreversible pulpitis or pulpal necrosis has been consistently found in histologic studies of teeth extracted because of severe periodontal disease.[8,20,40] It has been suggested that the presence of an intact layer of cementum may protect the pulp from injurious elements produced by plaque microbiota.[1] Severe breakdown of the pulp apparently does not occur until periodontitis has reached a terminal state—that is, when bacterial plaque has involved the main apical foramina.[20] The pulp has a good capacity for defense as long as the blood supply via the apical foramina is intact. Therefore retrograde periodontitis, if it occurs, is exceedingly rare.[14,15,40]

DIFFERENTIATION OF PERIODONTAL AND PULPAL LESIONS

The Signs and Symptoms of Periodontitis

The signs and symptoms of periodontitis are described in Chapters 26 to 28 of this text. Periodontitis is a chronic inflammatory lesion, which begins in the marginal gingiva and extends apically causing attachment loss and periodontal pocket formation In general the progression rate of attachment loss is slow, unless an acute incident such as a periodontal abscess occurs.

Teeth with chronic periodontal lesions are commonly free of acute symptoms. The patient may indeed be unaware of the condition, with the exception of bleeding on brushing and flossing, or bad breath, until sufficient attachment is lost, resulting in increased tooth mobility. The pocket may be tender to probing and extensive deposits may be present on the root(s) of the tooth/teeth. Probing is usually accompanied by bleeding and in deeper pockets with suppuration. However, significant discomfort is not elicited by percussion or thermal stimuli. Increased tooth mobility may occur if sufficient attachment has been lost. Dental radiographs usually disclose the extent of attachment loss, which should correlate with clinical probing data.

The Signs and Symptoms of Pulpal Disease

The pulp has the ability to respond to stimulation through enamel or dentin, or directly to the pulp. Higher nerve centers interpret these sensations as pain. There is some evidence that the pulp may also sense temperature and touch,[27] although the ability to discriminate between hot and cold may be affected by age.[19] The character of the pain may vary with its source. Pulpal sensation initiation by the stimulation of dentin is usually fast, sharp, and severe and is mediated by A-delta myelinated fibers. Sensation from the core of the pulp is initiated by smaller unmyelinated C fibers. This pain has been described as being slower, duller, and more diffuse.[27]

The only symptom a patient with reversible pulpitis may report is a sensitivity to hot or cold fluids. The period of discomfort is usually brief. Teeth in which the inflammation is confined to the pulp chamber respond normally to percussion and palpation. Thermal stimuli or percussion applied to teeth with irreversible pulpitis can provoke severe pain. This pain may be intense and is commonly described as bright or throbbing. When provoked, a significant period and/or the use of medications may be required before the pain is ameliorated. The progression of inflammation alters the response of the tooth to pulp testing. If the inflammatory process extends to involve the periodontal ligament, then the affected tooth can become tender to pressure, biting, or light tapping with an instrument. Necrosis of the pulp can result in bony resorption. Thus pulp death may result in radiolucency at the apex of the tooth, in the furcation,[15,41] or at points along the root (see Fig. 65-1). The ability of inflammatory periodontal disease to affect the pulp is much less certain.[8,40] Dental radiographs usually document the presence of apical or lateral lesions. However, it should be remembered that some inflamed and/or necrotic pulps are asymptomatic and the patient is unaware of their existence.

DIFFERENTIATION BETWEEN PULPAL AND PERIODONTAL ABSCESSES

Periodontal abscesses (see Chapter 22) are not usually severely painful lesions. They occur in the pocket or sulcus at the level of the connective tissue attachment, so there is little or no elevation of the periosteum to cause significant pain. The patient becomes aware of a sore or tender area in the gingiva and may notice swelling of the tissues to form a lump. This area may be sensitive to touch, mastication, or toothbrushing and/or flossing. Any stimulus to the site can indeed be painful. The formation of a fistula is less common than with apical periodontitis. If a fistula does form, it may be found in both the gingiva and mucosa. The path of the sinus tract can be determined by carefully placing a fine gutta percha point into the fistula and then making a radiograph. The point communicates with and stops within the periodontal pocket. Careful probing confirms the presence of the pocket, and dilation of the sulcus commonly results in drainage.

Acute apical abscesses commonly communicate directly with the external soft tissue surface by a sinus tract and a stoma through the oral mucosa or gingiva (Fig. 65-2). Before the completion of the tract, the patient commonly experiences acutely painful symptoms as a result of the involvement of the periodontal ligament. The tract may exit through the periodontium and dissect along the root to empty into the gingival sulcus and the interfurcal area. It then goes through the periodontal ligament of an adjacent tooth or into an existing periodontal pocket (see Fig. 65-1). When the latter occurs, the resulting defect is a true *combined lesion.*[14,31,35]

Acute apical abscesses can extend to involve the adjacent periodontium. The sinus tract that forms usually extends from the apex of the tooth to the buccal [word missing]; hence, the mandible and maxillary curvature results in thin plates of bone at these sites. Although palatal or lingual tracts do occur, they occur at a much lower frequency than buccal tracts. During formation of a sinus tract, the patient may experience extreme pain because of involvement of the periodontal ligament and the elevation of the periosteum. Perforation of the plate is accompanied by swelling, pus formation, and collection under the periosteum. The swelling that results can lead to substantial alterations in the appearance of the face, as substantial volumes of pus may be confined in the lesion. Ultimately, drainage is established via a stoma. As long as the sinus remains open and drainage occurs, the symptoms and signs may be diminished. The acute inflammatory response may then take on the characteristics of a chronic lesion.

The endodontic sinus tract is usually a narrow, constricted lesion directed from the apex of the tooth laterally. In the absence of inflammatory periodontal disease, a tract emptying into the sulcus exerts little effect on the

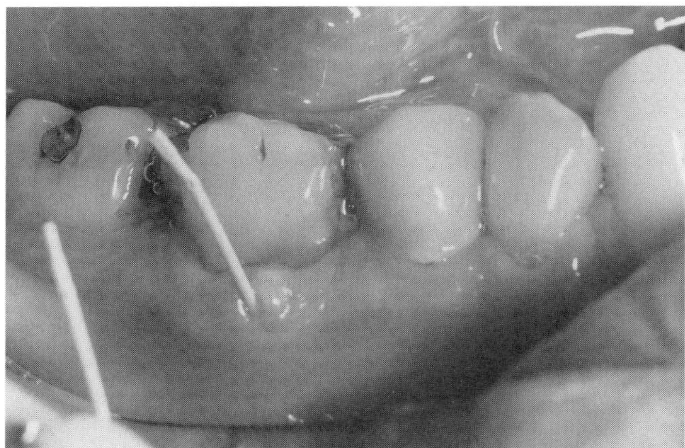

Fig. 65-2 Gutta percha point inserted into a stoma located near the junction of the gingiva and oral mucosa on a mandibular first molar. This molar tested nonvital.

remainder of the sulcus. Prichard stated that the "pulpal lesion does not change its character and become marginal periodontitis when it reaches the bony crest or gingival margin, and the pulp does not immediately or inevitably become infected when bone resorption from marginal periodontitis reaches the apex."[31] Both endodontic and periodontal lesions may, however, result in attachment loss that affects the furcation[15,31] and/or the apex of the tooth.[25]

THERAPEUTIC MANAGEMENT OF PULPAL AND PERIODONTAL DISEASE

Patients with pulpal disease may have a healthy periodontium, gingivitis, or varying amounts of attachment loss (periodontitis) on the affected or adjacent teeth. A host of other dental problems may also exist. Therefore, appropriate treatment varies with the presence, nature, and extent of involvement of the diseases.

ENDODONTIC LESION PRIMARY

Patients with pulpal disease present only diagnostic and treatment decisions relative to the endodontic lesion. Débridement of the pulp chamber and canal, as well as the completion of appropriate endodontic therapy, are sufficient to result in healing of the lesion (Fig. 65-3, *A and B*). Pulpal abscesses and apical lesions generally resolve with conventional therapy, although apical surgery may be required in certain instances. Periodontal treatment is not required in the absence of any periodontal involvement.

Occasionally, an abscess of pulpal origin, through an apical or lateral canal, may establish drainage through the periodontal ligament and erupt into the furcation or the gingival sulcus.[12,15,31,34] The signs and symptoms of this process are identical to the initial signs and symptoms of abscesses establishing a path in a more horizontal direction, with the exception that a fistula is not evident. Therefore it becomes necessary to separate the signs and symptoms of pulpal disease from those associated with a periodontal abscess. The patient's history, periodontal probing, radiographs, and pulpal testing are therefore consistent with pulpal disease. Root canal treatment resolves any tract or stoma that is present.

INDEPENDENT PERIODONTAL AND ENDODONTIC LESIONS

Patients with pulpal disease may also present with inflammatory periodontal disease. Gingivitis or early periodontitis, other than tenderness, bleeding on brushing, or probing, commonly results in little discomfort. Pulpal disease, however, is associated with more noxious signs and symptoms. The progress of periodontitis is slow, with the exception of acute disease such as periodontal abscesses or necrotizing ulcerative gingivitis. Therefore the prompt management of the pulpal lesion is the primary concern. Pulpal extirpation and filling of the canals is the proper course of therapy, since extirpation of the pulp usually leads to the elimination of the patient's acute symptoms. Although residual sensitivity to percussion or movement of the tooth may persist for a period, therapy for gingivitis or early periodontitis may

A

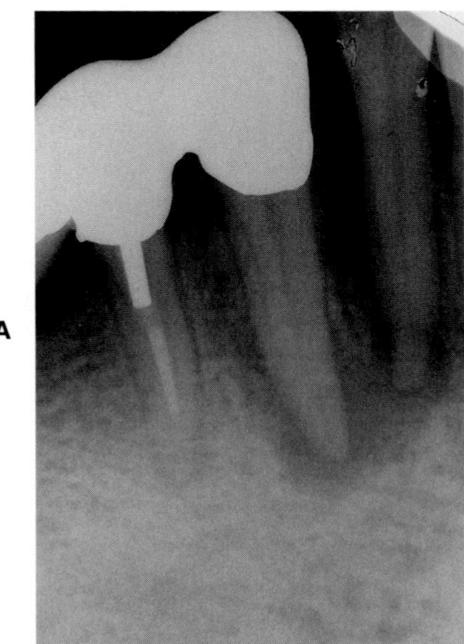

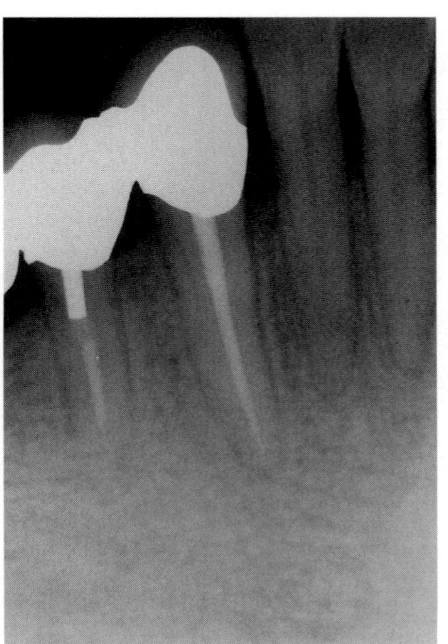

B

Fig. 65-3 Radiographs of suspected combined lesion (perio-endo lesion) on a maxillary cuspid and lateral incisor. **A,** Notice the advanced bone loss on the distal of the lateral incisor and the possible extension of the apical lesion to involve the maxillary canine. **B,** Posttreatment response. This canine was treated by a root canal procedure only. The lesion was of pulpal origin, and repair occurred following pulp extirpation and treatment.

be delayed until the acute symptoms of pulpal disease are alleviated.

A different scenario may result if a patient with chronic periodontitis experiences a loss of pulpal vitality. Such a patient may simultaneously have the clinical signs and symptoms of both periodontitis and apical periodontitis. The extent to which each can affect the tooth is both independent and variable. The involvement of the apical periodontium by a pulpal lesion may obscure the symptoms of periodontitis. Therefore the ability to determine the independence of the two lesions on any tooth or area is a key consideration in the sequence of therapy. Most commonly the lesions are independent and do not communicate (Fig. 65-4, *A–D*).

Rarely a patient may present with abscesses of both pulpal and periodontal origin (Fig. 65-5, *A–C*). As the apical lesion tends to be the most painful lesion, endodontic therapy is normally initiated before or at the same appointment at which the periodontal abscess is drained. Again, the patient's history and thorough probing allows a determination of the extent of each problem and the independence of the two defects. Endodontic therapy results in the resolution of the endodontic lesion. It will, however, have little or no effect on the periodontal pocket (see Fig. 65-5, *C*), and appropriate periodontal therapy will be required for a successful result.[16,17,31]

COMBINED LESIONS (PERIO-ENDO)

The true combined lesion results from the development and extension of an endodontic lesion into an existing periodontal lesion (pocket).[14,31] Such lesions may present with the characteristics of both diseases, which may complicate diagnosis and treatment sequencing (Fig. 65-6, *A and B*). A thorough history and careful clinical and radiographic examinations are required to identify and accurately assess the contribution of each lesion to the patient's dental problems and to derive a treatment sequence that is likely to produce an optimal therapeutic result. Usually the developing periapical lesion extends coronally to connect with a preexisting, chronic, wide-based periodontal pocket. On rare occasions a developing periodontal lesion, associated with a developmental groove, may extend apically to connect with an apical or

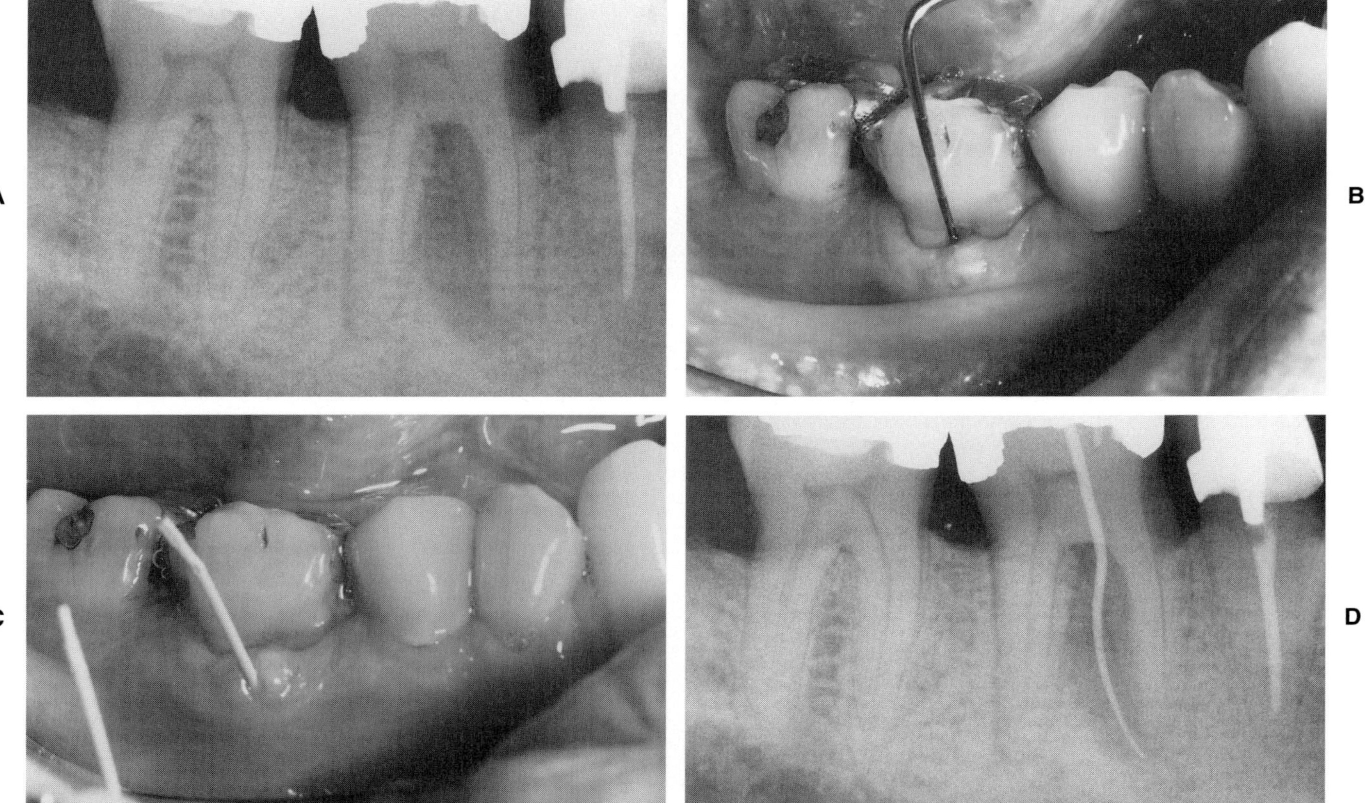

Fig. 65-4 Independent periodontal and endodontic lesions. **A,** Radiograph of the mandibular left molars. Note the radiographic appearance of bone loss on the first and second molars, a possible cervical enamel projection on the first molar, and a large interradicular area of reduced bone density. **B,** Periodontal probe inserted in buccal furcation of no. 19. Note the adjacent stoma. Observe that the sulcus depth is 3 mm at this site. **C,** Gutta percha point inserted into the facial stoma. **D,** Note the gutta percha point enters the furcation defect and extends to the apex of the mesial root of the molar. Although the molar displays signs consistent with periodontitis, the interradicular defect is purely of endodontic origin.

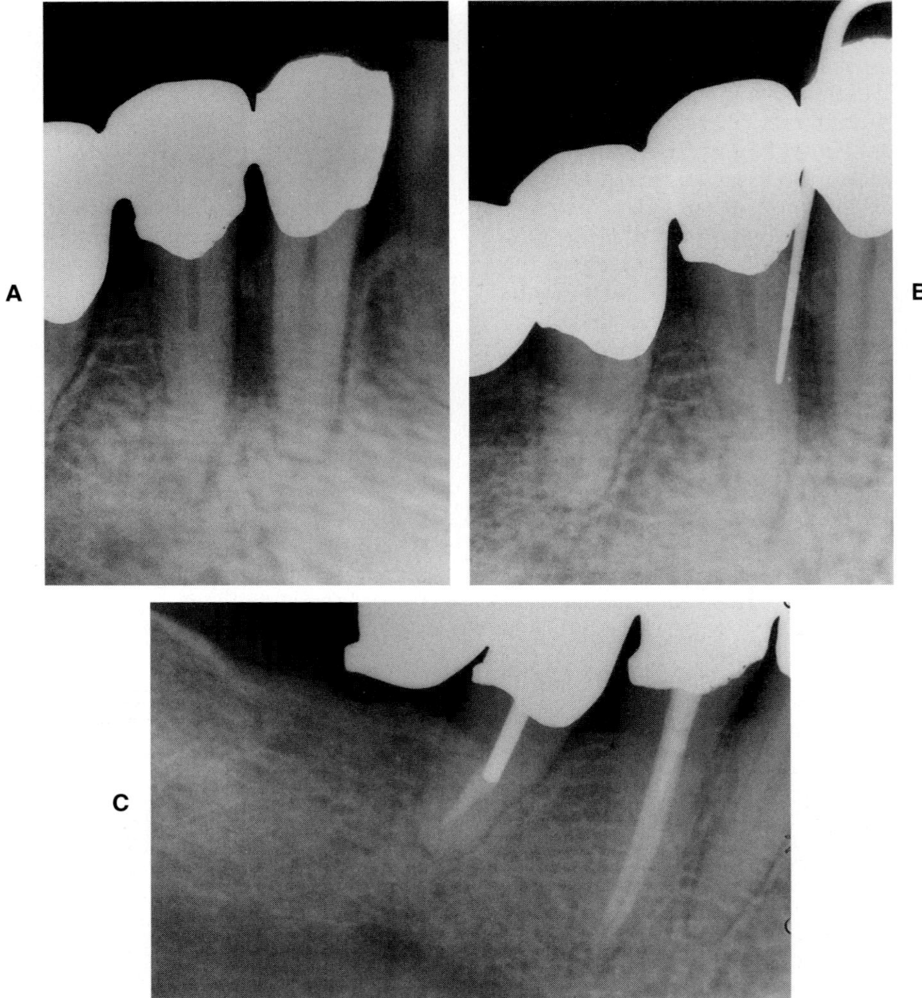

Fig. 65-5 Independent periodontal-endodontic abscesses. **A,** Radiograph of a mandibular left cuspid-bicuspid area. The patient presented with a large abscess involving all three teeth. Note the signs of marginal bone loss on the teeth, along with the area of decreased bone density at the mesial of the mandibular left first bicuspid and the apparent calcification of the pulp canals. **B,** Radiograph with periodontal probe inserted into the mesio-lingual sulcus. There was, however, no communication with the mesial radiolucent area. **C,** Radiograph taken 6 months postendodontic treatment. Note the resolution of the mesial radiolucent area. The periodontal abscess was débrided, but the residual bony deformities remain.

lateral endodontic lesion. It also has been suggested that if periodontitis progresses to involve a lateral canal or the apex of a tooth, then a secondary pulpal infection may be induced. This is referred to as *retrograde pulpitis*. Retrograde pulpitis, if it exists, is quite rare.[8,14,15,35,40]

The pain from the loss of pulpal vitality is the most common presenting complaint of patients with combined lesions. The symptoms reported are those most commonly found with pulpal disease. Thermal pulp testing provides information relative to the status of the pulp, and dental radiographs can confirm the presence of apical changes and the extent of bone loss. Careful probing confirms the presence and morphology of any periodontal pocket and permits the location of the communication with the apical lesion. The periodontal portion of the defect commonly has plaque, calculus, and/or root roughness as a finding.[31] This contaminated root surface and the associated osseous defect is the major complication to treatment of combined lesions.

The extent to which the periodontal lesion contributes to the loss of bone is a key consideration in diagnosis and treatment planning. Endodontic treatment is highly predictable,[36] and when appropriately performed, the alterations in radiographic appearance and clinical probing disappear (Fig. 65-3). The periodontal component of a combined lesion is a more difficult problem. It cannot resolve as long as the endodontic lesion is present, yet effective endodontic treatment cannot eliminate the periodontal pocket. Even with periodontal treatment, the periodontal defect commonly does not resolve to the same extent that the endodontic lesion does (Fig. 65-6, *A and B*). The ability to eliminate the periodontal component of the defect ultimately dictates treatment of the tooth. If the majority of the bony support has been lost from periodontitis, regardless of the predictability of endodontic therapy, the tooth may have a hopeless prognosis.

Once the decision to retain the tooth is made, endodontic therapy should precede attempts at periodontal pocket elimination.[14] After successful endodontics, the residual periodontal pocket that remains can be more predictably treated. The periodontal therapeutic objectives vary with the extent and configuration of the residual periodontal lesion. The elimination of etiologic factors, alterations in the depth and configuration of the pocket, and the facilitation of restorative dentistry may all be legitimate objectives. Thus periodontal treatment may include scaling and root planing, as well as various surgical treatments. If the endodontic lesion requires apical surgery, then the surgical treatment of both apical and periodontal lesions may be accomplished simultaneously.

PROGNOSIS OF COMBINED LESIONS

With proper treatment the healing of an endodontic lesion is highly predictable. However, the prognosis for teeth with combined lesions varies with the extent that each lesion contributes to the loss of attachment. Lesions resulting from pulpal disease tend to resolve with endodontic therapy, whereas the repair/regeneration of attachment loss from periodontitis is less predictable. The long-term prognosis for a tooth with a combined lesion is therefore closely related to the extent and configuration of the periodontal attachment loss. With advanced horizontal attachment loss, even an optimal endodontic result may not be sufficient to retain the tooth as a functioning member of the dentition. If the periodontal lesion is an advanced, multiwalled bony defect, the success of therapy likely depends on the ability to fill or regenerate attachment to obliterate the defect. Therefore the decision to treat and retain teeth with combined periodontal and endodontic lesions should be carefully considered in regard to the overall dental treatment plan as the time and cost of combined defect treatment may be considerable.

POTENTIAL COMPLICATIONS TO ENDODONTIC THERAPY

As with any therapeutic modality, complications may arise during endodontic treatment. Some are of an iatrogenic nature such as perforations of the floor of the pulp chamber or the root during access, canal instrumentation or preparation for a post (Fig. 65-7). These accidents may result in periodontal defects, and treatment should be instituted as soon as the perforation occurs. The healing of the lesion that occurs in the periodontium depends on whether bacterial infection can be excluded from the wound area by obturation of the site of perforation.[4,29] If the perforation occurs in the cervical area of the tooth, a surgical flap approach may provide sufficient access to expose the perforation and allow a successful seal. However, because of the difficulty in sealing a lateral perforation of the root, a guarded prognosis should be given to such a tooth.

Additional problems are root resorption and vertical root fracture. Resorption may be of an internal or external nature. External resorption may follow impact injuries such as luxation or tooth avulsion and is most commonly seen after reimplantation.

Vertical root fractures are fractures oriented more or less longitudinally toward the apex of the tooth. The cause and prevalence of such fractures is not clearly established. However, such fractures may result during canal obturation, pin or post placement, or cementation of intracoronal restorations.[23,24] In some cases, they appear to

A

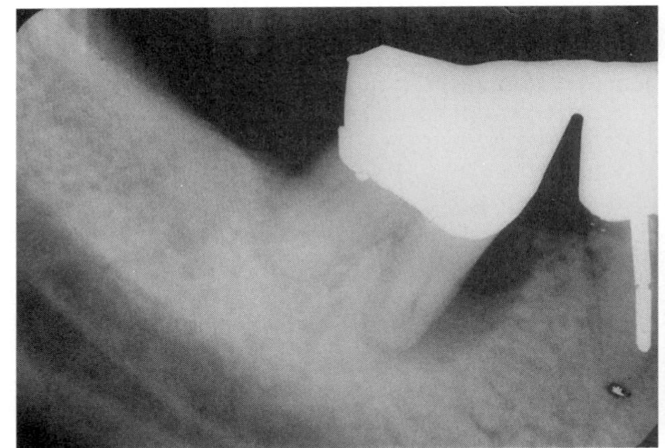

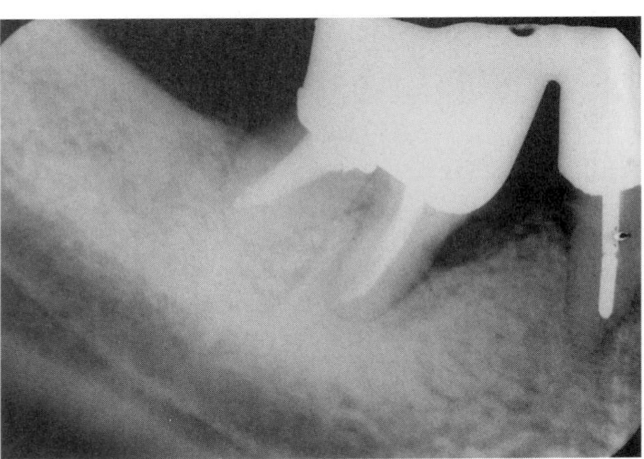

B

Fig. 65-6 Periodontal-endodontic lesion on a mandibular second molar. **A,** Pretreatment radiograph of a deep combination one- and two-walled bony defect on the mesial root of the second molar. Note the apparent involvement of the apex of the mesial root. **B,** Postendodontic therapy. The performance of the root canal has resulted in repair of the endodontic component of the defect. The periodontal component of the defect shows little change. The residual bony defect will require periodontal therapy. This is a "true" perio-endo lesion.

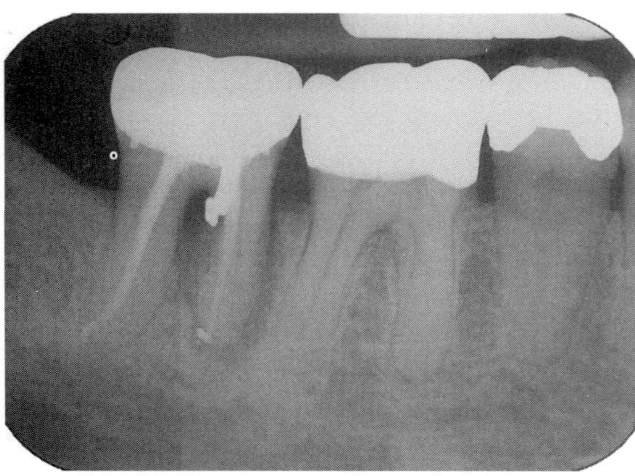

Fig. 65-7 Radiograph of mandibular right molar area. Endodontic perforation into the furcation area on the mesial root of a mandibular second molar. The curvature and deep distal fluting on the mesial root of mandibular molars increases the risk of inadvertant root perforation.

A

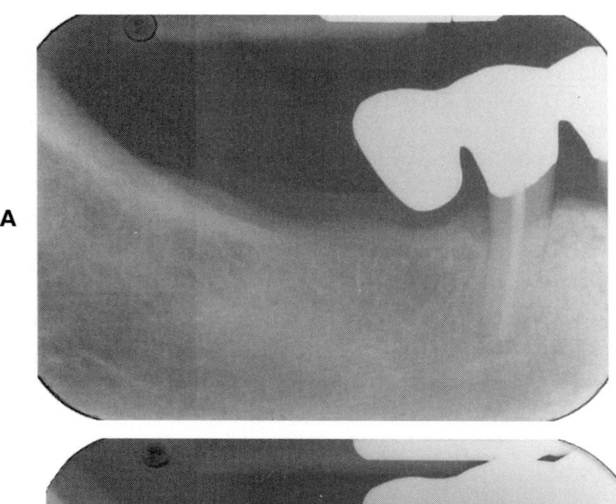

B

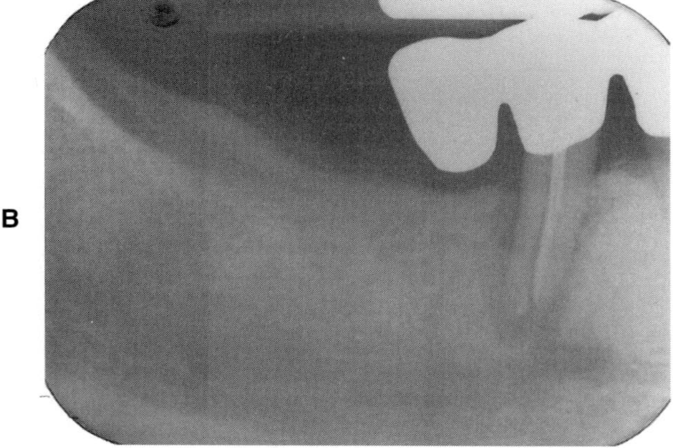

Fig. 65-8 Vertical root fractures. **A,** Radiograph of mandibular left second bicuspid with a cantilevered pontic. This tooth shows evidence of periodontal attachment loss at the mesial and distal surfaces and an apparent widening of the periodontal ligament space. **B,** Radiograph of the same bicuspid six months later. Note the advanced loss of attachment and the radiographic signs of a vertical root fracture (separation of fragments). The sectioning of the bridge and removal of the tooth was required.

A

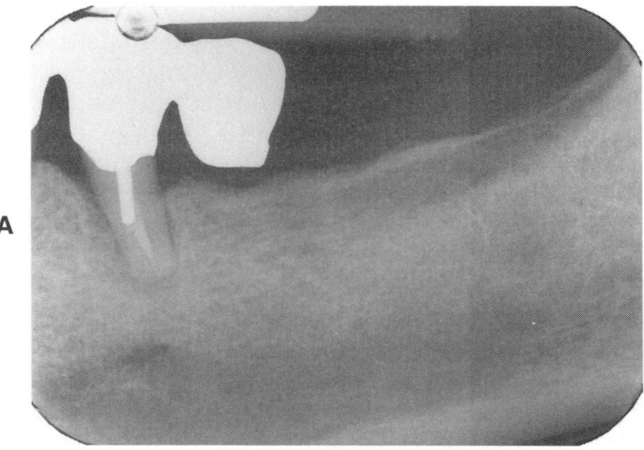

B

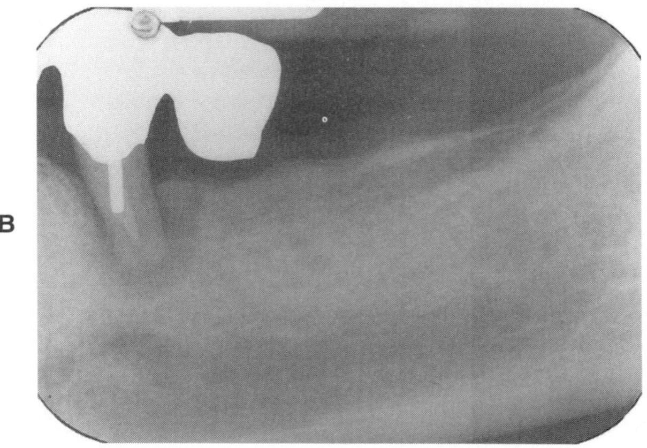

Fig. 65-9 Radiographs of vertical root fracture. **A,** Radiograph of the mandibular right second molar in the same patient as Fig. 65-8. The bicuspid, supporting a cantilevered pontic, has an endodontic post in the root. It also has radiographic evidence of loss of periodontal attachment and widening of the periodontal ligament space. Note the apical halolike radiolucency. **B,** Radiograph of no. 29 taken 10 months later showing advanced attachment loss around the apical area of the root and evidence of vertical root fracture. This tooth also required extraction.

occur spontaneously. They appear to occur more commonly in teeth treated with endodontics than in nonendodontically treated teeth. It has been postulated that endodontic treatment may result in the teeth becoming more brittle and less resistant to forces of mastication.

These fractures may occur years after endodontic treatment[23] and are not readily visible in radiographs unless the fragments are separated (Fig. 65-8, *A and B*). It has been suggested that a thin, halolike apical radiolucency is an indication of vertical root fracture[30] (Fig. 65-9, *A and B*). Fractures are often inferred from symptoms of pain or tenderness on mastication or the development of a localized periodontal defect or sinus tract that cannot be explained by other clinical findings. Both the application of an iodine stain or plaque-disclosing solution and indirect illumination are also useful diagnostic measures. However surgical exposure and direct visual examination is sometimes required to confirm the fracture. Vertical root fracture generally results in a hopeless prognosis for the affected root.

RESTORATIVE IMPLICATIONS OF ENDODONTIC THERAPY

Ultimately, most root canal–treated teeth require restorations. Although the initial success rate for endodontics is quite high,[36] the long-term retention and function is dependent on, to a great extent, the ability to adequately restore the tooth. Restoration is complicated by the extent of crown loss from caries, fracture, and the size and placement of the access to the pulp chamber.[18] Additional factors are the type of restoration to be used, the configuration and number of the pulp canals, root form, and the need for a post and core.[7,11,24,32,37] Although severely decayed and/or fractured teeth can often be successfully treated endodontically, such teeth may require periodontal surgery and yet be difficult or impossible to restore. Complex interdisciplinary treatment should be confined to teeth that are of critical importance to the overall treatment plan after due consideration of alternate treatment methods.

REFERENCES

1. Armitage GC, Ryder MI, Wilcox SE: Cemental changes in teeth with heavily infected root canals. J Endodon 1983; 9(2):127.
2. Baumgartner JC: Endodontic microbiology. In: Walton RE, Torabinejad M (eds): Principles and Practice of Endodontics, ed 3. Philadelphia, Saunders, 2002.
3. Baumgartner JC, Falkler WA: Bacteria in the apical 5 mm of infected root canals. J Endodon 1991; 17(8):380.
4. Beavers RA, Bergenholtz G, Cox CF: Periodontal wound healing following intentional root perforation in permanent teeth of Macaca mulatta. Int J Endodont 1986; 19:36.
5. Bergenholtz G, Lekholm U, Liljenberg B, et al: Morphometric analysis of chronic inflammatory periapical lesions in root-filled teeth. Oral Surg Oral Med Oral Pathol 1983; 55(3):295.
6. Bergenholtz G, Lindhe J: Effect of soluble plaque factors on inflammatory reaction in the dental pulp. Scand J Dent Res 1975; 83:153.
7. Brannstrom M, Lind PO: Pulpal response to early dental caries. J Dent Res 1965; 44:1045.
8. Czarnecki R, Schilder H: A histological evaluation of the human pulp in teeth with varying degrees of periodontal disease. J Endodon 1979; 5(8):242.
9. DeDeus QD: Frequency, location, and direction of the lateral, secondary and accessory canals. J Endodon 1975; 1:361.
10. Gharbia S, Haapasalo M, Shah HN, et al: Characterization of *Prevotella intermedia* and *Prevotella nigrescens* isolates from periodontal and endodontic lesions. J Periodontol 1994; 65:56.
11. Gutmann JL: Preparation of endodontically treated teeth to receive a post-core restoration. J Prosthet Dent 1977; 38:413.
12. Gutmann JL: Prevalence, location and patency of accessory canals in the furcation region of permanent molars. J Periodontol 1978; 49:21.
13. Haapasalo M: Bacteroides spp in dental root canal infections. Endodont Dent Traumatol 1989; 5:1.
14. Harrington GW: The perio-endo question: differential diagnosis. Dent Clin N Amer 1979; 23(4):673.
15. Harrington G, Steiner D: Endodontic and periodontal interrelationships. In: Walton RE, Torabinejad M (eds): Principles and Practice of Endodontics, ed 3. Philadelphia, Saunders, 2002.
16. Hiatt W: Periodontal pocket elimination by combined endodontic-periodontic therapy. Periodontics 1963; 1:152.
17. Hiatt WH, Amen C: Periodontal pocket elimination by combined therapy. Dent Clin N Amer 1964; 9(1):133.
18. Johnson J, Schwartz H, Blackwell R: Evaluation and restoration of endodontically treated posterior teeth. J Am Dent Assn 1976; 93:597.
19. Kollman W, Mijatovic E: Age dependent changes in thermoperception in human anterior teeth. Arch Oral Biol 1985; 30:711.
20. Langeland K, Rodriques H, Dowden W: Periodontal disease, bacteria and pulpal histopathology. Oral Surg Oral Med Oral Pathol 1974; 37(2):257.
21. Lin LB, Langeland K: Light and electron microscopic study of teeth with carious pulp exposures. Oral Surg Oral Med Oral Pathol 1981; 51(3):292.
22. Lowman JV, Burke RS, Pelleu GB: Patent accessory canals: incidence in moral furcation region. Oral Surg Oral Med Oral Pathol 1973; 36(4):580.
23. Meister F, Lommel TJ, Gerstein H: Diagnosis and possible causes of vertical root fracture. Oral Surg Oral Med Oral Pathol 1980; 49(3):243.
24. Milot P, Stein R: Root fracture in endodontically treated teeth related to post selection and crown design. J Prosthet Dent 1992; 68:428.
25. Moller AJR, Fabricius L, Dahlen G, et al: Influence on periapical tissues of indigenous oral bacteria and necrotic pulp tissue in monkeys. Scand J Dent Res 1981; 89:475.
26. Mumford JM: Pain perception threshold on stimulating human teeth and the histological condition of the pulp. Br Dent J 1967; 123:427.
27. Nahri MVO: The characteristics of interdental sensory units and their responses to stimulation. J Dent Res 1985; 54:654.
28. Nilsen R, Johannessen AC, Skaug N, et al: In situ characterization of mononuclear cells in human dental periapical inflammatory lesions using monoclonal antibodies. Oral Surg Oral Med Oral Pathol 1984; 58(2):160.
29. Petersson K, Hasselgren G, Tronstad L: Endodontic treatment of experimental root perforations in dog teeth. Endod Dent Traumatol 1986; 1:22.
30. Pitts DL, Natkin E: Diagnosis and treatment of vertical root fractures. J Endodon 1983; 9(8):338.
31. Prichard JF, Simon P: Combined periodontal pulpal problems. In: Prichard JF (ed): The Diagnosis and Treatment of Periodontal Disease in General Dental Practice. Philadelphia, Saunders, 1979.
32. Ross R, Nicholls J, Harrington G: A comparison of strains generated during placement of five endodontic posts. J Endodont 1991; 17(9):450.
33. Seltzer S, Bender IB, Ziontz M: Interrelationship of the pulp and periodontal disease. Oral Surg Oral Med Oral Pathol 1963; 16:1474.
34. Simon JHS, Glick DH, Frank AL: The relationship of endodontic-periodontic lesions. J Periodontol 1972; 43:202.
35. Simring M, Goldberg M: The pulpal pocket approach: Retrograde periodontitis. J Periodontol 1964; 35:22.
36. Sjogren U, Hagglund B, Sundqvist G, et al: Factors affecting the long-term results of endodontic treatment. J Endodont 1990; 16:498.
37. Sorenson J, Englemen M: Ferrule design and fracture resistance of endodontically treated teeth. J Prosthet Dent 1990; 63:529.

38. Sundqvist G, Johansson E, Sjogren U: Prevalence of black pigmented Bacteroides species in root canal infections. J Endodon 1989; 15(1):13.
39. Walton RE, Garnick JT: The histology of periapical inflammatory lesions in permanent molars in monkeys. J Endodon 1986; 12(2):49.
40. Torabinejad M, Kiger RD: A histologic evaluation of dental pulp tissue of a patient with periodontal disease. Oral Surg Oral Med Oral Pathol 1985; 59(2);198.
41. Torabinejad M: Pulp and periradicular pathosis. In: Walton RE, Torabinejad M (eds): Principles and Practice of Endodontics, ed 3. Philadelphia, Saunders, 2002.
42. Van Hassel HJ: Physiology of the human dental pulp. Oral Surg Oral Med Oral Pathol 1971; 32:126.
43. Vertucci TJ, Williams RG: Furcation canals in the human mandibular first molar. Oral Surg Oral Med Oral Pathol 1974; 38(2):308.
44. Yanagisawa S: Pathologic study of periapical lesions. I. Periapical granulomas: clinical histopathologic and immunohistopathologic studies. J Oral Path 1980; 9:288.

Periodontal Plastic and Esthetic Surgery

Henry H. Takei and Robert R. Azzi

CHAPTER

CHAPTER OUTLINE

TERMINOLOGY

The term *mucogingival surgery* was initially introduced in the literature by Friedman[30] to describe surgical procedures for the correction of relationships between the gingiva and the oral mucous membrane with reference to three specific problems: those associated with attached gingiva, shallow vestibules, and a frenum interfering with the marginal gingiva. With the advancement of periodontal surgical techniques, the scope of nonpocket surgical procedures increased, encompassing now a multitude of areas that were not addressed in the past. Recognizing this, the 1996 World Workshop renamed mucogingival surgery as *periodontal plastic surgery,*[2] a term originally proposed by Miller in 1993, and broadened to include the following areas[1,2]:

Periodontal-prosthetic corrections
Crown lengthening
Ridge augmentation
Esthetic surgical corrections
Coverage of the denuded root surface
Reconstruction of papillae
Esthetic surgical correction around implants
Surgical exposure of unerupted teeth for orthodontics

Periodontal plastic surgery is defined as the surgical procedures performed to correct or eliminate anatomic, developmental, or traumatic deformities of the gingiva or alveolar mucosa.[1,2] The term *mucogingival therapy* is a broader one, since it also includes nonsurgical procedures such as papilla reconstruction by means of orthodontics or restorative dentistry. Periodontal plastic surgery includes only the surgical procedures of mucogingival therapy.

This chapter deals only with the periodontal plastic surgical techniques that were traditionally included in the definition of mucogingival surgery—that is, widening attached gingiva; deepening of shallow vestibules; and resection of aberrant frena. Other aspects of periodontal plastic surgery such as periodontal-prosthetic surgery, esthetic surgery around implants, and surgical exposure of teeth for orthodontics are covered in Chapters 53, 70, and 74.

OBJECTIVES

The three objectives of periodontal plastic surgery to be addressed in this chapter are as follows:

1. Problems associated with attached gingiva
2. Problems associated with shallow vestibule
3. Problems associated with aberrant frenum

Problems Associated with Attached Gingiva

The ultimate goal of mucogingival surgical procedures is the creation and/or widening of attached gingiva around teeth and implants.[2] The width of the attached gingiva varies in different individuals and on different teeth of the same individual (see Chapter 31). Attached gingiva is not synonymous with keratinized gingiva because the latter also includes the free gingival margin.

The width of the attached gingiva is determined by subtracting the depth of the sulcus or pocket from the distance between the crest of the gingival margin to the mucogingival junction.

The original rationale for mucogingival surgery was predicated on the assumption that a minimal width of attached gingiva was required for optimal gingival health to be maintained. However, several studies have challenged the view that a wide attached gingiva is more protective against the accumulation of plaque than a narrow or a nonexistent zone. No minimum width of attached gingiva has been established as a standard necessary for gingival health. Persons who practice excellent oral hygiene may maintain healthy areas with almost no attached gingiva.

However, those individuals whose oral hygiene practices are less than optimal can be helped by the presence of keratinized gingiva and vestibular depth, which provide room for easier placement of the toothbrush and to avoid brushing on mucosal tissue. To improve esthetics, the objective is the coverage of the denuded root surface. The maxillary anterior area, especially the facial aspect of the canine, often presents extensive recession. In an individual with a high smile line, this recession may create an esthetic defect. The coverage of the denuded root for esthetic purposes also widens the zone of attached gingiva. There is also a need for a wider zone of attached gingiva around teeth that serve as abutments for fixed or removable partial dentures, as well as in ridge areas in relation to dentures. Teeth with subgingival restorations and narrow zones of keratinized gingiva have higher gingival inflammation scores than teeth with similar restorations and wide zones of attached gingiva.[68] Therefore, in such cases, techniques for widening the attached gingiva are considered preprosthetic periodontal surgical procedures.

Widening the attached gingiva accomplishes the following three objectives:

1. Enhances plaque removal around the gingival margin
2. Improves esthetics
3. Reduces inflammation around restored teeth

Problems Associated with a Shallow Vestibule

Another objective of periodontal plastic surgery is the creation of some vestibular depth when this is lacking. Gingival recession displaces the gingival margin apically, thus reducing vestibular depth, which is measured from the gingival margin to the bottom of the vestibule. With minimal vestibular depth, proper hygiene procedures are jeopardized. The sulcular brushing technique requires the placement of the toothbrush at the gingival margin, which may not be possible with reduced vestibular depth.

Minimal attached gingiva with adequate vestibular depth may not require surgical correction if proper atraumatic hygiene is practiced with a soft brush. Minimal amounts of keratinized attached gingiva with no vestibular depth usually benefit from mucogingival correction. Adequate vestibular depth may also be necessary for proper placement of removable prostheses.

Problems Associated with an Aberrant Frenum

The final objective of periodontal plastic surgery is to correct frenal or muscle attachments. If there is adequate gingiva coronal to the frenum, there is usually no need to surgically remove it. A frenum that encroaches on the margin of the gingiva may interfere with plaque removal and tension on this frenum may tend to open the sulcus. In these cases, surgical removal of the frenum is indicated.

ETIOLOGIC FACTORS OF MARGINAL TISSUE RECESSION

The most common cause for these defects is abrasive and traumatic toothbrushing habits. Teeth positioned buccally tend to have greater recession. Recession of the gingival tissue and bone exposes the cemental surface, which allows abrasion and "ditching" of the cervical area.

Periodontal inflammation and the resultant loss of attachment results in reduced attached gingiva. Advanced periodontal involvement in areas of minimal attached gingiva result in the base of the pocket extending close to, or apical to, the mucogingival junction.

Frenal and muscle attachments that encroach on the marginal gingiva distend the gingival sulcus, fostering plaque accumulation, increasing the rate of progression of periodontal recession, and causing their recurrence after treatment (Fig. 66-1, *A–C*). The problem is more common on facial surfaces, but it may also occur on the lingual surface[4] (see Fig. 66-1, *D*).

Orthodontic tooth movement through a thin buccal osseous plate leading to a dehiscence beneath a thin gingival tissue can cause recession and/or loss of the gingiva (Fig. 66-2).[36,80]

FACTORS THAT AFFECT THE OUTCOME OF PERIODONTAL PLASTIC SURGERY

Irregularity of Teeth

Abnormal tooth alignment is an important cause of gingival deformities that require corrective surgery and likewise, an important factor in determining the outcome of treatment. The location of the gingival margin, width of the attached gingiva, and alveolar bone height and thickness are all affected by tooth alignment. On teeth that are tilted or rotated labially, the labial bony

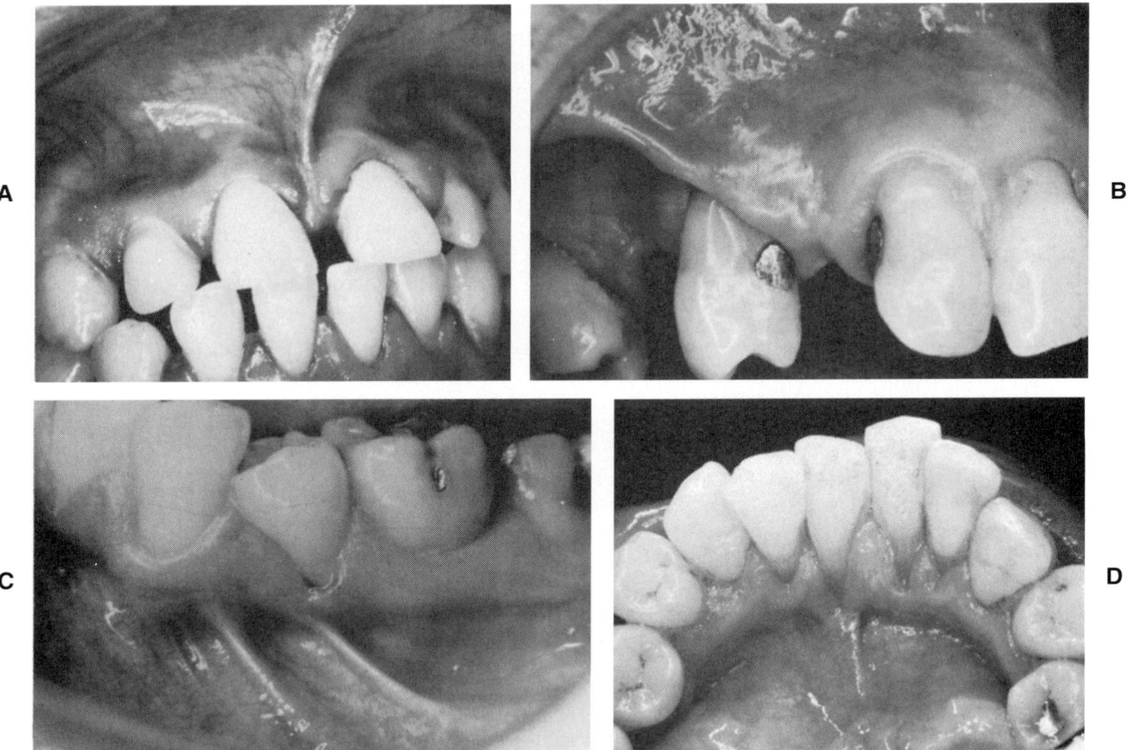

Fig. 66-1 High frenum attachments. **A,** Frenum between maxillary central incisors. **B,** Frenum on the mesial surface of the maxillary second premolar. **C,** Frenum attached to a pocket wall on a mandibular first premolar. **D,** Frenum attached to a pocket wall on the lingual surface of an incisor.

plate is thinner and located farther apically than on the adjacent teeth; therefore the gingiva is recessed so that the root is exposed.[80] On the lingual surface of such teeth, the gingiva is bulbous, and the bone margins are closer to the cementoenamel junction (CEJ). The level of gingival attachment on root surfaces and the width of the attached gingiva after mucogingival surgery are affected as much by tooth alignment as by variations in treatment procedures.

Orthodontic correction is indicated when mucogingival surgery is performed on malposed teeth in an attempt to widen the attached gingiva or to restore the gingiva over denuded roots. If orthodontic treatment is not feasible, the prominent tooth should be reduced to within the borders of the alveolar bone, with special care taken to avoid pulp injury.

Roots covered with thin bony plates present a hazard in mucogingival surgery. Even the most protective type of flap, a partial-thickness flap, creates the risk of bone resorption on the periosteal surface.[38] Resorption in amounts that ordinarily are not significant may cause loss of bone height when the bone plate is thin or tapered at the crest.

The Mucogingival Line (Junction)

Normally, the mucogingival line in the incisor and canine areas is located approximately 3-mm apical to the

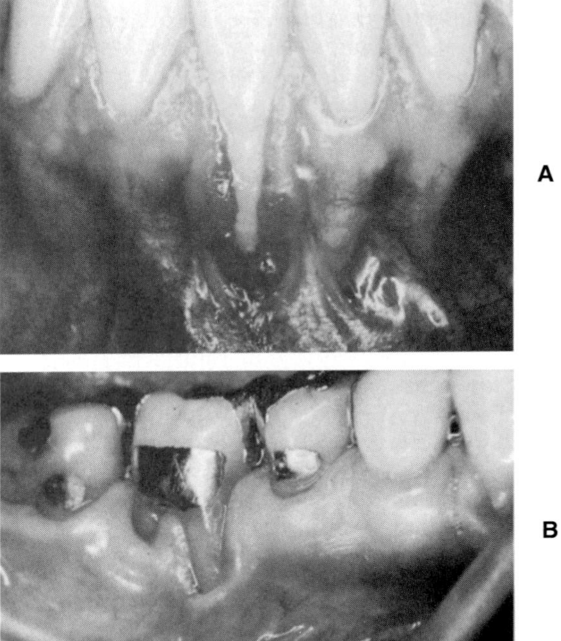

Fig. 66-2 **A,** Gingival recession and extreme inflammation around a lower central incisor. **B,** Advanced recession of mesiobuccal root of a first lower molar.

crest of the alveolar bone on the radicular surfaces and 5-mm interdentally.[69] In periodontal disease and on malposed, disease-free teeth, the bone margin is located farther apically and may extend beyond the mucogingival line. The distance between the mucogingival line and the CEJ before and after periodontal surgery is not necessarily constant. After inflammation is eliminated, there is a tendency for the tissue to contract and draw the mucogingival line in the direction of the crown.[23]

TECHNIQUES FOR INCREASING ATTACHED GINGIVA

To simplify and to better understand the techniques and the result of the surgery, the following classifications are presented:

Gingival augmentation apical *to the area of recession.* A graft, either pedicle or free, is placed on a recipient bed apical to the recessed gingival margin. No attempt is made to cover the denuded root surface where there is gingival and bone recession.

Gingival augmentation coronal *to the recession (root coverage).* A graft (either pedicle or free) is placed covering the denuded root surface. Both the apical and coronal widening of attached gingiva enhance oral hygiene procedures, but only the latter can correct an esthetic problem. For preprosthetic purposes, the combination of widening keratinized gingiva apical and coronal to the recession would satisfy this objective. Consideration of the objectives as apical, coronal, or both provides a better understanding of the techniques required to achieve the goals.

Widening of the keratinized attached gingiva (apical or coronal to the area of recession) can be accomplished by numerous techniques such as the free gingival autograft, free connective tissue autograft, and lateral pedicle flap, which can be used for either objective.

Gingival Augmentation Apical to Recession

Techniques for this procedure include the following: free gingival autograft, free connective tissue autograft,[3] and apically positioned flap

Free Gingival Autografts. Free gingival grafts are used to create a widened zone of attached gingiva. They were initially described by Bjorn[5] in 1963 and have been extensively investigated since that time.

THE CLASSIC TECHNIQUE

Step One: Prepare the Recipient Site. The purpose of this step is to prepare a firm connective tissue bed to receive the graft. The recipient site can be prepared by incising at the existing mucogingival junction with a #15 blade to the desired depth, blending the incision on both ends with the existing mucogingival line (Color Figs. 66-1 and 66-2). Periosteum should be left covering the bone.

Another technique consists of outlining the recipient site with two vertical incisions from the cut gingival margin into the alveolar mucosa (Fig. 66-3).

Extend the incisions to approximately twice the desired width of the attached gingiva, allowing for 50% contraction of the graft when healing is complete. The amount of contraction depends on the extent to which the recipient site penetrates the muscle attachments. The deeper the recipient site, the greater is the tendency for the muscles to elevate the graft and reduce the final width of the attached gingiva. The periosteum along the apical border of the graft is sometimes penetrated in an effort to prevent postoperative narrowing of the attached gingiva.

Insert a #15 blade along the cut gingival margin and separate a flap consisting of epithelium and underlying connective tissue without disturbing the periosteum. Extend the flap to the depth of the vertical incisions.

If a narrow band of attached gingiva remains after the pockets are eliminated, it should be left intact, and the recipient site should be started by inserting the blade at the mucogingival junction instead of at the cut gingival margin.

Suture the flap where the apical portion of the free graft will be located. Three to four independent gut sutures are placed. The needle is first passed as a superficial mattress suture perpendicular to the incision and then on the periosteum parallel to the incision (Fig 66-4).

Make an aluminum foil template of the recipient site to be used as a pattern for the graft (see Fig. 66-3, *C and D*).

Grafts can also be placed directly on bone tissue. For this technique, the flap should be separated by blunt dissection with a periosteal elevator. Reported advantages of this variant are less postoperative mobility of the graft, less swelling, better hemostasis,[24] and 1.5 to 2 times less shrinkage.[41,42] However, a healing lag is observed for the first 2 weeks.[12,15,28]

Step Two: Obtain the Graft from the Donor Site. The classic or conventional-free gingival graft technique consists of transferring a piece of keratinized gingiva of approximately the size of the recipient site. To avoid the large wound that this procedure sometimes leaves in the donor site, some alternative methods have been proposed. The original technique is described first, followed by several of the most common variants. For the classic technique (see Fig. 66-3 and Color Figs. 66-1 and 66-2), a partial thickness graft is used. The palate is the usual site from which donor tissue is removed. The graft should consist of epithelium and a thin layer of underlying connective tissue. Place the template over the donor site (see Fig. 66-3, *D*), and make a shallow incision around it with a #15 blade. Insert the blade to the desired thickness at one edge of the graft. Elevate the edge and hold it with tissue forceps. Continue to separate the graft with the blade, lifting it gently as separation progresses to provide visibility. Placing sutures at the margins of the graft helps control it during separation and transfer and simplifies placement and suturing to the recipient site.[3]

Proper thickness is important for survival of the graft. It should be thin enough to permit ready diffusion of nutritive fluid from the recipient site, which is essential in the immediate posttransplant period. A graft that is too thin may necrose and expose the recipient site.[53,57] If the graft is too thick, its peripheral layer is jeopardized because of the excessive tissue that separates it from new

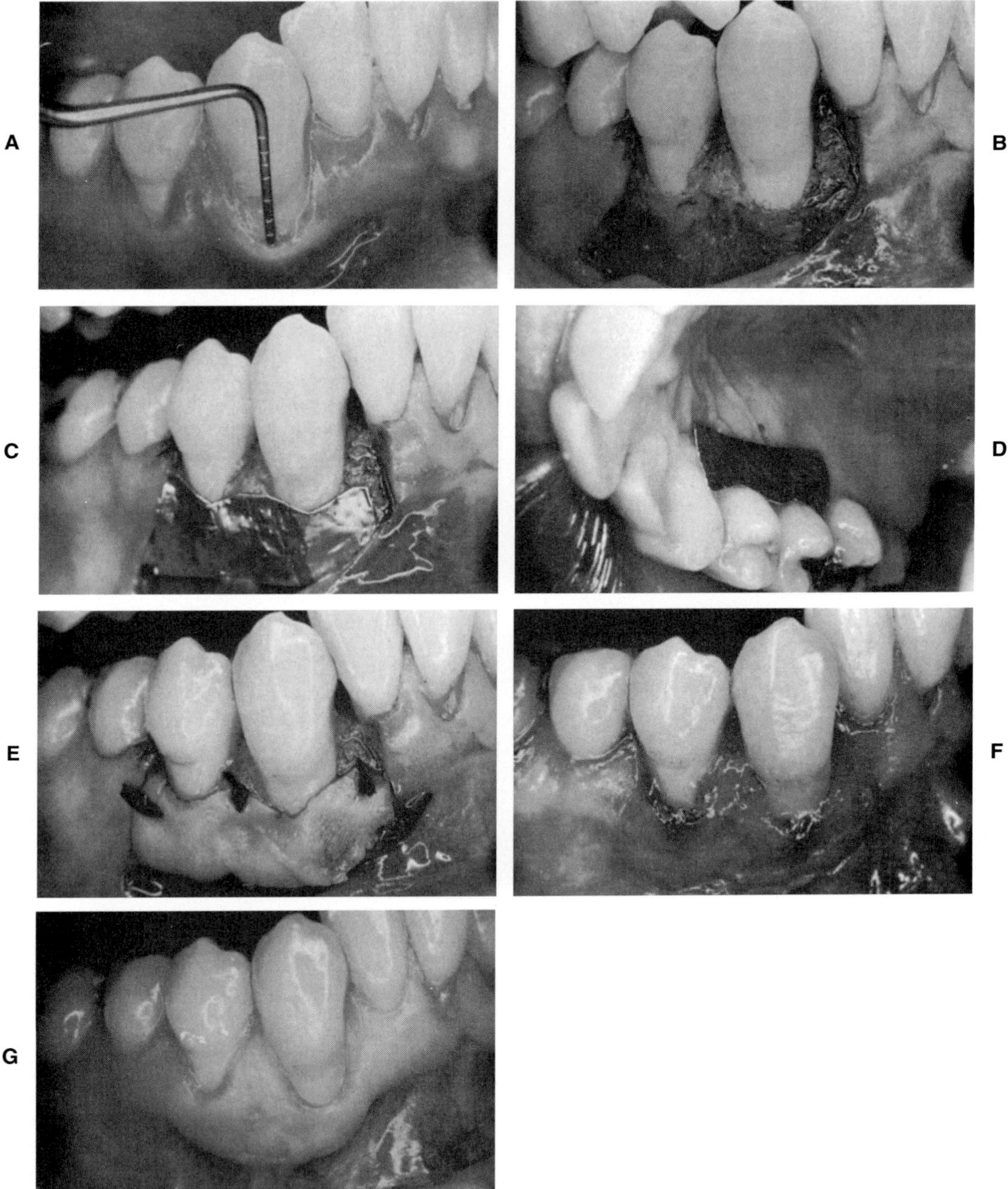

Fig. 66-3 Free gingival graft. **A,** Before treatment; sulcus extends into alveolar mucosa. **B,** Recipient site prepared for free gingival graft. **C,** Aluminum foil template of the desired graft. **D,** Template used to outline the graft in the donor site. **E,** Graft transferred. **F,** After 2 weeks. **G,** After 1 year, showing widened zone of attached gingiva.

circulation and nutrients. Thick grafts may also create a deeper wound at the donor site, with the possibility of injuring major palatal arteries.[77] The ideal thickness of a graft is between 1.0 and 1.5 mm.[53,57] After the graft is separated, remove loose tissue tabs from the undersurface. Thin the edge to avoid bulbous marginal and interdental contours. Special precautions must be taken with grafts from the palate.

The submucosa in the posterior region is thick and fatty and should be trimmed so that it will not interfere with vascularization. Grafts tend to reestablish their original epithelial structure so that mucous glands may occur in grafts obtained from the palate.

A thick graft can be thinned by holding it between two wet wooden tongue depressors and slicing it longitudinally with a sharp #15 blade.

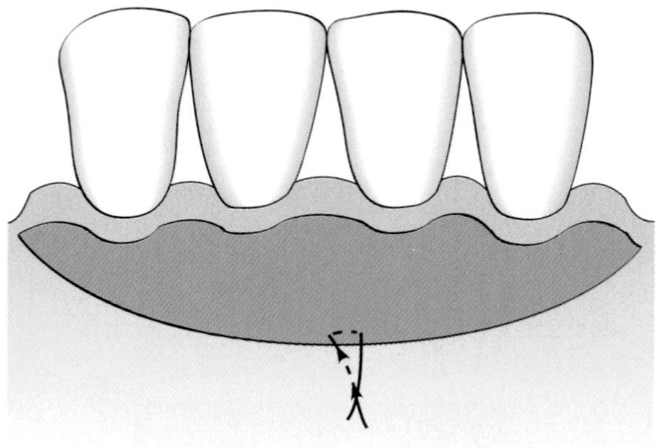

Fig. 66-4 Diagram of graft bed suture.

Step Three: Transfer and Immobilize the Graft. Remove the sponge from the recipient site; reapply it, with pressure if necessary, until bleeding is stopped. Remove the excess clot. A thick clot interferes with vascularization of the graft.[54]

Position the graft and adapt it firmly to the recipient site. A space between the graft and the underlying tissue (dead space) retards vascularization and jeopardizes the graft. Suture the graft at the lateral borders and to the periosteum to secure it in position (see Fig. 66-3, *E* and Color Figs. 66-1 and 66-2). Before suturing is completed, elevate the unsutured portion and cleanse the recipient bed beneath it with an aspirator to remove clots or loose tissue fragments. Press the graft back into position and complete the sutures. The graft must be immobilized. Any movement interferes with healing. Avoid excessive tension, which can distort the graft from the underlying surface. Every precaution should be taken to avoid trauma to the graft. Tissue forceps should be used delicately, and a minimum number of sutures used to avoid unnecessary tissue perforation.

Step Four: Protect the Donor Site. Cover the donor site with a periodontal pack for 1 week and repeat if necessary. Retention of the pack on the donor site can be a problem. If facial attached gingiva was used, the pack may be retained by locking it through the interproximal spaces onto the lingual surface. If there are no open interdental spaces, the pack can be covered by a plastic stent wired to the teeth. A modified Hawley retainer is useful to cover the pack on the palate and over edentulous ridges.

VARIANT TECHNIQUES. The following variants to the classic technique are described in this section: accordion technique, strip technique, or a combination of both. All are modifications of the free grafts:

The **accordion technique** has been described by Rateitschak and colleagues.[61] It attains expansion of the graft by alternate incisions in opposite sides of the graft.

The **strip technique** developed by Han and associates[37] consists of obtaining two or three strips of gingival donor tissue about 3- to 5-mm wide and long enough to cover the entire length of the recipient site (Fig. 66-5). These strips are placed side by side to form one donor tissue and sutured on the recipient site. The area is then covered with aluminum foil and surgical pack. The advantages of this technique are the rapid healing of the donor site. The epithelial migration of the close wound edges (3 to 5 mm) allows rapid epithelization of the open wound. The donor site usually does not require any suturing and heals uneventfully in 1 week.

In some cases, a **combination technique** can be performed as follows. Remove a strip of tissue from the palate, about 3- to 4-mm thick, place it between two wet tongue depressors, and split it longitudinally with a sharp #15 blade. Both will be used as free grafts. The superficial portion consists of epithelium and connective tissue and the deeper portion consists only of connective tissue. These donor tissues are placed on the recipient site as in the strip technique. The minimal donor site wound by obtaining two donor tissues from one site is the advantage of this technique.

HEALING OF THE GRAFT. The success of the graft depends on survival of the connective tissue (see Fig. 66-3 and Color Fig. 66-1). Sloughing of the epithelium occurs in most cases, but the extent to which the connective tissue withstands the transfer to the new location determines the fate of the graft. Fibrous organization of the interface between the graft and the recipient bed occurs within 2 to several days.[67]

The graft is initially maintained by a diffusion of fluid from the host bed, adjacent gingiva, and alveolar mucosa.[32] The fluid is a transudate from the host vessels and provides nutrition and hydration essential for the initial survival of the transplanted tissues. During the first day, the connective tissue becomes edematous and disorganized and undergoes degeneration and lysis of some of its elements. As healing progresses, the edema is resolved and degenerated connective tissue is replaced by new granulation tissue.

Revascularization of the graft starts by the second[6] or third day.[43] Capillaries from the recipient bed proliferate into the graft to form a network of new capillaries and anastomose with preexisting vessels.[43]

Many of the graft vessels degenerate and are replaced by new ones, and some participate in the new circulation. The central section of the surface is the last to vascularize, but this is complete by the tenth day.

The epithelium undergoes degeneration and sloughing, with complete necrosis occurring in some areas.[13,56] It is replaced by new epithelium from the borders of the recipient site. A thin layer of new epithelium is present by the fourth day, with rete pegs developing by the seventh day.

The fact that heterotopically placed grafts maintain their structure (keratinized epithelium), even after the grafted epithelium has become necrotic and has been replaced by neighboring areas of nonkeratinized epithelium, suggests that there exists a genetic predetermination of the specific character of the oral mucosa that is dependent on stimuli that originate in the connective tissue.[44] This is the basis for the technique that uses grafts composed only of connective tissue obtained from areas where it is covered by keratinized epithelium.[10,22,28]

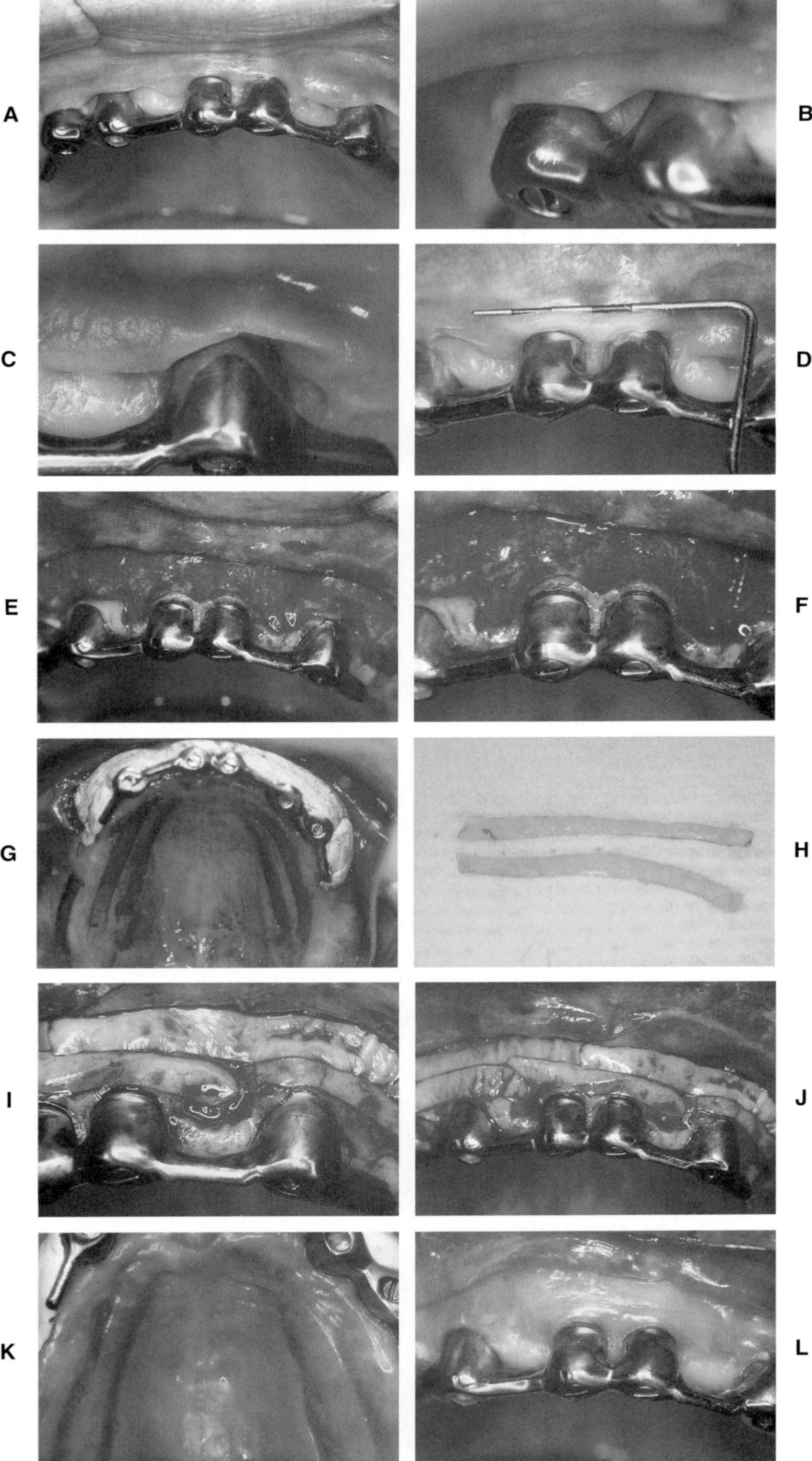

Fig. 66-5 Free gingival graft: strip technique. **A–D,** Mucosal tissue around implants. **E and F,** Recipient site prepared. **G,** Donor site with strips of free graft removed. **H,** Donor strips of free graft. **I and J,** Strips placed side by side on recipient site. **K,** Donor area one week after graft removal. **L,** Healing of recipient site after three months. Note good keratinized, attached gingiva.

As seen microscopically, healing of a graft of intermediate thickness (0.75 mm) is complete by 10.5 weeks; thicker grafts (1.75 mm) may require 16 weeks or longer.[33] The gross appearance of the graft reflects the tissue changes within it. At the time of transplantation, the graft vessels are empty, and the graft is pale. The pallor changes to an ischemic grayish white during the first 2 days until vascularization begins and a pink color appears. The plasmatic circulation accumulates and causes softening and swelling of the graft, which are reduced when the edema is removed from the recipient site by the new blood vessels. Loss of epithelium leaves the graft smooth and shiny. New epithelium creates a thin, gray, veil-like surface that develops normal features as the epithelium matures.

Functional integration of the graft occurs by the seventeenth day, but the graft is morphologically distinguishable from the surrounding tissue for months. The graft eventually blends with adjacent tissues, but sometimes, although pink, firm, and healthy, it is somewhat bulbous.

This ordinarily presents no problem, but if the graft traps plaque or is esthetically unacceptable, thinning of the graft may be necessary.

Thinning the surface of the grafted tissue does reduce the bulbous condition, because the surface epithelium tends to proliferate again. The graft should be thinned by making the necessary incisions to elevate it from the periosteum, removing tissue from its undersurface, and suturing it back in place.

ACCOMPLISHMENTS OF FREE GINGIVAL GRAFTS. Free gingival grafts effectively widen the attached gingiva. Several biometric studies have analyzed the width of the attached gingiva after the placement of a free gingival graft.[11,38,41] After 24 weeks, grafts placed on denuded bone shrink 25%; whereas grafts placed on periosteum shrink 50%.[49] The greatest amount of shrinkage occurs within the first 6 weeks.

The placement of a gingival graft does not, per se, improve the status of the gingiva.[26,27,75] Therefore the indication for a free gingival graft should be based on the presence of progressive gingival recession and inflammation. When recession continues to progress after a period of a few months with good plaque control, a graft can be placed to prevent further recession and loss of attached gingiva.

Other materials have been used to replace gingival tissue in gingival extension operations. Attempts with lyophilized dura mater[66] and sclera[51] have not been satisfactory. The use of irradiated free gingival allografts showed satisfactory results,[64] but further research is necessary before they can be considered for clinical use.

Free autogenous gingival grafts have been found to be useful for covering nonpathologic dehiscences and fenestrations. *Nonpathologic* refers to openings of the bone through the tooth surface not previously exposed to the oral environment and found in the course of flap surgery.[25]

The use of free gingival autografts to cover denuded roots is described in the section entitled "Gingival Augmentation Coronal to the Recession."

FREE CONNECTIVE TISSUE AUTOGRAFTS. The connective tissue technique was originally described by Edel[28] and is based on the fact that the connective tissue carries the genetic message for the overlying epithelium to become keratinized. Therefore only connective tissue from a keratinized zone can be used as a graft.

This technique has the advantage that the donor tissue is obtained from the undersurface of the palatal flap, which is sutured back in primary closure; therefore healing is by first intention. There is less discomfort for the patient postoperatively at the donor site. In cases where resective flap surgery is planned for the palate, the connective tissue removed to thin the palatal flap can be used as the graft tissue to augment areas of recession. Fig. 66-6 shows a case in which the free connective tissue graft technique was used.

Another advantage is that better esthetics can be achieved because of a better color match of the grafted tissue to adjacent areas.

The Apically Positioned Flap. This technique uses the apically positioned flap, either partial thickness or full thickness, to increase the zone of keratinized gingiva. A step-by-step description of the surgical technique for apically positioned flaps is given in Chapter 61, and the procedure is shown in Fig. 66-7.

ACCOMPLISHMENTS OF THE APICALLY POSITIONED FLAP. The apically positioned flap operation increases the width of the keratinized gingiva but cannot predictability deepen the vestibule with attached gingiva.

Adequate vestibular depth must be present before the surgery to allow apical positioning of the flap. The edge of the flap may be located in three positions in relation to the bone:

1. *Slightly coronal to the crest of the bone.* This location attempts to preserve the attachment of supracrestal fibers; it may also result in thick gingival margins and interdental papillae with deep sulci and may create the risk of recurrent pockets.
2. *At the level of the crest (see Fig. 66-7,* C*).* This results in a satisfactory gingival contour, provided that the flap is adequately thinned.
3. *Two millimeters short of the crest (see Figs. 66-7,* D*; Fig. 66-8).* This position produces the most desirable gingival contour and the same posttreatment level of gingival attachment, as is obtained by placing the flap at the crest of the bone.[31] New tissue covers the crest of the bone to produce a firm, tapered gingival margin.

Placing the flap short of the crest increases the risk of a slight reduction in bone height,[21] but this is compensated for by the advantages of a well-formed gingival margin.

OTHER TECHNIQUES. The following techniques are briefly presented only because of their historical interest. The vestibular extension technique, originally described by Edlan and Mejchar,[29] produces statistically significant widening of attached nonkeratinized tissue. This increase in width in the mandibular area reportedly persists in patients observed for periods of up to 5 years.[29,65,76] Currently, this technique is of historical interest only.

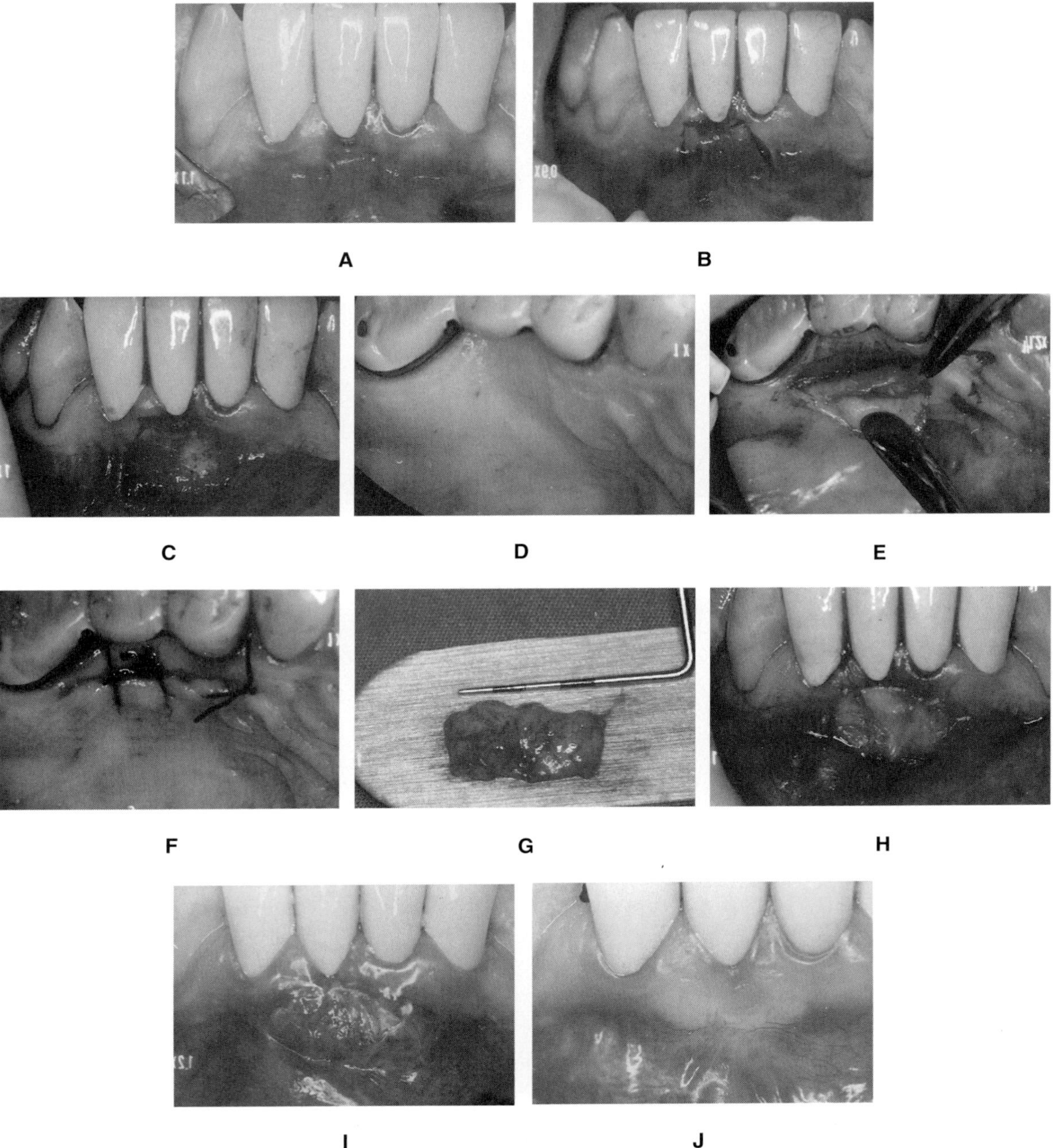

Fig. 66-6 Free connective tissue graft. **A,** Lack of keratinized, attached gingiva buccal to central incisor. **B,** Vertical incisions to prepare recipient site. **C,** Recipient site prepared. **D,** Palate from which connective tissue will be removed for donor tissue. **E,** Removal of connective tissue. **F,** Donor site sutured. **G,** Connective tissue for graft. **H,** Free connective tissue placed at donor site. **I,** Ten days postoperative healing. **J,** Final healing at 3 months. Note wide keratinized, attached gingiva.

The *fenestration operation* was designed to widen the zone of attached gingiva with a minimum loss of bone height.[62,63] It has also been called *periosteal separation.*[19] It used a partial thickness flap, except in a rectangular area at the base of the operative field, where the periosteum is removed, exposing the bone. This is the area of fenestration. Its purpose is to create a scar that is firmly bound to the bone.[16] It prevents separation from the bone and postsurgical narrowing of the attached zone. Results obtained with this technique are not as predictable as with the free gingival graft; therefore it is not widely performed except for small, isolated areas.

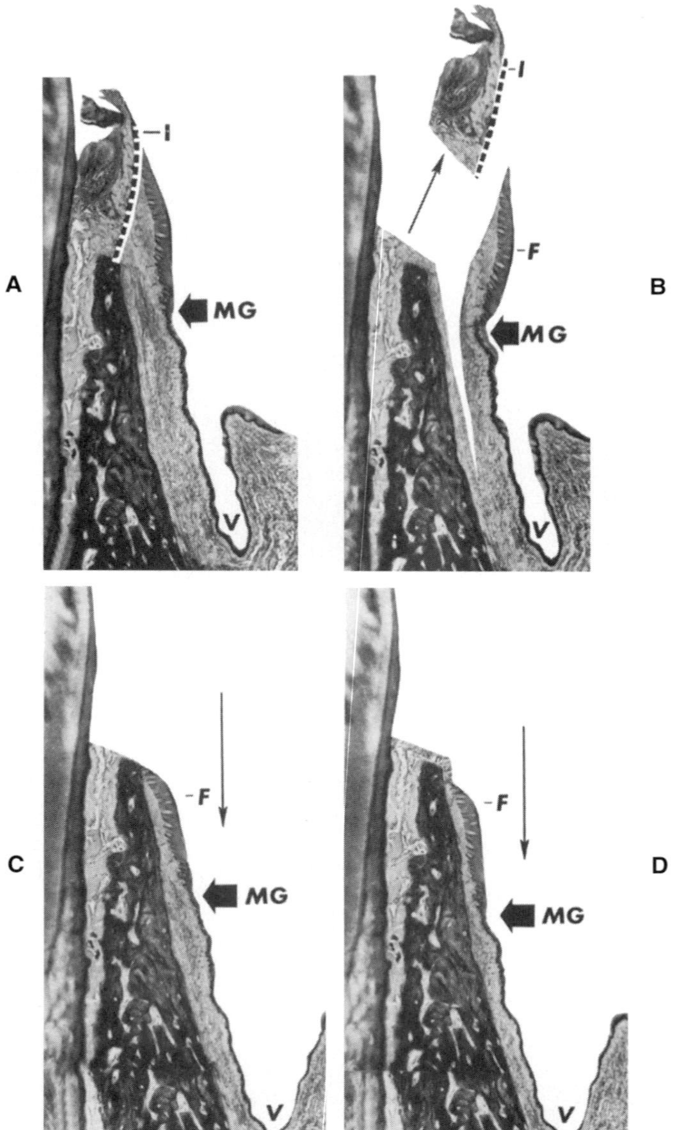

Fig. 66-7 Apically positioned partial-thickness flap. **A,** Internal bevel incision *(I)* separates inner wall of periodontal pocket. *MG,* Mucogingival junction; *V,* vestibular fornix. **B,** Partial-thickness flap *(F)* separated, leaving periosteum and a layer of connective tissue on the bone. The inner wall of the periodontal pocket *(I)* is removed, and the tooth is scaled and planed. **C,** Partial-thickness flap *(F)* positioned apically with the edge of the flap at the crest of the bone. Note that the vestibular fornix is also moved apically. **D,** Partial-thickness flap *(F)* displaced apically with the edge of the flap several millimeters below the crest of the bone.

Gingival Augmentation Coronal to Recession (Root Coverage)

The understanding and knowledge of the different stages and condition of gingival recession is necessary for predictable root coverage. Several classifications of denuded roots have been proposed. In the 1960s, Sullivan and Atkins[71] classified gingival recession into four morphologic categories: 1) shallow-narrow, 2) shallow-wide, 3) deep-narrow, and 4) deep-wide.

This early classification was helpful to better categorize the lesion but did not enable the clinician to predict the outcome of therapy. The predictability of root coverage can be enhanced by the presurgical examination and the correlation of the recession by using the classification proposed by Miller.[50] The following is his classification (Fig. 66-9):

Class I. This includes marginal tissue recession that does not extend to the mucogingival junction. There is no loss of bone or soft tissue in the interdental area. This type of recession can be narrow or wide.

Class II. Class II consists of marginal tissue recession that extends to or beyond the mucogingival junction.

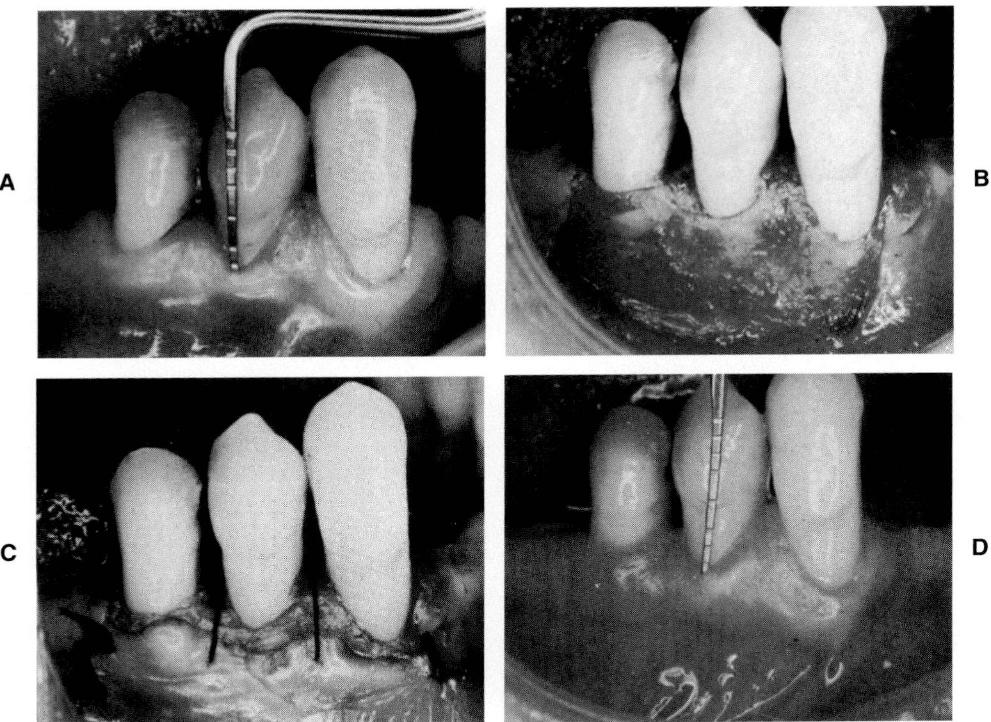

Fig. 66-8 Apically positioned partial-thickness flap. **A,** Before treatment, the base of pocket extends to the mucogingival line. **B,** Mucosal flap separated from the periosterum; teeth scaled and smoothed. **C,** Flap replaced below the crest of the bone. **D,** Eight months after treatment. Note the shallow sulcus and the widened zone of attached gingiva. Compare with **A.**

There is no loss of bone or soft tissue in the interdental area. This type of recession can be subclassified into wide and narrow.

Class III. In Class III, there is marginal tissue recession that extends to or beyond the mucogingival junction; in addition, there is bone and/or soft tissue loss interdentally or there is malpositioning of the tooth.

Class IV. There is marginal tissue recession that extends to or beyond the mucogingival junction with severe bone and soft tissue loss interdentally and/or severe tooth malposition.

Prognosis. In general, the prognosis for Classes I and II is good to excellent; whereas for Class III, only partial coverage can be expected. Class IV has a very poor prognosis with present-day techniques.

The following is a list of techniques used for gingival augmentation coronal to the recession (root coverage):

1. Free gingival autograft
2. Free connective tissue autograft
3. Pedicle autografts
   - Laterally (horizontally) positioned
   - Coronally positioned
   - Semilunar pedicle (Tarnow)
4. Subepithelial connective tissue graft (Langer)
5. Guided tissue regeneration
6. Pouch and tunnel technique

Some of the techniques used for widening the attached gingiva apical to the area of recession can also be used for root coverage. Both the free gingival and connective tissue autografts used for apical widening can be used for coronal augmentation by incorporating some modifications. In using the free grafts for root coverage, the recipient bed surrounding the denuded root surface must be extended wider to allow for better blood supply to the donor free graft since a portion of the donor tissue overlies the root surface that has no blood supply.

Free Gingival Autograft. In the last decade, successful and predictable root coverage has been reported using free gingival autografts.[51,52]

THE CLASSIC TECHNIQUE. Miller[52] applied the classic free gingival autograft described previously with a few modifications. The technique is as follows:

Step One: Root Planing. Root planing is performed, with application of saturated citric acid for 5 minutes with a cotton pledget, burnishing it on the root. The advantage of citric acid application has not been confirmed by other studies.[40]

Step Two: Prepare the Recipient Site. Make a horizontal incision in the interdental papillae at right angles to create a margin against which the graft may have a butt joint with the incision. Vertical incisions are made at the proximal line angles of adjacent teeth, and the retracted tissue is excised. Maintain an intact periosteum in the apical area.

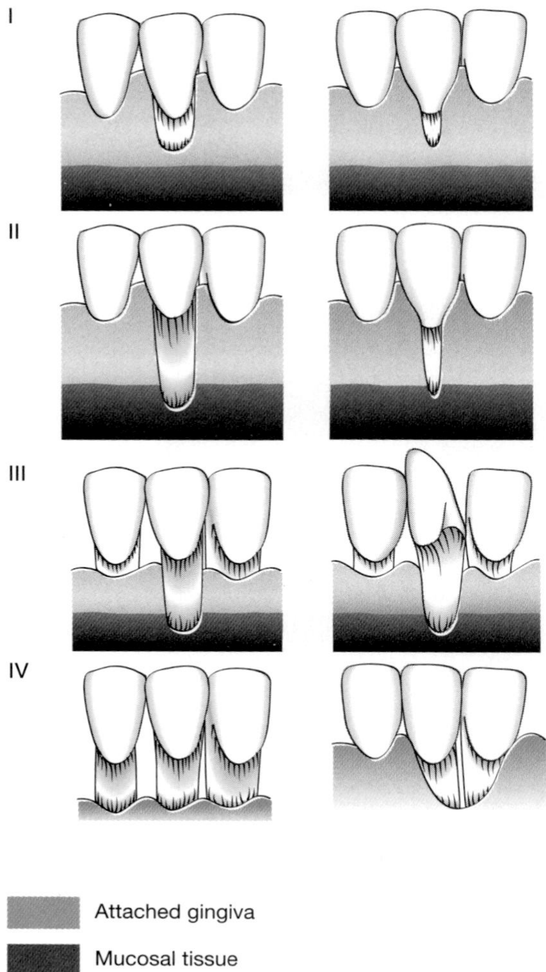

Fig. 66-9 P. D. Miller's classification of denuded roots.

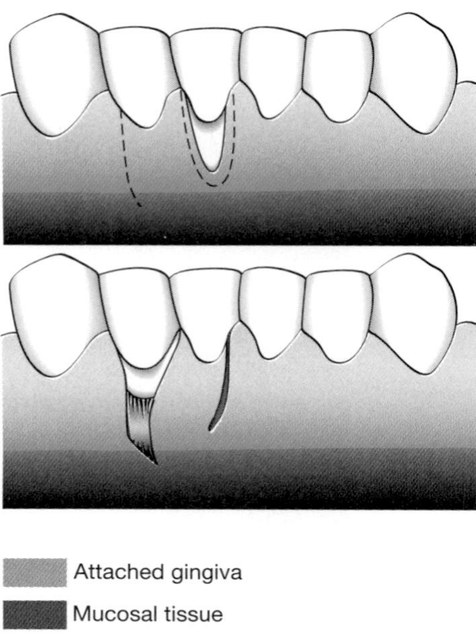

Fig. 66-10 Laterally positioned flap for coverage of denuded root. *Top,* Incisions removing the gingival margin around the exposed root and outlining flap. *Bottom,* After the gingiva around exposed root is removed, flap is separated, transferred, and sutured.

Steps Three and Four. Refer to the step-by-step technique described for the classic gingival graft earlier in this chapter.

This technique results in predictable coverage of the denuded roots but may present esthetic color discrepancies with the adjacent gingiva due to a lighter color.

Free Connective Tissue Autograft. This technique was described by Levine in 1991.[46] The difference between this technique and the previous one is that the donor tissue is connective tissue. It consists of the following steps (see Fig. 66-6).

CONNECTIVE TISSUE TECHNIQUE

Step One: Divergent Vertical Incisions. Divergent vertical incisions are made at the line angles of the tooth to be covered, creating a partial-thickness flap to at least 5 mm apical to the receded area.

Step Two: Suturing. Suture the apical mucosal border to the periosteum using gut suture.

Step Three: Scaling and Planing. Thoroughly scale and plane the root surface, reducing any prominence of the root surface.

Step Four: Obtaining the Graft. From the palate, obtain a connective tissue graft. The donor site is sutured after the graft is removed.

Step Five: Transferring the Graft. Transfer the graft to the recipient site and suture it to the periosteum with gut suture. Good stability of the graft must be attained with adequate sutures.

Step Six: Covering the Graft. Cover the grafted site with dry aluminum foil and periodontal dressing.

Pedicle Autograft

LATERALLY (HORIZONTALLY) DISPLACED. This technique, originally described by Grupe and Warren in 1956,[35] was the standard technique for many years and is still indicated in some cases. The laterally positioned flap can be used to cover isolated, denuded roots that have adequate donor tissue laterally and vestibular depth. The following is a step-by-step procedure for this technique.

Step One: Prepare the Recipient Site. Make an incision, resecting the gingival margin around the exposed roots (Figs. 66-10 and 66-11). Remove the resected soft tissue and scale and plane the root surface (see Fig. 66-11, *C*).

Step Two: Prepare the Flap. The periodontium of the donor site should have a satisfactory width of attached gingiva and minimal loss of bone and without dehiscences or fenestrations. A full-thickness or partial-thickness flap may be used, but the latter is preferable because it offers the advantage of more rapid healing in the donor site and reduces the risk of loss of facial bone height, particularly if the bone is thin or the presence of a dehiscence or a fenestration is suspected. However, if the gingiva is thin, partial thickness may not be sufficient for flap survival.

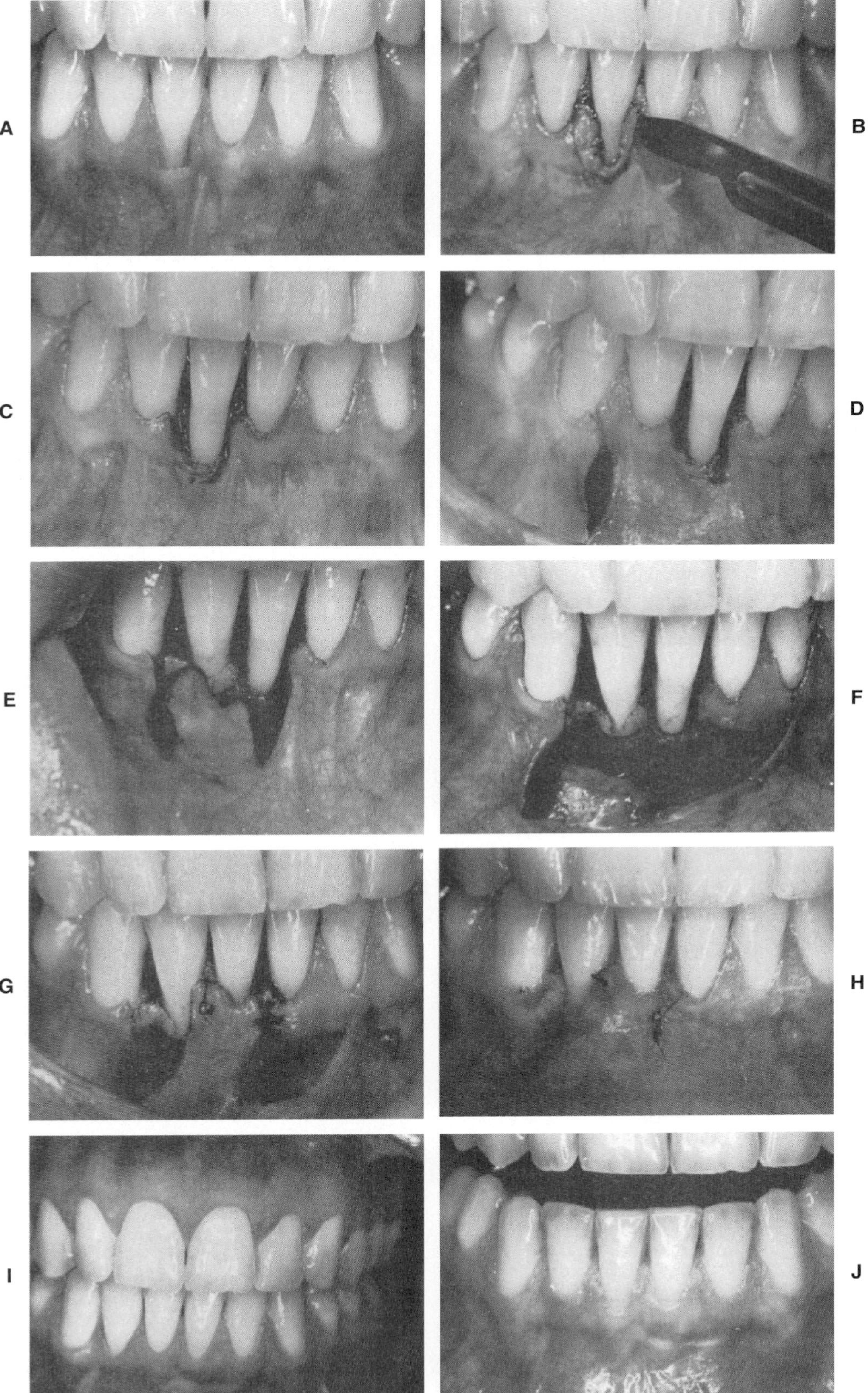

Fig. 66-11 Horizontally displaced flap combined with relocation of frenum attachment. **A,** Gingival defect of central incisor. **B,** Defect incised. **C,** Gingiva removed and tooth scaled and planed. **D,** Vertical incision on the canine for sliding flap. **E,** Sliding flap detached. Note high frenum attachment between the central incisors. **F,** Frenum detached and resected to level of vestibular fornix. **G,** Sliding flap positioned laterally on central incisor and fixed lateral and suspensory suture. **H,** One week after operation. Sutures to be removed. **I,** Five weeks after operation. **J,** Seven years after treatment. Note the preservation of gingival position and contour.

With a #15 blade, make a vertical incision from the gingival margin to outline a flap adjacent to the recipient site. Incise to the periosteum and extend the incision into the oral mucosa to the level of the base of the recipient site (see Fig. 66-11, *D*). The flap should be sufficiently wider than the recipient site to cover the root and provide a broad margin for attachment to the connective tissue border around the root. The interdental papilla at the distal end of the flap, or a major portion of it, should be included to secure the flap in the interproximal space between the donor and the recipient teeth.

Make a vertical incision along the gingival margin and interdental papilla and separate a flap consisting of epithelium and a thin layer of connective tissue, leaving the periosteum on the bone.

It is sometimes necessary to make a releasing incision to avoid tension on the base of the flap that can impair the circulation when the flap is moved (see Fig. 66-11, *E*). To do this, make a short oblique incision into the alveolar mucosa at the distal corner of the flap, pointing in the direction of the recipient site (see Fig. 66-11, *F*).

Step Three: Transfer the Flap. Slide the flap laterally onto the adjacent root, making sure that it lies flat and firm without excess tension on the base. Fix the flap to the adjacent gingiva and alveolar mucosa with interrupted sutures. A suspensory suture may be made around the involved tooth to prevent the flap from slipping apically (see Fig. 66-11, *F*).

Step Four: Protect the Flap and Donor Site. Cover the operative field with aluminum foil and a soft periodontal pack, extending it interdentally and onto the lingual surface to secure it. Remove the pack and sutures after 1 week (see Fig. 66-11, *H*).

VARIANT TECHNIQUES. There are many variations in the incisions for this operation. A common one is the use of converging oblique incisions over the recipient site and a vertical or oblique incision at the distal end of the donor site so that the transposed flap is slightly wider at its base. In another modification, the

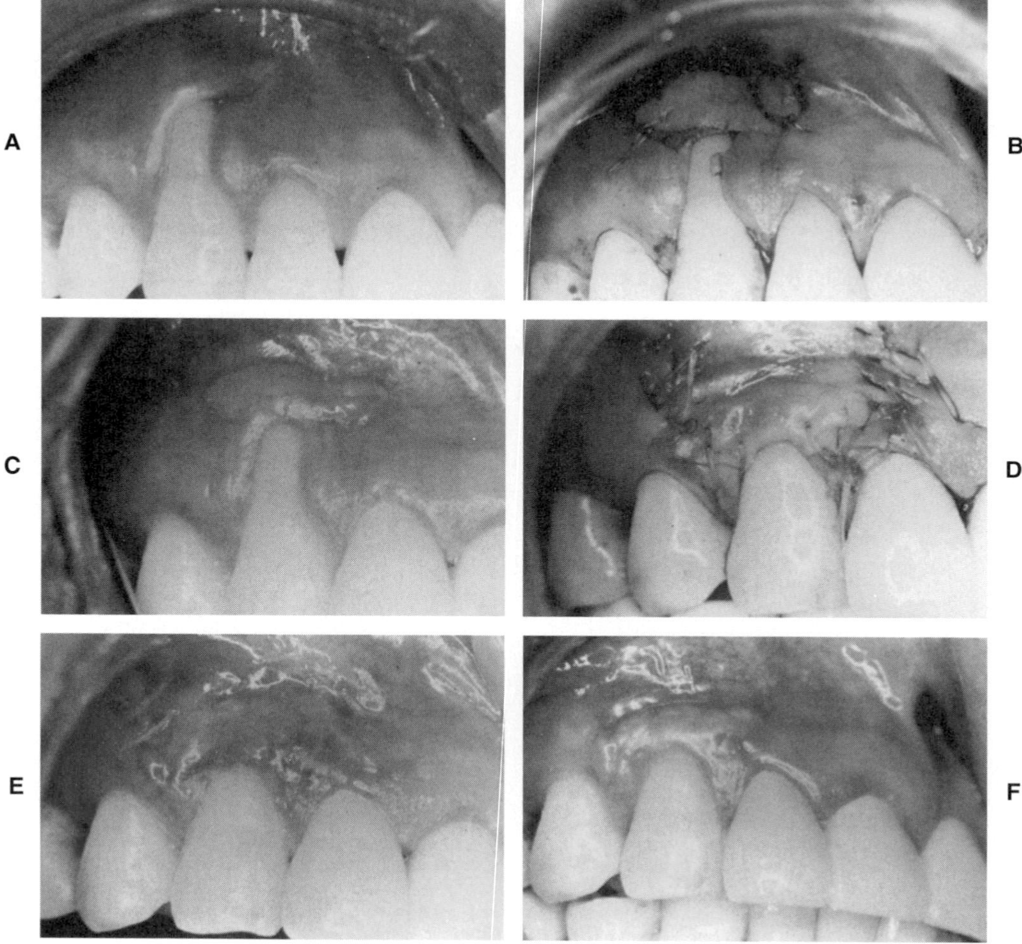

Fig. 66-12 Coronally positioned flap. **A,** Preoperative view. Note the recession and the lack of attached gingiva. **B,** After placement of a free gingival graft. **C,** Three months after placement of the graft. **D,** Flap including the graft, positioned coronally and sutured. **E,** After 2 weeks of healing. **F,** Six months later. Note the root coverage and the presence of attached gingiva. Compare with **A.** (Courtesy Dr. T. J. Han, Los Angeles, Calif.)

marginal attachment at the donor site is preserved to reduce the likelihood of recession and marginal bone resorption, but this requires a donor site with a wider zone of attached gingiva.

Sliding partial-thickness grafts from neighboring edentulous areas (pedicle grafts)[34] can be used to restore attached gingiva on teeth adjacent to edentulous spaces with denuded roots and a small, vestibular fornix, often complicated by tension from a frenum. The so-called double papilla flap attempts to cover roots denuded by isolated gingival defects with a flap formed by joining the contiguous halves of the adjacent interdental papillae.[18,39] Results with this technique are often poor because blood supply is impaired by suturing the two flaps over the root surface.

ACCOMPLISHMENTS OF THE PEDICLE AUTOGRAFT. Coverage of the exposed root surface with the sliding flap operation has been reported to be 60%,[32] 61%, and 72%.[61] Histologic studies in animals have reported 50% coverage.[17,79]

The extent to which the flap establishes a new attachment to the root with the formation of new cementum and the embedding of new connective tissue fibers has not been settled. New attachment on artificially denuded roots in experimental animals[79] and in some clinical studies in humans has been reported,[70,72] but it does not occur consistently enough to be predictable.

In the donor site, there is uneventful repair and restoration of gingival health and contours, with some loss of radicular bone (0.5 mm) and recession (1.5 mm) reported with full-thickness flaps.

Coronally Displaced Flap. The purpose of the coronally displaced flap operation is to create a split-thickness flap in the area apical to the denuded root and position it coronally to cover the root. Two techniques are available for this purpose.

FIRST TECHNIQUE FOR CORONALLY DISPLACED FLAP

Step One. With two vertical incisions, delineate the flap. These incisions should go beyond the mucogingival junction. Make an internal bevel incision from the gingival margin to the bottom of the pocket to eliminate the diseased pocket wall. Elevate a mucoperiosteal flap using careful sharp dissection.

Step Two. Scale and plane the root surface.

Step Three. Return the flap and suture it at a level coronal to the pretreatment position. Cover the area with a periodontal pack, which is removed along with the sutures after 1 week. The pack is replaced for an additional week if necessary.

VARIATIONS TO FIRST TECHNIQUE. Results with the coronally displaced flap technique are not often favorable[36] owing to the presence of insufficient keratinized gingiva. To solve this and increase the chance of success, a gingival extension operation with a free autogenous graft can be performed. (This technique was described earlier in this chapter.) This creates several millimeters of attached keratinized gingiva apical to the denuded root (Fig. 66-12, *C*).

Two months after this operation, a second-stage operation is performed, coronally positioning the flap that includes the free autogenous graft. The use of citric acid with a pH 1.0 for conditioning the root surface has been suggested[47] (see Fig. 66-12).

A significant degree of reduction in recession treated by this double-step operation was reported after 2 years by Bernimoulin and colleagues[4] and confirmed by other authors.[14,48,49]

SECOND TECHNIQUE FOR CORONALLY DISPLACED FLAP. Tarnow has described the semilunar coronally repositioned flap to cover denuded root surfaces.[73] It is performed as follows (Fig. 66-13).

Step One. A semilunar incision is made following the curvature of the receded gingival margin and ending about 2 to 3 mm short of the tip of the papillae. This is very important, as the flap derives all of its blood supply from the papillary areas. The incision may have to reach the alveolar mucosa if the attached gingiva is narrow.

Step Two. Perform a split-thickness dissection coronally from the incision and connect it to an intrasulcular incision.

Step Three. The tissue will collapse coronally, covering the denuded root. It is then held in its new position for a few minutes with moist gauze; there is no need to suture or to pack.

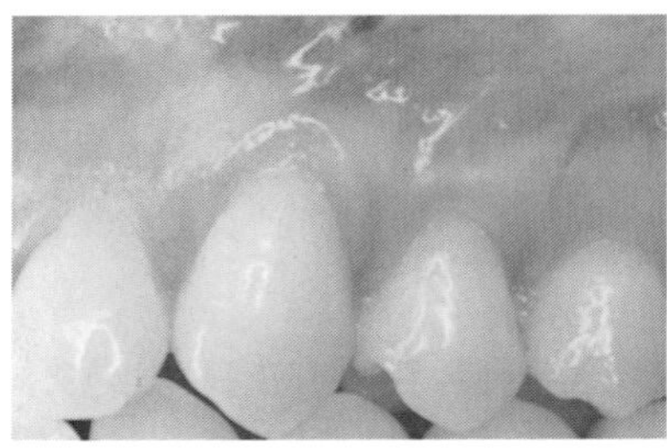

A

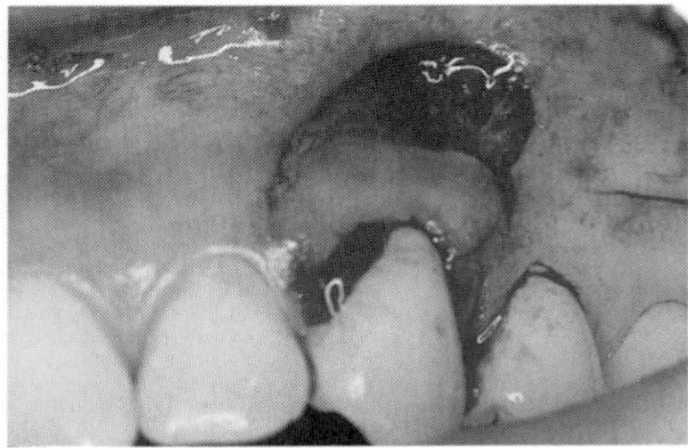

B

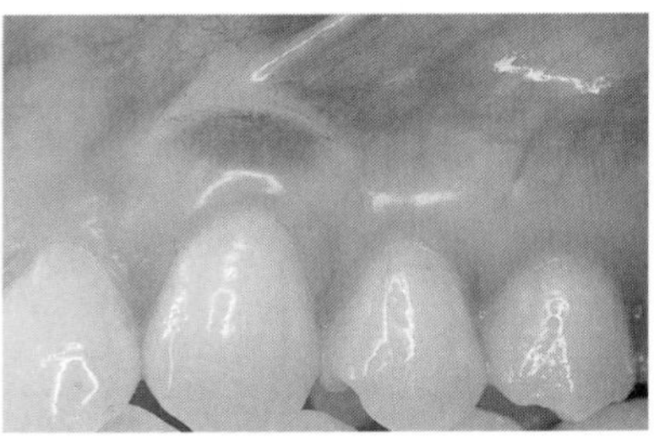

C

Fig. 66-13 Semilunar coronally positioned flap. **A,** Slight recession in facial of the upper left canine. **B,** After thorough scaling and root planing of the area, a semilunar incision is made and the tissue separated from the underlying bone. The flap collapses, covering the recession. **C,** Appearance after 7 weeks. Note coverage of the previous root denudation. (Courtesy Dr. Steven Kwan, Los Angeles, Calif.)

This technique is very simple and predictably provides 2 to 3 mm of root coverage. It can be performed on several adjoining teeth, but even though the incision may be continuous, extreme care should be exercised not to dissect the blood supply. The Tarnow technique is successful for the maxilla, particularly in covering root left exposed by the gingival margin receding from a recently placed crown margin. It is not recommended for mandibular teeth.

SUBEPITHELIAL CONNECTIVE TISSUE GRAFT (LANGER). This procedure is indicated for larger and multiple defects with good vestibular depth and gingival thickness to allow a split thickness flap to be elevated. Adjacent to the denuded root surface, the donor connective tissue is sandwiched between the split flap. It was described by Langer and Langer in 1985.[45] Similar approaches had been previously reported by Perez-Fernandez[58] and Raetzke.[60] The technique is as follows (Fig. 66-14).

Step One. Raise a partial-thickness flap with a horizontal incision 2 mm away from the tip of the papilla and two vertical incisions 1- to 2-mm away from the gingival margin of the adjoining teeth (Fig. 66-14). These incisions should extend at least one half to one tooth wider mesiodistally than the area of gingival reces-

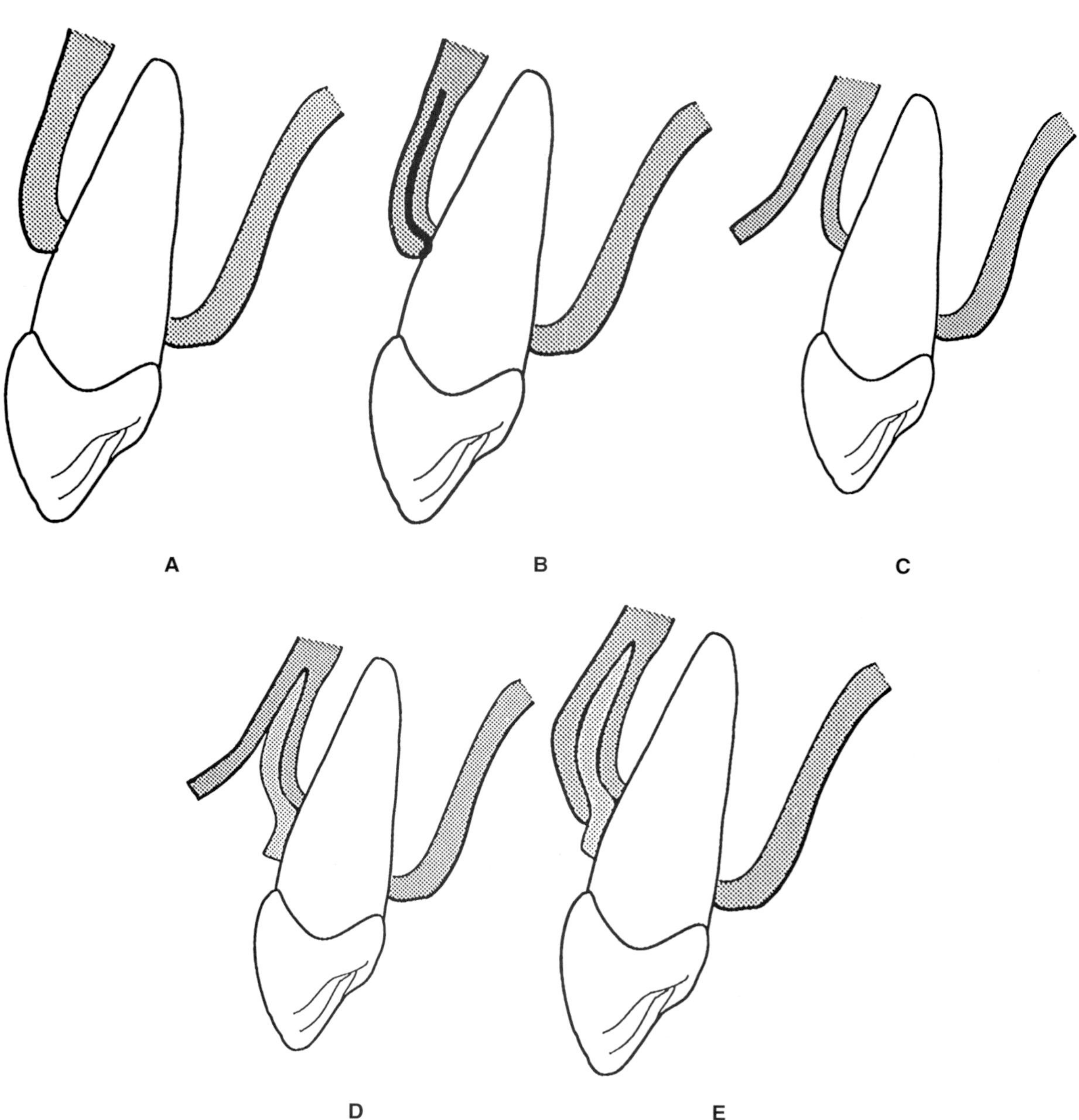

Fig. 66-14 Subepithelial connective tissue graft for root coverage. **A–E,** Sagittal view. **A,** Preoperative view of facial recession on maxillary central incisor. **B,** Split-thickness incision for recipient site. **C,** Split-thickness flap reflected. **D,** Connective tissue placed over denuded root surface. Note apical portion of donor tissue is placed between the split flap. **E,** Recipient flap is closed.

Continued

sion. Extend the flap to the mucobuccal fold without perforations that could affect the blood supply.

Step Two. Thoroughly plane the root, reducing its convexity.

Step Three. Obtain a connective tissue graft from the palate by means of a horizontal incision 5 to 6 mm from the gingival margin of molars and premolars (Fig. 66-15). The connective tissue is carefully removed and all adipose and glandular tissue removed. The palatal wound is sutured in a primary closure.

Step Four. Place the connective tissue on the denuded root(s). Suture it with resorbable sutures to the periosteum.

Step Five. Cover the graft with the outer portion of the partial-thickness flap and suture it interdentally (see Fig. 66-14). At least one half to two thirds of the connective tissue graft must be covered by the flap for the exposed portion to survive over the denuded root.

Step Six. Cover the area with tinfoil and surgical pack. After 7 days, the dressing and sutures are removed. The esthetics are favorable with this technique since the donor tissue is connective tissue (see Fig. 66-15, *F*). The donor site heals by primary intention, with considerably less discomfort than after a free gingival graft.

A variant of the subepithelial connective tissue graft, called a *subpedicle connective tissue graft,* was described by Nelson in 1987.[55] This technique uses a pedicle over the connective tissue that covers the denuded root surface. Therefore the blood supply is increased over the donor tissue.

GUIDED TISSUE REGENERATION TECHNIQUE FOR ROOT COVERAGE. Pini-Prato and colleagues[59] have described a technique based on the principle of guided tissue regeneration. Theoretically, guided tissue regeneration (GTR) should result in reconstruction of the attachment apparatus, along with coverage of the denuded root surface. This technique consists of the following steps (Figure 66-16).

Step One. A full-thickness flap is reflected to the mucogingival junction continuing as a partial-thickness flap 8 mm apical to the mucogingival junction.

Step Two. A microporous membrane is placed over the denuded root surface and the adjacent tissue. It is trimmed and adapted to the root surface and covers at least 2 mm of marginal periosteum.

Step Three. A suture is passed through the portion of the membrane that will cover the bone. This suture is knotted on the exterior and tied to bend the

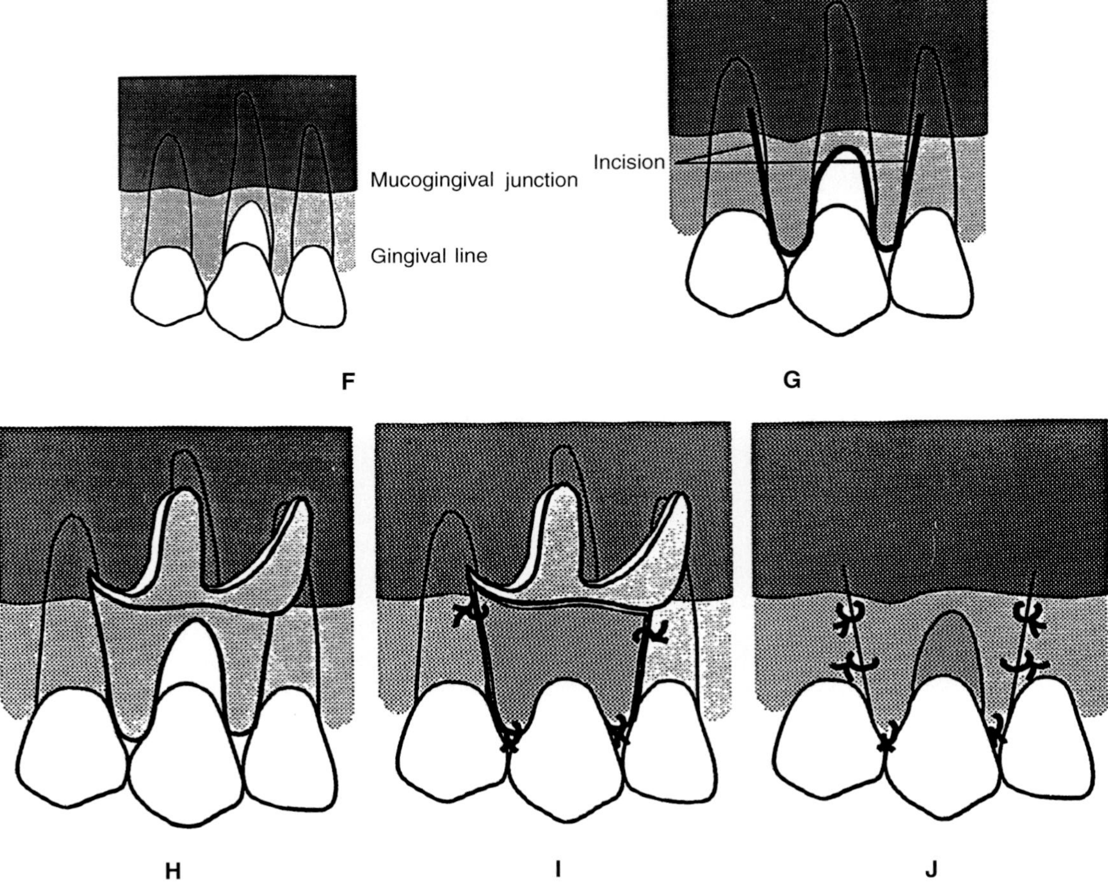

Fig. 66-14 cont'd Subepithelial connective tissue graft for root coverage. **F–J,** Facial view. **F,** Facial view of gingival recession. **G,** Vertical incisions to prepare recipient site. **H,** Split-thickness flap reflected. **I,** Connective tissue sutured over denuded root surface. **J,** Split-thickness flap sutured over donor connective tissue.

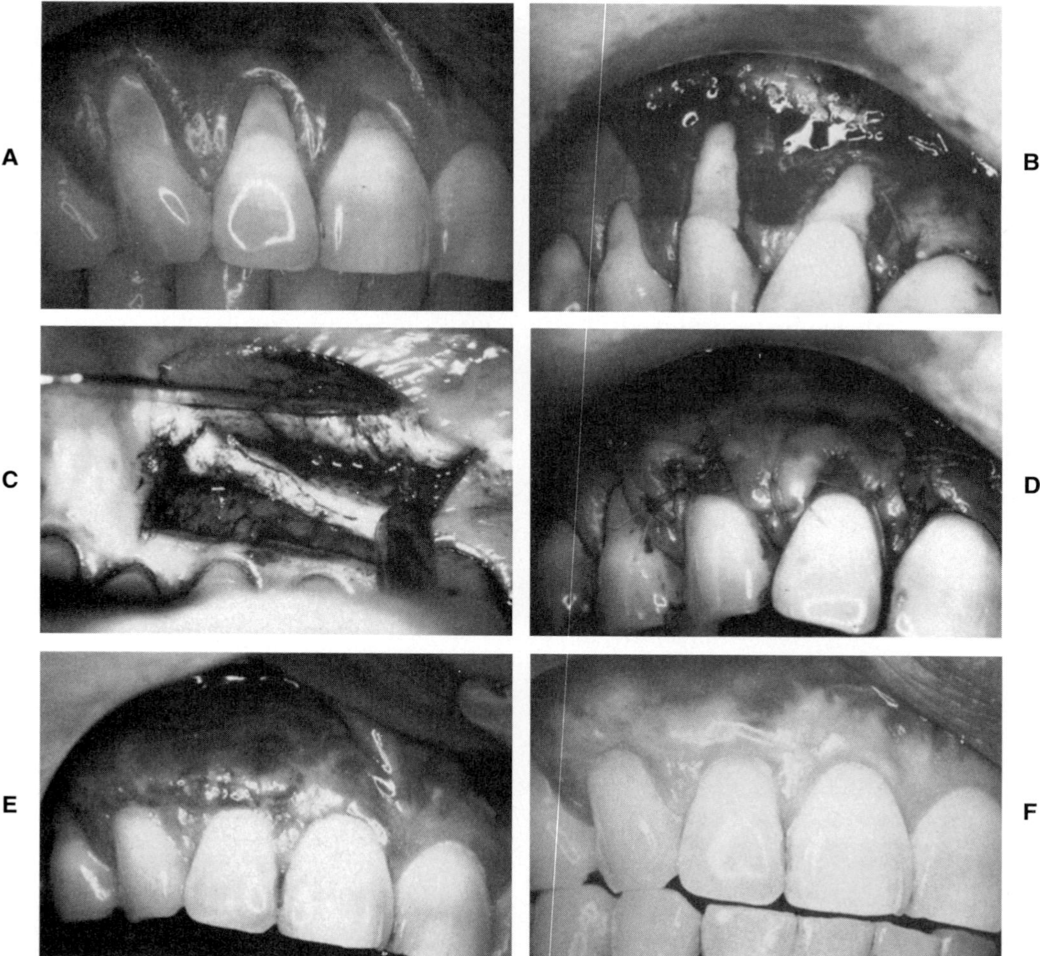

Fig. 66-15 The Langer technique for root coverage. **A,** Preoperative view. Note the recession on teeth no. 6 to 8. **B,** Split-thickness flap elevated on teeth no. 6 and 7. Note that the interdental papillae are not included in the flap, nor is the gingival margin area of tooth no. 8, which was treated by means of a coronally positioned flap. **C,** Palatal flap and the removal of the connective tissue graft. **D,** The graft placed under the flap and covering receded areas approximately to the cementoenamel junction. Sutures in place. **E,** After 1 week of healing. **F,** Roots covered after complete healing. Note the thickness of the tissue in the area covered and excellent color. (Courtesy Dr. T. J. Han, Los Angeles, Calif.)

membrane, creating a space between the root and the membrane. This space allows the growth of tissue beneath the membrane.

Step Four. The flap is then positioned coronally and sutured. Four weeks later, a small envelope flap is performed, and the membrane is carefully removed. The flap is then again positioned coronally to protect the growing tissue and sutured. One week later, these sutures are removed.

Tinti and colleagues[74] have used titanium-reinforced membranes to create space beneath the membrane. Resorbable membranes have also been used to achieve root coverage. The inability to create space between the resorbable membrane and the denuded root, due to its softness, may present a problem, even though there is the advantage of not necessitating a second surgery.

Clinical studies comparing this technique with the coronally positioned flap have shown that the GTR technique is better when the recession is greater than 4.98 mm apico-oronally.[59] Histologically, one case reported 3.66 mm of new connective tissue attachment associated with 2.48 mm of new cementum and 1.84 mm of bone growth.[20]

POUCH AND TUNNEL TECHNIQUE. To minimize incisions and reflection of flaps and to provide abundant blood supply to the donor tissue, the placement of subepithelial donor connective tissue into pouches beneath papillary tunnels allows for intimate contact of donor tissue to the recipient site. [81] After positioning the graft, the coronal placement of the recessed gingival margins completely covers the donor tissue. Therefore the esthetic result is excellent. This technique is especially effective for the maxillary anterior area where vestibular depth is adequate and there is good gingival thickness (Fig. 66-17). One of the advantages to this technique is the thickening of the gingival margin

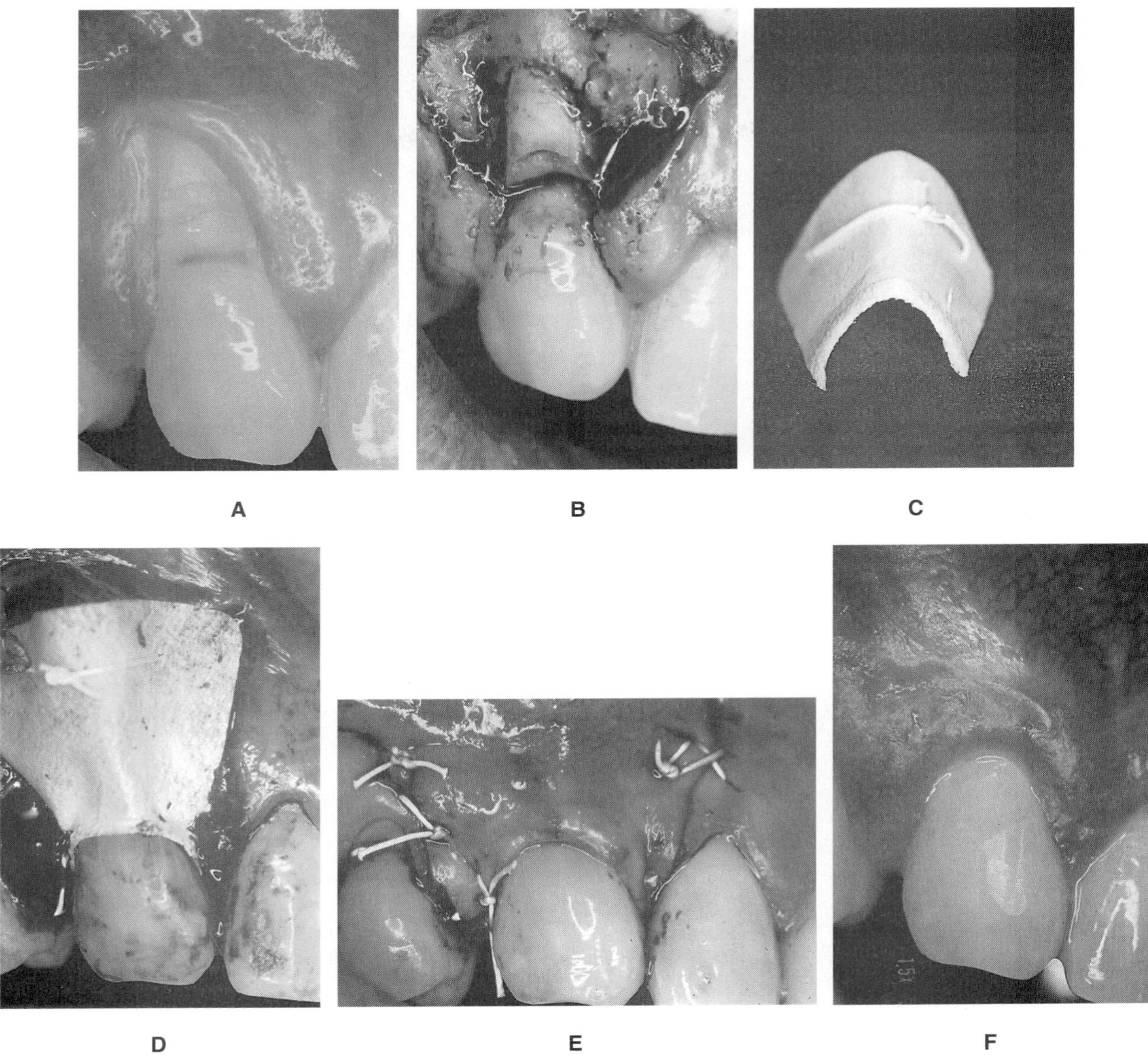

Fig. 66-16 Guided tissue regeneration technique for root coverage. **A,** Marked recession in the upper right cuspid. **B,** Incisions made and flap elevated. **C,** Membrane trimmed and bent with suture. **D,** Membrane placed on exposed root and covering bone margin. **E,** Sutures in place. **F,** After healing, the root is completely covered. (Courtesy Dr. Carlo Tinti, Milano, Italy.)

after healing. The thicker gingival margin is more stable to allow for the possibility of "creeping reattachment" of the gingival margin. The use of small, contoured blades enables the surgeon to incise and split the gingival tissues to create the recipient pouches and tunnels (Fig. 66-18). This technique consists of the following steps (see Fig. 66-17).

Step One. Using a no. 15C or 12D blade, a sulcular incision is made around the teeth adjacent to the recession. This incision separates the junctional epithelium and the connective tissue attachment from the root.

Step Two. Using either a curette or a small blade such as the no. 15C, a tunnel is created beneath the adjacent buccal papilla, into which the connective tissue is placed.

Step Three. A split-thickness pouch is created apical to the papilla, which has been tunneled, and the adjacent radicular surface. This pouch may extend 10- to 12-mm apical to the recessed gingival margin and papilla and 6- to 8-mm mesial and distal to the denuded root surface.

Step Four. The size of the pouch that includes the area of the denuded root surface is measured so an equivalent size connective tissue donor can be procured from the palate.

Step Five. Using sutures, curettes, and elevators, the connective tissue is placed under the pouch and tunnel with a portion covering the denuded root surface.

Step Six. The mesial and distal ends of the donor tissue are secured by gut sutures. The gingival margin of

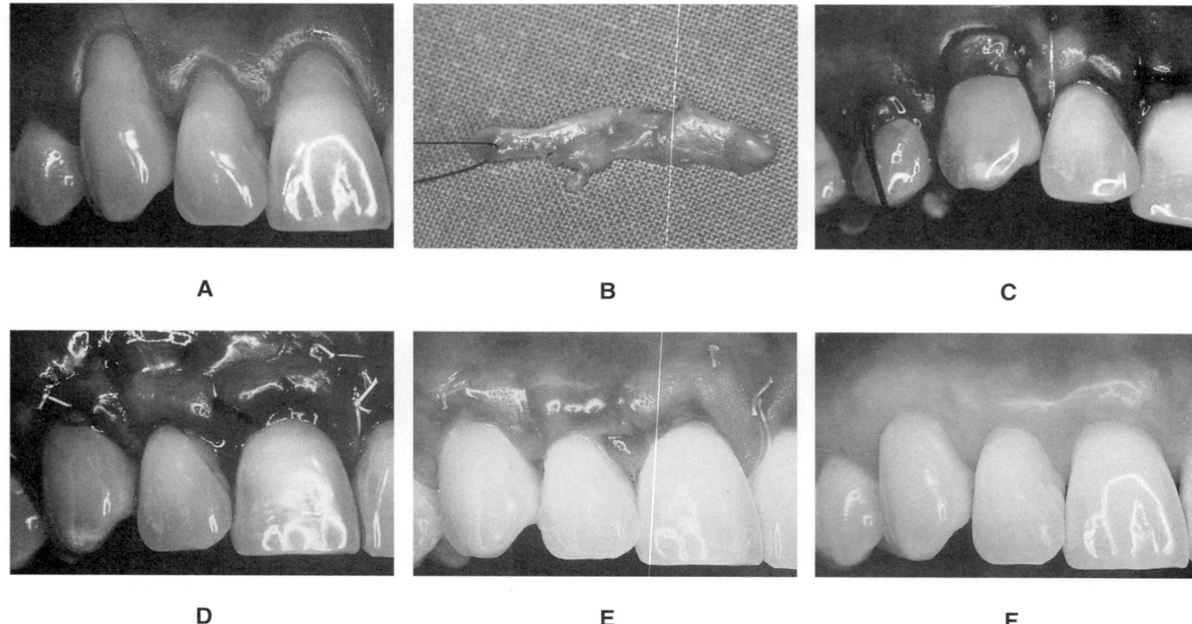

Fig. 66-17 Pouch and tunnel technique for root coverage. **A,** Preoperative view. Note gingival recession. **B,** Donor connective tissue from palate. **C,** Donor tissue placed in pouch and tunnel. **D,** Facial gingiva is sutured coronally to cover donor tissue. **E,** Two week postoperative healing. **F,** Final healing three months. Note root coverage and thick marginal gingiva.

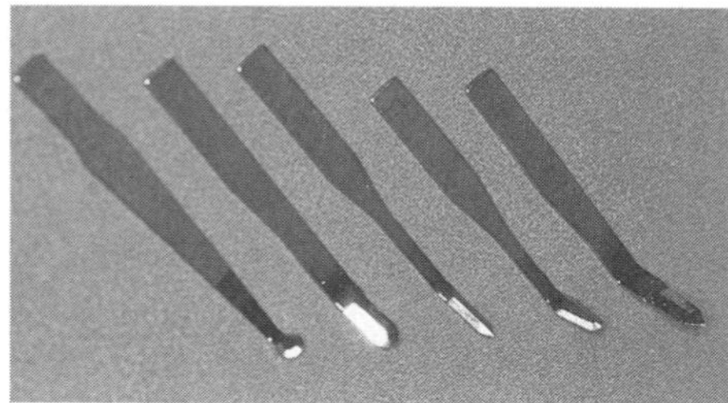

Fig. 66-18 Small, contoured blades used for periodontal plastic surgery.

the flap is coronally placed and secured by horizontal mattress sutures that extend over the contact of the two adjacent teeth. If the teeth are not in contact, a small amount of composite material may be placed temporarily between the two teeth to allow the placement of the suture over the closed contact.

Step Seven. Other holding sutures are placed through the overlying gingival tissue and donor tissue to the underlying periosteum to secure and stabilize the donor tissue beneath the gingiva.

Step Eight. A periodontal dressing is used to cover the surgical site.

TECHNIQUES TO DEEPEN THE VESTIBULE

The presence of adequate vestibular depth is important for both oral hygiene and retention of prosthetic appliances. Numerous surgical techniques have been proposed to accomplish this objective. The classic clinical studies in the early 1960s by Bohannan[7,8,9] indicated that deepening of the vestibule by nonfree graft procedures were not successful when evaluated years later. Predictable deepening of the vestibule can only be accomplished by the use of free autogenous grafts and its variants. Discussion on free grafts are covered in this chapter.

TECHNIQUES FOR THE REMOVAL OF THE FRENUM

A frenum is a fold of mucous membrane, usually with enclosed muscle fibers, that attaches the lips and cheeks to the alveolar mucosa and/or gingiva and underlying periosteum. A frenum becomes a problem if the attachment is too close to the marginal gingiva. Tension on the frenum may pull the gingival margin away from the tooth. This condition may be conducive to plaque accumulation and inhibit proper brushing of the teeth.

Frenectomy or Frenotomy

The terms *frenectomy* and *frenotomy* signify operations that differ in degree. Frenectomy is complete removal of the frenum, including its attachment to underlying bone, and may be required in the correction of an abnormal diastema between maxillary central incisors. Frenotomy is the incision of the frenum. Both procedures are used, but frenotomy generally suffices for periodontal purposes—that is, relocating the frenal attachment so as to create a zone of attached gingiva between the gingival

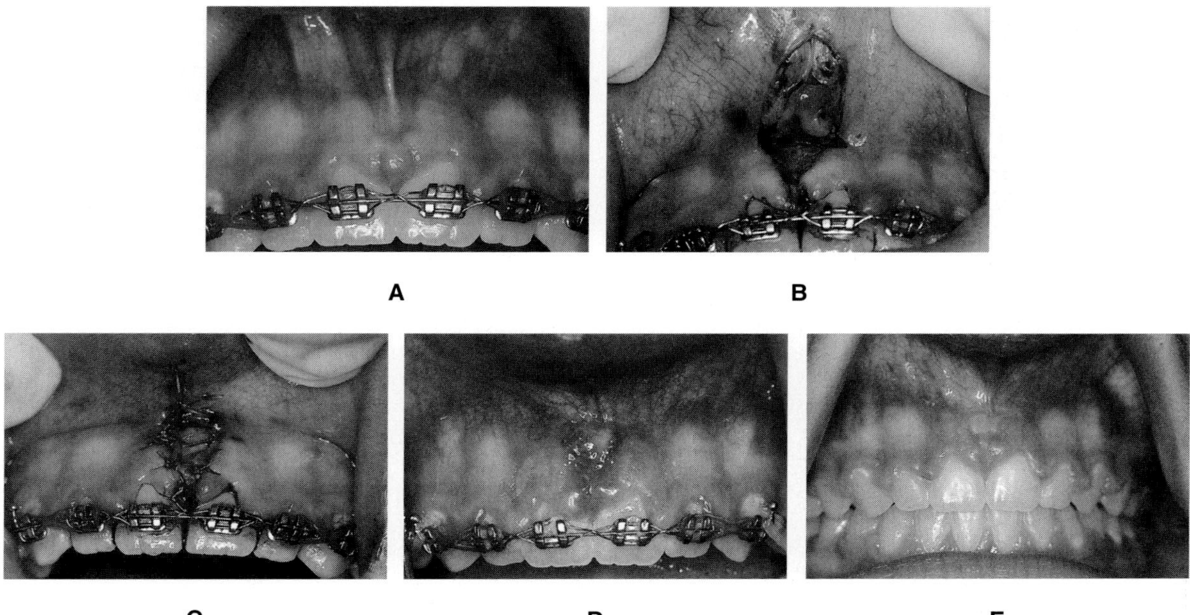

Fig. 66-19 Removal of the frenum. **A,** Preoperative view of frenum between the two maxillary central incisors. **B,** Removal of the frenum from both the lip and gingiva. **C,** The site is sutured after it is placed over the wound. **D,** Postoperative view after two weeks. **E,** Postoperative view after three months.

margin and the frenum. Frenectomy and frenotomy are usually performed in conjunction with other periodontal treatment procedures but occasionally are done as separate operations. Frenal problems occur most often on the facial surface between the maxillary and mandibular central incisors and in the canine and premolar areas.[78] (see Fig. 66-1, *D*). They occur less often on the lingual surface of the mandible.

Technique for the Removal of the Frenum. If the vestibule is deep enough, the operation is confined to the frenum. It is often necessary to deepen the vestibule to provide space for the repositioned frenum. This is accomplished as follows (Fig. 66-19):

1. After anesthetizing the area, engage the frenum with a hemostat inserted to the depth of the vestibule.
2. Incise along the upper surface of the hemostat, extending beyond the tip.
3. Make a similar incision along the undersurface of the hemostat.
4. Remove the triangular resected portion of the frenum with the hemostat. This exposes the underlying brushlike fibrous attachment to the bone.
5. Make a horizontal incision, separating the fibers, and bluntly dissect to the bone.
6. If necessary, extend the incisions laterally and suture the labial mucosa to the apical periosteum. Sometimes the area is covered with a free gingival or connective tissue graft.
7. Clean the field of operation and pack with gauze sponges until bleeding stops.
8. Cover the area with dry aluminum foil and apply the periodontal pack.
9. Remove the pack after 2 weeks and repack if necessary. One month is usually required for the formation of an intact mucosa with the frenum attached in its new position.

High frenal attachments on the lingual surface are uncommon. To correct these without involving the structures in the floor of the mouth, approximately 2 mm of the attachment is separated from the mucosa with a periodontal knife at weekly intervals until the desired level is reached. The area is covered with a periodontal pack in the intervals between treatments.

CRITERIA FOR SELECTION OF TECHNIQUES

Different techniques have been presented for solving mucogingival problems outlined in this chapter. The proper selection of the numerous techniques must be based on the predictability of success which, in turn, is based on the following criteria (see also Box 66-1):

1. *Surgical site free of plaque, calculus, and inflammation:* Periodontal plastic surgical procedures should be undertaken in a plaque- and inflammation-free environment to enable the clinician to manage gingival tissue that is firm. Meticulous, precise incisions and flap reflection cannot be achieved when the tissue is inflamed and edematous. Careful and thorough scaling, root planing, and meticulous plaque removal by the patient must be accomplished before any surgical procedure.

BOX 66-1

Criteria for Selection of Techniques for Solving Mucogingival Problems

Surgical site free of plaque, calculus, and inflammation
Adequate blood supply to the donor tissue
Anatomy of the recipient and donor site
Stability of the grafted tissue to the recipient site
Minimal trauma to the surgical site

2. *Adequate blood supply:* To obtain the maximum amount of blood supply to the donor tissue, gingival augmentation apical to the area of recession will provide a better blood supply than coronal augmentation, since the recipient site is entirely periosteal tissue. Root coverage procedures present a portion of the recipient site (denuded root surface) without blood supply. Therefore if esthetics is not a factor, gingival augmentation apical to the recession may be more predictable. A pedicle-displaced flap has a better blood supply than a free graft, with the base of the flap intact. Therefore, in root coverage, if the anatomy is favorable, the pedicle flap or any of its variants may be the best procedure.

   The subepithelial connective tissue graft (Langer) and the pouch and tunnel techniques use a split flap with the connective tissue sandwiched in between the flap. This flap design maximizes the blood supply to the donor tissue. If large areas require root coverage, these sandwich-type recipient sites provide the best flap design for blood supply.
3. *Anatomy of the recipient and donor sites:* The anatomy of the recipient and donor sites are an important consideration in selecting the proper technique. The presence or absence of vestibular depth is an important anatomic criteria at the recipient site for gingival augmentation. If gingival augmentation is indicated apical to the area of recession, there must be adequate vestibular depth apical to the recessed gingival margin to provide space for either a free or pedicle graft. If a vestibule is necessary, only a free graft can accomplish this objective apical to the recession.

   Mucogingival techniques such as free gingival grafts and free connective tissue grafts can be used to create vestibular depth and widen the zone of attached gingiva. Other techniques require vestibular depth to be present before the surgery. These procedures include pedicle grafts (lateral and coronal); subepithelial connective tissue graft (Langer); and pouch and tunnel procedures.

   The availability of donor tissue is another anatomic factor that must be considered. Pedicle displacement of tissue necessitates the presence of an adjacent donor site that presents gingival thickness and width. Palatal tissue thickness is also necessary for the connective tissue donor autograft. Gingival thickness is also required at the recipient site for techniques using split thickness, sandwich-type flap, or the pouch and tunnel techniques.
4. Stability of the grafted tissue to the recipient site: Good communication of the blood vessels from the grafted donor tissue to the recipient site requires a stable environment. This necessitates sutures that stabilize the donor tissue firmly against the recipient site. The least amount of sutures and maximum stability should be achieved.
5. Minimal trauma to the surgical site: Like all surgical procedures, periodontal plastic surgery is based on the meticulous, delicate, and precise management of the oral tissues. Unnecessary tissue trauma due to poor incisions, flap perforations, tears, traumatic and excessive placement of sutures can lead to tissue necrosis. The selection of proper instruments, needles, and sutures are mandatory to minimize tissue trauma. The use of sharp, contoured blades (see Fig. 66-18); smaller diameter needles; and resorbable, monofilament sutures are all important factors in achieving atraumatic surgery.

SUMMARY

New techniques are constantly being developed and are slowly incorporated into periodontal practice. The practitioner should be aware that, at times, new methods are published without adequate clinical research to ensure the predictability of the results and the extent to which the techniques may benefit the patient. Critical analysis of newly presented techniques should guide our constant evolution toward better clinical methods.

REFERENCES

1. American Academy of Periodontology: Proceedings of the World Workshop in Clinical Periodontics. Annals of Periodontology. Chicago, 1989, The Academy.
2. American Academy of Periodontology: Proceedings of the World Workshop in Periodontics. Annals of Periodontology. Chicago, 1996, The Academy.
3. Becker NG: A free gingival graft utilizing a presuturing technique. Periodontics 1967; 5:194.
4. Bernimoulin JP, Loscher B, Muhlemann HR: Coronally repositioned periodontal flap. J Clin Periodontol 1975; 2:1.
5. Bjorn H: Free transplantation of gingiva propia. Sveriges Tandlak T 1963; 22:684.
6. Brackett RC, Gargiulo AW: Free gingival grafts in humans. J Periodontol 1970; 41:581.
7. Bohannan H: Studies in the alteration of vestibular depth. I. Complete denudation. J Periodontol 1962; 33:120.
8. Bohannan H: Studies in the alteration of vestibular depth. II. Periosteum retention. J Periodontol 1962; 33:120.
9. Bohannan H: Studies in the alteration of vestibular depth. III. Vestibular incision. J Periodontol 1963; 34:208.
10. Broome WC, Taggart EJ Jr: Free autogenous connective tissue grafting. J Periodontol 1976; 47:580.
11. Caffesse RG, Albano E, Plot C: Injertos gingivalis libres en perros: analisis biometrico. Rev Asoc Odontol Argent 1972; 60:517.
12. Caffesse RG, Burgett FG, Nasjleti CE, et al: Healing of free gingival grafts with and without periosteum. Part I. Histologic evaluation. J Peridontol 1979; 50:586.
13. Caffesse RG, Carraro JJ, Carranza FA Jr: Injertos givgivales libres en perros: estudio clinico e histologico. Rev Asoc Odontol Argent 1972; 60:465.
14. Caffesse RG, Guinard E: Treatment of localized gingival recessions. II. Coronally repositioned flap with a free gingival graft. J Periodontol 1978; 49:358.

15. Caffesse RG, Nasjleti CE, Burgett FG, et al: Healing of free gingival grafts with and without periosteum. II. Radioautographic evaluation. J Periodontol 1979; 50:595.
16. Carranza FA Jr, Carraro JJ, Dotto CA, et al: Effect of periosteal fenestration in gingival extension operations. J Periodontol 1966; 37:335.
17. Chacker FM, Cohen DW: Regeneration of gingival tissues in non-human primates. J Dent Res 1960; 39:743.
18. Cohen DW, Ross SE: The double papillae repositioned flap in periodontal therapy. J Periodontol 1968; 39:65.
19. Corn H: Periosteal separation—Its clinical significance. J Periodontol 1962; 33:140.
20. Cortellini P, Clauser C, Pini-Prato GP: Histologic assessment of new attachment following the treatment of a human buccal recession by means of a guided tissue regeneration procedure. J Periodontol 1993; 64:387.
21. Costich ER, Ramfjord SP: Healing after partial denudation of the alveolar process. J Periodontol 1968; 39:127.
22. Donn BJ Jr: The free connective tissue autograft: a clinical and histologic wound healing study in humans. J Periodontol 1978; 49:253.
23. Donnenfeld OW, Glickman I: A biometric study of the effects of gingivectomy. J Periodontol 1966; 37:447.
24. Donnenfeld OW, Marks R, Glickman I: The apically repositioned flap: a clinical study. J Periodontol 1964; 35:381.
25. Dordick B, Coslet JG, Seibert JS: Clinical evaluation of free autogenous gingival grafts placed on alveolar bone. II. Coverage of non-pathologic dehiscences and fenestrations. J Periodontol 1976; 47:568.
26. Dorfman HS, Kennedy JE, Bird WC: Longitudinal evaluation of free autogenous gingival grafts. J Clin Periodontol 1980; 7:316.
27. Dorfman HS, Kennedy JE, Bird WC: Longitudinal evaluation of free autogenous gingival grafts. A four-year report. J Periodontol 1974; 1:185.
28. Edel A: Clinical evaluation of free connective tissue grafts used to increase the width of keratinized gingiva. J Clin Periodontol 1974; 1:185.
29. Edlan A, Mejchar B: Plastic surgery of the vestibulum in periodontal therapy. Int Dent J 1963; 13:593.
30. Friedman N: Mucogingival surgery. Texas Dent J 1957; 75:358.
31. Friedman N, Levine HL: Mucogingival surgery: current status. J Periodontol 1964; 35:5.
32. Gargiulo AW, Arrocha R: Histo-clinical evaluation of free gingival grafts. Periodontics 1967; 5:285.
33. Gordon HP, Sullivan HC, Atkins JH: Free autogenous gingival grafts. Part II, supplemental findings—Histology of the graft site. Periodontics 1968; 6:130.
34. Grupe HE: Modified technique for the sliding flap operation. J Periodontol 1966; 37:491.
35. Grupe HE, Warren RF Jr: Repair of gingival defects by a sliding flap operation. J Periodontol 1956; 27:92.
36. Hall WB: Pure mucogingival problems. Etiology, treatment and prevention. Chicago, Quintessence, 1984.
37. Han TJ, Takei HH, Carranza FA Jr: The strip gingival autograft technique. Int J Periodont Restor Dent 1993; 13:181.
38. Hangorsky V, Bissada NF: Clinical assessment of free gingival graft effectiveness on the maintenance of periodontal health. J Periodontol 1980; 51:274.
39. Harvey PM: Management of advanced periodontitis. Part I, Preliminary report of a method of surgical reconstruction. NZ Dent J 1965; 61:180.
40. Ibbott CG, Oles RD, Laverty WH: Effects of citric acid treatment on autogenous free graft coverage of localized recession. J Periodontol 1985; 56:662.
41. James WC, McFall WT Jr: Placement of free gingival grafts on denuded alveolar bone. Part I. Clinical evaluations. J Periodontol 49:283, 1978.
42. James WC, McFall WT Jr, Burkes EJ: Placement of free gingival grafts on denuded alveolar bone. II. Microscopic observations. J Periodontol 1978; 49:291.
43. Janson WA, Ruben MP, Kraamer GM, et al: Development of the blood supply to split-thickness free gingival autografts. J Periodontol 1969; 40:707.
44. Karring T, Ostergaard E, Löe H: Conservation of tissue specificity after heterotopic transplantation of gingiva and alveolar mucosa. J Periodont Res 1971; 6:282.
45. Langer B, Langer L: Subepithelial connective tissue graft technique for root coverage. J Periodontol 1985; 56:715.
46. Levine RA: Covering denuded root surface with the subepithelial connective tissue graft. Compendium Continuing Education Dent 1991; 12:568.
47. Liu WWJ, Solt CW: A surgical procedure for the treatment of localized gingival recession in conjunction with root surface citric acid conditioning. J Periodontol 1980; 51:505.
48. Matter J: Free gingival graft and coronally repositioned flap. A 2-year follow-up report. J Clin Periodontol 1979; 6:437.
49. Matter J, Cimasoni G: Creeping attachment after free gingival grafts. J Periodontol 1976; 47:574.
50. Miller PD Jr: A classification of marginal tissue recession. Int J Periodont Restor Dent 1985; 5:9.
51. Miller PD Jr: Root coverage using a free soft tissue autograft following citric acid application. Part I. Technique. Int J Periodont Restor Dent 1982; 2:65.
52. Miller PD Jr: Root coverage using a free soft tissue autograft following citric acid application. III. A successful and predictable procedure in areas of deep wide recession. Int J Periodont Restor Dent 1985; 5:15.
53. Mormann W, Schaer F, Firestone AC: The relationship between success of free gingival grafts and transplant thickness. J Periodontol 1981; 52:74.
54. Nabers J: Free gingival grafts. Periodontics 1966; 4:243.
55. Nelson SW: The subpedicle connective tissue graft—a bilaminar reconstructive procedure for the coverage of denuded root surfaces. J Periodontol 1987; 58:95.
56. Oliver RC, Löe H, Karring T: Microscopic evaluation of the healing and revascularization of free gingival grafts. J Periodontol 1968; 3:84.
57. Pennel BM, Tabor JC, King KO, et al: Free masticatory mucosa graft. J Periodontol 1969; 40:162.
58. Perez-Fernandez A: Injerto submucoso libre de encia. Una nueva perspectiva. Bol Inform Dent 1982; 42:63.
59. Pini-Prato G, Tinti C, Vincenzi G, et al: Guided tissue regeneration versus mucogingival surgery in the treatment of human buccal gingival recession. J Periodontol 1992; 63:919.
60. Raetzke PB: Covering localized areas of root exposure employing the "envelope" technique. J Periodontol 1985; 56:397.
61. Rateitschak KH, Rateitschak EM, Wolff HF, et al: Color Atlas of Periodontology. New York, Thieme, 1985.
62. Robinson RE: Periosteal fenestration in mucogingival surgery. J West Soc Periodontol 1961; 9:107.
63. Rosenberg MM: Vestibular alterations in periodontics. J Periodontol 1960; 31:231.
64. Rubenstein HS, Ruben MP, Levy C, et al: Evidence for successful acceptance of irradiated free gingival allografts in dogs. J Periodontol 1975; 46:195.
65. Schmid MO: The subperiosteal vestibule extension—literature review, rationale and technique. J West Soc Periodontol 1976; 24:89.
66. Schoo WH, Copes L: Use of palatal mucosa and lyophilized dura mater to create attached gingiva. J Clin Periodontol 1976; 3:166.
67. Staffileno H, Levy S, Gargiulo A: Histologic study of cellular mobilization and repair following a periosteal retention operation via split thickness mucogingival flap surgery. J Periodontol 1969; 40:311.

68. Stetler KJ, Bissada NF: Significance of the width of keratinized gingiva on the periodontal status of teeth with submarginal restorations. J Periodontol 1987; 58:696.
69. Strahan JD: The relation of the mucogingival junction to the alveolar bone margin. Dent Practit Dent Record 1963; 14:72.
70. Sugarman EF: A clinical and histological study of the attachment of grafted tissue to bone and teeth. J Periodontol 1969; 40:381.
71. Sullivan HC, Atkins JC: Free autogenous gingival grafts. III. Utilization of grafts in the treatment of gingival recession. Periodontics 1968; 6:152.
72. Sullivan HC, Carman D, Dinner D: Histological evaluation of the laterally positioned flap. IADR Abstracts 1971; 467:169.
73. Tarnow DP: Semilunar coronally repositioned flap. J Clin Periodontol 1986; 13:182.
74. Tinti C, Vincenzi GP: Expanded polytetrafluoroethylene titanium-reinforced membranes for regeneration of mucogingival recession defects. A 12-case report. J Periodontol 1994; 65:1088.
75. Trey E, Bernimoulin JP: Influence of free gingival grafts on the health of the marginal gingiva. J Clin Periodontol 1980; 7:381.
76. Wade AB: Vestibular deepening by the technique of Edlan and Meejchar. J Periodont Res 1969; 4:300.
77. Ward VJ: A clinical assessment of the use of the free gingival graft for correcting localized recession associated with frenal pull. J Periodontol 1974; 45:78.
78. Whinston GJ: Frenotomy and mucobuccal fold resection used in periodontal therapy. NY Dent J 1956; 22:495.
79. Wilderman MN, Wentz FM: Repair of a dentogingival defect with a pedicle flap. J Periodontol 1965; 36:218.
80. Woofter C: The prevalence and etiology of gingival recession. Perodont Abstr 1969; 17:45.
81. Zabalegui I, Sicua A, Cambra J, et al: Treatment of multiple adjacent gingival recessions with the tunnel subepithelial connective tissue graft. A clinical report. Int J of Perio Rest Dent 1999; 19:199.

SUGGESTED READINGS

1. American Academy of Periodontology: Glossary of Periodontal Terms, ed 3. Chicago, The Academy, 1992.
2. Albano EA, Caffesse RC, Carranza FA Jr: A biometric analysis of laterally displaced pedicle flaps. Rev Asoc Odontol Argent 1969; 57:351.
3. Ariaudo AA, Tyrrell HA: Elimination of pockets extending to or beyond mucogingival junction. Dent Clin North Am 1960; 4:67.
4. Becker BE, Becker W: Use of connective tissue autografts for treatment of mucogingival problems. Int J Periodont Restor Dent 1986; 6:89.
5. Bergenholtz A, Hugoson A: Vestibular sulcus extension surgery in cases with periodontal disease. J Periodont Res 1967; 2:221.
6. Bhaskar SN, Cutright DE, Perez B, et al: Full and partial thickness pedicle grafts in miniature swine and man. J Periodontol 1971; 42:66.
7. Carranza FA Jr, Carraro JJ: Effect of removal of periosteum on postoperative result of mucogingival surgery. J Periodontol 1963; 34:223.
8. Carranza FA Jr, Carraro JJ: Mucogingival techniques in periodontal surgery. J Periodontol 1970; 41:294.
9. Carraro JJ, Carranza FA Jr, Albano EA, et al: Effect of bone denudation in mucogingival surgery in humans. J Periodontol 1964; 35:463.
10. Corn H: Edentulous area pedicle graft in mucogingival surgery. Periodontics 1964; 2:229.
11. Dordick B, Coslet JG, Siebert JS: Clinical evaluation of the free autogenous gingival grafts placed on alveolar bone. I. Clinical predictability. J Periodontol 1976; 47:559.
12. Friedman N: Mucogingival surgery: the apically repositioned flap. J Periodontol 1964; 35:5.
13. Grant DA: Experimental periodontal surgery; sequestration of alveolar bone. J Periodontol 1967; 38:409.
14. Guinard EA, Caffesse RG: Localized gingival recessions II. Treatment. J West Soc Periodontol 1977; 25:10.
15. Guinard EA, Caffesse RG: Treatment of localized gingival recessions, Part I: lateral sliding flap. J Periodontol 1978; 49:351.
16. Hawley CE, Staffileno H: Clinical evaluation of free gingival grafts in periodontal surgery. J Periodontol 1970; 41:105.
17. Maynard JB: Coronal positioning of a previously placed autogenous gingival graft. J Periodontol 1977; 48:151.
18. Miller PD Jr: Root coverage with the free gingival graft. Factors associated with incomplete coverage. J Periodontol 1987; 58:674.
19. Miller PD Jr, Allen EP: The development of periodontal plastic surgery. Periodontol 2000 1996; 2:7.
20. Miller PD Jr: Regenerative and reconstructive periodontal plastic surgery, mucogingival surgery. Dent Clin North Am 1988; 32:287.
21. Miyasato M, Crigger M, Egelberg J: Gingival conditions in areas of minimal and appreciable width of keratinized gingiva. J Clin Periodontol 1977; 4:200.
22. Nabers CL: Repositioning the attached gingiva. J Periodontol 1954; 25:38.
23. Nabers CL: When is gingival repositioning an indicated procedure? J West Soc Periodontol 1957; 5:4.
24. Neach K: The use of allogenic sclera and autogenous gingiva as free gingival grafts. Thesis, University of California at Los Angeles, 1978.
25. Pennel B, King KO, Higgason JD, et al: Retention of periosteum in mucogingival surgery. J Periodontol 1965; 36:39.
26. Pini-Prato G, Clauser C, Magnani C, et al: Resorbable membrane in the treatment of human buccal recession. A nine-case report. Int J Perio Rest Dent 1995; 15:258.
27. Ramfjord SP, Costich ER: Healing after exposure of periosteum on the alveolar process. J Periodontol 1968; 39:199.
28. Rateitschak KH, Egli U, Fingeli G: Recession: a four-year longitudinal study after free gingival graft. J Clin Periodontol 1979; 6:158.
29. Redondo VF, Bustamante A, Carranza FA Jr: Evaluacion biometrica de la tecnica de extension gingival con fenestracion periostica. Rev Asoc Odontol Argent 1968; 56:346.
30. Robinson RE, Agnew RG: Periosteal fenestration at the mucogingival line. J Periodontol 1963; 34:503.
31. Roth H: Some speculations as to predictable fenestrations prior to mucogingival surgery. Periodontics 1965; 3:29.
32. Smith RM: A study of the intertransplanatation of alveolar mucosa. Oral Surg 1970; 29:328.
33. Smith RM: A study of the intertransplantation of gingiva. Oral Surg 1970; 29:169.
34. Smukler H: Laterally positioned mucoperiosteal pedicle grafts in the treatment of denuded roots. J Periodontol 1976; 47:590.
35. Spengler DE, Hayward JR: Study of sulcus extension wound healing in dogs. J Oral Surg 1964; 22:413.
36. Staaffileno H: Palatal flap surgery: mucosal flap (split thickness) and its advantages over the mucoperiosteal flap. J Periodontol 1969; 40:547.
37. Staffileno H, Levy S, Gargiulo A: Histologic study of cellular mobilization and repair following a periosteal retention operation via split thickness mucogingival flap surgery. J Periodontol 1966; 37:117.

38. Staffileno H, Wentz F, Orban B: Histologic study of healing of split-thickness flap surgery in dogs. J Periodontol 1962; 33:56.
39. Sullivan HC, Atkins JC: Free autogenous gingival grafts, Part I: principles of successful grafting. Periodontics 1968; 6:5.
40. Sullivan HC, Atkins JC: The role of free gingival grafts in periodontal therapy. Dent Clin North Am 1969; 13:33.
41. Tavtigian R: The height of the facial radicular alveolar crest following apically positioned flap operations. J Periodontol 1970; 41:412.
42. Wennstrom J, Lindhe J, Nyman S: Role of keratinized gingiva for gingival health. J Clin Periodontol 1981; 8:311.
43. Wennstrom J, Lindhe J, Nyman S: The role of keratinized gingiva in plaque-associated gingivitis in dogs. J Clin Periodontol 1982; 9:75.
44. Wilderman MN: Exposure of bone in periodontal surgery. Dent Clin North Am 1964; 8:23.
45. Wood DL, Hoag PL, Donnenfeld OW, et al: Alveolar crest reduction following full and partial thickness flaps. J Periodontol 1972; 43:141.

Recent Advances in Surgical Technology

Dennis A. Shanelec and Leonard S. Tibbetts

CHAPTER

Chapter Outline

The use of magnification in periodontics is not an isolated development. It is part of a broader trend in medicine and dentistry toward the application of minimally invasive techniques for procedures that previously required extensive surgical incisions.[2,3,10,13] *Microsurgery* is defined as a refinement in operative technique by which visual acuity is enhanced through the use of the surgical operating microscope. It is a methodology, through which surgical techniques are modified to accommodate the improved motor coordination made possible through magnification.[12] In addition to clinical microsurgery, magnification in periodontics may be applied to diagnostic and nonsurgical procedures as a result of the improved visual acuity and motor coordination.

MAGNIFICATION SYSTEMS

A variety of simple and complex magnification systems are available to dentists, ranging from simple loupes to prism telescopic loupes and surgical microscopes. Each magnification system has its specific advantages and limitations. Although magnification improves the accuracy of clinical and diagnostic skills, it requires an understanding of optical principles that govern all magnification systems. The assumption that more magnification is better must always be weighed against a decrease in field of view and depth of focus that can occur as magnification increases. This is a problem more common with dental loops than with surgical operating microscopes.

Magnifying Loupes

Dental loupes are by far the most common system of optical magnification used in periodontics. Loupes are fundamentally two monocular telescopes with side-by-side lenses converged to focus on the operative field. The magnified image they form has stereoscopic properties by virtue of their convergence. A convergent lens optical system is also called a *Keplerian optical system.*

Although dental loupes are widely used, they have a considerable disadvantage. The clinician's eyes must converge to view the operative field. This may result in eyestrain, fatigue, and even pathologic vision changes, especially after prolonged use of poorly fitted loupes.

Three types of Keplerian loupes are commonly used in periodontics: simple or single-element loupes, compound loupes, and prism telescopic loupes. Each type may differ widely in optical sophistication and individual design.

Simple Loupes. Simple loupes consist of a pair of single meniscus lenses (Fig. 67-1). Simple loupes are primitive magnifiers with limited capabilities. Each lens is limited to just two refracting surfaces. Only increasing their lens diameter or thickness can increase their magnification. Size and weight limitations make simple loupes impractical for magnification beyond 1.5 diameters. Another disadvantage of simple loupes is that they are highly affected by spherical and chromatic aberration, which distorts the shape and color of, objects being viewed.

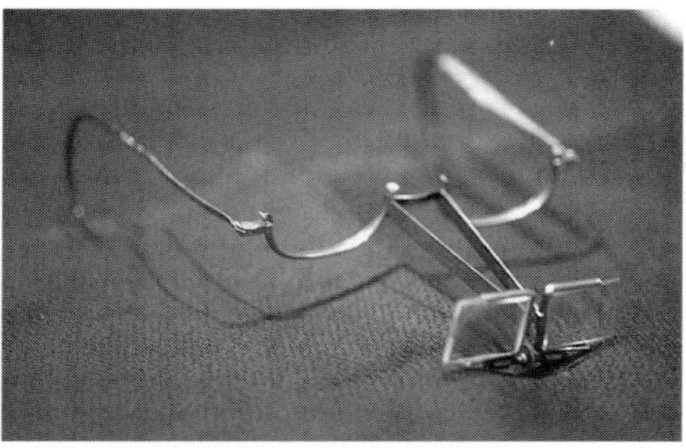

Fig. 67-1 Simple loupes.

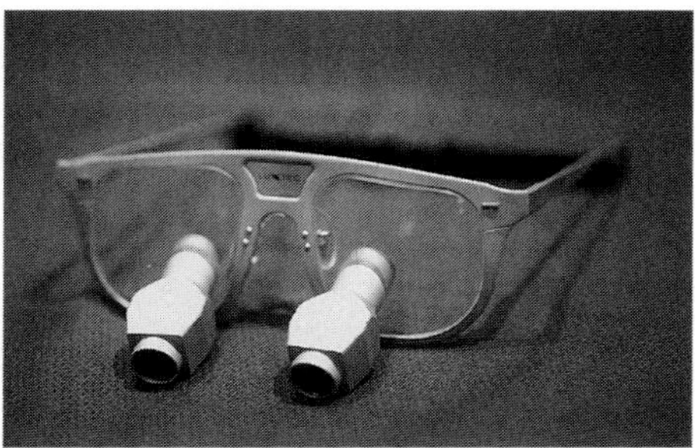

Fig. 67-3 Eyeglass-mounted prism loupes.

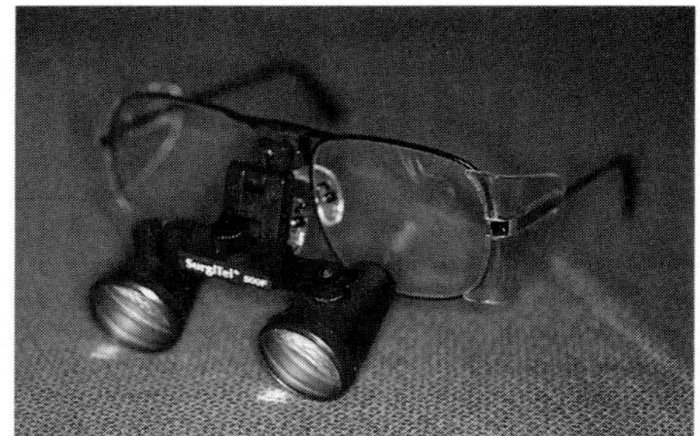

Fig. 67-2 Compound loupes.

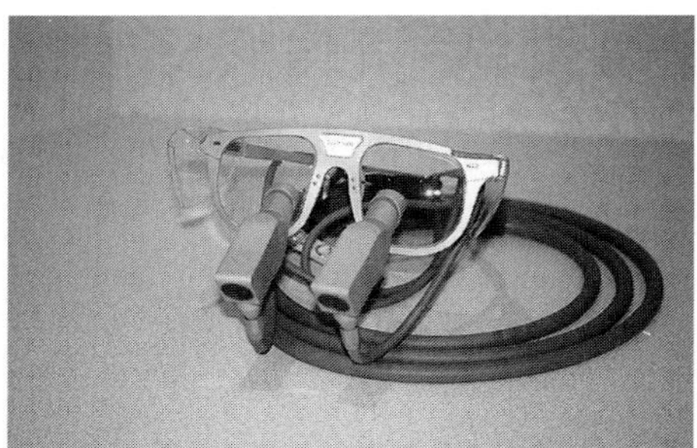

Fig. 67-4 Coaxial lighted prism loupes.

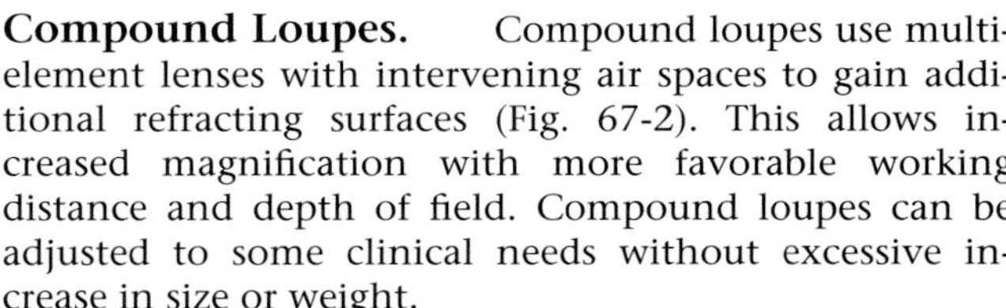

Compound Loupes. Compound loupes use multi-element lenses with intervening air spaces to gain additional refracting surfaces (Fig. 67-2). This allows increased magnification with more favorable working distance and depth of field. Compound loupes can be adjusted to some clinical needs without excessive increase in size or weight.

In addition to offering improved optical performance, compound lenses can be achromatic. This is an optical feature that clinicians should always choose when selecting magnifying loupes. Achromatic lenses consist of two glass lenses, joined together with clear resin. The specific density of each lens counteracts the chromatic aberration of its paired lens to produce a color-correct image. Multi-element compound loupes become optically inefficient at magnifications above 3.0 diameters.

Prism Telescopic Loupes. The most advanced type of loupe magnification currently available is the prism telescopic loupe. Such loupes employ Schmidt or rooftop prisms to lengthen the light path through a series of switchback mirror reflections within the lens elements. This arrangement literally folds light so that the barrel of the telescopic loupes can be shortened. Prism loupes produce better magnification, wider depths of field, longer working distances, and larger fields of view than other types of loupes. The barrels of prism loupes are short enough to be mounted on either eyeglass frames (Fig. 67-3) or headbands. However, the increased weight of prism telescopic loupes with magnification above 3× makes headband mounting more comfortable and stable than eyeglass frame mounting. Recent innovations in prism telescopic loupes include coaxial fiberoptic lighting incorporated in the lens elements to improve illumination (Fig. 67-4).

Magnification Range of Surgical Loupes

Dental loupes provide a limited range of magnification (1.5× to 10×). Those delivering magnification of less than 2.5× are usually inadequate for the visual acuity necessary for periodontal microsurgery. Those providing magnification of more than 4.5× are awkward to use because of their small field of view, shallow depth of focus, and excessive weight. The latter makes it quite difficult for a surgeon to maintain a stable visual field.

For some periodontal procedures, prism telescopic loupes with magnification of 4× provide an adequate combination of magnification, field of view, and depth of focus. However, the surgical operating microscope provides much higher magnification and superior optical properties than any of the loupe optical systems previously discussed.

The Operating Microscope

The surgical operating microscope provides superior magnification and better optical performance compared with dental loupes (Fig. 67-5). Although the microscope is expensive, it is durable and can withstand an entire clinical career. An operating microscope requires a period of adjustment to reach clinical proficiency, but it offers far better clinical performance and versatility than loupes. Operating microscopes designed for use in dentistry employ Galilean optical principles[1] and have binocular eyepieces joined by offsetting prisms with parallel optical axes. Galilean optics allows stereoscopic viewing of the operative field without eye convergence. This positions the eyes as if they were focused on infinity to permit a relaxed viewing of the operative field without eyestrain or fatigue. The operating microscope incorporates fully coated optics with achromatic lenses to provide the highest optical resolution with the most efficient illumination.

Perhaps the greatest advantage of the surgical operating microscope is its ability allow the dentist to easily change working magnification to a level appropriate for the clinical task at hand.[5] Operating microscopes have a rotating variable magnification element that easily varies magnification to match the immediate surgical demands. Some operating microscopes incorporate electronic foot-controlled focus and magnification for further convenience. Because the optical elements of surgical microscopes are more sophisticated than those found in loupes, depth-of-focus and field-of-view characteristics are quite enhanced.

The periodontal surgeon must establish adequate working distance between the surgical field and the microscope objective lens. This permits the surgical assistant to retract tissues and to irrigate or evacuate the surgical site. Such assistant aided control of surgical access is essential for microsurgical visibility. Assistant eyepiece attachments are available for all surgical microscopes and can greatly aid the progress of microsurgical procedures. Surgical microscopes are available with objective lenses with various working distances. The useful range in dentistry is 250 to 350 mm. Because operating with indirect mirror vision adds 100 to 150 mm to the working distance, a ready means of changing working distances is valuable. Quick-change objective lenses are available for many surgical microscopes.

For practical use in periodontics, the surgical microscope must have both maneuverability and stability. Microscope mountings are available for ceiling, wall, or floor. Inclining eyepieces also lend flexibility to the clinical use of the surgical microscope in periodontics. Maneuverability must always be sufficient to meet the clinical requirements for visual access to the various posterior regions of the oral cavity and the anatomic tissues dealt with during periodontal microsurgery. Optical performance of most microscope lenses is almost identical. Maneuverability is, therefore, more important than optical configuration in choosing an appropriate microscope for periodontal microsurgery procedures.

Illumination of the microsurgical field is an extremely important consideration. Periodontists are accustomed to lateral illumination from side-mounted dental lights. Clinicians who work with loupes often require a headlamp to compensate for the decreased light-gathering ability of loupes compared with normal vision. Coaxial fiberoptic illumination had been a major advantage of the operating microscope over surgical loupes. Coaxial lighting positions the light source exactly parallel to the microscope's optical axis. With coaxial lighting, no shadows are produced. The surgeon can view perfectly the deepest reaches of the oral cavity, including into subgingival pockets and angular bony defects. Definitive visualization of root surface deposits and irregularities is only possible at magnification levels provided by a surgical microscope. Through the microscope, surgeons can view normal and abnormal periodontal anatomy never before possible. Clinical decisions can be made based on certain visual knowledge of altered or normal anatomy rather than based on blind educated guesses.

Documentation of periodontal procedures has become increasingly important for dental-legal reasons as well as for patient and professional education. The surgical operating microscope is ideal for documenting periodontal pathology and procedures of all types; 35-mm slides can easily be produced using a beam splitter camera attachment (Fig. 67-6). With a foot-operated shutter control, the surgeon can compose the photographic field as the procedure unfolds without interrupting the surgery. In addition, the photographic slide represents the surgical field exactly as seen by the surgeon, as opposed to a photographer's view produced over the surgeon's shoulder as he or she works. Excellent video documentation is also available through the operating microscope using a video beam splitter attachment. High-resolution cameras with video and slide printers are currently replacing 35-mm camera photography in many microsurgical disciplines. High-resolution digital video cameras bring new capabilities for live or recorded video of periodontal procedures for educational purposes.

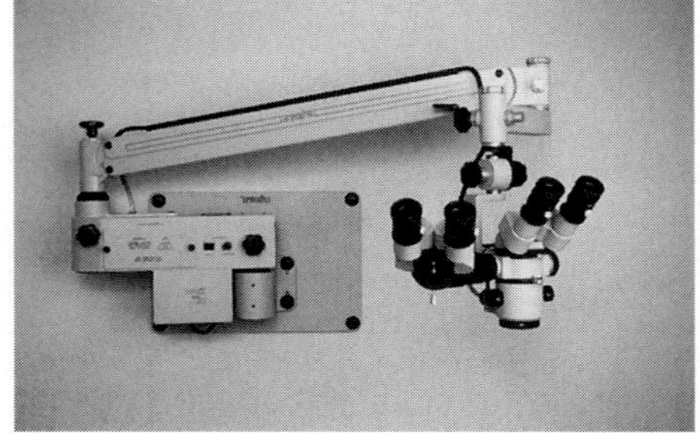

Fig. 67-5 Surgical operating microscope.

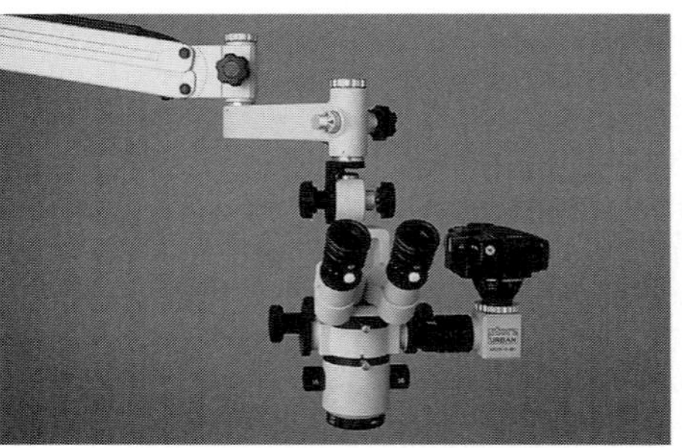

Fig. 67-6 Microscope camera and beam splitter.

PERIODONTAL MICROSURGERY

In recent years periodontics has seen increasing employment of procedures requiring progressively more intricate surgical skills. Regenerative and resective surgical procedures, periodontal plastic surgery, and dental implants all demand clinical performance levels that challenge the technical motor skills of periodontal surgeons beyond a range possible with unassisted vision.

Periodontal microsurgery introduces the potential for a less invasive surgical approach in periodontics. This is exemplified by a lessened need for vertical releasing incisions and smaller surgical sites. Periodontal surgeons, like other microsurgeons, continue to be surprised by the extent to which reduced incision size and surgical retraction are directly related to reduced postoperative pain and rapid healing.[15]

Root Preparation

The importance of root débridement is recognized universally as an essential component of periodontal therapy.[4,7,8,11] Research in clinical dentistry has shown that magnification-enhanced vision more ideally accomplishes the established clinical goals of endodontic and restorative dentistry. In periodontics, studies demonstrate that root débridement, performed without magnification, was incomplete. When débrided roots were examined with the aid of a microscope, substantial deposits remained. It may be inferred that magnification-enhanced vision in periodontics may permit more definitive root débridement.

Among the primary aims of periodontal surgery is visual access to the root surface for plaque and calculus removal and for removing pathologically altered tooth structure. Magnification greatly improves the surgeon's ability to create a clean, smooth root surface (Fig. 67-7). The root surface represents one opposing edge of the periodontal wound. Root planing is, therefore, analogous to establishing a clean, right-angled, soft tissue incision. Magnification permits preparation of both hard and soft tissue wound surfaces so they may be joined together according to the commonly held microsurgical principle of butt-joint wound approximation. This encourages primary wound healing and enhanced periodontal regeneration. Wound healing studies show epithelial anastomosis of microsurgically joined surgical wounds in animals within 48 hours.[6,14]

Surgery Under Magnification. Viewing periodontal surgery under magnification cannot help but impress the periodontal surgeon with the coarseness of conventional surgical manipulation. What appears to the unaided eye as gentle handling is revealed, under magnification, as gross crushing and tearing of delicate tissues. Periodontists have always attempted to treat the surgical site atraumatically and to achieve primary wound closure. However, the limits of normal vision dictate the extent to which this goal was possible. Periodontal microsurgery is the natural transition from conventional surgical principles to a surgical ethic in which the microscope is employed to permit more accurate and atraumatic handling tissues to enhance wound healing.

Microsurgical Instruments. In addition to the use of magnification and reliance on atraumatic technique, microsurgery entails the use of specially constructed microsurgical instruments designed specifically to minimize trauma. An important characteristic of microsurgical instruments is their ability to create clean incisions that prepare wounds for healing by primary intention. Microsurgical incisions are established at a 90-degree angle to the surface using ophthalmic microsurgical scalpels (Fig. 67-8). Microscopy permits easy identification of ragged wound edges for trimming and freshening. For primary wound closure, microsutures in the range of 6-0 to 9-0 are needed to approximate the wound edges (Fig. 67-9). Microsurgical wound apposition minimizes gaps or voids at the wound edges. This encourages rapid healing with less postoperative inflammation and with less pain.

Figures 67-10 through 67-15 illustrate periodontal surgery cases treated using microsurgical techniques.

Ergonomics. The ergonomics of hand position and body posture is closely related to the improved motor skills made possible by a microsurgical approach to therapy. Studies show that motor coordination is greatly improved when surgeons use microsurgical instruments specifically designed to employ a precision grip of the hand. Microsurgical instruments are circular in cross

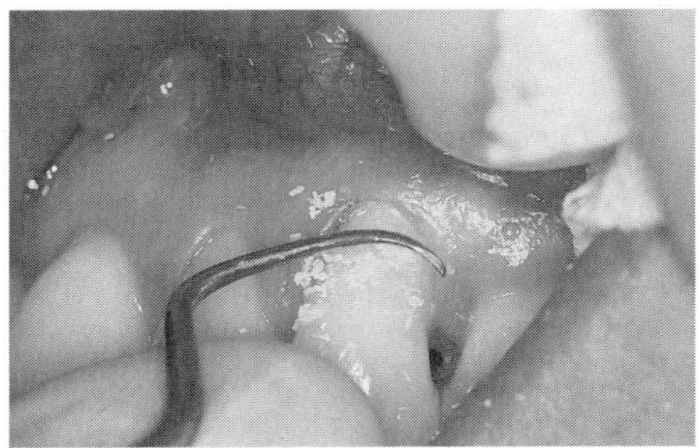

Fig. 67-7 Magnified root planing.

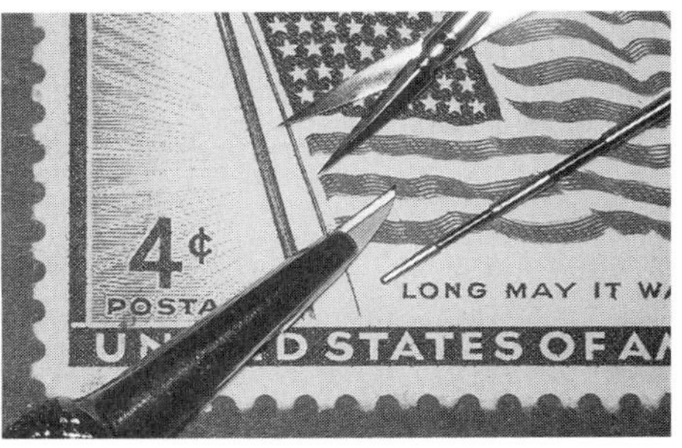

Fig. 67-8 Castroviejo microsurgical scalpel.

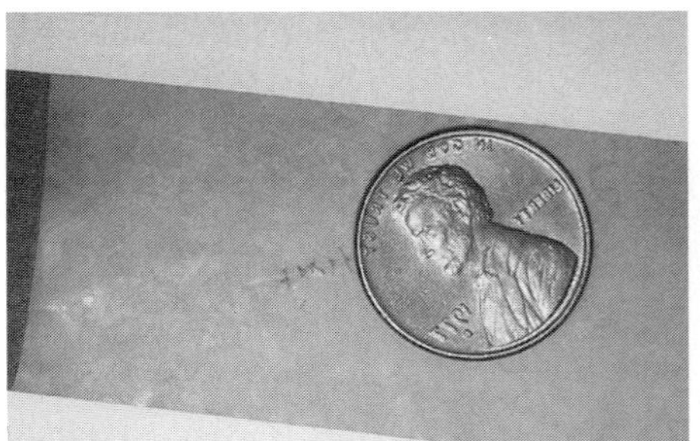
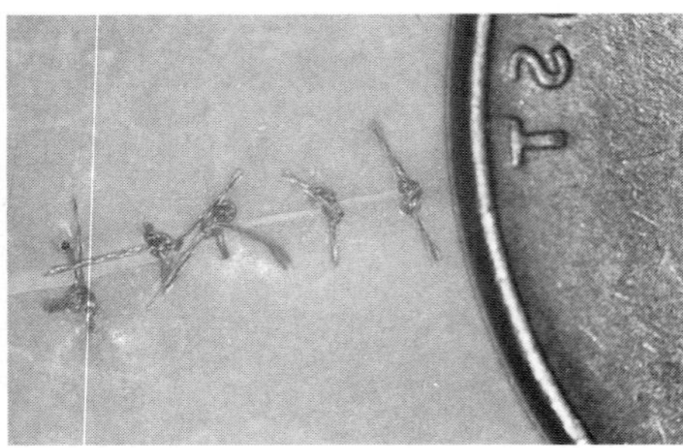

Fig. 67-9 Microsurgical suturing.

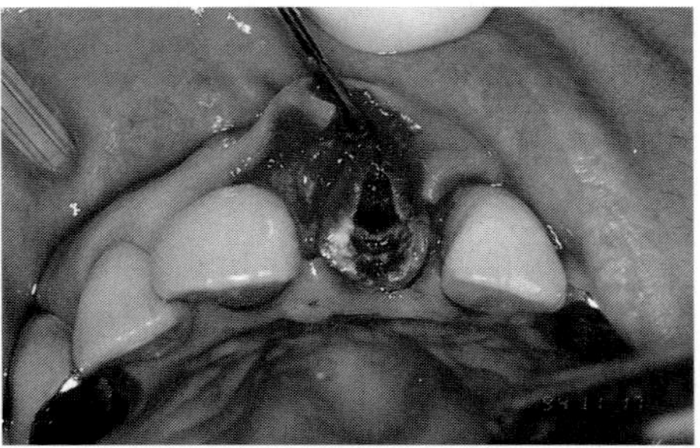

Fig. 67-10 Microsurgical extraction: presurgery.

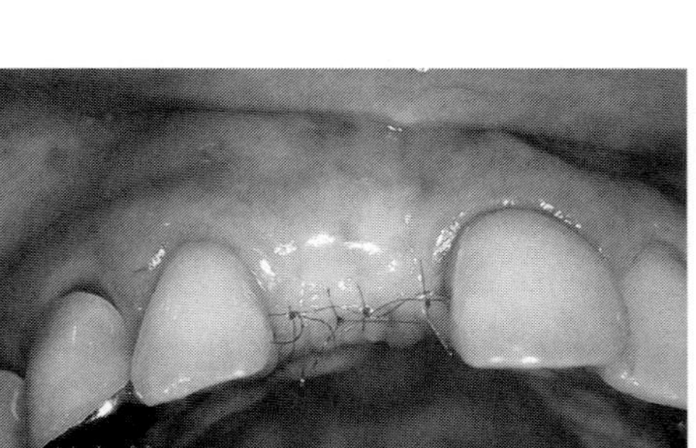

Fig. 67-11 Microsurgical extraction: microsurgical view.

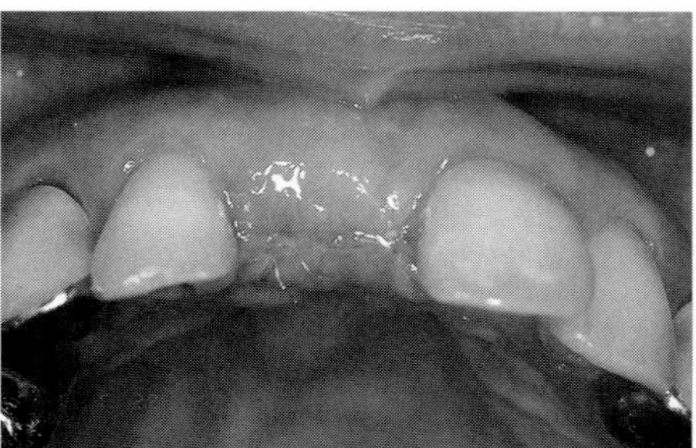

Fig. 67-12 Microsurgical extraction graft: 1 week postsurgery.

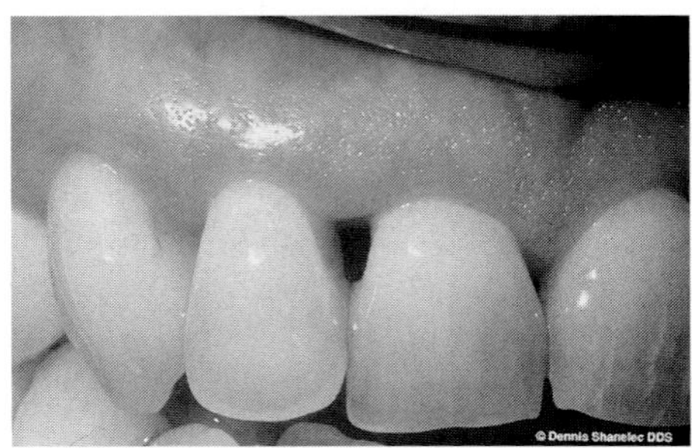

Fig. 67-13 Papilla reconstruction: presurgery.

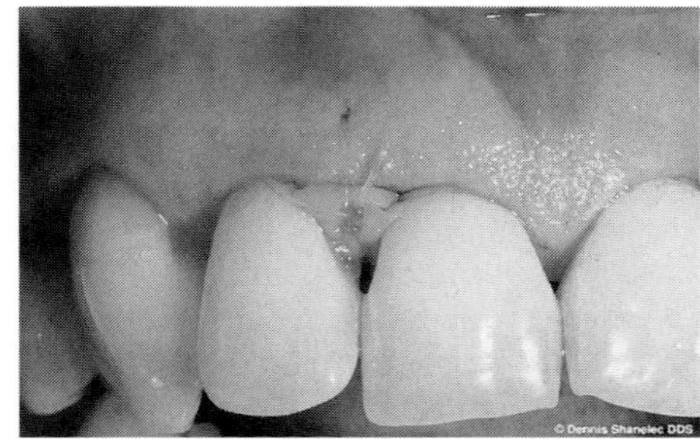

Fig. 67-14 Papilla reconstruction: microsurgical view.

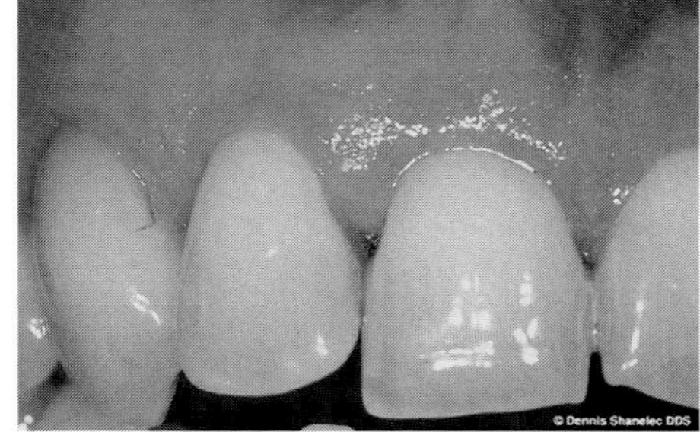

Fig. 67-15 Papilla reconstruction: postsurgery.

section to permit precise rotational movements. They are manufactured of titanium because of its strength, lightness, and nonmagnetizing characteristics. The various postural and ergonomic ways of reducing unwanted hand movements results in more precise surgeries and greatly reduces surgical fatigue and the development of spinal and occupational pathology. In the long term, this beneficial ergonomic aspect of microscopy may be the most influential in its adoption by the dental profession at large.

SUMMARY

Microsurgery offers new possibilities for periodontal surgery that can improve therapeutic results for a variety of procedures. Its benefits include improved cosmetics, rapid healing, minimal discomfort, and enhanced patient acceptance. Periodontics of the future will see increasing use of magnification in all areas of practice, including implantology.

REFERENCES

1. Apotheker H, Jako GJ: A microscope for use in dentistry. J Microsurg 1981; 3:7.
2. Banowsky LH: Basic microvascular techniques and principles. Urology 1984; 23:495.
3. Daniel RK: Microsurgery: Through the looking glass. N Engl J Med 1979; 300:1251.
4. Hirshfeld L, Wasserman B: A long-term survey of tooth loss in 600 treated periodontal patients. J Periodontol 1978; 49:225.
5. Hoerenz P: The operating microscope. I. Optical principles, illumination systems and support systems. J Microsurg 1980; 1:367.
6. Klopper P, Muller JH, Van Hattum AH: Microsurgery and Wound Healing. Amsterdam, Excerpta Medica, 1979.
7. Loos B, Nylund K. Claffey N, et al: Clinical effects of root debridement in molar and nonmolar teeth. A 2-year follow-up. J Clin Periodontol 1989; 16:498.
8. Nordland P, Garrett S, Kiger R, Vanooteghem R, et al: The effect of plaque control and root debridement in molar teeth. J Clin Periodontol 1987; 14:445.
9. Owen ER: Practical microsurgery. I. A choice of optical aids. Med Aust 1971; 1:244.
10. Pecora G, Andreana S: Operating microscope in endodontic surgery. Oral Surg Med Pathol 1993; 75:751.
11. Pihlstrom BL, Ortiz-Campos C, McHugh RB: A randomized four-year study of periodontal therapy. J Periodontol 1981; 52:227.
12. Serafin D: Microsurgery: Past, present and future. Plast Reconstr Surg 1979; 66:781.
13. Shanelec DA: Optical principles of loupes. Calif Dent Assoc J 1992; 20:25.
14. Van Hattum A, James J, Klopper PJ, et al: Epithelial migration in wound healing. Virchows Archiv B Cell Path 1979; 30:221–230.
15. Way L: Changing therapy for gallstone disease. N Engl J Med 1990; 323:1273.

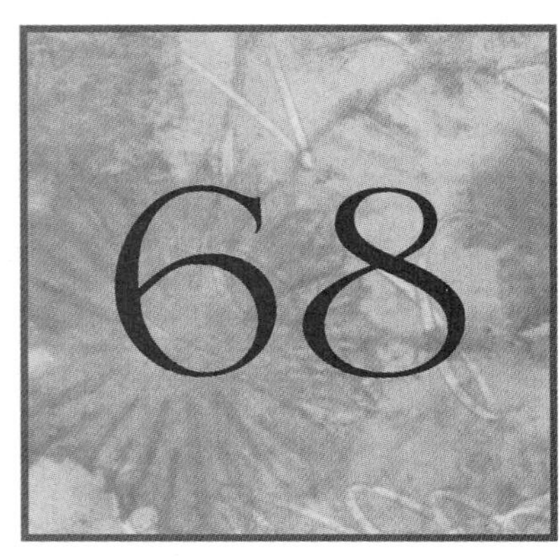

Biologic Aspects of Dental Implants

CHAPTER 68

George W. Bernard, Fermin A. Carranza, and Sascha A. Jovanovic

CHAPTER OUTLINE

Developing artificial replacements for missing teeth has been an elusive goal for more than 1500 years. A fine, dark stone, shaped like a tooth, was found implanted in a Mayan skull in Central America from 600 AD, and there are reports of implant attempts in ancient Egypt and the Middle East.[40] Interest in developing artificial teeth anchored to the jaws has continued to the present.

The present surge in the use of implants was initiated in 1952 by Branemark, who conducted extensive experimental and clinical studies.[8–10] Branemark and associates described the relationship between titanium and bone, for which they coined the term *osseointegration,* as the "direct structural and functional connection between ordered, living bone and the surface of a load-carrying implant."[4,8]

BIOMATERIALS

Many biologically compatible materials can be used for the manufacturing of implants. Currently, interest is centered on metals and metal alloys, but research continues with biomaterials such as ceramics and carbons, as well as polymers and composites.

Metals and Metal Alloys

Metallic biomaterials have been extensively used, particularly titanium and alloys of titanium, aluminum, and vanadium.[8–10] Early work also tested combinations of cobalt, chromium, and molybdenum, as well as iron, chromium, and nickel. Precious metals such as gold and platinum and their alloys are less frequently used. The most widely used dental implant material is titanium and its alloy; the most available clinical and experimental data concern this material.[5,15]

Ceramics and Carbons

This group includes aluminum oxide (alumina and sapphire) ceramics, carbon, and carbon-silicon compounds.[32] Hydroxyapatite has been proposed as a solid material, and as a surface coating, it is also widely used. Because coatings are used on load-bearing metals, there

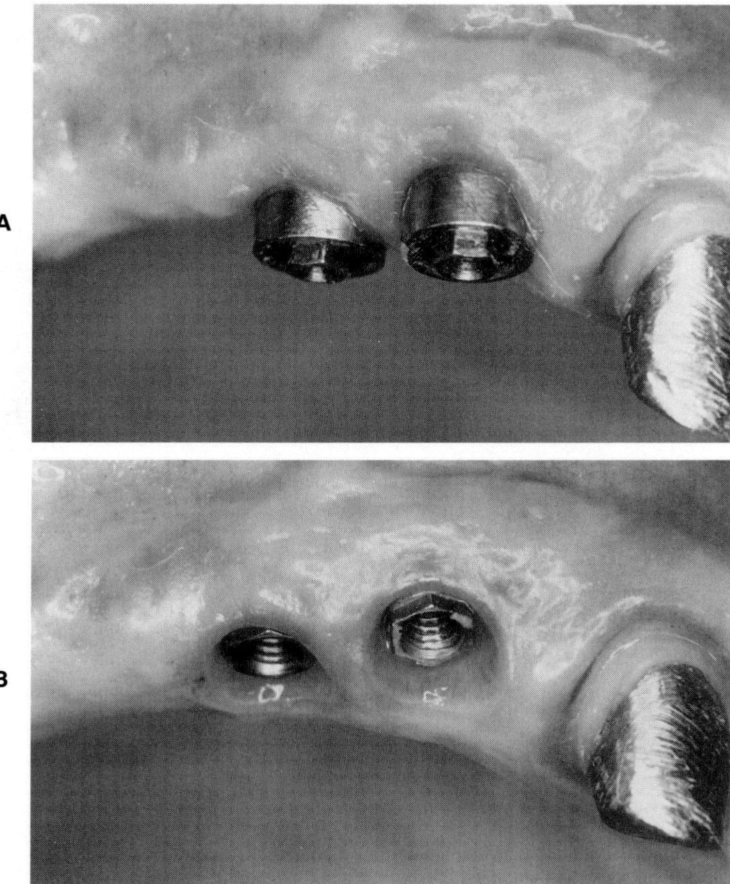

Fig. 68-1 **A,** Clinically normal gingival mucosa next to two implants. **B,** Normal epithelium lining the implant after removal of the cover screw.

is a need for high interfacial shear strength and resistance to resorption.

Polymers and Composites

These include cross-linked polymers such as polymethylmethacrylate, silicone rubber, and polyethylene. They are not in general use at present, but technologic developments may bring an increased use of these materials in the future.[34,35]

THE PERIIMPLANT MUCOSA

The mucosal tissues around intraosseous implants form a tightly adherent band consisting of a dense collagenous lamina propria covered by stratified squamous keratinizing epithelium (Figs. 68-1 and 68-2).[26] In general, the term *biologic width/height* is being used when describing the soft tissue dimensions around implants.[17]

The implant-epithelium junction is analogous to the junctional epithelium around natural teeth, in that the epithelial cells attach to the titanium implant by means of hemidesmosomes and a basal lamina.[21,22,25] Evidence for an adhesive junctional epithelium attachment to ceramic implants has also been presented.[32,33]

> This evidence supports the concept that a viable biologic seal can exist between the epithelial cells and the implants.

A sulcus forms around the implant lined with a sulcular epithelium. The depth of a normal, noninflamed or minimally inflamed sulcus around an intraosseous implant has not yet been accurately determined but is assumed to be between 1.5 and 2.0 mm.[7,14,17,31] Studies on sulcus and pocket depth around normal teeth have determined that the penetration of the probe, particularly if inflammation is present, will be stopped by the first attached collagen fibers. Because these are not present around implants, the probe would be expected to attain deeper measurements.[18] Bleeding on gentle probing rarely occurs in healthy mucosal tissues around implants. The presence of bleeding indicates the presence of plaque-induced inflammation,[43] although false-negative results have been reported.[31]

The sulcus around an implant is lined with sulcular epithelium that is continuous apically with the junctional epithelium. Normal tissues around implants have an

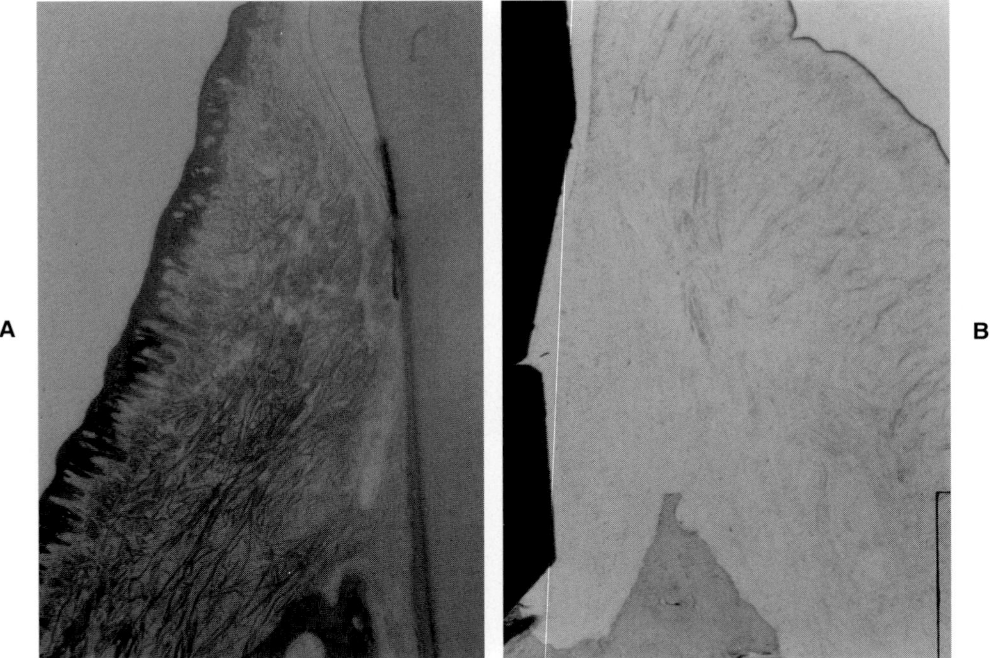

Fig. 68-2 **A,** Micrograph showing normal periodontium surrounding a tooth. **B,** Micrograph showing normal periimplant tissues.

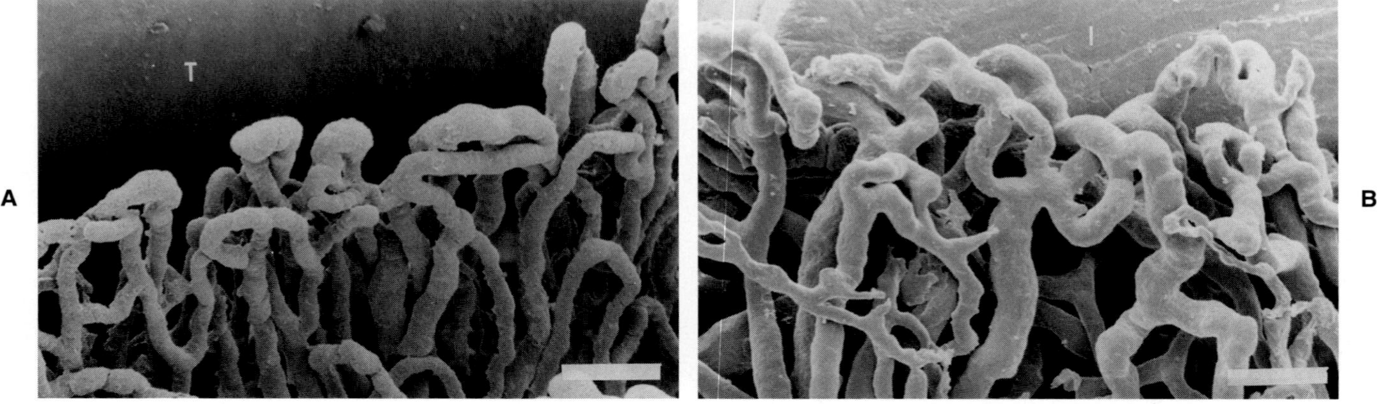

Fig. 68-3 Microvascular topography surrounding a tooth **(A)** and an implant **(B).** Bar = 5 μm. (Courtesy Drs. N. Selliseth and K. Selvig; Bergen, Norway.)

intact epithelial lining and about the same number of inflammatory cells as are found around a nature tooth.[1,6,29]

Capillary loops in the connective tissue under the junctional and the sulcular epithelia appear to be anatomically similar to those found in the normal periodontium (Fig. 68-3).[6,39] Some investigators, however, have found reduced vascularity close to the implant surface compared with that around teeth and are of the opinion that this may make periimplant tissues more vulnerable to pathogenic insults.[14,31]

Although some investigators have suggested that the amount of inflammation is not affected by the quality of periimplant soft tissues, others have found an increased chance of periimplant mucositis in patients without keratinized mucosa. [7,33,43]

Collagen fibers are nonattached and run parallel to the implant surface, owing to the lack of cementum. This is an important difference between periimplant and periodontal tissues.[6] However, some reports have suggested that microscopic irregularities and porosities like those found on plasma-sprayed titanium surfaces may favor the appearance of fibers oriented perpendicularly to the implant surface[11,14,37] and in turn, orient fibroblasts in specific directions.[24]

The marginal portion of the periimplant mucosa contains significantly more collagen and fewer fibroblasts

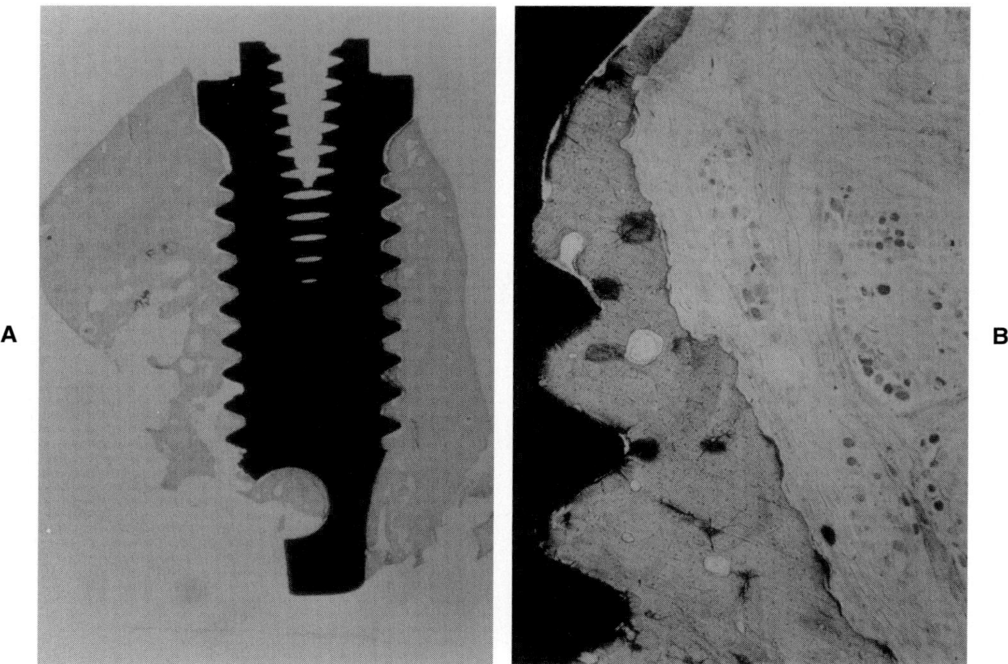

Fig. 68-4 Periimplant supporting tissues around an implant at the light microscopy level. **A,** Topographic view. **B,** Higher magnification showing direct apposition of bone and implant.

than the corresponding gingival tissue, which may indicate that tissue turnover in the periimplant mucosa is less rapid than that in the gingiva.[6]

THE IMPLANT-BONE INTERFACE

The relationship between endosseous implants and bone consists of one of two mechanisms: **osseointegration,** when the bone is in intimate but not ultrastructural contact with the implant, or **fibrosseous integration,** in which soft tissues such as fibers and/or cells, are interposed between the two surfaces.

The proponents of the fibrosseous system of implant retention suggest that the presence of a dense collagenous tissue between implant and bone may act as an osteogenic membrane.[42] However, there is no wide support for this concept.

The osseointegration concept proposed by Branemark et al[8] and called *functional ankylosis* by Schroeder[36] states that there is an absence of connective tissue or any nonbone tissue in the interface between the implant and the bone. A more accurate term, *microinterlock,* is used in orthopedic implantology, where tissue and implant are juxtaposed, providing a bioinert fixation with surface porosities, grooves, or beads.[16] It is important to note that *osseointegration* refers to the direct contact of bone and implant at the *light microscope level* (Fig 68-4). Furthermore, even with this definition, osseointegration never occurs on 100% of the implant surface. Successful cases have between 30% and 95% of the implant surface, as measured by light microscopy, in contact with bone.

Under the light microscope, bone appears to be in direct contact with the implant. By virtue of its excellent regenerative potential, bone is seen to grow around the ridges and grooves of screw-type implants and through the openings of blade- and hollow cylinder-type implants. Remodeling of bone occurs constantly as part of the normal physiology of bone and continues to occur after the implant has been placed.

Histologic sections of the bone-implant interface, however, are usually thick (20 to 150 μm) and do not permit an accurate view of the interface. These thick sections have been the primary standard of viewing the interface and may have led to the premature definition of the interface as an osteointegrative one.

Although some ultrastructural investigations have reported mineralized matrix in direct contact with titanium without the presence of any amorphous layer,[2,3,27] others have reported the interposition of connective tissue.[19,35,38]

Reports using conventional transmission and high-voltage electron microscopy have contradicted the direct bone-to-implant results. These studies suggested a close approximation of calcified tissue to the implant surface but found no conclusive evidence of any molecular bonds between the metal oxide surface of titanium and the adjacent bone.[41] An amorphous, cell-free layer, ranging in width from 20 to 1000 nm and composed of glycosaminoglycans and proteoglycans, has been reported to be interposed between bone and titanium.[38] There may also be a lamina limitans-like line[38] that is 50 nm thick and a layer of noncalcified collagen adjacent to the titanium surface. Complete mineralization is seen only 2000 nm (2 μm) from the metal.[38]

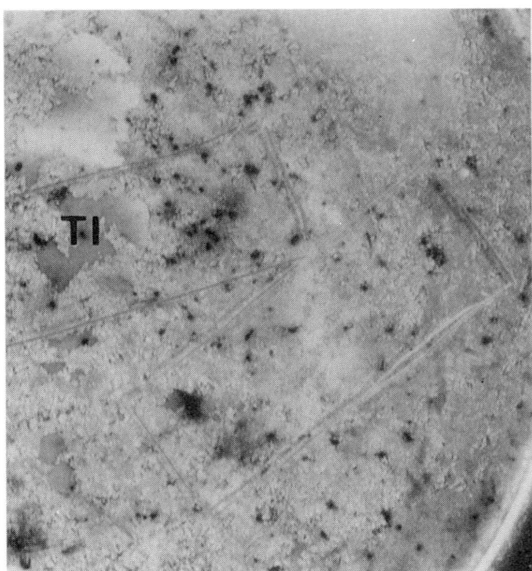

Fig. 68-5 Petri dish with many dark bone colonies. Evaporated titanium (TI) in areas denuded of cells. Original magnification ×1.

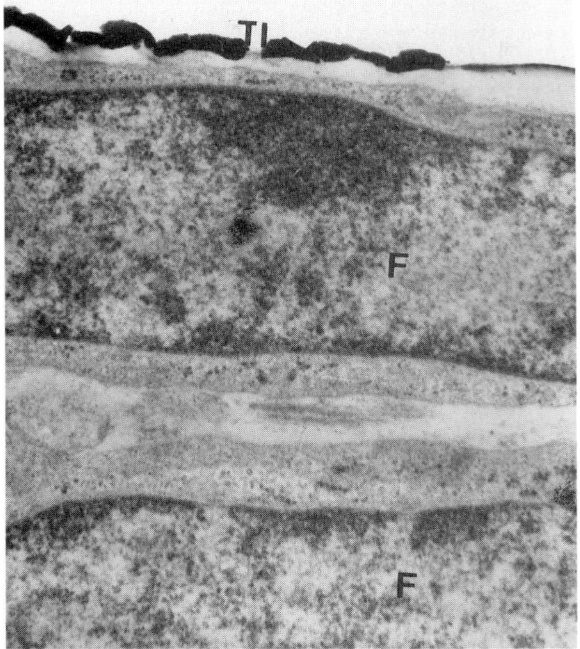

Fig. 68-6 Transmission electron micrograph of the interface of bone colonies on evaporated titanium (TI). Portions of two fibroblasts (F) are seen with a clear zone between the innermost cells and the titanium. Original magnification ×20,000.

An in vitro technique devised by Holden and Bernard[23] has provided a reproducible system to analyze the bone-implant interface. With this technique Petri dishes are coated with titanium, titanium alloy, or cobalt/chrome, and then bone is grown on the thinly coated implant materials. Semi-thin (2 μm) and thin (80 nm) sections can then be prepared and analyzed using light and transmission electron microscopy.

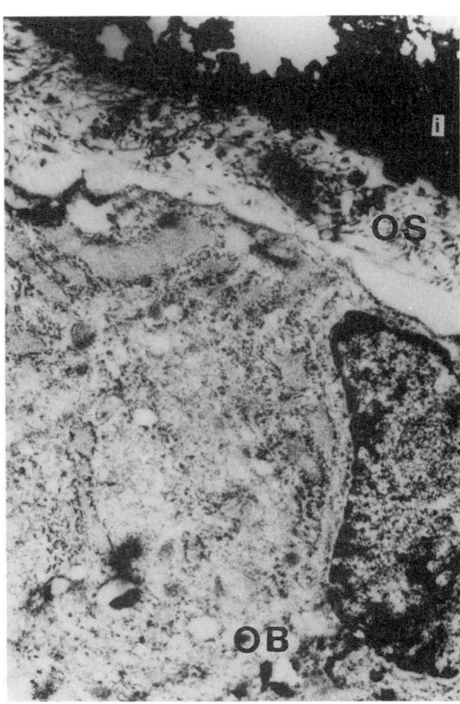

Fig. 68-7 Transmission electron micrograph showing a portion of an osteoblast (OB) and osteoid with initial calcification (OS) juxtaposed to the hydroxyapatite surface of the implant (i). Original magnification ×18,000.

The compatibility of bone and titanium can be demonstrated by the large number of bone colonies that grow on titanium (Fig. 68-5); a lesser amount grow on titanium alloy, and almost none grow on cobalt/chrome.

Electron microscopy of the bone-titanium interface using this technique shows that there is always connective tissue between the implant and the bone (Fig. 68-6). A carbohydrate-rich adhesive substrate is invariably found on the metal adjoining the fibroblasts in vitro. With in vivo studies, as with in vitro, bone is never found in direct contact with titanium.[19,35]

Plasma-sprayed hydroxyapatite in Petri dishes is even more receptive to bone growth than titanium, forming larger and more numerous colonies. At the interface with hydroxyapatite, fibroblasts and osteoblasts can be demonstrated (Fig. 68-7). Where osteoblasts have developed, collagen is seen in the interface with hydroxyapatite molecularly bonded with the implant hydroxyapatite.[20]

The absence of cementum on the implant surface prevents the attachment of collagen fibers to the implants. This lack of cementum is interpreted as being due to the absence of cementum progenitor cells in the area receiving the implant.[30] When these cells are available, cementum can form on the implant surface, and a functional collagen attachment can attach to it. Buser and associates have described the presence of a distinct layer of cementum on the implant surface and a periodontal ligament with fibers oriented perpendicularly when the implant was placed close to retained roots that had a periodontal ligament.[12]

Increasing the surface area on the implant would increase the tissue implant contact to increase implant stability.[13,28,44] Acid etching and blasting are two techniques used to enhance implant surface topography with micro- to macroscopic hills, valleys, and indentations. When pure titanium surfaces are roughened with 22 μm or 150 μm aluminum oxide blasting, removal torque of the implant from the bone was significantly increased with both blasted surfaces. This demonstrated that the increase of blasted surface topography observed after 1 year increased bone fixation compared with machined surfaces. The increased surface created by blasting substantiated earlier findings of grit blasting and acid etching to increase the surface of the implants. Buser et al[12] used morphometric histologic analysis to conclude that grit-blasted and acid-etched surfaces increase bone opposition.

It is important to note that when undecalcified bone interfaces with titanium, whether in vivo or in vitro, electron microscopy has always shown connective tissue interposed between the two surfaces.

This brings up two considerations. In the first place, inflammatory cells are potential constituents of connective tissue, and improper loading of the implant may trigger an inflammatory response leading to bone resorption. The second is possibly a positive factor in that connective tissue may provide a cushioning structure between the hard surfaces of metal and bone. Furthermore, hydroxyapatite surfaces of implants have true osseointegration but only in a macular fashion with connective tissue in the intervening sites. There is also reason to believe that plasma-sprayed hydroxyapatite with less than optimal crystallinity may not have a long half-life, although long-term studies have not been reported.

REFERENCES

1. Adell R, Lekholm U, Branemark P-1, et al: Marginal tissue reactions at osseointegrated titanium fixtures. Swed Dent J 1985; 28(suppl):175.
2. Albrektsson T, Branemark P-1, Hanson HA, et al: Ultrastructural analysis of the interface zone of titanium and gold implants. Adv Biomater 1982; 4:167.
3. Albrektsson T, Branemark P-1, Hanson HA, et al: The interface zone of inorganic implants in-vivo: Titanium implants in bone. Ann Biomed Eng 1983, 11:1.
4. Albrektsson T, Branemark P-1, Hanson HA, Lindstrom J: Osseointegrated titanium implants. Acta Orthrop Scand 1981; 52:155.
5. Albrektsson T, Sennerby L: Direct bone anchorage of oral implants: Clinical and experimental considerations of the concept of osseointegration. Int J Prosthodont 1990; 3:30.
6. Berglundh T, Lindhe J, Jonsson K, et al: The topography of the vascular system in the periodontal and periimplant tissues in the dog. J Clin Periodontol 1994; 21:189.
7. Berglundh T, Lindhe J, Ericsson I, et al: The soft tissue barrier at implants and teeth. Clin Oral Implant Res 1991; 2:81.
8. Block M, Kent J: Factors associated with soft and hard tissue compromise of endosseous implants. J Oral Maxillofac Surg 1990; 48:1160.
9. Branemark P-I, Adell R, Breine U, et al: Intraosseous anchorage of dental prosthesis. I. Experimental studies. Scand J Plast Reconstr Surg 1969; 3:81.
10. Branemark P-I, Hunsson BO, Adell R, et al: Osseointegrated implants in the treatment of the edentulous jaw. Scand J Plast Reconstr Surg 1977; 16(suppl):11.
11. Branemark P-I, Zarb GA, Albrektsson T: Tissue-integrated prostheses. In Branemark P-I, Zarb GA, Albrektsson T: Osseointegration in Clinical Dentistry. Chicago, Quintessence Publishing, 1985.
12. Buser, D, Nydegger T, Oxland T, et al: Influence of surface characteristics on the interface shear strength between titanium implants and bone. A biomechanical study in the maxilla of miniature pigs. J Biomed Res 1999a; 45:75.
13. Buser D, Schenk R, Steinemann S, et al: Influences of surface characteristics on bone integration of titanium implants. A histomorphometric study in miniature pigs. J Biomed Materials Res 1991; 25:889.
14. Buser D, Warre K, Karring T: Formation of a periodontal ligament around titanium implants. J Periodontol 1990; 61:597.
15. Buser D, Weber HP, Donath K, et al: Soft tissue reactions to non-submerged implants. J Periodontol 1990; 61:597.
16. Buser D, Weber HP, Lang NP: Tissue integration of non-submerged implants. 1-year results of a prospective study with 100 ITI hollow-cylinder and hollow screw implants. Clin Oral Implant Res 1990; 1:33.
17. Cochran DL, Hermann JS, Schenk R, et al: Biological width around titanium implants. A histometric analysis of the implanto-gingival junction around unloaded and loaded nonsubmerged implants in the canine mandible. J Periodontol 1997; 68:186.
18. Dienn MG, Maxian SH: Biomaterials used in orthopedic surgery. In Greco RS (Ed): Implantation Biology. Boca Raton, Fla, CRC Press, 1994.
19. Elisha J, Bernard GW: The bone/ceramic hydroxyapatite interface following in vitro bone formation. Unpublished manuscript. Los Angeles, University of California, Los Angeles, 1989.
20. Ericsson I, Lindhe J: Probing depths at implants and teeth. J Clin Periodontol 1993; 20:263.
21. Falez F, Bernard G, Perugia L, et al: Valutazione quatitativa e qualitativa dell interfaccia osso-ceramica. Giornale Italiano di Ortop e Traumat 1994; 85:661.
22. Golijanin L, Bernard GW: Biocompatability of implant metals in bone tissue culture. J Dent Res 1988; 67:367.
23. Gould TR, Brunette DM, Westbury C: The attachment mechanism of epithelial cells to titanium in vitro. J Periodont Res 1981; 16:611.
24. Gould TR, Westbury C, Brunette DM: Ultrastructural study of the attachment of human gingiva to titanium in vivo. J Prosthet Dent 1984; 52:418.
25. Holden C, Bernard GW: Ultrastructural in-vitro characterization of a porous hydroxyapatite/bone cell interface. J Oral Implantol 1990; 16:86.
26. Inoue T, Cox JE, Pilliar RM, et al: Effect of the surface geometry of smooth and porous-coated titanium alloy on the orientation of fibroblasts in vivo. J Biomed Mater Res 1987; 21:107.
27. James RA, Schultz R: Hemidesmosomes and the adhesion of junctional epithelial cells to metal implants. J Oral Implantol 1974; 3:294.
28. Klokkevold, PR, Nishimura, RD, Adachi M, et al: Osseointegration enhanced by chemical etching of the titanium surface: A torque removal study in the rabbit. Clin Oral Implants Res 1997; 8:442.
29. Lekholm U, Ericsson I, Adell R, et al: The condition of the soft tissues at tooth and fixture abutment supporting fixed bridges. J Clin Periodontol 1986; 13:558.

30. Linder L, Albrektsson T, Branemark P-I, et al: Electron-microscopic analysis of the bone-titanium interface. Acta Orthop Scand 1983; 54:45.
31. Lindhe J, Berglundh T, Ericsson I, et al: Experimental breakdown of periimplant and periodontal tissues. A study in the beagle dog. Clin Oral Implant Res 1992; 3:9.
32. Listgarten MA, Buser D, Steinemann SG, et al: Light and transmission electron microscopy of the intact interfaces between non-submerged titanium-coated epoxy resin implants and bone or gingiva. J Dent Res 1992; 71:364.
33. Listgarten MA, Lang NP, Schroeder HE, et al: Periodonal tissues and their counterparts around endosseous implants. Clin Oral Implant Res 1991; 2:1.
34. McKinney Jr RV, Steflik DE, Koth DL: The biologic tissue response to dental implants. In McKinney Jr RV (ed): Endosteal Dental Implants. St. Louis, Mosby, 1991.
35. Meffert R: In the soft tissue interface in dental implantology. Dental Implants NIH Consensus Development Conference, Boston, MA, 1988.
36. Peppas NA, Lnager R: New challenges in biomaterials. Science 1994; 263:1715.
37. Pilloni A, Falez F, Bernard GW: Iddrossiapatite e osteoconduzione: Effetto sulle cellule staminale pluripotenti midollari. Proceedings of the First World Congress on Osseointegration, Venice, 1994.
38. Schroeder A, Sutter F, Krekeler G: Orale implantologie, allegemeine grundlagen und ITI-Hohlzylindersystem. G Thieme, Stuttgart, 1988.
39. Schroeder A, van de Zypen E, Stich H, et al: The reaction of bone, connective tissue and epithelium to endosteal implants with titanium-sprayed surfaces. J Maxillofac Surg 1981; 9:15.
40. Selliseth NJ, Selvig K: Personal communication, June 1994.
41. Sennerby L, Ericsson LE, Thomsen P, et al: Structure of the bone/titanium interface in retrieved clinical oral implants. Clin Oral Implant Res 1992; 2:103.
42. Steflik MA, McKinney Jr RV: History of implantology. In McKinney Jr RV (ed): Endosteal dental implants. St. Louis, Mosby, 1991.
43. Steinemann SG, Eulenberg J, Maesuli PA, et al: Adhesion of bone to titanium. Adv Biomater 1986; 6:409.
44. Wennerberg A, Ektessebi A, Albrektsson T, et al: A one-year follow up of implants of differing surface roughness placed in raffet bone. Int J Oral Maxillofac Implants 1997; 12:486.
45. Weiss CM: A comparative analysis of fibro-osteal and osteal integration and other variables that affect long term bone maintenance around dental implants. J Oral Implant 1987; 13:467.
46. Wennstrom J, Bengazi F, Lekholm U: The influence of the masticatory mucosa on the periimplant soft tissue condition. Clin Oral Implant Res 1994; 5:1.

Clinical Aspects of Dental Implants

Sascha A. Jovanovic

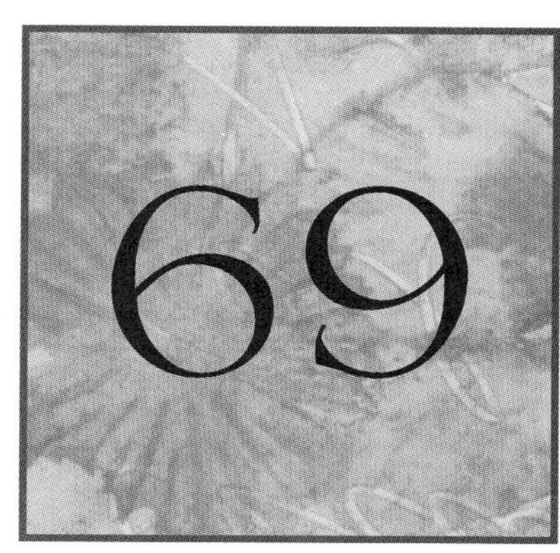

CHAPTER

Chapter Outline

The fundamental work of Branemark and associates in the 1960s demonstrated that commercially pure titanium implants can be anchored to the jawbone and used successfully for tooth replacement in edentulous arches. Controlled clinical research showed excellent long-term results achieved after appropriate selection of cases, adequate preparation of biomaterials, and careful handling of patients' soft and hard tissues. The relationship between the bone and the implant was called *osseointegration* (see Chapter 68). Branemark presented his research for the first time in North America at the conference held in Toronto, Ontario, Canada, in 1982, and his findings were unanimously considered a breakthrough in dental prosthetics and oral rehabilitation and the opening of a new era in clinical dentistry.

Since the mid-1980s, clinical and laboratory research in dental implantology has resulted in the development of numerous implant systems and different techniques for surgical placement and subsequent prosthetic reconstruction. This chapter presents some basic concepts in implant dentistry and will attempt to clarify the indications, advantages, and disadvantages of the various systems.

CLINICAL MANAGEMENT OF DENTAL IMPLANTS

To achieve an osseointegrated dental implant with a high degree of predictability,[10–12] the implant must be 1) sterile, 2) made of a highly biocompatible material such as titanium, 3) inserted with an atraumatic surgical technique that avoids overheating of the bone during preparation of the recipient site, 4) placed with initial stability, and 5) not functionally loaded during the healing period of 4 to 6 months.

When these clinical guidelines are followed, successful osseointegration occurs predictably for submerged[10] and nonsubmerged[34] dental implants. Well-controlled studies of patients with good plaque control and appropriate occlusal forces have demonstrated that osseointegrated implants show little change in bone height around the implant.[1] After an initial remodeling in the first year that results in 1.0 to 1.5 mm of bone reduction,[1] the bone level around healthy functioning implants remains stable for many years, allowing implants to be a predictable means for tooth replacement. The first patient with osseointegrated implants was treated in 1965 in Sweden, and long-term studies have shown excellent survival rates of implants over 20 years.[2]

Bone quality at the recipient site influences the interface between bone and implant.[21] Compact bone offers a much greater surface area for mineralized tissue-to-implant contact than cancellous bone. Clinical studies have shown that areas of the jaw exhibiting thin layers of cortical bone and large cancellous spaces, such as the posterior maxilla, have significantly lower success rates than areas of denser bone structures.[21] The best results are obtained when contact between bone and implant is most intimate at implant placement.

The surgical preparation of the tissues at the recipient site may also markedly affect healing. Drilling of the bone without proper cooling results in production of temperatures that inflict thermal injury to the tissues and an increased failure rate to osseointegrate.[38]

Indications and Contraindications

The treatment indications for dental implants are extensive and can include patients with partially and fully edentulous arches, as well as patients with maxillofacial deformities. Many patients can benefit from the osseointegration procedure as long as they fulfill specific requirements for surgical and prosthetic rehabilitation. Patients who are unable to wear removable dentures and have adequate bone for the placement of dental implants are especially good candidates.

However, each patient must be evaluated individually according to rigorous clinical parameters. Important criteria are oral hygiene, periodontal health (in partially edentulous patients) or history of periodontal health in an edentulous patient, jaw relationship, tooth positions, tooth restorations present, level of decay activity, cause for previous tooth loss, amount of bone quantity and quality available, and patient motivation. In addition, a restorative treatment plan needs to establish that the patient is a good candidate for tooth replacement with implants or if conventional prosthetic means are better suited for the patient. It is conceivable that a patient may not be a good candidate at the time of consultation, but that further dental treatment can prepare the patient for implant placement.

Patients must be in good general health. Uncontrolled or even controlled diabetes, chronic steroid therapy, high-dose irradiation, and smoking and alcohol abuse[6,16] can increase the occurrence of early and late implant complications. A thorough physical examination is mandatory if any questions arise about the health status of the patient.[11]

The overall preoperative requirement regarding the local health of oral tissues is that no pathologic conditions are present in any of the hard or soft tissues of either jaw. All oral lesions, including periodontal inflammation, should be treated in advance and evaluated at a later date for resolution. The presence of nontreated or unsuccessfully treated periodontal disease is a contraindication to implant placement, since the bacterial flora in periodontitis can jeopardize the healing of the implant sites. Only when the periodontitis has been resolved can implant treatment be considered. The quality and quantity of soft tissue present in the anticipated implant site is also important, since keratinized, attached mucosa has better functional and aesthetic results for implant restorations.

After the patient has gone through the initial screening of being a good implant candidate, based on good general health, good oral health, and appropriate restorative needs, the amount of available bone is the next most important criteria for selection. The minimal width of the jawbone needs to be 6 mm, and the minimal height should be 10 mm. These dimensions are based on an implant with a diameter of 4 mm and should be used as a guide and not as an absolute term. These bone dimensions have to be evaluated in a 3-dimensional view, since the implant has to be placed in the appropriate prosthetic position. Minimum requirements of bone might be available in the anticipated implant site, but they might not be in the appropriate location to place an implant necessitating a grafting procedure.[35]

Although the traditional implant placement calls for a healed ridge, implant placement immediately after extraction has been attempted with success.[23,37] Covering the implant with a barrier membrane placed under the flap or placing a bone graft significantly increases the success rate of implants placed in extraction sockets.[23,37] Immediate placement of implants in extraction sockets of single-rooted maxillary and mandibular teeth has been documented in cases of severe periodontal breakdown, root fractures, or endodontic failures, provided the following conditions are met:

1. After tooth extraction, the alveolar socket must have sufficient residual bone walls.
2. The extraction socket must be free of pathosis.
3. The available soft tissue should allow primary closure.
4. Apical to the socket, a sufficient volume of healthy jawbone must be available to ensure good initial stabilization of the implant.

If the amount of bone is not sufficient to place an implant, the advanced bone augmentation surgery described in Chapter 71 can be employed. It is important to note that procedures to enhance the amount of bone have increased risks and failure rates and need the clinician to gain more training and experience before commencing these reconstructive procedures.

Selection of Cases and Preoperative Diagnosis

The possibility of implant installation can be determined after studying the jaw structures that are present.[11] Wide variations in jaw anatomy are encountered, and it is therefore important to analyze the anatomy of the maxillofacial and intraoral region via clinical and radiographic examinations before any surgery is started.

The preoperative diagnosis is necessary to predict the amount of bone available for implant placement and to evaluate presurgically whether the patient is a suitable candidate for implant treatment. Clinical examination of the jawbone consists of palpation and probing through the soft tissue (intraoral bone mapping) to assess the thickness of the soft tissues at the proposed surgical site. Appropriate radiographic procedures, including periapical and panoramic views, lateral cephalometric views, and orthopantomograms can help identify vital structures such as the floor of the nasal cavity, maxillary sinus, mandibular canal, and mental foramen.

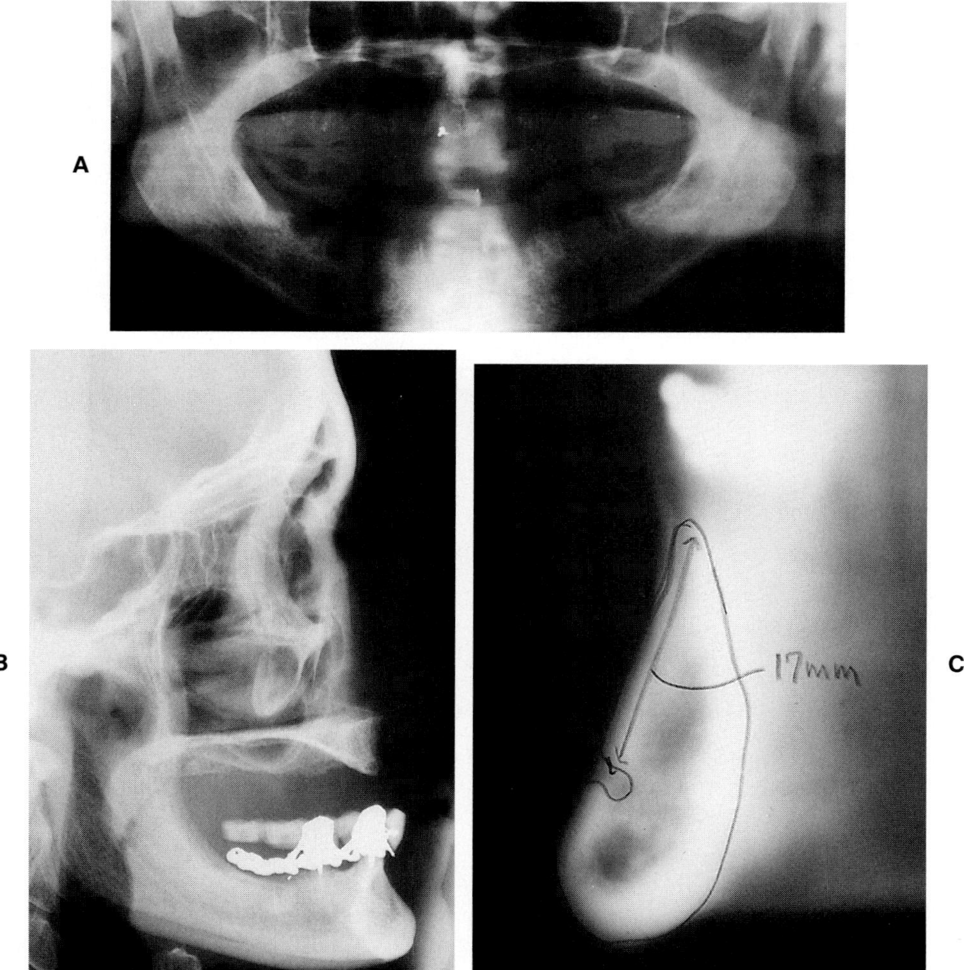

Fig. 69-1 Different radiographic procedures used in implant dentistry. **A,** Panoramic radiograph. **B,** Lateral cephalometric radiograph. **C,** Tomogram of mandibular premolar area.

When only periapical radiographs are used, such findings are severely limited.

The orthopantomogram allows a more comprehensive view of the mandible and maxilla. In the totally edentulous patient, the lateral cephalometric view is very beneficial, especially in the mandible, because it shows angulation, thickness, and vertical bone height. With newer diagnostic techniques such as conventional linear tomograms (Fig. 69-1, *C*) and computed tomographic (CT) scans (Fig. 69-2), it is possible to go beyond the standard two-dimensional radiographs mentioned previously.[32] Exact cross-sectional (three-dimensional) radiographic views of residual bone are possible via specialized software programs. This technology is costly and has increased risk for radiation, but it allows a more predictable diagnosis, since it demonstrates whether there is inadequate height and width of bone and the location of vital anatomic structures.[30] Newer clinical data show that even the quality of bone in an anticipated implant site can be evaluated.

VARIOUS IMPLANT SYSTEMS

Several implant systems are used for tooth replacement. These differ mainly in biomaterial, design, and surgical procedure. The four most often used biomaterials are commercially pure titanium, micro-enhanced pure titanium, plasma-sprayed titanium surfaces, and plasma-sprayed hydroxyapatite surfaces.

The three main implant designs are the screw-shaped implant form, cylinder-shaped form, and tapered screw-shaped form.

Surgical procedures can be performed in two interventions (two-stage) or in one stage. In the two-stage procedure, the first operation is for implant insertion and the second operation, several months later, is for uncovering the implant, and attaching a prosthetic abutment. Implants requiring a one-stage procedure are inserted and left exposed to the oral environment; they are not loaded, however, during the healing period. Chapter 70 describes in detail the surgical procedures for one-stage and two-stage implant placement.

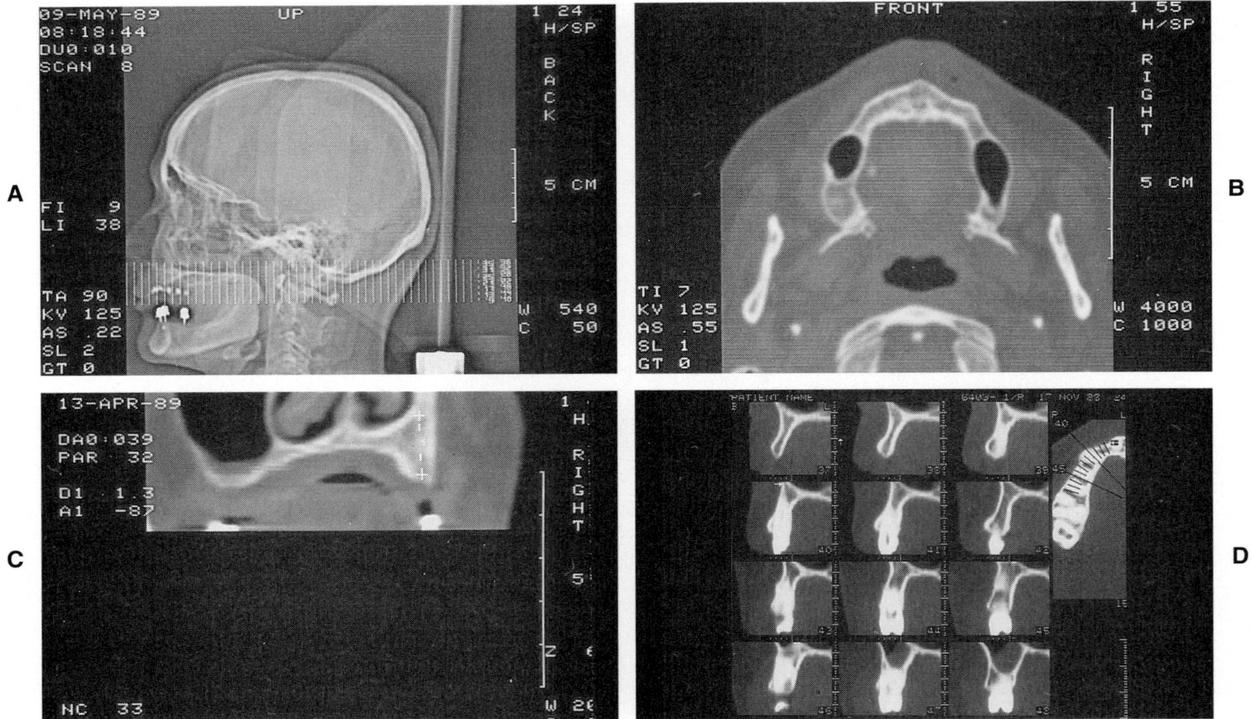

Fig. 69-2 Computed tomographic scans. **A,** Sagittal view. **B,** Occlusal view. **C,** Cross-sectional view. **D,** Cross-sectional reformatted view.

Most implant systems offer a variety of implant lengths (7 to 20 mm) and widths (3.25 to 6 mm) to accommodate the available bone quantity. In addition, they include an internally or externally irrigated precision drill set, as well as precisely matched components for surgical and prosthetic needs.

More than 50 different types of implants are available worldwide. Many systems use the term *osseointegration* but lack short- and long-term data to support their claims.[3,36] For this reason, only implant systems with appropriate clinical and experimental research are presented in the following descriptions (Table 69-1).

Nobel Biocare System

The Branemark system consists of a screw-shaped dental implant, made of commercially pure titanium and applied in a two-stage surgical procedure. The titanium implant surface is machined and forms and maintains an oxide layer without apparent breakdown or corrosion under physiologic conditions. This system was developed by Branemark in Sweden in the early 1960s, and the term *osseointegration* was coined to designate the relationship of the implant to the bone *at the light microscopic level.* Recently, a new surface treatment to the implant has been added by increasing the thickness of the oxide layer (Ti-unite).

The Branemark implant is by far the most extensively researched system, with long-term prospective follow-up studies carried out in fully edentulous and partially edentulous patients. The major advantage of this system is its excellent long-term data (>20 years) and its very meticulous testing in the preclinical stage.[1,11] New implant designs and surfaces have been added to the system in recent years and have increased success rates in poor quality bone sites.

The Steri-Oss system[33] is part of the Nobel Biocare product line and has a large variety of different implant designs and implant surfaces. The most used implant of this system is a tapered titanium screw (Replace), which comes in an acid-etched, TPS and HA coating.

International Team for Oral Implantology (ITI) System

In Switzerland, Schroeder and colleagues initiated clinical and experimental studies evaluating one-stage hollow cylinder implants in the early 1970s.[34] They demonstrated that one-stage implants can also result in direct bone-to-implant contact and in 1976, called this phenomenon **functional ankylosis.** The ITI implant system[13] has shown good results in long-term retrospective studies on fully edentulous patients and in short-term prospective studies on partially edentulous patients.

This implant system can accommodate several different designs, from the original hollow cylinder (Fig. 69-3, *right*) to a full-body screw design. The initial surface characteristics (plasma-sprayed titanium coating) have changed in the recent years to a sand-blasted, acid-etched surface.[14,15] Because this implant system

TABLE 69-1

Principal Features of Commonly Used Implant Systems

System	Design	Number of Surgery Stages	Surface	Indication	ADA Accepted	Follow-up Since
Nobel Biocare (Branemark)	Screw and tapered screw	Two	Pure Ti machined and Ti-unite	Full/partial edentulism	Yes	1965
ITI Straumann	Screw, cylinder, and basket	One	Ti plasma-sprayed and SLA	Full/partial edentulism	Yes	1977*
Nobel Biocare (Steri-Oss)	Screw, cylinder, and tapered screw	Two and one	Acid-etched, Ti and HA plasma-sprayed	Full/partial edentulism	Yes	1988
Integral	Cylinder, screw	Two	HA plasma-sprayed	Full/partial edentulism	Yes	1985
Paragon/ Core-Vent	Screw, cylinder, hollow basket	Two	Acid-etched Ti + HA plasma-sprayed	Full/partial edentulism	Yes	1984
Friadent	Tapered cylinder and screw	Two	Acid-etched Ti	Full/partial edentulism	Yes	1991
Astra	Screw	Two	Pure Ti blasted	Full/partial edentulism	Yes	1990
3i	Screw, cylinder	Two and one	Osseotite and Ti + HA plasma-sprayed	Full/partial edentulism	Yes	1990

* Follow-up of the new-generation ITI dental implant since 1986.

ADA, American Dental Association; *HA,* hydroxyapatite; *ITI,* International Team for Oral Implantology; *3i,* Implant Innovations, Inc.; *Ti,* titanium.

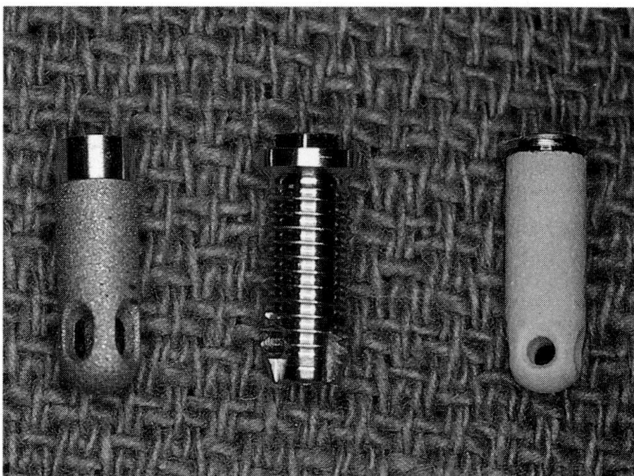

Fig. 69-3 Different implant designs. *Left,* IMZ. *Center,* Branemark (Nobelpharma). *Right,* Integral-hydroxyapatite.

protrudes through the mucosa from the day of insertion, it does not require a second intervention, but there is an increased risk of premature loading during the healing period and the danger of titanium showing in the marginal mucosal area.

3i (Implant Innovations) System

The 3i implant system[27] was developed by Lazzara and Beaty in 1988 and has gone through several changes and additions since its early phase. The system is based on the research of Branemark and colleagues and includes a 2-stage commercially pure titanium screw and cylinder with either an acid etched, a plasma-sprayed titanium-coated (TPS) or a plasma-sprayed hydroxyapatite (HA)-coated surface. Recently one-stage implant was introduced to the market, which is largely based on the research of Schroeder and colleagues.[34] Another implant concept was recently introduced by roughening the middle and more apical part of the implant for better bone integration and keeping the coronal part a smooth surface for better maintenance properties. The system went into clinical trials in 1990, and several retrospective studies of its implant survival have been reported.[27]

Astra Dental Implant System[19,20]

Another implant system presenting significant research and clinical studies was developed in the 1980s in Sweden. It consists of a self-tapping screw made of pure titanium and is characterized by a conical abutment that fits tightly into the coronal part of the implant. The system has a titanium oxide–blasted surface and a special single-tooth implant with a wider microthreaded, tapered collar. The screw-shaped titanium implants are presented with a titanium oxide–blasted coating.

Other Systems

The Paragon/Core-vent system,[18] Integral System,[25] IMZ system,[5,26] Friadent system, and the TPS system[4] offer a variety of implant designs, from screw-shaped to cylinder type, as well as implant surface characteristics, from machined pure titanium to HA to plasma-sprayed titanium coatings. These systems have been developed since the early to mid-1980s and resemble some of the previously described systems. Some long-term follow-up data of their clinical results are available.

Hydroxyapatite coated implants have been recommended for compromised bone sites, because the HA coating accelerates bone apposition to the implant surface in the early healing period and significantly improves the anchorage in bone (see Chapter 70). However, long-term results have reported that the HA coating is biologically unstable over time and shows signs of resorption in histologic studies.[22] This might be one of the factors responsible for controversial data about the increasing rate of complications reported after a 3- to 5-year functional period.[9,25]

IMPLANT RECONSTRUCTION AND AESTHETICS

The patients who seem to benefit most from dental implants are those with fully edentulous arches. In these patients, removable and fixed implant prosthetic devices can restore almost normal stomatognathic function. The original design of the edentulous arch was a fixed bone–anchored bridge that used five to six implants in the anterior area of the mandible or the maxilla and a cantilever through the premolar area. Most implant bridges currently used are screwed into place and can easily be removed by loosening the fixation screws. This adds a retrievability characteristic to the treatment, which increases the overall comfort and reliability for the patient.

Another treatment option for the rehabilitation of an edentulous arch is the overdenture retained by clips to a bar splinting two to six implants. This treatment results in less prosthesis stability but is still far superior to conventional complete dentures (see Chapter 72).[39]

Partially edentulous patients with single or multiple missing teeth represent another viable treatment population for osseointegrated implants, but the remaining natural dentition (i.e., its occlusal schemes, periodontal health status, vertical dimension problems, and aesthetics) introduces an additional challenge to achieve a long-lasting, successful rehabilitation.[28] In general, osseointegrated implants can support a freestanding fixed partial denture. Adjacent natural teeth are not necessary for additional support. However, the close proximity of anatomic structures and the limited bone quantity require special attention to diagnosis and treatment planning.[7] The major advantage of implant-supported restorations in partially edentulous patients is that they are less invasive to adjacent teeth (i.e., preparation of abutment teeth becomes unnecessary), and larger edentulous spans can be restored with fixed bridges.[31] Obtaining ideal aesthetic results, however, poses interesting and difficult challenges for the restorative/surgical team.[7]

The **single-tooth restoration** (Fig. 69-4) requires detailed planning and careful management to achieve perfect harmony among implant position, bone level, soft tissue aesthetics, and tooth form and color.[17,24] The replacement of single missing teeth with implants has two major advantages over replacement with conventional fixed prostheses. First, there is no need to prepare adjacent teeth, and second, the ridge will be maintained by the implant. The primary candidates for single-tooth implants are all anterior teeth, from central incisor to second premolar in the maxilla and mandible provided that no lateral forces are induced by the single standing implant. Molar replacements with single implants are less indicated, owing to the high stresses generated in the posterior region of the mouth and the insufficient force distribution over one implant, leading to potential bone resorption.

Early on, the UCLA (University of California, Los Angeles) abutment[29] was developed by Beumer and colleagues to allow direct connection between the implant-supported restoration and the top of the implant, thereby eliminating the need for the transmucosal abutment cylinder and improving the aesthetic result dramatically, since porcelain rather than titanium emerges from the tissues. Similar techniques have since evolved, and aesthetically pleasing implant restorations are a reality. No significant difference in fully implant-supported bridges or implant-and-tooth–supported bridges have been found in the short term, but the fully implant-supported bridges may have a better long-term outlook.

Although 10-year data for the partially edentulous patient are still missing, the less invasive dental implant approach is promising and is increasingly preferred by patients and their treatment teams.

Complications

Less than 10% of implants will show some form of complication over the life of the implant.[8] Complications can be detected during the treatment phase (early onset) and/or during the maintenance phase (late onset). When a dental implant demonstrates any degree of mobility *after* the healing period, it is considered a failure. Implant mobility suggests a fibrous connective tissue interface that does not function well over time. When this mobility is detected, the implant, with its surrounding fibrous capsule, must be removed. After an appropriate healing time it is possible to place another implant.

During the maintenance phase, once osseointegration is established, complications can be divided into adverse tissue reactions such as mucosal inflammation and progressive bone loss and mechanical problems such as component fractures or screw loosenings (see Chapter 73).

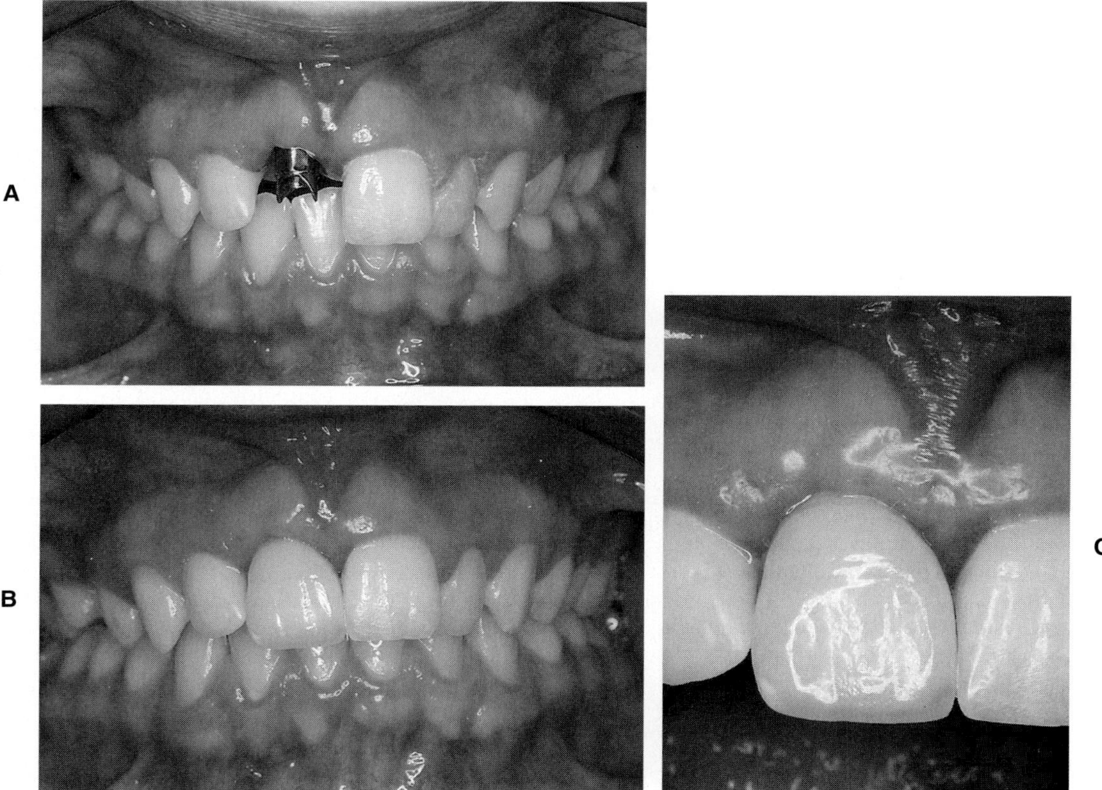

Fig. 69-4 Single tooth replacement. **A,** Implant in place. **B,** Metalloceramic crown. **C,** Close-up view.

Maintenance Phase

Proper oral hygiene and appropriate occlusal forces are critical for long-term function of an implant prosthesis, as poor hygiene and occlusal trauma have been related to marginal bone loss. Plaque control should be started immediately after the implant is exposed to the intraoral environment and monitored over time. Implant superstructures are often bulky and overcontoured, which makes traditional home care procedures more difficult. In addition, implant patients usually have a history of less than ideal home care, which has resulted in their partially or totally edentulous state. Patient recalls should be at 3-month intervals for the first year and then on a semiannual basis. However, some patients may require more frequent follow-up care. Recall visits should include an evaluation of oral hygiene compliance, occlusal harmony, implant and prosthesis stability, overall soft and hard peri-implant tissue health, and radiographic follow-up.

REFERENCES

1. Adell R, Lekholm U, Rockler B, et al: A 15-year study of osseointegrated implants in the treatment of the edentulous jaw. Int J Oral Surg 1981; 10:387.
2. Adell R, Eriksson B, Lekholm U, et al: A long term follow-up study of osseointegrated implants in the treatment of totally edentulous jaws. Int J Oral Maxillofac Implants 1990; 5:347.
3. Albrektsson T, Zarb G, Worthington P, et al: The long-term efficacy of currently used dental implants. A review and proposed criteria of success. Int J Oral Maxillofac Implants 1986; 1:11.
4. Babbush CA, Kent JN, Misiek DJ: Titanium-plasma-sprayed (TPS) screw implants for the reconstruction of the edentulous mandible. J Oral Maxillofac Surg 1986; 44:274.
5. Babbush CA, Shimura M: Five-year statistical and clinical observations with the IMZ two-stage osteointegrated implant system. Int J Oral Maxillofac Implants 1993; 8:245, 1993.
6. Bain CA, Moy PK: The association between the failure of dental implants and cigarette smoking. Int J Oral Maxillofac Implants 1993; 8:609.
7. Belser UC, Buser D, Hess D, et al: Aesthetic implant restorations in partially edentulous patients—a critical appraisal. Periodontology 2000 1998; 17:132.
8. Berman CL: Osseointegration, complications, prevention, recognition, treatment. Dent Clin North Am 1989; 33:635.
9. Block MS, Gardiner D, Kent JN, et al: Hydroxapatite-coated cylindrical implants in the posterior mandible: 10-year observations. Int J Oral Maxillofac Implants 1996; 11:626.
10. Branemark P-I, Breine U, Adell R, et al: Intraosseous anchorage of dental prostheses. I. Experimental studies. Scand J Plast Reconstr Surg 1969; 3:81.
11. Branemark P-I, Zarb GA, Albrektsson T: Tissue-integrated prostheses. Chicago, Quintessence, 1985.
12. Brunski JB: Biomechanics of oral implants: Future research directions. J Dent Educ 1988; 52:775.
13. Buser D, Mericske-Stern R, Bernard JP, et al: Long-term evaluation of non-submerged ITI implants. I. 8-year life table

analysis of a prospective multi-center study with 2359 implants. Clin Oral Implant Res 1997; 8:161.

14. Buser D, Schenk R, Steinemann S, et al: Influence of surface characteristics on bone integration of titanium implants. A histomorphometric study in miniature pigs. J Biomed Mat Res 1991; 25:889.
15. Buser D, Nydegger T, Oxland T, et al: Influence of surface characteristics on the interface shear strength between titanium implants and bone. A biomedical study in the maxilla of miniature pigs. J Biomed Res 1999; 45:75.
16. DeBruyn H, Collaert B: The effect of smoking on early implant failure. Clin Oral Implant Res 1994; 5:260.
17. Ekfeldt A, Carlsson GE, Börjesson G: Clinical evaluation of single-tooth restorations supported by osseointegrated implants: a retrospective study. Int J Oral Maxillofac Implants 1994; 9:179.
18. Evian CI: A comparison of hydroxyapatite-coated Micro-vent and pure titanium Swede-vent implants. Int J Oral Maxillofac Implants 1996; 11:639.
19. Gotfredsen K, Holm B, Sewerin I, et al: Marginal tissue response adjacent to Astra Dental implants supporting overdentures in the mandible. A 2-year follow-up study. Clin Oral Implant Res 1993; 4:83.
20. Gotfredsen K, Wennerberg A, Johansson C, et al: Anchorage of TiO^2-blasted, HA-coated, and machined implants: an experimental study with rabbits. J Biomed Mat Res 1995; 29:1223.
21. Jaffin RA, Berman CI: The excessive loss of Branemark implants in type IV bone. A 5-year analysis. J Periodontol 1991; 62:2.
22. Johnson BW: HA-coated dental implants: Long-term consequences. 1992; Calif Dent Assoc J 20:33.
23. Jovanovic S, Buser D: Guided bone regeneration in dehiscence defects and delayed extraction sockets. In Buser D, Dahlin C, Schenk RK (eds): Guided Bone Regeneration in Implant Dentistry. Chicago, Quintessence, 1994.
24. Jovanovic S, Paul S, Nishimura R: Anterior implant-supported reconstructions: a surgical challenge. Pract Perio Aesthet Dentistry 1999; 11:5:551.
25. Kent J, Block M: Biointegrated hydroxyapatite coated dental implants: 5 year clinical observations. J Am Dent Assoc 1990; 121:138.
26. Kirsch A, Ackermann KL: The IMZ osteointegrated implant system. Dent Clin North Am 1989; 33:733.
27. Lazzara R, Siddiqui AA, Binon P, et al: Retrospective multicenter analysis of 3I endosseous dental implants placed over a 5-year period. Clin Oral Impl Res 1996; 7:73.
28. Lekholm U, van Steenberghe D, Herrmann I, et al: Osseointegrated implants in the treatment of partially edentulous jaws: a prospective 5-year multicenter study. Int J Oral Maxillofac Implants 1994; 9:627.
29. Lewis SG, Beumer J, Perri GR, et al: The UCLA abutment. J Oral Maxillo-Fac Implants 1989; 3:183.
30. Mecall R, Rosenfeld A: Influence of residual ridge resorption pattern on fixture placement and tooth position. III. Presurgical assessment of ridge augmentation requirements. Intl J Perio Res Dentistry 1996; 16:322.
31. Pylant T, Triplett RG, Key MC, et al: A retrospective evaluation of endosseous titanium implants in the partially edentulous patient. Intl J Oral Maxillofac Implants 1992; 7:195.
32. Reddy MS, Mayfield-Donahoo T, Vanderven FJJ, et al: A comparison of the diagnostic advantages of panoramic radiography and computed tomography scanning for placement of root form dental implants. Clin Oral Implant Res 1994; 5:229.
33. Saadoun AP, LeGall ML: Clinical results and guidelines on Steri-Oss endosseous implants. Int J Periodont Restor Dent 1992; 12:487.
34. Schroeder A, van der Zypen E, Stich H, et al: The reactions of bone, connective tissue, and epithelium to endosteal implants with titanium-sprayed surfaces. J Maxillofac Surg 1981; 9:15.
35. Shanaman RH: The use of guided tissue regeneration of facilitate ideal prosthetic placement of implants. Intl J Perio Res Dentistry 1992; 12:257.
36. Van Steenberghe D, Quirynen M, Naert I: Survival and success rates with oral endosseous implants. In Lang NP, Karring T, Lindhe J (eds): International Implant Dentistry. Proceedings of 3rd European Workshop in Periodontology. Berlin, Quintessence, 1999.
37. Warrer K, Gotfredsen K, Hjørting-Hansen E, et al: Guided tissue regeneration ensures osseointegration of dental implants placed in extraction sockets. Clin Oral Implant Res 1991; 2:166.
38. Watanabe F, Tawada Y, Komatsu S, et al: Heat distribution in bone during preparation of implant sites: heat analysis by real-time thermography. Int J Oral Maxillofac Implants 1992; 7:213.
39. Zitzmann N, Marinello C: Treatment plan for restoring the edentulous maxilla with implant-supported restorations: removable overdenture versus fixed partial denture design. J Prosthet Dentistry 1999; 82:188.

Surgical Aspects of Dental Implants

Thomas J. Han and Kwang-Bum Park

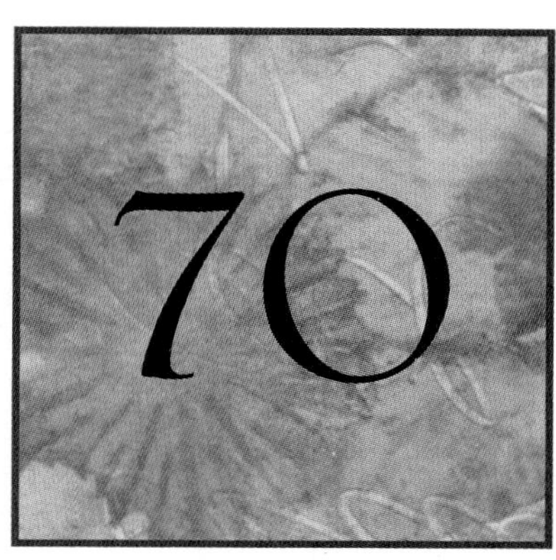

CHAPTER

CHAPTER OUTLINE

CONSIDERATIONS OF FIXTURE DESIGN AND SURFACE CHARACTERISTICS FOR IMPLANT SURGERY

The root form implant surgical techniques are mostly based on the researches performed on the biologic, physiologic, and mechanical aspects of the Nobelpharma implant system developed by Per-Ingvar Branemark and colleagues in Sweden approximately three decades ago. Since then, many different designs of root form implants have been studied, and presently more than 50 implant manufacturers exist worldwide.

The root form implants can be divided according to their body shapes (macrodesign) and surface topography (microdesign).

Screw-Threaded and Threadless, Cylinder-Shaped Implants (Macrodesign)

In consideration of surgical protocol, the root form implants can be divided into two basic groups: one has threads, and the other is threadless and in cylinder form (Fig. 70-1). The first type is threaded into the bone recipient site like a screw with a handpiece or wrench after drilling a hole slightly smaller in diameter than the implant. The cylinder-shaped, threadless implants are tapped into a recipient hole that is similar to the diameter of the implant body. The threaded implants are more widely used today because they usually provide superior initial stability in bone, and vertical positioning of the implant during placement can be more precisely controlled. The high initial stability is crucial when considering placing a provisional restoration on the implant immediately after implant placement. In dense bone, it may be necessary to "tap" the bone for easier placement. Some threaded implants are shaped conically to minimize apical bone fenestration, and these are useful in placing implants into anterior extraction sockets immediately (Fig. 70-2).

Surface Topography of Implant (Microdesign)

It is generally believed that the textured surfaces accelerate the initial healing phase through the adsorption of bioactive components of bone, and a stronger bond between implants and bone is achieved faster.[5,9,13] Titanium plasma-sprayed (TPS) and hydroxyapatite (HA) surfaces are considered highly textured surfaces (Fig. 70-3, *A, B*). Although these surfaces achieve secondary stability and integration earlier, progressive bone loss can occur if the rough surface of the implant becomes exposed to oral fluid and microorganisms. Therefore when using these types of surface implants, care must be taken to ensure complete submersion of the rough surface in bone with sufficient crestal bone thickness around the implant. Thinner crestal bone can resorb during function, and the subsequent exposure of the rough surface to oral

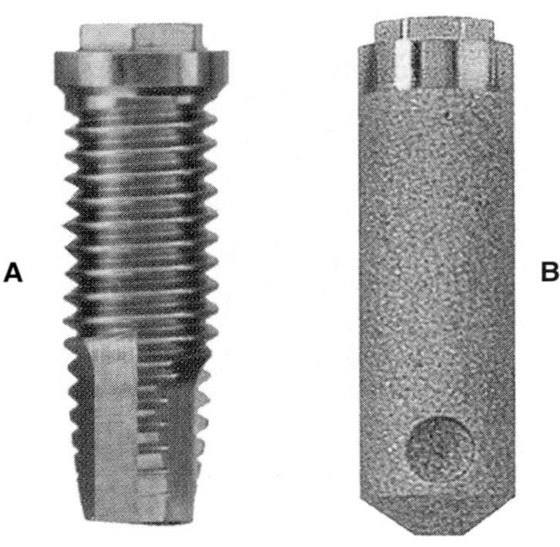

Fig. 70-1 Two basic groups of the root form implants (Macrodesign). One is with threads **(A),** and the other is threadless **(B).**

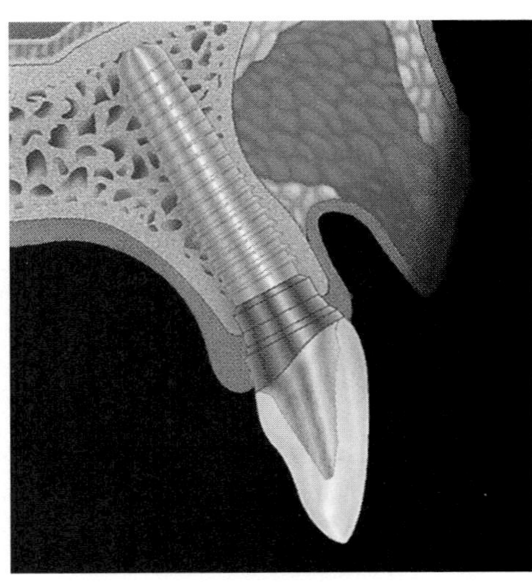

Fig. 70-2 A conically shaped, threaded implant is helpful to minimize apical bone fenestration and also useful in placing implants into extraction sockets immediately. (Courtesy Nobel Biocare, Yorba Linda, Calif.)

fluid can initiate progressive bone loss and result in eventual failure of the implant. Smooth surface implant is much more resistant to bacterial contamination and progressive bone loss, but it provides weaker secondary stability and consequently has a lower success rate in soft or grafted bone (Fig. 70-3, *C*). Therefore medium-textured implants with blasted/etched (for example, RBM surface of Lifecore system, SLA surface of ITI system) or etched/etched (for example, Osseotite surface of 3i system, Etched titanium implant of Steri-Oss system) surfaces have gained favor recently because they have stronger bonding capacity with minimal likelihood of progressive bone loss due to bacterial contamination (Fig. 70-3, *D*).

ONE-STAGE VERSUS TWO-STAGE IMPLANT SURGERIES

The most threaded endosseous implant can be placed either as one stage, meaning the coronal portion stays exposed through gingiva during the healing period (Fig. 70-4, *A, B*), or two stage, meaning the top of the implant is completely submerged under gingiva (see Fig. 70-4, *C*). In two-stage implant surgery, the head of the implant needs to be surgically exposed with a second surgery. Some implants, notably from the ITI system, TG implant of 3i system, and Lifecore single-stage system are specifically designed to have the coronal portion of the implant extend through the gingiva during the healing period (see Fig. 70-4, *A*).[6] However, most other systems require attaching a healing abutment to the implanted fixture before it can be used in one-stage surgery (see Fig. 70-4, *B*).

The advantages of the one-stage surgical approach are that the mucogingival management around the implant is easier, patient comfort increases because less surgeries are involved, and the esthetic management is easier in many cases. However, if extensive bone loss occurs at the implant site, vertical bone augmentation is necessary, interproximal bone of the adjacent teeth is lacking, and/or bone quality is poor, then the two-stage surgical approach is recommended.

Because some fundamental differences in flap management for both two-stage and one-stage endosseous implant surgeries exist, the two surgical techniques are described separately.

In the two-stage implant surgical approach, the first-stage surgery ends by suturing the soft tissues over the implant so that it remains excluded from the oral cavity. *In the mandible, the implants are left undisturbed for 2 to 3 months, whereas in the maxilla, they remain covered for approximately 4 to 6 months because of slower healing due to less dense bone.* During this period, the healing bone makes direct contact with the implant surface (osseointegration) and sometimes grows to its occlusal surface, even covering it.[4] In the second-stage surgery, the buried implant is uncovered, and a titanium abutment is connected to allow access to the implant from the oral cavity. The restorative dentist then proceeds with the prosthodontic aspects of the implant therapy.

In the one-stage implant surgical approach, a second intervention is not needed because the implant is left exposed after the first surgery. Again the implants are left unloaded and undisturbed for a period similar to the implants placed in the two-stage approach.

Regardless of the type of surgical approach, the implant must be placed in healthy bone to achieve osseointegration, and an atraumatic and aseptic technique must be followed to avoid damage to vital structures. Generally, implant surgery is done under local anesthesia, but oral or intravenous (IV) sedation can also be used if necessary. The surgical site should be kept aseptic and the patient appropriately prepared and draped for an intraoral surgical procedure. The patient should rinse with chlorhexidine gluconate for 30 seconds immediately before the procedure. Every effort should be made to mini-

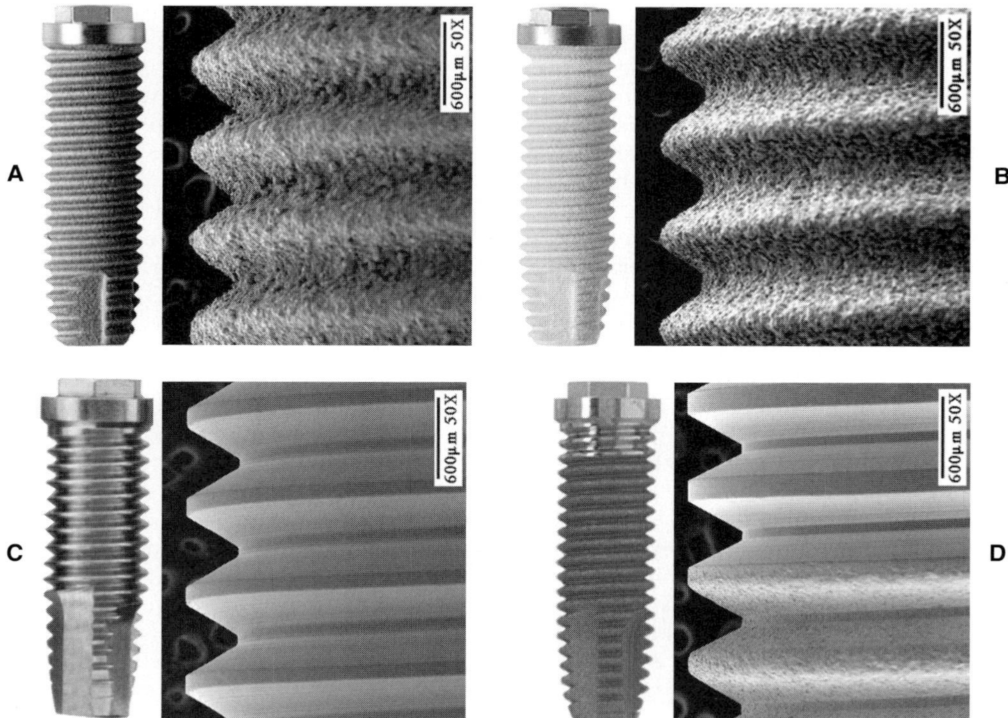

Fig. 70-3 Surface topography of implant (microdesign). **A,** Highly textured implant with TPS (titanium plasma-sprayed) surface. **B,** Highly textured implant with hydroxyapatite-coated surface. **C,** Implant with smooth machined surface. **D,** Medium textured implant with blasted/etched surface. (Courtesy 3i/Implant Innovations, Inc., Palm Beach Gardens, Fla.)

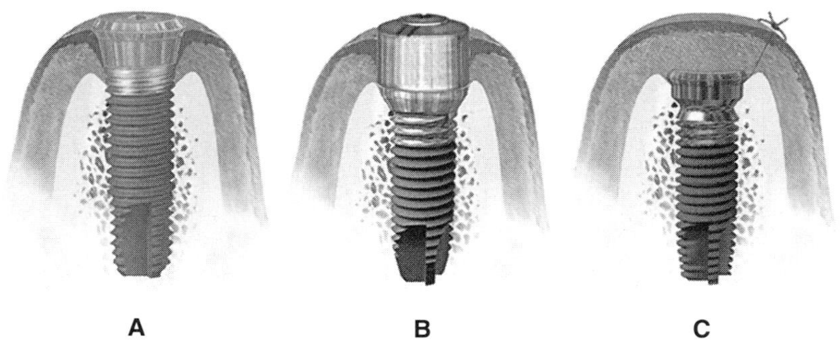

Fig. 70-4 One-stage implant versus two-stage implant surgeries. **A,** One-stage surgery with the implant designed so that the coronal portion of the implant extends through the gingiva. **B,** One-stage surgery with implant designed to be used for two-stage surgery. A healing abutment is connected to the implanted fixture during the first stage surgery. **C,** In the two-stage surgery, the top of the implant is completely submerged under gingiva. (Courtesy Lifecore Biomedical, Chaska, Minn.)

mize the risk of contamination of the implant surfaces by such items as gloves, instruments, suction tubing, or saliva.

This chapter presents general surgical considerations and guidance on some of the most commonly used implant systems. The great variety of implant systems with their own specific armamentarium makes it advisable in each case to follow the detailed, step-by-step description usually found in the manufacturer's manual.

Two-Stage Endosseous Implant Surgery

First-Stage Surgical Technique

FLAP DESIGN AND INCISION. Two types of incisions—crestal or remote—can be used. In the latter, the incision is made away from the implant site, usually 1 to 2 mm inferior to the mucogingival junction. A back-action chisel or a periosteal elevator is then used to reflect a mucoperiosteal (full-thickness) flap. For the crestal design flap, the incision is made along the crest of the ridge, bisecting the existing zone of keratinized mucosa (Fig. 70-5, *A*).

The remote incision has the advantage of covering the implant without sutures over its top. The crestal incision, however, is preferred in most instances because it results in less bleeding, easier flap management, less edema, less ecchymosis, less vestibular change postoperatively, faster healing, and easier denture reline.[17] Sutures placed over the implant generally do not interfere with proper healing. When extensive bone augmentation is planned, a remote incision with layer suturing technique is used to minimize the incidence of bone graft exposure.

FLAP ELEVATION. A full-thickness flap is raised buccally and lingually to the level of the mucogingival junction, exposing the alveolar ridge of the implant sites (see Fig. 70-5, *B*). Elevated flaps may be sutured to the buccal mucosa or the opposing teeth to keep the surgical site open during the surgery.

If a bone augmentation technique, with or without membranes, is anticipated, the flap can be extended by making a partial-thickness flap beyond the mucogingival junction. This lengthens the flap while providing flexibility to close it without tension after the implantation and ridge augmentation procedure (see Fig. 70-5, *C, D*).

For a knife-edge alveolar process with sufficient alveolar height and distance from vital structures such as the sinuses or the inferior alveolar nerve or mental nerves, a suitable round bur is used to recontour the bone to provide a reasonably flat bed for the implant site (see Fig. 70-5, *B*).

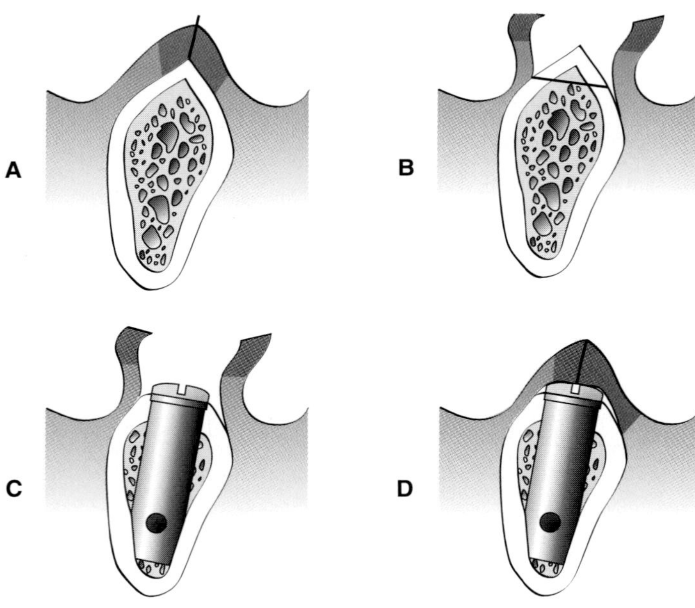

Fig. 70-5 A, Crestal incision made along the crest of the ridge, bisecting the existing zone of keratinized mucosa. **B,** A full-thickness flap is raised buccally and lingually to the level of the mucogingival junction. A sharp ridge can be surgically contoured to provide a reasonably flat bed for the implant. **C,** A partial-thickness flap is raised apically from the mucogingival junction to provide extension of the flap. **D,** Crestal flap closure without tension.

IMPLANT PLACEMENT. Once the implant site is prepared, a surgical guide or stent is placed intraorally, and a small round bur or spiral drill is used to mark the implant sites. The stent is then removed, and the sites are checked for their appropriate faciolingual location. Slight modifications may be necessary to avoid obvious ridge defects.

The site is then marked to a depth of 1 to 2 mm, breaking through the cortical bone (Fig. 70-6, *A*). A small spiral drill, usually 2 mm in diameter and marked to indicate appropriate depth, is used next to establish the depth and align the axis of the implant recipient site (see Fig. 70-4, *B*). This drill may be externally or internally irrigated. In either case, the spiral drill is used at a speed if approximately 800 to 1000 rpm with copious irrigation to prevent overheating the bone.

If the vertical height of the bone is reduced during the ridge preparation, this must be taken into account when selecting the length of the implant. When multiple implants are used to support one prosthesis, a paralleling or direction-indicating pin should be used to align subsequent implants correctly. The relationship to neighboring vital structures can be determined by taking a periapical radiograph with a radiographic marker placed at the bottom of the prepared site. Implants should be at least 3 mm apart to ensure sufficient room for adequate oral hygiene once the prosthesis is in place.

The next step is to use a series of drills to systematically widen the size to accommodate the selected size of the implant. The shapes of the drills may slightly differ among systems, but their general purpose is to prepare a recipient site that is accurate in size, both in diameter and in length, for the selected implant without unduly traumatizing the surrounding bone.

Usually after the 2-mm spiral drill, a pilot drill with 2-mm diameter at the lower part and wider diameter at the upper part is used to enlarge the osteotomy site to allow easy insertion of the following drill. Then a wider diameter spiral drill can be used to drill to the depth reached with the 2-mm spiral drill. When it is necessary to place the height of the cover screw slightly under the crestal bone to avoid a risk of premature exposure from the pressure of the temporary denture and minimize the thread exposure due to the inclined ridge, the countersink drilling is recommended (see Fig. 70-6, *E*). Implant therapy in posterior areas of the mouth often requires wide diameter implants. When a large-diameter drill is used for site preparation, it is necessary to reduce the drilling speed to approximately 500 rpm to prevent overheating the bone. Copious external irrigation is mandatory, and internal irritation is helpful.

Regardless of the system used, it is very important that the final diameter drilling be accomplished with a steady hand, without wobbling. Some techniques help accomplish this. If the final drill hits the bottom of the recipient site before reaching the desired depth, the added hand pressure necessary to achieve the proper depth often causes wobbling and funneling of the recipient site. This is especially true with cannon drills that have been used for the cylinder-type implant. To minimize this effect, during the preparation of the recipient site with the smaller-diameter drill, the operator should

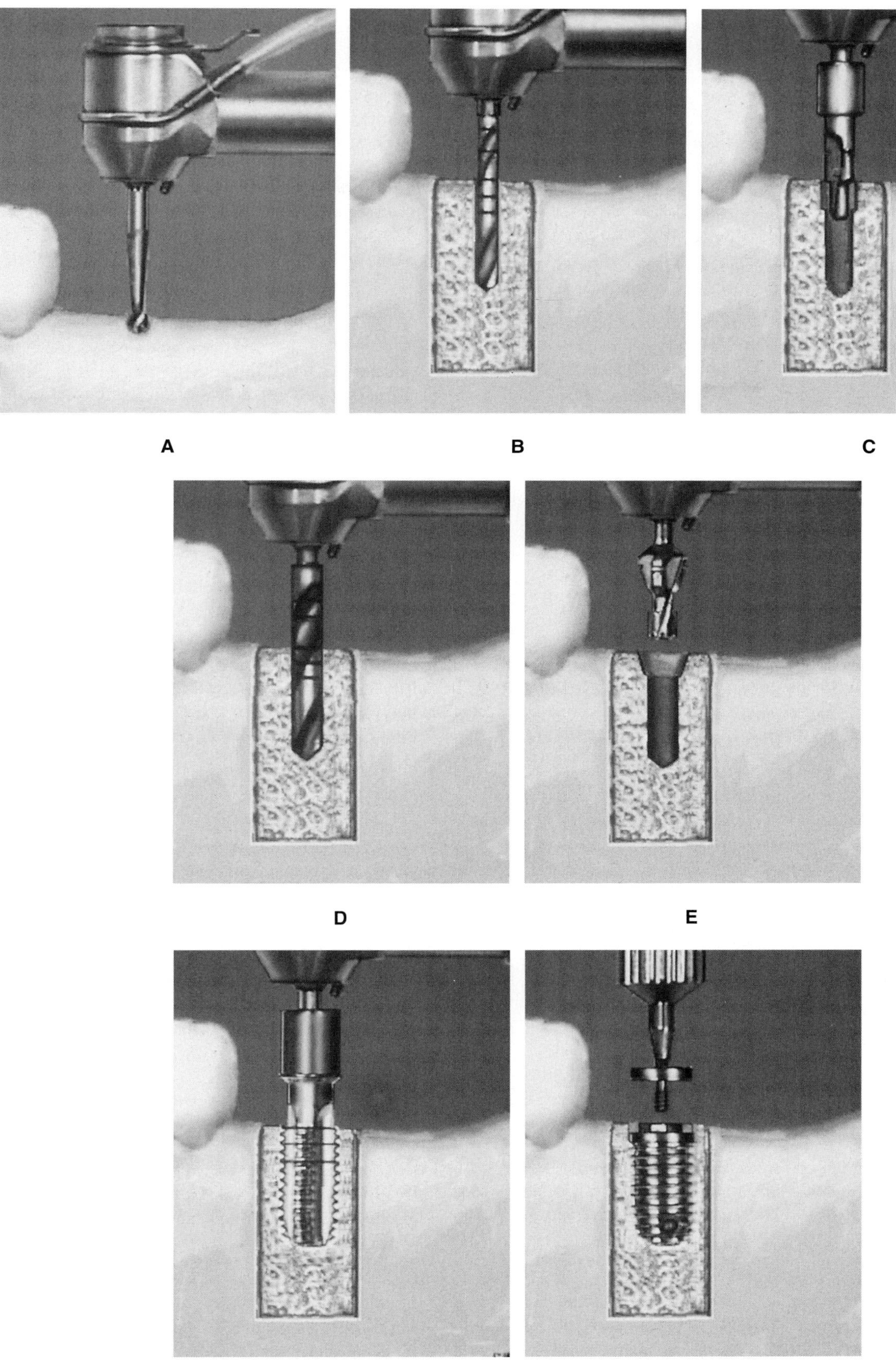

Fig. 70-6 **A,** Initial site preparation for screw-type implant. **B,** Use of a 2-mm drill to establish depth and align the implant. **C,** A wider-diameter pilot drill is used to increase the size of the recipient site. **D,** A final-size drill is used to finish the preparation of the recipient site. **E,** A countersink drill is used to widen the entrance of the recipient site. **F,** A tap is used to create screw threads. **G,** The implant is screwed into the recipient site, and the cover screw is placed. (Courtesy 3i/Implant Innovations, Inc., Palm Beach Gardens, Fla.)

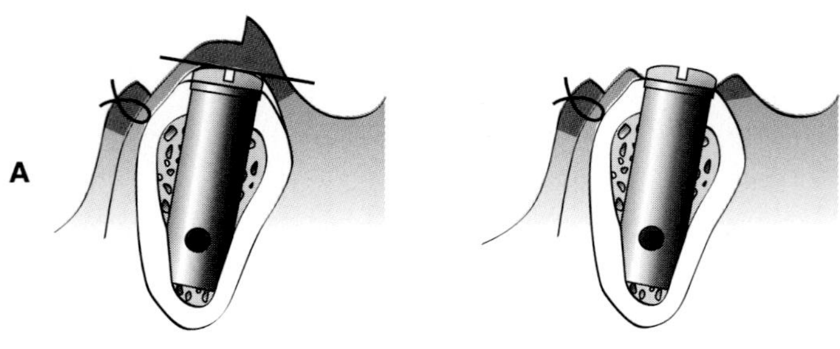

Fig. 70-7 **A,** A partial-thickness flap is apically sutured to the periosteum, and excess connective tissue coronal to the cover screw is excised by gingivectomy. **B,** A sharp blade is used to eliminate all tissue coronal to the cover screw.

drill to approximately 0.5 mm deeper than needed. This allows the desired depth to be reached with the final drill without touching the bottom.

In addition, if the final drill is inserted at an inaccurate angle, the result is funneling of the coronal portion of the implant site. To minimize this when drilling multiple implant sites, the operator should always keep a direction indicator in adjacent site. For single implant cases, some type of direction reference guide should be used. When dealing with very dense bone, a precise recipient site can be achieved more predictably if there is minimal diameter change from drill to drill. For example, going from 3.0 to 5.0 mm is far more difficult than going from 3.0 to 3.3 to 4.2 to 5.0 mm.

For the placement of threaded implants, a tapping procedure may be necessary. With self-tapping implants becoming increasingly popular, there is less need for a tapping procedure, but in very dense bone or when placing longer implants, it is prudent to use a tap (see Fig. 70-6, *F*). When dealing with a very soft bone (e.g., in posterior maxillary areas), tapping is not recommended.

It is important to create a recipient site accurate in size and angulation. In partially edentulous cases, a limited opening of the mouth may prevent appropriate positioning of the drills in posterior edentulous areas. Therefore a combination of longer drills or shorter drills, with or without extensions, may be necessary. Anticipating these needs facilitates the procedure and improves the results.

CLOSURE OF THE FLAP. Once the implants are screwed in and the cover screws are placed (Fig. 70-6, *G*), proper closure of the flap over the implant is very important. One suturing technique that consistently provides the desired result is a combination of inverted mattress and interrupted sutures. The inverted mattress sutures keep the bleeding edges of the flap close together, while the interrupted sutures seal the edges. However, the most important aspect of flap management at this stage is *closure of the flap without tension.* It is better to use a suture that does not require removal during the postoperative visit, such as a 4.0 chromic gut suture.

POSTOPERATIVE CARE. Patients are premedicated with antibiotics (amoxicillin, 500 mg tid) starting immediately before the surgery and continuing for at least 1 week afterward (see Chapter 55). Swelling is likely to occur, and the patient should apply ice packs extraorally intermittently for the first 24 hours. Chlorhexidine gluconate mouthrinses should be used twice daily because oral hygiene and plaque control will be difficult to perform. Adequate pain medication should be prescribed (see Chapter 55). Patients should have a liquid or semisoft diet for the first few days and then gradually return to a normal diet. Patients should also refrain from tobacco and alcohol use for 1 to 2 weeks postoperatively.

Color Fig. 70-1 shows all steps of first-stage implant placement surgery in a clinical case.

Second-Stage Surgical Technique.

The objectives of the second-stage surgery are as follows:

1. To expose the submerged implant without damaging the surrounding bone.
2. To control the thickness of the soft tissue surrounding the implant.
3. To preserve or create attached keratinized tissue around the implant.
4. To facilitate oral hygiene.
5. To ensure proper abutment seating.

Thin soft tissue with an adequate amount of keratinized attached gingiva, along with good oral hygiene, ensures healthier periimplant soft tissues and better clinical results. The need for keratinized tissue is somewhat controversial, depending on the type of implant prosthesis and location of the implant. But one long-term study indicated that, at least in the posterior mandible and in partially edentulous cases, the presence of keratinized tissue is strongly correlated with soft and hard tissue health.[3]

In areas with sufficient zones of keratinized tissue, either the gingiva covering the head of the implant can be punched out or a full-thickness flap technique that places a band of keratinized tissue on both sides of the implants is used. If deficient keratinized tissue is available, the following partial-thickness flap-gingivectomy technique can be used to predictably fulfill the objection of the second-stage surgery listed previously.

PARTIAL-THICKNESS FLAP-GINGIVECTOMY TECHNIQUE

Flap Design and Incisions. The initial incision is made approximately 2 mm coronal to the facial mucogingival junction, with vertical incisions both mesially and distally (Color Fig. 70-2, *A, B*). When dealing with anterior implants, the flap design should preserve the adjacent papilla.

Flap Elevation and Apical Displacement. A partial-thickness flap is then raised in such a manner that a relatively firm periosteum remains. The flap, containing a band of keratinized tissue, is then placed facial to the emerging head of the implant fixture and fixed to the periosteum with 5.0-gut suture (Fig. 70-7; see also Color Fig. 70-2, *C*). If the initial amount of keratinized tissue is less than 2 mm, the flap may be started from the lingual part of the ridge, positioning facially the entire band of keratinized tissue. When a partial-thickness flap is apically displaced in this manner, not exposing the alveolar bone, a band of attached keratinized tissue is maintained or created around the implants.

Gingivectomy. Once the flap is positioned facially, the excess tissue coronal to the cover screw is excised, usually using a gingivectomy technique (see Fig. 70-7 and Color Fig. 70-2, *D*). However, if a gingivectomy technique would compromise the lingual keratinized tissue around the implant(s), a similar partial-thickness flap can be made on the lingual side.

Once the excess tissue coronal to the cover screw is removed, the outline of the cover screw is visible. A sharp blade is used to eliminate all tissues coronal to the cover screw (see Fig. 70-7, *B* and Color Fig. 70-2, *E*). The cover screw is then removed, the head of the implant is thoroughly cleaned of any soft or hard tissue overgrowth, and the healing abutments or standard abutments are placed on the fixture (see Color Fig. 70-2, *F*). The fit of the implants to the healing abutments can often be visually evaluated.

Postoperative Care. Once the implant is exposed, it is important to remind the patient of the need for good oral hygiene around the implant. A chlorhexidine rinse is highly recommended for at least the initial 2 weeks while the tissues are healing. At this time, there should not be any direct pressure to the area from dentures. Fabrication of the suprastructure can begin in about 2 weeks.

Color Fig. 70-2, *G* and *H* shows the postoperative results in a clinical case after 2 to 3 weeks and 4 months, respectively.

MAXILLARY ANTERIOR SECOND-STAGE SURGERY. The partial-thickness gingivectomy technique can be used in maxillary edentulous cases in which implant overdenture is the restorative goal. However, when placing individual implant dentition or an implant fixed bridge where maximal gingival vertical height is important for esthetic reasons, the soft tissue thickness should be maintained as much as possible. Therefore the partial-thickness gingivectomy technique should not be used. When the amount of keratinized tissue is sufficient, the punch biopsy technique can be used. If the flap reflection is necessary, vertical incisions should be avoided if at all possible. When the vertical incision is necessary, it should be made at least one tooth away from the implant site to minimize the facial clefting or indentation in esthetic areas.

One-Stage Endosseous Implant Surgery

In the two-stage surgical approach, the implant is placed flush with the bone crest, and the soft tissue covering is purposely kept thick to minimize the chances of a premature exposure of the cover screws. In the one-stage surgical approach, the implant or the healing abutment protrudes about 2 to 3 mm from the bone crest, and the flaps are adapted around the implant. In posterior areas of the mouth, the flap is thinned and sometimes placed apically to increase the zone of keratinized attached gingiva.

Surgical Technique

FLAP DESIGN AND INCISIONS. The flap design for the one-stage surgical approach is always a crestal incision bisecting the existing keratinized tissue. Vertical incisions may be needed in one or both ends. Facial and lingual flaps in posterior areas should be carefully thinned before total reflection to minimize the soft tissue thickness. The soft tissue is not thinned in anterior or other aesthetic areas of the mouth to prevent the metal collar from showing. Full-thickness flaps are elevated facially and lingually.

PLACEMENT OF THE IMPLANT. The implant site preparation to place the implants in one surgery is identical in principle to the two-stage implant surgical approach. The only difference is that the implant or the healing abutment extension of the implant is placed in such way that the head of the implant protrudes about 2 to 3 mm from the bone crest.

CLOSURE OF THE FLAP. The keratinized edges of the flap are tied with independent sutures around the implant. When keratinized tissue is abundant, scalloping around the implant(s) provides better flap adaptation.

POSTOPERATIVE CARE. The postoperative care for one-stage surgical approach is same as that for the two-stage surgical approach.

ADJUNCTIVE ADVANCED SURGICAL TECHNIQUES

Oral implantology is often complicated by anatomic limitations of the jaw. Advanced surgical techniques are designed to overcome these difficulties, but often these procedures are very technique sensitive and expensive and have a high degree of postoperative morbidity. It is important to carefully weigh the benefits versus the risks of these procedures. Consider that if the patient has functioned relatively well with a conventional prosthesis before the implants were considered, it may be wise to continue with the traditional type of tooth replacement rather than perform surgical correction of unfavorable anatomic conditions.

One of the most often encountered anatomic limitations in both jaws is a narrow ridge. *Bone augmentation techniques* using the principle of guided bone regeneration and various kinds of bone graft material are indicated.[11] However, the regenerated bone is weaker and requires that the stability of the initial and early loaded stages come from integration with the preexisting bone. If most of the implant surface is exposed and an extensive amount of bone needs to regenerate to cover the implant, the risk of deintegration during the early-loaded stage is higher.

A new approach to implant therapy in esthetic areas combines surgical and restorative procedures to *provisionalize the implant immediately after implantation into extraction socket.* Simultaneous perigingival bone grafting is often performed. The obvious advantage of this approach is to increase the patient's satisfaction esthetically and phonetically during the provisional period, and studies have shown that an immobile immediate provisional restoration can enhance soft tissue management.[1,2,7,14–16] When a provisional restoration similar in shape and size to the natural tooth is placed in the extraction socket, it can support the periimplant mucosa and thus maintain the papillary height and gingival outline and form throughout the osseointegration period.[10,16]

Another common anatomic limitation of the maxillary arch is *excessive pneumatization of the maxillary sinus,* leaving a very thin inferior wall or floor of the maxillary sinus. Various techniques are available for elevating the floor of the sinus and augmenting the bone to accommodate the length of the implants.[8,12,18] These techniques are generally successful and, if done properly, benefit the patient. The sinus lift-augmentation can be performed as an initial separate procedure or combined in one intervention with the placement of the implants. To accomplish both objectives in one operation, the height of bone must be sufficient (usually greater than 5 mm) to provide the initial stability of the implant. In addition, if the existing bone height is sufficient but the bone is very soft, it is better to perform the sinus lift and implantation in separate interventions. When the sinus lift and the implantation are done in two stages, the bone should be allowed to mature for approximately 6 months before placing the implants. The implants are usually placed in a one-stage approach.

In the partially edentulous mandibular arch with severely resorbed ridges, a *mandibular nerve repositioning* is an option.[8] This procedure requires extensive manipulation of the mandibular nerve and often results in extended periods of paresthesia and dysesthesia of the lower lip. In most cases, the patient returns to normal sensation in about 6 months. Patients should be carefully selected for these procedures and clearly informed in writing of all possible side effects.

REFERENCES

1. Bain CA, Weisgold AS: Customized emergence profile in the implant crown—A new technique. Compendium 1997; 18(1):41.
2. Biggs WF: Placement of a custom implant provisional restoration at the second-stage surgery for improved gingival management: A clinical report. J Prosthet Dent 1996; 75(3):231.
3. Block MS, Kent JN: Factors associated with soft and hard tissue compromise of endosseous implants. J Oral Maxillofac Implants 1990; 48:1153.
4. Branemark P-I, Zarb G, Albrektsson I: Tissue-integrated prosthesis. In: Osseointegration in Clinical Dentistry. Chicago, Quintessence, 1987.
5. Buser D, Nydegger T, Hirt HP, et al: Removal torque values of titanium implants in the maxilla of miniature pigs. Int J Oral Maxillofac Implants 1998; 13(5):611.
6. Buser D, Weber HP, Bragger U: The treatment of partially edentulous patients with ITI hollow-screw implants: Presurgical evaluation and surgical procedures. Int J Oral Maxillofac Implants 1990; 5:165.
7. Chee WWL, Donovan T: Use of provisional restorations to enhance soft-tissue contours for implant restorations. Compendium 1998; 19(5):481.
8. Cranin AN: Atlas of Oral Implantology. New York, Thieme Medical, 1993.
9. Ericsson J, Johansson CB, Bystedt H, et al: A histomorphometric evaluation of bone-to-implant contact on machine-prepared and roughened titanium dental implants. A pilot study in dog. Clin Oral Implant Res 1994; 5:202.
10. Garber DA, Salama, MA, Salama H: Immediate total tooth replacement in the external root resorption case. World Dentistry 2000. www.worlddent.com.
11. Jovanovic SA, Giovannoli JL: New bone formation by the principle of guided tissue regeneration for periimplant osseous lesions. J Parodontologie 1992; 11:29.
12. Kent JN, Block MS: Simultaneous maxillary sinus floor bone grafting and placement of hydroxyapatite-coated implant. J Oral Maxillofac Implants 1989; 47:238.
13. Klokkevold P, Nishimura T, Adachi M, et al: Osseointegration enhanced by chemical etching of the titanium surface. Clin Oral Implant Res 1997; 8:442.
14. Lewis S, Parel S, Faulkner R: Provisional implant supported fixed restorations. Int J Oral Maxillofac Implants 1995; 10:319.
15. Markus SJ: Interim esthetic restorations in conjunction with anterior implants. J Prosthet Dent 1999; 82(2):233.
16. Nowzari H, Chee W, Tuan A, et al: Clinical and microbiological aspects of the Sargon Immediate load implant. Compendium 1998; 19(7):686.
17. Scharf DR, Tarnow DP: The effect of crestal versus mucobuccal incisions on the success rate of implant osseointegration. Int J Oral Maxillofac Implants 1993; 8:187.
18. Wood RM, Moore DI: Grafting of the maxillary sinus with intraorally harvested autogenous bone prior to implant placement. J Oral Maxillofac Implants 1988; 3:209.

Advanced Implant Surgery and Bone Grafting Techniques

Perry R. Klokkevold and Sascha A. Jovanovic

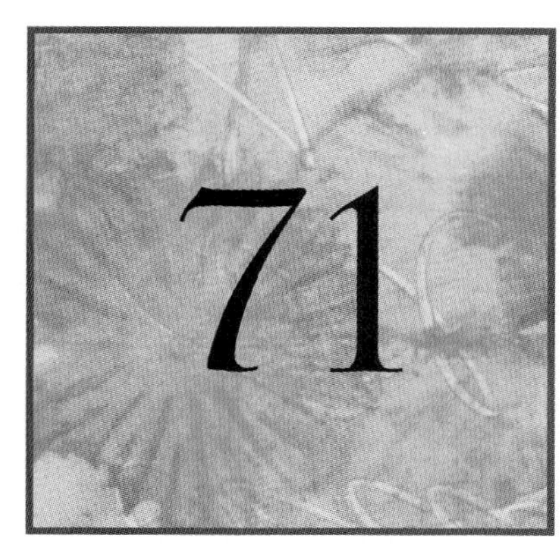

CHAPTER

CHAPTER OUTLINE

The use of dental implants in the partially and fully edentulous patient with deficient jawbones creates a new demand for bone reconstruction before or simultaneously with implant therapy, especially when natural esthetics is required. The most critical aspect of creating an implant restoration is the surgical placement of the implant in a prosthetically driven position so as to restore the natural position and emulate the natural emergence of a tooth from the soft tissues. Implants placed without regard for prosthetic position often result in dental restorations that are functionally and esthetically compromised, and patients are left with a less-than-optimal end result.

Periodontal bone loss, tooth extraction, and long-term use of removable appliances typically result in advanced alveolar bone loss that prevents the placement of implants in an optimal prosthetic position. Fortunately, continuous innovations in surgical techniques along with advances in the biologic understanding of bone regenerative techniques have resulted in advanced implant procedures and an increased predictability to reconstruct alveolar ridge defects.[27,40]

Conventional implant surgery, as described in Chapter 70, is based on adequate bone volume and quality in the desired implant location. The time-tested protocol allows for adequate remodeling and maturation of bone, with healing periods of 4 and 6 months for the mandible and maxilla, respectively. Advanced implant procedures often challenge these original conventions by placing implants in areas with inadequate bone volume, simultaneously augmenting bone and restoring or loading implants after shorter healing periods. This chapter presents an overview of advanced implant surgical and bone augmentation procedures currently used to overcome anatomic deficiencies for the optimal placement of dental implants.

GUIDED BONE REGENERATION

Much of what can be achieved with implant surgery and bone augmentation procedures is directly related to our achievements and understanding of guided bone regeneration. Historically, augmentation or "regeneration" of alveolar bone lost as a result of tooth extraction, resorption, or trauma presented a significant challenge for clinicians. Allowed to heal without the intervention of regenerative procedures, extraction site defects (especially those lacking a self-supporting bone structure) healed with fibrous connective tissue or scar formation and often did not fill with bone. The surrounding soft tissues collapsed, leaving an anatomic deficiency with respect to the natural tooth position. If a removable prosthetic appliance was used, the alveolar ridge resorbed even more.

Periodontal studies during the last several decades have led to new techniques and a new treatment approach referred to as *guided tissue regeneration (GTR).* Briefly, this concept is based on the principle that specific cells contribute to the formation of specific tissues. Exclusion of the faster-growing epithelium and connective tissue from a periodontal wound for a period of 6 to 8 weeks allows the slower growing tissues to occupy the space adjacent to the tooth. Osteoblasts, cementoblasts, and periodontal ligament cells are then afforded the opportunity to regenerate a new periodontal attachment (new bone and new connective tissue fibers inserted into newly formed cementum) on the previously diseased root surface. See Chapter 63 for a complete discussion on the concepts of GTR as it relates to periodontal regeneration.

The same basic principle of GTR has been applied to alveolar bone defects to regenerate new bone.[12] Using a canine model, Schenk and co-workers demonstrated with histology that bone regeneration in membrane-protected defects healed in a sequence of steps that simulated bone formation after tooth extraction.[48] They found that after blood clot formation, bone regeneration was initiated by the formation of woven bone initially along new blood vasculature at the periphery of the defect. The new vascular supply emanated from surgically created perforations in the cortical bone. The woven bone was subsequently replaced by lamellar bone, which resulted in mature bone anatomy. Ultimately, bone remodeling occurred with new secondary osteons being formed. This concept employed the same principles of specific tissue exclusion but was not associated with teeth. Hence the term applied to this technique was *guided bone regeneration (GBR).* Because the objective of GBR is to regenerate a single tissue, namely bone, it is theoretically easier to accomplish than GTR, which strives to regenerate multiple tissues in a complex relationship.

It is interesting to note that long before the current concepts of guided bone regeneration were introduced, Murray and Roschlau demonstrated that when a cavity with a source of osteoblasts and a blood supply was isolated from adjacent soft tissues, it could fill with bone, whereas if the space were not protected, it would fill with fibrous connective tissue.[42] In addition to this observation, they suggested that a bone graft placed in the space might interfere with bone formation because the graft would need to be resorbed before bone could occupy the space.

Bone is a unique tissue that has the capacity to completely regenerate itself. However, due to its rigid calcified structure, bone has specific requirements that must be respected to achieve regeneration. Because the calcified structure of bone is not conducive to perfusion, new bone formation is critically dependent on establishing an adequate blood supply via new vasculature while maintaining rigid fixation or stabilization for bone formation. Any movement of the segments of bone relative to one another (even micromotion) during healing results in disruption of the blood supply and a change in the type of tissue formed in the site from bone to fibrous connective tissue. Table 71-1 lists the biologic requirements for bone regeneration along with the associated component of GBR surgical procedures needed to accomplish bone regeneration.

TABLE 71-1

Requirements for Bone Regeneration

Biologic Requirements	Surgical Procedure
Blood supply	Cortical perforations
Stabilization	Fixation screws, membrane tacks
Osteoblasts	Autogenous bone graft
Confined space	Barrier membrane
Space maintenance	Tenting screws, bone graft materials
Wound coverage	Flap management, tension-free suturing

Barrier Membranes

Barrier membranes are bio-inert materials that serve to protect the blood clot and prevent soft tissue cells (epithelium and connective tissue) from migrating into the bone defect, allowing osteogenic cells to be established. Membranes have been manufactured from biocompatible materials that are nonresorbable and resorbable in nature. The ideal properties of a barrier membrane are 1) biocompatibility, 2) space maintenance, 3) cell-occlusiveness, 4) good handling properties, and 5) resorbability. Advantages and disadvantages of the resorbable versus nonresorbable membranes are described here.

Nonresorbable Barrier Membranes. Various nonresorbable materials have been used as barrier membranes, including latex and teflon. Teflon, an expanded polytetrafluoroethylene membrane (e-PTFE, Gore-Tex Periodontal and Bone Regenerative Membranes, Gore and Associates, Flagstaff, AZ), has been used extensively as a barrier membrane in both GTR and GBR procedures. A variety of shapes and sizes have been designed to custom fit around teeth and osseous defects. These barrier membranes are nonresorbable and thus require a subsequent surgical procedure to remove them. The advantage of a nonresorbable barrier membrane is its ability to maintain separation of tissues over an extended time. Unless the barrier is exposed, it can remain in place for several months to years. Typically, GBR membranes are removed after 6 to 12 months.

The disadvantage of a nonresorbable barrier membrane is that if it becomes exposed, it will not heal spontaneously. Exposed membranes become contaminated with oral bacteria, which may lead to infection of the site and result in bone loss. Hence exposed membranes must be removed. Early removal may also result in less bone regeneration.

Space can be maintained under a barrier membrane with bone graft material or tenting screws, thereby facilitating the regeneration of increased bone volume. Stiffer or titanium-reinforced (TR) membranes (Gore and Associates, Flagstaff, AZ) with space-maintaining capabilities have been demonstrated to regenerate bone without bone grafts or tenting apparatus.[38,49] Stiffer membranes are able to promote significant amounts of new bone and maintain sufficient space without the addition of supportive devices. Ridge augmentation can be enhanced with a titanium-reinforced membrane in conjunction with implant placement in localized bone defects.[23]

Resorbable Barrier Membranes. There has been a recent surge of interest regarding the use of resorbable membranes. Co-polymers of polylactide and polyglycolide (PLA/PGA) or collagen have been used to construct biodegradable membranes. The primary advantage of a resorbable membrane is the elimination of a surgical reentry for a membrane removal. In the case of subsequent implant placement procedure (or exposure surgery), this may not be a significant advantage.

A possible disadvantage is that most resorbable membranes degrade before bone formation is completed and the degradation process is associated with varying degrees of inflammation.[65] Fortunately, the mild inflammatory reaction caused by bioresorbable membranes does not seem to interfere with osteogenesis. Another disadvantage is that resorbable membranes are quite pliable. The lack in stiffness results in a collapse of the membrane into the defect area.[48]

Human histology demonstrating the effectiveness of resorbable membranes is lacking, and further clinical research is needed before conclusions can be made about their use in bone regeneration. At the present time, it can be stated that biodegradable membranes have the potential to support bone formation if they are supported by bone graft material to resist collapse and if they are long-lasting enough to maintain their barrier function for extended periods in small to moderate bone defects.[28,29]

Bone Graft Materials

Unlike other tissues, bone has the unique capacity to regenerate itself completely. The major limiting factor is maintenance of space for bone formation. Bone graft materials have been used to facilitate bone formation within a given space by occupying that space and allowing the subsequent bone growth (and graft replacement) to take place. The biologic mechanisms that support the use of bone graft materials are osteoconduction, osteoinduction, and osteogenesis (Table 71-2).

Osteoconduction is the formation of bone by osteoblasts from the margins of the defect on the bone graft material. Materials that are osteoconductive serve as a scaffold for bone growth. They do not inhibit bone formation, nor do they induce bone formation. They simply allow the normal formation of bone by osteoblasts into the grafted defect along the surface of the graft material. Osteoconductive bone graft materials facilitate bone formation by bridging the gap between the existing bone and a distant location that otherwise would not be occupied by bone.

Osteoinduction involves new bone formation via stimulation of osteoprogenitors from the defect (or from the vasculature) to differentiate into osteoblasts and begin forming new bone. This induction of the bone-forming process by cells that would otherwise remain inactive occurs via cell mediators that "turn on" these bone forming cells. The most widely studied of these is the family of bone morphogenic proteins (BMPs).

Osteogenesis occurs when living osteoblasts are part of the bone graft as in autogenous bone transplantation. Given an adequate blood supply and cellular viability, these transplanted osteoblasts form new centers of ossification within the graft. Hence in addition to the bone formation from osteoblasts that already exist in the defect, osteoblasts that have been added as part of the bone graft also form ossification centers and contribute to the total capacity for bone formation.

Numerous bone graft materials have been used to aid in the reconstruction of bone defects. These range from allografts (derived from the same species) to xenografts (derived from a different species) and alloplast or synthetic graft materials. At a minimum, bone graft materials should be osteoconductive. Bone graft materials that are osteoinductive are believed to be more advantageous than those that are only osteoconductive. Decalcified, freeze-dried bone allograft (DFDBA) is thought to have osteoinductive effects because it retains some of the original BMPs within the donor tissue matrix.[62]

In contrast to this view, several recent reports have suggested that bone augmentation with DFDBA is not osteoinductive because it does not contain the BMPs necessary to induce bone formation.[4,7] Schwartz et al reported that variations in the amount of bone formation induced by DFDBA may be related to the source and processing of the bone.[51] In addition to processing

TABLE 71-2

Biologic Properties of Various Bone Graft Materials (Grouped by Source Type)

	Osteoconductive	Osteoinductive	Osteogenic
Alloplast	Yes	No	No
Xenograft	Yes	No	No
Allograft	Yes	Yes/No	No
Autograft	Yes	Yes	Yes

variations, it has been demonstrated that young donor bone results in significantly greater quantities of BMPs retained in the bone allograft matrix as compared with older donor bone.[52] Hence the source of donor bone can greatly influence its osteoinductive capacity.

Bone graft materials help maintain space under a barrier membrane to facilitate the formation of bone within a confined space. Perhaps a more important requirement of bone graft materials is that they should facilitate the ingrowth of neovascularization and migration of osteoprogenitors. Because the size of the bone graft particles determine the resultant space available (between particles) for osseous formation, it has been carefully selected according to this concept. The typical size of bone graft particles ranges from 100 to 1000 μm, which is conducive to the ingrowth of bone. Bone forms in cones called *osteons* with a central blood supply. The dimension of these cones (100μ radius) is determined by the distance that the central vasculature can supply nutrients to cells.

Autogenous Bone Harvesting

As compared with other bone graft materials, autogenous bone is thought to be the best bone graft as it is osteoinductive and osteogenic in addition to being osteoconductive. Intraoral sources of autogenous bone include edentulous spaces, maxillary tuberosity, mandibular ramus, mandibular symphysis, and extraction sites. Bone from a recent extraction site (within 6 to 12 weeks) may have the advantage of increased osteogenic activity as compared with other sites, which are more static and undergoing little or no osteogenesis. The maxillary tuberosity provides a more cellular source of autogenous bone as compared with other sites. However, the trabecular nature of this site provides a lesser quantity of mineralized matrix and the resultant total volume of bone available for grafting is often inadequate. For greater amounts of bone, it is more desirable to harvest bone from the mandibular ramus or symphysis. This bone, which is typically more cortical, can be harvested and used as a block graft or ground or shaved into small fragments and used as a particulate graft.

Despite the fact that the mandibular ramus and symphysis offer good sources of bone for grafting, clinicians are sometimes reluctant to harvest bone from these sites due to an increased risk of morbidity from the surgical procedure. Risks of surgery in the mandibular symphysis region include postoperative bleeding, bruising, wound dehiscence, damage to lower incisors, disfigurement, and injury to nerves. Nerve injury is perhaps the most significant concern because it has the potential to be a long-term, annoying alteration in sensation of the lower lip, chin, anterior teeth, and gingiva for the patient. A more serious risk is the alteration of facial appearance. This is a particular risk when the facial muscles are completely elevated from the bone beyond the inferior border of the mandible. A condition referred to as "witch's chin" can occur when the facial muscles and overlying skin of the chin fall, causing a disfiguring sag of facial tissues after surgery.

Hunt and Jovanovic[17] presented a retrospective analysis of 48 chin graft harvesting procedures. They emphasized maintaining a 5-mm margin of safety between graft harvest sites and the lower incisors, the inferior border of the chin, and the mental foramen. Using both trephine and custom block harvesting techniques, they reported minimal postoperative complications. In the 48 procedures, postoperative sequelae included bruising of lower face (48/48), bruising of upper neck (6/48), paresthesia of lower lip and incisors (6/48). No patients (0/48) experienced facial disfigurement or muscle prolapse (chin droop). Three of the six patients with paresthesia experienced transient symptoms and recovered completely within 2 months, whereas symptoms persisted longer than 6 months in the other 3 patients. Not surprisingly, the larger harvest defects (trephined 6-rings) resulted in a higher incidence of paresthesia, which was longer lasting than that of the smaller defects (trephined 4-rings). Harvesting bone in a custom-shaped "block" did not result in paresthesia, presumably because these harvest sites were smaller than the 4-ring and 6-ring trephine-harvested sites.

Observation of the following basic principles can minimize the risk of postoperative morbidity:

1. Carefully evaluate the harvest site for potential risks. A critical radiographic evaluation prior to surgery can identify individuals with inferior alveolar nerve branches that extend anterior beyond the mental foramen.
2. Use extreme care in making incisions laterally toward the mental nerve, and dissect the area with blunt instruments to locate the foramen.
3. Do not elevate and reflect muscle attachments beyond the inferior border of the mandible.
4. Limit bone cuts to an area at least 5 mm away from the tooth apices, the inferior border of the mandible, and the mental foramen. Do not extend cuts or harvest bone deeper than 6 mm, and do not include both labial and lingual cortical plates.
5. Suture the wound in layers (muscle and overlying mucosa separately) to prevent postoperative wound separation.

Whenever harvesting autogenous bone, regardless of site or method used, it is important to use techniques that prevent overheating and maintain viability of the bone cells. Exceeding 47° C (116.6° F) is known to cause bone necrosis. Thus use of drills, trephines, or saws to cut bone should always be done with profuse irrigation to keep instruments and bone cooled.

Flap Management for Ridge Augmentation

Soft tissue management is a critical aspect of bone augmentation procedures. Incisions, reflection, and manipulation should be designed to optimize blood supply and wound closure. The design and management of mucoperiosteal flaps must consider the increased dimensions of the ridge after augmentation as well as esthetics and approximation of the wound margins. The surgical procedure needs to be executed with utmost care to preserve the maximum vascularity to the flap and minimize tissue injury.[1]

Several flap techniques maintain a submerged position of bone grafts and barrier membranes during the entire healing process, including a remote or displaced incision.[8,25] The advantage of a remote incision is that the wound opening is positioned away from the graft. A conventional crestal incision can be used, even in large supracrestal defects, as long as periosteal releasing incision and coronal advancement of the flap achieve the tension free closure.[31,58] Most reports suggest removing sutures approximately 10 to 14 days after surgery. It is also suggested that no prosthesis be inserted for 2 to 3 weeks after surgery to avoid pressure over the wound during the early healing period.

General concepts for flap management associated with ridge augmentation include the following:

1. Whenever possible, it is desirable to make incisions remote relative to the placement of barrier membranes (e.g., vertical releasing incisions at least one tooth away from the site to be grafted). In the anterior maxilla, keeping vertical incisions remote is also an esthetic advantage.
2. Full mucoperiosteal flap elevation at least 5 mm beyond the edge of the bone defect is desirable.
3. The use of vertical incisions, although often required for surgical access, should be minimized whenever possible.
4. Use of periosteal releasing incision to give the flap elasticity and permit tension-free suturing is essential. This permits complete closure without stress on the wound margins.
5. Avoid postoperative trauma to the surgical site (i.e., no removable appliance should be inserted over the wound for a postoperative period of 2 weeks or more).
6. Wound closure should incorporate a combination of mattress sutures to approximate connective tissues and interrupted sutures to adapt wound edges.

LOCALIZED RIDGE AUGMENTATION

Patients often present for implant planning after tooth loss and alveolar ridge resorption. In these cases, the clinician is obligated to perform advanced augmentation procedures to reconstruct lost bone and place implants in a prosthetically driven position.

Surgical reconstructive procedures for the preparation and placement of dental implants have become more numerous and complex. Depending on the size and morphology of the defect, various augmentation procedures can be used. These procedures have been categorized according to the deficient dimension (i.e., horizontal or vertical). Methods used to augment horizontal as well as vertical bone deficiencies include particulate bone grafts and monocortical block grafts. Barrier membranes can be used along with bone grafts to reconstruct all types of alveolar bone defects. Recently, distraction osteogenesis has been described to regain bone in a vertical direction.

All the proven principles of guided bone regeneration and flap management must be followed to achieve good results. These include generating a blood supply; maintaining a stable, protected space for bone growth; and achieving tension-free flap closure.

Horizontal Bone Augmentation

A deficiency in the horizontal dimension of bone may be minimal, such as a dehiscence or fenestration of an implant surface, or it may be more significant such that the implant would have more than one axial surface exposed while having some bone along the entire vertical length. Dehiscence defects can usually be managed simultaneously with implant placement because most of the implant is covered and stabilized by native bone. If the horizontal deficiency is large and the implant placement would result in significant exposure, it may be better to reconstruct the bone prior to implant placement (staged implant placement).

Although reconstruction of deficient ridges with bone grafts alone (i.e., without barrier membrane) has proved to be effective, variable resorption of the grafted bone has been reported. Preliminary results in a 1- to 3-year study using autografts harvested from the maxillary tuberosity showed an increased ridge width, but resorption of 50% of the graft volume was also noted.[59]

Buser[8] investigated the lateral ridge augmentation procedure using an autograft from the retromolar or symphysis area covered by a membrane in 40 consecutively treated patients and showed that no clinical signs of resorption of the block graft were observed. Emphasis was given to a remote incision technique, perforation of the cortex, stable placement of corticocancellous autografts, precise adaptation and stabilization (with miniscrews) of the e-PTFE membranes, and a tension-free primary soft tissue closure. After 7 to 13 months, the sites were reopened for membrane removal and implant placement. Approximately 38 of 40 patients exhibited excellent ridge augmentation, with two sites showing some soft tissue encapsulation of the grafted bone.

Nevins[44] and Doblin[13] demonstrated case report results that the use of freeze-dried bone allografts with membranes increased the amount of new bone, even in the presence of a membrane exposure. The biopsies showed viable bone cells and visible osteocytes in lacunae, and a 9-month specimen showed no remainder of allograft material. On the other hand, there are some contradictory results using DFDBA and membrane combinations.[2,6,7]

Particulate Bone Graft. Advantages of particulate bone grafts (or bone chips) are that the smaller pieces of bone demonstrate more rapid ingrowth of blood vessels (revascularization), larger osteoconduction surface, more exposure of osteoconductive growth factors, and easier biologic remodeling when compared with a bone block. However, particulate grafts often lack a rigid structure and are easier displaced then block grafts.

Harvesting autologous particulated bone grafts can be performed from any edentulous jaw site, either in smaller particle sizes or in larger block size. If the bone has been harvested in block size, a bone mill is necessary to particulate the bone and prepare the bone to be transplanted into the bone defect.

Particulate grafts are indicated in defects with multiple osseous walls or single bone walls and when implants are placed simultaneously with the bone augmentation procedure. If a bone defect does not have sufficient osseous walls to contain the graft and if an implant is placed simultaneously, a barrier membrane is secured along the periphery with tacks or screws. This bone graft–implant–membrane combination becomes an environment that is stable and supports bone formation.

Monocortical Block Graft. Horizontal alveolar deficiencies can easily be reconstructed with a monocortical block bone graft. The technique uses a cortical block of bone harvested from a remote site and used to increase the width of bone. The block graft taken from an intraoral (e.g., mandibular symphysis or ramus) or extraoral (e.g., iliac crest or tibia) site is fixated to the prepared recipient site with screws. The graft can be separated from overlying soft tissues with a barrier membrane or simply covered with the mucoperiosteal flap. Fixation hardware (i.e., screws and plates) should be removed after an adequate period of healing (approximately 6 months). The disadvantage of this technique is the biologic limitation of revascularizing large bone blocks. It therefore is crucial to have sufficient osteogenic cells in the residual surface of the surrounding bone and to limit this technique to horizontal augmentation and only minimal vertical defects.

Fig. 71-1 shows the use of a monocortical block graft to reconstruct a horizontal deficiency in the posterior right mandible. The patient presented with a loss of the buccal cortical plate of bone after a traumatic extraction of endodontically treated tooth #29. The surgical extraction also resulted in a nonrestorable cut into the mesial root of tooth #30. Recommended treatment included extraction of tooth #30 with monocortical block graft to reconstruct the buccal defect of site #29.

PROCEDURE. After local anesthesia, an incision was made in keratinized tissue along the crest and around the molar tooth (#30) with a vertical releasing incision mesial to the first bicuspid (#28). A full-thickness flap was elevated to expose the alveolar bone. All soft tissues were thoroughly removed from the recipient site prior to bone grafting. After simple forceps delivery of tooth #30, the defect to be grafted was measured to determine the size of block graft to harvest from the mandibular symphysis. Several bleeding points were created using a small round bur.

The autogenous monocortical block graft was harvested from the mandibular symphysis (see Autogenous Bone Harvesting). It was cut to an appropriate size and mortised to intimately fit the recipient site (defect). Once properly positioned, the graft was fixated with two fixation screws (Leibinger, Kalamazoo, MI) that passed through the graft and into the remaining native alveolar bone. A periosteal releasing incision was used to sever the periosteum from anterior to posterior and facilitate coronal advancement of the mucogingival flap.

After 6 months of healing, a full-thickness mucoperiosteal flap was elevated to expose the alveolar bone sites #29 and 30. Minimal resorption of the monocortical block graft is evident. Notice the position of the head of the fixation screws (especially the posterior screw), which are more protruded than the bone (see Fig. 71-1, *H, I*).

The fixation screws are removed and the sites are prepared in the usual manner for the placement of two screw-type, wide-diameter implants (Implant Innovations, Inc., Palm Beach Gardens, FL). Care is taken to avoid preparing the grafted site too wide or too far labially because the grafted bone may be vulnerable to fracture or resorption (see Fig. 71-1, *J*).

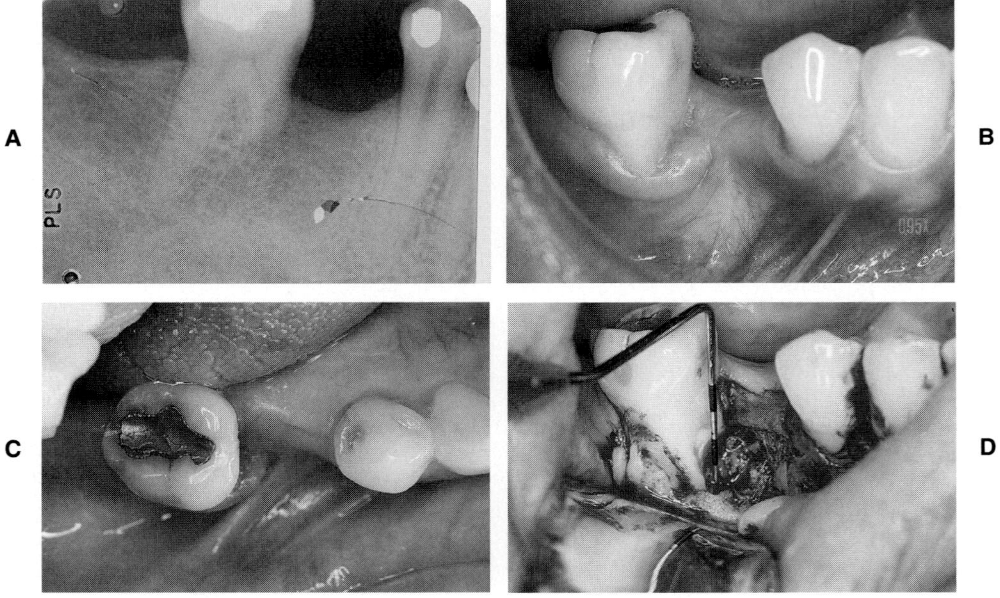

Fig. 71-1 The use of a monocortical block graft to reconstruct a horizontal deficiency in the posterior right mandible. **A,** Periapical radiograph shows missing tooth #29 and severed mesial root #30. **B and C,** Labial and occlusal views, respectively, of site reveals deficient alveolar ridge buccal side of #29. **D,** Full-thickness flap reflection reveals the extent of missing bone in the buccal aspect of site #29 as well as the periodontal defect and damaged mesial root #30. *Continued*

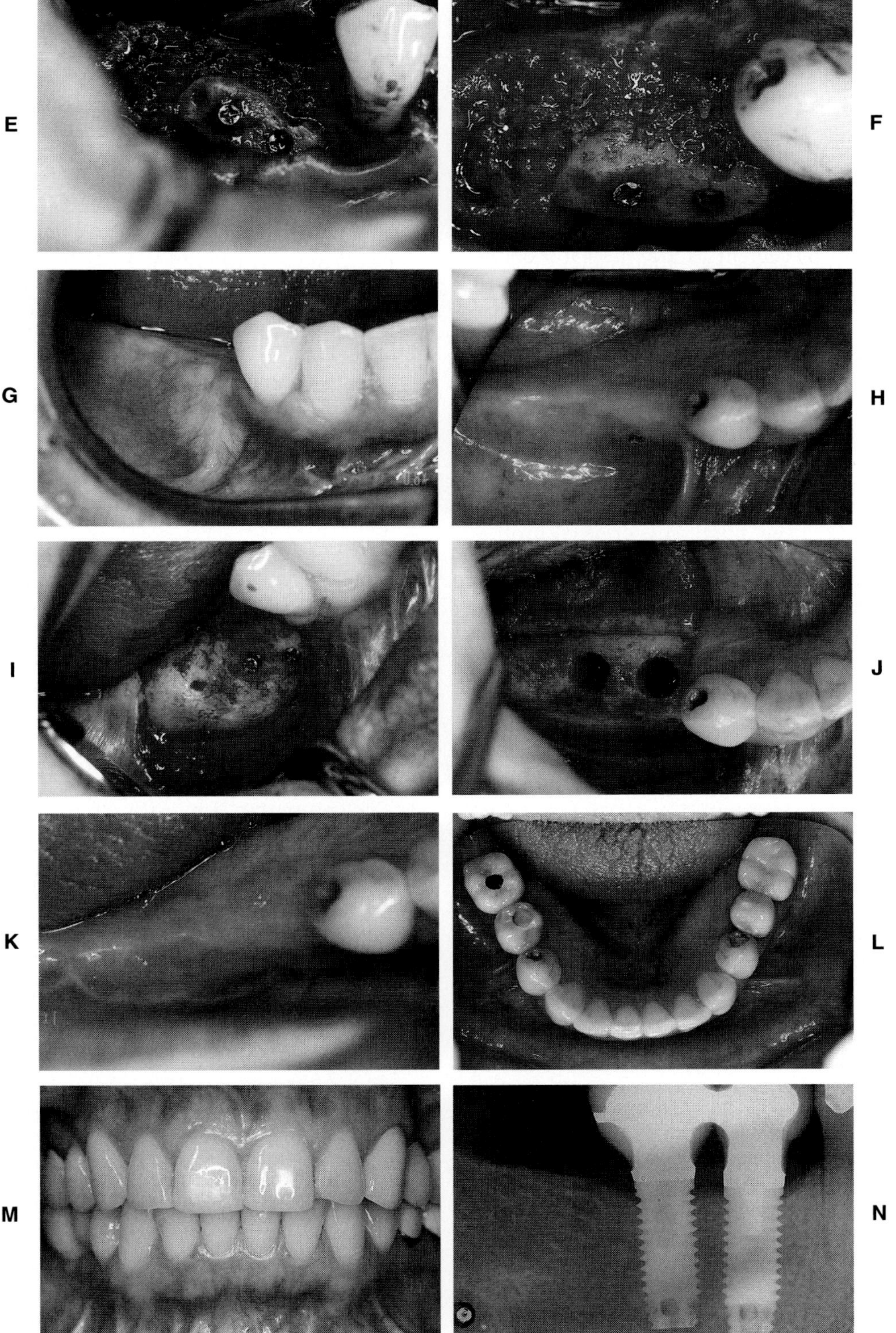

Fig. 71-1, cont'd The use of a monocortical block graft to reconstruct a horizontal deficiency in the posterior right mandible. **E and F,** Autogenous monocortical bone block graft secured to native alveolar bone with fixation screws. **G,** Good tissue healing after block graft with evidence of a widened alveolar ridge. **H,** After 6 months of healing, the posterior fixation screw is observed protruding through the mucosa. **I,** Full-thickness flap reveals that bone resorption has resulted in exposure of part of the fixation screw. **J,** Osteotomy prepared for wide-diameter implants, taking care to avoid making the labial bone "graft" too thin. **K,** Complete closure and good healing of wound after implant placement. **L and M,** Clinical photos of completed restorations. **N,** Final radiograph shows good restoration contours on wide-diameter implants.

SIMULTANEOUS IMPLANT PLACEMENT AND GUIDED BONE REGENERATION

Large alveolar bone defects need to be augmented prior to implant placement and require a healing period of 6 months or longer. In selected cases, it is possible to perform a bone augmentation procedure simultaneously with the implant placement. It is essential to achieve good implant stability in the existing native bone so that endosseous integration can occur.

A very predictable osseous defect to manage with simultaneous implant placement is the implant dehiscence or fenestration defect. Fenestrations are exposures of the implant's axial surface that do not include the coronal aspect of the implant. Dehiscence defects are those that expose a part of the axial surface including the coronal aspect of the implant while maintaining sufficient bone volume around all remaining implant surfaces. In a dehiscence defect, the implant remains within the confines of the existing bone.

Fenestration and dehiscence defects have been managed with barrier membranes or simply with flap closure. Bone grafts have also been used. The only controlled comparison studies between a membrane treatment and a periosteal flap coverage of exposed implant surfaces in humans demonstrated that the membrane treatment was far superior with regard to bone fill.[10] Another controlled study in humans evidenced better results in the membrane groups; 4 of 6 sites treated with a membrane resulted in 95% to 100% elimination of the dehiscence and total coverage of the threads. In the control sites, only 2 out of 6 sites showed moderate to complete bone fill.[45] All other clinical studies are in the form of case report studies.[40] Fig. 71-2, *M* demonstrates coverage of an implant dehiscence using a barrier membrane. Admittedly, without a biopsy, it cannot be determined whether the tissue covering the implant is bone or firm connective tissue.[25,26]

A 1-year multicenter study evaluating 55 dehisced implants in 45 patients, treated by membrane alone, demonstrated an average bone fill of 82%.[11] The average initial defect size was 4.6 mm. The 1-year follow-up of these implants demonstrated a favorable response to loading. Of the 55 implants a total of 6 failed, corresponding to a cumulative survival rate of 84.7% in the maxilla and 95% in the mandible, which is similar to previously published results.

A clinical report on the use of titanium-reinforced (TR) membranes demonstrated the biologic potential to fill a large protected space in 4 patients. The dehisced implant sites ranged from 5 to 12 mm (mean 8.2 mm). They were covered with a TR membrane alone. Reentry after 7 to 8 months of submerged healing found complete bone coverage of the implants. Radiographic evaluation demonstrated the implants functioning with normal crestal bone support after 1 year.[23]

No clinical comparisons are available in the literature evaluating the placement of bone grafts with or without membranes on dehisced implant surfaces. Most evidence supports the use of graft materials in conjunction with membrane treatment, especially the use of freeze-dried bone allografts (FDBA) in conjunction with GBR. In a study with 40 patients, 110 implants were placed in conjunction with barrier membranes and FDBA grafts; a success rate of 96.8% was achieved with complete bone fill (defined as >90% fill of dehiscence). This study reported an exposure rate of 29% of the membranes, but little effect on the bone regeneration was noted.[47]

Another study evaluated the treatment of dehiscence type bone defects associated with the placement of implants into fresh extraction sockets.[30] Augmentation procedures were conducted with demineralized FDBA particles and e-PTFE membranes. Complete flap closure resulted in complete bone regeneration. Histologic evaluation revealed remnants of the graft material and large areas of vital bone tissue as evidenced by distinct osteocytes. Both woven bone and lamellar bone were observed in direct contact with graft particles. In a 1-year postgrafting biopsy, DFDB particles were still present and osteoblasts were observed engaged in bone formation. Fig. 71-2, *L, M* demonstrates a simultaneous GBR and implant placement in a dehiscence defect.

Supracrestal/Vertical Bone Augmentation

Supracrestal or vertical bone augmentation (Fig. 71-3) presents the greatest challenge in terms of regenerating bone for implant placement. The available evidence related to GBR–associated and supracrestal implant placement is limited.

Some published studies have evaluated the effect of space creation by a membrane alone or with an autograft. In one clinical study, 5 patients were treated with a supracrestal exposure of 3 to 7 mm (average of 4.67 mm) and showed a clinical bone gain of 0.5 to 4 mm (average of 2.97 mm) after 9 months.[58] The second study evaluated the treatment of an average supracrestal implant exposure of 2.7 mm in a dog study and resulted in a histometric supracrestal bone gain of 0.9 to 4.0 mm with good bone-to-implant contact.[24] The space underneath the membranes in the two studies was filled with new bone 64% and 70%, respectively.

Another experimental dog study evaluated implants with supracrestal implant dehiscence. The membrane resulted in 83% of the defect fill with new bone and a higher interface contact than other graft treatments with or without membrane. The incorporation of bone grafts covered by membranes demonstrated that graft sites without membranes around implants tended to be less well preserved then membrane-covered sites. The membrane treatment preserved the bone graft volume by 70% or greater. The membrane also helped increase bone-implant contact of the incorporated bone graft.[10] All three studies showed that supracrestal bone formation up to 3 mm is predictable using the GBR technique with a membrane–blood clot combination.

Simion[58] and Jovanovic[24] used a titanium reinforced membrane for vertical bone regeneration around dental implants. No supportive bone substrates were used, except a careful fill of space with a blood clot by perforating the bone surface or injecting it with venous blood. Although the ridge defects varied—one had a wide resorbed bone base and the other a narrow resorbed bone base—significant supracrestal bone regeneration was evident in both studies. The variation in supracrestal bone regeneration achieved (3.3 mm versus 1.82 mm) in these studies might be explained by the difference in residual bone base at the beginning of the study and the difference in method used to evaluate the results (clinical versus histomorphometric). Recent studies showed that supracrestal bone formation is more predictable using a TR membrane and bone graft filler material. Therefore at present, an advanced surgical reconstruction technique for vertical bone gain is always combined with an autograft material and a nonresorbable TR membrane. (See Fig. 71-3, *A–G*). A recent 5-year clinical study has demonstrated that vertically augmented bone can be maintained with loaded implant restoration.[57]

Distraction Osteogenesis

This surgical technique has been developed to increase vertical bone height in the deficient jaw site and is in contrast to the more conventional method of bone grafting with or without membranes. Under the proper circumstances, most cells in bone can differentiate into osteogenic or chondrogenic cells needed for repair. The process of generating new bone by stretching, referred to as *distraction osteogenesis,* was introduced by Ilizarov.[18,19]

Based on experimental and clinical studies over 35 years, distraction osteogenesis can provide a surgeon with the possibility of treating extremities, small bones in hands and feet using external fixation devices. Recently, new intraoral devices for vertical bone growth of the alveolar process have been developed and successfully applied before dental implant placement. Other important advantages of distraction osteogenesis are that no second surgical site is needed to harvest bone and the newly created bone has native bone at the crest, which can withstand forces better than fully regenerated bone.

The application for vertical bone augmentation has shown a broad use in the preprosthetic surgical indication with good predictability, although limitations have been encountered to develop horizontal bone growth with this method. A frequent need for secondary bone grafting is seen in the extremely resorbed jaw.

MANAGEMENT OF EXTRACTIONS

Because tooth extraction (or tooth loss) often results in alveolar ridge resorption or collapse, preservation of bone volume at the time of extraction is a desirable goal. A majority of the bone loss after extraction occurs within the first 6 to 24 months.[9] Therefore when clinicians are afforded the opportunity to intervene at the time of extraction, the preservation of alveolar bone should be initiated. A conservative approach to the management of extraction sites can eliminate or significantly reduce the necessity of advanced bone augmentation procedures.

When extracting a tooth and preparing for implant placement, it is highly desirable to prevent alveolar bone resorption. Experimental animal studies have shown that the use of a barrier membrane enhances the predictability of bone fill in the extraction site and therefore maintains original bone volume when compared with mucoperiosteal flap coverage alone.[6] Clinical studies have also demonstrated the benefits of a regenerative approach to tooth extraction.[35,36,43] These authors found that a nonresorbable barrier membrane resulted in minimal resorption of alveolar ridge size and shape.

Although earlier studies have proposed the concept of treating extraction sites without flap closure (i.e., an exposed membrane used to cover the graft), recent studies concluded that complete wound closure over the physical barrier might be associated with greater bone fill.[5,55]

The timing of implant placement relative to the time of extraction has been debated by many clinicians. Depending on the quantity, quality, and support of existing bone as well as the preferences of the clinician and patient, the placement of implants after tooth extraction can be immediate, delayed, or staged. By definition, immediate implant placement occurs at the time of extraction. Delayed implant placement is performed approximately 2 months postextraction to allow for soft tissue healing. Staged implant placement allows for substantial bone healing within the extraction site that typically requires 4 to 6 months or longer.

Immediate Implant Placement

The primary advantage of immediate implant placement is the reduction of the healing time.[34,41,50,63] Because the implant is placed at the time of extraction, the bone-to-implant healing begins immediately with extraction site healing. Another advantage is that the normal bone healing, which generally occurs within the extraction site, takes effect around the implant. This bone-forming activity may enhance the bone-to-implant contact as compared with an implant placed in a less osteogenically active site. Possible disadvantages of immediate implant placement include the need for mucogingival surgeries and bone grafting around the implant.

When a two-stage implant is placed at the time of tooth extraction, the mucogingival flap must be advanced to completely cover the implant (exception = one-stage implants). It may also be necessary to graft bone into the extraction site in areas that do not contact the implant to avoid soft tissue invasion around the implant.[50] A 1-year study of 49 immediate extraction site implants treated by a membrane alone demonstrated a 93.6% bone fill. After 1 year (postloading), the implant success rate was 93.9%.[5]

The placement of 21 transmucosal implants in immediate extraction sites treated with a barrier membrane were tested for the implant success rate and the bone fill. Of 21 transmucosal implants, 20 yielded complete bone fill and coverage of the entire plasma-coated implant surface.[32] More clinical review is needed before it can be suggested to treat more advanced bone defects with transmucosal implants. Until then, submerging implants is preferred.[22]

A clinical report on the use of resorbable collagen membranes around extraction site implants demonstrated a variable degree of bone fill in 9 patients.[46] More clinical review of the use of resorbable membranes for GBR is required because evidence is insufficient to properly evaluate the predictability.

Text continued on p. 917

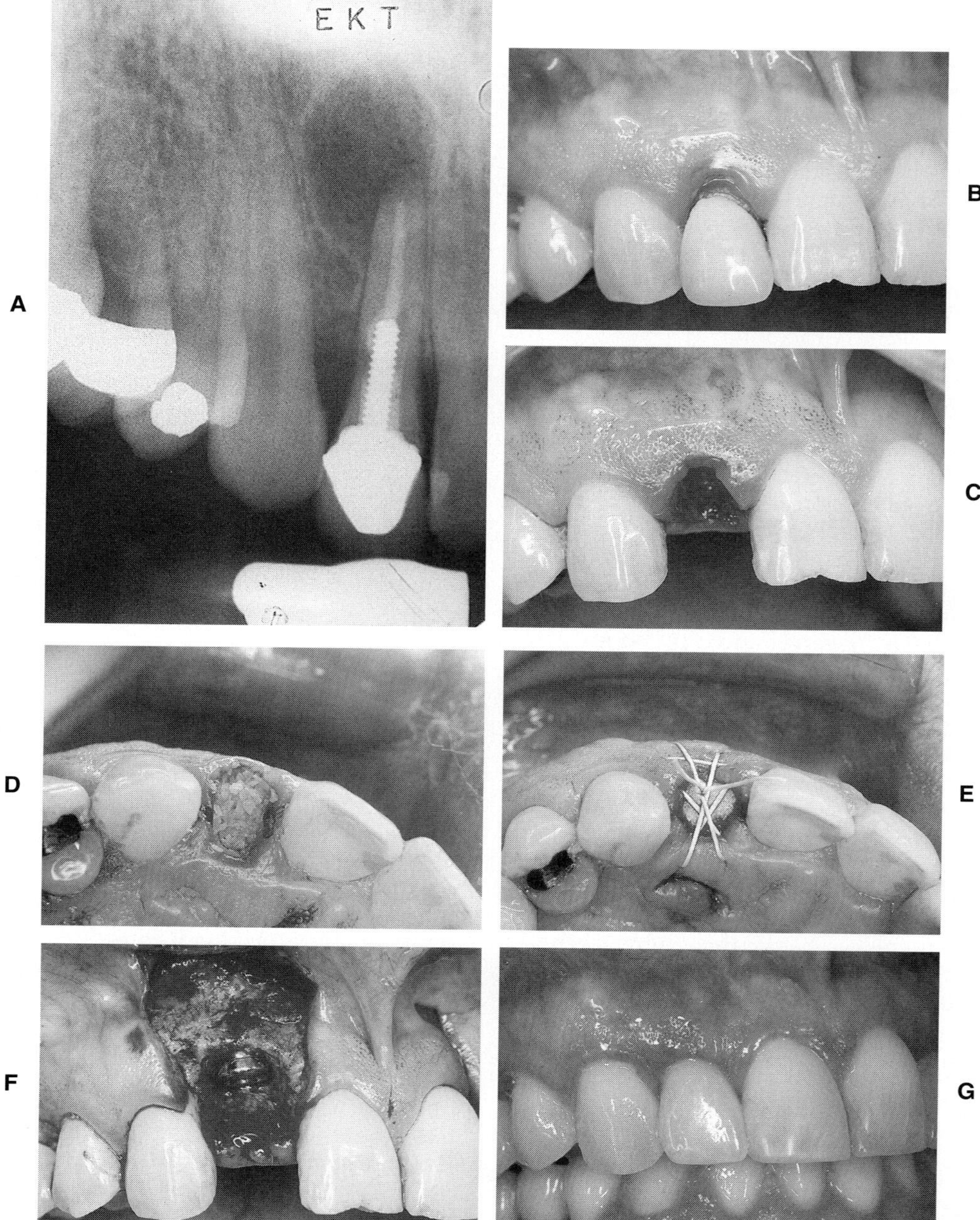

Fig. 71-2 The use of a staged **(A–H)** and delayed **(I–O)** implant placement after extraction of two maxillary lateral incisors in one individual. **A,** Periapical radiograph of tooth #7 with a large radiolucent lesion around the apex and periodontal bone loss along the distal interproximal area. **B,** Preoperative photograph of tooth #7 with gingival recession and marginal inflammation. **C,** Atraumatic extraction #7 without tissue incision or tissue elevation. Palpation reveals no facial bone present at the time of extraction. **D,** DFDB allograft condensed into extraction site. **E,** e-PTFE barrier membrane positioned over graft and held in place with sutures. **F,** Six months after the extraction/graft, the implant is placed. Notice the implant is completely covered with bone. **G,** Final restoration. **H,** Final radiograph of delayed implant placement. **I,** Periapical radiograph of tooth #10. **J,** Preoperative photograph of tooth #10 with exposed gingival margin. **K,** Atraumatic extraction #10 without tissue incision or tissue elevation. Palpation reveals no facial bone present and a dehiscence is expected. **L,** Two months after extraction, the implant is placed with dehiscence defect. **M,** Guided bone regeneration accomplished with e-PTFE barrier membrane positioned over the dehiscence. **N,** Final restoration. **O,** Final radiograph. (**A, B, C, F, G, J, M, N, and O,** From Klokkevold PR, Han TJ, Camargo PM: Aesthetic management of extractions for implant site development: Delayed versus staged implant placement. Pract Perio Aesthet Dent 1999; 11(5):603.)

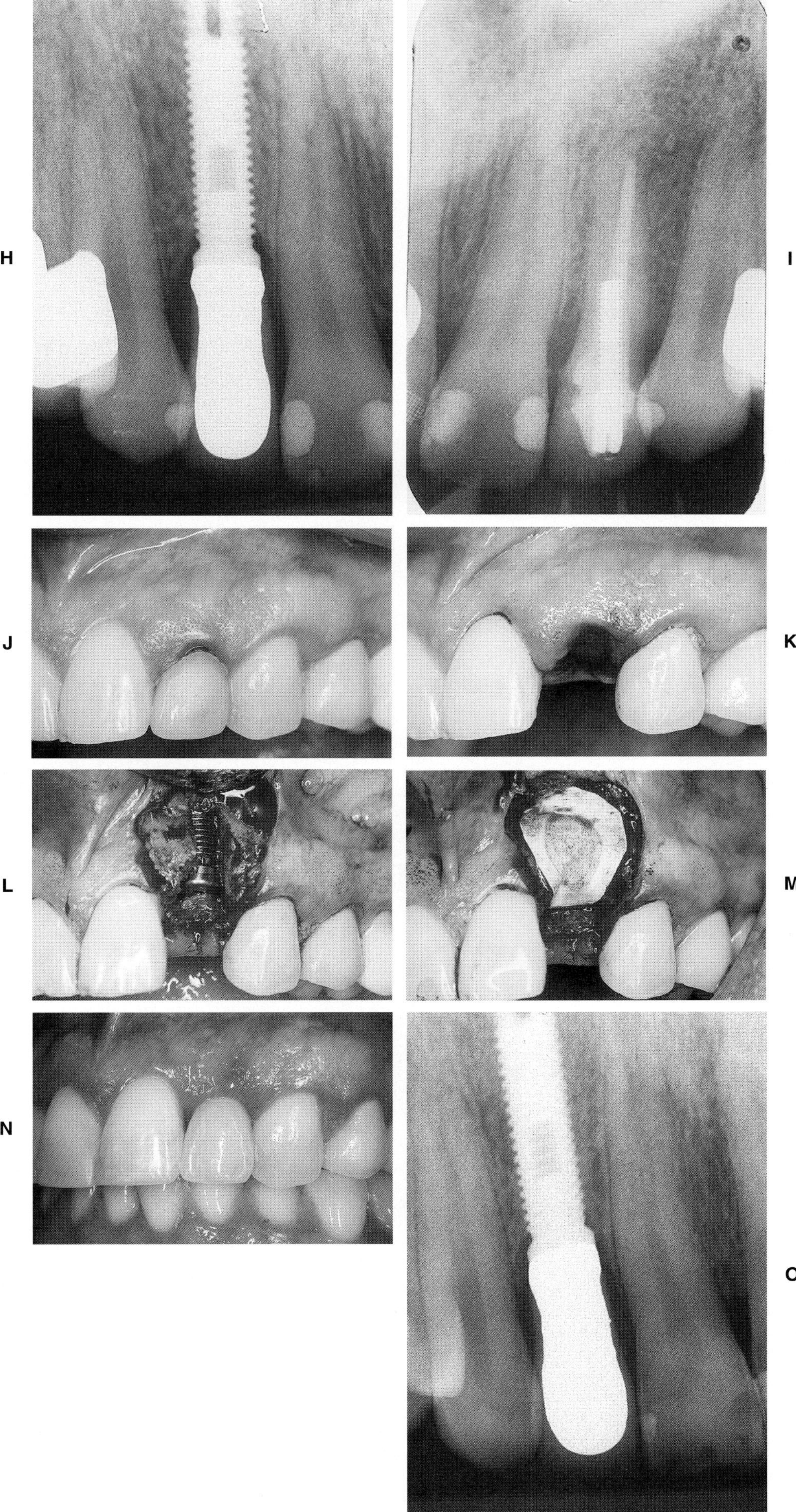
H
I
J
K
L
M
N
O

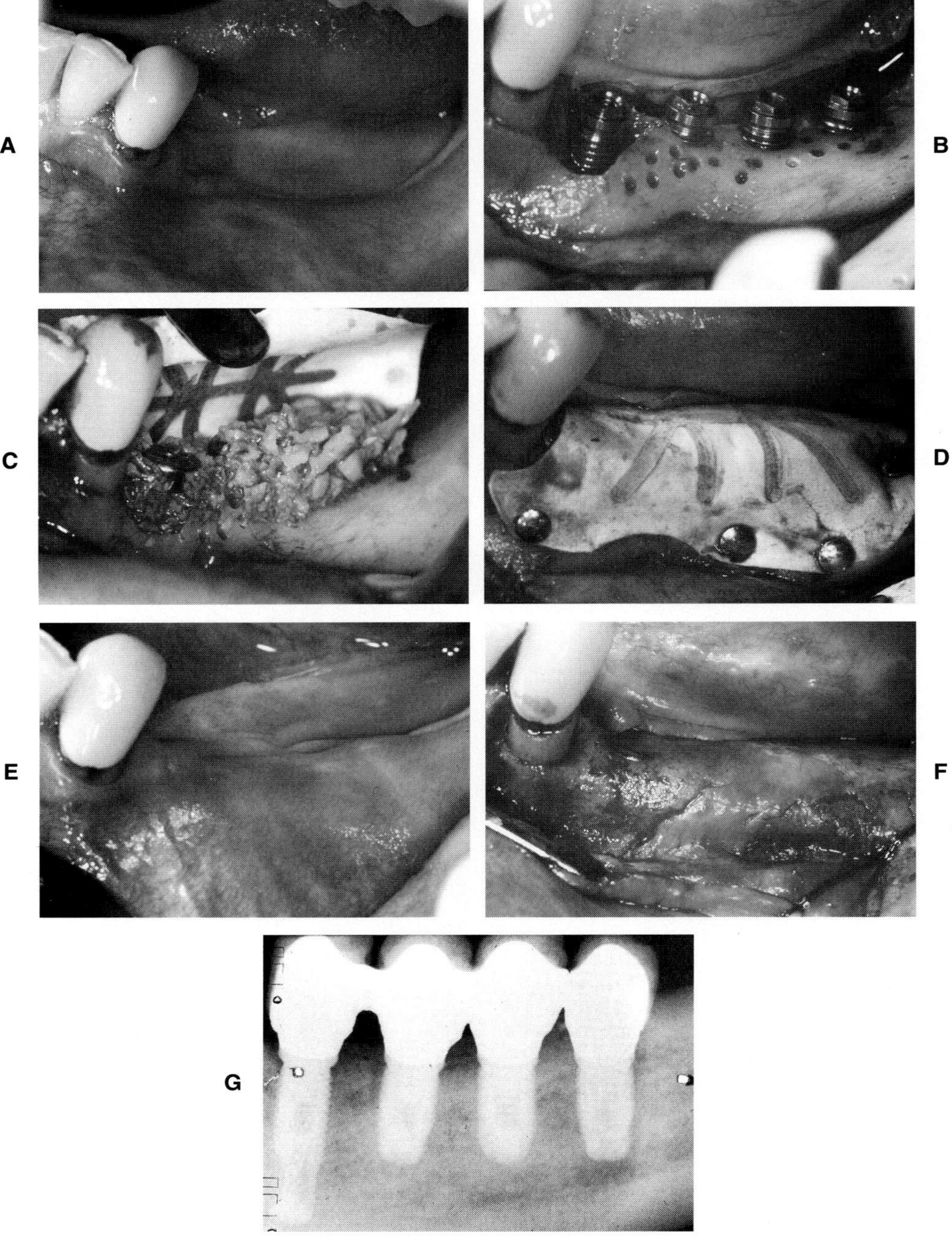

Fig. 71-3 Vertical bone augmentation. **A,** Partially edentulous patient with a vertically resorbed posterior mandible, with 5 mm from the mandibular canal to the bone crest. Note the normal periodontal level around the anterior teeth. **B,** After full-thickness flap elevation and implant placement, a supracrestal position of 2 to 4 mm was achieved. The most anterior implant was 15 mm in length (mesial to the mental foramen) and the three posterior implants were 8.5 mm. Note the perforations in the cortical bone to open the marrow spaces and allow for blood supply. **C,** After an autogenous bone graft was harvested from the ramus and particulated, a nonresorbable, titanium-reinforced e-PTFE membrane (TR-9Y) was trimmed and fixated with two pins on the lingual to act as an envelope for the bone graft. **D,** The membrane was closed on the buccal and fixated with four pins. Note the safety margin between the membrane and the tooth and the mental foramen of a minimum of 2 mm. **E,** Closure of the surgical site by periosteal release of the buccal and lingual flap. After advancement of the buccal flap and the lingual floor of the mouth, tension-free closure was achieved with a horizontal mattress and interrupted sutures. During an uneventful healing of 7 months, no prostheses was inserted. **F,** After full-thickness flap elevation and membrane removal, a vertical and horizontal bone gain of more than 5 mm was evident. Note that the vertical augmentation procedure with guided bone regeneration achieved vertical and horizontal bone reconstruction around the previously exposed implant surfaces. **G,** Radiograph after 1 year of loading shows normal maintenance of bone structures around the implants.

If inadequate bone exists to stabilize the implant, immediate implant placement is not recommended. Finally, there is potential for preexisting infections associated with the tooth to adversely affect the healing and implant success. Acute or subacute infection is a contraindication to immediate implant placement.

In a study of 30 patients, the use of autografts alone in 54 simultaneous extraction site implants was highly effective for implants placed completely within the envelope of bone. The study showed that extraction sites, including those with a buccal dehiscence, could be treated with autografts alone. Because ungrafted sites were not evaluated, the absolute need to graft small defects adjacent to implants was not ascertained by this study.[3] In another study, implants placed in extraction sockets were tested for their potential to regenerate bone with allograft alone, a membrane alone, and a combination treatment. Reentry confirmed 100% thread coverage in all but one implant in the no-wall group treated with DFDB alone.[15]

A clinical study of 5 patients evaluated different treatment modalities for extraction site implants together with bone graft combinations. It was demonstrated that non-spacemaking defects are best treated with a combination of a barrier membrane with an autograft or allograft and achieve better results than a nonreinforced membrane without graft.[56]

Delayed Implant Placement

A delayed implant placement shares some of the advantages afforded by immediate implant placement, namely extraction site preservation, and offers some additional advantages. Unlike immediate implant placement, which is deficient of soft tissue for coverage, the delayed implant placement technique allows time for soft tissue healing.[22] The delayed placement technique still reduces the length of treatment time by several months because it is not necessary to wait for complete bone healing. Furthermore, because bone formation is active within the first few months after tooth extraction, the delayed technique may facilitate more osteogenesis adjacent to the implant. The primary advantage of delayed implant placement is that by allowing for soft tissue healing and closure of the extraction site, mucogingival flap advancement is not necessary. This alleviates the need for additional surgeries to correct mucogingival discrepancies. Delayed implant placement also allows time for resolution of infections that may have been present within the extraction site. As with immediate implant placement, similar limitations of bone support and implant stability exist. The normal osseous healing that occurs within the first 2 months does not significantly affect the anatomy of the alveolar ridge. Hence limitations in bone support after 2 months of healing are similar to those that exist at the time of extraction.

Staged Implant Placement

A staged implant placement allows adequate time for osseous healing. This may be complete osseous healing of an extraction site without a bone graft (if circumferential bone support is good) or with a bone graft. Staged implant placement, by definition, allows for complete hard and soft tissue healing and permits the placement of implants into prosthetically driven positions with adequate coverage by hard and soft tissues.[53] This eliminates the necessity of mucogingival flap advancement, allows for the resolution of preexisting infections, and prevents soft tissue invasion. Furthermore, by using an extended healing period, the grafted bone also has the opportunity to become vascularized. Bone grafts performed simultaneously with implant placement do not share this advantage. The primary disadvantage of staged implant placement is the length of time required for bone healing.

Surgical Technique. Delayed and staged implant placement techniques are demonstrated in one individual using two extraction sites with similar bone morphologies in the anterior maxilla (see Fig. 71-2). Both techniques facilitate the esthetic placement of implants into prosthetically driven positions. They maintain alveolar bone volume, reduce the need for advanced bone augmentation and eliminate the need for subsequent mucogingival surgery. The timing and management of delayed versus staged implant placement techniques vary as described in the following section.

To decide which implant placement method to use, the quantity and location of bone surrounding the tooth should be assessed. Once the patient has been anesthetized, a periodontal probe can be used to "sound" for the level of bone support through the soft tissue. Using this method, the bone levels surrounding the tooth can be mapped. Bone support that surrounds the extraction site can also be evaluated and confirmed after tooth removal by palpation, probing, and direct (internal) visualization.

If the tooth to be extracted has sufficient bone support on all surfaces, then the extraction site can be expected to fill with bone without any additional augmentation procedures except when the labial bone is very thin. A simple extraction followed by a healing period of 4 to 6 months would be sufficient for complete osseous healing. Subsequently, an implant could be placed in the usual manner without the need for bone augmentation. Conversely, if little or no bone exists on the labial surface, it should be anticipated that the site would require bone augmentation to facilitate placement of the implant. In this case, bone grafting at the time of extraction can be used to maintain the alveolar ridge dimensions occupied by the tooth.

Tooth extraction is managed with an atraumatic surgical technique that uses a narrow, flat instrument (Periotome, Hu-Friedy Mfg. Co., Inc., Chicago, IL) directed apically into the sulcus to sever the periodontal ligament and slightly expand the adjacent periodontal tissues. The tooth is elevated and removed with forceps using a gentle, rotational movement. Buccolingual forces are avoided to prevent damaging the integrity of the labial bone. No incisions are made, and care is taken to avoid soft tissue reflection. In this manner, soft tissues maintain their structural anatomy, and the periosteum (blood supply to the bone) remains intact. If the tooth has multiple roots, curved roots, or other anatomic features that make removal difficult, it may be necessary to cut the tooth using a high-speed drill and remove it in smaller pieces. It is important to cut only tooth structure and avoid cutting (overheating) bone when using high-speed drills. The bone within the extraction site is completely debrided of soft tissue with surgical curettes. After debridement, the extraction site is thoroughly irrigated with sterile saline. At this point, bone level and support is evaluated and a decision is made whether to bone graft the site and when to place the implant, immediate, delayed, or staged.

SINUS ELEVATION AND SINUS BONE GRAFTING

Rehabilitation of the edentulous posterior maxilla with osseointegrated implants often represents a clinical challenge because of the insufficient bone volume resulting from enlargement of the maxillary sinus and crestal bone resorption. In situations where the interarch distance is normal or moderately reduced, grafting of the maxillary sinus is indicated. In this procedure, the lateral wall of the maxillary sinus membrane is elevated prior to grafting of the new sinus-floor cavity. In cases demonstrating sufficient crestal bone height, a sinus lift approach can be taken through the implant osteotomy. Several recent clinical studies and reports have attempted to evaluate the maxillary sinus augmentation procedures using a variety of bone grafting materials such as autogenous bone from iliac crest or the oral cavity, as well as bone substitutes such as freeze-dried demineralized bone, resorbable and nonresorbable hydroxyapatite, and xenografts. However, only a few studies have critically evaluated the long-term clinical outcome of this procedure, and most of these have used a small study population.

Short- to long-term clinical studies on the survival of dental implants placed into grafted sinuses demonstrate a similar or even higher survival rate reported in previous studies for implants placed in the maxilla without a sinus augmentation procedure.[21] The results of these studies support the clinical predictability of maxillary sinus augmentation procedures for the rehabilitation of the edentulous posterior maxilla with implant-supported prostheses. It should not be underestimated that the sinus graft is a technique-sensitive procedure, which requires surgical and prosthodontic skills. Complications can include tearing of the sinus membrane, infection of the graft, or loss of implants.

THE ROLE OF GROWTH FACTORS IN BONE AUGMENTATION

Another adjunct to regenerative therapy is osteogenic stimulating substrates to enhance bone formation. One group is the bone morphogenetic proteins (BMPs), belonging to the transforming growth factor β (TGF-β) superfamily. Of this family, recombinant human bone morphogenetic protein (rhBMP-2) has shown significant signs of bone-enhancing potential.

Recently, studies showed substantial preclinical data of rapid new bone formation using rhBMP-2 in critical size defects. The potential of combining barrier membranes and rhBMP-2 for osteogenesis is evident.

The inductive capacity of recombinant human rhBMP-2 was demonstrated by impregnating a polymer carrier and placing the substrate in critical-sized rat mandibular defects with or without a barrier membrane.[37] The study evaluated 12- and 24-day healing times and showed a bony union of the defects for BMP treated sites. The membrane by itself took up to 6 weeks before full healing was evident. The authors concluded that rhBMP-2 can be used with or without a barrier membrane but that the membrane might function as a space maintainer.

Platelet-Rich Plasma: Growth Factor Enhancement for Bone Grafts

In recent years, a new approach to enhance the vitality of bone grafts has been introduced by using platelet-rich plasma (PRP).[39] PRP is an autologous source of platelet-derived growth factors and transforming growth factors that is obtained by sequestering and concentrating platelets by centrifugation. The patient's own blood is withdrawn and separated into its three basic components. The PRP is the important content, which contains a high mixture of platelets and a concentration of growth factors. This PRP mixture is added to the autologous bone graft and has shown to increase the quality of and reduce the time needed for bone regeneration. Clinical and experimental studies are scarce but suggest that this technique holds promise for large bone defects or bone defects with low osteogenic potential. Extrapolation to the effect PRP might have on other bone filler materials cannot be made at this time.

Complications of Localized Ridge Augmentation

Advanced procedures such as GBR and bone grafting to increase the bone volume in deficient alveolar ridges have been successful and have enabled the placement of implants into prosthetically driven positions.[53] Unfortunately, these advanced procedures carry an increased risk of morbidity and can require secondary surgeries to correct soft tissue changes resulting from the procedure.[64] For example, keratinized tissues that have been advanced to cover an increased volume of bone create unaesthetic and non–load-bearing mucogingival discrepancies. The subsequent corrective surgeries required to correct mucogingival discrepancies add surgical time and complexity to the implant therapy.

Surgical complications are reported for a variety of bone reconstructive techniques.[14] The use of bone grafts from the hip to rehabilitate extremely resorbed maxilla has reported exposure of bone transplants in up to 30% of the cases.[61] The exposure rate usually correlates with an increased loss of transplanted tissue. Fenestration defects have the least risk and immediate extraction sites have the highest risk for membrane exposure.

A recent review of the literature assessed the number and types of complications associated with bone reconstructive procedures for endosseous implants. The review of literature (published from 1976 to 1994) included 2315 implants in 733 autogenous block, particulate, and various other bone graft materials. Complications reported included bleeding, postoperative infection, bone fracture, nerve dysfunction, perforation of the mucosa, loss of a portion of the bone graft, pain, decubital ulcers, sinusitis, and wound dehiscence. Wound dehiscence seemed to have the most deleterious effect on implant survival.[60] This finding emphasizes the importance of flap management as discussed previously.

Typical findings include less bone fill with an early exposure and membrane removal as compared with retaining the membrane without exposure for 6 to 8 months.[25,55] Buccolingual ridge deficiencies were treated in a prospective study involving 19 patients using e-PTFE membranes and miniscrews as fixation and tenting devices. The group of defects, which healed uneventfully, yielded upon reentry a 90% to 100% bone regeneration compared with the maximal volume of the space defined by the membrane placement. In the exposed membrane group, the percentage of regenerated bone ranged from 0% to 62%. When a late membrane removal was performed (i.e., 3 to 5 months postsurgically), the regeneration varied between 42% and 62%. The authors concluded that the length of membrane healing and size of the defect played a significant role in the amount of new bone formation.[33]

Other authors have reported successful bone fill in situations where the membranes had to be removed because of an early exposure.[44,54] The use of a bone graft material under the membrane might account for the difference in results. This was confirmed in a clinical study evaluating 36 patients with 23 TPS implants and 20 HA-coated implants placed in immediate extraction sites and treated with membrane alone or membrane in combination with DFDB grafts.[16] When the effect of membrane exposure on bone gain was compared with membranes that remained covered, a significant difference was seen between the covered membrane group and the exposed membrane group but no difference with the exposed membrane/DFDB group. A significantly greater fill of the osseous defects at the grafted sites was noted. The authors concluded that the regeneration of bone around the implants appeared most dependent on the anatomy of the bony defect at the time of implant placement.

Although the effect or amount of regenerated bone with regard to membrane exposure is somewhat contradictory, the aim should be to keep the membranes covered during the healing period so that the risk of infection and soft tissue and esthetic problems can be eliminated. Again, the importance of flap management for ridge augmentation procedures should be stressed.

It can be concluded that the selection of a localized ridge augmentation procedure depends on the size and dimension of the osseous defect. In cases of advanced bone resorption, ridge augmentation before implant placement may be a better choice. It seems reasonable to conclude that the predictability for bone formation is better in horizontal ridge augmentation procedures when compared with vertical ridge augmentation. This conclusion was also made for total maxillary and mandibular ridge reconstruction with calvarial bone grafts because the implant survival rate was increased in cases with horizontal grafting when compared with vertical grafting techniques.[14]

LONG-TERM RESULTS OF IMPLANTS PLACED WITH/AFTER BONE AUGMENTATION PROCEDURES

Long-term data (more than 3 years) of the outcome of the membrane technique is scarcely available, and the few reports that have addressed the question of how regenerated bone behaves under functional loading with dental implants have shown a favorable result. A canine study showed that implants placed in regenerated bone have a normal interaction with the surrounding bone, resulting in direct bone-to-implant contact within 3 months. A loading period of 6 months demonstrated that the regenerated bone is capable of bearing functional load and reacts similarly to nonloaded regenerated bone sites. Regenerated bone sites that did not receive an implant demonstrated bone atrophy beneath the membrane.

One-year clinical follow-up data is available for implants placed in extraction sites with dehiscence or fenestration-type defects grafted with bone using a membrane-technique. All were comparable to normal implant sites.[5,11] A multicenter study determining the predictability of implants placed in immediate extraction sockets and augmented by e-PTFE membranes showed an implant survival rate of 93% after 1 year of loading.[5] Nonstandardized radiographs were evaluated for bone loss after an average loading of 7.5 months.

Dehiscence type defects were analyzed in 2 separate studies. Dahlin[11] demonstrated in a multicenter study that implants with regenerated bone withstood loading for 1- to 2-year evaluation periods and demonstrated a cumulative survival rate of 84.7% in the maxilla and 95% in the mandible, which is in line with previously published work with the Branemark implant-type.

Jovanovic[25] treated 19 dehisced implants with a membrane technique and demonstrated a 6- to 12-month loading result of 100% implant survival. Radiographic analysis demonstrated an average of 1.73-mm mesiodistal bone loss. Differences between studies are related to the measurement method because the choice of a reference point can add or subtract 0.6 mm. If subtracted, a total crestal bone level remains of 1.13 mm, which is in line with other long-term studies of implant loading.

Simion et al[57] demonstrated in a 1- to 5-year clinical follow-up that vertically regenerated bone can be loaded by dental implants successfully and that the periimplant bone structures are maintained similar to implants placed in native, nonregenerated bone.

CONCLUSIONS

Bone augmentation and advanced implant surgery procedures have been described that allow clinicians to reconstruct alveolar bone deficiencies and replace missing teeth with dental implants in a prosthetically driven position with natural appearance and function. The predictable outcome of these procedures is dependent on several biologic principles that must be followed. Diagnosis, treatment planning, careful execution of the surgical treatment, postoperative follow-up, and appropriate implant loading are all important factors in achieving success.

REFERENCES

1. Bahat O, Handelsman M: Periodontal reconstructive flaps—Classification and surgical considerations. Int J Perio Rest Dent 1991; 11(6):481.
2. Becker W, Becker BE, Caffesse R: A comparison of demineralized freeze-dried bone and autologous bone to induce bone formation in human extraction sockets. J Periodontol 1994; 65(12):1128.
3. Becker W, Becker BE, Polizzi G: Autogenous bone grafting of bone defects adjacent to implants placed into immediate extraction sockets in patients: A prospective study. Int J Oral Maxillofac Implants 1994; 9(4):389.
4. Becker W, Clokie C, Sennerby L, et al: Histologic findings after implantation and evaluation of different grafting materials and titanium micro screws into extraction sockets: Case reports. J Periodontol 1998; 69(4):414.
5. Becker W, Dahlin C, Becker BE, et al: The use of e-PTFE barrier membranes for bone promotion around titanium implants placed into extraction sockets: A prospective multicenter study. Int J Oral Maxillofac Implants 1994; 9(1):31.
6. Becker W, Schenk R, Higuchi K, et al: Variations in bone regeneration adjacent to implants augmented with barrier membranes alone or with demineralized freeze-dried bone or autologous grafts: A study in dogs. Int J Oral Maxillofac Implants 1995; 10(2):143.
7. Becker W, Urist MR, Tucker LM, et al: Human demineralized freeze-dried bone: Inadequate induced bone formation in athymic mice. A preliminary report. J Periodontol 1995; 66(9):822.
8. Buser D, Dula K, Hirt HP, et al: Lateral ridge augmentation using autografts and barrier membranes: a clinical study with 40 partially edentulous patients. J Oral Maxillofac Surg 1996; 54(4):420.
9. Carlsson GE, Persson G: Morphologic changes of the mandible after extraction and wearing of dentures. A longitudinal, clinical and x-ray cephalometric study covering 5 years. Odontol Rev 1967; 18:27.
10. Dahlin C, Andersson L, Linde A: Bone augmentation at fenestrated implants by an osteopromotive membrane technique. A controlled clinical study. Clin Oral Implants Res 1991; 2(4):159.
11. Dahlin C, Lekholm U, Becker W, et al: Treatment of fenestration and dehiscence bone defects around oral implants using the guided tissue regeneration technique: A prospective multicenter study. Int J Oral Maxillofac Implants 1995; 10(3):312.
12. Dahlin C, Linde A, Gottlow J, et al: Healing of bone defects by guided tissue regeneration. Plast Reconstr Surg 1988; 81:672.
13. Doblin JM, Salkin LM, Mellado JR, et al: A histologic evaluation of localized ridge augmentation utilizing DFDBA in combination with e-PTFE membranes and stainless steel bone pins in humans. Int J Periodontics Restorative Dent 1996; 16(2):120.
14. Donovan MG, Dickerson NC, Hanson LJ: Maxillary and mandibular reconstruction using calvarial bone grafts and Branemark implants: A preliminary report. Int J Oral Maxillofac Surg 1994; 52(6):588.
15. Gelb DA: Immediate implant surgery: Three-year retrospective evaluation of 50 consecutive cases. Int J Oral Maxillofac Implants 1993; 8(4):388.
16. Gher ME, Quintero G, Assad D: Bone grafting and guided bone regeneration for immediate dental implants in humans. J Periodontol 1994; 65(9):881.
17. Hunt D, Jovanovic S: Autogenous bone harvesting: A clinical graft technique for particulate and amniocortical bone blocks. Int J Periodont Rest Dent 1999; 19:165
18. Ilizarov GA: The tension-stress effect on the genesis and growth of tissues. Part 1. The influence of stability of fixation and soft tissue preservation. Clin Orthop 1989; 238:249.
19. Ilizarov GA: The tension-stress effect on the genesis and growth of tissues. Part 2. The influence of the rate and frequency of distraction. Clin Orthop 1989; 239:263.
20. Jensen OT, Greer RO Jr, Johnson L, et al: Vertical guided bone-graft augmentation in a new canine mandibular model. Int J Oral Maxillofac Implants 1995; 10(3):335.
21. Jensen OT, Shulman LB, Block M, et al: Report of the sinus conference of 1996. Int J Oral Maxillofac Implants 1998; 13 (supplement).
22. Jovanovic SA, Buser D: Guided bone regeneration in dehiscence defects and delayed extraction sockets. In: Buser D, Dahlin C, Schenk RK: Guided Bone Regeneration in Implant Dentistry. Chicago, Quintessence, 1994.
23. Jovanovic SA, Nevins M: Bone formation utilizing titanium-reinforced barrier membranes. Int J Periodont Rest Dent 1995; 15(1):56.
24. Jovanovic SA, Schenk RK, Orsini M: Supracrestal bone formation around dental implants: An experimental dog study. Int J Oral Maxillofac Implants 1995; 10:23.
25. Jovanovic SA, Spiekermann H, Richter EJ: Bone regeneration around titanium dental implants in dehisced defect sites: a clinical study. Int J Oral Maxillofac Implants 1992; 7:233.
26. Klokkevold PR, Han TJ, Camargo PM: Aesthetic management of extractions for implant site development: Delayed versus staged implant placement. Pract Periodontics Aesthet Dent 1999; 11(5):603–.
27. Klokkevold PR, Newman MG: Current status of dental implants: A periodontal perspective. Int J Oral Maxillofac Implants 2000; 15(1):56.
28. Kostopoulos L, Karring T: Guided bone regeneration in mandibular defects in rats using a bioresorbable polymer. Clin Oral Implants Res 1994; 5:66.
29. Kostopoulos L, Karring T: Augmentation of the rat mandible using guided tissue regeneration. Clin Oral Implants Res 1994; 5(2):75.
30. Landsberg C, Grosskopf A, Weinreb M: Clinical and biological observations of demineralized freeze-dried bone allografts in augmentation procedures around dental implants. Int J Oral Maxillofac Implants 1994; 9:586.
31. Landsberg CJ: The reversed crestal flap: A surgical modification in endosseous implant procedures. Quintessence 1994; 25:229.
32. Lang NP, Bragger U, Hammerle CH, et al: Immediate transmucosal implants using the principle of guided tissue regeneration. I. Rationale, clinical procedures and 30-month results. Clin Oral Implants Res 1994; 5(3):154.
33. Lang NP, Hammerle CH, Bragger U, et al: Guided tissue regeneration in jawbone defects prior to implant placement. Clin Oral Implants Res 1994; 5(2):92.
34. Lazzara RJ: Immediate implant placement into extraction sites: Surgical and restorative advantages. Int J Periodont Rest Dent 1989; 9(5):332.
35. Lekovic V, Camargo P, Klokkevold P, et al: Preservation of alveolar bone in extraction sockets using bioabsorbable membranes. J Periodontol 1998; 69:1044.

36. Lekovic V, Kenney EB, Weinlaender M, et al: A bone regenerative approach to alveolar ridge maintenance following tooth extraction. Report of 10 cases. J Periodontol 1997; 68(6):563.
37. Linde A, Hedner E: Recombinant bone morphogenetic protein-2 enhances bone healing, guided by osteopromotive e-PTFE membranes: An experimental study in rats. Calcified Tissue International 1995; 56:549.
38. Linde A, Thoren C, Dahlin C: Creation of new bone by an osteopromotive membrane technique. Int J Oral Maxillofac Surg 1993; 51:892.
39. Marx RE, Carlson ER, Eichstaedt RM, et al: Platelet rich plasma. Oral Surg Oral Med Oral Pathol Oral Radiol Endod 1998; 85:638.
40. Mellonig JT, Nevins M: Guided bone regeneration of bone defects associated with implants: an evidence-based outcome assessment. Int J Periodontics Restorative Dent 1995; 15(2):168.
41. Missika P, Abbou M, Rahal B: Osseous regeneration in immediate post-extraction implant placement: A literature review and clinical evaluation. Pract Periodont Aesthet Dent 1997; 9(2):165.
42. Murray G, Roschlau W: Experimental and clinical study of new growth of bone in a cavity. Amer J Surg 1957; 93:385.
43. Nemcovsky CE, Serfaty V: Alveolar ridge preservation following extraction of maxillary anterior teeth. Report on 23 consecutive cases. J Periodontol 1996; 67(4):390.
44. Nevins M, Mellonig JT: The advantages of localized ridge augmentation prior to implant placement: a staged event. Int J Periodontics Restorative Dent 1994; 14(2):96.
45. Palmer RM, Floyd PD, Palmer PJ: Healing implant dehiscence defects with and without expanded polytetrafluoroethylene membranes: A controlled clinical and histological study. Clin Oral Implants Res 1994; 5(2):98.
46. Parodi R, Santarelli G, Carusi G: Application of slow-resorbing collagen membrane to periodontal and peri-implant guided tissue regeneration. Int J Periodontics Restorative Dent 1996; 16(2):174.
47. Rominger JW, Triplett RG: The use of guided tissue regeneration to improve implant osseointegration [see comments]. J Oral Maxillofac Surg 1994; 52(2):106.
48. Sandberg E, Dahlin C, Linde A: Bone regeneration by the osteopromotive technique using bioabsorbable membranes. An experimental study in rats. Int J Oral Maxillofac Surg 1993; 51:1106.
49. Schenk RK, Buser D, Hardwick WR: Healing pattern of bone regeneration in membrane-protected defects. Int J Periodont Rest Dent 1994; 9(1):13.
50. Schwartz-Arad D, Chaushu G: Placement of implants into fresh extraction sites: 4 to 7 years retrospective evaluation of 95 immediate implants. J Periodontol 1997; 68(11):1110.
51. Schwartz Z, Mellonig JT, Carnes DL Jr, et al: Ability of commercial demineralized freeze-dried bone allograft to induce new bone formation. J Periodontol 1996; 67(9):918.
52. Schwartz Z, Somers A, Mellonig JT, et al: Ability of commercial demineralized freeze-dried bone allograft to induce new bone formation is dependent on donor age but not gender. J Periodontol 1998; 69(4):470.
53. Shanaman RH: The use of guided tissue regeneration to facilitate ideal prosthetic placement of implants. Int J Periodont Rest Dent 1992; 12(4):257.
54. Shanaman RH: A retrospective study of 237 sites treated consecutively with guided tissue regeneration. Int J Periodont Rest Dent 1994; 14(4):292.
55. Simion M, Baldoni M, Rossi P, et al: A comparative study of the effectiveness of e-PTFE membranes with and without early exposure during the healing period. Int J Periodontics Restorative Dent 1994; 14(2):166.
56. Simion M, Dahlin C, Trisi P, et al: Qualitative and quantitative comparative study on different filling materials used in bone tissue regeneration: A controlled clinical study. Int J Periodontics Restorative Dent 1994; 14(3):198.
57. Simion M, Jovanovic SA, Tinti C, et al: Long-term evaluation of osseointegrated implants inserted at the time or after vertical ridge augmentation. Clin Oral Impl Res 2001; 12:35.
58. Simion M, Trisi P, Piattelli A: Vertical ridge augmentation using a membrane technique associated with osseointegrated implants. Int J Periodontics Restorative Dent 1994; 14(6):496.
59. ten Bruggenkate CM, Kraaijenhagen HA, van der Kwast WAM: Autogenous maxillary bone grafts in conjunction with placement of I.T.I. endosseous implants. A preliminary report. Int J Oral Maxillofac Surg 1992; 21:81.
60. Tolman DE: Advanced residual ridge resorption: Surgical management. Int J Prosthodont 1993; 6(2):118.
61. Tolman DE: Reconstructive procedures with endosseous implants in grafted bone: A review of literature. Int J Oral Maxillofac Implants 1995; 10:275.
62. Urist MR: Bone formation by autoinduction. Science 1965; 150:893.
63. Wilson TG Jr, Schenk R, Buser D, et al: Implants placed in immediate extraction sites: A report of histologic and histometric analyses of human biopsies. Int J Oral Maxillofac Implants 1998; 13(3):333.
64. Yildirim M, Hanisch O, Spiekermann H: Simultaneous hard and soft tissue augmentation for implant-supported single-tooth restorations [see comments]. Pract Periodontics Aesthet Dent; 9(9):1023.
65. Zellin G, Gritli-Linde A, Linde A: Healing of mandibular defects with different biodegradable and non-biodegradable membranes: An experimental study in rats. Biomaterials 1995; 16(8):601.

Prosthetic Aspects of Dental Implants

Ting-Ling Chang, Eleni Roumanas, Sascha A. Jovanovic, and John Beumer III

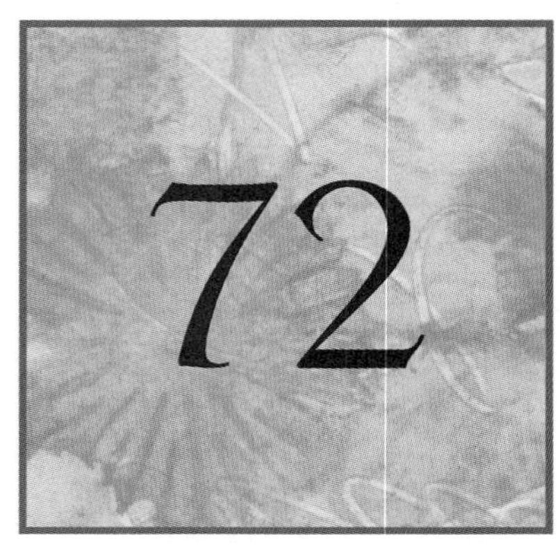

CHAPTER

CHAPTER OUTLINE

Controlled clinical research in implant prosthodontics showed excellent long-term results achieved after appropriate case selection, good occlusal harmony and oral hygiene, and careful handling of patients' soft and hard tissues. With these results the placement of implants has become one of the most beneficial surgical procedures performed in connection with prosthodontic procedures and treatment modalities. It has also provided a high psychologic impact and improvement of quality of life for completely and partially edentulous patients.

After the first year of implant function, loss of marginal bone is small around most oral implants. However, clinical studies have shown a correlation between insufficient oral hygiene, occlusal overload, and progression of bone loss around dental implants. In general, occlusal loading can affect the prognosis of both implants and prosthetic reconstructions in implant dentistry. The occlusal load may exceed the mechanical or biologic load-bearing capacity of the osseointegrated oral implants or the prosthesis, causing either a mechanical failure or failure in the osseointegration. If this happens, the load can be defined as an overload.

IMPLANT BIOMECHANICS

It is becoming clear that a knowledge of implant biomechanics is essential if implant-supported restorations are to be employed predictably. The load-bearing capacity of implants supporting the restoration must exceed the loads anticipated during function. If the loads applied exceed load-bearing capacity of the implants, implant overload may be the result, and a resorption remodeling response of the bone around the implants is provoked.[1,8]

Several factors affect the load-bearing capacity of implants (Fig. 72-1), including implant length, the number of implants used, their arrangement, and their angulation in relation to the plane of occlusion.[2,15] The quality of the bone implant interface (bone anchorage, or bone appositional index) also greatly influences the load-bearing capacity of implant-supported restorations.[21,18,19,22]

The bone appositional index is particularly influential (see Fig. 72-1). For example, bone anchorage of implants in the posterior maxilla is particularly poor compared with the anterior mandible. As one progresses posteriorly in the maxilla, the trabecular bone is less dense, the cortical layer is thinner, and as a result the bone appositional index in the posterior maxilla may be one third to one half

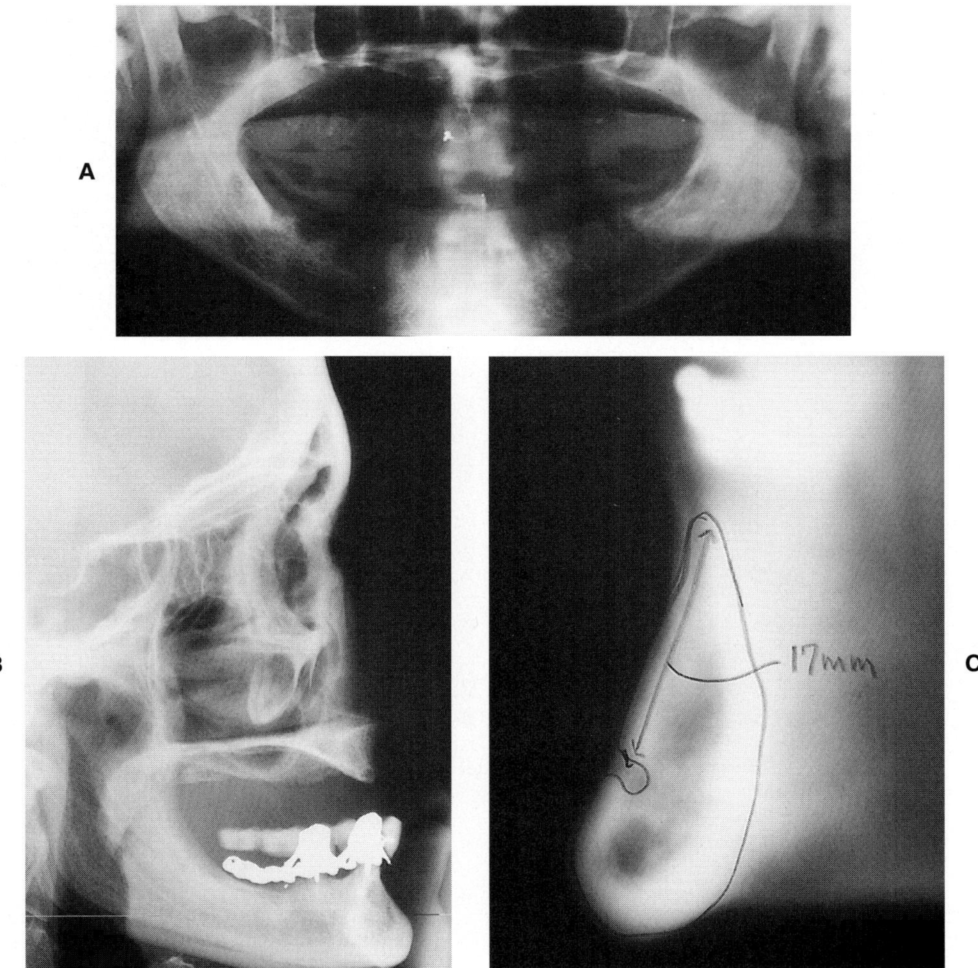

Fig. 72-1 Different radiographic procedures used in implant dentistry. **A,** Panoramic radiograph. **B,** Lateral cephalometric radiograph. **C,** Tomogram of mandibular premolar area.

of that achieved in the anterior mandible. In addition, pneumatization of the maxillary sinus limits the lengths of implants used, further reducing the load-carrying capacity of implants placed in this region.

The number of implants used obviously affects load-bearing capacity (see Fig. 72-1). In the 1980s and early 1990s, many posterior quadrants of the maxilla were restored with one or two implants, and in some patients these implant restorations supported 3 or 4 dental units. In many instances, soon after loading, a distinct pattern of bone loss was observed that led to loss of the implants in many patients. Additional implants significantly improve the biomechanics of these implant-supported fixed partial dentures. Today, when restoring the posterior quadrant of the maxilla, an implant is placed for every tooth restored. There is no unanimous opinion on the number of implants to be used, and extreme positions are championed, such as installing as many implants as possible. However, in general, the tendency at present is to reduce the number of implants.

The angulation of implants (see Fig. 72-1) in relation to the plane of occlusion and the direction of the occlusal load is also an important factor in predicting the success-failure rates of implants used to restore posterior quadrants. In the 1980s, prior to the utilization of the sinus lift and graft, many implants placed in the posterior maxilla exhibited excessive buccal angulations. In addition, many implants placed in the mandible presented with excessive distal angulations. A high percentage of such implants exhibited signs of implant overload (i.e., bone loss around the neck of implants that was progressive and irreversible) after delivery of the prosthesis.

Minor discrepancies in angulation are probably not clinically significant, but if loads are at an angle of 20 degrees or more to the long axis of the implant, load magnification can result, provoking a resorptive remodeling response of the adjacent bone.[2] The combination of short implants in poor-quality bone, where occlusal loads are delivered at angles of 20 degrees or greater along the long axis of the implants, make implants

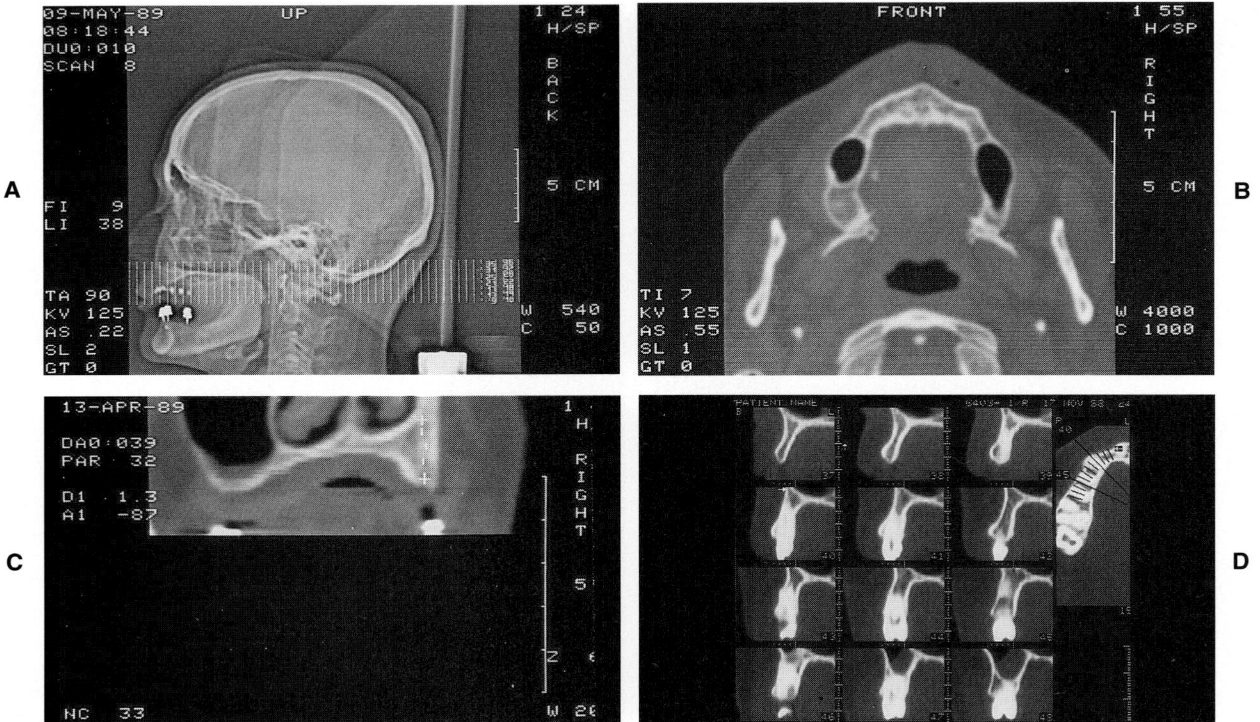

Fig. 72-2 Computed tomographic scans. **A,** Sagittal view. **B,** Occlusal view. **C,** Cross-sectional view. **D,** Cross-sectional reformatted view.

prone to implant overload, leading to progressive and irreversible bone loss and implant failure.

In clinical situations, the risk of implant overload can be minimized by limiting the width of the occlusal table of the implant-supported fixed partial denture, flattening the cusp angles, avoiding the use of cantilevered restorations, and restoring the anterior guidance provided by the residual anterior dentition. In addition, designing the restoration so that it is independent of the natural dentition simplifies the biomechanics.

EDENTULOUS MAXILLA

Although a conventional denture may be satisfactory for most edentulous maxillas, implants may be desirable in some situations. When a conventional maxillary denture is only marginally stable, the patient may not be aware of the problem when the conventional mandibular denture is even more unstable. If the mandible is restored with a stable implant-assisted overlay denture, the patient becomes aware of the deficiency of the maxillary denture and requests the same type of stability for the maxillary restoration. Another indication for implants in the maxilla may be to offset the potentially destructive effects on the premaxillary area when an edentulous maxilla is opposed by a mandible with natural anterior teeth.

Many patients may feel a psychologic need for either a palateless denture or better retention. The four implant–assisted, palateless overlay denture ideally addresses the needs of most patients (Fig. 72-2). It is usually unsatisfactory to construct a fixed prosthesis in the completely edentulous maxilla unless an unusual amount of alveolar bone is present. The usual resorption pattern of the alveolus places the gingival margin of a fixed restoration too far superiorly, too far palatally, or both. Even if the patient has a low smile line, a lack of lip support just beneath the nose can be unsightly. Most patients are best served with implant-assisted overlay dentures.

EDENTULOUS MANDIBLE

Implant-assisted overlay dentures are most commonly employed. An implant-assisted denture is designed so that most of the masticatory load is borne by the primary denture-support areas (retromolar pad, buccal shelf). A common practice is to place two implants in the anterior mandible with a connecting bar. The denture is retained by two clips over the bar. When an occlusal force is applied posteriorly, the denture rotates around the bar, directing the force into the primary denture support areas (Box 72-1).

Fixed implant–supported prostheses require four to six implants arranged in an appropriate arc of curvature (Fig. 72-3). Many patients prefer this option for psychologic reasons, but the mastication efficiency provided by this prosthesis is little better than that provided by an implant-assisted overlay denture. However, evidence suggests that such fixed restorations tend to stop resorption

BOX 72-1

Implant Biomechanics

Load-Bearing Capacity
Implant
  Number
  Length
  Arrangement
  Angulation
Quality of bone-implant interference

Anticipated Load (Affected by)
Occlusal factors
  Cusp angles
  Width of occlusal table
Guidance type
  Anterior guidance
  Group function
Cantilevers
Connection to natural dentition
Parafunctional habits (bruxism)

of the body of the posterior mandible and in some cases enable regeneration of the bone in this region.

PARTIALLY EDENTULOUS PATIENTS: POSTERIOR QUADRANTS

Anatomic Limitations

Anatomic limitations may prevent placement of implants of adequate length in the posterior quadrants. In the posterior quadrants of the maxilla, the maxillary sinus limits the lengths used, and in the mandible the inferior alveolar nerve limits the lengths of the implants used. In the posterior quadrant of the maxilla, the bone-implant interface or the bone anchorage for osseointegrated implants is compromised because the bone quality is poor. Primary anchorage for an implant placed in this region is provided by the implant engaging the cortical bone of the floor of the sinus and the cortical bone on the alveolar ridge. There is generally very little bone implant interface along the course of the implant, and if the tip is not properly anchored in the cortical bone in the floor of the sinus, the implant may fail during occlusal loading. The use of implants with rougher surfaces may improve the bone anchorage in poor-quality bone but still may not provide all patients with sufficient anchorage to support unilateral implant-supported fixed partial dentures if the implants are too short.

Because many patients possess insufficient bone in the posterior maxillary quadrant to receive an implant of suitable length, bone augmentation of the alveolar ridge or maxillary sinus has been suggested.[12,22] Free bone grafts taken from the chin, iliac crest, or other locations, often mixed with bone substitutes, are now being used to supplement the existing bone at these sites.[23]

Augmented posterior maxillary sites created by elevating the sinus membrane and placing bone grafts in this region appears to be most successful in supporting implants, particularly if a minimum of 5 mm of residual bone is available over the sinus with which to anchor the neck of the implant. The success rates, however, appear to decrease when less than 5 mm of bone is available over the sinus, presumably because a majority of the site is composed of grafted bone.

In the mandible, the limiting factor with respect to implant placement is the presence of the inferior alveolar nerve. Based on clinical data, the authors feel the minimum length for implants used to restore posterior mandibular quadrants, regardless of implant width, is 10 mm. Implants less than 10 mm should not be used

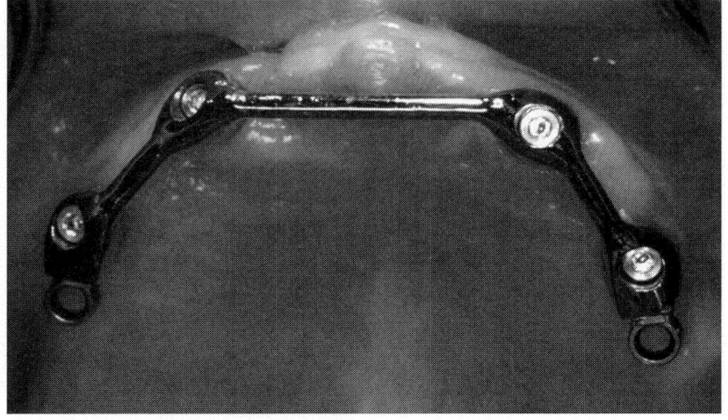
A

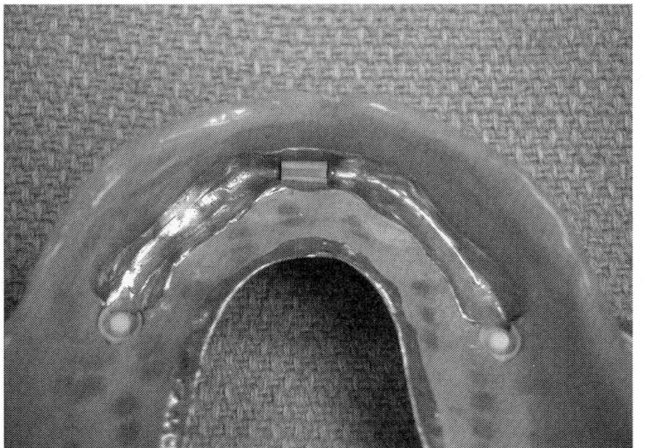
B

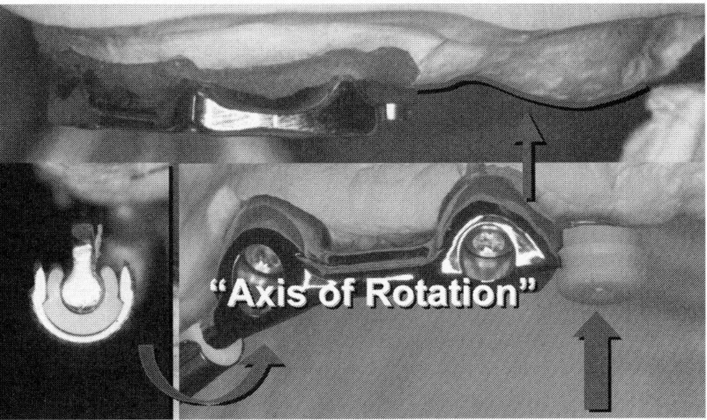

C

Fig. 72-3 A and B, Four-implant, palateless, overlay assisted design. **C,** When posterior occlusal forces are applied, the denture rotates around the bar clip anteriorly and resilient attachment *(arrow)* allows the denture to be compressed to primary denture support areas posteriorly *(arrow).*

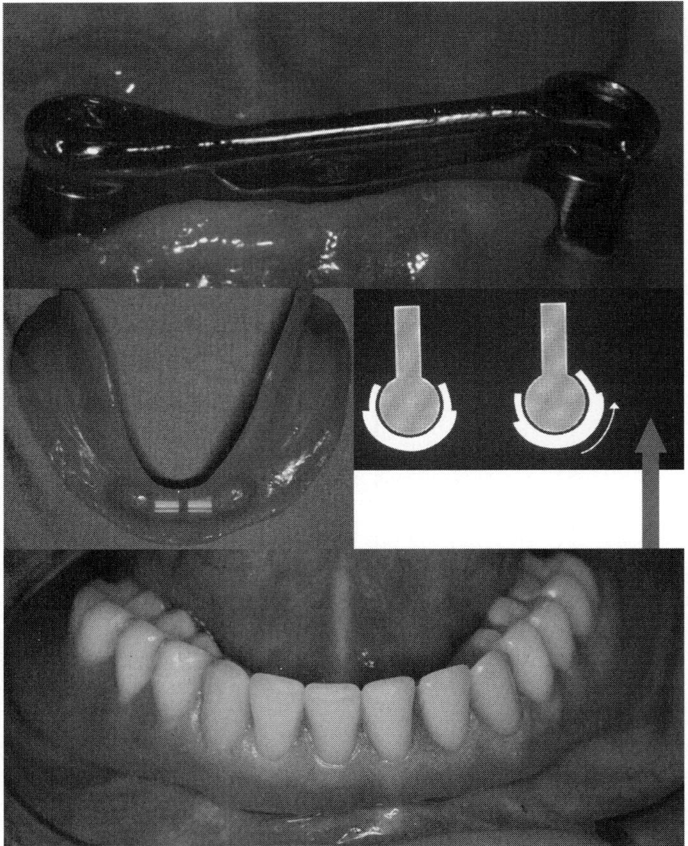

Fig. 72-4 Implant-assisted overlay denture using a bar clip design. When the patient applies occlusal force posteriorly, the overlay denture rotates around the bar and the load is absorbed by primary denture-bearing surfaces posteriorly.

because the bone anchorage of the implant is not sufficient to support posterior occlusal forces. These factors, in combination with the linear configuration of the implants, suggest that 10 mm is the minimal length that should be used for implant supported fixed partial dentures used to restore posterior mandibular quadrants.

When bone for placement of a 10-mm implant is insufficient, some clinicians have recommended that the inferior alveolar nerve be dissected out of its canal and lateralized.[3,10] Implants can then be used to extend all the way to the inferior border of the mandible, providing bicortical stabilization. The implant success rates obtained with this technique are very high, but unfortunately the risk of injury to the inferior alveolar nerve is significant. In some reports the incidence of permanent nerve injury can be as high as 25%.[4,6] Therefore the authors recommend that this technique not be used. If the patient has a reasonable dentition anteriorly, a distal extension removable partial denture is still a good option. It should be remembered that the mastication efficiency of patients fitted with properly extended and properly designed distal extension removable partial dentures is equivalent to that of patients fitted with implant-supported fixed partial dentures restoring distal extension areas.[14]

Distraction osteogenesis offers a new approach for creating bony sites that possess sufficient width and vertical height. In most instances, however, after completion of distraction osteogenesis, the horizontal dimension of the site must be enhanced with bone grafting. No long-term clinical results of this procedure are available.

Linear Configurations and Implant Overload

When implants are arranged in a linear fashion, the biomechanics with respect to anticipated bone response are quite unfavorable as compared with a configuration where the implants are arranged in a curvilinear fashion with significant anterior-posterior spread, particularly when loads are *not* applied along the long axis of the implant. In the 1980s, conventional dogma stated that once an implant became "osseointegrated," it did not matter whether occlusal loads were applied axially. However, as more clinical follow-up data and animal research data become available, it is increasingly obvious that in some clinical situations—namely, implant-supported fixed partial dentures restoring posterior quadrants—nonaxial loads can cause sufficient load magnification at the bone-implant interface to lead to bone resorption and eventually a higher rate of implant failure.

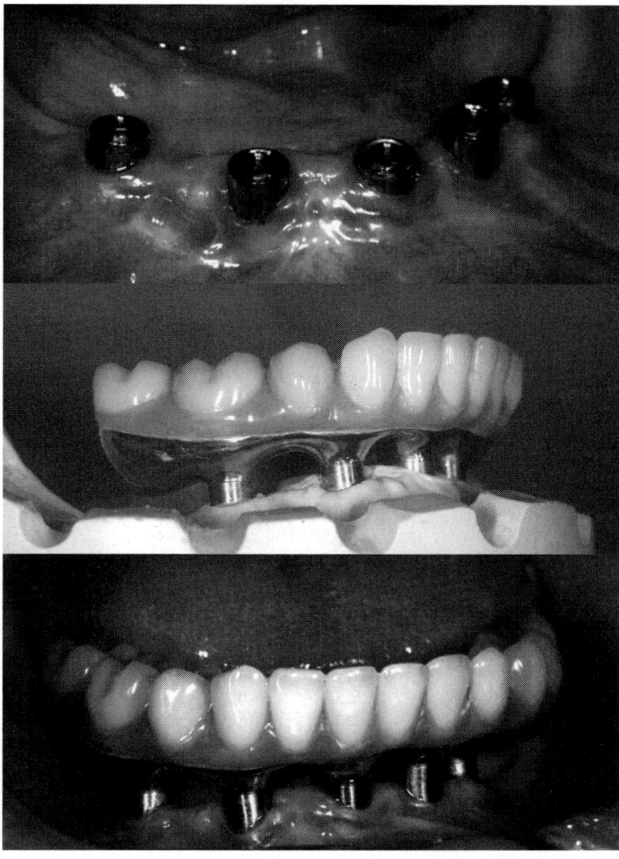

Fig. 72-5 Fixed hybrid prosthesis fabricated from denture teeth and acrylic resin with a nonprecious metal support structure.

Brunski proposed the following hypothesis with regard to the biologic mechanisms initiated in bone when an implant was overloaded.[1] He proposed that excessive occlusal loads lead to microdamage (e.g., fractures, cracks, and delamination) of the bone adjacent to the implant, which provokes a resorptive remodeling response. This results in increased porosity of the affected bone. A vicious cycle ensues in which continued loading leads to more microdamage, porosity, and bone loss until the implant fails (Fig. 72-5).

Nonaxial loads, which cause load magnification, can lead to implant overload, which in turn precipitates a resorptive remodeling response of the bone around the neck of the implants. The bone loss appears to be progressive and can lead to implant failure. Linear implant configurations in the posterior mandible and posterior maxilla are particularly prone to bone loss when loads are not applied axially. Implants should be positioned so that occlusal loads can be directed axially. The response is not universal, however, and is probably dependent on the bone anchorage of the implant, length of the implant, magnitude of the occlusal loads applied to the implants, and whether the implant supported restoration is used for incising or masticating the food bolus. Therefore the authors believe every attempt should be made to surgically position implants in the posterior quadrants so that occlusal forces can be directed axially or along the long axis of the implant. If implants are positioned in such a way, the restoration is very easy and cost effective to fabricate and the implants have a better long-term prognosis.

The use of cantilevered implant-supported restorations in posterior quadrants of the mandible or maxilla is strongly discouraged. Cantilever extensions result in load magnification and can cause overloading of the implant next to the cantilever extension, which in turn may lead to bone loss and implant failure.

When connecting implants to the natural dentition, the authors recommend it be done in a rigid fashion, either with rigid, screw-retained attachments or copings secured with permanent cement (see Fig. 72-5). The case for such rigid connections has been eloquently made by Gulbransen.[7] He showed that if implants are connected to the natural dentition with a rigid system of attachment, the implant failure and complication rates, such as screw loosening, were dramatically reduced. In addition, the well-documented phenomenon of intrusion of the natural tooth abutment associated with the use of semiprecision attachments is prevented.

BOX 72-2

Implant Overload and Bone Resorption: Possible Mechanisms

Excessive occlusal loads
Resultant microdamage (fractures, cracks, and delaminations)
Resorptive remodeling response of bone
Increased porosity secondary to remodeling
Vicious cycle of continued loading, with more microdamage and more porosity until implant fails

Adapted from Brunski J, Puelo D, Nanci A: Biomaterials and biomechanics of oral and maxillofacial implants: Current status and future developments. Int J Oral Maxillofac Imp 2000; 15.

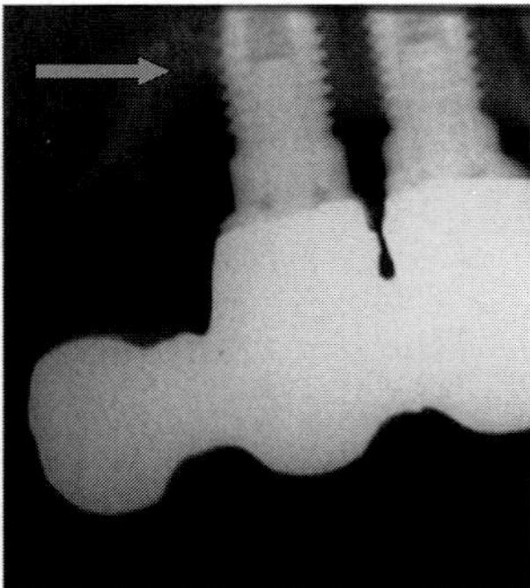

Fig. 72-6 Cantilevers in the posterior quadrants of partially edentulous patients should be discouraged. Note bone loss *(arrows)*.

IMMEDIATE OR EARLY LOADING: POSTERIOR QUADRANTS

Immediate or early loading of osseointegrated implants is generally not recommended when implants are used to restore posterior quadrant defects in partially edentulous patients. When an implant is placed into bone, the initial bone anchorage is not very good and if it is loaded and as a result becomes mobile, it fails to osseointegrate; in other words, a fibrous connective tissue capsule develops around the body of the implant. The biologic processes required to achieve osseointegration takes about 4 months in humans (Box 72-2). Some evidence suggests that implants with acid-etched surfaces resulting in a specific surface morphology may result in the expression of specific genes that promote more rapid healing of the bone around implants.[16,17] However, these animal studies are yet to be confirmed by human follow-up studies. Immediate or early loading may be feasible when implants are placed in good-quality bone (i.e., anterior mandible) and are used to retain implant-assisted overlay dentures. However, when they are placed in posterior quadrants of partially edentulous patients where the bone sites are less dense and all the occlusal loads are born by the implants, immediate or early loading is inadvisable.

BOX 72-3

Biologic Processes

The following biologic processes need to be completed before an implant is firmly anchored in bone. This process takes 4 months in humans.

- Blood clot
- Angiogenesis
- Osteoprogenitor cell migration
- Woven bone formation
- Deposition of lamellar bone
- Secondary remodeling of woven bone with lamellar

In summary, every effort should be made to design implant-supported restorations that are not subject to implant overload. A summary of the strategies are found in Fig. 72-4. If the clinician follows this prescription and also places implants in tooth positions, 1) proper emergence profiles can be developed, 2) space is available interproximately for hygienic access, 3) the clinician has better control over the occlusal anatomy (narrowed occlusal table and flat cusp angles), 4) occlusal loads are delivered axially, and 5) abutment selection is simplified (Fig. 72-6).

SINGLE-TOOTH IMPLANTS IN THE POSTERIOR QUADRANTS

Standard-diameter implants have been used to restore single tooth defects in the posterior quadrants of the maxilla and mandible with mixed results. In the 1980s, clinicians attempted to restore mandibular first molar sites with conventional 3.75- or 4.0-mm diameter implants. Unfortunately, the results were quite disappointing. In some patients, occlusal overload led to loss of bone around the implant, and implant fixtures fractured in other patients. However, these occurrences were rare. The most common problem observed was loosening of the screw retaining the restoration. This is caused by the fact that the diameter of the head of the implant is much smaller than the size of the occlusal surface. Tipping of the restoration during function eventually leads to stretching and loosening of the screw securing the crown to the implant fixture. The buccal-lingual width of the crown can be controlled and the dimension kept to a minimum. However, clinicians do not have control over the mesiodistal dimension because this space must be filled. When the bolus of food becomes positioned on the mesial side of the crown, tipping forces are generated that eventually lead to loosening of the screw retaining the crown. The use of wide-diameter implants resolves the screw-loosening complication (Box 72-4). If the first molar is lost and suitable abutments are available on both sides, a conventional, three-unit, fixed partial denture is still the preferred option. This restoration is cost

BOX 72-4

Strategies to Avoid Implant Overload

The following strategies are used to avoid implant overload in the posterior quadrants of partially edentulous patients. When these conditions cannot be met, removable partial dentures are recommended.

- Place implants perpendicular to the occlusal plane. (Note that the occlusal plane is not flat [i.e., curve of Wilson, curve of Spee].)
- In mandibular extension defects, when in doubt, always add a third implant.
- In maxillary extension defects, use at least three implants.
- Avoid the use of cantilevers in linear configurations.
- If you are required to attach to the natural dentition, do so with a rigid attachment system.
- Control occlusal factors (i.e., cusp angles and width of occlusal table) and restore anterior guidance if required.
- Avoid the use of short implants (less than 10 mm).

effective and quite predictable. In distal extension areas restoring one molar tooth, the authors recommend that two conventionally sized implants be placed close together. This restoration is biomechanically sound and can be designed to allow adequate hygiene access.

Single implants can be used with a high rate of success in the mandibular and bicuspid area. The bone implant interface achieved in this area is good and the size of the occlusal surface is generally small. Likewise, the success rate in the maxillary bicuspid region has been good. However, the authors recommend the use of implants 13 mm in length or longer to restore these sites because the bone-implant interface is not ideal in these regions.

IMPLANTS IN THE ESTHETIC ZONE

Implants placed in the anterior quadrants of partially edentulous patients enjoy a high success rate and high satisfaction rate with patients. In the anterior region, the forces and bending moments acting on the implant-supported replacement are normally less and the bone volume is greater than in the posterior region. Therefore it may be possible to reduce the number of implants in the anterior region to a few longer implants, such as replacing four incisors with two implants and a four-unit fixed prostheses. The bone sites are generally favorable in quality and quantity, although there may be deficiencies in labial lingual and apicocoronal dimension in the maxilla in patients. These areas, however, can be predictably augmented with autogenous bone grafts with or without barrier membranes.[11] The quality of the esthetic result is dependent on restoration of bone and soft tissue contours and proper implant positioning (Fig. 72-7). The rule of thumb has been to place the implant in the tooth position in a mesiodistal, buccolingual, and apicocoronal position.[13] A number of reviews recommend placing implants after esthetic three-dimensional considerations in the anterior region. This is called *prosthetically driven implant placement* and may be preceded by prosthetically driven site development. If the neighboring teeth demonstrate intact periodontal tissue support, the implant head is placed about 2 to 3 mm below the anticipated buccal gingival margin. The implant-supported restoration should contour the soft tissue and emerge with a profile in the same dimensions as the natural tooth and with physiologic contours.

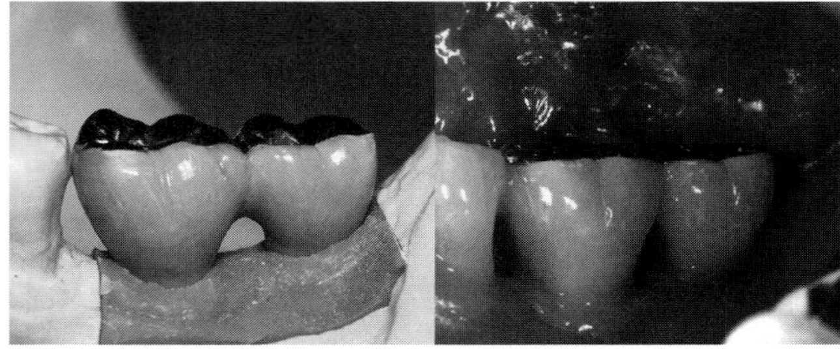

Fig. 72-7 Guidelines for restoring posterior quadrants. Embrasures must be large enough for proxy brush access, occlusal table must be narrowed, posterior cusp angles flattened, proper emergence profiles developed, and anterior guidance restored.

REFERENCES

1. Brunski J, Puelo D, Nanci A: Biomaterials and biomechanics of oral and maxillofacial implants: Current status and future developments. Int J Oral Maxillofac Imp 2000; 15.
2. Cho G: Personal communication, 1992.
3. Davis H, Rydevik B, Lundborg S, et al: Mobilization of the inferior alvelor nerve to allow placement of osseintegratable fixtures. In: Worthington P, Branemark PI (eds): Advanced Osseointegration Surgery Applications in the Maxillofacial Region. Chicago, Quintessence, 1992.
4. Davis H: Neurologic complications in implant surgery. American Associations of Oral and Maxillofacial Surgeons, 1992 Clinical Congress—Study Guide, 1992; 42.
5. De Bruyn H, Collaert B: The effect of making an early implant failure. Clin Oral Implant Res 1994; 5:260.
6. Ehrenfeld N, Roser M, Altenmuller E: Transposition of the inferior alveolar nerve in preprosthetic surgery. Proceedings of the 6th International Congress of Preprosthetics Surgery. Palm Springs, CA, 1995.
7. Gulbransen H: Unpublished data, 1995.
8. Hoshaw S, Brunski J, Cochran C: Mechanical loading of Branemark implants affects interfacial bone modeling and remodeling. Int J Oral Maxillofac Implants 1994; 9:345.
9. Jemt T, Lekholm U, Adell R: Osseointegrated implants in the treatment of partially edentulous patients: A preliminary study of 876 consecutively placed fixtures. Int J Oral Maxillofac Implant 1989; 4:211.
10. Jensen O, Nock D: Inferior alveolar nerve repositioning in conjunction with placement of osseointegrated implants: A case report. Oral Surg Oral Med Oral Path Oral Radiol 1987; 63:263.

11. Jovanovic SA, Spiekermann H, and Richter EJ: Bone regeneration on dehisced titanium dental implants. A clinical study. Int J Oral Maxillofac Implants 1992; 7:233.
12. Jovanovic S, Schenk R, Orsini M, et al: Supracrestal bone formation around dental implants: an experimental dog study. Int J Oral Maxillofac Implants 1995; 10:23.
13. Jovanovic SA, Paul S, Nishimura R: Anterior implant-supported reconstructions: A surgical challenge. Practic Periodont Aesthet Dent 1999; 11:5:551.
14. Kapur K, Deupree R, Frechette AR, et al: Veterans Administrations cooperative dental implant study. Comparisons between fixed partial dentures supported by blade vent implants and removable partial dentures. Part III: Comparision of masticatory scores between two treatment modalities. J Prosthet Dent 1991; 65:272.
15. Kinni B, Hokanas S, Caputo A: Force transfer by osseointegration. Int J Oral Maxillofac Implants 1998, 1:11.
16. Ogawa T, Ozawa S, Shih JH, et al: Biomechanical evaluation of osseous implants having different surface topographies. J Dent Res 2000; 79:1857.
17. Ogawa T, Ozawa S, Sukotjo C, et al: Bone matrix-related gene response to implants and their surface topography in vivo. Proceed Int Cong Maxillofac Prosthet 2000; 117 (abstract).
18. Rangert B, Krogh P, Langer B, et al: Bending overload and implant fracture. A retrospective clinical analysis. Int J Oral Maxillofac Implants 1995; 10:326.
19. Rangert B, Jemt T, Jorneus L: Forces and moments on Branemark implants. Int J Oral Maxillofac Implants 1989; 4:241.
20. Rangert B, Sullivan R, Jemt T: Load factor control for implants in the posterior partially edentulous segment. Int J Oral Maxillofac Implants 1997; 12:360.
21. Richter E: In vivo vertical forces on implant. Int J Oral Maxillofac Implants 1995; 10:99.
22. Simion M, Jovanovic SA, Trisi P, et al: Vertical ridge augmentation around dental implants using a membrane technique and bone auto or allografts in humans. Int J Periodont Restor Dent 1998, 18:9.
23. Tolman D: Reconstructive procedures with endosseous implants in grafted bone: A review of the literature. Int J Oral Maxillofac Implants 1995; 10:275.

Diagnosis and Treatment of Periimplant Complications

Sascha A. Jovanovic

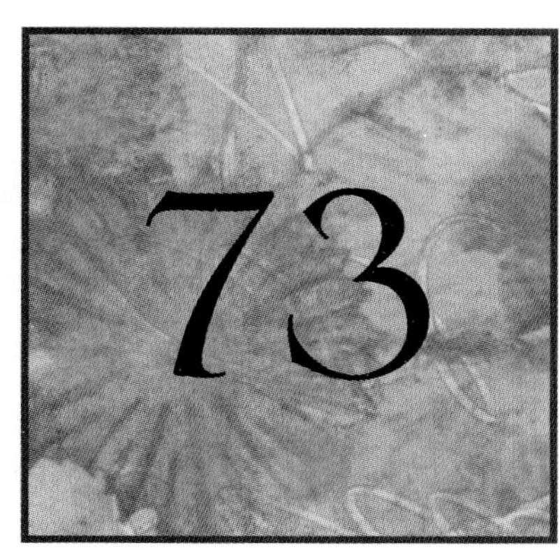

CHAPTER

CHAPTER OUTLINE

Despite the long-term predictability of osseointegrated implants,[1,3,11] biologic, biomechanical, and esthetic complications can occur in a small percentage of cases. Pathologic changes of the periimplant tissues can be placed in the general category of *periimplant disease*.[31] Inflammatory changes, which are confined to the soft tissue surrounding an implant, are diagnosed as *periimplant mucositis*.[31] Progressive periimplant bone loss in conjunction with a soft tissue inflammatory lesion is termed *periimplantitis*.[31] Periimplantitis begins at the coronal portion of the implant, while the more apical portion of the implant maintains an osseointegrated status.[24,30,34,55] This means that the implant is not clinically mobile until the late stages when bone loss has progressed to involve the complete implant surface.[19,45] Technical failures can occur in a small percentage of cases in the form of implant, abutment, and screw fractures and loosening of fixation screws. Esthetic complications may occur in patients with high esthetic expectations and less than optimal implant placement and restorative treatment results.

The invaluable help of Dr. Karl Donath, University of Hamburg, Department of Oral Pathology, Germany, with the histologic aspects of this chapter is gratefully acknowledged.

INCIDENCE

Few studies have reported the frequency of occurrence of periimplant disease.[16,21,52,57,58,63,64] Most long-term studies present an average of the marginal bone loss around implants, and therefore individual implant sites with periimplant disease are not reported.[1] It is important to note that mean crestal bone around an implant decreases 0.9 to 1.6 mm during the first year of implant function. In the follow-up period, mean annual rates of bone loss decrease to 0.05 to 0.13 mm.[1,3,11]

Recent clinical data showed that after a period of implant function, bone loss around implants can develop and even progress to levels at which the implant is at risk for failure. Implant designs and surface characteristics can influence the amount of periimplant marginal bone loss.[22,48] Under experimental periimplantitis conditions, the character of the implant surface influenced the amount of periimplant tissue breakdown.[22]

Titanium plasma-sprayed (TPS)-coated implants (TPS-screw) in a clinical retrospective study demonstrated periimplant bone loss exceeding 4 mm in 4% to 15% and probing depth exceeding 5 mm in 5% to 20% of the implants.[52]

Machined titanium implants (Branemark) showed in a 2-year follow-up study on maxillary overdentures that 6% had a partial marginal radiolucency, but the amount of bone loss in millimeters was not reported.[57]

TPS International Team for Oral Implantology (ITI)-implants demonstrated a mean radiographic change in periimplant bone levels of less than 1.1 mm in the first year of function.[64] However, the percentages of implant sites with bone level changes of more than 0.5 mm between years 1 and 2 was 7% and bone level changes of more then 1 mm were 4%.

Hydroxyapatite (HA)-coated implants showed a significant number of implants experiencing moderate (1 to 3 mm) bone loss, whereas a smaller number of implants demonstrated severe bone loss.[16] Further data is necessary because case reports have been published demonstrating an alarming amount of bone loss. Thus the overall frequency of periimplantitis appears to be in the range of 5% to 10%.

Implants with a smooth coronal titanium neck and nonsplinted maxillary implants have shown increased

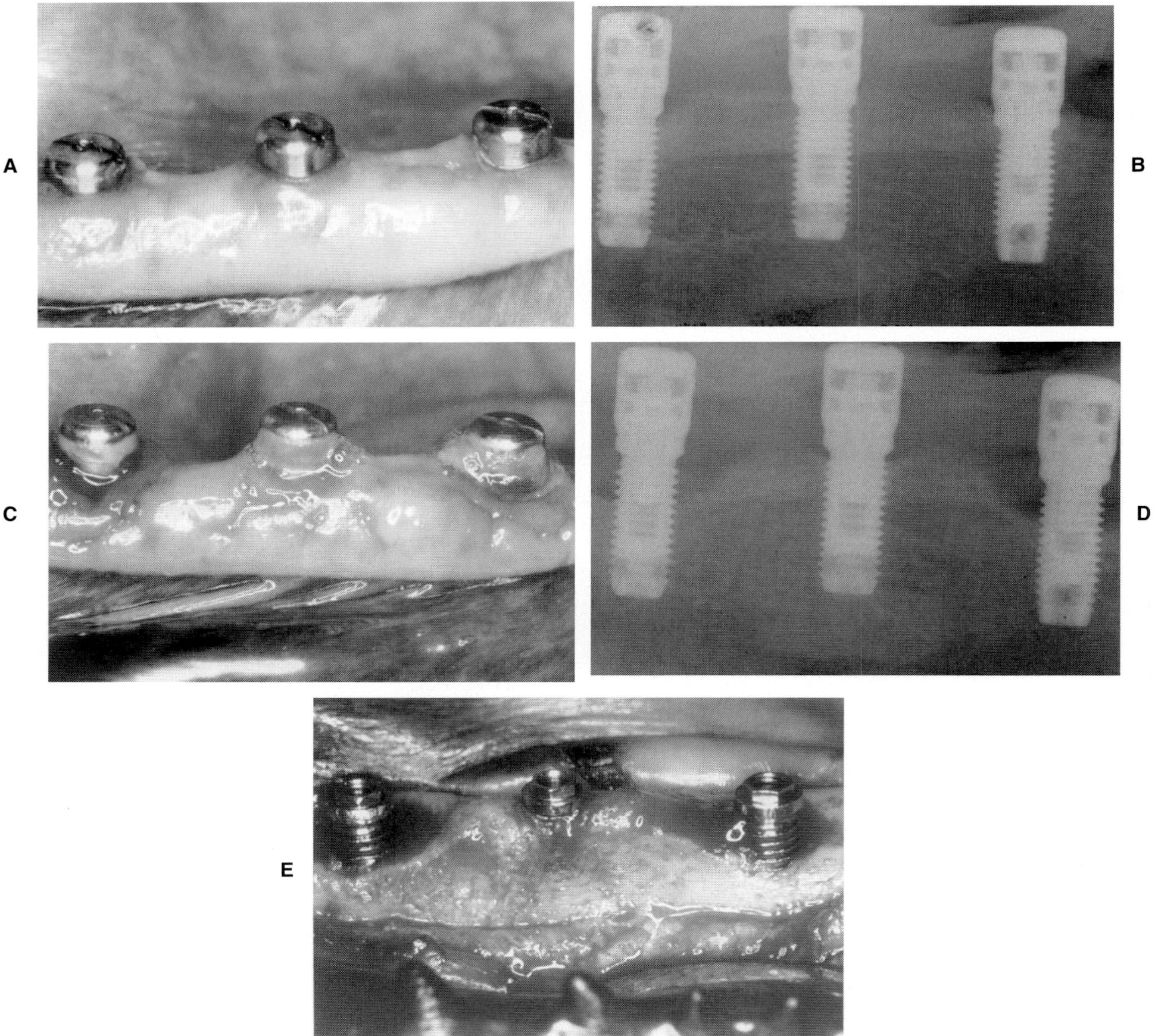

Fig. 73-1 Experimental periimplantitis in beagle dogs. Clinical picture **(A)** and radiograph **(B)** of three Branemark implants in place, 6 months after abutment connection. **C to E,** Six months after placement of a ligature to induce plaque accumulation in implants at left and at right; the middle implant represents a nonligated control. **C,** Clinical picture showing inflammatory changes. **D,** Radiograph depicting the resultant bone loss. **E,** Actual bone loss shown after raising a flap.

periimplant bone loss during the functional phase.[48] This bone loss is attributed to the nonfunctional characteristic of smooth or polished titanium, which does not maintain bone integration during the loading period. Nonsplinted implants are at risk for overloading, especially in the maxilla and in sites with high stress zones and few implants.

Soft tissue complications such as periimplant mucositis and hyperplasia were noted in 21% to 28% of the jaws during the first period of clinical experience with osseointegration[63] but decreased to a low degree in recent years. The improvement was attributed to improved oral hygiene methods and changes in prosthetic designs.

Depending on the severity of the periimplant bone loss, morphology of the bone defect, and implant surface, there is the potential to arrest the progression of the disease process, and in selected cases, to regenerate the lost bone tissue.

Patients with a history of periodontitis may represent a group of individuals with an elevated risk of developing periimplantitis. This view is based on the evident susceptibility to periodontitis, and the potential for transmission of periodontal pathogens from teeth to implants.[39]

ETIOLOGY

The two major etiologic factors associated with resorption of crestal periimplant bone tissue are bacterial infection and biomechanical factors associated with an overloaded implant site.[27,44]

Bacterial Infection

If plaque accumulates on the implant surface, the subepithelial connective tissue becomes infiltrated by large number of inflammatory cells and the epithelium appears ulcerated and loosely adherent. When the plaque front continues to migrate apically, the clinical and radiographic signs of tissue destruction are seen around both implants and teeth (Fig. 73-1); however, the size of the soft tissue inflammatory lesion and the bone loss is larger around implants. In addition, the implant lesions extend into the supracrestal connective tissue and approximate/populate the bone marrow (Fig. 73-2) while the lesions associated with teeth do not. These studies suggest that plaque-associated soft tissue inflammation around implants may have more serious implications than marginal inflammation around teeth with a periodontal ligament (Fig. 73-3). One reason for the increased inflammation around an implant might be the low-vascularity soft tissue band and the difference in collagen/fibroblast ratio of gingival tissue, which affects the defense mechanisms around an implant as compared with those seen in tissues around teeth with a periodontal ligament.[24,34,55] In addition, different implant surface characteristics influence the amount of periimplant tissue breakdown and inflammation; specifically, HA-coated implants seem to have increased bone loss when compared with titanium implants (Fig. 73-4).[16,21,22]

Subgingival bacterial flora associated with clinically inflamed implant sites is quite different to that seen around "healthy" implants. These microbial shifts are very similar to those occurring around natural teeth, and

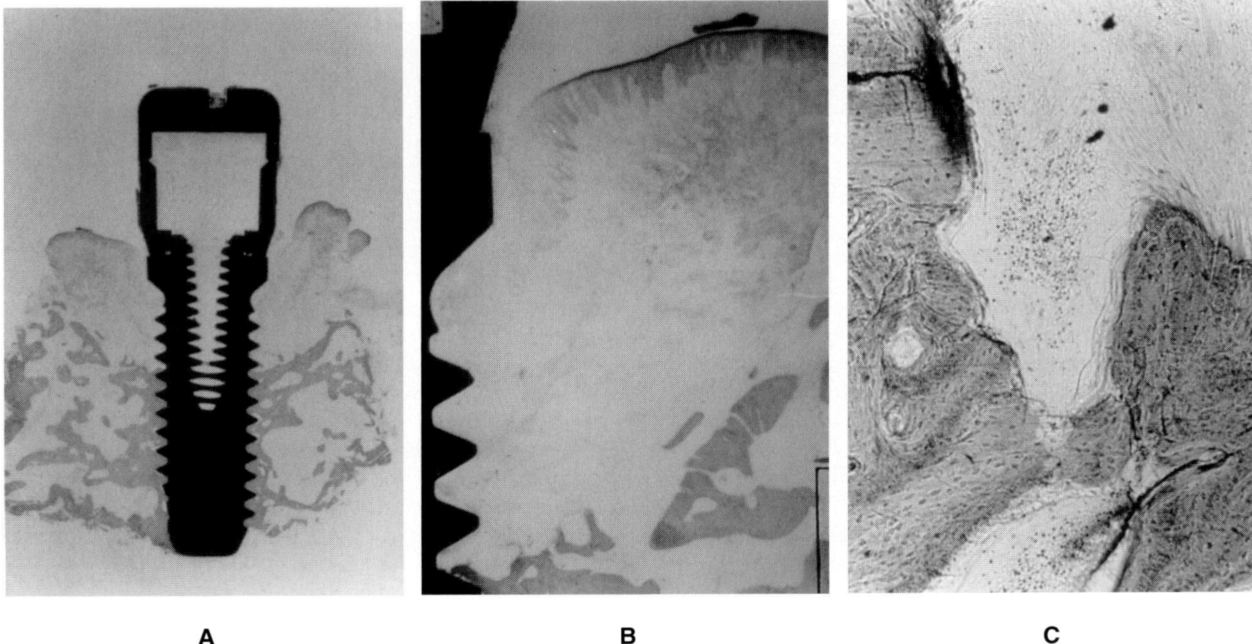

Fig. 73-2 Microscopic view of experimental periimplantitis in a beagle dog. **A,** Low-power view of the implant in situ, showing vertical bone loss. Note that osseointegration persists in deeper portions of the implant. **B,** Higher-power view of the area of bone loss next to the implant. **C,** Higher-power view showing extension of inflammation into bone.

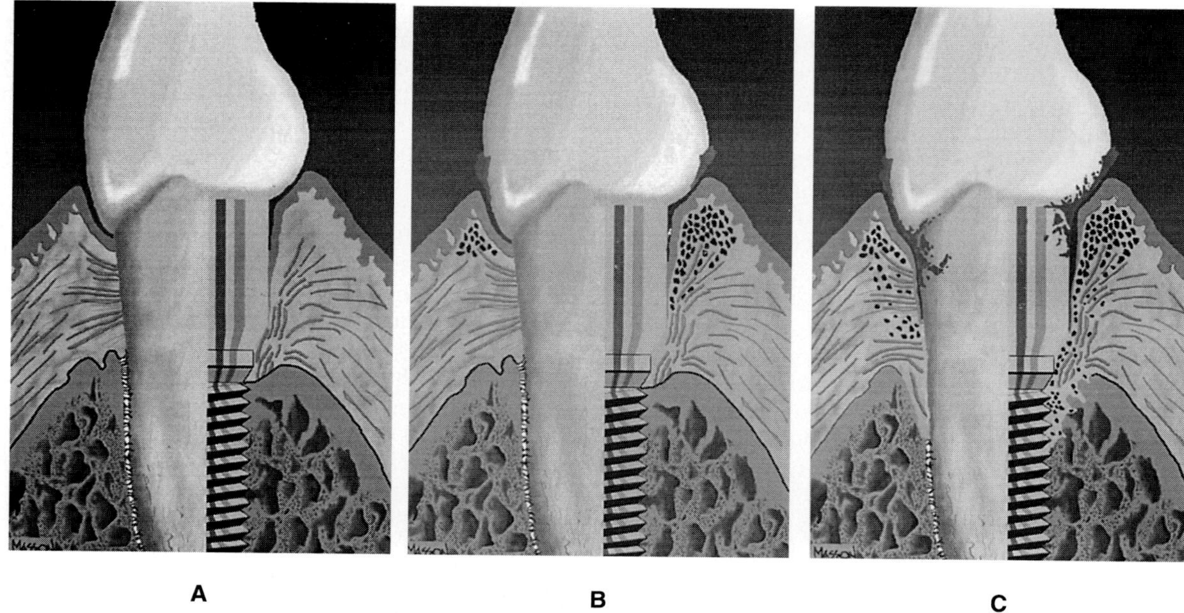

Fig. 73-3 Diagrammatic representation of periodontitis *(left)* and periimplantitis *(right)*. **A,** Normal tissues. **B,** Initial inflammatory involvement of soft tissues, representing gingivitis and mucositis stage. **C,** Destruction of supporting structures.

no bacterial flora in chronic periodontitis and periimplantitis seem to have great similarities.[7,23,33,40,42,50]

It is possible that these organisms are the direct cause of the periimplant breakdown, but proof is not available. Nevertheless, a subepithelial inflammatory response occurs and undoubtedly plays a role in continuing the inflammatory changes that cause this breakdown to progress.[24,28,30,55] A marked difference has been documented between the bacterial morphotypes of the totally edentulous and the partially edentulous mouth.[4,46] The so-called periodontal pathogens were decreased in the implant sulci of the totally edentulous mouth. This might indicate a higher susceptibility for periimplantitis in the partially edentulous mouth.

Biomechanical Factors

Experimental and clinical evidence supports the concept that excessive biomechanical forces may lead to high stress or microfractures in the coronal bone-to-implant contact and thus lead to loss of osseointegration around the neck of the implant.[17,34,48,53,61] Although overload is clinically difficult to define and measure, the role of overloading is likely to increase in four clinical situations:

1. The implant is placed in poor quality bone.
2. The implant's position or the total amount of implants placed does not favor ideal load transmission over the implant surface.
3. The patient has a pattern of heavy occlusal function associated with parafunction.
4. The prosthetic superstructure does not fit the implants precisely.

It is important to note that the cause for periimplant crestal bone loss can be multifactorial and that both bacterial infection and biomechanical factors can be contributing factors. Each factor should be identified and eliminated before treatment of the implant site is initiated. Other etiologic factors such as traumatic surgical techniques, smoking, inadequate amount of host bone resulting in an exposed implant surface at the time of placement, and a compromised host response can act as co-factors in the development of periimplant disease.

TECHNICAL IMPLANT FAILURES

In clinical reality, fatigue of implant materials, weakness in prosthetic design and dimensions, and other factors may result in implant fractures.[1,6] Balshi listed three categories of causes that may explain implant fractures: design and material, nonpassive fit of the prosthetic framework, and physiologic or biomechanical overload.[6]

Fractures may occur in a few cases out of thousands of patients treated with oral implants and cannot completely be avoided. The occurrence of implant fractures can be kept to a minimum through the use of quality controlled implant designs and the consideration of physical principles and biomechanical characteristics of various materials and prosthesis design. Patients with bruxism seem to be at higher risk for such events and therefore need to be screened and informed accordingly.[5,6]

Abutment Loosening and Fracture

Screw loosening has been reported to occur quite frequently in screw-retained fixed partial dentures. Screw-

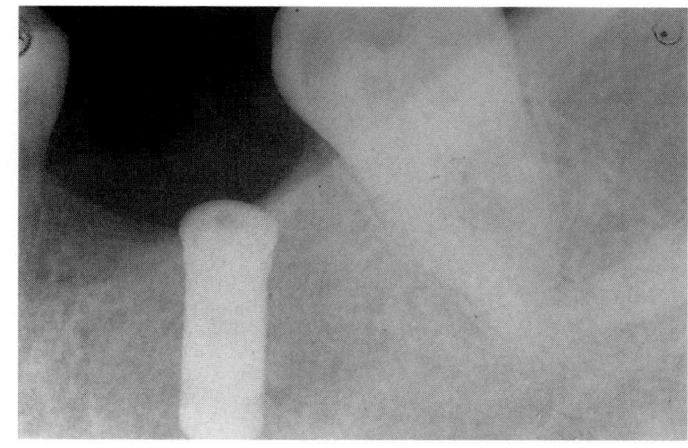

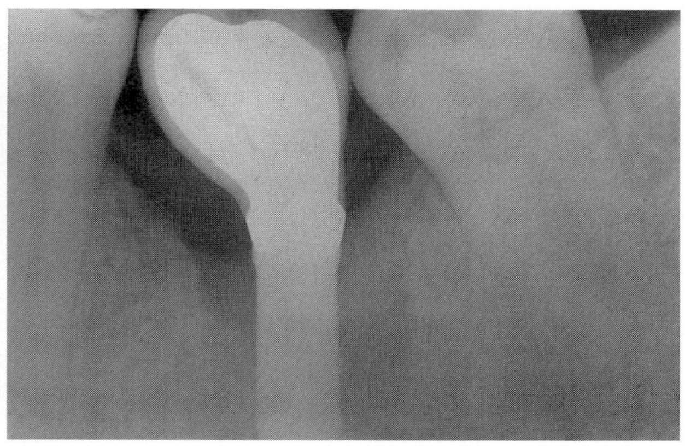

Fig. 73-4 Rapid destruction of bone after placement of an implant. **A,** Normal supporting tissues after placement of the implant. **B,** Advanced bone loss 12 months later.

retained single crowns may also be prone to technical complications. Reports have shown anywhere from 6% to 49% screw loosening at the first annual check-up.[20,41] Newer abutment designs and higher torque levels used to insert abutment screws have helped reduce the rate of screw loosenings.

Abutment screw fractures are less frequent but remain clinical hazards that are not always easily resolved. If the fractured abutment is buried within the internal threads of the implant, it may be impossible to retrieve the screw. Such an implant may then be left buried beneath the mucosa. In some instances, screw retrieval sets can be used successfully to salvage implants with deep broken fragments.

It is important to note that any of the previously mentioned technical implant failures are caused by stress and should be addressed at an early stage of onset.

Esthetic Complications

Implant placement in the esthetic zone requires precise three-dimensional tissue reconstruction and ideal implant placement. This reconstructive procedure enables the restorative dentist to develop a natural emergence profile of the implant crown. If the amount of available bone does not allow for ideal implant placement and the implant is positioned too apical, buccal, or interproximal, a prosthetic profile will be developed with unesthetic dimensions. The same is true if a bone reconstruction procedure shows a compromised result and the implant is still placed but in an inappropriate position.

If crown form, dimension, shape, and gingival harmony around the implants are not ideal, the patients consider the implants/restorations as complications because the result does not represent a natural profile. Often these implants need to be removed, the case reevaluated, and if possible, retreated.

Appropriate treatment planning and execution keeps esthetic complications to a minimum, although it should be noted that anterior implant work is very technique sensitive and time consuming.

DIAGNOSIS OF PERIIMPLANT TISSUE BREAKDOWN

A number of clinical parameters used to evaluate periodontal conditions have also been used to assess periimplant conditions. These parameters include the evaluation of oral hygiene, periimplant marginal tissues, and bone-implant interface.

Successful implants generally allow probe penetration of approximately 3 to 4 mm, and the location of the periimplant bone level can be expected to be about 1 mm apical to the position of the probe tip.

The long-term success of dental implants depends on the continued health of periimplant hard and soft tissues and an appropriate force distribution to the implants.[44,51] Soft tissue health should be established by obtaining a high level of patient compliance for plaque removal and having a prosthesis design that follows perioprosthetic guidelines.

The rationale to prefer attached, masticatory mucosa surrounding an implant, especially in the partially edentulous mouth, is based on the different microbial composition between the partially and totally edentulous mouth, the risk for bacterial seeding from adjacent periodontal pockets, the weak soft tissue adherence around the perigingival area of an implant, and the increased inflammatory response around implants undergoing bacterial infection.[4,8,12,24,34,46]

Radiographs reveal the periimplant bone status as well as the marginal bone level. Periapical intraoral radiographs should be obtained because panoramic radiographs have a lower discrimination power. Baseline radiographs should be taken at functional loading (i.e., insertion of the prosthesis). Direct digital imaging may have the potential to replace conventional radiology.

Biomechanical forces on implants are influenced by an adequate number of implants, favorable implant positions for load distribution, and the establishment of an appropriate occlusion.[51,53]

To diagnose a compromised implant site, soft tissue measurements using manual or automated probes have

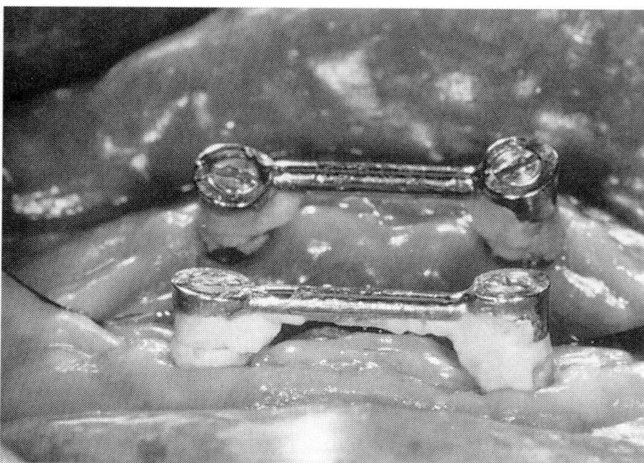

Fig. 73-5 Plaque and debris accumulation around implants, with resultant inflammation.

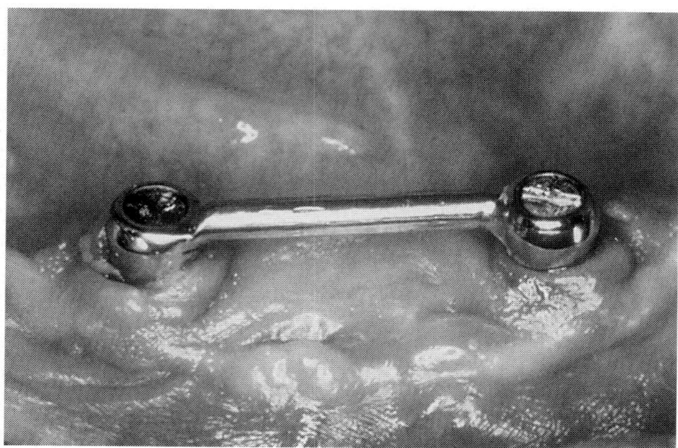

Fig. 73-6 Periimplant disease, resulting in soft tissue swelling and inflammation.

been suggested. Although some reports say that probing is contraindicated, careful monitoring of probing depth and clinical attachment level over time seems useful in detecting changes of the periimplant tissue.[13,52,61,62] Radiographic procedures to assess perimplant bone level have been shown to be useful. Standardized radiography, both with and without computerized analysis, have been documented in a number of studies (see Fig. 73-4).[1,9,11,24,52]

Aside from pocket formation and radiographic bone destruction, suppuration, calculus build-up (Fig. 73-5), swelling (Fig. 73-6), color changes, and bleeding upon gentle probing have been documented as signs of periimplant disease.[40,44]

Mobility has been extensively described to detect early and late failures after loading of the implants with the superstructure.[1,44,48] However, mobility should only be used as an absolute diagnostic information for lack of osseointegration. The current electronic diagnostic tools for measuring mobility are not sensitive enough to detect mobility changes in osseointegrated implants undergoing marginal bone loss.

Microbial monitoring is useful in evaluating the periimplant health condition and the microbial composition of a periimplantitis site. This information then can potentially be used to determine the etiology of the breakdown and select a specific antibiotic regimen.[7,38,44]

REMOVAL OF FAILED IMPLANTS

In cases in which osseointegration has been reduced severely and bone loss has extended into the apical half of the implant, or in which the implant demonstrates mobility, implant removal should be considered (Box 73-1).[3,43] After the implants are removed, the ridge defects can be reconstructed to their original level using bone graft and membrane techniques. This treatment usually enables the clinician to place new implants in a previously compromised situation.

INITIAL PHASE OF PERIIMPLANTITIS TREATMENT

Occlusal Therapy

When excessive forces are considered the main etiologic factor for periimplant bone loss, treatment involves an analysis of the fit of the prosthesis, the number and position of the implants, and an occlusal evaluation. Prostheses design changes, improvement of implant number and position, and occlusal equilibration can contribute to arrest the progression of periimplant tissue breakdown.

Antiinfective Therapy

The nonsurgical treatment of periimplant bacterial infection involves the local removal of plaque deposits with plastic instruments and polishing of all accessible surfaces with pumice[59]; subgingival irrigation of all periimplant pockets with 0.12% chlorhexidine; systemic antimicrobial therapy for 10 consecutive days; and improved patient compliance with oral hygiene until a healthy periimplant site is established.[38,62] As in the treatment of periodontal disease, this initial phase of therapy may be sufficient to reestablish gingival health or may need to be followed by a surgical approach (Box 73-2).

The implant surface is contaminated with soft tissue cells, bacteria, and bacterial byproducts.[24,29,34] Bacterial adherence is enhanced by the microirregularities of implant surfaces,[47] and as long as the contamination is present, wound healing is compromised. Therefore if regeneration of new bone and reosseointegration is to occur, the defect must first be debrided and the contaminated implant surface prepared. *Reosseointegration* can be defined as the growth of new bone in direct contact to the previously contaminated implant surface without an intervening band of organized connective tissue.[25]

For implant surface preparation, mechanical devices and chemotherapeutics have been evaluated in vitro and in vivo.[14,45] Conventional hand and ultrasonic instru-

BOX 73-1

Indications for Implant Removal

Severe periimplant bone loss (>50% of implant length)
Bone loss involving implant vents or holes
Unfavorable advanced bone defect (one wall)
Rapid, severe bone destruction (within 1 year of loading)
Nonsurgical or surgical therapy ineffective
Esthetic area precluding implant surface exposure

BOX 73-2

Indications for Nonsurgical Therapy

Mucosal inflammation detected by clinical signs
Radiographic bone level stable

ments are not suitable for the preparation and detoxification of the implant surface. Mechanical instrumentation may damage the implant surface if performed with metal instruments harder than titanium.[39] The method of choice involves the use of a high-pressure air powder abrasive (mixture of sodium bicarbonate and sterile water). This method removes microbial deposits completely from titanium surfaces, does not change the surface topography significantly, and does not adversely affect cell adhesion.[14,45] There have been some warnings for the potential of air-emphysema when using high pressure air spray instrumentation in the surgical site.[12] Clinical case reports have shown successful treatment of periimplant disease with a protocol for detoxification using an air-powder abrasive.[26,35]

Preparation of the implant surface has also been achieved by applying chemotherapeutic agents. Different agents[15,65,66] have been evaluated for this purpose, and it has been reported that the use of a super saturated solution of citric acid for 30 to 60 seconds has the highest potential for removal of endotoxins from both HA- and titanium-implant surfaces. Clinical case reports have also shown the succesful treatment of periimplant disease using only chemotherapeutic agents as a detoxification protocol.[32,37]

Irradiation with a soft laser for elimination of bacteria associated with periimplantitis has also shown promising results in the destruction of bacterial cells.[22]

SURGICAL TECHNIQUES FOR TREATMENT OF PERIIMPLANTITIS

Once the inflammatory process in the periimplant tissues is under control, an attempt may be made to improve or reestablish osseointegration.

The surgical techniques presently advocated to control periimplant lesions are modified from techniques used to treat bone defects around teeth. The type and size of bone defect has to be identified before deciding on the appropriate treatment modality. Therefore probing and sounding of the defects is done using local anesthesia, and radiographs are evaluated so that the surgical treatment plan is finalized immediately prior to beginning the procedure. This forms the basis to determine whether the implant will be removed or a resective type of surgery or a regenerative procedure will be used. The resective therapy is used to reduce pockets, correct negative osseous architecture and rough implant surfaces, and increase the area of keratinized gingiva if needed. The regenerative therapy is also used to reduce pockets but with the ultimate goal of regeneration of lost bone tissue.

As in the treatment of certain types of periodontitis, systemic antibiotics have been advocated as a supportive regimen during the treatment phase of periimplant disease.[26,32,38] This may be especially important due to the close proximity of the inflammatory lesion to the implant and the bone marrow (see Fig. 73-2, *C*).[24,42] Antibiotics frequently used without sensitivity testing are doxycycline and metronidazole.[26,32,38] If bacterial sensitivity testing is done, the antibiotic regimen is determined by the laboratory result.

Morphology of Osseous Defects

The pattern of bone destruction caused by periimplant disease varies and in general depends on the amount of bone present at the time of implant placement and the length and severity of the pathologic insult. The bone defects can be divided into four main groups.

Group I demonstrates moderate horizontal bone loss with a minimal intrabony component. This group of implants is usually covered by a thin buccal and lingual/palatal bone crest at time of placement and is at an early stage of periimplant breakdown.

Group II presents moderate to severe horizontal bone loss with a minimal intrabony component. This group of implants is an advanced condition of the implants in Group I.

Group III demonstrates minimal to moderate horizontal bone loss with an advanced circumferential intrabony lesion. These implants are initially covered by a thin coronal bone crest with a wider apical bone base. Frequently the pattern of bone loss has a symmetric feature, with a circular trough of uniform width and depth occurring around the circumference of the implant.

Group IV presents more complicated implant defects with moderate horizontal bone loss with an advanced circumferential intrabony lesion; additionally, the buccal and/or lingual plate has been lost (Fig. 73-7). These implants usually demonstrated a thin bone plate at the time of implant placement, which resorbed under the pathologic conditions.

Implant Surface in the Defect Area. The surface of the implant is a source of controversy and might play a role in the choice of treatment. HA-coated implants have clinical and histologic evidence that resorption of the surface by inflammatory phagocytosis is present under the influence of marginal bacterial inflammation (Fig. 73-8).[21,22,29] The treated and detoxified periimplantitis-affected sites show continued phagocytosis of the HA surface.[22] Until further experimental and clinical data are available, a careful and conservative approach should be employed when treating HA-coated implants affected by periimplant disease.

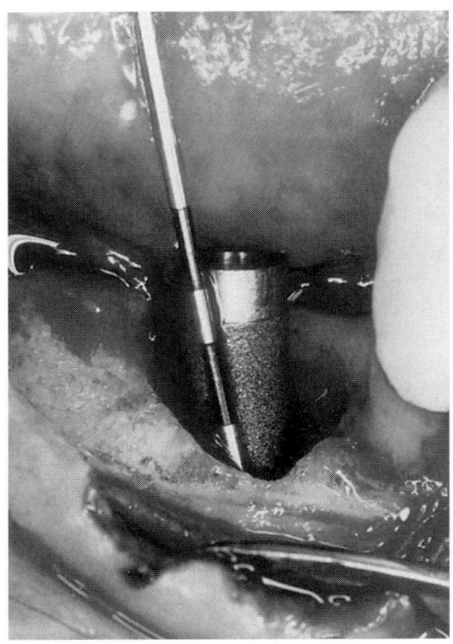

Fig. 73-7 Advanced type IV bone loss around implants.

Titanium implants show little to no resorption of the surface.[24,34] As long as the inflammatory lesion around a titanium implant can be arrested, surgical treatment of selected cases seems indicated.

Periimplant Resective Therapy

The type of osseous defect should be identified before deciding on the treatment modality (Box 73-3). Apically positioned flap techniques and osseous resective therapy are used to correct horizontal bone loss and moderate vertical (≤3 mm) bone defects and reduce overall pocket depth (Fig. 73-9).[27,35,60]

Full-thickness or split-thickness flap management are used to access the surgical area. With the flap raised, degranulation of the osseous defect is performed. Care should be taken to avoid contact between the implant and metal instruments. An implant surface can now be prepared with chemicals and air abrasives. Implant surface preparation is performed by applying the air spray of the air-powder abrasive for a maximum of 60 seconds on the implant surface, followed by copious irrigation with saline solution. Then the application of supersaturated citric acid is applied for 30 seconds, followed again by irrigation with saline solution.

Surface Polishing/Implantoplasty. The long-term goal of the surgical treatment of periimplant breakdown is to arrest the progression of the disease and achieve a maintainable site for the patient. For this purpose, all implant surfaces that are smooth and clean coronal to the bone level are preferred. Therefore surfaces with threads or roughened topography, such as HA, are indicated for alterations with high-speed diamond

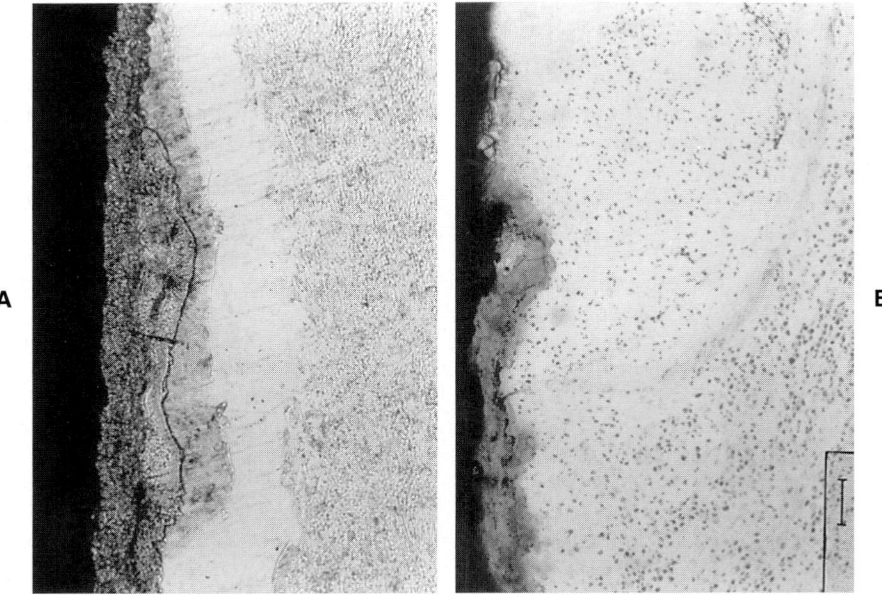

Fig. 73-8 Light microscopic view of resorption of the surface of a HA-coated implant surrounded by inflammatory cells (Toluidine blue stain). **A,** Early stage of calculus buildup on HA surface, showing dense inflammatory infiltrate. **B,** Late stage of inflammation around HA surface, resulting in partial resorption.

burs and polishers to produce a smooth continuous surface (see Fig. 73-9, *B*).[27,35] Copious irrigation for cooling purposes is used while the implant topography is modified. Surface modifications are performed only during a resective type of surgery and not during a regenerative procedure, where the metal particles could interfere with the regeneration of bone tissue. If a rough implant surface or moderate bone defect still exists after a bone regeneration procedure, a reentry surgical procedure after a minimal healing time of 6 months can be performed. During this second surgical intervention, a resective approach with a modification of the implant surface can be applied. Periimplant bone defects with predominately horizontal or one-wall topographies treated with surgical resective techniques result in healthy shallow pockets postsurgery.[62]

Periimplant Regenerative Therapy

An increasing number of reports have shown successful treatment of periimplant bone defects around functioning dental implants.[2,26,27,32,37] To accomplish regeneration of lost bone tissue and reosseointegration, guided bone regeneration (GBR) and bone graft techniques have been suggested.[27,37] In several experimental and clinical studies, the GBR principle using a nonresorbable expanded polytetrafluoroethylene membrane has been used for healing of bone defects seen at the time of implant placement[13,25] and around failing implants.[22,26,32]

Regeneration of bone seems to be enhanced if the area is isolated from the oral environment. Therefore it is recommended to remove the implant prosthesis 4 to 8 weeks prior to the regenerative surgical procedure to allow optimal compliance with oral hygiene procedures and the soft tissue to collapse and heal over the implant site with a newly attached cover screw in place. Thus at the time of regenerative surgery, a more intact soft tissue flap can be helpful to seal off the periimplant tissues during the healing period. A crestal incision is then used for the flap design.

If it is not possible to remove the prosthesis beforehand, a sulcular incision is used to raise a full-thickness flap and evaluate the surgical site. With the flap raised, degranulation of the osseous defect is performed with curettes while extreme care is taken not to contaminate the implant surface.

The surgical therapy includes implant surface preparation by air-powder abrasive for 30 to 60 seconds and the application of an oversaturated citric acid solution for 30 to 60 seconds. Consecutively, an elaborate rinse of the surgical area is performed with saline solution. To achieve increased access of osteogenic cells to the defect, the bone surface is prepared by roughening and penetrations with small round burs.

A membrane is then trimmed to extend 3 to 4 mm beyond the margins of the bone defect and secured with fixation screws. The flap is closed primarily over the site with mattress and interrupted sutures. Care is taken not to have any tension on the flap and therefore periosteal release can be used to advance the flap. Postoperatively the patients are instructed to rinse twice daily for 2 weeks with 0.12% chlorhexidine solution, and a systemic antibiotic is prescribed.[28] The sutures are removed after 14 days. The membrane is left undisturbed, if a submerged condition is maintained, for at least 4 to 6 months (Box 73-4). At that time the membrane is removed and the abutment secured (Color Fig. 73-1). If the membrane becomes exposed before this time, chlorhexidine application is continued to control infection of the healing tissues over the defect. If exudation is present, immediate removal of the membrane is advised. Otherwise, exposed membranes are usually removed 4 weeks after the perforation occurs.

BOX 73-3

Indications for Resective Therapy

Moderate to severe horizontal bone loss
One- and two-wall bone defects
Implant position in unesthetic area

A 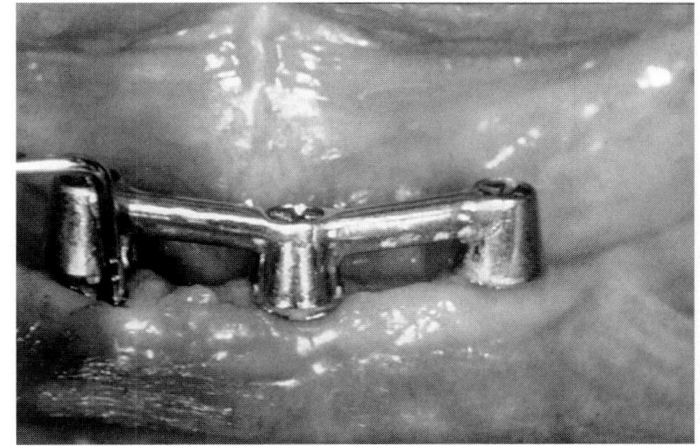

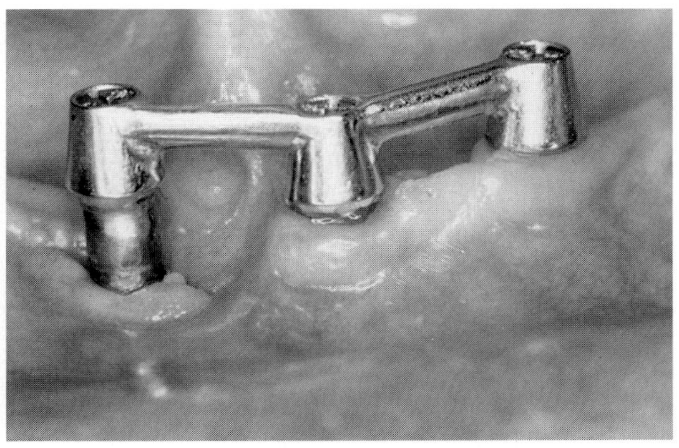 B

Fig. 73-9 Treatment of periimplantitis by resective surgical therapy and implantoplasty. **A,** Before treatment. **B,** After treatment.

BOX 73-4

Indications for Submerged Regenerative Therapy

Implant allowing complete closure with flap
Moderate to severe circumferential intrabony defects
Two- and three-wall bone defects
Detoxification of implant surface possible

BOX 73-5

Indications for Pergingival Regenerative Therapy

One-stage implant or nonretrievable prostheses
Moderate to severe circumferential intrabony defects
Three-wall bone defects
Detoxification of implant surface possible

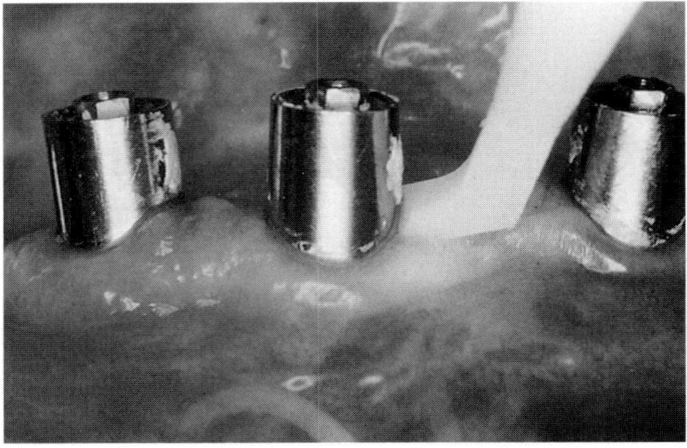

Fig. 73-10 Professional plaque removal around implants as part of maintenance care.

When one-stage implants are treated or the prosthesis has to be maintained in place, a pergingival GBR therapy is applied (Box 73-5). The membrane is perforated with a 3-mm hole and slid over the implant. The membrane should ensure complete coverage and isolation of the vertical bone defect. The flap is then sutured closely to the implant neck.

With a pergingival healing environment present, the removal of membranes has to occur 6 to 8 weeks after surgery. This is necessary due to the accumulation of plaque on the membrane and the potential risk of membrane and periimplant infection. Postoperative maintenance care is the same as for the submerged GBR therapy.

Various *bone graft materials* can be used in conjunction with GBR therapies. Graft materials such as HA demineralized freeze-dried bone, and autogenous bone have been suggested as support for the membrane.

Demineralized freeze-dried bone and HA have been used as a supporting graft material for the membrane therapy, but with inconclusive results.[37,56] The allograft bone undergoes patterns of incorporation similar to those of autografts, but the incorporation tends to be slower and less complete.[56]

Until more supportive results for allografts or synthetic graft materials are demonstrated, the use of intraoral autogenous bone grafts are preferred.[25] These bone grafts have been extensively evaluated in the surgical literature and have shown their potential to be revascularized and eventually to be replaced by the patient's own bone. Furthermore, the bone grafts stabilize the blood clot, support the membrane, and above all, totally exclude disease transmission. The removal of the bone graft brings minimal morbidity to the intraoral donor site, and the surgical cost is minimal. However, remodeling occurs slowly and, depending on the size and quality of the graft, revascularization may require up to 1 year.

A recent study evaluated the use of recombinant human bone morphogenetic protein (rhBMP-2) in experimental periimplantitis sites. Within the newly formed bone, reosseointegration averaged 40% in rhBMP-2 defects as compared with control defects.[18]

Although incomplete surface decontamination seems to be the major obstacle for growth of bone on previously exposed implants, the biologic requirements for direct regrowth of bone still need investigation.

MAINTENANCE

After surgical intervention, all patients are placed on a close recall schedule (Fig. 73-10). It is advised to schedule maintenance visits at least every 3 months. This allows for monitoring of plaque levels, soft tissue inflammation, and changes in the level of the bone. The importance of the maintenance procedures should never be underestimated by either the patient or the therapist.

REFERENCES

1. Adell R, Lekholm U, Rockler B, et al: A 15-year study of osseointegrated implants in the treatment of the edentulous jaw. Int J Oral Surg 1981; 10:387.
2. Adell R, Lekholm U, Branemark PI, et al: Marginal tissue reaction at osseointegrated titanium fixtures. Swed Dent J 1985; 28:175.
3. Albrektsson T, Zarb G, Worthington P, et al: The long-term efficacy of currently used dental implants. A review and prognosis criteria for success. Int J Oral Maxillofac Implants 1986; 1:11.
4. Apse P, Ellen RP, Overall CM, et al: Microbiota and crevicular fluid collagenase activity in the osseointegrated dental implant sulcus: A comparison of sites in edentulous and partially edentulous patients. J Periodont Res 1989; 24:96.
5. Balshi TJ: Preventing and resolving complications with osseointegrates implants. Dent Clin North Am 1989; 33:821.
6. Balshi TJ: An analysis and management of fractured implants: a clinical report. Int J Oral Maxillofac Implants 1996; 11:660.
7. Becker W, Becker BE, Newman MG, et al: Clinical and microbiologic findings that may contribute to dental implant failure. Int J Oral Maxillofac Implants 1980; 5:31.
8. Block M, Kent J: Factors associated with soft and hard-tissue compromise of endosseous implants. J Oral Maxillofac Surg 1990; 48:1160.
9. Bragger U, Burgin W, Fourmousis J, et al: Image processing for the evaluations of dental implants. Dentomaxillofac Radiol 1992; 21:208.

10. Brown FH, Ogletree RC, Houston GD: Pnuemoparotitis associated with the use of an air-powder prophylaxis unit. J Periodontology 1992; 63:642.
11. Buser D, Weber HP, Bragger U, et al: Tissue integration of one stage ITI implants: 3-year results of a longitudinal study with hollow-cylinder and hollow-screw implants. Int J Oral Maxillofac Implants 1991; 6:405.
12. Buser D, Weber HP, Donath K, et al: Soft tissue reactions to non-submerged unloaded titanium implants in beagle dogs. J Periodontol 1992; 63:226.
13. Dahlin C, Sennerby L, Lekholm U, et al: Generation of new bone around titanium implants using a membrane technique: an experimental study in rabbits. Int J Oral Maxillofac Implants 1989; 4:19.
14. Dohm GJ, Stender E, Foitzik CH: Die Reinigung von Implantatoberflachen mit Strahl- und Zahnsteinentfernungsgeraten. Dtsch Z Zahnarztl Implantol 1986; 2:133.
15. Ericsson I, Persson LG, Glanz PO, et al: The effect of antimicrobial therapy on periimplantitis lesions. An experimental study in the dog. Clin Oral Impl Res 1996; 7:320.
16. Golec TS, Krauser JT: Long-term retrospective studies on hydroxyapatite-coated endosteal and subperiosteal implants. Dent Clin North Am 1992; 36:39.
17. Hadeen G, Ismail Y, Garrana H, et al: Three-dimensional finite element stress analysis of Nobelpharma and Core-Vent implants and their supporting structures. J Dent Res 1998; 67:286 [abstract].
18. Hanisch O, Tatakis DN, Boskovic MM, et al: Bone formation and re-osseointegration in periimplantitis defects following surgical implantation of rhBMP-2. Int J Oral Maxillofac Implants 1997; 12:604.
19. James RA: Periodontal considerations in implant dentistry. J Prosth Dent 1973; 30:202.
20. Jemt T: Fixed implant-supported prosthesis in the edentulous maxilla. A five year follow-up report. Clin Oral Impl Res 1994; 5:142.
21. Johnson B: HA-coated dental implants: long term consequences. Calif Dent Assoc J 1992; 20:33.
22. Jovanovic SA, Kenney EB, Carranza FA, et al: The regenerative potential of plaque-induced periimplant bone defects treated by a submerged membrane technique. An experimental study. Int J Oral Maxillofacial Impl 1993; 8:13.
23. Jovanovic SA, James RA, Lessard G: Bacterial morphotypes and PGE_2 levels from the pergingival site of dental implants with intact and compromised bone support. J Dent Res 1988; 67:28 [abstr].
24. Jovanovic SA: Plaque-induced periimplant bone loss in mongrel dogs. A clinical, microbial, radiographic and histological study. University of California, Los Angeles, master's of science thesis, 1994.
25. Jovanovic SA, Spiekermann H, Richter EJ: Bone regeneration on titanium dental implants with dehisced defect sites. A clinical study. Int J Oral Maxillofac Implants 1992; 7:233.
26. Jovanovic SA, Spiekermann H, Richter EJ, et al: Guided tissue regeneration around titanium dental implants. In: Laney WR, Tolmen DE (eds.): Tissue Integration in Oral, Orthopedic and Maxillofacial Reconstruction. Chicago, Quintessence, 1992.
27. Jovanovic SA: The management of periimplant breakdown around functioning osseointegrated dental implants. J Periodontol 1993; 64:1176.
28. Koth DL, McKinney RV, Steflik DE: Microscopic study of hygiene effect on periimplant gingival tissues. J Dent Res 1986; 65:186.
29. Krauser J, Berthold P, Tamery I, et al: A SEM study of failed endosseous root formed dental implants. J Dent Res 1991; 70:274 [abstract].
30. Lang NP, Bragger U, Walther D, et al: Ligature-induced periimplant infection in cynomolgus monkeys. I. Clinical and radiographic findings. Clin Oral Impl Res 1993; 4:2.
31. Lang NP, Karring T: Proceedings of the 1st European Workshop on Periodontology. Chicago, Quintessence, 1994.
32. Lehmann B, Bragger U, Hammerle CHF, et al: Treatment of an early failure according to the principles of guided tissue regeneration. Clin Oral Implant Res 1992; 3:43.
33. Lekholm U, Ericsson I, Adell R, et al: The condition of the soft tissues at tooth and fixture abutments supporting fixed bridges. A microbiological and histological study. J Clin Periodontol 1986; 13:558.
34. Lindhe J, Berglundh T, Ericsson I, et al: Experimental breakdown of periimplant and periodontal tissues. A study in the beagle dog. Clin Oral Implant Res 1992; 3:9.
35. Lindquist LW, Rockler B, Carlsson GE, et al: Bone resorption around fixtures in edentulous patients treated with mandibular fixed tissue-integrated prostheses. J Prosthet Dent 1988; 59:59.
36. Lozada J, James R, Boskovic M, et al: Surgical repair of periimplant defects. J Oral Implant 1990; 16:42.
37. Matarasso S, Quaremba G, Coraggio F, et al: Maintenance of implants: An in vitro study of titanium implant surface modifications subsequent to the application of different prophylaxis procedures. Clin Oral Impl Res 1996; 7:64.
38. Meffert RM: Treatment of the ailing, failing implants. J Calif Dent Assoc 1992; 20:42.
39. Mombelli A, Lang NP: Antimicrobial treatment of periimplant infections. Clin Oral Impl Res 1992; 3:162.
40. Mombelli A, Marxer M, Gaberthuel T, et al: The microbiota of osseointegrated implants in patients with a history of periodontal disease. J Clin Periodontol 1995; 22:124.
41. Mombelli A, Van Oosten M, Schurch E, et al: The microbiota associated with successful or failing osseointegrated titanium implants. Oral Microbiol Immunol 1987; 2:145.
42. Naert I, Quirynen M, van Steenberghe D, et al: A study of 589 consecutive implants supporting complete fixed prosthesis. Part II: Prosthetic aspects. J Prosthet Dent 1992; 68:949.
43. Nakou M, Mikx FH, Oosterwaal PJM, et al: Early microbial colonization of perimucosal implants in edentulous patients. J Dent Res 1987; 66:1654.
44. Nevins M, Mellonig JT: Enhancement of the damaged edentulous ridge to receive dental implants: A combination of allograft and the Gore-Tex membrane. Int J Periodont Rest Dent 1992; 12:97.
45. Newman M, Flemmig T: Periodontal considerations of implants and implant associated microbiota. J Dent Educ 1988; 52:737.
46. Philip L, Parham PL Jr, Charles M, et al: Effects of air-powder abrasive system on plasma-sprayed titanium implant surfaces: An in vitro evaluation. J Oral Implant 1989; 15:78.
47. Quirijnen M, Listgarten MA: The distribution of bacterial morphotypes around natural teeth and titanium implants ad modum Branemark. Clin Implant Res 1990; 1:8.
48. Quirijnen M, Marechal M, Busscher HJ, et al: The influence of surface free energy and surface roughness on early plaque formation. J Clin Periodontol 1990; 17:138.
49. Quirijnen M, Naert I, van Steenberghe D: Fixture design and overload influence marginal bone loss and fixture success in the Branemark system. Clin Oral Impl Res 1992; 3:104.
50. Quirijnen M, van Steenberghe D, Jacobs R, et al: The reliability of pocket probing around screw-type implants. Clin Oral Impl Res 1991; 2:186.
51. Rams TE, Link C: Microbiology of failing dental implants in humans: Electron microscopic observations. J Oral Implant 1983; 11:93.
52. Rangert B, Jemt T, Jorneus L: Forces and moments on Branemark implants. Int J Oral Maxillofac Implants 1989; 4:241.

53. Richter EJ, Jansen V, Spiekermann H, et al: Langzeitergebnisse von IMZ-und TPS-Implantaten im interforaminalen Bereich des zahnlosen Unterkiefers. Dtsch Zahnarztl Z 1992; 47:449.
54. Roberts WE, Garetto LP, de Castro RA: Remodeling of devitalized bone threatens periosteal margin integrity of endosseous titanium implants with treated or smooth surfaces: indications for provisional loading and axilliary directed occlusion. J Indiana Dent Assoc 1989; 68:19.
55. Sanz M, Newman M, Nachnani S, et al: Characterization of the subgingival microbial flora around endosteal dental implants in partially edentulous patients. Int J Oral Maxillofac Implants 1990; 5:247.
56. Schou S, Holmstrup P, Stoltze K, et al: Ligature-induced marginal inflammation around osseointegrated implants and ankylosed teeth. Clinical and radiographic observations in cynomolgus monkeys. Clin Oral Impl Res 1993; 4:12.
57. Simion M, Dahlin C, Trisi P, et al: Qualitative and quantiative comparative study on different filling materials used in bone regeneration. Int J Period Rest Dent 1994; 14:199.
58. Smedberg J-I, Lothigius E, Bodin I, et al: A clinical and radiological two-year follow-up study of maxillary overdentures on osseointegrated implants. Clin Oral Impl Res 1993; 4:39.
59. Smithloff M, Fritz M: The use of blade implants in a population of partially edentulous adults. A 15-year report. J Periodontol 1987; 58:589.
60. Stefani LA: The care and maintenance of the dental implant patient. J Dent Hyg 1988; 62:447.
61. Strub JR: Langzeitprognose von enossalen oralen Implantaten unter spezieller Beruchsichtigung von periimplantaren, materialkundlichen und okklusalen Gesichtspunkten. Habilitationsschriften der ZMK. Berlin, Quintessenz Verlags-GmbH, 1986.
62. Strub JR, Gaberthuel TW, Grunder U: The role of attached gingiva in the health of periimplant tissue in dogs. Part I. Clinical Findings. Int J Perio Rest Dent 1991; 11:317.
63. Thompson-Neal D, Evans G, Meffert R: Effects of various prophylactic treatments on titanium, sapphire, and hydroxyapatite-coated implants: An SEM study. Int J Periodont Restor Dent 1989; 9:301.
64. Tolman DE and Laney WR. Tissue-integrated prosthesis complications. Int J Oral Maxillofac Implants 1992; 7:477.
65. Weber HP, Buser D, Fiorellini JP, et al: Radiographic evaluation of crestal bone levels adjacent to nonsubmerged titanium implants. Clin Oral Impl Res 1992; 3:181.
66. Zablotsky M, Diedrich, D, Meffert R, et al: The ability of various chemotherapeutic agents to detoxify the endotoxin infected HA-coated implant surface. Int J Oral Implant 1991; 8:45.
67. Zablotsky M, Diedrich D, Meffert R: Detoxification of endotoxin-contaminated titanium and hydroxyapatite-coated surfaces utilizing various chemotherapeutic and mechanical modalities. Implant Dent 1992; 1:154.

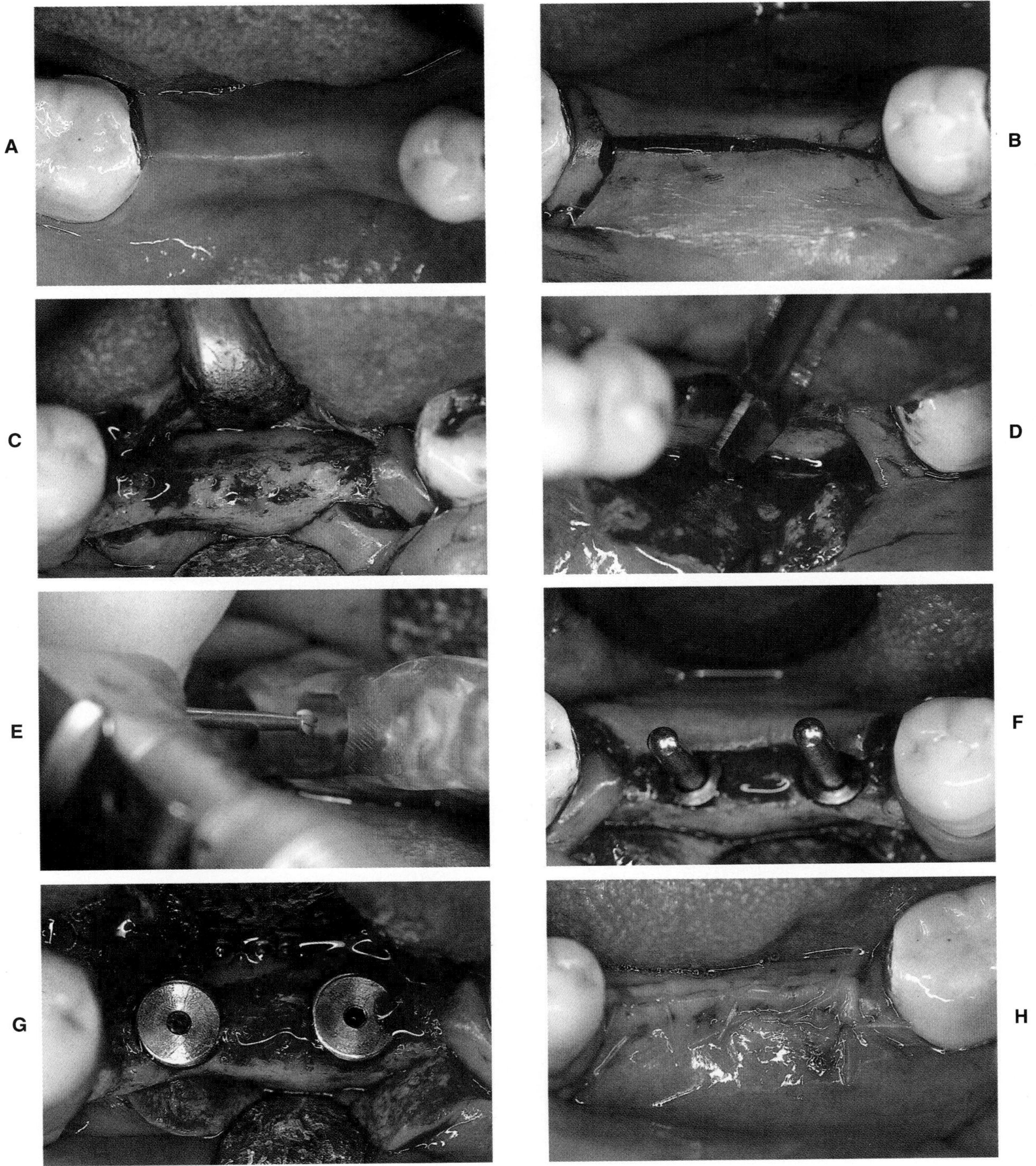

Color Fig. 70-1 First-stage surgery. **A,** A partial edentulous ridge. A presurgical and prosthodontic treatment has been completed. **B,** Mesial and vertical incisions are connected by a crestal incision. Notice that bands of gingival collars remain adjacent to teeth. **C,** Minimal flap reflection is used to expose the alveolar bone. Sometimes a ridge modification is necessary to provide a flap recipient bed. **D,** A buccal flap is partially dissected at the apical portion to provide a flap extension. This is a very critical step to ensure a tension-free closure of the flap after the implant placement. **E,** It is important to use the surgical stent to determine the mesial-distal, buccal-lingual, and proper angulation of the implant placement. **F,** Frequent use of the guide pins ensures the parallelism of the implant placement. **G,** After the placement of two Nobelpharma implants, the cover screws are placed. The cover screws should be flush with the rest of the ridge to minimize the chance of exposure. This is especially important if a partial denture is to be worn during the healing phase. **H,** Suturing completed. Both regular interrupted and inverted mattress sutures are used intermittently to ensure tension-free, tight closure of the flaps.

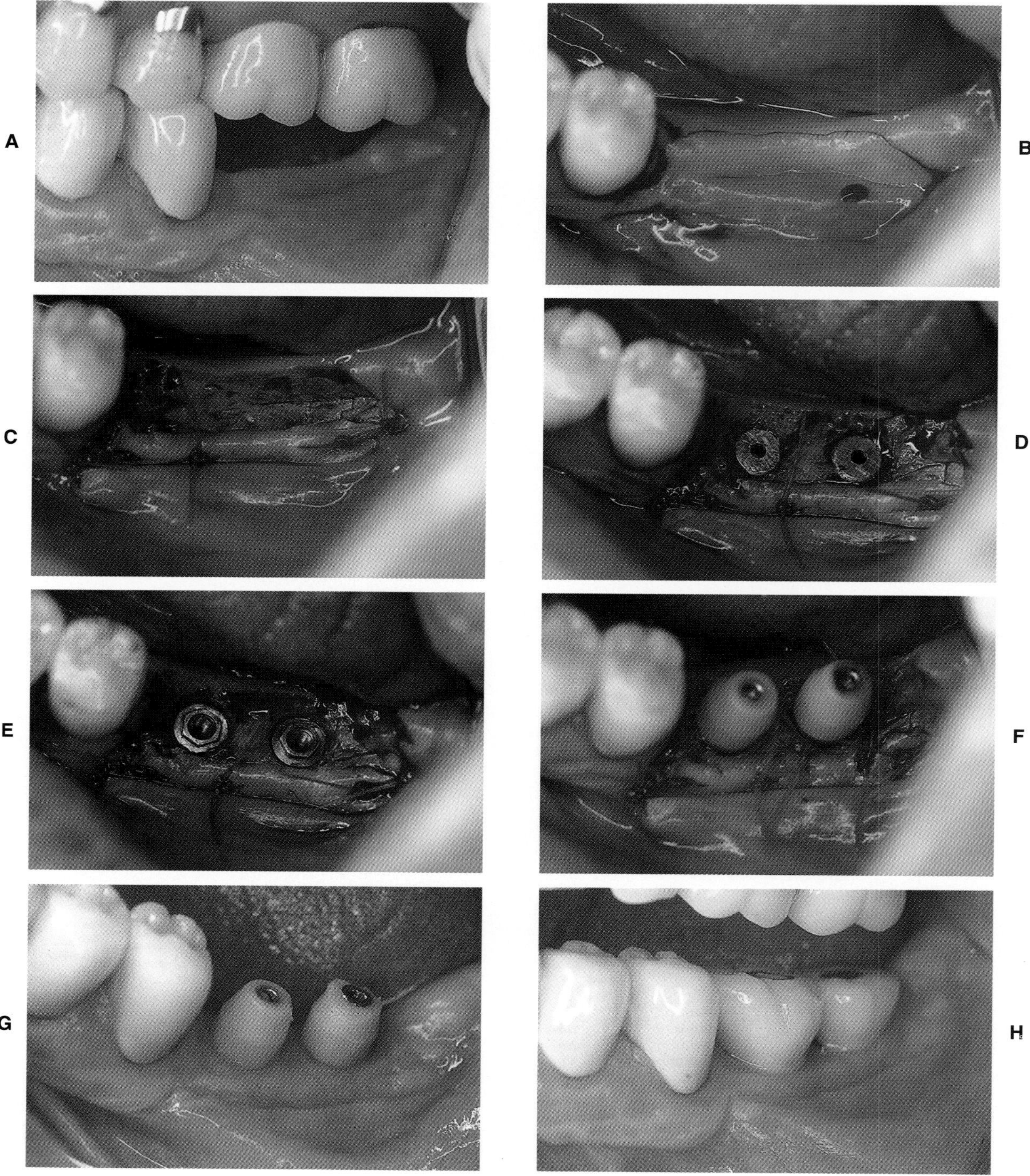

Color Fig. 70-2 Second-stage surgery. **A,** Two endosseous implants were placed 4 months previously and are ready to be exposed. Notice the narrow band of keratinized tissue. **B,** Two vertical incisions are connected by crestal incision. If facial keratinized tissue is insufficient, it is necessary to locate the crestal more lingually so that there is a minimum of 2 to 3 mm of keratinized band. **C,** A buccal partial-thickness flap is sutured to the periosteum apical to the emerging implants. **D,** Gingival tissue coronal to the cover screws is excised using the gingivectomy technique. **E,** The cover screws are removed and the heads of the implants are cleared. **F,** Abutments are placed. Visual inspection ensures intimate contact between the abutments and the implants. **G,** Two- to three-week healing after second-stage surgery. **H,** Four months after the final restoration. Notice the healthy band of keratinized attached gingiva around the implants.

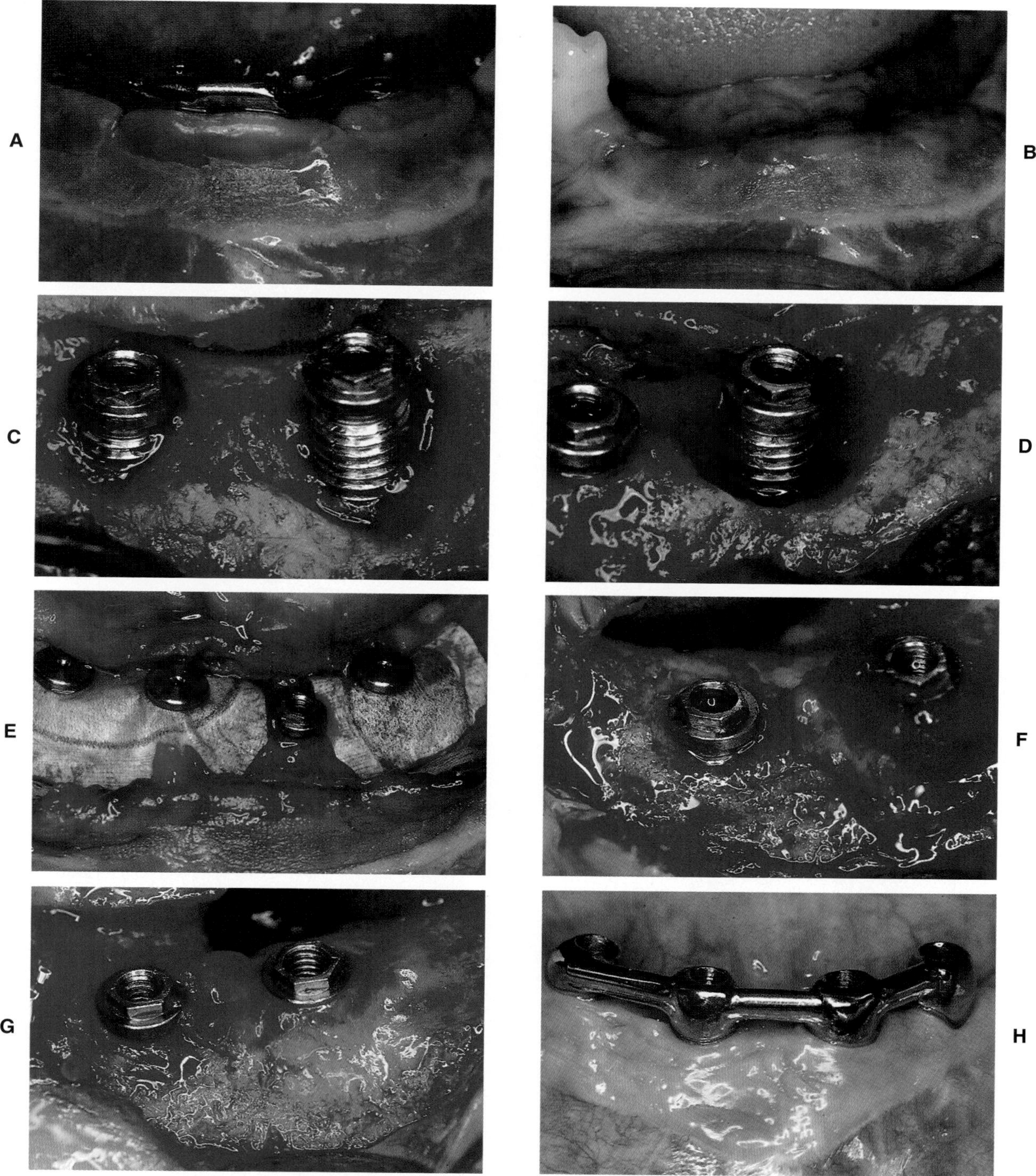

Color Fig. 73-1 Reconstructive treatment of periimplantitis. **A,** Four osseointegrated implants used for retention of an overdenture in an edentulous lower jaw. Moderate to severe periimplantitis, with soft tissue hyperplasia and deep pockets around all implants. There was radiographic evidence of progressive bone loss around three of the four implants. **B,** A submerged regenerative therapy was initiated by removal of the abutments 6 months before surgery, and a 1-week period of systemic antibiotic coverage was instituted. Note the improved soft tissue appearance. **C and D,** Elevated flap, showing bone loss around three of the four implants. The defects consisted of horizontal bone loss and shallow-to-deep circumferential vertical defects around the implants. The defects were carefully degranulated by hand, and the implant surfaces were detoxified with supersaturated citric acid and an air abrasive for 30 to 60 seconds and then flushed with sterile water. Bone surfaces were roughened and penetrated with small, round burs. **E,** Two membranes placed over the periimplant bone defects, allowing a blood clot to form underneath. Note the close adaptation of the membranes to the periphery of the bone defects, acting as a tent over the defects. **F and G,** After an uneventful healing period of 4 months, the surgical sites are exposed and the membranes removed. Note the osseous regeneration in the minimal soft tissue retraction around all implants.

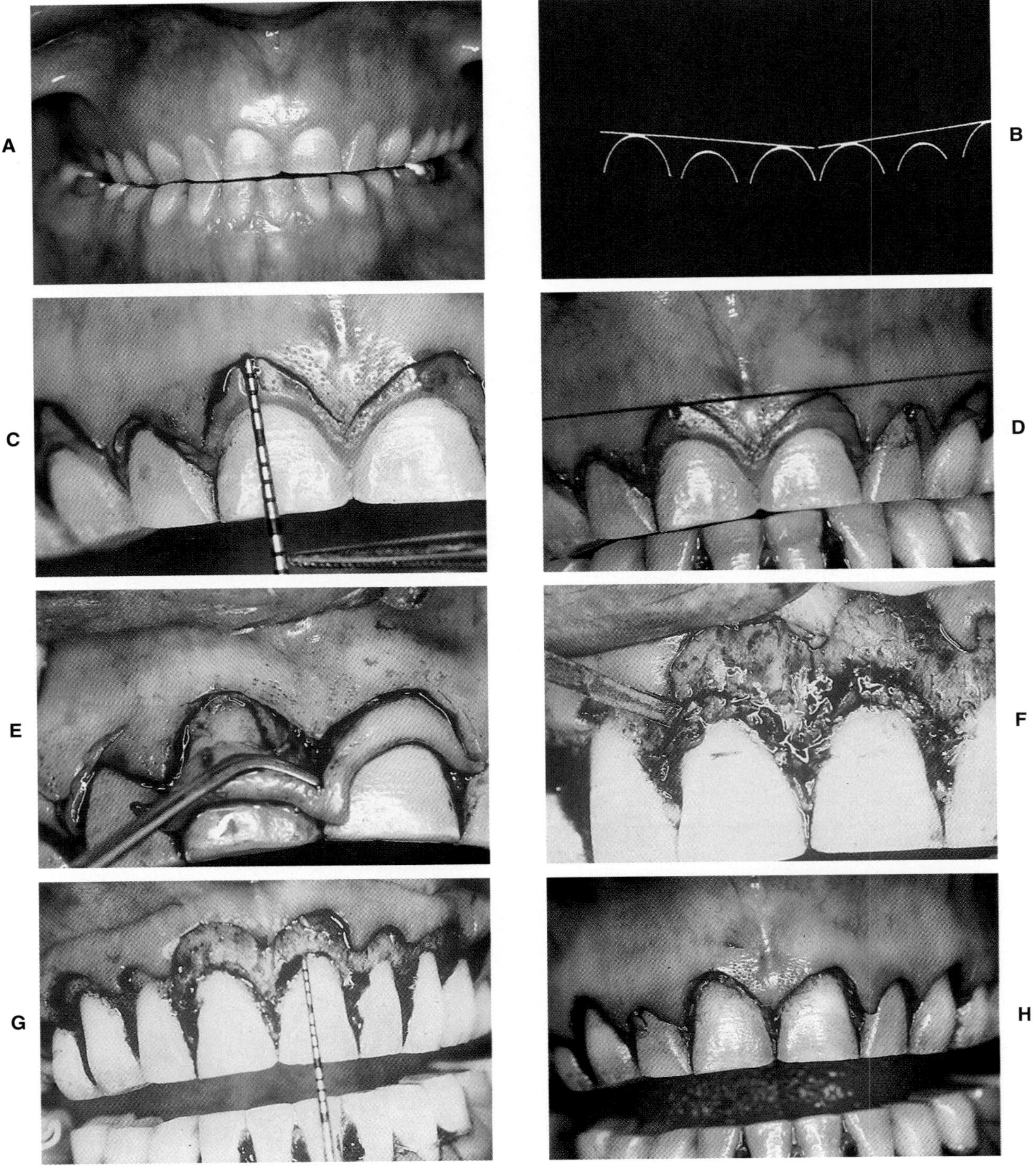

Color Fig. 74-1 Crown lengthening of the maxillary anterior dentition. **A,** Before treatment. Note the short clinical crown that is inadequate for full crown restorations. The facial gingival symmetry is also uneven. The gingival margin of the two lateral incisors is apical to the two cuspids and even with the two central incisors. **B,** The ideal gingival symmetry. The apical gingival margins for the two central incisors and cuspids are even and apical to that of the lateral incisors. **C,** Measurement taken for crown lengthening. **D,** The incision for the flap, following the ideal symmetry. **E,** Removal of tissue prior to flap reflection. **F,** Bone removal with a chisel, following ideal symmetry and measurement. **G,** Measurement taken after bone removal. **H,** The flap positioned for suturing.

Continued

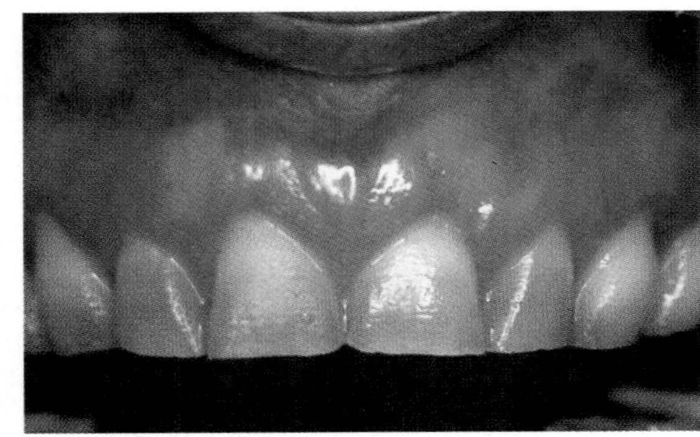

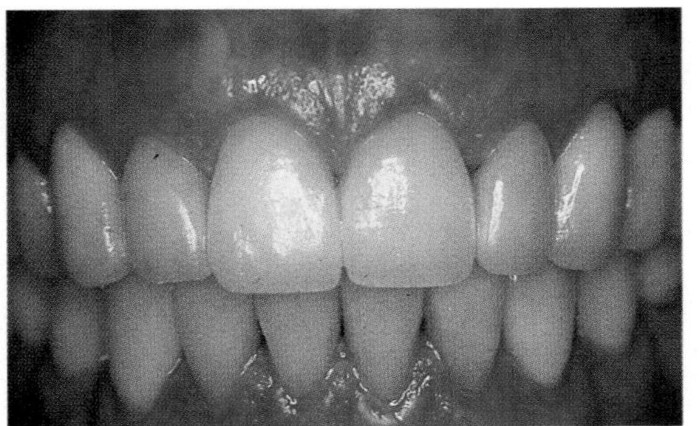

Color Fig. 74-1, cont'd **I,** Healing after 3 months. The crown is ready for restorations. **J,** The final restoration. Note the ideal symmetry.

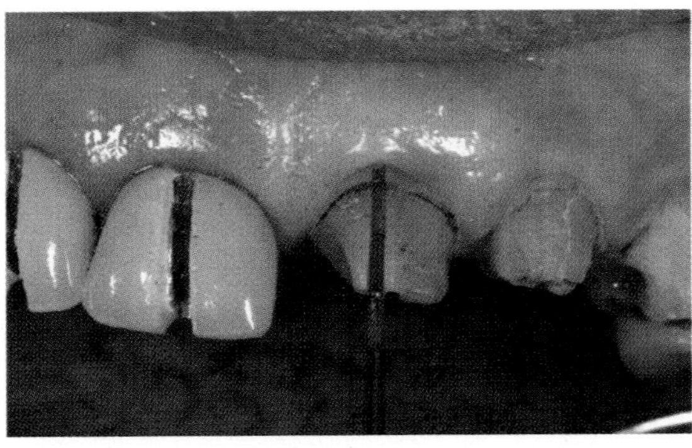

Color Fig. 75-1 Depth from the attachment to the level of the margin is greater than 3 mm. This patient had an altered eruption pattern and a sulcus of more than 3 mm at the time these restorations were placed.

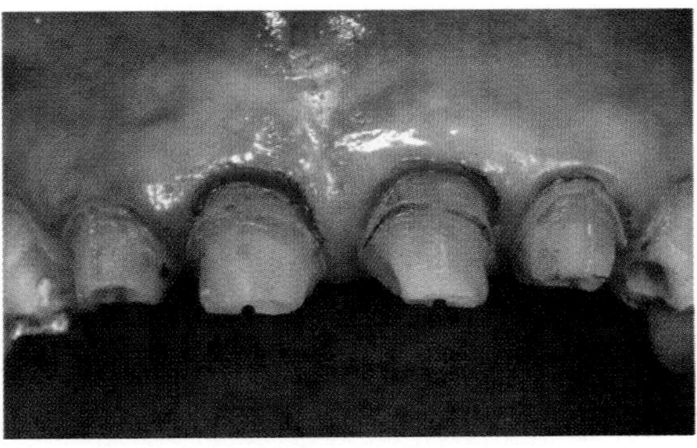

Color Fig. 75-2 Two options were available to appropriately manage treatment: 1) place the original margins half the depth of the sulcus, in which case the recession that occurred would not have exposed them; or 2) perform a gingivectomy, creating a 1- to 1.5-mm sulcus. This was the option chosen when the restorations were redone. The margins were then placed 0.5 mm below tissue after the gingivectomy.

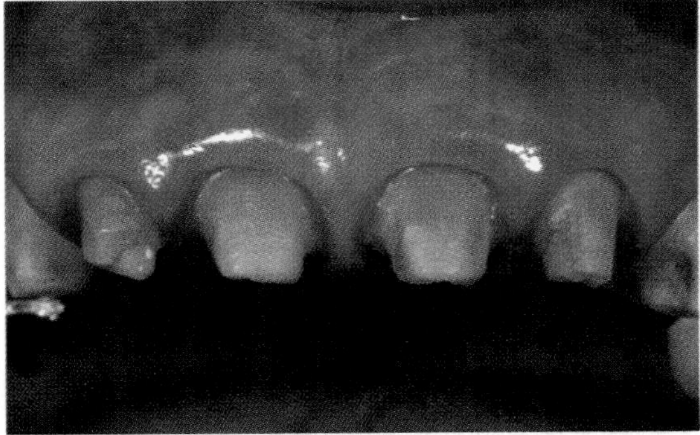

Color Fig. 75-3 At 6 weeks after the gingivectomy and preparation of the teeth. Note the tissue level and that the tissue is rebounding coronally over the margins. This is a common finding when a pure gingivectomy is done.

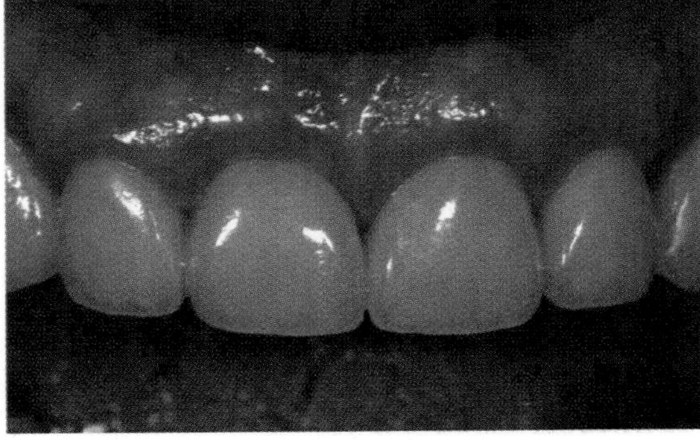

Color Fig. 75-4 A 4-year recall photograph after placement of the final restorations. Note the tissue level has been maintained with a sulcus depth of 2 mm on the facial.

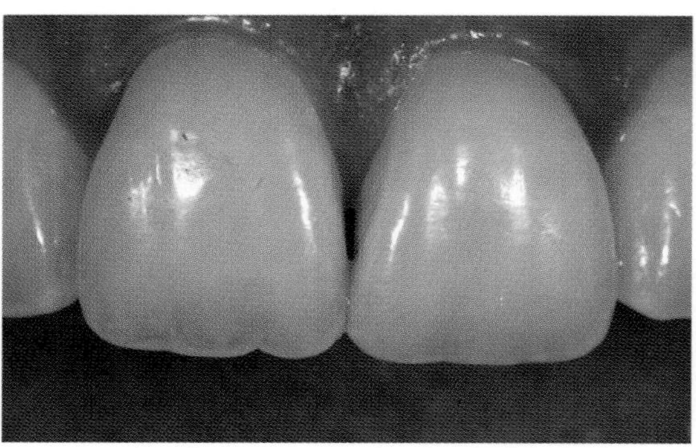

Color Fig. 75-5 This patient has parallel roots, has recently completed orthodontics, and is unhappy with the open gingival embrasure between her centrals. An evaluation of papillary heights finds them all at an equal level. This can only mean that the open embrasure is the result of an overly tapered tooth form.

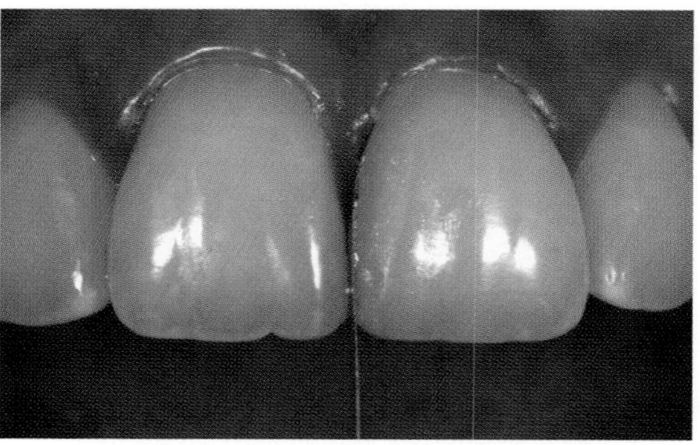

Color Fig. 75-6 One method of correctly altering tooth form. A metal matrix band has been shaped to the desired tooth form and placed 1 to 1.5 mm below the tip of the papilla. Restorative material then was added to the tooth against the matrix band, forming the new mesial surface of the left central incisor.

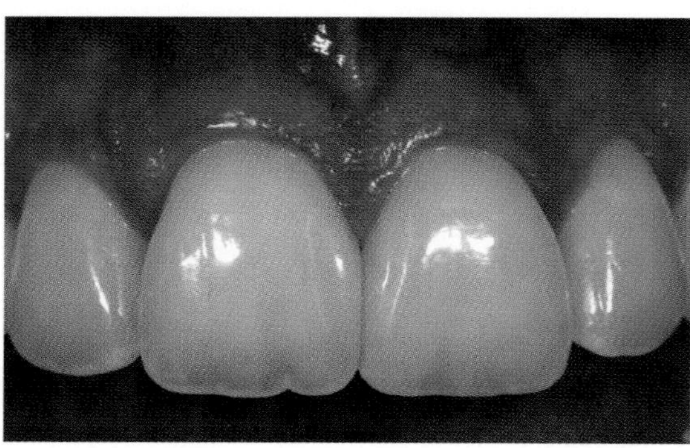

Color Fig. 75-7 A 1-year recall photograph after restoring the mesial surfaces of the right and the left central incisors, moving the contact to the tip of the papilla and carrying the restorations 1 to 1.5 mm below the papilla, blending them into the tooth and making an easily cleaned area.

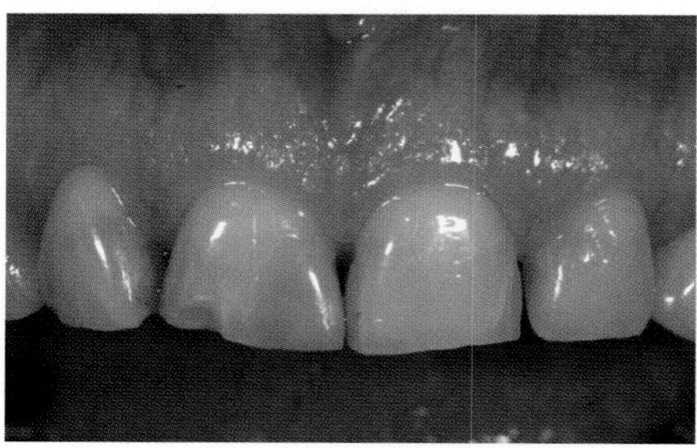

Color Fig. 75-8 A patient who will have the right central incisor extracted due to periodontal disease. The patient is choosing to have a fixed partial denture rather than an implant as the method of replacement. An ovate pontic will be used to maintain the papillary form after the removal of this central incisor.

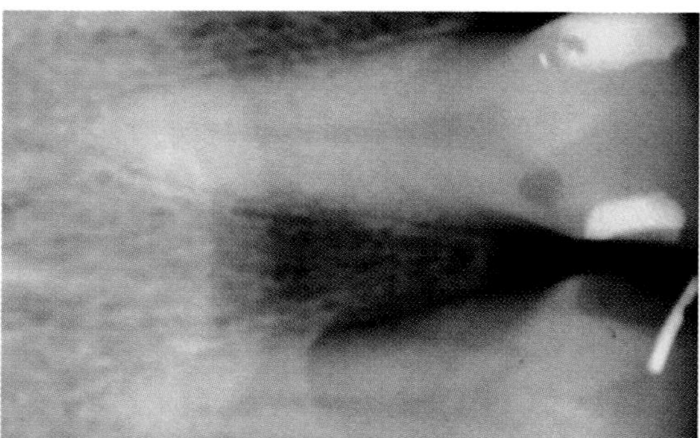

Color Fig. 75-9 Note radiographically the presence of the palatal well due to a deep palatal groove on this right central incisor. Two attempted periodontal surgeries have failed to correct this, and it still probes 10 mm with suppuration.

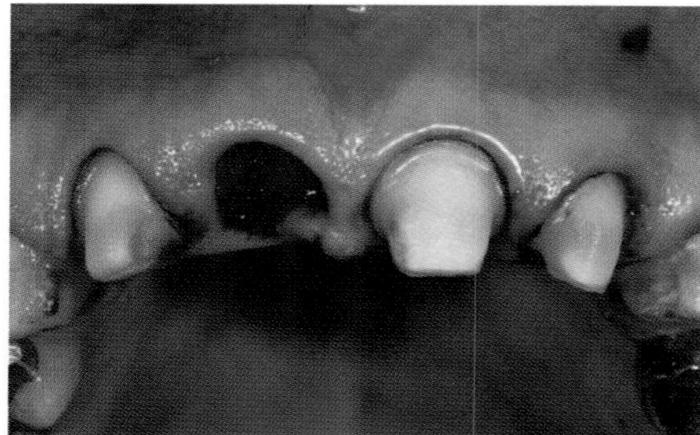

Color Fig. 75-10 Because the patient desired to alter the esthetics of her remaining anterior teeth, all the anterior teeth were prepared before removal of the right central incisor.

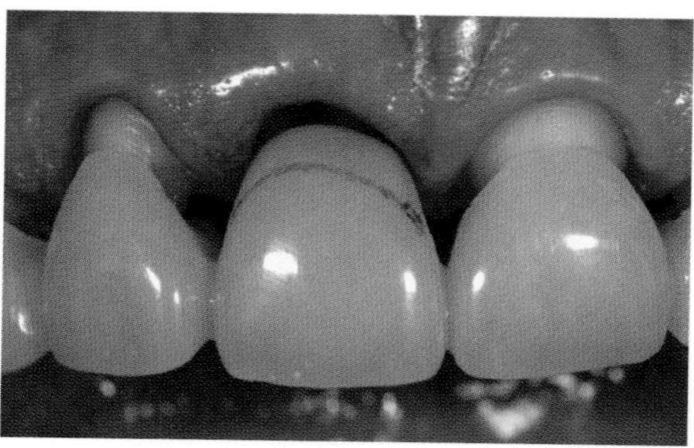

Color Fig. 75-11 The key to maintenance of the interproximal papilla is that the ovate pontic extend 2.5 mm into the extraction site on the day of extraction. This will maintain gingival embrasure form and therefore maintain interproximal papilla height.

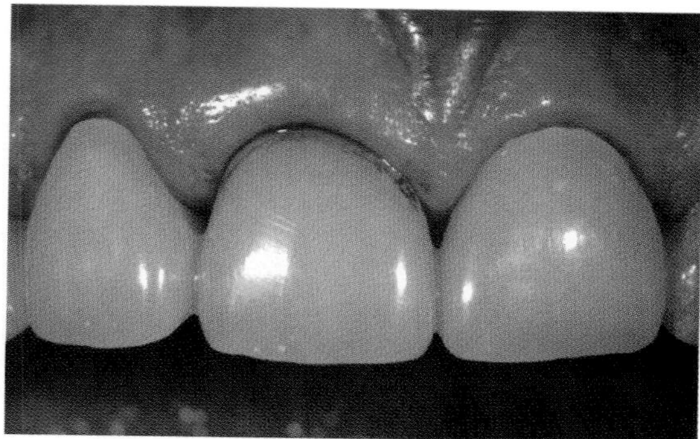

Color Fig. 75-12 Note that when the provisional is seated on the day of extraction, 2.5 mm of temporary extend upward into the extraction socket. Also note the open gingival embrasures present to allow space for the papilla to rebound coronally.

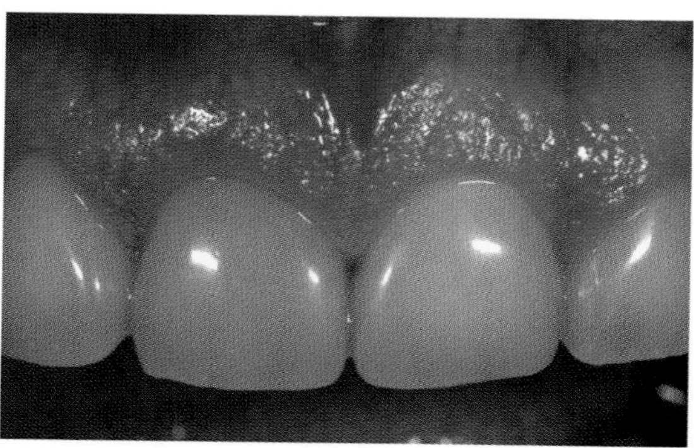

Color Fig. 75-13 9 months after placement of the provisional restoration. At 4 weeks after placement, the pontic was shortened to extend 1.5 mm into the extraction site to facilitate oral hygiene. Note maintenance of papillary form and free gingival margin height, predictable in this patient because she has excellent interproximal and facial bone.

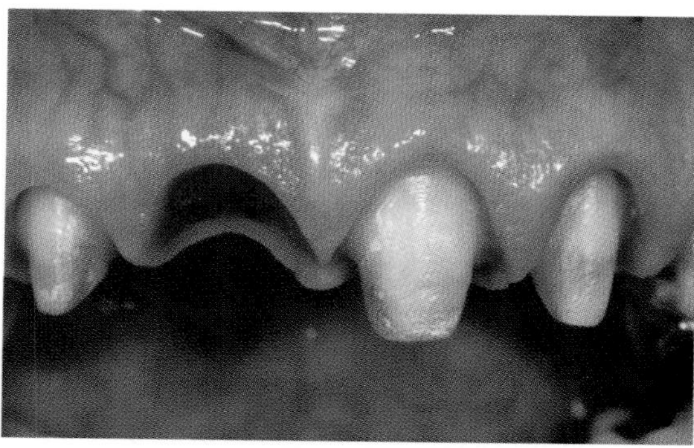

Color Fig. 75-14 The ovate pontic after removal of the provisional and prior to final impressions. Note that papillary form has been maintained because of the ovate pontic maintaining gingival embrasure volume.

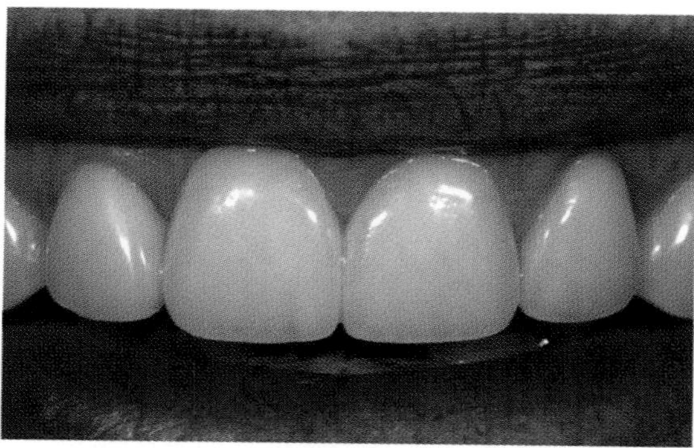

Color Fig. 75-15 A 2-year recall photograph of the final fixed prosthesis. Note how the final ovate pontic also has maintained papillary form.

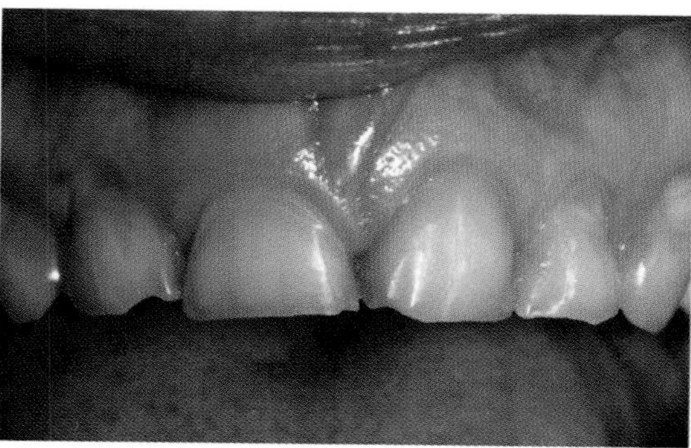

Color Fig. 75-16 A patient who is unhappy with the appearance of her maxillary teeth and the discrepancies of tissue height and tooth form.

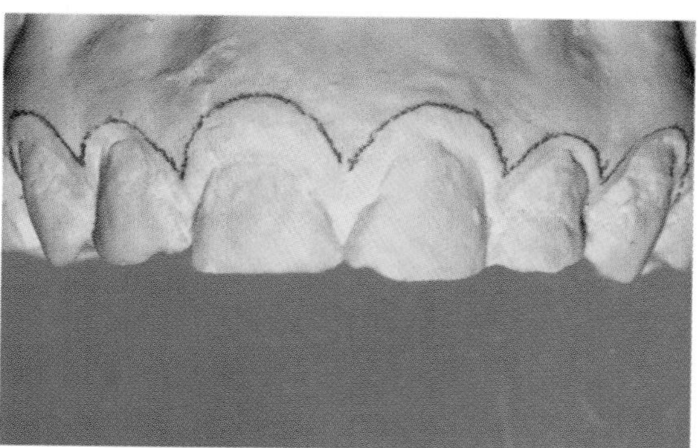

Color Fig. 75-17 To create a surgical guide, a stone model is modified by drawing the desired soft tissue profile with a red wax pencil.

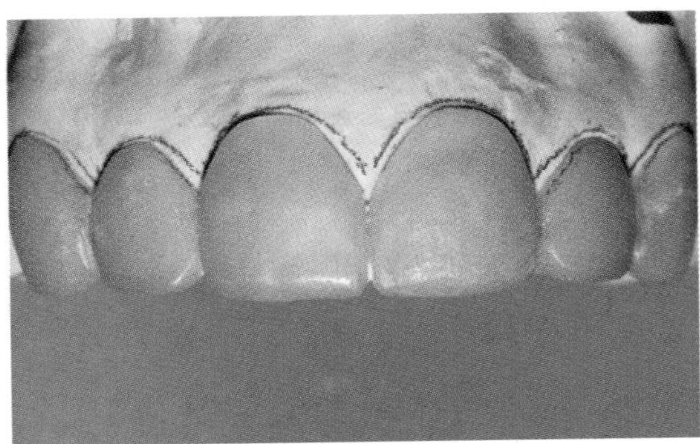

Color Fig. 75-18 A composite resin surgical guide is fabricated on this stone model, extending to the line drawn. This guide can be taken to the mouth for try-in and verification by the patient.

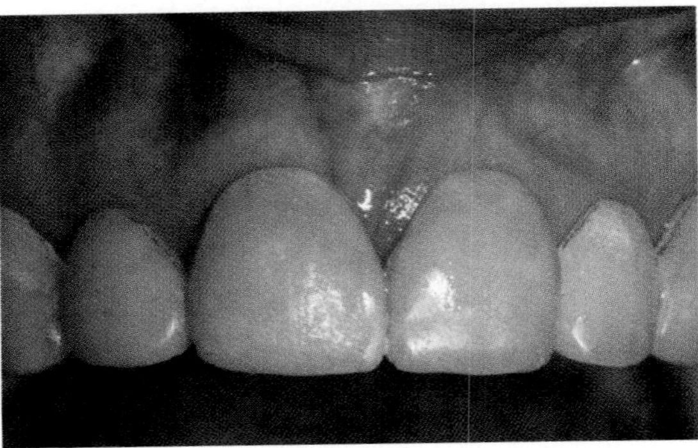

Color Fig. 75-19 A photograph taken the day the surgical guide was tried in. The patient approved the new length of the maxillary anterior teeth and the form created by altering the soft tissue profile.

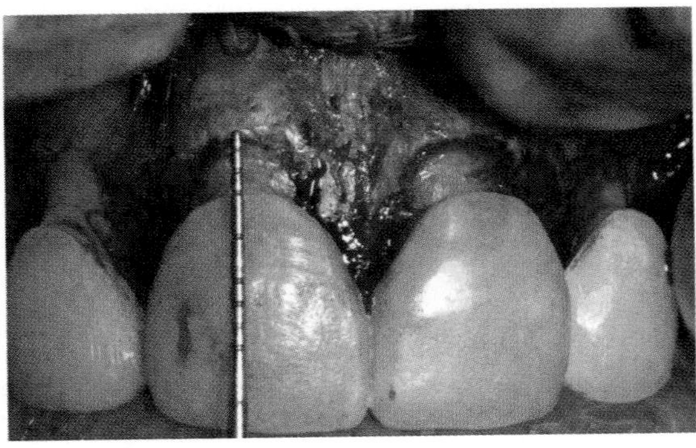

Color Fig. 75-20 By placing the surgical guide during the surgery, it is possible to recognize where the bone needs to be placed. The surgical guide represents the desired final free gingival margin position and can be used as a reference for osseous recontouring. This patient had an average biologic width of 2 mm. Allowing an additional 1 mm for sulcus depth, the desired distance between the bone and free gingival margin will be 3 mm. With this knowledge, the periodontist can use the guide and remove bone until it is 3 mm from the position of the guide on each tooth.

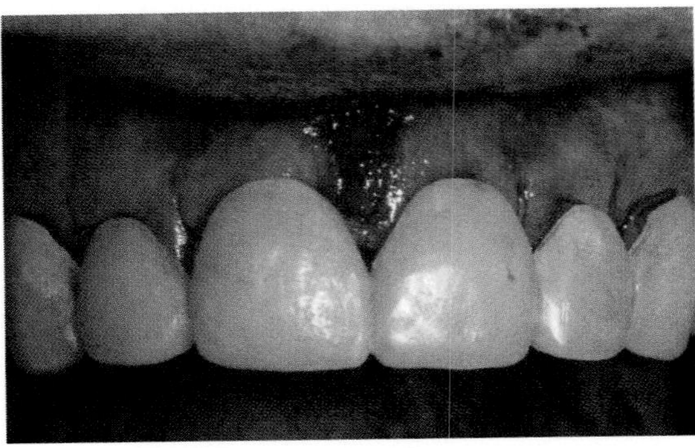

Color Fig. 75-21 The surgical guide is also useful during suturing. Because the guide represents the desired free gingival margin position, it is possible to suture to the level of the guide, knowing that the surgery has now recreated biologic width and a 1-mm sulcus. This shortens the amount of time necessary for healing and eliminates the need to wait for tissue rebound prior to restorative dentistry.

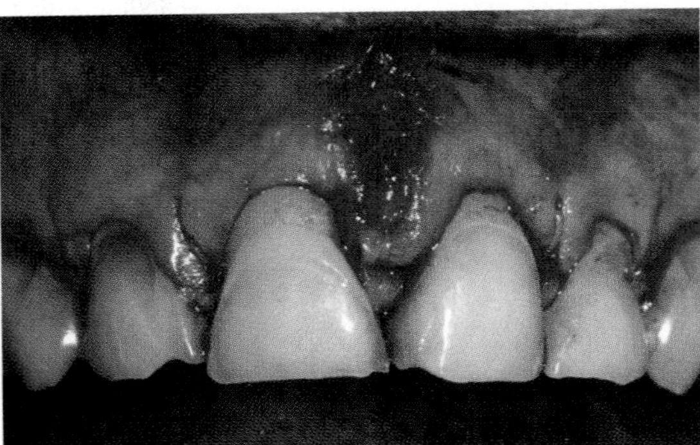

Color Fig. 75-22 The soft tissue profile as seen the day of surgery with the guide removed. Note that in this patient, the interproximal papillae were not changed because the interproximal papilla form and height were deemed acceptable.

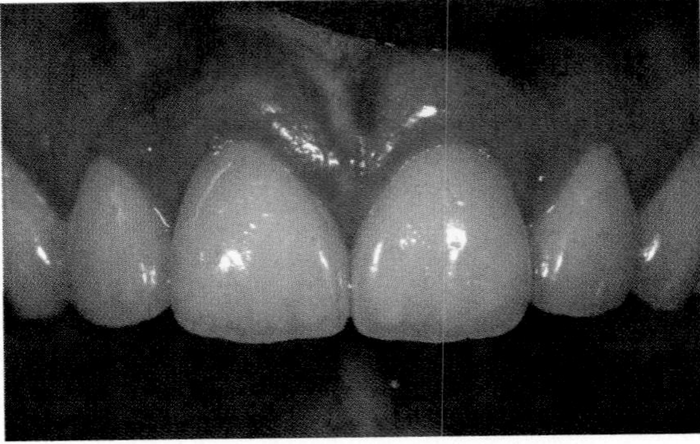

Color Fig. 75-23 A photograph taken 4 years after placement of the final restorations. Note the excellent soft tissue health and the attainment of the desired free gingival margin and papillary form.

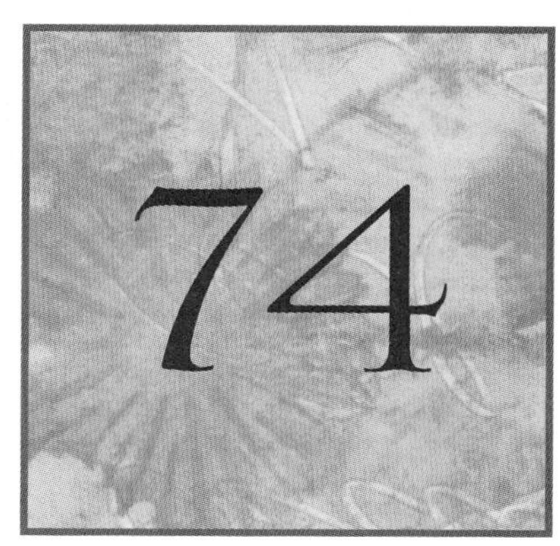

CHAPTER 74

Preparation of the Periodontium for Restorative Dentistry

Henry H. Takei, Robert R. Azzi, and Thomas J. Han

CHAPTER OUTLINE

Active periodontal disease must be treated and controlled prior to any restorative dentistry. If restorative dentistry is performed on teeth where the periodontal prognosis is not determined and disease not treated, the loss of the restored tooth can occur. Restorative dentistry must be performed on a periodontium free of inflammation and pockets, without any mucogingival involvement, and with the contour and shape of the periodontium corrected for a good functional and esthetic restorative result. Implant dentistry also requires site development and preparation, not only for bone where it may be lacking but also for the augmentation of gingival soft tissues. The following are reasons why periodontal disease must be eliminated prior to restorative dentistry:

1. To locate and determine the gingival margins of restorations properly, the position of the healthy and stable gingival margin must be established prior to tooth preparation. Margins of restorations covered by inflamed gingiva shrinks after periodontal treatment.
2. The position of teeth is frequently altered in periodontal disease. Resolution of inflammation and regeneration of periodontal ligament fibers after treatment cause the teeth to move again, often back to their original position. Restorations designed for teeth before the periodontium is treated may produce injurious tensions and pressures on the treated periodontium.
3. Inflammation of the periodontium impairs the capacity of abutment teeth to meet the functional demands made on them. Restorations constructed to provide beneficial functional stimulation to a healthy periodontium become a destructive influence when superimposed on existing periodontal disease, shortening the life of the teeth and the restoration.
4. Partial prostheses constructed on casts made from impressions of diseased gingiva and edentulous mucosa do not fit properly when periodontal health is restored. When the inflammation is eliminated, the contour of the gingiva and adjacent mucosa is altered. Shrinkage creates spaces beneath the pontics of fixed bridges and the saddle areas of removable prostheses. Resultant plaque accumulation leads to inflammation of the mucosa and gingiva of the abutment teeth.

5. Discomfort from tooth mobility interferes with mastication and function. Periodontal treatment can reduce mobility with the elimination of edema in the periodontal ligament and regeneration of bone.

Furthermore, the aims of periodontal treatment are not limited to elimination of periodontal pockets and restoration of gingival health. *Treatment should also create the gingivomucosal environment and osseous topography necessary for the proper function of single-tooth restorations and fixed and removable partial prostheses.*

In patients with mutilated dentitions and extensive periodontal disease, the sequence of treatment can be modified as follows:

1. "Hopeless" teeth are extracted, followed by construction of a temporary partial denture. Temporary crowns are prepared with provisional margins.
2. Periodontal therapy is performed.
3. Approximately 2 months after periodontal treatment, when gingival health is restored and the location of the gingival sulcus is established, the preparations are modified to relocate the margins in proper relation to the healthy gingival sulcus, and final restorations are constructed.

Current periodontal and restorative therapy must also address the esthetic demands of the patient. A stable, healthy gingival margin and adequate exposure of the clinical crown is mandatory prior to crown preparation. This is necessary to prevent the exposure of the crown margin and root surface after the crown is placed. If there is not adequate clinical crown exposure for the retention of the crown, the margin of the crown may be placed in the junctional epithelium and the connective tissue attachment, resulting in gingival inflammation and subsequent bone loss. These situations require crown lengthening surgery. Fixed bridges in the anterior areas requires pontic placement on edentulous ridges that are not resorbed to avoid unesthetic pontics. Ridge augmentation would be necessary. Therefore the goal of these procedures is not treatment of a periodontal condition but instead preparation of the mouth for the ensuing esthetic, restorative, or prosthetic therapy. These surgical techniques are called *preprosthetic periodontal surgery* and include procedures such as crown lengthening and ridge augmentation. This chapter discusses Phase I therapy to control and treat the inflammatory phase of periodontal disease prior to restorative treatment and preprosthetic periodontal surgery.

PHASE I THERAPY

The specific goal of Phase I therapy is the control of active dental disease (see Chapters 47 and 48). Therefore when this phase of therapy is completed, patients should be in a state of dental health with active caries no longer present and active destruction of the periodontium under control. This results in elimination of the acute inflammatory response associated with periodontal destruction. Thus the status of the gingival tissues should be such that further restorative procedures of a more complex nature can be carried out without detrimental effects from unhealthy gingiva.

Obtaining control of periodontal inflammation during Phase I therapy results in restorations of a much higher quality than would be obtained if restoration were carried out in an environment of gingival inflammation. The presence of an acute inflammatory response in the gingiva causes ulceration of the epithelium that lines the gingival pocket and an increase in vascularity and edema of the tissues immediately beneath this epithelium. There is a possibility of continual bleeding and exudation of inflammatory tissue fluid into the gingival crevice and into the environment of restorative dental procedures. Therefore it is of utmost importance that all areas of the gingiva showing hemorrhage and significant amounts of inflammatory exudates be brought to an improved state of health before any restorative procedures other than emergency control of dental caries are carried out.

The removal of etiologic factors causing gingival inflammation results in a return to a healthy gingival state within 1 or 2 weeks. Thus plaque control, calculus removal, and the correction of any inadequate dental restorations in the gingival environment should be important initial procedures.

PERIODONTAL SURGERY

Restorative Considerations in Periodontal Surgery

Periodontal surgery is necessary in some patients. These periodontal surgical procedures should be carried out with due regard for the restorative needs of the patient. Therefore the final level of the periodontium should allow good access to all restorative marginal regions, and any necessary increase in clinical crown length should be obtained by postsurgical positioning of the periodontal tissues. If restorative procedures necessitate the resolution of mucogingival inadequacies, the appropriate surgical procedure should be completed before restorative therapy is begun.

Routine periodontal surgery procedures aimed at the correction of periodontal and mucogingival defects are described in previous chapters. Some of these surgical procedures may be modified because of the restorative or prosthetic needs of the patient. In addition, the goal of some procedures is not treatment of a periodontal condition, but preparation of the mouth for the ensuing restorative or prosthetic therapy.

Preprosthetic Periodontal Surgery

Management of Mucogingival Problems. It often is necessary to carry out a free soft tissue autograft in the patient who has a mucogingival defect associated with gingival inflammation and requires a dental restoration in the immediate environment of the gingiva (Fig. 74-1). The procedure for this free soft tissue autograft is presented in Chapter 66. Periodontal plastic surgery should be carried out at least 2 months before placement of the dental restorations. This allows time for mature tissue to form in the gingival margin so that restorative procedures do not cause a return of clinical inflammation. Augmentation of keratinized gingiva provides stability of the free gingival margin and surrounding gingival tissues

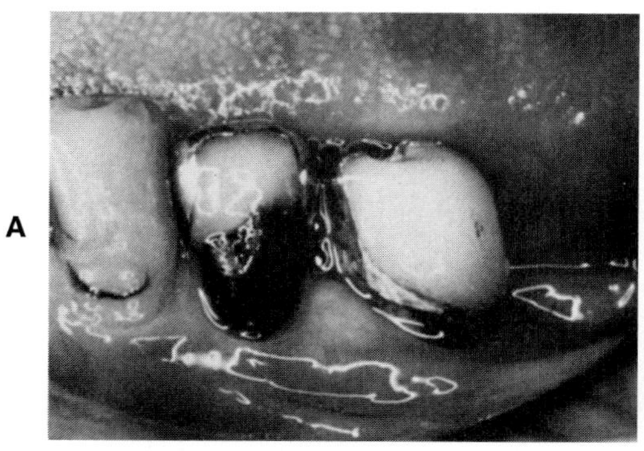

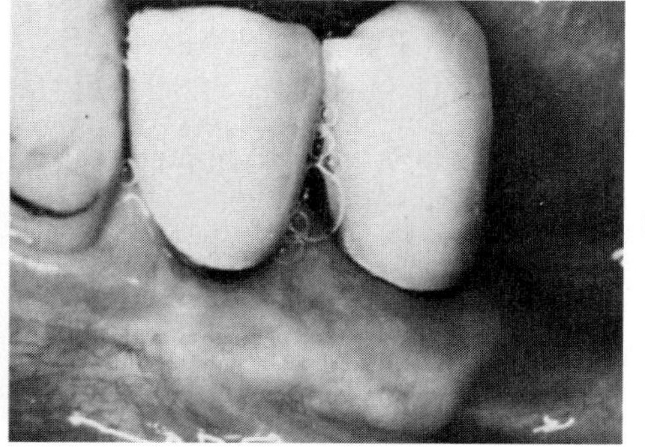

Fig. 74-1 Mucogingival problems. **A,** Preoperative mucogingival problem. The gingiva in the region where a crown margin is to be placed is inadequate. The presence of a plaque-enhancing margin necessitates the development of an adequate band of gingiva. **B,** Postoperative soft tissue autograft, 6 months after mucogingival surgery and placement of restoration. Note the adequate band of gingiva.

so that the dental restoration can be placed in an environment in which gingival health can be maintained.

Crown-Lengthening Procedures. In situations in which a tooth has a short clinical crown deemed inadequate for the retention of a required cast restoration, it is necessary to increase the size of the clinical crown using periodontal surgical procedures. These crown-lengthening procedures enable the dentist performing the restoration to develop an adequate area for crown retention without extending the crown margins deep into the periodontal tissues, referred to as the *biologic width.*[2] As discussed in Chapter 75, the term *biologic width* is used to describe the junctional epithelium and connective tissue that attach to the root surface. Studies have indicated that the average lengths of the connective tissue attachment and junctional epithelium are 1.07 and 0.97 mm, respectively.[1] Therefore the average length of the biologic width is about 2 mm (Fig. 74-2). The healthy gingival sulcus coronal to the junctional epithelium, which is not attached to the tooth surface, has an average depth of 0.69 mm. The biologic width usually remains constant. If the restorative margin is placed into this area, the crestal bone will be lost to reestablish the biologic width. The other consequence of margin placement into this area is gingival inflammation and pocket formation. A detailed discussion of biologic width and margin placement is presented in Chapter 75. The surgical procedure to expose adequate clinical crown to prevent the placement of the crown margin into the area of the biologic width is termed *crown-lengthening surgery.* A gingivectomy technique can be used to eliminate the tissue that forms the pocket or sulcus wall; such tissue may be overgrown (gingival pocket) and may interfere with the intended restorative procedures. This technique does not lengthen the clinical crown and therefore is not considered true crown-lengthening surgery. By definition, the clinical crown is that portion of the tooth coronal to the alveolar crest. Therefore the bone margin must be removed to lengthen it. This is accomplished with an apically positioned flap and osteoectomy (Color Fig. 74-1), which means that tooth-supporting bone is removed. The removal of bone is usually not necessary around the

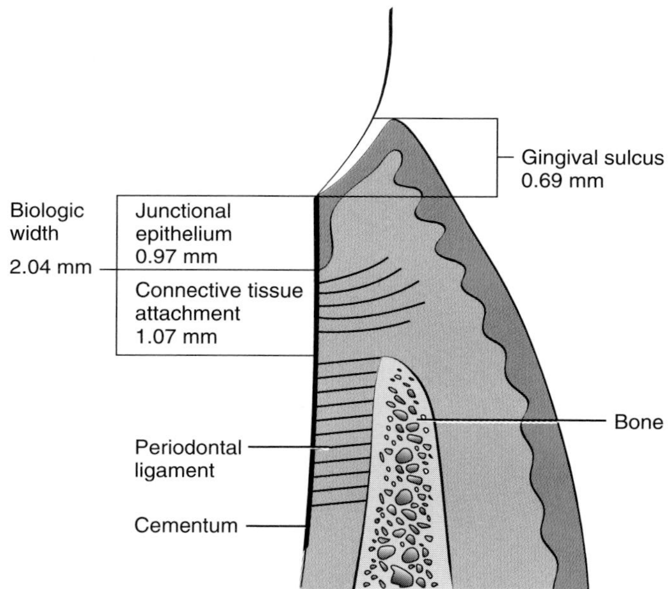

Fig. 74-2 The dentogingival junction. Note the area of biologic width composed of junctional epithelium and connective tissue attachment.

entire circumference of the tooth but, if undertaken, should be done with great caution. *It is essential that there be at least 3 mm between the most apical extension of the restoration margin and the alveolar bone crest.* This space allows sufficient room for the supracrestal collagen fibers that are part of the periodontal support mechanism, as well as providing a gingival crevice of 2 to 3 mm. If this guideline is used, the margin of the crown is finally positioned at its correct level, approximately halfway down the gingival crevice. Chapter 75 presents the clinical evaluation and determination of methods used for assessing the biologic width. Failure to allow sufficient space between the crown margin and the alveolar crest height means that the finished restoration is positioned deep in the periodontal tissues and results in increased inflammation and pocket formation.

Color Fig. 74-1 presents crown-lengthening surgery of the maxillary anterior area. Extensive loss of tooth structure has occurred, and crown-lengthening surgery is necessary prior to crown preparation. This area not only requires crown lengthening but also proper symmetry and shape of the gingival tissues for esthetic objectives. Because the gingival tissue outline follows that of the underlying bone, the removal of the bone must achieve an esthetic symmetry. A surgical template constructed prior to surgery helps determine the amount of bone removal and the contour that must be incorporated to achieve a good esthetic symmetry. Chapter 62 addresses this technique. Chisels are used to sculpt the outline of the bone removal. For proper esthetic symmetry, the height of the central incisors and the cuspids are equal and apical to the lateral incisors. The flap to expose the bone is initially full thickness at the crestal area but converted to a split thickness flap so that the flap may be positioned apically during closure. Holding sutures are used to position the flap, and closing sutures are placed at the papilla for flap closure. The final result (see Color Fig. 74-1, *J*) was both functionally and esthetically acceptable to the patient.

Ridge Augmentation Procedures. These procedures are aimed at correcting the excessive loss of alveolar bone that sometimes occurs in the anterior region as

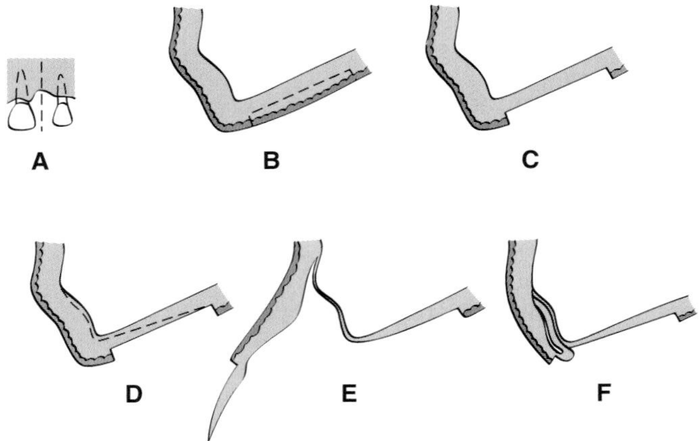

Fig. 74-3 The roll technique for ridge augmentation. **A and B,** The epithelial surface is removed on the palatal surface. **C,** The split-thickness flap is directed toward the facial aspect. **D,** The split thickness flap is reflected. **E and F,** The portion of the split thickness flap with the epithelium removed is folded to augment the

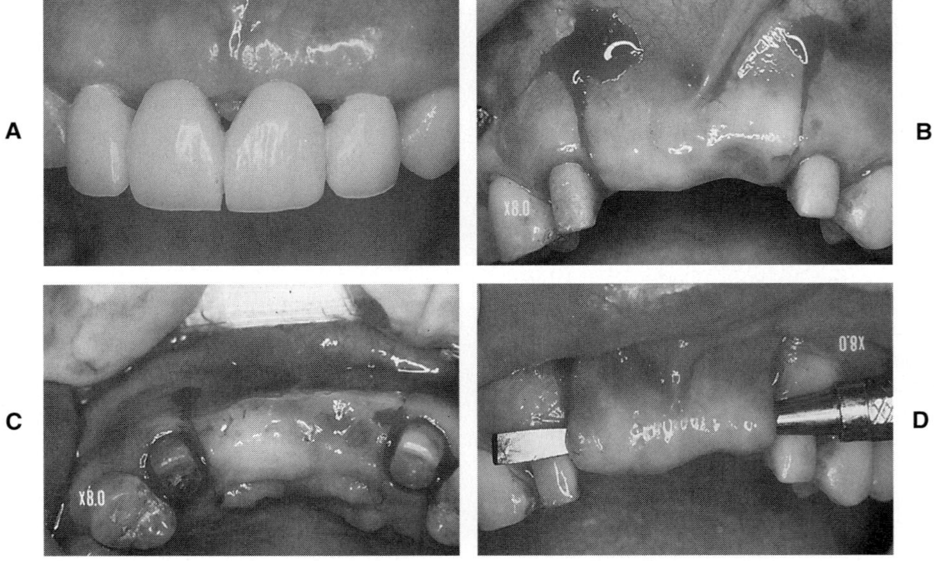

Fig. 74-4 Vertical and horizontal ridge augmentation using the connective tissue tunnel technique. **A,** Preoperative view of the maxillary anterior area. Note the deficient ridge. **B,** Vertical incisions at both ends of the deficient ridge after the bridge is removed. **C,** The vertical incision is extended to the palatal areas to augment vertically. **D,** A split thickness tunnel is created at the recipient site.

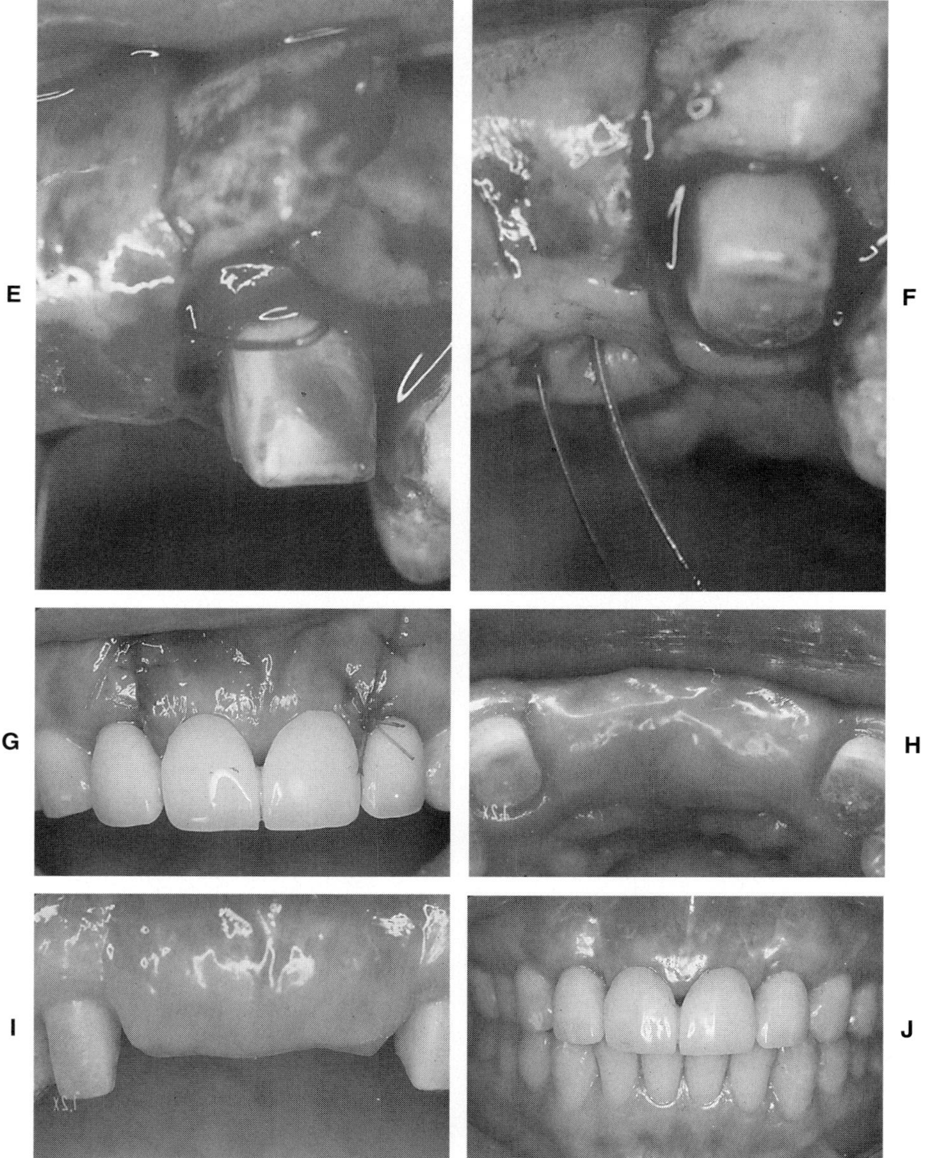

Fig. 74-4, cont'd E, Two separate subepithelial connective tissues are inserted into the tunnel at both ends. **F,** Sutures placed from the palatal surface are used to position the connective tissue in the tunnel. **G,** The recipient site is sutured. **H,** Four months postoperative. Horizontal augmentation. **I,** Four months postoperative. Vertical augmentation. **J,** The final result with the fixed restoration in place.

a consequence of advanced periodontal disease, advanced periapical bone loss, traumatic tooth extractions, and external trauma. This excessive bone loss may create a difficult esthetic problem and complicate the prosthetic reconstruction.

In fixed prosthetic replacement, the large space may result in either a long pontic or a space between the apical end of the pontic and the resorbed ridge. These osseous defects may occur in a coronoapical or buccolingual direction. In many situations, it can occur in both directions simultaneously.

Several surgical procedures have been developed to correct these ridge discrepancies. The roll technique was reported by Abrams to manage moderate tissue loss in the buccolingual direction. Fig. 74-3 illustrates this surgical procedure. Initially, the epithelium on the palatal side of the defect is removed (see Fig. 74-3, *A*). After a split-thickness incision, the flap denuded of the epithelial covering is rolled beneath the buccal split flap. The rolled portion of the palatal split flap augments the ridge in a buccal direction. Ridge defects that are more extensive can be augmented using subepithelial connective donor tissue from the palate, which is placed in pouches or tunnels created at the recipient site. Fig. 74-4 illustrates a case using connective tissue donor graft placed in a tunnel. Vertical incisors at the two ends of the defect and a tunnel made in both the horizontal and vertical directions create a recipient site that provides excellent blood supply to the donor tissue. This tissue is positioned with gut sutures from the palatal side. The vertical augmentation achieved by this surgery provides an excellent soft tissue environment for an esthetic fixed restoration (see Fig. 74-4, *J*). Larger defects may require bone grafts in the form of a monocortical block using fixation screws or particulate bone grafts held in place with a titanium-supported membrane. These procedures are discussed in Chapter 66.

REFERENCES

1. Gargiulo A, Wentz F, Orban B: Dimensions and relations of the dentogingival junction in humans. J Periodontol 1961; 32:261.
2. Rosenberg E, Garber D, Evian C: Tooth lengthening procedures. Comp Cont Ed Gen Dent 1980; 1:161.

Periodontal-Restorative Interrelationships

Frank M. Spear and Joseph P. Cooney

CHAPTER

CHAPTER OUTLINE

The relationship between periodontal health and the restoration of teeth is intimate and inseparable. For restorations to survive long term, the periodontium must remain healthy so that the teeth are maintained. For the periodontium to remain healthy, restorations must be critically managed in several areas so that they are in harmony with their surrounding periodontal tissues. To maintain or enhance the patient's esthetic appearance, the tooth/tissue interface must present a healthy natural appearance, with gingival tissues framing the restored teeth in a harmonious manner. This chapter reviews the key areas of restorative management necessary to optimize periodontal health and therefore the esthetics and function of restorations.

BIOLOGIC CONSIDERATIONS

Margin Placement and Biologic Width

Restorative clinicians must understand the role of biologic width in preserving healthy gingival tissues and controlling the gingival form around restorations. They must also apply this information in the positioning of restoration margins, especially in the esthetic zone where a primary treatment goal is to mask the junction of the margin with the tooth. A clinician is presented with three options for margin placement: supragingival, equigingival (even with the tissue), and subgingival locations.[70] The supragingival margin has the least impact on the periodontium. Classically, this margin location has been applied in nonesthetic areas due to the marked contrast in color and opacity of traditional restorative materials against the tooth. With the advent of more translucent restorative materials, adhesive dentistry, and resin cements, the ability to place supragingival margins in esthetic areas is now a reality (Figs. 75-1 and 75-2). Therefore whenever possible, these restorations should be chosen not just for their esthetic advantages but for their favorable periodontal impact as well. The use of equigingival margins traditionally was not desirable because they were thought to retain more plaque than supragingival or subgingival margins and therefore result

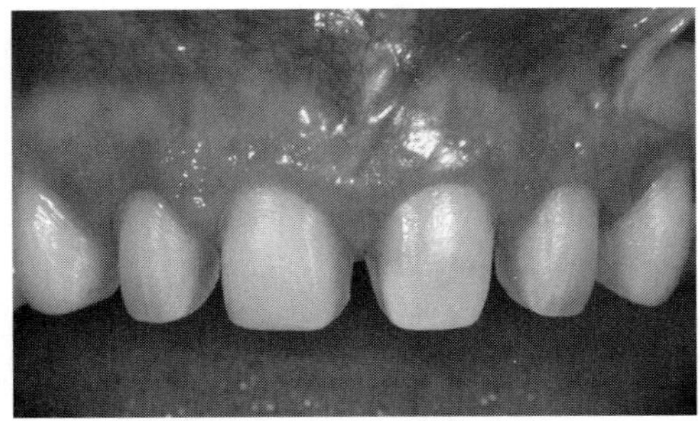

Fig. 75-1 With the advent of adhesive dentistry and ultrathin ceramic veneers, it now is possible to prepare restorations equigingival without visible margins. The preparations for six porcelain veneers with the margins placed at the level of tissue are shown.

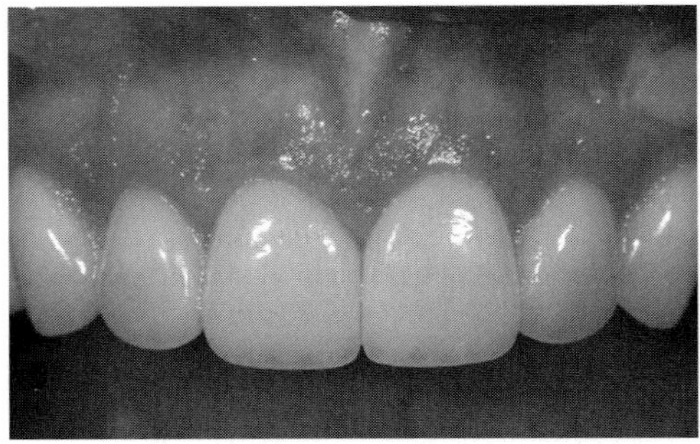

Fig. 75-2 The completed veneers. Note the invisible gingival finish line, even though the margin has not been carried below tissue.

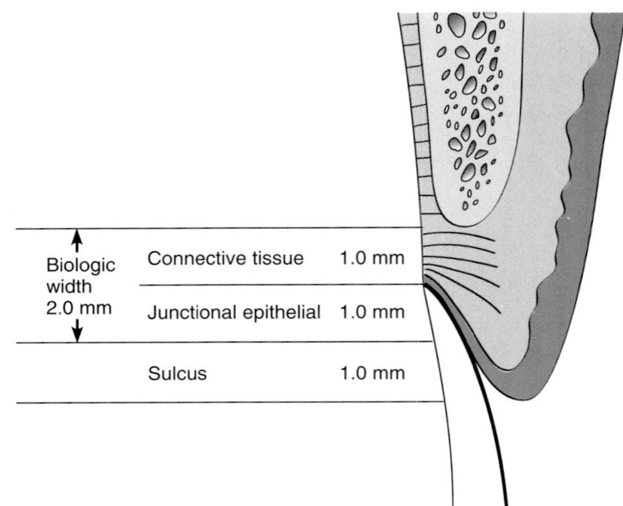

Fig. 75-3 Average human biologic width: Connective tissue attachment 1 mm in height; epithelial attachment 1 mm in height; sulcus depth of approximately 1 mm. The combined connective tissue attachment and epithelial attachment or biologic width equals 2 mm.

in greater gingival inflammation. There was also the concern that any minor gingival recession would create an unsightly margin display. These concerns are not valid today, not only because the restoration margins can be esthetically blended with the tooth but also because restorations can be finished easily to provide a smooth, polished interface at the gingival margin. From a periodontal viewpoint, both supragingival and equigingival margins are well tolerated. The greatest biologic risk occurs when placing subgingival margins.[44] These margins are not as accessible as supragingival or equigingival margins for finishing procedures, and in addition, if the margin is placed too far below the gingival tissue crest, it violates the gingival attachment apparatus.

The dimension of space that the healthy gingival tissues occupy above the alveolar bone is now identified as the *biologic width*. Most authors credit Gargiulo, Wentz, and Orban's study on cadavers with establishing the dimensions of space required by the gingival tissues.[19] They found that in the average human, the connective tissue attachment occupies 1.07 mm of space above the crest of the alveolar bone and that the junctional epithelium below the base of the gingival sulcus occupies another 0.97 mm of space above the connective tissue attachment. The combination of these two measurements constitutes the biologic width (Fig. 75-3). Clinically, this information is applied to diagnose biologic width violations when the restoration margin is placed 2 mm or less away from the alveolar bone and the gingival tissues are inflamed with no other etiologic factors evident.

Restorative considerations frequently dictate the placement of restoration margins beneath the gingival tissue crest. Restorations may need to be extended gingivally to create adequate resistance and retentive form in the preparation, to make significant contour alterations because of caries or other tooth deficiencies, or to mask the tooth/restoration interface by locating it subgingivally. When the restoration margin is placed too far below the gingival tissue crest, it impinges on the gingival attachment apparatus and creates a violation of biologic width.[49] Two different responses can be observed from the involved gingival tissues (Fig. 75-4). One possibility is that bone loss of an unpredictable nature and gingival tissue recession occur as the body attempts to recreate room between the alveolar bone and the margin to allow space for tissue reattachment. This is more likely to occur in areas where the alveolar bone surrounding the tooth is very thin. Trauma from restorative procedures can play a major role in causing this fragile tissue to recede. Other factors also have been presented in the literature as influencing the likelihood of recession. These variables include whether the gingiva is thick and fibrotic or thin and fragile and whether the periodontium is highly scalloped or flat in its gingival form. It has been found that highly scalloped thin gingiva is more prone to recession than a flat periodontium with thick fibrous tissue.[48]

The more common finding with deep margin placement is that the bone level appears to remain unchanged, but gingival inflammation develops and persists. To restore gingival tissue health, it is necessary to clinically establish space between the alveolar bone and the margin.

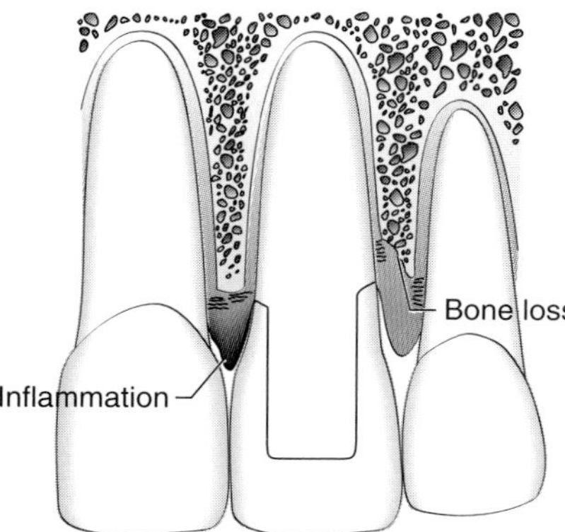

Fig. 75-4 Ramifications of a biologic width violation if a restorative margin is placed within the zone of the attachment. On the mesial of the left central, bone has not been lost, but gingival inflammation occurs. On the distal of the left central, bone loss has occurred and a normal biologic width has been reestablished.

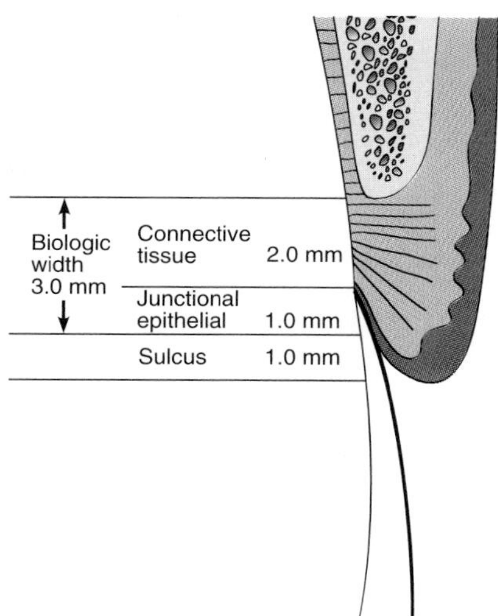

Fig. 75-5 Possible variations exist in biologic width. Connective tissue attachments and epithelial attachments may be variable. In this example the connective tissue attachment is 2 mm in height, the epithelial attachment 1 mm in height, and the sulcus depth 1 mm, for a combined total tissue height above bone of 4 mm. However, the biologic width is 3 mm. This is just one variation that can occur from the average depicted in Fig. 75-3.

This can be accomplished either by surgery to alter the bone level or by orthodontic extrusion to move the restoration margin farther away from the bone level.

Evaluation of Biologic Width

Radiographic interpretation can identify interproximal violations of biologic width. However, with the more common locations on the mesiofacial and distofacial line angles of teeth, radiographs are not diagnostic because of tooth superimposition. If a patient experiences tissue discomfort when the restoration margin levels are being assessed with a periodontal probe, it is a good indication that the margin extends into the attachment and that a biologic width violation has occurred. A more positive assessment can be made clinically by measuring the distance between the bone and the restoration margin using a periodontal probe. The probe is pushed through the anaesthetized attachment tissues from the sulcus to the underlying bone. If this distance is less than 2 mm at one or more locations, a diagnosis of biologic width violation can be confirmed. This assessment is completed circumferentially around the tooth to evaluate the extent of the problem. However, biologic width violations can occur in some patients in whom the margins are located more than 2 mm above the alveolar bone level.[23] In 1994, Vacek et al also investigated the biologic width phenomenon.[71] Although their average width finding of 2 mm was the same as that previously presented by Gargiulo et al, they also reported a range of different, patient-specific biologic widths. They reported biologic widths as narrow as 0.75 mm in some individuals, whereas others had biologic widths as tall as 4.3 mm (Fig. 75-5). This information dictates that specific biologic width assessment should be performed for each patient to determine whether they need additional biologic width in excess of 2 mm for restorations to be in harmony with their gingival tissues. The biologic, or attachment, width can be identified for each individual patient by probing under anesthesia to the bone level (referred to as "sounding to bone") and subtracting the sulcus depth from the resulting measurement. This measurement must be performed on teeth with healthy gingival tissues and should be repeated on more than one tooth to ensure an accurate assessment. The technique allows the variations in sulcus depths found in individual patients to be assessed and factored into the diagnostic evaluation. The information obtained is then used to definitively diagnose biologic width violations, the extent of correction needed, and the parameters for placement of future restorations.

Correction of Biologic Width Violations

Biologic width violations can be corrected by either surgically removing bone away from proximity to the restoration margin or orthodontically extruding the tooth and thus moving the margin away from the bone. Surgery is the more rapid of the two treatment options.[58] It is also preferred if the resulting crown lengthening will create a more pleasing tooth length. In these situations, the bone should be moved away from the margin by the measured distance of the ideal biologic width for that patient, with an additional 0.5 mm of bone removed as a safety zone.

Gingival recession is a potential risk after removal of bone.[7] If interproximal bone is removed, there is a high likelihood of papillary recession and the creation of an unesthetic triangle of space below the interproximal contacts. If the biologic width violation is on the interproximal, or if the violation is across the facial surface and the gingival tissue level is correct, then orthodontic

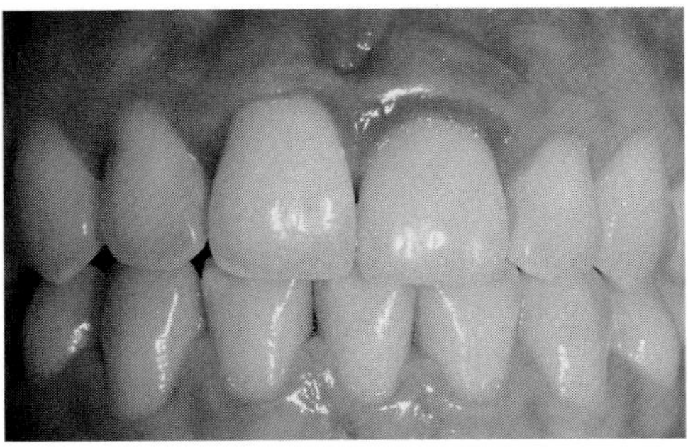

Fig. 75-6 The left central incisor was fractured in an accident 12 months ago and restored at that time. The patient is unhappy with the appearance of the tissue surrounding the restoration.

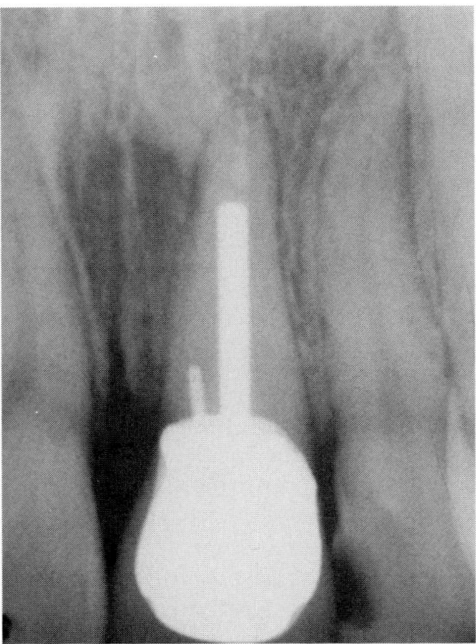

Fig. 75-7 A radiograph reveals a biologic width violation on the mesial surface interproximally. Removal of interproximal bone would create an esthetic deformity. This patient is better treated with orthodontic extrusion.

extrusion is indicated (Figs. 75-6 to 75-9).[28] The extrusion can be performed in two ways. By applying low orthodontic extrusion force, the tooth is erupted slowly, bringing the alveolar bone and gingival tissue with it. The tooth is extruded until the bone level has been carried coronal to the ideal level by the amount that needs to be removed surgically to correct the attachment violation. The tooth is stabilized in this new position and then treated with surgery to correct the bone and gingival tissue levels. Another option is to carry out rapid orthodontic extrusion whereby the tooth is erupted the desired amount over several weeks.[32] During this period, a supercrestal fiberotomy is performed weekly in an effort to prevent the tissue and bone from following the tooth. The tooth is then stabilized for at least 12 weeks to confirm the position of the tissue and bone, and any coronal creep can be corrected surgically.

Margin Placement Guidelines

When determining where to place restorative margins relative to the periodontal attachment, it is recommended that the patient's existing sulcus depth be used as a guideline in assessing the biologic width requirement for that patient. The base of the sulcus can be viewed as the top of the attachment, and therefore variations in attachment height are accounted for by assuring that the margin is placed in the sulcus and not in the attachment.[4,37,38,57] The variations in sulcular probing depth are then used to predict how deeply the margin can safely be placed below the gingival crest. With shallow probing depths (1 to 1.5 mm), extending the preparation more than 0.5 mm subgingivally will risk violating the attachment. This assumes that the periodontal probe penetrates an average of 0.5 mm into the epithelial attachment in healthy gingiva. With shallow probing depths, future recession is unlikely because the free gingival margin is located close to the top of the attachment. Deeper sulcular probing depths provide more freedom in locating restoration margins farther below the gingival crest. However, in most circumstances, the deeper the gingival sulcus, the greater the risk of gingival

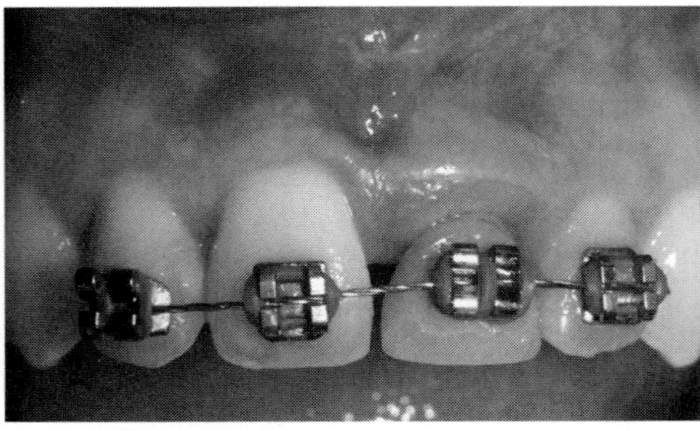

Fig. 75-8 After orthodontic eruption. The tooth has been erupted 3 mm to move the bone and gingiva coronally 3 mm on the left central. It is now possible to surgically reposition the bone to the correct level and position the gingiva to the correct level, reestablishing normal biologic width.

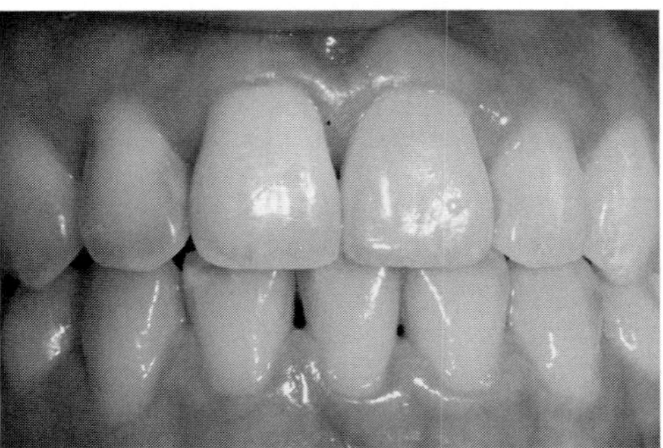

Fig. 75-9 A 1-year recall photograph after orthodontic extrusion, osseous surgery, and placement of a new restoration. Note the excellent tissue health after the re-establishment of biologic width.

recession. The first step in using sulcus depth as a guide in margin placement is to manage gingival health. Once the tissue is healthy, the following three rules can be used to place intracrevicular margins.

1. If the sulcus probes 1.5 mm or less, place the restoration margin 0.5 mm below the gingival tissue crest. This is especially important on the facial aspect and prevents a biologic width violation in a patient who is at high risk in that regard.
2. If the sulcus probes more than 1.5 mm, place the margin one half the depth of the sulcus below the tissue crest. This places the margin far enough below tissue so that it still is covered if the patient is at higher risk of recession.
3. If a sulcus greater than 2 mm is found, especially on the facial aspect of the tooth, then evaluate to see whether a gingivectomy could be performed to lengthen the teeth and create a 1.5-mm sulcus. Then the patient can be treated using Rule 1.

The rationale for Rule 3 is that deep margin placement is more difficult and the stability of the free gingival margin is less predictable when a deep sulcus exists. Reducing the sulcus depth created a more predictable situation in which to place an intracrevicular margin. It is not guaranteed that the tissue will remain at the corrected level, however, because some gingival rebound can occur after gingivectomy. However, it ensures that the restorative margins are not exposed and visible in the patient's mouth (Fig. 75-10 and Color Figs. 75-1 to 75-4).

Clinical Procedures in Margin Placement

The placement of supragingival or equigingival margins is simple because they require no tissue manipulation. With regard to overall tooth preparation, the amount reduced incisally or occlusally, facially, lingually, and interproximally will be dictated by the choice of restorative materials. Prior to extending subgingivally, the preparation should be completed to the free gingival margin facially and interproximally. This allows the margin of the tooth preparation to be used as a reference for subgingival extension once the tissue is retracted (Fig. 75-11).

Tissue Retraction

Once the supragingival portion of the preparation is completed, it is necessary to extend below the tissue.[6,24] The preparation margin must now be extended to the appropriate depth in the sulcus, applying the guidelines presented previously. In this process, the tissue must be protected from abrasion, which will cause hemorrhage and can adversely affect the stability of the tissue level around the tooth. Access to the margin is also required for the final impression, and a clean, fluid controlled environment is desired. Tissue management is achieved with gingival retraction cords, using the appropriate size to achieve the displacement required. Thin, fragile gingival tissues and shallow sulcus situations usually dictate that smaller diameter cords be chosen to achieve the desired tissue displacement.

For a Rule 1 margin, the cord should be placed so that the top of the cord is located in the sulcus at the level where the final margin will be established, which will be 0.5 mm below the previously prepared margin (Fig. 75-12). On the interproximal aspects of the tooth, the cord will usually be 1 to 1.5 mm below the tissue height because the interproximal sulcus is often 2.5 to 3 mm in depth. With this initial cord in place, the preparation is extended to the top of the cord, with the bur angled to the tooth so that it will not abrade the tissue (Fig. 75-13). This process protects the tissue, creates the correct axial reduction, and establishes the margin at the desired subgingival level. To create space and allow access for a final impression, it is now necessary to pack a second retraction cord. The second cord is pushed so that it displaces the first cord apically and sits between the margin and the tissue (Fig. 75-14). For the final impression, the top cord only is removed, leaving the margins visible and accessible to be recorded with the impression material (Fig. 75-15). The initial cord remains in place in the sulcus until the provisional restoration is completed.

As an alternative to additional retraction cords, electrosurgery can be used to remove any overlying tissue in

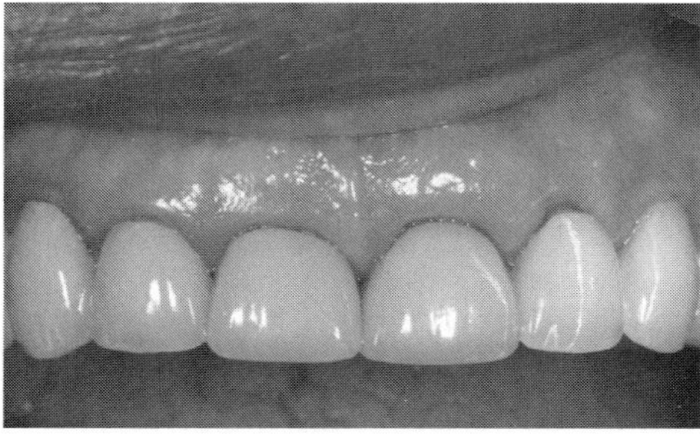

Fig. 75-10 A 78-year-old woman presents with the maxillary anterior restorations placed 6 months earlier. She is unhappy with the exposed margins and notes that the margins were covered the day the restorations were placed.

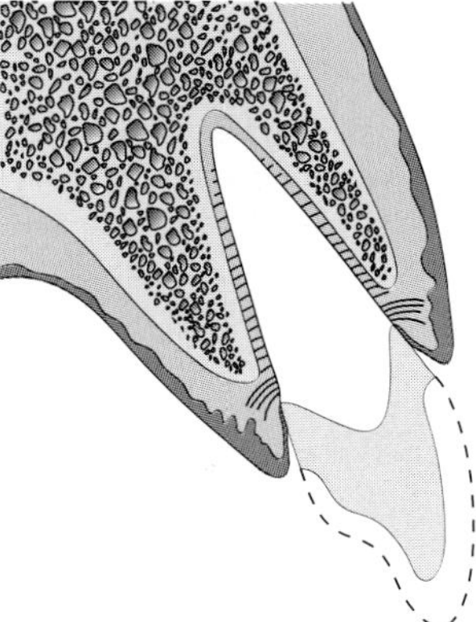

Fig. 75-11 To provide a reference position for margin placement after tissue retraction, the margin of the tooth preparation is initially established level with the free gingival margin.

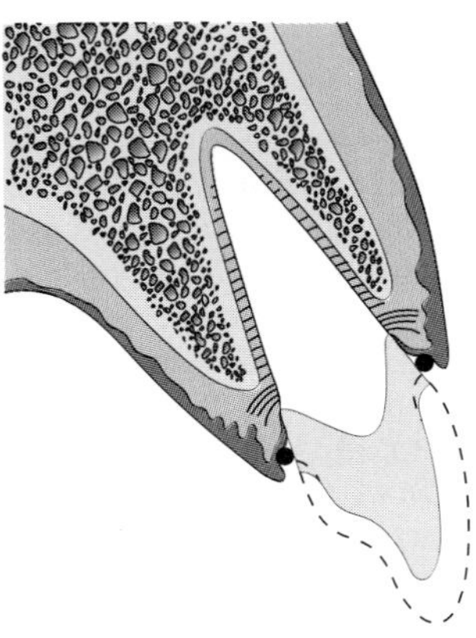

Fig. 75-12 The second step in margin placement is to place a single layer of deflection cord below the previously prepared margin to the desired final margin level. Here, a single cord has been placed 0.5 mm below the previously prepared margin.

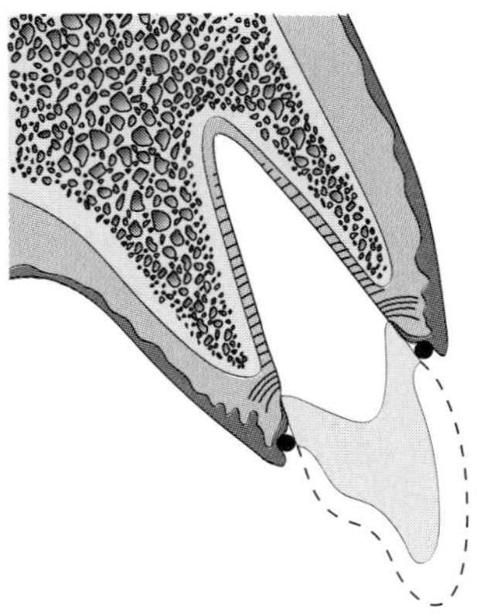

Fig. 75-13 The margin of the preparation is now extended apically to the top of the retraction cord; this represents the correct placement of the margin below the previously nonreflected free gingival margin.

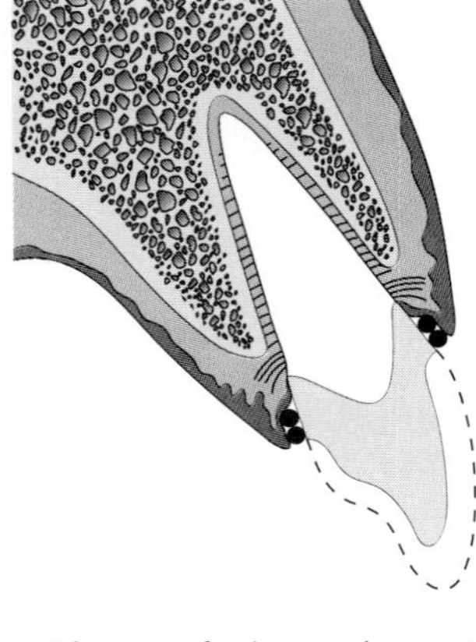

Fig. 75-14 To provide space for impression material, a second impression cord is now placed on top of the first deflection cord. This impression cord is placed so that it is between the margin of the preparation and the gingiva to create adequate space for impression material after removal of the cord.

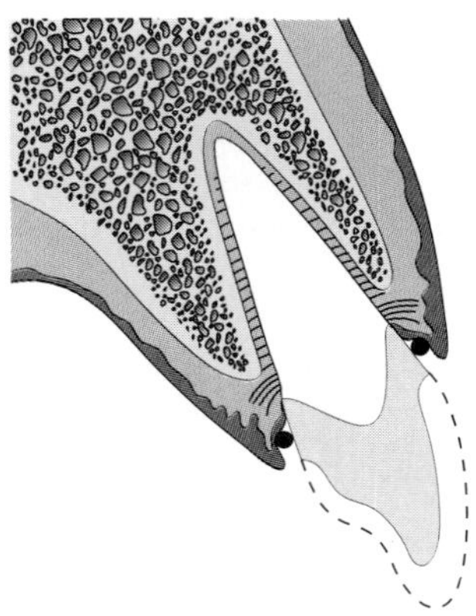

Fig. 75-15 The ideal situation after removal of the impression cord. The deflection cord is still in place maintaining the open sulcus but has been displaced apically another .05 mm by the placement of the impression cord, exposing tooth structure apical to the margin so that it can be captured in the impression.

the retraction process. A fine wire-tip electrode is held parallel to the tooth and against the margin in the sulcus and moved through the overhanging tissue, opening up the margin and the retraction cord to visual access (Figs. 75-16 to 75-19). The electrosurgery tip sits on top of the retraction cord in place in the sulcus. This controls the vertical position of the tip and results in the removal of the least tissue needed for access.

For Rule 2 situations where the sulcus is deeper, two larger diameter cords are used to deflect the tissue prior to extending the margin apically (Figs. 75-20 to 75-22). The top of the second cord is placed to identify the final margin location at the correct distance below the previously prepared margin, which was at the gingival tissue crest level. The margin is lowered to the top of the second cord (Fig. 75-23) and then a third cord is placed in preparation for the impression (Figs. 75-24 and 75-25). In the deep sulcus patient where the margin may be 1.5 to 2 mm below the tissue crest, electrosurgery is often necessary to remove overhanging tissue. To avoid altering the gingival tissue height, it is important to hold the electrosurgery tip parallel to the preparation (Fig. 75-26).

Provisional Restorations

Three critical areas must be effectively managed to produce a favorable biologic response to provisional restorations.[3,75] The marginal fit, contour, and surface finish of the interim restorations must be appropriate to maintain the health and position of the gingival tissues during the time interval until the final restorations are delivered. Provisional restorations that are poorly adapted at the

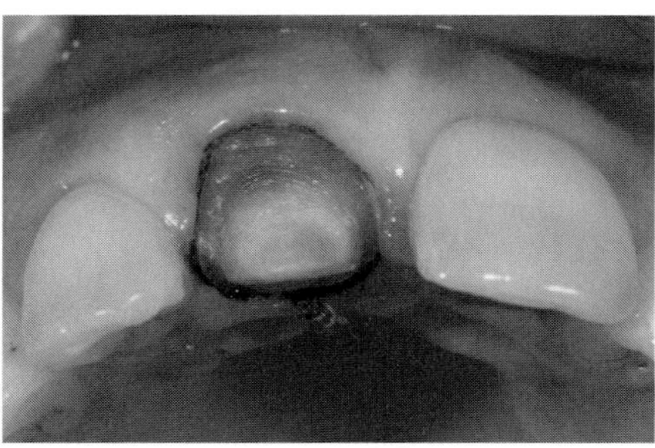

Fig. 75-16 The deflection cord and the impression cord are in place. The soft tissue is falling over the margins of the preparation. In this situation, if the impression cord were removed, the impression would not capture the margins in the areas where the tissue is overhanging.

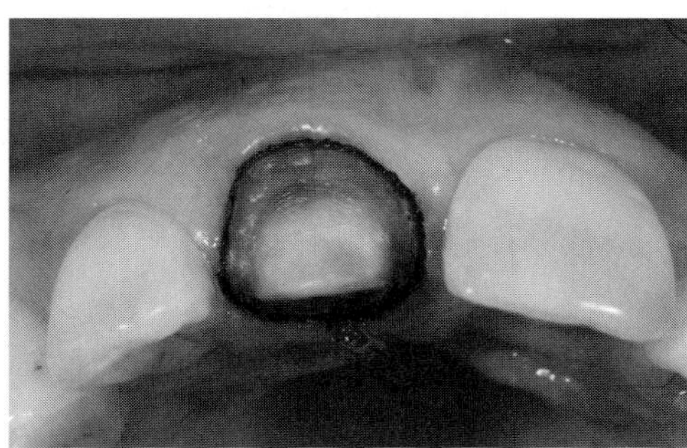

Fig. 75-17 The overhanging tissue has been removed and space created for the impression material with electrosurgery. Note that the deflection cord and the impression cord are still in place. The impression cord is now visible completely around the tooth, allowing easy access for the impression material to the margin after removal of the impression cord.

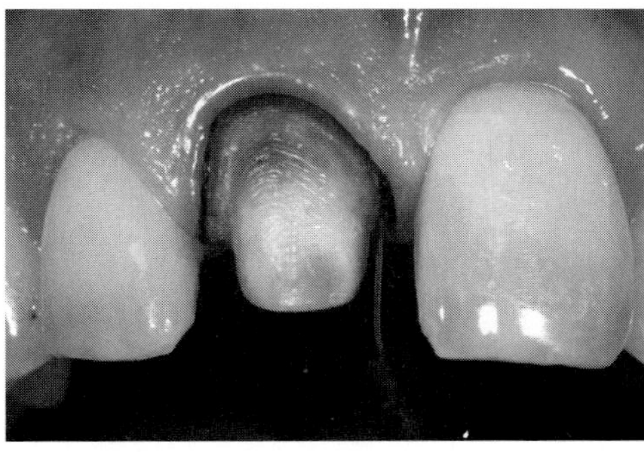

Fig. 75-18 With electrosurgery, the fine wire electrode tip is held parallel to the tooth preparation and rests on the cord as the tip is moved around the tooth.

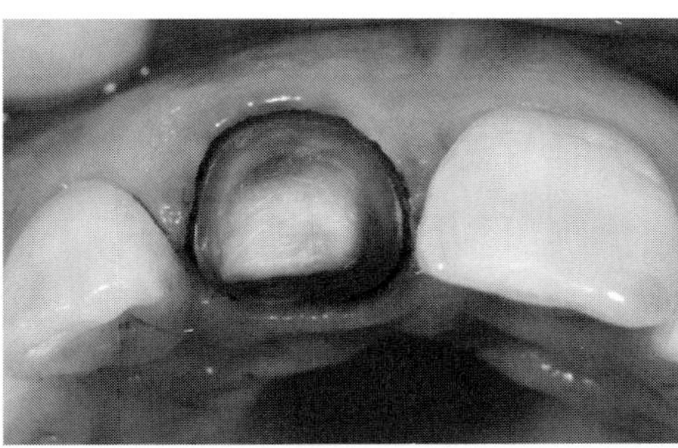

Fig. 75-19 After removal of the impression cord, an adequate space is created for the impression material, with no soft tissue overhanging the margins to trap or tear the impression material. Note the first or deflection cord is still in place.

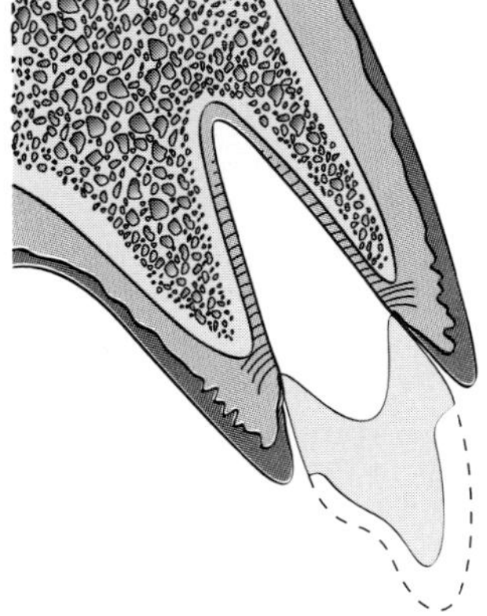

Fig. 75-20 The first step in margin placement for the patient with altered eruption or a deep sulcus is to prepare to the existing free gingival margin, just as in the Rule 1 patient.

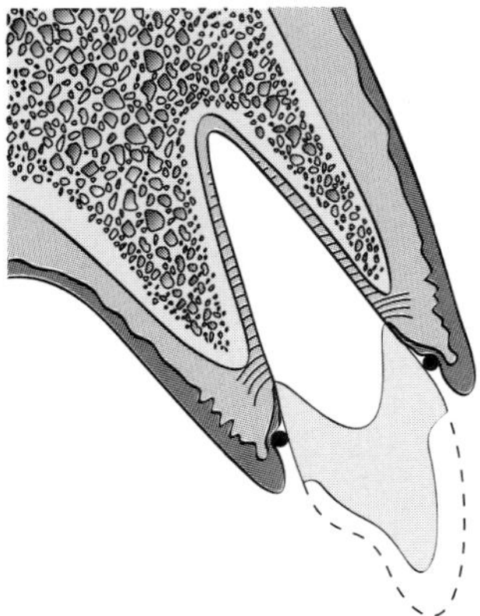

Fig. 75-21 The second step for the patient with altered eruption is to place the deflection cord. Note that the placement of a single deflection cord does not provide adequate deflection of the tissue to allow the margin to be carried below tissue without abrading the gingiva with the bur.

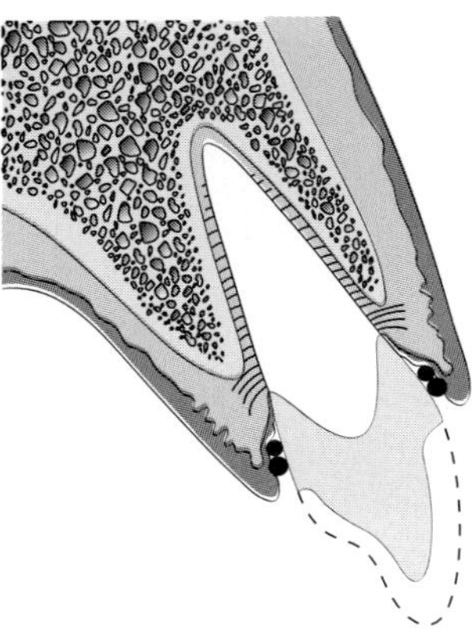

Fig. 75-22 The third step for the patient with altered eruption and a deep sulcus is to place a second, larger-diameter deflection cord on top of the first deflection cord. Combined, these two cords allow adequate deflection to open up the sulcus so that the margin can be carried below tissue without abrading the gingiva.

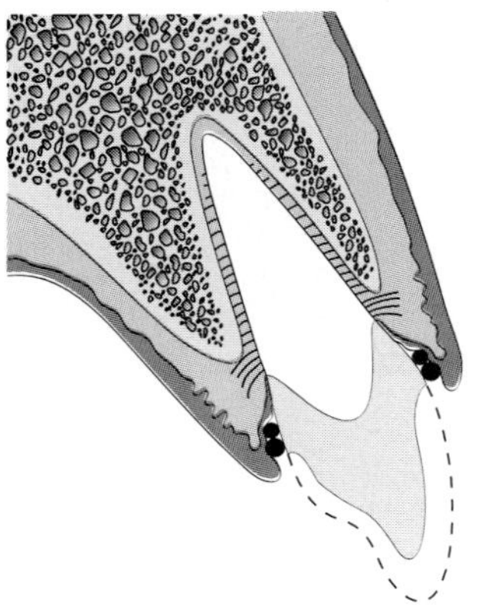

Fig. 75-23 The preparation is now extended to the top of the second deflection cord, finalizing margin location.

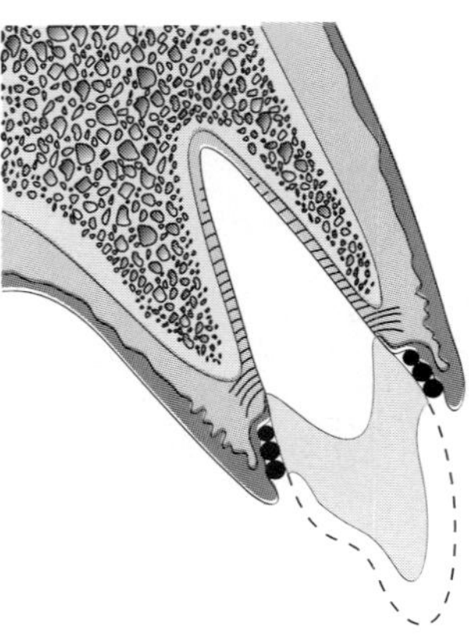

Fig. 75-24 After the extension of the margin to the top of the deflection cord, a third layer of cord is applied that will act as the impression cord. This impression cord should be placed so that it fits between the free gingival margin and the margin of the preparation. Its placement will also apically displace the previously two placed deflection cords.

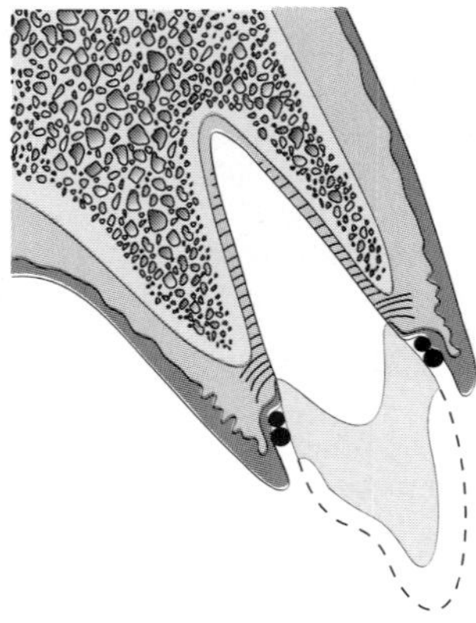

Fig. 75-25 Removal of the impression cord creates an adequate space for the impression material to capture the margin and 0.5 mm of tooth structure below the margin where the impression cord had displaced the first two cords.

margins, are overcontoured or undercontoured, and have rough or porous surfaces can cause inflammation, overgrowth, or recession of gingival tissues. The outcome can be unpredictable and lead to unfavorable changes in the tissue architecture that can compromise the success of the final restoration.

Marginal Fit

Marginal fit has clearly been implicated in producing an inflammatory response in the periodontium. It has been shown that the level of gingival inflammation can increase, corresponding with the level of marginal opening.[16] Margins that are significantly open (several tenths of a millimeter) are capable of harboring large numbers of bacteria and may be responsible for the inflammatory response seen. However, the quality of marginal finish and the margin location relative to the attachment are far more critical to the periodontium than is the difference between a 20 μm fit versus a 100 μm fit.[44,47,60]

Crown Contour

Restoration contour has been described as extremely important to the maintenance of periodontal health.[27,76] Ideal contour provides access for hygiene and has the fullness to create the desired gingival form and a pleasing visual tooth contour in esthetic areas. Evidence from hu-

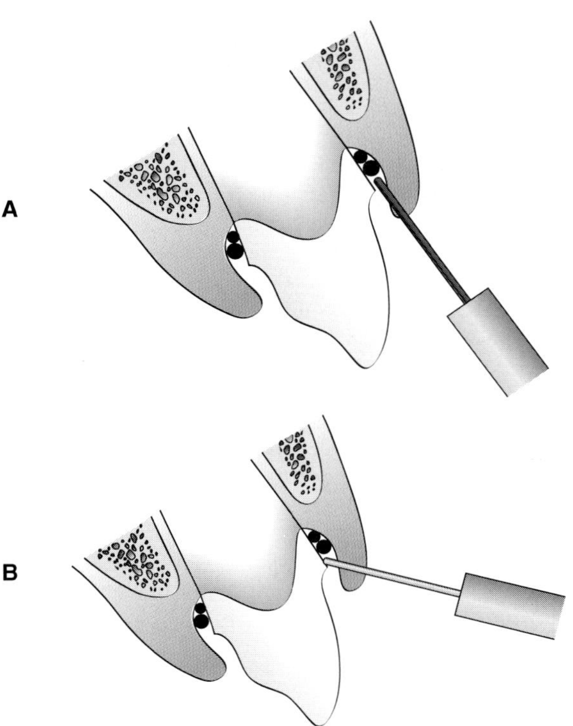

Fig. 75-26 If it is necessary to use electrosurgery, either in the normal or altered eruption patient, the correct inclination of the electrosurgery tip is important. **(A)** illustrates the electrosurgery tip being held parallel to the preparation and resting on the previously placed retraction cord. This removes a minimal amount of tissue, and the presence of the retraction cord protects the attachment from the electrosurgery. **(B)** represents the incorrect inclination of the electrosurgery tip. The tip is leaning away from the preparation. This inclination results in excess tissue removal.

man and animal studies clearly demonstrates a relationship between overcontouring and gingival inflammation; however, at the same time, undercontouring produces no adverse periodontal effect.[50,52] The most frequent cause of overcontoured restorations is inadequate tooth preparation by the dentist, which forces the technician to produce a bulky restoration to provide room for the restorative material. In areas of the mouth where esthetics are not critical, a flatter contour is always acceptable.

Subgingival Debris

Leaving debris below the tissue during restorative procedures can create an adverse periodontal response. The cause can be the retraction cord, impression material, provisional material, or either temporary or permanent cement.[56] The diagnosis of debris as the cause of gingival inflammation can be confirmed by examination of the sulcus surrounding the restoration with an explorer, removal of any foreign bodies, and monitoring of the tissue response. It may be necessary to provide tissue anesthesia for patient comfort during the procedure.

Hypersensitivity to Dental Materials

Inflammatory gingival responses have been reported related to the use of nonprecious alloys in dental restorations.[53] Typically, the responses have occurred to alloys containing nickel, although the frequency of these occurrences has been debated.[51] Hypersensitivity responses to precious alloys are extremely rare, and these alloys provide an easy solution to the problems encountered with the nonprecious alloys. More importantly, tissues respond more to the differences in surface roughness of the material rather than the composition of the material.[1,67] The rougher the surface of the restoration subgingivally, the greater the plaque accumulation and gingival inflammation. In clinical research, porcelain, highly polished gold, and highly polished resin all show similar plaque accumulation. Regardless of the restorative material selected, a smooth surface is essential on all materials subgingivally.

ESTHETIC CONSIDERATIONS IN GINGIVAL TISSUE MANAGEMENT

Interproximal Embrasure Form

The interproximal embrasure created by restorations and the form of the interdental papilla have a unique and intimate relationship.[62,63] The ideal interproximal embrasure should house the gingival papilla without impinging on it and also extend the interproximal tooth contact to the top of the papilla so that no excess space exists to trap food or be esthetically displeasing. Papillary height is established by the level of the bone, the biologic width, and the form of the gingival embrasure. Changes in the shape of the embrasure can have an impact on the height and form of the papilla. The tip of the papilla behaves differently than the free gingival margin on the facial aspect of the tooth. Whereas the free gingival margin averages 3 mm above the underlying facial bone, the tip of the papilla averages 4.5 to 5 mm above the interproximal bone (Fig. 75-27). This means that if the papilla is farther above the bone than the facial tissue but has the same biologic width, the interproximal area will have a 1.0 to 1.5 mm deeper sulcus than is found on the facial. In 1982, Van-der-Veldon published results of a study in which he completely removed healthy papillae to the bone level and found that it routinely regenerated 4 to 4.5 mm of total tissue above bone, with an average sulcus depth of 2 to 2.5 mm.[73] The height above bone that the papilla wants to maintain was indirectly confirmed by Tarnow, who studied the relationship of the papilla between the interproximal contact and the underlying bone.[68] When the gingival level of the interproximal tooth contacts measured 5 mm or less to the alveolar bone, the papilla always filled the space. When the contact was 6 mm from bone, only 56% of the papillae could fill the space. Finally, when the contact was 7 mm from bone, only 37% of the papillae could fill the spaces. Knowing that there is an individual variability to the required biologic width, this information relative to the papilla is applied by locating the lowest point of the interproximal contact in relation to the top of the epithelial attachment. The ideal contact should be 2 to 3 mm coronal to the attachment, which coincides with the depth of the average interproximal sulcus. As in assessing the facial tissues for margin location, this technique requires that the tissue is healthy to allow accurate probing. If the sulcus measures greater than 3 mm, there is some risk of papillary recession with restorative procedures.

The clinician is most frequently presented with a normal or shallow sulcus with a papilla that appears too short, rather than a tall papilla with a deep sulcus. Management of this situation is best approached by viewing the papilla as a balloon of a certain volume that sits on the attachment. This balloon of tissue has a form and height dictated by the gingival embrasure of the teeth. If the embrasure is too wide, the balloon flattens out and becomes blunted, with a shallow sulcus (Fig. 75-28). If the embrasure is the ideal width, the papilla has a pointed form and a sulcus of 2.5 to 3 mm and is healthy. If the embrasure is too narrow, the papilla may grow out to the facial and lingual, form a col, and become inflamed. This information is applied when evaluating an individual papilla with an open embrasure. The papilla in question is compared with the adjacent papillae. If they are all on the same level and the other areas do not have open embrasures, then the problem is one of gingival embrasure form. If however, the papilla in the area of concern is apical to the adjacent papillae, evaluate the interproximal bone levels. If the bone under that papilla is apical to the adjacent bone levels, the problem is due to bone loss. If the bone is at the same level, the open embrasure is due to the embrasure form of the teeth and not a periodontal problem with the papilla.

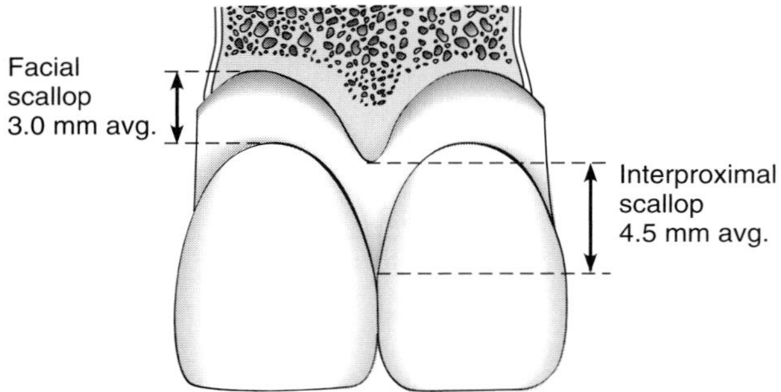

Fig. 75-27 A comparison of the behavior of the interproximal papilla relative to bone and the free gingival margin relative to bone in the average human. There is a 3-mm scallop from the facial bone to the interproximal bone. However, on average, a 4.5 to 5 mm gingival scallop exists between the facial tissue height and the interproximal papilla height. This extra scallop of 1.5 to 2 mm of gingiva compared with bone is the result of the extra soft tissue height above the attachment interproximally.

Restorative Correction of Open Gingival Embrasures

There are two causes of open gingival embrasures. Either the papilla is inadequate in height due to bone loss, or the interproximal contact is located too high coronally. If a high contact has been diagnosed as the cause of the problem, there are two potential reasons. If the root angulation of the teeth diverges, the interproximal contact is moved coronally, resulting in the open embrasure. Chapter 53 discusses correction of this problem. However, if

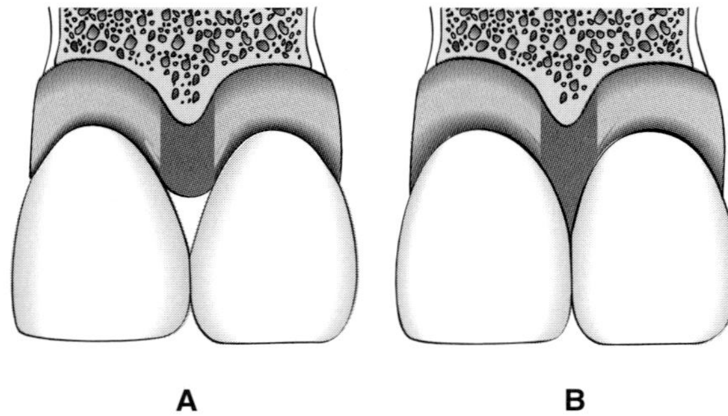

Fig. 75-28 The relationship between gingival embrasure volume and papillary form. **A,** The gingival embrasure of the teeth is excessively large due to a tapered tooth form. Because of the large embrasure form, the volume of tissue sitting on top of the attachment is not molded to the shape of a normal papilla but rather has a blunted form and a shallower sulcus. **B,** An ideal tooth form where the same volume of tissue sits on top of the attachment as in **A.** But because of the more closed embrasure form from the teeth in **B,** the papilla completely fills the embrasure and has a deeper sulcus averaging 2.5 to 3 mm. Note that the ideal contact position is 3 mm coronal to the attachment.

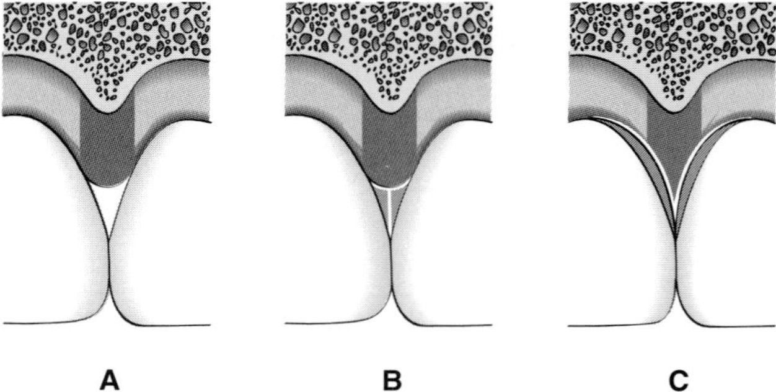

Fig. 75-29 Methods of altering gingival embrasure form. **A,** The typical open gingival embrasure due to excessively tapered tooth form. **B,** A common method employed by restorative dentists to correct the embrasure, whereby material is added supragingivally. This closes the embrasure by moving the contact to the tip of the papilla but results in overhangs that cannot be cleaned using dental floss. Removing these overhangs restoratively reopens the embrasure. **C,** The correct method of closing the gingival embrasure, whereby the margins of the restoration are carried 1 to 1.5 mm below the tip of the papilla. Note that this does not encroach on the attachment because the average interproximal sulcus probes 2.5 to 3 mm. This allows easy cleaning because of the convex profile. It also reshapes the papilla to a more pleasing profile esthetically.

the roots are parallel, the papilla form is normal, and an open embrasure exists, then the problem is probably related to tooth shape, specifically, an excessively tapered form. Restorative dentistry can correct this problem by moving the contact point to the tip of the papilla. To accomplish this, the margins of the restoration must be carried subgingivally 1 to 1.5 mm, and the emergence profile of the restoration is designed to move the contact point toward the papilla while blending the contour into the tooth below the tissue (Fig. 75-29). This can be accomplished easily with direct bonded restorations because the soft tissue can clearly be seen (Color Figs. 75-5 to 75-7). For indirect restorations, the desired restoration contours and embrasure form should be established in the provisional restorations, and the gingival tissues are allowed to adapt for 4 to 6 weeks before the tissue contour information is relayed to the laboratory to be used in the final restorations.

Management of Gingival Embrasure Form with Periodontal Recession

Management of the gingival embrasure form for patients who have experienced gingival recession varies depending on whether the treatment is either in the anterior or posterior regions of the mouth.[31] In esthetic areas, it is necessary to carry the interproximal contacts apically toward the papilla to eliminate the presence of large open embrasures. With multiple unit restorations, it also is possible to bake porcelain papillae directly on the restoration using tissue-colored ceramics. In the posterior areas where the interroot widths are significantly greater, it is often impossible to carry the proximal contacts to contact the tissue without creating large overhangs on the restorations. In these situations, the contact should be moved far enough apically to minimize any large food traps while still leaving an embrasure of a convenient size to be accessed with an interdental brush for hygiene. It should be noted that developing excessively long interproximal contacts, whether on anterior or posterior teeth, always creates rectangular, somewhat unesthetic tooth forms.

Pontic Design

Classically, four options should be considered in evaluating pontic design: sanitary, ridge-lap, modified ridge-lap, and ovate pontic designs (Fig. 75-30). Regardless of design, the pontic should provide an occlusal surface that stabilizes the opposing teeth, allows for normal mastication, and does not overload the abutment teeth. The restorative material for all four designs can be either glazed porcelain, polished gold, or polished resin. There is no difference in biologic response of the tissue from contact with the restoration, regardless of the material chosen, as long as it has a smooth surface finish.[26,54,64] The key differences between the four pontic designs relate to the esthetics and access for hygiene procedures. The primary method for cleaning the undersurface of pontics is to draw dental floss mesiodistally along the undersurface. The shape of this undersurface determines the ease with which plaque and food debris can be removed in the process. The sanitary and ovate pontics have convex undersurfaces that facilitate cleaning. The ridgelap and modified ridgelap designs have concave surfaces that are more difficult to access with dental floss. Although the sanitary pontic design provides the easiest access for hygiene procedures, it is rarely used due to its unesthetic form and a variable acceptance of the open contour by patients.

The ovate pontic is the ideal pontic form.[62] It is created by forming a receptor site in the edentulous ridge with either a diamond bur or electrosurgery. The site is shaped to create either a flat or concave contour so that when the pontic is created to adapt to the site, it will have a flat or convex outline. The depth of the receptor site is dependent on the esthetic requirements of the pontic. In highly esthetic areas such as the maxillary

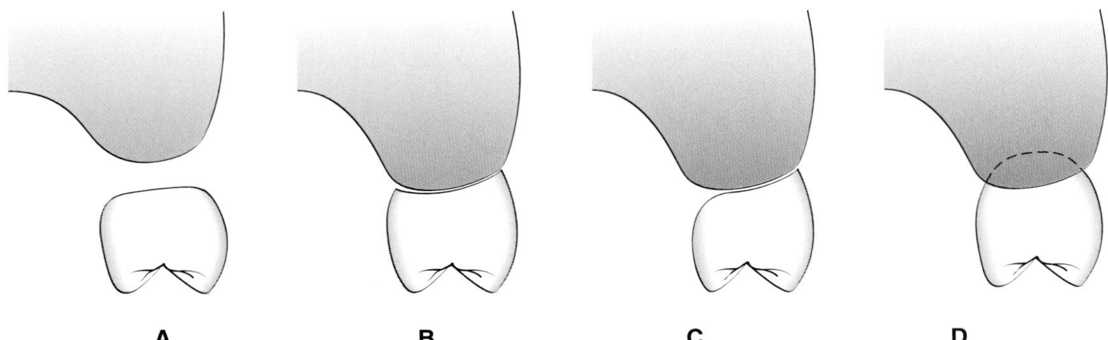

Fig. 75-30 Four options to designing the shape of a pontic. **A,** The sanitary pontic where the tissue surface of the pontic is 3 mm from the underlying ridge. **B,** The ridge lap pontic where the tissue surface of the pontic straddles the ridge much like a saddle. The entire tissue surface of the ridge lapped pontic is convex and very difficult to clean. **C,** The modified ridge lap pontic. The tissue surface on the facial is concave, following the ridge. However, the lingual saddle has been removed to allow access for oral hygiene. **D,** The ovate pontic. The pontic form fits into a receptor site within the ridge. This allows the tissue surface of the pontic to be convex and also optimizes esthetics.

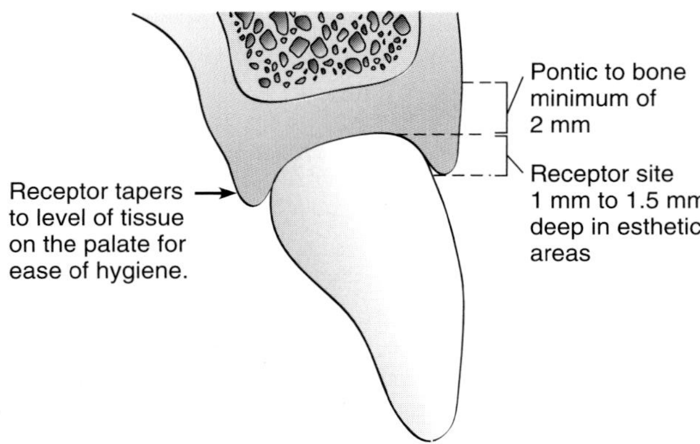

Fig. 75-31 The ideal shape and form of an ovate pontic in the esthetic area. The receptor site has been created 1 to 1.5 mm apical to the free gingival margin on the facial. This creates the illusion of the pontic erupting from the tissue. On the palatal, the pontic is tapered so that the receptor site is not extended below tissue. This allows for easier access for oral hygiene. Note that when the receptor site is created, the bone must be a minimum of 2 mm from the most apical portion of the pontic.

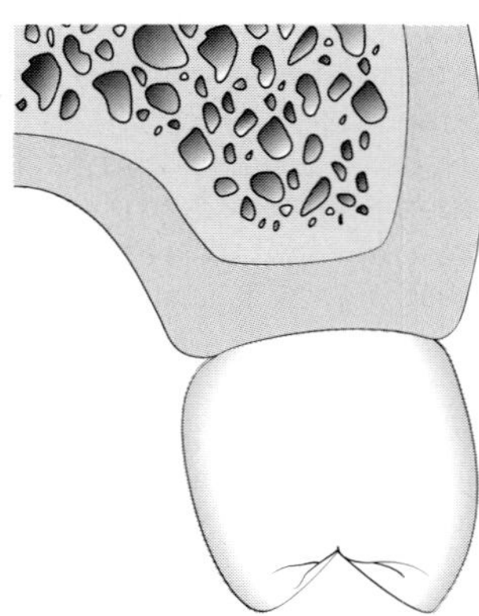

Fig. 75-32 An option for creating an ovate pontic receptor site in less esthetic areas of the mouth. Rather than creating the receptor site so that the pontic extends into the ridge, it is possible to create a flattened receptor site where the pontic sits flush with the ridge. This makes oral hygiene easier.

anterior region, it is necessary to create a receptor area that is 1 mm to 1.5 mm below the tissue on the facial aspect. This creates the appearance of a free gingival margin and produces optimum esthetics (Fig. 75-31). This site can then be tapered to the height of the palatal tissue to facilitate hygiene access from the palatal side. In the posterior areas, a deep receptor site can complicate hygiene access. In these situations, the ideal site has the facial portion of the pontic at the same level as the ridge, and then the site is created as a straight line to the lingual side of the pontic. This removes the convexity of the ridge and produces a flat, easily cleansable tissue surface on the pontic (Fig. 75-32).

When the ridge is being surgically modified, it is important to know the thickness of soft tissue above the bone. This measurement is obtained by probing to the bone through the anesthetized tissue. If the tissue is removed to less than 2 mm in thickness, significant rebound in ridge height may occur. If it is necessary to reduce the tissue height to less than 2 mm above the bone to create the desired pontic form, then some bone must be removed to achieve the desired result.

It is important when considering an ovate pontic to realize that certain soft tissue ridge parameters must exist to optimize the ovate pontic form. The ridge height needs to match the ideal height of the interproximal papillae where interproximal embrasures are planned, either between pontics or next to abutment teeth. The gingival margin height must also be at the ideal level or the pontic will appear too long. Finally, the ridge tissue must be facial to the ideal cervical facial form of the pontic so that the pontic can be made to emerge from the tissue. If any of these three areas are inadequate, some form of ridge augmentation is needed to produce a ridge on which an adequate receptor site can be created (Fig. 75-33). Any ridge augmentation procedures should be completed prior to or in conjunction with fabricating an ovate pontic. When constructing the final restorations, the contours of the developed ovate pontic receptor site can be conveyed to the laboratory by capturing a soft tissue impression 4 to 6 weeks after the site has been created.

The ovate pontic can serve another important periodontal function by maintaining the interdental papilla next to abutment teeth after extraction.[62] When a tooth is removed, the gingival embrasure form is lost. The normal response of the papilla to this loss of embrasure form is to recede 1.5 to 2 mm, which corresponds to the additional soft tissue existing above bone on the interproximal compared with the facial. However, this recession can be prevented. By inserting the correct pontic form 2.5 mm into the extraction site on the day the tooth is removed, the gingival embrasure form and papilla can be maintained. At 4 weeks, the 2.5-mm extension can be reduced to a 1.0 to 1.5 mm extension to facilitate hygiene. This procedure can maintain the papilla next to the abutment teeth as long as the bone on the abutment tooth is at a normal level (Color Figs. 75-8 to 75-15).

The full-ridge lap pontic is an outdated design that straddles the convexity of the ridge buccolingually and creates an undersurface that is entirely concave and cannot be cleaned. It is not recommended for use in any situations. However, a modified ridge lap design can be an acceptable design if inadequate ridge exists to create an ovate pontic. With the modified ridge lap design, the pontic follows the convexity of the ridge on the facial but stops on the lingual crest of the ridge without extending down the lingual side of the ridge. Whereas the facial aspect of the undersurface has a concave shape, adequate access for oral hygiene is allowed by the more open lingual form.

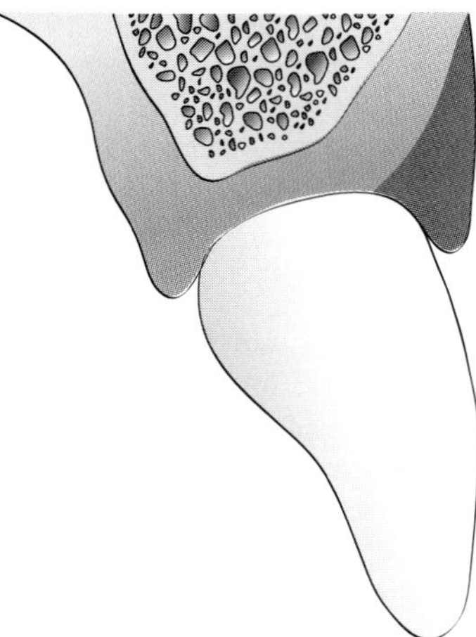

Fig. 75-33 Ridge considerations when an ovate pontic is desired. For an ovate pontic to be properly created, the soft tissue ridge must be labial to the desired cervical portion of the pontic. When the pontic is facial to the ridge, it is not possible to create what appears to be a free gingival margin correctly. The shaded area represents the necessary amount of tissue that would be augmented to produce an ideal ovate pontic in this particular site.

OCCLUSAL CONSIDERATIONS

The importance of occlusion and its role in dentistry has been decreasing significantly over the past 20 years. Occlusal trauma as a factor in periodontal disease and its role in orofacial pain has been deemphasized in numerous papers.[9,15,35,36,45,46,55,66,72] However, the role occlusion plays in restorative dentistry is becoming reemphasized. The increase in the utilization of dental implants and nonmetallic cosmetic restorations has resulted in an increased concern with force management. These restorations are more sensitive to occlusal trauma with subsequent structural failure than are traditional restorations on teeth. Consequently, for the restorative dentist wanting a high degree of predictability in their final result, understanding occlusion is critical. The clinician must know how to create an occlusion with the following guidelines as a goal:

1. There should be even simultaneous contacts on all teeth during centric closure. This distributes the force of closure over all the teeth instead of the few teeth that may touch first.
2. When the mandible moves from centric closure, some form of canine or anterior guidance is desirable, with no posterior tooth contacts. This combination of anterior guidance and posterior disclusion reduces the ability of the elevator muscles to contract and distributes the force of the movement onto the anterior teeth, which receive less force due to the class III lever system that is being applied in this situation. It has been shown that due to the class III lever action, the anterior teeth receive approximately one ninth the force of a second molar.[25,61]
3. The anterior guidance needs to be in harmony with the patient's neuromuscular envelope of function. Harmony of this relationship is demonstrated by a lack of fremitus and mobility on the anterior teeth, the ability of the patient to speak clearly and comfortably, and the patient's general sense of comfort with the overbite, overjet, and guidance created during chewing and when holding their head in an upright posture.
4. The occlusion should be created at a vertical dimension that is stable for the patient. It is generally accepted that the patient's existing vertical dimension is an equilibrium between the eruptive forces of their teeth and the repetitive contracted length of their elevator muscles. It has been demonstrated that vertical dimension can be altered with no sense of pain from muscles and joints.[9,11,22,30] However, if this alteration lengthens the pterygomasseteric sling beyond its ability to adapt, the patient will not maintain the vertical change and will close the occlusal vertical dimension by intruding the teeth.[12,34,41–43]
5. When managing a pathologic occlusion or when restoring a complete occlusion, a repeatable condylar reference position is needed. *Centric relation,* defined as the most superior condylar position, provides such a starting point.[21] Centric relation has been shown to be reproducible over multiple appointments, allowing the clinician to create the occlusion indirectly on an articulator and return it to the same reference position in the mouth.[14,39,40,74] It is the only position that has been shown to shut off lateral pterygoid muscle contraction.[20] Because it is a border position, any mandibular movement will result in the condyle moving inferiorly. Therefore it is the only position from which an interference-free occlusion can be created.

To manage the occlusion as described here, the clinician must be able to make accurate casts, use a face-bow, and create centric relation records so that the information can be transferred to a suitable articulator. Although the details of these procedures are beyond the scope of this chapter, they are a routine part of any restorative treatment plan and must be mastered for the clinician to achieve predictable long-term restorative success.

SPECIAL CONSIDERATIONS

Restoration of Root-Resected Teeth

Although the availability of implant therapy has greatly reduced the frequency with which root-amputated teeth are saved, they are still a viable mode of treatment. Structural challenges are created in restoring these teeth because of the amount of tooth structure lost in the resection process (Fig. 75-34). Conservative tooth preparation maintains as much of the remaining tooth as possible, but the resulting supragingival or minimally prepared subgingival finish lines requires additional metal display in the final restoration. A cast post and core may be indicated to create an adequate foundation for the final restoration. Because the remaining roots are often very thin mesiodistally, it is difficult to cement prefabricated posts and have adequate bulk to place a foundation core on the mesial and distal of the post. This problem is avoided with the one-piece cast post and core restoration.

Another area of concern when restoring these teeth is the development of appropriate contours for hygiene access. The primary concern is to avoid any excessively heavy convexities of contour that would prevent access (Figs. 75-35 and 75-36). Facially and lingually, the contours should be essentially a straight line from the margin coronally, whereas interproximally, the contour emerges from the margin as a straight line or is slightly convex as it slopes up to the contact point. The interproximal areas of root-amputated and -hemisected teeth often present with surface concavities on the root trunk, and these areas cannot be adequately cleaned with floss because it will bridge across the concavity. The gingival embrasure form created in the restoration must be fluted into these areas so that the surfaces can be accessed with an interdental brush.

Esthetics is usually not a major concern unless the tooth in question is a maxillary molar with a mesiobuccal root amputation and the patient has a broad smile. The solution is to create an artificial mesiobuccal root with normal crown contour coronal to it and a furcation made out of restorative material that is easily cleaned with an interdental brush.

Splinting

Splinting therapy may be applied with bonded external appliances, intracoronal appliances, or indirect cast restorations to connect multiple teeth together with the goal of improving tooth stability. Unstable teeth may be due to a lack of periodontal support from bone loss, a lack of support from tooth loss, or the need to splint abutment teeth to support pontics. Indications for splinting are mobility of teeth that is increasing or impairs patient comfort, migration of teeth, or prosthetics where multiple abutments are necessary. Before considering splinting, the etiology of the instability must be identified.[2] Excessive occlusal forces from parafunction or deflective tooth contacts are frequent causes of excessive mobility. Whenever the occlusion is the cause, occlusal therapy is always performed first. The mobility is then evaluated over time to determine whether it resolves before splinting is considered. In addition, any inflammation of the periodontal supporting apparatus must be controlled before making a decision on splinting because inflammation can produce mobility in the presence of normal occlusal forces and normal periodontal support. When the teeth are splinted, all the teeth in the splint share the occlusal load to some extent.[17] The rigidity of the splint and the number of teeth used determines how the forces are distributed. The most common indication to splint mobile teeth is to improve patient comfort and provide better control of the occlusion if the anterior teeth are mobile. It is critical that adequate crown length on the teeth is being splinted so that the interproximal connectors do not impinge on the interdental papilla. Also, adequate space is needed between the connector and the papilla for access with dental floss anteriorly and an interproximal brush on posterior teeth.

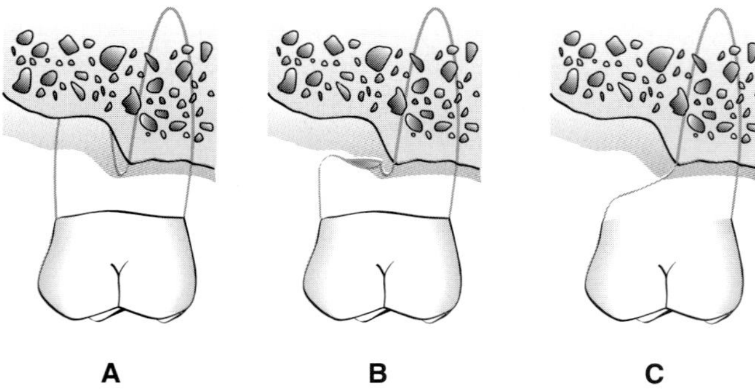

Fig. 75-34 **A,** A maxillary molar with a Class 3 furcation and bone loss surrounding the distal buccal root. **B,** The contour created when the distal buccal root is removed but the coronal contour has not yet been reshaped. Note the overhang, which can trap food and plaque and create gingival inflammation. **C,** The correct contour after the restoration or reshaping of the tooth. Note this illustration is only of the facial portion of the tooth. The palatal portion of the crown and the palatal root do not appear. Note how the contour has been altered to allow easy access for an interdental brush to the gingival tissue and the tooth in the area where the root was removed.

Anterior Esthetic Surgery

The importance of gingiva in relation to anterior esthetics has been well documented.[10,29,59,65] Various methods for altering gingival levels have been described, including gingivectomy, apically displaced flaps with osseous recontouring, and the use of orthodontics to position the gingival apically or coronally by intruding or extruding the teeth.[5,13,33,69] Whenever an alteration in gingival levels is contemplated, the expected outcome must be communicated to the patient to determine whether the planned surgery is acceptable. Computer imaging can be used to provide the patient with a visual plan for the

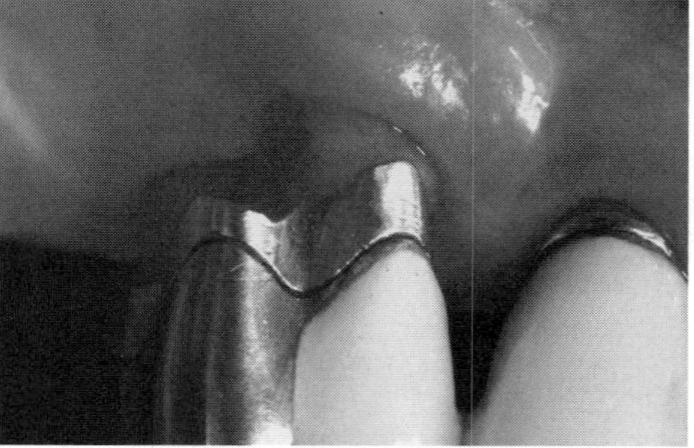

Fig. 75-35 A photograph taken 6 weeks after the removal of the distal buccal root on this maxillary first molar. Note the crown contour has not been altered yet and the presence of a large overhang that easily traps debris.

final esthetic result.[18] However, the imaging process does not allow the dentist or patient to include the dynamics of lip movement in the evaluation of the proposed changes. Computer imaging provides enough information to accurately depict the final outcome when the planned surgery will alter the gingiva on one or two teeth while leaving the gingival levels of adjacent teeth in their existing position.

However, when the surgery will involve many or all of the anterior teeth and result in moving gingiva several millimeters, to the extent that a flap will be raised and bony levels altered, an additional guide is desirable before surgery. Constructing these guides directly on a stone cast is the easiest and least time-consuming method. Before constructing the guide, treatment planning is completed to determine the desired incisal edge position and gingival level of the tissues. This establishes the amount of tooth display at rest and at full smile. The information is transferred to a stone cast of the patient's teeth, and the desired shape of the gingival margins for each tooth is drawn on the cast. The existing incisal edge position of each tooth is used as a reference in establishing the desired gingival level. A composite or acrylic resin veneer is then constructed on the cast, extending gingivally to the desired tissue position. The veneer guide also can be extended incisally to the desired incisal edge position so that that information also can be included in the veneer. The veneer is trimmed, polished, and tried in the patient's mouth. When the patient approves the gingival levels established with the guide, the desired gingival correction can be completed using the veneer guide as a surgical template. In addition to locating the initial incisions at the correct level, the guide also can be employed after flap reflection to aid in the bony recontouring, ensuring adequate biologic width and sulcus depth at the new gingival position. The surgeon replaces the flap at closure to the gingival level established with the guide. Employing an esthetic template in this manner optimizes the predictability of the surgical therapy and establishes the ideal tissue framework to complete the esthetic restorations (Color Figs. 75-16 to 75-23).

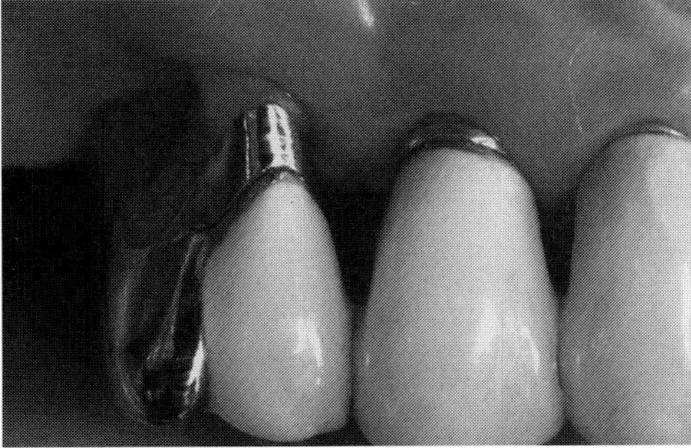

Fig. 75-36 The correct modification of the crown form seen in Fig. 75-35. The roof of the furcation of the remaining distal buccal root has been completely removed and the crown reformed to allow easy access to the remaining roots and soft tissue.

REFERENCES

1. Adamczyk E, Speichowics E: Plaque accumulation on crowns made of various materials. Int J Prosthodont 1990; 3:285.
2. Amsterdam M: Periodontal prosthesis: Twenty-five years in retrospect. Alpha Omegan 1974; 67:30.
3. Amsterdam M, Fox L: Provisional splinting: Principles and techniques. Dent Clin North Am 1959; 4:73.
4. Armitage GC, Svanberg GK, Löe H: Microscopic evaluation of clinical measurements of connective tissue attachment levels. J Clin Periodontol 1977; 4:173.
5. Becker W, Ochsenbein C, Becker B: Crown lengthening: The periodontal-restorative connection. Compend Contin Educ Dent 1998; 19(3):239.
6. Benson BW, Bomberg TJ, Hatch RA, et al: Tissue displacement in fixed prosthodontics. J Prosthet Dent 1986; 55(2):175.
7. Bragger U, Laachenauer D, Lang NP: Surgical lengthening of the clinical crown. J Clin Periodontol 1992; 19:58.
8. Carlsson G, De Boever J: Epidemiology. In: Zarb G, Carlsson G, Sessle B, et al (eds): Epidemiology. Copenhagen, Munksgaard, 1994.
9. Carlsson GE, Ingerval B, Kocak G: Effect of increasing vertical dimension on the masticatory system in subjects with natural teeth. J Prosthet Dent 1979; 41(3):284.
10. Chiche GJ, Pinault A: Esthetics of anterior fixed prosthodontics. Chicago, Quintessence, 1994.
11. Christensen J: Effect of occlusion-raising procedures on the chewing system. Dent Pract Dent Rec 1970; 20(7):233.
12. Dahl BL, Krogstad O: Long-term observations of an increased occlusal face height obtained by a combined orthodontic/prosthetic approach. J Oral Rehabil 1985; 12(2):173.
13. Dolt A, Robbins J: Altered passive eruption: An etiology of short clinical crowns. Quintessence Int 1997; 28(6):363.
14. Downs DH: An investigation into condylar position with leaf gauge and bimanual manipulation. J Gnathol 1988; 7:75.
15. Ericsson I, Lindhe J: Effect of longstanding jiggling on experimental periodontitis in the beagle dog. J Clin Periodontol 1982; 9(6):497.
16. Felton DA, Kanoy Be, Bayne SC, et al: Effect of in vivo crown margin discrepancies on periodontal health. J Prosthet Dent 1991; 65:357.
17. Foucher RR, Bryant RA: Bilateral fixed splints. Int J Periodont Restor Dent 1983; 5:9.
18. Ganz CH, Brisman SA, Tauro V: Computer video imaging: Computerization, communication, and creation. QDT Yearbook 1989; 64.
19. Gargiulo AW, Wentz FM, Orban B: Dimension and relations of the dentogingival junction in humans. J Periodontol 1961; 32:262.
20. Gibb CH, Mahan PE, Wilkenson TM, et al: EMG activity of the superior belly of the lateral pterygoid muscle in relation to other jaw muscles. J Prosthet Dent 1984; 51(5):691.
21. The Glossary of Prosthodontic Terms, ed 6. St Louis, Mosby, 1994.
22. Gross MD, Ormianer Z: A preliminary study on the effect of occlusal vertical dimension increases on mandibular postural rest position. Int J Prosthodont 1994; 7(3):216.
23. Günay H, Seeger A, Tschernitschek H, et al: Placement of the preparation line and periodontal health—A prospective 2-year clinical study. Int J Periodont Restor Dent 2000; 20:173.
24. Hansen PA, Tira DE, Barlow J: Current methods of finish line exposure by practicing prosthodontists. J Prosthodont 1999; 8(3):163.
25. Hatcher DC, Faulkner MG, Hay A: Development of mechanical and mathematic models to study temporomandibular joint loading. J Prosthet Dent 1986; 55(3):377.
26. Henry PJ, Johnson JF, Mitchell DF: Tissue changes beneath fixed partial dentures. J Prosthet Dent 1966; 16:937.

27. Hochman N, Yaffe A, Ehrlich J: Crown contour variation in gingival health. Compendium 1983; 4:360.
28. Ingber JS: Forced eruption. II. A method of treating nonrestorable teeth—Periodontal and restorative considerations. J Periodontol 1995; 47:203.
29. Kay HB: Esthetic considerations in the definitive periodontal prosthetic management of the maxillary anterior segment. Int J Periodont Restor Dent 1982; 2(3):44.
30. Kohno S, Bando E: Die funcktionelle anpassung der kaumuskulatur bei starker beisshenbung (Functional adaptation of masticatory muscles as a result of large increases in the vertical dimension). Dtsch Zahnãrtzl Z 1983; 38:759.
31. Kois JC, Spear FM: Periodontal prosthesis: Creating successful restorations. J Am Dent Assoc 1992; 123:108.
32. Kozlovsky A, Tal H, Lieberman M: Forced eruption combined with gingival fiberotomy. A technique for clinical crown lengthening. J Clin Periodontol 1991; 18:330.
33. Lie T: Periodontal surgery for the maxillary anterior area. Int J Peridont Restor Dent 1992; 12(1):73.
34. Lindauer SJ, Gay T, Rendell J: Effect of jaw opening on masticatory muscles: EMG-force characteristics. J Dent Res 1993; 72(1):51.
35. Lindhe J, Ericsson I: The influence of trauma from occlusion on progression of experimental periodontitis in dogs. J Clin Periodontol 1982; 53(9):562.
36. Lindhe J, Svanberg G: Influence of trauma from occlusion on progression of experimental periodontitis in the beagle dog. J Clin Periodontol 1974; 1(1):3.
37. Listgarten MA, Mao R, Robinson PJ: Periodontal probing and the relationship of the probe tip to periodontal tissues. J Periodontol 1976; 47:511.
38. Listgarten MA: Periodontal probing: What does it mean? J Clin Periodontol 1980; 7:165.
39. Long JH: Locating centric relation with a leaf gauge. J Prosthet Dent 1973; 29(6):608.
40. McKee JR: Comparing condylar position respectability for standardized versus nonstandardized methods of achieving centric relation. J Prosthet Dent 1997; 77(3):280.
41. MacKenna BR, Türker KS: Jaw separation and maximum incising force. J Prosthet Dent 1983; 49(5):726.
42. Manns A, Mirallees R, Guerrs F: The changes in electrical activity of the postural muscles of the mandible upon varying the vertical dimension. J Prosthet Dent 1981; 45(4):438.
43. Manns A, Spreng M: EMG amplitude and frequency at different muscular elongations under constant masticatory force or EMG activity. Acta Physiol Lat Am 1977; 27(5):259.
44. Marcum JS: The effect of crown margin depth upon gingival tissue. J Prosthet Dent 1967; 17:479.
45. Meitner S: Co-destructive factors of marginal periodontitis and repetitive mechanical injury. J Dent Res 1975; (c):78.
46. National Institutes of Health Technology: Assessment conference statement: Management of temporomandibular disorders, 29 April–1 May 1996. Oral Surg Oral Med Oral Pathol Oral Radiol Endod 1997; 83:177.
47. Newcomb GJ: The relationship between the location of subgingival crown margins and gingival inflammation. J Periodontol 1974; 45:151.
48. Olsson M, Lindhe S: Periodontol characteristics in individuals with varying forms of the upper central incisors. J Clin Periodontol 1991; 18:78.
49. Parma-Benfenati S, Fugazzoto PA, Ruben MP: The effect of restorative margins on the postsurgical development and nature of the periodontium. Part I. Int J Periodont Restor Dent 1985; 6:31.
50. Parkinson CF: Excessive crown contours facilitate endemic plaque niches. J Prosthet Dent 1976; 35:424.
51. Pelton L: Nickel sensibility in the general population. Contact Derm 1979; 5:27.
52. Perel ML: Axial crown contours. J Prosthet Dent 1971; 25:642.
53. Pierce LH, Goodkind RJ: A status report of possible risks in base metal alloys and their components. J Prosthet Dent 1989; 62:234.
54. Podshadley AG: Gingival response to pontics. J Prosthet Dent 1968; 19:51.
55. Polson AM, Meitner SW, Zander HA: Trauma and progression of marginal periodontitis in squirrel monkeys. III. Adaptation of interproximal alveolar bone to repetitive injury. J Periodont Res 1976; 11(5):279.
56. Price C, Whitehead FJH: Impression material as foreign bodies. Br Dent J 1972; 133:9.
57. Robinson PJ, Vitek RM: The relationship between gingival inflammation and the probe resistance. J Periodont Res 1975; 14:239.
58. Rosenburg ES, Garber DA, Evian CL: Tooth lengthening procedures. Compend Contin Educ Dent 1980; 1:161.
59. Rufenache CR: Fundamentals of esthetics. Chicago, Quintessence, 1990.
60. Sillness J: Treated with dental bridges. III. The relationship between the location of the crown margin and the periodontal condition. J Periodont Res 1970; 5:225.
61. Smith DM, McLachlan KR, McCall WD Jr: A numerical model of temporomandibular joint loading. J Dent Res 1986; 65(8):1046.
62. Spear FM: Maintenance of the interdental papilla following anterior tooth removal. Pract Periodont Aesthet Dent 1999; 11(1):21.
63. Spear FM, Mathews DM, Kokich VG: Interdisciplinary treatment: Integrating orthodontics with periodontics, endodontics, and restorative dentistry. Seminar Orthodont 1997; 3(1).
64. Stein RS: Pontic-residual ridge relationship: A research report. J Prosthet Dent 1966; 16:251.
65. Studer S, Zellweger U, Scharer P: The esthetic guidelines of the mucogingival complex for fixed prosthodontics. Pract Periodontics Aesthet Dent 1996; 8(4):333.
66. Suvinen T, Hanes K, Gerchman J, et al: Psychophysical subtypes of temporomandibular disorders. J Orofac Pain 1997; 11:200.
67. Swartz ML, Phillips RW: Comparison of bacterial accumulations on rough and smooth surfaces. J Periodontol 1957; 28:304.
68. Tarnow DP, Magner AW, Fletcher P: The effects of the distance from the contact point to the crest of bone on the presence or absence of the interproximal dental papilla. J Periodontol 1992; 63:995.
69. Townsend CL: Resective surgery: An esthetic application. Quintessence Int 1993; 24(8):535.
70. Tylman SD: Theory and Practice of Crown and Bridge Prosthodontics, ed 5. St Louis, Mosby, 1965.
71. Vacek JS, Gher ME, Assad DA, et al: The dimensions of the human dentogingival junction. Int J Periodont Restor Dent 1994; 14(2):155.
72. Vallon D: Studies of occlusion adjustment therapy in patients with craniomandibular disorders (thesis). Malmö, Lund University. Swed Dent J 1997; suppl 124.
73. Van-der-Veldon U: Regeneration of the interdental soft tissue following denudation procedures. J Clin Periodont 1982; 9(6):455.
74. Wood DP, Elliott RW: Reproducibility of the centric relation bite registration technique. Angle Orthod 1994; 64:211.
75. Yuodelis RA, Faucher R: Provisional restorations: An integrated approach to periodontics and restorative dentistry. Dent Clin North Am 1980; 24:285.
76. Yuodelis RA, Weaver JD, Sapko S: Facial and lingual contours of artificial complete crowns and their effect on the periodontium. J Prosthet Dent 1973; 29:61.

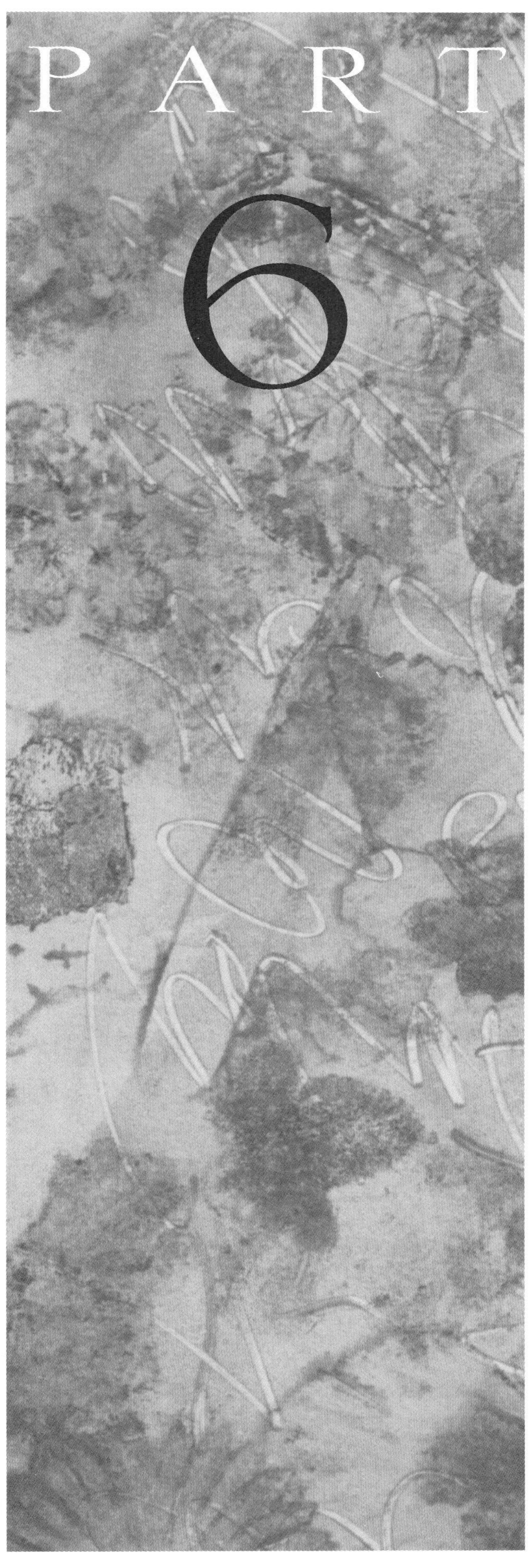

Periodontal Maintenance Phase

Henry H. Takei

The successful management of periodontal disease requires a positive program directed at maintaining and improving the results of treatment as well as preventing the development of new disease. The gradual microbial recolonization of tooth surfaces begins soon after plaque is eliminated; therefore the measures to stop recolonization also must be a constant effort on the part of the patient, following the professional instructions and guidance and including periodic professional care visits. This part also presents the overwhelming evidence that has been accumulated about the effectiveness of periodontal therapy.

Supportive Periodontal Treatment

Robert L. Merin

CHAPTER

CHAPTER OUTLINE

Preservation of the periodontal health of the treated patient requires as positive a program as that required for the elimination of periodontal disease. After Phase I therapy is completed, patients are placed on a schedule of periodic recall visits for maintenance care to prevent recurrence of the disease (Figs. 76-1 and 76-2).

Transfer of the patient from active treatment status to a maintenance program is a definitive step in total patient care that requires time and effort on the part of the dentist and staff. Patients must be made to understand the purpose of the maintenance program, and the dentist must emphasize that preservation of the teeth is dependent on it. Patients who are not maintained in a supervised recall program subsequent to active treatment show obvious signs of recurrent periodontitis (e.g., increased pocket depth, bone loss, and tooth loss).[4,7] The more often patients present for recommended supportive periodontal treatment (SPT), the less likely they are to lose teeth.[61] In fact, one study found that tooth loss is three times as common in treated patients who do not return for regular recall visits as in those who do[24]; another showed that patients with inadequate SPT after successful regenerative therapy have a 50-fold increase in risk of probing attachment loss as compared with those with regular recalls.[14] Motivational techniques and reinforcement of the importance of the maintenance phase of treatment should be considered prior to performing definitive periodontal surgery.[7] Studies have shown that few patients display complete compliance with recommended maintenance schedules[1,34,36,60,62] (Fig. 76-3). *It is meaningless simply to inform patients that they are to return for periodic recall visits without clearly explaining the significance of these visits and describing what is expected of patients between visits.*

The maintenance phase of periodontal treatment starts immediately after the completion of Phase I therapy (see Figs. 76-1 and 76-2). While the patient is in the maintenance phase, the necessary surgical and restorative procedures are performed. This ensures that all areas of the mouth retain the degree of health attained after Phase I therapy.

RATIONALE FOR SUPPORTIVE PERIODONTAL TREATMENT

Studies have shown that even with appropriate periodontal therapy, some progression of disease is possible.[18,21,37,42,55] One likely explanation for the recurrence of periodontal disease is *incomplete subgingival plaque removal.*[58] If subgingival plaque is left behind during scaling, it regrows within the pocket. The regrowth of

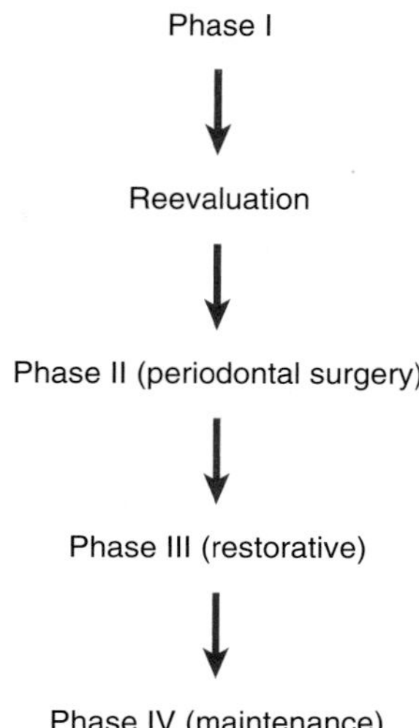

Fig. 76-1 Incorrect sequence of periodontal treatment phases. Maintenance phase should be started immediately after the reevaluation of Phase I.

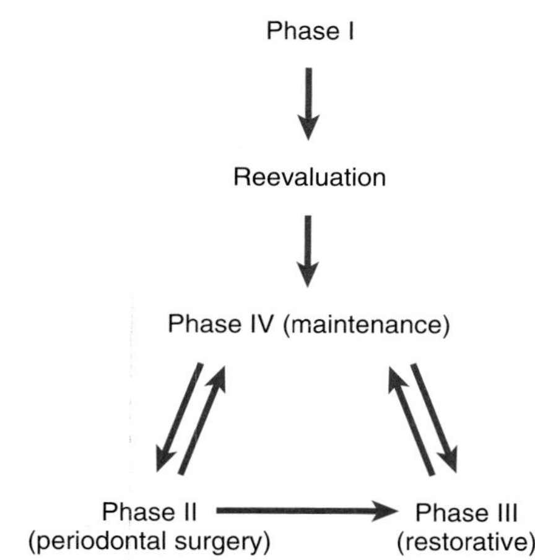

Fig. 76-2 Correct sequence of periodontal treatment phases.

subgingival plaque is a slow process compared with that of supragingival plaque. During this period (perhaps months), the subgingival plaque may not induce inflammatory reactions that can be discerned at the gingival margin. The clinical diagnosis may be further confused by the introduction of adequate supragingival plaque control because the inflammatory reactions caused by the plaque in the soft tissue wall of the pocket are not likely to be manifested clinically as gingivitis. Thus inadequate subgingival plaque control can lead to continued loss of attachment, even without the presence of clinical gingival inflammation.

Bacteria are present in the gingival tissues in chronic and aggressive periodontitis cases.[10,13,39,44] Eradication of intragingival microorganisms may be necessary for a stable periodontal result. Scaling, root planing, and even flap surgery may not eliminate intragingival bacteria in some areas.[16] These bacteria may recolonize the pocket and cause recurrent disease.

Bacteria associated with periodontitis can be transmitted between spouses and other family members.[2,56] Patients who appear to be successfully treated can become infected or reinfected with potential pathogens. This is especially likely in patients with remaining pockets.

Another possible explanation for the recurrence of periodontal disease is the microscopic nature of the dentogingival unit healing after periodontal treatment. Histologic studies have shown that after periodontal procedures, tissues usually do not heal by formation of new connective tissue attachment to root surfaces[11,49,50] but result in a long junctional epithelium. It has been speculated that this type of dentogingival unit may be weaker and inflammation may rapidly separate the long junctional epithelium from the tooth. Thus treated periodontal patients may be predisposed to recurrent pocket formation if maintenance care is not optimal.

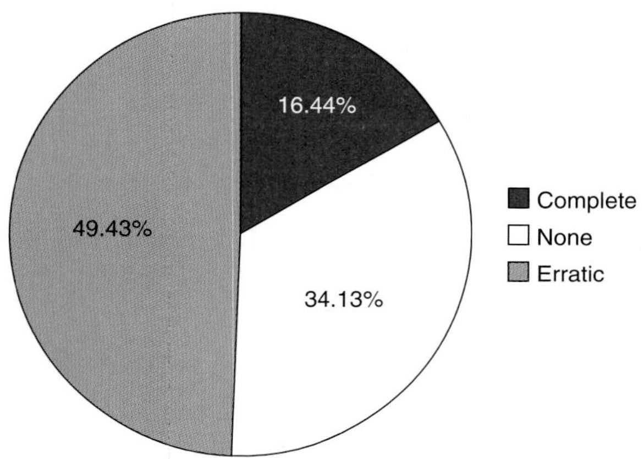

Fig. 76-3 Compliance with maintenance therapy in 961 patients studied for 1 to 8 years. (Adapted from Wilson TG Jr, Glover ME, Schoen J, et al: Compliance with maintenance therapy in a private periodontal practice. J Periodontol 1984; 55:468.)

Subgingival scaling alters the microflora of periodontal pockets.[35,41,47] In one study,[35] a single session of scaling and root planing in patients with chronic periodontitis resulted in significant changes in subgingival microflora. Reported alterations included a decrease in the proportion of motile rods for 1 week, a marked elevation in the proportion of coccoid cells for 21 days, and a marked reduction in the proportion of spirochetes for 7 weeks.

Another study reported that subgingival bacteria had not returned to pretreatment proportions after 3 to 6 months.[47] However, the rate of return of the pretreatment microbial flora varied among patients. These findings indicate that mechanical debridement produces a relatively long-lasting effect on the microbial flora and that the different groups of microorganisms return to baseline values after varying time periods.

BOX 76-1

Maintenance Recall Procedures

Part I: Examination (approximate time: 17 minutes)[54]
- Medical history changes
- Oral pathologic examination
- Oral hygiene status
- Gingival changes
- Pocket depth changes
- Mobility changes
- Occlusal changes
- Dental caries
- Restorative and prosthetic status

Part II: Treatment (approximate time: 35 minutes)[54]
- Oral hygiene reinforcement
- Scaling
- Polishing
- Chemical Irrigation

Part III: Schedule next procedure (approximate time: 1 minute)[54]
- Schedule next recall visit
- Schedule further periodontal treatment
- Schedule or refer for restorative or prosthetic treatment

A
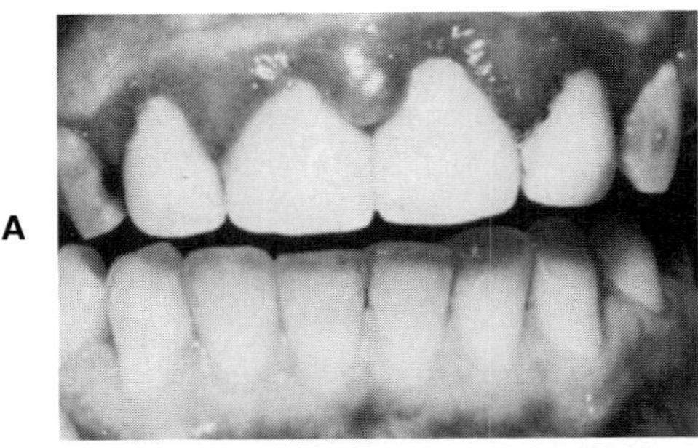

B
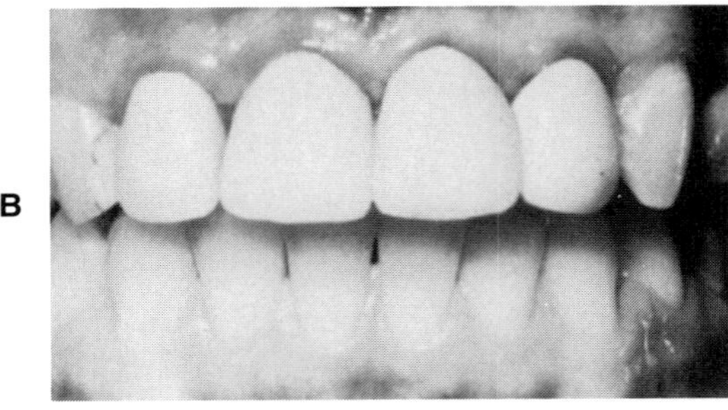

Fig. 76-4 A, Hyperplastic gingivitis related to crown margins and plaque accumulation in a 27-year-old woman. **B,** Four months after treatment, there is significant improvement. However, some inflammation around crown margins still exists, which cannot be resolved without replacing the crowns.

There is reason to believe that both the mechanical debridement performed by the therapist and the motivational environment provided by the appointment are necessary for good maintenance results. Patients tend to reduce their oral hygiene efforts between appointments.[4,62] Knowing that their hygiene will be evaluated causes them to perform better oral hygiene in anticipation of the appointment.

In one study, the proportion of spirochetes obtained in baseline samples of subgingival flora was highly correlated with clinical periodontal deterioration over a period of 1 year.[27] However, subsequent reports in the same longitudinal study concluded that the arbitrary assignment of treated periodontitis patients to 3-month maintenance intervals appears to be as effective in preventing recurrences of periodontitis as assignment of recall intervals based on microscopic monitoring of the subgingival flora.[28,29] Microscopic monitoring was found not to be a reliable predictor of future periodontal destruction in patients on 3-month recall programs, presumably because of the alteration of subgingival flora produced by subgingival instrumentation.

In conclusion, there is a sound scientific basis for recall maintenance because subgingival scaling alters the pocket microflora for variable but relatively long periods.

MAINTENANCE PROGRAM

Periodic recall visits form the foundation of a meaningful long-term prevention program. The interval between visits is initially set at 3 months but may be varied according to the patient's needs.

Periodontal care at each recall visit comprises three parts (Box 76-1). The first part is concerned with examination and evaluation of the patient's current oral health. The second part includes the necessary maintenance treatment and oral hygiene reinforcement. The third part involves scheduling the patient for the next recall appointment, additional periodontal treatment, or restorative dental procedures. The time required for a recall visit for patients with multiple teeth in both arches is approximately 1 hour,[45] which includes time for greeting the patient, setting up, and cleaning up.

Examination and Evaluation

The recall examination is similar to the initial evaluation of the patient discussed in Chapter 30. However, because the patient is not new to the office, the dentist primarily looks for changes that have occurred since the last evaluation. Analysis of the current oral hygiene status of the patient is essential. Updating of changes in the medical history and evaluation of restorations, caries, prostheses, occlusion, tooth mobility, gingival status, and periodontal pockets are important parts of the recall appointment. The oral mucosa should be carefully inspected for pathologic conditions (Figs. 76-4 to 76-9).

Radiographic examination must be individualized[30] depending on the initial severity of the case and the findings at the recall visit (Table 76-1). These are compared with findings on previous radiographs to check the bone height and look for repair of osseous defects, signs of trauma from occlusion, periapical pathologic changes, and caries.

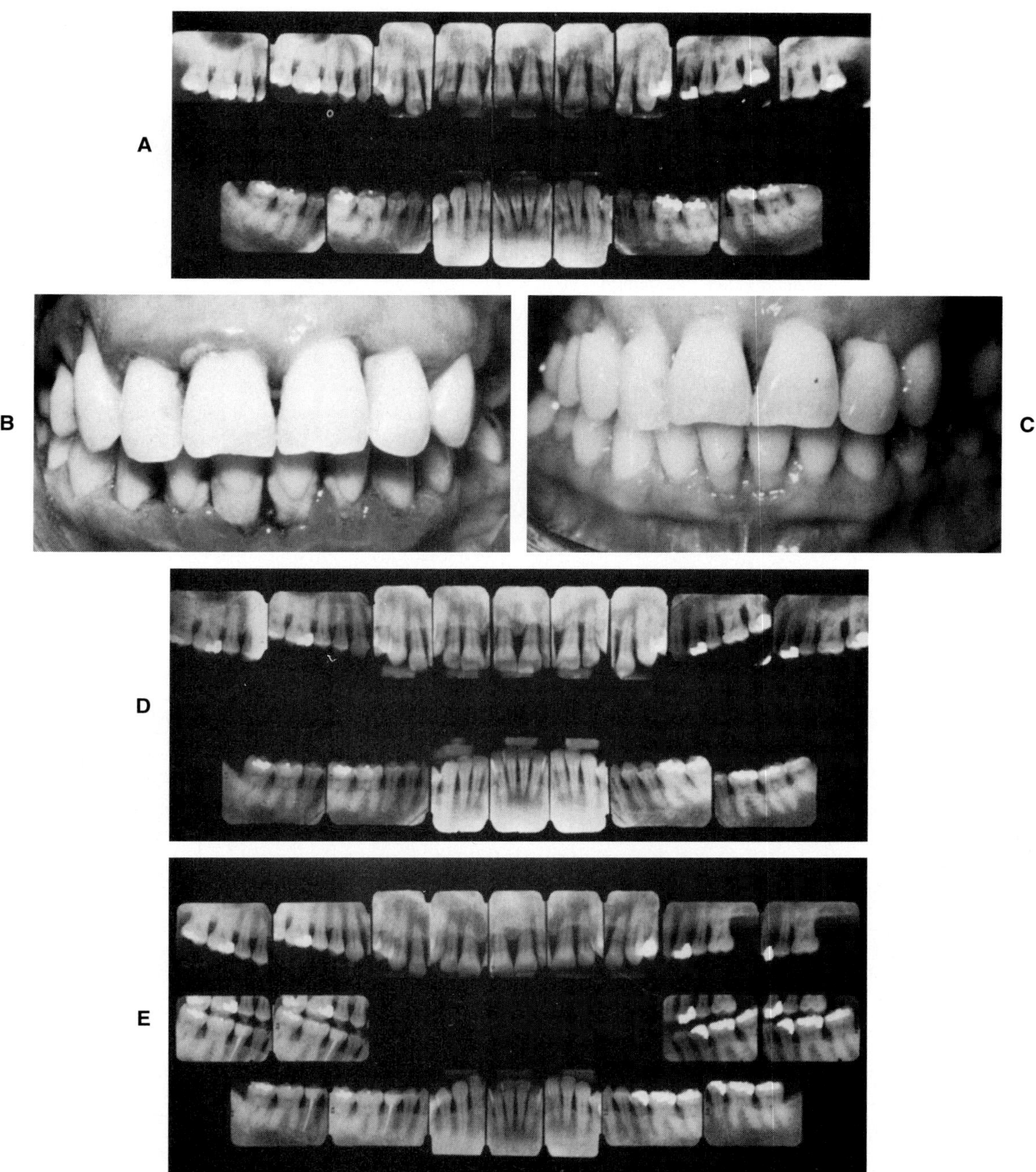

Fig. 76-5 **A,** The patient was 38 years old when these original radiographs were taken and was treated with a combination of surgical and nonsurgical therapy. This individual is a classic class C maintenance patient. **B,** Pretreatment photographs. Note the inflammation and heavy calculus deposits. **C,** Photograph taken 10 years after treatment. **D,** Radiographs taken 5 years after treatment. **E,** Radiographs taken 10 years after treatment. The radiographic appearance is as good as can be expected in such a severe case. Teeth #15 and #17 were extracted 8 years after treatment.

Checking of Plaque Control

To assess the effectiveness of their plaque control, patients should perform their hygiene regimen immediately before the recall appointment. Plaque control must be reviewed and corrected until the patient demonstrates the necessary proficiency, even if additional instruction sessions are required. Patients instructed in plaque control have less plaque and gingivitis than uninstructed patients,[4,53,54] and the amount of supragingival plaque affects the number of subgingival anaerobic organisms.[15,48]

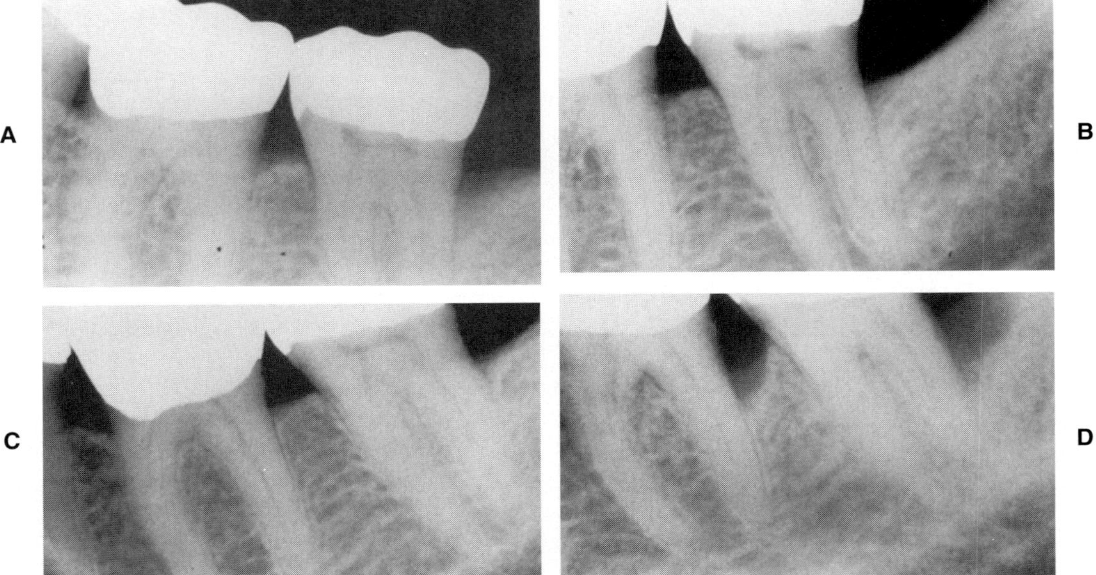

Fig. 76-6 This series of radiographs clearly shows the importance of maintenance therapy. **A,** Original radiograph of a 58-year-old man. Note the deep distal bone loss on tooth #18 and the moderate distal lesion of tooth #19. Surgical treatment that included osseous grafting was performed. **B,** Radiograph 14 months after surgical therapy. The patient had recall maintenance performed every 3 to 4 months. **C,** Appearance $3\frac{1}{2}$ years after surgery, with regular recalls every 3 to 4 months. **D,** Appearance after 2 years without recalls (7 years after surgery). Note the progression of the disease on the distal surfaces of teeth #18 and #19.

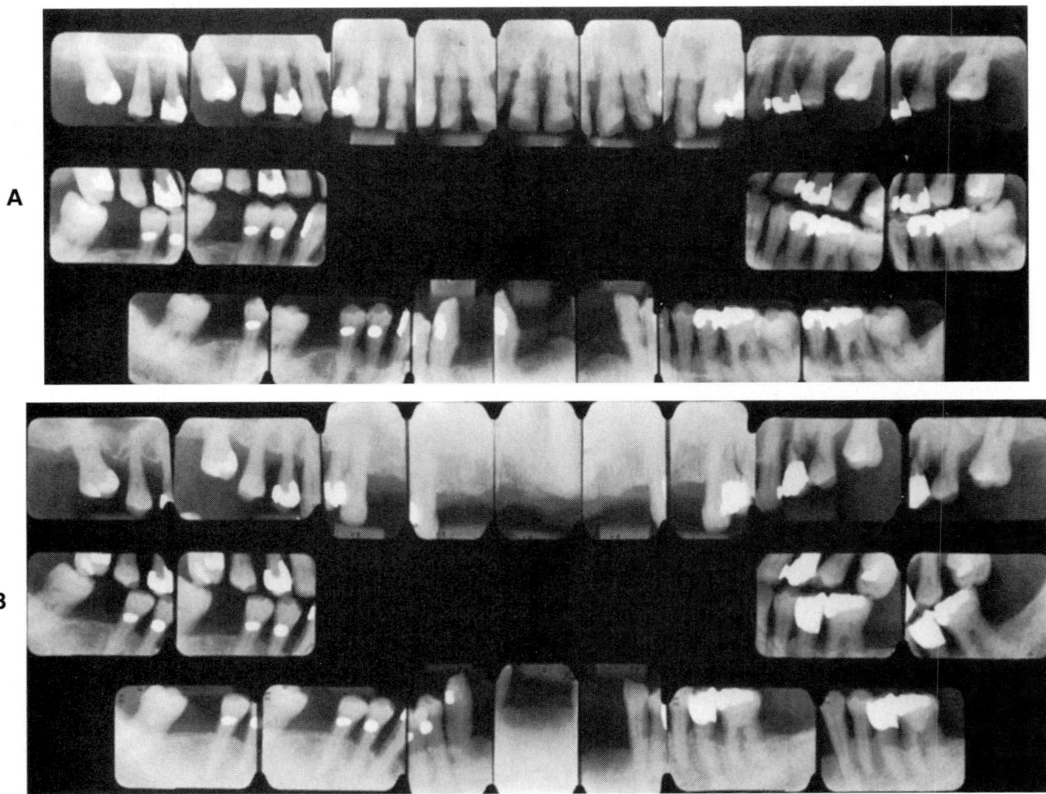

Fig. 76-7 Advanced cases sometimes do better than expected when the patient complies with maintenance therapy. **A,** Initial radiographs showing a very advanced case. The maxillary arch had extractions and nonsurgical treatment. A plastic treatment partial denture was placed and was expected to grow into a full denture within a few years. The mandibular arch was treated with periodontal surgery, and a permanent metal and plastic removable partial denture was placed. **B,** Radiographs taken 8 years later. The patient performed good oral hygiene and had 3-month recalls. Teeth #12 and #15 required extraction.

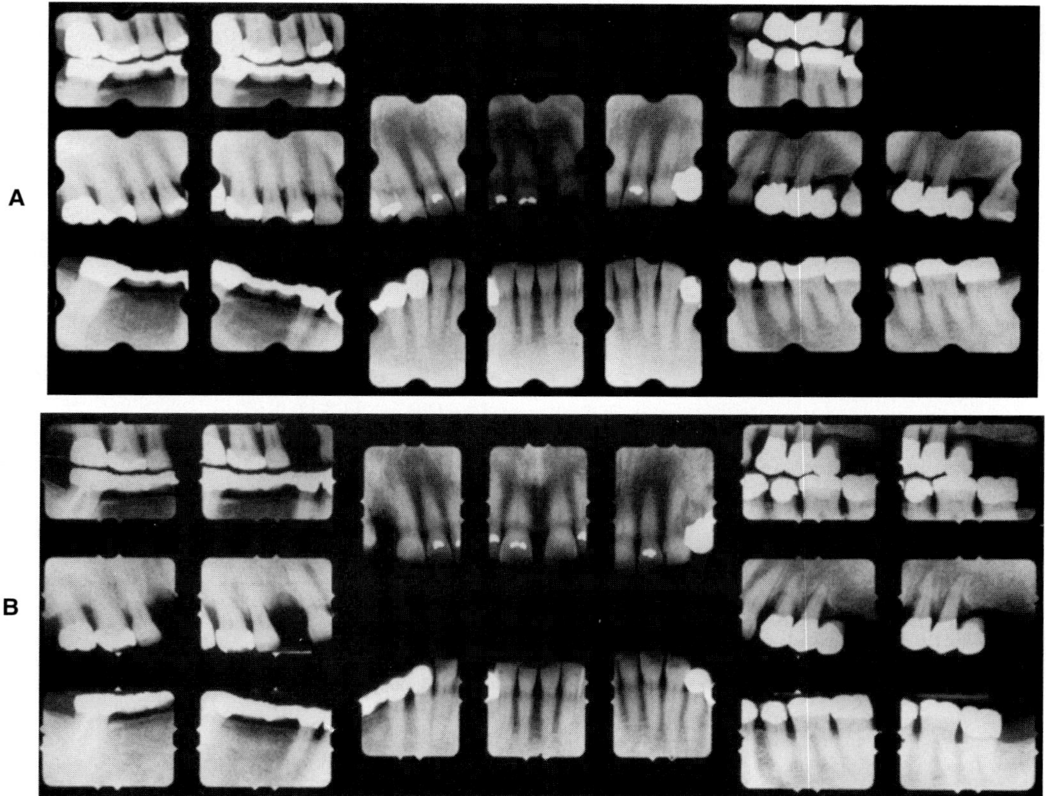

Fig. 76-8 **A,** Initial radiographs. The patient was advised to have localized areas of periodontal surgery and periodontal recall every 3 months. However, the patient did not comply and only had dental cleanings once or twice yearly. **B,** Radiographs 4 years later. Note the loss of teeth #5 and #15 and the increased bone loss of several premolars and molars.

Treatment

The required scaling and root planing are performed, followed by an oral prophylaxis (see Chapter 47). Care must be taken not to heavily instrument normal sites with shallow sulci (1 to 3 mm deep) because studies have shown that repeated subgingival scaling and root planing in initially normal periodontal sites result in significant loss of attachment.[26] Irrigation with antimicrobial agents is performed in maintenance patients with remaining pockets.[25,31,45]

Recurrence of Periodontal Disease

Occasionally, lesions may recur. This often can be traced to inadequate plaque control on the part of the patient or failure to comply with recommended SPT schedules. It should be understood, however, that it is the dentist's responsibility to teach, motivate, and control the patient's oral hygiene technique, and the patient's failure is the dentist's failure. Surgery should not be undertaken unless the patient has shown proficiency and willingness to cooperate by adequately performing his or her part of therapy.[7,51,60]

Other causes for recurrence are the following:

1. Inadequate or insufficient treatment that has failed to remove all the potential factors favoring plaque accumulation (see Fig. 76-4). Incomplete calculus removal in areas of difficult access is a common source of problems.
2. Inadequate restorations placed after the periodontal treatment was completed.
3. Failure of the patient to return for periodic checkups (see Fig. 76-6). This may be due to the patient's conscious or unconscious decision not to continue treatment or to the failure of the dentist and staff to emphasize the need for periodic examinations.
4. Presence of some systemic diseases that may affect host resistance to previously acceptable levels of plaque.

A failing case can be recognized by the following:

1. Recurring inflammation revealed by gingival changes and bleeding of the sulcus on probing.
2. Increasing depth of sulci, leading to the recurrence of pocket formation.
3. Gradual increases in bone loss as determined by radiographs.
4. Gradual increases in tooth mobility as ascertained by clinical examination.

Cases that do not respond to adequate therapy or recur for unknown reasons are referred to as *refractory periodontitis* (see Chapters 27 and 40).

TABLE 76-1

Radiographic Examination of SPT Recall Patients*[35,63,72]

Patient Condition	Type of Examination
Patients with clinical caries or high-risk factors for caries.	Posterior bitewing examination at 12- to 18-month intervals.
Patients with no clinical caries and no high-risk factors for caries.	Posterior bitewing examination at 24- to 36-month intervals.
Patients with periodontal disease not under good control.	Periapical and/or vertical bitewings of problem areas every 12 to 24 months; full-mouth series every 3 to 5 years.
Patients with history of periodontal treatment with disease under good control.	Bitewing examination every 24 to 36 months; full-mouth series every 5 years.
Patients with root form dental implants.	Periapical or vertical bitewings at 6, 12, and 36 months after prosthetic placement, then every 36 months unless clinical problems arise.
Transfer periodontal or implant maintenance patients.	Full-mouth series if a current set is not available. If a full-mouth series has been taken within 24 months, then radiographs of implants and periodontal problem areas should be taken.

* Radiographs should be taken when they are likely to affect diagnosis and patient treatment. The recommendations in this table are subject to clinical judgment and may not apply to every patient.

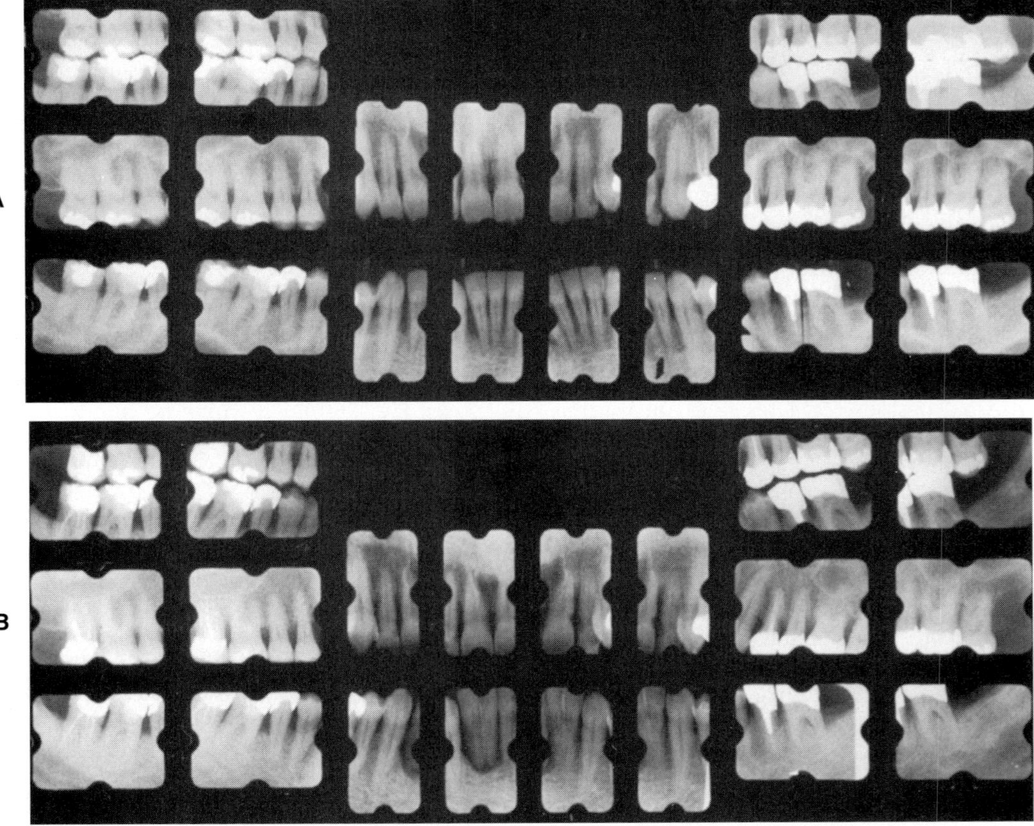

Fig. 76-9 **A,** Initial radiographs. The patient was advised to have localized areas of periodontal surgery and periodontal recall every 3 months. However, the patient did not comply and had no treatment other than emergency care and occasional dental cleanings. **B,** Radiographs 7 years later. Note the advanced bone loss and caries on many teeth.

TABLE 76-2

Symptoms and Causes of Recurrence of Disease

Symptom	Possible Causes
Increased mobility	Increased inflammation Poor oral hygiene Subgingival calculus Inadequate restorations Deteriorating or poorly designed prostheses Systemic disease modifying host response to plaque
Recession	Toothbrush abrasion Inadequate keratinized gingiva Frenum pull Orthodontic therapy
Increased mobility with no change in pocket depth and no radiographic change	Occlusal trauma due to lateral occlusal interference Bruxism High restoration Poorly designed or worn-out prosthesis Poor crown-to-root ratio
Increased pocket depth with no radiographic change	Poor oral hygiene Infrequent recall visits Subgingival calculus Poorly fitting partial denture Mesial inclination into edentulous space Failure of new attachment surgery Cracked teeth Grooves in teeth New periodontal disease
Increased pocket depth with increased radiographic bone loss	Poor oral hygiene Subgingival calculus Infrequent recall visits Inadequate or deteriorating restorations Poorly designed prostheses Inadequate surgery Systemic disease modifying host response to plaque Cracked teeth Grooves in teeth New periodontal disease

The decision to retreat a periodontal patient should not be made at the preventive maintenance appointment but should be postponed for 1 to 2 weeks.[10] Often the mouth looks a great deal better at that time, owing to the resolution of edema and the resulting improved tone of the gingiva. A summary of the symptoms of recurrence of periodontal disease and their probable causes can be found in Table 76-2.

CLASSIFICATION OF POSTTREATMENT PATIENTS

The first year after periodontal therapy is important in terms of indoctrinating the patient in a recall pattern and reinforcing oral hygiene techniques. In addition, it may take several months to accurately evaluate the results of some periodontal surgical procedures. Consequently, some areas may have to be retreated because the results may not be optimal. Furthermore, the first-year patient often has etiologic factors that may have been overlooked and may be more amenable to treatment at this early stage. For these reasons, *the recall interval for first-year patients should not be longer than 3 months.*

The patients who are on a periodontal recall schedule are a varied group. Table 76-3 lists several categories of maintenance patients and a suggested recall interval for each. Patients can improve or relapse to a different classification with a reduction in or exacerbation of periodontal disease. When one dental arch is more involved than the other, the patient's periodontal disease is classified by the arch that is in worse condition.

In summary, maintenance care is a critical phase of therapy. *The long-term preservation of the dentition is closely associated with the frequency and quality of recall maintenance.*

TABLE 76-3

Recall Intervals for Various Classes of Recall Patients

Merin Classification	Characteristics	Recall Interval
First year	First-year patient—routing therapy and uneventful healing or	3 months
	First-year patient—difficult case with complicated prosthesis, furcation involvement, poor crown-to-root ratios, or questionable patient cooperation	1 to 2 months
Class A	Excellent results well maintained for 1 year or more Patient displays good oral hygiene, minimal calculus, no occlusal problems, no complicated prostheses, no remaining pockets, and no teeth with less than 50% of alveolar bone remaining	6 months to 1 year
Class B	Generally good results maintained reasonably well for 1 year or more, but patient displays some of the following factors: 1. Inconsistent or poor oral hygiene 2. Heavy calculus formation 3. Systemic disease that predisposes to periodontal breakdown 4. Some remaining pockets 5. Occlusal problems 6. Complicated prostheses 7. Ongoing orthodontic therapy 8. Recurrent dental caries 9. Some teeth with less than 50% of alveolar bone support 10. Smoking 11. Positive genetic test	3 to 4 months (decide on recall interval on the basis of the number and severity of negative factors)
Class C	Generally poor results following periodontal therapy and/or several negative factors from the following list: 1. Inconsistent or poor oral hygiene 2. Heavy calculus formation 3. Systemic disease that predisposes to periodontal breakdown 4. Remaining pockets 5. Occlusal problems 6. Complicated prostheses 7. Recurrent dental caries 8. Periodontal surgery indicated but not performed for medical, psychologic, or financial reasons 9. Many teeth with less than 50% of alveolar bone support 10. Condition too far advanced to be improved by periodontal surgery 11. Smoking 12. Positive genetic test 13. More than 20% of pockets bleed on probing	1 to 3 months (decide on recall interval on the basis of the number and severity of negative factors; consider retreating some areas or extracting the severely involved teeth)

REFERRAL OF PATIENTS TO THE PERIODONTIST

The majority of periodontal care belongs in the hands of the general dentist. This is because of the overwhelming number of patients with periodontal disease and the intimate relationship between periodontal disease and restorative dentistry.

For various reasons, an ever-greater number of periodontal maintenance patients are expected in future years. The number of caries per capita has dwindled since the mid-1970s by about 50%, and some evidence suggests that this decline will continue.[45] As more people retain their teeth throughout their lifetimes and the proportion of older people in the population increases, more teeth will be at risk of periodontal disease. Hence the prevalence of patients requiring SPT is likely to increase in the future.

This expected increase in the number of periodontal patients will necessitate a greater understanding of periodontal problems and an increased level of expertise for the solution of such problems on the part of the general practitioner of dentistry. However, specialists always will be needed to treat particularly difficult cases, patients with systemic health problems, dental implant patients, and situations in which a complex prosthetic construction requires absolute assurance of reliable results.

The question remains where to draw the line between the cases to be treated in the general dental office and those to be referred to a specialist varies for different practitioners and patients. The diagnosis indicates the type of periodontal treatment required. If periodontal destruction necessitates surgery on the distal surfaces of second molars, extensive osseous surgery, or complex regenerative procedures, the patient is usually best treated by a specialist. On the other hand, patients who require localized gingivectomy or flap curettage usually can be treated by the general dentist.

It is immediately obvious that some patients should be referred to a specialist, whereas most patients clearly have problems that can be treated by a general dentist. However, for a third group of patients, it will be difficult to decide whether treatment by a specialist is required. Any patient who does not plainly belong in the second of these categories should be considered a candidate for referral to a specialist.[38]

The decision to have the general practitioner treat a patient's periodontal problem should be guided by a consideration of the degree of risk that the patient will lose a tooth or teeth for periodontally related reasons.

The most important factors in the decision are the extent and *location of the periodontal deterioration.* Teeth with pockets of 5 mm or more, as measured from the cementoenamel junction, may have a prognosis of rapid decline. The location of the periodontal deterioration is also an important factor in determining the risk of tooth loss. Teeth with furcation lesions may be at risk even when more than 50% of bone support remains. Therefore cases in which strategically important teeth fall into these categories are usually best treated by specialists.

An important question remains: *Should the maintenance phase of therapy be performed by the general practitioner or the specialist?* This should be determined by the amount of periodontal deterioration present. Class A recall patients should be maintained by the general dentist, whereas Class C patients should be maintained by the specialist (see Table 76-3). Class B patients can alternate recall visits between the general practitioner and the specialist (Fig. 76-10). The suggested rule is that the *patient's disease should dictate whether the general practitioner or the specialist should perform the maintenance therapy.*

TESTS FOR DISEASE ACTIVITY

Periodontal patients, even though they have received effective periodontal therapy, are at risk of disease recurrence for the rest of their lives.[20,21] In addition,

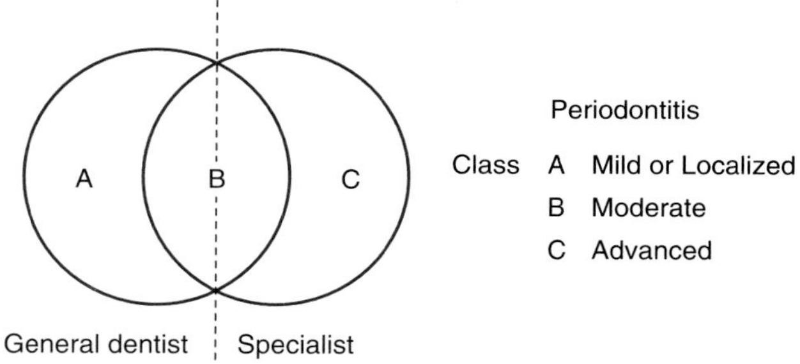

Fig. 76-10 Scheme for determining which practitioner should perform periodontal maintenance in patients with different degrees of periodontitis.

many pockets in furcation areas may not have been eliminated by surgery. At present, the best way of determining areas that are losing attachment uses a well-organized charting system[43,59]; some computerized systems offer the possibility of easy retrieval and comparison of past findings.

Comparison of sequential probing measurements gives the most accurate indication of rate of loss of attachment.[3] A number of other clinical and laboratory variables have been correlated with disease activity (see Chapter 34). At present, no accurate method of identifying disease activity exists, and clinicians rely on the information provided by combining probing, bleeding on probing, and sequential attachment measurements.[22,28,59] Patients whose disease is clearly refractory are candidates for bacterial culturing and antibiotic therapy in conjunction with additional mechanical therapy.

Tests will undoubtedly be developed in the future to help determine disease activity. The clinician must be able to interpret whether a test may be useful in determining disease activity and future loss of attachment.[8] Tests should be adopted only when they are based on research that includes a critical analysis of the sensitivity, specificity, disease incidence, and predictive value of the proposed test.

MAINTENANCE FOR DENTAL IMPLANT PATIENTS

Patients with implants are susceptible to a form of bone loss called *periimplantitis,* and evidence suggests that such patients may be more prone to plaque-induced inflammation with bone loss than those with natural teeth[6,46,57] (see Chapter 73).

The overall periodontal condition in partially edentulous implant patients can influence the clinical condition around implants.[9] The microflora of implants in partially edentulous patients differs from that in edentulous patients.[5] The implant microflora is similar to tooth microflora in the partially edentulous mouth. Periodontal and implant maintenance are linked because maintenance of a tooth microflora consistent with periodontal health is necessary to maintain implant microflora consistent with periimplant health.[5] Because periimplantitis is difficult to treat,[19] it is extremely important to treat periodontal disease prior to implant placement and provide good supportive therapy with implant patients.

In general, procedures for maintenance of patients with implants are similar to those with natural teeth[33,52,17,23], with three differences:

1. Special instrumention that will not scratch the implants are used for calculus removal on the implants.
2. Acidic fluoride prophylactic agents are avoided.
3. Nonabrasive prophy pastes are used.

During the phase after uncovering the implants, patients must use ultrasoft brushes, chemotherapeutic rinses, tartar control pastes, irrigation devices, and yarn-like materials to keep the implants and natural teeth clean. Patients often are afraid to touch the implants but must be encouraged to keep the areas clean.

Special instruments should be used on the implants during recall appointments.[17,33] Metal hand instruments and ultrasonic and sonic tips should be avoided because they can alter the titanium surface. Only plastic instruments or specially designed gold-plated curettes should be used for calculus removal because the implant surfaces can be easily scratched. The rubber cup with flour of pumice, tin oxide, or special implant polishing pastes should be used on abutment surfaces with light, intermittent pressure.[32]

Although daily use of topically applied antimicrobials is advised,[33] acidic fluoride agents should not be used because they cause surface damage to titanium abutments.[40]

When prosthetics must be unscrewed and removed for maintenance, it is best done in the office responsible for placing the prosthetics. Each time the prosthetics are reattached, a slight change in the occlusion occurs. Time must be allowed for occlusal corrections.

REFERENCES

1. Ainamo J, Ainamo A: Risk assessment of recurrence of disease during supportive periodontal care. J Clin Periodontol 1996; 23:232.
2. Alaluusua S, Asikainen S, Lai CH: Intrafamilial transmission of Actinobacillus actinomycetemcomitans. J Periodontol 1991; 62:207.
3. Armitage GC: Diagnosing periodontal diseases. In: Perspectives on Oral Antimicrobial Therapeutics. Littleton, MA, PSG Publishing Co, 1987.
4. Axelson P, Lindhe J: The significance of maintenance care in the treatment of periodontal disease. J Clin Periodontol 1981; 8:281.
5. Bauman GR, Mills M, Rapley JW, et al: Plaque-induced inflammation around implants. Int J Oral Maxillofac Implants 1992; 7:330.
6. Bauman GR, Rapley JW, Hallmon WW, et al: The peri-implant sulcus. Int J Oral Maxillofac Implants 1993; 8:273.
7. Becker W, Becker BE, Berg LE: Periodontal treatment without maintenance. A retrospective study in 44 patients. J Periodontol 1984; 155:505.
8. Bennett WI: Screening for bowel cancer. Harvard Med School Health Lett 1986; 11:6.
9. Bragger U, Burgin WB, Hammerle CH, et al: Associations between clinical parameters assessed around implants and teeth. Clin Oral Implants Res 1997; 8:412.
10. Carranza FA Jr, Saglie FR, Newman MG, et al: Scanning and transmission electron microscope study of tissue invading microorganisms in localized juvenile periodontitis. J Periodontol 1983; 54:598.
11. Caton JG, Zander HA: The attachment between tooth and gingival tissues after periodic root planing and soft tissue curettage. J Periodontol 1979; 50:462.
12. Chace R: Retreatment in periodontal practice. J Periodontol 1977; 48:410.
13. Christersson LA, Albini B, Zambon JJ, et al: Tissue localization of *Actinobacillus actinomycetemcomitans* in human periodontitis. I. Light, immunofluorescence and electron microscopic studies. J Periodontol 1987; 58:529.
14. Cortellimi P, Pini-Prato G, Torretti M: Periodontal regeneration of human infrabony defects. V. Effects of oral hygiene on long-term stability. J Clin Periodontal 1994; 21:606.
15. Dahlen G, Lindhe J, Sato K, et al: The effect of supragingival plaque control on the subgingival microbiota in subjects with periodontal disease. J Clin Periodontol 1992; 19:802.
16. Egloff E, Saglie FR, Newman MG: Intragingival bacteria subsequent to scaling and root planing. Abstract. J Dent Res 1986; 65:269.
17. Eskow RN, Smith VS: Preventive periimplant protocol. Compendium Cont Ed 1999; 20:137.
18. Greenwell H, Bissada NB, Wittwer JW: Periodontics in general practice: Perspectives on periodontal diagnosis. J Am Dent Assoc 1989; 119:537.
19. Grunder U, Hürzeler MB, Schüpbach P, et al: Treatment of ligature-induced peri-implantitis using guided tissue regeneration: A clinical and histologic study in the beagle dog. Int J Oral Maxillofac Implants 1993; 8:282.
20. Halazonetis TD, Smulow JB, Donnenfeld W, et al: Pocket formation 3 years after comprehensive periodontal therapy. A retrospective study. J Periodontol 1985; 56:515.
21. Hirschfeld L, Wasserman B: A long-term survey of tooth loss in 600 treated periodontal patients. J Periodontol 1978; 49:225.
22. Lang NP, Joss A, Orsanic T, et al: Bleeding on probing. J Clin Periodontol 1986; 13:590.
23. Lang NP, Nyman SR: Supportive maintenance care for patients with implants and advanced restorative therapy. Periodontology 2000 1994; 4:119.
24. Lietha-Elmer E: Langsfritsgie Ergebnisse reglemassig betreuter und unbetreuter Parodontosepatienten. Schweiz Monatsschr Zahnheilkd 1977; 87:613.
25. Lindhe J, Heijl L, Goodson JM, et al: Local tetracycline delivery using hollow fiber devices in periodontal therapy. J Clin Periodontol 1979; 6:141.
26. Lindhe J, Nyman S, Karring T: Scaling and root planing in shallow pockets. J Clin Periodontol 1982; 9:415.
27. Listgarten MA, Hellden L:. Relative distribution of bacteria at clinically healthy and periodontally diseased sites in humans. J Clin Periodontol 1978; 5:115.
28. Listgarten MA, Schifter CC, Sullivan P, et al: Failure of a microbiological assay to reliably predict disease recurrence in a treated periodontitis population receiving regularly scheduled prophylaxes. J Clin Periodontol 1986; 13:768.
29. Listgarten MA, Sullivan P, George C, et al: Comparative longitudinal study of 2 methods of scheduling maintenance visit: 4-year data. J Clin Periodontol 1989; 16:105.
30. Matteson SR, Bottomley W, Finger H, et al: The selection of patients for x-ray examinations: Dental radiographic examinations. DHHS publication no. FDA 88-8273. Washington, DC, Department of Health and Human Services, October 1987.
31. Mazza JE, Newman MG, Sims TN: Clinical and antimicrobial effect of stannous fluoride on periodontitis. J Clin Periodontol 1981; 8:213.

32. McCollum J, O'Neal RB, Brennan WA, et al: The effect of titanium implant abutment surface irregularities on plaque accumulation in vivo. J Periodontol 1992; 63:802.
33. Meffert RM, Langer B, Fritz ME: Dental implants: A review. J Periodontol 1992; 63:859.
34. Mendoza AR, Newcomb GM, Nixon KC: Compliance with supportive periodontal therapy. J Periodontol 1991; 62:731.
35. Mousques T, Listgarten MA, Phillips RW: Effect of scaling and root planing on the composition of human subgingival microflora. J Periodont Res 1980; 15:144.
36. Novaes AB Jr, Novaes AB: Compliance with supportive periodontal therapy. Part 1. Risk of non-compliance in the first 5-year period. J Periodontol 1999; 70:679.
37. Oliver RC: Tooth loss with and without periodontal therapy. Periodont Abstracts 1969; 17:8.
38. Parr RW, Pipe P, Watts T: Periodontal Maintenance Therapy. Berkeley, CA, Praxis Publishing, 1974.
39. Pertuiset JH, Saglie FR, Lofthus J, et al: Recurrent periodontal disease and bacterial presence in the gingiva. J Periodontol 1987; 58:553.
40. Probster L, Lin W, Juttemann H: Effect of fluoride prophylactic agents on titanium surfaces. Int J Oral Maxillofac Implants 1992; 7:390.
41. Rosenberg ES, Evian CI, Listgarten MA: The composition of the subgingival microbiota after periodontal therapy. J Periodontol 1981; 52:435.
42. Ross IF, Thompson RH, Galdi M: The results of treatment: A long term study of 180 patients. Parodontologie 1971; 25:125.
43. Ryan RJ: The accuracy of clinical parameters in detecting periodontal disease activity. J Am Dent Assoc 1985; 111:753.
44. Saglie FR, Newman MG, Carranza FA Jr, et al: Immunohistochemical localization of *Actinobacillus actinomycetemcomitans* in sections of gingival tissue in localized juvenile periodontitis. Acta Odont Lat Am 1984; 1:40.
45. Schallhorn RG, Snider LE: Periodontal maintenance therapy. J Am Dent Assoc 1981; 103:227.
46. Schou S, Holmstrup P, Reibel J, et al: Ligature-induced marginal inflammation around osseointegrated implants and ankylosed teeth: Stereologic and histologic observations on cynomolgus monkeys. J Periodontol 1993; 64:529.
47. Slots J, Mashimo P, Levine MJ, et al: Periodontal therapy in humans. I. Microbiological and clinical effects of a single course of periodontal scaling and root planing, and of adjunctive tetracycline therapy. J Periodontol 1979; 50:495.
48. Smulow JB, Turesky SS, Hill RG.: The effect of supragingival plaque removal on anaerobic bacteria in deep pockets. J Am Dent Assoc 1983; 107:737.
49. Stahl SS: Repair potential of the soft tissue-root interface. J Periodontol 1977; 48:545.
50. Stahl SS, Witkin GJ, Heller A, et al: Gingival healing. IV. The effects of home care on gingivectomy repair. J Periodontol 1969; 40:264.
51. Sternlich HC: Evaluating long-term periodontal therapy. Tex Dent J 1974; 92:4.
52. Stewart RT: Personal communication, 1986.
53. Suomi JD, Greene JC, Vermillion JR, et al: The effect of controlled oral hygiene procedures on the progression of periodontal disease in adults: Results after the third and final year. J Periodontol 1971; 42:152.
54. Suomi JD, West JD, Chang JJ, et al: The effect of controlled oral hygiene procedures on the progression of periodontal disease in adults: Radiographic findings. J Periodontol 1971; 42:562.
55. Tonetti MA, Muller-Campanile V, Lang NP: Changes in the prevalence of residual pockets and tooth loss in treated periodontal patients during a supportive maintenance care program. J Clin Periodontol 1998; 25:1008.
56. Van Steenbergen TJM, Petit MDA, van-der-Velden U, et al: Transmission of *Porphyromonas gingivalis* between spouses. J Clin Periodontol 1993; 20:340.
57. Van Steenberghe D, Klinge B, Linden U, et al: Periodontal indices around natural and titanium abutments: A longitudinal multicenter study. J Periodontol 1993; 64:538.
58. Waerhaug J: Healing of the dentoepithelial junction following subgingival plaque control. J Periodontol 1978; 49:119.
59. Wilson TG, Kornman KS: Retreatment. Periodontology 2000 1996; 12:119.
60. Wilson TG Jr: Compliance. A review of the literature. J Periodontol 1987; 58:706.
61. Wilson TG Jr, Glover ME, Malik AK, et al: Tooth loss in maintenance patients in a private periodontal practice. J Periodontol 1987; 58:231.
62. Wilson TG Jr, Glover ME, Schoen J, et al: Compliance with maintenance therapy in a private periodontal practice. J Periodontol 1984; 55:468.

Results of Periodontal Treatment

Robert L. Merin

CHAPTER

CHAPTER OUTLINE

The prevalence of periodontal disease, the high tooth mortality rate resulting from it, and the potential for multiple systemic health complications aggravated by chronic periodontitis raise an important question: Is periodontal treatment effective in preventing and controlling the chronic infection and progressive destruction of periodontal disease? Current concepts of evaluating health care require a scientific basis for treatment. This is referred to as **evidence-based therapy.** *Evidence is now overwhelming that periodontal therapy is effective in preventing periodontal disease, slowing the destruction of the periodontium, and reducing tooth loss.*

PREVENTION AND TREATMENT OF GINGIVITIS

For many years, the belief that good oral hygiene is necessary for the successful prevention and treatment of gingivitis has been widespread among periodontists. In addition, worldwide epidemiologic studies have confirmed a close relationship between the incidence of gingivitis and lack of oral hygiene.[5,6]

Conclusive evidence on the relation of oral hygiene and gingivitis in healthy dental students was shown by Löe and co-workers.[17,34] After 9 to 21 days without performing oral hygiene measures, experimental subjects with previously excellent oral hygiene and healthy gingiva developed heavy accumulations of plaque and generalized mild gingivitis. When oral hygiene techniques were reinstituted, the plaque in most areas disappeared in 1 or 2 days, and gingival inflammation in these areas disappeared approximately 1 week after the plaque was removed. Thus gingivitis is reversible and can be resolved by daily effective plaque removal.

A number of long-term studies have shown that gingival health can be maintained by a combination of effective oral hygiene maintenance and scaling procedures.[1,2,8,10,11,18,32,33]

A 3-year study was conducted on 1248 General Telephone workers in California to determine whether progression of gingival inflammation is retarded in an oral environment in which high levels of hygiene are maintained.[32,33] Experimental and control groups were computer matched on the basis of periodontal and oral hygiene status, past caries experience, age, and gender. During the study period, several procedures were instituted to ensure that the oral hygiene status of the experimental group was maintained at a high level. Subjects were given a series of frequent oral prophylaxis treatments combined with oral hygiene instruction. Subjects in the control group received no attention from the study team except for annual examinations. They were advised to continue their usual daily practices and accustomed visits for professional care. After 3 years, the

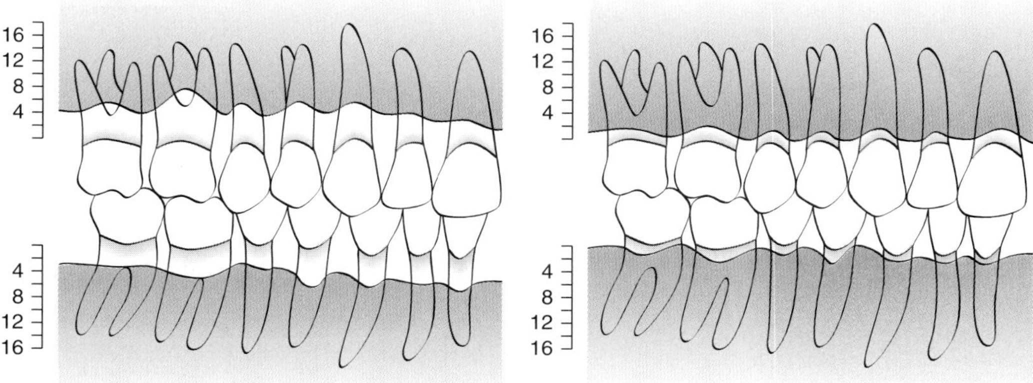

Fig. 77-1 *Left,* Mean periodontal support of teeth of Sri Lankan tea laborers at approximately 40 years of age. *Right,* Mean periodontal support of teeth of Norwegian academicians at approximately 40 years of age. (From Löe H, Anerud A, Boysen H, et al: The natural history of periodontal disease in man. J Periodontol 1978; 49:607.)

increase in plaque and debris in the control group was four times as great as that in the experimental group. Similarly, gingivitis scores were much higher in control subjects than in the matching experimental group. Therefore *chronic marginal gingivitis can be controlled with good oral hygiene and dental prophylaxis.*

PREVENTION AND TREATMENT OF LOSS OF ATTACHMENT

Although periodontal therapy has been used for more than 100 years, it is only since the mid-1970s that a number of studies have been conducted to determine the effect of treatment on reducing the progressive loss of periodontal support for the natural dentition.

Prevention of Loss of Attachment

A longitudinal investigation to study the natural development and progression of periodontal disease was conducted by Löe and co-workers.[15,16] The first group, established in Oslo, Norway in 1969, consisted of 565 healthy male nondental students and academicians between 17 and 40 years of age. The principal reason for selecting Oslo as a study site was that this city had had a preschool, school, and postschool dental program offering systematic preventive, restorative, endodontic, orthodontic, and surgical therapy on an annual recall basis for all children and adolescents, complete with a documented attendance record, for the previous 40 years. Members of the study population had had maximum exposure to conventional dental care throughout their lives. A second group, established in Sri Lanka in 1970, consisted of 480 male tea laborers between 15 and 40 years of age. They were healthy and well built by local standards, and their nutritional condition was clinically fair. The workers had never been exposed to any programs relative to the prevention or treatment of dental diseases. Toothbrushing was unknown, and dental caries was virtually nonexistent.

The results of this study are quite interesting. The Norwegian group, as the members approached 40 years of age, had a mean individual loss of attachment of slightly above 1.5 mm, and the mean annual rate of attachment loss was 0.08 mm for interproximal surfaces and 0.10 mm for buccal surfaces. As the Sri Lankans approached 40 years of age, the mean individual loss of attachment was 4.50 mm, and the mean annual rate of progression of the lesion was 0.30 mm for interproximal surfaces and 0.20 mm for buccal surfaces. Fig. 77-1 shows a graphic interpretation of the difference between the two groups. This study suggests that without interference, periodontal lesions progress continually and at a relatively even pace.

Further analysis of the Sri Lankan laborers[15] showed that they were not all losing attachment at the same rate (Figs. 77-2 and 77-3). Virtually all gingival areas showed inflammation, but attachment loss varied tremendously. Based on interproximal loss of attachment and tooth mortality, three subpopulations were identified: individuals with rapid progression (RP) of periodontal disease (8%), individuals with moderate progression (MP) (81%), and individuals who exhibited no progression (NP) of periodontal disease beyond gingivitis (11%). At age 35, the mean loss of attachment in the RP group was 9 mm; in the MP group, 4 mm; and in the NP group, less than 1 mm. At the age of 45, the mean loss of attachment in the RP group was 13 mm and in the MP group, 7 mm. It is obvious that under natural conditions and in the absence of any therapy, 89% of the Sri Lankan laborers had severe periodontitis that progressed at much greater rates than in the Norwegian group.

In the previously discussed study of General Telephone workers in California, loss of attachment was measured clinically and alveolar bone loss was measured radiographically.[29,30] After 3 years, the control group showed loss of attachment at a rate more than $3\frac{1}{2}$ times that of the matching experimental group during the same period (Fig. 77-4). In addition, subjects who received frequent oral prophylaxis and were instructed in

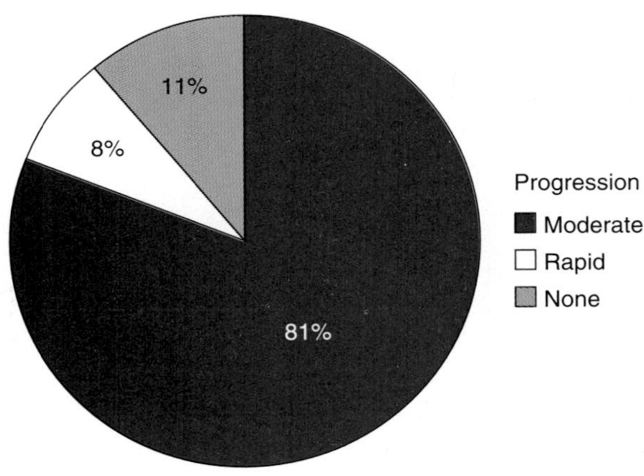

Fig. 77-2 Progression of periodontal disease in an untreated population. (Data from Löe H, Anerud A, Boysen H, et al: Natural history of periodontal disease in man. J Clin Periodontol 1986; 13:431.)

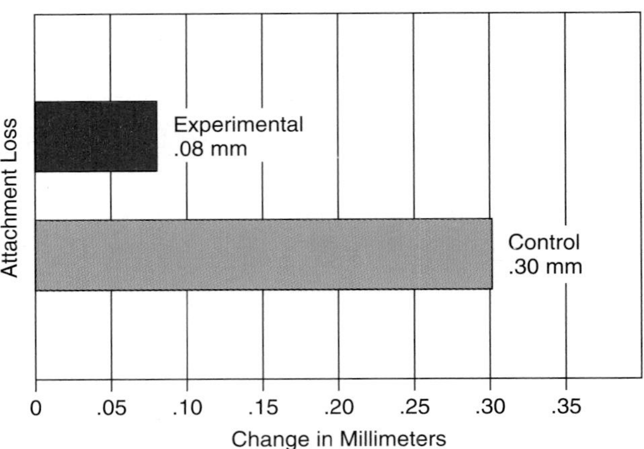

Fig. 77-4 Change in mean attachment level from baseline to third-year examination for experimental and control groups. (From Suomi JD, West JD, Chang JJ, et al: The effect of controlled oral hygiene procedures on the progression of periodontal disease in adults: Radiographic findings. J Periodontol 1971; 42:152.)

Mean Loss of Attachment at Various Ages (mm)

Age	Progression Group	
	Rapid	**Moderate**
35	9	4
45	13	7

Fig. 77-3 Loss of attachment in untreated Sri Lankan laborers. (Data from Löe H, Anerud A, Boysen H, et al: Natural history of periodontal disease in man. J Clin Periodontol 1986; 13:431.)

good oral hygiene practices showed less bone loss radiographically after 3 years than did control subjects. *It is clear that loss of attachment can be reduced by good oral hygiene and frequent dental prophylaxis.*

Treatment of Loss of Attachment

A longitudinal study of patients with moderate to advanced periodontal disease conducted at the University of Michigan showed that the progression of periodontal disease can be stopped for a period of 3 years postoperatively regardless of the modality of treatment.[24-27] With long-term observations, the average loss of attachment was only 0.3 mm over 7 years.[24] These results indicated a more favorable prognosis for treatment of advanced periodontal lesions than previously assumed.

Another study was conducted in 75 patients with advanced periodontal disease to determine the effect of plaque control and surgical pocket elimination on the establishment and maintenance of periodontal health.[13] This study showed that no further alveolar bone loss occurred during the 5-year observation period. The meticulous plaque control practiced by the patients in this study was considered a major factor in the excellent results produced. After 14 years, results for 61 of the initial 75 individuals were reported.[14] Repeated examinations demonstrated that treatment of advanced forms of periodontal disease resulted in clinically healthy periodontal conditions and that this state of health was maintained in most patients and sites during the 14-year period. A more detailed analysis of the data revealed, however, that a small number of sites in a few patients lost a substantial amount of attachment. Approximately 43 surfaces in 15 different patients were exposed to recurrent periodontal disease of significant magnitude. The frequency of sites that lost more than 2 mm of attachment during the 14 years of maintenance was 0.8% to 0.1% per year.

Neither of these studies used a control group because failing to treat advanced periodontal patients cannot be justified for ethical reasons. However, in a study in private practice, an effort was made to find and evaluate patients with diagnosed moderate to advanced periodontitis who had not followed through with recommended periodontal therapy.[3] Thirty patients ranging in age from 25 to 71 years were evaluated after periods ranging from 18 to 115 months. All these untreated patients had progressive increases in pocket depth and radiographic evidence of progressive bone resorption.

In a study of the progression of periodontal disease in the absence of therapy, two different populations were monitored.[12] One group of 64 Swedish adults with mild to moderate periodontal disease and one group of 36 American adults with advanced destructive disease were monitored but not treated for 6 years and 1 year, respectively. During the course of 6 years, 11.6% of all sites in the Swedish population (1.9% per year) showed attachment loss of greater than 2 mm, and the corresponding figure for the American population was 3.2% per year.

TABLE 77-1

Average Loss of Teeth during a 5-Year Period as Compared with Normal Loss of Teeth in 1428 Men and Women Ages 20 through 59

	GRADE OF ORAL HYGIENE		
	Good	Fairly Good	Not Good
"Normal" loss of teeth (estimate based on data recorded at initiation of study period)	1.1	1.4	1.8
Actual loss of teeth during 5-year period	0.4	0.6	0.9

From Lovdal A, Arno A, Schei O, et al. Combined effect of subgingival scaling and controlled oral hygiene on the incidence of gingivitis. Acta Odontol Scand 1961; 19:537.

TABLE 77-2

Tooth Mortality After Treatment of Advanced Periodontitis in 104 Patients with 2604 Teeth Treated over a 10-Year Period

Teeth Lost*	Reason
2	Pulpal disease
3	Accidents
4	Prosthetic considerations
14	For example, the desire of one patient for a maxillary denture for cosmetic reasons
30	Periodontal
53	All reasons

* 2% of the teeth were lost during the study period.
Adapted from data in Ramfjord SP, Knowles JW, Nissle RR, et al: Longitudinal study of periodontal therapy. J Periodontol 1973; 44:66.

Thus the frequency of sites with disease progression was 20 to 30 times higher in untreated groups of patients than in the treated and well-maintained groups described in the preceding discussion.[13] *Thus treatment is effective in reducing loss of attachment.*

TOOTH MORTALITY

The ultimate test for the effectiveness of periodontal treatment is whether the loss of teeth can be prevented. Enough studies from both private practice and research institutions are now available to document that loss of teeth is retarded or prevented by therapy.

The combined effect of subgingival scaling every 3 to 6 months and controlled oral hygiene was evaluated over a 5-year period in 1428 factory workers in Oslo.[18] Tooth loss was significantly reduced in all patients. This study showed that frequent subgingival scalings reduce tooth loss even when oral hygiene is not good (Table 77-1).

The previously mentioned longitudinal study conducted at the University of Michigan included 104 patients with a total of 2604 teeth.[24-27] After 1 to 7 years of treatment, 53 teeth were lost for various reasons (Table 77-2). Approximately 32 teeth were lost during the first and second years after initiation of treatment. The remaining 21 teeth were lost in a random pattern over the next 6 years. Therefore the loss of teeth owing to advanced periodontal disease after treatment was minimal (1.15%).

Another study was undertaken to test the effect of periodontal therapy in cases of advanced disease.[13,14] The subjects were 75 patients who had lost 50% or more of their periodontal support (Fig. 77-5). Treatment consisted of oral hygiene measures, scaling procedures, extraction of untreatable teeth, periodontal surgery, and prosthetics if indicated. After completion of periodontal treatment, a 5-year period followed during which none of the patients showed any further loss of periodontal support. No teeth were extracted in the 5-year posttreatment period. It should be pointed out that the patients in this study were selected because of their capacity to meet high requirements of plaque control after repeated instruction in oral hygiene techniques. This fact does not detract from the validity of the study but tends to show the etiologic importance of bacterial plaque. The results indicate that periodontal surgery coupled with a detailed plaque control program not only temporarily cures the disease but also reduces further progression of periodontal breakdown, even in patients with severely reduced periodontal support. After 14 years, 61 of the original patients were still in the study.[13] Recurrence of destructive periodontal disease in isolated sites of the dentition resulted in loss of a certain number of teeth during the observation period (Fig. 77-6). In the 6 to 10 years after active therapy, one tooth in each of three different patients was lost, and during the final observation period (11 to 14 years), three teeth in one patient, two teeth in each of three patients, and one tooth in each of four patients had to be extracted because of recurrent periodontal disease. In addition, three teeth in each of three different patients and one tooth in each of five patients were extracted owing to the development of extensive caries, periapical lesions, or other endodontic complications. During the entire course of the study, the total loss was 30 teeth (for all reasons) out of 1330 teeth. The tooth mortality rate was therefore 2.3%.

Several studies in private practice have attempted to measure frequency of tooth loss after periodontal therapy. In one study, 180 patients who had been treated for chronic destructive periodontal disease were evaluated.[28,29] The average age of the patients before treatment was 43.7 years. A total of 141 teeth were lost. From the beginning of treatment to the time of the survey, the majority of patients lost no teeth (Fig. 77-7). Three patients out of 180 (1.7%) lost 35 teeth, approximately

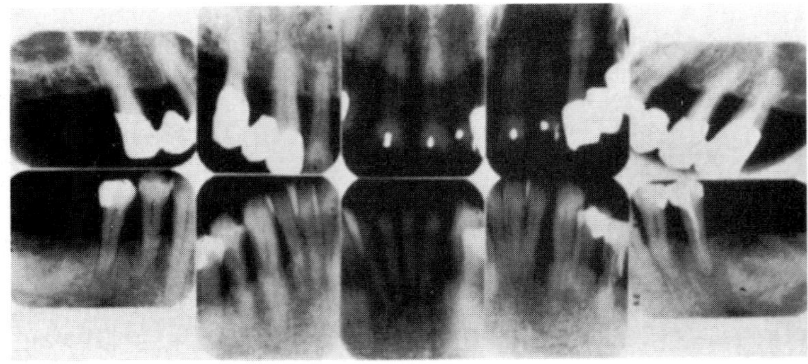

Fig. 77-5 Radiographs taken 5 years after typical periodontal treatment. Note the advanced bone loss, in spite of which teeth were retained in a healthy condition for the duration of the study. (From Lindhe J, Nyman S: The effect of plaque control and surgical pocket elimination on the establishment and maintenance of periodontal health. A longitudinal study of periodontal therapy in cases of advanced disease. J Clin Periodontol 1975; 2:67.)

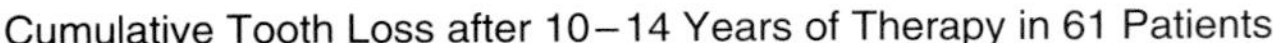

Cumulative Tooth Loss after 10–14 Years of Therapy in 61 Patients

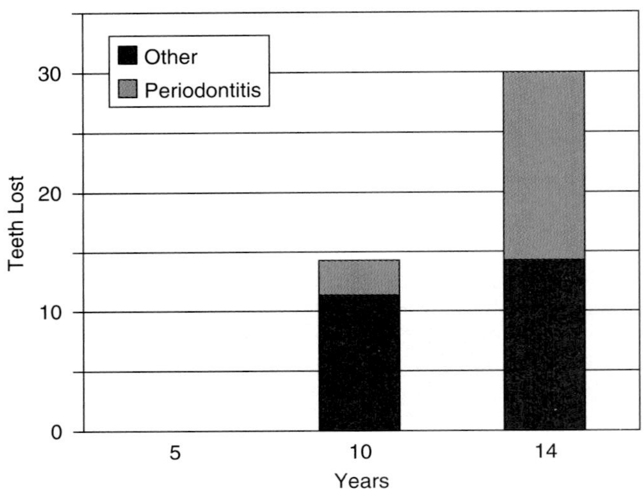

Fig. 77-6 Tooth loss in treated patients with very advanced periodontal disease. (Data from Lindhe J, Nyman S: Long-term maintenance of patients treated for advanced periodontal disease. J Clin Periodontol 1984; 11:504.)

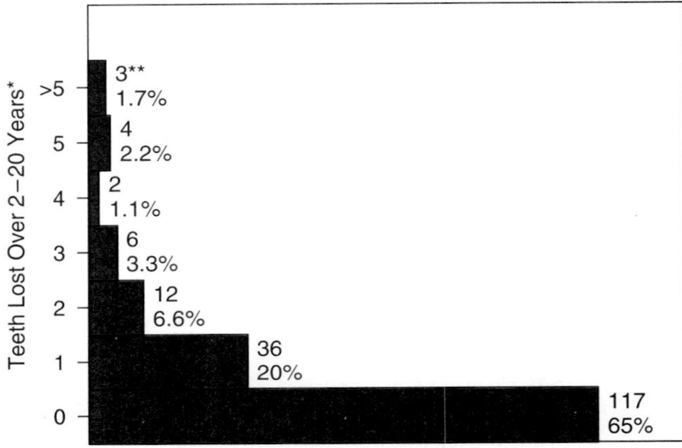

Fig. 77-7 Tooth mortality. (Adapted from Ross IF, Thompson RH, Galdi M: The results of treatment. A long term study of one hundred and eighty patients. Parodontologie 1971; 25:125.)

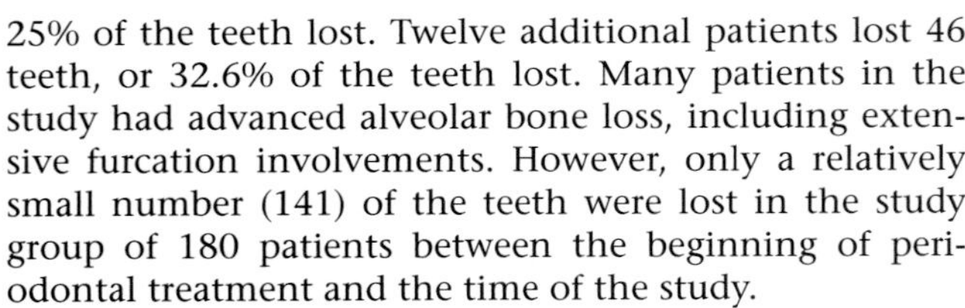

25% of the teeth lost. Twelve additional patients lost 46 teeth, or 32.6% of the teeth lost. Many patients in the study had advanced alveolar bone loss, including extensive furcation involvements. However, only a relatively small number (141) of the teeth were lost in the study group of 180 patients between the beginning of periodontal treatment and the time of the study.

The teeth were lost for several reasons including periodontal disease, caries, and other nonperiodontal causes.* The length of time after treatment varied from 2 to 20 years, with an average of 8.6 years. Of considerable significance is the large number of teeth (81 teeth, or 57.5%) lost by a few patients (15 patients, or 8.4%). Even when this group is considered with the remaining 165 patients, it may be seen that the periodontal care provided helped to retain most teeth, as the average tooth loss was slightly less than one tooth (0.9) over the 10 years after treatment.

In a follow-up study, the long-term results of periodontal therapy were evaluated after 15 to 34 years (average of 22.2 years).[4] The average tooth loss at this time was 1.6 teeth per 10 years. Patients were classified into three groups according to tooth loss. Approximately 62% had an average tooth loss of 0.45 per 10 years and were

* U.S. Health Surveys conducted in the 1960s indicated that an average of 4.3 teeth were lost after age 35 in the general population.[9]

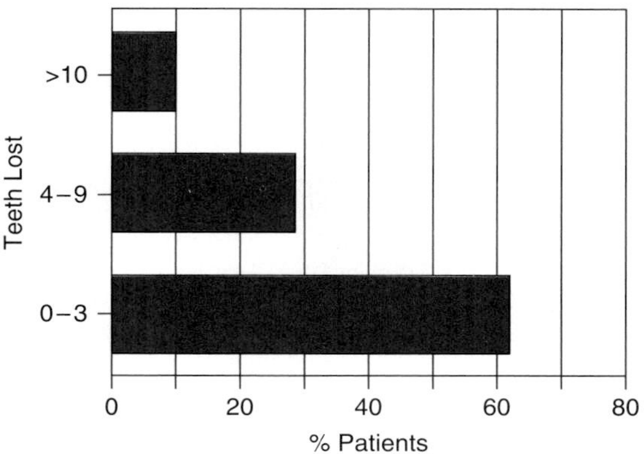

Fig. 77-8 Tooth mortality 15 to 34 years after initiation of therapy (average of 22.2 years). Average tooth loss is 1.6 teeth per 10 years. Compare with the same study population in Fig. 77-7. As the treated population ages, the rate of bone loss appears to increase. (Adapted from Goldman MJ, Ross IF, Goteiner D: Effect of periodontal therapy on patients maintained for 15 years or longer. J Periodontol 1986; 57:347.)

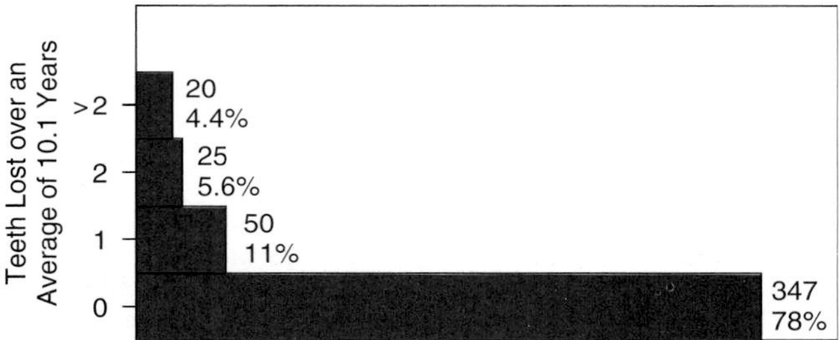

Fig. 77-9 Tooth mortality in 442 periodontal patients treated over 10 years. (Courtesy Dr. R. C. Oliver, Rio Verde, Ariz.)

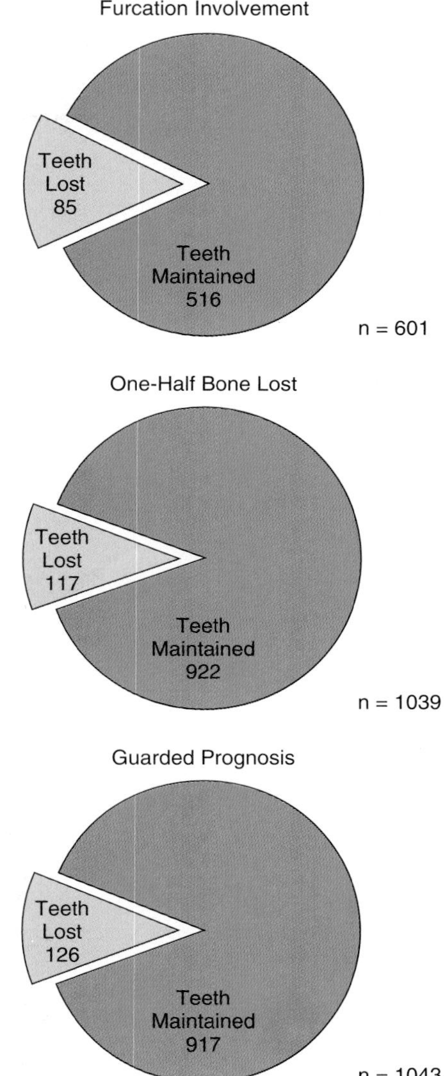

Fig. 77-10 Loss of teeth with advanced periodontal disease over 10 years. (Courtesy Dr. R. C. Oliver, Rio Verde, Ariz.)

considered "well maintained"; 28% lost an average of 2.6 teeth per 10 years and were considered "downhill"; and 10% lost an average of 6.4 teeth per 10 years and were considered "extreme downhill" (Fig. 77-8).

Another study included all patients in a practice who had been treated 5 or more years previously and had received regular preventive periodontal care since that time.[23] The 442 patients had an average of 10.1 years since treatment. Two thirds of the patients were older than 40 at the time of treatment. These patients had been seen every 4.6 months, on average, for their preventive periodontal care, which consisted of oral hygiene instruction and prophylaxis (Figs. 77-9 and 77-10).

The total tooth loss owing to periodontal disease was 178 of more than 11,000 teeth available for treatment. More important, 78% of the patients did not lose a single tooth after periodontal therapy, and 11% lost only one tooth. Considering that more than 600 teeth had furcation involvements at the time of the original treatment and that well over 1000 teeth had less than half of the alveolar bone support remaining, the tooth loss was low. During the same average 10-year period after periodontal therapy, only 45 teeth were lost through caries or pulpal involvement. Even more surprising are the statistics over an average 10-year period for teeth with a less-than-optimal prognosis. Only 85 (14%) of a total of 601 teeth with furcation involvement were lost, and 117 (11%) of 1039 teeth with half or less of the bone remaining were lost. Of the 1043 teeth listed as having a guarded prognosis for any reason by the clinician performing the initial examination, only 126 (12%) were lost over this 10-year average period. The average tooth mortality rate was 0.72 tooth lost per patient per 10 years.

In a third study in private practice, 600 patients were followed for between 15 and 53 years after periodontal therapy[7] (Table 77-3; Figs. 77-11 and 77-12). The majority (76.5%) had advanced periodontal disease at the start of treatment. There were 15,666 teeth present, for an

TABLE 77-3

Tooth Mortality in Treated Periodontitis Patients

Average Number of Teeth Lost per 10 Years with Periodontal Treatment*	Study
Hirschfeld and Wasserman[7]	1.0
McFall[19]	1.4
Oliver[23]	0.72
Ross et al[29]	0.9
Goldman et al[4]	1.6
McLeod et al[20]	1.5

* Tooth mortality adjusted to 10 years by chapter author.

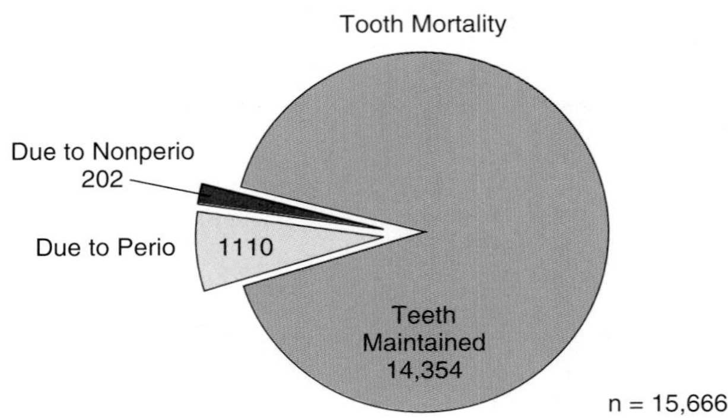

Fig. 77-12 Loss of teeth in 600 patients over 15 to 53 years. (Data from Hirschfeld L, Wasserman B: A long-term survey of tooth loss in 600 treated periodontal patients. J Periodontol 1978; 49:225.)

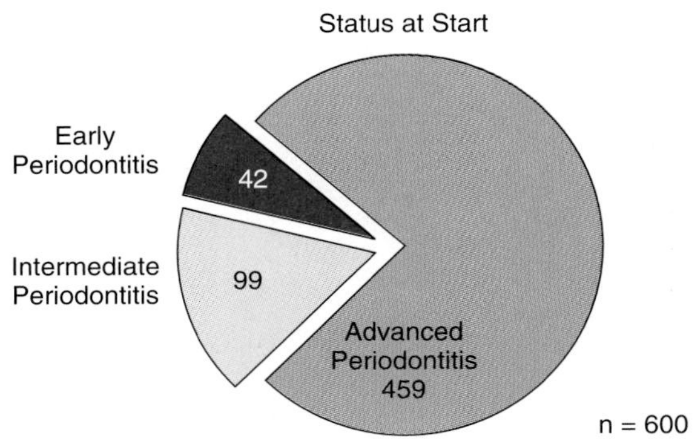

Fig. 77-11 Status at start of study of 600 patients reported by Hirschfeld and Wasserman. (Data from Hirschfeld L, Wasserman B: A long-term survey of tooth loss in 600 treated periodontal patients. J Periodontol 1978; 49:225.)

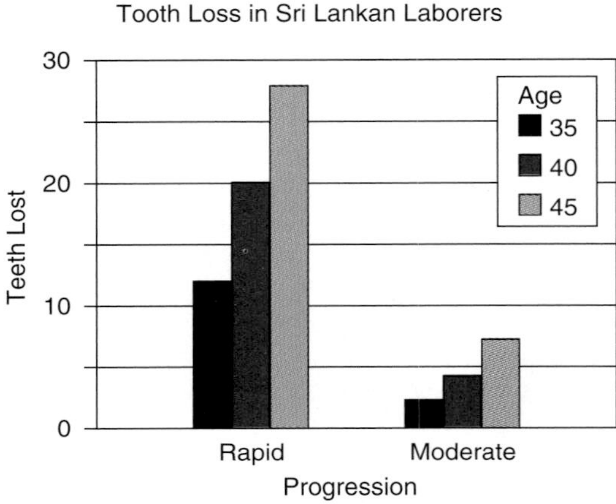

Fig. 77-13 Tooth loss in a population with untreated periodontal disease. (Data from Löe H, Anerud A, Boysen H, et al: Natural history of periodontal disease in man. J Clin Periodontol 1986; 13:431.)

average of 26 teeth per patient. During the follow-up period (average of 22 years), a total of 1312 teeth were lost owing to all causes. Of this number, 1110 were lost for periodontal reasons. The average tooth mortality rate per patient was 2.2 teeth; when this is converted to a 10-year rate, an average of one tooth was lost per 10 years in each patient. During this period of observation, 666 teeth with a questionable prognosis were lost out of a total of 2141. This means that 31% of the teeth with a questionable prognosis were lost over 22 years of treatment. A total of 1464 teeth with furcation involvement were treated, and 31.6% were lost during the period of study. Approximately 83% of the patients lost fewer than three teeth over the 22-year average treatment period and were classified as well maintained. The remaining 17 percent of the patients were divided into two groups: downhill (4 to 9 teeth lost) or extreme downhill (10 to 23 teeth lost). Thus 17% of the patients studied accounted for 69% of the teeth lost owing to periodontal causes. This study also showed that relatively few teeth are lost after periodontal therapy. In addition, relatively few of the teeth with guarded prognosis, including those with furcation involvement, are lost, and a small percentage of patients lose most of the teeth.

Two studies give insight into tooth mortality in untreated patients. The studies of Löe and co-workers in Sri Lankan laborers[15] showed that after the age of 35, an average of 5 and 16 teeth were lost per 10 years in the moderate progression and rapid progression groups, respectively (Fig. 77-13). In a previously discussed study in private practice,[3] an effort was made to find and evaluate patients with diagnosed moderate to advanced periodontitis who did not follow through with recommended periodontal therapy. Patients with untreated periodontal disease were losing teeth at a rate greater than 0.61 tooth per year (6.1 teeth per 10 years). A total of 83 teeth were lost in 30 patients, but the investigators excluded one patient who had lost 25 teeth. Including this patient would have increased the tooth loss in untreated patients to an even higher rate. When Tables 77-3 and 77-4 are compared, it is obvious that tooth mortality is much greater in untreated groups.

In summary, the prevalence of periodontal disease and the high tooth mortality rate resulting from the disease have raised the need for effective

TABLE 77-4

Tooth Mortality in Untreated Periodontitis Patients

Study	Average Number of Teeth Lost per 10 Years without Periodontal Treatment
Becker et al[3]	6
Löe et al[15] (moderate progression)	5
Löe et al[15] (rapid progression)	16

treatment. There is now strong evidence that periodontal disease can contribute to numerous health problems including pregnancy complications, heart disease, stroke, and diabetes.[21,22,30,31] Available treatment is effective in preventing the disease and stopping the progression of bone destruction after periodontitis is present. In addition, overwhelming evidence suggests that periodontal therapy greatly reduces tooth mortality. Every dental practitioner should be familiar with the philosophy and techniques of periodontal therapy. Failure to diagnose and treat periodontal disease or to make periodontal treatment available to patients causes unnecessary dental problems and tooth loss and places the patient at risk for systemic health problems.

REFERENCES

1. Axelsson P, Lindhe J: Effect of controlled oral hygiene procedures on caries and periodontal disease in adults. Results after 6 years. J Clin Periodontol 1981; 18239.
2. Bay I, Moller IJ: The effect of a sodium monofluorophosphate dentifrice on the gingiva. J Periodont Res 1968; 3:103.
3. Becker W, Berg L, Becker EB: Untreated periodontal disease: A longitudinal study. J Periodontol 1979; 50:234.
4. Goldman MJ, Ross IF, Goteiner D: Effect of periodontal therapy on patients maintained for 15 years or longer. J Periodontol 1986; 57:347.
5. Greene JC: Periodontal disease in India: Report of an epidemiological study. J Dent Res 1960; 39:302.
6. Greville TNE: United States life tables by dentulous or edentulous condition, 1971, and 1957–58. Publication no. (HRA) 75-1338. Washington, DC, U.S. Department of Health, Education, and Welfare, August 1974.
7. Hirschfeld L, Wasserman B: A long-term survey of tooth loss in 600 treated periodontal patients. J Periodontol 1978; 49:225.
8. Hoover DR, Lefkowitz W: Reduction of gingivitis by toothbrushing. J Periodontol 1955; 36:193.
9. Kelly JE, Van Kirk LE Jr, Garst CC: Decayed, missing and filled teeth in adults. United States 1960–1962. Public Health Service Publication no. 1000, Series 11, No. 23. Washington, DC, February 1967.
10. Ladavalya MRN, Harris R: A study of the gingival and periodontal conditions of a group of people in Chieng Mai province. J Periodontol 1959; 30:219.
11. Lightner LM, O'Leary JT, Drake RB, et al: Preventive periodontic treatment procedures: Results over 46 months. J Periodontol 1971; 42:555.
12. Lindhe J, Haffajee AD, Socransky SS: Progression of periodontal disease in adult subjects in the absence of periodontal therapy. J Clin Periodontol 1983; 10:433.
13. Lindhe J, Nyman S: Long-term maintenance of patients treated for advanced periodontal disease. J Clin Periodontol 1984; 11:504.
14. Lindhe J, Nyman S: The effect of plaque control and surgical pocket elimination on the establishment and maintenance of periodontal health. A longitudinal study of periodontal therapy in cases of advanced disease. J Clin Periodontol 1975; 2:67.
15. Löe H, Anerud A, Boysen H, et al: Natural history of periodontal disease in man. J Clin Periodontol 1986; 13:431.
16. Löe H, Anerud A, Boysen H, et al: The natural history of periodontal disease in man. J Periodontol 1978; 49:607.
17. Löe H, Theilade E, Jensen SB: Experimental gingivitis in man. J Periodontol 1965; 36:177.
18. Lovdal A, Arno A, Schei O, et al: Combined effect of subgingival scaling and controlled oral hygiene on the incidence of gingivitis. Acta Odontol Scand 1961; 19:537.
19. McFall WT Jr: Tooth loss with and without periodontal therapy. Periodont Abstracts 1969; 17:8.
20. McLeod DE, Lainson PA, Spivey JD: The effectiveness of periodontal treatment as measured by tooth loss. JADA 1997; 128:316.
21. Meskin LH: Focal infection: Back with a bang! JADA 1998; 129:8.
22. Offenbacher S, Lieff S, Beck JD: Periodontitis-associated pregnancy complications. Pregnancy Neonatal Med 1988; 3:82.
23. Oliver RC: Personal communication, 1977.
24. Ramfjord SP, Knowles JW, Nissle RR, et al: Longitudinal study of periodontal therapy. J Periodontol 1973; 44:66.
25. Ramfjord SP, Knowles JW, Nissle RR, et al: Results following three modalities of periodontal therapy. J Periodontol 1975; 46:522.
26. Ramfjord SP, Nissle RR: The modified Widman flap. J Periodontol 1974; 45:601.
27. Ramfjord SP, Nissle RR, Shick RA, et al: Subgingival curettage versus surgical elimination of periodontal pockets. J Periodontol 1968; 39:167.
28. Ross IF, Thompson RH: A long-term study of root retention in the treatment of maxillary molars with furcation involvement. J Periodontol 1978; 49:238.
29. Ross IF, Thompson RH, Galdi M: The results of treatment. A long term study of one hundred and eighty patients. Parodontologie 1971; 25:125.
30. Slavkin HC: Does the mouth put the heart at risk? JADA 1999; 130:109.
31. Stamm JW (ed): Proceedings of the Sunstar-Chapel Hill Symposium 1997 on Periodontal Diseases and Human Health: New directions in periodontal medicine. Ann Periodontol 1998; 3:1.
32. Suomi JD, West JD, Chang JJ, et al: The effect of controlled oral hygiene procedures on the progression of periodontal disease in adults: Radiographic findings. J Periodontol 1971; 42:152.
33. Suomi JD, Greene JC, Vermillion JR, et al: The effect of controlled oral hygiene on the progression of periodontal disease in adults: Results after the third and final year. J Periodontol 1971; 42:152.
34. Theilade E, Wright WH, Jensen SB, et al: Experimental gingivitis in man. II. J Periodont Res 1966; 1:1.

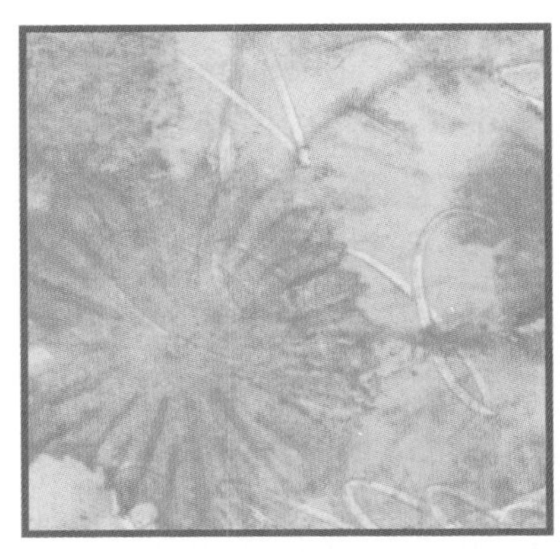

Internet Resources in Periodontics

E. Barrie Kenney

APPENDIX

Appendix Outline

Humans have an unquenchable thirst for knowledge. Since civilization began, communities have developed information networks using the best available technology. For millennia, this meant the conveyance of written, spoken, and graphic information directly by individuals specialized in the most effective transmission methods. Thus in 490 BCE the war news of Athenian victory at the battle of Marathon was carried by trained athletes to the Greek leaders. From this grew courier-based operations that used specialized methods to move packets of information across the planet. In the 19th century, horseback-based networks were connected to ship and railway-based systems in a complex mail network, which dramatically increased the number of people who could share communications.

The transmission problems were improved in each historical era, thus upgrading access, but there was also the problem of storage of information. Before the invention of printing with movable type in the 15th century, knowledge was written by individuals one copy at a time and kept solely in centralized information banks such as libraries, which were under strict controls by rulers, religious leaders, or other authoritarian groups. This resulted in two dramatic restrictions. First, only the privileged few whom were acceptable to the controlling elite, could read, and had geographic proximity could benefit. Secondly, the ruling elite controlled the nature of information and only allowed credence for that which was in support of their dogmas. This crippled scientific progress, and for centuries, false information survived. A good example of this is the perpetuation of false anatomic concepts. For centuries it was accepted that the human mandible was made up of two bones with a suture in the middle. This obvious mistake survived until Vesalius in the 16th century published his results of human dissection. He was ostracized by the ruling authorities of his time for using information gathered by observations from cadavers, even though his findings were true.

Networks became the keys to universal access when human-based methods were replaced by wire and cable connections. The use of telegraph to send Morse-encoded, binary-based information was an early example of a digital system of communications. However, analog systems using telephones, radio, and television gave immediate worldwide coverage that provided generalized sharing of knowledge but still with an overriding authority that could control content. The use of digital data together with decentralization and uncontrollable access to

The web addresses of host sites are often changed, and thus the sites listed in this chapter may not be current in the future.

multitudes of information sources make the Internet a truly revolutionary step in human development.

DEVELOPMENT OF THE INTERNET

At the end of the 20th century, this new era in communications has made management of information the primary focus of scientific, commercial, and personal interactions of society. The Internet and the World Wide Web have revolutionized information technology by providing universal global accessibility to scientific knowledge. No longer is it possible or necessary to restrict knowledge to an elite *cognoscenti* of intellectuals. No longer is geographic isolation or social restriction an insurmountable barrier to access to humanity's accumulated information base. Anyone with a simple digital processor and a connection to a telephone line or a network is immediately part of the World Wide Web. The full human resource is now able to participate and contribute to humanity's information base.

The prominence of information technology (IT) has come about by a combination of technologic progress and development of a conceptual model for unrestricted interaction between Internet users. An egalitarian ethos also drives this and has given access to the new methodologies to all wishing to use them. The electronic innovations are no more important than the conceptualized planning, which assured universal applicability to the networks that make up the information superhighway. It is a remarkable quality of the Internet that it has developed an administration that is decentralized, voluntary, and not under the direct control of agencies nor governments. This has resulted in enormous uncontrolled growth and complexity, which usually are not seen in human institutions. Networks that started as elite prerogatives of computer specialists working for the U.S. military gave rise to wider-ranging clusters of computers used by university-based scientists, which then grew to involve educators and commercial and industrial corporations, and then spread to all who desired connectivity with the advent of the personal computer.

The interconnectivity of computers was made possible by several innovative breakthroughs, but probably the most important was the use of packet switching as a means of conveying data. This utilization of digital data overcame the inadequacy of the circuit-switched telephone system. Packet switching involved the breaking down of data into datagrams, packages of information that contained the origin and forwarding electronic addresses of each packet. This meant that even if the first attempt at computer to computer linkage failed, the message could be resent by the original source. The first two computers to exchange host-to-host communications were those at the University of California, Los Angeles (UCLA) Network Measuring Center and the Augmentation of the Human Intellect project at Stanford University. This occurred in September 1968. Two more computers were connected later in 1968; one at the University of California, Santa Barbara involved in mathematics, and one at the University of Utah concerned with three-dimensional modeling. These formed the basis for a network called *ARPANET,* which was sponsored by the Advanced Research Projects Agency. The original ARPANET was designed to serve the needs of the military by providing a network of communications between computers that was decentralized and could maintain command and control of missiles and bombs after a nuclear attack, even if significant components of the system were destroyed or inoperable. The U.S. Department of Defense funded many military- and university-based research projects to develop this strategic connectivity, and its access was limited to those research contractors and employees. The next major achievement was the introduction of the first e-mail program in 1972. By this time, 23 host computers were included in the network. The ARPANET computers were all connected by special landlines capable of handling 50 kilobits of information per second. This was superseded in 1988 when the ARPANET was disbanded and T3 lines capable of 45 megabits per second were used for connectivity. By this time there were several networks and the number of host computers had grown to 56,000.

During the 1980s, the National Science Foundation started its own network named CSNET, which connected a selected group of computer scientists. At the same time, other U.S. government agencies such as NASA and the Department of Defense began their own computer-connected networks.

Eventually, the concept of an Internet composed of many independent and different networks allowed the initial ARPANET to be connected to a multitude of other networks, including those based on coaxial cable (ethernet) or radio and satellite links. These computer-to-computer systems were initially based on large complex research computers, and only later did simplifications of the electronic protocols allow the use of desktop computers such as the personal computer. Thus by 1985 an increasing number of people were using the Internet for electronic communication. By this time, this technology had spread from being the specialized domain of computer research scientists into involvement of a wide group of scientists, educators, and government agencies such as the National Science Foundation. Federal agencies shouldered the costs of research, development, and infrastructure development.

DEVELOPMENT OF THE WORLD WIDE WEB

Although the origins of the Internet began in the U.S., the wide-ranging facilitation was made possible by the development of the World Wide Web. This concept came to fruition in 1989, when Tim Berners-Lee developed a system to use hypertext to provide online access to specific pieces of information stored in large computers. This development of browser technology was founded by the Conseil European Pour La Recherche Nucleaire (CERN) in Switzerland, and they made the software available to the public.

Whereas the Internet is the system of host computers, routers, telephone lines, satellite, wireless, and cable connections accessed from a home computer, the *World Wide Web* refers to the abstract universe of information accessible on the Internet and is composed of data in documents, photographs, graphics, sounds, and videos.

TABLE 1

Development of the Internet

Year	Number of Host Computers
1968	4
1972	23
1983	213
1985	1961
1990	313,000
1995	6,642,000
2000	97,758,400

TABLE 2

Number of Internet Users in December 2000: Top 10 Countries

Country	Number of Users (Millions)
United States	135.7
Japan	26.4
Germany	19.1
United Kingdom	17.9
China	15.8
Canada	15.2
South Korea	14.8
Italy	11.6
Brazil	10.6
France	9.0

From www.cyberatlas.Internet.com.

CONNECTIVITY ON THE INTERNET

By the end of 2000, more than 99 million host computer sites were on the Internet. This number grew from the original 4 in 1968 to 213 in 1983 to 313,000 in 1990 (Appendix Table 1). These host sites generally have a server computer that can handle multitudes of requests at the same time. These requests for data are managed by processing similar requests just a few nanoseconds apart so that the end users get continuous seamless access. There are now 275.5 million users of the Internet. The U.S. and Canada make up almost half the users worldwide, with more than 50% of American homes having access to the Internet (Appendix Table 2). It is possible to view the growth of hosts and users of the Internet in real time at the site http://www.netsizer.com.

Connection to the Internet is made via an internet service provider (ISP), which has high-speed access to all the networks. These ISPs may be related to a university or combined with telephone companies or exist as stand-alone commercial entities.

The type of connection determines the speed of transmission of data to the individual user computer. A standard telephone wire and modem can give 56 kilobits per second. New technology using telephone lines to transmit digitalized data (digital subscriber line, or *DSL*) increases the speed of transmission over a range of 250 kilobits per second to as high as 7 megabits per second. DSL also allows simultaneous use of the wire for normal analog telephone conversations.

Coaxial cable connections currently used for cable television transmission have the capacity to carry up to 2 megabits per second; this is about 35 times faster than a 56k modem. Networks of fiber optic cables are currently being deployed in some cities to link homes as well as trunk lines connecting cities, countries, and continents. These give significant improvement over the widely used, telephone-wired 56k modem, with possible speeds of up to 5 gigabits.

The air transmission of digitalized data using either satellite or cellular phone networks allows downloads transmission speeds of 400 kilobits per second to 1 megabit per second.

These new, high-speed technologies are replacing the widely used telephone modem connections. The increased band width of data transmission results in more acceptable download times to the users' computers, thus increasing the utilization of complex data sets inherent in movies and complex graphics. This will result in wider use of different media by most host computer sites.

PERIODONTAL AND DENTAL APPLICATIONS

Computers are widely used in dentistry to manage clinical practices, and most dental offices in the U.S. now use computer-based programs for billing, account management, insurance claims, patient recall scheduling, and in some cases for patient appointments. General office accounting activities such as payroll, taxation, and retirement accounts may also be part of the computer-based practice management systems. However, the use of office computers by dentists for Internet activities is much less, and dentists are more likely to have an Internet connection at home than in the office. At present, the percentage of dentists with home-based connectivity is most likely higher than the national average of more than 50% of American homes.

As mentioned previously, the vast majority of domestic Internet connections are via telephone cables and use a standard modem. Consequently, most of the online material in periodontics is textual with photographs or simple graphics. Future advances in bandwidth using the whole spectrum of methodologies such as coaxial cable, fiber optics, and digital satellite systems will result in more sophisticated use of media in periodontal applications.

More than 86,000 dental host sites are available on the World Wide Web. These cover a wide range of topics and sponsors, but the most common sites are those developed by individual practitioners. These private practice sites are directed toward marketing each practice to prospective patients. As such they represent the individual dentist's or periodontist's view of his or her practice. Most commonly they contain biographic data of the practitioners, a description of the services offered, and directives on how to find the office. Patient education material may also be included on the site as well as opportunities to use electronic mail to communicate with the dentist and staff. The production of these sites is either done by the periodontist using increasingly manageable software or produced by professional companies specializing in designing web pages for small businesses.

ONLINE DENTAL EDUCATION

Dental education has used the Internet for continuing education courses originating in universities, professional organizations, and private companies. Periodontics has always been prominent in these endeavors, and in 1999 periodontal online courses were the largest subject group in dentistry. Some of the earliest educational sites in periodontics were the site established at the University of Lund by Dr. Rolf Attström and associates (this site is now called *Periodontology from Sweden and Denmark* and comes from the Center for Oral Health Sciences at Malmö University and the School of Dentistry at Copenhagen at http://www.odont.ku.dk/basic periodontology/main.html) and the UCLA Periodontics Information Center supported by the Tarrson Endowed Chair in Periodontics at www.dent.ucla.edu/pic.

Commercial companies were also involved in the beginning offerings of online courses, with periodontal programs for dentists, dental hygienists, and periodontists. Colgate offers access to its publication *Oral Care Report* and continuing education credit can be obtained by answering questions. This is offered in conjunction with the Harvard School of Dental Medicine. The home pages can be found at http://www.colgate.com/Pro/index.html. Continuing education courses are available on such commercial sites as Procter & Gamble, which offers courses for dentists, dental hygienists, dental assistants, and office managers at http://www.dentalcare.com.

Most of these online continuing educational courses are available free for preview, but it is usually necessary to pay a fee if the health professional wishes to receive documentation of course completion. To verify an individual's mastery of the subject material, many courses have a postcourse examination that is taken online. Completion of this test allows participants to receive credit for satisfactory completion of the course. This may be used to satisfy continuing educational requirements for maintenance of state dental licenses in the U.S. or to be recognized by professional organizations such as the British Royal College of Surgeons.

Payment of tuition for these Internet courses is handled online using the students' credit cards. Security of these transactions is protected by commercial services, which process the credit card data with state-of-the-art security encryption that is almost impossible to intercept and translate. The initial consumer reticence to offer credit card data to online businesses essentially has been overcome by general acceptance that online financial transactions are more secure than direct, store-based, credit card purchases.

Since the inception of the UCLA Periodontics Information Center in 1996, many dentists have used this site for continuing education. Between 100 and 250 users come to this site each day (Appendix Box 1). There they get involved in a wide variety of courses ranging from periodontal examination procedures to management of patients with hypertension. This site has worldwide use, with 60% of the viewers coming from outside the U.S. People from many large and small countries are frequent users, including from those countries with relatively high access to the Internet such as Canada, Germany, Japan, Brazil, Australia, and the United Kingdom, and participants from other countries where Internet services are not widely used, such as India, Vietnam, Russia, Egypt, and Peru. It is a remarkable example of global access that so many widely placed practitioners can experience periodontal education from just one source. In any given month, the domains of more than 60 countries use this Internet periodontal site.

BOX 1

Typical Daily Log for Use of UCLA Periodontics Information Website

Number of individual users: 221
Average number of pages viewed per user: 4.4
Data transferred in kilobytes: 28,978

University-based dental education is now beginning to use Internet-based courses to supplement the conventional teaching programs of the dental curriculum. Many universities including UCLA now require entering students to purchase a laptop computer and have access to the Internet. This gives students the ability to review course material outside of the classroom and individualize their educational experience. Computer-based laboratory and clinical teaching, with students using their laptop computers connected to Internet outlets in the laboratory or clinical cubicle, expands the educational opportunities by allowing each student to select specific topics and spend as much time as they wish to master the content. At UCLA, significant university funds have been spent to give all schools and departments Internet access via high-speed landlines and to wire clinics and the preclinical laboratories for personalized access.

In the immediate future, dental schools and others will be more universally involved in teledentistry, with site-to-site connections by either satellite or coaxial and fiber optic cables. This permits conferencing across continents with both voice and visual connectivity so that lectures, laboratory clinical demonstrations, and patient-centered learning can be shared. Dental schools are already using these links. Recently, a teleconference between the faculties of the UCLA School of Dentistry, the University of California, San Francisco School of Dentistry, and a government agency in Washington, D.C. was able to facilitate the development of a joint research grant proposal.

In 2000, at least 68 dental schools had home pages. These dental schools' web sites provide information on curricula, faculty, and enrollment requirements to prospective students. At UCLA it is possible to apply for postdoctoral educational programs in periodontics via the Internet. At present, more than one third of completed applications arrive electronically. This results in quicker receipt of enrollment data and allows for the immediate request of any additional material.

PROFESSIONAL ORGANIZATIONS ON THE INTERNET

Periodontal professional organizations throughout the world have a presence on the World Wide Web. The American Academy of Periodontology has developed a broad spectrum of information available at http://www.perio.org. Visitors to this site can access information on periodontal disease and treatment in segments designed for patient education. Pages also are devoted to members, with courses, practice administration information, a buyer's guide with direct links to dental companies and manufacturers, classified advertisements and bulletin boards, educational and career opportunities, and links to the Journal of Periodontology and the American Board of Periodontology.

The European Federation of Periodontology, at www.efp.net/organizations.html, gives information on meetings, with online registration for Europerio available. This site also gives educational guidelines and curricula for periodontal programs for training specialists, dentists, and hygienists. Current news is also listed with a link to the *Journal of Clinical Periodontology.* Periodontal societies of various European countries also list their addresses and officers on this site.

Several European countries have their periodontal societies with web sites, e.g., the British Society of Periodontology at www.derweb.ac.uk/bsp/, the Irish Society of Periodontology at http://homepages.iob.re/˜perio/index.html, the Belgium Society of Periodontology at http://users.swing.be/FDB/sbp-bvp/, the Swiss Society of Periodontology at http://users.swing.be/FDB/sbp-bvp, and the Nederlandse Vereniginy voor Paradontologie at http://www.nvvp.org. These all give lists of members and officers, patient-oriented information, and schedules of meetings and current news in periodontics. Similar sites have been established in other geographic regions such as the Sociedad de Periodoncia de Chile at http://www.free cl/spoch/spch.regalem.htm#b.

RETRIEVAL OF SCIENTIFIC DATA ON THE WORLD WIDE WEB

Access to scientific journal articles is also an important part of online services in the field of periodontics. Some individual journals offer Internet access to complete articles to subscribers. In some cases, this is included in the regular subscription. In other cases, an additional payment is required and a separate online subscription is yet another method of utilization. Some examples are the *Journal of Periodontology* accessed through the American Academy of Periodontology site at http://www.perio.org or directly at http://www.perio.org/journal.html. The *Journal of Clinical Periodontology* can be accessed via the European Federation of Periodontology or directly at http://www.efp.net/jcp.html. Information on the *Journal of Periodontal Research* is reached at http://www.munksgaard.dk/. The *International Journal of Oral and Maxillofacial Implants* has a site at http://www.quint.pub.com.

The U.S. National Library of Medicine has a free service to medical and dental literature via Medline. This gives users the ability to search by author, topic, and journal and to download abstracts of selected articles (www.ncbi.nim.nih.gov/PubMed). Essentially all of the important periodontal, dental, and medical journals are viewable at the National Library of Medicine site. More than 11 million citations are stored in their servers' database, which also gives online access to participating online journals. Another web site at the National Library of Medicine is called Grateful Med (http://igm.nlm.nih.gov), which includes Medline as well as many other databases. Some examples are Chem ID, with a file of 344,000 chemical compounds of interest to health scientists; DIRLINE, with 16,000 records of health and biomedical information on courses associated with health care organizations; CATLINE, a database of 786,000 monographs and manuscripts going back to the 15th century; BIOETHICSLINE, with 53,000 entries concerned with ethics; and two sites devoted to information on AIDS, AIDSLINE and AIDSTRIALS. POPLINE has data on family planning, SPACELINE has data from NASA, and TOXLINE has toxicologic data. This Grateful Med site is the most comprehensive portal to health-related scientific data.

The pace of growth of information technology ensures that networks will spread wider and wider in the coming years. At present, 160,000 new connections to the Internet are made everyday, and the number of host sites continues to show dramatic growth (Appendix Fig. 1). This has important implications for periodontics. New proven procedures will be used by more clinicians in much shorter time periods than previously. The race to solve the problems of treatment prevention and control of human periodontal disease now has a much more optimistic time for the finish line.

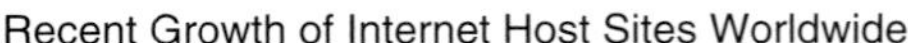

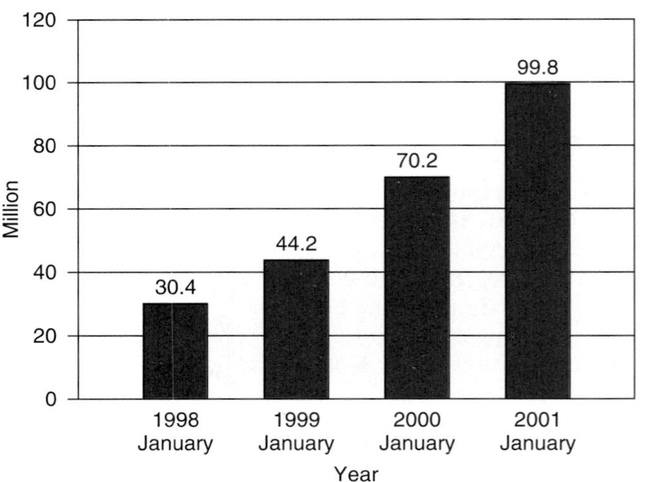

CONCLUSIONS

It is obvious that these scientific search sites offer everyone an enormous opportunity to retrieve the whole range of information relevant to periodontics. The Internet and World Wide Web provide the means for a complete understanding of current knowledge in our field.

In the immediate future, more nonspecialist dentists will become skilled in periodontal therapy, and these skills will be improved by continuing educational programs using the World Wide Web and national and international teleconferencing and teleclinics. Patient data will be digitalized and shared by network connectivity. Patients who desire to understand their own periodontal conditions will become sophisticated consumers, searching for the most accessible and acceptable clinical expertise. Universities and professional and commercial organizations will become more dependent on distance learning and less oriented toward traditional, geographic-based education. Periodontics and all scientific-based specialties will grow at a rate not previously seen nor anticipated. The hope for a cure for periodontal disease and other human maladies is much closer to fruition because of the acceleration of scientific knowledge bought about by dedicated intellectualism and a commitment to information technology.

Index

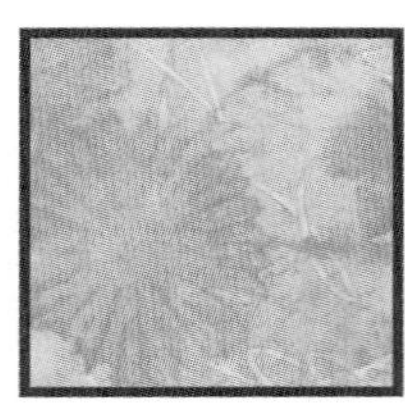

E

M

Q

R

S

T

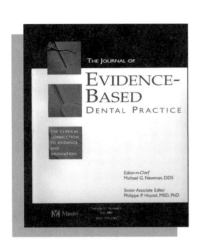

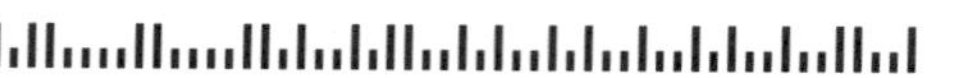